Cerebrovascular Disease

CEREBROVASCULAR DISEASE

Editor-in-Chief

H. Hunt Batjer, M.D.

Division of Neurological Surgery
Northwestern University Medical School
Chicago, Illinois

Associate Editors

Louis R. Caplan, M.D.

Department of Neurology
New England Medical Center
Boston, Massachusetts

Lars Friberg, M.D.

Department of Clinical Physiology
and Nuclear Medicine
Rigshospitalet
Copenhagen, Denmark

Ralph G. Greenlee, Jr., M.D.

Department of Neurology
The University of Texas
Southwestern Medical Center
Dallas, Texas

Thomas A. Kopitnik, Jr., M.D.

Department of Neurological Surgery
The University of Texas
Southwestern Medical Center
Dallas, Texas

William L. Young, M.D.

Departments of Anesthesiology,
Radiology, and Neurological Surgery
College of Physicians & Surgeons
of Columbia University
New York, New York

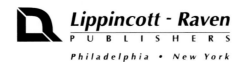

Lippincott - Raven
P U B L I S H E R S

Philadelphia • New York

Acquisitions Editor: Elizabeth Greenspan
Developmental Editor: Ann Sydor
Manufacturing Manager: Dennis Teston
Production Manager: Lawrence Bernstein
Production Editor: Bob Berkel
Cover Designer: Diana Andrews
Indexer: Kathy Pitcoff
Compositor: Maryland Composition, Inc.
Printer: Quebecor–Kingsport

Printed in the United States of America

9 8 7 6 5 4 3 2 1

Library of Congress Cataloging-in-Publication Data

Cerebrovascular disease / editor, H. Hunt Batjer ; associate editors,
    Louis Caplan . . . [et al.].
        p. cm.
    Includes bibliographical references and index.
    ISBN 0-397-51661-4
    1. Cerebrovascular disease. I. Batjer, H. Hunt.
    [DNLM: 1. Cerebrovascular Disorders. WL 355 C41338 1996]
RC388.5.C664 1996
616.8′1—dc20
DNLM/DLC
for Library of Congress   96-13565
                                                        CIP

*To my mentors, Duke Samson and Charles Drake, who made this possible,
and to my three girls Janet, Hannah, and Devon who make this worthwhile.*

Foreword

Apoplexy, the perception of stroke by the ancient Greeks, used even a generation before Hippocrates, meant both to be 'struck dumb' in the mind and 'paralysed' in the body. In modern times, poignantly, Francis Murphey expressed it so, "there is nothing in the field of medicine to equal the disability and loss of human dignity as a stroke."

The human calamity of stroke has kindled the interest and enquiry of physicians since ancient times but only in the late 19th Century did the first preventive measure appear with occasional carotid occlusion for a large intracranial aneurysm. The landmark for change occurred with Moniz' introduction of cerebral angiography in 1927, although remarkably, it was adopted slowly in Europe and only burgeoned in North America after the war, partially because of concern for the contrast agents. When the carotid artery in the neck was shown to be a common source of stroke, endarterectomy followed in succession to anticoagulation in the early 1950's and intracranial surgery for aneurysm began its evolution.

Although there has been a dramatic decline in ischemic and hemorrhagic (excepting aneurysmal) stroke over the last three decades from management of the risk profile, they remain the most common neurological threats to mental and physical incapacitation world wide and third among the causes of death after heart disease and cancer.

Quite remarkable advances have occurred, even in the last 5 years, in the understanding and treatment of cerebrovascular disorder and disease. In this timely comprehensive multi-authored volume, Dr. Batjer has brought together the experience and authority of nearly 200 of those eminently involved in all aspects of the brain and its vessels in stroke, with particular emphasis on advances in medical, surgical, and endovascular management, mostly in prevention, but including new concepts and strategies that may, in selected patients, modify the outcome of the evolving stroke.

Charles Drake, M.D.

Contents

Section I: The Cerebral Vasculature in Health and Disease

Extracranial Vascular Disease

Intracranial Vascular Disease and Stroke Management

Perioperative Considerations—AVM

Intracranial Aneurysm

Contributors

Robert J. Adams, M.S., M.D.
Professor of Neurology
Co-Director, Cerebrovascular Section
Principal Investigator, STOP Study
Department of Neurology
Medical College of Georgia
Augusta, Georgia 30912-3235

Andrei V. Alexandrov, M.D.
Research Fellow
Western New York Neuroscience Center
State University of New York at Buffalo
100 High Street
Buffalo, New York 14203

Robert W. Androux, M.D.
Fellow, Department of Radiology
Northwestern University Medical School
710 North Fairbanks Court
Chicago, Illinois 60611-2909

Issam A. Awad, M.D., M.Sc., F.A.C.S., M.A.
  (hon.)
Professor, Section of Neurological Surgery
Department of Surgery
Yale University School of Medicine
333 Cedar Street, TMP 405
New Haven, Connecticut 06510

Julian E. Bailes, Jr., M.D.
Associate Professor, Department of Neurosurgery
Chief, Cerebrovascular Surgery
Medical College of Pennsylvania and
  Hahnemann University
Allegheny General Hospital
420 East North Avenue, Suite 302
Pittsburgh, Pennsylvania 15212-9986

Christopher J. Baker, M.D.
Department of Neurosurgery
Columbia University College of Physicians and
  Surgeons
Columbia-Presbyterian Medical Center
710 West 168th Street
New York, New York 10032-2603

Kristy Z. Baker, M.D.
Department of Anesthesiology
Columbia University College of Physicians and
  Surgeons
Columbia-Presbyterian Medical Center
710 West 168th Street
New York, New York 10032-2603

Lucia Balos-Miller, M.D.
Assistant Professor, Department of Pathology
State University of New York at Buffalo
Buffalo General Hospital,
100 High Street
Buffalo, New York 14203

Gordon H. Baltuch, M.D., Ph.D., F.R.C.S. (C)
Fellow, Department of Neurology
Centre Hospitalier Universitaire Vaudois
Lausanne, Switzerland 1011

Daniel L. Barrow, M.D.
MBNA/Bowman Professor and Chairman
Department of Neurosurgery
Emory University School of Medicine
1365 B Clifton Road NE, Suite B2200
Atlanta, Georgia 30322

H. Hunt Batjer, M.D.
Michael Marchese Professor and Chief
Division of Neurological Surgery
Department of Surgery
Northwestern University Medical School
233 East Erie Street, Suite 614
Chicago, Illinois 60611

José Biller, M.D.
Professor and Chairman
Department of Neurology
Indiana University Medical Center
545 Barnhill Drive, Emerson Hall, 125
Indianapolis, Indiana 46202-5124

Randolph C. Bishop, M.D.
Division of Neurosurgery
University of Alabama at Birmingham
1813 Sixth Avenue South
Birmingham, Alabama 35294-3295

Julien Bogousslavsky, M.D.
Professor, Department of Neurology
University of Lausanne
Centre Hospitalier Universitaire Vaudois
CH 1011 Lausanne, Switzerland

Rance A. Boren, M.D.
Assistant Instructor, Department of Neurology
The University of Texas Southwestern Medical
School
5323 Harry Hines Boulevard
Dallas, Texas 75235-8897

Larry D. Brace, M.S., Ph.D.
Associate Professor of Pathology and Laboratory
Medicine
Director of Hematology and Head of
Coagulation
Department of Pathology, College of Medicine
University of Illinois at Chicago
840 South Wood Street, Rm. 201
Chicago, Illinois 60612-7312

Robin L. Brey, M.D.
Associate Professor of Medicine
Division of Neurology
University of Texas Health Science Center
7703 Floyd Curl Drive
San Antonio, Texas 78284-7883

Joseph P. Broderick, M.D.
Associate Professor
Department of Neurology
University of Cincinnati Medical Center
231 Bethesda Avenue, Room 4010
Cincinnati, Ohio 45267-0525

Thomas Brott, M.D.
Professor, Department of Neurology
University of Cincinnati College of Medicine
231 Bethesda Avenue
Cincinnati, Ohio 45267-0525

Adam P. Brown, M.D.
Attending Neurosurgeon,
New Hanover Regional Medical Center
Coastal Neurosurgical Associates, Private
Practice
1908 Meeting Court
Wilmington, North Carolina 28401

Askiel Bruno, M.D.
Associate Professor,
Department of Neurology
Indiana University School of Medicine
541 Clinical Drive, R365
Indianapolis, Indiana 46202-5111

Louis R. Caplan, M.D.
Professor of Neurology and Medicine
Chairman of Neurology, Tufts University Medical
School
Neurologist-in-Chief
New England Medical Center
750 Washington Street
Boston, Massachusetts 02111

Gregory J. Castiglia, M.D.
Assistant Clinical Instructor
Department of Neurosurgery
State University of New York at Buffalo
School of Medicine and Biomedical Sciences
3 Gates Circle
Buffalo, New York 14209

Michael Cawley, M.D.
Resident, Department of Neurosurgery
Emory University School of Medicine
1365 Clifton Road NE, Suite 2220B
Atlanta, Georgia 30322

Richard K.T. Chan, M.B.B.S. (Singapore),
M.R.C.P. (UK)
Senior Clinical Fellow
Department of Clinical Neurological Sciences
University of Western Ontario
339 Windermere Road
London, Ontario N6A 5A5 Canada

James P. Chandler, M.D.
Division of Neurological Surgery
Department of Surgery
Northwestern University Medical School
233 East Erie Street, Suite 614
Chicago, Illinois 60611

David P. Chason, M.D.
Associate Professor, Division of Neuroradiology
Department of Radiology
The University of Texas Southwestern Medical
Center
5323 Harry Hines Boulevard
Dallas, Texas 75235-8896

Mary Ann Cheng, M.D.
Instructor
Department of Anesthesiology
Washington University School of Medicine
660 South Euclid Avenue, Campus Box 8054
St. Louis, Missouri 63110

Marc I. Chimowitz, M.B., Ch.B.
Associate Professor
Department of Neurology
Emory University School of Medicine
1364 Clifton Road, NE
Atlanta, Georgia 30322

G. Patrick Clagett, M.D.
Professor of Surgery
Chairman, Vascular Surgery Division
Department of Surgery
The University of Texas Southwestern Medical
 Center
5323 Harry Hines Boulevard
Dallas, Texas 75235-9157

Caetano Coimbra, M.D.
Assistant Professor
Department of Neurological Surgery
The University of Texas Southwestern Medical
 Center
5161 Harry Hines Boulevard
Dallas, Texas 75235-8855

Thomas J. Cummings, M.D.
Resident
Department of Neurosurgery
Wayne State University
4201 St. Antoine 6E-UHC
Detroit, Michigan, 48201

Mark D. D'Alise, M.D.
Chief Resident
Department of Neurological Surgery
The University of Texas Southwestern Medical
 Center
5323 Harry Hines Boulevard
Dallas, Texas 75235-8855

Ralph G. Dacey, Jr., M.D.
Huang Professor and Chairman of Neurological
 Surgery
Department of Neurological Surgery
Washington University School of Medicine
660 South Euclid, Campus Box 8057
St. Louis, Missouri 63110

Renato Da Pian, M.D.
Professor, Department of Neurosurgery
Verona City Hospital
37100 Verona, Italy

Carlos A. David, M.D.
Department of Neurological Surgery
Univeristy of Miami School of Medicine
1501 NW Ninth Ave
Miami, Florida 33136

Ted M. Dawson, M.D., Ph. D.
Assistant Professor
Department of Neurology and Neuroscience
Johns Hopkins University School of Medicine
600 North Wolfe Street, Path 2-210
Baltimore, Maryland 21287

Valina L. Dawson, Ph. D.
Assitant Professor
Departments of Neurology, Neuroscience, and
 Physiology
Johns Hopkins University School of Medicine
600 North Wolfe Street, Path 2-210
Baltimore, Maryland 21287

Arthur L. Day, M.D.
Professor, Department of Neurosurgery
University of Florida Health Center, Box 100265
 JHMHC
Gainesville, Florida 32610

R.A. de los Reyes, M.D.
Associate Professor, Department of Neurosurgery
Beth Israel Medical Center-North Division
170 East End Avenue
New York, New York 10128

Robert J. Dempsey, M.D.
Professor and Chairman, Department of
 Neurological Surgery
University of Wisconsin Hospital and Clinics
600 Highland Avenue H4/338
Madison, Wisconsin 53792

Colin P. Derdeyn, M.D.
Assistant Professor of Radiology
Mallinckrodt Institute of Radiology
Washington University School of Medicine
510 South Kingshighway
St. Louis, Missouri 63110

Nicoloas de Tribolet, M.D.
Chairman, Department of Neurosurgery
University Hospital of Lausanne-CHUV
Lausanne 1011, Switzerland

Fernando G. Diaz, M.D., Ph.D.
Professor and Chairman, Department of
 Neurological Surgery
Wayne State University
4201 St. Antoine Boulevard
Detroit, Michigan 48201

Bruce H. Dobkin, M.D.
Professor, Department of Neurology
University of California at Los Angeles
Reed Neurologic Research Center
Los Angeles, California 90095

Vinko V. Dolenc, M.D., Ph.D.
Professor, Department of Neurosurgery
University of Ljubljana Hospital Center
Zalośka 7
1105- Ljubljana, Slovenia

Christopher F. Dowd, M.D.
Associate Professor of Radiology and
*   Neurological Surgery*
Department of Radiology
University of California at San Francisco
*   Medical Center*
505 Parnassus Avenue, Rm L352
San Francisco, California 94143-0628

Charles G. Drake, M.D., F.R.C.S.C.
Professor Emeritus, Division of Neurosurgery
Department of Neurological Surgery
University of Western Ontario
339 Windermere Road
London, Ontario N6A 5A5 Canada

Gary R. Duckwiler, M.D.
Associate Professor, Department of
Interventional Neuroradiology/Radiology
University of California at Los Angeles
10833 Le Conte Avenue
Los Angeles, California 90024

John G. Ferguson, M.D.
Director of Clinical Epidemiology
Memphis Vascular Research Foundation
910 Madison Avenue, Suite 710
Memphis, Tennessee 38103

Robert D. G. Ferguson, M.D.
Clinical Associate Professor,
University of Tennessee, Memphis
Director, Interventional Neuroradiology,
Baptist Memorial Hospital
Director, Memphis Vascular Research
*   Foundation*
930 Madison Avenue, Suite 364
Memphis, Tennessee 38103

R. Fern, M.D.
Department of Neurology
University of Washington School of Medicine
1959 NE Pacific Street
Seattle, Washington 98195

Matthew E. Fink, M.D.
Chairman, Department of Neurology
Beth Israel Medical Center-North Division
170 East End Avenue
New York, New York 10128

Seth P. Finklestein, M.D.
Associate Professor
Department of Neurology
Harvard Medical School
Massachusetts General Hospital
32 Fruit Street
Boston, Massachusetts 02114

Winfield S. Fisher III, M.D.
Associate Professor
Department of Neurosurgery
University of Alabama at Birmingham
514 MEB
1816 Sixth Avenue South, UAB Station
Birmingham, Alabama 35294-3295

James L. Fleckenstein, M.D.
Associate Professor
Department of Radiology
The University of Texas Southwestern Medical
*   Center*
5323 Harry Hines Boulevard
Dallas, Texas 75235-8896

Lars Friberg, M.D.
Department of Clinical Physiology and Nuclear
*   Medicine*
KF 4011 Rigshospitalet
Blegdamsvej 9
DK-2100 Copenhagen, Denmark

William A. Friedman, M.D.
Professor and Associate Chairman
Department of Neurosurgery
University of Florida
P.O. Box 100265, UHMHC
Gainesville, Florida 32610-0265

R. Tyler Frizzell, M.D., Ph.D.
Department of Neurological Surgery
University of Boise
222 North Second Street #307
Boise, Idaho 83702

Anthony J. Furlan, M.D.
Director, Cerebrovascular Center,
Head, Section of Adult Neurology
The Cleveland Clinic Foundation
9500 Euclid Avenue
Cleveland, Ohio 44195-0001

Julio H. Garcia, M.D.
Professor, Department of Pathology
Case Western Reserve University
Cleveland, Ohio
Henry Ford Hospital
2799 West Grand Boulevard
Detroit, Michigan 48202-2689

Bhuwan P. Garg, M.B.B.S.
Associate Professor
Department of Pediatric Neurology
Indiana University Medical Center
James Whitcomb Riley Hospital for Children
702 Barnhill Drive, Rm 1757
Indianapolis, Indiana 46202-5124

Bruce L. Gewertz, M.D.
Dallas B. Phemister Professor and Chairman
Department of Surgery
The University of Chicago Medical Center
5841 South Maryland Avenue
Chicago, Illinois 60637-1470

Kevin J. Gibbons, M.D.
Assistant Professor
Department of Neurosurgery
State University of New York at Buffalo
School of Medicine and Biomedical Sciences
Director of Skull Base Surgery
Millard Fillmore Hospital
3 Gates Circle
Buffalo, New York 14209

Cole A. Giller, M.D., Ph.D.
Assistant Professor
Department of Neurosurgery and Radiology
The University of Texas Southwestern Medical
*   School*
5323 Harry Hines Boulevard
Dallas, Texas 75235-8855

Michael I. Ginsburg, M.D.
Assistant Professor, Division of Neuroradiology
Department of Radiology
The University of Texas Southwestern Medical
*   Center*
5323 Harry Hines Boulevard
Dallas, Texas 75235-8896

Albert Gjedde, M.D., D.Sc.
MRC (Denmark) Professor of Brain Research
Åarhus University Medical Institutions
Adjunct Professor of Neurology and
*   Neurosurgery*
McGill University, Montreal Canada
Director, The Positron Emission Tomography
*   Center*
at Åarhus Kommunehospital
Nørrebrogade 44
DK-8000 Åarhus C, Denmark

Camillo R. Gomez, M.D.
Director, Comprehensive Stroke Center
Associate Professor, Department of Neurology
University of Alabama at Birmingham
1202 Jefferson Tower
625 South 19th Street
Birmingham, Alabama 35294

Vickie Gordon, M.S.N., N.P.
Department of Neurosurgery
Wayne State University School of Medicine
Harper Hospital, Detroit Medical Center
4160 John R, Suite 930
Detroit, Michigan 48201

M. Sean Grady, M.D.
Associate Professor
Department of Neurological Surgery
University of Washington, Harborview Medical
*   Center*
325 Ninth Avenue, Box 359766
Seattle, Washington 98104

Ralph G. Greenlee Jr., M.D.
Professor, Departments of Neurology
and Neurosurgery
The University of Texas Southwestern Medical
*   Center*
5323 Harry Hines Boulevard
Dallas, Texas 75235-8897

Jeffrey I. Greenstein, M.D.
Matthew T. Moore Professor and Chair
Department of Neurology
Temple University Hospital
3401 North Broad Street
Philadelphia, Pennsylvania 19140

Guido Guglielmi, M.D.
Professor, Department of Radiological Sciences
University of California at Los Angeles
School of Medicine, Box 951721
Los Angeles, California 90095-1721

Jing Guo, M.D.
Associate Professor
Department of Neurosurgery
Beijing General Railway Hospital
Bei Feng Wo, Hai Dan District
Beijing 100038, Peoples Republic of China

Lee R. Guterman, Ph.D., M.D.
Assistant Professor
Department of Neurosurgery
State University of New York at Buffalo
School of Medicine and Biomedical Sciences
3 Gates Circle
Buffalo, New York 14226

Vladimir Hachinski, M.D., F.R.C.P.(C),
**   M.Sc.(DME), D.Sc.(Med.)**
Richard and Beryl Ivey Professor and Chair
Department of Clinical Neurological Sciences
University of Western Ontario
London Health Sciences Center
339 Windermere Road
London, Ontario N6A 5A5 Canada

Werner Hacke, M.D.
Professor, Department of Neurology
University of Heidelberg
Im Neuenheimer Feld 40
Heidelberg, Germany D-69120

Mark N. Hadley, M.D.
Associate Professor
Department of Neurological Surgery
University of Alabama at Birmingham
1813 Sixth Avenue South
Birminghm, Alabama 35294

Stephen J. Haines, M.D.
Professor, Department of Neurosurgery
University of Minnesota
420 Delaware Street Southeast, Box 96 UMHC
Minneapolis, Minnesota 55455

Van V. Halbach, M.D.
Professor, Departments of Radiology and
*   Neurological Surgery*
University of California at San Francisco
*   Medical Center*
505 Parnassus Avenue, Rm L352
San Francisco, California 94143-0628

Daniel F. Hanley, M.D.
Associate Professor, Director of the
*   Neurosciences Critical Care Unit*
Departments of Anesthesiology/Critical Care
*   Medicine, Neurology, and Neurosurgery*
Johns Hopkins Medical Institutions, Meyer 8-140
600 North Wolfe Street
Baltimore, Maryland 21287-7840

Cathy M. Helgason, M.D.
Professor, Department of Neurology
Director, Cerebrovascular Service
University of Illinois College of Medicine
912 South Wood Street, Rm 855N
Chicago, Illinois 60612

Scott Henson, M.D.
Department of Neurosurgery
Virginia Neurological Institute
Charlottesville, Virginia 22908

Roberto C. Heros, M.D.
Professor and Co-Chairman,
Department of Neurosurgery
University of Miami
1501 NW Ninth Avenue
Miami, Florida 33136

Grant B. Hieshima, M.D.
Clinical Professor of Radiology and Neurological
*   Surgery*
Department of Radiology
University of California at San Francisco
*   Medical Center*
505 Parnassus Avenue, Rm L352
San Francisco, California 94143-0628

Randall T. Higashida, M.D.
Clinical Professor of Radiology and
*   Neurosurgery*
Division of Interventional Neurovascular
*   Radiology*
Department of Radiology
University of California at San Francisco
*   Medical Center*
505 Parnassus Avenue, Room L352
San Francisco, California 94143-0628

Hector W. Ho, M.D.
Division of Neurological Surgery
Department of Surgery
Northwestern University Medical School
233 East Erie Street, Suite 614
Chicago, Illinois 60611

Khang-Loon Ho, M.D.
Department of Pathology
Henry Ford Hospital
2799 West Grand Boulevard
Detroit, Michigan 48202

L. Nelson Hopkins, M.D.
Professor of Radiology
Professor and Chairman, Department of
*   Neurosurgery*
State University of New York at Buffalo
School of Medicine and Biomedical Sciences
3 Gates Circle
Buffalo, New York 14209

Michael Bruce Horowitz, M.D.
Instructor
Departments of Neurosurgery and Radiology
The University of Texas Southwestern Medical
*   Center*
5323 Harry Hines Boulevard
Dallas, Texas 75235-8896

Joseph H. Introcaso, M.D., D.M.D.
Assistant Professor, Division of Neuroradiology
Department of Radiology
Northwestern University Medical School
Northwestern Memorial Hospital
710 North Fairbanks Court
Chicago, Illinois 60611

Shailendra Joshi, F.F.A.R.C.S.(I), M.D.
Fellow, Department of Anesthesiology
Columbia-Presbyterian Medical Center
630 West 168th Street, MH-4GN
New York, New York 10032

Charles A. Jungreis, M.D.
Associate Professor of Radiology and
*   Neurological Surgery*
Division of Neuroradiology, Department of
*   Radiology*
University of Pittsburgh Medical Center
200 Lothrop Street
Pittsburgh, Pennsylvania 15213-2582

Abraham Kader, M.D.
Assistant Professor
Department of Neurosurgery
Albert Einstein College of Medicine
111 East 210 Street
Bronx, New York 10467

Daniel S. Kanter, M.D.
Instructor in Neurology, Harvard Medical School
Medical Director, Neurology-Neurosurgery
*   Intensive Care Unit*
Brigham and Women's Hospital
75 Francis Street
Boston, Massachusetts 02115

Neal F. Kassell, M.D.
Distinguished Professor and Vice-Chairman
Department of Neurosurgery
University of Virginia
Health Sciences Center, Box 212
Charlottesville, Virginia 22908

Shigeaki Kobayashi, M.D., Ph.D.
Professor, Department of Neurosurgery
Shinshu University School of Medicine
Asahi 3-1-1
Matsumoto 390, Japan

Eberhard Kochs, M.D., M.Sc.
Professor of Anesthesiology
Klinikum Rechts der Isar
Technische Universität München
Ismaniger Strasse 22
Munich, 81675, Germany

Thomas A. Kopitnik Jr., M.D.
Associate Professor, Department of Neurological
*   Surgery*
The University of Texas Southwestern Medical
*   Center*
5323 Harry Hines Boulevard
Dallas, Texas 75235

Rashmi U. Kothari, M.D.
Assistant Professor, Department of Emergency
*   Medicine*
University of Cincinnati College of Medicine
231 Bethesda Avenue
Cincinnati, Ohio 45267-0001

Guiseppe Lanzino, M.D.
Resident, Department of Neurosurgery
University of Virginia Health Sciences Center
*   Box 212*
Charlottesville, Virginia 22908

Donald W. Larsen, M.D.
Associate Professor, Interventional
*   Neuroradiology Section*
Department of Radiology
University of Miami School of Medicine
(R-109), P.O. Box 016960
Miami, Florida 33101

Richard E. Latchaw, M.D.
Professor of Radiology and Neurosurgery
Chief, Interventional Neuroradiology Section
Department of Radiology
University of Miami School of Medicine
(R-109), P.O. Box 016960
Miami, Florida 33101

Richard Leblanc, M.D., M.Sc., F.R.C.S.C.
Associate Professor, Departments of Neurology
*   and Neurosurgery*
McGill University and Montreál Neurological
*   Institute*
3801 University Street
Montreál, Quebec H3A 2B4 Canada

Laurance I. Lee, M.D.
Assistant Director
Department of Interventional Neuroradiology
Baptist Memorial Hospital
910 Madison Avenue, Suite 364
Memphis, Tenessee 38103

Peter D. Le Roux, M.B., Ch.B, M.D.
Assistant Professor
Department of Neurosurgery
New York University
550 First Avenue
New York, New York 10016

Nicholas S. Little, M.B.B.S., F.R.A.C.S.
Fellow, Department of Neurological Surgery
Mayo Clinic
200 First Street SW
Rochester, Minnesota 55905

Christopher M. Loftus, M.D.
Professor, Department of Neurosurgery
The University of Iowa College of Medicine
1844 JPP 200 Hawkins Drive
Iowa City, Iowa 52242

R. Loch MacDonald, M.D., Ph.D.
Assistant Professor
Department of Surgery
University of Chicago
5841 South Maryland Avenue
Chicago, Illinois 60637

Michael T. Madison, M.D.
Assistant Professor of Radiology and
*   Neurosurgery*
Chief, Interventional Neuroradiology Division
Neuroradiology Section, Department of
*   Radiology*
University of Minnesota Hospital and Clinic
Harvard and East River Roads, SE
Minneapolis, Minnesota 55455

Marc D. Malkoff, M.D.
Associate Professor, Departments of
Neurology, Neurosurgery, and Anesthesiology
Director, Neurointensive Care Service
Indiana University Medical Center
550 University Boulevard, Room 3542
Indianapolis, Indiana 46202-5250

J. Nozipo Maraire, B.A., M.D.
Resident, Department of Neurology
Yale University Hospital
333 Cedar Street TMP 4
New Haven Connecticut 06571

Michael P. Marks, M.D.
Assistant Professor
Departments of Radiology and Neurosurgery
Stanford University Medical Center
300 Pasteur Drive, S-047
Stanford, California 94305

Neil A. Martin, M.D.
Professor, Division of Neurosurgery
Head, Neurovascular Surgery Section
University of California at Los Angeles School of
*   Medicine*
10833 LeConte Avenue
Los Angeles, California 90095

Marc R. Mayberg, M.D.
Professor, Department of Neurological Surgery
University of Washington Medical Center
1959 NE Pacific Street
Seattle, Washington 98195

Cameron G. McDougall, M.D.
Department of Radiology
University of California at San Francisco
*   Medical Center*
505 Parnassus Avenue, Rm L352
San Francisco, California 94143-0628

Dianne B. Mendelsohn, M.D.
Professor of Neuroradiology
Department of Radiology
The University of Texas Southwestern Medical
*   Center*
5171 Harry Hines Boulevard
Dallas, Texas 75235-8896

Joel R. Meyer, M.D.
Director of Magnetic Resonance Neuroimaging
and Interventional Radiology, Evanston Hospital
Assistant Professor
Departments of Radiology and Neurology
Northwestern University Medical School
710 North Fairbanks Court
Chicago, Illinois 60611

Marek A. Z. Mirski, M.D., Ph.D.
Medical Director, Queens Neuroscience Institute
Associate Professor of Surgery and Medicine
University of Hawaii Medical School
1301 Punch Bowl Street, Tower 4D
Honolulu, Hawaii 96813

Jorge Moncayo, M.D.
Fellow in Stroke Studies
Department of Neurology
University of Lausanne
Centre Hospitalier Universitaire Vaudois
CH 1011 Lausanne, Switzerland

Patricia M. Moore, M.D.
Associate Professor, Department of Neurology
Wayne State University School of Medicine
4201 St. Antoine 6E-UHC
Detroit, Michigan 48201

Richard B. Morawetz, M.D.
J.G. Galbraith Professor of Neurosurgery
Director, Division of Neurosurgery
Department of Surgery
The University of Alabama at Birmingham
1813 Sixth Avenue South
Birmingham, Alabama 35294

Jacques J. Morcos, M.D., F.R.C.S.(Eng.)
**   F.R.C.S.(Ed.)**
Assistant Professor
Department of Neurosurgery
University of Miami/Mount Sinai Medical Center
4300 Alton Road, 4-Greene
Miami Beach, Florida 33140

Howard Morgan, M.D., M.A., F.A.C.S.
Associate Professor, Department of Neurological
*   Surgery*
The University of Texas Southwestern Medical
*   Center*
5323 Harry Hines Boulevard
Dallas, Texas 75235-8855

Michael A. Murphy, M.D.
Department of Neurological Surgery
The University of Texas Southwestern Medical
*   Center*
5323 Harry Hines Boulevard
Dallas, Texas 75235-8896

David W. Newell, M.D.
Associate Professor
Department of Neurological Surgery
University of Washington, Harborview Medical
*   Center*
325 Ninth Avenue
Seattle, Washington 98104

John W. Norris, M.D.
Professor, Department of Neurology
University of Toronto
Toronto, Ontario M4N 3M5 Canada

Eugene Ornstein, Ph.D., M.D.
Associate Professor
Department of Anesthesiology
College of Physicians and Surgeons
Columbia University
630 West 168th Street
New York, New York 10032

Michihiko Osawa, M.D.
Assistant Professor
Department of Neurosurgery
Shinshu University School of Medicine
Asahi 3-1-1, Matsumoto
Nagano, 390 Japan

John N. Oshinski, Ph.D.
Assistant Professor
Department of Radiology
Emory University School of Medicine
1364 Clifton Road NE
Atlanta, Georgia 30322

Alberto Pasqualin, M.D.
Assistant Professor, Department of Neurosurgery
School of Medicine, University of Verona
Verona City Hospital
Piazzale Stefani
37100 Verona, Italy

Sydney John Peerless, M.D., F.R.C.S.C.
Director of the Mercy Neuroscience Institute
Clinical Professor, Department of Neurological
*   Surgery*
University of Miami
3661 South Miami Avenue, Suite 209
Miami, Florida 33133

Michael S. Pessin, M.D.
Professor, Department of Neurology
Tufts University School of Medicine
New England Medical Center Hospital
750 Washington Street, Box 314
Boston, Massachusetts 02111

David G. Piepgras, M.D.
Professor, Department of Neurologic Surgery
Mayo Clinic
200 First Street SW
Rochester, Minnesota 55905

John Pile-Spellman, M.D.
Associate Professor of Radiology and
*   Neurosurgery*
Director, Interventional Neuroradiology
College of Physicians and Surgeons
Columbia University
177 Fort Washington Avenue, MHB 8 South
*   Knuckle*
New York, New York 10032

R. Michael Poole, M.D.
Assistant Professor
Department of Neurology
University of Rochester
Rochester General Hospital
1425 Portland Ave
Rochester, New York 14621

William J. Powers, M.D.
Associate Professor
Departments of Neurology and Radiology
Washington University School of Medicine
East Building Imaging Center
4525 Scott Avenue, Campus Box 8225
St. Louis, Missouri 63110

Patrick Pullicino, M.D., Ph.D.
Associate Professor, Department of Neurology
Buffalo General Hospital
100 High Street
Buffalo, New York 14203

Phillip D. Purdy, M.D.
Professor of Radiology and
Associate Professor of Neurology and
*   Neurological Surgery*
Department of Radiology
The University of Texas Southwestern Medical
*   Center*
5323 Harry Hines Boulevard
Dallas, Texas 75235-8896

Ronald G. Quisling, M.D.
Professor of Neuroradiology
Department of Radiology
University of Florida Medical Center
Box 100374 JHMHC
Gainesville, Florida 32610

Bruce R. Ransom, M.D., Ph.D.
Professor and Chair
Department of Neurology
University of Washington School of Medicine
1959 NE Pacific Street, Room RR650
Seattle, Washington 98195

Robert A. Ratcheson, M.D.
The Harvey Huntington Brown, Jr. Professor and
Chairman, Department of Neurological Surgery
Director of Neurological Surgery
Case Western Reserve University
University Hospitals of Cleveland
11100 Euclid Avenue
Cleveland, Ohio 44106-2602

Mark B. Renfro, M.D.
Neurosurgery Resident
Department of Neurosurgery
University of Florida
1600 SW Archer Road
Gainesville, Florida 32610

Albert L. Rhoton, Jr., M.D.
R.D. Keene Family Professor and Chairman
Department of Neurological Surgery
University of Florida College of Medicine,
Shands Hospital
1600 SW Archer Road, Room M-219
P.O. Box 100265
Gainesville, Florida 32610-0265

Daniele Rigamonti, M.D.
Associate Professor
Department of Neurosurgery
John Hopkins University
600 North Wolfe Street/M. Bldg. 5-181
Baltimore, Maryland 20205

Mark B. Rorick, M.D.
Department of Neurology
MetroHealth Medical Center
Case Western Reserve University
Cleveland, Ohio 44109-1998

Richard A. Roski, M.S., M.D., F.A.C.S.
Genesis Medical Center
1351 West Central Park, Suite 2100
Davenport, Iowa 52804-1889

Eric J. Russell, M.D., F.A.C.R.
Professor and Acting Chairman, Department of
Radiology
and Chief, Section of Neuroradiology
Northwestern University Medical School
710 North Fairbanks Court
Chicago, Illinois 60611

Michael Salcman, M.D.
Clinical Professor of Neurosurgery
120 Sister Pierre Drive, Suite 107
Towson, Maryland 21204

Duke S. Samson, M.D.
Professor and Chairman
Department of Neurological Surgery
Lois C.A. and Darwin E. Smith Distinguished
Chair
The University of Texas Southwestern Medical
Center
Department of Neurological Surgery
5323 Harry Hines Boulevard
Dallas, Texas 75235-8855

Jeffrey L. Saver, M.D.
Assistant Professor of Clinical Neurology and
Neurology Director of the University of
California at Los Angeles Stroke Center
Department of Neurology
University of California at Los Angeles Medical
Center
710 Westwood Plaza
Los Angeles, California 90095

Stefan Schwab, M.D.
Department of Neurology
University of Heidelberg
Im Neuenheimer Feld 400
Heidelberg Germany D-69120

Lee H. Schwamm, M.D.
Clinical Assistant in Neurology
Harvard Medical School
Neurological Intensive Care Unit
Massachusetts General Hospital
32 Fruit Street
Boston, Massachusetts 02114

Renato Scienza, M.D.
Department of Neurosurgery
Bolzano City Hospital
L. Böhler Street nr. 5
Bolzano, Italy 39100

Warren R. Selman, M.D.
Professor and Vice Chairman, Department of
Neurological Surgery
Case Western Reserve University
University Hospitals of Cleveland
11100 Euclid Avenue
Cleveland, Ohio 44106-2602

Souvik Sen, M.D., M.S.
Chief Resident, Department of Neurology
Temple University Hospital
3401 North Broad Street
Philadelphia, Pennsylvania 19140

Christopher I. Shaffrey, M.D.
Department of Neurosurgery
Virginia Neurological Institute
Charlottesville, Virginia 22908

Marc E. Shaffrey, M.D.
Associate Professor, Department of
Neurosurgical Science
University of Virginia Health Sciences Center,
Box 212
Charlottesville, Virginia 22908

David H. Shafron, M.D.
Department of Neurological Surgery
University of Florida Health Center, Box 100265
Gainesville, Florida 32610

Ze'ev Shenkman, M.D.
Lecturer, Department of Anesthesiology and
Critical Care Medicine
Hadassah University Hospital and the Hebrew
University
Jerusalem, Israel

Patricia Silva, M.D.
Neuroradiologist
Departamento de Neuroimagen y Terapía
Endovascular
Instituto Nacional de Neurología y Neurocirugia
Insurgentes Sur No.3877
Mexico City, Mexico 14269

Michael B. Sisti, M.D.
Assistant Professor
Department of Neurological Surgery
Columbia University College of Physicians and
Surgeons
710 West 168th Street, Rm 414
New York, New York 10032-2603

Stephen L. Skirboll, M.D.
Resident, Department of Neurological Surgery
University of Washington, Harborview Medical
Center
325 Ninth Avenue Box 359766
Seattle, Washington 98104

Robert A. Solomon, M.D.
Professor, Department of Neurological Surgery
Columbia University
710 West 168th Street
New York, New York 10032-2603

Robert F. Spetzler, M.D.
Director, Barrow Neurological Institute
J.N. Harber Chairman of Neurolgical Surgery
Professor, Section of Neurosurgery, University of
Arizona at Tucson
Division of Neurological Surgery
Barrow Neurological Institute
350 West Thomas Road
Phoenix, Arizona 85013-4496

Bennett M. Stein, M.D.
Byron Stookey Professor and Chairman
Department of Neurological Surgery
Columbia University College of Physicians and
Surgeons
710 West 168th Street, Rm 204
New York, New York 10032-2603

Gary K. Steinberg, M.D., Ph.D.
Associate Professor and Chairman
Department of Neurosurgery
Stanford University School of Medicine
300 Pasteur Drive, Room S-006
Stanford, California 94305-5327

Thorsten Steiner, M.D.
Doctor of Medicine
Department of Neurology
University of Heidelberg
Im Neuenheimer Feld 400
Heidelberg Germany D-69120

Philip E. Stieg, M.D., Ph.D.
Assistant Professor of Surgery, Associate Chief
Division of Neurosurgery
Brigham and Women's Hospital/Harvard
Medical School
75 Francis Street
Boston, Massachusetts 02115

Constantino Takis, M.D.
New England Medical Center
750 Washington Street
Boston, Massachusetts 02111

Rafael J. Tamargo, M.D.
Assistant Professor and Co-director
of the Division of Vascular Neurology
Department of Neurosurgery
Johns Hopkins Hospital
600 North Woolfe Street, Meyer 7-113
Baltimore, Maryland 21287-7713

Yuichiro Tanaka, M.D.
Assistant Professor, Department of Neurosurgery
Shinshu University School of Medicine
Asahi 3-1-1, Matsumoto 390 Japan

Robert W. Tarr, M.D.
Assistant Professor, Department of Radiology
Case Western Reserve University
Co-Director, Cerebrovascular Center
University Hospitals of Cleveland
11100 Euclid Avenue
Cleveland, Ohio 44106-2602

Philip A. Teal, B.Sc., M.D., F.R.C.P.(C)
Assistant Clinical Professor
Department of Neurology
University of British Columbia
Vancouver Hospital
943 West Broadway Suite 510
Vancouver, BC V5Z 4E1 Canada

René Tempelhoff, M.D.
Associate Professor of Anesthesiology and
* Neurological Surgery*
Washington University School of Medicine
660 South Euclid Avenue #8054
St. Louis, Missouri 63110-1093

John B. Terry, M.D.
Senior Clinical Fellow
Neurosciences Critical Care Unit
Johns Hopkins Hospital
600 North Wolfe Street
Baltimore, Maryland 21287-7839

Daryl W. Thompson, M.D.
Dept of Neurology
The Cleveland Clinic Foundation
9500 Euclid
Cleveland, Ohio 44195-0001

Shwe Z. Tun, M.D.
Assistant Professor, Department of Neurology
Director, Cerebrovascular Disease Center
Temple University School of Medicine
3401 North Broad Street
Philadelphia, Pennsylvania 19140

D. Hal Unwin, M.D.
Associate Professor
Department of Neurology
The University of Texas Southwestern Medical
* School*
5323 Harry Hines Boulevard
Dallas, Texas 75235-8897

Antoine Uské, M.D.
Privat Docent, Maître D'Enseignement et de
* Recherche*
Chief, Section of Neuroradiology
Department of Radiology
University of Lausanne
Centre Hospitalier Universitaire Vaudois
Rue Du Bugnon 11
Lausanne, Switzerland CH-1011

Anton Valavanis, M.D., Ph.D.
Professor of Neuroradiology
Institut for Neuroradiologie
University Hospital Zurich
Frauenklinikstrasse 10
CH-8091 Zurich, Switzerland

Fernando L. Vale, M.D.
Resident Physician
Department of Neurosurgery
University of Alabama Hospitals at Birmingham
1813 Sixth Avenue South
511 Medical Education Building
Birmingham, Alabama 35294

R. James Valentine, M.D.
Associate Professor, Division of Vascular
* Surgery*
Department of Surgery,
The University of Texas Southwestern Medical
* Center*
5323 Harry Hines Boulevard
Dallas, Texas 75235-9031

Harry V. Vinters, M.D., F.R.C.P.(C)
Chief of Neuropathology
Professor, Department of Pathology and
* Laboratory Medicine*
University of California at Los Angeles Medical
* Center*
Los Angeles, California 90095-1732

Fernando Viñuela, M.D.
Professor, Radiological Sciences
Chief, Therapeutic Neuroradiology
Department of Radiology
University of California at Los Angeles
School of Medicine and Medical Center, Box
* 951721*
Los Angeles, California 90095-1721

Stephen G. Waxman, M.D., Ph.D.
Professor and Chairman, Department of
* Neurology*
Yale School of Medicine
P.O. Box 208018, 333 Cedar Street
New Haven, Connecticut 06520-8018

Jesse Weinberger, M.D.
Professor, Department of Neurology
The Mount Sinai School of Medicine
Box 1052, One Gustave Levy Place
New York, New York 10029-6574

Bryce Weir, M.Sc., M.D.C.M., F.R.C.S.(C),
** F.A.C.S., F.R.C.S.Ed. Hon.**
Maurice Goldblatt Professor of Surgery and
* Neurology*
Chief, Section of Neurosurgery
Director, Brain Research Institute
The University of Chicago Medical Center
5841 South Maryland Avenue
Chicago, Illinois 60637

Christian Werner, M.D.
*Associate Professor, Department of
 Anesthesiology*
Klinikum Rechts der Isar
Technische Universität München
Ismaniger Strasse 22
Munich, 81675, Germany

Harvey Ira Wilner, M.D., F.A.C.R.
Associate Professor
Department of Radiology
Wayne State University
4201 St. Antoine
Detroit, Michigan, 48201

H. Richard Winn, M.D.
Professor and Chairman
Department of Neurological Surgery
University of Washington School of Medicine
Harborview Medical Center,
325 Ninth Avenue, Box 359766
Seattle, Washington 98104

Robert J. Wityk, M.D.
*Assistant Professor, Departments of Neurology
 and Medicine*
*The Johns Hopkins University School of
 Medicine*
Sinai Hospital of Baltimore
2401 West Belvedere Avenue
Baltimore, Maryland 21215

Charles W. Wyble, M.D.
Resident, Department of Surgery
The University of Chicago Medical Center
5841 South Maryland Avenue
Chicago, Illinois 60637-1470

William L. Young, M.D.
*Associate Professor, Departments of
Anesthesiology, Radiology, and Neurological
 Surgery*
*College of Physicians and Surgeons of Columbia
 University*
630 West 168th Street, Box 46
New York, New York 10032

Mario Zuccarello, M.D.
Associate Professor
Department of Neurosurgery
Mayfield Clinic
222 Piedmont Avenue #3100
Cincinnati, Ohio 45219

Preface

Cerebrovascular Disease represents an enormous effort on behalf of many of the most outstanding neuroscientists in the world. From the inception of this project, it has been my goal as well as that of the associate editors to produce a work under a single cover that will serve clinicians and scientists as both a freshly up-to-date resource for their daily work as well as a set of clinical and scientific principles that will retain lasting value and usefulness. The authorship is as diverse clinically and scientifically as it is dispersed geographically. Leading scholars in the fields of neurology, neurophysiology, neurosurgery, neuroradiology, neuropathology, critical care, and molecular biology have succinctly reported their perspectives and hopes for the future in the management of these conditions, which represent a leading cause of death and disability.

The volume is organized so as to relate to the readership the complete story of cerebrovascular disorders. The specific topics presented span the gamut from fundamental anatomy and physiology to current medical and surgical treatment alternatives and finally to the implications of modern biological research. The editors have made every attempt to include the highest level of authorship from the multiple disciplines involved in studying and treating these conditions. Significant weight has been attached to the specific treatment modalities appropriate for the complete range of ischemic and hemorrhagic stroke disorders.

The volume concludes with a section dealing with socioeconomic and ethical issues. At first glance, such a section might appear provincial and specifically related only to current issues faced by North American physicians. On the most fundamental level however, each of these issues must be successfully negotiated in all countries and in all regions of the world. Each country has a finite resource that may be made available to the care of its citizens. Health professionals and health scientists have the responsibility to ensure that these resources are allocated such that the public receives optimal care and that such care be constantly improving.

It is my sincerest hope that the reader finds this work as interesting and exciting as I have. Great care has been taken to ensure that the important material presented is as user friendly as possible. We now have the information and technology available to allow the next generation of clinicians and scientists to make great strides in many of these conditions which at present are poorly and empirically treated.

H. Hunt Batjer, M.D.

Acknowledgments

I would like to thank Elizabeth Greenspan, our editor at Lippincott-Raven, for her encouragement and tenacity in the achievement of such a high quality and timely volume. I am indebted to the associate editors for their numerous personal contributions and for their insights into the neurosciences, which have enriched their work.

SECTION I
The Cerebral Vasculature in Health and Disease

The first chapters of this book deal with normal cerebrovascular anatomy and physiology as well as the basic pathological elements of the most frequently occurring cerebrovascular diseases. Knowledge about intra- and extracranial vascular anatomy and its multiple variations have largely been gathered with traditional anatomical methods. Over the past two decades, however, new and largely non-traumatic examination techniques have contributed substantially to our knowledge about the physiology of the intact, living human brain.

Magnetic resonance imaging (MRI) has not only developed into a refined morphological method providing us with tremendous accurate details of the brain tissue, but also with non-invasive, angiographic images with continuous improvement of quality. Through the past few years of the 1990's, the development of flow sensitive MR techniques and fast-echo planar imaging have also provided us with the ability to examine intravascular flow and functions of localized brain areas. Similarly, the radioisotope methods of positron emission tomography (PET) and single photon emission tomography (SPECT) have become available at more medical centers, and they have enhanced our knowledge about crucial elements of normal cerebrovascular physiology and changes found in cerebrovascular disease. SPECT, of course, being the most widespread, cheapest, and easiest applicable method for clinical examinations. Finally, the transcranial Doppler (TCD) method has proven to be a useful functional method, particularly for monitoring interventional procedures for selected cerebrovascular diseases; though the TCD method is less sensitive for primary diagnostic purposes. The techniques have provided substantial new knowledge widely reflected in the chapters of this book. It is difficult to imagine future cerebrovascular research, least of all handling just the slightest complicated clinical condition, without them.

Regional cerebral blood flow (rCBF) has been the most prominent parameter used, not only to describe the cerebrovascular blood supply, but also as a sensitive marker for local brain function. For decades it has been assumed that there is a direct coupling between changes in cerebral glucose and oxygen metabolism and changes in rCBF, however, new and controversial results have emerged from studies of regulation of the normal brain's metabolism (Chapter 2). rCBF rises during neuronal activation, but not necessarily parallel with changes in glucose and oxygen consumption. Although these findings are not completely understood, controversial suggestions have arisen; that non-oxidative neuronal metabolism may act as a ''kick starter'' and the lactate produced may influence rCBF regulation (Chapter 2).

Chapters 3 through 9 constitute exhaustive descriptions of causes for cerebrovascular disease; atherosclerosis and hypertension being the most common and extensively studied causes. Many aspects of the microvascular disease syndromes still remain to be explored and understood. Patterns of chances of recovery from focal ischemic damage to brain tissue begin to emerge, although the cellular mechanisms are not fully understood (Chapter 10). Early start of rehabilitation after a cerebrovascular event seems to provide the most successful outcome at this point. Probably, the cerebrovascular responses to anesthesia is, overall, the most serious concern held by the anesthesiologist (Chapter 11). Many drugs act unfavorably on intracranial pressure, and the manipulation of CBF may be necessary.

Gene therapy (Chapter 12) is such a novel approach that doctors graduating from medical school just a few years ago were not even taught about this field. The fundamental rationale and methods for gene therapy are interesting. The initial hurdle is to identify patients with genetic risk for cerebrovascular disease; a far from trivial task. Gene therapy, however, still remains a future possibility for treatment of some selected cerebrovascular disease states.

Lars Friberg, M.D.

Cerebrovascular Disease, edited by H. Hunt Batjer.
Lippincott-Raven Publishers, Philadelphia © 1997.

CHAPTER 1

The Extracranial and Intracranial Vessels: Normal Anatomy and Variations

Mark B. Renfro, Arthur L. Day, and Albert L. Rhoton

Blood supply to the brain is provided by two carotid and two vertebral arteries. The carotid or anterior circulation supplies most of the supratentorial parenchyma (which includes the majority of the cerebral hemispheres), whereas the vertebrobasilar or posterior circulation supplies all of the infratentorial structures (the brain-stem and cerebellum) and the occipital and mesial temporal structures supratentorially. Each arterial system originates within the chest and has lengthy cervical segments prior to penetrance of the skull base to enter the subarachnoid space.

CAROTID SYSTEM (ANTERIOR CIRCULATION)

Common Carotid Artery

The right common carotid artery (CCA) begins at the bifurcation of the innominate (brachiocephalic) artery, whereas the left originates in the thorax from the aortic arch (Fig. 1). Both arteries emerge from the base of the neck behind the sternoclavicular articulations to run upward and backward toward the angle of the mandible, under cover of the sternocleidomastoid muscle. Near the upper border of the thyroid cartilage each CCA divides into its two terminal branches, the internal and external carotid arteries. The region of this bifurcation contains two important sensory structures: (a) the carotid body, which represents a specialized vascular chemoreceptor that stimulates respiration in response to a fall in arterial po_2 or a rise in pco_2, and (a) the carotid sinus, which is a focal dilatation of the artery (carotid bulb) that contains the baroreceptors that reflexively regulate blood pressure. Both of these receptor areas project primarily into the glossopharyngeal nerve, although some connections with the vagus, hypoglossal, or superior cervical ganglion

may also exist. Throughout its course, each CCA is enclosed in a carotid sheath, a layer of connective tissue that also contains the internal jugular vein and the vagus nerve. Usually there are no branches from the CCA before its bifurcation, although the ascending pharyngeal or superior thyroid may arise from this vessel when its bifurcation is at higher levels.

A normal pattern of origin of the common carotid arteries from the aortic arch is seen in 65–70% of patients (1). Variations are generally of minor clinical importance and most often involve an anomalous origin of the left CCA from the innominate artery or the right CCA from the aorta. The most frequently encountered CCA bifurcation site corresponds to approximately the C4-5 vertebral level, although the bifurcation may occur as high as Cl or as low as T2. Such variations are often of clinical importance when planning a surgical procedure. Krayenbuhl and Yasargil found that 48.1% of bifurcations occurred at C4-5, 34.2% at C3-4, and 13% at C5-6 (2). The bifurcation level is typically one or two cervical levels higher in children than in adults (1,2).

External Carotid Artery

The external carotid artery (ECA) is the smaller of two terminal CCA branches and extends from the bifurcation until its terminal branching into the superficial temporal and internal maxillary arteries (Fig. 2). The ECA typically has eight branches, each of which is primarily distributed to parts outside the skull. Throughout their courses, these branches are accompanied by numerous sympathetic fibers that regulate facial vascular tone and sweating.

Several ECA branches supply the dura of the basal and lateral brain surfaces (3,4). Meningeal branches from the ascending pharyngeal artery enter the skull through the foramen lacerum, jugular foramen, and hypoglossal canal to supply much of the posterior fossa dura. The occipital artery has

M. B. Renfro, A. L. Day, and A. L. Rhoton: Department of Neurological Surgery, University of Florida, Gainesville, Florida 32610

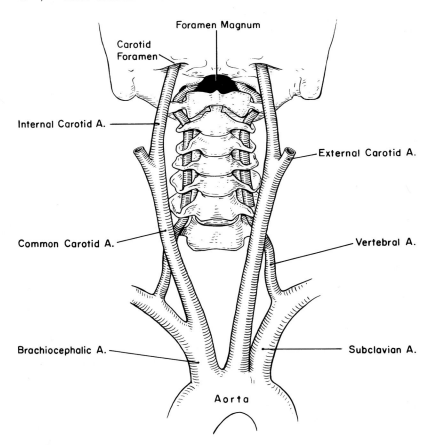

FIG. 1. Origin and extracranial course of cerebral vessels *(anterior view)*: normal anatomy.

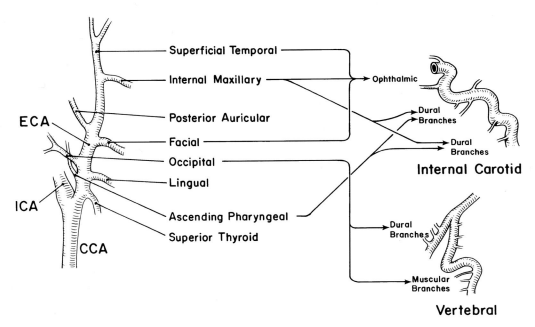

FIG. 2. External carotid artery (ECA): branches and intracranial communications. Arrows indicate potential connections with intracranial structures via anastomoses with internal carotid (ICA) and vertebral arteries. CCA, common carotid artery.

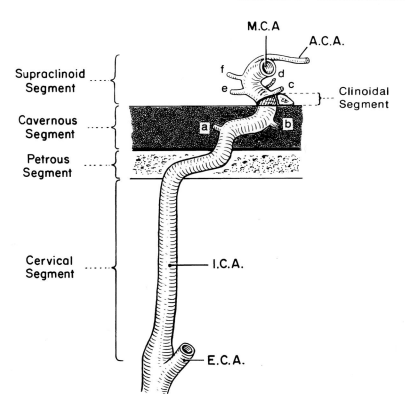

FIG. 3. Internal carotid artery (ICA): segments and branches. Major branches include (A) meningohypophyseal trunk, (B) artery of the inferior cavernous sinus (C) ophthalmic artery, (D) superior hypophyseal artery, (E) posterior communicating artery, (F) anterior choroidal artery and terminal branches. ACA, anterior cerebral artery; MCA, middle cerebral artery; ECA = external carotid artery.

meningeal branches that also supply the posterior fossa dura after entering the skull through the jugular foramen and condylar canal. The internal maxillary artery, through its middle and accessory meningeal artery branches, penetrate the skull through the foramen spinosum and foramen ovale to vascularize most of middle and anterior cranial fossae dura.

Congenital abnormalities of the ECA are usually of little clinical significance, as the excellent transfacial collateral circulation from ipsilateral and contralateral sources prevents any facial arterial insufficiency, even with complete absence of this vessel. The abundant anastomoses between the external carotid and the intracranial circulation may provide an important source of collateral blood flow to the brain (Fig. 2) (3–5).

Internal Carotid Artery

The larger of the two CCA branches, the internal carotid artery (ICA), provides blood supply to the cerebral hemispheres, ipsilateral eye, and parts of the forehead and nose. The ICA is classically divided into four segments: cervical, petrosal, cavernous, and supraclinoid or subarachnoid (Fig. 3) (6).

Segments

Cervical

This segment begins at the CCA bifurcation, then ascends without branching posterior and medial to the ECA until it enters the temporal bone at the skull base. During its course, the ICA is frequently crossed, in ascending order, by the common facial vein, the hypoglossal nerve, the occipital artery, the digastric (posterior belly) and stylohyoid muscles, and the posterior auricular artery. In its upper course the ICA lies deep to the parotid gland, with the external carotid located anterolaterally. The stylopharyngeus muscle and its associated glossopharyngeal nerve, the pharyngeal branch of the vagus, and the stylohyoid ligament pass between the two arteries in this area. The internal jugular vein, which initially ran lateral to the artery, now lies behind it. The 9th, 10th, 11th, and 12th cranial nerves all normally pass between the artery and vein at this level. Throughout this segment, the artery is accompanied by sympathetic fibers that project to the pupillodilator and superior tarsal muscles of the ipsilateral eye.

Excessive or accentuated curvatures within the cervical segment (usually within 3–5 cm of the bifurcation) are commonplace and can be divided into three groups: (a) tortuosity, ie, any S- or C-shaped elongation or undulation, (b) coiling elongation or redundancy resulting in an exaggerated S-shaped curve or circular configuration, and (c) kinking angulation of one or more portions of the vessel generally associated with stenosis (7). Tortuosity and coiling are often bilateral, may be present in children, and are generally regarded as congenital conditions that tend to increase with age, with any eventual manifestations being dependent on the resilience and function of the perivascular connective tissue within the affected artery. Kinking is usually a condition of older adults and is associated with arteriosclerosis (1,7).

Total absence of the ICA is rare, but variations in size are commonplace. Most differences in caliber are direct reflections of the area of brain that it ultimately supplies (8). A larger ICA would be expected when one carotid supplies both distal anterior cerebral artery territories, a situation that occurs when the ipsilateral proximal anterior cerebral is large while the corresponding contralateral vessel is hypoplastic. Similar but less noticeable caliber differences may also occur when the posterior cerebral artery is fed primarily from the carotid system rather than from the vertebrobasilar circuit (a "fetal" posterior communicating artery).

Petrous

This segment begins when the artery enters the carotid canal within the petrous portion of the temporal bone, directly anterior to the jugular foramen and behind the eustachian tube, and ends where the vessel enters the cavernous sinus (Fig. 4) (9). At its point of entrance, the ICA is surrounded by a tough fibrous ring of periosteum that firmly anchors the vessel to the skull base. During its course, the petrous segment can be divided into a vertical or ascending portion, a genu, and a horizontal portion. The vertical portion ascends in the temporal bone, then angles sharply in an anteromedial direction at the genu to form the horizontal portion. The artery then courses forward and medially through the carotid canal until it reaches the petrous apex, where it ascends from its bony canal medial to the Gasserian ganglion and superior to the foramen lacerum to enter the middle cranial fossa. Common branches of the petrous segment include the vidian artery, which passes to the pterygoid canal, a caroticotympanic artery that enters the tympanic cavity, and a periosteal branch.

Within the petrous segment, the ICA is surrounded by a periosteal sheath, a small plexus of veins, and a periarterial neural plexus originating from the cervical sympathetic plexus. The horizontal portion has several important relationships to surrounding structures in the floor of the middle fossa. The greater superficial petrosal nerve passes superiorly and parallel to the vessel as it runs from the geniculate ganglion to the pterygoid canal within the facial hiatus. The tensor tympani muscle and bony eustachian tube, located below the floor of the middle fossa, lay anterior and lateral, and also course parallel to the vessel. The cochlea, encased in dense bone anterior to the internal auditory canal, sits posterior to the genu and horizontal portions of the artery, and its proximity (average 2 mm) places it at risk for injury during exposure of the petrous ICA during vascular bypass or skull base procedures. The bony roof of the horizontal portion may be incomplete, exposing parts of the artery extradurally prior to its entrance into the cavernous sinus.

Cavernous

The cavernous segment of the ICA begins at the foramen lacerum as the vessel ascends from the carotid canal to enter the posterior inferior cavernous sinus (Fig. 5) (10). The artery is briefly directed upward toward the posterior clinoid process, then runs forward and horizontally, lateral to the sphenoid sinus. The segment terminates by penetrating the

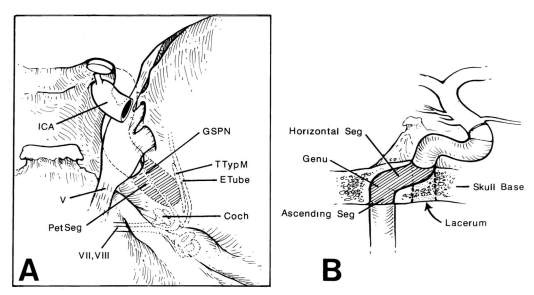

FIG. 4. Internal carotid artery (ICA): *petrous segment* (PetSeg), dorsal **(A)** and lateral **(B)** views. Note artery course within temporal bone, the three divisions of this segment (ascending, genu, and horizontal segments), and ICA relationship to eustachian tube (E tube), tensor typani muscle (T Typ M), greater superficial petrosal nerve (GSPN), and cochlea (coch). V, trigeminal nerve; VII, facial nerve; VIII, auditovestibular nerve; lacerum, foramen lacerum

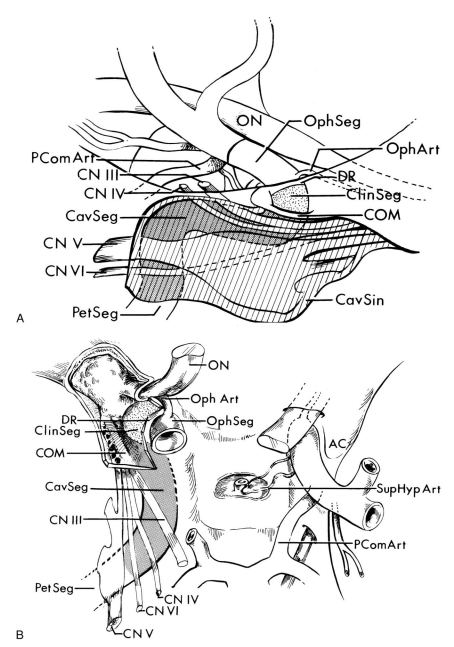

FIG. 5. Internal carotid artery (ICA): *cavernous segment*, (CavSeg), lateral (A) and dorsal (B) views. Note the two portions of the carotid artery traditionally considered to be within the cavernous sinus (CavSin), the CavSeg and clinoidal segment (ClinSeg). The CavSeg (shaded ICA segment) lies within the large venous channel of the cavernous sinus (obliquely striped region). The ClinSeg (stippled ICA segment) corresponds to the anterior vertical segment of the cavernous carotid artery, but lies outside the venous lumen. Both segments lie below the dural ring and outside the subarachnoid space. DR, dural ring; COM, carotid-oculomotor membrane; ON, optic nerve; OS, optic strut; AC, anterior clinoid process; OphSeg, ophthalmic segment; PetSeg, petrous segment; OphArt, ophthalmic artery; PComArt, posterior communicating artery; SupHypArt, superior hypophyseal artery; CN III, oculomotor nerve; CN IV, trochlear nerve; CN V, trigeminal nerve; CN VI, abducens nerve.

dura medial to the anterior clinoid process to enter the sub-arachnoid space. The intracavernous ICA is classically divided into five parts: (a) the posterior vertical segment, (b) the posterior bend, (c) the horizontal segment, (d) the anterior bend, and (e) the anterior vertical segment (10,11).

The most consistent cavernous ICA branches are the meningohypophyseal trunk and the inferolateral (artery of the inferior cavernous sinus) trunks. The meningohypophyseal trunk arises from the posterior bend of the intracavernous ICA and typically gives rise to three branches: (a) the tentorial artery (artery of Bernasconi–Cassinari), which supplies the tentorium, (b) the inferior hypophyseal artery, which passes medial to the pituitary gland, and (c) the dorsal meningeal artery, which supplies the dura over the upper clivus. The inferolateral trunk usually arises from the horizontal portion of the artery and passes laterally above the abducens nerve to supply the cranial nerves and dura of the inferior cavernous sinus, as well as the dura of the middle fossa floor from the cavernous sinus lateral to foramens ovale and spinosum. In pathologic states, these vessels may provide extensive communications with external carotid branches or arteries from the contralateral side.

McConnell's capsular artery may occasionally originate within the intracavernous ICA segment (present in about 8% of specimens) arising from the medial portion of the horizontal segment and passing medial to the pituitary gland (11). The ophthalmic artery may also arise from distal portions of the cavernous segment (4–8% of specimens), and in such instances the artery reaches the orbit through the superior orbital fissure or, less commonly, through a foramen located within the optic strut (10,11).

The cranial nerves that mediate ocular motility and facial sensation pass in close proximity to the cavernous carotid artery. The oculomotor, trochlear, and upper divisions of the trigeminal nerves lie within the dura of the lateral cavernous sinus wall, whereas the abducens nerve actually courses within the sinus between the carotid artery medially and the outer sinus wall laterally. Sympathetic fibers traverse the cavernous sinus as a grossly visible plexus on the carotid artery. Some of these fibers jump to the abducens nerve before joining the trigeminal nerve to ultimately enter the orbit, whereas the remainder continue upwards with the ICA to enter the subarachnoid space.

The intracavernous ICA segment is classically considered to be completely surrounded by the venous blood and dural sheaths of the cavernous sinus. As the distal portion of the anterior vertical segment ascends and courses medial to the anterior clinoid process, however, a distinct portion of the ICA can be delineated that is within neither the cavernous sinus nor the subarachnoid space (11–13). This segment, termed the clinoidal segment, is defined inferiorly by a thin layer of periosteum reflected off the inferior-medial edge of the anterior clinoid process. Bridging from the ICA to the oculomotor nerve, this sheet of periosteum (called the carotid-oculomotor membrane or membranous ring) separates the clinoidal segment from the venous walls of the cavernous sinus. The clinoidal segment is limited superiorly by the dural reflections (the dural ring) from the superomedial edge of the anterior clinoid process that encircle and attach to the ICA and then pass medial along the inferior and posterior edge of the optic canal to fuse with the dura of the diaphragma sellae. The dural ring marks the true point of penetrance of the ICA into the subarachnoid space (14–16).

Supraclinoid (Intracranial or Subarachnoid)

As the ICA spans the cavernous and supraclinoid segments, it assumes an S-shaped configuration on lateral view that is referred to as the carotid siphon. The supraclinoid carotid artery begins where the artery emerges through the dural ring from the clinoidal segment, thereby forming the distal half of the siphon (Fig. 6). The artery enters the subarachnoid space medial to the anterior clinoid process, just inferior to the optic nerve, and then passes posteriorly, superiorly, and laterally to the side of the optic chiasm. The vessel then angles forward as it nears the anterior perforated substance at the medial end of the Sylvian fissure, where it bifurcates into the anterior and medial cerebral arteries (6). The supraclinoid portion of the ICA can be divided into three

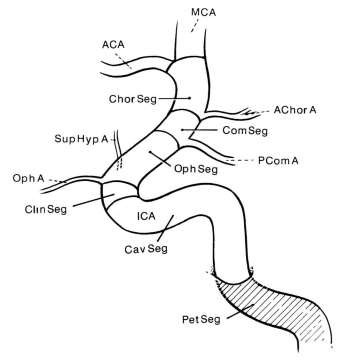

FIG. 6. Internal carotid artery (ICA): *intracranial segments.* In order of origin, segments include petrous segment (PetSeg), cavernous segment (CavSeg), clinoidal segment (ClinSeg), ophthalmic segment (OphSeg), communicating segment (ComSeg), choroidal segment (ChorSeg) and branches (OphA, ophthalmic artery, SupHypA, superior hypophyseal artery, PComA, posterior communicating artery, AChorA, anterior choroidal artery, ACA, anterior cerebral artery, MCA, middle cerebral artery).

segments: ophthalmic, communicating, and choroidal, based on the site of origin of the ophthalmic, posterior communicating, and anterior choroidal arteries, respectively (6).

Ophthalmic Segment

The ophthalmic segment is the longest subarachnoid portion of the ICA, beginning at the dural ring and ending at the origin of the posterior communicating artery (Fig. 6) (6). Two named branches typically arise from the ophthalmic segment, the ophthalmic and superior hypophyseal arteries. The ophthalmic artery usually arises from the dorsal or dorsomedial ICA surface, immediately beneath the lateral aspect of the overlying optic nerve, and courses anteriorly through the optic canal to the orbit. The artery initially runs lateral to the optic nerve, but eventually it crosses obliquely over the top of the optic nerve within the optic canal to enter the medial side of the orbit. Branches of the ophthalmic artery include (a) the central retinal artery, which supplies the eye, (b) the lacrimal artery, which supplies the lacrimal gland and upper and lower eyelids, (c) the anterior and posterior ethmoidal arteries, which course medial to enter the ethmoids and anterior skull base giving rise to ethmoidal, nasal, and meningeal branches, and (d) the supraorbital and supratrochlear arteries, which pass to the face and anastomose freely with branches from the external carotid artery (17,18).

Several large perforating vessels also arise from the ophthalmic segment, the largest of which has been named the superior hypophyseal artery. These perforators usually arise from the medial or ventromedial surface of the ICA and supply a portion of the dura around the cavernous sinus, the superior aspect of the pituitary gland and stalk, and the optic nerves and chiasm (19–21).

Communicating Segment

The communicating ICA segment extends from (and includes) the origin of the posterior communicating artery and ends at the anterior choroidal artery takeoff (Fig. 6) (21). The posterior communicating artery (PComA) typically arises from the posterior ICA surface, passes posteriorly and medially above the sella turcica and oculomotor nerve, and then joins the posterior cerebral artery to complete the posterior aspect of the circle of Willis. Embryologically the PComA and posterior cerebral artery are both derived from the carotid system. During development, however, the PComA ceases its growth, and the posterior cerebral artery becomes annexed into the vertebrobasilar system. When the PComA remains the major contributor to the posterior cerebral artery (22% of cases), it is termed a "fetal" PComA (22). In such situations, the PComA courses posterolaterally either above or lateral to the oculomotor nerve. Infundibular widening at the PComA origin are found in 6.5% of normal cerebral angiograms, and debate exists as to whether this dilatation represents a normal variation or a preaneurysmal lesion (23).

Numerous perforating arteries off the PComA (collectively called the anterior thalamoperforating arteries) course superiorly to the premamillary part of the floor of the third ventricle, the posterior perforated substance, and the interpeduncular fossa. These vessels supply the thalamus, hypothalamus, subthalamus, and internal capsule, and some may also supply the optic chiasm, optic tract, and pituitary stalk.

Choroidal Segment

The choroidal segment extends from the anterior choroidal artery origin to the terminal ICA bifurcation (Fig. 6). The anterior choroidal artery (AChorA) arises from the posterior ICA surface and its initial or cisternal portion runs posteriorly, inferior to the optic tract and lateral to the PComA, to reach the lateral margin of the cerebral peduncle (Fig. 7) (6,24,25). Branches of the cisternal segment supply the optic tract, cerebral peduncle, lateral geniculate body, and temporal lobe. At the anterior margin of the lateral geniculate body, the AChorA crosses the optic tract from medial to lateral to reach a position near the uncus. The plexal segment of the AChorA begins here as the vessel penetrates the choroidal fissure to supply the choroid plexus in the temporal horn and lateral ventricle. This segment may also provide blood supply to parts of the internal capsule, thalamus, lateral geniculate body, cerebral peduncle, and optic tract. Perforating branches frequently arise from choroidal ICA segment, distal to the AChorA origin, and supply the anterior perforated substance, optic chiasm, and uncus.

Terminal Branches

Anterior Cerebral Artery

The anterior cerebral artery (ACA), the smaller of the two terminal ICA branches, arises from the ICA bifurcation below the anterior perforated substance (Fig. 8). Each ACA then passes medially and anteriorly above the optic nerves and chiasm to join its contralateral counterpart just anterior to the lamina terminalis at the anterior communicating artery, thereby completing the anterior portion of the circle of Willis (26,27). The proximal portion on the ACA, lying between its origin and the anterior communicating artery (AComA), is called the A1 segment. Numerous perforators off the A1 segment enter the medial anterior perforated substance to supply the septal region and hypothalamus (21).

The A2 segments of the ACA span, together in parallel in the longitudinal fissure between the two hemispheres, from the anterior communicating artery to the rostrum of the corpus callosum (27). Multiple small perforators arise from this segment, entering the lamina terminalis and anterior forebrain below the corpus callosum to supply the anterior hypothalamus, septum pellucidum, medial portion of the

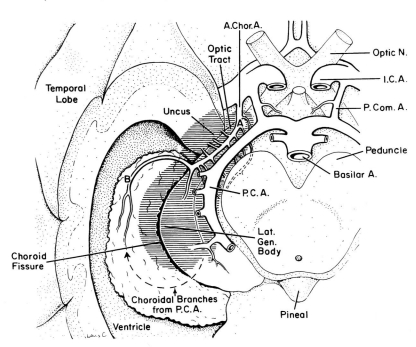

FIG. 7. *Anterior choroidal artery* (AChorA): branches and distribution, inferior view. **A:** cisternal segment; **B:** plexal segment; horizontally striped area is parenchymal regions normally supplied by AChorA and its branches. ICA, internal carotid artery; PComA, posterior communicating artery; PCA, posterior cerebral artery.

anterior commissure, pillars of the fornix, and anteroinferior part of the striatum (27). The recurrent artery of Heubner arises from the proximal A2 segment in two-thirds of cases (the remainder arising more proximally from the A1 segment). This artery doubles back on its parent vessel and accompanies the middle cerebral artery into the Sylvian fissure prior to entering the anterior perforated substance (28). Heubner's artery supplies the anterior part of the caudate nucleus, the anterior third of the putamen, the outer portion of the globus pallidus, and the anterior limb of the internal capsule.

The distal portion of the ACA (also called the pericallosal artery) makes a smooth curve around the genu of the corpus callosum and passes posteriorly in the pericallosal cistern, giving rise to numerous and variable cortical branches (29). The first cortical branch is usually the orbitofrontal artery, which supplies the medial portion of the orbital gyri, the gyrus rectus, and the olfactory bulb and tract. The next named branch, the frontopolar artery, passes anteriorly to supply the inferior, medial, and anterior surfaces of the frontal pole.

The most prominent pericallosal branch is the callosomarginal artery, which when well formed lies in the sulcus immediately above the cingulate gyrus. Proceeding posteriorly in parallel with the pericallosal artery, cortical branches from both vessels supply the entire anterior two thirds of the medial cerebral hemispheres, including the corpus callosum, cingulate gyrus, paracentral lobule, and precuneus. After leaving the interhemispheric fissure, branches of the ACA course laterally to supply the superior frontal gyrus and the superior parts of the precentral and postcentral gyri.

Asymmetry between the two A1 segments is the most common variation occurring within the circle of Willis. Uni-lateral hypoplasia (arterial diameter <1.5 mm) is not infrequent and often correlates with an intracranial aneurysm of the AComA complex (30,31). The caliber of the AComA correlates well with the differences in the diameter of the right and left A1 segments. With large differences in size, the AComA is larger, carries greater flow volumes from the dominant A1 into the A2 segments, and is more prone to aneurysm development. Variations in the distal ACA include triplication of the A2 segment (the arteria termatica of Wilder), failure of pairing of the distal ACA known as an azygous ACA, crossover of branches from one hemisphere to another, and bihemispheric branches (32–34).

Middle Cerebral Artery

The middle cerebral artery (MCA), the larger of the two terminal branches of the ICA, is approximately twice the diameter of the ACA. The MCA originates at the medial end of the Sylvian fissure, lateral to the optic chiasm, posterior to the division of the olfactory tract into the medial and lateral olfactory striae, and inferior to the anterior perforated substance (Fig. 9). The MCA can be divided into four segments: (a) the M1 or sphenoidal segment, (b) the M2 or insular segment, (c) the M3 or opercular segment, and (d) the M4 or cortical segment (35).

The M1 segment is a direct continuation of the ICA, coursing horizontally, laterally, and slightly forward within the Sylvian fissure and ending at the limen insulae where the vessel makes a 90° turn (the genu). During its course, the M1 segment typically bifurcates into two arterial trunks running in parallel, creating both pre- and postbifurcation portions of this segment. The M1 segment gives off multiple small perforators (lenticulostriate arteries) that penetrate the

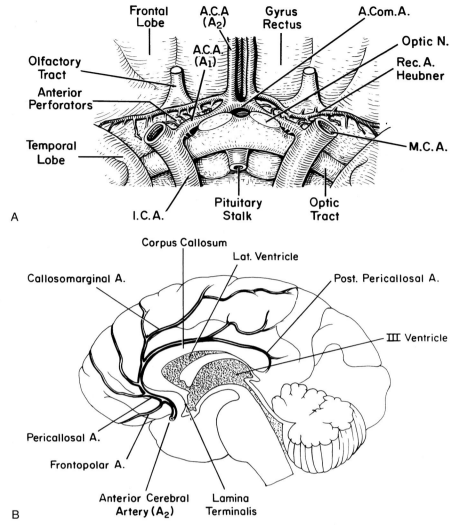

FIG. 8. *Anterior cerebral artery* (ACA): branches and distribution, basal-frontal **(A)** and midsagittal **(B)** views. A1, precommunicating segment; A2, postcommunicating segment; AComA, anterior communicating artery; ICA, internal cerebral artery; MCA, middle cerebral artery.

anterior perforated substance to supply the internal capsule, the body and head of the caudate nucleus, and the lateral part of the globus pallidus. The M1 segment may also give off early cortical branches distributed to the frontal and temporal lobes (35).

The M2 segment begins at the genu where the MCA bends sharply to run superior and posterior over the insular surface in the deep Sylvian fissure. The M2 segment is classically composed of two major divisions (a superior and inferior trunk) that ultimately supply the frontal and temporal sides, respectively, of the peri-Sylvian area.

The M3 segment begins as branches off the superior or inferior divisions of M2 and end as the vessels reach the superficial Sylvian fissure surface. Each branch undergoes a series of turns to reach the cortical surface. Those that supply the supra-Sylvian cortical surfaces course upward over the insular surface, turn 180°, and then pass down over

the medial surface of the frontoparietal operculum. These branches then take a second 180° turn at the external surface of the Sylvian fissure where they course around the inferior margin of the frontoparietal operculum and pass superiorly on the lateral surface of the frontal and parietal lobes. Those arteries supplying cortical areas below the Sylvian fissure turn superiorly and pass over the medial temporal operculum before turning inferior at the edge of the Sylvian fissure to course over the temporal lobe.

The M4 segment begins at the external surface where the vessels leave the Sylvian fissure and course over the cortical surface of the cerebral hemispheres. The cortical territory supplied by the MCA includes the lateral two thirds of the cerebral hemispheres (frontal, parietal, occipital, and temporal), all of the insular and opercular surfaces, the lateral orbital surface of the frontal lobe, the temporal pole, and the lateral inferior surface of the temporal lobe.

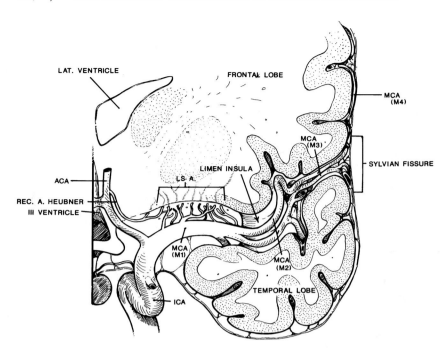

FIG. 9. *Middle cerebral artery* (MCA): branches and distribution, anterior **(A)** and lateral **(B)** views. M1, segment including main MCA trunk(s) to limen insulae; M2, segments including superior and inferior trunks overlying insular surface; M3, segments including portions of MCA exiting from M2 trunks to external cortical surface; M4, cortical branches; LSA, lenticulostriate arteries; ICA, internal carotid artery; ACA, anterior cerebral artery; Rec A Heubner, recurrent artery of Heubner.

Variations of the MCA are less frequent than with other intracranial arteries (36,37). A duplicate MCA represents a second parallel M1 trunk that arises from the ICA and an accessory MCA is an M1 trunk that arises from the ACA. Both variants send cortical branches to cortical areas usually supplied by the MCA.

Anterior Perforating Arteries

The anterior perforating arteries are a series of small penetrating vessels that enter the brain through the anterior perforated substance (APS) (Fig. 10). A rhomboid-shaped area within the Sylvian fissure, the APS is bounded anteriorly by the lateral and medial olfactory striae, posteriorly by the optic tract and temporal lobe, laterally by the limen insula, and medially by the interhemispheric fissure (21). The anterior perforating arteries may originate from the ICA (distal to the AChorA origin), the AChorA (branches of the cisternal segment), the MCA (lenticulostriate arteries from the M1 and proximal M2 segments), and the ACA (branches from the A1 segment and recurrent artery of Heubner). These vessels supply the cerebral structures directly above and posterior to the APS, including the frontal horn of the lateral ventricle, the caudate nucleus, the putamen, the internal capsule, the globus pallidus, and the thalamus. Because these

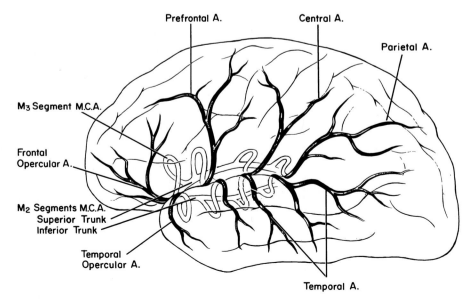

FIG. 10. Anterior perforating arteries: origin and distribution. **A:** surface anatomy, basal view, demonstrating site of entry of branches into anterior perforated substance. A, anterior cerebral artery (A1) perforators; B, anterior cerebral artery (A1) and recurrent artery of Heubner's branches; C, recurrent artery of Heubner's branches; D, lenticulostriates; E, internal carotid and anterior choroidal artery perforators. **B:** Cross-section through basal ganglia: relationship of anterior perforating arteries to deep cerebral structures. Horizontally shaded areas, normal autonomous regions supplied by perforators from various carotid branches: ICA, internal carotid artery; AChorA, anterior choroidal artery; LSA, lenticulostriate arteries; ACA, anterior cerebral artery.

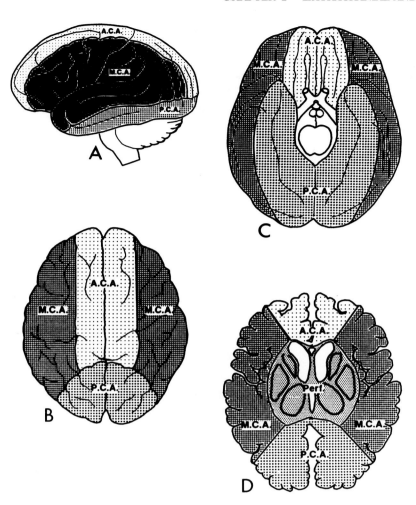

FIG. 11. Arterial supply of cerebrum, including lateral view (**A**), superior view (**B**), basal view (**C**), and horizontal section through basal ganglia and thalamus (**D**). Lines bordering adjacent vascular territories represent watershed zones. Perf., perforators from internal carotid and basilar arteries and branches; ACA, anterior cerebral artery; MCA, middle cerebral artery; PCA, posterior cerebral artery.

perforators are generally end-arteries, there is minimal overlap and anastomosis with vessels in the other vascular territories.

Distribution

The ICA and its branches provide most of the blood supply to the cerebrum (Fig. 11). Since the MCA can be considered as the direct and terminal projection of the ICA, obstruction of an ICA will commonly produce flow abnormalities within and often restricted to the MCA territory. In some instances, however, the circle of Willis connections are of sufficient size to allow an ICA thrombosis without causing any detectable cerebral parenchymal damage.

Following an ICA occlusion, the other ICA branches are generally spared by the extensive collateral system that protects against total destruction of the entire hemisphere. The eye will rarely be affected, as the ipsilateral ECA will supply the ophthalmic circulation through branches from the facial, superficial temporal, or maxillary arteries. The ACA territories are also usually spared due to collateral flow from the opposite ICA through the AComA. The mesial and inferior temporal lobe and the occipital lobe will generally be spared, as these areas are typically supplied by the posterior cerebral artery arising from the vertebrobasilar circuit.

VERTEBRAL AND BASILAR ARTERIES (POSTERIOR CIRCULATION)

Vertebral Artery

Segments

The vertebral artery (VA), the first and largest branch of the subclavian artery, can be divided into four segments: (a) initial, or soft tissue segment, (b) the intervertebral segment, (c) the horizontal segment, and (d) the intracranial segment (Figs. 1 and 12).

Initial

The initial segment passes upwards and posteriorly behind the CCA, between the longus colli and the scalenus anticus

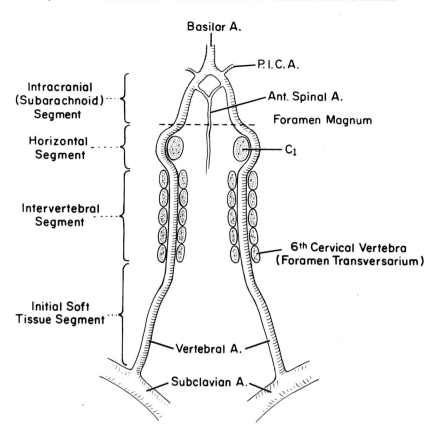

FIG. 12. *Vertebral artery* (VA): segments and branches. PICA, posterior interior cerebellar artery; CI, first cervical vertebra, Ant Spinal A, anterior spinal artery.

muscles anteriorly and the transverse process of the seventh cervical vertebra posteriorly. On the left side it is crossed anteriorly by the thoracic duct. The segment ends as the artery enters the foramen transversarium of the sixth or, less commonly, the fifth or seventh cervical vertebra. There are no branches from this segment.

Intervertebral

The intervertebral or osseous segment ascends within the foramina transversaria of the upper six cervical vertebra. Throughout its course the artery is surrounded by the vertebral venous plexus. The vessel initially courses straight upward until it reaches the axis, where it angles sharply outward to reach the laterally placed foramina (38). As it ascends, this segment is located lateral to the uncinate processes of the cervical vertebrae and anterior to the ventral rami of the cervical nerves.

Branches include meningeal, muscular, and radicular arteries. A meningeal branch often arises from the distal portion of the intervertebral segment, passes through the C2–3 intervertebral foramen, and ascends in the spinal canal to supply the anterior foramen magnum dura. Muscular branches supply the deep neck muscles and often anastomose with branches of the occipital artery. The radicular arteries are small branches that enter the spinal canal through the intervertebral foramina and provide collateral flow to the anterior and posterior spinal arteries.

Horizontal

The horizontal portion begins as the VA emerges from the foramen transversarium of the atlas. The artery then courses medially in a groove on the upper surface of the posterior arch of the atlas, immediately posterior to the lateral mass of C1. This groove is frequently transformed into a bony canal that surrounds a short portion of the artery (39–41). After passing medially, the artery angles forward to enter the spinal canal anterior and lateral to the cervicomedullary junction. Several small meningeal branches arise from this segment to supply the posterior fossa dura and anastomose with other VA and ECA meningeal branches.

The paired posterior spinal arteries usually arise from the horizontal segment of the VA, but they may also arise inside the dura or from the posterior inferior cerebellar artery. Once in the subarachnoid space these branches course medially, posterior to the dentate ligament, and divide into an ascending branch to the medulla and a descending branch to the posterior spinal cord surface.

Intracranial

The intracranial segment begins as the artery pierces the dura just inferior to the lateral edge of the foramen magnum. Here the dura forms a funnel-shaped foramen around a 4- to 6-mm length of the artery, through which also traverse the first cervical nerve and the posterior spinal artery (40). The initial portion of the segment ascends anterior to the first dentate ligament, posterior spinal artery, and spinal portion of the accessory nerve, then passes through the foramen magnum anterior to the hypoglossal rootlets. The VA then courses anterior and medial to the anterior surface of the medulla and unites with the contralateral VA to form the basilar artery. Branches from this segment include the anterior spinal and posterior inferior cerebellar arteries.

Variations in the VA origin are frequent and have been reported from the aorta, common carotid, external carotid, intercostal, and inferior thyroid arteries (42–44). Inequality in diameter between the two vessels is also quite common. In one series, the left VA was dominant in 51% of cases, the right vessel was larger in 41%, and the two were equal in 8% (45). The VA may occasionally terminate at the posterior inferior cerebellar artery origin and not contribute to basilar artery flow.

Branches

Anterior Spinal Artery

The anterior spinal artery arises from the union of the paired anterior ventral spinal arteries that originate from the distal portion of the intracranial segment of the VA (Fig. 12). The vessel descends through the foramen magnum on the ventral surface of the medulla and spinal cord in the anteromedian fissure. On the medulla, it supplies the pyramids and their decussation, the medial lemniscus, the interolivary bundles, the hypothalamic nuclei and nerves, and the posterior longitudinal fasciculus (46). The caudal extension of this artery (with frequent contribution from segmental vessels) provides the blood supply to the anterior two thirds of the spinal cord.

Posterior Inferior Cerebellar Artery

The posterior inferior cerebellar artery (PICA) is the largest VA branch and has the most complex and variable course of all the cerebellar arteries (Figs. 12–15) (47). The vessel most commonly arises from the VA near the inferior olive at the anterolateral brainstem surface, but it may also originate from the extradural VA or less commonly from the occipital artery. The PICA course can be divided into several segments: (a) the anterior medullary segment begins at the PICA–VA junction and passes to the lateral aspect of the medulla, in close proximity to the hypoglossal nerve rootlets, (b) the lateral medullary segment passes to the posterolateral medulla and extends to the rootlets of the glossopharyngeal, vagal, and accessory nerves, (c) the tonsillomedullary segment extends from these rootlets, turns downward to form a caudally convex loop that parallels the medial portion of the tonsil, then turns upward and ascends toward the roof of the fourth ventricle, (d) the telovelotonsillar segment be-

gins at the midportion of the tonsil and extends rostrally to form a convex (cranial) loop near the roof of the fourth ventricle, and (e) this segment runs through a cleft between the vermis medially and the tonsil and cerebellar hemispheres laterally to extend onto the vermis and inferior hemispheres as the cortical segment (47).

The first and second segments of the PICA supply the lateral surface of the caudal medulla. Branches to the tonsil and choroid plexus of the fourth ventricle arise from the tonsillomedullary and telovelotonsillar segments, while the terminal cortical segment typically divides into a medial branch that supplies the inferior vermis and lateral branches that supply the inferior (suboccipital) surface of the cerebellar hemispheres.

Distribution

The neurologic manifestations of unilateral VA occlusion can be quite variable and benign, as the opposite VA is often large enough to provide blood supply for the entire basilar system. In addition, branches from the thyrocervical trunk or occipital artery may provide collateral blood flow to the VA distal to the occlusion. Neurologic deficits can result with interruption of flow at specific locations. Blockage of the subclavian artery proximal to the VA origin can result in a phenomenon known as subclavian steal. In such cases, exercise of the ipsilateral arm can cause reversal of blood flow from the vertebral basilar system into the arm resulting in symptoms of basilar insufficiency. VA occlusion with simultaneous obstruction of the PICA origin results in damage to the lateral medulla and posterior inferior cerebellar surface (Wallenberg's syndrome).

Basilar Artery (BA)

Formed by the union of the two VAs at the pontomedullary junction, the basilar artery (BA) ascends on the anterior surface of the pons, within the prepontine cistern (Figs. 13B,14B,14C). The distal portion of the BA passes between the oculomotor nerves and terminates by dividing into two posterior cerebral arteries within the interpeduncular cistern near the pontomesencephalic junction. During its course, the BA gives off several paired and circumferential tributaries that supply the brainstem, cerebellum, and cerebral cortex, including the anterior inferior cerebellar, the superior cerebellar, the posterior cerebral, and, occasionally, a separate internal auditory artery (Fig. 13). Small perforating arteries also arise from the upper 1 cm of the BA that supply the ventral and lateral portions of the pons and upper brainstem.

Variation in the level of bifurcation of the basilar artery can occur as far rostral as the mamillary bodies and as far caudal as 1.3 cm below the pontomesencephalic junction (22). Variations in the BA itself most frequently involve short segments of duplication or island formation and, except for occasional association with aneurysm formation, are

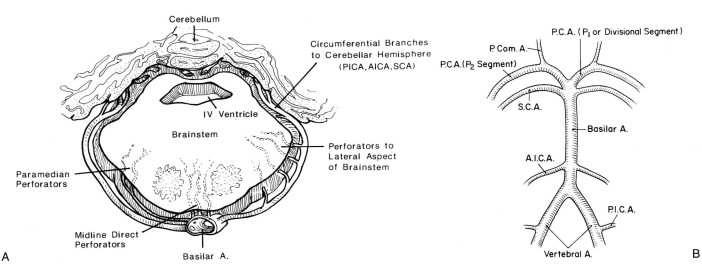

FIG. 13. *Basilar and vertebral arteries*: typical arrangement, nomenclature for arteries to brainstem, cerebellum, and occipital lobes. **(A)** course of perforating and circumferential arteries and **(B)** major paired circumferential arteries. PICA, posterior inferior cerebellar artery, AICA, anterior inferior cerebellar artery, SCA, superior cerebellar artery, PCA, posterior cerebral artery, PComA, posterior communicating artery; P1, precommunicating segment PCA; P2, postcommunicating segment PCA.

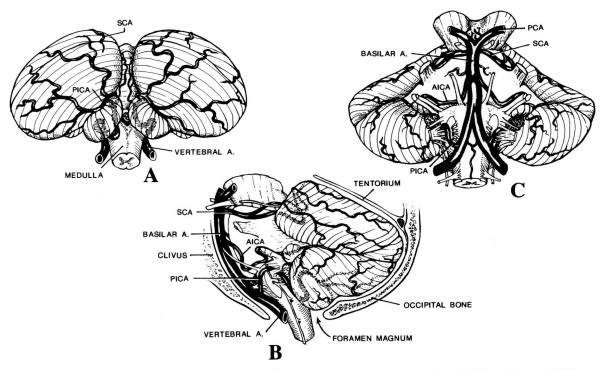

FIG. 14. Blood supply to the *cerebellar surfaces*, including posterior **(A)**, lateral **(B)**, and ventral **(C)** view. Suboccipital surface is supplied mainly by the posterior inferior cerebellar artery (PICA), petrosal surface by the anterior inferior cerebellar artery (AICA), and tentorial surface by the superior cerebellar artery (SCA). PCA, posterior cerebral artery.

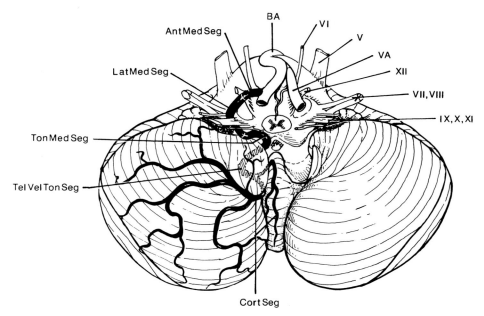

FIG. 15. *Posterior inferior cerebellar artery* (PICA): segments and course, inferior view. In order of origin, segments include anterior medullary segment (AntMedSeg), lateral medullary segment (LatMedSeg), tonsillomedullary segment (TonMedSeg), telovelotonsillar segment (TelVelTonSeg), and cortical segment (CortSeg). BA, basilar artery; VA, vertebral artery; V, trigeminal nerve; VI, abducens nerve; VII, facial nerve; VIII, auditovestibular nerve; IX, glossopharyngeal nerve; X, vagus nerve; XI, spinal accessory nerve; XII, hypoglossal nerve.

rarely of clinical significance (22). The BA branches are much more variable, particularly in regard to their caliber. For instance, the PCA may remain as a major carotid branch, and the ipsilateral PComA may be very hypoplastic, thus greatly limiting communications between the anterior and posterior circuits. Similar alterations in caliber are also seen between the PICA and the anterior inferior cerebellar artery (AICA). A dominant AICA will often be associated with an absent BA origin of the labyrinthine artery, and the ipsilateral PICA territory will be smaller. Conversely, an enlarged PICA is usually accompanied by a smaller AICA (47).

Branches

Anterior Inferior Cerebellar Artery

The smallest of the three cerebellar arteries, the AICA arises from the first or middle third of the BA and encircles the pons near the pontomedullary sulcus (Figs. 14 and 16) (48). During its proximal course, the AICA sends off numerous penetrating branches that supply the lower two thirds of the pons and the upper part of the medulla. Lateral to the abducens nerve the artery typically splits into rostral and caudal trunks that pass around the brainstem either above, below, or between the facial and vestibulocochlear nerves. The largest of the two branches, the rostral trunk, loops near the internal auditory meatus and

then passes back to the surface of the middle cerebellar peduncle above the flocculus. The trunk terminates in the horizontal fissure and supplies the upper part of the petrosal cerebellar surface. The caudal trunk passes downward and medially near the lateral recess and supplies the lower pons, pontomedullary sulcus, supraolivary fossa, the glossopharyngeal and vagal nerves, and a small inferior portion of the petrosal cerebellar surface (48,49). The AICA typically has three additional branches related to the internal auditory canal, including the internal auditory, recurrent perforating, and the subarcuate arteries.

Superior Cerebellar Artery

The superior cerebellar artery (SCA) is the most rostral of the paired infratentorial arteries, originating from the BA at the pontomedullary junction just proximal to the posterior cerebral artery (Figs. 14 and 17) (50). During its course, the SCA can be divided into four segments: (a) the anterior pontine segment courses laterally on the ventral pontine surface, lying inferior to the oculomotor nerve that separates it from the proximal portion of the posterior cerebral artery; (b) the ambient segment begins at the lateral border of the pons and runs posteriorly in the infratentorial portion of the ambient cistern, paralleling the course of the trochlear nerve, posterior cerebral artery, basal vein of Rosenthal, and the free edge of the tentorium; (c) the ambient segment commonly divides into rostral and caudal trunks that ultimately

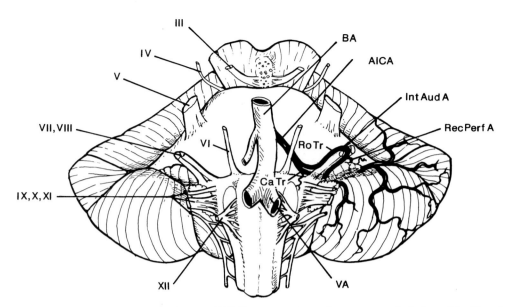

FIG. 16. *Anterior inferior cerebellar artery* (AICA): segments and course, ventral view. Significant portions include rostral (RoTr) and caudal (CaTr) trunks, recurrent perforator branches to the brainstem (RecPerfA), and the internal auditory artery (IntAudA). BA, basilar artery; VA, vertebral artery; III, oculomotor nerve; IV, trochlear nerve; V, trigeminal nerve; VI, abducens nerve; VII, facial nerve; VIII, auditovestibular nerve; IX, glossopharyngeal nerve; X, vagus nerve; XI, spinal accessory nerve; XII, hypoglossal nerve.

reach the superior (tentorial) surface of the cerebellum; and (d) the quadrigeminal segment courses within the quadrigeminal cistern and provides arterial supply to the tectum (50).

Several classes of branches arise from the SCA: (a) perforating arteries that supply the upper ventrolateral pons, (b) precerebellar arteries that supply the deep cerebellar nuclei, inferior colliculus, and superior medullary velum, and (c) cortical arteries that project to the superior vermis and hemispheres. The vermian arteries typically originate from the rostral trunk, whereas the cerebellar hemispheres receive flow from both the rostral and caudal trunks (50).

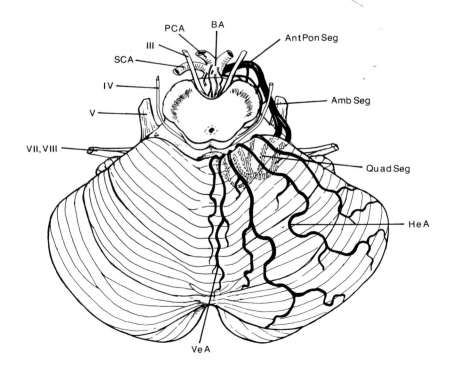

FIG. 17. *Superior cerebellar artery* (SCA): segments and course, superior view. Significant portions include the anterior pontine segment (AntPonSeg), the ambient segment (AmbSeg), the quadrigeminal segment (QuadSeg), and cortical branches (HeA, hemispheric; VeA, vermian). BA, basilar artery; PCA, posterior cerebral artery; III, oculomotor nerve; IV, trochlear nerve; V, trigeminal nerve; VI, abducens nerve; VII, facial nerve; VIII, auditovestibular nerve.

Posterior Cerebral Artery

The posterior cerebral artery (PCA) arises as the terminal BA branch. Its course may be divided into four segments: (a) The P1 segment, spanning from the PCA origin to the PComA, courses laterally, anterior to the mesencephalon, posterior to the clivus, and superior to the oculomotor nerve. (b) The P2 segment begins at the PComA and courses posteriorly within the ambient cistern to the pulvinar, inferior to the optic tract and basal vein of Rosenthal. (c) The P3 segment begins at the pulvinar and courses posteriorly in the lateral aspect of the quadrigeminal cistern to the anterior limit of the calcarine fissure (51). The two P3 segments approach each other at the midline, inferior to the corpus callosum splenium and posterior to the colliculi. (d) The P4 segment incorporates the terminal cortical branches projecting to the medial occipital lobes surface (Figs. 11 and 18) (22,51).

Branches of the PCA may be categorized into three types: (a) central, which supply the brainstem, (b) ventricular, which supply the choroid plexus, and (c) cerebral, which supply the occipital lobes and portions of the temporal and parietal lobes. The central branches are divided into direct perforating and circumflex arteries. The direct perforating branches arise from the parent trunk and pass directly into the brainstem, including the posterior thalamoperforating arteries arising from the P1 segment and the thalamogeniculate

and peduncular perforating arteries arising from the P2 segment. The circumflex arteries are short and long branches that encircle the brainstem for variable distances before entering the parenchyma.

The ventricular arteries consist of the medial posterior choroidal artery (MPChA) and the lateral posterior choroidal artery (LPChA). The MPChA typically arises from the P1 or P2 segments, encircles the midbrain medial to the PCA, then turns forward lateral to the pineal gland to enter the roof of the third ventricle. It supplies the third ventricular choroid plexus, then enters the lateral ventricle through the foramen of Monro and supplies part of the lateral ventricle choroid plexus. The LPChA most commonly arises from the P2 segment distal to the MPChA origin, then courses laterally to enter the choroidal fissure where it then divides into anterior and posterior branches. The anterior branch passes forward to supply a portion of the temporal horn choroid plexus, whereas the posterior branch courses around the pulvinar to supply the choroid plexus of the trigone and lateral ventricle (51).

The cerebral branches of the PCA include the inferior temporal, parieto-occipital, calcarine, and splenial branches. The inferior temporal arteries arise from the P2 segment and are called the hippocampal, anterior, middle, posterior, and common temporal arteries. These vessels supply the inferior temporal lobe surface and may also send branches through the choroidal fissure into the temporal horn choroid plexus. One of two terminal PCA branches, the parieto-occipital artery, runs in the parieto-occipital fissure to supply the posterior parasagittal region, cuneus, precuneus, lateral occipital gyrus, and occasionally the precentral and superior parietal lobules. The other terminal PCA branch, the calcarine artery, courses in the calcarine fissure to reach the occipital pole, supplying branches to the lingual and inferior cuneus gyrus and the visual cortex. The splenial (posterior pericallosal) artery usually arises from the parieto-occipital branch but may also originate from the P2 or P3 segment, calcarine artery, LPChA, or MPChA. This artery passes anteriorly over the splenium to anastomose with the anterior pericallosal artery. The territory supplied by the PCA therefore encompasses the posterior portions of the cerebral hemisphere (primarily serving vision and memory) as well as critical areas of the thalamus, midbrain, choroid plexus, and walls of the lateral and third ventricle (22,51).

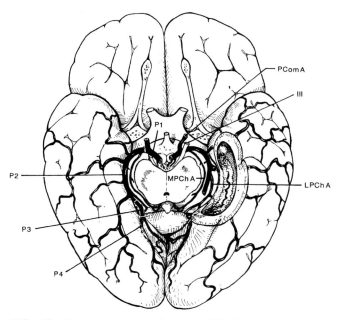

FIG. 18. *Posterior cerebral artery* (PCA): segments and branches, inferior view. P1, segment from PCA origin to posterior communicating artery (PComA); P2, segment from PComA to posterior brainstem surface; P3, segment spanning quadrigeminal cistern; and P4, cortical branches to occipital and parietal lobes. III, oculomotor nerve; LPChA, lateral posterior choroidal artery; MPChA, medial posterior choroidal artery.

Posterior Perforating Arteries

This group of vessels includes branches originating from the upper 1 cm of the BA, the PComA, the P1 segment, and less commonly the ICA and AChorA. Collectively, these perforators supply the region of the diencephalon and midbrain, including the optic tract and lateral geniculate body, the medial lemniscus and thalamus, the internal capsule and cerebral peduncle, the hypothalamic connections to the mamillary bodies, the extraocular nerves and midbrain nuclei, the anterior and posterior hypothalamus, the midbrain reticular formation, the cerebellothalamic circuits in the midbrain and thalamus, and the hypothalamic-pituitary axis (22).

Distribution

The BA and its branches provide blood supply to all of the structures within the posterior fossa, as well as to the mesencephalon, thalamus, occipital lobes, and inferomedial temporal lobes. Since the posterior circulation typically has multiple collateral pathways, BA obstructions can have various outcomes dependent on the degree of collateral flow. The larger cerebellar arteries (PICA, AICA, and SCA) form a system of leptomeningeal collaterals that can bypass a blocked BA. The ICA may also provide blood flow to the cerebellum and brainstem through the PComA into PCA and SCA branches.

COLLATERAL CIRCULATION

Circle of Willis

The circle of Willis is a polygonal anastomotic ring of arteries located in the subarachnoid space surrounding the optic chiasm and pituitary stalk (Fig. 19). Anteriorly, the circle is composed of the two ICAs, the two A1 segments, and the AComA. Posteriorly, the circle is made up by the two P1 segments and the two PComAs. When intact, the circle of Willis allows theoretical communication between both the anterior and posterior circuits (via PComA) and the two cerebral hemispheres (via AComA). Functionally significant hypoplasia of the AComA or PComA is common, however, and a classic "normal" anastomotic ring of communications is found in <50% of brains (52,53).

During arteriography, little mingling of dye is normally seen outside the expected territory of the injected vessel. Following large vessel obstruction, however, the anastomotic channels become crucial, and hypoplasia of a portion of the circle may have major adverse neurological sequelae (30). Hypoplasia of the AComA, a common variant, may reduce crossover capabilities following an ICA occlusion by restricting available collateral blood flow from the opposite side through the anterior circle of Willis. Similarly, the occipital lobe would more likely be spared from infarction following BA thrombosis if a widely patent PComA is present.

ICA-BA Anastomoses

Aside from the PComA (a universally present channel), connections between the carotid and vertebrobasilar circulations are uncommon. Occasionally, however, embryonal channels may persist that serve as major connections be-

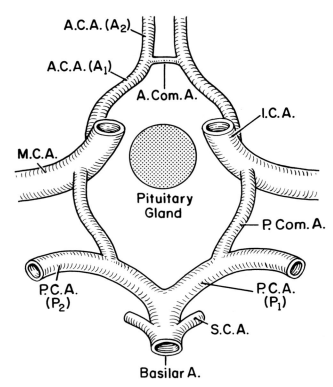

FIG. 19. Normal circle of Willis. ICA, internal carotid artery; AComA, anterior communicating artery; MCA, middle cerebral artery; A1, precommunicating segment ACA; A2, postcommunicating segment ACA; PComA, posterior communicating artery; PCA, posterior cerebral artery; Pl, precommunicating segment PCA; P2, postcommunicating segment PCA; SCA, superior cerebellar artery.

tween the two circuits (Fig. 20). Such anastomoses may explain the rare development of posterior circulation symptoms with anterior circulation disease and may account for simultaneous filling of the VA during carotid arteriography (1,54).

The largest and most common of these anastomoses is the persistent trigeminal artery, which is identified in 0.1–0.4% of all arteriograms (2,55). The vessel arises from the distal horizontal portion of the petrous ICA, passes through or around the sella contents, and joins the BA between the SCA and AICA origins (56). When large, this communication may supply most of the blood flow to the BA, and in such cases, the vertebral and proximal BAs are correspondingly small or absent.

The rarest of the persistent embryonal connections is the otic (acousticofacial or acoustic) artery. This vessel arises more proximally from the horizontal petrous ICA, runs through the internal auditory canal with the 7th and 8th cranial nerves, and joins the proximal BA between the AICA and PICA takeoffs (57).

The second most common congenital carotid–basilar communication is the primitive hypoglossal artery. This vessel originates from the upper cervical ICA around the C1 or C2 vertebral level, enters the posterior fossa via the anterior

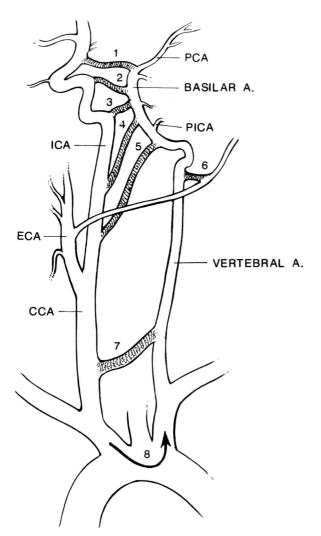

FIG. 20. Carotid–vertebrobasilar anastomoses: shaded areas represent possible channels that could allow opacification of vertebrobasilar (posterior) circuit during selective carotid arteriography: (1) posterior communicating artery, (2) trigeminal artery, (3) otic artery, (4) hypoglossal artery, (5) proatlantal intersegmental artery, (6) occipital–vertebral arterial anastomoses, (7) cervical intersegmental artery, and (8) retrograde filling into subclavian artery. CCA, common carotid artery; ECA, external carotid artery; ICA, internal carotid artery; OA, occipital artery; PCA, posterior cerebral artery; SCA, superior cerebellar artery; AICA, anterior inferior cerebellar artery; PICA, posterior inferior cerebellar artery.

condylar foramen, and joins the BA just distal to the junction of the two VAs (1).

ICA-VA Connections

Communications between the ICA and VA are rare. Such connections include the proatlantal and cervical intersegmental arteries (Fig. 20). The proatlantal variant is more common and connects the cervical ICA with the horizontal portion of the ipsilateral VA (1,58). The rare intersegmental artery connects the ICA with the intervertebral segment of the VA.

ECA–VA Connections

The vertebral artery may communicate with the carotid system via the ascending pharyngeal and occipital ECA branches. Following proximal VA occlusion, the occipital artery may provide distal flow to terminal VA segments through intramuscular communications. These anastomoses may also keep the ICA patent following CCA occlusion by providing VA flow into the ECA–ICA junction via reversed flow in the occipital artery.

Leptomeningeal Connections

Pial anastomoses often connect the cortical irrigation zones between the major cerebral vessel territories. These anastomoses generally occur between branches of different major trunks and are rare between branches of the same artery (59). Supratentorially, most occur between the ACA and MCA and between the MCA and PCA territories. Similar connections also occur between the cerebellar cortical arteries (SCA, AICA, and PICA).

The leptomeningeal collaterals are composed of arteries with small diameters and high resistance. Because these boundary or watershed zones depend on both arterial systems for flow maintenance, these regions are particularly susceptible to injury following generalized flow reduction (low cardiac output, carbon monoxide poisoning, etc.). Although occasionally well-developed arteriographically, these channels are rarely sufficient to prevent damage following proximal major vessel occlusion (60).

ECA–ICA Anastomoses

The ICA most frequently occludes in the proximal cervical segment, and in such cases, communications between the ECA and ICA may be crucial in maintaining intracranial flow (Fig. 2) (5). The ophthalmic artery is the largest and most significant conduit of this type. Following ICA occlusion, the ophthalmic artery receives blood flow by several different ECA pathways. The reversed flow within the ophthalmic artery subsequently fills the proximal subarachnoid ICA segment.

Meningeal branches from the ECA (the middle meningeal, accessory meningeal, and ascending pharyngeal arteries) may also connect with the inferolateral trunk (artery of the inferior cavernous sinus) and the dorsal meningeal artery of the meningohypophyseal trunk to then provide blood flow to the cavernous ICA segment. Unlike the ophthalmic artery, these channels do not usually provide substantial intracranial flow following ICA obstruction. Their presence, however, may be of importance in patients with moyamoya disease (61).

REFERENCES

1. Lie TA. *Congenital Anomalies of the Carotid Arteries*. Amsterdam: Excerpta Medica, 1968.
2. Krayenbuhl H, Yasargil MG. *Die zerebrale angiographe*. 2nd ed. Stuttgart: Verlag, 1965.
3. Hawkins TD. The collateral anastomoses in cerebrovascular occlusion. *Clin Radiol* 1966;17:203–219.
4. Kaplan HA. Collateral circulation of the brain. *Neurology* 1961;11:9–15.
5. Countee RW, Vijayanathan T. External carotid artery in internal carotid artery occlusion: angiographic, therapeutic, and prognostic considerations. *Stroke* 1979;10:450–460.
6. Gibo H, Lenkey C, Rhoton AL. Microsurgical anatomy of the supraclinoid portion of the internal carotid artery. *J Neurosurg* 1981;55:560–574.
7. Weibel J, Fields WS. Tortuosity, coiling, and kinking of the internal carotid artery. Etiology and radiographic anatomy. *Neurology* 1965;15:7–18.
8. Leher HZ. Relative calibre of the cervical internal carotid artery: normal variation with the circle of Willis. *Brain* 1968;91:339–348.
9. Paullus W, Pait TG, Rhoton AL Jr. Microsurgical exposure of the petrous portion of the carotid artery. *J Neurosurg* 1977;47:713–726.
10. Harris FS, Rhoton AL Jr. Anatomy of the cavernous sinus: a microsurgical study. *J Neurosurg* 1976;45:169–180.
11. Inoue T, Rhoton AL Jr, Theele D, et al. Surgical approaches to the cavernous sinus: a microsurgical study. *Neurosurgery* 1990;26:903–932.
12. Nutik SL. Removal of the anterior clinoid process for exposure of the proximal intracranial carotid artery. *J Neurosurg* 1988;69:529–534.
13. Perneczky A, Knosp E, Vorkapic P, et al. Direct surgical approach to infraclinoid aneurysms. *Acta Neurochir* 1985;76:36–44.
14. Nutik S. Ventral paraclinoid carotid aneurysms. *J Neurosurg* 1988;69:340–344.
15. Knosp E, Muller G, Perneczky A. The paraclinoid carotid artery: anatomical aspects of a microsurgical approach. *Neurosurgery* 1988;22:896–901.
16. Kobayashi S, Kyoshima K, Gibo H, et al. Carotid cave aneurysms of the internal carotid artery. *J Neurosurg* 1989;70:216–221.
17. Hollinshead WH. *Anatomy for Surgeons. vol 1. The Head and Neck.* 3rd ed. New York: Harper and Row, 1982.
18. Williams P, Warwick R, eds. *Gray's Anatomy*. 35th ed. Philadelphia: WB Saunders, 1980.
19. Dawson BH. The blood vessels of the human optic chiasma and their relation to those of hypophysis and hypothalamus. *Brain* 1958;81:207–217.
20. Gibo H, Kobayashi S, Kyoshima K, et al. Microsurgical anatomy of the arteries of the pituitary stalk and gland as viewed from above. *Acta Neurochir* 1988;90:60–66.
21. Rosner SS, Rhoton AL Jr, Ono M, et al. Microsurgical anatomy of the anterior perforating arteries. *J Neurosurg* 1984;61:463–485.
22. Saeki N, Rhoton AL Jr. Microsurgical anatomy of the upper basilar artery and the posterior circle of Willis. *J Neurosurg* 1977;46:563–578.
23. Hassler O, Salzman GF. Angiographic and histologic changes in infundibular widening of the posterior communicating artery. *Acta Radiol* 1963;1:321–323.
24. Rhoton AL Jr, Fuji K, Fradd B. Microsurgical anatomy of the anterior choroidal artery. *Surg Neurol* 1979;12:171–187.
25. Fuji K, Lenkey C, Rhoton AL Jr. Microsurgical anatomy of the choroidal arteries: lateral and third ventricles. *J Neurosurg* 1980;52:165–188.
26. Critchley M. The anterior cerebral artery and its syndromes. *Brain* 1930; 53:120–165.
27. Perlmutter D, Rhoton AL Jr. Microsurgical anatomy of the anterior cerebral–anterior communicating–recurrent artery complex. *J Neurosurg* 1976;45:259–272.
28. Heubner O. Zur Topographie der ernahrungsgebrete der einzelnen hirn-arnterien. *Cent Med Wissen* 1872;52:816–821.
29. Perlmutter D, Rhoton AL Jr. Microsurgical anatomy of the distal anterior cerebral artery. *J Neurosurg* 1978;49:204–228.
30. Stehbens WE. *Pathology of the Cerebral Blood Vessels*. St. Louis: CV Mosby, 1972.
31. Wilson G., Riggs HE, rupp C. The pathologic anatomy of ruptured cerebral aneurysms. *J Neurosurg* 1954;11:128–134.
32. Alpers BJ, Berry RG. Circle of Willis in cerebrovascular disorders. *Arch Neurol* 1963;8:398–402.
33. Baptista AG. Studies on the arteries of the brain. II. The anterior cerbral artery: some anatomic features and their clinical implications. *Neurology* 1963;13:825–835.
34. Laitinen L, Snellman A. Aneurysms of the pericallosal artery: a study of 14 cases verified angiographically and treated mainly by surgical attack. *J Neurosurg* 1960;17:447–458.
35. Gibo H, Carver C, Rhoton AL Jr, et al. Microsurgical anatomy of the middle cerebral artery. *J Neurosurg* 1981;54:151–169.
36. Jain KK. Some observations on the anatomy of the middle cerebral artery. *Can J Surg* 1964;7:134–139.
37. Teal JS, Rumbaugh CL, Bergeron R, et al. Anomalies of the middle cerebral artery 1: accessory artery, duplication and early bifurcation. *AJR Radium Ther Nucl Med* 1973;118:567–575.
38. Hutchinson EC, Yates PO. The cervical portion of the vertebral artery: a clinicopathological study. *Brain* 1956;79:319–331.
39. Lamberty GH, Zivonovics S. The retro-articular vertebral artery ring of the atlas and its significance. *Acta Anat* 1963;55:186–194.
40. De Olivera E, Rhoton AL Jr, Peace D. Microsurgical antomy of the region of the foramen magnum. *Surg Neurol* 1985;24:293–352.
41. Radojevic S, Negovanovic B. La gouttiere et les anneuaux osseaux de l'artere vertebrale de l'atlas. *Acta Anat* 1963;55:186–194.
42. Brash JC. Blood-vascular and lymphatic systems. In: Brash JC, Jamieson EB, eds. *Cunningham's Textbook of Anatomy*. London: Oxford University Press, 1943;1177.
43. Flynn RE. External carotid origin of the dominant vertebral artery. *J Neurosurg* 1968;29:300–301.
44. Taveras JM, Wood EH. *Diagnostic Neuroradiology*. Baltimore: Williams and Willkins, 1964.
45. Stopford JSB. The arteries of the pons and medulla oblongata. *J Anat Physiol* 1915;50:131–164.
46. Margaretten I. Syndromes of the anterior spinal artery. *J Neurosurg* 1923;58:127–133.
47. Lister JR, Rhoton AL Jr, Matsushima T, et al. Microsurgical anatomy of the posterior inferior cerebellar artery. *Neurosurgery* 1982;10:170–199.
48. Martin RG, Grant JL, Peace D, et al. Microsurgical relationships of the anterior inferior cerebellar artery and the facial-vestibulocochlear nerve complex. *Neurosurgery* 1980;6,3–507.
49. Matsushima T, Rhoton AL Jr, Lenkey C. Microsurgical anatomy of the fourth ventricle: 1. Microsurgical anatomy. *Neurosurgery* 1982;11:631–667.
50. Hardy DG, Peace DA, Rhton AL Jr. Microsurgical anatomy of the superior cerebellar artery. *Neurosurgery* 1980;6:10–28.
51. Zeal AA, Rhoton AL Jr. Microsurgical anatomy of the posterior cerebral artery. *J Neurosurg* 1978;48:534–551.
52. Pallie W, Samarasinghe DD. A study in the quantification of the circle of Willis. *Brain* 1962;85:559–578.
53. Stehbens WE. Aneurysms and anatomical variation of cerebral arteries. *Arch Pathol* 1963;75:45–64.
54. Stern J, Correll JW, Bryan N. Persistent hypoglossal artery and persistent trigeminal artery presenting with posterior fossa transient ischemic attacks: report of two cases. *J Neurosurg* 1978; 49:614–619.
55. Fields WS, Bruetman ME, Weibel J. Collateral circulation of the brain. *Monogr Surg Sci* 1965;2:183–259.
56. Saltzman GF. Patent primitive trigeminal artery studied by cerebral angiography. *Acta Radiol* 1959;51:329.
57. Reynolds AF, Stovring J, Turner PT. Persistent otic artery. *Surg Neurol* 1980;13:115– 117.
58. Sukamoto S, Hori Y, Utsumi S et al. Proatlantal intersegmental artery with absence of bilateral vertebral arteries: case report. *J Neurosurg* 1981;54:122–124.
59. Vander Eecken HM. *The Anastomses Between the Leptomeningeal Arteries of the Brain*. Springfield: Charles C Thomas, 1959.
60. Meyer JS, Circulatory changes following occlusion of the middlecerebral artery and their relationship to function. *J Neurosurg* 1958;15:653–673.
61. Karwasawa J, Kikuchi H, Furuse S, et al. Treatment of moya-moya disease with STA-MCA anastomosis. *J Neurosurg* 1978;49:679–688.

Cerebrovascular Disease, edited by H. Hunt Batjer.
Lippincott-Raven Publishers, Philadelphia © 1997.

CHAPTER 2

The Relation Between Brain Function and Cerebral Blood Flow and Metabolism

Albert Gjedde

THE FLOW–METABOLISM COUPLE

The brain consumes 20% of the body's glucose and oxygen and receives 20% of its blood supply in the service of brain function. The relationship between these variables has puzzled scientists since the discovery of the circulation. Thus, Descartes (1) formulated a mechanistic relationship between the activity of the mind and the activity of the brain:

> I [show] what changes must take place in the brain to produce waking, sleep, and dreams; how light, sounds, odours, tastes, heat, and all the other qualities of external objects impress it with different ideas by means of the senses; how hunger, thirst, and the other internal affections can likewise impress upon it divers ideas; what must be understood by the common sense (sensus communis) in which these ideas are received, by the memory which retains them, by the fantasy which can change them in various ways, and out of them compose new ideas, and which, by the same means, distributing the animal spirits through the muscles, can cause the members of such a body to move in as many different ways, and in a manner as suited, whether to the objects that are presented to its senses or to its internal affections, as can take place in our own case apart from the guidance of the will.

The circulation of the blood was hypothesized by William Harvey during his studies in Padua in 1598–1602 and was quickly accepted by Descartes following publication of Harvey's work in 1628. According to Descartes, a simple hydraulic mechanism linked the circulation to the brain's activity (1):

> The arteries . . . proceed from the heart in the most direct lines, and . . . , according to the rules of mechanics, which are the same with those of nature, when many objects tend at once to the same point where there is not sufficient room for all (as is the case with the parts of the blood which flow forth from the left cavity of the heart and tend towards the

A. Gjedde: Department of Neurology and Neurosurgery, McGill University, Montreal, Canada H3A 2B4; and PET Center at Aarhus General Hospital, Aarhus, Denmark 8000.

brain), the weaker and less agitated parts must necessarily be driven aside from that point by the stronger which alone in this way reach it.

The mechanism linking neuronal activity to the circulation is generally claimed to constitute a flow–metabolism couple. The purpose of this couple is said to be to satisfy the principle of Roy and Sherrington (2), according to whom

> the chemical products of cerebral metabolism contained in the lymph which bathes the walls of the arterioles of the brain can cause variations of the calibre of the cerebral vessels: That in this reaction the brain possesses an intrinsic mechanism by which its vascular supply can be varied locally in correspondence with local variations of functional activity.

The Roy–Sherrington principle has been interpreted to mean that blood flow changes must be a function of a tight coupling between cellular energy requirements and the supplies of glucose and oxygen to the brain, although the hypothetical mechanism underlying such a couple has never been revealed unequivocally. At the very least, it must be the purpose of such a homeostatic mechanism to maintain a constant concentration of adenosine triphosphate (ATP), the chemical that ties the processes that deplete the energy potential of brain tissue to the processes that restore it. The mechanism must take into account that the processes that restore ATP are sensitive, directly or indirectly, to the depletion of ATP (feedback), whereas the opposite is not the case: ATP depletion is not self-limiting (eg, in the case of failure of restorative processes to prevent the loss of ATP; feedforward). Thus, ATP depletion proceeds until it is complete (3).

In contravention of the Roy–Sherrington principle, recent reports claim a mismatch between changes of blood flow and glucose consumption, on the one hand, and oxygen utilization, on the other, during functional activation of regions of the human brain. These claims follow a speculation by van den Berg and Bruntink (4) who reviewed studies of glucose metabolism and concluded that the rate of oxidative metabolism in the brain of rodents is close to the normal physiologic limit, ie, prolonged stimulation or other abnormal intervention would be required to raise the oxygen consumption above this limit.

In support of this speculation, evidence for focal (or global) increases of oxidative metabolism during physiologic stimulation of brain tissue is rare. As recently as 1989, an authoritative review of brain energy metabolism gave seizures in the rat as the only example of raised oxidative brain metabolism (5).

Although it is unclear as to why a limit should exist, limits to work-related changes of oxidative metabolism do exist in other organs, specifically heart and skeletal muscle. The claim to mismatches between changes of blood flow and oxygen consumption in brain is now believed to represent a significant departure from the principle formulated by Roy and Sherrington. Any new hypothetical mechanism must include an explanation of the mismatches between changes of blood flow, glucose consumption, and oxygen utilization that occur under normal physiologic circumstances.

BRAIN ENERGY METABOLISM

The work of the brain is difficult to define or to measure. The work is assumed to be predominantly electrochemical. At least 50% of the awake brain's energy metabolism is believed to subserve the restoration of ions that leak through neuronal membranes, allowing the neurons to maintain ion gradients (6). This claim is supported by numerous observations: The oxygen consumption of cerebral cortex slices devoid of functional activity is about half of the brain metabolism in vivo. In coma and persistent vegetative state in humans, conditions associated with absent function of cerebral gray matter, oxygen and glucose consumption rates are 33–50% of the normal average (7,8). Barbiturate anesthesia and coma both reduce brain metabolism to about 50% of the awake average in humans (9) and rats (10).

Conversely (in brain slices), the earliest studies showed that aerobic and anaerobic metabolism can be increased by electrical stimulation (11). In isolated rabbit vagus nerve, oxygen consumption is about 0.5 μmol hg^{-1} min^{-1}, or close to one third of the human cerebral average. When maximally and repetitively stimulated, the oxygen consumption increased by 60% (12). More recently, in posterior pituitary in vitro, Mata et al measured a 30% increase of glucose consumption at 10-Hz electrical stimulation (13).

In intact brain in vivo Bowers and Zigmond (14) and Yarowsky and Ingvar (15) observed substantial increases of 2-deoxyglucose-derived radioactivity (a measure of glucose metabolism) in rat superior cervical ganglion by antidromic stimulation of the external carotid nerve with electrical pulses at 5–15 Hz. In spinal cord in vivo Kadekaro et al. observed a linear increase of glucose metabolic rate from 0.2 to 0.5 μmol hg^{-1} min^{-1} when the frequency of electrical stimulation of sciatic nerve increased from 5 to 15 Hz (16).

The conventional link between the function of nervous tissue and the electrochemical work of the brain is provided by the sodium theory, which explains excitation of nervous system tissue by the existence of sodium, potassium, and chloride as free ions in the intracellular space and the presence of special ion transporters in the plasma membrane that maintain the concentrations of these ions. The theory ascribes the electrical properties of the membrane to diffusion potentials established by specific membrane conductances (17).

Electrochemical work is translatable in terms of information transfer (18). The information transfer of the brain can be calculated tentatively from the work required to maintain the ion gradients associated with the functional activity of the brain. According to one calculation, a single binary decision, ie, a unity bit, requires a minimum energy expenditure of 3×10^{-24} kJ. The brain tissue hydrolysis of about 5 μmol ATP g^{-1} min^{-1} has a free energy of about 3×10^{-6} kJ μmol^{-1}. Assuming an upper limit of thermodynamic efficiency, human brain tissue has the capacity to perform binary decisions at the maximum rate of 10^{11} megabytes g^{-1} s^{-1}, or about 10^6 teraflops s^{-1} for one whole brain. Considering that the largest computer devised by man has a capacity of about 1 teraflop s^{-1}, a million of these would be required to match the functional work and coincident energy flow of a single human brain.

ATP Hydrolysis

Stimulation of the brain to work by appropriate excitation is a function of the tissue's ability to transport sodium, potassium, and other ions such as calcium and hydrogen. As early as 1962, Whittam estimated that 40% of the metabolism of the brain subserved the transport of sodium and potassium (19). By blocking ion transport in isolated crab nerves, oxygen consumption was reduced by 50%. Similarly, blocking sodium transport with ouabain, which inactivates Na$^+$,K$^+$–ATPase, was shown to reduce the oxygen consumption of the isolated rabbit vagus nerve preparation referred to above by 40% (12). More recently, in the isolated posterior pituitary also referred to above, the stimulation-induced increase of metabolism was abolished after ouabain treatment (13).

According to these and numerous other studies, the increased conductances of sodium and potassium underlying excitation are matched by increases of active ion pumping to maintain constant ion concentrations. For example, the P type (for plasma membrane), Na$^+$, K$^+$–ATPase, combines with ATP, Mg^{2+}, Na$^+$, and K$^+$ to form an enzyme–substrate association during which the enzyme is phosphorylated and Mg^{2-} and ADP are released (20). As the phosphorylated enzyme splits into inorganic phosphate and the original enzyme, Na$^+$, and K$^+$ are translocated in the appropriate directions according to this simplified reaction scheme:

$$\text{ATPMg}^{2-} + \text{H}_2\text{O} \leftrightarrow \text{ADPMg}^- + \text{H}_2\text{PO}_4^-$$

Excitation- and inhibition-induced changes of sodium and potassium ion concentrations stimulate the Na^+,K^+–ATPase activity. One recently discovered stimulus is the cotransport of sodium and transmitter molecules from the synaptic cleft, which increases the intracellular content of sodium. This reuptake mechanism for glutamate stimulates ATP hydrolysis in astrocytes (21).

ATP Synthesis

Recent observations (22–24) suggest that in heart and brain a 2- to 10-fold variation of the rate of physiologic work is associated with a minimal change of ATP, inorganic phosphate, magnesium ions, and pH. In the heart, the work was measured as cardiac output; in brain the work was induced by administration of amphetamine, which led to a 4-fold increase of blood flow, as also shown in previous work (25,26). Amphetamine has been shown not only to elevate blood flow but to stimulate oxygen and glucose consumption in regions of the rat brain (27,28). In the study by Berntman et al. (27), oxygen consumption rose 30–95%, depending on the dose and strain of rat, accompanied by increases of pyruvate and lactate.

The mechanism underlying the remarkable ability of brain tissue to vary blood flow and metabolism several fold with little change of the ATP concentration is unknown. Many of the conventional explanations of cellular energetics are irrelevant because they assume feedback of signals from altered concentrations of nucleotide and other intermediates. In the absence of such changes, the regulation must involve a change in fluxes through near-equilibrium reactions that require adjustment of enzyme affinities by second or third messengers of neurotransmission rather than changes in substrate levels.

Although numerous mechanisms are known to influence ATP synthesis, there is little agreement on the specific mechanism by which ATP synthesis is stimulated by functional activation of brain tissue in vivo, in the absence of an actual overall change of ATP content. Four processes of ATP regeneration are possible targets of such a mechanism. They include the hydrolysis of cytosolic phosphocreatine, aerobic glycolysis in the cytosol, phosphorylation of mitochondrial creatine, and oxidative phosphorylation of mitochondrial ADP.

Creatine Kinase

Creatine kinase (CK) occupies a pivotal role in the regulation of the oxidative metabolism of the brain. CK catalyzes the reversible reaction:

$$PCr^{2-} + ADPMg^- + H^+ \leftrightarrow Cr + ATPMg^{2-}$$

The enzyme exists both in a form dissolved in cytosol, which differs in composition among the tissues and has a brain-predominant subtype known as BB-CK because it consists of two brain-specific elements, and a form bound to the inner mitochondrial membrane known as Mi-CK. The function of the different CKs is subject to debate. However, there is agreement that the cytosolic creatine kinase reaction is near equilibrium in living human brain (29,30).

When the near-equilibrium of cytoplasmic creatine kinase is perturbed, the reaction buffers any increase of ADP by increased phosphorylation of ADP to ATP. The reaction is accompanied by loss of hydrogen ions and hence, in principle, leads to alkalosis. Cytoplasmic phosphocreatine is replenished by mitochondrial CK where it is regenerated by hydrolysis of ATP. Phosphocreatine diffuses an order of magnitude faster than the adenine nucleotides but the significance of this PCr–Cr shuttle is in dispute, as is the near-equilibrium status of Mi-CK. Recent simulations show that the shuttle maintains cytosolic ATP intact for almost a minute following excitation. The reason for the subsequent failure of perfect ATP homeostasis may be a rate limitation of the CK transphosphorylation in the mitochondria (30a).

Glycolysis

Glycolysis is the breakdown of glucose to pyruvate and lactate. Under anaerobic conditions, most of the glucose leaves the glycolytic chain as lactate. Under aerobic conditions (aerobic glycolysis) the amount of glucose that leaves the glycolytic chain as pyruvate depends on the activity of the tricarboxylic acid cycle. As a term, aerobic glycolysis therefore vaguely covers any oxygen/glucose consumption ratio below normal under aerobic conditions.

Phosphate and citrate ions, AMP, ammonium and hydrogen ions, and phosphocreatine itself, are among the classic regulators of the glycolytic enzymes *hexokinase* (HK) and *phosphofructokinase-1* (PFK-1) in the brain. In vitro, phosphate ion activity and phosphocreatine concentration both change upon stimulation of the cytosolic creatine kinase reaction, and both may contribute to the enhancement of glycolysis under controlled conditions.

While the classical list of regulators does not include Mg^{2+}, changes in concentration of Mg^{2+} may accompany increased ATP turn-over and increased creatine kinase activity. However, in vivo these regulators seem to change little during amphetamine stimulation of brain tissue, which leads to increased glycolysis as measured by the 2-deoxyglucose method and increased oxygen consumption as measured by arteriovenous difference (24,25).

The two enzymes HK and PFK-1 catalyze the irreversible phosphorylation of glycolytic intermediates at the expense of ATP. Four moles ATP is generated during the second stage of glycolysis for a net return of 1 mol ATP and two hydrogen ion equivalents per mol pyruvate in the reaction,

$$C_6H_{12}O_6 + 2ADP + 2P_i + 2NAD^+ \rightarrow 2C_3H_3O_3^- + 2ATP + 4H^+ + 2NADH$$

in which four hydrogen ion equivalents are liberated.

Pyruvate occupies a pivotal role because it participates in three different reactions in brain tissue. Pyruvate may be reduced by conversion to lactate, transported into mitochondria, or transported out of brain by the monocarboxylate transporter in cell membranes and the endothelium of brain capillaries. Hydrogen ions and the pyruvate are cotransported into the matrix of the mitochondrion by a *proton symporter* (31,32). The regulation of this transporter has not been described. As a proton symporter it would appear to be regulated in part by proton-motive forces in the cells. As the first committed step in the delivery of nutrient to the mitochondrion, the pyruvate transport seems to qualify as a potential site for the regulation of oxidative metabolism of the brain.

In aerobic and anaerobic glycolysis, the near-equilibrium reaction catalyzed by *lactate dehydrogenase* (LDH) is strongly balanced toward lactate:

$$2C_3H_3O_3^- + 2H^+ + 2NADH \leftrightarrow 2C_3H_5O_3^- + 2NAD^+$$

In this reaction, only half of the hydrogen ions produced during glycolysis are neutralized. The other half participate in the generation of lactic acid. The net yield is 2 mol ATP per mol glucose converted to lactic acid.

Since lactate is continuously produced in resting brain tissue (Table 3), the LDH reaction is near, not at, equilibrium. The transport of lactate across the cell membranes and across the blood–brain barrier drives the lactate generation. In the absence of such transport, the pyruvate-lactate concentrations would rise until pyruvate transport into mitochondria and pyruvate export across the blood–brain barrier matched its rate of generation, and no lactate would be generated.

The lactate/pyruvate ratio depends on the prevailing isozymes of LDH (LD1–LD5), as well as on the NAD/NADH ratio and pH, because the K_m of LDH for pyruvate varies with subtype, the aerobic heart form LD1 (H4) having the highest K_m (and hence the lowest affinity), and the anaerobic muscle and liver form LD5 (M4) the lowest K_m (ie, highest affinity). The brain has several forms of which the aerobic forms LD2 and LD3 predominate (32a).

The consequences of the presence of the LDH isozymes have remained an enigma but one will be postulated here: The effect of the LDH reaction is to provide the tissue with a flexible pyruvate-lactate pool the size of which depends on the specific isozymes and that responds to the oxidation status and proton-motive force of the cytosol. In theory, the individual property of the isozyme LD1 renders it particularly suited for tissue of high oxidative capacity because this enzyme allows the most rapid buildup of pyruvate by contraction of the pyruvate-lactate pool size to the lowest possible equilibrium lactate/pyruvate ratio.

The differences between the isozymes appear to be less pronounced at 37°C than at lower temperatures and they are subject to local factors that affect the combined pyruvate-lactate pool size.

Oxidative Phosphorylation

At steady state, brain metabolism has a respiratory quotient of unity, consistent with almost complete oxidation of glucose (33–35). Respiration is defined as the oxidation of cytochrome c by molecular oxygen, which serves as the ultimate electron acceptor. The oxidation is catalyzed by cytochrome a-a$_3$, known as *cytochrome oxidase*:

$$6O_2 + 24[e^-]\text{cytochrome c} \rightarrow 12O^{2-} + \text{cytochrome c}$$

It is on this reaction that much of the discussion hinges. How is it speeded up when the need arises? When is there a need? Is the reaction speeded up by more oxygen, more $[e^-]$cytochrome c, or higher activity of the enzyme? While oxygen is provided by the circulation, $[e^-]$cytochrome c is regenerated by the nicotinamide (NADH) and flavin (FADH$_2$) adenine dinucleotides in complex reactions catalyzed by proteins functioning as a *cytochrome reductase*. In these reactions, hydrogen ions escape to the outside of the inner membrane,

$$10NADH + 2FADH_2 + \text{cytochrome c} \rightarrow 10NAD^+ + 2FAD + 14H^+ + 24[e^-]\text{cytochrome c}$$

Per mole glucose, 2 mol NAD^+ is reduced in glycolysis, and 2 mol NAD^+ is reduced by the oxidation of pyruvate by the pyruvate dehydrogenase complex. The remainder of the NAD^+ and all of the FAD are reduced by the tricarboxylic acid (TCA) cycle dehydrogenases (Table 1):

$$6NAD^+ + 2FAD + 8TCA\text{-}H_2 \rightarrow 8TCA + 6NADH + 2FADH_2 + 6H^+$$

where TCA symbolizes the Krebs cycle intermediates. Via the regeneration of guanine triphosphate (GTP), two turns of the cycle leads to the nonoxidative phosphorylation of 2 mol ATP per mol glucose:

$$2C_3H_3O_3^- + 8TCA + 2GDP + 4P_i + 2NAD^+ + 6H_2O \rightarrow 6CO_2 + 8TCA\text{-}H_2 + 2GTP + 2NADH$$

Thus, per mol glucose, 20 hydrogen ion equivalents are extruded from the matrix and join the 4 hydrogen ion equivalents generated in the cytosol. The 24 hydrogen ion equivalents provide the driving force for the rephosphorylation of ADP. In this way, 3 mol ATP for each mole NADH oxidized to NAD^+, and 2 mol ATP for each mole FADH$_2$, are formed from ADP and P$_i$ by the proton-driven F-type ATPase (ATP synthase F0F1) in the inner membrane of the mitochondrial cristae, named for its discoverer Ephraim ("F") Racker. The transfer of protons into the matrix allows the hydrogen and oxide ions to form water:

$$34ADP + 34P_i + 24H^+ + 12O^{2-} \rightarrow 34ATP + 12H_2O$$

The ADP is transported into, and the ATP out of, the matrix by means of exchange diffusion mediated by the *ATP-ADP translocase* in the inner mitochondrial membrane.

The steady-state production of ATP and lactate can now be calculated from the stoichiometric relationships:

TABLE 1. *Potential sites of regulation of oxidative metabolism in vivo*

Location	Substrate	Type	Enzyme or transporter
Cytosol	ADP	Near-equilibrium	Creatine kinase (BB-CK)
	Glucose	Facilitated diffusion	glut-1 (blood–brain barrier)
	Glucose	Facilitated diffusion	glut-3 (neuronal membranes)
	Glucose	Irreversible	Hexokinase/PFK-1
	Pyruvate	Near-equilibrium	LDH (primarily LD_{2-3})
	Pyruvate	Facilitated diffusion	MCT (blood–brain barrier)
Mitochondria	Pyruvate	Cotransport, unsaturated	Proton symporter
	Pyruvate	Irreversible	Pyruvate dehydrogenase complex
	Isocitrate	Irreversible	NAD-linked ICDH
	2-Oxoglutarate	Irreversible	OGDH complex
	Oxygen	Passive diffusion	Oxygen transport
	Oxygen	Irreversible	Cytochrome oxidase
	ADP	Reversible	ATP synthase
	ADP	Exchange diffusion	ADP-ATP translocase
	ATP	Nonequilibrium?	Creatine kinase (Mi-CK)

PFK, phosphofructokinase; LDH, lactate dehydrogenase; MCT, monocarboxylate acid transporter; NAD, nicotinamide adenine dinucleotide; ICDH, isocitrate dehydrogenase; OGDH, oxoglutarate dehydrogenase; CK, creatine kinase.

$$J_{ATP} = 2CMR_{glc} + 6CMR_{O_2} \qquad (1)$$

$$J_{lact} = 2CMR_{glc} - \tfrac{1}{3}CMR_{O_2} \qquad (2)$$

where J_{ATP} is the ATP production and J_{lact} the lactate production. Equations (1) and (2) confirm that brain energy metabolism is largely synonymous with oxygen consumption.

REGULATION OF OXIDATIVE METABOLISM IN BRAIN

The steps that contribute to the regulation of oxidative metabolism in the brain in vivo are listed in Table 1. The purpose of these reactions is to provide the mitochondria with sufficient ADP, P_i, NADH, $FADH_2$, and oxygen to synthesize ATP and transfer it to the cytosol in sufficient quantities. The substrates can be divided into three groups including (a) oxygen, (b) ADP and P_i, and (c) glucose, pyruvate, and NADH-$FADH_2$.

The search for the control of brain oxidative metabolism has focused on reactions far from equilibrium because convention holds that near-equilibrium reactions cannot effectively regulate the net flux of metabolites. Were neurons controlled metabolically as skeletal muscle cells, convention would also claim that the rate of oxidative phosphorylation must be determined by the concentration of free ADP in the cytosol, with a maximum determined by the maximum oxidative capacity of the cell.

Oxygen

The near-equilibrium hypothesis of Erecinska and Wilson (3) assigns the rate limitation of brain oxidative metabolism to the irreversible reaction between cytochrome c and oxygen. According to this hypothesis, the sensitivity of oxidative phosphorylation to cytosolic ADP is subordinated a more general regulation by the cytosolic energy charge. In this hypothesis, the "near-equilibrium" refers to the entire electron transport chain and hence also to the ATP synthase reaction. According to the hypothesis, the apparent K_m of cytochrome oxidase toward oxygen is adjusted according to the [ADP][P_i]/[ATP] ratio in the cytosol. The hypothesis predicts that increases of this ratio change the properties of cytochrome oxidase in such a way that cytochrome c continues to react with oxygen at a rate that matches the rate of cytosolic ATP utilization. The activity of cytochrome oxidase must change to accommodate the prevailing concentration of oxygen.

The oxygen concentration reflects the balance between the delivery of oxygen and cytochrome oxidase activity. In reality, therefore, the near-equilibrium hypothesis assigns the regulation of oxygen consumption to the regulation of oxygen delivery (Fig. 1).

Although the brain tissue oxygen concentration is a function of the relationship between the delivery of oxygen and the rate of cytochrome oxidation, its influence on oxidative metabolism is poorly understood despite a century of speculation and research. Only recently was it realized that oxygen transport from blood to brain tissue is significantly limited by the hemoglobin binding and possibly by other factors as well, including a specific resistance at the endothelium of brain capillaries (36,37). The diffusion limitation imposed by the hemoglobin binding renders oxygen transport, reflected in the extraction fraction, somewhat insensitive to blood flow increases (38) such that blood flow must increase disproportionately to raise oxygen transport.

The relationship between blood flow and oxygen delivery is shown in Fig. 1. The relationship equals the relationship between blood flow and oxygen consumption when the tissue tension is negligible compared to the average capillary tension. In this case, the average oxygen tension of arterial blood drives most of the oxygen delivery.

Oxygen Delivery and Extraction Fraction as Function of Blood Flow

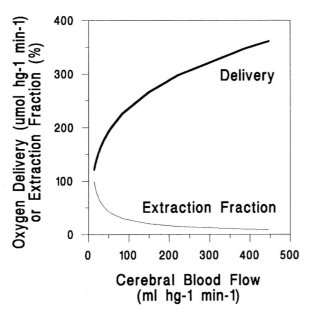

FIG. 1. Relationship between blood flow and oxygen delivery to brain tissue, equal to the oxygen consumption if the oxygen tension is negligible in brain tissue. The figure shows decline of oxygen extraction which follows increase of blood flow and drives increase of oxygen consumption. Extraction fraction equals fraction of deoxyhemoglobin in venous blood. Decline of extraction fraction is measure of relative decline of fraction of deoxygenated blood in cerebral veins when blood flow increases. The unidirectional oxygen delivery was calculated from the following equations:

$$J_{O_2} = FE_{O_2}C_{O_2} \qquad (7)$$

where J_{O_2} is the oxygen delivery, F blood flow, E_{O_2} the unidirectional oxygen extraction fraction, equal to the net oxygen extraction fraction when the tissue oxygen tension is negligible, and C_{O_2} the arterial oxygen concentration. The delivery is also a function of the average capillary oxygen tension:

$$J_{O_2} = LP_{cO_2} \qquad (8)$$

where L is the average tissue conductivity of oxygen transport between the capillary lumen and the mitochondria, and P_{cO_2} the average capillary oxygen tension. The net extraction defines the average capillary hemoglobin saturation with oxygen, assuming even distribution of the oxygen delivery along the capillary length:

$$S_{O_2} = 1 - \frac{E_{O_2}}{2} \qquad (9)$$

Finally, the average capillary oxygen tension and average capillary hemoglobin saturation with oxygen were related by the equation of the oxygen dissociation curve:

$$S_{O_2} = \frac{1}{1 + \left[\dfrac{P_{50}}{P_{cO_2}}\right]^{2.8}} \qquad (10)$$

If more oxygen is needed, paradoxically the oxygen extraction must decline in order to raise the average capillary oxygen tension to the magnitude required to drive more oxygen into the tissue. The relationship shown in Fig. 1 assumes that there is no absolute recruitment of the capillary bed capable of reducing the diffusion distances in the tissue or increasing the intrinsic permeability of the capillary endothelial wall. It is the current consensus that recruitment of capillaries in brain tissue is relative, ie, that it occurs by reduction of capillary transit times toward greater homogeneity of transit times and a lower average transit time rather than by an absolute increase of the number of perfused capillaries (39). Because the capillary surface area remains the same, relative recruitment does not benefit barrier-limited transport, like that of oxygen.

On the basis of the near-equilibrium hypothesis and the relationship shown in Fig. 1, Gjedde et al. proposed that blood flow in the absence of recruitment could sometimes fail to rise sufficiently to raise oxygen delivery measurably (36). On the one hand, this proposal invoked a limitation peculiar to brain because restricted oxygen supply is no longer considered the reason for the inappropriately named oxygen debt in skeletal muscle during exercise (39–44). On the other hand, the proposal offered an explanation of why the oxygen consumption of brain tissue fails to rise during some stimulations. Kuwabara et al. found the oxygen consumption in brain to remain unchanged in the presence of both increased blood flow and increased capillary diffusion capacity during vibrotactile stimulation of sensorimotor cortex (45). Because oxygen tension in the tissue must go up when blood flow rises without a parallel increase of oxygen consumption, this experiment proved that deficient oxygen supply is not the explanation for the limited oxygen consumption in the brain under these circumstances.

Using rat heart mitochondria as a model, LaNoue et al. showed that near-equilibrium of oxidative phosphorylation exists when respiration is slow (state 4) but that mitochondrial ATP synthesis occurs far from equilibrium when respiration is normal or fast (state 3) (46). These observations cause the near-equilibrium hypothesis of the regulation of oxidative metabolism in normally and rapidly respiring brain tissue to probably be wrong as well.

---

where P_{50} is the hemoglobin half-saturation oxygen tension. Using the corresponding values of blood flow and oxygen consumption listed in Table 3, C_{O_2} equal to 9 mM, P_{50} equal to 26 mm Hg, and negligible oxygen tension in the tissue, the extraction fraction is 0.47, the average capillary oxygen tension is 40 mm Hg, and the average tissue conductivity is 4.7 μmol mm Hg^{-1} min^{-1}. The conductivity was used to calculate oxygen delivery at the blood flow values shown in Fig. 1. Of course, oxygen delivery is the upper limit of oxygen consumption and equal to oxygen consumption only if the tissue oxygen tension is negligible compared to the average capillary tension.

ADP and Pi

Although a single rate-limiting step is not likely to be responsible for the regulation of oxidative phosphorylation in state 3 respiration of brain tissue, Groen et al. showed that the mitochondrial ATP-ADP translocase possessed increasing control strength with increasing rates of mitochondrial respiration in rat liver mitochondria (30% of the entire control strength at maximum rate of respiration) (47), as predicted by the translocase hypothesis of Klingenberg (48). This hypothesis assigns the major rate limitation to the ADP–ATP translocase.

In skeletal muscle in vitro and in certain conditions in vivo, cytosolic concentrations of ADP and Pi influence oxidative phosphorylation (49), and the relationship between the cytosolic ADP concentration and the rate of oxidative phosphorylation obeys the Michaelis–Menten equation (50). For human skeletal muscle tissue in vivo (51), phosphocreatine hydrolysis is associated with a significant increase of ADP in the absence of oxygen. As discussed above, ADP does not appear to rise in physiologically activated brain tissue in vivo. For this reason alone, limits in the translocation of ADP into the mitochondria do not explain limits in oxygen consumption.

Glucose, Pyruvate, and NADH–FADH$_2$

Neither the cytosolic phosphorylation potential nor the ADP-ATP translocase activity is likely to contribute to the regulation of oxidative phosphorylation metabolism in brain if ADP and ATP concentrations do not actually change during neuronal excitation. Instead, the hexokinase and PFK-1 reactions and the mono- and dicarboxylate transporters of the mitochondrial inner membrane may be responsible for much of the control.

Glucose itself is not rate limiting for brain oxidative metabolism (52,53). Glucose is the source of pyruvate and enters neurons by the glut-1 and glut-3 transporters of the blood–brain barrier and neuronal membranes, respectively. Glucose is transported so freely into neurons that the glucose concentration everywhere is the same substantial fraction of the plasma glucose (54).

The monocarboxylate carrier of pyruvate ultimately provides the mitochondrial electron carriers with NADH and FADH$_2$. Pyruvate enters the mitochondrial matrix as pyruvic acid by cotransport (symport) with hydrogen ions but transport into mitochondria is not obligatory. In the cytosol of brain cells, pyruvate can follow other paths, ie, it may undergo export from brain as pyruvate, or reduction to lactate and export from brain as lactate. Both lactate and pyruvate are transported by the monocarboxylic acid transporter (MCT) of the blood–brain barrier and neuronal membranes (32,55). These alternate paths influence the concentration of pyruvate.

The change of the cytosolic pyruvate concentration induced by an increase of the rate of glycolysis can be approximated by the equation accounting for all three paths available to pyruvate:

$$\Delta C_{pyr}(t) = 2 \frac{\Delta CMR_{glc}}{\left[\sum \frac{T_{max}}{K_t}\right]} \left(1 - e^{-t\left[\sum \frac{T_{max}}{K_t}\right]\left[1 + \frac{C_{lact}}{C_{pyr}}\right]}\right) \quad (3)$$

where ΔCMR_{glc} represents the increase of glycolysis, $\sum T_{max}/K_t$ the sum of the clearances of pyruvate into the matrix and across the endothelium (assuming C_{pyr} always to be small relative to K_t), and C_{lact}/C_{pyr} the near-equilibrium lactate/pyruvate ratio, approximately equal to the ratio between the K_m values of the two substrates.

The lower the ratio between LDH's affinities for pyruvate and lactate, the more rapid the approach to a new steady state, with a time constant of $[1 - (K_m^{lact}/K_m^{pyr})]/[\sum T_{max}/K_t]$. As noted above, the brain has several isozymes of LDH, including MH$_3$ (LD2), which has a low K_m^{lact}/K_m^{pyr} ratio and causes pyruvate to rise quickly for a given increase of glycolysis, and M$_2$H$_2$ (LD3), which has a lower ratio and causes pyruvate to rise more slowly.

Once pyruvate enters the matrix, calcium may play a role in the oxidation of pyruvate by activating the nonequilibrium mitochondrial dehydrogenases (pyruvate dehydrogenase complex, NAD$^+$-linked isocitrate dehydrogenase, and 2-oxoglutarate dehydrogenase complex), which supply the NADH (56).

The possibility that the pyruvic acid symporter may be rate limiting for oxidative metabolism in tissue other than brain was explored initially by Halestrap (57). Halestrap and Armston concluded that this was not the case in liver (58). However, Shearman and Halestrap discovered that ''pyruvate transport is rate-limiting for pyruvate oxidation by heart mitochondria in State 3,'' the state of activation also in brain cells (59). It is therefore a reasonable but untested hypothesis that pyruvate transport into brain mitochondria may limit oxidative metabolism when the activation-induced increase of cytosolic pyruvate is incomplete.

RESTING ENERGY DETERMINATION OF BRAIN TISSUE

The brain tissue metabolite stores (Table 2) represent about 1 minute's worth of ATP turnover, including ATP itself. Half of the ATP turnover represents ion pumping necessary to match the sodium and potassium leaks through brain cell membranes; in turn, these leaks reflect the sodium, potassium, and chloride permeability–surface area products consistent with the resting membrane potential.

Turnover of ATP and Lactate

Representative resting or average steady-state values of energy metabolism and blood flow of the human brain (60) are listed in Table 3, together with the steady-state turnover rates of ATP and lactate, calculated from Eqs. (1) and (2). Blood flow and metabolic rates were all measured by posi-

TABLE 2. *Average metabolites in human brain*

	Cytosol		Glycolytic equivalents	
Metabolite	Conc. (mM)	Content (μmol g^{-1})	ATP (μmol g^{-1})	Lactate (μmol g^{-1})
PCR	5.0	4.0	4.0	
Glycogen	3.0	2.4	3.6	3.6
Glucose	1.2	1.0	2.0	2.0
ATP	2.2	1.7	1.7	
ADP	1.2×10^{-2}	1.0×10^{-2}	5.0×10^{-3}	
AMP	7.1×10^{-5}	5.6×10^{-5}		
Pyruvate	0.16	0.13		0.1
Lactate	2.9	2.3		2.3
Total			11.3	8.0

From Olesen (65), Roth and Weiner (29). The "glycolytic equivalent" is the ATP reserve that each metabolite would represent in case of complete depletion.

tron emission tomography (PET) of the distribution of labeled tracers. Blood flow was measured after intravenous bolus injection of [^{15}O]water (61). Oxygen consumption was measured after single-breath inhalation of [^{15}O]O$_2$ (62). Glucose consumption was measured after intravenous bolus injection of [^{18}F]fluorodeoxyglucose (60). The values agree with previous and current determinations (63,64). The molar oxygen/glucose ratio was 5.6, indicating that 93% of the glucose fuels oxidative phosphorylation, not far from the 87% value reported by Himwich and Himwich (34). The corresponding ATP turnover calculated from Eq. (1) is 10 μmol g^{-1} min^{-1} and the lactate production is 0.05 μmol g^{-1} min^{-1}.

The maximal transport capacity (T_{max}) of the monocarboxylic acid transporter of the blood–brain barrier is 0.1–0.2 μmol g^{-1} min^{-1} with a Michaelis constant of 1–2 μmol g^{-1} min^{-1}, close to the average lactate content of brain (see Table 2). The efflux is therefore half of the T_{max}.

The average rate of pyruvate generation in the brain is about 0.6 μmol g^{-1} min^{-1}, calculated from the glycolytic rate. The resulting pyruvate concentration in brain tissue of living humans is unknown, but Olesen measured the pyruvate and lactate concentrations in brain tissue biopsies obtained at surgery (65). The least perturbed concentrations in near-normal tissue were twice the concentrations measured in rat brain (66) with a ratio of 18 (see Table 2).

The K_m of the transport of pyruvic acid into mitochondria is 0.3–0.5 μmol g^{-1} min^{-1}, ie, considerably higher than the cytosolic pyruvate concentration, consistent with a symporter T_{max} of 3 μmol g^{-1} min^{-1}. Since the blood–brain

barrier T_{max} and K_t of pyruvate are about equal to those of lactate (67), the export of pyruvate to the circulation is about one tenth that of lactate (34). This is consistent with the average combined pyruvate-lactate pool size being 10- to 20-fold larger than the pyruvate pool size itself in brain tissue.

Ion Permeabilities

The energy released by the hydrolysis of 5 μmol ATP g^{-1} min^{-1} (half the ATP turnover) is sufficient to transport 15 μmol Na$^+$ g^{-1} min^{-1}. The half-life of sodium in the cells is then less than a minute, and considerably less than the 20-minute half-life of sodium in active (stimulated) squid axons (68). Also, the sodium ion flux through nerve membrane per unit tissue weight appears to be one or more orders of magnitude less than the sodium ion flux estimated from the average metabolism of nervous tissue (69). These considerations suggest that the major leakage of sodium occurs in dendrites, rather than in cell bodies, or axons, in which the density of sodium channels and the ratio between the membrane surface area and intracellular volume are both low (70).

The apparent average sodium permeability–surface area product in the steady state can be calculated from the sodium flux by means of Goldman's flux equation (71). On the basis of the concentrations listed in Table 4, an assumed average steady-state membrane potential, an assumed sodium flux calculated from the measured ATP turnover, and the 3:2 ratio between the net sodium and potassium fluxes in the steady state, the permeability-surface area products of sodium and potassium of Table 5 were calculated by means of Goldman's flux equation. Details of this calculation were given by Gjedde (72).

To estimate the chloride permeability, it was necessary to use a simplified form of the equation derived by Goldman (73) and Hodgkin and Katz (68) from the constant field theory. The equation yielded the membrane potential difference on the basis of the permeability-weighted individual concentrations of sodium, potassium, and chloride. In the steady state, the chloride flux matched the difference between the sodium and potassium fluxes, rendering the total ion flux electroneutral (see Table 5).

TABLE 3. *Average physiologic variables of human cerebral cortex*

Somatosensory cortex	Average	Ref.
CMR$_{glc}$ [μmol g^{-1} min^{-1}]	0.30	
CMR$_{O_2}$ [μmol g^{-1} min^{-1}]	1.60	45
CBF [ml g^{-1} min^{-1}]	0.45	
ATP turnover [μmol g^{-1} min^{-1}]	10	Eq. (1)
Lactate flux [μmol g^{-1} min^{-1}]	0.05	Eq. (2)

CMR, cerebral metabolic rate; CBF, cerebral blood flow.

TABLE 4. *Ion concentrations in nerve cells*

		Ion				
		Sodium		Potassium		Chloride
Variable	Unit	E&S	M	E&S	M	M
Equililbrium potential	mV	+41	+40	−84	−100	−75
Intracellular concentration	mM	27	30	80	140	8
Extracellular concentration	mM	133	150	3	3	130

From Erecinska and Silver (5) (E&S), McCormick (73a) (M).

ENERGY DEMAND DURING NEURONAL ACTIVATION

Depolarization of neuronal membranes leads to increased oxygen uptake (73). Although the exact mechanism is unknown, the finding is important because cells may depolarize without a change of the ATP requirement, as shown in Table 5, in which the ion fluxes and hence ATP requirement at two different membrane potentials (−65 and −55 mV) are identical. This identity is accomplished by a moderate increase of sodium conductance paired with substantial declines of potassium and chloride conductances (74).

In contrast, the following analysis of energy demand during excitation is based entirely on steady-state consideration of either sodium and potassium or chloride, assuming states *during* which there are no changes of permeabilities, concentrations, or turnover rates. The transition from one steady state to another is therefore ignored. The values are intended as averages for a homogeneous tissue of vaguely cortical composition, and no distinction is made between neurons and glia.

Metabolic Cost of Membrane Depolarization

The Goldman–Hodgkin–Katz constant field equation predicts the changes of the membrane potential that occur when ion permeabilities change. Using the permeabilities calculated in Table 5, the corresponding membrane potentials were calculated (Fig. 2A, C). The membrane potentials reflect changes of both sodium and potassium (adjusted to preserve the 3:2 flux ratio required by the P-type Na,K–ATPase), or chloride, permeability. The resulting Na,K–ATPase activity was calculated as the flux required to preserve ion homeostasis. The glucose demand was in turn calculated as the nutrient delivery required to compensate for a steady-state ATPase activity of this magnitude by oxidative phosphorylation.

Figure 2B reveals the metabolic consequence of sodium and potassium leakage: for an arbitrary depolarization from −70 to −60 mV, the ATP turnover must increase fourfold from 2.5 to 9 μmol g^{-1} min^{-1} to preserve ion homeostasis. With a sodium ion transport–stimulated glucose metabolic rate of 0.15 μmol g^{-1} min^{-1}, the total glucose demand would be expected to increase from 0.2 to 0.4 μmol g^{-1} min^{-1} to fuel this turnover of ATP. For further depolarization to a firing level of −55 mV, the glucose supply would have to increase to as much as 0.6 μmol g^{-1} min^{-1} to fuel an ATP turnover of 20 μmol g^{-1} min^{-1}. In the absence of oxygen (or with no increase of oxygen consumption), the glucose supply would have to increase to as much as 10 μmol g^{-1} min^{-1}, a 30-fold increase.

Increased chloride permeability, presumed to underlie the inhibition mediated by GABA$_A$ receptors, can be predicted to increase membrane polarization (Fig. 2D). Since the metabolic consequences of chloride leakage are not known with certainty, the predicted metabolic requirement for this ion reflects only the change of the membrane potential according to Goldman's flux equation. The requirement increased much less than calculated for the tissue stimulated by sodium and potassium permeability.

Sources of ATP During Neuronal Activation

To satisfy the need for increased energy turnover during neuronal excitation, additional nutrients must be supplied from tissue stores or from the circulation. With no additional nutrients and no net loss of ATP, the PCr, glycogen, and glucose concentrations sustain a 100% rise of ATP turnover for less than a minute. This will cause the sum of pyruvate and lactate levels to rise threefold, unless oxidative phosphorylation increases (see Table 2).

TABLE 5. *Ion movements across nerve cell membranes*

		Ion		
Variable	Unit	Sodium	Potassium	Chloride
Transmembrane leakage	μmol g^{-1} min^{-1}	15	10	5
PS product at −65 mV	ml g^{-1} min^{-1}	0.038	0.404	0.549
PS product at −55 mV	ml g^{-1} min^{-1}	0.044	0.285	0.246

From Gjedde (72), assuming 50% of ATP turnover dedicated to ion transport, calculated from the concentrations listed in Table 4 (M). PS, permeability–surface area.

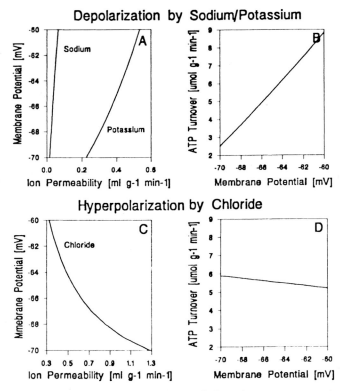

FIG. 2. Upper row: A. *Left panel:* Steady-state neuronal membrane potential change as function of altered sodium and potassium ion permeabilities. Abscissa: Ion permeability <ml g^{-1} min^{-1}). Ordinate: membrane potential (mV), calculated from the Goldman–Hodgkin–Katz constant field equation by Gjedde (72). B. *Right panel:* Steady-state neuronal ATP requirement as function of membrane depolarization caused by increased sodium and potassium permeability. Ordinate: Steady-state ATP requirement (μmol g^{-1} min^{-1}), calculated from steady-state ion flux. Abscissa: Membrane potential (mV). Calculated from the Goldman–Hodgkin–Katz constant field equation on the basis of assumed changes of sodium and potassium ion permeabilities. **Lower row:** *C.* Left panel: Steady-state neuronal membrane potential change as function of altered chloride ion permeability. Abscissa: Ion permeability (ml g^{-1} min^{-1}). *Ordinate:* Membrane potential (mV), calculated from the Goldman–Hodgkin–Katz constant field equation. D. *Right panel:* Steady-state neuronal ATP requirement as function of membrane depolarization caused by increased chloride ion permeability. Ordinate: Steady-state ATP requirement (μmol g^{-1} min^{-1}), calculated from steady-state ion flux. Abscissa: Membrane potential (mV), calculated from the Goldman–Hodgkin–Katz constant field equation on the basis of calculated changes of chloride ion permeability. (From ref. 74.)

Hydrolysis of Phosphocreatine

Contrary to the classical view, studies on heart and brain cells in vitro and in vivo fail to reproduce the decline of ATP observed during increased work of skeletal muscle in vivo (75). During experimental excitation of rat brain by amphetamine, phosphocreatine is converted to ATP so efficiently that no drop of ATP is detected by phosphorus nu-

clear magnetic resonance (24). The near-equilibrium state of the creatine kinase reaction would seem to make it of little use if ATP and ADP concentrations do not change. However, Roth and Weiner demonstrated that a substantial reduction of the concentration of PCr (5 mM) is compatible with minimal change of ATP and ADP when measured changes of Mg^{2+} and pH are taken into account (29). This decline of PCr may be as much as threefold the turnover of ATP in 1 minute and hence allows a threefold increase of ATP hydrolysis with little or no change of the ATP concentration during the first minute.

Erecinska and Silver calculated that hydrolysis of 5 mM PCr could raise the pH of brain tissue by as much as 0.3 units at the prevailing buffering capacity (5). This finding was anticipated by Chesler and Kraig who found that astrocytes become more alkaline when depolarized during brain activation (76,77). The change is observed in several kinds of cells in which a rise in pH correlates with an increase in metabolic activity (78).

Glycolytic Rate

Alkalinization of brain tissue by hydrolysis of phosphocreatine may stimulate glycolysis at the PFK step, as in skeletal muscle (79). The extracellular glucose concentration in brain determined by means of glucose-sensitive microelectrodes placed in brain tissue of live rats showed slight decreases during physiologic activation (55). Studies in humans confirm that excitation of cerebral cortex leads to significant increase of the glucose phosphorylation rate (Table 6). Because many of these studies were complicated by the long circulation of tracer fluorodeoxyglucose required to determine glucose consumption accurately (10), Kuwabara et al. and Ribeiro et al. shortened the method from 45 to 20 minutes, with the same result (60,80).

When not coupled to oxidative phosphorylation, even tiny increases of energy demand require substantial increases of the glucose supply (81,82). In the absence of an increase of oxidative phosphorylation, the 50% increase of the glucose phosphorylation rate observed by Fox et al. (81) (see Table 6) adds 0.3 μmol g^{-1} min^{-1} to the lactate production, a sevenfold increase. Thus, a 3% increase of ATP generation caused a 600% increase of lactate flux. Continued lactate production of this magnitude doubles the lactate concentration in 7 minutes, unless oxidative metabolism begins.

The lactate increase must be driven by an increase of the pyruvate concentration with which it is in near-equilibrium. In turn, increased lactate drives up the lactate efflux. When maximally stimulated, the rate of pyruvate generation can rise to 3–4 μmol g^{-1} min^{-1} (83,84), which is several fold the calculated maximum velocity of pyruvate oxidation and close to the calculated T_{max} of the pyruvic acid symporter. The pyruvate concentration must rise for the rate of pyruvate removal to match the generation of pyruvate. The pyruvate increase raises the pyruvate transport into the matrix,

TABLE 6. *Neuronal activation of brain metabolism*

Stimulus	Duration (min)	Supply (%)			Products (μmol g^{-1} min^{-1})	
		ΔCBF	ΔCMRglc	ΔCMRO$_2$	ΔJ_{ATP}	ΔJ_{lact}
Somatosensory	1[a]	28	[17]*	9**	0.96**	0.05
	1[b]	31	[18]*	13**	1.35**	0.03
	1[c]	18	[8]*	0	0.04	0.04
	20[d]	18	8	[0]*	0.04	0.04
	20[c]	18	[8]*	0	0.04	0.04
	45[e]	27	17	[0]*	0.10	0.10
Photic	30[f]	43	27	0	0.15	0.15
	45[g]	49	51	5**	0.76**	0.26
Checkerboard	5[h]	25	[28]*	28	2.83	0.008
	10[h]	26	[29]*	29	2.93	0.009

From [a]Fox & Raichle (91), [b]Seitz & Roland (92), [c]Fujita et al. (92a), [d]Kuwabara et al. (45), [e]Ginsberg et al. (82), [f]Ribeiro et al. (80), [g]Fox et al. (81), [h]Marrett et al. (98).
* Values deduced from other studies. ** CMR$_{O_2}$ increase not significant. CBF, cerebral blood flow; CMR, cerebral metabolic rate.

but the greater the equilibrium lactate/pyruvate ratio, the more slowly this rise of pyruvate occurs. For a pyruvate transport $\Sigma T_{max}/K_t$ ratio of 6 min^{-1} (from typical values) and an equilibrium C_{lact}/C_{pyr}7 ratio of 15, for the increase of tissue pyruvate during an increase of glucose consumption becomes:

$$\Delta C_{pyr}(t) = 0.33 \Delta CMR_{glc}(1 - e^{-0.375t}) \qquad (4)$$

according to which the half-time of approach to a new steady-state pyruvate concentration is approximately 2 minutes. The half-time depends on the equilibrium C_{lact}/C_{pyr} ratio and hence on the kinetic properties of the prevailing LDH isozymes. Lactate efflux through the capillary endothelium further increases the half-time, as do both pyruvate transport and decreases of the NAD$^+$/NADH ratio.

It is interesting that Dóra et al. observed that physiologic

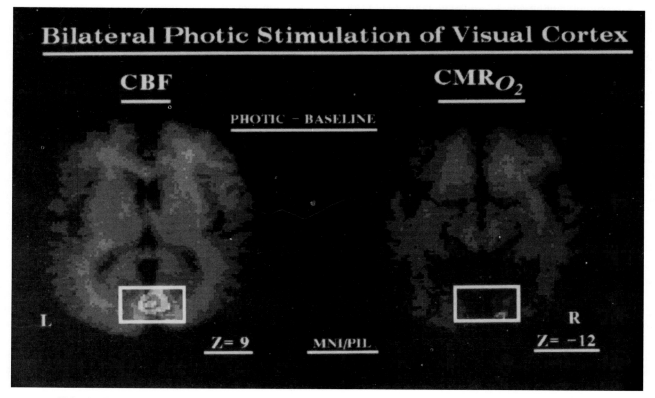

FIG. 3. Absent focal increase of oxygen consumption in visual cortex of healthy human volunteers viewing a photic stimulus. Left panel shows significant blood flow increase, right panel absent increase of oxygen consumption. (From ref. 80.)

stimulation of feline cortex in vivo resulted in significant reduction of the NAD$^+$/NADH ratio (85). In this case, it appears that the NADH generated during glycolysis delayed the rise of pyruvate by stimulating the conversion to lactate. It is particularly interesting in this context that a massive addition of pyruvate (10 mM) to stimulated hearts in vitro inhibited the decline of the NAD$^+$/NADH ratio (86), most likely by providing enough pyruvate to immediately saturate the symporter and kick-start oxidative phosphorylation. Thus, insufficient accumulation of pyruvate may prevent the activation of oxidative phosphorylation and instead stimulate oxidation of NADH in the cytosol. The lactate concentration in working dog skeletal muscle is directly rather than inversely proportional to the rate of oxygen consumption, as expected if a specific pyruvate level were required to sustain a given rate of oxygen consumption (87).

The locus of the measured changes of glucose metabolism has been the subject of much discussion. There is evidence that the site of increased glucose metabolism is presynaptic (88), which is also in some studies the predominant location of lactate dehydrogenase (89). Mitochondria, on the other hand, have been observed to be particularly concentrated and reactive in postsynaptic structures (90).

Oxygen Consumption

It has been surmised for some time that oxidative phosphorylation cannot match the sevenfold increase of pyruvate production seen under the most extreme circumstances of glycolytic stimulation in the mammalian brain (4). With important exceptions, recent measurements of oxygen consumption during sensory stimulation of human cerebral cortex generally show little or no change of oxygen consumption of the human brain during brief cortical stimulation (81,91,92) (see Table 6).

With the single-inhalation method of measuring oxygen consumption, changes of blood flow and oxygen consumption were compared during 30 minutes of vibrotactile stimulation of one hand's fingers. In primary sensory cortex, the blood flow change was 18% both at the onset of stimulation and after 20 minutes of stimulation, but oxygen consumption did not increase at any time (92a). Similarly, Fig. 3 shows the absent change of oxygen consumption during 10 minutes of photic stimulation of visual cortex (80).

In the absence of increased oxygen consumption, increased blood flow must lead to elevated capillary and tissue oxygen tensions (see Fig. 4). Using the constants derived from Fig. 1, Fig. 4 shows that tissue oxygen increases when the capillary oxygen increases, if the blood flow elevation occurs without an increase of the oxygen consumption. This proves that oxidative metabolism is not stimulated merely by increase of tissue oxygen.

The average capillary and venous deoxyhemoglobin declines by half when blood flow doubles. Deoxyhemoglobin is paramagnetic. The decline has been claimed to give rise to the so-called BOLD (blood oxygenation level–dependent) magnetic resonance signal changes during functional activa-

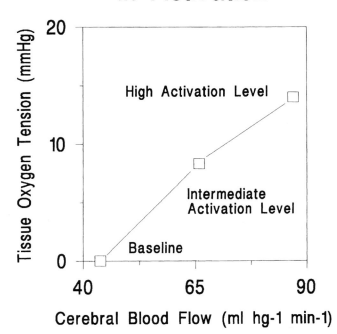

FIG. 4. Tissue oxygen tension as a function of blood flow elevation in the absence of any elevation of oxygen consumption. Calculated from constants listed in the legend to Fig. 1. Tissue oxygen tensions were calculated from a rearrangement of Eq. (7) above:

$$Pt_{O_2} = Pc_{O_2} - (J_{O_2}/L) \tag{11}$$

where Pt_{O_2} is the average tissue oxygen tension at the distal end of the diffusion path.

tion of brain tissue (93–96). In a tissue of average composition (of which 20% of the vascular volume is arteries and arterioles, 10% capillaries, and 70% venules and veins), the vast majority (93%) of such a signal would originate in cerebral venules and veins, as also suspected in practice (97). The 93% is a constant obtained from the ratio

$$\frac{0.7 \, E_{O_2}}{0.1 \, \dfrac{E_{O_2}}{2} + 0.7 \, E_{O_2}} \tag{5}$$

because the average oxygen saturation equals $1 - E_{O_2}/2$ in capillaries and $1 - E_{O2}$ in veins. The fraction can be recalculated for any assumed proportions of capillaries and veins.

Contrary to the results of no change of oxygen consumption, Marrett et al discovered that stimulation of visual cortex with a reversing checkerboard pattern for 5 or 10 minutes caused significant increase of oxygen consumption (98) (see Fig. 5). The reported values of CMR$_{O_2}$ and the calculated ATP flux have been listed in Table 6 and correlated in Fig. 6 to illustrate the dependency of ATP generation on oxidative phosphorylation. Tentative conclusions can be drawn from these observations:

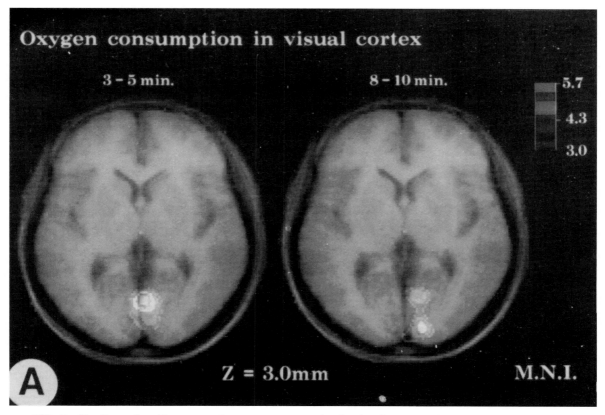

FIG. 5. Significant focal increase of oxygen consumption in visual cortex of healthy human volunteers visually stimulated by reversing checkerboard pattern. (From ref. 98.)

1. The discrepancy between the result of different types of sensorimotor stimulation suggests that the ultimate increase of oxygen consumption depends significantly on the biochemical peculiarities of the neuronal pathway mediating the response to the stimulus (89). In skeletal muscle cells, the content of cytochrome oxidase reflects the maximal level of oxygen consumption habitually required by specific cells (99). In these cells, neural input regulates the categorization of muscle cells into types I, IIa, or IIb. This observation suggests that transient increases of energy metabolism above the habitual level of activity cannot, or need never, be accompanied by increased oxygen consumption, eg, during vibrotactile stimulation of primary sensory cortex or photic stimulation of visual cortex (80).

2. The reason for the slow initial rise of oxygen consumption may be the inability (or absent need) to raise the cytosolic pyruvate concentration rapidly in the presence of a lactate leak. If pyruvate transport were indeed rate limiting in state 3 activation (59), the consumption of oxygen would depend on the cytosolic pyruvate concentration and hence on the rate of glycolysis as described by Eq. (4):

$$\Delta CMR_{O_2}(t) = 5.6\Delta CMR_{glc} (1 - e^{-0.375t}) \quad (6)$$

according to which the half-time of change is 2 minutes

for a lactate/pyruvate ratio of 15 (but as much as 14 minutes for a ratio of 100).

Blood Flow

"Peaks," or foci, of blood flow change in response to specific stimulation have been documented with considerable certainty (see Table 6). However, the table reveals that the link between the changes of blood flow and the generation of additional ATP is markedly variable, with ratios between the relative changes ranging from unity to 20. It is not known as to which specific aspect of neuronal excitation is reflected in the blood flow increase. The findings suggest that the (initial) blood flow changes are unrelated to the direct satisfaction of the energy demand by oxidative phosphorylation because little extra oxygen is being used and hence minimal increase of net energy turnover is evident.

The factors that control the blood flow of the brain are not known with uncertainty. The best known of the blood flow stimulants is carbon dioxide but there is almost universal agreement that carbon dioxide itself is not the regulator of blood flow changes that occur in response to functional activation of brain tissue (100). This agreement finds support in the evidence that acidosis and increased synthesis of carbon dioxide are not among the primary metabolic consequences of functional activation of brain tissue.

ATP-O2 Couple

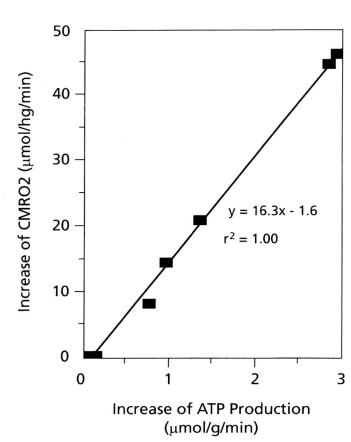

FIG. 6. ATP–oxygen couple. Association between increase of ATP generation and increase of oxygen consumption measured in published studies listed in Table 6. ATP flux was calculated by means of Eq. (1) in text. Abscissa: Calculated increase of ATP flux (μmol hg^{-1} min^{-1}). Ordinate: Measured change of oxygen consumption (μmol hg^{-1} min^{-1}).

Lactate-CBF Couple

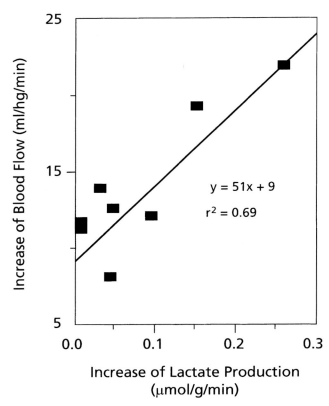

FIG. 7. Lactate–flow couple. Association between increase of lactate generation and increase of blood flow in published studies listed in Table 6. Lactate flux was calculated by means of Eq. (2) in text. Abscissa: Calculated increase of lactate flux (μmol g^{-1} min^{-1}). Ordinate: Measured blood flow change (ml g^{-1} min^{-1}).

A multitude of factors appear capable of stimulating blood flow changes of brain tissue. On the one hand, none of the classical factors seems to be the actual link between functional activation and blood flow change. On the other hand, the blocking of the vascular receptors suspected of being involved in the synthesis of nitric oxide abolishes functionally induced blood flow increases. Apparently, some blood flow stimulators act by means of nitric oxide, including acetylcholine (100).

Focal changes of cortical blood flow induced by sensory stimulation can be eliminated by blocking endothelial acetylcholine receptors (101), including those involved in mediating synthesis of the endothelium-derived relaxation factor (EDRF) nitric oxide. Yet the underlying neuronal activation is unimpeded, as indicated by increased glycolysis (101).

Skeletal muscle studies suggest that a correlation exists between the increase of blood flow and the increase of lactate (40). Laptook et al showed that lactate may contribute to the regulation of cerebral blood flow (102). The blood flow changes listed in Table 6 vary positively with the rate of lactate generation calculated by means of Eq. (2) (Fig. 7).

The detailed relationships among acetylcholinergic activity, synthesis of nitric oxide, generation of lactate, and functionally induced blood flow changes of brain tissue are largely unknown. The elucidation of these relations is among the most pressing items on the neuroscientific agenda of the future.

THE FLOW–METABOLISM COUPLE REVISITED

There are few facts in evidence of a rigid association in vivo between changes of oxygen consumption, glucose combustion, and blood flow in the human brain. The claim that blood flow must somehow satisfy equally the demand for oxygen and glucose during excitation is therefore without foundation. It is important to note that Roy and Sherrington measured neither glucose nor oxygen consumption (2). They observed pial vasodilatation after administration of postmortem brain extracts to living animals. They surmised that a metabolite had caused the dilatation and that metabolite might be lactate.

The theoretical analysis suggests that the cerebral energy demand reflects the steady-state level of membrane polarization. Substantial increases of net energy turnover are required neither for neuronal inhibition caused by increased chloride conductance nor for increased action potential frequency per se. Increased energy turnover is not required to sustain hyperpolarization caused by decreased conductance of sodium or increased conductance of potassium.

Increased energy supply is only required to maintain reduced dendritic and/or somatic membrane polarization, caused by increases of both sodium and potassium conductances.

The J_{ATP}/J_{lact} ratio divides the responses into two types possibly related to the responses of hypothetical ''red'' and ''white'' neurons (Fig. 8). Some studies show little or no increase of net energy turnover during cortical stimulation but greatly increased blood flow. Except in the case of photic stimulation, the generated lactate was no more than could be transported by the blood–brain barrier. The cases of greatly increased blood flow were associated with a low ATP/lactate flux ratio, possibly characteristic of white neurons or terminals of low oxidative capacity.

Conversely, during the checkerboard stimulation of visual cortex, the energy demand rose greatly but lactate production remained minimal because of the simultaneous rise of oxygen consumption. In this case, the ATP/lactate flux ratio was in the high range. The increased oxygen supply satisfied a need for increased ATP turnover, possibly characteristic of the excitation of red neurons or dendrites of high oxidative capacity.

These conclusions provide no clue to the mechanism underlying a putative flow–lactate couple in white neurons. If not accompanied by capillary recruitment, blood flow increases have a moderate effect on glucose and oxygen delivery. This may not be true of lactate removal because the cerebral venous lactate concentration is inversely proportional to blood flow. The evidence suggests that the rise of pyruvate accompanying an excessive rise of lactate ultimately may cause oxidative phosphorylation to kick in to inhibit further lactate generation and thus to reduce the need for further glucose delivery and blood flow removal of lactate. This would occur only if blood flow were not sufficient to remove the lactate and prevent the rise of pyruvate. The tissue lactate level at which this would occur would be under the control of the LDH isozyme profile and could therefore differ for different metabolic categories of cells. Additional modulation could be offered by calcium entry into the mitochondria and the ADP concentration.

This conclusion suggests that regional peaks of increased blood flow and increased oxygen consumption under some circumstances could be dissociated by the different metabolic needs of different sections of neuronal networks. Paradoxically, the regions with the highest oxidative capacity could be those with the least need for increased blood flow.

ACKNOWLEDGMENTS

The author's work summarized in this chapter was supported by the Medical Research Council of Canada grants SP-5, PG-41, and SP-30, and by the Medical Research Council of Denmark grants 94-1233 and 94-1234.

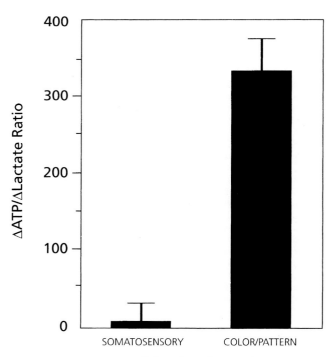

"White" and "Red" Neurons

FIG. 8. "White" and "red" neurons in human brain in vivo. Based on ratio between ATP and lactate production increases during excitation, stimulus and/or cells fall into two metabolic categories, one with average ratio <20 and one with average ratio >300. Ordinate: Ratio between change of ATP production and change of lactate generation.

REFERENCES

1. Descartes R. Discours de la Méthode, 1637, Leiden, quoted from Discourse on the Method, *Library of the Future*, 3rd ed., Ver. 4.3 (Electronically Enhanced Text), c 1991–1995 World Library.
2. Roy CS, Sherrington CS. On the regulation of the blood supply of the brain. *J Physiol (Lond)* 1890;11:85–108.
3. Erecinska M, Wilson DF. Regulation of cellular energy metabolism. *J Membrane Biol* 1982;70:1–14.

4. van den Berg CJ, Bruntink R. Glucose oxidation in the brain during seizures: experiments with labeled glucose and deoxyglucose. In: Hertz L, Kvamme E, McGeer EG, Schousboe A, eds. *Glutamine, Glutamate and GABA in the Central Nervous System*. New York: Alan R Liss, 1983;619–624.

5. Erecinska M, Silver I. ATP and brain function. *J Cereb Blood Flow Metab* 1989;9:2–19.

6. Hertz L, Schousboe A. Ion and energy metabolism of the brain at the cellular level. *Int Rev Neurobiol* 1975;18:141–211.

7. Shalit MN, Beller AJ, Feinsod M, Drapkin AJ, Cotev S. The blood flow and oxygen consumption of the dying brain. *Neurology* 1970; 20:740–748.

8. Levy DE, Sidtis JJ, Rottenberg DA, Jarden JO, Strother SC, Dhawan V, Ginos JZ, Tramo MJ, Evans AC, Plum F. Differences in cerebral blood flow and glucose utilization in vegetative versus locked-in patients. *Ann Neurol* 1987;22:673–682.

9. Brodersen P, Jorgensen EO. Cerebral blood flow and oxygen uptake, and cerebrospinal fluid biochemistry in severe coma. *J Neurol Neurosurg Psychiatry* 1974;37:384–391.

10. Sokoloff L, Reivich M, Kennedy C, DesRosiers MH, Patlak CS, Pettigrew KD, Sakurada O, Shinohara M. The [^{14}C]deoxyglucose method for the measurement of local cerebral glucose utilization: theory, procedure, and normal values in the conscious and anesthetized albine rat. *J Neurochem* 1977;28:897–916.

11. McIlwain H. Metabolic response in vitro to electrical stimulation of section. *Biochem J* 1951;49:382–393.

12. Ritchie JM. The oxygen consumption of mammalian non-myelinated fibres at rest and during activity. *J Physiol (Lond)* 1967;188:309–329.

13. Mata M, Fink DG, Gainer H, Smith CB, Davidsen L, Savaki HE, Schwarts WJ, Sokoloff L. Activity-dependent energy metabolism in rat posterior pituitary primarily reflects sodium pump activity. *J Neurochem* 1980;34:213–215.

14. Bowers C, Zigmond R. Localization of neurons in the rat superior cervical ganglion that project into different postganglionic trunks. *J Comp Neurol* 1979;185:381–391.

15. Yarowsky PJ, Ingvar DH. Neuronal activity and energy metabolism. *Fed Proc* 1981;40:2353–2362.

16. Kadekaro M, Crane AM, Sokoloff L. Differential effects of electrical stimulation of sciatic nerve on metabolic activity in spinal cord and dorsal root ganglion in the rat. *Proc Natl Acad Sci USA* 1985;82: 6010–6013.

17. Hodgkin AL, Huxley A. A quantitative description of membrane current and its application to conductance and excitation in nerve. *J Physiol (Lond)* 1952;117:500–544.

18. Morowitz HJ. *Foundations of Bioenergetics*. New York: Academic Press, 1978.

19. Whittam R. The dependence of the respiration of brain cortex on active cation transport. *Biochem J* 1962;82:205–212.

20. Skou JC. Further investigations on a Mg^{2+}– Na^{+}–activated adenosine-triphosphatase, possibly related to the active, linked transport of Na^{+} and K^{+} across the nerve membrane. *Biochim Biophys Acta* 1960; 42:6–23.

21. Pellerin L, Magistretti PJ. Glutamate uptake into astrocytes stimulates aerobic glycolysis: a mechanism coupling neuronal activity to glucose utilization. *Proc Natl Acad Sci USA* 1994;91:10625–10629.

22. Balaban RS, Kantor HL, Katz LA, Briggs RW. Relation between work and phosphate metabolites in the in vivo paced mammalian heart. *Science* 1986;232:1121–1123.

23. Detre JA, Koretsky AP, Williams DS, Ho C. Absence of pH changes during altered work in the in vivo sheep heart: a ^{31}P-NMR investigation. *J Mol Cell Cardiol* 1990;22:543–553.

24. Detre JA, Williams DS, Koretsky AP. Nuclear magnetic resonance determination of flow, lactate, and phosphate metabolites during amphetamine stimulation of the rat brain. *Nucl Magn Res Biomed* 1990; 3:272–278.

25. Berntman L, Carlsson C, Hägerdal M, Siesjö BK. Excessive increase in oxygen uptake and blood flow in the brain during amphetamine intoxication. *Acta Physiologica Scand* 1976;97(2):264–266.

26. Carlsson C, Hägerdal M, Siesjö BK. Influence of amphetamine sulphate on cerebral blood flow and metabolism. *Acta Physiol Scand* 1975;94:128–129.

27. Berntman L, Carlsson C, Hägerdal M, Siesjö BK. Circulatory and metabolic effects in the brain induced by amphetamine sulphate. *Acta Physiol Scand* 102(3):310–23, 1978

28. Silva AC, Zhang W, Williams DS, Koretsky AP. Multi-slice MRI of rat brain perfusion during amphetamine stimulation using arterial spin labeling. *Magn Reson Med* 1995;33:209–14.

29. Roth K, Weiner MW. Determination of cytosolic ADP and AMP concentrations and the free energy of ATP hydrolysis in huan muscle and brain tissues with ^{31}P NMR spectroscopy. *Magn Reson Med* 1991; 22:505–511.

30. Mora BN, Narasimhan PT, Ross BD. ^{31}P magnetization transfer studies in the monkey brain. *Magn Reson Med* 1992;26:100–115.

30a. Fedosov SN. Creatine-creatine phosphate shuttle modeled as two-compartment system at different levels of creatine kinase activity. *Biochim Biophys Acta* 1994;1208(2):238–246.

31. Halestrap AP. The mitochondrial pyruvate carrier. *Biochem J* 1975; 148:85–96.

32. Poole RC, Halestrap AP. Transport of lactate and other monocarboxylates across mammalian plasma membranes. *Am J Physiol* 1993;264: C761–82.

32a. Murrell W, Crane D, Masters C. Ontongenic activities and interactions of the lactate dehydrogenase isozymes with cellular structure in the guinea pig. *Mech Aging Dev* 1993;69(1–2):37–52.

33. Himwich HE, Fazekas JF. Effect of hypoglycemia on metabolism of brain. *Endocrinology* 1937;21:800–807.

34. Himwich WA, Himwich HE. Pyruvic acid exchange of brain. *J Neurophysiol* 1946;9:133–136.

35. Gibbs EL, Lennox WG, Nims LF, Gibbs FA. Arterial and cerebral venous blood; arterial-venous differences in man. *J Biol Chem* 1942; 144:325–332.

36. Gjedde A, Ohta S, Kuwabara H, Meyer E. Is oxygen diffusion limiting for blood-brain transfer of oxygen? In: Lassen NA, Ingvar DH, Raichle ME, Friberg L, eds. *Brain Work and Mental Activity*. Alfred Benzon Symposium 31. Copenhagen: Munksgaard, 1991;177–184.

37. Kassissia IG, Goresky CA, Rose CP, Schwab AJ, Simard A, Huet PM, Bach GG. Tracer oxygen distribution is barrier-limited in the cerebral microcirculation. *Circ Res* 1995;77:1201–1211.

38. Honig CR, Connett RJ, Gayeski TE. O$_2$ transport and its interaction with metabolism; a systems view of aerobic capacity. *Med Sci Sports Exerc* 1992;24:47–53.

39. Kuschinsky W, Paulson OB. Capillary circulation in the brain. *Cerebrovasc Brain Metab Rev* 1992;4:261–286.

40. Connett RJ, Gayeski TE, Honig CR. Energy sources in fully aerobic rest–work transitions: a new role for glycolysis. *Am J Physiol* 1985; 248:H922.

41. Ye JM, Colquhoun EQ, Hettiarachchi M, Clark MG. Flow-induced oxygen uptake by the perfused rat hindlimb is inhibited by vasodilators and augmented by norepinephrine: a possible role for the microvasculature in hindlimb thermogenesis. *Can J Physiol Pharmacol* 1990;68: 119–125.

42. McCully KK, Kakihira H, van den Borne K, Kent-Braun J. Noninvasive measurements of activity-induced changes in muscle metabolism. *J Biomechan* 1991;24(Suppl 1)153–161.

43. Ohira Y, Tabata I. Muscle metabolism during exercise: anaerobic threshold does not exist. *Ann Physiol Anthropol* 1992;11:319–323.

44. Reeves JT, Wolfel EE, Green HJ, Mazzeo RS, Young AJ, Sutton JR, Brooks GA. Oxygen transport during exercise at altitude and the lactate paradox: lessons from Operation Everest II and Pike's Peak. *Exerc Sport Sci Rev* 1992;20:275–296.

45. Kuwabara H, Ohta S, Brust P, Meyer E, Gjedde A. Density of perfused capillaries in living human brain during functional activation. *Progr Brain Res* 1992;91:209–215.

46. LaNoue KF, Jeffries FM, Radda GK. Kinetic control of mitochondrial ATP synthesis. *Biochemistry* 1986;25:7667–7675.

47. Groen AK, Wanders RJA, Westerhoff HV, van der Meer R, Tager JM. Quantification of the contribution of various steps to the control of mitochondrial respiration. *J Biol Chem* 1982;257:2754–2757.

48. Klingenberg M. The ADP-ATP translocation in mitochondria, a membrane potential controlled transport. *J Membrane Biol* 1980;56: 97–105.

49. Chance B, Williams CM. The respiratory chain and oxidative phosphorylation. *Adv Enzymol* 1956;17:65–134.

50. Chance B, Leigh JS, Clark BJ, Maris J, Kent J, Nioka S, Smith D. Control of oxidative metabolism and oxygen delivery in human skeletal muscle: a steady-state analysis of the work/energy cost transfer function. *Proc Natl Acad Sci USA* 1985;82:8384–8388.

51. Blei ML, Conley KE, Kushmerick MJ. Separate measures of ATP utilization and recovery in human skeletal muscle. *J Physiol (Lond)* 1993;465:203–222.

52. Gjedde A. Modulation of substrate transport to the brain. *Acta Neurol Scand* 1983;67:3–25.

53. Gjedde A. Blood–brain glucose transfer. In: Bradbury MWB, ed. *Physiology and Pharmacology of the Blood–Brain Barrier, Volume 103: Handbook of Experimental Pharmacology.* New York: Springer-Verlag, 1992;65–115.

54. Silver IA, Erecinska M. Extracellular glucose concentration in mammalian brain: continuous monitoring of changes during increased neuronal activity and upon limitation in oxygen supply in normo-, hypo-, and hyperglycemic animals. *J Neurosci* 1994;14:5068–5076.

55. Oldendorf WH. Carrier-mediated blood-brain barrier transport of short-chain monocarboxylic organic acids. *Am J Physiol* 1973;224:1450–1453.

56. Denton RM, McCormack JG. Ca transport by mammalian mitochondria and its role in hormone action. *Am J Physiol* 1985;249:543.

57. Halestrap AP. Stimulation of pyruvate transport in metabolizing mitochondria through changes in the transmembrane pH gradient induced by glucagon treatment of rat. *Biochem J* 1978;172:389–398.

58. Halestrap AP, Armston AE. A re-evaluation of the role of mitochondrial pyruvate transport in the hormonal control of rat liver mitochondrial pyruvate metabolism. *Biochem J* 1984;223:677–685.

59. Shearman MS, Halestrap AP. The concentration of the mitochondrial pyruvate carrier in rat liver and heart mitochondria determined with alpha-cyano-β-(1-phenylindol-3-yl) acrylate. *Biochem J* 1984;223:673–676.

60. Kuwabara H, Evans AC, Gjedde A. Michaelis–Menten constraints improved cerebral glucose metabolism and regional lumped constant measurements with [^{18}F]fluoro-deoxyglucose. *J Cereb Blood Flow Metab* 1990;10:180–189.

61. Ohta S, Meyer E, Thompson CJ, Gjedde A. Oxygen consumption of the living human brain measured after a single inhalation of positron emitting oxygen. *J Cereb Blood Flow Metab* 1992;12:179–192.

62. Ohta S, Meyer E, Gjedde A. Cerebral [^{15}O]water clearance in humans determined by PET. I. Theory and normal values. *J Cereb Blood Flow Metab.* In press.

63. Kety SS. The physiology of the human cerebral circulation. *Anesthesiology* 1949;10:610–614.

64. Lassen NA. Cerebral blood flow and oxygen consumption in man. *Physiol Rev* 1959;39:183–238.

65. Olesen J. Total CO_2, lactate, and pyruvate in brain biopsies taken after freezing the tissue in situ. *Acta Neurol Scand* 1970;46:141–148.

66. Granholm L, Kaasik AE, Nilsson L, Siesj BK. The lactate/pyruvate ratios of cerebrospinal fluid of rats and cats related to the lactate/pyruvate, ATP/ADP, and the phosphocreatinine/creatine ratios of brain tissue. *Acta Physiol Scand* 1968;74:398–409.

67. Cremer JE, Cunningham VJ, Pardridge WM, Braun LD, Oldendorf WH. Kinetics of blood–brain barrier transport of pyruvate, lactate and glucose in suckling, weanling and adult rats. *J Neurochem* 1979;33:439–446.

68. Hodgkin AL, Katz B. The effect of sodium ions on the electrical activity of the giant axon of the squid. *J Physiol (Lond)* 1949;108:37–77.

69. Hurlbut WP. Ion movements in nerve. In: Bittar EE, ed. *Membranes and Ion Transport, vol. 2.* New York: Wiley-Interscience; 1970;95–143.

70. Creutzfeldt OD. Neurophysiological correlates of different functional states of the brain. In: Ingvar DH, Lassen NA, eds. *Brain Work. The Coupling of Function, Metabolism and Blood Flow in the Brain.* Alfred Benzon Symposium 7. Copenhagen: Munksgaard, 1975;21–46.

71. Goldman DE. Potential, impedance, and rectification in membranes. *J Gen Physiol* 1943;27:37–60.

72. Gjedde A. The energy cost of neuronal depolarization. In: Gulyas B, Ottoson D, Roland PE, eds. *Functional Organization of the Human Visual Cortex.* Oxford: Pergamon Press, 1993;291–306.

73. Erecinska M, Nelson D, Chance B. Depolarization-induced changes in cellular energy production. *Proc Natl Acad Sci USA* 1991;88:7600–7604.

73a. McCormick DA. Membrane properties and neurotransmitter actions. In: Shepherd G, ed. *The Synaptic Organization of the Brain*, 3rd Ed., Oxford University Press, New York, 1990;32–66.

74. Gjedde A. Interpreting physiology maps of the living human brain. In: Uemura K, Lassen NA, Jones T, Kanno I, eds. *Quantification of Brain Function: Tracer Kinetics and Image Analysis in Brain PET.* Amsterdam: Elsevier, 1993;187–196.

75. Balaban RS. Regulation of oxidative phosphorylation in the mammalian cell. *Am J Physiol* 1990;258:C377–C389.

76. Chesler M, Kraig RP. Intracellular pH of astrocytes increases rapidly with cortical stimulation. *Am J Physiol* 1987;253:R666

77. Chesler M, Kraig RP. Intracellular pH transients of mammalian astrocytes. *J Neurosci* 1989;9:2011–2019.

78. Kraig RP. Astrocytic acid–base homeostasis in cerebral ischemia. In: Schurr A, Rigor BM, eds. *Cerebral Ischemia and Resuscitation.* Boca Raton: CRC Press, 1990;89–99.

79. Connett RJ. Glycolytic regulation during aerobic rest-to-work transition in dog gracilis muscle. *J Appl Physiol* 1987;63:2366–2374.

80. Ribeiro L, Kuwabara H, Meyer E, Fujita H, Marrett S, Evans A, Gjedde A. Cerebral blood flow and metabolism during nonspecific bilateral visual stimulation in normal subjects. In: Uemura K, Lassen NA, Jones T, Kanno I, eds. *Quantification of Brain Function: Tracer Kinetics and Image Analysis in Brain PET.* Amsterdam: Elsevier, 1993;217–224.

81. Fox PT, Raichle ME, Mintun MA, Dence CE. Nonoxidative glucose consumption during focal physiological activity. *Science* 1988;241:462–464.

82. Ginsberg MD, Chang JY, Kelley RE, Yoshii F, Barker WW, Ingento G, Boothe TE. Increases in both cerebral glucose utilization and blood flow during execution of a somatosensory task. *Ann Neurol* 1988;23:152–160.

83. Robin ED, Murphy BJ, Theodore J. Coordinate regulation of glycolysis by hypoxia in mammalian cells. *J Cell Physiol* 1984;118:287–290.

84. Gjedde A. On the measurement of glucose in brain. *Neurochem Res* 1984;9:1667–1671.

85. Dóra E, Gyulai L, Kovách AGB. Determinants of brain activation-induced cortical NAD/NADH responses in vivo. *Brain Res* 1984;299:61–72.

86. Williamson JR. Glycolytic control mechanisms. I. Inhibition of glycolysis by acetate and pyruvate in the isolated, perfused rat heart. *J Biol Chem* 1965;240:2308–2321.

87. Connett RJ, Gayeski TE, Honig CR. Lactate production in a pure red muscle in absence of anaoxia: mechanisms and significance. *Adv Exp Med Biol* 1983;159:327–335.

88. Eisenberg HM, Kadekaro M, Freeman S, Terrell ML. Metabolism in the globus pallidus after fetal implants in rats with nigral lesions. *J Neurosurg* 1993;78:83–89.

89. Borowsky IW, Collins RC. Metabolic anatomy of brain: A comparison of regional capillary density, glucose metabolism and enzyme activities. *J Comp Neurol* 1989;288:401–413.

90. Ribak CE. The histochemical localization of cytochrome oxidase in the dentate gyrus of the rat hippocampal. *Brain Res* 1981;212:169–174.

91. Fox PT, Raichle ME. Focal physiological uncoupling of cerebral blood flow and oxidative metabolism during somatosensory stimulation in human subjects. *Proc Natl Acad Sci USA* 1986;83:1140–1144.

92. Seitz RJ, Roland PE. Vibratory stimulation increases and decreases the regional cerebral blood flow and oxidative metabolism: a positron emission tomography (PET) study. *Acta Neurol Scand* 1992;86:60–67.

92a. Fujita H, Meyer E, Kuwabara H, Evans AC, Gjedde A. Cerebral blood flow and oxidative metabolism remain uncoupled during chronic vibrotactile stimulation in humans. *J Cereb Blood Flow Metab* 1993a;13, Suppl 1:S798.

93. Ogawa S, Lee TM, Nayak AS, et al. Oxygenation-sensitive contrast in magnetic resonance imaging of rodent brain at high magnetic fields. *Magn Reson Med* 1990;14:68–78.

94. Ogawa S, Lee TM, Kay AR, Tank DW. Brain magnetic resonance imaging with contrast dependent on blood oxygenation. *Proc Natl Acad Sci USA* 1990;87:9868–72.

95. Kwong KK, Belliveau JW, Chesler DA, Goldberg IE, Weisskoff RM, Poncelet BP, Kennedy DN, Hoppel BE, Cohen MS, Turner R, et al.

Dynamic magnetic resonance imaging of human brain activity during primary sensory stimulation. *Proc Natl Acad Sci USA* 1992;86:5675–5679.

96. Ogawa S, Menon RS, Tank DW, Kim SG, Merkle H, Ellermann JM, Ugurbil K. Functional brain mapping by blood oxygenation level–dependent contrast magnetic resonance imaging. A comparison of signal characteristics with a biophysical model. *Biophys J* 1993;64:803–812.

97. Menon RS, Ogawa S, Hu X, Strupp JP, Anderson P, Ugurbil K. BOLD based functional MRI at 4 Tesla includes a capillary bed contribution: echo-planar imaging correlates with previous optical imaging using intrinsic signals. *Magn Reson Med* 1995;33:453–459.

98. Marrett S, Fujita H, Meyer E, Ribeiro L, Evans AC, Kuwabara H, Gjedde A. Stimulus specific increase of oxidative metabolism in human visual cortex. In: Uemura K, Lassen NA, Jones T, Kanno I, eds. *Quantification of Brain Function: Tracer Kinetics and Image Analysis in Brain PET*. Elsevier: Amsterdam, 1993;217–224.

99. Pette D. Metabolic heterogeneity of muscle fibres. *J Exp Biol* 1985;115:179–189.

100. Villringer A, Dirnagl U. Coupling of brain activity and cerebral blood flow: basis of functional neuroimaging. *Cerebrovasc Brain Metabol Rev* 1995;7:240–276.

101. Ogawa M, Magata Y, Ouchi Y, Fukuyama H, Yamauchi H, Kimura J, Yonekura Y, Konishi J. Scopolamine abolishes cerebral blood flow response to somatosensory stimulation in anesthetized cats: PET study. *Brain Res* 1994;650:249–252.

102. Laptook AR, Peterson J, Porter AM. Effects of lactic acid infusions and pH on cerebral blood flow and metabolism. *J Cereb Blood Flow Metab* 1988;8:193–201.

Cerebrovascular Disease, edited by H. Hunt Batjer.
Lippincott-Raven Publishers, Philadelphia © 1997.

CHAPTER 3

Pathology of Cervical and Intracranial Atherosclerosis and Fibromuscular Dysplasia

Harry V. Vinters

This chapter describes the distinctive neuropathologic features and pathogenesis of (a) atherosclerosis and (b) fibromuscular dysplasia of extracranial and intracranial arteries. Both of these vasculopathies, the former much more common than the latter, must be considered in two distinctive frameworks: (a) the general features of the relevant disease process, considering especially the pathogenetic roles of cellular and molecular events in affected blood vessel walls, and (b) unique characteristics of the disease processes as they affect arteries supplying the brain and spinal cord; the latter cannot be considered in isolation from effects of the arteriopathies on an end organ (the brain) with unique metabolic needs, deprivation of which may have dire consequences for various aspects of central nervous system (CNS) function.

Any contribution on pathologic features of the cerebral blood vessels must pay tribute to the 1972 monograph of Stehbens (1), which remains the most authoritative and comprehensive work on the subject, one that provides an exhaustive review of the relevant literature up to the time of its publication. Other texts (2–4) have provided detailed reviews and illustrations of the clinicopathologic (specifically neuropathologic) features of large vessel disease.

ATHEROSCLEROSIS

Cellular Pathology and Pathogenesis

A detailed consideration of the molecular and cell biology of atherosclerosis, the major cause of ischemic stroke, myocardial infarcts, and gangrene of the extremities, as well as strategies for its prevention, while beyond the scope of this

chapter, is extensively reviewed annually by key workers in the field (5–10). The relative roles of cholesterol, low-density lipoproteins and other lipids, endothelial injury, platelets and monocytes/macrophages (particularly as a source of active components, including growth factors and vasoregulatory molecules, that may stimulate smooth muscle cell proliferation in the vessel wall), prostaglandins, and fibromuscular hyperplasia (to be distinguished from dysplasia; see below), interplay of which results in vascular lesions that we recognize as atheromatous plaques (Fig. 1) have been dissected in detail using both in vitro systems (especially with blood vessel–derived endothelium and smooth muscle in tissue culture) and animal models. Molecular understanding of this systemic disease has progressed to the point where modification of the genes that determine the progression of atherosclerosis may soon lead to therapeutic agents that can potentially cause its regression or prevent it entirely (7). Atherosclerotic lesions that are usually associated with symptomatic ischemia in an end organ (eg, the brain) are in general calcified, heavily laden with lipids including lipid-laden macrophages/histiocytes and cholesterol (manifest in tissue sections as clefts), ulcerated (with focal denudation of endothelium), and significantly stenotic (the range of microscopic features noted in cerebral atherosclerosis is illustrated in Fig. 2). A luminal thrombus or mural thrombus may be present in association with the plaque, especially when the plaque has become ulcerated (Fig. 1).

Neuropathologic Features

The neuropathologist usually encounters features of severe atheromatous disease in either a surgical specimen (ie, derived from a carotid endarterectomy) or at the time of necropsy. In a patient who dies of ischemic stroke and comes to autopsy, examination of the complete internal carotid arteries is mandatory; the vertebral arteries should be studied

H. V. Vinters: Section of Neuropathology, Department of Pathology and Laboratory Medicine, Brain Research Institute and Mental Retardation Research Center, UCLA Medical Center, Los Angeles, California 90095.

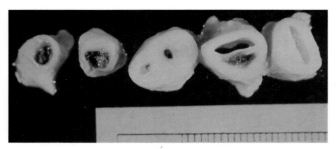

FIG. 1. Autopsy specimen of common carotid artery (including carotid bifurcation, three sections on the right) and internal carotid artery (two sections at left). Scale marker is in units of 1 mm. Note severe eccentric atheroma in all sections of the vessel, with associated recent thrombosis of the internal carotid (at left).

throughout their extraspinal length. The role of extracranial atherosclerosis in the causation of ischemic stroke has been well documented (11) and has led to the performance of carotid endarterectomies as a measure used to prevent completed ischemic strokes in individuals who have experienced warning transient ischemic attacks or incomplete strokes (12,13). Carotid endarterectomy specimens removed from patients with threatened stroke in this vascular territory reflect the dynamic state of the intimal surface in such patients vessels (14), often showing thrombus (in varying states of organization) attached to deendothelialized ulcerative plaque, intraluminal necrotic material, foamy histiocytes, and even foreign body giant cells being shed into the lumen. Any of these materials may act as the source(s) of artery-to-artery emboli to distal sites in the brain. Even vessels that appear (clinically and by angiography) to be occluded by thrombus can act as a source of subsequent distal emboli, presumably through collateral circulation (15).

The severely atherosclerotic carotid artery (bifurcation, internal and external) (see Fig. 1) is extremely unstable (16). The progression of atherosclerosis at this site, as elsewhere, is best demonstrated by serial cerebral angiography. There is debate as to what factors most influence plaque instability, though intraplaque hemorrhage and reparative neovascularization are probably of importance, based on large series in which the carotid endarterectomy specimen was carefully examined by histopathology (16,17). Quantitative biophysical evaluations of carotid bifurcation arteries removed at autopsies have been effectively utilized to evaluate which hemodynamic conditions are most consistently associated with the development of intimal atherosclerotic disease (18), ie, events that precede the plaque becoming symptomatic.

A series of papers from Norway in the late 1960s (19–22) provided vital autopsy data on the significance of cerebral and extracranial atherosclerosis in the causation of ischemic stroke in a necropsy population of almost 1000 patients, representing 40% of all patients who died in Oslo during a 6-month period. The crucial information in this invaluable series of reports must be interpreted in the light of more current strategies used to prevent or treat atherosclerosis (7,8,10), which would probably markedly influence the results obtained. Nevertheless, the conclusions derived from the meticulous postmortem evaluations of all brains and the full extent of the carotid and vertebral arteries (excluding only the extracranial vertebral arteries) provided an incomparable dataset. Approximately 5% of patients (including 30 men and 22 women with a mean age of 74 years) had spontaneous thromboembolic occlusion of a carotid artery, of whom two showed bilateral carotid occlusions. The vast majority of the occlusions were complete, and right- and left-sided vessels were equally affected. Just under half of the occlusions appeared to have originated in the extracranial carotid artery, with the remainder in its intracranial portion. Of the occlusions that could be classified, >80% were thrombotic whereas the rest were judged to be embolic; almost all of the embolic occlusions had occurred in the intracranial carotid artery and all had originated in the heart. Almost all patients with carotid occlusions showed other evidence of severe cardiovascular disease, ie, almost half of the affected individuals had suffered a previous myocardial infarct.

Cerebral infarcts were discovered in >75% of those with carotid occlusions. Large infarcts were more likely to be found in patients with intracranial carotid occlusions, a correlation attributed to blockage of the collateral circulation through the circle of Willis. Over half of all infarcts found were noted to comprise the entire middle cerebral artery (MCA) territory, sometimes extending into the anterior cerebral (ACA) and posterior cerebral (PCA) areas of supply within the cerebral hemispheres. By contrast, watershed infarcts were noted in just under a fifth of those with ischemic lesions. Platelet aggregates or emboli in various stages of development were found in small parenchymal and leptomeningeal arteries in all types of infarcts encountered; many were thought to have arisen in carotid thrombi, which in turn had formed at foci of severe atherosclerosis. Of interest is that carotid occlusions had produced clinical neurologic symptoms in just under 80% of patients. This supports the author's experience of (not infrequently) finding asymptomatic carotid occlusions in patients judged to be neurologically intact during life.

Consideration was given in this series to the prevalence and severity of stroke among all individuals who came to necropsy, independent of the presence or absence of occlusion of the great vessels (20,22). Some evidence of ischemic cerebrovascular disease was discovered in a total of one third of the nearly 1000 total autopsied patients. Almost 90% of large, recent infarcts were caused by grossly identifiable thromboemboli. The combination of atherosclerotic vascular stenoses and episodic circulatory failure was judged to be responsible for less than a fifth of cerebral infarcts. Based on analysis of symptomatic patients with ischemic lesions, it was concluded that 15% of cases with recent and 6% of cases with old lesions could be attributed to extracranial carotid occlusions and stenoses.

Of the 320 patients with evidence of ischemic stroke at necropsy, >60% had experienced clinical symptoms. Almost half of the 320 patients had deep lacunar infarcts, assessed as being regions of ischemic necrosis <0.5 cm in maximal dimension (the pathogenesis of lacunes is discussed in greater detail below). Thrombotic and other nonembolic infarcts were distributed throughout the brain, whereas embolic infarcts tended to occur much more commonly in the MCA territory. A total of 58 of 138 recent cerebral infarcts were hemorrhagic. In general, this exhaustive Scandinavian study re-emphasized the importance of careful neuropathologic study of straightforward stroke patients who come to autopsy; detailed inspection of the full extent of the great vessels and cardiac chambers is particularly likely to be diagnostically rewarding in such individuals, especially when the etiology of a stroke syndrome in a given patient appears at first to be elusive.

The incidence and severity of intracranial atherosclerosis (ie, that involving the circle of Willis and its major branches) has been examined in other autopsy series. For instance, a Polish study (23) based on necropsies on 600 unselected patients with an age range of 11–99 years found the following:

1. More than two thirds of all autopsies showed significant cerebral atherosclerosis, which was classified as mild (29.8% of total cases examined), moderate (11.5%), or severe (27.3%), without a significant sex difference.
2. Not surprisingly, the extent and severity of atheroma increased with age (24), beginning in the third decade of life.
3. The most severely involved vessels were the internal carotid, anterior and posterior portions of the basilar artery (with relative sparing of its midportion), and the middle cerebral arteries in the Sylvian fissure. The spectrum of gross morphologic features of cerebral atherosclerosis (from the author's own experience) is illustrated in Fig. 3.

Studies that have looked at comparative neuropathologic features of cerebral atherosclerosis among ethnic groups have revealed that there are significant variations in the disease process between, for example, North American and Japanese populations. In the former, examined using a Minnesotan population, atherosclerotic lesions were found primarily in the large-caliber vessels of the circle of Willis, whereas among the Japanese (examined in Kyushu, Fukuoka) atherosclerosis was much more likely to have occurred also in the smaller caliber vessels (25). While age of onset for cerebral atherosclerosis (as judged by its earliest occurrence in necropsy material) was similar in North American and Japanese populations, its progression and severity were greater among the Japanese (25).

Miller Fisher et al., in a detailed autopsy study of the entire vertebrobasilar (including intraspinal) and carotid arterial systems in 178 patients from the fourth through the ninth decade (26), showed that (a) atherosclerosis of the carotid arteries was usually less severe than that in the aorta but greater than that noted in the vertebral and cerebral arteries, and tended to be more focal in the carotid system; (b) 40% of patients showed some degree of stenosis whereas almost 10% of individuals had occlusion of a vessel in the neck and six patients had intracranial vascular occlusion; (c) symptomatic occlusion was more commonly extracranial in the carotid system but intracranial in the vertebral system; (d) stenosis of the carotid and vertebral arteries was asymptomatic; (e) hypertension aggravated cerebral atherosclerosis in general and basilar artery stenosis in particular; (f) the presence of lacunar infarcts correlated with both hypertension and atherosclerosis; and (g) the severity of (intracranial) atherosclerosis was similar in anterior and posterior portions of the circle of Willis.

Further investigations of the incidence and severity of cerebral atherosclerosis (and related parenchymal brain lesions) utilizing epidemiologic and autopsy data have been carried out among Japanese men living in Honolulu, Hawaii and a comparable cohort in Hiroshima, Japan (27). Though atherosclerosis of the major branches of the circle of Willis was more severe in the Honolulu group, intraparenchymal arteriosclerosis, with histologic features among small arteries that included intimal hyperplasia and subintimal foam cell and cholesterol cleft deposition, was more common in men studied in the Hiroshima cohort. The latter group also showed a higher incidence of cerebral infarcts, though the two cohorts had a similar incidence of cerebral hemorrhage. The higher incidence of ischemic lesions in the Hiroshima group was attributed to the higher frequency of intraparenchymal arteriosclerosis among these men (27). Correlation of cerebral atherosclerosis severity with autopsy-verified cerebral infarcts and hemorrhages (in a study also carried out among male participants in the Honolulu Heart Program) (28) strongly implicates the former arteriopathy as being strongly associated with both of the latter types of stroke. This clinical study also indicates a strong trend toward *decreasing* cerebral atherosclerosis in this population over the years 1965–1983.

An autopsy investigation of cerebrovascular diseases and their underlying vascular lesions among 724 patients over the age of 40 who came to autopsy in Hisayama, Japan (29) confirmed the association of morphologically verified cerebral atherosclerosis with both cerebral infarcts and hemorrhages, with the correlation being especially significant in patients with large infarcts and less so in patients with small infarcts or primary cerebral hemorrhage. All of these investigations highlight the still crucial role of detailed autopsies in addressing the natural history, pathogenesis, and complications of cerebral atherosclerosis in varying populations. The obvious drawback to autopsy-based studies is that the arteriopathy is studied at a finite point in time.

Events within atherosclerotic cerebral and extracranial (carotid, vertebral) artery walls that lead to ischemic stroke are similar to those that are hypothesized to occur within coronary arteries resulting in myocardial ischemia. In a de-

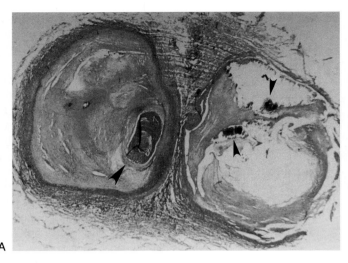

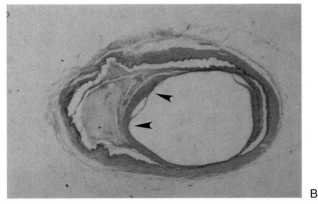

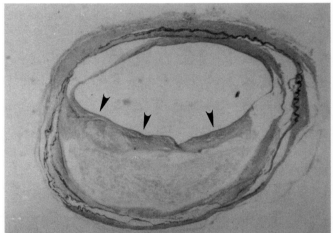

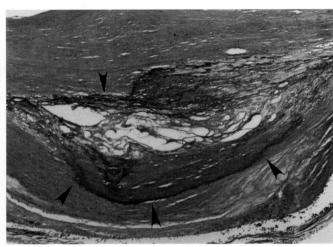

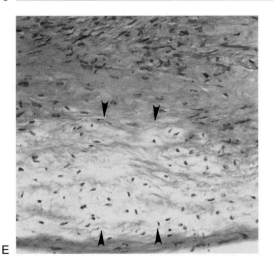

FIG. 2. Histopathology of cerebral atherosclerosis and atherosclerosis involving the great vessels in the neck. **A:** Very low-power micrograph [from hematoxylin-and-eosin (H&E)–stained section] of carotid bifurcation, showing severe complicated atheroma in both of its branches. Branch at left shows severe eccentric intimal fibromuscular hyperplasia, with a tiny residual lumen (arrow). Branch at right also shows extensive fibromuscular hyperplasia, and abundant plaque calcification (arrows), which has resulted in fragmentation of the specimen during cutting, so that residual lumen size (if any remains) is impossible to evaluate. **B, C:** Cross-sections of two arteries (stained with a technique to demonstrate elastica) from an 85-year-old man with Alzheimer's disease and multiple lacunar infarcts. Elastica is demonstrated in both sections as a wavy continuous line of varying staining intensity internal to the media. There is artifactual separation of the plaque from the elastica, which occurs during tissue preparation. Both vessels (B, right MCA; C, left MCA) show eccentric atheromatous plaques (arrows in both panels) characterized by fibromuscular hyperplasia and (especially in panel C) underlying cholesterol clefts indicating lipid deposition. (Magnification panels B,C ×22.) Remaining panels (for this figure) represent sections of vessels removed at necropsy from a 78-year-old man with atherosclerotic cardiovascular disease who died after a right carotid endarterectomy. **D:** Section of right internal carotid artery shows severe atherosclerotic/fibromuscular thickening of the vessel wall and a dense zone of calcification (arrowheads). Lumen of vessel is at top (H&E ×75). **E:** Noncalcified atheromatous plaque shows two relatively distinct regions: arrowheads indicate a relatively paucicellular zone, probably composed of glycosaminoglycans; the region closer to the vessel lumen (at top of micrograph) shows more typical fibromuscular hyperplasia (H&E × 190).

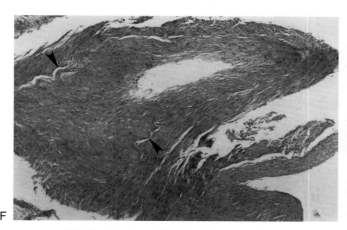
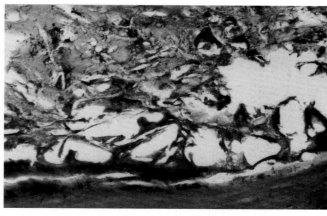

FIG. 2. *Continued.* **F:** Smaller artery shows relatively concentric intimal hyperplasia without calcification or obvious lipid deposition in the atherosclerotic regions. Arrowheads indicate elastica (H&E ×75). **G:** Cleft-like spaces noted within atheromatous plaque represent cholesterol that has dissolved during tissue processing. Such clefts are often surrounded by foreign body giant cells. Adjacent portion of the plaque shows particulate dark material probably representing calcium (H&E ×190).

tailed histopathologic study of segments of thrombosed intracranial arteries performed on eight patients who died within 28 days of brain infarction, occlusive thrombi were found in six instances and mural thrombi in two; thrombi had most commonly developed at or immediately distal to the sites of maximal stenosis. Arteries that had undergone thrombosis showed plaque rupture (three cases), intramural hemorrhage (one), ulceration (one), and thrombosis without plaque rupture or intramural hemorrhage (three cases) (30). Two patients showed occlusive emboli distal to the site of thrombosis, indicating the occurrence of intracranial artery-to-artery thromboembolism. An important conclusion of this work was that intraplaque hemorrhage or plaque rupture is not a requirement for arterial thrombosis (30). The same group (31) has demonstrated atheromatous embolism in cerebral arteries with internal diameters of 50–300 μm in a variety of stroke patients. A common antecedent for such emboli was cardiovascular surgery and/or catheterization in individuals with coronary or thoracic aortic atherosclerosis; common sequelae included hemorrhagic infarcts in either single-vessel territories (when atheromatous emboli were large enough to occlude major arteries) or in border zones between territories of supply (when the emboli were present in smaller parenchymal or leptomeningeal arteries).

The consequences of severe atherosclerotic disease within individual major cerebral arteries has been reviewed in several excellent clinical papers with radiographic correlation (32–34). These often highlight the importance of propagation of thrombotic material from the internal carotid artery into both the MCA and ACA. Furthermore, the occurence of lacunar infarcts in patients with large vessel atherosclerosis (eg, affecting the MCA) (32) highlights the probable importance of large vessel disease in the causation of small regions of ischemia, which previously had been thought to result largely from intraparenchymal cerebral microvascular disease, though the association of lacunae with atherosclerosis was

commented on frequently by Miller Fisher in the 1970's (26,35–37). For masterful reviews and discussions of the clinicopathologic consequences of vertebrobasilar artery atherosclerosis and thrombosis, readers are referred to the classic studies of Kubik and Adams (38) and Castaigne et al. (39), which remain timely decades after their initial publication.

Fusiform Aneurysms

Rarely, severe atheromatous disease of branches of the circle of Willis (especially the basilar artery) may eventuate in ectasia or fusiform enlargement of the vessel, leading to development of aneurysmal dilatation that may produce symptoms by compression of adjacent structures, eg, the brainstem (40–42). Cross-sectional analysis of such aneurysms at necropsy shows that they manifest severe complicated atherosclerotic changes with mural hemorrhage, rupture, and infiltration by acute and chronic inflammatory cells (40). Their luminal portions often show laminated mural thrombus and they may become entirely occluded, resulting in brainstem and cerebellar infarcts. Unlike saccular/berry aneurysms, which are especially common in younger women, fusiform aneurysms occur more commonly in elderly men (41).

Atherosclerosis in Berry Aneurysms and Arteriovenous Malformations

Both saccular/berry aneurysms and cerebral arteriovenous malformations (AVMs) may develop superimposed atherosclerotic changes on their luminal aspects. In the case of berry aneurysms (43), immunohistochemical studies show that the atherosclerotic change consists of smooth muscle cell proliferation, with an admixture of small numbers of macrophages and lymphocytes. Macrophages and some

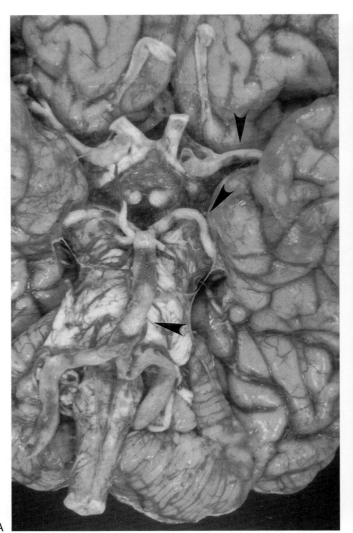

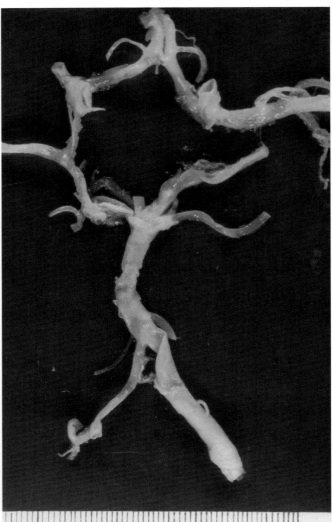

A   B

FIG. 3. A: Basal view of the brain in a 75-year-old man who died of nonneurologic disease. Note patchy but focally severe atherosclerosis, which manifests as opacification of the major vessels (eg, areas highlighted by arrowheads). The severity and extent of atherosclerosis is more clearly documented by dissecting the basal vessels from the brain (see next three panels). **B–D:** Panels show varying degrees of atherosclerotic change on circles of Willis removed from fixed (autopsy) brains of three patients. **B:** A 46-year-old man with familial Mediterranean fever and systemic amyloidosis; vessels are relatively free of atheroma (translucent) though with patchy atheroma, eg, in the left vertebral artery and at the basilar tip.

smooth muscle cells in the atheromatous regions expressed major histocompatibility complex (MHC) class II antigen.

Significant numbers of lymphocytes and natural killer (NK) cells were found to be present at sites of aneurysmal rupture. Progression of atherosclerotic changes within the aneurysmal sac correlated with aneurysm growth, and the authors hypothesized that there may even be a role for atherosclerosis in the formation of such aneurysms; the occurrence of symptomatic berry aneurysms in a patient population that generally shows minimal systemic atherosclerosis would tend to argue against this.

Encephalic AVMs, but not other types of cerbral vascular malformations (eg, cavernous hemangiomas), also usually

show marked fibromuscular hyperplasia on the intimal aspects of their lumina; usually, the degree of intimal hyperplasia varies markedly among vascular channels, as does the caliber and lumen diameter among the channels themselves (44), which are lined by arteries, veins, and arterialized [thickened] veins. Most commonly, the intimal hyperplasia appears as a cushion of spindle cells (Fig. 4), most of them (as shown by immunohistochemistry using anti–smooth muscle actin antibodies) with the phenotype of smooth muscle cells (45). Of biologic interest is the observation that despite the focally prominent intimal fibromuscular thickening in these loci, complicated atheroma is almost never observed within the cushions, ie, their endothelial lining re-

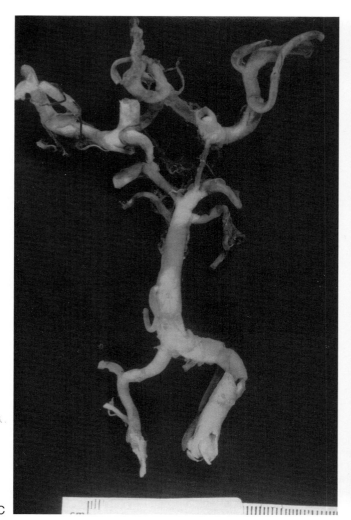
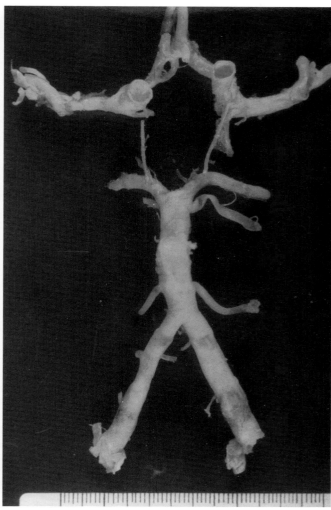

C

D

FIG. 3. C: An 80-year-old female with a history of transient ischemic attacks (but no cerebral infarcts at autopsy) and pathologically confirmed Alzheimer's disease. Note prominent atheroma throughout the basilar artery but especially at its tip, the left vertebral artery, both internal carotid arteries, and the proximal MCAs. **D:** A 90-year-old woman who died of bronchoalveolar lung carcinoma but was free of neurologic disease. Vertebrobasilar and carotid arteries show severe diffuse atherosclerotic change. By comparison to panels A and B, the basilar artery demonstrates early fusiform enlargement.

mains intact, macrophages are rarely (Fig. 4) seen within the atherosclerotic regions, they do not develop ulceration, and although the media of AVM component vessels can become heavily calcified, the atherosclerotic foci/intimal cushions are almost always devoid of calcification.

Increasingly, iatrogenic therapeutic embolization is carried out on encephalic AVMs using a variety of synthetic materials (45,46). Some of these (especially cyanoacrylates) appear to insinuate themselves into intimal atherosclerotic cushions and then become surrounded by smooth muscle cell layers with an endothelial covering (46).

FIBROMUSCULAR DYSPLASIA

By comparison to cerebrovascular atherosclerosis (considering its occurrence in both intracranial and extracranial

loci), fibromuscular dysplasia (FMD) is a rare cause of neurologic disability related to stroke. The author has never encountered (or recognized!) an example in over 12 years of practice. Appropriately, and since the relevant pathologic literature is more circumscribed, discussion of this entity will be less extensive. Renal artery FMD has been estimated to occur in over 1% of consecutive necropsies (47), so this personal experience may be a function of not having diligently sought the lesion in carotid arteries removed postmortem. However, FMD is more often a radiographic than a pathologic diagnosis, and the condition is not uniformly fatal; indeed, many patients make an excellent recovery (48,49). Various surgical modalities may be used to treat FMD of the internal carotid artery (ICA), with varying success (50).

First described almost 60 years ago, FMD is defined (47)

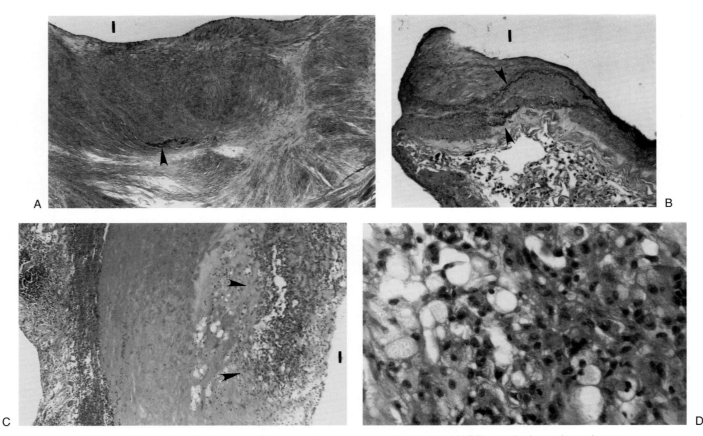

FIG. 4. Atherosclerotic change within an arteriovenous malformation (AVM); surgical specimen from a 52-year-old man. In panels A–C, "I" indicates lumen of a vascular channel; A and B stained with an elastic stain, C and D with H&E. **A:** Note massive fibromuscular hyperplasia; arrowhead indicates a fragment of elastica (×75). **B:** Arrowheads indicate fragmentation and reduplication of elastica, a characteristic feature of AVMs. There is intimal fibromuscular hyperplasia superficial to the fragmented elastica (×190). **C:** Arrowheads indicate chronic inflammatory cells in a region of fibromuscular hyperplasia (×75). **D:** Magnified view of region highlighted by arrowheads in C, showing mononuclear inflammatory cells including histiocytes, the latter a distinctly unusual feature of atherosclerotic change within AVMs (×490).

as an idiopathic, systemic vascular disease characterized by nonatherosclerotic abnormalities of smooth muscle and fibrous and elastic tissue present in arteries of small and medium size. Cephalic vessels are said to be affected in 25% of reported cases; they are the second most common location (after the renal arteries) in which FMD occurs. The ICA is almost always affected in patients with cephalic FMD; the vertebral artery much less often. Bilateral ICA disease is seen in approximately 60–85% of cases, usually involving the midportion of the artery. Intracranial vessels are almost never the site of FMD.

Vessel wall involvement is either medial (>90% of cases), intimal (approximately 5%), or adventitial (rare) (47). FMD may lead to ischemic stroke secondary to vascular stenosis or (rarely) occlusion and is thought to be the cause of many cases of spontaneous arterial dissections in the neck, including as many as 20% of patients with dissections of the carotid artery. Vertebral artery dissections with FMD have been shown to be the probable cause of cerebellar in-

farcts in children and young adults (51). FMD has been noted to occur in association with connective tissue disorders including Marfan's syndrome (52), eg, in a 26-year-old woman with this condition who experienced an aortic dissection that extended into the right ICA and at necropsy months later was found to have carotid FMD with moderately severe cystic medial necrosis of the aorta (Fig. 5). More recently, a retrospective analysis (53) suggested that patients with α_1-antitrypsin deficiency may have a high incidence of FMD and that FMD itself may be a relatively nonspecific disorder.

The fundamental cellular abnormality at sites of involvement is smooth muscle cell hyperplasia or (conversely) thinning, destruction of the elastica, fibrosis, and in general disorganization of component elements of the arterial wall (47). Many features of severe complicated atherosclerosis (eg, calcification, lipid and macrophage deposition in the vessel wall) are conspicuous by their absence, and no features to suggest an inflammatory/infectious origin for the condition

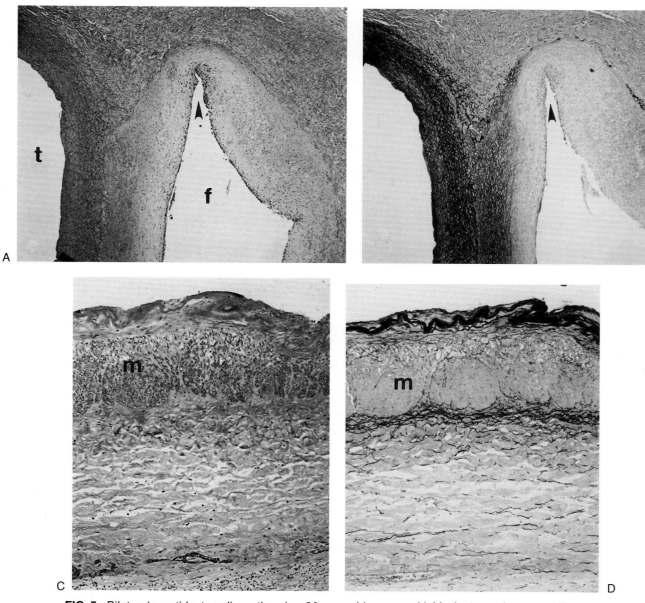

FIG. 5. Bilateral carotid artery dissections in a 26-year-old woman with Marfan's syndrome and fibromuscular dysplasia (FMD) (for details, see ref. 52). **A, B:** Right internal carotid artery showing advancing point of dissection in outer media (arrow). False lumen (f) is lined by flattened endothelium. True vessel lumen (t) is bordered by intact intima and inner media with parallel bundles of elastic fibers. **C, D:** Left internal carotid artery showing FMD in the arterial media and nodules of disordered smooth muscle (M) cell proliferation in the media, with paucity of medial elastic fibers. (Panels A and C stained with H&E; B and D with Lawson's elastica–van Gieson stain; all panels × 50). (From ref. 52.)

have been identified in histopathologic specimens. It has been suggested, however, that FMD may be etiologically related to segmental arterial mediolysis (SAM) (54), which occurs mainly in coronary and splanchnic arteries; SAM may be related to vasospasm, which in turn has been ascribed to focal endothelial paracrine dysfunction (54).

FMD may be associated with aneurysms of either the extracranial or intracranial arteries (55–58). Histopathologic studies of such aneurysms are extraordinarily rare, though an

excellent report by Miyauchi and Shionoya (55) has shown typical features of FMD in the aneurysm wall (Fig. 6).

ACKNOWLEDGMENTS

Work related to cerebrovascular disease in the author's laboratory was supported in part by PHS Grant AG 12435. I am grateful to Ms. Carol Appleton for excellent photo-

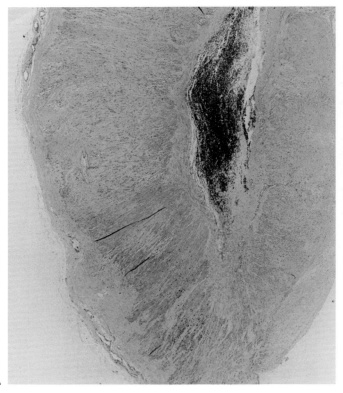
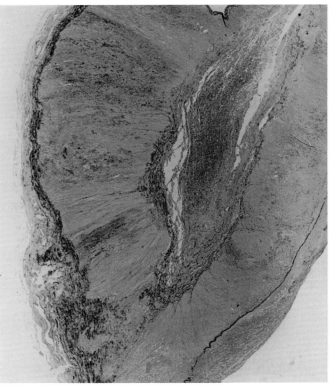

A   B

FIG. 6. Aneurysm of extracranial internal carotid artery caused by fibromuscular dysplasia (FMD). (For details of the case, see ref. 55.) Both panels show sections of the aneurysm with characteristic histopathology of FMD (medial type). A, H&E; B, elastic stain. (Panel B from ref. 55.)

graphic assistance, and to Drs. Masayuki Miyauchi (Yokkaichi City, Japan) and Wouter Schievink (Rochester, MN) for sharing micrographs from their publications. Dr. Shannon Venance provided helpful review of the manuscript.

REFERENCES

1. Stehbens WE. *Pathology of the Cerebral Blood Vessels.* St. Louis: CV Mosby, 1972.
2. Barnett HJM, Mohr JP, Stein BM, Yatsu FM, eds. *Stroke: Pathophysiology, Diagnosis, and Management.* 2nd ed. New York: Churchill Livingstone, 1992.
3. Toole JF. *Cerebrovascular Disorders.* 3d ed. New York: Raven Press, 1984.
4. Fisher M, ed. *Clinical Atlas of Cerebrovascular Disorders.* London: Mosby-Wolfe, 1994.
5. Ross R. The pathogenesis of atherosclerosis—an update. *N Engl J Med* 1986;314:488–500.
6. Levine GN, Keaney JF Jr, Vita JA. Cholesterol reduction in cardiovascular disease. Clinical benefits and possible mechanisms. *N Engl J Med* 1995;332:512–521.
7. Ross R. The pathogenesis of atherosclerosis: a perspective for the 1990s. *Nature* 1993;362:801–809.
8. White RA, Cavaye DM. Pathology of arterial disease: influence of morphology and distribution of lesions on interventional therapy. *J Cardiovasc Surg* 1993;34:105–113.
9. Slyper AH. Low-density lipoprotein density and atherosclerosis. Unraveling the connection. *JAMA* 1994;272:305–308.
10. O Keefe JH Jr, Lavie CJ Jr, McCallister BD. Insights into the pathogenesis and prevention of coronary artery disease. *Mayo Clin Proc* 1995; 70:69–79.
11. Barnett HJM. Transient cerebral ischemia. Pathogenesis, prognosis and management. Annals Royal College Phys & Surg Canada 1974;7: 153–173.
12. Marler JR. Carotid endarterectomy clinical trials. *Mayo Clin Proc* 1989; 64:1026–1029.
13. Barnett HJM, Eliasziw M, Meldrum HE. Drugs and surgery in the prevention of ischemic stroke. *N Engl J Med* 1995;332:238–248.
14. Barnett HJM, Peerless SJ, Kaufmann JCE. Stump of internal carotid artery a source for further cerebral embolic ischemia. *Stroke* 1978;9: 448–456.
15. Barnett HJM. Delayed cerebral ischemic episodes distal to occlusion of major cerebral arteries. *Neurology* 1978;28:769–774.
16. Bornstein NM, Norris JW. The unstable carotid plaque. *Stroke* 1989; 20:1104–1106.
17. Bornstein NM, Krajewski A, Lewis AJ, Norris JW. Clinical significance of carotid plaque hemorrhage. *Arch Neurol* 1990;47:958–959.
18. Zarins CK, Giddens DP, Bharadvaj BK, Sottiurai VS, Mabon RF, Glagov S. Carotid bifurcation atherosclerosis. Quantitative correlation of plaque localization with flow velocity profiles and wall shear stress. *Circ Res* 1983;53:502–514.
19. Torvik A, Jörgensen L. Thrombotic and embolic occlusions of the carotid arteries in an autopsy material. 1. Prevalence, location and associated diseases. *J Neurol Sci* 1964;1:24–39.
20. Jörgensen L, Torvik A. Ischaemic cerebrovascular diseases in an autopsy series. 1. Prevalence, location and predisposing factors in verified thrombo-embolic occlusions, and their significance in the pathogenesis of cerebral infarction. *J Neurol Sci* 1966;3:490–509.
21. Torvik A, Jörgensen L. Thrombotic and embolic occlusions of the carotid arteries in an autopsy series. 2. Cerebral lesions and clinical course. *J Neurol Sci* 1966;3:410–432.
22. Jörgensen L, Torvik A. Ischaemic cerebrovascular disease in an autopsy series. 2. Prevalence, location, pathogenesis, and clinical course of cerebral infarcts. *J Neurol Sci* 1969;9:285–320.
23. Mossakowski MJ, Kraśnicka Z, Iwanowski L. Atheroma of the larger

arteries of the brain in a Polish population: a study of 600 cases. *J Neurol Sci* 1964;1:13–23.

24. Vinters HV, Mah VH. Vascular diseases. In: Duckett S, ed. *The Pathology of the Aging Human Nervous System*. Philadelphia: Lea and Febiger, 1991;20–76.

25. Resch JA, Okabe N, Loewenson RB, Kimoto K, Katsuki S, Baker AB. Pattern of vessel involvement in cerebral atherosclerosis. A comparative study between a Japanese and Minnesota population. *J Atheroscler Res* 1969;9:239–250.

26. Fisher CM, Gore I, Okabe N, White PD. Atherosclerosis of the carotid and vertebral arteries—extracranial and intracranial. *J Neuropathol Exp Neurol* 1965;24:455–476.

27. Mitsuyama Y, Thompson LR, Hayashi T, Lee KK, Keehn RJ, Resch JA, Steer A. Autopsy study of cerebrovascular disease in Japanese men who lived in Hiroshima, Japan, and Honolulu, Hawaii. *Stroke* 1979; 10:389–395.

28. Reed DM, Resch JA, Hayashi T, MacLean C, Yano K. A prospective study of cerebral artery atherosclerosis. *Stroke* 1988;19:820–825.

29. Masuda J, Tanaka K, Omae T, Ueda K, Sadoshima S. Cerebrovascular diseases and their underlying vascular lesions in Hisayama, Japan—a pathological study of autopsy cases. *Stroke* 1983;14:934–940.

30. Ogata J, Masuda J, Yutani C, Yamaguchi T. Mechanisms of cerebral artery thrombosis: a histopathological analysis on eight necropsy cases. *J Neurol Neurosurg Psychiatry* 1994;57:17–21.

31. Masuda J, Yutani C, Ogata J, Kuriyama Y, Yamaguchi T. Atheromatous embolism in the brain: A clinicopathologic analysis of 15 autopsy cases. *Neurology* 1994;44:1231–1237.

32. Bogousslavsky J, Barnett HJM, Fox AJ, Hachinski VC, Taylor W, for the EC/IC Bypass Study Group. Atherosclerotic disease of the middle cerebral artery. *Stroke* 1986;17:1112–1120.

33. Gacs G, Fox AJ, Barnett HJM, Viñuela F. Occurrence and mechanisms of occlusion of the anterior cerebral artery. *Stroke* 1983;14:952–959.

34. Lhermitte F, Gautier JC, Derouesńe C. Nature of occlusions of the middle cerebral artery. *Neurology* 1970;20:82–88.

35. Mohr JP. Lacunes. *Stroke* 1982;13:3–11.

36. Miller VT. Lacunar stroke. A reassessment. *Arch Neurol* 1983;40:129–134.

37. Miller Fisher C. Capsular infarcts. The underlying vascular lesions. *Arch Neurol* 1979;36:65–73.

38. Kubik CS, Adams RD. Occlusion of the basilar artery: a clinical and pathological study. *Brain* 1946;69(Pt. 2):73–121.

39. Castaigne P, Lhermitte F, Gautier JC, Escourolle R, Derouesńe C, Der Agopian P, Popa C. Arterial occlusions in the vertebro-basilar system. A study of 44 patients with post-mortem data. *Brain* 1973;96:133–154.

40. Shokunbi MT, Vinters HV, Kaufmann JCE. Fusiform intracranial aneurysms. Clinicopathologic features. *Surg Neurol* 1988;29:263–270.

41. Nijensohn DE, Saez RJ, Reagan TJ. Clinical significance of basilar artery aneurysms. *Neurology* 1974;24:301–305.

42. Slade WR Jr. Massive basilar artery aneurysms. *Vasc Surg* 1974;8:74–81.

43. Kosierkiewicz TA, Factor SM, Dickson DW. Immunocytochemical studies of atherosclerotic lesions of cerebral berry aneurysms. *J Neuropathol Exp Neurol* 1994;53:399–406.

44. Martin NA, Vinters HV. Arteriovenous malformations. In: Carter LP, Spetzler RF, eds. *Neurovascular Surgery*. New York: McGraw-Hill, 1995;875–903.

45. Schweitzer JS, Chang BS, Madsen P, Viñuela F, Martin NA, Marroquin CE, Vinters HV. The pathology of arteriovenous malformations of the brain treated by embolotherapy. II. Results of embolization with multiple agents. *Neuroradiology* 1993;35:468–474.

46. Vinters HV, Lundie MJ, Kaufmann JCE. Long-term pathological follow-up of cerebral arteriovenous malformations treated by embolization with bucrylate. *N Engl J Med* 1986;314:477–483.

47. Healton EB. Cerebrovascular fibromuscular dysplasia. In: Barnett HJM, Mohr JP, Stein BM, Yatsu FM, eds. *Stroke: Pathophysiology, Diagnosis, and Management*, 2nd ed. New York: Churchill Livingstone, 1992;749–760.

48. Sandmann J, Hojer C, Bewermeyer H, Bamborschke S, Neufang KFR. Die fibromuskuläre dysplasie als ursache zerebraler insulte. *Nervenarzt* 1992;63:335–340.

49. Furie DM, Tien RD. Fibromuscular dysplasia of arteries of the head and neck: imaging findings. *AJR* 1994;162:1205–1209.

50. Moreau P, Albat B, Thevenet A. Fibromuscular dysplasia of the internal carotid artery: long-term surgical results. *J Cardiovasc Surg* 1993;34:465–472.

51. Díez-Tejedor E, Muñoz C, Frank A. Cerebellar infarction in children and young adults related to fibromuscular dysplasia and dissection of the vertebral artery. *Stroke* 1993;24:1096.

52. Schievink WI, Björnsson J, Piepgras DG. Coexistence of fibromuscular dysplasia and cystic medial necrosis in a patient with Marfan's syndrome and bilateral carotid artery dissections. *Stroke* 1994;25:2492–2496.

53. Schievink WI, Björnsson J, Parisi JE, Prakash UBS. Arterial fibromuscular dysplasia associated with severe alpha$_1$-antitrypsin deficiency. *Mayo Clin Proc* 1994;69:1040–1043.

54. Slavin RE, Saeki K, Bhagavan B, Maas AE. Segmental arterial mediolysis: a precursor to fibromuscular dysplasia? *Mod Pathol* 1995;8:287–294.

55. Miyauchi M, Shionoya S. Aneurysm of the extracranial internal carotid artery caused by fibromuscular dysplasia. *Eur J Vasc Surg* 1991;5:587–591.

56. Bour P, Taghavi I, Bracard S, Frisch N, Fiévé G. Aneurysms of the extracranial internal carotid artery due to fibromuscular dysplasia: Results of surgical management. *Ann Vasc Surg* 1992;6:205–208.

57. Itoyama Y, Fujioka S, Takaki S, Morioka M, Hide T, Ushio Y. Occlusion of internal carotid artery and formation of anterior communicating artery aneurysm in cervicocephalic fibromuscular dysplasia. Follow-up case report. *Neurol Med Chir (Tokyo)* 1994;34:547–550.

58. Abdul-Rahman AM, Abu-Salih HS, Brun A, Kin H, Ljunggren B, Mizukami M, Moquist-Olsson I, Sahlin Ch, Svendgaard NAa, Thulin C-A. Fibromuscular dysplasia of the cervico-cephalic arteries. *Surg Neurol* 1978;9:217–222.

Cerebrovascular Disease, edited by H. Hunt Batjer.
Lippincott-Raven Publishers, Philadelphia © 1997.

CHAPTER 4

Cerebral Microvascular Disease

Patrick Pullicino, Lucia Balos-Miller, and Andrei Alexandrov

HISTORY

The term *lacune* means "empty space." It was first used by Dechambre in 1838 to describe small cavities caused by the resorption of small deep areas of infarcted brain. Shortly after, Durand-Fardel noted that some small cerebral cavities contain a small blood vessel and are not infarcts but enlarged perivascular spaces (EPVSs). In the late 19th century, other causes of small deep cavities were discovered, including small resorbed hemorrhages and postmortem autolysis, but because there was no clear understanding of pathogenesis these different lesions were frequently mistaken for one another (1). Confusion between small deep infarcts and EPVSs was probably one of the main reasons for researchers being so slow to unravel the clinical manifestations of lacunar infarcts.

Marie's important work on different cavitary states (2) distinguished lacunar infarcts from other causes of small brain cavities and established the morphologic characteristics of lacunar infarcts and the fact that they can cause an isolated hemiparesis. Although Marie knew that lacunar infarcts had an ischemic basis, he still did not fully understand their pathogenesis. He suggested that some lacunar infarcts were caused by an inflammation of the perivascular lymphatic sheaths around patent central arteries (so-called *vaginalite destructive*). This shows that he still did not clearly distinguish EPVS from small deep infarcts.

The historical reasons for the confusion between EPVS and lacunar infarcts are relevant today because these lesions are still occasionally confused in the literature (3). First, small deep infarcts and EPVS have a similar appearance macroscopically (they also have a similar appearance on imaging studies). Second, it was not clear whether small deep

infarcts could have a patent central artery as was held by Ferrand (1). (It is now known that the artery supplying a lacunar infarct is occluded. The central artery may fall out during tissue processing of an EPVS or not be included in the plane of section. If the lack of a central artery is the sole criterion used to differentiate infarcts from EPVS, confusion may arise.) Third, terminology was imprecise: "lacune" was applied to any small deep space and its usage was never clearly restricted, and "état criblé" was used for both multiple lacunar infarcts and EPVS. The term "lacune" still has no generally accepted definition and is widely used nowadays for both lacunar infarcts and EPVS (1).

MILLER FISHER'S WORK

Knowledge about lacunar infarcts was fragmentary until Miller Fisher. By combining careful clinical observation with a painstaking histopathologic search for small arterial lesions, Fisher not only established the cause of lacunar infarcts—occlusions of small arteries—and the nature of these occlusions (4), but he also described the main clinical syndromes that they produced (5). Fisher single-handedly established a firm pathologic basis for the clinical diagnosis of small deep cerebral infarcts. It could be said that his work took the study of lacunar infarction out of its "dark ages."

Fisher and a few colleagues used the technique of serial sectioning to study the entire course of a penetrating artery from its origin at the parent large artery to the site of occlusive arterial disease in 68 infarcts. This technique necessitated the preparation, staining, and individual examination of several hundred microscopic sections for each infarct studied. Thus the study of one lacunar infarct might take several months to complete. Fisher's work showed that lacunar infarcts were most often due to occlusion of a penetrating artery (81%) but they could also be due to a tight penetrating artery stenosis (15%). Only occasionally was there no arterial pathology (4%) (1).

Fisher described a pathology he called "segmental arterial disorganization" or "lipohyalinosis," which affected arter-

P. Pullicino and A. Alexandrov: Stroke Program, Department of Neurology, State University of New York at Buffalo, Buffalo General Hospital, Buffalo, New York 14203.

L. Balos-Miller: Division of Neuropathology, Department of Pathology, State University of New York at Buffalo, Buffalo General Hospital, Buffalo, New York 14203.

ies with diameters less than 200 μm and was seen only in the brains of hypertensives. He thought that lipohyalinosis was the small arterial counterpart of large artery atherosclerosis because it stained with fat stains. Fisher initially took lipohyalinosis to be the most common arterial pathology underlying lacunar infarcts but his later work showed that atherosclerotic narrowing within and around the origins of penetrating arteries (microatheroma) was more common, and this pathology could be seen in the absence of hypertension.

In 20 of the lacunar infarcts he studied with serial sections, Fisher and colleagues also published detailed clinical data that had enabled him to determine that the most frequent clinical presentation of a lacunar infarct was a "pure" motor hemiparesis (without clinical signs outside the motor system) (6) and that lacunar infarcts could cause several other clinical syndromes (7–10) (see below). Fisher did not, however, show that these "lacunar" syndromes were specific to lacunar infarcts.

The "Lacunar Hypothesis"

Three main concepts or conclusions were drawn from Fisher's work: (a) a lacunar infarct results from occlusion of a single penetrating artery (the "lacunar hypothesis"); (b) the presence of a lacunar infarct can be reliably predicted from the presence of clinical lacunar syndromes; and (c) a specific penetrating artery pathology (lipohyalinosis or microatheroma) is the cause of lacunar infarcts. Although these conclusions are true of the lacunar infarcts studied by Fisher, it has become clear that they are an oversimplification of the pathology, pathogenesis, and clinical features of small artery disease. Although an important fundamental concept, the lacunar hypothesis is of little use as a working definition of lacunar infarction. It is currently impossible to image single penetrating artery occlusions; thus the in vivo diagnosis of a lacunar infarct cannot be made in this way. Second, modern imaging has shown that cortical infarcts occasionally give rise to lacunar syndromes and the clinical lacunar syndromes are sometimes produced by nonvascular lesions. Third, although microatheroma is probably the most common pathology underlying lacunar infarcts, the pathogenesis of small deep infarcts is probably as varied as that of large infarcts and may include large artery disease as well as systemic conditions (1).

DEFINITIONS

In this chapter, a lacunar infarct is a pathologically verified cavitary infarct that appears to result from ischemia in the territory of a single penetrating artery. A lacune is any small cavitary space of vascular origin. A small deep infarct is a subcortical presumed infarct seen on imaging. A presumed lacunar infarct is a small deep infarct in a patient with a clinical lacunar syndrome corresponding to the anatomic site of the infarct. Subcortical arteriosclerotic encephalopathy (SAE) describes a histologic appearance of white matter ischemic rarefaction secondary to small artery disease. White matter low attenuation (WMLA) is the typical CT appearance of SAE. Binswanger's disease is the clinical dementia syndrome caused by extensive SAE.

PATHOLOGY: CEREBRAL ALTERATIONS DUE TO ARTERIAL DISEASE

There are few different types of histologic alteration seen in the cerebrum or brainstem secondary to vascular disease. Neither the histologic characteristics nor the size of a cerebral lesion differentiate between a small or large vessel occlusion: small ischemic lesions may arise from occlusion of a single penetrating artery or occlusion of a large artery with distal reduction of flow. There is a continuum of cerebral histologic alteration due to ischemia ranging from an isolated focal loss of neurons to cavitary infarction with loss of all tissue elements. Minor focal ischemic episodes may result in focal loss of neurons sensitive to hypoxia such as Purkinje cells or hippocampal pyramidal cells without any noticeable abnormality on imaging studies. At the other extreme, a severe, prolonged interruption of blood flow will result in an area where all the tissue elements are totally destroyed, and as the damaged tissue is removed a cavity results.

Ischemic Rarefaction

In between these two extremes ischemia may cause a variable rarefaction of all tissue elements with demyelination and axonal, neuronal, and oligodendroglial loss associated with astrocytosis. This rarefaction may vary in extent and severity and may contain small foci of frank cavitary infarction. Ischemic rarefaction is particularly prevalent in the periventricular white matter (SAE) but it may also be seen in the pons (11). Since infarction implies death of all tissue elements and formation of a cavity, "noncavitary" infarction (12) should really be considered a focal form of ischemic rarefaction.

Enlarged Perivascular Spaces

EPVSs are cavitary lesions with a patent central artery. These lesions may be mistaken for lacunar infarcts on gross brain sections or imaging if they are single and large (Fig. 1) or for the lacunar state (état lacunaire) if they are small and multiple. Histologically they can be differentiated from infarcts by the presence of a patent central artery and the absence of surrounding ischemic brain tissue with astrocytosis.

Posthemorrhagic Cavities

A cavitary space may be the end result of a small hemorrhage rather than an infarct, and such lesions will show hemosiderin-containing macrophages in their walls.

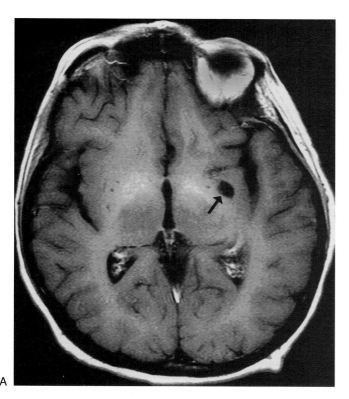

A

FIG. 1. A: Axial T1-weighted MR scan showing an oval hypointensity in the left subinsular region, thought to be a lacunar infarct. **B:** Macrophotograph of the same brain at autopsy shows a large perivascular space containing two lenticulostriate arteries. AC indicates anterior commissure; WM indicates subinsular white matter; P indicates putamen. (From ref. 3 with permission of the American Heart Association, Inc.)

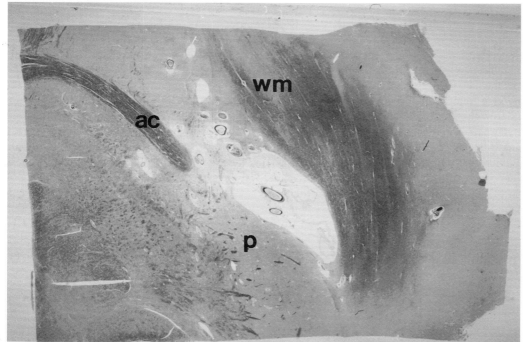

B

PATHOLOGY: TYPES OF SMALL ARTERIAL DISEASE

Hyaline Arteriosclerosis

Hyaline arteriosclerosis is one of the most common types of small arterial pathology. Hyaline deposits are seen in the media and may extend to all layers of the small arterial walls. There is also hypertrophy of the media and thickening of the intima with a concentric increase in connective tissue that is more prominent in hypertensives but may be seen in normotensives. These changes result in rigidity of the wall and narrowing of the lumen, but ectasia may also be seen. Hyaline arteriolosclerosis is the most frequent microvascular

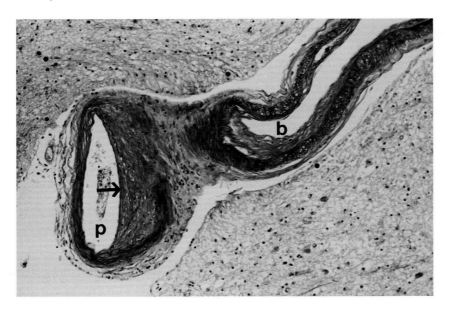

FIG. 2. Microatheroma. Proximal penetrating artery (P) at a branch point in a hypertensive, demonstrating an atheromatous plaque *(arrow)* with extension into the proximal part of the branch B.

pathology in diabetes, occurring more frequently than in nondiabetics

Atherosclerosis

Atherosclerosis does not normally affect arteries less than 2 mm in diameter but small deep infarcts may be produced in three different ways: (a) atheroma in the parent large artery may block the orifices of the penetrating arteries (luminal atheroma); (b) atheroma may involve the origin of the penetrating artery at its junction with the parent artery (junctional atheroma); or (c) in hypertensives or diabetics typical atheroma may involve the proximal part of penetrating arteries, particularly at branch points (microatheroma) (Fig. 2).

Atherosclerosis is characterized by a focal thickening of the intima by the deposition of lipids and the formation of fibrous tissue. Eccentric plaques enlarge, thicken, and tend to become confluent, and the media also becomes involved. The plaque may cause arterial stenosis and may be complicated by ulceration or hemorrhage. Thrombosis may superimpose and occlude the artery.

Lipohyalinosis

Segmental arterial disorganization or "lipohyalinosis" is a focal pathology of small arteries typically less than 200 μm in diameter and almost totally restricted to hypertensives. Lipohyalinosis may be the small artery counterpart of atherosclerosis because it stains with lipid stains (4). The process starts in the media just below the intima (subintima) with the appearance of fibrinoid that stains readily with eosin. Subsequently, the alteration becomes more extensive and the integrity of the media and the elastica is lost. The lumen

of the vessel becomes occluded with fibrous connective tissue or fibrinoid (Fig. 3).

Microaneurysms

Small arterial aneurysms have been recognized since they were first reported by Charcot and Bouchard in 1868. Lipohyalinosis has also been called the angionecrosis-aneurysm phenomenon because it was suggested that lipohyalinosis could cause a loss of integrity of the arterial wall and a dilatation of the wall to form a microaneurysm (4). These microaneurysms have been demonstrated both by microangiography and histopathologically in surgical specimens following operation for evacuation of hypertensive intracerebral hematomas. Rupture of these aneurysms is generally thought to be the cause of hypertensive intracerebral hemorrhage. Recently, Challa et al. (13) have shown that tight coils and loops are common in small penetrating arteries in hypertensives and suggested that they might have been mistaken for microaneurysms in the past. Challa et al. did, however, confirm the occasional occurrence of the type of aneurysm associated with degeneration of small arterial walls.

Amyloid Angiopathy

Amyloid angiopathy mostly affects arteries of the outer cerebral cortex and causes stiffening, fragility, and narrowing of the vessels. Amyloid angiopathy may reduce blood flow and lead to an SAE-like pathology in the white matter.

Vasculitis

Vasculitides such as polyarteritis nodosa and granulomatous angiitis of the central nervous system may affect small

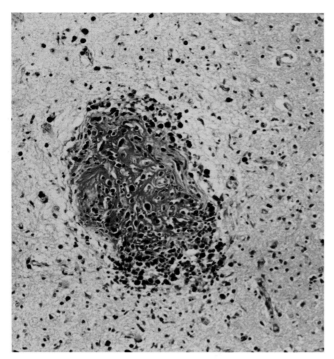

FIG. 3. Lipohyalinosis. Small penetrating artery in a 64-year-old poorly controlled hypertensive showing complete obliteration of the arterial lumen with foamy and hemosiderin-laden macrophages and fibroblast proliferation characteristic of segmental arterial disorganization.

arteries. In polyarteritis nodosa a segmental fibrinoid necrosis of the wall is seen. In granulomatous angiitis of the central nervous system the vasculitis is characterized by a predominantly mononuclear cell infiltrate, and branch points of vessels are preferentially affected. Amphetamines and cocaine may also cause a vasculitis.

RISK FACTORS FOR SMALL DEEP INFARCTS

Hypertension

Fisher found the frequency of hypertension in patients with lacunar infarct to be nearly 100% (14), and since then hypertension has been recognized as the main risk factor for lacunar infarction. The incidence of hypertension in presumed lacunar infarcts seen on computed tomography (CT) is lower, however, and ranges from 44% to 65% (1). This frequency is similar to that found in the autopsy study by Tuszynski et al.–64% (15). The differences between Fisher's figure and the subsequent figures may relate to the less stringent definition of hypertension used by Fisher (>140/90 mm Hg) and the higher frequency of lacunar infarcts due to lipohyalinosis than to microatheroma in Fisher's material. Microatheroma is less closely linked to hypertension than is lipohyalinosis. Several studies have shown that hypertension is more common in patients with lacunar infarction than

with nonlacunar infarction, and hypertension seems to be the only risk factor for which this is true.

Diabetes Mellitus

Diabetes is probably a risk factor for lacunar infarction, although it does not seem to be a greater risk factor than for nonlacunar infarcts. This is also true of age, male sex, ischemic heart disease, cigarette smoking, and the occurrence of a transient ischemic attack. In diabetics the major risk factor for lacunar infarction is hypertension, which frequently coexists. There is no evidence of synergism between hypertension and diabetes on the frequency of lacunar infarction (16).

Other risk factors for stroke, such as alcohol consumption and fibrinogen level, have not been shown to be risk factors for lacunar infarction. Patients with presumed lacunar infarction have been found to have higher concentrations of high-density lipoprotein (HDL)–cholesterol than patients with cortical infarction, but hyperlipidemia has not been clearly established as a risk factor for lacunar infarction. It has also been shown that patients with lacunar infarction have a higher hematocrit than patients with thrombotic or embolic stroke, but this is only significant in the presence of systolic hypertension. The angiotensin-converting enzyme (ACE) gene may be a risk factor for lacunar infarction (17).

PATHOGENESIS OF SMALL DEEP INFARCTS

Although microatheroma and lipohyalinosis are probably the most frequent causes of lacunar infarction, case reports have linked several conditions to small deep infarcts or presumed lacunar infarcts but have not established these as risk factors in case control studies.

Cardiogenic Embolism

Cardiogenic embolism is not a major cause of lacunar infarction, although it has been established as an occasional cause. Tuszynski et al. (15) have found lacunar infarcts at autopsy in patients with rheumatic heart disease and nonbacterial thrombotic endocarditis. Patients with obvious cardiac emboligenic lesions (prosthetic cardiac valves, left ventricular mural thrombus) have been reported with small deep infarcts in the region of the top of the basilar, an infarct location suggestive of embolism.

Artery-to-Artery Embolism

Artery-to-artery embolism is an established but probably infrequent cause of lacunar infarction. Lacunar and small deep infarcts have been reported as complications of arch or coronary angiography, resulting from cholesterol embolism from an aortic dissection (18). There may be an association

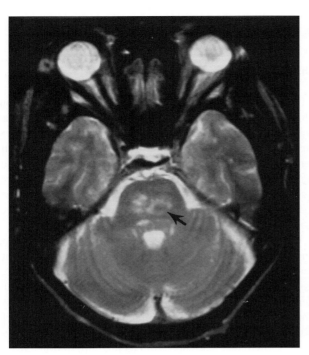

A

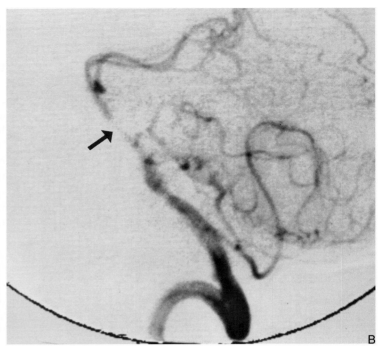

B

FIG. 4. A 75-year-old hypertensive with pure motor hemiparesis. **A:** Axial T2-weighted image shows a hemorrhagic small deep infarct in the left dorsal basis pontis *(arrow)* with right-sided patchy hyperintensity probably due to ischemic rarefaction. **B:** Angiogram shows a tight midbasilar atherosclerotic stenosis.

between carotid stenosis and asymptomatic small deep infarcts.

Large Artery Disease

The involvement of large intracranial arteries by atherosclerosis is probably underestimated as a cause of presumed lacunar infarction (19). Bogousslavsky et al. found that 10 (63%) of 16 patients with small deep infarcts of undetermined cause had a relevant stenosis of the large parent artery (middle cerebral or basilar). This is potentially of great clinical importance because a lacunar syndrome may be the first indication of a critical large artery stenosis (Fig. 4).

Hypoperfusion

Fisher established that penetrating arteries supplying a lacunar infarct may be stenosed but not occluded, making it likely that these infarcts resulted from hypoperfusion (20). Small deep infarcts at the upper lateral borders of the lateral ventricles, which are in a deep watershed territory, are seen in association with ipsilateral carotid occlusion and are called low-flow infarcts (21). Hypoperfusion caused by narrowing of small, white-matter, long penetrating arteries is probably the cause of SAE. Hemodynamically significant cardiac disease may interact with stenosis of intracerebral small arteries to increase the risk of hypoperfusion injury (1).

Coagulopathies

Small deep infarcts may occasionally be seen in systemic lupus erythematosus, antiphospholipid antibody syndrome, and other coagulopathies such as factor V deficiency (1).

CLINICAL PRESENTATION OF SINGLE LACUNAR INFARCTS

Many lacunar infarcts are asymptomatic. This is partly a function of size, in that the majority of smaller lacunar infarcts caused by occlusion of penetrating arteries less than 200 μm in diameter are silent whereas larger lacunar infarcts are frequently symptomatic. Location is also important; lacunar infarcts in the posterior limb of the internal capsule are usually symptomatic whereas single lacunar infarcts in the basal ganglia tend to be silent.

Transient ischemic attacks are frequent prior to lacunar infarcts, and small artery disease may be the most frequent cause of transient ischemic attacks. Lacunar infarcts often have a gradual or stepwise onset with transient ischemic attacks, or a progressive or fluctuating course, most likely due to hypoperfusion distal to a stenosed penetrating artery (1).

"Classical" Lacunar Syndromes

The hallmark and most frequent presentation of a lacunar infarct is hemiparesis without aphasia or sensory or visual deficit (pure motor hemiparesis, PMH). In about 40% of cases the face, arm, and leg are not involved symmetrically (22). PMH can be produced by a lacunar infarct in the posterior limb of the internal capsule, pontine base, cerebral peduncle, or medullary pyramid. The most frequent site is the posterior limb of the internal capsule and the next most frequent location is the basis pontis; the ratio of PMH in these two sites is 7:3. Repeated transient attacks of PMH (so-called "capsular warning syndrome") suggests stenosis of a penetrating artery supply to the posterior limb of the internal capsule and carries a high likelihood of subsequent infarction (23).

The second most frequent lacunar syndrome is ataxic hemiparesis (7), which is a combination of cerebellar limb ataxia and hemiparesis on the same side of the body. Ataxic hemiparesis may occur with infarcts at sites where the corticospinal tract and the corticopontine fibers are close together (posterior limb of internal capsule, cerebral peduncle, or pontine base) or where the corticospinal tract and the cerebellothalamocortical tract are close (lateral thalamus, corona radiata, posterior limb of internal capsule). The most frequent sites are pontine base and posterior limb of the internal capsule or corona radiata. Gait ataxia and slight hemihypesthesia are often associated with it. If the hemiparesis is severe the limb ataxia may not be seen till strength improves. There are three variants of the ataxic hemiparesis syndrome: (a) the dysarthria–clumsy hand syndrome (8) (severe dysarthria; clumsy ataxic hand especially on writing, with or without tongue deviation; facial weakness; dysphagia; ipsilateral hyperreflexia; and Babinski sign) indicative of a basis pontis lacunar infarct; (b) homolateral ataxia and crural paresis (leg weakness with ipsilateral arm and leg ataxia) indicating a posterior limb of internal capsule infarct; (c) hypesthetic ataxic hemiparesis (prominent sensory signs present) indicating an infarct in the region of the posterolateral thalamus or the posterior limb of the internal capsule affecting the thalamus.

The other two "classical" lacunar syndromes are pure sensory stroke (10), most frequently seen with a small lacunar infarct in the posterior ventral thalamus but also with pontine infarcts, and sensorimotor stroke (9), most often seen with infarcts in the posterior internal capsule that involve the lateral thalamus.

In addition to these four "classical" lacunar syndromes, Fisher has reviewed at least 70 syndromes due to small deep infarcts (5), the number and variety of which makes clear that relying solely on the four classical syndromes is insufficient for making a clinical diagnosis of lacunar infarct. A lacunar infarct should be suspected when a clinical picture can be explained by a small lesion affecting contiguous anatomic structures and a small deep infarct in an appropriate location can be confirmed by imaging. The diagnosis of presumed lacunar infarct does not just depend on a knowledge of clinical syndromes but also on a thorough knowledge of neuroanatomy and the availability of high-quality imaging.

CLINICAL PRESENTATION OF DISEASE OF MULTIPLE SMALL ARTERIES

Patients with a single lacunar infarct tend to have recurrent lacunar infarcts rather than large infarcts (24). The most frequent location for multiple lacunar infarcts are the putamen and basis pontis (14,15). Frontal white matter rarefaction associated with small arterial pathology (with a histologic picture of SAE) almost routinely accompanies multiple lacunar infarcts (25). The clinical picture in patients with multiple lacunar infarcts is due to both the SAE and the infarcts. The two most frequent clinical pictures seen are cognitive impairment and pseudobulbar palsy (1). Signs of presumed frontal origin such as lack of volition, emotional lability, gait abnormality, urinary incontinence, and akinetic mutism are also frequent (26). However, only about 30% of patients with multiple lacunar infarcts meet strict criteria for dementia. The classical lacunar state with multiple lacunar infarcts causing a short-stepped gait (marche à petits pas) is rare nowadays.

Binswanger's Disease

Extensive SAE is the predominant abnormality histologically in patients with pathologically verified Binswanger's disease but multiple small deep infarcts are also frequent (27). The clinical picture in patients with Binswanger's disease overlaps with that of patients with multiple lacunar infarcts outlined above. A slowly progressing or fluctuating dementia without cortical signs, often punctuated by focal neurologic deficits, is typical. The features of the dementia vary, however, and the patient may have pseudobulbar palsy and pyramidal signs or other focal deficits (1).

CLINICORADIOLOGIC CORRELATION

Different Small Artery Lesions Seen on Magnetic Resonance/Computed Tomography

Reliance on histopathologic correlation for the diagnosis of lacunar infarction has decreased very much because of the ease of obtaining in vivo imaging correlation. However, imaging is much less precise than pathology in establishing the nature of a small deep lesion. A presumptive diagnosis of lacunar infarction should only be made if a clinical lacunar syndrome and a presumed small deep infarct both fit the same anatomic location. It is not yet possible to image single penetrating arteries reliably and thus never possible to confirm single penetrating artery disease in vivo. In addition, the imaging appearance of different small arterial ischemic lesions is fairly uniform, making in vivo differentiation of pathogenesis difficult. Thus it may be difficult on imaging to differentiate a cavitary presumed lacunar infarct from noncavitary ischemic rarefaction (such as in SAE), from wallerian degeneration or gliosis, or from an EPVS. The tendency to call all small focal lesions on imaging "lacunes" and assume they are lacunar infarcts should be avoided.

Presumed Lacunar Infarcts

Forty-nine to fifty-eight percent of patients with a clinical lacunar syndrome have compatible small deep infarcts on CT and 74–89% have them on magnetic resonance imaging (MRI), although MR and especially CT may be normal in the early period after a stroke. CT is poor at detecting small deep infarcts in the brainstem. In the first few days, edema causes acute lacunar infarcts to appear larger than the actual area of infarction. In addition, acute infarcts are less hypointense on T1 images and less bright on T2 images, making differentiation from focal ischemic rarefaction more difficult. After the acute stage, cavitary lacunar infarcts appear as focal round or oval areas of reduced attenuation on CT and as focal hypointensities on T1-weighted MR. They are hyperintense on proton density and T2-weighted MR images. Hemorrhagic lacunar infarcts may be hyperintense on T1 images and hypointense on T2 images (1). Enhancement of a small deep infarct may help to differentiate recent infarcts from longstanding infarcts.

According to Fisher, lacunar infarcts vary in diameter from 2 mm to 20 mm in diameter (volume: 0.03–33 ml) (28). Presumed lacunar infarcts seen on MRI have a mean volume of 0.8 ml (29). The volume of presumed lacunar infarcts varies according to the syndrome produced: sensorimotor stroke 1.7 ml, pure motor hemiparesis 1.2 ml, ataxic hemiparesis 0.6 ml, and pure sensory stroke 0.2 ml. Theoretically, an infarct of a single lateral lenticulostriate artery may reach 42 mm by 16 mm (about 92 ml in volume), which is the size of the ramification zone of its branches (30). Small ischemic lesions such as EPVS, low-flow "infarcts," and foci of ischemic rarefaction have a size range similar to that of small deep infarcts. The dimensions of larger presumed lacunar infarcts overlap with those of deep infarcts due to the occlusion of multiple penetrating arteries (striatocapsular infarcts). Thus the size of an infarct is not a good indicator of the pathogenesis or of single penetrating artery involvement. The larger a small deep infarct, however, the more likely it is that multiple penetrating arteries are involved and that the parent large artery is the site of the causative pathology.

EPVSs are occasionally mistaken for small deep infarcts because they have a similar shape and signal characteristics on T1 and heavily weighted T2 images (3). They may be differentiated from lacunar infarcts because, unlike infarcts, they are not hyperintense on proton density images. Typical locations for EPVSs are the subcortical white matter of the vertex or trigone or the inferior putaminal region where they may reach 10 mm in diameter (Fig. 1).

Foci of ischemic rarefaction/SAE are either minimally hypointense or isointense with brain on T1-weighted images and hyperintense on T2 images. The T1 characteristics may thus differentiate cavitary infarction and noncavitary ischemic rarefaction, but it may be difficult to detect a recent small deep infarct in a patient with confluent white matter hyperintensities due to SAE (Fig. 5). Focal areas of demyelination, gliosis, or wallerian degeneration have similar imaging characteristics to ischemic rarefaction/SAE.

Low-flow "infarcts" are small focal lesions seen adjacent to the lateral ventricles ipsilateral to a carotid occlusion (21) (Fig. 6). They are not typically hypointense on T1 MR images implying that they are focal areas of ischemic rarefaction and not cavitary infarcts.

INVESTIGATIONS

A patient presenting with one of the four classical lacunar syndromes is likely to have a small focal subcortical hemispheric or brainstem infarct. A CT within 24 hours of the stroke may show a recent small deep infarct but is often normal. CT will help to exclude occasional cortical or nonischemic lesions. Because all of the four classical lacunar syndromes may arise from both a hemispheric and a brainstem location, an MR scan is helpful in detecting a recent brainstem infarct even if the CT shows a compatible hemispheric infarct. Since a lacunar syndrome may occasionally be the first indication of potentially life-threatening large artery (vertebral, basilar, or middle cerebral) disease (31) (Figs. 4 and 7), MR should be combined with MR angiography.

Patients with a lacunar syndrome who have no evidence of intracranial large artery disease on angiography and who are hypertensive are likely to have small artery disease (microatheroma or lipohyalinosis). If the patient is normotensive microatheroma is most likely. Potential causes of embolism such as cardiac valvular disease and atrial fibrillation have to be considered in normotensives, however, especially if the infarct location is suggestive of embolism (thalamic or top-of-the-basilar location). Patients with presumed lacunar infarcts probably do not need routine echocardiography because the yield is likely to be low (32). The yield of carotid Doppler is low in patients with presumed lacunar infarct (33), but there appears to be an association of tight carotid stenosis with asymptomatic small deep infarcts (34) or low-flow infarcts (21), so that Doppler should be performed on every patient in whom the infarct location suggests low-flow infarcts (Fig. 6).

Other investigations such as antiphospholipid antibody screen, coagulation profile, or search for lupus or other collagen vascular disease may be needed in occasional cases and should be determined by the clinical picture.

MEDICAL MANAGEMENT

Risk Factor Control

Control of known risk factors such as hypertension and smoking are the mainstays of prevention against progression of microvascular disease and recurrent stroke in patients with

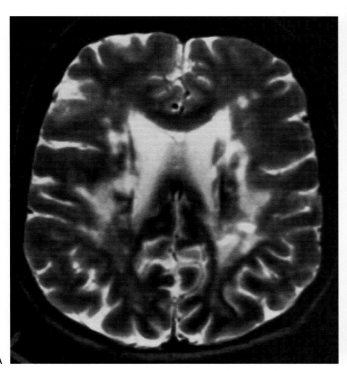
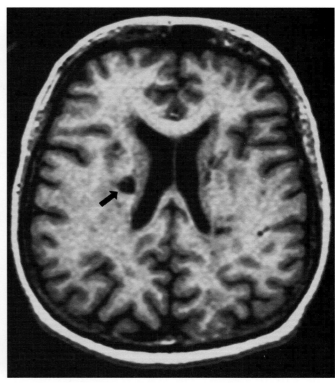

A

B

FIG. 5. A 57-year-old hypertensive woman with left pure motor hemiparesis. **A:** T2-weighted image shows confluent white matter hyperintensities, with no clear indication of a focal infarct. **B:** SPGR image shows a clearly defined focal hypointensity in the right corona radiata due to a presumed lacunar infarct.

presumed lacunar infarction. It has not been established that hypertension control actually reduces the rate of recurrent stroke in patients with an initial presumed lacunar infarct, though it is likely (1). Meyer et al. have shown that control of risk factors may lead to improved cognition in patients with vascular dementia who have WMLA and small deep infarcts on CT because of microvascular disease (35).

Antiplatelet Agents

Aspirin and ticlopidine reduce the risk of recurrence of all sub-types of infarction. Patients with lacunar infarcts tend to have recurrent lacunar infarcts rather than large infarcts (24,36) and thus may respond differently to antiplatelet agents than patients with large infarcts. The French antiplatelet drug study (37) showed that 1000 mg of aspirin with or without 225 mg/day dipyridamole reduced the rate of stroke recurrence ($p < 0.05$). Sixteen percent of the patients in this study had presumed lacunar infarcts, and there was a similar reduction in the recurrent stroke rate in the lacunar group as with other stroke types, although the numbers were too small to reach statistical significance. Several other studies have shown that aspirin is effective in ''minor'' stroke. In the French study, only 30% of patients with minor stroke had presumed lacunar infarcts, so although an aspirin effect on

minor stroke may indicate a possible effect on lacunar infarct patients, minor stroke is not the same as lacunar infarction and probably includes strokes of differing pathogenesis.

A subgroup analysis of the TASS study (38) showed that ticlopidine is effective in reducing the risk of recurrent stroke in patients with a completed minor stroke and was a little more effective than aspirin. On the basis of a small retrospective analysis, Weisberg (36) suggested that high-dose (600–1300 mg) aspirin and ticlopidine are more effective in preventing recurrent stroke in patients with an initial lacunar infarct than low-dose (325 mg or less) aspirin, but his data were not statistically significant. Meyer et al. have shown that both aspirin (325 mg) and ticlopidine improve cerebral perfusion and cognition in patients with vascular dementia (35).

Heparin

The use of heparin in lacunar stroke in progression was suggested by Miller Fisher's finding that sometimes the culminating event in the development of a lacunar infarct was a thrombus superimposed on an atheromatous stenosis of a penetrating artery (20). One small trial of four patients did not show any therapeutic effect of heparin in this situation (39). If large artery disease is found to be the cause of lacunar

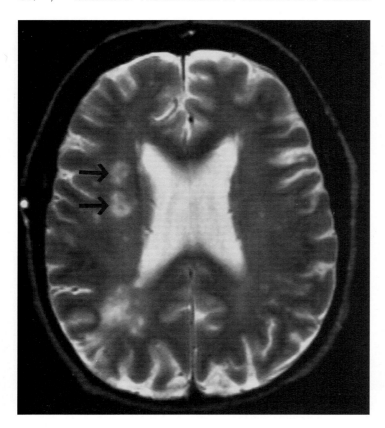

FIG. 6. Axial T2-weighted image showing two low-flow "infarcts" *(arrows)* in a patient with an ipsilateral carotid artery occlusion. (From ref. 1.)

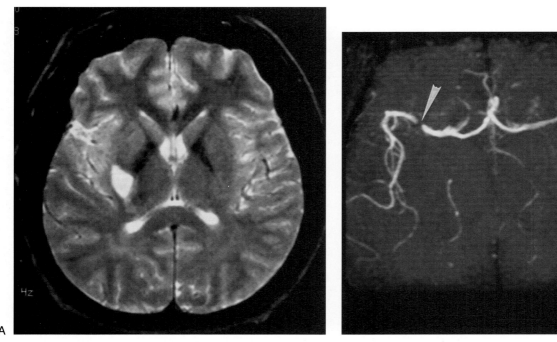

A

B

FIG. 7. A 29-year-old man with sudden left-sided weakness and dysarthria and transient cardiac murmur. **A:** Axial T2-weighted MR scan showing lateral lenticulostriate territory infarct involving the posterior lentiform nucleus and region of posterior limb of internal capsule. **B:** Three-dimensional time-of-flight MR angiogram showing focal discontinuity *(arrow)* in the signal from the right middle cerebral artery due to probable embolic stenosis. (From ref. 41.)

stroke in progression (Fig. 4), heparinization is probably indicated.

Coumarin

There are no data to support the use of coumarin to prevent recurrent small artery infarcts. The ongoing National Institutes of Health warfarin-aspirin study may provide data about this.

Hemodilution

Frey (40) has reported that nine of ten patients with presumed lacunar infarction treated with hemodilution improved. However, his series was uncontrolled.

REFERENCES

1. Pullicino PM, Caplan LR, Hommel M. *Cerebral small artery disease.* New York: Raven Press, 1993.
2. Marie P. Des foyers lacunaires de désintégration et de différents autres états cavitaires du cerveau. *Rev Med* 1901;21:281–298.
3. Pullicino PM, Miller LL, Alexandrov AV, Ostrow PT. Infraputaminal "lacunes": clinical and pathological correlations. *Stroke* 1995;26:1598–1602.
4. Fisher CM. The arterial lesions underlying lacunes. *Acta Neuropathol* 1969;12:115.
5. Fisher CM. Lacunar infarcts a review. *Cerebrovasc Dis* 1991;1:311–320.
6. Fisher CM, Curry HB. Pure motor hemiplegia of vascular origin. *Arch Neurol* 1965;13:30–44.
7. Fisher CM. Ataxic hemiparesis. A pathologic study. *Arch Neurol* 1978;35:126–128.
8. Fisher CM. A lacunar stroke. The dysarthria clumsy hand syndrome. *Neurology* 1967;17:614–617.
9. Mohr JP, Kase CS, Meckler RJ, Fisher CM. Sensorimotor stroke due to thalamocapsular ischemia. *Arch Neurol* 1977;34:739–741.
10. Fisher CM. Thalamic pure sensory stroke: a pathologic study. *Neurology* 1978;28:1141–1144.
11. Pullicino P, Ostrow P, Miller L, Snyder W, Munschauer F. Pontine ischemic rarefaction. *Ann Neurol* 1995;37:460–466.
12. Dozono K, Ishii N, Nishihara Y, Horie A. An autopsy study of the incidence of lacunes in relation to age, hypertension and atherosclerosis. *Stroke* 1991;22:993–996.
13. Challa VR, Moody DM, Bell MA. The Charcot–Bouchard aneurysm controversy: impact of a new histologic technique. *J Neuropathol Exp Neurol* 1992;51:264–271.
14. Fisher CM. Lacunes: small deep cerebral infarcts. *Neurology* 1965;15:774–784.
15. Tuszynski MH, Petito CK, Levy DE. Risk factors and clinical manifestations of pathologically verified lacunar infarctions. *Stroke* 1989;20:990–999.
16. Pullicino P, Zammit A. Small deep cerebral infarcts: is there synergism between hypertension and diabetes? *J Stroke Cerebrovasc Dis* 1993;3:189–192.
17. Markus HS, Barley J, Lunt R, et al. Angiotensin-converting enzyme gene deletion polymorphism. A new risk factor for lacunar stroke but not carotid atheroma. *Stroke* 1995;26:1329–1333.
18. Laloux P, Brucher JM. Lacunar infarctions due to cholesterol emboli. *Stroke* 1991;22:1440–1444.
19. Bogousslavsky J, Regli F, Maeder P. Intracranial large artery disease and "lacunar" infarction. *Cerebrovasc Dis* 1991;1:154–159.
20. Fisher CM. Capsular infarcts. The underlying vascular lesions. *Arch Neurol* 1979;36:65–73.
21. Weiller C, Ringelstein EB, Reiche W, Buell U. Clinical and hemodynamic aspects of low flow infarcts. *Stroke* 1991;22:1117–1123.
22. Richter RW, Brust JCM, Bruun B, Shafer SQ. Frequency and course of pure motor hemiparesis: a clinical study. *Stroke* 1977;8:58–60.
23. Donnan GA, O'Malley HM, Quang L, Hurley S, Bladin PF. The capsular warning syndrome: pathogenesis and clinical features. *Neurology* 1993;43:957–962.
24. Boiten J, Lodder J. Prognosis for survival, handicap and recurrence of stroke in lacunar and superficial infarction. *Cerebrovasc Dis* 1993;3:221–226.
25. Fukuda H, Kobayashi S, Okada K, Tsunematsu T. Frontal white matter lesions and dementia in lacunar infarction. *Stroke* 1990;21:1143–1149.
26. Ishii N, Nishihara Y, Imamura T. Why do frontal lobe symptoms predominate in vascular dementia with lacunes. *Neurology* 1986;36:340–345.
27. Caplan LR, Schoene WC. Clinical features of subcortical arteriosclerotic encephalopathy (Binswanger disease). *Neurology* 1978;28:1206–1215.
28. Fisher CM. Lacunar strokes and infarcts: a review. *Neurology* 1982;32:871–876.
29. Hommel M, Besson G, Le Bas JF, et al. Prospective study of lacunar infarction using magnetic resonance imaging. *Stroke* 1990;21:546–554.
30. Marinkovic SV, Milisavljevic MM, Kovacevic MS, Stevic ZD. Perforating branches of the middle cerebral artery. *Stroke* 1985;16:1022–1029.
31. Caplan LR. Intracranial branch atheromatous disease: a neglected, understudied and underused concept. *Neurology* 1989;39:1246–1250.
32. Goldby AJ, Bracci PM, Comess KA, DeRook FA, Albers GW. Low yield of clinically significant transesophageal echocardiographic findings in patients with lacunar stroke. *J Stroke Cerebrovasc Dis* 1995;5:39–43.
33. Tegeler CH, Shi F, Morgan T. Carotid stenosis in lacunar stroke. *Stroke* 1991;22:1124–1128.
34. Norris JW, Zhu CZ. Silent stroke and carotid stenosis. *Stroke* 1992;23:483–485.
35. Meyer JS, Terayama Y, Takashima S, Mortel KF. Longitudinal outcome among patients with ischemic vascular dementia. *J Stroke Cerebrovasc Dis* 1993;3:90–101.
36. Weisberg LA. Retrospective analysis of aspirin and ticlopidine in preventing recurrent stroke following an initial lacunar infarct. *J Stroke Cerebrovasc Dis* 1995;5:44–48.
37. Bousser MG, Eschwege E, Haguenau M, et al. "AICLA" controlled trial of aspirin and dipyridamole in the secondary prevention of atherothrombotic cerebral ischemia. *Stroke* 1983;14:5–14.
38. Harbison JW. Ticlopidine versus aspirin for the prevention of recurrent stroke: analysis of patients with minor stroke from the Ticlopidine Aspirin Stroke Study. *Stroke* 1992;23:1723–1727.
39. Dobkin BH. Heparin for lacunar stroke in progression. *Stroke* 1983;14:421–423.
40. Frey JL. Hemodilution therapy for lacunar stroke: treatment results in 10 consecutive cases. *J Stroke Cerebrovasc Dis* 1992;2:136–145.
41. Pullicino P, Alexandrov A, Lee Kwen P. Anterior choroidal artery territory. *Brain.* 1995;118:1353–1355.

Cerebrovascular Disease, edited by H. Hunt Batjer.
Lippincott-Raven Publishers, Philadelphia © 1997.

CHAPTER 5

Pathology of Intracranial Aneurysms and Vascular Malformations

Fernando Vale and Mark N. Hadley

ANEURYSMS

Intracranial aneurysms have been classified into six types according to their etiology, shape, and histologic characteristics. These are (a) saccular or berry, (b) atherosclerotic-fusiform, (c) inflammatory/infectious, (d) tumor-related (eg, choriocarcinoma), (e) traumatic, and (f) dissecting.

Rare microaneurysms of the deep perforating brain vessels occur in patients with hypertension, moya-moya disease, and other uncommon intracranial vascular disorders and have been named Charcot–Bouchard aneurysms. These obscure aneurysmal lesions will not be discussed in this chapter, which will focus primarily on the origin, growth, and pathophysiology of intracranial saccular aneurysms.

INCIDENCE

Autopsy studies reveal that the incidence of ruptured and unruptured intracranial aneurysms is approximately 5% in the general population (1). The highest frequency of aneurysms is among individuals in their fourth through sixth decades of life, ie, the years when most intracranial aneurysms become symptomatic. Women are more commonly affected than men. The female-to-male ratio ranges around 2–3:1, but there is a male predominance below age 40 (1). Multiple aneurysms have been reported in 15–31% of patients and are more frequently located in the middle cerebral artery distributions. Although the numbers vary according to the series, approximately 85–90% of intracranial aneurysms originate in the anterior circulation, more commonly in the anterior communicating artery complex (30%), and at the

origin of the posterior communicating artery (25%) (Fig. 1). Middle cerebral artery aneurysms represent about 20% of all intracranial saccular vascular lesions. Between 5% and 15% of all intracranial aneurysms are located in the posterior cerebral circulation including the posterior cerebral arteries, basilar artery, and vertebral arteries.

Cerebral aneurysms are rarely discovered in children. In this population, intracranial aneurysms are most commonly located at the internal carotid artery bifurcation and at the trifurcation of the middle cerebral artery. Pediatric aneurysms tend to be peripheral in location and giant in size (more than 2.5 cm) (1). These notable differences of location and size between pediatric patients with aneurysms and adults suggest different mechanisms regarding aneurysm formation and rupture.

Aneurysmal subarachnoid hemorrhage occurs clinically in 10 patients per 100,000 population per year (2). Ruptured intracranial aneurysms account for 75–80% of all spontaneous hemorrhages. A sentinal hemorrhage occurs in approximately 30–60% of patients presenting with subarachnoid hemorrhage (SAH) due to aneurysm rupture. It is believed that 10% of patients die before reaching the hospital following SAH. The 30-day mortality for aneurysmal SAH approaches 45%. Rebleeding followed by vasospasm is the most common cause of morbidity and mortality after the original SAH. The impact on society of SAH due to aneurysm rupture is extremely high as approximately 50% of surviving patients are left with disability, some profoundly neurologically impaired.

The natural history of unruptured intracranial aneurysms is not well known. The annual risk of rupture is estimated to be 1–2% per year. It is suggested that the risk of rupture correlates with increasing aneurysm size, but it is known that smaller aneurysms, those less than 10 mm in size, do rupture and produce catastrophic results. In this context it is important to understand the pathogenesis of aneurysm for-

F. Vale and M. N. Hadley: Division of Neurosurgery, University of Alabama at Birmingham, Birmingham, Alabama 35294.

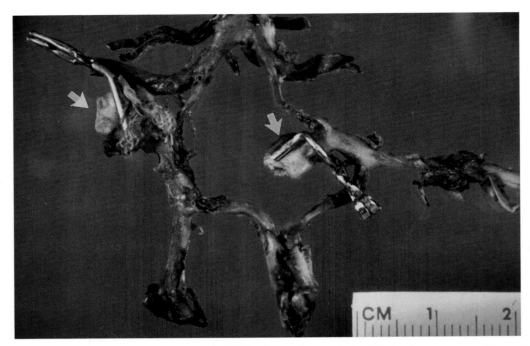

FIG. 1. Anatomic specimens of the circle of Willis. Arrow demonstrates bilateral aneurysms at the origin of the posterior communicating artery.

mation and their rupture. Only with this background can clinicians attempt to prevent, or at least diminish, the loss of life and permanent disability associated with spontaneous intracranial SAH.

SACCULAR ANEURYSMS

Saccular (berry) aneurysms account for approximately 90% of all intracranial aneurysms (3). They have been subdivided according to their size. Small aneurysms are those less than one cm in diameter, whereas large aneurysms are between 1 and 2.5 cm in diameter. Giant aneurysms are those greater than 2.5 cm in diameter. This classification does not allow categorization regarding the clinical risk of rupture. To understand the pathogenesis of aneurysms it is important to review their histologic characteristics.

Histology of Cerebral Arteries and Saccular Aneurysms

Saccular aneurysms are seldom reported outside the intracranial vasculature. Knowledge of the normal anatomy of the cerebral arteries is essential to the study of formation and growth of aneurysms. Cerebral arteries consist of three layers: (a) the tunica intima is the innermost layer and is lined by a monolayer of endothelial cells; (b) the tunica media is the middle layer and is predominantly muscular; and (c) the tunica adventitia is the outermost layer and is a thin

collagenous covering. The tunica intima contains abundant collagen and an internal elastic lamina that separates the intima from the tunica media (1,3). In contrast to the extracranial arteries, the intracranial vasculature lacks an external elastic lamina between the tunica media and adventitia. In about 80% of intracranial arteries a tunica media defect can be found at the apex of arterial bifurcations. These defects are also common in the lateral angles of both intracranial and extracranial arteries in humans and animals. Cerebral arteries lack perivascular support and have thin walls when compared to their counterparts in the extracranial systemic circulation (2). These anatomic differences in structure between intracranial and extracranial arterial walls represent an anatomic predisposition for the genesis of intracranial aneurysms in humans.

Intracranial saccular aneurysms are typically located at the apex of arterial bifurcations. When rupture occurs, the site of rupture is commonly at the fundus. The inner surface of the aneurysm sac is usually smooth, but sometimes the endothelial monolayer is incomplete and adherent blood clots can be found. The neck and fundus of the saccular aneurysm are usually thin. The thickness of the aneurysm wall correlates with aneurysm radius in a linear fashion (4). When the sac is small, it is usually transparent and consists of acellular hyaline tissue. In contrast, if the sac is large, there is variable thickness of connective tissue within the wall often associated with inflammatory cells. Reactive healing and wall thickening become prominent with the increasing diameter of the sac. Occasionally, part of the aneurysm wall will reveal necrosis and inflammatory changes. Partial thrombosis is common, especially in large aneurysms. Uncommonly, thrombosis within the aneurysm may occlude the lumen and result in self-cure.

Microscopically, the intima of a saccular aneurysm consists of degenerated cells and interendothelial gaps. Intimal hyperplasia is a common occurrence and is associated with thick fibrotic aneurysm walls. These walls lack a tunica media and an internal elastic lamina. Fragmentary remnants may be identified (Fig. 2). Usually the tunica media and the internal elastic lamina stop abruptly at the neck of the sac. The presence of immature collagen with degeneration of the reticular network has been demonstrated in the aneurysm wall (2). Fibroblasts with fibrin deposits and small lymphocytes can be seen. Calcifications, without ossification, and a prominent vasa vasorum can sometimes be found. Atherosclerotic changes are commonly found in the tunica intima. They consist of smooth muscle proliferation, lipid-laden macrophages, cholesterol clefts, and ulceration (1). Very early berry aneurysm vessel wall changes such as mural thinning and microevaginations of the intima into the medial raphe are difficult to demonstrate histologically in surgical or autopsy specimens.

Giant aneurysms are frequently thrombosed or nearly so. They may not be visualized on angiography if the lumen is occluded. Pathologic examination of a giant aneurysm and its contents typically reveals a laminated thrombus and an aneurysm wall that is thick and focally calcified. Organization of the clot may not occur and often there is little macrophage invasion (5). Giant serpentine aneurysms are pathologically defined as partially or incompletely thrombosed aneurysms that contain tortuous vascular channels.

It has been postulated that both the internal elastic lamina and the tunica media must be absent or weakened for intracranial aneurysm formation to occur. It is not known as to which layer is the more critical and which factors predispose to arterial wall damage. A variety of theories have been offered to explain intracranial aneurysm formation.

Theories of Aneurysm Formation

Medial Defect Theory

A postmortem study by Forbus (6) in 1930 documented his observations on the intracranial vasculature and its pathologic variations. He found that about two thirds of the arterial wall specimens had medial wall defects. He called these arterial wall defects "locus minoris resistantiae" and postulated that they were the framework for intracranial aneurysm formation. Forbus assumed that these defects were congenital in origin, but did not discount the importance of a defective elastic lamina. He claimed that the combination of a muscularis defect and degeneration of the elastic lamina were necessary for aneurysm formation. He assumed that overstretching of the arterial wall at the apices secondary to hemodynamic stress was an important factor in the genesis of an aneurysmal sac. This theory has been frequently labeled the "congenital theory."

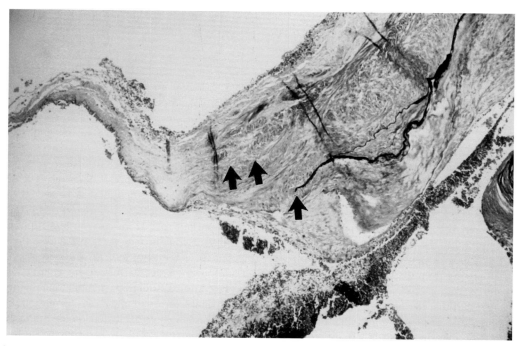

FIG. 2. Histology of a saccular aneurysm. Note the discontinuity of the elastic lamina *(arrow)* and the muscular layer *(double arrow)*. (Courtesy of Dr. Cheryl Palmer, Associate Professor of Neuropathology.)

Elastic Lamellar Theory

Because medial wall defects are common in the general population, Glynn proposed that aneurysm formation was dependent on focal degeneration of the elastica (7). To prove his point, he demonstrated that arterial walls composed only of intima and elastica withstood pressures up to 600 mm Hg without distention. He assumed that degeneration of the elastic lamina was caused by atherosclerosis or hemodynamic factors.

Carmichael (8) theorized that both tunica media and elastic lamina defects must be present for aneurysms to form. He felt that the elastica defect was likely to be secondary to atherosclerosis and that the medial defect was congenital in origin. Even when both lesions were present, the development of an aneurysm could sometimes be stalled by fibrosis of the intima.

Degenerative Theory

Stehbens (9,10) rejected Forbus's medial defect theory for a variety of reasons, including (a) the prevalence of medial wall defects increases with age, (b) medial wall defects occur at bifurcations of small and large arteries, whereas aneurysms occur more frequently at large arterial bifurcations, (c) saccular aneurysms are rarely found at extracranial bifurcations in humans or in animals, even though medial defects are very common in the extracranial circulation, and (d) medial wall defects also occur in the lateral angles of vessel bifurcations where aneurysm formation is extremely uncommon. He suggested that degeneration of the arterial wall secondary to hemodynamic stress and other local degenerative factors were responsible for aneurysm formation.

He described three types of preaneurysmal lesions: (a) funnel-shaped arterial dilatation, which consisted of attenuation of the media, degeneration of the elastica and attenuation of the adventitia; (b) areas of arterial wall thinning, described as thin and transparent vessel walls with focal attenuation of the adventitia, and absent media and elastic lamina; and (c) small vessel wall evaginations, described as microscopic lesions of a bulging intima through a medial wall defect (9).

Other Theories

Bremer (11) suggested that intracranial aneurysms are the result of failure of atrophy of the primitive capillary plexus. Against this theory is the fact that no "primitive" vessels have been identified arising from the wall of an intracranial aneurysm.

Drennan (12) suggested that the origin of small vestigial vessels may constitute a weak spot for subsequent intracranial aneurysm formation. No such vessels have been found clinically or on pathologic study.

Congenital variations of the circle of Willis have been suggested as a theoretical basis for intracranial aneurysm formation. Most investigators, however, feel that the mechanism of aneurysm formation in this instance is increased hemodynamic stress on arterial bifurcations secondary to augmented collateral blood flow.

Factors in Aneurysm Formation and Rupture

Hemodynamic Factors

Intraarterial hemodynamic stress can be classified into three main categories: (a) axial stream, (b) water-hammer effect, and (c) turbulence. These three factors likely act together in the pathogenesis of intracranial aneurysms, but the individual contribution of each to aneurysm rupture is not well known.

Physicists have determined that fluid flows through a straight tube in a stream-like fashion. They have documented that there are several layers of fluid flow, of which the central or axial stream is faster than the peripheral stream. Assuming that the geometric configuration of the cerebral arteries is comparable to a straight tube, then the axial stream of intraarterial blood will hit the apices of the arterial forks with greater force than will the peripheral stream. The apex of an arterial bifurcation will thus be subjected to an increased amount of hemodynamic stress compared to adjacent but less apical arterial wall segments. The greater the angle of the arterial bifurcation, the greater the stress and "wear-and-tear" on the apex portion of the arterial wall. Dissipation of the kinetic energy of the fluid stream at the apex results in structural fatigue and might be an important factor in the origin of aneurysms (3).

The water-hammer effect occurs as a consequence of the pulsatile nature of intraarterial blood flow. When two or more aneurysms are present in the same arterial distribution, the pulsations in the more distal aneurysm sac are damped. The proximal aneurysm tends to rupture more frequently in this situation, unless it has become thrombosed. These observations and others suggest that arterial pulsations play an important potential role in the genesis and rupture of intracranial aneurysms (1).

When a critical velocity of fluid flow is exceeded in a straight tube, turbulence will occur. Turbulence increases the wall stress and potential distention of the tube or conduit. Mathematical calculations suggest that turbulence may play an important role in the growth and rupture of intracranial aneurysms, but its clinical significance remains unclear. Turbulence can further weaken aneurysmal walls and probably contributes to saccular aneurysm enlargement (1).

Two clinical situations demonstrate the importance of hemodynamic stress in aneurysm formation. First, it has been demonstrated that occlusion of an intracranial vessel will foster collateral circulation and aneurysm formation secondary to the augmented blood flow and hemodynamic stress associated with the collateral flow (9). In the second situation, poststenotic arterial dilatation induced by hemodynamic stress is often associated with compensatory arterial wall changes similar to those found in the sacs of intracranial aneurysms. Wall thickening due to increased deposition of connective tissue, sometimes immature, and injury to the elastica have been identified histologically.

Arterial Hypertension

The incidence of systemic hypertension among patients with aneurysmal subarachnoid hemorrhage is not well defined, mainly because many truly hypertensive patients remain undetected. Through an increase in hemodynamic stress at arterial bifurcations, hypertension can aggravate any structural weakness of an intracranial vessel wall. The role of systemic hypertension in the genesis of intracranial aneurysm formation and rupture is supported by the variety of clinical associations and studies following: (a) there is an increased frequency of intracranial aneurysms in diseases associated with systemic hypertension such as coarctation of the aorta and polycystic kidney disease; (b) clinical studies have demonstrated that hypertensive individuals with a subarachnoid hemorrhage have an increased incidence of multiple aneurysms compared to nonhypertensive patients with subarachnoid hemorrhage (14); and (c) in experimental models, animals treated with β-aminoproprionitrile (which causes a defect in the linkage between elastin and collagen in the arterial wall) and induced hypertension have an increased incidence of intracranial aneurysm formation (13).

Despite what appears to be an obvious association between hypertension and intracranial aneurysms, autopsy studies have found no difference in the incidence of intracranial aneurysms among known hypertensive patients and nonhypertensive individuals. Age-matched control studies demonstrate an incidence and severity of systemic hypertension in patients without aneurysms similar to those hypertensive patients with aneurysms (15). The question that remains unanswered is what effect sudden stress-related or exertional elevations in blood pressure associated with lifting, defecation, coitus, and so forth have among normotensive patients who harbor intracranial saccular berry aneurysms. The clinical data suggest a role for hypertension in the genesis of intracranial aneurysms and their rupture, yet the specific significance of that role remains to be elucidated.

Atherosclerosis

Histologic findings in aneurysmal vessel walls support the concept that atherosclerosis is a factor in the pathogenesis of aneurysm formation. A higher incidence of multiple aneurysms has been found in patients with severe atherosclerosis compared to individuals without advanced arteriosclerotic vascular disease. There is, however, no conclusive evidence that atheromatous plaques affect the growth or rupture of intracranial saccular aneurysms (see atherosclerotic aneurysms).

Age, Gender, and Genetic Factors

The incidence of aneurysmal subarachnoid hemorrhage increases with age, but it is not known at what specific age aneurysms originate. Old age seems to be a risk factor for intracranial aneurysm formation but not for aneurysm rupture. It is not known as to how much time elapses between the development of a berry aneurysm and its eventual rupture. Current data support degeneration of the arterial wall by hemodynamic stress, atherosclerosis, and hypertension as the cause of aneurysms discovered in the elderly. In children, intracranial aneurysms are rare and seldom discovered incidentally. This suggests a higher relative risk of aneurysm rupture in younger patients and indicates a different pathogenic mechanism for their formation and rupture compared to middle- and late-aged patients (2).

Epidemiologic studies indicate that women are more often affected by aneurysmal subarachnoid hemorrhage than men. Hormonal factors have been suggested as the cause. Clinical studies have documented an increased risk for hemorrhage among females who use oral contraceptives. Other studies have demonstrated a higher incidence of intracranial saccular aneurysms in women than in men. These data suggest that aneurysm formation is more likely in females than males, and this probably accounts for their reported higher incidence of subarachnoid hemorrhage. It not known as to whether or not females have a greater predisposition for rupture compared to males (2).

Familial cases of intracranial aneurysms due to autosomal transmission have been described. Aneurysm frequency higher than that documented among the general population (up to 6.8%) has been recognized among blood relatives of patients found to have an SAH due to an intracranial saccular aneurysm. Younger age at the time of aneurysm rupture, multiple aneurysms, and unusual aneurysm location are features that suggest genetic transmission. Recently, an association between the histocompatibility antigens (known as the HLA system) and intracranial aneurysms has been detected. HLA-DR2 and HLA-B7 antigens have been identified with increased frequency in a subgroup of patients who harbor intracranial aneurysms (2). The estimated relative risk of harboring an intracranial saccular aneurysm in these patients is 2.5–4.7 higher than that reported for the general population.

Connective Tissue Disorders

Two types of collagen predominate in vascular structures: type I and type III collagen. Type I fibers are the key to the tensile strength of the vessel wall, whereas type III fibers play an important role in the regulation of collagen fibril and fiber structure (2). The resultant reticular framework formed by type I and type III collagen is important for vessel wall and intimal proliferation and repair. A deficiency of type III fibers has been identified in the vascular wall of some surgical specimens. Altered mechanical properties of vessels that are associated with the presence of immature collagen and a deficiency in reticular fibers has been postulated to contribute to aneurysm enlargement and rupture (16). Several studies have demonstrated alterations in vessel wall extensibility at physiologic blood pressures in patients with type III collagen deficiency. Patients with Ehlers–Danlos syndrome type IV suffer from a generalized deficiency of type III collagen. These patients have an increased propensity for arterial fragility and aneurysm formation.

Associated Diseases

Two disease entities have been associated with an increased risk of intracranial aneurysm formation: (a) coarctation of the aorta and (b) polycystic kidney disease. A factor common to both disorders appears to be accelerated systemic hypertension. No other systemic or vessel wall abnormality has been identified in these patients. This association suggests that the hemodynamic stress imposed by consistently high blood pressure is an important factor in the pathogenesis of intracranial aneurysm formation (9).

In others diseases like Marfan's syndrome and pseudoxanthoma elasticum the incidence of intracranial aneurysms is no greater than that in age-matched controls. However, the unusual location of intracranial aneurysms in patients with these disorders suggests some association with these disease processes and with aneurysm formation. Intracranial saccular aneurysms have been reported in association with fibromuscular hyperplasia, findings that have been discussed in another chapter.

An increased incidence of intracranial aneurysms has been reported among patients with arteriovenous malformations. The incidence of associated intracranial aneurysms in this group of patients is approximately 3–9% (1). These findings support the concept that aneurysm origin may be fostered by local hemodynamic factors.

Other Factors

Smoking has been associated with a 3–5 times higher risk of subarachnoid hemorrhage compared to that in age-matched nonsmoking controls. Alcohol consumption and oral contraceptive use also have been considered deleterious factors that favor aneurysm formation, but their specific roles remain unclear (17).

The size of the cerebral blood vessels must be an important factor in aneurysm formation. Spinal arteries have the same histologic architecture as intracranial arteries yet the incidence of aneurysm formation in these vessels is low. Only in situations in which there is enlargement of the spinal arteries (arteriovenous malformation and coarctation of the aorta) are aneurysms found (10).

Growth and Rupture of Saccular Aneurysms

The inability of the vessel wall, mainly the intima, to proliferate, repair, and respond to damage produced by hemodynamic stress and environmental factors leads to focal weakening of the arterial wall. Mechanical fatigue and injury fostered by ischemia (likely secondary to disruption of the vasa vasorum) is the probable final common pathway in aneurysm formation and enlargement. Each of the factors discussed above contributes somewhat to aneurysm formation and growth (Fig. 3).

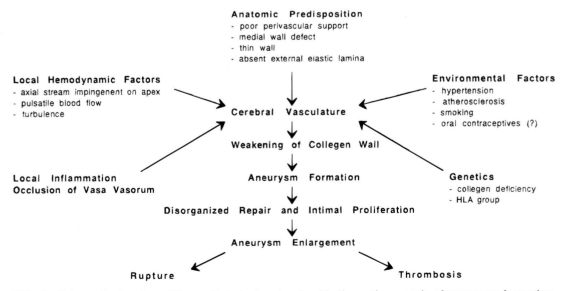

FIG. 3. Schematic drawing of the multiple factors involved in the pathogenesis of aneurysm formation.

Aneurysm rupture is the terminal event in aneurysm development. Rupture cannot be explained simply by mechanical distention and the law of Laplace (tension = pressure × radius) (10). Mathematical models based on static mechanics, using the variables of blood pressure, wall strength, and total wall substance, predict a critical aneurysmal sac diameter of 8 mm and 40 μm of wall thickness for rupture (18). It is common clinical practice for aneurysms smaller than the above dimensions to cause catastrophic subarachnoid hemorrhage. Mechanical models aside, current evidence supports the concept that vascular wall injury and fatigue caused by age and degenerative changes, aggravated by hemodynamic stress, hypertension, and congenital variations of the circle of Willis, are important features in aneurysm rupture.

Clinical correlations and experimental studies indicate that intracranial aneurysms have a multifactorial origin. The unique features of the intracranial vasculature including their lack of perivascular support, thin walls, medial wall defects, and absence of an external elastic lamina may predispose them to aneurysm formation. However, for saccular aneurysms to develop there must be an injured, weakened, or absent internal elastic lamina and tunica media (1). This suggests that hemodynamic stresses, hypertension, atherosclerosis, and other vessel wall degenerative changes are important elements in the pathogenesis of intracranial aneurysms. Current evidence favors hemodynamically induced degenerative vascular disease as the most important factor in the formation and rupture of saccular aneurysms.

ATHEROSCLEROTIC FUSIFORM ANEURYSMS

In patients with advanced atherosclerotic vascular disease, fusiform dilatation of the intracranial arteries is a common finding. Atherosclerotic plaques increase in frequency in the arterial wall of older patients as their systemic atherosclerosis progresses in severity. Although atherosclerotic changes are detected in all aneurysms, including the saccular type, the earliest stages of atherogenesis, ''fatty streaks,'' are usually not found. The absence of these early changes is probably related to the advanced stage of the patient's disease by the time of diagnosis. The arterial walls of the arteriosclerotic vessels stretch and dilate due to the replacement of smooth muscle fibers with fibrous tissue. Histologically, calcium deposits, necrosis, cholesterol crystals, and lipid deposition have been identified in the vessel wall. Macrophages, lymphocytes, and other inflammatory cells are interspersed within the dense connective tissue matrix of the atherosclerotic aneurysm wall.

The lumen of the vessel may be increased in size (ectasia) and when the dilatation is extreme it results in fusiform aneurysm formation. The supraclinoid segment of the internal carotid artery (ICA) and the basilar artery are the two most frequent locations for fusiform aneurysm formation. Clinical symptoms may result from compression of adjacent structures or transient ischemic attacks, presumably secondary to embolization. Hemorrhage from rupture of a fusiform aneurysm may also occur (5).

DISSECTING ANEURYSMS

Dissecting aneurysms of the intracranial vessels are uncommon and are usually the result of head injury or blunt trauma to the neck, especially the craniocervical junction. The basilar, vertebral, and middle cerebral arteries and the intracranial portions of the ICA are the most commonly involved vessels. Dissecting lesions are produced by penetration of circulating blood within the substance of the arterial wall. Dissections have been described between the intima and the media and between the tunica media and tunica adventitia. Clinically, subadventitial dissections are more commonly associated with subarachnoid hemorrhage, whereas subintimal dissections are typically associated with luminal occlusion by intramural hematoma formation (19).

INFLAMMATORY, BACTERIAL, AND OTHER MYCOTIC ANEURYSMS

Streptococcus viridans and *Staphylococcus aureus* are the most common organisms associated with bacterial aneurysm formation. Approximately 3–10% of patients with infective endocarditis will develop infective aneurysms of the distal middle, anterior, or posterior cerebral arteries. Multiple aneurysms are identified in approximately 20% of cases. Autopsy studies reveal that the infective organisms spread from an infected emboli to a point in the vessel distal to the site of occlusion. Inflammation and necrosis occurs in the vessel wall within 24 hours and are often more severe in the tunica adventitia (5). These aneurysms may have a fusiform morphology and are usually very friable, which makes surgical intervention very difficult.

Fungal aneurysms may also form in the distal branches of the intracranial circulation. Nasal sinus infections and fungal endocarditis are the most frequent sources of infection. *Aspergillus* is the most common organism. A variety of fungal organisms can contribute to opportunistic mycotic aneurysm formation including *Nocardia* and *Coccidioides immitis*. Necrosis and inflammation within the vessel wall with growing fungal hyphae are seen on pathologic examination (5). Aneurysm rupture with extensive hemorrhage and disruption of the brain parenchyma frequently occurs.

Local vessel wall inflammatory changes have been described in patients with aneurysms in association with conditions such as polyarteritis nodosa, lupus, and other autoimmune diseases. It is proposed that aneurysm formation in patients with these diseases relate to hyperactivity of the immune system. Focal angiitis with inflammatory cells and marked destruction of the vessel wall secondary to the release of lysosomal enzymes have been described histologically (20).

VASCULAR MALFORMATIONS

Intracranial vascular malformations have been divided into five different types according to the configuration of the vascular channels, the continuity with the cerebral vasculature, and the relationship between the vessels and the intervening brain parenchyma. These types are as follows: (a) arteriovenous, (b) cavernous, (c) capillary telangiectases, (d) venous, and (e) mixed malformations (Table 1). These malformations are not neoplastic and originate as a result of abnormal embryonic development of the intracranial vascular network.

The incidence of these malformations is close to 5% in the general adult population (21). Approximately 90% of intracranial vascular malformations are clinically silent. Malformations of the venous type are the most common in the central nervous system (CNS) and are the most benign with respect to clinical symptoms. The arteriovenous type is the most biologically aggressive, and often causes symptoms secondary to hemorrhage, ischemia (''steal''), and mass effect. The spontaneous thrombosis of intracranial vascular malformations has been documented and is usually accompanied with disappearance on angiography.

Although most intracranial vascular malformations remain stable in size, there is an important percentage that will enlarge. Growth most commonly occurs in arteriovenous and cavernous malformations (22). The incremental increases in the size of these lesions appears to be related to enlargement of the component vessels and/or to recruitment of adjacent vascular supply. The cause of rupture of these malformations is not well known, but does not appear to be related to hypertension, physical activity, stress, or other patient physical feature (21).

Cerebral angiography plays an important role in the diagnosis of vascular malformations of the brain. A small subgroup of intracranial vascular malformations cannot be visualized angiographically. The term ''cryptic'' has been used to describe these angiographically occult malformations. The majority of cavernous and capillary-type malformations are angiographically occult. Some small arteriovenous and venous malformations may be angiographically occult as well. Patients with occult vascular malformations may present with seizures, neurologic deficits, headaches, or hemorrhage. Magnetic resonance imaging (MRI) is an excellent way to image the angiographically occult lesion in these patients.

ARTERIOVENOUS MALFORMATIONS

Arteriovenous malformations (AVM) are one of the most familiar intracranial vascular malformations to the clinician because they are most often symptomatic (Fig. 3). Patients with AVMs present with hemorrhage, seizures, ischemia, or symptoms related to mass effect. Bleeding from AVMs is most common between the ages of 10 and 30 years; after 60 years of age hemorrhage is rare. Males are affected twice as often as females. Subarachnoid and intracerebral hemorrhage associated with seizures are the most common presenting feature. Chronic recurrent headache is a frequent complaint. Large AVMs may produce progressive neurologic deficits due to shunting of blood through the abnormally dilated vascular channels of the AVM, directing nutrient blood supply away from adjacent neural tissue (steal). Approximately 90% of arteriovenous malformations are located supratentorially. They are usually supplied by branches of the middle cerebral artery and their most common locations are the frontal and temporal lobes. They are usually triangular in shape with their base toward the meninges and the apex toward the ventricular system (23). Intracranial saccular aneurysms are associated with high-flow arteriovenous malformations in about 7–10% of the cases.

AVMs are a conglomerate of abnormal arteries and veins with minimal intervening gliotic brain parenchyma, commonly described as a ''bag of worms'' (Fig. 4). The size of the vessels of an AVM may vary greatly. Some vessels have thin collagenous walls like veins, whereas others possess the muscular and elastic laminae of arteries. Histologically, the larger vascular channels resemble veins in that they contain a small amount of muscularis and lack elastica. Sometimes

TABLE 1. *Classification of vascular malformations*

Vascular malformations	Histology	Clinical presentation
Arteriovenous malformations	Clusters of abnormal arteries and veins "Hypertrophied arteries and arterialized veins" No capillary bed in the parenchyma Minimal intervening brain tissue	Hemorrhage (40–50%) Seizures (15–30%) Headaches (20%) Focal deficit (10%)
Cavernous malformations	Compact mass of sinusoidal channels No intervening parenchyma	Seizures (40–70%) Hemorrhage (10–30%) Focal deficit/space-occupying lesion (20–40%)
Capillary telangiectases	Collection of capillary-type vessels Intervening normal parenchyma	Incidental finding Hemorrhage rare
Venous malformations	Collection of anomalous veins Intervening normal brain parenchyma	Incidental finding Hemorrhage or thrombosis rare
Mixed malformations	Combination of two or more of the above lesions	

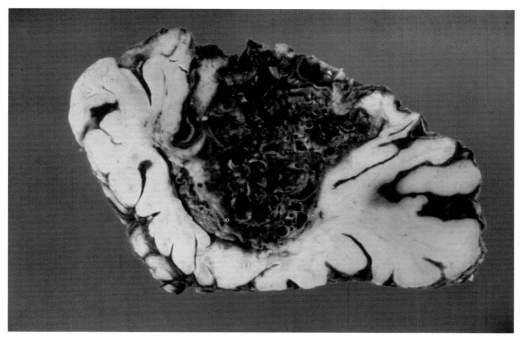

FIG. 4. Arteriovenous malformation involving the cerebral parenchyma commonly described as "bag of worms."

the walls of the arteries are thinner than normal allowing visualization of the flowing blood on direct inspection.

Evidence of prior hemorrhage is found in the majority of AVMs. Hemosiderin-laden microphages are almost always present in the periphery of the lesion. Mineralization of blood breakdown products is found in approximately 10% of cases. AVMs of the cortical surface are often associated with thickened and opacified leptomeninges. Inflammation and extensive thrombosis can sometimes be observed. The marked gliosis of the surrounding brain parenchyma characteristic of these lesions is probably the result of hypoperfusion and ischemia (steal) of the tissue secondary to the low-resistance, high-flow vascular shunt of the AVM (21). Residual arterial ectasia and dilatation after occlusion or removal of an AVM suggests that the arteries contributing to the AVM are abnormal as they approach the malformation and do not autoregulate properly.

The most reasonable theory for the pathogenesis of AVMs seems to be a congenital absence of the intervening capillary bed between arteries and veins. The resultant high-flow, relatively low-resistance "shunt" of blood in these malformations increases the intraluminal pressure of the venous side vessels and causes as a consequence, venous ectasia and the formation of "hybrid" vessels, with both venous and arterial characteristics ("arterialized veins") (Fig. 5).

CAVERNOUS MALFORMATIONS

Cavernous-type intracranial vascular malformations occur randomly throughout the brain tissue, the leptomeninges, and/or the lining of the ventricular system (22). They represent roughly 5–20% of all CNS vascular malformations (24).

Approximately 16% of patients with cavernous malformations will have multiple lesions. A familial incidence, especially in Hispanics, has been described that follows an autosomal dominant pattern (25). Most of these lesions are supratentorial near the Rolandic region or basal ganglia, but 15% to 20% are infratentorial, most commonly in the pons. Clinically, they present with focal neurologic deficits, seizures, signs of increased intracranial pressure (obstructive hydrocephalus), or hemorrhage. Early reports referred to them as part of the group of "cryptic" malformations (as capillary telangiectases and small AVMs) because of the difficulty in identifying them on cerebral angiography (26). These malformations are not well visualized on arteriography because they lack direct arterial input.

Cavernous malformations are composed of clusters of sinusoidal vascular channels with thin walls devoid of elastin and smooth muscle. They appear as a discrete, purplish, mulberry-like mass. No intervening brain parenchyma is found within the nidus of the lesion, only at the periphery. The sinusoidal channels are often filled with thrombus of varying degrees of organization (Fig. 6). Microscopically there is evidence of subclinical hemorrhage with numerous hemosiderin-laden macrophages in the adjacent tissue. Calcification may occur in larger malformations.

Seizures are the presenting symptoms in 40–70% of the patients harboring these lesions. In most of these individuals the lesions are located in temporal and frontal lobe parenchyma. The incidence of hemorrhage from a cavernous malformation is less than that associated with AVMs and is estimated to occur in approximately 10–30% of patients (24).

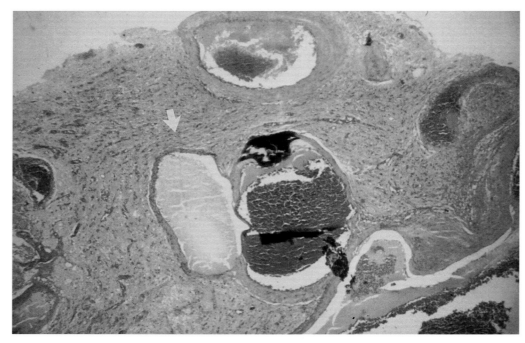

FIG. 5. Microscopic appearance of an arteriovenous malformation. The presence of "arterial veins" is demonstrated (arrow).

CAPILLARY TELANGIECTASES

Most capillary malformations are not visualized with angiography and are most frequently discovered at autopsy (22). These malformations are typically found in the pons and, less frequently, in the white matter. Macroscopically, they appear as a pink–red circular lesion that may be mistaken for a cluster of petechiae. Microscopically, they are a collection of dilated capillaries lined by a single layer of endothelial cells devoid of smooth muscle or elastic fibers

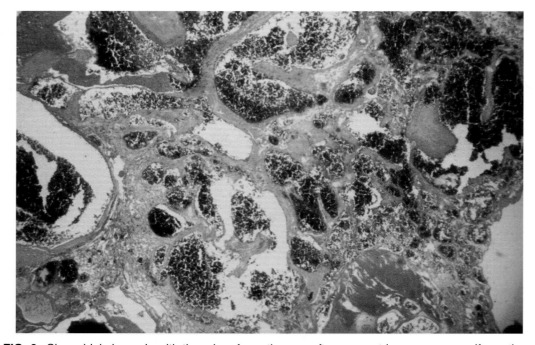

FIG. 6. Sinusoidal channels with thrombus formation are often present in cavernous malformations.

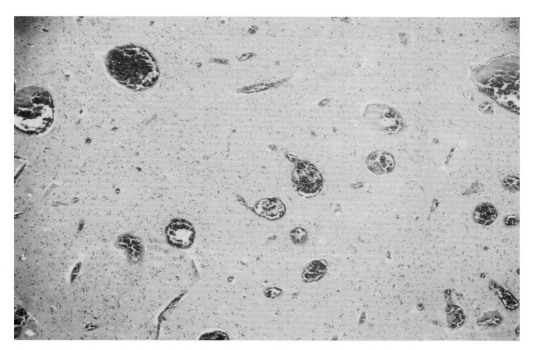

FIG. 7. Capillary telangiectasia. Dilated capillaries with normal intervening brain parenchyma are seen.

(27) (Fig. 7). The capillaries are separated from each other by brain parenchyma with normal architecture. Gliosis, mineralization, and/or hemorrhage are rare but have been reported. Capillary telangiectases have been observed in the brain of patients with hereditary Osler–Weber–Rendu disease (23).

New clinical and radiographic evidence suggests that cavernous malformations and capillary telangiectases represent two extremes within the same spectrum of vascular malformations. Both lesions are derived from capillary vessels and are frequently present within the same patient. A key discriminating feature has been distinguishing the presence of normal brain tissue among capillary telangiectases compared to the absence of brain parenchyma and the characteristic hemosiderin stain found in the brain tissue surrounding the cavernous malformation. The term ''cerebral capillary malformation'' has been suggested as descriptive of these combined lesions (28).

VENOUS MALFORMATIONS

Venous malformations are the most common vascular malformation of the CNS (21). These malformations are more common in the spinal cord and spinal meninges than in the intracranial compartment (23). Venous angiomas are composed of anomalous veins separated by normal brain tissue. The walls of the veins are thickened and hyalinized and are usually devoid of smooth muscle and elastic tissue. Although histologically abnormal, they function as the ve-

nous outflow for normal cerebral tissues. There is no direct arterial input to these lesions.

Venous malformations usually originate in the deep white matter, where typically veins of the caliber of venous malformation will not be found. It is unusual to find areas suggestive of hemorrhage (macro- or micro-) or gliosis in association with these malformations. Although spontaneous thrombosis of venous malformations has been reported, hemorrhage from a venous malformation is distinctly uncommon. Associated gliosis and mineralization have rarely been described.

The angiographic appearance of a venous malformation is typical. The arterial and capillary phase are normal, but the venous phase reveals an arcade of veins described as caput medusae.

A variant of the venous malformation has been called a varix. This is a single dilated vein with histologic findings consistent with thickened, fibrotic, and hyalinized walls (21).

VEIN OF GALEN ANEURYSMS

A vein of Galen aneurysm represents a unique entity within the intracranial vascular system. Although initially thought to be an arteriovenous malformation, a vein of Galen aneurysm is now considered to be a direct arteriovenous fistula between choroidal and/or quadrigeminal arteries and a venous sac (Fig. 8). The arteries involved in this entity are not developmentally related to the involved veins. Essentially it is an extracerebral, but intraarachnoidal vascular

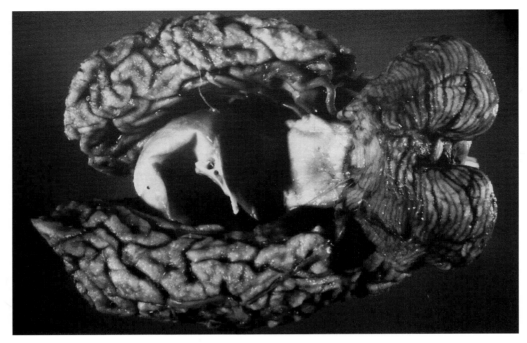

FIG. 8. Pathologic specimen of a large "vein of Galen" aneurysm.

malformation with retention of fetal anatomic features. This high-flow system will produce symptoms secondary to cardiac failure (neonates), head enlargement, mass effect (hydrocephalus), and/or hemorrhage. Persistence of the embryonic median prosencephalic vein of Markowski is currently the accepted theory for this condition (29). Even though the nomenclature "vein of Galen aneurysm" is anatomically incorrect, it remains a generally accepted descriptive term in clinical practice.

ARTERIOVENOUS FISTULAS

Dural arteriovenous fistulas are characterized by a direct communication of the intracranial arteries to the venous system without intervening capillaries. Experimental studies support the idea that tears in the internal elastic lamina are responsible for fistula formation. Endothelial discontinuities are also found in the areas of the elastic tears. Apparently, hemodynamic stress appears to propagate and perpetuate the communication (30). Dural arteriovenous fistulas shunt blood to the dural sinuses from meningeal and extracranial arteries. Dural fistulas commonly affect women over the age of 40 and predominantly involve the transverse sinuses. Abnormalities of the sinuses are frequent in these cases. The etiology of a dural fistula is controversial, but recent evidence suggests that at least some are acquired (31). Commonly dural fistulas resolve spontaneously but associated symptoms including headaches, seizures, and/or bruits may require definitive treatment. Dural fistulas may also present with SAH and progressive neurologic deficit.

REFERENCES

1. Sekhar LN, Heros RC. Origin, growth, and rupture of saccular aneurysms: a review. *Neurosurgery* 1981;8:248–260.
2. Ostergaard JR. Risk factors in intracranial saccular aneurysms: aspects on the formation and rupture of aneurysms, and development of cerebral vasospasm. *Acta Neurol Scand* 1989;80:81–98.
3. Yong-Zhong G, van Alphen HA. Pathogenesis and histopathology of the saccular aneurysms: review of the literature. *Neurol Res* 1990;12:249–255.
4. Steiger HJ, Aaslid R, Keller S, Reulen HJ. Growth of aneurysms can be understood as passive yield to blood pressure. An experimental study. *Acta Neurochir* 1989;100:74–78.
5. Weller RO. Spontaneous intracranial hemorrhage. In: Adams JH, Duchen LW, eds. *Greenfield's neuropathology.* New York: Oxford Clinic Press, 1992;282–301.
6. Forbus WD. On the origin of miliary aneurysms of the superficial cerebral arteries. *Bull Johns Hopkins Hosp* 1930;47:239–284.
7. Glynn LE. Medial defects in the circle of Willis and their relation to aneurysm formation. *J Pathol Bact* 1940;51:213–222.
8. Carmichael B. The pathogenesis of non-inflammatory cerebral aneurysms. *J Pathol* 1950;35:347–368.
9. Stehbens WE. Etiology of intracranial berry aneurysms. *J Neurosurg* 1989;70:823–831.
10. Stehbens WE. Pathology and pathogenesis of intracranial berry aneurysms. *Neurol Res* 1990;12:29–34.
11. Bremer JL. Congenital aneurysms of the cerebral arteries: An embryonic study. *Arch Pathol* 1943;35:819–831.
12. Drennan AM. Discussion. *Edinb Med J* 1933;38:721–757.
13. Hashimoto N, Handa H, Hazama F. Experimentally induced cerebral aneurysms in rats: Part III. *Surg Neurol* 1979;11:299–304.
14. Andrews RJ, Spiegel PK. Intracranial aneurysms *J Neurosurg* 1979;51:27–32.
15. McCormick WF, Schmalstieg EJ. The relationship of arterial hypertension to intracranial aneurysms. *Arch Neurol* 1977;34:285–287.
16. Hegedus K. Pattern of reticular fibers of the major cerebral arteries in cases of unexplained subarachnoid haemorrhage. *J Neurol* 1986;233:44–47.
17. Misra BK, Whittle IR, Steers JW, Sellar RJ. De novo saccular aneurysms. *Neurosurgery* 1988;23:10–14.

18. Canham PB, Ferguson GG. A mathematical model for the mechanics of saccular aneurysms. *Neurosurgery* 1985;17:291–295.

19. Sasaki O, Ogawa H, Koike T, Koizumi T, Tanaka R. A clinicopathological study of dissecting aneurysms of the intracranial vertebral artery. *J Neurosurg* 1991;75:874–882.

20. Sasaki T, Morimoto T, Utsumi S. Cerebral transmural angiitis and ruptured cerebral aneurysms in patients with systemic lupus erythematosus. *Neurochir* 1990;33:132–135.

21. Mccormick WF. Pathology of vascular malformations of the brain. In: Wilson CB, Stein BM, eds. *Intracranial arteriovenous malformations.* Baltimore: Williams and Wilkins, 1984;44–63.

22. Burger P, Scheithauer B, Vogel FS, eds. *Surgical pathology of the nervous system and its coverings.* 3rd ed. New York: Churchill Livingstone, 1991.

23. Garcia J, Anderson M. Circulatory disorders and their effects on the brain. In: Davis R, Robertson D, eds. *Textbook of neuropathology.* Baltimore: Williams and Wilkins, 1991;625–635.

24. Farmer JP, Cosgrove GR, Villemure JG, Meagher-Villemure K, Tampieri D, Melanson D. Intracranial cavernous angiomas. *Neurology* 1988;38:1699–1704.

25. Rigamonti D, Hadley MN, Drayer BP, et al. Cerebral cavernous malformations: incidence and familial ocurrence. *N Engl J Med* 1988;319:343–347.

26. Robinson JR, Awad IA, Masaryk TJ, Estes ML. Pathological heterogeneity of angiographically occult vascular malformations of the brain. *Neurosurgery* 1993;33:547–555.

27. McCormick WF. The pathology of vascular (''arteriovenous'') malformations. *J Neurosurg* 1966;24:807–812.

28. Rigamonti D, Johnson PC, Spetzler RF, Hadley MN, Drayer BP. Cavernous malformations and capillary telangiectasia: a spectrum within a single pathological entity. *Neurosurgery* 1991;28:60–64.

29. Raybaud CA, Strother CM, Hald JK. Aneurysms of the vein of Galen: embryonic considerations and anatomical features relating to the pathogenesis of the malformation. *Neuroradiology* 1989;31:109–128.

30. Jones GT, Stehbens WE, Martin BJ. Ultrastructural changes in arteries proximal to short-term experimental carotid-jugular arteriovenous fistulae in rabbits. *Int J Exp Pathol* 1994;75:225–232.

31. Graer DA, Dolman CL. Radiological and pathological aspects of dural arteriovenous fistulas. *J Neurosurg* 1986;64:962–967.

Cerebrovascular Disease, edited by H. Hunt Batjer.
Lippincott-Raven Publishers, Philadelphia © 1997.

CHAPTER 6

Physiology of Hypertensive Cardiovascular Disease: Effects on the Brain

Daryl W. Thompson and Anthony J. Furlan

Hypertension is the most prevalent cardiovascular disorder in the United States (1). It is also the most modifiable risk factor for cerebrovascular disease. However, despite being so common, the complex physiology of hypertension is not completely understood, and the etiology remains elusive. The effect of hypertension on cerebrovascular disease morbidity and mortality is more potent than its effects on other vascular beds, such as the cardiovascular and peripheral vascular systems. Hypertensive cerebrovascular disease may manifest as large vessel cerebral infarction, small vessel cerebral infarction, and cerebral hemorrhage.

The association between blood pressure and stroke persists with advancing age (2). Isolated systolic hypertension, which is prevalent after the age of 65 years, is also a substantial risk factor for stroke (3). At any level of blood pressure, various cardiac impairments (including coronary heart disease, cardiac failure, atrial fibrillation, and ventricular hypertrophy) more than double the risk of stroke.

NORMAL PHYSIOLOGY OF ARTERIAL PRESSURE

The body has several systems involved in the regulation of arterial pressure. Arterial pressure is directly related to cardiac output and peripheral vascular resistance. Cardiac output is defined as a product of the stroke volume multiplied by heart rate. Four important factors that determine cardiac performance are preload, afterload, contractility, and heart rate. The term *preload* is defined as the initial resting force stretching the cardiac muscle prior to contraction; it correlates with end-diastolic volume. The term *afterload* refers to the resistance against which the heart must contract. It is the load resisting shortening as the muscle is stimulated,

and it roughly correlates with arterial pressure or impedance against which the heart has to work. Changes in preload and afterload are closely related. Thus, as the arterial pressure is increased, the ventricle has greater difficulty ejecting blood, eventually causing left ventricular hypertrophy as a compensatory response.

Large arteries contribute importantly to total cerebral vascular resistance and are major determinants of local microvascular pressure. The resistance of large arteries and the cerebral microvascular pressure are affected by several physiologic stimuli. A response can be elicited by changes in systemic blood pressure, increases in cerebral metabolism, activity of sympathetic nerves, and humoral stimuli such as circulating vasopressin and angiotensin. Stimuli such as sympathetic stimulation and vasopressin produce selective responses of large arteries and thereby regulate microvascular pressure without a significant change in cerebral blood flow (4).

Most of the vascular resistance is generated by changes in the caliber of the blood vessels. Small alterations in the caliber of the vessel can produce marked changes in resistance to blood flow since resistance is inversely related to the radius of the vessel raised to the fourth power. On a cellular level, the changes in the caliber of blood vessels are mediated by the release of vasoactive substances from the endothelium. The endothelium is capable of producing potent vasorelaxing factors. One example is nitric oxide, previously known as endothelium-derived relaxing factor (EDRF). Nitric oxide is the principal vasorelaxing factor produced by the endothelium. It is derived from the amino acid L-arginine and has a short half-life (seconds). In oxygenated environments, nitric oxide decomposes rapidly to form mixtures of nitrite and nitrate. Nitric oxide is continuously released from the endothelium, and if its synthesis is blocked experimentally, a sharp rise in arterial pressure occurs. The endothelium also produces powerful vasoconstrictive factors such as endothelin 1 and angiotensin II. Under

---

D. W. Thompson and A. J. Furlan: Department of Neurology, The Cleveland Clinic Foundation, Cleveland, Ohio 44195.

normal conditions, the opposing forces of vasorelaxing and vasoconstricting forces achieve a state of equilibrium and normal vascular tone is maintained (5,6).

Neuronal and hormonal systems act very rapidly in response to transient hemodynamic disturbances, whereas regulatory systems related to renal and blood volume act more slowly and cause chronic adaptive changes. The vasomotor center, located in the lateral medulla, plays an important role in the generation of neurogenic vasomotor tone and the maintenance of arterial pressure (7). Neuronal regulation of the circulatory system occurs chiefly by means of modulating the frequency of impulses transmitted by sympathetic vasoconstrictor fibers innervating the vascular smooth muscle of resistance vessels. An increase in frequency of these impulses enhances the release of norepinephrine from nerve fiber endings, thus producing vasoconstriction, whereas a decrease in the discharge frequency of these fibers results in vasodilatation (8). Electrical stimulation of the medullary reticular formation and adjacent periventricular gray matter experimentally produces elevation of arterial blood pressure and cardiac acceleration, probably as a consequence of activating sympathetic effectors.

Stimulation in the region of the obex and in a wide area medial and ventral to the sympathetic area produces a slowing of the heart rate. The output of the medullary vasomotor center is modulated by input from the baroreceptors in the carotid sinuses and aortic arch. A sudden rise in arterial pressure causes the baroreceptors to increase their frequency of firing, thereby inhibiting the medullary sympathetic vasomotor center and exciting the vagal center. The combined response of these systems to a sudden rise in arterial pressure consists of a decrease in peripheral vascular resistance, slowing of the heart rate, and reduction in myocardial contractility, which acts to restore arterial pressure to the baseline level. However, if this system is chronically subjected to elevated levels of arterial pressure, the baroreceptors rapidly adapt and decrease their frequency of firing despite a persistently elevated arterial pressure. Therefore, although the baroreceptor reflex effectively responds to acute changes in arterial pressure, elevations over sustained periods prevent the reflex from being effective (36). Complete removal of baroreceptor inhibition produces a sharp increase in arterial pressure that if sustained is referred to as neurogenic hypertension (9).

The major arterial chemoreceptors are located in the aortic arch just medial to the carotid sinuses. Reduced PO_2, increased PCO_2, or a reduction in pH stimulates the chemoreceptors. Their principal role is regulating respiration, but they also can influence the medullary vasomotor center. Under conditions of hypoxia, these chemoreceptors can elicit powerful peripheral vasoconstriction.

PATHOPHYSIOLOGY OF HYPERTENSION

The changes in vascular resistance to hemodynamic and humoral stimuli are relatively short-term adaptations. The long-term adaptive responses to sustained alterations in physiologic or pathophysiologic conditions are mediated primarily by changes in the vascular architecture. Three types of changes are found in blood vessels associated with sustained hypertension. These are structurally adaptive changes, degenerative alterations, and atherosclerosis (10). It remains unclear as to whether these changes cause hypertension or simply sequelae of hypertension.

Hypertension and atherosclerosis are characterized by trophic changes that occur in the vascular wall (11,12). One of the earliest morphologic changes in the development of an atherosclerotic lesion is the appearance of mononuclear cells. At least 90% of these cells are blood monocytes. They leave the circulation and diapedese between endothelial cells to take up residence in the subendothelial space. These monocytes convert to macrophages and accumulate cholesteryl esters that appear foamy on histologic sections; hence, they have been named foam cells. Macroscopically, macrophage foam cells initially appear as a fatty streak. With time, the number of foam cells may increase to eventually deform the overlying endothelium causing microscopic separations. Exposure of the subendothelial content and extracellular matrix elicits the body's inflammatory response to injury. The exposed sites attract platelets that release mitogenic substances and other products to attract other components of the inflammatory response. The mitogenic substances stimulate excessive proliferation of smooth cells that also migrate into the subendothelial space. The expanding lesion of smooth muscle and foam cells initially expands outward from the subendothelial space to the adventitia but eventually turns inward to encroach on the vascular lumen (13). Approximately two thirds of the tissue volume of the atherosclerotic lesion is constituted by smooth muscle cells and smooth muscle cell products; the remainder are the lipid components. Reduction in blood flow may result either from luminal narrowing or from the formation of thrombi on the surface of the atherosclerotic lesion. Clinically, atherosclerotic stenoses or occlusions of predominantly extracranial arteries cause transient ischemic attacks or cerebral infarcts due to thrombosis, artery-to-artery embolism, or distal hemodynamic perfusion insufficiency.

Endothelial cells and smooth muscle cells make up the cell population of the normal tunica intima. In response to hemodynamic changes in the circulation, hypertensive vascular remodeling may result in medial hypertrophy of these cells. The increase in smooth muscle mass may amplify the vasoconstrictive response to neural and hormonal stimuli and may perpetuate hypertension by accentuating systemic vascular resistance. After prolonged exposure to hypertension, the endothelium becomes functionally abnormal impairing the release of nitric oxide to regulate arterial tone (14,15).

Degenerative changes, such as defective collagen, in the small intracerebral arteries can lead to plasma extravasation and focal brain edema, lacunar infarcts, and intracerebral hemorrhages. Hypertension also predisposes to the formation of saccular aneurysms and, subsequently, subarachnoid hemorrhages.

HYPERTENSION AND LACUNAR INFARCTS

Hypertensive cerebrovascular disease affects mainly the small arteries and arterioles. Lacunar infarcts are usually due to an occlusion of a single perforating artery by a lipohyalinotic process associated with arterial hypertension. Lacunae measure less than 0.3–0.5 cm. Larger lacunae (0.5–1.5 cm) may also be caused by arterial hypertension, but may also be due to cardioembolism or atherosclerosis of a parent vessel of a perforating artery (16).

The major histopathologic features of lacunar disease are hypertrophy of the muscular layers and proliferation of the intima, often with some hyaline changes in the arterial wall. The walls of the vasculature become less compliant and the lumens narrow, impeding blood flow. If flow is sustained below a critical level, the tissue supplied by that vessel becomes ischemic and eventually infarcts. Once infarction occurs, necrotic neurons, glia, and blood vessels are removed by polymorphonuclear leukocytes and macrophages. Removal of the cellular debris is followed by the growth of capillaries and proliferation of reactive astrocytes at the margin of the infarct, ultimately resulting in a cavity surrounded by a zone of gliosis.

HYPERTENSION AND INTRACEREBRAL HEMORRHAGE

Hypertension is the major risk factor for intracerebral hemorrhage and is present in about 50% of patients with intracerebral hemorrhage (17–20). Microaneurysm (Charcot–Bouchard) rupture is believed to be the usual cause of intracerebral hemorrhage associated with hypertension. Microaneurysms arise from the weakened walls of vessels with lipohyalinosis, providing a unifying lesion for lacunar infarcts and hemorrhages. In contrast, Kurata and colleagues reported that hypertension was responsible for only 11% of 80 cases of intracerebral hemorrhages in their series. Vascular malformation was the most common etiology in 68% of their cases (21).

Challa and colleagues provided an alternative explanation when they reported that cerebral micrographs from 35 hypertensive and 20 normotensive patients did not reveal any microaneurysms; instead, vessels contained many tight coils and twists. The investigators postulated that flow through tortuous vessels generates considerable turbulence, which promotes intimal hypertrophy and the development of atherosclerosis (22).

DIRECT IMPACT OF THE HEART ON THE BRAIN

Cerebrovascular disease is associated with various cardiovascular risk factors. The major cardiac sequelae of hyper-

tension include left ventricular hypertrophy (LVH), myocardial infarction, and congestive heart failure (23). All are independent risk factors for cerebrovascular disease. Left ventricular hypertrophy is an ominous result of hypertension and is a serious risk factor for cerebrovascular disease, coronary disease, and cardiac failure. With excessive increase in afterload, preload is inadequate; however, the sympathetic nervous system can be activated to increase contractility. Hypertrophy appears to be the mechanism by which the heart maintains a normal cardiac output when presented with a stress that cannot be easily overcome despite maximal use of preload reserve and autonomic augmentation of contractility. The response to this sustained increase in afterload is ventricular hypertrophy. However, the cost of this compensatory mechanism is high. Similar to hypertension, the development of LVH is often asymptomatic with deadly consequences (24,25). Left ventricular hypertrophy, as evidenced by electrocardiography criteria, is associated with a 3- to 15-fold increase of cardiovascular events, especially cardiac failure and stroke.

The most common clinical manifestations of chronic hypertension are coronary heart disease and congestive heart failure. These long-term effects of hypertension are major causes of mortality in patients with cerebrovascular disease. The underlying causes are contractile impairment due to myocyte loss, reduced compliance due to myocardial fibrosis, and acceleration of atherosclerotic coronary lesions.

TREATMENT STRATEGIES

The results of many major clinical trials provide convincing evidence that judicious treatment of hypertension significantly reduces the rate of morbidity and mortality from stroke (26–32). The primary goals of therapy should be to reverse structural arterial changes and to preserve or restore tissue viability and function. In particular, angiotensin-converting enzyme (ACE) inhibitors can reverse structural arterial changes, increase arterial compliance, and produce a more pronounced decrease in systolic than in diastolic blood pressure (34).

In recent years, experimental studies have shown that regression of hypertensive cardiac hypertrophy can be induced by long-term treatment with ACE inhibitors, calcium channel blockers, β-receptor blockers, and antisympathetic drugs. However, vasodilators and diuretics, which stimulate adrenoreceptor activity and increase angiotensin II levels, were found to be less effective in reversing LVH (33,34).

There is experimental evidence to suggest that sustained activation of the renin-angiotensin system has a proatherogenic effect. Blockade of this system by ACE inhibition in patients with moderate heart failure reduces the rate of myocardial infarction and reinfarction. An activated renin-angiotensin system downregulates the endothelial production of nitric oxide. Nitric oxide exerts many potentially antiatherogenic effects on endothelium, platelets, and low-density lipoproteins. Hypertension-induced chronic distention of elastic arteries upregulates the local renin-angiotensin system in these arteries and thereby downregulates nitric oxide production. Enhanced local synthesis of the trophic factor angiotensin II and reduced production of the antitrophic factor nitric oxide appear to cooperate in the trophic adaptation of the distended vessel wall to the enhanced load but with the disadvantage of enhanced susceptibility of atheroma development. Chronic blockade of the renin-angiotensin system by ACE inhibitors or by angiotensin receptor type 1 antagonists normalizes a reduced endothelial production of nitric oxide in several models, partially by a bradykinin-dependent mechanism (35).

CONCLUSIONS

Approximately 60 million Americans have one or more forms of cardiovascular disease, claiming almost 1 million lives annually (1). Hypertension is the most prevalent and preventable form of cardiovascular disease, affecting one in four U.S. adults. Unfortunately, almost 80% of these persons are on inadequate or no treatment and 35% do not know that they have hypertension. No vascular system is more favorably affected by the control of hypertension than the cerebrovascular system. However, stroke remains a leading cause of mortality in the United States and a leading cause of serious disability. In addition to continuing to raise awareness about cardiovascular diseases, advances in the medical treatment of hypertension based on a better understanding of the underlying mechanisms are vital.

REFERENCES

1. *Heart and Stroke Facts: 1995 Statistical Supplement*. Dallas: American Heart Association, 1995.
2. Bikkina M, Levy D, Evans JC, Larson MG, Benjamin EJ, Wolf PA, Castelli WP. Left ventricular mass and risk of stroke in an elderly cohort. The Framingham Heart Study. *JAMA* 1994;272(1):3–6.
3. SHEP Cooperative Research Group. Prevention of stroke by antihypertensive drug treatment in older persons with isolated systolic hypertension: final results of the Systolic Hypertension in the Elderly Program. *JAMA* 1991;265:3255–3264.
4. Faraci FM, Heistad DD, Regulation of large cerebral arteries and cerebral microvascular pressure. *Circ Res* 1990;66(1):8–17.
5. Conger JD. Endothelial regulation of vascular tone. *Hosp Practice* (Office Edition) 1994;29(10):117–122,125–126.
6. Tolins JP, Shultz PJ, Raij L. Role of endothelium-derived relaxing factor in regulation of vascular tone and remodeling. Update on humoral regulation of vascular tone. *Hypertension* 1991;17 (6 Pt 2): 909–916.
7. Brody JB, Varner KJ, Vasquez EC, Lewis SJ. Central nervous system and pathogenesis of hypertension: sites and mechanisms. *Hypertension* Supplement 1991(18)3:III7–12.
8. Ferrario CM, Averill DB. Do primary dysfunctions in neural control of arterial pressure contribute to hypertension? *Hypertension* 1991;18(3 Suppl):I38–51.
9. Biagioni I, Whetsell WO, Jobe J, Nadeau JH. Baroflex failure in a patient with central nervous system lesions involving the nucleus tractus solitarii. *Hypertension* 1994;23(4):491–5.
10. Johansson BB. Vascular mechanisms in hypertensive cerebrovascular disease. *J Cardiovasc Pharmacol* 1992;19 Suppl 3:S11–15.
11. Harrison DG. Physiological aspects of vascular endothelial cell interac-

tions in hypertension and atherosclerosis. *Acta Anaesthesiol Scand* 1993₅Suppl 99:10–15.
12. Lithell H. Pathogenesis and prevalence of atherosclerosis in hypertensive patients. *Am J Hypertens* 1994;7(7 pt. 2):2S–6S.
13. Bondjers G, Glukhova M, Hansson GK, Postnov YV, Reidy MA, Schwartz SM. Hypertension and atherosclerosis. Cause and effect, or two effects with one unknown cause? *Circulation* 1991;84 (6 Suppl): VI 2–16.
14. Briner VA, Luscher TF. Role of vascular endothelial abnormalities in clinical medicine: atherosclerosis, hypertension, diabetes, and endotoxemia. *Adv Inter Med* 1994;39:1—2.
15. Dzau VJ, Gibbons G. Does hypertension potentiate atherosclerosis via vascular hypertrophy? *J Cardiovasc Pharmacol* 1991;17 Suppl 2:S34.
16. Lodder J, Boiten J. Incidence, natural history, and risk factors in lacunar infarction. *Adv Neurol* 1993;62:213–227.
17. Wityk RJ, Caplan LR. Hypertensive intracerebral hemorrhage. Epidemiology and clinical pathology. *Neurosurgery Clinics of North America*. 1992;3(3):521–532.
18. Sacco SE, Whisnant JP, Broderick JP, Phillips SJ, O'Fallon WM. Epidemiological characteristics of lacunar infarcts in a population. *Stroke* 1991;22(10):1236–1241.
19. Horowitz DR, Tuhrim S, Weinberger JM, Rudolph SH. Mechanisms in lacunar infarction. *Stroke* 1992;23(3):325–327.
20. Dozono K, Ishii N, Nishihara Y, Horie A. An autopsy study of the incidence of lacunes in relation to age, hypertension, and arteriosclerosis. *Stroke* 1991;22(8):993–996.
21. Kurata A, Miyasaka Y, Kitahara T, Kan S, Takagi H. Subcortical cerebral hemorrhage with reference to vascular malformations and hypertension as causes of hemorrhage. *Neurosurgery* 1993;32(4):505–511.
22. Challa VR, Moody DM, Bell MA. The Charcot-Bouchard aneurysm controversy: impact of a new histologic technique. *J Neuropathol Exp Neurol* 1992;51:264–271.
23. Kannel WB. Hypertension as a risk factor for cardiac events—epidemiologic results of long-term studies. *J Cardiovasc Pharmacol* 1993;21 Suppl 2:S27–37.
24. Kannel WB. Left ventricular hypertrophy as a risk factor: the Framingham experience. *J Hypertens* Suppl 1991;9(2):S3–8.
25. Devereux RB, Roman MJ, Ganau A, de Simone G, Okin PM, Kligfield P. Cardiac and arterial hypertrophy and atherosclerosis in hypertension. *Hypertension* 1994;23(6 pt 1):802–809.
26. Veterans Administration Cooperative Study Group on Antihypertensive Agents. Effects of treatment on morbidity in hypertension: results in patients with diastolic blood pressures averaging 115–129 mm Hg. *JAMA* 1967;202:1028–1034.
27. Veterans Administration Cooperative Study Group on Antihypertensive Agents. Effects of treatment on morbidity in hypertension, III: influence of age, diastolic pressure, and prior cardiovascular disease; further analyses of side-effects. *Circulation* 1972;45:991–1004.
28. Management Committee. Treatment of mild hypertension in the elderly. *Med J Aust* 1981;2:398–402.
29. Medical Research Council Working Party. MRC trial of treatment of mild hypertension: principal results. *BMJ* 1985;291:97–104.
30. Daughtery SA, Berman R, Entwisle G, Haerer AF. Cerebrovascular events in Hypertension Detection and Follow-up Program. *Prog Cardiovasc Dis.* 1986; 29(suppl 1):63–72.
31. Hypertension Detection and Follow-Up Cooperative Group. Five-year findings of the Hypertension Detection and Follow-up Program. *JAMA* 1979;242:2562, 2572.
32. National Heart Foundation of Australia. Treatment of mild hypertension in the elderly. *Med J Aust* 1981;247:633.
33. Betocchi S, Chiariello M. Effects of calcium antagonists on left ventricular structure and function. *J Hypertens* Suppl 1993;11(1):S33–-37.
34. Dahlof B. The importance of the renin-angiotensin system in reversal of left ventricular hypertrophy. *J Hypertens* Suppl 1993;11(3):S29–35.
35. Holtz J, Goetz RM. Vascular renin-angiotensin-system, endothelial function and atherosclerosis? *Basic Res Cardiol* 1994;89 Suppl 1: 71–86.
36. Reid JL. Hypertension and the brain. *Br Med Bull* 1994;50(2):371–380.
37. Reid JL. Hypertension and stroke: opportunities for prevention and prospects for protection. *J Hypertens Suppl* 1993;11 Suppl 5:S2–6.
38. Phillips SJ, Whisnant JP. Hypertension and the brain. The National High Blood Pressure Education Program. *Arch Intern Med* 1992; 152(5):938–945.

39. Williams JL, Furlan AJ. Cerebral vascular physiology in hypertensive disease. *Neurosurg Clin North Am* 1992;3(3):509–520.

40. Heistad DD, Baumbach GL. Cerebral vascular changes during chronic hypertension: good guys and bad guys. *J Hypertens* Suppl 1992;10(7): S71–75.

41. Naraghi R, Gaab MR, Walter GF, Kleineberg B. Arterial hypertension and neurovascular compression at the ventrolateral medulla. A comparative microanatomical and pathological study. *J Neurosurg* 1992;77(1): 103–112.

42. Strandgaard S, Paulson OB. Cerebrovascular consequences of hypertension. *Lancet* 1994;344 (8921):519–521.

43. Lodder J, Bamford JM, Sandercock PA, Jones LN, Warlow CP. Are hypertension or cardiac embolism likely causes of lacunar infarction? *Stroke* 1990;21(3):375–381.

44. Georgiou D, Brundage BH. Regression of left ventricular mass in systemic hypertension. *Clin Cardiol* 1992;15(1):5–16.

45. Franks PF, Bulpitt PF, Hartley K, Bulpitt CJ. Myocardial infarction and stroke during treatment of hypertensive patients with different diuretic regimens. *J Hum Hypertens* 1991;5(1):45–77.

46. Shimada K, Miyashita H, Kawamoto A, Matsubayashi K. Nishinaga M, Kimura S, Ozawa T. Pathophysiology and end-organ damage in elderly hypertensives. *J Hypertens* Suppl 1994;12(6):S7–12.

47. Alter M, Friday G, Lai SM, O'Connell J, Sobel E. Hypertension and risk of stroke recurrence. *Stroke* 1994;25(8):1605–1610.

48. Simon AC, Pithois-Merli I, Levenson J. Physiopharmacological approach to mechanical factors of hypertension in the atherosclerotic process. *J Hum Hypertens* 1991;5 Suppl 1:15–21.

49. Campbell JH, Tachas G, Black MJ, Cockerill G, Campbell GR. Molecular biology of vascular hypertrophy. *Basic Res Cardiol* 1991;86 Suppl 1:3–11.

50. Pauletto P. Scannapieco G. Pessina AC. Sympathetic drive and vascular damage in hypertension and atherosclerosis. *Hypertension* 1991;17 (4 Suppl):III75–81.

51. MacMahon S. Blood pressure reduction and the prevention of stroke. *J Hypertens* Suppl 1991;9(7):S7–10.

Cerebrovascular Disease, edited by H. Hunt Batjer.
Lippincott-Raven Publishers, Philadelphia © 1997.

CHAPTER 7

Pathology of Hypertensive Cerebral Angiopathy

Khang-Loon Ho and Julio H. Garcia

Arterial hypertension (HTN), defined in different ways by various investigators, is a major risk factor for stroke (1). Many clinicopathologic studies suggest that HTN is causally associated with about 50% of all intracerebral hemorrhages (ICHs) (2). But by what mechanism? Attempts to answer this question have focused on analysis of the pathoanatomic changes induced by chronic HTN; the reason for this is that these changes are more amenable to structural evaluation than the pathophysiologic mechanism of the acute phase of HTN. Our understanding of the mechanism by which chronic HTN alters the normal central nervous system (CNS) circulation derives from epidemiologic investigations, autopsy studies, and clinical trials. The development of new imaging techniques, such as positron emission tomography (PET) and diffusion-weighted magnetic resonance imaging (DW-MRI), and the availability of animal models of HTN permit rigorous scientific study of the effects of acute HTN on the CNS vasculature. As a result of these observations, some of the traditional interpretations of the HTN-related phenomena have been drastically modified.

Arterial HTN affects in the brain primarily the resistance vessels or small arteries (<200 μm in diameter) that undergo segmental constriction in response to sustained increases in intraluminal pressure. The long-term effect of this constriction is the replacement of the smooth muscle cells by collagen fibers. This change is thought to be related to abnormalities in endothelial permeability that lead to one of two undesirable results: leakage of circulating macromolecules or development of brain edema as a result of abnormalities in the mechanisms controlling water transport. The various derangements responsible for the occurrence of brain edema, brain hemorrhage, and leakage of circulating macromolecules, although ultimately related to abnormalities involving intraparenchymal arterioles, may occur independently of one

another and in response to diverse neurogenic, mechanical, and chemical effectors.

The material covered in this chapter is divided into two parts; the initial portion summarizes information pertaining to the definition of structural abnormalities, attributed to HTN, involving intraparenchymal cerebral blood vessels. After a brief mention of the brain parenchymal lesions that accompany hypertensive arteriopathies, we summarize important modern mechanistic concepts that are derived primarily from animal observations.

ARTERIAL AND ARTERIOLAR DISEASE (SMALL BLOOD VESSEL DISEASE OR MICROANGIOPATHY)

A wealth of epidemiologic evidence indicates that HTN is the most important modifiable risk factor for transient ischemic attacks, ischemic stroke, and focal intracerebral hemorrhage. Epidemiologic observations and laboratory experimentation show that HTN predisposes to stroke by (a) accelerating atherosclerosis in the aortic arch and in the large cervicocranial arteries, (b) causing structural alterations in the small-diameter penetrating cerebral arterioles, and (c) promoting cardiac diseases that may be complicated by stroke. Chronic diabetes mellitus and advanced aging aggravate the progress of HTN-related processes. The prevalence of cerebral infarcts and hemorrhages, and the severity of the resulting neurologic deficits, have decreased significantly over the past two decades, presumably because of the aggressive treatment of asymptomatic HTN.

Cerebral arteriolosclerosis describes structural changes affecting perforating arterial vessels (<500 μm in diameter), such as the lenticulostriate branches of the anterior and middle cerebral arteries and the thalamoperforating branches of the basilar artery (3). Two types of arterial vessels penetrate the brain: (a) Those endowed with an internal elastic lamina

K.-L. Ho and J. H. Garcia: Department of Pathology, Henry Ford Hospital, Detroit, Michigan 48202.

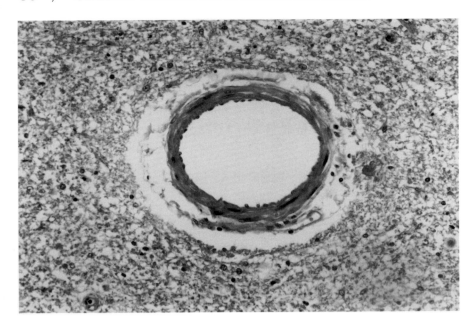

FIG. 1. Normal penetrating brain arteriole without internal elastic lamina and with a tunica media composed of one to two layers of smooth muscle cells. (Hematoxylin-eosin ×33.)

and a tunica media composed of three or four layers of smooth muscle cells are called arteries; their internal diameter ranges between 100 and 400 μm. (b) Those devoid of continuous elastic lamina and having a tunica media composed of one or two layers of smooth muscle cells are called arterioles (Fig. 1); most arterioles measure 100 μm or less in diameter. Both penetrating arteries and arterioles arise directly from large parent arteries such as the basilar artery whose diameter can be as large as 6–8 mm. Long penetrating arteries, destined to the deep brain structures, do not anastomose with neighboring arteries; this pattern of nonanastomosing vessel is called "end artery." The anatomic characteristics of these vessels may expose them to intraluminal pressures that scarcely reach arteries or arterioles of similar caliber located in the cerebral cortex (4). Cortical vessels are thought to be protected from abrupt pressure changes by a gradual stepdown in the caliber of their parent vessels. This difference may account for the low incidence of hypertensive arteriopathic changes in the superficial cerebral vessels (5).

MICROATHEROMA

In patients with chronic HTN, the perforating arteries are typically involved by atherosclerosis, a process characterized by subintimal proliferation of fibroblasts and deposits of lipid-laden macrophages (microatheroma). In contrast, perforating arterioles are susceptible to developing structural changes that involve the smooth muscle cells of the tunica media. Atherosclerosis of the cervico-cranial arteries in most normotensive persons involves the origin of the internal carotid arteries, the basilar artery, and the proximal portion of the middle cerebral arteries. Among hypertensives and diabetics microatheroma may spread distally to the small cerebral arteries located over the convexity of the hemi-

spheres; chronic, advanced HTN is accompanied by the formation of atheromatous plaques that sometimes involve the orifice and initial segment of penetrating arteries with a diameter of 300–700 μm (Fig. 2). Lenticulostriate branches, thalamogeniculate branches, anterior choroidal artery, Heubner's recurrent artery, thalamoperforating branches, and paramedian and short circumferential basilar artery branches are all susceptible to developing microatheroma. The lumen of the involved artery is either narrowed or occluded by an atheromatous plaque that may be located within the parent artery blocking the branch orifice, extend into the branch from the parent artery (junctional plaque), or originate at the branch's orifice (6). Microdissection, hemorrhage within plaques (Fig. 3), and platelet and platelet-fibrin plugs could all play roles in narrowing or obstructing the penetrating branches and causing lacunar infarcts. This type of stenosis or occlusion affecting penetrating arteries was identified in 6 of 11 small blood vessels located near capsular lacunar infarcts studied in serial sections (7).

LIPOHYALINOSIS

Fisher introduced the term *lipohyalinosis* to include all previously used designations: fibrinoid necrosis, hyaline atherosclerosis, atherosclerosis of small arteries, hyaline change, plasmatic vascular destruction, hyalinosis, angioneurosis, and fibrinoid arteritis (8,9). Lipohyalinosis therefore includes a continuum of structural alterations that stretch from the earliest thickening of the vessel wall to progressive narrowing, thrombosis, and fibrinoid necrosis. Lipohyalinosis is closely related to the hypertensive vascular lesions seen elsewhere in the body rather than being a hypertensive lesion unique to the brain. The structural changes of lipohyalinosis involve the cerebral penetrating arterial ves-

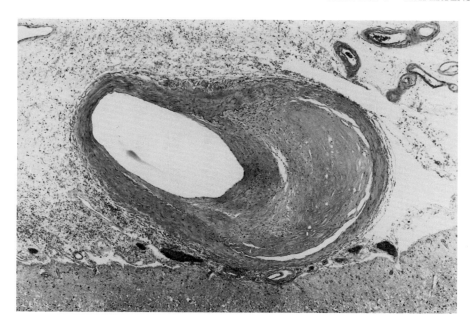

FIG. 2. Microatheroma in a penetrating artery. The plaque is located near the take off from the parent artery and the eccentric growth of the plaque has narrowed the lumen. (Hematoxylin-eosin ×5.)

sels; the lesions have combined features of both arterial (lipidoses, atheroma) (Figs. 4 and 5) and arteriolar (hyalinization) (Fig. 6) disease.

''Hyaline'' describes the glassy, acellular appearance of the vessel wall as seen by conventional light microscopy. The tunica media is thickened by deposits of connective tissue, particularly collagen, and by accumulations of plasma protein. This combination of lesions in a single vascular bed reflects the fact that the progression of both processes (hyalinization and atheromatous lipid deposit) is influenced by a common factor, ie, arterial HTN. The diameter of the

penetrating arteries involved by lipohyalinosis ranges from 80 to 300 μm, and the sites where these changes are most common include caudate, putamen, thalamus, internal capsule, pons, and cerebellum; these are the same sites where hypertensive hemorrhages and lacunar infarctions are most common.

FIBRINOID NECROSIS

The occurrence of fibrinoid necrosis and lipohyalinosis in the cerebral vessels has different implications. Lipohya-

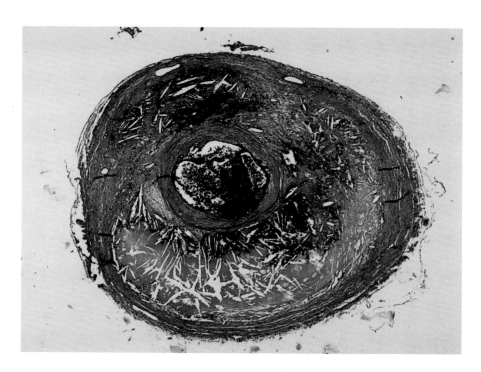

FIG. 3. Hemorrhage within the atheromatous material of a penetrating artery showing marked concentric narrowing of the lumen. (Hematoxylin-eosin × 8.)

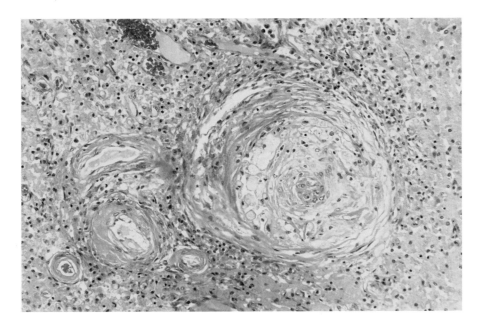

FIG. 4. Lipohyalinosis in a penetrating artery of the lenticulostriate group. The lumen of the largest vessel in this photomicrograph is almost completely obliterated by an aggregate of lipid-laden macrophages. (Hematoxylin-eosin ×40.)

linosis is common in chronic, longstanding HTN, whereas fibrinoid necrosis is seen only in acute, malignant HTN. Fibrinoid necrosis describes a bright, eosinophilic, finely granular material deposited in the tunica media of intraparenchymal arteries (Fig. 7). The deposit represents a combination of necrotic smooth muscle cells and extravasated plasma proteins. The mechanism by which fibrinoid necrosis develops may involve impairment of the cerebral autoregulation as a result of sustained HTN; this loss of autoregulation may lead to a subsequent breakdown of the blood–brain barrier accompanied by necrosis of the smooth muscle layers. Fibrinoid necrosis involving cerebral arterioles is the most characteristic vascular change observed in patients with hy-

pertensive encephalopathy. In this condition, the vascular changes involving the brain parallel in frequency, severity, and type those present in the arterioles of the kidney and the retina. Similar types of changes, including fibrinoid necrosis and fibrin thrombosis, occur in the cerebral microvessels of spontaneously hypertensive rats (10).

MICROANEURYSM

Several studies completed during the past 100 years have clarified various aspects of the cerebral miliary aneurysms (microaneurysms), originally described by Charcot and

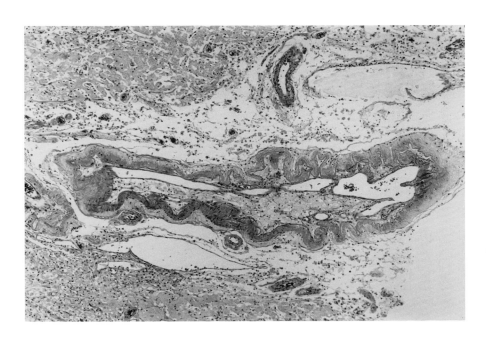

FIG. 5. Longitudinal section of a penetrating artery showing segmental adhesions of the vessel wall (probably remnants of a thrombus) and irregular narrowing of the lumen secondary to extensive subintimal lipid deposits. (Hematoxylin-eosin ×16.)

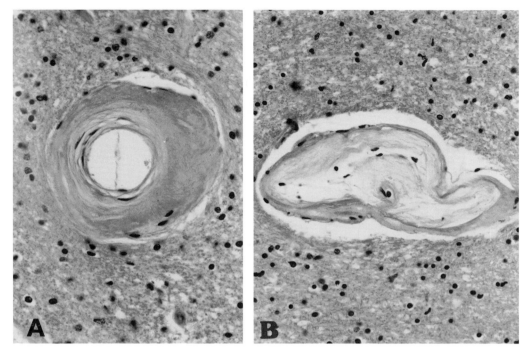

FIG. 6. Hyalinosis in penetrating arterioles has resulted in concentric narrowing of the lumen **(A)** and complete luminal occlusion **(B)**. (Hematoxylin-eosin ×80.)

Bouchard in 1868, as being a common finding in the brains of hypertensive patients; however, several points remain controversial. Fisher (9) classified cerebral microaneurysms, associated with hypertension, into four types: (a) Miliary saccular aneurysms (300–1100 μm in diameter) involve arteries measuring 40–100 μm in diameter (Fig. 8). These aneurysms are symmetric, their walls are devoid of endothelial lining, and the sac's wall is composed of a thin layer

of collagenous fibers. These aneurysms are most frequently found in the same areas where intracerebral hemorrhage is common. (b) Miliary aneurysms occur in vessels with lipohyalinosis (lipohyalinotic aneurysm) (Fig. 9); they have variable shape, ie, can be fusiform or globular, symmetric or asymmetric. These aneurysms can involve either the entire circumference of a vessel or only a segment. The dilated portion of the vascular wall may measure up to ten times

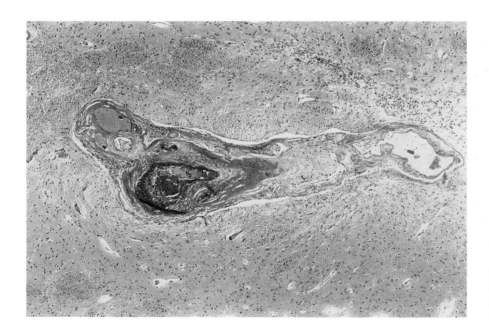

FIG. 7. Lipohyalinosis in a penetrating arteriole of the thalamoperforating group with superimposed fibrinoid necrosis. (Hematoxylin-eosin ×10.)

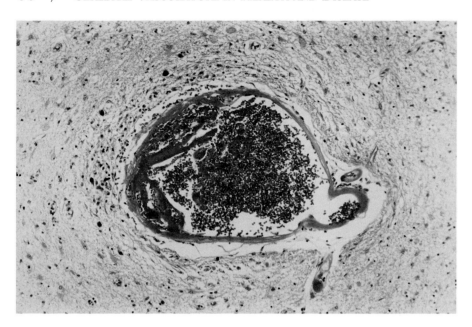

FIG. 8. Saccular microaneurysm with extravasated red blood cells, hemosiderin pigment, and astrogliosis of the surrounding brain parenchyma. (Hematoxylin-eosin ×33.)

the diameter of the parent artery. The involved vessels range between 80 and 300 μm in diameter; however, the aneurysms' actual size ranges from 0.5 mm to 1.5 mm. The involved vascular wall is thickened (hyalinized) and a dilated lumen is usually not visible. Lipohyalinotic microaneurysms are common in the cerebral cortex and are especially numerous in the boundary zones between adjacent major arterial territories. These aneurysms are often associated with deposits of hemosiderin pigment in the surrounding tissues, suggesting the previous occurrence of small leakages of blood from the aneurysm; the role of these aneurysms causing massive hypertensive hemorrhage remains unclear.

(d) Fusiform miliary aneurysms (Fig. 10) are found in penetrating arteries with an average diameter of 150 μm. The thin-walled sac, measuring up to 700–800 μm in diameter, is usually filled with fresh fibrin thrombi. Fusiform aneurysms are seldom associated with hypertensive intracerebral hemorrhages. (d) Bleeding globes, fibrin globes, or pseudoaneurysms consist of masses of red blood cells and platelets wrapped in concentric layers of fibrin and reticulin (collagen) fibers (Fig. 11), thus remaining attached to the tunica adventitia of leaky arteries. The fibrin probably serves as a limiting membrane that tethers the bleeding globe to the parent artery. These fibrin globes are chiefly found in the

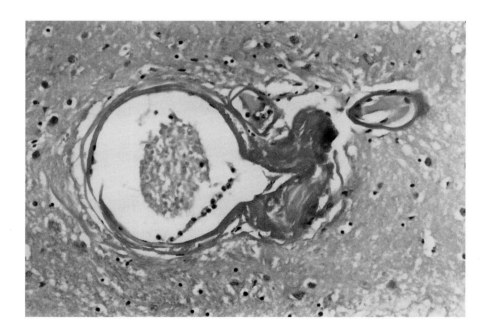

FIG. 9. Lipohyalinotic microaneurysm arising from an arteriole with severe mural hyalinosis. (Hematoxylin-eosin ×60.)

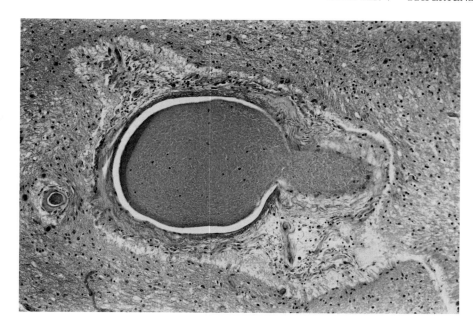

FIG. 10. This type of symmetric thin-walled aneurysm (about 600 μm in diameter) probably is not associated with arterial hypertension. (Hematoxylin-eosin ×5.)

region where large intracerebral hemorrhages are common and often are located near sites of angionecrosis or fibrinoid necrosis. The diameter of bleeding globes ranges from 0.3 mm to 1 cm.

Although the existence of the microaneurysms associated with HTN has been challenged, several studies have shown a correlation between the sites where intracerebral hemorrhages are common and the topographic distribution of microaneurysms (11,12). However, the prevalence of microaneurysms of the Charcot–Bouchard type has been disputed; using a histochemical stain that labels endothelial cells with a radiodense lead sulfide precipitate, together with microradiography, Challa et al. (13) concluded that microaneurysms are uncommon; these authors opine that vessels with coils, twists, and overlapping loops have been radiographically misinterpreted as microaneurysms.

PARENCHYMAL BRAIN LESIONS IN ARTERIAL HYPERTENSION

Large brain infarcts among hypertensives are more common at those sites where atheromatous changes are more severe. Large infarcts in the brainstem (with special involvement of the pons) can be a frequent complication of atherosclerosis of the basilar artery.

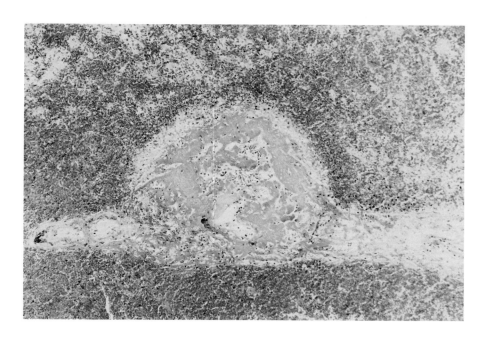

FIG. 11. This bleeding globe (fibrin globe) was found at the periphery of a large intracerebral hemorrhage in a hypertensive patient. (Hematoxylin-eosin ×25.)

Small brain infarcts (<1.5 cm in diameter) are common at locations where small blood vessel disease is frequent; these sites include the basal ganglia, the thalamic nuclei, the internal capsule, the pons, and the corona radiata. Because of their small size, these deep-seated infarcts may not be clearly visible in neuroimaging studies until they become cavitary. Their cavitary appearance may account for their designation as lacunar lesions; *lacuna* (Greek meaning a hole, a gape, or a hiatus) is a descriptive pathologic term whose current use can be traced to Fisher (8). The uncritical and therefore confusing use of the term lead Poirier and others (14) to distinguish three types of lacunae: type I corresponds to old and small infarcts (<15–20 mm in diameter), made of irregular cavities and surrounded by astrocytic gliosis; type II corresponds to old, small hemorrhages (<15–20 mm in diameter); these are cavities with relatively smooth edges containing hemosiderin-laden macrophages; and type III lacunae are dilated perivascular spaces that are centered by one or more normal or hyalinized arterioles. Etat lacunaire (lacunar status) is the French designation for a structural abnormality consisting of multiple type I lacunae that are usually located in either the basal ganglia or the thalamus. In contrast, état criblé applies to a lesion in which numerous type III lacunae are confluent (Fig. 12). These two conditions may coexist in the same specimen. In two autopsy studies, over 50% of the brain specimens with lacunar infarcts had multiple small lesions in the deeper structures of the brain (15,16).

Lacunar infarcts are thought to result from obstruction of a single penetrating artery; the resulting clinical manifestations vary widely (17,18). Fisher distinguished two causes of local small vessel obstruction: lipohyalinosis, mainly found in hypertensive patients with small, multiple, and usually asymptomatic lacunae; and microatheromatous disease, which occurred in cases with larger, usually symptomatic lacunae (7,18,19). Caplan also drew attention to the microatheromatous cause of small vessel obstruction, particularly at or near the orifices (6). The limited pathologic evidence available suggests that microatheroma is the most frequent cause of symptomatic individual lacunar infarcts (6,7,17–20). Microatheroma and lipohyalinosis are considered the reactions elicited by different parts of the arterial system to different degrees or different durations of HTN, although the association with HTN is less convincing in cases of single symptomatic lacunae than in cases of lacunar state. Two clinically distinct lacunar infarct entities have been recognized and the role of HTN in the genesis of lacunar infarct has recently been questioned (21,22). Embolism originating from cardiac, aortic, and carotid sources is a potential cause of lacunar infarction; this observation was prompted by the fact that HTN was not evident in a substantial number of patients with lacunar infarcts (12,22,23).

Intracerebral hemorrhages are also common among patients with HTN (12,24). Large intracerebral hemorrhages usually produce devastating clinical manifestations. Small intracerebral hemorrhage (<1.5 cm in diameter) may produce discrete clinical syndromes often mimicking classic lacunar syndromes (24). The sites where these hemorrhages tend to occur are the same where arteriolosclerosis is frequent and where lacunar lesions are found: basal ganglia, thalamus, pons, cerebellum, and deep cerebral white matter. One hundred years after the original publication by Charcot and Bouchard followed by clinical, histopathologic, and epidemiologic studies, many questions remain concerning the cause of hypertensive brain hemorrhages. None of the proposed causes of hypertensive brain hemorrhage such as preceding brain infarct, circulating angionecrotic factor, rupture of vein, coalescence of petechiae, and effects of angiospasm

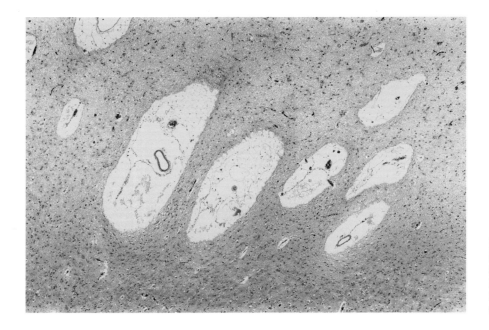

FIG. 12. The cribriform state (état criblé) of the cerebral white matter corresponds to a cluster of dilated perivascular spaces, each containing one or two hyalinized arterioles. (Hematoxylin-eosin ×10.)

have found universal acceptance. Strong circumstantial evidence for the relationship between hypertensive brain hemorrhage and microaneurysms was provided by a study of hypertensive ($n = 100$) and normotensive ($n = 100$) brains (11). Microaneurysms existed in 46 of the hypertensive and 7 of the nonhypertensive individuals. Furthermore, both microaneurysms and hemorrhages occurred predominantly in hypertensives; aneurysms were found in each patient with hemorrhage, and aneurysms and hematomas had a common topographic distribution in the brain.

The results of serial brain sections obtained from samples of two patients who died with hypertensive brain hemorrhage were reported by Fisher (9). He did not find support for aneurysms as the cause of the hemorrhages and noted: "The conclusion must be drawn that the same type of hypertensive vascular disease (lipohyalinosis) under some circumstances evokes ischemia and under others tends to bleeding." Electron microscopy (25), immunohistochemical, and high-resolution microangiographic studies (13) have all questioned the relationship between microaneurysms and hypertensive brain hemorrhage.

SUBCORTICAL LEUKOENCEPHALOPATHY

HTN is thought to play a pathogenetic role in the development of periventricular white matter lesions by promoting arteriolosclerosis, which in turn impairs autoregulation, rendering the periventricular white matter vulnerable to ischemia during episodes of relative hypoperfusion (26). The advent of improved neuroimaging methods has resulted in the frequent detection of cerebral white matter alterations, which are especially common among persons older than 60 years; the descriptive term *leukoaraiosis* has been suggested for white matter changes that are visible either with computed tomography (CT) or with MRI (27,28).

Morphologists have long recognized the existence of these changes under the designation of subcortical leukoencephalopathy. The pathologic features of this condition include diffuse rarefaction of the white matter with sparing of the subcortical U fibers. The pattern of myelin "loss" and oligodendroglial disintegration can be homogeneous or patchy and is mostly symmetric in the two hemispheres. There might be numerous small infarcts as well as perivascular dilatation (état criblé) varying from a few millimeters to a centimeter in diameter; these lesions are frequently scattered throughout the white matter. Severe microangiopathy of the small arteries and arterioles (ie, lipohyalinosis) is frequently observed in the white matter and basal ganglia. In addition to arterial HTN, several conditions have been associated with this white matter abnormality; these include radiation encephalopathy and cerebral amyloid angiopathy. The common link among these entities is believed to be arteriolosclerosis, a condition that is thought to induce subliminal and intermittent ischemia to the white matter; leakage of circulating macromolecules may constitute an added factor causing white matter injury. In addition to the vascular changes, episodic hypotensive crises, as may occur in patients suffering from congestive heart failure, could render the periventricular white matter sufficiently hypoperfused as to induce the structural changes typical of subcortical leukoencephalopathy.

In addition to localized brain lesions, high-blood pressure crises may also induce generalized brain disturbances in a clinical syndrome of hypertensive encephalopathy (HEP) (1,5,29). Uncommon since the advent of effective antihypertensive therapy, HEP occurs as a result of a sudden, sustained rise in blood pressure above the upper limits of cerebral autoregulation. Causes of HEP include acute glomerulonephritis, renal vascular HTN, chronic renal failure, and abrupt blood pressure rises (characteristically on the order of 250/150 mm Hg) in patients with chronic HTN. The clinical manifestations of HEP are severe headache, impaired consciousness, nausea and vomiting, vision disturbances, fleeting focal neurologic symptoms, seizures, and retinopathy (papilledema, hemorrhages, and exudates). CT and MRI findings include diffuse or multifocal edema, small ischemic infarcts, and an occasional intracerebral hemorrhage or a large cerebral infarct. The pathologic changes observed in autopsy specimens represent the extreme in a spectrum of abnormalities: fibrinoid necrosis of arterioles, thrombosis of arterioles and capillaries, microinfarcts, and petechiae. The brainstem is most severely affected; this is followed by the basal ganglia, the cerebral white matter, the cerebral cortex, and the spinal cord (5). Vascular and brain parenchymal lesions of a comparable nature and severity have been observed in spontaneously hypertensive stroke-prone rats (30).

PATHOPHYSIOLOGY OF THE MICROCIRCULATION IN ARTERIAL HYPERTENSION

The cerebral microcirculation may be involved in arterial HTN, directly or indirectly, by several functional abnormalities that induce structural alterations and alter the regulatory mechanisms of brain perfusion (31). The cerebral microcirculation is regulated by various complex mechanisms that include (a) neurogenic influence mediated by adrenergic vasoconstrictor and vasodilator fibers; (b) chemical regulation involving circulating metabolites in particular CO_2; (c) myogenic responses to changes in intravascular pressure; and (d) myogenic responses to metabolic changes in neural tissue.

Chronic HTN produces hypertrophy of the tunica muscularis of the arteries and arterioles, probably through the trophic effect of the sympathetic nervous system (32,33). Medial hypertrophy increases vascular wall thickness and reduces the diameter of the vascular lumen. These vascular changes are advantageous in enhancing the capacity to withstand a high intramural pressure by reducing tension in arterial walls, maintaining autoregulation of cerebral blood flow, and preserving the integrity of the blood–brain barrier. Focal disturbances of the blood–brain barrier occur when these adaptive mechanisms are no longer sufficient to compensate for the increased pressure. The extravasation of plasma constituents is an important step in the development of degenerative changes in the arterial wall.

The cerebral endothelium may become abnormally permeable to circulating macromolecules by several mechanisms (34):

1. *Enhanced transcytosis.* As demonstrated by quantitative studies conducted in several experimental models of arterial hypertension, twice as many endothelial vesicles exist in permeable arteriolar segments as there are in the nonpermeable vascular segments.
2. *Opening of endothelial junctional sites.* Passage of plasma proteins between endothelial junctions is a rare occurrence in the early phase of arterial HTN.
3. *Tubular channels.* During periods of increased protein permeability, pinocytotic vesicles may fuse to form transendothelial tubular channels that serve as a conduit for the transfer of proteins from the luminal to the abluminal side.
4. *Loss of the net negative charge of the endothelium,* particularly the terminal sialic acid group on the luminal side of the plasma membrane. The breakdown of the blood–brain barrier to proteins allows blood constituents to interact directly with constituents of the tunica media. Of special importance are substances that may be released from platelets such as thromboxane and serotonin (35); both of these compounds have a vasoconstrictor effect.

Forty percent of the total vascular resistance in the CNS can be traced to the intraparenchymal arteries measuring >200 μm in diameter. Chronic HTN increases the resistance in these vessels while it protects the arterioles and capillaries. Cerebral blood flow does not change in chronic HTN; this is probably explained by the dual effect of angiotensin, which simultaneously induces constriction and dilatation of arterial microvessels. Once the autoregulatory responses are exhausted on the basis of chronic arterial HTN, cerebral arteries dilate; deleterious effects such as altered endothelial permeability may begin during this stage of vasodilation.

Recent studies have shown that endothelial cells can release substances with vasoactive properties (31). Activation of these endothelial mechanisms triggers release of substances that produce local vasodilatation [endothelium-derived relaxing factors (EDRF)] or those that induce vasoconstriction [endothelium-derived constricting factors (EDCF)] in arteries and arterioles of the brain. In chronic HTN, these mechanisms are impaired and create an imbalance between vasorelaxing and vasoconstricting factors that favors vasoconstriction. Alterations in endothelial vasoactive mechanisms during chronic HTN may contribute to increased incidence of vasospasm, ischemia, and stroke during chronic HTN (36).

Given the same type of arterial occlusion, brain infarcts are more common and larger in hypertensive animals than in appropriately matched normotensive controls. This is thought to be a reflection of the altered responses that collateral anastomic vessels develop in chronic hypertensive subjects (37). The combination of impairment of endothelial activation mechanism with the altered collateral anastomosis may conspire to increase the size of an ischemic brain lesion induced by hypoperfusion whether occlusive or hypotensive in origin (37).

REFERENCES

1. Phillips SJ, Whisnant JP. Hypertension and the brain. *Arch Intern Med* 1992;152:938–945.
2. Wityk RJ, Caplan LR. Hypertensive intracerebral hemorrhage. Epidemiology and clinical pathology. *Neurosurg Clin North Am* 1992;3:521–532.
3. Pullicino PM. The course and territories of cerebral small arteries. In: Pullicino PM, Caplan LT, Hommel M, eds. *Cerebral small artery disease.* Advances in neurology vol 62. New York: Raven Press, 1993;11–39.
4. Harper SL, Bohlen HG. Microvascular adaptation in cerebral cortex of adult spontaneously hypertensive rats. *Hypertension* 1984;6:408–419.
5. Chester EM, Agamanolis DP, Banker Q, Victor M. Hypertensive encephalopathy: a clinicopathologic study of 20 cases. *Neurology* 1978;28:928–939.
6. Caplan LS. Intracranial branch atheromatous disease: a neglected, understudied, and underused concept. *Neurology* 1989;39:1246–1250.
7. Fisher CM. Capsular infarcts. The underlying vascular lesions. *Arch Neurol* 1979;36:65–73.
8. Fisher CM. Lacunes, small deep cerebral infarcts. *Neurology* 1965;15:774–784.
9. Fisher CM. Cerebral miliary aneurysms in hypertension. *Am J Pathol* 1971;66:313–330.
10. Ogata J, Fujishima M, Tamaki K, et al. Stroke-prone spontaneously hypertensive rats as an experimental model of malignant hypertension. *Acta Neuropathol* 1980;51:179–184.
11. Cole FM, Yates PO. Pseudo-aneurysms in relationship to massive cerebral hemorrhage. *J Neurol Neurosurg Psychiatry* 1967;30:61–66.
12. Caplan LR. Hypertensive intracerebral hemorrhage. In: Kase CS, Caplan LR, eds. *Intracerebral hemorrhage.* Boston: Butterworth-Heinemann, 1994;99–116.
13. Challa VR, Moody DM, Bell MA. The Charcot–Bouchard aneurysm controversy: impact of a new histologic technique. *J Neuropathol Exp Neurol* 1992;51:264–271.
14. Poirier J, Derouesne C. Le concept de lacune cérébrale de 1838 â nos jours. *Rev Neurol* 1985;141:3–17.
15. Chamorro A, Sacco RL, Mohr TR, et al. Clinical-computed tomographic correlations of lacunar infarction in the Stroke Data Bank. *Stroke* 1991;22:175–181.
16. Dozono K, Ishii N, Nishihara Y, Horil A. An autopsy study of the incidence of lacunes in relation to age, hypertension, and arteriosclerosis. *Stroke* 1991;22:993–996.
17. Fisher CM. Thalamic pure sensory stroke: a pathologic study. *Neurology* 1978;28:1141–1144.
18. Fisher CM. Lacunar strokes and infarcts: a review. *Neurology* 1982;32:65–73.
19. Fisher CM. The arterial lesions underlying lacunes. *Acta Neuropathol* 1969;12:1–15.
20. Fisher CM. Bilateral occlusion of basilar artery branches. *J Neurol Neurosurg Psychiatry* 1977;40:1182–1189.
21. Boiten J, Lodder J, Kessels F. Two clinically distinct lacunar infarct entities. A hypothesis. *Stroke* 1993;24:652–656.
22. Lodder J, Boiten J. Incidence, nature, history, and risk factors in lacunar infarction. In: Pullicino PM, Caplan LT, Hommel M, eds. *Cerebral small artery disease.* Advances in neurology vol. 62. New York: Raven Press, 1993:213–228.
23. Kappelle LJ, Van Gijn J. Lacunar infarcts. *Clin Neurol Neurosurg* 1986;88:3–17.

24. Kim JS, Lee JH, Lee MC. Small primary intracerebral hemorrhage. Clinical presentation of 28 cases. *Stroke* 1994;25:1500–1506.

25. Takebayashi S, Kaneko M. Electron microscopic studies of ruptured arteries in hypertensive intracerebral hemorrhage. *Stroke* 1983;14: 28–36.

26. Matsushita K, Kurijama Y, Nagatsuka K, Nakamura M, Sawada T, Omal T. Periventricular white matter lucency and cerebral blood flow autoregulation in hypertensive patients. *Hypertension* 1994;23: 565–568.

27. Hachinski VC, Potter P, Merskey H. Leuko-araiosis. *Arch Neurol* 1987; 44:21–23.

28. Van Swieten JC, Van den Hout JHW, Van Ketel BA, Hijdia A, Wokke JHJ, Van Gijn J. Periventricular lesions in the white matter on magnetic resonance imaging in the elderly: a morphometric correlation with arteriolar sclerosis and dilated perivascular spaces. *Brain* 1991;114: 761–774.

29. Healton EB, Brust JC, Feinfeld DA, et al. Hypertensive encephalopathy and the neurologic manifestations of malignant hypertension. *Neurology* 1982;32:127–132.

30. Fredriksson K, Nordborg C, Kalimo H, et al. Cerebral microangiopathy in stroke-prone spontaneously hypertensive rats. *Acta Neuropathol* 1988;75:241–252.

31. Williams JL, Furlan AJ. Cerebral vascular physiology in hypertensive disease. *Neurosurg Clin North Am* 1992;3:509–520.

32. Baumbach GL, Heistad DD. Remodeling of cerebral arterioles in chronic hypertension. *Hypertension* 1989;13:968–972.

33. Baumbach GL, Mayhan WG, Heistad DD. Protective effects of sympathetic nerves during hypertension. In: Owman C, Hardebo JE, eds. *Neurol regulation of brain circulation*. Cambridge: Elsevier, 1986; 607–615.

34. Nag S. Morphologic aspects of blood–brain barrier dysfunction. *Proceedings XIth International Congress of Neuropathology* Sasaki Printing and Publishing Co. Ltd. Tokyo, Japan. 1990;769–772.

35. Nayhan WG, Faraci FM, Heistad DD. Responses of cerebral arterioles to adenosine 5'-diphosphate, serotonin, and the thromboxane analogue U-46619 during chronic hypertension. *Hypertension* 1988;12:556–561.

36. Heistad DD, Lopez JAG, Baumbach GL. Hemodynamic determinants of vascular changes in hypertension and atherosclerosis. *Hypertension* 1991;17:3–7.

37. Baumbach GL, Heistad DD. Cerebral circulation in chronic arterial hypertension. *Hypertension* 1988;12:89–95.

Cerebrovascular Disease, edited by H. Hunt Batjer.
Lippincott-Raven Publishers, Philadelphia © 1997.

CHAPTER 8

Hypertensive Encephalopathy

Robert J. Wityk and Michael S. Pessin

Hypertensive encephalopathy refers to a constellation of generalized and focal neurologic symptoms associated with severe, sustained hypertension that completely or partially resolves upon lowering of blood pressure. Headache, confusion, visual disturbances, convulsions, and papilledema are common manifestations of the disorder. The term *hypertensive encephalopathy* was first used by Oppenheimer and Fishberg in 1928 in describing a patient with transient neurologic symptoms associated with surges of markedly elevated blood pressure (1). Volhard had earlier proposed that severe hypertension was the cause of uremic convulsions and distinguished this syndrome from other neurologic complications of the uremia (2). Subsequent authors, however, were less precise and studies of hypertensive encephalopathy often included patients with hypertension associated with acute ischemic or hemorrhagic stroke. A clearer picture has emerged from pathologic studies and the widespread clinical use of computed tomography (CT) and magnetic resonance imaging (MRI) to identify associated structural lesions.

With the advent of effective antihypertensive therapy, hypertensive encephalopathy should be rare. There are few epidemiologic studies of hypertensive encephalopathy, however, to document the incidence of this condition or trends over time. Jellinek mentions in 1964 that hypertensive encephalopathy was becoming a rarity due to the lessening incidence of acute nephritis (3). In 1982, Healton reported only 5 patients with hypertensive encephalopathy (of 34 patients with malignant hypertension) seen over a 3-year period (4). National statistics, however, show an increase in hospital admissions in the 1980s for malignant hypertension (5).

Increasingly, other conditions associated with elevated

blood pressure or focally increased cerebral perfusion are recognized as having features similar to hypertensive encephalopathy (6). Eclampsia, for example, has been considered as a form of hypertensive encephalopathy. The hyperperfusion syndrome after carotid endarterectomy, malignant edema after repair of an arteriovenous malformation, and encephalopathy associated with some drugs may share similar pathophysiologic mechanisms, although they have not been as well recognized.

CLINICAL FEATURES

Hypertensive encephalopathy described in the older literature was often a consequence of acute glomerulonephritis (Bright's disease) or eclampsia, but the typical patient seen at the present time usually has a history of poorly controlled chronic hypertension. Medical non-compliance and abrupt discontinuation of antihypertensive medications often leads to rebound hypertension. Acute, severe hypertension causing encephalopathy can also occur with drug abuse (particularly cocaine) (7), with the use of sympathomimetic drugs (eg, phenyl-propanolamine) (8), with the tyramine reaction in patients taking monoamine oxidase inhibitors, and in patients with renal failure who are started on erythropoietin (9).

Patients complain of generalized headache, nausea, and vomiting. Confusion and drowsiness may develop insidiously. In severe cases, patients may be stuporous or comatose, presumably due to increased intracranial pressure. In many early case reports, however, coma was probably due to intracerebral hemorrhage and focal mass effect (10). Visual disturbances ranging from blurred vision, difficulty in reading, scintillating scotoma, to the extreme of cortical blindness (uremic amaurosis) are characteristic findings in hypertensive encephalopathy and eclampsia (3,11). Imaging studies (see below) demonstrate that the occipital white matter has a predilection for development of signal abnormalities in patients with hypertensive encephalopathy and eclampsia, which may explain the frequent association of

R. J. Wityk: Department of Medicine, Sinai Hospital of Baltimore, Baltimore, Maryland 21215, and Department of Neurology, The Johns Hopkins University School of Medicine, Baltimore, Maryland 21287.

M. S. Pessin: Department of Neurology, New England Medical Center, 750 Washington Street, Boston, Massachusetts 02111, and Department of Neurology, Tufts University School of Medicine, Boston, Massachusetts 02111.

visual symptoms. Patients with prominent visual symptoms will have occipital slowing on electroencephalography (3).

Focal neurologic deficits may be present, but they are often mild in severity and may resolve rapidly with control of blood pressure. Significant deficits, such as hemiparesis, suggest associated ischemic stroke or parenchymal hemorrhage. Shiokawa reported a patient with hypertensive encephalopathy in the setting of acute basal ganglia hemorrhage (12). Reduction of blood pressure resulted in prompt improvement of headache and encephalopathy without change in the focal neurologic deficits related solely to the hemorrhage. Clearly, distinguishing cognitive changes due to hypertensive encephalopathy from the effects of a focal brain lesion is difficult in most cases, and caution is advised in blood pressure management.

Focal or generalized seizures are common and may be the first manifestation of hypertensive encephalopathy. The seizures tend to be self-limited and typically do not recur once effective blood pressure treatment is initiated.

Examination of the fundus may reveal hypertensive retinopathy with arteriovenous nicking, hemorrhages, and exudates. Papilledema is a helpful diagnostic finding, but hypertensive encephalopathy can be present in the absence of papilledema (3,13). Neurologic findings may include visual field deficits, a mild degree of focal weakness, aphasia, hyperreflexia, and bilateral Babinski signs. Clonus is a common finding in eclamptics. Meningismus may be present to a mild degree.

Lumbar puncture is not recommended if increased intracerebral pressure is suspected, unless there is a suspicion of meningitis. Spinal fluid analysis may show a lymphocytic pleocytosis or a mild elevation of protein. Cerebrospinal fluid (CSF) pressure may be markedly elevated (up to 560 mm H_2O) in some, but not all, patients (10,14), making it unreliable for the diagnosis of hypertensive encephalopathy. Griswold reported elevated intracranial pressure in three pediatric patients with hypertensive encephalopathy as measured by a subdural monitoring device (15). Simultaneous measurement of arterial and intracranial pressure allowed optimization of cerebral perfusion pressure during blood pressure reduction.

PATHOLOGY AND PATHOPHYSIOLOGY

Chester and colleagues reported the pathologic findings in 20 patients with hypertensive encephalopathy (10). All patients were black, despite the fact that twice as many whites had autopsies during the years of the study. The time interval between the clinical manifestations of hypertensive encephalopathy and the time of post-mortem examination was not stated. Nevertheless, a clear pattern of neuropathologic abnormalities was seen. Most patients had cortical or lacunar infarcts and atherosclerosis of the vessels of the circle of Willis. Multiple petechial hemorrhages were common.

Microscopically, the most prominent feature was fibrinoid necrosis of the walls of arterioles, often with associated fibrin thrombus in the lumen. Other vessels showed patchy involvement with hyalinization or fibrous thickening of the vessel wall. Miliary zones of infarction were seen in the brain tissue surrounding many of the affected vessels. Fibrinoid necrosis was also noted in other organs, particularly the retina and kidney.

Volhard initially suggested that hypertensive encephalopathy was due to widespread vasospasm (2). Early studies in animals demonstrated constriction of pial vessels and a multifocal breakdown of the blood–brain barrier with severe hypertension (16). Based on these studies, Byrom suggested that widespread cerebral vasospasm resulted in multiple focal regions of cerebral edema (16). In the later stages, cerebral edema caused increased intracranial pressure and was responsible for global neurologic dysfunction and mortality. Chester and colleagues challenged this hypothesis and suggested the symptoms of hypertensive encephalopathy were a consequence of the multiple, widely distributed miliary infarcts and petechial hemorrhages seen in their pathologic studies (10). Cerebral edema was conspicuously absent in their material, in contrast to findings of other investigators (16,17). Chester's study has been criticized, however, because the temporal relationship between the manifestations of hypertensive encephalopathy and the time of autopsy was unclear (17). One of the earliest microscopic findings in an experimental model of hypertensive encephalopathy is an increased rate of pinocytosis in the vascular endothelium, which would allow significant passage of fluid and macromolecules into the brain (18). These changes occur prior to the breakdown of endothelial tight junctions.

Current concepts of cerebral autoregulation suggest a dynamic state in which constriction or dilatation of resistance vessels in the brain would be protective by maintaining constant cerebral blood flow within a wide range of blood pressures (19,20). Hypertensive encephalopathy is hypothesized to occur when the upper limits of cerebral autoregulation is exceeded, leading to dilatation and injury of cerebral arterioles (19,21,22). Cerebral autoregulation is thought to be effective for mean arterial pressures between 50 and 150 mm Hg, but wide interindividual variations are likely. Patients with chronic hypertension, for example, appear to have a shift of the autoregulatory curve to high values (19,20), so that higher mean blood pressures are tolerated, but lowering of blood pressure to a normal range may be deleterious.

The few studies of cerebral perfusion during hypertensive encephalopathy have shown mixed results. Using a Xe-133 technique, Skinhoj and Strandgaard found increased cerebral blood flow in one patient with hypertensive encephalopathy and two patients with transient increases of blood pressure above the presumed limit of cerebral autoregulation (22). Using an animal model, Dinsdale found a marked increase in cerebral blood flow simultaneous with a sudden surge in systemic blood pressure, followed 5 minutes later by relative hypoperfusion in watershed areas when blood pressure returned to normal (23). Schwartz reported one patient studied by single-photon-emission computed tomography (SPECT) imaging who had bilateral occipital hyperperfusion during hypertensive encephalopathy with normalization of findings 10 days later (24). Breakdown of cerebral autoregulation may be a patchy process, with areas of maintained vasoconstriction scattered among regions of hyperperfusion. With continued vascular injury and formation of luminal thrombi, perfusion to some regions of the brain may decrease.

IMAGING STUDIES

A number of case reports and small series demonstrate consistent features on CT or MRI in patients with hypertensive encephalopathy and eclampsia (11,13,24–31). The most common finding on CT is bilateral, symmetric white matter hypodensity (edema) that resolves over days to weeks with control of blood pressure and resolution of the clinical syndrome. In some patients, CT also shows obliteration of sulci and compression of the lateral ventricles. The white matter abnormality can be diffuse, but in many cases white matter hypodensity is most prominent or entirely confined to the posterior regions. White matter lesions are better appreciated on MRI, showing bright signal on T2-weighted images. T1-weighted images may be normal or show signs of diffuse cerebral swelling. Patchy, small, T2-bright lesions not apparent on CT may also be seen in cortical and subcortical regions. Findings on MRI will also resolve over several weeks with appropriate therapy. In young women with eclampsia, the MRI is otherwise normal, but in older patients with chronic hypertension one commonly sees evidence of previous lacunar or cortical infarcts. The signal characteristics on CT and MRI as well as the reversible nature of the abnormalities suggest focal cerebral edema as the cause of the abnormalities (13,28). The predilection for CT and MRI abnormalities in the occipital regions is unexplained. Differences in sympathetic innervation of the anterior and posterior circulations may be a factor (24).

There are few data concerning vascular studies in patients with hypertensive encephalopathy. A few reports of angiography in patients with postpartum eclampsia demonstrate probable vasospasm, but in these cases the lesions likely represent a primary vasculopathy or are due to vasoconstrictive drugs (eg, ergonovine) (32,33). One study used transcranial Doppler (TCD) to measure middle cerebral artery velocities in pregnant women during infusion of angiotensin II (34). Mean flow velocities increased significantly during angiotensin II infusion and were related to increases in systemic blood pressure. Although logistically difficult, serial TCD studies of patients with eclampsia or acute hypertensive encephalopathy would be of interest to determine whether measurements of flow velocity or changes in velocity would be clinically meaningful in patient management.

TREATMENT

By definition, much of the deleterious effect of hypertensive encephalopathy can be alleviated with reduction of blood pressure to a range in which cerebral autoregulation is capable of controlling cerebral perfusion. Reduction of mean arterial pressure by 25% will often be effective. Further reductions within the first 24 hours of treatment may lead to hypoperfusion in patients with chronic hypertension and an altered autoregulatory curve (19). Rapid and excessive reduction in blood pressure has resulted in ischemic cerebral infarction, particularly in watershed regions (35). Patients with focal lesions (ischemic infarct or parenchymal hemorrhage) have disrupted autoregulation in the region around the lesion and may develop worsening ischemia around the lesion from excessive reduction in blood pressure.

A wide variety of agents are available for rapid blood pressure control (36,37). Intravenous labetolol, sometimes combined with an angiotensin-converting enzyme (ACE) inhibitor or a diuretic, is often effective and can be used for maintenance therapy (36,38). Neither β blockers nor ACE inhibitors increase cerebral blood flow and therefore have a favorable hemodynamic profile for use in patients with increased intracranial pressure (38). Intravenous esmolol can be used in patients with labile blood pressure in whom the need for rapid reversal of the antihypertensive effect is anticipated. Intravenous nitroprusside remains the most potent antihypertensive agent for refractory patients (39). Concerns have been raised about the use of a potential cerebral vasodilator in patients with increased intracranial pressure (40), but in situations of sustained excessive blood pressure elevation that do not respond to other agents, the effectiveness of nitroprusside in reducing blood pressure outweighs potential side effects.

Use of diazoxide, recommended in earlier reports, has waned due to the unpredictable nature of the response and potential for excessive reduction in blood pressure (17,36). Oral or sublingual nifedipine may also cause excessive, rapid reduction in blood pressure and should be used cautiously (41). The hypotensive effect of nifedipine appears to be greatest in patients with hypovolemia. One study suggested that sublingual captopril was as effective as sublingual nifedipine in the treatment of hypertensive emergencies (42). Clonidine is also an effective antihypertensive agent but is generally not used in patients with hypertensive encephalopathy due to the potential for sedation, which may interfere with the neurologic examination (43).

ECLAMPSIA

Eclampsia is a complication of pregnancy that typically occurs in the third trimester in primigravidas. Preeclampsia refers to the constellation of weight gain, proteinuria, and elevation of blood pressure from baseline. The term "eclampsia" is used when malignant hypertension develops associated with neurologic symptoms. As described earlier, common symptoms include headache, confusion, drowsiness, and visual disturbance. Seizures may occur in the absence of other neurologic findings or symptoms other than headache. Hemispheric white matter edema may be transiently present on CT, resolving with treatment of blood pressure (Fig. 1). Because many women with eclampsia have normal blood pressures prior to pregnancy, the elevation of blood pressure with eclampsia may appear modest compared to chronically hypertensive patients. Nevertheless, in otherwise healthy young women the cerebral autoregulatory curve is shifted to a lower range than patients with chronic hypertension, and an acute elevation of blood pressure to 140/100 may easily exceed the upper limits of autoregulation.

The pathogenesis of eclampsia is uncertain and potential mechanisms and accumulated data are summarized in several reviews (44–46). The treatment is urgent delivery of the fetus, which results in rapid improvement of blood pressure and neurologic abnormalities in 24–48 hours in most cases. Hydralazine is the preferred antihypertensive medication in eclamptics. In the United States, intravenous magnesium is routinely used by obstetricians, although debate continues about the effectiveness of this medication (46). Seizures in eclamptics tend to be self-limited. Although magnesium has some anticonvulsant effects, patients in status epilepticus should be treated with standard anticonvulsant medications, including benzodiazepines and phenytoin (46).

HYPERPERFUSION SYNDROME AFTER CAROTID ENDARTERECTOMY

The hyperperfusion syndrome is an uncommon but well-described complication after carotid endarterectomy (47–51). In a typical case, the patient develops an intense, throbbing headache on the side of the endarterectomy hours or days after the surgery (52). Confusion and either fluctuating or elevated blood pressure may occur. Patients can develop focal motor seizures in the arm contralateral to the side of surgery. Focal motor signs, including arm and face weakness, slurred speech, aphasia, or hemianopia, may be present with or without seizures. In some patients, the onset of symptoms is abrupt and the presence of impaired consciousness and vomiting suggests intracerebral hemorrhage (53).

Imaging studies may be normal or may show patchy hypodensity on CT, consistent with edema, and that is sometimes severe in the hemisphere ipsilateral to the surgery (51). The

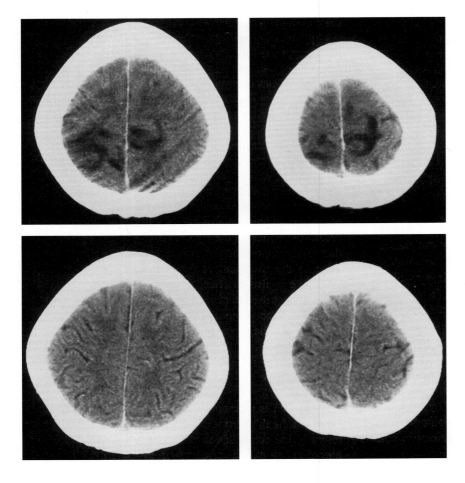

FIG. 1. A 15-year-old primigravida was admitted near term with progressive hypertension, proteinuria, and generalized seizures. Neurologic examination was notable for a left pronator drift and bilateral Babinski signs. Initial head CT scan *(top)* revealed bilateral frontoparietal hypodensities. The seizures stopped and the neurologic examination returned to normal after delivery. Repeat head CT scan *(bottom)* 8 days after the first showed resolution of the hypodensities.

cerebral edema seen on CT is often mistaken for infarction but resolves with reduction of blood pressure. In two reported patients, TCD studies showed markedly increased flow velocity in the middle cerebral artery (51). Rapid neurologic deterioration suggests basal ganglia or lobar hemorrhage. The electroencephalogram may show periodic lateralized epileptiform discharges (PLEDs) over the affected hemisphere (49). Reocclusion of the carotid artery is often suspected, but vascular studies confirm the patency of the vessel and absence of distal embolization. Pathologic findings in the affected hemisphere include fibrinoid necrosis of arterioles and cerebral edema (48).

Patients with high-grade carotid stenosis or occlusion maintain cerebral perfusion in the ipsilateral hemisphere by compensatory vasodilatation. Studies using acetazolamide and either TCD or scintigraphic cerebral perfusion techniques demonstrate limited or lost ability to further vasodilate in the hemisphere ipsilateral to the carotid lesion, suggesting that the cerebral vessels on that side are maximally dilated (54). Removal of the carotid occlusive lesions rapidly exposes that hemisphere to full systemic blood pressure. Sundt reported a twofold increase in cerebral blood flow in some patients after endarterectomy (47). Cerebral autoregulation may not respond quickly enough to prevent hyperperfusion; alternatively, cerebral autoregulation may be set lower in the hemisphere ipsilateral to an occlusive carotid lesion, resulting in unilateral hypertensive encephalopathy (47,48).

A similar process may occur in a patient with an arteriovenous malformation (AVM) and arterial steal of blood from normal surrounding brain by the AVM. Spetzler reported the development of malignant cerebral edema in a patient after technically successful resection of an enlarging AVM (55). Using the term ''normal perfusion pressure breakthrough,'' they proposed that return of normal blood flow resulted in hyperperfusion because of chronic impairment of cerebral autoregulation in the brain tissue surrounding the AVM.

REFERENCES

1. Oppenheimer BS, Fishberg AM. Hypertensive encephalopathy. *Arch Intern Med* 1928;41:264–278.
2. Volhard F, Fahr KT. *Die Brightsche Nierenkrankheit: Klinik, Pathologie und Atlas.* Berlin: Julius Springer, 1914.
3. Jellinek EH, Painter M, Prineas J, Russell RR. Hypertensive encephalopathy with cortical disorders of vision. *Q J Med* 1964;33:239–256.
4. Healton EB, Brust JC, Feinfeld DA, Thomson GE. Hypertensive encephalopathy and the neurologic manifestations of malignant hypertension. *Neurology* 1982;32:127–132.
5. Prisant LM, Carr AA, Hawkins DW. Treating hypertensive emergencies. Controlled reduction of blood pressure and protection of target organs. *Postgrad Med* 1993;93:92–96.
6. Macfarlane R, Moskowitz, MM, Sakas DE, Tasdemiroglu E, Wei EP, Kontos HA. The role of neuroeffector mechanisms in cerebral hyperfusion syndromes. *Neurosurgery* 1991;75:845–855.
7. Grewal RP, Miller BL. Cocaine induced hypertensive encephalopathy. *Acta Neurologica* 1991;13:279–281.
8. Pentel P. Toxicity of over-the-counter stimulants. *JAMA* 1984;252:1898–903.
9. Raine AE, Roger SD. Effects of erythropoietin on blood pressure. *Am J Kidney Dis* 1991;18(Suppl 1):76–83.
10. Chester EM, Agamanolis DP, Banker BQ, Victor M. Hypertensive encephalopathy: a clinicopathologic study of 20 cases. *Neurology* 1978; 28:928–939.
11. Marra TR, Shah M, Mikus MA. Transient cortical blindness due to hypertensive encephalopathy. Magnetic resonance imaging correlation. *J Clin Neuro-ophthalmol* 1993;13:35–37.
12. Shiokawa O, Lau AH, Sadoshima S, Fujishima M. Transient encephalopathy related to rapidly and markedly elevated blood pressure in acute stage of hypertensive cerebral hemorrhage. Relationship to hypertensive encephalopathy: a case report. *Angiology* 1988;39:996–1000.
13. Fisher M, Maister B, Jacobs R. Hypertensive encephalopathy: diffuse reversible white matter CT abnormalities. *Ann Neurol* 1985;18:268–270.
14. Taylor RD, Corcoran AC, Page IH. Increased cerebrospinal fluid pressure and papilledema in malignant hypertension. *Arch Intern Med* 1954; 93:818–824.
15. Griswold WR, Viney J, Mendoza SA, James HE. Intracranial pressure monitoring in severe hypertensive encephalopathy. *Crit Care Med* 1981;9:573–576.
16. Byrom FB. The pathogenesis of hypertensive encephalopathy and its relation to the malignant phase of hypertension. *Lancet* 1954;2:201–211.
17. Dinsdale HB. Hypertensive encephalopathy. *Stroke* 1982;13:717–719.
18. Nag S, Robertson DM, Dinsdale HB. Cerebral cortical changes in acute experimental hypertension. An ultrastructural study. *Lab Invest* 1977; 36:150–161.
19. Strandgaard S, Olesen J, Skinhoj E, Lassen NA. Autoregulation of brain circulation in severe arterial hypertension. *BMJ* 1973;1:507–510.
20. Paulson OB, Strandgaard S, Edvinsson L. Cerebral autoregulation. *Cerebrovasc Brain Metab Rev* 1990;2:161–192.
21. Lassen NA, Agnoli A. The upper limit of autoregulation of cerebral blood flow. On the pathogenesis of hypertensive encephalopathy. *Scand J Clin Lab Invest* 1972;30:113–116.
22. Skinhoj E, Strandgaard S. Pathogenesis of hypertensive encephalopathy. *Lancet* 1973;1:461–462.
23. Dinsdale HB, Robertson DM, Haas RA. Cerebral blood flow in acute hypertension. *Arch Neurol* 1974;31:80–87.
24. Schwartz RB, Jones KM, Kalina P, et al. Hypertensive encephalopathy: findings on CT, MR imaging, and SPECT imaging in 14 cases. *AJR* 1992;159:379–383.
25. Rail DL, Perkin GD. Computerized tomographic appearance of hypertensive encephalopathy. *Arch Neurol* 1980;37:310–311.
26. Beeson JH, Duda EE. Computed axial tomography scan demonstration of cerebral edema in eclampsia preceded by blindness. *Obstet Gynecol* 1982;60:529–532.
27. Colosimo J C., Fileni, A., Guerrini, P. CT findings in eclampsia. *Neuroradiology* 1985;27:313–317.
28. Crawford S, Varner MW, Digre KB, Servais G, Corbett JJ. Cranial magnetic resonance imaging in eclampsia. *Obstet Gynecol* 1987;70:474–477.
29. Hauser RA, Lacey DM, Knight MR. Hypertensive encephalopathy. Magnetic resonance imaging demonstration of reversible cortical and white matter lesions. *Arch Neurol* 1988;45:1078–1083.
30. Gibby WA, Stecker MM, Goldberg HI, et al. Reversal of white matter edema in hypertensive encephalopathy. *Am J Neuroradiol* 1989;10:S78.
31. Weingarten K, Barbut D, Filippi C, Zimmerman RD. Acute hypertensive encephalopathy: findings on spin–echo and gradient-echo MR imaging. *AJR* 1994;162:665–670.
32. Barinagarrementeria F, Cantu C, Balderrama J. Postpartum cerebral angiopathy with cerebral infarction due to ergonovine use. *Stroke* 1992; 23:1364–1366.
33. Will AD, Lewis KL, Hinshaw JDB, et al. Cerebral vasoconstriction in toxemia. *Neurology* 1987;37:1555–1557.
34. Kyle P, De Swiet M, Buckley D, Serra V, Redman C. Noninvasive assessment of the maternal cerebral circulation by transcranial Doppler ultrasound during angiotensin II infusion. *Br J Obstet Gynecol* 1993; 100:85–91.
35. Graham DI. Ischaemic brain damage of cerebral perfusion failure after treatment of severe hypertension. *BMJ* 1975;4:739.
36. Ferguson RK, Viasses PH. Hypertensive emergencies and urgencies. *JAMA* 1986;225:1607–1613.

37. Kaplan NM. Treatment of hypertensive emergencies and urgencies. *Heart Dis Stroke* 1992ₛ:373–378.

38. Wilson DJ, Wallin JD, Vlachakis ND, et al. Intravenous labetalol in the treatment of severe hypertension and hypertensive emergencies. *Am J Med* 1983;75:95–102.

39. Cohn JN, Burke LP. Nitroprusside. *Ann Intern Med* 1979;91:752–757.

40. Egol AB, Snyder JV, Grenvik A. Hypertensive encephalopathy. *Stroke* 1983;14:1009–1010.

41. Wachter RM. Symptomatic hypotension induced by nifedipine in the acute treatment of severe hypertension. *Arch Intern Med* 1987;147:556–558.

42. Angeli P, Chiesa M, Caregaro L, et al. Comparison of sublingual captopril and nifedipine in immediate treatment of hypertensive emergencies. *Arch Intern Med* 1991;151:678–682.

43. Ferguson RK, Vlasses PH. How urgent is "urgent" hypertension? *Arch Intern Med* 1989;149:257–258.

44. Sibai B. Eclampsia. In: Goldstein P, Stern BJ, eds. *Neurological disorders of pregnancy.* Second Revised Ed. Mount Kisco, NY: Futura, 1992:1–24.

45. Donaldson JO. Eclampsia. In: Donaldson JO. *Neurology of pregnancy.* Philadelphia: WB Saunders, 1989:269–310.

46. Donaldson JO. Eclamptic hypertensive encephalopathy. *Semin Neurol* 1988;8:230–233.

47. Sundt J Thorale M., Sharbrough FW, Piepgras DG, Kearns TP, Messick J Joseph M., O'Fallon WO. Correlation of cerebral blood flow and electroencephalographic changes during carotid endartectomy. *Mayo Clin Proc* 1981;56:533–543.

48. Bernstein M, Fleming JFR, Deck JHN. Cerebral hyperperfusion after carotid endarterectomy: a cause of cerebral hemorrhage. *Neurosurgery* 1984;15:50–56.

49. Reigel MM, Hollier LH, Sundt J, Thoralf M, Piepgras DG, Sharbrough FW, Cherry KJ. Cerebral hyperfusion syndrome: A neurologic dysfunction after carotid endarterectomy. *J Vasc Surg* 1987;5:628–634.

50. Piepgras DG, Morgan MK, Sundt J Thoralf M, Yanagihara T, Mussman LM. Intracerebral hemorrhage after carotid endarterectomy. *J Neurol* 1988;68:532–536.

51. Breen JC, Caplan LR, DeWitt LD, Belkin M, Mackey WC, O'Donnell TP. Brain edema after carotid surgery. *Neurology* 1996;46:175–181.

52. Leviton A, Caplan L, Salzman E. Severe headache after carotid endarterectomy. *Headache* 1975;15:207–210.

53. Caplan LR, Skillman J, Ojemann R, Fields WS. Intracerebral hemorrhage following carotid endarterectomy: a hypertensive complication. *Stroke* 1978;9:457–460.

54. Powers WJ. Cerebral hemodynamics in ischemic cerebrovascular disease. *Ann Neurol* 1991;29:231–240.

55. Spetzler RF, Wilson CB, Weinstein P, Mehdorn M, Townsend J, Telles D. Normal perfusion pressure breakthrough theory. *Clin Neurosurg* 1978;25:651–672.

Cerebrovascular Disease, edited by H. Hunt Batjer.
Lippincott-Raven Publishers, Philadelphia © 1997.

CHAPTER 9

Cardiac Manifestation of Cerebrovascular Events

Richard K. T. Chan and Vladimir Hachinski

HISTORICAL BACKGROUND

The idea of a brain–heart axis is not new. In the early 19th century, Magendie proposed that the heart, like many viscera, is under neurologic control with respect to its nutrition (1). Discovery of the autonomic nervous system and subsequent clarification of the functions of the sympathetic and vagus nerves confirmed his theory. However, the idea of an injured brain causing cardiac damage was recognized only recently.

The association between intracranial disease and electrocardiographic changes was first noted by Aschenbrenner and Bodechtel in 1938 (2). In 1947, Byer et al. reported electrocardiographic changes in patients with recent cerebrovascular events (3). Of their six patients, one had ''cerebral hemorrhage,'' one had ''hypertensive encephalopathy,'' and three had ''cerebrovascular accident.'' (No clinical data were available on the last patient.) The electrocardiograms (ECGs) of all the patients showed large upright T waves and prolonged Q-T intervals in the standard limb leads. Since then, other investigators had described similar ECG changes in cases of subarachnoid hemorrhage, intracerebral hemorrhage, cerebral venous thrombosis, and cerebral neoplasm (4–11). More recently, there were also reports of cardiac arrhythmia and sudden unexpected death among patients with recent cerebrovascular events (12) or epilepsy (13). Subtle myocardial damage, termed focal myocytolysis, was often found in the patients who died (14). The term ''neurogenic heart disease'' was coined for this syndrome.

In this chapter, we will elaborate on the clinical and pathologic findings in this syndrome. We will also explore the possible pathogenetic mechanism, based on currently available experimental and clinical data. The final section will be

a brief discussion on the management issues facing clinicians today.

CLINICAL MANIFESTATION

The syndrome of neurogenic heart disease is often asymptomatic. Electrocardiographic changes and/or elevations of ''cardiac enzymes''—often uncovered as part of a routine screen—are the more common modes of presentation. In some patients, sudden unexpected death, presumably from cardiac arrhythmia, is the presenting feature (15). In a study of 100 stroke patients who died within 7 days after the onset of symptoms, 14% had no important pathologic findings outside the nervous system at the time of postmortem examination (16). The unexpected deaths are likely results of cardiac arrhythmias.

''Cardiac'' Enzymes

The serum aspartate transaminase (AST or SGOT), lactate dehydrogenase (LDH), and total creatine phosphokinase (CPK) activities may be elevated, either in isolation or in combination. About 40% of patients with subarachnoid hemorrhage had elevated serum AST, and 30–40% had elevated total CPK levels (8,17). Increases in at least two of the cardiac enzymes were seen in about 8% of patients with an ischemic stroke (18). Using elevated CPK level as the only criterion, Dubo et al. found the abnormality in 71% of patients with cerebral infarction (19).

By themselves the elevated activity levels do not always imply cardiac damage because these enzymes are also found in brain tissue. However, the relatively cardiospecific CPK-MB fraction, which is more suggestive of myocardial injury, is also abnormal in a significant proportion of patients. Elevation of the CPK-MB fraction was seen in approximately 40% and 10% of patients with subarachnoid hemorrhage and

R. K. T. Chan and V. Hachinski: Department of Clinical Neurological Sciences, University of Western Ontario, London, Ontario, N6A 5A5 Canada.

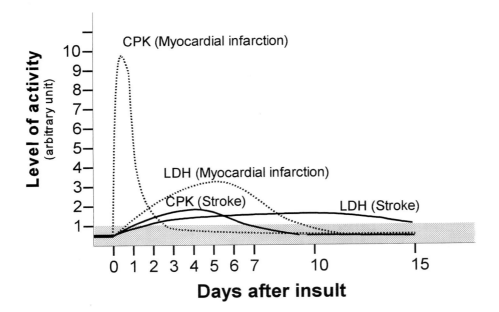

FIG. 1. Schematic diagram showing changes in the cardiac enzymes activity after acute myocardial infarction and acute stroke. CPK, creatinine phosphokinase; LDH, lactic dehydrogenase.

ischemic stroke, respectively (17,18). Elevation of the CPK-MB fraction has been associated with a higher mortality rate in patients with ischemic stroke (20).

With neurogenic heart disease, all three enzymes' activities rose gradually in the first 4–5 days after the acute insult suggesting continuing low-grade myocardial necrosis (8,18,19). The levels usually returned to normal range within 2 weeks (21). This cardiac enzyme profile is quite different compared to acute myocardial infarction, where the most rapid rise in CPK level occurs in the first 24–48 hours (Fig. 1). The elevated activities are due to leakage of the respective enzymes from the damaged myocardial cells. The magnitude of elevation is usually small when compared to acute transmural myocardial infarction.

Depolarization–Repolarization Abnormalities

Electrocardiographic changes are common manifestation of neurogenic heart disease. Some 40–60% of patients with subarachnoid hemorrhage and 80% of patients with intracerebral hemorrhage, as well as 15% of patients with ischemic strokes, had new ECG changes (6–8). Nearly all types of ECG changes had been reported and they are shown in Table 1. The most often encountered abnormalities are prolonged Q-T interval, large inverted T wave, and prominent U wave. These are most pronounced in the anterolateral leads. With the possible exception of prolonged QT interval, the changes are usually transient, lasting no longer than 2 weeks. Changes in the QRS complex can occur but they are less common. These changes are consistent with non-Q (or subendocardial) infarction and will be interpreted as such by an electrocardiographer who is unaware of the clinical situation. Surgery had been denied to patients with subarachnoid hem-

orrhage due to these ECG abnormalities, although the hearts were free of frank infarction at autopsy (6).

Cardiac Rhythm Disturbances

Cardiac arrhythmias are frequently encountered in patients with an acute central nervous system insult (22). About 75% of patients have some disturbances of cardiac rhythm in the acute stages of their illness (23). Patients with hemispheric pathology are more likely to have cardiac arrhythmia compared to those with brainstem lesions, especially those with pathology in the right cerebral hemisphere (24). The arrhythmias may or may not be accompanied by the ECG changes mentioned above.

All types of rhythm abnormalities have been reported (Table 2). Fortunately, most of these are the relatively benign sinus tachycardia and premature atrial or ventricular contractions that are of little physiologic or clinical significance. Atrial fibrillation and flutter also occur frequently.

TABLE 1. *Spectrum of ECG changes in cerebrovascular events*

Depolarization-repolarization abnormality
Peaked P wave
"Pathologic" q wave
Prolonged Q-T interval[a]
Depressed or raised (coved) S-T segment
Wide T wave[a]
Tall and peaked, or deep and inverted, T wave[a]
U wave[a]
Conduction abnormality
First-, and second-, and/or third-degree AV block
Intraventricular conduction defect
Arrhythmias (see Table 2)

[a] Commonly observed abnormalities.

TABLE 2. *Arrhythmias associated with cerebrovascular events*

Sinus dysrhythmias
    Sinus bradycardia
    Sinus tachycardia
Supraventricular dysrhythmias
    Atrial premature contractions
    Atrial fibrillation/flutter
    Supraventricular tachycardia
    Sick sinus syndrome
Ventricular dysrhythmias
    Ventricular premature contractions
    Ventricular bigeminy
    Ventricular tachycardia
    Torsade de pointes
    Ventricular fibrillation

Of concern are the "malignant arrhythmias." Included within this group are ventricular tachycardia and ventricular fibrillation. Torsade de pointe, a specific polymorphic form of ventricular tachycardia, has been associated with prolonged QT interval as mentioned in the preceding section. All of these arrhythmias are mostly unpredictable, of sudden onset, and lead to severe hemodynamic compromise. They are believed to be the cause of sudden unexpected death among patients with cardiac and cerebrovascular diseases.

PATHOLOGIC CHANGES IN THE HEART

The hearts of patients who died of cerebrovascular events and had associated cardiac manifestation may appear normal on gross inspection. In approximately 12% of cases one may find subendocardial hemorrhages (14,25). With careful and meticulous histologic examination, focal myocytolysis can often be seen (9,26). They are characterized by their multiplicity, seemingly random locations, and loss of sarcoplasm and striations of the affected myocytes. The sarcolemma, stroma, muscle nuclei, and lipofuscin granules are relatively intact. These lesions may be surrounded by mononuclear cells. Under the electron microscope these lesions are seen near the intracardiac nerves. The cell architecture is disrupted although the ribosomes and mitochondria are preserved. The affected myocytes appear hypercontracted. This contrasts sharply with typical myocardial infarction where confluence coagulative necrosis is the predominant histologic finding. In coagulative necrosis, the cells die in a state of relaxation, often with polymorphonuclear cellular infiltration.

The changes described above are not specific to cerebrovascular diseases. Other diseases, such as intracranial neoplasm or meningitis, may also produce these changes (27). They have been described in patients with pheochromocytoma (28–30), cocaine abusers, and patients who received high-dose catecholamine for a prolonged period (L-epinephrine myocarditis) (31,32). Patients who died of "insulin shock" may also manifest the same pathologic changes (33).

Experimentally, reperfusion of myocardium after a period of ischemia and reoxygenation of hypoxic myocardium also induced similar changes (34).

AUTONOMIC INNERVATION OF THE HEART

To understand the pathogenesis of neurogenic heart disease, one must be familiar with the autonomic nervous input to the heart. The heart derives its parasympathetic autonomic innervation from the vagus nerves. They arise from the dorsal motor nuclei, emerge from the lateral surface of the medulla oblongata, and leave the intracranial cavity via the jugular foramina. The fibers destined to innervate the heart eventually synapse with the postganglionic neurons in the sinoatrial node and, to a lesser extent, the atrioventricular node. Physiologic stimulation of the vagus nerves produced bradycardia. The dorsal nuclei of the vagus nerves are under hypothalamic influence, particularly from the anterior and medial regions of the hypothalamus. Stimulation of certain cortical areas in the frontal lobe can also produce parasympathetic responses. After reviewing the literature available to him, Fulton suggested that the orbitofrontal areas house the cortical representation of the vagus nerve (35). More recently, stimulation of the medial frontal cortex was also shown to have a similar effect (36). The pathway linking these frontal cortical areas to the dorsal nucleus of the vagus nerves are not well understood.

The cell bodies of the postganglionic sympathetic nerve fibers to the heart are located in the inferior cervical and the upper five or six thoracic sympathetic ganglia. Of these, the inferior cervical ganglion is often fused with the first thoracic sympathetic ganglion and is known by the term "stellate ganglion." Physiologic stimulation of the stellate ganglion causes an increase in heart rate and blood pressure.

Like the parasympathetic division, the sympathetic division is also under the influence of the hypothalamus. Electrical stimulation of the posterior and lateral regions of the hypothalamus consistently produces sympathetic responses. Cortical representation of the sympathetic division has only been described recently (37). Both animal and human studies suggest that this cortical representation lies in the insular cortex. Stimulation of the insular cortex led to various degree of heart blocks and death from asystole in rats (38). Evidence also suggests that the sympathetic functions of the insular cortices are lateralized. The results from various studies from our center suggest the right insular cortex is dominant in regard to the sympathetic innervation of the heart. In a rat model of ischemic stroke, increased postganglionic sympathetic nerve activities and blood catecholamine levels were seen after occlusion of the right, but not the left, middle cerebral artery (39). In epileptic humans undergoing temporal lobectomy, intraoperative stimulation of the right insular cortex caused increased heart rate and blood pressure (40). In another study involving human subjects, inactivation of the right cerebral hemisphere by intracarotid amobarbital injections were associated with attenuation of the heart rate variability. This attenuation did not occur with injection into the left internal carotid artery. The observation suggests the sympathetic tone arises from the right cerebral hemisphere (unpublished data). In a recent case report, Svigelj et al. described a patient with various types of cardiac arrhythmias associated with an intracerebral hematoma in the right insular cortex from a ruptured aneurysm. The arrhythmias abated when the hematoma was evacuated and the aneurysm clipped (41).

In summary, increased parasympathetic discharges can be caused by physiologic or functional changes in the orbital or medial frontal cortex and the hypothalamus. Increased sympathetic discharges to the heart, on the other hand, may occur following similar changes in the (right) insular cortex, hypothalamus, or the stellate ganglion.

PATHOGENESIS

Initially, the cardiac manifestations were attributed to concomitant myocardial ischemia or infarction because cerebrovascular disease and coronary artery disease share many risk factors. However, many patients who had the typical ECG changes or cardiac enzymes elevation had normal heart and coronary artery at postmortem examination. The similarities between the pathologic changes in the heart and the lesions observed in catecholamine-induced cardiac damage suggest a causative role of the catecholamines. Plasma catecholamine levels are often elevated in humans with acute stroke, and they can also be reproduced in laboratory animals (42–44). In rats with iatrogenic intracranial hemorrhage, focal myocytolysis can be prevented by an adrenergic antagonist, such as propranolol (45). In animal studies, the cardiac changes were only slightly attenuated, but not prevented, by removal of the adrenal glands. Since adrenal glands are the major sources of circulating catecholamine, the result suggests that the latter are not by themselves the initiating factor.

We now believe that local catecholamines are responsible for the cardiac damage. Norepinephrine, an adrenergic agonist with both α and β activities, is the neurotransmitter utilized by the sympathetic nerves in the heart. Stimulation of the sympathetic ganglia or cardiac nerves in animals has been shown to produce focal myocytolysis. β-Adrenergic antagonists prevent the formation of these lesions (45). Intense sympathetic stimulation results in accumulation of norepinephrine that becomes cardiotoxic. This explains the distribution of these lesions close to the intracardiac nerves.

The means by which norepinephrine causes myocardial damage is not entirely clear. Under normal circumstances, activation of β-adrenergic receptors stimulates the production of 3′,5′-cyclic adenosine monophosphate (cAMP). In turn, cAMP causes the opening of the calcium channels resulting in the influx of calcium and efflux of potassium ions. The increase in intracellular calcium promotes actin–myosin interaction with subsequent muscle contraction. The calcium ions are then rapidly sequestered and relaxation ensues.

With continuous β-adrenergic activation, the calcium channels may fail to close. The cells remain contracted until all energy stores are exhausted and die from intracellular metabolic derangement (46).

The repolarization abnormalities most likely occur on the basis of diffuse, focal myocardial damage secondary to sympathetic activation. In theory, with intense sympathetic stimulation, the efflux of potassium ions may account for the peaked T wave. The continuous influx of calcium, on the other hand, will impair the repolarization process resulting in wide T wave. The prolonged Q-T interval is probably a combination of widened T waves and mergence of T and U waves (46). When the cells die, they become electrically silent and the ECG reverts to normal. In cases where the damage is more extensive, permanent ECG changes, including appearance of Q waves, may occur. The pathogenesis of U wave is not clear.

The pathogenesis of the cardiac arrhythmias is not clearly understood. Increased sympathetic and/or parasympathetic discharges to the heart increases the risk of cardiac arrhythmia. Much of the early literature shows conflicting results. Recent work suggests that cardiac arrhythmias occur only when both the sympathetic and parasympathetic divisions of the autonomic nervous system are stimulated. Manning and Cotton found that cardiac arrhythmias can only be produced by simultaneous stimulation of the vagus nerve and right stellate ganglion, but not either in isolation, in anesthetized cats (6). In another experiment, ventricular tachycardia was more common in pigs that have high parasympathetic and sympathetic tones compared to pigs with isolated elevated sympathetic tone only (47).

From the preceding section, lesions in the right insular cortex or the hypothalamus clearly produce activation of the sympathetic and parasympathetic divisions of the autonomic nervous system. However, some cerebrovascular diseases that do not affect these locations can also produce similar cardiac changes. In these cases, the changes are probably produced by the effect of raised intracranial pressure. Smith and Ray demonstrated activation of the sympathetic nervous system by raising the intracranial pressure in dogs. This effect was not seen when the spinal cord was transected at the C2 level, suggesting that the neural impulses originated from the brain. The effect was also blunted by atropine administration (48). It is believed that the ECG changes and cardiac arrhythmias are the results of compression of the hypothalamus and brainstem (49). In subarachnoid hemorrhage, the cardiac changes probably result from raised intracranial pressure as well as focal lesions in the hypothalamus. It is not uncommon to find microinfarcts within the hypothalamus after a subarachnoid hemorrhage. Presumably, they are the results of occlusion of the penetrating vessels that supply the hypothalamus from the region of the circle of Willis (50).

CLINICAL MANAGEMENT

Neurogenic heart disease is not rare. With subarachnoid hemorrhage, ECG changes are associated with a high mortal-

TABLE 3. *Presumed risk factors for the development of malignant cardiac arrhythmia*

Factor	High risk	Moderate to low risk
Type of lesion	Subarachnoid hemorrhage	Intracerebral hemorrhage
		Cerebral infarction
Location of lesion	Right cerebral hemisphere (especially right insular cortex)	Left cerebral hemisphere
Size of lesion	Large	Brainstem
Intracranial pressure	High	Medium to small
ECG changes:		Normal
QT interval	Prolonged	
QRS changes	Present	Normal
Serum CPK-MB	Elevated	Absent
Preexisting ischemic heart disease	Present	Normal
		Absent

CPK-MB, creatine phosphokinase

ity rate (27). Whether the ECG changes are manifestations of the severity of the subarachnoid hemorrhage or the excessive mortality was attributed to the cardiac changes is not known. In ischemic stroke, our clinical experience has shown that 6% of patients died unexpectedly in the first 30 days after their acute stroke, many of whom had minor or improving neurologic deficits (51).

The main problem concerning neurogenic heart disease lies with its prognosis. Unlike myocardial infarction, focal myocytolysis does not appear to adversely affect the hemodynamic status of the patient. However, not unlike myocardial infarction, there is an increased propensity for dysrhythmia and sudden death. Should we therefore treat both conditions in the same way? There is no easy answer.

At the very least, all patients with acute intracranial pathology must have a 12-lead ECG and cardiac enzymes measurement performed at the time of admission. In an ideal situation, such patients should also be monitored by continuous ECG to detect the occurrence of any malignant arrhythmias during the susceptible period. Therein lies the difficulty. This approach requires the use of an intensive care or telemetry facility and the cost could be prohibitive. In a smaller medical center, this facility might not even be available. To add to this, we do not know the length of the susceptible period and prolonged monitoring, though desirable, may not be feasible. Until more clinical data are made available, we suggest that selected individuals with cerebrovascular disease be monitored based on the presumed risk of developing a malignant arrhythmia (Table 3).

Subarachnoid Hemorrhage

These patients require intensive monitoring, not only neurologically but by means of continuous ECG monitoring. As many as 70% of patients with subarachnoid hemorrhage develop new ECG changes. In smaller centers, the patient should be transferred to another facility with an intensive care unit once his or her condition is stabilized.

Intracerebral Hemorrhage and Ischemic Stroke

In patients with massive intracerebral hemorrhage or cerebral infarction, the ECG depolarization or rhythm changes are likely a reflection of the severe intracranial pathology. When the prognosis for survival is considered poor, it is probably justifiable to observe the patient in a general neurologic care facility, allowing sudden death from cardiac arrhythmia to become a means of merciful deliverance.

When the hematoma or area of infarction is located near the hypothalamus (as in most cases of hypertensive basal ganglia hemorrhage) or in the right insular cortex, and the patient's prognosis is considered good, then the patient should be monitored continuously in a telemetry facility. Any ECG changes should be managed in accordance with the current standard of care, eg, monitoring in the coronary care unit if the ECG shows a pattern consistent with infarction or occurrence of life-threatening arrhythmias.

Based on the experimental data, hemorrhage or infarct involving other areas of the cerebrum does not appear to be a significant risk factor for neurogenic heart disease. Small, slit hemorrhages in the cerebral gray matter also fall in this category. In these cases, continuous monitoring is still recommended because raised intracranial pressure may still cause cardiac changes. When the facility is limited or unavailable, it is probably sufficient to manage these patients in the general neurologic or neurosurgical floor with regular 12-lead ECGs and cardiac enzyme assays as necessary.

Once an ECG abnormality or arrhythmia is recognized, the treatment is fairly standard. The distinction of neurally induced cardiac damage and myocardial infarction is difficult. Under most situations, differentiation is probably academic because management is essentially similar. There will be times, however, when one needs to confirm or rule out concomitant myocardial infarction. As an example, the physician may want to assess the risk of surgery for a patient who is to undergo surgery for subarachnoid or intracerebral hemorrhage. For myocytolysis, the risk of death from the surgery is unknown. In view of the myocardium's sensitivity to sympathetic activity, the risk is likely to be high even when there is no evidence of coexisting coronary artery disease. Nonetheless, the ECG changes should not preclude any life-saving surgery when it is needed. Patients with ischemic stroke who have new ECG changes suggesting ischemia or infarct is another situation where the physician may be concerned. A cardiac thrombus from a recent myocardial infarction with secondary cardioembolism needs to be excluded.

Unfortunately, there is no good clinical test available to discriminate myocardial infarction from myocytolysis at this time. The following features suggest focal myocytolysis rather than classical myocardial infarction:

1. Young age
2. No past history of myocardial infarction or angina pectoris
3. Lack of typical angina or myocardial infarction symptoms
4. Presence of significant intracranial lesions, including cerebral infarction, intracerebral hemorrhage, subarachnoid hemorrhage, or severe cerebral contusion
5. ECG changes were transient with complete restoration to baseline
6. No or mild elevation of serum CPK activity, even serially
7. Absence of significant hemodynamic disturbances

The presence of significant hemodynamic compromise with typical chest pain strongly suggests myocardial infarction. Dipyridamole thallium^{201} scintigraphy may be useful to exclude significant coronary ischemia or infarction. Transthoracic two-dimensional echocardiography may also be used to demonstrate focal hypokinesia or akinesia from myocardial damage. Unfortunately, these tests only confirm the presence or absence of significant myocardial ischemia or infarct, and they cannot differentiate lesions that are acute or remote. Furthermore, these tests do not exclude concomitant focal myocytolysis when there are focal abnormalities.

Sinus dysrhythmias and supraventricular dysrhythmias without associated hemodynamic changes can be safely observed. Similarly, atrial ectopics and unifocal ventricular ectopics are often benign and need no specific treatment. In the case of atrial fibrillation or flutter, it is important to establish whether the abnormality has been longstanding, especially if an embolic stroke is suspected. If the atrial fibrillation or flutter is of recent onset, they are frequently transient and treatment may not be necessary if the ventricular response rate and the hemodynamic status are satisfactory.

The ventricular tachycardias, including torsade de pointe, need to be treated aggressively with standard antiarrhythmic agents. Ventricular fibrillation once recognized requires immediate electrical defibrillation followed by antiarrhythmic agents to prevent recurrence. Once started, it is not known as to how long the drugs should be given. In the absence of significant coronary artery disease, they may be discontinued after the susceptible period. In subarachnoid hemorrhage, the susceptible period appears to be within the first 72 hours

after the initial bleed. The susceptible period for other cerebrovascular events has not been established.

Most general neurologists may be uncomfortable managing these cardiac events, and further education will be needed. Until such time, the neurologist may wish to work with a cardiologist with good knowledge of neurogenic heart syndrome to optimize the patient's management.

FUTURE DIRECTIONS

It has been 50 years since Byer et al. reported ECG changes after cerebrovascular events. Since then, experimental works have confirmed the observations and clarify, to a certain extent, the pathogenetic mechanisms. However, it is painfully clear that this has not translated into practical clinical knowledge as far as management of patients is concerned.

To justify continuous monitoring or treatment (or otherwise) of this syndrome, one needs to know the natural history and prognosis. The neurogenic heart syndrome is no longer considered rare. The current challenge is to identify the risk factors that predispose any individuals to life-threatening malignant arrhythmias. This will involve a prospective study of a large number of patients with acute cerebrovascular insult. Parameters that aid in the determination of the parasympathetic/sympathetic tone, such as heart rate variability, may prove useful.

The other issue that needs further clarification is the susceptible period for sudden death following an acute stroke. Current data show that the risk of sudden death remains unchanged in the first 30 days after acute stroke. It is vital to learn how long this susceptible period is. Knowing this susceptible period will help the clinician determine the period of time for which patients require close cardiac monitoring. Also, it will help in defining the period of antiarrhythmic treatment. Since sudden death after acute stroke is a relatively uncommon occurrence, a multicenter prospective study may be required to answer this question.

To protect patients against malignant ventricular arrhythmia, we may consider empirical treatment with antiarrhythmic agents. β-Adrenergic blockers would be the logical choice given the experimental data presented above. Animal studies have shown the cardioprotective effect of propranolol (45,52). Considering the success of β-adrenergic blockers in acute myocardial infarction in reducing arrhythmia and sudden death, there is sufficient rationale to initiate a trial to study the cardioprotective effect of β-adrenergic blockers in patients with cerebrovascular events. Diltiazem and amiodarone may also be considered, although we need more experimental data before a full-scale human study can be proposed (53).

CONCLUSION

There is powerful evidence to suggest that intracranial pathology, including the vascular diseases, can adversely affect the heart both anatomically and physiologically. The effect appears to be mediated by the autonomic system. Although it is known that patients may develop ECG changes, dysrhythmias, or sudden death, there is no objective means to predict their occurrences. Intensive monitoring would be ideal but may not be practical. We need more studies to clarify the natural history and the role of empirical prophylactic therapy in this syndrome before firm management guidelines can be formulated.

REFERENCES

1. Magendie F. L'influence de la cinquiema paire des nerfs sur la nutrition et les fonctions de l'oeil. *J Physiol Exp Pathol 1824;*4:176–179.
2. Aschenbrenner R, Bodechtel G. Ueber EKG veranderungen bei hirntumorkranken. *Klin Wschr* 1938;17:298–302.
3. Byer E, Ashman R, Toth LA. Electrocardiograms with large, upright T-waves and long Q-T intervals. *Am Heart J* 1947;33:796–806.
4. Burch GE, Meyers R, Abildskov JA. A new electrocardiographic pattern observed in cerebrovascular accidents. *Circulation* 1954;9:719–723.
5. Beard EF, Robertson JW, Robertson RCL. Spontaneous subarachnoid hemorrhage simulating acute myocardial infarction. *Am Heart J* 1959;58:755–759.
6. Cropp GJ, Manning GW. Electrocardiographic changes simulating myocardial ischemia and infarction associated with spontaneous intracranial hemorrhage. *Circulation* 1960;22:25–38.
7. Fentz V, Gormsen J. Electrocardiographic patterns in patients with cerebrovascular accidents. *Circulation* 1962;25:22–28.
8. Hunt D, McRae C, Zapf P. Electrocardiographic and serum enzyme changes in subarachnoid hemorrhage. *Am Heart J* 1969;77:479–488.
9. Hammermeister KE, Reichenbach DD. QRS changes, pulmonary edema, and myocardial necrosis associated with subarachnoid hemorrhage. *Am Heart J* 1969;78:94–100.
10. Hugenholtz PG. Electrocardiographic abnormalities in cerebral disorders. Report of six cases and review of the literature. *Am Heart J* 1962;63:451–461.
11. Harrison MT, Gibb BH. Electrocardiographic changes associated with a cerebrovascular accident. *Lancet* 1964;2:429–430.
12. Oppenheimer SM, Cechetto DF, Hachinski VC. Cerebrogenic cardiac arrhythmias: cerebral electrocardiographic influences and their role in sudden death. *Arch Neurol* 1990;47;513–519.
13. Leestma JE, Walczar T, Hughes JR, Kalekar MS, Teas SS. A prospective study on sudden unexpected death in epilepsy. *Ann Neurol* 1989;26:195–203.
14. Koskelo P, Punsar S, Sipila W. Subendocardial haemorrhage and ECG changes in intracranial bleeding. *BMJ* 1964;1:1479–1480.
15. Natelson BH, Chang Q. Sudden death: a neurocardiologic phenomenon. *Neurol Clin* 1993;11:293–308.
16. Down M, Glassenberg M. Mortality factors in patients with acute stroke. *JAMA* 1973;224:1493–1495.
17. Fabinyi G, Hunt D, McKinley L. Myocardial creatine kinase isoenzyme in serum after subarachnoid haemorrhage. *J Neurol Neurosurg Psychiatry* 1977;40:818–820.
18. Norris JW, Hachinski VC, Myers MG, Callow J, Wong T, Moore RW. Serum cardiac enzymes in stroke. *Stroke* 1979;10:548–553.
19. Dubo H, Park DC, Pennington RJT, Kalbag RM, Walton JN. Serum-creatine-kinase in cases of stroke, head injury, and meningitis. *Lancet* 1967;2:743–748.
20. Dimant J, Grob D. Electrocardiographic changes and myocardial damage in patients with acute cerebrovascular accidents. *Stroke* 1977;8:448–455.
21. Acheson J, James DC, Hutchinson EC, Westhead R. Serum-creatine-kinase levels in cerebral vascular disease. *Lancet* 1965;1:1306–1307.
22. Norris JW, Froggatt GM, Hachinski VC. Cardiac arrhythmias in acute stroke. *Stroke* 1978;9:392–396.
23. Valeriano J, Elson J. Electrocardiographic changes in central nervous system disease. *Neurol Clin* 1993;11:257–272
24. Lane RD, Wallace JD, Petrosky PP, Schwartz GE, Gradman AH. Su-

praventricular tachycardia in patients with right hemispheric strokes. *Stroke* 1992;23:362–366.
25. Greenhoot JH, Reichenbach DD. Cardiac injury and subarachnoid hemorrhage: a clinical, pathological, and physiological correlation. *J Neurosurg* 1969;30:521–531.
26. Connor RCR. Heart damage associated with intracranial lesions. *BMJ* 1968;3:29–31.
27. Rudehill A, Olsson GL, Sundqvist K, Gordon E. ECG abnormalities in patients with subarachnoid hemorrhage and intracranial tumors. *J Neurol Neurosurg Psychiatry* 1987;50:1357–1381.
28. Kline IK. Myocardial alterations associated with pheochromocytomas. *Am J Pathol* 1961;38:539–544.
29. Van Vliet PD, Burchell HB, Titus JL. Focal myocarditis associated with pheochromocytoma. *N Engl J Med* 1966;274:1102–1108.
30. Reichenbach D, Benditt EP. Catecholamines and cardiomyopathy. *Hum Pathol* 1970;1:125–150
31. Piscatelli RL, Fox LM. Myocardial injury from epinephrine overdosage. *Am J Cardiol* 1968;21:735–737.
32. Szakas J, Cannon A. L-Norepinephrine myocarditis. *Am J Clin Pathol* 1958;30:425–434.
33. Schlesinger MJ, Reiner L. Focal myocytolysis of the heart. *Am J Pathol* 1955;31:443–459.
34. Hearse DJ, Humphrey SM, Chain EG. Abrupt reoxygenation of the anoxic potassium arrested perfused rat heart: a study of myocardial enzyme release. *J Mol Cell Cardiol* 1973;5:395–407.
35. Fulton JF. *Functional localization in the frontal lobes and cerebellum.* London: Oxford University Press, 1949:66.
36. Skinner JE. Neurocardiology: brain mechanism underlying fatal cardiac arrhythmias. *Neurol Clin* 1993;11:325–351.
37. Cechetto DF. Experimental cerebral ischemic lesions and autonomic and cardiac effects in cats and rats. *Stroke* 1993;24[suppl I]:I6–I9.
38. Oppenheimer SM, Wilson JX, Guiraudon C, Cechetto DF. Insular cortex stimulation produces lethal cardiac arrhythmias: a mechanism of sudden death? *Brain Res* 1991;550:115–121.
39. Hachinski VC, Oppenheimer SM, Wilson JX, Guiraudon C, Cachetto DF. Asymmetry of sympathetic consequences of experimental stroke. *Arch Neurol* 1992;49:697–702.
40. Oppenheimer SM, Gelb AW, Girvin JP, Hachinski VC. Cardiovascular effects of human insular stimulation. *Neurology* 1992;42:1727–1732.
41. Svigelj V, Grad A, Tekavcic I, Kiauta T. Cardiac arrhythmia associated with reversible damage to insula in a patient with subarachnoid hemorrhage. *Stroke* 1994;25:1053–1055.
42. Myers MG, Norris JW, Hachinski VC, Sole MJ. Plasma norepinephrine in stroke. *Stroke* 1981;12:200–204.
43. Hachinski VC, Smith KE, Silver MD, Gibson CJ, Ciriello J. Acute myocardial and plasma catecholamine changes in experimental stroke. *Stroke* 1986;17:387–390.
44. Smith KE, Hachinski VC, Gibson CJ, Ciriello J. Changes in plasma catecholamine levels after insula damage in experimental stroke. *Brain Res* 1986;375:182–185.
45. Hunt D, Gore I. Myocardial lesions following experimental intracranial hemorrhage: prevention with propranolol. *Am Heart J* 1972;83:232–236.
46. Samuels MA. Neurogenic heart disease: a unifying hypothesis. *Am J Cardiol* 1987;60:15J–19J.
47. Skinner JE, Mohr DN, Kellaway P. Sleep-stage regulation of ventricular arrhythmias in the unanaesthetized pig. *Circ Res* 1975 37:342–349.
48. Smith M, Ray CT. Cardiac arrhythmias, increased intracranial pressure, and the autonomic nervous system. *Chest* 1972;61:125–133.
49. Jachuck SJ, Ramani PS, Clark F, Kalbag. Electrocardiographic abnormalities associated with raised intracranial pressure. *BMJ* 1975;1:242–244.
50. Doshi R, Neil-Dwyer G. Hypothalamic and myocardial lesions after subarachnoid haemorrhage. *J Neurol Neurosurg Psychiatry* 1977;40:821–826.
51. Silver FL, Norris JW, Lewis AJ, Hachinski VC. Early mortality following stroke: a prospective review. *Stroke* 1984;15:492–496.
52. Schwartz PJ, Vanoli E, Zara D, Zaza A, Zuanetti G. The effect of antiarrhythmic drugs in life threatening arrhythmias induced by the interaction between acute myocardial ischemia and sympathetic hyperactivity. *Am Heart J* 1985; 109: 937–948.
53. Schwartz PJ, Priori SG, Vanolie, Zaza A, Zuanetti G. Efficacy of diltiazem in two experimental models of sudden death. *J Am Coll Cardiol* 1986;8:661–668.

Cerebrovascular Disease, edited by H. Hunt Batjer.
Lippincott-Raven Publishers, Philadelphia © 1997.

CHAPTER 10

Neurological Recovery

Bruce H. Dobkin

Most patients who survive an acute ischemic or hemorrhagic stroke have at least some lessening of their neurologic impairments and related functional disabilities in the subsequent 3–12 months. The mechanisms that permit improvements are beginning to be understood. Clinicians can potentially manipulate these basic mechanisms with biological and rehabilitative interventions that enhance recovery of function (1).

NATURAL HISTORY OF RECOVERY

Prospective studies of patients with acute stroke have documented the incidence of neurologic deficits and the natural history of changes in these physical and cognitive impairments. Changes are perhaps more evident over time in functional disabilities for self-care skills, mobility, and community activities that arise from impairments. Mild to moderate impairments and disabilities can respond to rehabilitation therapies.

The Nature of Postinjury Changes

To consider how patients change over time after injury, some definitions are helpful. Table 1 distinguishes between *recovery*, *sparing*, and *compensation*. Several other general terms elaborate on the mechanisms of recovery. *Restitution* of function is relatively independent of external variables such as physical and cognitive stimulation. It includes the biochemical events that tend to recover in neural tissue. *Substitution* depends on external stimuli such as rehabilitative interventions. It includes the functional adaptations of defective but partially restored neural networks that compensate for components lost or disrupted by the injury.

These distinctions, both for the behaviors we observe in

B. H. Dobkin: Department of Neurology, Neurologic Rehabilitation and Research Unit, University of California, Los Angeles, California 90095-6975.

our patients and for the biological mechanisms that might account for the behaviors, can be difficult to make clinically. Motor functions can appear to have recovered when in fact residual neural activity is actually supporting behavioral plasticity. For example, the hemiplegic patient might be able to walk well enough to get about in the community, but a formal gait analysis could reveal biomechanical adaptations and a new pattern of muscle activation in the affected leg. Studies of animal models are especially useful for understanding neural and behavioral plasticity. After a unilateral pyramidal lesion in the monkey, the ability to reach for food gradually improves and can appear to have fully recovered. A closer analysis by slow motion videotaping of the movement reveals better control of the proximal than the distal limb. The animal reaches with a grasp, brings the pellet to its mouth without the normal supination of the hand and forearm, turns its head to chase after the food, and cannot easily release its grip (2). The hand-to-mouth pattern of the hemiparetic patient is often similar to this alternate strategy.

Course of Common Impairments and Disabilities

A community-based, prospective study assessed 680 patients at the onset of an acute stroke. The investigators found a hemiparesis in 88% with equal numbers graded mild (functionally insignificant), moderate, and severe (little or no movement) (3). At 1 month, 26% had no impairment and 39% were graded as mild. Motor impairment on this broad scale at 6 months was rated as none for 39% of survivors, mild for 36%, moderate for 10%, and severe for 14%. Presenting with a mild, compared to a severe, motor impairment made it ten times more likely that full recovery would follow.

A prospective study in Bristol's Frenchay Health District followed 976 patients with an acute stroke and reexamined survivors at 3 weeks and at 6 months (4). Of the 453 cases assessed within 7 days of the stroke, 17% had no paralysis and 31% had a severe paralysis of arm and leg. At 6 months, 47% of survivors had no measurable weakness in the arm or leg, much like the results of the Framingham Study. Only

TABLE 1. *Terminology for postinjury gains*

Recovery: complete return of identical functions that were lost or impaired
Restitution: tendency of a neural network to recover after an interruption as a consequence of internal biological events
Substitution: functional adaptation of a defective but partially restored neural network that depends on external stimulation
Sparing: adequate function via residual neural pathways
Compensation: functional adaptation for an impairment or disability

From Ref. 44.

9% had profound weakness. Of those with paralysis of the arm or leg at 3 weeks after onset, no one achieved normal strength at 6 months. Scores of limb movement significantly correlated with functional outcomes on the Barthel Index. The study found that 47% of survivors were functionally independent and 21% showed moderate to severe dependence at 6 months after their stroke. Activities of daily living recovered in a consistent order at 3 weeks and at 6 months. The evolution of gains went from walking to dressing, stair climbing, and then bathing (5).

The ability to ambulate is an important outcome after stroke. A community-based population study that prospectively followed 800 acute stroke survivors initially found that 51% were unable to walk, 12% walked with assistance, and 37% were independent (6). Within the same facility, all who needed rehabilitation received services for an average total stay of 35 days (SD = 41). At discharge, 22% could not walk, 14% walked with assistance, and 64% of survivors walked independently. About 80% of those who were initially nonwalkers reached their best walking function within 6 weeks and 95% within 11 weeks. In patients who walked with assistance, 80% reached best function within 3 weeks and 95% within 5 weeks. Independent walking was achieved by 34% of the survivors who had been dependent and 60% of those who initially required assistance. Recovery of ambulation correlated directly with leg strength. These measures of recovery refer to the level of independence for walking modest distances. They do not reflect walking speed, which is often one third to one half as fast as normal, or to endurance, which is also limited after hemiplegic stroke.

Upper extremity function is another important outcome. A community study that assessed upper extremity strength and function with Barthel Index subscores for grooming and feeding found that the best function was achieved by 95% within 9 weeks (7). Patients with mild paresis improved by 6 weeks. With severe paresis they reached best function by 11 weeks. Full function was achieved by 79% of those with mild paresis, but only 18% with severe paresis. These and other studies suggest that arm and hand function for most patients tend to improve for up to 12 weeks. Patients who have fair function by 3 months can improve for up to a year in some specific tasks. Those who reach full recovery usually do so by 8 weeks.

The sensitivity of measures of initial impairments and sub-

sequent recovery, especially for cognitive and behavioral deficits, will depend on the testing method and the scales employed. Some general statements about recovery can be made. For example, in a longitudinal study of 41 patients starting within a week of a right cerebral infarction, arm and leg weakness recovered in about 40% by week 16, sensory extinction in 80% by week 46, hemianopsia in 65% by week 33, unilateral spatial neglect on drawing in 70% by week 13, anosognosia and neglect in nearly all by week 20 with half of those affected recovering by week 10, motor impersistence in all by week 55 with 45% recovering by week 8, and prosopagnosia and constructional apraxia on the block design and Rey figure in 80% by week 20 (8). Patients with smaller lesions (less than 6% of right hemisphere volume), hemorrhages, or who were younger tended to recover faster for some of these impairments. The length of time for the recovery of many of these behaviors is consistent with the notion that gains after a stroke can proceed for impairments that have a diffuse neural substrate for reorganization.

Multivariate statistical analyses have been attempted on both the acute stroke and the rehabilitation populations to establish predictors of neurologic and functional outcome. Mortality and functional recovery at 6 months were related to leg and arm power and function, a weighted mental status score similar to the Mini–Mental Status Examination, level of consciousness, score on a line cancellation test for perceptual neglect, and electrocardiographic abnormalities within 48 hours of a stroke (9). These predicted functional outcome with 67% accuracy and death with 83% accuracy. Poor strength and cognition, hemineglect, and incontinence tend to predict poorer outcomes.

POTENTIAL MECHANISMS OF RECOVERY

A variety of mechanisms can account for the improvements that follow a cerebral injury. Table 2 outlines major categories that have been investigated in human and animal studies. These mechanisms of neuroplasticity usually overlap and tend to depend on each other. They also interact with many other variables. For example, recovery from an acquired brain injury appears to partly depend on the premorbid strength of connections in neural networks. Thus, after stroke and traumatic brain injury, a higher premorbid level of education predicts better cognitive and functional outcomes. These provide some protection against losing what was learned and increase the ability of the subject to relearn. Age, number of lesions, timing of sequential lesions, and genetic factors also contribute to the degree of neurologic restoration (10,11).

Recovery of Neuronal Excitability

Improvements in initial clinical impairments evolve as reversibly injured, edematous, and metabolically depressed tissue regains its normal properties. With this, the cellular activities and the excitability of neurons, axons, and glia

TABLE 2. *Potential mechanisms for substitution or restitution of function*

A. *Network Plasticity*
    1. Recovery of neuronal excitability
        Resolution of cellular toxic-metabolic dysfunction
        Resolution of edema; resorption of blood products
        Resolution of diaschisis
    2. Activity in partially spared pathways
    3. Alternate behavioral strategies
    4. Representational mutability of neuronal assemblies
        Expansion of representational maps
        Recruitment of cells not ordinarily involved in an activity
    5. Recruitment of parallel and subcomponent pathways
        Altered activity of the distributed functions of cortical and subcortical neural networks
        Activation of pattern generators, eg, for stepping
        Inhibition and disinhibition of functional groups of neurons
        Recruitment of networks not ordinarily involved in an activity
    6. Dependence on task-related stimulation
B. *Neuronal Plasticity*
    1. Altered efficacy of synaptic activity
        Activity-dependent unmasking of previously ineffective synapses
        Learning and memory tied to activity-dependent changes in synaptic strength
        Increased neuronal responsiveness from denervation hypersensitivity
        Change in number of receptors
        Change in neurotransmitter release and uptake
    2. Synaptic sprouting
    3. Axonal and dendritic regeneration
        Signaling gene expression for cell viability, growth, and remodeling proteins
        Modulation by neurotrophic factors
        Actions of chemoattractants and inhibitors in the milieu
    4. Remyelination
    5. Transsynaptic degeneration
    6. Ion channel changes on fibers for impulse conduction
    7. Actions of neurotransmitters and neuromodulators

From Ref. 44.

recover and the functions of partially spared pathways resume. For example, as the local toxic and compressive effects of an intracerebral hemorrhage resolve, patients who have survived the initial insult tend to improve to a greater degree than patients who experienced an ischemic infarction of the same size at that location. Progressive neurologic deficits in patients with vasospasm after a subarachnoid hemorrhage can be rapidly reversed with induced hypervolemia and hypertension that restore perfusion pressure. After an ischemic stroke, functional brain imaging by positron emission tomography (PET) has revealed patterns of cerebral perfusion and oxygen metabolism that provide an early indication as to whether or not tissue and clinical recovery are likely (12). Most of the proposed pharmacologic interventions to improve the perfusion of ischemic tissue and to halt the cascade of cellular events that lead to neuronal death aim to both prevent worsening and improve impairments.

Recovery can also follow the reversal of diaschisis, which includes the notion of a transsynaptic functional deactivation of neural tissue that is remote from the injured region. On PET studies, this deactivation would be reflected by hypometabolism of, for example, the dorsolateral frontal cortex that receives direct and indirect projections from the damaged caudate and anterior limb of the internal capsule after an infarction in the distribution of the recurrent artery of Heubner. Diaschisis has also been related to the disruption of the modulation of cortical neurons by neurotransmitters from subcortical and brainstem sources that have been disconnected by an infarction or hemorrhage. Among their activities, the cholinergic projections serve as a gate for behaviorally relevant sensory information. Noradrenergic projections increase the signal-to-noise ratio and modulate resistance to distraction. Dopaminergic projections relate a reward to the cognitive effort. Histaminergic projections and serotonergic projections play roles in attention, mood, motivation, learning, and vigilance (13).

Alternate Behavioral Strategies

The method used to carry out a movement or other activity after stroke is often one that works around the impairment. In the simplest instance, a patient uses the normal left hand when the right arm is plegic. A hemiparetic gait or feeding with the affected upper limb can appear rather normal, but the activity is often carried out with motor modifications and assistive aides. Rehabilitative efforts stress this type of relearning and compensation. For example, investigators constructed life table analyses of the probability of recovering mobility in a study of patients undergoing stroke rehabilitation (14). The patients were divided into three categories of impairment and examined at 2-week intervals until they reached a plateau in recovery. Over 90% of patients with a pure motor (M) deficit became independent in walking 150 feet by week 14, but only 35% of those with motor and proprioceptive (SM) loss by week 24, and 3% of those with motor, sensory, and hemianoptic deficits (SMH) by week 30. However, with the addition of physical assistance, the probability of walking over 150 feet increased to 100% with M impairment by week 14 and to over 90% in those with SM and SMH deficits by week 28 poststroke.

Even these behavioral adaptations are likely to be mediated in part by spared pathways, the distributed functions of motor and cognitive networks, and mechanisms of learning.

Activity in Partially Spared Pathways

Descending and ascending tracts might be partially spared after a stroke. Even when magnetic resonance imaging (MRI) suggests Wallerian degeneration of a pathway, some of the axons could be intact. For example, MRI combined with PET has revealed an island of spared striate cortex in a patient with occipital infarctions who had blindsight (15).

Functional imaging could identify other spared nodes in the neural networks for cognitive and motor tasks. The severity of a chronic hemiparesis in subjects who had suffered a stroke has been correlated with the magnitude of shrinkage of the cerebral peduncle measured by computerized tomography. Sparing of more than 60% of the peduncle, including the medial portion, predicted the recovery of a precision grip and, to a lesser degree, the force of the grip (16). The typical hemiplegic posture of elbow, wrist, and finger flexion followed 60% shrinkage, which roughly corresponded to a loss of 88% of the descending fibers. After a surgical lesioning of a cerebral peduncle, very good motor function was found despite the intactness of only 17% of the axis cylinders in the ipsilateral medullary pyramid and retrograde degeneration of 90% of the precentral giant cells of Betz (17). Thus, a relatively modest percentage of residual axons can orchestrate a motor activity.

A few of the descending pathways might provide a margin of redundancy for at least partial restitution or substitution. From 70% to 90% of pyramidal fibers decussate into the lateral corticospinal tract and 10–30% remain uncrossed, forming the ventral corticospinal tract (18). The fibers of the ventral tract synapse especially with motoneurons for axial and girdle muscles. Thus, the primary motor cortex has connections that could modulate some proximal and distal ipsilateral as well as contralateral movements. Functional imaging studies show that the ipsilateral motor areas can play a role in recovery after a cerebral infarction (19).

The red nuclei help control the extremities and digits for skillful steering and fractionated movements and appear to considerably overlap the spinal projections of the motor cortex (20). The several motor cortices project directly and by collaterals to the ipsilateral red nucleus. These midbrain neurons, which also receive cerebellar projections, might independently subserve aspects of motor control for the distal limbs after a hemispheric injury (21). Other corticomotoneurons project directly and by collaterals to the upper medullary medial reticular formation. They overlap the descending reticulospinal pathway to the same spinal cord gray matter. The vestibulospinal and reticulospinal tracts connect to bilateral spinal motoneurons associated mostly with axial and girdle muscles.

Within several pathways, then, there is some potential to allow partial sparing or reorganization of their motor functions, especially for axial and proximal movements. Recovery of an adequate excitatory input to spinal motoneurons could depend on an increase in the strength of output from undamaged cortical and brainstem neurons that also descend onto spinal neurons to the same muscle.

Representational Mutability of Neuronal Assemblies

Cortical motor and sensory neurons adapt quickly to changing demands. In the adult and developing animal and in humans, the topographic maps of motor neuronal representations for movements and sensory representations of dermatomes are capable of physiologic and structural reorganization (22). Electrophysiologic and metabolic imaging experiments also reveal changes in the cortical maps for visual, auditory, and olfactory representations induced by central and peripheral lesions and by experience. Manipulations that lead to alterations in cortical somatosensory maps also change the organization of representational maps in the thalamus, brainstem, and spinal cord. This apparently ubiquitous property of adult cortical output and receptive fields offers insight into the training and other input conditions that might optimize remodeling and, in turn, the recovery of motor control and higher cognitive activities.

For example, a group of patients who had recovered from hand weakness following a stroke limited to the posterior limb of the internal capsule were studied by PET as they tapped their fingers (23). The hand area of the contralateral sensorimotor cortex was activated. In addition, the PET study showed a 1-cm extension of activation that corresponded to a spread from the hand area into the cortex that normally subserved the face. This metabolically visualized enlargement of the contiguous cortical sensorimotor field is consistent both with many animal studies that have revealed the multiple representations of muscles and movements within the motor cortex and with the mutability of neuronal representational maps (24–26). Cortical representational changes are especially likely to arise during training paradigms that involve learning and the acquisition of specific skills. For example, the more a set of neurons was activated by a sensory stimulus when a primate learned to perform a task with repeated use of the same skin surface, the more widespread the cortical sensory representation became for the most stimulated area of skin (27). This activity-dependent plasticity could be critical to understanding how impairments might lessen and skilled movements might be regained.

Recruit Parallel and Subcomponent Pathways

Motor and cognitive functions are controlled by networks whose components are distributed throughout cortical and subcortical regions (28). Regions that contribute to a motor or a cognitive activity are not so much functionally localized as they are functionally specialized.

For example. each of six cortical motor areas has a separate and independent set of inputs from adjacent and remote regions, as well as parallel, separate outputs to the brainstem and spinal cord (29). The roles of these multiple generators for movement and their interaction with their subcortical components are just beginning to be understood. The subcortical components might explain how locomotion improves despite damage to the cortical pathways. The brainstem, particularly the reticular formation, is one of the most important structures for the automatic and volitional control of features of posture and movement. Interacting with the cortex, deep cerebellar nuclei, substantia nigra, and globus pallidus, the brainstem contains a convergent region for locomotion. In animal models, stimulation of several midbrain and pontine groups of nuclei will elicit stepping and modulate the rate of stepping. These regions help control spinal motor circuits that themselves are capable of generating features of automatic stepping (30). For walking, the motor cortex needs only to establish a goal; then preset neural routines in the brainstem and spinal cord are capable of carrying out the details of automatic stepping. These parameters include the timing, intensity, and duration of the sequences of muscle activity for walking.

Intact circuits for task subroutines could enable improvements and new motor learning after a neurologic injury. Mountcastle proposed, "The remarkable capacity for improvement of function after partial brain lesions is viewed as evidence for the adaptive capacity of such distributed systems to achieve a goal, albeit slowly and with error, with the remaining neural apparatus" (31).

Activation and subtraction studies with PET and functional magnetic resonance imaging (fMRI) have broadened our understanding of some of the specific operations within the distributed neural systems for movement, language, and other aspects of cognition (32). They show how the nature of a task, such as its difficulty, whether it is internally or externally cued, and how it is learned, alters what cerebral regions come into play (33,34). For example, functional neuroimaging studies show that the recovery of prelearned finger movements requires the activation of the same primary sensorimotor and supplementary motor (SMA) cortices as the learning of a novel, difficult task (34). Functional imaging of the motor areas during the rehabilitative training of an important task could potentially be used to show whether or not critical tissue for learning is activated by the training strategy.

Regional cerebral blood flow (rCBF) studies by PET in a group of patients who recovered from a motor stroke revealed the adaptations of a neural network. About 3 months after a striatocapsular infarction, patients were tested under the conditions of rest, repeated thumb-to-finger opposition of the recovered right hand, and the same movement for the left hand (35). During the motor task with either hand, the contralateral motor cortices and ipsilateral cerebellum were activated to the same degree as in normals. However, for the patients with recovered hand function, rCBF was greater than in normal subjects in the bilateral ventral premotor, SMA, anterior insula, and parietal cortices, as well as in the ipsilateral premotor cortex and basal ganglia and the contralateral cerebellum. These nonprimary cortical motor areas seem to have served a compensatory function. Indeed this series of PET studies of hand recovery after subcortical stroke has revealed at least three mechanisms for recovery: sparing of pathways in the case of anterior limb capsular lesions; representational expansion with posterior capsular lesions; and activation of distributed pathways that would not ordinarily have been as metabolically active (23,35,36).

Cognitive functions are represented by neural networks that also show great adaptability. This plasticity is derived from their anatomically distributed, parallel processing, as well as from the projections of neurotransmitters from sub-

cortical nuclei that modulate arousal, motivation, and emotional impact (13,37). In addition, patterns of connectivity within a network reveal circuitry that possesses great flexibility (38). A further potential for compensation after disruption of a network derives from the finding that multiple associational, sensory, and motor areas of the brain contain some of the learned features of, for example, what we later recognize, though a particular modality may carry the highest weight and be especially important (39). Many cognitive rehabilitation strategies have been developed based on the notion that impairments might be ameliorated by tapping into one or more of the distributed grids of functional specialization that remain connected.

APPROACHES TO ENHANCING RECOVERY

Studies of dynamic neuronal cell assemblies suggest that specific training paradigms and drugs that increase local synaptic activity might optimize remodeling and in turn improve sensorimotor and higher cognitive activities. If the movement or sensory stimulation is part of an act that is important to the subject, the task is more likely to lead to widespread neuronal activation, to enlarge its representation, and to play a role in restitution of function. Goal-oriented training would also appear to be a means to induce the activation of the distributed pathways that might participate in partial recovery of function. Nonuse of a limb, as when compensating for impaired use of a hemiparetic hand with the normal one, would be expected to undermine the level of improvement of the affected hand.

Pharmacologic interventions might also enhance recovery. Noradrenergic and dopaminergic agents appear capable of reducing diaschisis in experimental settings (40). Some agents could replace a depleted neurotransmitter, provide a mediator for cortical representational plasticity, stimulate a subcomponent pathway of a network, such as a spinal circuit for stepping, and modulate other substances such as growth factors. Some drugs have clear-cut mechanisms of action. For example, the conduction of action potentials along demyelinated axons could be partially restored by 4-aminopyridine, which blocks potassium channels, prolongs the action potential, and improves impulse conduction (41,42). Muscle also has considerable plasticity. Fiber features are altered by thyroid and growth hormones and testosterone and β_2 agonists (43), which may stimulate muscle growth or prevent disuse atrophy.

Biological interventions (Table 2) might become practical tools in the future (44). Studies in animal models show that certain neurotrophic factors can protect injured neurons, prevent retrograde and transsynaptic degeneration after neuronal damage, and regenerate axons. Antibodies to neurite growth inhibitors can increase axonal elongation. Other manipulations of the axon's environment can guide it to target neurons to make functional connections. Transplants of critical neurons and neurotransmitter-producing cells might also enhance recovery along a particular network.

SUMMARY

Multiple groups of neurons that represent aspects of a sensorimotor or cognitive behavior can expand their representations to neighboring cells that then participate in the behavior. Task-oriented movements and learning paradigms with optimal reinforcement schedules should increase the coupling of neuronal assemblies for a sensorimotor function. Assemblies that provide features for the performance of a task are often highly distributed and function in parallel pathways, which can potentially carry out some aspects of the behavior mediated by injured pathways. These neuronal assemblies are also connected to other assemblies by relative hierarchical controls. Many of the details of motor activities, such as stepping, can be carried out by components of the hierarchy and can be evoked with little cortical input. Goal-oriented behaviors, along with paradigms that optimize learning, will induce representational plasticity and could help reorganize output from the anatomic networks that participate in a behavior. Rehabilitation, pharmacologic, and biological interventions might be developed to induce this plasticity and enhance neurologic recovery.

REFERENCES

1. Dobkin B. Neuroplasticity: key to recovery after central nervous system injury. *West J Med* 1993;159:56–60.
2. Whishaw I, Pellis S, Gorny B, Pellis V. The impairments in reaching and the movements of compensation in rats with motor cortex lesions: an endpoint, videorecording and movement notation analysis. *Behav Brain Res* 1991;42:77–91.
3. Bonita R, Beaglehole R. Recovery of motor function after stroke. *Stroke* 1988;19:1497–1500.
4. Wade D, Hewer R. Motor loss and swallowing difficulty after stroke: frequency, recovery, and prognosis. *Acta Neurol Scand* 1987;76:50–54.
5. Wade D, Langton Hewer R. Functional abilities after stroke: measurement, natural history and prognosis. *J Neurol Neurosurg Psychiatry* 1987;50:177–182.
6. Jorgensen H, Nakayama H, Raaschou H, Olsen T. Recovery of walking function in stroke patients: the Copenhagen Stroke Study. *Arch Phys Med Rehab* 1995;76:27–32.
7. Nakayama H, Jorgensen H, Raaschou H, Olsen T. Recovery of upper extremity function in stroke patients: the Copenhagen Stroke Study. *Arch Phys Med Rehab* 1994;75:394–398.
8. Hier D, Mondlock J, Caplan L. Recovery of behavioral abnormalities after right hemisphere stroke. *Neurology* 1983;33:337–350.
9. Fullerton K, Mackenzie G, Stout R. Prognostic indices in stroke. *Q J Med* 1988;66:147–162.
10. Geschwind N. Mechanisms of change after brain lesions. In: Nottebohm F, ed. Hope for a new neurology. *Ann NY Acad Sci* 1985;457:1–11.
11. Irle E. Lesion size and recovery of function: some new perspectives. *Brain Res Rev* 1987;12:307–320.
12. Marchal G, Serrati C, Baron J, et al. PET imaging of cerebral perfusion and oxygen consumption in acute ischaemic stroke: relation to outcome. *Lancet* 1993;341:925–927.
13. Mesulam M-M. Large-scale neurocognitive networks and distributed processing for attention, language, and memory. *Ann Neurol* 1990;28:597–613.
14. Reding M, Potes E. Rehabilitation outcome following initial unilateral hemispheric stroke: life table analysis approach. *Stroke* 1988;19:1354–1364.
15. Fendrich R, Wessinger C, Gazzaniga M. Technical notes: sources of blindsight. *Science* 1993;261:493–495.
16. Warabi T, Inoue K, Noda H, Murakami S. Recovery of voluntary movement in hemiplegic patients. *Brain* 1990;113:177–189.
17. Bucy P, Keplinger J, Siqueira E. Destruction of the "pyramidal tract" in man. *J Neurosurg* 1964;21:385–398.
18. Nathan P, Smith M. Effects of two unilateral cordotomies on the mobility of the lower limbs. *Brain* 1973;96:471–494.
19. Brion J-P, Demeurisse G, Capon A. Evidence of cortical reorganization in hemiparetic patients. *Stroke* 1989;20(8):1079–1084.
20. Schieber M. How might the cortex individuate movements? *Trends Neurosci* 1990;13:440–445.
21. Kennedy P. Corticospinal, rubrospinal and rubro-olivary projections: a unifying hypothesis. *Trends Neurosci* 1990;13:474–479.
22. Asanuma C. Mapping movements within a moving motor map. *Trends Neurosci* 1991;14:217–218.
23. Weiller C, Ramsay S, Wise R, Frackowiak R. Individual patterns of functional reorganization in the human cerebral cortex after capsular infarction. *Ann Neurol* 1993;33:181–189.
24. Merzenich M, Recanzone G, Jenkins W, Nudo R. How the brain functionally rewires itself. In: Arbib M, Robinson J, eds. *Natural and artificial parallel computations.* Cambridge, MA: MIT Press, 1990:170–198.
25. Jenkins W, Merzenich M, Recanzone G. Neocortical representational dynamics in adult primates: implications for neuropsychology. *Neuropsychologia* 1990;28:573–584.
26. Recanzone G, Merzenich M, Jenkins W, Grajski K, Dinse H. Topographic reorganization of the hand representation in cortical area 3b of owl monkeys trained in a frequency-discrimination task. *J Neurophysiol* 1992;67:1031–1056.
27. Recanzone G, Merzenich M, Schreiner C. Changes in the distributed temporal response properties of SI cortical neurons reflect improvements in performance on a temporally based tactile discrimination task. *J Neurophysiol* 1992;5:1071–1091.
28. Brooks V. *The neural basis of motor control.* New York: Oxford University Press, 1986:330.
29. Strick P. Anatomical organization of multiple motor areas in the frontal lobe. In: Waxman S, ed. *Functional recovery in neurological disease.* New York: Raven Press, 1988:293–312.
30. Hodgson JA, Roy R, de Leon R, Dobkin B, Edgerton VR. Can the mammalian lumbar spinal cord learn a motor task? *Med Sci Sports Med* 1994;26:1491–1497.
31. Mountcastle V. An organizing principle for cerebral function: the unit module and the distributed system. In: Schmitt F, Worden F, eds. *The Neurosciences Fourth Study Program.* Cambridge: MIT Press, 1977:21.
32. Posner M. Seeing the mind. *Science* 1993;262:673–674.
33. Rao S, Binder J, Bandettini P. Functional magnetic resonance imaging of complex human movements. *Neurology* 1993;43:2311–2318.
34. Remy P, Zilbovicius M, Leroy-Willig A, et al. Movement- and task-related activations of motor cortical areas: a positron emission tomographic study. *Ann Neurol* 1994;36:19–26.
35. Weiller C, Chollet F, Friston K, Wise R, Frackowiak R. Functional reorganization of the brain in recovery from striatocapsular infarction in man. *Ann Neurol* 1992;31:463–472.
36. Chollet F, DiPiero V, Wise R, Frackowiak R. The functional anatomy of motor recovery after stroke in humans: a study with positron emission tomography. *Ann Neurol* 1991;29:63–71.
37. McCormick D. Cholinergic and noradrenergic modulation of thalamo-cortical processing. *Trends Neurosci* 1989;12:215–220.
38. Morecraft R, Geula C, Mesulam M-M. Architecture of connectivity within a cingulo-fronto-parietal neurocognitive network for directed attention. *Arch Neurol* 1993;50:279–284.
39. Damasio A. Category-related recognition defects as a clue to the neural substrates of knowledge. *Trends Neurosci* 1990;13:95–98.
40. Boyeson M, Jones J, Harmon R. Sparing of motor function after cortical injury. *Arch Neurol* 1994;51:405–414.
41. Davis F, Stefoski D, Rush J. Orally administered 4-AP improves clinical signs in multiple sclerosis. *Ann Neurol* 1990;27:186–192.
42. Waxman S, Ritchie J. Molecular dissection of the myelinated axon. *Ann Neurol* 1993;33:121–136.
43. Gupta K, Shetty K, Agre J, et al. Human growth hormone effect on serum IGF-I and muscle function in poliomyelitis survivors. *Arch Phys Med Rehab* 1994;75:889–894.
44. Dobkin B. *Neurologic Rehabilitation.* Contemporary Neurology Series. Philadelphia: FA Davis, 1996.

Cerebrovascular Disease, edited by H. Hunt Batjer.
Lippincott-Raven Publishers, Philadelphia © 1997.

CHAPTER 11

Cerebrovascular Responses to General Anesthesia and the Modern "Neuroanesthetic"

Christian Werner and Eberhard Kochs

Rational delivery of general anesthesia and sedation to neurosurgical patients is based on the maintenance of coupling between cerebral metabolism and cerebral blood flow (CBF) while achieving hypnosis, amnesia, analgesia, low central sympathetic tone, and a "relaxed brain." The administration of anesthetics and narcotics is associated with substantial changes in CBF, cerebral oxygen consumption ($CMRO_2$), and intracranial pressure (ICP). In the presence of an intracranial pathology (such as intracranial space–occupying lesion, intracranial hemorrhage, cerebral vasospasm, or trauma), the CBF autoregulation, cerebrovascular reactivity to CO_2 and drugs, as well as the physiologic intracranial pressure volume relation are frequently impaired or abolished.[1] Any uncritical use of anesthetic or narcotic agents may produce cerebral ischemia and increases in ICP, which in turn may increase neuronal injury and worsen neurologic damage. It is therefore important to know the effects of anesthetic agents and their impact on CBF, $CMRO_2$, and ICP in both physiologic and pathologic conditions.

Numerous studies have investigated the effects of anesthetics and narcotics on CBF, $CMRO_2$, and ICP in laboratory animals and humans. However, the data from these studies are often controversial. Several factors may account for the lack of consistency of investigations assessing the anesthetic effects on CBF and $CMRO_2$.

1. *Differences in the CBF measurement technique* (eg, microspheres vs. Kety–Schmidt techniques vs. autoradiography). Investigations of CBF are comparable only with other investigations of that region of interest. For example, cortical CBF is physiologically different from global or hemispheric CBF and will be changed as a function of regionally specific anesthetic effects.

2. *Species differences.* Resting CBF decreases over time in dogs and goats anesthetized with constant concentrations of volatile agents whereas CBF increases over time in primates under identical conditions. Additionally, human studies are usually performed in a select patient population, which does not represent normal conditions.

3. *Baseline tone.* Cerebrovascular responses to anesthetic agents are related to the baseline cerebrovascular tone, which is a function of both the baseline cerebral metabolism and the background anesthetic condition. This explains why differences in baseline conditions between animal and/or human studies may produce different results (1).

INHALATIONAL ANESTHETICS

In general, the inhalational anesthetics halothane, isoflurane, sevoflurane, and desflurane depress cerebral metabolism in a dose-dependent fashion. However, inhalational anesthetics produce direct cerebral vasodilatation with increasing concentrations of the volatile agent while reducing cerebral metabolism in a dose-dependent fashion. For years this effect has been considered an "uncoupling" between CBF and cerebral metabolism. However, a more recent view of the issue of flow/metabolism uncoupling suggests that local CBF and local cerebral glucose consumption are still coupled with increasing concentrations of isoflurane (2). This is based on autoradiographic studies in rats that show that flow remains coupled to the degree of cerebral metabolic depression with isoflurane whereas the relation between flow and metabolism is reset along a different line

---

[1] Intracranial compliance is something of a misnomer, although it is widely used. Compliance, rigorously defined, is change in volume for a given change in pressure (DV/DP), as might be applicable to pulmonary mechanics. In the case of the brain, we usually are concerned with the inverse of this relationship, ie, the change in pressure for a given change in volume (DP/DV). The inverse of compliance is properly termed elastance. For the sake of simplicity, we have used the common parlance rather than the more technically precise term.

C. Werner and E. Kochs: Department of Anesthesiology, Technische Universität München, 81675 Munich, Germany.

at each respective minimal alveolar concentration (MAC) level (2). The cerebrovascular dilatation induced by volatile anesthetics may result in increases in cerebral blood volume and ICP, which is most pronounced in the presence of nitrous oxide (N_2O). In contrast to most volatile anesthetic agents, such as halothane, isoflurane, sevoflurane, desflurane, and enflurane, the cerebral metabolism appears to be unaffected or stimulated with N_2O.

Halothane and Isoflurane

Isoflurane has a long record of safe use in patients undergoing intracranial surgery. Compared to halothane, isoflurane has a relatively low blood/gas partition coefficient that allows for appropriate control during the induction and emergence from anesthesia. Both halothane and isoflurane are associated with adequate hemodynamic stability during normovolemia. As with volatile anesthetics, however, halothane and isoflurane have the potential to elevate cerebral blood volume and ICP.

Several studies have shown that halothane or isoflurane anesthesia is associated with a decrease in cerebrovascular resistance that results in an increase in CBF (1,3). This increase in CBF is not due to cerebral metabolic stimulation because both agents reduce cerebral metabolism, isoflurane more than halothane. In N_2O-anesthetized cats, isoflurane (0.5–1.5 MAC) produced a dose-dependent decrease in $CMRO_2$ that was similar to that of halothane (4). However, the cortical CBF was unchanged with isoflurane regardless of the anesthetic dose. In contrast, both isoflurane and halothane increased CBF in barbiturate-anesthetized rabbits (1). These results suggest that the cerebrovascular effects of isoflurane and halothane are dependent on the status of cerebral metabolism prior to their administration. When the baseline cerebral metabolism is not markedly depressed (N_2O background anesthesia), halothane and isoflurane decrease cerebral metabolism with only minor changes in CBF. With barbiturate background anesthesia, halothane and isoflurane produce significant cerebral vasodilatation and increase CBF.

Differences in CBF between isoflurane and other volatile anesthetics may also be due to regionally specific effects of the various volatile anesthetics and differences in the tissue regions measured by different CBF techniques. Measurements of cortical CBF using the xenon-133 injection technique have shown that CBF was increased with halothane but unchanged with isoflurane despite decreases in cerebral vascular resistance (4). In contrast, autoradiographic measurements found substantial differences in regional CBF between isoflurane and halothane. Although hemispheric CBF was similar between the two agents, neocortical CBF was higher with halothane and subcortical CBF was higher with isoflurane (5).

Increasing concentrations of isoflurane reduce cerebral metabolism until cortical electrical activity is maximally suppressed (EEG isoelectricity) (1,3,6). The cerebral metabolic depression appears to be greater with isoflurane compared to halothane, which does not cause complete EEG suppression (4). With EEG isoelectricity, further increase in the isoflurane concentration had no effect on cerebral metabolism. At high isoflurane concentrations (4 MAC), brain biopsy analyses revealed normal concentrations of ATP, phosphocreatine, and normal energy charges (6). This indicates that isoflurane can abolish cerebral cortical activity without adversely affecting the cerebral metabolic pathways.

The cerebrovascular responses to changes in Pa_{CO_2} are maintained with halothane and isoflurane. Studies in rats have shown that CO_2 reactivity was similar for both agents although halothane appeared to selectively vasodilate cortical vessels (7). In cats, the CO_2 reactivity was even greater during 1 MAC isoflurane compared to 1 MAC halothane (8). This is consistent with studies in dogs showing cerebral vasoconstriction to hypocapnia with 1 and 2 MAC isoflurane (9). However, CO_2 reactivity to hypercapnia may be impaired or abolished at isoflurane concentrations >2 MAC due to the preexisting cerebral vasodilatation. In dogs subjected to 3 hours of isoflurane anesthesia, cerebral CO_2 reactivity was decreased over time as was normocapnic CBF (10). In contrast, studies in primates constantly exposed to 1 MAC isoflurane have shown that CBF increased over time whereas cerebral metabolism did not change (11). This indicates the substantial impact of species differences on measurements of CBF. In cats and dogs, CBF autoregulation was maintained within the mean arterial blood pressure range of 85–120 mm Hg with 1 MAC isoflurane but was impaired with 1 MAC halothane. However, increases in CBF occurred with increases in cerebral perfusion pressure during 2 MAC isoflurane, indicating an impaired CBF autoregulation with higher concentrations of isoflurane (12).

Animal studies have shown that isoflurane produces less brain surface protrusion and less increase in ICP at 0.5, 1.0, and 1.5 MAC isoflurane compared to halothane (4,13). This effect appears to be consistent with the substantial increases in cortical CBF seen with halothane but not isoflurane anesthesia. In fentanyl/droperidol-anesthetized hypocapnic baboons, administration of isoflurane did not significantly change CBF or cerebral blood volume (14). However, the combination of isoflurane with N_2O may increase cerebral blood volume and ICP even in the presence of hypocapnia (15,16). This suggests that increases in ICP seen with isoflurane are related to the preexisting cerebrovascular tone induced by normocapnia or N_2O. In rabbits subjected to cryogenic brain injury, halothane anesthesia was associated with less edema formation in the vicinity of the insult compared to isoflurane, although the animals may have differed in the severity of the lesion and intracranial hypertension (17).

In humans, the effects of isoflurane and halothane on CBF and cerebral metabolism appear to be similar to the results from studies in laboratory animals. In neurosurgical patients, isoflurane anesthesia (0.65–1.5 MAC) produced only minor changes in cortical CBF whereas administration of halothane (0.65–1.5 MAC) was associated with substantial increases in cortical CBF (18—20). This is consistent with data from patients undergoing carotid endarterectomy where CBF within the territory of the middle cerebral artery was higher with halothane than with isoflurane (21). In contrast, the reduction in cerebral metabolism was more pronounced with isoflurane at any given MAC level (19–21). Measurements of the regional distribution of CBF in humans during 1 MAC isoflurane vs. 1 MAC halothane anesthesia have confirmed autoradiographic studies where subcortical CBF was higher with isoflurane whereas cortical CBF was higher with halothane (22). Cerebrovascular CO_2 reactivity was maintained with isoflurane and halothane anesthesia in clinically relevant concentrations in normal subjects (22) or in patients with intracranial mass lesions or cerebrovascular occlusive disease (23–25). In contrast to the animal studies, administration of constant isoflurane concentrations did not change CBF as a function of time (24).

In normocapnic neurosurgical patients, administration of isoflurane was associated with increases in ICP, but this effect was reversible with the induction of hypocapnia or infusion of barbiturates (26,27). The available data suggest that inhalation of isoflurane in concentrations less than 1 MAC and in combination with hypocapnia is not associated with clinically relevant increases in ICP.

Sevoflurane and Desflurane

Sevoflurane and desflurane are relatively new inhalational anesthetic agents with lower blood/gas partition coefficients than isoflurane. The low solubility of these inhalational anesthetics is associated with more rapid uptake and elimination, promising fast induction and emergence from anesthesia.

The effects of sevoflurane on CBF, cerebral metabolism, and ICP appear to be similar to those of isoflurane. In spontaneously ventilating rats receiving 1 MAC sevoflurane anesthesia, CBF was increased 35% compared to the awake state (28). However, increases in CBF with sevoflurane may have been due to the hypercapnic effect induced by the anesthetic state. In morphine/N_2O-anesthetized rabbits, 1 MAC sevoflurane or isoflurane produced a 50% reduction in $CMRO_2$ parallel to EEG burst suppression with no evidence of spike or seizure activity (29). Global and cortical CBF were unchanged during anesthesia with 0.5 or 1.0 MAC sevoflurane or isoflurane. This suggests ''uncoupling'' between cerebral metabolism and CBF with sevoflurane. However, ICP was increased with the administration of sevoflurane and isoflurane, indicating a nonlinear relation between CBF and cerebral blood volume (29).

In dogs, desflurane (0.5–2.0 MAC) produced a dose-related decrease in $CMRO_2$ (30). The cerebral metabolic suppression with desflurane was associated with suppression of cortical electrical activity similar to burst suppression seen with isoflurane. The cerebrovascular responses to desflurane

were related to the status of cerebral perfusion pressure. CBF was unchanged when cerebral perfusion pressure decreased with increasing concentrations of desflurane. In contrast, CBF increased when cerebral perfusion pressure was maintained using phenylephrine infusion. This suggests that CBF autoregulation is impaired with desflurane in concentrations >1 MAC. Desflurane-induced systemic hypotension (mean arterial blood pressure 40 mm Hg) decreased CBF 60% and $CMRO_2$ 21% (31). However, normal cerebral metabolite concentrations of high-energy phosphates taken at the end of the hypotensive challenge suggest that CBF was still adequate to meet cerebral metabolic demands. In desflurane-anesthetized dogs (0.5–1.5 MAC) with and without systemic hypotension, cerebrovascular CO_2 reactivity to hypocapnia ($Paco_2$ 20 mm Hg) was maintained, although attenuation occurred at higher MAC levels (32). Desflurane may increase ICP by at least two mechanisms: general cerebrovascular dilatation (30) and/or imbalance between the formation and reabsorption of cerebrospinal fluid (33).

In hyperventilated neurosurgical patients, CBF during use of 1.0 MAC desflurane was similar compared to using 1.0 MAC isoflurane (24). CBF did not change when desflurane or isoflurane concentrations were increased to 1.5 MAC. Cerebrovascular reactivity to CO_2 was maintained with both anesthetics within the $Paco_2$ range of 25–35 mm Hg. This is consistent with results from patients with ischemic cerebrovascular disease and 0.88 MAC sevoflurane anesthesia, where cerebrovascular CO_2 reactivity was maintained within a $Paco_2$ range of 35–45 mm Hg (34). In these patients, CBF remained unchanged within the mean arterial blood pressure range of 89–113 mm Hg, indicating preserved CBF autoregulation. In patients with supratentorial mass lesions, cerebrospinal fluid pressure measured in the lumbar subarachnoid space may increase during 1 MAC desflurane anesthesia but not during 1 MAC isoflurane anesthesia (35).

Nitrous Oxide

N_2O is one of the oldest and most commonly administered anesthetic adjuvants. It possesses characteristics that make it an excellent supplemental anesthetic/analgesic: it is inexpensive, easy to deliver, and has a low blood/gas partition coefficient that results in a rapid onset and recovery. Early reports have suggested that N_2O acts as an analgesic agent with only minimal cerebrovascular effects. However, recent studies indicate that N_2O may increase CBF, cerebral blood volume, and ICP and should be avoided as a supplemental anesthetic/analgesic in patients with decreased intracranial compliance.

In awake goats and rats, inhalation of 70% N_2O produced regionally specific increases in CBF and $CMRO_2$ (36,37). In contrast, experiments in rabbits anesthetized with halothane, isoflurane, or fentanyl/pentobarbital have shown that the administration of 70% N_2O was associated with increases in

CBF during normocapnia and hypocapnia whereas cerebral metabolism was unchanged, regardless of the background anesthetic or the status of $Paco_2$ (38). This is consistent with experiments in halothane- or isoflurane-anesthetized, normocapnic rats and dogs where 0.5 MAC N_2O resulted in substantial increases in CBF with both background anesthetics while cerebral glucose consumption remained unchanged (39–41). These data indicate that N_2O is a potent cerebral vasodilator that can increase CBF by mechanisms other than cerebral metabolic activation. However, the vasodilatation induced by N_2O is related to the preexisting cerebrovascular tone induced by the background anesthetic. Likewise, N_2O may also increase ICP. In rabbits anesthetized with halothane, isoflurane, or fentanyl/pentobarbital, the administration of 70% N_2O was associated with an increase in ICP during normocapnia and hypocapnia (38).

In awake, normocapnic humans, middle cerebral artery flow velocity was increased during inhalation of 30% or 60% N_2O (42). This supports regional CBF data in humans, showing increases in CBF with inhalation of 50% N_2O during normocapnia and hypocapnia (43). In contrast, CBF increased 43% during normocapnia but was unchanged during hypocapnia in isoflurane-anesthetized patients (44). In this study, $CMRO_2$ was unchanged with the administration of N_2O. These data support results from animal studies, further reinforcing the interaction between the cerebrovascular responses to N_2O and the background anesthetic technique. While cerebrovascular CO_2 reactivity may be reduced during N_2O inhalation, the regional distribution of CBF is related to the level of $Paco_2$ (43). During hypocapnia, inhalation of 50% N_2O increased CBF to frontal, parietal, and temporal brain structures as well as to the thalamus and basal ganglia compared to hypocapnic CBF without N_2O (43). Several clinical reports indicate that N_2O increases ICP (45,46). The increase in ICP seen with the administration of N_2O appears to be mitigated by the induction of hypocapnia or the infusion of cerebral vasoconstrictors. This suggests that the increase in ICP is related to increases in CBF and cerebral blood volume, as suggested by animal experiments.

Patients with intracranial pathology but normal ICP may be ventilated using N_2O. To be conservative, however, N_2O should probably be avoided in those patients expected to have reduced intracranial compliance (eg, head injury, emergent reoperations for bleeds).

NONNARCOTIC INTRAVENOUS AGENTS

Intravenous anesthetic agents such as barbiturates, etomidate, and propofol are widely used in neurosurgical patients for induction and maintenance of anesthesia. In general, with the exception of ketamine, intravenous anesthetics are considered to be cerebral vasoconstrictors, although this effect appears to be secondary to the cerebral metabolic depression induced by these drugs. Intravenous anesthetics reduce ICP or have little effect on it (except ketamine), providing con-

trolled ventilation to prevent hypercapnia. There is experimental evidence that their use may improve neurologic outcome following focal cerebral ischemia, making continuous infusion of intravenous anesthetics during neurosurgical procedures an attractive technique. However, infusion of intravenous anesthetics may be associated with hemodynamic instability and prolonged emergence from anesthesia.

Barbiturates

In dogs, infusion of thiopental produced dose-dependent decreases of $CMRO_2$ and suppression of spontaneous EEG until induction of EEG burst suppression (47). The cerebral metabolic and functional depression was paralleled by increases in cerebral vascular resistance and concomitant decreases in CBF. A similar reduction in CBF and $CMRO_2$ has been reported with phenobarbital and pentobarbital. With the induction of stable EEG isoelectricity (ie, maximum suppression of cortical functional activity), additional barbiturate did not change $CMRO_2$ or CBF. This indicates that coupling of CBF and $CMRO_2$ is maintained with barbiturate infusion. Cerebrovascular reactivity to CO_2 is qualitatively maintained but quantitatively reduced as a function of increases in cerebrovascular resistance due to the barbiturate. In contrast to time-dependent changes in the cerebrovascular responses to CO_2 during halothane or isoflurane anesthesia, CO_2 reactivity does not change with barbiturates over time (10).

The experimental data support studies in volunteers (48) whereby infusion of thiopental (10–55 mg/kg total dose) was associated with 50–55% decreases in $CMRO_2$ and CBF compared to historical controls. Cerebrovascular CO_2 reactivity was also maintained. Patients with increased ICP may thus benefit from bolus applications of barbiturates as well as from transient hyperventilation with barbiturate background anesthesia since the reduction in intracranial blood volume can reduce ICP (49). However, barbiturate infusion may lead to cerebral ischemia in patients with elevated ICP whenever mean arterial blood pressure is decreased to an extent where cerebral perfusion pressure is critically reduced.

Etomidate

Studies in dogs have shown that etomidate produces a dose-dependent reduction in $CMRO_2$ and CBF, until EEG burst suppression is induced (50). In contrast to the barbiturates, etomidate decreased CBF and $CMRO_2$ in a nonlinear fashion. Near-maximum reduction of CBF was induced by low rates of etomidate infusion (0.02 mg/kg/min); further increase in the rate of infusion (0.3 mg/kg/min) produced progressive suppression of $CMRO_2$ until EEG burst suppression. However, this was not associated with further decreases in CBF despite an increased total dose. This suggests that etomidate decreases canine CBF by direct cerebral vasoconstriction rather than neuronal metabolic suppression alone, but these results have not been confirmed. Unlike barbiturates, etomidate changes cerebral metabolism in a regionally specific fashion. Autoradiographic studies in laboratory animals have shown reductions of cerebral glucose consumption predominantly in frontal and parietal brain areas whereas only minor changes were measured in occipital tissue regardless of the anesthetic dose (51).

In contrast to studies in dogs, clinically relevant concentrations of etomidate (0.02–0.06 mg/kg/min) produced concomitant decreases in $CMRO_2$ and CBF in patients (52). The cerebrovascular reactivity to CO_2 was maintained with etomidate. Systemic hemodynamic depression was less pronounced with etomidate compared to barbiturate infusion. Studies in head-injured patients have shown that etomidate administration decreases ICP with only minor reductions in mean arterial blood pressure or cerebral perfusion pressure (53). Etomidate has a short beta-elimination half-life and is hence useful for continuous infusion in the ICU. However, its use for prolonged sedation has been prevented by its ability to inhibit 2-β hydroxylase enzyme in the adrenal cortex and thereby inhibit corticosteroid synthesis. Whether clinically significant inhibition of the enzyme occurs with a single dose is not clear.

Propofol

Propofol, similar to barbiturates, produces a dose-dependent reduction of $CMRO_2$ and CBF until induction of EEG burst suppression (54,55). With the induction of EEG isoelectricity, further increases in the propofol plasma concentration did not change $CMRO_2$ or CBF. Cerebral metabolic suppression appears to be the major mechanism for a reduction in CBF. Studies in laboratory animals have shown that the cerebrovascular reactivity to CO_2 is maintained even with high doses of propofol (48 mg/kg/hr) (54). In dogs, propofol infusion of 48 mg/kg/hr was associated with impaired CBF autoregulation when cerebral perfusion pressure was decreased from 76 ± 14 mm Hg to 42 ± 11 mm Hg (54). In contrast, studies in rats found CBF autoregulation maintained within a mean arterial blood pressure range of 50–140 mm Hg with doses as high as 120 mg/kg/hr (56).

In cardiac patients, propofol infusion (12 mg/kg/hr) was associated with parallel decreases in global $CMRO_2$ and global CBF (57). This is consistent with studies in healthy volunteers anesthetized with propofol (7.8 ± 1.5 mg/kg/hr) where cerebral metabolic depression was higher in cortical (-58%) compared to subcortical tissue (-48%) (58). Studies in healthy humans have shown that propofol infusion (<200 μg/kg/min with or without N_2O) is associated with preserved CBF autoregulation within a mean arterial blood pressure range of 66–115 mm Hg (59). Cerebrovascular reactivity to CO_2 was also maintained with propofol (3–12 mg/kg/hr) (57). Propofol reduces ICP in a fashion comparable to that of barbiturates or etomidate (60,61). However,

propofol may critically reduce cerebral perfusion pressure due to decreases in systemic vascular resistance. This response is related to the propofol dose, speed of infusion, and preexisting volume status of the patients. Infusion of propofol may be associated with the occurrence of opisthotonus, or substantial EEG beta activity at times when the patient would be considered clinically to be "awake." Some authors have suggested that propofol is proconvulsant; however, evidence is weak and most would suggest that propofol has potent anticonvulsant effects, although its use may interfere with recording of EEG spikes (62).

BENZODIAZEPINES

The benzodiazepines produce many of the characteristics considered mandatory for the "anesthetic state." All benzodiazepines have hypnotic, sedative, anxiolytic, centrally acting muscle relaxant, amnestic, and anticonvulsant properties. In addition, the effects of benzodiazepines can be reversed by the specific competitive antagonist flumazenil. There is also experimental evidence that benzodiazepines may increase the tolerance of the brain during hypoxic or ischemic challenges. Due to the pharmacokinetic properties of currently available benzodiazepines, recovery from sedation or anesthesia following benzodiazepine infusion may be prolonged. However, more rapid emergence would be possible with agents that are more short acting.

In laboratory animals, benzodiazepines induce a dose-dependent reduction in CBF secondary to cerebral metabolic suppression (63). However, benzodiazepines appear to have some direct vasoconstrictor effects on cerebral vessels within the low-dose range. Studies in dogs have shown that the infusion of midazolam (0.2 mg/kg) produced decreases in CBF without changing $CMRO_2$ (64). This uncoupling between CBF and $CMRO_2$ was not associated with electrophysiologic or biochemical evidence of cerebral ischemia. In contrast, infusion of higher doses of midazolam (2–10 mg/kg) was associated with a parallel reduction of CBF and $CMRO_2$ (65). The cerebrovascular effects of benzodiazepines appear to be independent of background anesthesia using N_2O.

In surgical patients, midazolam produced concomitant decreases in $CMRO_2$ and CBF when fentanyl was given as a background narcotic agent (66). CBF autoregulation and cerebrovascular CO_2 reactivity are maintained with benzodiazepines. Decreases in CBF following benzodiazepine infusion are not associated with substantial changes in cerebral blood volume. This hypothesis is consistent with clinical observations where ICP did not change in patients with a normal ICP following midazolam; in contrast, ICP was decreased following midazolam in patients with intracranial hypertension (67).

Flumazenil reverses the sedative effect of benzodiazepines as well as the depression of CBF, cerebral metabolism, and ICP. Therefore, acute benzodiazepine reversal may be deleterious in patients with high baseline ICP.

NARCOTICS

The synthetic opioids fentanyl, alfentanil, sufentanil, and the new short-acting narcotic agent remifentanil have been used extensively in patients with intracranial pathology as they provide potent analgesia with maintained hemodynamic stability. The effects of all narcotics can be reversed by the μ-receptor antagonist naloxone or by the agonist-antagonist nalbuphine. Recent studies in laboratory animals and humans indicate variable changes in CBF and ICP with infusion of narcotic agents. The variability of narcotic effects on CBF and ICP appears to be related to the use of different background anesthetics and changes in mean arterial blood pressure rather than to differences in species.

In vivo experiments in piglets using the cranial window technique have shown that fentanyl, alfentanil, and sufentanil produce dose-dependent pial arteriolar vasoconstriction (68). This effect appears to be mediated by opioid receptors and is independent of the analgesic effect of the drug. These morphometric studies are consistent with data from N_2O-anesthetized rats, where $CMRO_2$ and CBF were reduced with fentanyl (25–400 μg/kg) or sufentanil (5–160 μg/kg) regardless of the status of arterial blood pressure (69,70). CBF and ICP were also decreased in isoflurane/N_2O anesthetized dogs following infusion of remifentanil (0.5–1.0 μg/kg/min) (71). In contrast, studies in awake or lightly anesthetized (0.1% halothane) dogs (without N_2O) have shown that fentanyl (50–100 μg/kg) or sufentanil (10–200 μg/kg) may increase CBF (72,73). In these experiments, increases in CBF were completely blocked by the presence of N_2O (73). These controversial results suggest that the responses of CBF to opioid infusion are related to the preexisting cerebral vascular tone induced by N_2O (36). In dogs and rats, cerebrovascular reactivity to changes in arterial CO_2 and cerebral and spinal cord blood flow autoregulation are maintained with opioids (74,75).

The effects of narcotic agents on ICP are controversial. ICP was constant following 2 μg/kg sufentanil and controlled mean arterial blood pressure in piritramide-anesthetized dogs with and without decreased intracranial compliance (76). In contrast, ICP was increased in halothane-anesthetized rabbits with cryogenic brain injury given 20 μg/kg sufentanil (77). In healthy human volunteers, CBF did not change with sufentanil infusion (0.5 μg/kg) (78). However, higher doses of sufentanil (<15 μg/kg total dose) were associated with decreases in CBF and $CMRO_2$ in patients undergoing carotid or cardiac surgery (79). This suggests that decreases in CBF occurred secondary to cerebral metabolic depression. In patients undergoing carotid endarterectomy with sufentanil (1.5–2.0 μg/kg bolus followed by a continuous infusion of 0.2–0.3 μg/kg/hr) (80) or resection of supratentorial masses with remifentanil (1 μg/kg/10 min)

(81), CO_2 reactivity was maintained. Studies in midazolam-sedated, head-injured patients with intracranial hypertension found no increases in ICP with sufentanil (0.5–3.0 μg/kg) as long as mean arterial blood pressure was maintained constant (82,83). In contrast, studies in patients with head injury and normal or elevated ICP have shown that ICP may increase with fentanyl (3.0 μg/kg) or sufentanil (0.6–3.0 μg/kg) (83,84,85). However, increases in ICP were always associated with concomitant decreases in mean arterial blood pressure. This suggests that all increase in ICP is due to an appropriate autoregulatory decrease in cerebral vascular resistance secondary to decreased cerebral perfusion pressure. With decreases in cerebral perfusion pressure secondary to systemic hypotension, cerebral vasodilatation occurs to maintain CBF constant. This autoregulatory decrease in cerebral vascular resistance is associated with an increase in cerebral blood volume that in turn increases ICP. Taken together, the available data suggest that narcotic agents can be used in patients with decreased intracranial compliance or high ICP as long as arterial blood pressure is supported and maintained in normal range.

Antagonism of narcotic effects using naloxone or nalbuphine may increase CBF and $CMRO_2$ and rapid reversal of narcosis. Hence, such a pharmacologic intervention should be undertaken with care in patients with decreased intracranial compliance.

KETAMINE

The phencyclidine derivative ketamine is a noncompetitive N-methyl-D-aspartate (NMDA) receptor antagonist with the thalamoneocortical projection system as the primary site of action. Ketamine induces regional neuronal excitation and produces a cataleptic state with dose-related unconsciousness and analgesia. Ketamine has never been considered an attractive anesthetic agent in neurosurgical patients because it produces regionally specific stimulation of cerebral metabolism and increases CBF and ICP. However, recent experiments suggest that in animal models of incomplete cerebral ischemia and brain injury ketamine may reduce infarct size. This experimental protective effect appears to be related to decreases in Ca^{2+}-influx and maintenance of brain tissue magnesium due to the NMDA and quisqualate receptor blockade by ketamine.

Studies in dogs have shown that ketamine (2.0 mg/kg) reduces CBF in the presence of the cerebral vasodilator N_2O (86). In contrast, studies in rats without background anesthesia found increases in CBF with ketamine (100 mg/kg IP) (87). This suggests that the cerebrovascular effects of ketamine are related to the preexisting cerebrovascular tone induced by background anesthetics. Cerebrovascular CO_2 reactivity was maintained regardless of the baseline cerebrovascular resistance. There are several mechanisms by which ketamine may increase CBF. Ketamine induces a dose-dependent respiratory depression with consecutive mild hypercapnia in spontaneously ventilating subjects. This produces vasodilatation based on the intact cerebrovascular CO_2 reactivity. Ketamine also induces regional neuroexcitation. This leads to stimulation of cerebral glucose consumption in the limbic, extrapyramidal, auditory, and sensory–motor systems (87). This regional neuroexcitation with consecutive increases in cerebral metabolism produces an increase in CBF that can be blocked with the infusion of barbiturates or benzodiazepines. However, increase in CBF with ketamine (1 mg/kg) may also occur during normocapnia and without any change in cerebral metabolism (88). This indicates some additional direct cerebral vasodilating action of ketamine (89).

Infusion of ketamine alters intracranial volume and ICP. Studies in spontaneously ventilating pigs with and without intracranial hypertension have shown that ketamine (0.5–5.0 mg/kg) produces an increase in $Paco_2$ and ICP (90). In contrast, identical experiments with mechanical ventilation and controlled $Paco_2$ found no changes in ICP following ketamine infusion. This shows that increases in ICP are related to inadequate ventilation with consecutive hypercapnia and increases in intracranial blood volume (91). However, mechanical ventilation may not be sufficient to control ICP following ketamine administration. Experiments in mechanically ventilated dogs indicate that ketamine (2 mg/kg) increases cerebral blood volume and ICP even in the presence of normoventilation, a response that is reversible with hyperventilation or the administration of diazepam (91).

Studies in patients have shown that ketamine (2.0 mg/kg) reduces CBF in the presence of cerebral vasodilators such as halothane or N_2O (92). In contrast, studies in unanesthetized humans found increases in CBF with ketamine (2–3 mg/kg) (93,94). This observation is consistent with animal studies and suggests that the cerebrovascular effects of ketamine are related to the preexisting cerebrovascular tone induced by background anesthetics.

Studies in humans with and without intracranial pathology confirm the data from animal experiments. In patients, increases in ICP appear to be most pronounced when baseline ICP is elevated and when the infusion of ketamine induces hypercapnia and the resulting increase in cerebral blood volume (90). This supports the view that infusion of ketamine is not indicated in patients with intracranial hypertension.

α_2-ADRENERGIC AGONISTS

Clonidine and dexmedetomidine are α_2-adrenergic agonists available as oral or intravenous agents. The clinical effects of clonidine and the more potent dexmedetomidine are predominantly related to stimulation of α_2-adrenergic receptors that reduce secretion of norepinephrine from presynaptic sympathetic nerve terminals. The reduction in central and peripheral sympathetic tone results in systemic antihypertensive responses, sedation, analgesia, and increased tolerance of the brain to ischemic episodes. In the rat, stimu-

lation of α_2 receptors was associated with a reduction of the minimal alveolar concentration (MAC) for halothane, by 48% with clonidine and by approximately 90% with dexmedetomidine (95,96). These results are consistent with clinical studies showing a reduction in the requirements of barbiturates and isoflurane with perioperative administration of dexmedetomidine (97,98). The increasing clinical interest in α_2-adrenergic agonists is due to experimental and clinical observations showing excellent hemodynamic stability associated with substantial reductions in the concentrations and side effects of intravenous and volatile anesthetics. Intravenous α_2-adrenergic agonists are not yet available in the United States, and experimental evidence for perioperative hemodynamic stability combined with analgesia and brain protection must be shown in humans prior to a definitive clinical recommendation.

Experiments in barbiturate-anesthetized cats have shown that the infusion of clonidine (20 μg/kg) produced a 37% reduction in CBF (99). In the same experiments, CBF autoregulation was maintained within a mean arterial blood pressure range of 60–180 mm Hg. This is in contrast to studies in dogs where infusion of dexmedetomidine (10 μg/kg), a more potent α_2-adrenergic agonist, produced decreases in CBF only in the presence of isoflurane and halothane but not with barbiturates. This indicates that the changes in CBF induced by α_2-adrenergic agonists are related to the baseline cerebrovascular dilatation induced by volatile anesthetics. However, $CMRO_2$ did not change regardless of the background anesthetic (100,101). The uncoupling between cerebral metabolism and CBF did not induce cerebral ischemia. Cerebrovascular reactivity to CO_2 is preserved with clonidine (99) or dexmedetomidine (100) but may be reduced by >50% compared to subjects without α_2-adrenergic stimulation. This is likely related to the increased cerebral vascular tone induced by clonidine or dexmedetomidine, which in part antagonizes the vasodilating stimulation of CO_2. The cerebral vasoconstriction of α_2-adrenergic agonists affects both the arterial and the capacitance vessels with consecutive reductions in cerebral blood volume. This is suggested by studies in dogs with subarachnoid hemorrhage showing dose-related decreases in ICP with the α_2-adrenergic agonist xylazine (102). In contrast, experiments in rabbits with low and high intracranial compliance states demonstrated no decreases in ICP following dexmedetomidine (20–320 μg/kg) (103).

SUMMARY

This chapter shows that all of the anesthetic agents and adjuvants currently available for neuroanesthetic practice present advantages and disadvantages. The uncritical application of any anesthetic or narcotic agent may produce increases in ICP and cerebral ischemia in turn may worsen neurologic outcome. Neuroanesthetic management requires flexibility and modification based on the knowledge of the effects of drugs on CBF, CMRO$_2$, and ICP in both physiologic and pathologic conditions according to the individual status of the patient.

The inhalational anesthetics isoflurane, sevoflurane, and desflurane depress cerebral metabolism in a dose-dependent fashion. However, inhalational anesthetics produce direct cerebral vasodilatation with increasing concentrations of the volatile agent. This "uncoupling" between CBF and cerebral metabolism may result in increases in cerebral blood volume and ICP that are most pronounced in the presence of N$_2$O. In contrast, cerebral metabolism appears to be unaffected or stimulated by N$_2$O. As with the other inhalational anesthetics, CBF is increased with N$_2$O. The administration of hypnotics, benzodiazepines, opioids, and α_2-agonists is associated with a reduction in CBF, which occurs secondary to cerebral metabolic suppression. The exception is α_2-agonists, which decrease CBF related to decreases in central sympathetic tone. Ketamine infusion induces regionally specific changes in CBF and cerebral metabolism with areas of the brain showing stimulation and areas showing suppression in CBF and cerebral metabolism. Nonnarcotic intravenous agents reduce ICP but may reduce mean arterial blood pressure and therefore may decrease cerebral perfusion pressure despite the reduction in ICP. Narcotic agents may increase ICP in parallel to decreases in cerebral perfusion pressure. This response appears to be due to autoregulatory cerebral vasodilatation. Ketamine may increase ICP, particularly in normocapnic subjects. However, the induction of hypocapnia attenuates the raise in ICP seen with ketamine. The infusion of α_2-adrenergic agonists produces a transient reduction in ICP.

REFERENCES

1. Drummond JC, Todd MM, Scheller MS, Shapiro HM. A comparison of the direct vasodilating potencies of halothane and isoflurane in the New Zealand white rabbit. *Anesthesiology* 1986;65:462–467.
2. Maekawa T, Tommasino C, Shapiro HM, Keifer-Goodman J, Kohlenberger RW. Local cerebral blood flow and glucose utilization during isoflurane anesthesia in the rat. *Anesthesiology* 1986;65:144–151.
3. Stullken EH, Milde JD, Michenfelder JD, Tinker JH. The nonlinear responses of cerebral metabolism to low concentrations of halothane, enflurane, isoflurane and thiopental. *Anesthesiology* 1977;46:28–34.
4. Todd MM, Drummond JC. A comparison of the cerebrovascular and metabolic effects of halothane and isoflurane in the cat. *Anesthesiology* 1984;60:276–282.
5. Hansen TD, Warner DS, Todd MM, Vust LJ, Trawick DC. Distribution of cerebral blood flow during halothane versus isoflurane anesthesia in rats. *Anesthesiology* 1988;69:332–337.
6. Newberg LA, Milde JH, Michenfelder JD. The cerebral metabolic effects of isoflurane at and above concentrations that suppress cortical electrical activity. *Anesthesiology* 1983;59:23–28.
7. Young WL, Barkai AI, Prohovnik I, Nelson H, Durkin M. Effect of Paco$_2$ on cerebral blood flow distribution during halothane compared with isoflurane anaesthesia in the rat. *Br J Anaesth* 1991;67:440–446.
8. Drummond JC, Todd MM. The response of the feline circulation to Paco$_2$ during anesthesia with isoflurane and halothane and during sedation with nitrous oxide. *Anesthesiology* 1985;62:268–273.
9. McPherson RW, Brian JE, Traystman RJ. Cerebrovascular responsiveness to carbon dioxide in dogs with 1.4% and 2.8% isoflurane. *Anesthesiology* 1989;70:843–850.
10. McPherson RW, Derrer SA, Traystman RJ. Changes in cerebral CO$_2$

11. McPherson RW, Kirsch JR, Tobin JR, Ghaly RF, Traystman RJ. Cerebral blood flow in primates is increased by isoflurane over time and is decreased by nitric oxide synthase inhibition. *Anesthesiology* 1994; 80:1320–1327.
12. McPherson RW, Traystman RJ. Effects of isoflurane on cerebral autoregulation in dogs. *Anesthesiology* 1988;69:493–499.
13. Drummond JC, Todd MM, Toutant SM, Shapiro HM. Brain surface protrusion during enflurane, halothane, and isoflurane anesthesia in cats. *Anesthesiology* 1983;59:288–293.
14. Archer DP, Labrecque P, Tyler JL, et al. Measurement of cerebral blood flow and volume with positron emission tomography during isoflurane administration in the hypocapnic baboon. *Anesthesiology* 1990;72:1031–1037.
15. Archer DP, Labrecque P, Tyler JL, Meyer E, Trop D. Cerebral blood volume is increased in dogs during administration of nitrous oxide or isoflurane. *Anesthesiology* 1987;67:642–648.
16. Artru AA. Relationship between cerebral blood volume and CSF pressure during anesthesia with isoflurane or fentanyl in dogs. *Anesthesiology* 1984;60:575–579.
17. Kaieda R, Todd MM, Weeks JB, Warner DS. A comparison of the effects of halothane, isoflurane, and pentobarbital anesthesia on intracranial pressure and cerebral edema formation following brain injury in rabbits. *Anesthesiology* 1989;71:571–579.
18. Entrei C, Leszniewski W, Carlsson C. Local application of 133 Xenon for measurement of regional cerebral blood flow (rCBF) during halothane, enflurane, and isoflurane anesthesia in humans. *Anesthesiology* 1985;63:391–394.
19. Madsen JB, Cold GE, Hansen ES, Bardrum B. The effect of isoflurane on cerebral blood flow and metabolism in humans during craniotomy for small supratentorial tumors. *Anesthesiology* 1987;66:332–336.
20. Algotsson L, Messeter K, Nordström CH, Ryding E. Cerebral blood flow and oxygen consumption during isoflurane and halothane anesthesia in man. *Acta Anaesthesiol Scand* 1988;32:15–20.
21. Young WL, Prohovnik I, Correll JW, Ornstein E, Matteo RS, Ostapkovich N. Cerebral blood flow and metabolism in patients undergoing anesthesia for carotid endarterectomy. *Anesth Analg* 1989;68: 712–717.
22. Reinstrup P, Ryding E, Algotsson L, Messeter K, Asgeirsson B, Uski T. Distribution of cerebral blood flow during anesthesia with isoflurane or halothane in humans. *Anesthesiology* 1995;82:359–366.
23. Young WL, Prohovnik I, Ornstein E, Ostapkovich N, Sisti MB, Solomon RA, Stein BM. The effect of arteriovenous malformation resection on cerebrovascular reactivity to carbon dioxide. *Neurosurgery* 1990;27:257–267.
24. Ornstein E, Young WL, Fleischer LH, Ostapkovich N. Desflurane and isoflurane have similar effects on cerebral blood flow in patients with intracranial mass lesions. *Anesthesiology* 1993;79:498–502.
25. Young WL, Prohovnik I, Correll JW, Ostapkovich N, Ornstein E, Quest DO. A comparison of cerebral blood flow reactivity to CO$_2$ during halothane versus isoflurane anesthesia for carotid endarterectomy. *Anesth Analg* 1991;73:416–421.
26. Gordon E, Lagerkranser M, Rudehill A, von Holst H: The effect of isoflurane on cerebrospinal fluid pressure in patients undergoing neurosurgery. *Acta Anaesthesiol Scand* 1988;32:108–112.
27. Adams RW, Cucchiara RF, Gronert GA, Messick JM, Michenfelder JD: Isoflurane and cerebrospinal fluid pressure in neurosurgical patients. *Anesthesiology* 1981;54:97–99.
28. Crawford MW, Lerman J, Saldivia V, Carmichael FJ. Hemodynamic and organ blood flow responses to halothane and sevoflurane anesthesia during spontaneous ventilation. *Anesth Analg* 1992;75:1000–1006.
29. Scheller MS, Tateishi A, Drummond JC, Zornow MH. The effects of sevoflurane on cerebral blood flow, cerebral metabolic rate for oxygen, intracranial pressure, and the electroencephalogram are similar to those of isoflurane in the rabbit. *Anesthesiology* 1988;68:548–551.
30. Lutz LJ, Milde JH, Newberg Milde L. The cerebral functional, metabolic, and hemodynamic effects of desflurane in dogs. *Anesthesiology* 1990;73:125–131.
31. Newberg Milde L, Milde JH. The cerebral and systemic hemodynamic effects of desflurane-induced hypotension in dogs. *Anesthesiology* 1991;74:513–518.
32. Lutz LJ, Milde JH, Newberg Milde L. The response of the canine

reactivity over time during isoflurane anesthesia in the dog. *J Neurosurg Anesth* 1991;3:12–19.

cerebral circulation to hyperventilation during anesthesia with desflurane. *Anesthesiology* 1991;74:504–507.

33. Artru AA. Rate of cerebrospinal fluid formation, resistance to reabsorption of cerebrospinal fluid, brain tissue water content, and electroencephalogram during desflurane anesthesia in dogs. *J Neurosurg Anesth* 1993;5:178–186.

34. Kitaguchi K, Ohsumi H, Kuro M, Nakajima T, Hayashi Y. Effects of sevoflurane on cerebral circulation and metabolism in patients with ischemic cerebrovascular disease. *Anesthesiology* 1993;79:704–709.

35. Muzzi DA, Losasso TJ, Dietz NM, Faust RJ, Cucchiara RF, Milde LN. The effect of desflurane and isoflurane on cerebrospinal fluid pressure in humans with supratentorial mass lesions. *Anesthesiology* 1992;76:720–724.

36. Pelligrino DA, Miletich DJ, Hoffman WE, Albrecht RF. Nitrous oxide markedly increases cerebral cortical metabolic rate and blood flow in the goat. *Anesthesiology* 1984;60:405–412.

37. Baughman VL, Hoffman WE, Miletich DJ, Albrecht RF. Cerebrovascular and metabolic effects of N_2O in unrestrained rats. *Anesthesiology* 1990;73:269–272.

38. Kaieda R, Todd MM, Warner DS. The effects of anesthetics and $PaCO_2$ on the cerebrovascular, metabolic, and electroencephalographic responses to nitrous oxide in the rabbit. *Anesth Analg* 1989; 68:135–143.

39. Hansen TD, Warner DS, Todd MM, Vust LJ. Effects of nitrous oxide and volatile anaesthetics on cerebral blood flow. *Br J Anaesth* 1989; 63:290–295.

40. Reasoner DK, Warner DS, Todd MM, McAllister A. Effects of nitrous oxide on cerebral metabolic rate in rats anaesthetized with isoflurane. *Br J Anaesth* 1990;65:210–215.

41. Roald OK, Forsman M, Heier MS, Steen PA. Cerebral effects of nitrous oxide when added to low and high concentrations of isoflurane in the dog. *Anesth Analg* 1991;72:75–79.

42. Field LM, Dorrance DE, Krzeminska EK, Barsoum LZ. Effect of nitrous oxide on cerebral blood flow in normal humans. *Br J Anaesth* 1993;70:154–159.

43. Reinstrup P, Ryding E, Algotsson L, Berntman L, Uski T. Effects of nitrous oxide on human regional cerebral blood flow and isolated pial arteries. *Anesthesiology* 1994; 81: 396–402.

44. Algotsson L, Messeter K, Rosén I, Holmin T. Effects of nitrous oxide on cerebral haemodynamics and metabolism during isoflurane anaesthesia in man. *Acta Anaesthesiol Scand* 1992;36:46–52.

45. Phirman JR, Shapiro HM. Modification of nitrous oxide-induced intracranial hypertension by prior induction of anesthesia. *Anesthesiology* 1977;46:150–151.

46. Moss E, McDowall DG. ICP increases with 50% nitrous oxide in oxygen in severe head injuries during controlled ventilation. *Br J Anaesth* 1979;51:757–761.

47. Kassell NF, Hitchon PW, Gerk MK, Sokoll MD, Hill TR. Alterations in cerebral blood flow, oxygen metabolism, and electrical activity produced by high dose sodium thiopental. *Neurosurgery* 1980;7: 598–603.

48. Pierce EC, Lambertsen CL, Deutsch S, Chase PE, Linde HW, Dripps RD, Price HL. Cerebral circulation and metabolism during thiopental anesthesia and hyperventilation in man. *J Clin Invest* 1962;41: 1664–1671.

49. Shapiro HM, Galindo A, Wyte SR, Harris AB. Rapid intraoperative reduction of intracranial pressure with thiopentone. *Br J Anaesth* 1973; 45:1057–1062.

50. Newberg Milde L, Milde JH, Michenfelder JD. Cerebral functional, metabolic, and hemodynamic effects of etomidate in dogs. *Anesthesiology* 1985;63:371–377.

51. Davis DW, Mans AM, Biebuyck JF, Hawkins RA. Regional brain glucose utilization in rats during etomidate anesthesia. *Anesthesiology* 1986;64:751–757.

52. Cold GE, Eskesen V, Eriksen H, Amtoft O, Madsen JB. CBF and $CMRO_2$ during continuous etomidate infusion supplemented with N_2O and fentanyl in patients with supratentorial cerebral tumour. *Acta Anaesthesiol Scand* 1985;29:490–494.

53. Dearden NM, McDowell DG. Comparison of etomidate and althesin in the reduction of increased intracranial pressure after head injury. *Br J Anaesth* 1985;57:361–368.

54. Artru AA, Shapira Y, Bowdle TA. Electroencephalogram, cerebral metabolic, and vascular responses to propofol anesthesia in dogs. *J Neurosurg Anesth* 1992;4:99–109.

55. Ramani R, Todd MM, Warner DS. A dose-response study of the influence of propofol on cerebral blood flow, metabolism and the electroencephalogram in the rabbit. *J Neurosurg Anesth* 1992;4: 110–119.

56. Werner C, Hoffman WE, Kochs E, Schulte am Esch J, Albrecht RF. The effects of propofol on cerebral and spinal cord blood flow in rats. *Anesth Analg* 1993;76:971–975.

57. Stephan H, Sonntag H, Schenk HD, Kohlhausen S. Effects of disoprivan on cerebral blood flow, cerebral oxygen consumption, and cerebral vascular reactivity. *Anaesthesist* 1987;36:60–65.

58. Alkire MT, Haier RJ, Barker SJ, Shah NK, Wu JC, Kao J. Cerebral metabolism during propofol anesthesia in humans studied with positron emisson tomography. *Anesthesiology* 1995;82:393–403.

59. Craen RA, Gelb AW, Murkin JM, Chong KY. Human cerebral autoregulation is maintained during propofol air/O_2 anesthesia. *Anesthesiology* 1992;77:A220.

60. Pinaud M, Lelausque J-N, Chetanneau A, Fauchoux N, Ménégalli D, Souron R. Effects of propofol on cerebral hemodynamics and metabolism in patients with brain trauma. *Anesthesiology* 1990;73:404–409.

61. Ravussin P, Guinard JP, Ralley F, Thorin D. Effect of propofol on cerebrospinal fluid pressure and cerebral perfusion pressure in patients undergoing craniotomy. *Anaesthesia* 1988;43:37–41.

62. Ebrahim ZY, Schubert A, Van Ness P, Wolgamuth B, Awad I. The effect of propofol on the electroencephalogram of patients with epilepsy. *Anesth Analg* 1994;78:275–279.

63. Fleischer JE, Milde JH, Moyer TP, Michenfelder JD. Cerebral effects of high-dose midazolam and subsequent reversal with Ro 15-1788 in dogs. *Anesthesiology* 1988;68:234–242.

64. Nugent M, Artru AA, Michenfelder JD. Cerebral metabolic, vascular and protective effects of midazolam maleate. *Anesthesiology* 1982; 56:172–176.

65. Hoffman WE, Miletich DJ, Albrecht RF. The effects of midazolam on cerebral blood flow and oxygen consumption and its interaction with nitrous oxide. *Anesth Analg* 1986;65:729–733.

66. Forster A, Juge O, Morel D. Effects of midazolam on cerebral blood flow in human volunteers. *Anesthesiology* 1982;56:453–455.

67. Griffin JP, Cottrell JE, Shwiry B, Hartung J, Epstein J, Lim K. Intracranial pressure, mean arterial pressure, and heart rate following midazolam or thiopental in humans with brain tumors. *Anesthesiology* 1984;60:491–494.

68. Monitto CL, Kurth CD. The effect of fentanyl, sufentanil, and alfentanil on cerebral arterioles in piglets. *Anesth Analg* 1993;76:985–989.

69. Carlsson C, Smith DS, Keykhah MM, Englebach I, Harp JR: The effects of high-dose fentanyl on cerebral circulation and metabolism in rats. *Anesthesiology* 1982;57:375–380.

70. Keykhah MM, Smith DS, Carlsson C, Safo Y, Englebach I, Harp JR. Influence of sufentanil on cerebral metabolism and circulation in the rat. *Anesthesiology* 1985;63:274–277.

71. Hoffman WE, Cunningham F, James MK, Baughman VL, Albrecht RF. Effects of remifentanil, a new short-acting opioid, on cerebral blood flow, brain electrical activity, and intracranial pressure in dogs anesthetized with isoflurane and nitrous oxide. *Anesthesiology* 1993; 79:107–113.

72. Milde LN, Milde JH, Gallagher WJ. Cerebral effects of fentanyl in dogs. *Br J Anaesth* 1989;63:710–715.

73. Newberg Milde L, Milde JH, Gallagher WJ. Effects of sufentanil on cerebral circulation and metabolism in dogs. *Anesth Analg* 1990;70: 138–146.

74. McPherson RW, Traystman RJ. Fentanyl and cerebral vascular responsivity in dogs. *Anesthesiology* 1984;60:180–186.

75. Hoffman WE, Werner C, Kochs E, Segil L, Edelman G, Albrecht RF. Cerebral and spinal cord blood flow in awake and fentanyl-N_2O anesthetized rats: evidence for preservation of blood flow autoregulation during anesthesia. *J Neurosurg Anesth* 1992;4:31–35.

76. Van Hemelrijck J, Mattheussen M, Wüsten R, Lauwers T, van Aken H. The effect of sufentanil on intracranial pressure (ICP) in anesthetized dogs. *Acta Anaesthesiol Belg* 1989;40:239–245.

77. Sheehan PB, Zornow MH, Scheller MS, Peterson BM: The effects of fentanyl and sufentanil on intracranial and cerebral blood flow in rabbits with an acute cryogenic brain injury. *J Neurosurg Anesth* 1992; 4:261–267.

78. Mayer N, Weinstabl C, Podreka I, Spiss CK. Sufentanil does not increase cerebral blood flow in healthy human volunteers. *Anesthesiology* 1990;73:240–243.

79. Stephan H, Gröger P, Weyland A, Hoeft A, Sonntag H: Effects of high-dose sufentanil-O_2 anesthesia on cerebral blood flow, metabolism, and the cerebrovascular response to carbon dioxide in man. *Anaesthesist* 1991;40:153–160.

80. Young WL, Prohovnik I, Correll JW, Ostapkovich N, Ornstein E, Matteo RS, Baker KZ. A comparison of the cerebral hemodynamic effects of sufentanil and isoflurane in humans undergoing carotid endarterectomy. *Anesthesiology* 1989;71:863–869.

81. Baker KZ, Ostapkovich N, Jackson T, Ornstein E, Young WL. Cerebral blood flow reactivity is intact during remifentanil/N_2O anesthesia. *Anesth Analg* 1995;80:S27 (abstract)

82. Weinstabl C, Mayer N, Richling B, Czech T, Spiss CK. Effect of sufentanil on intracranial pressure in neurosurgical patients. *Anaesthesia* 1991;46:837–840.

83. Werner C, Kochs E, Bause H, Hoffman WE, Schulte am Esch J. The effects of sufentanil on cerebral hemodynamics and intracranial pressure in brain injured patients. *Anesthesiology* 1995;83:721–726.

84. Albanese J, Durbec O, Viviand X, Potie F, Alliez B, Martin C. Sufentanil increases intracranial pressure in patients with head trauma. *Anesthesiology* 1993;79:493–497.

85. Sperry RJ, Bailey PL, Reichman MV, Peterson JC, Petersen PB, Pace NL. Fentanyl and sufentanil increase intracranial pressure in head trauma patients. *Anesthesiology* 1992;77:416–420.

86. Kreuscher H, Grote J. The effect of the phencyclidine derivative ketamine (CI 581) on cerebral blood flow and cerebral oxygen uptake in dogs. *Anaesthesist* 1967;16:304–307.

87. Cavazzuti M, Porro CA, Biral GP, Benassi CG, Barbieri GC. Ketamine effects on local cerebral blood flow and metabolism in the rat. *J Cereb Blood Flow Metab* 1987;7:806–811.

88. Oren RE, Rasool NA, Rubinstein EH. Effect of ketamine on cerebral cortical blood flow and metabolism in rabbits. *Stroke* 1987;18:441–444.

89. Wendling WW, Daniels FB, Chen D, Harakal C, Carlsson C: Ketamine directly dilates bovine cerebral arteries by acting as a calcium entry blocker. *J Neurosurg Anesth* 1994;6:186–192.

90. Pfenninger E, Reith A. Ketamine and intracranial pressure. In: Domino EF, ed. *Status of Ketamine in Anesthesiology*. Ann Arbor, MI: NPP Books, 1990;109–118.

91. Artru AA, Katz RA. Cerebral blood volume and CSF pressure following administration of ketamine in dogs; modification by pre- or post-treatment with hypocapnia or diazepam. *J Neurosurg Anesth* 1989;1:8–15.

92. Herrschaft H, Schmidt H. Changes in the global and regional cerebral blood flow under the influence of propanidid, ketamine and sodium thiopental. *Anaesthesist* 1973;22:486–495.

93. Hougaard K, Hansen A, Brodersen P. The effect of ketamine on regional cerebral blood flow in man. *Anesthesiology* 1974;41:562–567.

94. Takeshita H, Okuda Y, Sari A. The effects of ketamine on cerebral circulation and metabolism in man. *Anesthesiology* 1972;36:69–7.

95. Bloor BC, Flacke WE. Reduction in halothane anesthetic requirement by clonidine, an alpha-adrenergic agonist. *Anesth Analg* 1982;61:741–745.

96. Segal IS, Vickery RG, Walton JK, Doze VA, Maze M. Dexmedetomidine diminishes halothane anesthetic requirements in rats through a postsynaptic alpha 2 adrenergic receptor. *Anesthesiology* 1988;69:818–823.

97. Aantaa R, Kanto J, Scheinin M, Kallio A, Scheinin H. Dexmedetomidine, an alpha 2 adrenoceptor agonist, reduces anesthetic requirements for patients undergoing minor gynecologic surgery. *Anesthesiology* 1990;73:230–235.

98. Aho M, Lehtinen A-M, Erkola O, Kallio A, Kortilla K. The effect of intravenously administered dexmedetomidine on perioperative hemodynamics and isoflurane requirements in patients undergoing abdominal hysterectomy. *Anesthesiology* 1991;74:997–1002.

99. Kanawati I, Yaksh TL, Anderson RE, Marsh RW. Effects of clonidine on cerebral blood flow and the response to arterial CO_2. *J Cereb Blood Flow Metab* 1986;6:358–365.

100. Fale A, Kirsch JR, McPherson RW. Alpha-2–adrenergic agonist effects on normocapnic and hypercapnic cerebral blood flow in the dog are anesthetic dependent. *Anesth Analg* 1994;79:892–898.

101. Zornow MH, Fleischer JE, Scheller MS, Nakakimura K, Drummond JC. Dexmedetomidine, an alpha-2-adrenergic agonist, decreases cerebral blood flow in the isoflurane-anesthetized dog. *Anesth Analg* 1990;70:624–630.

102. McCormick JM, McCormick PW, Zabramski JM, Spetzler RF. Intracranial pressure reduction by a central alpha-2 adrenoceptor agonist after subarachnoid hemorrhage. *Neurosurgery* 1993;32:974–979.

103. Zornow MH, Scheller MS, Sheehan PB, Strnat MAP, Matsumoto M. Intracranial pressure effects of dexmedetomidine in rabbits. *Anesth Analg* 1992;75:232–237.

Cerebrovascular Disease, edited by H. Hunt Batjer.
Lippincott-Raven Publishers, Philadelphia © 1997.

CHAPTER 12

Gene Therapy for Cerebrovascular Disease

David H. Shafron, R. Tyler Frizzel, and Arthur L. Day

Gene therapy is the introduction of genetic material into cells to provide temporary or permanent instructions for the prevention or treatment of illness. Gene transfer technology was introduced more than 50 years ago by Avery, who reported DNA-mediated bacterial transformation (1). The first workshop on gene therapy was held in 1971, and in 1988 the Recombinant DNA Advisory Committee of the National Institute of Health (NIH) approved guidelines for human gene therapy trials.

Much of the current progress in gene therapy has been fueled by discoveries associated with the Human Genome Project (2). Specific goals for the project were developed in 1990, including the construction of detailed human genetic maps, the improvement of physical maps of the human genome, improvement in the technology of DNA sequencing and information handling, and the definition of ethical, legal, and social issues.

Recently, methods of gene delivery have been developed that may be applicable to both the prevention and treatment of stroke. Current medical management of cerebrovascular disease typically involves the reduction of risk factors (hypertension, hyperlipidemia, obesity, diabetes, sedentary lifestyle, smoking) and some form of antiplatelet or anticoagulant drug therapy. Surgical intervention, including such techniques as carotid endarterectomy or extracranial–intracranial bypass procedures, may also be used to augment cerebral perfusion and reduce stroke risk. Despite these maneuvers, however, stroke continues to be a major cause of morbidity and mortality. The present chapter outlines the various forms of gene therapy that are currently being applied experimentally to the prevention and treatment of cerebrovascular disease, and discusses theoretical approaches that may have future applicability.

BASICS OF MOLECULAR BIOLOGY AND GENE TRANSFER

Just as physicians must understand cerebrovascular anatomy to gain insight into the pathophysiology of stroke, they must be familiar with basic gene anatomy and molecular biology in order to understand the potential role of gene therapy in the treatment of stroke. Deoxyribonucleic acid (DNA) is the molecule that contains the genetic information needed to code for all proteins. Every cell in the body contains within its nucleus an identical copy of the entire DNA sequence, which in humans is divided into 23 pairs of chromosomes. Each cell therefore has 46 chromosomes, which among them contain the complete DNA sequence for that individual. A gene is a relatively small section of the DNA sequence that contains the information needed to produce a single, unique peptide.

DNA is a complex molecule composed of nucleotide bases (adenine, thymine, guanine, and cytosine) attached to a deoxyribose sugar-phosphate backbone. Its shape is that of a double-stranded helix, resembling a twisting ladder; the sides of the ladder are the sugar-phosphate backbone, while the rungs are complementary pairs of the nucleotide bases (adenine-thymine and guanine-cytosine). The sequence of these bases along the molecule determines the ultimate protein product of the gene. Ribonucleic acid (RNA) differs from DNA in several ways. It is single-stranded, its sugar backbone is ribose (as opposed to deoxyribose), and its bases include adenine, guanine, cytosine, and uracil (instead of thymidine) (3).

The process by which the information contained in DNA is eventually used to make protein requires several discrete steps. The DNA composing a gene is first used as a template to produce RNA through a process called transcription. An enzyme, RNA polymerase, binds to the DNA and assembles ribonucleotides in a specific sequence (complementary to the DNA template) to produce messenger RNA (mRNA). This resulting mRNA is referred to as sense mRNA. After further modification, the mRNA leaves the nucleus and travels to the cytoplasm where it is used to manufacture a protein

D. H. Shafron and A. L. Day: Department of Neurological Surgery, University of Florida Health Center, Gainesville, Florida 32610

R. T. Frizzell: Department of Neurological Surgery, University of Boise, Boise, Idaho 83702

via a process called translation. In the cytoplasm, the mRNA molecule is bound by a ribosome, which "reads" the sequence of the mRNA and links amino acids together into a growing peptide (protein) chain based on the mRNA sequence. This peptide then undergoes a series of post-translational modifications to eventually become the desired end-product. Thus, via transcription and translation, the information contained within a gene is used to produce a certain protein (3).

The most common concept of genetic therapy is the modification of cellular protein production by adding a particular gene of interest to the cell nucleus, in hopes that it will be transcribed into mRNA and translated into a peptide chain. If a certain disease state were due to a genetic mutation resulting in an inability to manufacture a particular protein, the disease potentially could be cured or attenuated by inserting "correct" copies of the gene in question. This same approach could also be used to increase the production of certain beneficial proteins.

Other pathologic conditions arise from the relative overproduction of certain proteins. A genetic approach known as antisense technology targets this kind of problem [see review by Helene and Toulme (4) for a detailed discussion of antisense mechanisms]. Because mRNA is single-stranded, it retains the ability to be bound by a strand of complementary base pairs. If this were to occur, the resulting double-stranded RNA molecule could not be used for translation. Herein lies the essence of using the antisense approach to downregulate protein production. Exogenously manufactured antisense oligonucleotides, with a base sequence complementary to that of normal sense mRNA, can be introduced into a cell. These oligonucleotide strands will then bind to the normal message used by the cell for translation (3). Alternatively, a gene sequence may be inserted into a delivery vector (see subsequent discussion) in an inverted or antisense orientation and then introduced into a cell. The resulting antisense mRNA produced will have a base pair sequence that is complementary to the endogenous sense mRNA and can therefore block its translation.

Cloning represents the in vitro amplification of a particular DNA sequence, such as a gene (Fig. 1). The sequence of interest is inserted into a vector, or carrier, which is then placed into bacteria, usually *E. coli* (a process called bacterial transformation). As the bacteria multiply in culture, the inserted DNA sequence is exponentially amplified, and the latter can then be isolated. Vectors are DNA sequences that have been modified to carry genes or sequences of interest into cells. They can be broadly classified into two types: those derived from plasmids (as in Fig. 1) and those derived from viruses. Plasmids are small, circular segments of self-replicating extrachromosomal DNA that are normal constituents of bacterial cells. They contain genes that encode for nonvital but advantageous proteins, including those that confer resistance to antibiotics or heavy metals. By the addition and/or removal of different DNA segments, plasmids can be modified for the introduction of DNA into cells (5).

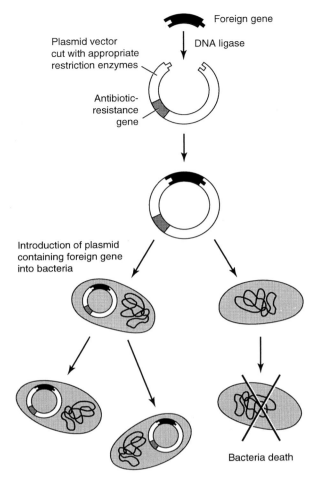

FIG. 1. Cloning of a gene using a plasmid vector. A plasmid is a circular piece of extrachromosomal DNA that can be a normal component of bacterial cells. It contains a variety of genes that code for proteins that confer advantageous properties (ie, antibiotic resistance). Because plasmids can be readily isolated, manipulated, and put back into bacterial cells, they can be exploited as vectors for gene delivery. The particular plasmid illustrated contains a gene that confers antibiotic resistance. The gene to be cloned (foreign gene) has been isolated from the host genome by use of restriction enzymes, which recognize and cleave DNA at certain base pair sequences. A plasmid vector has been opened using similar enzymes, and the gene is ligated, or spliced, into the plasmid using the enzyme DNA ligase. The recombinant plasmid is placed in bacteria, which are allowed to divide. Only the bacteria that have successfully incorporated the plasmid will survive when exposed to antibiotic. The surviving bacteria can be further screened for the foreign gene. Colonies that contain it can then be propagated in order to amplify the gene.

Cloning vectors can also be derived from modified viruses. A gene of interest is inserted into the viral genome, and this engineered virus is then used to infect bacterial cells. As these infected bacteria multiply, the sequence of interest is also amplified (5).

Transfection is the process of introducing exogenous genetic material (from small fragments to entire genes) into eukaryotic cells. Most transfection techniques involve the creation of holes or openings in the plasma membrane, allowing the foreign genetic material to enter; such methods include calcium phosphate precipitation, electroporation, and the use of liposome-based compounds. DNA can also be microinjected directly into the nucleus, or it can be coupled to a ligand that is then taken up by the cell. These processes are more commonly used to transfect cells in vitro, although some of them can be modified for in vivo use (6).

In the above discussion, vectors served as carriers of genetic information in order to clone, or amplify, a particular sequence in bacterial cells. In the context of gene therapy, vectors are primarily used to deliver a gene into a cell in order to alter in some way that cell's production of protein. Several common viral-derived vectors are used for gene delivery, including those based on modified adenovirus, adeno-associated virus (AAV), herpes simplex virus, and retroviruses (6,7). These vectors are often hybrids, or combinations, of viral and plasmid DNA.

When viruses infect a cell, they utilize cellular machinery to copy their genome and manufacture viral proteins in order to self-replicate. Wild-type AAV and retroviruses sometimes integrate their viral DNA into the host chromosome. Other viruses (ie, herpes and adenovirus) gain entry into the nucleus but do not integrate into the host DNA. By inserting a beneficial gene into a modified viral-derived vector (modified so as not to be pathologic), the gene can be delivered into a cell (in a process called transduction) in order to effect the production of the desired protein (Fig. 2). If that gene should be incorporated into the genome of a mitotic cell, then all progeny of that cell would contain this new gene. In essence, the genetic defect would be "corrected."

Although a discussion regarding the relative advantages and disadvantages of the available viral vectors is beyond the scope of this chapter, several important points regarding gene transfer into cells of the central nervous system, particularly neurons, should be mentioned. Retroviruses can only transduce actively dividing cells, so that retroviral vectors cannot be used for neuronal gene manipulation (6). Herpes is a naturally neurotropic virus, and recombinant herpes-based vectors have been very successful in neuronal transduction. Their use as gene delivery vectors, however, may be limited for several reasons. In the preparation of stocks of recombinant replication-defective herpesvirus, the removal of all replication-competent virus is difficult. In addition, even replication-defective herpesvirus can kill or injure cells (6,8).

AAV vectors are well suited for neuronal transduction. The wild-type virus is nonpathogenic and cannot replicate without coinfection with another virus (usually adenovirus). Recombinant AAV vectors have been created that do not contain any wild-type viral genes, thereby reducing pathogenicity in host tissue. AAV vectors transduce post-mitotic cells quite effectively and therefore have the potential to provide safe, long-term phenotypic correction in neurons (6,9).

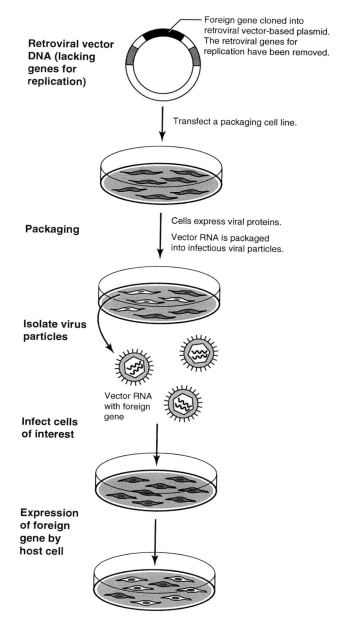

FIG. 2. The use of retrovirus vectors for gene delivery. A plasmid has been constructed based on the RNA genome of a retrovirus. Genes allowing for viral replication have been removed and the foreign gene of interest has been inserted into the plasmid. Cultures of packaging cells (specialized cells that contain the necessary machinery for the packaging of viral RNA into recombinant viral particles) are then transfected with the plasmid. The viral particles are isolated and used to infect cells of interest. The viral RNA is reverse-transcribed into DNA, which eventually integrates into the host chromosome. The foreign gene is then expressed by the host cell.

The techniques described above can be used to alter the protein production of the target tissue itself ie, the recombinant vector is delivered directly into cells in brain, endothelium, or other tissue. Grafting, an additional method for gene delivery into brain, deserves mention because of its success in animal models. In this paradigm, a recombinant vector is introduced into cultured cells (such as fibroblasts) that then produce the desired protein. These fibroblasts are subsequently implanted (grafted) into brain, where they function in a paracrine-like manner, releasing protein into the interstitial milieu for use by brain tissue (10).

GENE THERAPY APPROACHES TO THE TREATMENT OF STROKE

Several familial conditions associated with stroke have a discrete mutational genetic defect. In order to treat these conditions using gene therapy, the lacking gene must be placed in and expressed by a sufficient number of affected cells. This can be accomplished by transfecting a large population of cells or by altering a stem cell whose progeny would then carry the corrected genome. Diseases or risk factors without a clearly defined genetic or mutational defect (ie, hypertension) may also be treated with gene therapy. In still other conditions, gene therapy could be targeted to a specific anatomic abnormality that predisposes to stroke, thereby reducing some of the problems associated with the need for widespread manipulation (see discussion of endovascular gene therapy for vascular stenosis). Gene therapy also has the potential to reduce cellular injury in patients who sustain an ischemic event by interfering with the propagation of the excitotoxicity cascade.

Correcting large populations of cells in either widespread or discrete areas of the body represents one of the major obstacles in bringing gene therapy to the realm of clinical medicine. There are many other hurdles, such as those related to the control, regulation, and timing of transcription of implanted genes, as well as the possibility of disturbing the function of normal cellular genes or triggering neoplastic change in the cell (6).

The following sections describe disease states and clinical situations in which different genetic techniques could be used for the prevention or treatment of hemorrhagic or ischemic stroke. Although much of the discussion is by necessity theoretical and based on animal models, its purpose is to show how the various genetic strategies could be useful for treating patients with a wide variety of disorders predisposing to stroke or those in whom an ischemic event has occurred.

Genetic Predisposition to Stroke

Most patients who suffer strokes have multiple risk factors, often related to lifestyle and habit. A genetic predisposition to atherosclerotic disease does exist, however; hence the importance of family history in elucidating an individual's stroke risk. Most familial predispositions are polygenic, multifactorial entities and cannot presently be identified using modern neurogenetic techniques. Several conditions associated with stroke, however, appear to be due to a single genetic defect and are therefore potential candidates for gene

therapy. Some of these diseases have multiorgan system involvement, so that cure or palliation of the pathologic process utilizing genetic methods would therefore require correction on a diffuse basis.

Conditions in which aberrant protein expression is limited primarily to the hematopoietic system, for which gene delivery to primitive (bone marrow) progenitor cells could afford widespread correction, would be the most practical candidates for genetic therapy. Sickle cell disease, for example, is an autosomal recessive disease usually identified early in life and is due to a mutation in the β-hemoglobin gene. The mutation leads to changes in red blood cell morphology, predisposing to widespread arterial thrombosis. Patients are at increased risk for ischemic cerebral infarction as well as subarachnoid hemorrhage (11).

Several discrete genetic defects result in abnormal protein deposition in vessel walls, leading to structural weakness and a propensity for hemorrhage. Mutations in genes coding for cystatin C and amyloid precursor protein have each been identified as etiologies of the dementia and lobar hemorrhages associated with amyloid angiopathy (12,13).

Abnormalities in the clotting and thrombolysis cascades are important causes of stroke in young patients. Individuals with congenital deficiencies of either protein S or protein C, which have endogenous anticoagulant properties, are prone to widespread vascular occlusive disease (14).

Homocystinuria, an autosomal recessive disease characterized by stroke, ectopia lentis, and mental retardation, is due to a mutation in the gene for the enzyme cystathionine synthetase (15). The enzyme deficiency leads to accumulation of homocysteine in endothelial cells, causing a vascular injury that predisposes to stroke.

Neurofibromatosis type I (NF-1) is well known to neurosurgeons because of its association with central and peripheral nervous system neoplasia. Transmission is autosomal dominant, although a large percentage of cases are sporadic. The NF-1 gene is a tumor-suppressor gene located on chromosome 17 (16). Patients are at increased risk for several neurovascular complications, including vascular stenosis, occlusion, intracranial aneurysms, and arteriovenous fistulas of the cervical carotid and extracranial vertebral arteries (17).

Patients with the autosomal dominant form of polycystic kidney disease have a 10–40% incidence of cerebral aneurysms (18,19). This disease has been linked to a gene (PKD1) on chromosome 16, though the function of the normal gene is unclear (17).

Marfan's syndrome is an autosomal dominant disorder of connective tissue associated with many phenotypic changes, including vascular, cardiac, and skeletal defects. Patients are at increased risk for carotid and vertebral arterial dissections, as well as formation and rupture of intracranial aneurysms. These widespread manifestations are due to a mutation in the gene for fibrillin, an extracellular matrix protein found in a variety of connective tissues (17,20).

Ehlers–Danlos syndrome (EDS) is a connective tissue disorder characterized by hypermobile joints, bruising, and dystrophic scarring. EDS type IV is associated with a severe vasculopathy, predisposing to widespread arterial rupture, dissection, and intracranial aneurysm formation. Carotid-cavernous fistulas are especially common in these patients. The defective gene is COL3A, a component of type III collagen (17,21).

Fabry's disease is an X-linked recessive disease caused by mutations in the gene for α-galactosidase, a lysosomal enzyme. Endothelial cells accumulate glycolipids, leading to small vessel narrowing. Patients are at increased risk for cerebrovascular occlusive disease, predominantly lacunar infarction (22).

Cerebral cavernous malformations are endothelial-lined vascular channels that, although often asymptomatic, can lead to seizures, focal neurologic deficits, or intraparenchymal hemorrhage. Although most are solitary lesions occurring sporadically in the population, there are familiar cases in which there is a greater frequency of multiple lesions. Although the defective gene and protein are not yet known, recent linkage analyses in two affective kindreds have mapped the defect to a region on chromosome 7 (23).

Takayasu's arteritis is characterized by widespread vascular occlusive disease, predisposing affected individuals to ischemic stroke. The responsible gene is unknown, although there are associations with several human leukocyte antigen (HLA) haplotypes (24,25).

In the conditions described above, the introduction of the gene encoding for the defective or lacking structural or enzymatic protein has the potential to prevent or attenuate the pathologic effects of the disease, including stroke. However, limitations surrounding the need for correction on a diffuse basis must be kept in mind.

Gene delivery has already proven somewhat effective in the treatment of another hereditary condition with increased stroke risk. Many familial hyperlipidemias are associated with atherosclerotic disease, and a defective gene for the low-density lipoprotein (LDL) receptor is responsible for a subset of these patients. This condition has been partially treated in hyperlipidemic rabbits by transplanting genetically engineered hepatocytes that contain a correct gene (26,27). A human protocol was recently initiated in which hepatocytes from patients with familial hypercholesterolemia were genetically corrected ex vivo and transplanted back into the host. The first patient reported had a significant drop in the LDL/HDL (low-density lipoprotein/high-density lipoprotein) ratio, which remained stable for the entire follow-up period of 18 months (28).

Other Risk Factors for Stroke

Most stroke patients have multiple risk factors that while not necessarily familial can still be subjected to genetic modification. Hypertension, perhaps the most common risk factor for atherosclerotic disease and stroke, has a variety of causes. Whatever the etiology, correcting elevated blood pressure could be within the realm of gene therapy. Gyurko and colleagues (29) injected antisense oligonucleotides for either angiotensin II receptor mRNA or angiotensinogen mRNA into the cerebral ventricles of spontaneously hypertensive rats. Each approach successfully lowered mean arterial pressure in treated animals by downregulating renin-angiotensin activity. Introducing a gene that could code for an antisense mRNA on a continuous basis could hypothetically result in long-term down-regulation of this system, reducing blood pressure and stroke risk.

Vascular Stenosis

Smooth muscle cells proliferate in walls of blood vessels in response to endothelial cell injury. Such a reaction occurring in an atherosclerotic carotid artery, for example, can lead to stenosis, placing the brain at risk for thrombotic or embolic events. Endothelial damage and resultant smooth muscle proliferation may also occur in response to iatrogenic injury, such as angioplasty or endarterectomy. This smooth muscle proliferation is an attractive target for molecular biological strategies (30).

Nabel and colleagues (31) developed an endovascular, catheter-based system for introducing genetically modified endothelial cells to a local section of porcine femoral artery. After transfection with a marker gene (lac-z) these cells continued to produce the engineered gene product (β-glactosidase) for 4 weeks. Similarly, Wilson et al (32) reported on the use of Dacron carotid interposition grafts lined with autologous, genetically modified endothelial cells in a canine model. Such grafts produced the recombinant marker protein for at least 5 weeks postprocedure. Steg and colleagues (33) transfected rabbit endothelial and smooth muscle cells (in vivo) endovascularly with an adenoviral vector carrying a marker gene and demonstrated consistent expression. Riessen et al (34) successfully transfected rabbit arterial wall with naked (nonpackaged) DNA applied to a hydrogel-coated angioplasty balloon. The expression of the marker protein for up to 14 days posttransfection demonstrated the possibility of genetic modification of vessel walls without the use of viral-based vectors (34). All of these studies support the feasibility of genetically modifying a local segment of arterial wall for therapeutic or prophylactic purposes. Several different catheter-based systems applicable to endovascular gene therapy are shown in Fig. 3 (35–37).

A novel approach utilizing the herpesvirus thymidine kinase gene has been applied toward attenuating the process of vascular smooth muscle proliferation (38). Using an adenoviral vector, this gene was endovascularly delivered into the smooth muscle cells of injured porcine arteries, and the animals were subsequently treated with the antiviral drug ganciclovir. The thymidine kinase encoded by the delivered gene phosphorylates ganciclovir, forming a nucleoside analog that inhibits further DNA synthesis by the cell. This

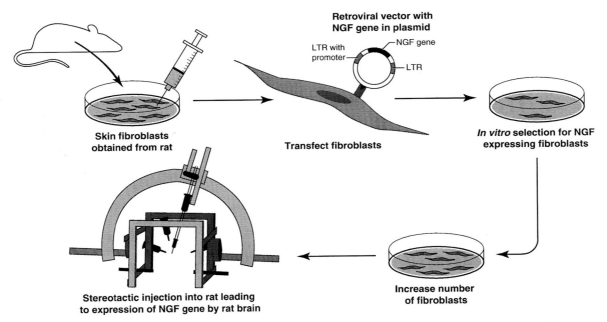

FIG. 3. Gene transfer utilizing a grafting technique. Primary skin fibroblasts were isolated from rats and using a retroviral vector construct were transfected with the gene for murine nerve growth factor (NGF). Those fibroblasts that then produced NGF were identified and allowed to proliferate in vitro. The NGF-producing cells were then stereotactically injected into the septal region of rats with fimbria-fornix lesions. The treated animals had reduced septal cell loss compared to controls and also had improved memory-based behavior (10).

strategy resulted in a 50–90% reduction of arterial wall thickness compared to controls. A similar approach performed in a rat carotid artery injury model also reduced injury-induced smooth muscle proliferation (39)

Another approach aimed at preventing restenosis was developed by Chang and colleagues (40), who delivered a modified retinoblastoma (Rb) gene into cultured aortic smooth muscle cells. The gene was modified such that the gene product (a classic tumor suppressor protein) was continuously active. The Rb protein activity inhibited cell cycle progression in smooth muscle cells and reduced cellular proliferation in response to growth factors in vitro. The same gene, when delivered into rat carotid and porcine femoral arterial wall following angioplasty, reduced subsequent smooth muscle proliferation and stenosis by 50%.

Nitric oxide produced within vascular endothelial cells relaxes blood vessels, inhibits vascular smooth muscle proliferation, and reduces platelet aggregation (41,42). von der Leyden and colleagues delivered the endothelial nitric oxide synthase (eNOS) gene into denuded rat carotid artery, reducing subsequent smooth muscle proliferation and neointimal formation (41). This group also delivered antisense oligonucleotides (directed at genes involved in cell cycle regulation) to balloon-injured arteries and demonstrated a reduction in cell proliferation and neointimal formation (43).

These studies reveal the efficacy of a single gene product in reducing postinjury stenosis. A "cocktail" of genes, delivered by a viral vector with an adequate "payload" capac-

ity, may prove to be more effective. Delivery systems for endovascular gene therapy of the cerebral vasculature (Fig. 3) obviously require further investigation.

Cerebral Ischemia

The previously described approaches are all aimed at preventing end-organ ischemia or infarction. Genetic manipulation might also have a role in reducing the extent of tissue damage once an ischemic event has occurred. When a thrombotic or embolic event eliminates cerebral perfusion, a central core of tissue is rendered ischemic and often quickly dies. At the margins of this core, however, there exists a penumbral region, an area of brain that has the potential for either recovery or delayed death. The cells in this region are electrically silent, as if in a state of suspended animation, but have not experienced the overt energy failure and the loss of ion homeostasis and membrane integrity that characterize the necrotic core (44,45). The brain encompassing the penumbra is at risk for death not only because of compromised blood flow but also as a result of its proximity to the infarcted core. Secondary excitotoxic mechanisms play a major role in incorporating the penumbral area into the infarct, and it is this process that may be amenable to genetic strategies.

Although the intricate details of the mechanisms involved in ischemic cell death are beyond the scope of this chapter [see reviews by Siesjo (46) and Hossmann (47)], it is important to review the basic events in order to understand how genetic strategies may prove useful. Glutamate is the major excitatory neurotransmitter within the central nervous system and under normal conditions plays a major role in cell–cell communication. When bound by glutamate, the NMDA receptor (a subtype of glutamate receptor so named because of its affinity for the ligand *N*-methyl-ᴅ-aspartate) conducts inward currents of sodium and, more importantly, calcium. Normally, NMDA neurotransmission is the basis for such processes as long-term potentiation (the physiologic correlate of learning and memory) and neuronal plasticity. Under pathologic conditions, however, glutamate mediates events involved in excitotoxic cell death (48,49). Neuronal death and injury, as occurs in and around the core of an infarct, causes the liberation of high levels of glutamate into the extracellular milieu, unleashing a cascade of events (mediated primarily but not exclusively through the NMDA receptor) which may ultimately injure or kill the cells in the penumbra (48,49).

Excessive intracellular calcium levels resulting from abnormal glutamate activity are caused by inward flux through ligand-gated (such as the NMDA receptor complex) and voltage-gated channels, as well as release from intracellular stores. High intracellular calcium levels activate an array of phospholipases, endonucleases, and proteases, causing breakdown of the cell membrane, nucleic acids, and structural and enzymatic proteins necessary for cellular viability. The resultant cellular injury liberates more glutamate, thus propagating a vicious cycle in which cells not killed by the initial event may ultimately die (50).

In the past several years the importance of other secondary events in the pathogenesis of excitotoxic injury (ie, the generation of nitric oxide and free radicals) and the natural cellular defenses (ie, heat shock response) has been established. As the characterization of these excitotoxic and protective mechanisms has progressed, genetic strategies that target these processes have also evolved rapidly.

An antisense approach devised to intervene early in the excitotoxic cascade was developed by Wahlestedt and colleagues (51). In an effort to downregulate NMDA receptor density, an 18-bp antisense oligonucleotide for the NMDA-R1 receptor subunit was delivered into the lateral ventricle of a rat every 12 hours for 2 days prior to permanent middle cerebral artery (MCA) occlusion. Infarct size was reduced by up to 40% compared to controls with the reduction primarily localized to the penumbral region. Pretreatment of neuronal cultures with this antisense oligonucleotide blocked calcium influx and neuronal death when the cultures were subsequently exposed to an NMDA receptor agonist.

Cerebral ischemia leads to increased brain production of nitric oxide (NO) (52). This molecule has been the subject of intense scrutiny in the past several years because of its multiple (and seemingly paradoxical) functions as a neurotransmitter, vascular relaxing agent, and mediator of excitotoxic cell injury. In addition, NO reduces platelet aggregation and can downregulate NMDA receptor activity (41). A rise in intracellular calcium levels stimulates the activity of nitric oxide synthase (NOS), resulting in increased NO production. A great deal of controversy initially arose surrounding NO's role in cerebral ischemia, as some groups found that NO synthase inhibition reduced experimental infarct size whereas others found that this approach increased infarct size [reviewed by Dalkara and Moskowitz (42)]. It is now known that there are three distinct forms of NOS: endothelial (eNOS), neuronal (nNOS), and an inducible form found in macrophages (iNOS). The balance in activity between these different forms determines to a large extent the effects that NO production will have in a particular experimental (and presumably clinical) situation. In addition, the redox state of the NO molecule influences its role in an ischemic event (53).

An increase in eNOS activity upregulates endothelial production of NO, leading to vascular relaxation and increased blood flow that would benefit an underperfused brain region (54). Increased nNOS activity, however, mediates (at least in part) excitotoxic brain injury (41,55). NO can interact with mitochondrial enzymes involved in electron transport and can also combine with the superoxide anion to form the oxidant peroxynitrite, an active free radical. At a neutral pH, peroxynitrite degrades to form nitrogen dioxide and the highly reactive hydroxyl radical, leading to lipid peroxidation, oxidation of proteins, and damage to nucleic acids (56). The discrepancy between the beneficial effects of eNOS vs. the deleterious effects of nNOS was the source of conflicting findings of the effects of NOS inhibition on infarct size in animal models (41). Preferential inhibition of one or the other form of NOS lead to the different results.

Recently, genetic strategies were employed to downregulate nNOS activity. Moskowitz's group (57) developed a mutant strain of mouse that does not express the nNOS gene (nNOS knockout mouse). When these animals were subjected to permanent MCA occlusion, the resultant infarcts were significantly smaller (15–38%) than those in mice with normal nNOS activity. Neurologic deficits were similarly reduced. When the knockout mice were treated with an eNOS inhibitor, infarct size was increased, showing the protective effects of eNOS activity. In a separate set of studies, this group also demonstrated that these knockout mice were more resistant to transient forebrain ischemia than controls.

The formation of free radicals plays a significant role in the pathogenesis of ischemic brain injury (56,58), particularly in association with reperfusion of brain after a period of arrested blood flow (56). Reperfusion overwhelms the injured brain's capacity to utilize oxygen normally, and the formation of reactive oxygen species (including the superoxide anion) exceeds endogenous scavenging mechanisms for proper free radical metabolism. Superoxide dismutase (SOD) is one such free radical scavenger that when given to an animal prior to a focal ischemia insult can reduce infarct size (59). Chan and colleagues have studied cerebral ischemia in a transgenic mouse strain that overexpresses a human form of SOD (CuZn-SOD). SOD levels in these animals were greater than three times those of nontransgenic litter mates. When subjected to temporary MCA occlusion followed by reperfusion, infarct volume in these mice was reduced by 26–36% compared to controls, depending on the model of ischemia used (60,61). Brain edema and neurologic deficits were also reduced in the transgenic animals. Penumbral antioxidant levels were significantly higher in transgenic animals, revealing the selective advantage that these mice have in the face of ischemia-reperfusion. Interestingly, the transgenic animals fared no better than controls in a permanent MCA occlusion model, indicating that free radicals may mediate injury when injured brain is subject to the increased oxidative stress associated with reperfusion (56,61).

The above studies suggest a neuroprotective effect of an endogenous class of molecules, the antioxidants. Another group of endogenous proteins, the heat shock proteins (HSPs), are receiving considerable attention for their possible role in cerebral response to ischemia (by convention *hsp* refers to the gene, hsp to the mRNA, and HSP to the gene product or protein). The heat shock response is a highly conserved cellular reaction to a variety of environmental and internal stresses, in which gene expression (and therefore protein production) is profoundly altered. During a period of stress, normal protein production drops precipitously, and HSP production is induced (62,63). HSPs are believed to bind to partially denatured proteins in injured cells to help stabilize them and prevent further unfolding (64). They may also act as chaperones, aiding protein translocation across cellular membranes (65). Transcription of *hsp* is rapidly induced in both focal and global ischemia models. In focal models, the location of HSP induction may define the ischemic penumbra where viable cells experience continued stress (62,66). In vitro studies have demonstrated that HSP production is associated with neuroprotection in response to excitotoxic insults (67). Such a protective role is assumed in animal models, as a prior ischemic stress not severe enough to cause infarction is neuroprotective when that animal is subsequently exposed to experimental infarction (68,69). This ischemic conditioning may be due, at least in part, to HSP induction.

A convincing demonstration of HSP neuroprotection was recently shown in preliminary studies (70). An adeno-associated viral vector was used to deliver the gene for a human HSP (*hsp*-72) into neuronal cultures. The cells transfected with this construct were more resistant to a hypoxic-ischemic insult than controls, implying a causal relationship between HSP production and subsequent neuroprotection.

Another class of genes, the immediate early genes (IEGs), are involved in the cellular response to cerebral ischemia. IEGs are proto-oncogenes that play a regulatory role in gene transcription. They are the first genes transcribed (and subsequently translated) in response to ischemia and other insults. Like the heat shock genes, IEGs are presumed to play a role in maintaining cellular homeostasis in the face of endogenous or environmental insults (71–73). These genes code

for proteins (eg, c-FOS and c-JUN) that bind to certain chromosomal regions and either stimulate or inhibit the transcription of specific genes. Like the HSPs, the exact role of the IEG proteins in cerebral ischemia is not well understood. The relationship and interaction between the HSP and IEG products are still being elucidated (72,74,75) as are the target genes to which IEG products bind (71).

One such class of target genes are those for trophic factors. Since the discovery of nerve growth factor (NGF) nearly a half century ago (76), many endogenous agents have been characterized that promote neuronal development and viability. These trophic factors are important not only in a developing nervous system but are also neuroprotective in response to excitotoxic injury (77–79). The exact mechanisms by which these factors promote survival is not clear, but at least part of their action involves stabilizing intracellular calcium levels (79). Exposing cultured neurons to one of these factors, basic fibroblast growth factor (bFGF), resulted in the down-regulation of an NMDA receptor, indicating one way by which they help to maintain calcium homeostasis (77,80). Other trophic agents, such as NGF, may mediate cytoprotection after an ischemic insult by promoting growth or inhibiting degradation of cytoskeletal neurofilaments (78).

Gene delivery of neurotrophic agents has been successful in conferring cytoprotection to a variety of insults. Gage's group utilized a retroviral vector to deliver the NGF gene to fibroblasts in vitro and then grafted these engineered fibroblasts into the septal area of rats (10). When these animals were subject to fimbrial transection (an insult that normally causes the loss of septal cholinergic neurons), they exhibited significantly less neuronal death than controls (Fig. 4). Recent preliminary studies showed that this strategy was also effective in conferring neuroprotection in a rat model of cerebral ischemia (81).

Transgenic mice that overexpress a bovine form of bFGF were created in order to assess this factor's ability to afford neuroprotection. When these mice were subjected to a hypoxic-ischemic insult, infarct size was significantly reduced compared to nontransgenic litter mates (82).

As discussed above, proto-oncogenes such as IEGs may mediate cellular stability in the face of an environmental challenge. A proto-oncogene involved in the pathogenesis of certain B-cell lymphomas, bcl-2, may also have a neuroprotective role. The BCL-2 protein promotes cultured cell survival in response to serum or growth factor deprivation (83). Although the mechanisms by which it acts have not been fully elucidated, it may reduce cellular damage mediated by toxic free radicals. In vitro studies have shown that neural cell lines transfected with a bcl-2 (using a retroviral vector) were more resistant to glutamate-induced excitotoxic death than controls (84).

In animal ischemia models, expression of BCL-2 has been shown to be neuroprotective. Transgenic mice that overexpress BCL-2 had infarct volumes half as large as nontransgenic litter mates. Interestingly, these animals also had 40–50% more neurons in the facial nucleus and retinal gan-

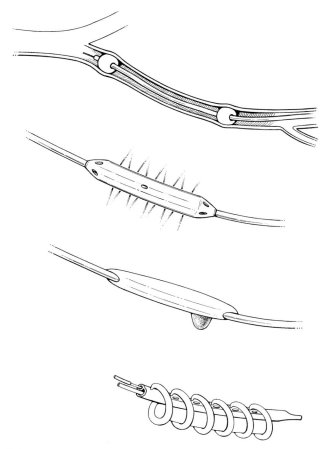

FIG. 4. Endovascular catheters for gene transfer. **A:** The Wolinsky double-balloon catheter has an infusion port between the balloons (35). **B:** The Wolinsky perforated balloon contains multiple"jet" ports and can deliver streams of liquid under pressure (36). **C:** The microporous balloon is similar to the Wolinsky perforated balloon but is covered by a microporous polycarbonate membrane, which reduces flow-related vascular injury (35). **D:** The dispatch catheter consists of a helical inflation coil wrapped around a nonporous urethane sheath, through which a dual-lumen shaft runs. One lumen is for drug infusion, and the other is used to inflate the coils. Inflation of the coils causes expansion of the underlying urethane sheath, allowing distal perfusion through the sheath. Drug is injected through the infusion port and exits through slits in the shaft between the inflation coils. Injected material is "trapped" in the space between the slits and the urethane sheath, and therefore has direct access to the vessel wall (37).

glion cell layer than controls, indicating the role that bcl-2 plays in programmed cell death and survival during development (85). The delivery of bcl-2 into rat brain by direct stereotactic injection (using a defective herpes vector) prior to a focal ischemic insult enhanced neuronal survival near the injection site (86).

Another approach to ameliorating ischemic insults has focused on cellular energy depletion due to excitotoxic stress. In the face of stress, considerable energy is utilized in an effort to maintain homeostasis. Using a defective herpesvirus vector, Sapolsky's group delivered a glucose transporter gene into both cultured neurons and in vivo and demonstrated that transfected tissues exhibited increased glucose uptake (87). This strategy provided cytoprotection in cultured neurons subsequently exposed to either hypoglycemia or glutamate, either of which can normally initiate the excitotoxic cascade (88).

The strategies discussed in this section involve some form of gene delivery to mediate a single step in either the excitotoxic cascade or the cellular response to such an insult. As our understanding of the various molecular events of ischemia increases, a greater variety of treatment options, including gene delivery, will be possible.

HUMAN GENE THERAPY TRIALS

Since 1989, more than 100 gene marking and gene therapy trials have been approved by the Recombinant DNA Advisory Committee (RAC) of the NIH and the Food and Drug Administration (FDA). High-risk patient groups such as those with lethal single-gene deficiencies, cancer, and AIDS have been the primary focus. Progress in the treatment of human disease is illustrated by adenosine deaminase (ADA) deficiency, a rare autosomal recessive disorder characterized by severe combined immunodeficiency (SCID) and eventual death from infection. Blaese (89) reported that two patients treated with "corrected" autologous T cells (which had been transfected in vitro with the ADA gene and reinfused) have demonstrated clinical and immunologic improvement. Oldfield's group (90) has treated patients with malignant brain tumors using the herpesvirus thymidine kinase (tk) gene model described above, delivered with a retroviral vector. After stereotactic injection into the tumor, the patients were treated with intravenous ganciclovir. Twelve of 19 lesions treated in this manner demonstrated a radiographically documented response (91).

The risk-to-benefit ratio for patients with vascular disease is higher than that of patients with cancer or AIDS, in whom treatment options and life expectancy are limited. Isner and associates recently performed endovascular gene therapy in a patient with a nonhealing ulcer and claudication in an attempt to stimulate angiogenesis and avoid amputation (92). Sixteen trillion copies of the gene for vascular endothelial growth factor (VEGF), an endogenously occurring mitogen that stimulates angiogenesis, were delivered through a percutaneous iliac artery catheter (Fig. 5). No follow-up data are available. To our knowledge, no endovascular, stereotactic, or intracerebroventricular delivery of genetic material has yet been performed in humans with cerebrovascular disease.

SUMMARY

Identification of patients with a genetically based risk for cerebrovascular disease remains a future challenge and will surely benefit from advances in the Human Genome Project.

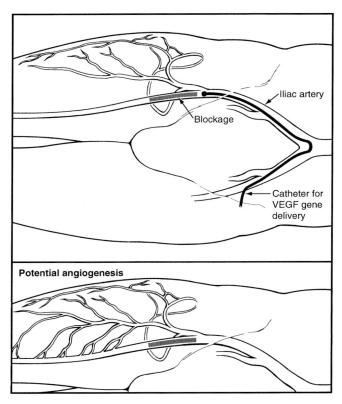

FIG. 5. Endovascularly delivered human gene therapy. A catheter was percutaneously placed into the iliac artery of a patient with arterial occlusion. Sixteen trillion copies of the gene for vasogenic endothelial growth factor (VEGF) were infused, in hopes of stimulating angiogenesis and avoiding limb amputation (92).

The current interest in the molecular biology of brain ischemia offers new strategies in the prevention and treatment of stroke. Techniques for endovascular gene transfer are becoming well established in cardiovascular research, and opportunities for cerebrovascular advances are ripe. The implications for the treatment of conditions such as carotid stenosis and postsubarachnoid hemorrhage vasospasm are obvious. Intraventricular and stereotactic gene transfers in animals have been successful, and long-term studies in larger animal models appear warranted. Stroke risk reduction in certain human genetic disease, however, presents significant obstacles associated with the need for widespread phenotypic correction. Human gene therapy for cerebrovascular disease should therefore only be initiated after safety and efficacy issues have been better defined.

REFERENCES

1. Morsey MA, Mitani K, Clemens P, Caskey T. Progress toward human gene therapy. *JAMA* 1993;270:2338–2345.
2. Collins F, Galas D. A new five-year plan for the U.S. human genome project. *Science* 1993;262:43–46.
3. Alberts B, Bray D, Lewis J, Raff M, Roberts K, Watson JD. *Molecular Biology of the Cell*, 2nd ed. New York: Garland Publishing, 1989
4. Helene C, Toulme JJ. Specific regulation of gene expression by antisense, sense, and antigene nucleic acids. *Biochim Biophys Acta* 1049:99–125, 1990
5. Ausubel FM, Brent R, Kingston RE, et al. (eds.). *Current Protocols in Molecular Biology*. New York: John Wiley and Sons, 1987.
6. Mulligan RC. The basic science of gene therapy. *Science* 1993;260:926–932.
7. Nabel EG. Gene therapy for cardiovascular disease. *Circulation* 1995;91:541–548.
8. Johnson PA, Miyanohara A, Levine F, Cahill T, Friedmann T. Cytotoxicity of a replication defective mutant of herpes simplex virus 1. *J Virol* 1992;66:2952–2955.
9. Kaplitt MG, Leone P, Samulski RJ, et al. Long-term gene expression and phenotypic correction using adeno-associated virus vectors in the mammalian brain. *Nat Genet* 1994;8:148–154.
10. Rosenberg MB, Friedmann T, Robertson RC, et al. Grafting genetically modified cells to the damaged brain: restorative effects of NGF expression. *Science* 1988;242:1575–1578.
11. Powers D, Wilson B, Imbus C, Pegelow C, Allen J. The natural history of stroke in sickle cell disease. *Am J Med* 1978;65:461–471.
12. Levy E, Carman MD, Fernandez-Madrid IJ, et al. Mutation of the Alzheimer's disease amyloid gene in hereditary cerebral hemorrhage, Dutch type. *Science* 1990;248:1124–1126.
13. Palsdottir A, Abrahamson M, Thorsteinsson L, et al. Mutation in cystatin C gene causes hereditary brain hemorrhage. *Lancet* 1988;2:603–604.
14. Devilat M, Toso M, Morales M. Children and strokes associated with protein C or S deficiency and primary antiphospholipid syndrome. *Pediatr Neurol* 1993;9:67–70.
15. Boers GHJ, Smals AGH, Trijbels FJM, et al. Heterozygosity for homocystinuria in premature peripheral and cerebrovascular occlusive arterial disease. *N Engl J Med* 1985;313:709–715.
16. Gutmann DH, Collins FS. The neurofibromatosis type 1 gene and its protein product, neurofibromin. *Neuron* 1993;10:335–343.
17. Schievink WI, Michels VV, Piepgras DG. Neurovascular manifestations of heritable connective tissue disorders: a review. *Stroke* 1994;25:889–903.
18. Fehlings MG, Gentili F. The association between polycystic kidney disease and cerebral aneurysms. *Can J Neurol Sci* 1991;18:505–509.
19. Ruggieri PM, Poulous AJ, Masaryk TJ, et al. Occult intracranial aneurysms in polycystic kidney disease: screening with MR angiography. *Radiology* 1994;191:33–39.
20. Pereira L, Levran O, Ramirez F, et al. A molecular approach to the stratification of cardiovascular risk in families with Marfan's syndrome. *N Eng J Med* 1994;331:148–153.
21. Schievink WI, Piepgras DG, Earnest F IV, Gordon H. Spontaneous carotid-cavernous fistulae in Ehlers–Danlos syndrome type IV: case report. *J Neurosurg* 1991;74:991–998.
22. Grewal RP. Stroke in Fabry's disease. *J Neurol* 1994;241:153–156.
23. Günel M, Awad IA, Anson J, Lifton RP. Mapping a gene causing cerebral cavernous malformation to 7q11.2-q21. *Proc Natl Acad Sci USA* 1995;92:6620–6624.
24. Wolkman OJ, Mann DL, Fauci AS. Association between Takayasu's arteritis and a B-cell alloantigen in North Americans. *N Engl J Med* 1982;306:464–465.
25. Dong RP, Kimura A, Numano F, et al. HLA-DP antigen and Takayasu arteritis. *Tissue Antigens* 1992;39:106–110.
26. Wilson JM, Chowdhury NR, Grossman M, et al. Temporary amelioration of hyperlipidemia in low density lipoprotein receptor-deficient rabbits transplanted with genetically modified hepatocytes. *Proc Natl Acad Sci USA* 1990;87:8437–8441.
27. Li J, Fang B, Eisensmith RC, et al. In vivo gene therapy for hyperlipidemia; phenotypic correction in Watanabe rabbits by hepatic delivery of the rabbit LDL receptor gene. *J Clin Invest* 1995;95:768–773.
28. Grossman M, Raper SE, Kozarsky K, et al. Successful ex vivo gene therapy directed to liver in a patient with familial hypercholesterolemia. *Nat Genet* 1994;6:323–324.
29. Gyurko R, Wielbo D, Phillips MI. Antisense inhibition of AT1 receptor mRNA and angiotensinogen mRNA in the brain of spontaneously hypertensive rats reduces hypertension of neurogenic origin. *Regul Pept* 1993;49:167–174.
30. Isner JM, Feldman LJ. Gene therapy for arterial disease. *Lancet* 1994;344:1653–1654.
31. Nabel EG, Plautz G, Boyce DM, Stanley JC, Nabel GJ. Recombinant

gene expression in vivo within endothelial cells of the arterial wall. *Science* 1989;244:1342–1344.

32. Wilson JM, Birinyi LK, Salomon RN, Libby P, Callow AD, Mulligan RC. Implantation of vascular grafts lined with genetically modified endothelial cells. *Science* 1989;244:1344–1346.

33. Steg PG, Feldman LJ, Scoazec JY, et al. Arterial gene transfer to rabbit endothelial and smooth muscle cells using percutaneous delivery of an adenoviral vector. *Circulation* 1994;90:1646–1656.

34. Riessen R, Rahimizadeh H, Blessing E, Takeshita S, Barry JJ, Isner JM. Arterial gene transfer using pure DNA applied directly to a hydrogel-coated angioplasty balloon. *Hum Gene Ther* 1993;4:749–758.

35. Riessen R, Isner JM. Prospects for site-specific delivery of pharmacologic and molecular therapies. *J Am Coll Cardiol* 1994;23:1234–1244.

36. Wolinsky H, Thung SN. Use of a perforated balloon catheter to deliver concentrated heparin into the wall of the normal canine artery. *J Am Coll Cardiol* 1990;15:475–481.

37. Mitchel JF, Fram D, Palme DF, et al. Enhanced intracoronary thrombolysis with urokinase using a novel, local drug delivery system. *Circulation* 1995;91:785–793.

38. Ohno T, Gordon D, San H, et al. Gene therapy for vascular smooth muscle proliferation after arterial injury. *Science* 1994;265:781–784.

39. Guzman RJ, Hirschowitz EA, Brody SL, Crystal RG, Epstein SE, Finkel T. In vivo suppression of injury-induced vascular smooth muscle cell accumulation using adenovirus-mediated transfer of the herpes simplex virus thymidine kinase gene. *Proc Natl Acad Sci USA* 1994;91:10732–10736.

40. Chang MW, Barr E, Seltzer J, et al. Cytostatic gene therapy for vascular proliferation disorders with a constitutively active form of the retinoblastoma gene project. *Science* 1995;262:518–522.

41. von der Leyden HE, Gibbons GH, Morishita R, et al. Gene therapy inhibiting neointimal vascular lesion: in vivo transfer of endothelial cell nitric oxide synthase gene. *Proc Natl Acad Sci USA* 1995;92:1137–1141.

42. Dalkara T, Moskowitz M. The complex role of nitric oxide in the pathophysiology of focal cerebral ischemia. *Brain Pathol* 1994;4:49–57.

43. Morishita R, Gibbons GH, Ellison KE, et al. Single intraluminal delivery of antisense cdc2 kinase and proliferating-cell nuclear antigen oligonucleotides results in chronic inhibition of neointimal hyperplasia. *Proc Natl Acad Sci USA* 1993;90:8474–8478.

44. Olsen TS, Larsen B, Herning M, Skriver EB, Lassen NA. Blood flow and vascular reactivity in collaterally perfused brain tissue. Evidence of an ischemic penumbra in patients with acute stroke. *Stroke* 1983;14:332–341.

45. Procter AW. Can we reverse the ischemic penumbra? Some mechanisms in the pathophysiology of energy-compromised brain tissue. *Clin Neuropharmacol* 1990;13(Suppl):S334–S39.

46. Siesjo BK. Pathophysiology and treatment of focal cerebral ischemia. *J Neurosurg* 1992;77:169–184.

47. Hossmann KA. Glutamate-mediated injury in focal cerebral ischemia: the excitotoxin hypothesis revised. *Brain Pathol* 1994;4:23–36.

48. Choi DW. Calcium-mediated neurotoxicity: relationship to specific channel types and role in ischemic damage. *Trends Neurosci* 1988;11:465–469.

49. Choi DW. Methods for antagonizing glutamate neurotoxicity. *Cerebrovasc Brain Metab Rev* 1990;2:105–147.

50. Choi DW, Hartley DM. Calcium and glutamate-induced cortical neuronal death. In: Waxman SG, ed. *Molecular and Cellular Approaches to the Treatment of Neurological Disease*. New York: Raven Press, 1993;23–34.

51. Wahlestedt C, Golanov E, Yamamoto S, et al. Antisense oligodeoxynucleotides to NMDA-R1 receptor channel protect cortical neurons from excitotoxicity and reduce focal ischaemic infarctions. *Nature* 1993;363:260–263.

52. Kader A, Frazzini VI, Solomon RA, Trifiletti RR. Nitric oxide production during focal cerebral ischemia in rats. *Stroke* 1993;24:1709–1716.

53. Lipton SA, Stamler JS. Actions of redox-related congeners of nitric oxide at the NMDA receptor. *Neuropharmacology* 1994;33:1229–1233.

54. Morikawa E, Moskowitz MA, Huang Z, Yoshida T, Irikura K, Dalkara T. L-arginine infusion promotes nitric oxide–dependent vasodilatation, increases regional blood flow, and reduces infarction volume in the rat. *Stroke* 1994;25:429–435.

55. Dawson TM, Dawson VL, Snyder SH. A novel neuronal messenger in brain: the free radical, nitric oxide. *Ann Neurol* 1992;32:297–311.

56. Chan PH. Oxygen radicals in focal cerebral ischemia. *Brain Pathol* 1994;4:59–65.

57. Huang Z, Huang PL, Panahian N, Dalkara T, Fishman MC, Moskowitz MA. Effects of cerebral ischemia in mice deficient in neuronal nitric oxide synthase. *Science* 1994;265:1883–1885.

58. Flamm ES, Demopoulos HB, Seligman ML, Poser RG, Ransohoff J. Free radicals in cerebral ischemia. *Stroke* 1978;9:445–447.

59. Liu TH, Beckman JS, Freeman BA, Hogan EL, Hsu CY. Polyethylene glycol-conjugated superoxide dismutase and catalase reduce ischemic brain injury. *Am J Physiol* 1989;256:H589–H593.

60. Yang G, Chan PH, Chen J, et al. Human copper-zinc superoxide dismutase transgenic mice are highly resistant to reperfusion injury after focal cerebral ischemia. *Stroke* 1994;25:165–170.

61. Kinouchi H, Epstein CJ, Mizui T, Carlson EJ, Chen SF, Chan PH. Attenuation of focal cerebral ischemic injury in transgenic mice overexpressing CuZn superoxide dismutase. *Proc Natl Acad Sci USA* 1991;88:11158–11162.

62. Nowak TS, Jacewicz M. The heat shock/stress response in focal cerebral ischemia. *Brain Pathol* 1994;4:67–76.

63. Sharp FR, Kinouchi H, Koistinaho J, Chan PH, Sagar SM. HSP70 heat shock gene regulation during ischemia. *Stroke* (Suppl I) 1993;24:I-72–I-75.

64. Beckmann RP, Mizzen LA, Welch WJ. Interaction of HSP70 with newly synthesized proteins: implications for protein folding and assembly. *Science* 1990;248:850–854.

65. Chirico WJ, Waters MG, Blobel G. 70K heat shock related proteins stimulate protein translocation into microsomes. *Nature* 1988;332:805–810.

66. Kinouchi H, Sharp FR, Koistinaho J, Hicks K, Kamii H, Chan PH. Induction of heat shock hsp70 mRNA and HSP70 kDa protein in neurons in the ''penumbra'' following focal cerebral ischemia in the rat. *Brain Res* 1993;619:334–338.

67. Rordorf G, Koroshetz WJ, Bonventre JV. Heat shock protects cultured neurons from glutamate toxicity. *Neuron* 1991;7:1043–1051.

68. Glazier SS, O'Rourke DM, Graham DI, Welsh FA. Induction of Ischemic tolerance following brief focal ischemia in rat brain. *J Cereb Blood Flow Metab* 1993;14:545–553.

69. Simon RP, Niiro M, Gwinn R. Prior ischemic stress protects against experimental stroke. *Neurosci Lett* 1993;163:135–137.

70. Lippman C, Welsh F, Kaplitt M, et al. AAV-vector mediated human hsp72 gene transfer into cultured cells. *Soc Neurosci Abstr* 1995;21:1805.

71. Kiessling M, Gass P. Stimulus-transcription coupling in focal cerebral ischemia. *Brain Pathol* 1994;4:77–83.

72. Takemoto O, Tomimoto H, Yanagihara T. Induction of c-fos and c-jun gene products and heat shock protein after brief and prolonged cerebral ischemia in gerbils. *Stroke* 1995;26:1639–1648.

73. Morgan JI, Curran T. Stimulus-transcription coupling in neurons: role of cellular immediate-early genes. *TINS* 1989;12:459–462.

74. Blumenfeld, KS, Welsh FA, Harris VA, Pesenson MA. Regional expression of c-fos and heat shock protein-70 mRNA following hypoxia-ischemia in immature rat brain. *J Cereb Blood Flow Metab* 1992;12:987–995.

75. Welsh FA, Moyer DJ, Harris VA. Regional expression of heat shock protein-70 mRNA and c-fos mRNA following focal ischemia in rat brain. *J Cereb Blood Flow Metab* 1992;12:204–212.

76. Levi-Montalcini R. The nerve growth factor 35 years later. *Science* 1987;237:1154–1162.

77. Finkelstein SP, Kemmou A, Caday CG, Berlove DJ. Basic fibroblast growth factor protects cerebrocortical neurons against excitatory amino acid toxicity in vitro. *Stroke* (Suppl I) 1993;24:I-141–I-143.

78. Tanaka K, Tsukahara T, Hashimoto N, et al. Effect of nerve growth factor on delayed neuronal death after cerebral ischemia. *Acta Neurochir (Wien)* 1994;129:64–71.

79. Mattson MP, Cheng B. Growth factors protect neurons against excitotoxic/ischemic damage by stabilizing calcium homeostasis. *Stroke* (Suppl I) 1993;24:I-136–I-140.

80. Mattson MP, Kumar K, Wang H, Michaelis EK. Basic FGF regulates the expression of a functional 71 kDa NMDA receptor protein that mediates calcium influx and excitotoxicity in cultured hippocampal neurons. *J Neurosci* 1993;13:4575–4588.

81. Pechan PA, Fujii M, Yoshida T, et al. Somatic gene therapy in rat global ischemia by grafting of NGF- and BDNF-secreting fibroblasts. *Soc Neurosci Abstr* 1995;21:513.

82. MacMillan V, Judge D, Wiseman A, Settles D, Swain J, Davis J. Mice expressing a bovine basic fibroblast growth factor transgene in the brain show increased resistance to hypoxemic-ischemic cerebral damage. *Stroke* 1993;24:1735–1739.

83. Mah S, Zhong L, Liu Y, Roghani A, Edwards R, Bredesen D. The proto-oncogene bcl-2 inhibits apoptosis in PC12 cells. *J Neurochem* 1993;60:1183–1186.

84. Zhong L, Kane D, Bredesen DE. BCL-2 blocks glutamate toxicity in neural cell lines. *Brain Res Mol Brain Res* 1993;19:353–355.

85. Martinou JC, Dubois-Dauphin M, Staple JK, et al. Overexpression of BCL-2 in transgenic mice protects neurons from naturally occurring cell death and experimental ischemia. *Neuron* 1994;133:1017–1030.

86. Linnik MD, Zahos P, Geschwind MD, Federoff HJ. Expression of bcl-2 from a defective herpes simplex virus–1 vector limits neuronal death in focal cerebral ischemia. *Stroke* 1995;26:1670–1674.

87. Ho DY, Mocarski ES, Sapolski RM. Altering central nervous system physiology with a defective herpes simplex virus vector expressing the glucose transporter gene. *Proc Natl Acad Sci USA* 1993;90:3655–3659.

88. Ho DY, Saydam TC, Fink SL, Lawrence MS, Sapolski RM. Defective herpes simplex virus vectors expressing the rat brain glucose transporter protect cultured neurons from necrotic insults. *J Neurochem* 1995;65:842–850.

89. Blaese RM. Development of gene therapy for immunodeficiency: adenosine deaminase deficiency. *Pediatr Res* 1993;33(1Suppl):S49–53.

90. Oldfield EH, Ram Z, Culver KW, Blaese RM, DeVroom HL, Anderson WF. Gene therapy for the treatment of brain tumors using intra-tumoral transduction with the thymidine kinase gene and intravenous ganciclovir. *Hum Gene Ther* 1993;4:39–69.

91. Blaese RM. Human gene therapy trials. Lecture at the University of Alabama, Birmingham, January 1995.

92. Kolata G. Novel bypass method: a dose of new genes. *The New York Times*, Dec 13, 1994:B5–6.

SECTION II
Cerebrovascular Diagnosis

The pathological conditions affecting the cerebral vasculature are diverse, and neurological symptoms and signs resulting from injury to cerebral vessels at times can be quite subtle. In accordance with classical neurological tradition, the role of the clinician is to recognize that injury has occurred, localize the level of the lesion, and then generate a cogent differential diagnosis of possible mechanisms. The technologies currently available to image the nervous system and its vascular supply are incredibly powerful. Routine angiography, CT, MR, Doppler, SPECT, and PET so enhance the evaluation of a patient with cerebrovascular disease as to render histopathologic examination unnecessary in many instances. Understandably, this has led to over-utilization of these diagnostic tools, the economic consequence of which threatens their wide-spread and easy access. Increasingly, it is the gate-keeper, be it physician, nurse, or hidden bureaucrat, who approves whether a patient may or may not receive a particular study.

This section provides a basis for understanding many of the technologies available for imaging of the central nervous system and its vasculature. Each chapter covers a particular modality, discusses the scientific basis for its technology, its clinical indications and limitations, and an overview of expected findings in various pathologic conditions related to cerebrovascular disease. Combined, the chapters are a superb overview of what has now become the specialty of neuroimaging.

Considering the power of modern neuroimaging, one might question the need for the clinical physician as a diagnostician. When confronted with a patient who has experienced a sudden neurologic event, why not order a predetermined set of imaging procedures to prove or disprove a diagnosis? The answer lies both in therapeutics and economics. It is the clinician's role to pick the appropriate diagnostic test at the appropriate point in the patient's illness while understanding the ways in which imaging modalities can be clinically misleading. Although the authoritative assistance of a neuroimaging specialist in performing and interpreting a particular test is invaluable, the managing clinician remains ultimately responsible for utilizing the results as a basis for treatment decisions. Therapy in vascular disease can be hazardous, be it medical or surgical. An example is the applica-tion of thrombolytic therapy in acute ischemic stroke. According to current standards, imaging procedures and initiation of therapy must be instituted in three to six hours. Lack of sophistication in obtaining a reliable history or performing a competent neurologic examination (in an often harried clinical setting) can result in unnecessarily exposing the patient to dangerous and expensive therapy. In the outpatient office, confronted with a capitated insurance program, the clinician must judiciously and knowledgeably limit ordering of procedures so as not to over-utilize this expensive technology. In summary, as with all other laboratory tests, imaging should be viewed not simply to confirm a diagnosis, but as an extension of the clinical examination in order to formulate and monitor therapeutic decisions.

It is appropriate, therefore, that this section begins with chapters on the history, physical examination, and differential diagnosis of the stroke patient. In recent years, no one has added more broadly to our knowledge of cerebrovascular disease in its clinical setting than Dr. Louis Caplan. His chapter should be read by all who treat stroke victims and order imaging procedures in the course of their care. Application of the principles and methods described in his chapter will provide a framework for the recognition of cerebrovascular embarrassment and develop discipline in ordering further diagnostic tests. The subsequent chapter by Moncayo and Bogousslavsky overviews the common physical findings in ischemic stroke. Particularly important is the emphasis on neurobehavioral signs, so often overlooked in the clinical encounter. The section concludes with an overview of the multiplicity of means available to monitor cerebral blood flow, cerebral perfusion pressure, cardiac output, and substrate delivery to the brain in critically ill patients. These measures often make the critical difference in clinical outcome. Clinical outcome measurements are becoming the standard by which the efficacy of therapy is judged and reimbursed. The ability to recognize and document neurologic deficits from the onset of an illness, minimize progression and document clinical outcome will increasingly impact the economics of medical practice. This section as a whole, explores some means by which this is feasible.

Ralph Greenlee, M.D.

Cerebrovascular Disease, edited by H. Hunt Batjer.
Lippincott-Raven Publishers, Philadelphia © 1997.

CHAPTER 13

History of Differential Diagnosis in Stroke

Louis R. Caplan

STROKE DIAGNOSIS STRATEGIES AND METHODS

Before delving into the details of focused history taking it is necessary to discuss the strategy and methods of clinical stroke diagnosis in order to place the role of the history in perspective. To be effective, the entire clinical encounter should be *hypothesis-driven*. At the very instant that the first clinical information about the patient becomes available, the clinician should begin to generate hypotheses that he or she will test repeatedly throughout the encounter. The first data may come from a variety of sources, eg, the patient, family members, another physician, a secretary, nurse, or other health care provider reading a consultation request. The information conveyed may contain a variety of different types of data, ie, past medical ills, how the acute symptoms occurred or evolved, laboratory or imaging data, and so forth. Irrespective of the nature and source of the data, the clinician should begin to generate hypotheses about the likely stroke mechanism (what is the patient's pathology), and the likely location of the brain and vascular lesions (where the pathology is located). The what and where hypotheses should be attacked concurrently, systematically, and sequentially as the clinical encounter progresses from the history to the general and neurologic examinations to selecting and interpreting imaging and laboratory data.

Data acquisition is not a passive recording of what the historian states. A patient who has a transient attack of numbness and weakness of the right hand will seldom spontaneously tell the clinician about an attack of transient monocular blindness in the left eye, thinking the two episodes to be completely unrelated. Even a prior attack of right leg weakness may similarly go unreported. The great majority of patients do not think anatomically or physiologically. Most have no idea how the brain works. Many have the idea that brain trouble mostly causes individuals to have a fit, go crazy, lose their intellect, or fall unconscious. They do not conceive of the brain as having the puppet strings that relate to movement, feeling, and special sensory input.

An alert clinician hearing the story of right-hand motor and sensory loss of function begins to think anatomically. Is the process in the left cerebral hemisphere, the left brainstem, the right spinal cord, or in the nerves of the right hand? The clinician asks questions to better define the location of the dysfunction within the nervous system. Was language affected? Could the patient speak, understand, read, write, and so forth during the event? If language was involved or if there was right-sided hemianopic-type visual loss the lesion would have to be in the left cerebral hemisphere. On the other hand, the presence of bilateral weakness, vertigo, or diplopia during the attack or in other attacks suggests a brainstem localization, and neck pain or pain in the right upper extremity would favor a spinal or local process. The technique of neurologic localization is akin to tracing the location of a car breakdown. Your son calls to say that his car is stuck and he wants you to come and help him. He has no idea where the car is. With your knowledge of the city and suburbs, you ask about the relation of the car to various cross streets and landmarks. By sequential questioning you may be able to place the car in a given vicinity depending very much on your son's observational abilities, recall, and knowledge of the neighborhoods through which he passed. Similarly, neurologic and neurosurgical clinicians, with their intimate knowledge of brain anatomy and physiology, actively query the patient about a variety of different symptoms that would help them define the exact location of the dysfunction in the brain as precisely as possible. Plumbers and car mechanics pursue similar strategies in locating the problem in your car and your water pipes. In the given patient with transient right-hand numbness and weakness, the clinician is able to determine that wrong words were used in the patient's conversation with his paramour during the attack, and so the lesion is surely in the left cerebral hemisphere and likely para-Sylvian and supra-Sylvian and in the vicinity of the Rolandic sulcus.

L. R. Caplan: Departments of Neurology and Medicine, Tufts University Medical School; Department of Neurology, New England Medical Center, Boston, Massachusetts 02111

Hypotheses about what is wrong are handled very similarly to ''where'' hypotheses. Our patient with transient left hemisphere dysfunction is a white man, 68 years old, and has angina pectoris and leg claudication. He smoked cigarettes for many years and stopped very recently only on his paramour's insistence. He never was told that he had hypertension or diabetes. Patients with this risk factor profile have a high frequency of having large artery atherosclerosis. In fact, we know that he has coronary artery and peripheral vascular occlusive disease. The most common site of large artery atherosclerosis in the cerebrovascular system of white men with systemic atherosclerosis is the internal carotid artery (ICA) in the neck at or near the carotid artery bifurcation. Recognizing that atherosclerotic ICA disease in the left neck is the most likely hypothesis, the clinician thinks of possible related symptoms such as transient monocular visual symptoms in the left eye and unaccustomed recent headaches. The clinician also realizes that the pathology could also be located within the more distal ICA in the high neck or carotid siphon, or in the middle cerebral artery (MCA). Alternatively, nonatherosclerotic pathologies such as dissection, embolism, and arterial aneurysms can also affect the vessels at these sites. The clinician thinks about the features of each of these conditions and each of these vascular sites and proceeds to acquire data that will influence each potential diagnostic hypothesis. Has there been recent head or neck trauma, sudden neck turning, active participation in sports, or unusual neck, face, or head pain? Positive responses favor arterial dissection or at least increase its probability whereas negative responses diminish its likelihood. This patient has angina pectoris, indicating the presence of coronary artery disease, and could have had a myocardial infarct, which might have been the source for an embolus to the left MCA. The clinician inquires if there has been recent unusual chest or jaw pain that might indicate a myocardial infarct. Have there been prior transient ischemic attacks (TIAs) or strokes in the right cerebral hemisphere or brainstem or sudden coolness and pain in a limb suggesting prior brain or systemic embolism? Positive responses increase the probability of a cardiogenic embolism. In the past months has there been an episode of sudden onset severe headache especially with vomiting and sudden cessation of activity? The presence of a prior small subarachnoid hemorrhage (SAH), a so-called warning leak, would enhance the remote possibility that an intracranial aneurysm is acting as a source of intraarterial embolism to cause the patient's TIA. All potential diagnoses should be considered by the clinician during the questioning. Even when one diagnosis seems very highly probable, the effective clinician will still consider potential alternatives and systematically test and exclude them. The technique of interrogation of a hypothesis is similar to that used in school to prove or disprove a geometric theorem. Assume the alternative possibility is true and then attempt to disprove it by reducing it to an absurdity—*reductio ad absurdem.*

Notice that in the foregoing discussion I have often used the words *probable* and *possible.* Clinical diagnoses are seldom absolute certainties, at least during the initial encounter before laboratory data are available. Usually there are some differential diagnostic possibilities in both the what and where categories. Diagnoses should be thought of in terms of probability. For example, in the patient described with risk factors for atherosclerosis who had an episode of transient left cerebral dysfunction, carotid atherosclerosis in the neck is surely the leading diagnosis, perhaps 75% likely, but cardiac origin embolism is still possible (20%). Aneurysm or other unusual intrinsic vascular disease within the ICA/MCA region is remote but still possible (5%). Of course, these are rough guesses at the probabilities but they serve a useful function because common events occur often and conditions with low probabilities occur much less often. I suggest that students, house officers, and neophytes in stroke diagnosis formally list on paper their differential what and where diagnoses and the probabilities of each after they have completed the initial history taking. They then should *stop and think* before the general and neurologic examinations. What findings could influence the likelihood of the listed diagnoses? A focal, long, and high-pitched bruit over the left carotid artery bifurcation in the neck would substantiate the presence of left carotid artery disease. Finding a Hollenhorst-type cholesterol embolus in the left optic fundus on ophthalmoscopy would also enhance the probability of carotid artery disease. Alternatively, unexpected fever, a heart murmur, and irregular heart rhythm, as well as peripheral finger and toe and retinal embolic lesions would increase by far the likelihood of a cardiac origin embolism. During the neurologic examination what findings would help the localization become more precise? Is there a visual field defect? Is there evidence now of aphasia and, if so, what type? Are the hand, arm, face, and leg equally involved with respect to numbness and weakness? The examination is greatly enhanced when the examiner is looking for various findings rather than conducting a rote or stereotyped performance. After the examination, the differential diagnoses lists and probabilities should be modified to reflect the physical findings. Sometimes new diagnoses might be suggested from the examination. For example, the unexpected finding of fever, a heart murmur, and a Janeway spot in the hand would raise the possibility of bacterial endocarditis, a diagnosis that might not have been thought of in the original history taking. The clinician will then go back to the patient and inquire about prior rheumatic fever, past murmurs, recent dental procedures, intravenous drug use, and other questions that might not have come up during the initial history taking. After the general and neurologic examinations, there should be a pause to *stop and think* again and plan the laboratory and imaging evaluation. What investigations will best distinguish between alternatives and prove or disprove each potential diagnosis? Of course, the most likely and most treatable diagnoses should be tested first. Laboratory tests are also chosen, interpreted, and considered sequentially because the results of the first tests strongly influence what tests should be ordered next (1,2).

How does the clinician make probability estimates and arrive at a final clinical diagnosis? Successful clinicians use two different strategies. The first strategy is *pattern matching*. We recognize Hilda because we know what Hilda looks like. We make a gestalt type of determination that the person in front of us is Hilda because she looks, talks, and walks like Hilda. We do not ordinarily go through an analysis adding up facial features, glasses, hair, figure, and so forth to arrive at a diagnosis of Hilda. Similarly, if the patient described with transient left cerebral dysfunction, a white man with atherosclerotic risk factors, had a left carotid bruit and a history of left amaurosis fugax, the pattern of left carotid artery disease would be unmistakable. Similarly, clinicians match the features in their individual patients with familiar patterns of the findings in patients with various stroke disease mechanisms and with the symptoms and signs relating to different brain sites.

The second technique is more complex and utilizes a Bayes theorem approach. Various data items are used to systematically calculate probabilities similar to the way a computer analysis might function. The Bayes theorem uses two types of data (2–4: (a) the incidence of each illness (in this case, stroke mechanisms) in the general population studied and (b) the incidence of a given finding in each stroke diagnosis. The findings from stroke data banks and registries indicate that on average about 80% of strokes are ischemic and 20% are due to hemorrhage (about 8–10% subarachnoid hemorrhage and 10–12% intracerebral hemorrhage) (2). If a clinician seeing a stroke patient in the emergency room knew nothing at all about stroke, a diagnosis of ischemic stroke would be correct four times in five. The frequency in the community factor in Bayes' theorem ensures that common diagnoses are given higher probability than uncommon ones. When you hear hoof beats in a city, horses are a more likely source than zebras or camels.

The other portion of Bayes' theorem uses individual clinical data items such as the presence or absence of risk factors, the course of the symptoms and signs, and the presence of other symptoms such as headache, vomiting, loss of consciousness, and seizures. If clinicians knew the frequency of each item, eg, hypertension, coronary artery disease, diabetes, smoking, sudden onset, occurrence during vigorous activity, headache preceding onset, vomiting, and so forth, in each of the stroke mechanism diagnoses, they could then calculate the probability of a patient having each of those conditions. The Harvard Stroke Registry (5) was designed at least partially to derive these probabilities, which could then be used in a computer diagnostic program based on Bayesian analysis (6). The various stroke conditions to be considered are diagrammed in a stroke differential diagnosis in Fig. 1. The published results of the Harvard Stroke Registry (5). The Lausanne Stroke Registry (7), the Stroke Data Bank (8), and other registries and data banks (2,6) provide inexperienced stroke clinicians with frequency estimates that can be used for judging probabilities of each of the diagnoses in Fig. 1. Remember, however, that one very powerful data

Stroke Differential Diagnosis

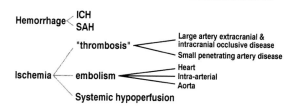

FIG. 1. Differential diagnosis of stroke mechanisms.

item can overpower all other items in a given patient (the so-called Mack truck phenomenon). For example, if a patient has a blood pressure of 270/170 the likelihood of intracerebral hemorrhage goes so high that all other diagnoses move way down the list. Similarly, a patient who has the sudden onset of the worst headache of his or her life during sexual intercourse has a very high probability of having had a subarachnoid hemorrhage no matter what the other data items reveal.

Listed in Table 1 are the methodologic rules suggested for stroke diagnosis. We are now ready to turn to a discussion of each of the various data items in the history taking encounter. I emphasize that the history is not a one-time endeavor performed only initially. Often patients during the first encounter are ill, tired, worried, and sometimes frightened, and they may not be able to concentrate or think clearly. Neurologic deficits such as aphasia, amnesia, and abulia may decrease their abilities as accurate historians. I have found it useful to return to key history items again and again during the care period because patients will often be able to give more accurate responses with further thought and effort and perhaps after some recovery of functions. I also strongly advocate utilizing sources other than the patient to derive all possible historical data. Spouses, children, friends, and the like can often provide very useful information. I usually have the others present when questioning the patient so that

TABLE 1. *Methodology and rules of stroke diagnosis*

1. Diagnoses are hypothesis-driven.
2. Vigorously pursue *what* (pathology and stroke mechanism) and *where* (the anatomic site of the dysfunction) diagnoses concurrently.
3. Diagnoses should be given probability estimates.
4. Diagnostic probabilities should be listed (on paper or mentally) and modified after each portion of the clinical encounter—history taking, general and neurologic examinations, and laboratory and imaging investigations.
5. Although each portion of the clinical encounter is performed sequentially, retaking of various history data items and reexaminations are important in testing new and modified *what* and *where* hypotheses.

they can add to or render their observations about the data the patient provides.

ECOLOGY: DEMOGRAPHY AND STROKE RISK FACTORS

Often the first information available to the clinician consists of very basic demographic data on the patient and elements of his or her past medical history that might relate to vascular disease. All of us can visualize being called at the office or on a car phone by someone asking us to see a patient with possible stroke in the emergency room. The voice on the other end of the line (or on a message machine) usually tells the age, race, and sex of the patient. Sometimes past medical ills are also relayed, such as the following: There is a 23-year-old street woman, a known drug user, who has collapsed on the street and has right-sided paralysis and can't talk. Demographic information and risk factors change the statistical probability of the various types of strokes being present. They seldom if ever allow definitive diagnosis. The young woman described above has a high probability, if she used cocaine or methamphetamine, of having a brain or subarachnoid hemorrhage or a drug-related ischemic stroke. If she used heroin, an ischemic stroke would be most likely. However, it is entirely possible that her stroke had nothing to do with her known risk factor—drugs. Perhaps, unknown to the caller, she also had rheumatic fever and has a cardiac origin embolism. She might have injured herself and had a carotid artery dissection. The past ills, demography, and present conditions can be thought of as "ecology" because they are the setting and environment in which the stroke developed. They allow clinicians to forecast the likely possibilities and probabilities of various diagnostic conditions in the given patient's milieu. In that way they should be thought of as yielding a priori odds of each diagnosis.

Demography

The *age* of the patient is a key data item. Clearly patients under 30 have a relatively low frequency of atherosclerotic cerebrovascular disease unless they have familial hyperlipidemia or have had juvenile diabetes or longstanding severe hypertension. Atherosclerotic ischemic strokes occur most often in the seventh and eighth decades of life and are much less common under age 50. Hypertension, in contrast, can be present in the young and may predispose to intracerebral hemorrhage at any age. Cardiogenic embolism from congenital heart disease and hemorrhage from vascular malformations are most common in the young and diminish in likelihood with age.

Sex is another important variable. Ischemic strokes are less common in premenopausal women than in similar aged men, but the frequency of ischemic stroke in women after the menopause is similar to that found in comparably aged men. Studies have shown that extracranial occlusive vascular disease involving the ICA in the neck and the vertebral artery in the neck is about twice as common in white men as in women (9). Intracranial arterial occlusive disease, on the other hand, is more common in women than in men.

Race is also an important determinant of the type of stroke mechanism and the distribution of occlusive lesions. Blacks tend to have more intracerebral hemorrhage than whites, perhaps in relationship to the prevalence of hypertension and the frequent lack of compliance and effective treatment of hypertension in blacks. In Cincinnati, the incidence of intracerebral hemorrhage under age 75 was 2.3 times higher in blacks as compared to white patients (10). Similarly, intracerebral hemorrhage is more common in patients of Chinese and Japanese heritage than in Caucasians.

White men, especially those with coronary artery and peripheral vascular disease, as well as hyperlipidemia, have a relatively high frequency of extracranial carotid and vertebral artery disease when compared to blacks and Asians, and women (9,11). Women of all races and black and Asian men have more frequent intracranial occlusive disease, especially involving the MCAs, than do white men (9,11). The distribution of vascular occlusive disease should affect diagnostic strategies. In white men with anterior circulation strokes, carotid duplex examination is often crucial. The same test has a very low yield in a black or Asian woman. Transcranial Doppler and intracranial magnetic resonance angiography (MRA) are more important than neck ultrasound testing in women, blacks, and Asians.

STROKE RISK FACTORS

Information about risk factors comes mostly from the history but some risk factors such as hypertension, diabetes, polycythemia, and hyperlipidemia might be recognized first on examination or only after laboratory testing. Stroke risk factors are discussed in detail in many texts under the heading of stroke prevention since modification of these risk factors is very important in decreasing the likelihood of stroke in individual patients and in the community. A very important reason for inquiring about the presence of any of these factors while taking the history is so that measures can be introduced during the acute care of the stroke patient to eliminate or minimize those factors that are potentially treatable and remedial. I will not discuss each of the potential risk factors at length here but will limit myself to general comments about their impact on diagnosis.

Risk factors are useful in diagnosis by changing the odds that an individual patient does or does not have a particular stroke mechanism. However, some risk factors impact on a number of different stroke mechanisms. For example, hypertension is a major cause of intracerebral hemorrhage and penetrating artery disease that underlies lacunar brain infarc-

TABLE 2. *Weighting of various demographic and risk factors*

Risk factor	Large artery atherosclerosis	Lacune	Embolism	ICH	SAH
Hypertension	+ +	+ + +		+ +	+
Severe hypertension		+		+ + + +	+ +
Coronary disease	+ + +		+ +		
Claudication	+ + +		+		
Atrial fibrillation			+ + + +		
Valvular heart disease			+ + + +		
Diabetes	+ + +	+	+		
Bleeding disorder				+ + + +	+ +
Smoking	+ + +		+		+ +
Cancer	+ +		+ +		+
TIAs	+ + + +	+ +	+	+	
Old age	+ + +	+		+	
Black or Asian origin	+	+ +		+ +	−

Modified from ref. 2.
TIA, transient ischemic attack.

tion. Hypertension is also a very potent risk factor for the development of both extracranial and intracranial large artery atherosclerosis. Hypertension also increases the probability of rupture in patients with aneurysms. The importance of a risk factor in given stroke mechanisms can be thought of in terms of weighting or loading onto that mechanism. Table 2 shows posited estimates of the weighting of the various risk factors.

In some situations the *absence* of a risk factor such as past or present hypertension is helpful diagnostically. If a young woman who develops a gradual onset hemiplegia in minutes is normotensive, then intracerebral hemorrhage becomes an unlikely diagnosis unless she uses drugs or has a bleeding disorder or vascular malformation. On the other hand, if her blood pressure were 220/125, then hypertensive intracerebral hemorrhage would be by far the leading diagnosis. If there are absolutely no risk factors present in a young patient who develops a focal neurologic syndrome, then causes other than stroke, eg, multiple sclerosis, tumor, infections or parainfections, should rise higher on the list of diagnostic possibilities.

Some individual risk factors often occur together and should best be thought of as a single factor. For example

angina pectoris, myocardial infarction, and peripheral vascular disease in the limbs are all tangible evidence of the presence of large artery atherosclerosis in the body. In the Harvard Stroke Registry, the presence of any of these individual items (grouped together as large artery atherosclerosis) was the single most important factor that impacted on the likely presence of carotid artery disease in the neck. The frequencies of atherosclerosis and other individual risk factors in the Harvard (5) and Michael Reese (12) Stroke registries are listed in Table 3. Coronary artery, peripheral arterial, and extracranial carotid and vertebral artery occlusive lesions often coexist and should be thought of as cotravelers because all are important manifestations of systemic atherosclerosis. Hyperlipidemia and hypertension are also often present in this group of patients with large artery atherosclerosis. The presence of large artery atherosclerosis as defined herein does not, however, predispose to intracranial atherosclerosis (except in relation to the intracranial vertebral and basilar arteries) unless there is also extensive extracranial disease. Most women, blacks, and Asians with MCA stenosis do not have evidence of coronary, peripheral vascular, or extracranial cerebrovascular disease, but they do have a higher incidence of hypertension and diabetes than in an age-matched

TABLE 3. *Incidence of some findings in the Harvard (5) and Michael Reese (12) stroke registries*

	Thrombosis*	Lacune	Embolism	ICH	SAH
HSR					
Atherosclerosis[a]	56%	37%	34%	11%	5%
Diabetes	26%	28%	13%	15%	2%
Past hypertension	55%	75%	40%	72%	19%
MRSR					
Angina pectoris	13%	8%	20%	5%	0%
Past MI	23%	16%	40%	12%	0%
Recent MI	7%	12%	12%	3%	0%
Past hypertension	75%	55%	55%	68%	44%

[a] Includes peripheral vascular disease, coronary disease, and bruits.
From ref. 2.
HSR, Harvard Stroke Registry; MRSR, Michael Reese Stroke Registry; ICH, intracerebral hemorrhage; SAH, subarachnoid hemorrhage; MI, myocardial infarction.

population. Smoking is a powerful risk factor for the presence of extracranial atherosclerosis. When combined with the use of oral contraceptives in women, smoking predisposes to subarachnoid hemorrhage and an unusual form of proximal extracranial occlusive disease that mimics Takayasu's, as well as to intracranial occlusive disease that sometimes mimics the moyamoya syndrome (13).

Not only the presence but also the *severity* of a risk factor should be considered. For example, very severe hypertension loads heavily on intracerebral hemorrhage. A patient who has very severe coronary and peripheral vascular occlusive disease has a very high likelihood of also having extracranial cerebrovascular disease. Although the use of Coumadin or other anticoagulants does load on intracranial hemorrhage (ICH), many patients take Coumadin because of atherosclerotic coronary or cerebrovascular occlusive lesions. However, the use of Coumadin plus an abnormally prolonged prothrombin time or a very high international normalized ratio (INR) would load very heavily on the diagnosis of intracranial hemorrhage. Anticoagulant-related ICH is especially important therapeutically because the condition must be treated quickly and aggressively due to the fact that bleeding often continues unless anticoagulation is reversed. Some diagnoses are very important to consider not because of the high probability of their occurrence but because of their impact on potential therapy. It is very important not to miss a treatable condition. Missing the diagnosis of a disorder that has no treatment is a far less important error.

PRIOR TRANSIENT ISCHEMIC ATTACKS AND STROKES

The presence of prior transient ischemic attacks is of great importance in the diagnosis of stroke mechanism. TIAs, especially if repeated and in the same vascular territory, indicate a local thrombo-occlusive process in the artery leading to the area of ischemia/infarction. Recent strokes leaving a neurologic deficit have the same significance as TIAs. The separation of brain ischemia by tempo into TIAs, reversible ischemic neurologic deficits (RINDs), and so-called completed strokes is arbitrary and practically useless. TIAs are common in both large artery extracranial and intracranial atherosclerosis and in penetrating artery disease, but the patterns and frequency are different. In large artery lesions, eg, carotid artery disease, spells are often varied and not stereotyped and may occur over a long duration (months). TIAs are somewhat less common in patients with penetrating artery disease–related ischemia, are stereotyped (always the same in different attacks), and usually occur during a period of hours or days. TIAs that represent ischemia in different vascular territories usually indicate cardiac origin embolism. TIAs consisting of focal neurologic brain dysfunction are never indicative of subarachnoid or intracerebral hemorrhage although warning leaks in the form of headaches do precede subarachnoid hemorrhage in a significant number of patients.

It is worth reemphasizing that a history of TIAs is not always easy to obtain. Several tactics can be suggested: (a) Inquire about *specific symptoms*. Have you ever had temporary trouble talking, walking, with your vision, in your hands, arms, legs, or one side of the body, or a temporary limp, etc.? First, clinicians should think of symptoms that would be likely in the vascular territory suspected of harboring the index event. For example, in the patient with transient right hand weakness and numbness, if the location was in the left cerebral hemisphere then aphasia, right visual field neglect, difficulty in reading and/or writing, and left monocular blindness might be associated. Inquire about these symptoms first. If the process were in the left brainstem, then vertigo, diplopia, left facial numbness or burning, gait ataxia, and left body symptoms and signs might be associated. Ask about these symptoms next. (b) Do not limit the inquiry to the time of the initial history taking; *ask and ask again* later. Patients are often sick, frightened, tired, distracted, and sometimes aphasic and amnestic initially. I have had the personal experience of obtaining a positive response with details from a patient who denied having TIAs the first three times that I asked. (c) Be sure to *ask other observers* if they know of any temporary spells. Sometimes patients are not aware of transient attacks or cannot characterize them well. Family members and significant others can sometimes provide useful accounts of spells that they witnessed. Sometimes the patient has told them of attacks and the patient can no longer recall or describe the spells to the physician at the time of questioning.

ONSET AND CLINICAL COURSE

The activity that the patient was engaging in at the onset of neurologic symptoms is less helpful than once thought. It was formerly posited that ischemia usually developed during the night while patients slept and the circulation was more sluggish, and those hemorrhages often occurred during vigorous physical activity. More recent studies show that stroke most often occurs in the morning after rising (16–18) and that the great majority of strokes of all kinds occur during ordinary activities of daily living. Occurrence during vigorous physical activity such as sports, running, or sex is very unusual in ischemic strokes and TIAs, although migrainous accompaniments that can mimic atherosclerotic-related ischemia do occur under those circumstances. Onset during sex, straining, or severe emotional duress (19,20) favors the diagnosis of hemorrhage, either subarachnoid or intracerebral. In the Michael Reese Stroke Registry only 10% of cases of ICH and 15% of cases of SAH occurred during stress (2,12). Some patients have their hemorrhages in the night presumably during sleep. Most hemorrhages develop during ordinary nonstressful activities. At times a sudden sneeze or cough, rising quickly after bending down, and rising at night to go to the bathroom (a matudinal embolus) precipitates brain embolism. Onset of stroke after a physical altercation, vigorous sports, or a motor vehicle accident suggests the possibility of traumatic vascular occlusion and arterial dissection. Onset of stroke during pregnancy and the puerperium should raise suspicion of venous dural sinus thrombosis as the mechanism of brain ischemia.

Characterization of the early course of symptoms and their later evolution is the single most important historical item. Each of the stroke mechanisms tabulated in Fig. 1 has its own characteristic course of illness and evolution. In *SAH*, the onset is instantaneous and always with headache often accompanied by a cessation of activity and vomiting. Focal neurologic symptoms are unusual at onset. *ICH* usually begins with parenchymatous symptoms depending on the area of brain into which the initial bleeding occurs. Then usually the bleeding increases gradually over minutes and the patient develops increasing neurologic signs. If the hematoma attains a large enough size, the mass effect increases pressure locally causing displacement of tissues and increases intracranial pressure. The pressure changes lead to headache, decrease in the level of consciousness, and vomiting [20]. Some patients with ICH are as bad as they will get when initially seen and the patient cannot provide an account of how the deficit developed.

In patients with *brain embolism*, irrespective of whether the source is from a cardiac, aortic, or proximal arterial site, the onset of neurologic symptoms is usually abrupt and is described as maximal at or shortly after onset. The embolus acutely blocks an intracranial artery explaining the sudden onset of neurologic symptoms. After onset, the patient's symptoms and signs may stabilize or improve. If the embolus moves distally blocking an important branch, then a stepwise increase in the deficit may occur. About 20% of patients with brain embolism have a stepwise increase in signs usually within the first 24–48 hours [21]. Another finding typical for embolism is the sudden clearing of a very severe neurologic deficit—so-called spectacular shrinking deficit [22].

Brain ischemia caused by a large artery or penetrating artery occlusive lesion with hypoperfusion is characterized by changing and fluctuating clinical symptoms. The situation is quite dynamic. Thrombi form and propagate and embolize but at the same time emboli pass and collateral circulation develops allowing reperfusion of ischemic zones with improvement in function. The clinical course may consist of transient attacks, stepwise, stuttering, or gradually increasing deficits, and fluctuations between normal and abnormal functioning. A sudden embolus in these patients arising from an atherosclerotic lesion can lead to a sudden onset or increase in focal neurologic signs.

The course of illness in patients with the various different stroke mechanisms is often characteristic. I encourage residents, fellows, and those physicians not experienced in the care of stroke patients to learn the importance of the clinical course by constructing a course-of-illness graph [1,23] in each stroke patient whom they see. Figure 2 shows examples of such graphs. The physician must obtain sufficient information at various points in time after the stroke onset in order to draw the graph. Unfortunately, obtaining information about the early development of the deficit is often diffi-

cult. Patients are inexperienced with neurologic signs and frequently do not test their own function. Patients often recognize that they have a problem only when they are involved in an activity that utilizes an impaired brain function. For instance, suppose a patient developed right-sided body numbness at about 9 a.m. At 10 a.m. he tried to read the newspaper and found that he could not see to the right and could not read. However, he could write, and continued to speak and understand spoken language well. Did the visual field abnormality and dyslexia begin at stroke onset or instead did it develop at 10 a.m. when he first looked at the newspaper? Sometimes it is difficult to tell.

Because patients cannot on their own tell you of the early course, I suggest a technique that I call walking through the events. I ask the patient to describe in detail their activities before and after the symptoms began. Usually the clinician must interrupt often to get the patient to describe in more detail the activities, what they entailed, and how they were performed. A recent example of this type of description was provided by a patient who developed right hand weakness while having breakfast tea. She tried to call her daughter. She walked to the phone, which was upstairs, and noticed no difficulty walking up the stairs. She was able to find the number in her address book and dial the number correctly with her left hand. She was able to converse normally and could clearly understand what her daughter was saying. She lay down on the bed to wait for her daughter to come; before lying down she washed her hands in the sink and was very surprised that she could now use the right hand normally. She took a brief nap and when she awakened to answer the door, she limped as she navigated the stairs and her right hand and arm were now quite weak and her voice was slurred. She had no headache, vomiting, or decrease in consciousness. This course of illness, with improvement and return to normal and then later worsening, is characteristic for brain ischemia related to an occlusive lesion. Brain embolism could also explain this course but would be less likely. The absence of headache or vomiting is inconsistent with SAH. Rapid improvement after a few minutes excludes ICH. By reviewing the minute-by-minute events and activities, the alert clinician can better judge the patient's deficits as they progressed over time. The information can then be conveyed visually by a course-of-illness graph, which is often more effective than verbal descriptions. "Stepwise" could mean one, two, or multiple steps that could vary in size (some large, some small) and time (eg, a short time before the second step and a longer time before the third). These features can readily be shown graphically. Different types of graphs can be used to display various features. Graphs 3a and 3b display the time course of a single deficit whereas graphs 3c and 3d display multiple deficits in 3c acquired sequentially and in 3d concurrently. The time element can be varied to show the course over minutes (graph 3a), days (graphs 3b and 3d), or weeks (graph 3c). When experienced stroke clinicians are shown a course-of-illness graph of a stroke patient they can usually pinpoint the stroke mechanism with a high degree of accuracy.

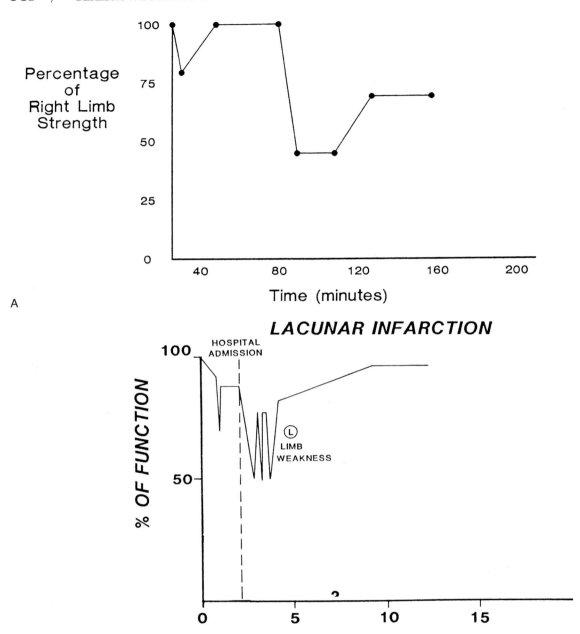

FIG. 2. Various course of illness graphs. **A:** Percentage of right limb strength is graphed during the first 3 hours after symptom onset in a patient with a left carotid artery occlusion. **B:** The severity of left limb weakness is graphed during the first 10 days after stroke onset in a patient with a capsular lacunar infarct.

OTHER SYMPTOMS: HEADACHE, SEIZURES, VOMITING, AND LOSS OF CONSCIOUSNESS

The symptoms discussed so far are all related to focal neurologic dysfunction. We now turn to associated ancillary symptoms that are found in some patients with cerebrovascular disease and strokes. These symptoms also weight the probabilities of different stroke mechanisms.

Headaches unusual for the patient may precede, accompany, or follow the onset of neurologic symptoms (2,24). Preceding headaches if of abrupt onset with high severity at onset may represent warning leaks in patients with SAH. These headaches are isolated, infrequent events, not daily headaches. Patients with large artery occlusive disease may also have unusual headaches that precede the occurrence of brain ischemic symptoms. These headaches are posited to

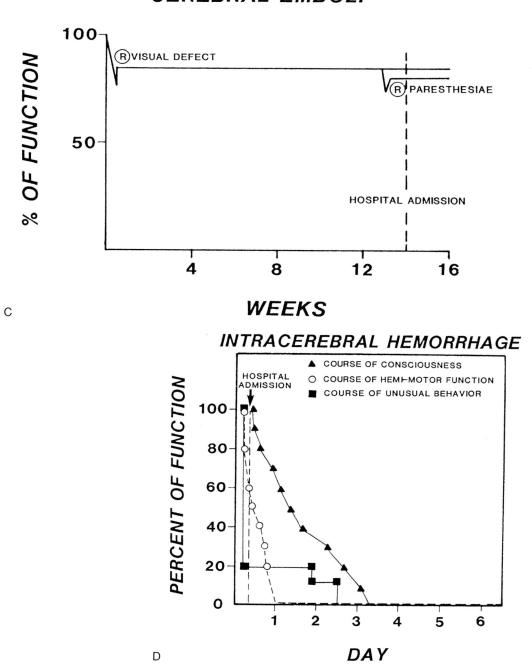

FIG. 2. *Continued.* **C:** Different neurologic abnormalities are shown during a period of weeks in a patient with cardiogenic brain embolism, first to the left occipital lobe, then to the left parietal region. Computed tomography showed embolic infarcts in three different vascular territories. **D:** Three different neurologic abnormalities are graphed over the first 3-1/2 days of hospitalization in a patient with a large right frontal lobe basal ganglionic hemorrhage.

result from vascular distention of collateral arteries. Some patients with hypertensive ICH have headaches, presumably related to hypertension, that precede their strokes. Brain embolism is not associated with premonitory headaches.

Headache at onset of stroke is invariable in patients with

SAH, and is common in patients with ICH in which it usually follows the onset of neurologic symptoms. Headache at onset is variable in patients with brain ischemia and relates to collateral artery dilatation and the presence of brain swelling. Data from the Michael Reese and University of Illinois

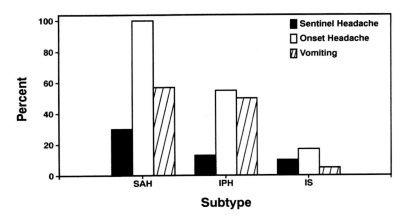

FIG. 3. Graph of frequencies of sentinel and onset headache and vomiting in the Michael Reese and University of Illinois Stroke Registries. (From ref. 24.)

Legend: SAH Subarachnoid
IPH Interparenchymal
IS Brain Ischemia

Stroke Registries show the relative frequency of warning and onset headaches (Fig. 3) (24). Headache may develop days after the stroke onset and occurs especially in patients who develop brain swelling. Large embolic and thrombotic brain infarcts and hematomas are the usual cause of delayed onset headaches.

Vomiting is a very important accompanying symptom. Vomiting is common in patients with posterior circulation vascular events irrespective of stroke mechanism. Vomiting is related to involvement of the vestibular system and its connections or distortion of the putative vomiting center in the floor of the fourth ventricle. Vomiting may also result from increased mass effect and is found in patients with cerebellar hemorrhages and infarcts. In contrast, vomiting is quite rare in patients with anterior circulation ischemia. In the Harvard Stroke Registry, vomiting occurred in only 2% of patients with anterior circulation embolism and in situ occlusive disease but was present in nearly half of the patients with anterior circulation distribution ICH (2,5). The combination of anterior circulation neurologic symptoms and vomiting is very strongly predictive of the presence of a hematoma. Vomiting is even more common at onset in patients with SAH and is explained by the sudden increase in intracranial pressure related to sudden influx of blood under arterial pressure into the subarachnoid space.

Loss of consciousness is common at onset in patients with large SAHs and develops after other neurologic signs in patients with large hematomas. Loss of consciousness is less common in patients with brain ischemia. When the ischemia involves the anterior circulation, loss of consciousness indicates a very large infarct with herniation. The decreased level of consciousness occurs in this situation 24–72 hours after stroke onset and only in patients with severe hemiplegia and other evidence of extensive cerebral hemisphere involvement. Decreased levels of consciousness are often found in patients with basilar artery occlusion causing bilateral pontine tegmental ischemia and in patients with pontine hemorrhages.

Seizures near stroke onset are most often found in patients with subcortical slit lobar hemorrhages and in patients with embolism to the cerebrum. Seizures are very rare at onset in patients with non-embolic brain ischemia. I believe that seizures are also rare in patients with SAH. The sudden influx of blood into the cranium causes abnormal motor behavior and postures that are often misinterpreted as seizures. Seizures are also very rare in patients with brainstem and cerebellar lesions.

Note that in this section interpretation of the diagnostic importance of one symptom, eg, headache and vomiting, is often aided by grouping data, eg, vomiting and stroke location. Vomiting has different diagnostic significance depending on whether the stroke involves the anterior or posterior circulation. Similarly, in patients with unaccustomed nearly daily moderately severe headache that is unusual for them without neurologic symptoms, the coexistence of hypertension is very important. Normotensive patients with warning headaches usually have an extracranial occlusive vascular lesion. In hypertensive patients, control of the blood pressure might alleviate headache and prevent the development of ICH.

HISTORY TAKING IS AN ART

With instruction, practice, and experience history taking can be learned and perfected. In patients with cerebrovascular disease the history often provides data that are not readily obtainable by other means. Although CT may be able to readily separate ischemic from hemorrhagic lesions and SAH from ICH, it often does not yield useful information about the cause of ischemia. Listen to your patients. They are trying to tell you their diagnosis if you will let them and if you know how to extract the information and to separate the chaff from the wheat.

REFERENCES

1. Caplan LR. *The Effective Clinical Neurologist.* Boston: Blackwell, 1990.
2. Caplan LR. *Stroke: A Clinical Approach.* 2nd ed. Boston: Butterworth-Heinemann, 1993.
3. Bayes T. An essay towards solving a problem in the doctrine of chances. *Phil Trans Roy Soc London* 1763;53:270–418. Reprinted in *Biometrika* 1935;45:296–315.
4. Winkler RL. *Introduction to Bayesian: Inference and Decision.* New York: Holt, Rinehart and Winston, 1972.
5. Mohr JP, Caplan LR, Melski J, et al. The Harvard Cooperative Stroke Registry: a prospective registry. *Neurology* 1978;28:754–762.
6. Caplan LR. *Brain Ischemia: Basic Concepts and Clinical Relevance.* London: Springer-Verlag, 1995;338–368.
7. Bogousslavsky J, Van Melle G, Regli F. The Lausanne Stroke Registry: analysis of 1000 consecutive patients with first stroke. *Stroke* 1988;19:1083–1092.
8. Foulkes MA, Wolf PA, Price TR, et al. The Stroke Data Bank: design, methods, and baseline characteristics. *Stroke* 1988;19:547–554.
9. Caplan LR, Gorelick PB, Hier DB. Race, sex, and occlusive vascular disease: a review. *Stroke* 1986;17:648–655.
10. Broderick JP, Brott T, Tomsick T et al. The risk of subarachnoid and intracerebral hemorrhage in blacks as compared to whites. *N Engl J Med* 1992;326:733–736.
11. Feldmann E, Daneault N, Kwan E, et al. Chinese–white differences in the distribution of cerebrovascular disease. *Neurology* 1990;40:1541–1545.
12. Caplan LR, Hier DB, D'Cruz I. Cerebral embolism in the Michael Reese Stroke Registry. *Stroke* 1983;14:530–536.
13. Levine SR, Fagan SC, Pessin MS, et al. Accelerated intracranial occlusive disease, oral contraceptives and cigarette use. *Neurology* 1991;41:1893–1901.
14. Caplan LR. TIAs: we need to return to the question, what is wrong with Mr Jones? *Neurology* 1988;38:791–793.
15. Caplan LR. Terms describing brain ischemia by tempo are no longer useful. A polemic (with apologies to Shakespeare). *Surg Neurol* 1993;40:91–95.
16. Marler J, Price TR, Clark GL, et al. Morning increase in onset of ischemic stroke. *Stroke* 1989;20:473–476.
17. Sloan M, Price TR, Foulkes MA, et al. Circadian rhythmicity of stroke onset: intracerebral and subarachnoid hemorrhage. *Ann Neurol* 1990;28:226–227.
18. Kelly-Hayes M, Wolf PA, Kase CS, et al. Temporal patterns of stroke onset. The Framingham study. *Stroke* 1995;26:1343–1347.
19. Caplan LR. Intracerebral hemorrhage revisited. *Neurology* 1988;38:624–627.
20. Kase CS, Caplan LR. *Intracerebral Hemorrhage.* Boston: Butterworth, 1994.
21. Caplan LR. Clinical diagnosis of brain embolism. *Cerebrovasc Dis* 1995;5:79–88.
22. Minematsu K, Yamaguchi T, Omae T. Spectacular shrinking deficit: rapid recovery from a major hemispheric syndrome by migration of an embolus. *Neurology* 1992;42:157–162.
23. Caplan LR. Course-of-illness graphs. *Hosp Pract* 1985;20:125–136.
24. Gorelick PB, Hier DB, Caplan LR. Headache in acute cerebrovascular disease. *Neurology* 1986;36:1445–1450.

Cerebrovascular Disease, edited by H. Hunt Batjer.
Lippincott-Raven Publishers, Philadelphia © 1997.

CHAPTER 14

The Neurologic Examination

Jorge Moncayo and Julien Bogousslavsky

Detailed clinical descriptions and clinicopathologic correlations of ischemic or hemorrhagic cerebral lesions were made mainly in the late 19th century and in the first half of the 20th century. Nevertheless, the neurologic examination of a patient with stroke is of fundamental importance in order to establish its topography and etiology and to initiate treatment. Also, the initial examination provides a clinical baseline, which is extremely useful when following the patient during the acute phase of stroke.

GENERAL ORIENTATION

The diagnosis of cerebral infarction is supported by the presence of previous transient ischemic attacks (TIAs), associated cardiovascular disease, and a neurologic deficit that is immediately or rapidly stabilized after onset. On the other hand, the presence of headache, vomiting, neck rigidity, decreased level of consciousness (somnolence or coma), seizures, and progressive onset of neurologic deficits supports the diagnosis of intracerebral hemorrhage. Large artery disease may be present if there is a history of previous TIAs or transient monocular blindness (TMB) in the same territory and an immediately complete neurologic deficit. Cardiac embolism may be suspected with a history of previous TIAs or infarcts in different arterial territories, abrupt onset, loss of consciousness at the onset, and an isolated branch artery syndrome. Lacunar infarct should be considered in an elderly patient with longstanding hypertension with proportional faciobrachiocrural hemiparesis, hemihypesthesia, or both as well as in the presence of dysarthria clumsy-hand syndrome, and ataxic hemiparesis (lacunar syndromes) without cognitive disturbances (except in the case of thalamic infarcts).

However, none of these criteria is absolute; eg, 8% of patients with cerebral hemorrhage report previous TIAs. A small deep hemorrhage may sometimes lead to pure motor hemiplegia or other lacunar syndromes. In clinical practice,

J. Moncayo and J. Bogousslavsky: Department of Neurology, Centre Hospitalier Universitaire Vaudois, Lausanne, Switzerland.

we have found that brain hemorrhage should be suspected when the neurologic picture does not fit the well-established vascular syndromes, suggesting that the underlying process may pass the boundaries of the usual arterial territories.

INITIAL EXAMINATION

In a patient with stroke, the initial basic clinical examination at the emergency room includes vital signs, level of consciousness, and ophthalmoscopic examination of the retina and optic disc, visual fields, pupils, and eye movements. Also, motor function including muscle tone, muscle strength, and sensory function including initially light touch, pinprick, position sense, stereognosis, and graphesthesia should be systematically tested when feasible. Cerebellar function, meningeal signs, gait, and observation of involuntary movements complete the initial examination. Higher cerebral functions and language function can be tested during this evaluation.

Vital Functions

High *blood pressure* values with a spontaneous decline pattern in the 2 weeks following stroke are found in patients with acute ischemic or hemorrhagic lesions, including those without a history of previous hypertension. *Respiratory function* can also be influenced by stroke: hemispheric strokes can produce contralateral reduced wall chest movements, reduced diaphragmatic excursion, or Cheyne–Stokes rhythm. Apneustic respiration occurs in patients with severe pontine lesions. Infrequently, lesions in the upper part of the pontine corticospinal tract produce loss of ability to alter voluntarily the breathing in the presence of preserved autonomic respiratory function (1). Central hypoventilation involving automatic and voluntary respiration may occur in lesions involving the nucleus ambiguus and the nucleus tractus solitarius. Loss of automatic respiration (Ondine's syndrome) and obstructive and mixed sleep apnea syndromes are observed in unilateral lateral medullary infarcts. *Dyspnea* is an unusual finding in stroke except when it is secondary to cardiac or pulmonary dysfunction. Periodic laryngeal dyspnea with alternating extreme abduction-adduction of the vocal cords and subsequent upper airway obstruction has been reported in bilateral opercular lesions (2). *Secondary cardiac dysrhythmia* including transient atrial fibrillation is found in over 5% of patients during the first hours following stroke. It is found mainly with parietoinsular and caudal brainstem lesions involving nuclei with arrhythmogenic capacity. *Fever* is rare in stroke and is occasionally related to brainstem lesions. More commonly, it indicates intercurrent infection. Noninfectious excessive sweating is found in ischemic or hemorrhagic brainstem lesions. *Transient unilateral hyperhidrosis* limited to the contralateral upper face, shoulder, or arm without other signs of autonomic dysfunction may occur in large infarcts of the middle cerebral artery (MCA) territory and in small infarcts of the frontal operculum (3), whereas *ipsilateral hypohidrosis* may occur in pontine and medullary infarctions (4). Focal areas of *decreased skin temperature* on the hemiparetic side are found in 5% of patients with large cortical, capsular, and pontine infarcts (5).

Visual Fields

Visual field deficits caused by stroke may be detected or at least suspected during the initial clinical examination. The optic tract and the temporal optic radiations (Meyer's loop) are involved in lesions of the choroidal anterior artery. The parietal lobe and the occipital cortex are involved in lesions of the MCA and posterior cerebral artery, respectively. Alterations of the visual field are summarized in Table 1.

Interestingly, the lateral geniculate nucleus (LGN) has an anatomic-vascular pattern that deserves particular attention. Actually, it is unique in that its supply comes from both the anterior (anterior choroidal artery) and posterior (posterior choroidal artery) circulation systems. Congruent and incongruent *homonymous horizontal sectoranopia* (HHS) may be observed in posterior choroidal artery infarction when this artery supplies the central part of the LGN (6). However, incongruent double *homonymous quadrantanopsia* may also occur in infarcts of the posterior choroidal artery territory. Moreover, *quadruple sectoranopia* with sparing of the horizontal meridian can be found with anterior choroidal artery territory infarction (7). Congruent *paracentral homonymous hemianopia* (homonymous paracentral scotoma) is observed in infarcts of the terminal territory of the lateral branch of the posterior choroidal artery, with damage being limited to a particular lamina of the LGN. A sectorial optic atrophy may subsequently develop.

Pupils

Asymmetric pupils may be due to oculomotor nerve or sympathetic involvement. Unilateral miosis with Horner's

TABLE 1. *Visual field deficits in stroke*

Topography	Visual field deficit
Optic chiasm	Bitemporal hernianopia (rarely)
Optic tract	Complete or incomplete contralateral incongruent HH
	Congruent paracentral HH
	Homonymous horizontal sectoranopia (HHS)
LGN	Congruent or incongruent HHS
	Incongruent HH with uni- or bilateral macular sparing
	Quadruple sectoranopia
	Incongruent double homonymous quadrantonopia
	Congruent paracentral HH
Optic radiation:	
Temporal loop	Incongruent contralateral HH or superior quadrantonopia
Parietal loop	Contralateral HH with macular sparing
	Complete inferior homonymous quadrantonopia (rarely)
Occipital cortex:	
Unilateral lesion	Congruent HH paracentral scotoma
	Unilateral altitudinal hemianopia
Anterior tip	Contralateral loss of temporal crescent
Posterior calcarine	Contralateral congruent HH with either macular sparing and contralateral temporal crescent
Tip of occipital lobe	Contralateral congruent HH scotoma
Bilateral lesions	HHS
	Upper or lower bilateral altitudinal hemianopia

HH, homonymous hemianopia; HHS, homonymous horizontal sectoranopia; LGN, lateral geniculate nucleus.

syndrome may be found in extensive MCA, hypothalamic, and brainstem infarctions. Bilateral miosis with preservation of the light reflex is observed in pontine lesions. Bilateral mydriasis is observed in mesencephalic infarction or hematoma. A loss of the pupillary reflex with preservation of the accommodation reflex is observed in pretectal infarcts. Rarely, corectopic pupils may be observed with mesencephalic infarction.

Eye Movements

Conjugate eye deviation (CED) toward the lesion is found in approximately 20% of patients with cerebral hemispheral stroke, especially on the right side. *Contralateral eye deviation* ("wrong way eyes") rarely occurs and is most common with thalamic hemorrhage. It is observed least often in patients with subcortical frontoparietal and lenticular hemorrhage (8). In infratentorial lesions, a *contralateral CED* (the patient looks at his or her hemiplegia) may be found in unilateral lesions of the pontine paramedian reticular formation (PPRF); however, it is more common in supratentorial lesions. Tonic CED ipsilateral to the affected side is noted in patients with lateral medullary infarct (ocular lateropulsion of Barré) and cerebellar hemispheral stroke.

Contralateral saccades and smooth pursuit movements are reduced during the acute phase of frontal or parietal stroke. *Slowing of ipsilateral saccadic movements* is seen in patients with partial lesions of the paramedian pontine reticular formation (PPRF). If the sixth nerve nucleus is involved, ipsilateral reflex movements are also lost. *Slow or absent vertical saccadic movements* are found in patients with lesions involving the rostral interstitial nucleus of the medial longitudinal fasciculus (riMLF). Simultaneous involvement of the interstitial nucleus of Cajal produces loss of the vertical oculocephalic reflex.

Ipsilateral hypermetric horizontal saccadic movements with hypometric saccades toward the contralateral side of the lesion are found in patients with lateral medullary infarct. Involvement of the climbing fibers (olivocerebellar pathway) with subsequent increased inhibition over the saccadic burst generator in the brainstem may be responsible. Moreover, impairment of *contralateral smooth pursuit movements* with normal pursuit movements towards the side of the lesion may be observed in these patients. *Microsaccadic eye movements* may be superimposed to horizontal pursuit movements (cogwheel pursuit) in patients with infarcts in the posterior inferior cerebellar artery (PICA) territory. *Contralateral hypermetric saccadic movements* with concomitant hypometria of the ipsilateral saccades is found in cerebellar infarction of the superior cerebellar artery (SCA) territory.

Fascicular *third-nerve palsy* from midbrain infarct may occur in isolation (Achard–Lévi syndrome) but also with contralateral hemiparesis (Weber's syndrome), contralateral hemiataxia (Claude's syndrome), and contralateral tremor (Benedikt's syndrome). However, lesions involving the oculomotor complex nucleus and related structures lead to other eye movement abnormalities (Table 2). Rarely, isolated bilateral ptosis by restricted lesions involving the central caudal nuclear complex are observed.

Monocular paresis of eye elevation (double-elevator paresis) is a combined paresis of the superior rectus and inferior oblique. It is observed with lesions in the rostral mesencephalon. This finding may be ipsi- or contralateral to the lesion. *Bilateral ptosis* with paresis of elevation of the contralateral eye and unilateral internuclear ophthalmoplegia (INO) ipsilateral to the side of the lesion can be observed with paramedian lower midbrain infarction (9). Involvement of the MLF before it reaches the oculomotor nucleus, the central caudal nucleus (lid elevator), and the prenuclear fibers from the posterior commissure to the ipsilateral nucleus of the contralateral superior rectus explains this finding. A *complete vertical gaze palsy* can be found in bilateral or, less often, unilateral lesions of the riMLF, posterior commissure, and interstitial nucleus of Cajal. Selective *upgaze palsy* or *downgaze palsy* is associated with bilateral ischemic or hemorrhagic lesions involving the posterior commissure, riMLF, and periaqueductal gray matter. The *one-and-a-half vertical*

TABLE 2. *Eye movement abnormalities in stroke*

Midbrain
  Isolated third oculomotor palsy (Achard–Lévi syndrome)
  Third oculomotor palsy with contralateral hemiparesis (Weber's syndrome), contralateral hemiataxia (Claude's syndrome), contralateral tremor (Benedikt's syndrome)
  Isolated bilateral ptosis
  Bilateral ptosis with paresis of elevation of the contralateral eye and unilateral INO
  Monocular paresis of eye elevation
  Selective upgaze or downgaze palsy
  Vertical gaze palsy
  One-and-a-half vertical syndrome
  Isolated fourth-nerve palsy

Pons
  Isolated abducens palsy
  Isolated abducens and facial palsy
  Unilateral abducens and facial nerve palsy with contralateral hemiparesis (Millard–Gubler's syndrome)
  One-and-a-half horizontal syndrome
  Unilateral and bilateral internuclear ophthalmoplegia
  Ocular bobbing

syndrome is an uncommon finding in patients with thalamomesencephalic infarction. In this case, upgaze palsy and monocular downgaze palsy or downgaze palsy and monocular upgaze palsy occurs (10). Rarely, *isolated fourth-nerve palsy* may be found in patients with stroke in the midbrain tectum, usually with Horner's syndrome on the side of the lesion (11).

Unilateral sixth- and seventh-nerve palsy with contralateral hemiparesis (Millard–Gubler's syndrome) and unilateral facial palsy with paralysis of the conjugate gaze to the affected side and contralateral hemiparesis (Foville's syndrome) are unusual in brainstem stroke. On the other hand, isolated abducens palsy or selective lesions of the abducens nerve and facial genu may occur in small pontine infarcts (Table 2).

Unilateral pontine lesions involving the PPRF cause an *ipsilateral conjugate gaze palsy*, while the *one-and-a-half horizontal syndrome* (conjugate gaze palsy on one side plus INO on the other side) is observed in lesions involving the ipsilateral PPRF and MLF. *Unilateral internuclear ophthalmoplegia* (INO) and occasionally *bilateral internuclear ophthalmoplegia* are related to stroke in the pons. *Ocular bobbing* may be observed in patients with pons lesions and with brainstem compression from a cerebellar hemorrhage. However, a ''paretic ocular bobbing'' has also been found in patients with extensive pontomesencephalic ischemic or hemorrhagic lesions (12).

Nystagmus

Nystagmus occurs somewhat frequently in brainstem and cerebellum stroke. Usually it is gaze-evoked, horizontal, and uni- or multidirectional.

Spontaneous *downbeat nystagmus* may occur with caudal brainstem or cerebellar lesions. Reports of *see-saw nystagmus* with a jerk waveform in unilateral midbrain infarction with a lesion involving mainly the interstitial nucleus of Cajal is rare and even rarer in patients with lateral medullary infarction (13).

Convergence-retraction nystagmus occurs in patients with midbrain infarction involving the posterior commissure. A pattern of dissociated vertical nystagmus with or without unilateral INO is rarely found in midbrain infarction (14). Probably, a disruption of the vestibular pathway traveling in the MLF toward the trochlear nucleus and the inferior rectus subnucleus in the oculomotor complex can explain this finding.

As *downbeat nystagmus,* primary position *upbeat nystagmus* can be found with caudal brainstem lesion. It is uncommon in stroke but may be seen in patients with lateral medullary infarct, probably due to involvement of the intercalatus nucleus (15). *Positional horizontal nystagmus* and *torsion nystagmus* may also develop in patients with lateral medullary infarct.

EXAMINATION OF MOTOR FUNCTION

Hemiparesis or hemiplegia of varying severity is common in patients with stroke. Faciobrachiocrural hemiplegia is found with large or deep MCA infarction, but it can also be due to pontine or anterior choroidal artery territory infarction. When isolated it is highly suggestive of lacunar infarction involving the internal capsule or pons. *Hemiparesis with crural predominance* is found in anterior cerebral artery territory (ACA) infarction and anterior junctional infarcts and is usually associated with transcortical motor aphasia in left-sided lesions. Rarely, hemiparesis with a faciobrachial predominance may be found in ACA infarction. A predominantly *proximal paresis of the arm* with greater difficulty in elevation and abduction may be observed with lesions limited to the premotor cortex in the MCA territory or the supplementary motor area in the ACA territory (16). Infarction in the territory of the cortical branches of the MCA usually leads to *hemiparesis with faciobrachial predominance*.

An unusual pattern of motor deficit, with *bilateral proximal brachial paresis* "man-in-the-barrel"), may be seen in bilateral anterior junctional infarcts involving the precentral gyri (17). On the other hand, when junctional infarct is mainly subcortical in the white matter a pattern of *cerebral paraparesis* may occur.

Small white-matter (centrum ovale) infarct may cause hemiparesis in any possible combination, including *isolated upper limb monoparesis*.

Unilateral lower cranial nerves palsy of supranuclear origin is found in corona radiata and capsular genu infarction (18). *Bilateral lower cranial nerves palsy* with marked dysarthria and facial-pharyngeal-lingual palsy sparing the emotional movements (automatic-voluntary dissociation) is found in bilateral frontal operculum or immediately deeper lesions. On the other hand, an inverse automatic-voluntary dissociation is rarely observed in patients with unilateral lesions involving the frontal cortex (supplementary motor area), internal capsule, anterolateral thalamus, or dorsal midbrain (19). Rarely, *facial diplegia with quadriplegia* is found in patients with bilateral simultaneous infarction of the internal capsule, a picture resembling locked-in state due to extensive damage to the basal pons or medulla.

Hemiparesis is uncommon in posterior cerebral artery infarctions, but it may occur when its midbrain territory is involved. Hemiparesis is not a feature of *lateral medullary infarct.* Rarely, contralateral hemiparesis by ventral extension of the infarct develops. More rarely, ipsilateral hemiplegia by extension of the infarct into the rostral spinal cord involving the corticospinal tract after the decussation (Opalski's syndrome) rarely develops.

Ipsilateral paralysis of the tongue with contralateral brachiocrural hemiparesis sparing the face may be found in medial medullary infarction.

SENSORY ABNORMALITIES

Hemihypesthesia with crural predominance and rarely with faciobrachial predominance is found in anterior cerebral artery (ACA) territory infarction. *Hemihypesthesia with faciobrachial predominance,* usually associated with hemiparesis, is characteristic of MCA territory infarct. However, a *pseudothalamic pattern* with predominantly elementary sensory loss in the hemibody, including the trunk and reaching the midline, may be found with a lesion of the inferoanterior portion of the parietal lobe (20). In some cases, it is associated with pain asymbolia. Similarly, sensory loss with a *pseudospinal* or *pseudoradicular pattern* is rarely found in patients with parietal stroke (21,22).

Pure sensory loss is not specific for a particular topographic pattern of lesion, although it is most commonly seen with lateral thalamic infarction. It is also observed with cortical, corona radiata, internal capsule, midbrain, and pons tegmentum lesions. Pure sensory stroke especially suggests lateral thalamic infarct when the face and the upper and lower limbs are involved to the same degree. Uncommonly, pure sensory stroke may herald a severe motor deficit due to large MCA infarction (23). Partial forms of pure sensory stroke may develop with lesions of the frontoparietal cortex, corona radiata, thalamus, midbrain, and pons. Sensory loss may be restricted to the perioral, intraoral, and hand and foot structures in any possible combination (cheiro-oral, cheiro-podal, cheiro-oral-podal syndromes). Rarely, sensory loss is limited to the oral cavity bilaterally (24). *Isolated pinprick and light touch loss* limited to the contralateral face may be caused by lateral pontine or midbrain tegmentum hemorrhage. A selective involvement of the main trigeminal nucleus or descending tract of the trigeminal nerve and involvement of the trigeminal tract in the inner portion of the medial lemniscus are the proposed mechanisms (25).

EXAMINATION OF CEREBELLAR FUNCTION

Ataxia and Cerebellar Signs

Limb incoordination associated with trunk ataxia, gait ataxia, and speech disturbances may be a prominent finding in patients with cerebellar or brainstem stroke. However, ataxia restricted to the upper limb, associated or not with negative myoclonus (asterixis), may be observed in patients with parietal stroke; a cortical or pseudothalamic pattern of sensory loss may coexist but not always. Interruption of the somatosensory or kinesthetic afferent pathways to primary sensory parietal areas or an impairment of sensorimotor efferent pathways may explain this type of parietal ataxia.

Ataxia associated with motor deficit is found in patients with cortical frontal, (ACA territory), centrum semiovale (MCA territory), internal capsule, midbrain, and pons infarction (ataxic hemiparesis). Hemiataxia may involve the entire hemibody or predominate in the upper or lower limb. An interesting pattern of ipsilateral ataxia mainly restricted to the upper limb with crural paresis is typical of superficial ACA infarct in the paracentral area although it has been previously attributed to deeper lesions (26). Uncommonly, strategic lesions in the internal capsule and upper midbrain may also produce isolated hemiataxia, sparing the corticospinal tract.

Approximately one fourth of patients with thalamic lesions exhibit ataxia. Several patterns of ataxia related to thalamic lesions have been identified: hypesthetic ataxic hemiparesis (HAH), ataxic hemiparesis (AH), and hemiataxia-hypesthesia (HH). The former is the most common type. It strongly suggests a lateral thalamic infarct, more exceptionally an anterior choroidal artery territory infarct. Variants of AH include dysarthria–clumsy hand syndrome caused by contralateral pontine lesion and ataxic tetraparesis associated with pontine or bilateral capsular stroke. Tetra-ataxia with or without hemiparesis can be found in paramedian lower midbrain infarction. Occasionally, it may be the only manifestation of midbrain infarction.

Infarct limited to the territory of the lateral branch of the posterior inferior cerebellar artery (lPICA) is characterized by ipsilateral limb ataxia involving the arm and leg without dysarthria, truncal ataxia, or alteration in eye movements. Limb ataxia, with trunk ataxia, nystagmus, and dysarthria, are the prominent signs in infarct in the territory of the SCA. Rarely, isolated axial lateropulsion is the only manifestation of an infarct involving the lateral branch of SCA, and gait ataxia may be observed as the only manifestation of upper midbrain infarction.

Abnormal Movements

Abnormal movements are rarely isolated manifestation of stroke. Usually they are associated with motor or sensory deficit. Contralateral hemichorea, hemiballismus, or hemidystonia can be observed in cortical, junctional, and basal ganglia stroke. Focal dystonia and tremor, usually restricted to the upper limb, may be found in basal ganglia and brainstem stroke. Unilateral asterixis mainly occurs in thalamic infarction, although it is not specific for a particularly stroke topography. Palatal myoclonus may be observed with caudal brainstem stroke. Stereotyped motor behaviors in the head, face, trunk, and nonparalyzed upper and lower limbs may be observed in approximately 10% of patients with large infarct in the ACA and MCA territories (27).

Gait Disorders

Thalamic astasia, characterized by an inability to stand or walk despite minimal weakness or marked sensory disturbance, may be found in thalamic stroke. Usually, it is associated with marked truncal instability (28). A disruption of the vestibulocerebellar projections from the fastigial nucleus to the posterior portion of the ventrolateral nucleus has been hypothesized.

EXAMINATION OF HIGHER CEREBRAL FUNCTIONS

Cerebral strokes may lead to many neuropsychological and behavioral disturbances (Table 3). Several of them have been associated with right-sided lesions, but this probably

---

TABLE 3. *Neurobehavioral disturbances in stroke*

Frontal lobe: Grasping, alien hand, loss of bimanual coordination, compulsive manipulation of tools, unilateral left ideomotor apraxia, tactile anomia, unilateral left agraphia, left-handed mirror writing, heminegligence, dyscalculia, inverted vision, urination behavior. Korsakoff-like picture. Perseverations, response to next-patient stimulation, delusions, reduplicative paramnesia of Pick, misidentification syndromes. Limb akinetic apraxia, motor impersistence, motor persistence

Parietal lobe: Anosognosia, asomatognosia, anosodiaphoria, denial of eye closure, constructional apraxia, dressing apraxia, autotopagnosia, tactile agnosia, contralateral hemianesthesia, pain asymbolia, Gertsmann's syndrome

Temporal lobe: Pure word deafness, cortical deafness, confusion, spatial hemineglect

Occipital lobe: Blindsight, central achromatopsia, akinetopsia, denial of blindness. Color anomia, pure alexia, optic aphasia, associative visual object agnosia, prosopagnosia, visual amnesia, visual hallucinations. Hemispatial neglect, constructional apraxia, disorientation to place, lack visual content of dreams, Balint's syndrome

Basal ganglia lesions: Caudate: Echopraxia, obsessive stereotypias, checking ritual, affective disinhibition
Genu of the internal capsule: abulia, confusion, inattention, and memory loss
Pallidum (bilateral lesions): apathy, loss of self-activation

Thalamic lesions: Loss of psychic self-activation, pure amnesia, pure word deafness

reflects a bias due to language abnormalities associated with left-sided brain damage. Although the frontal lobe is affected in a large proportion of strokes, the behavioral disturbances associated with frontal stroke have been little studied (29). A similar situation occurs with right temporal or occipital lobe dysfunction. Therefore, these may be overlooked during clinical examination because they are poorly recognized.

Aphasia

Broca's aphasia occurs with damage to the territory of cortical branches of the MCA involving the inferior left frontal gyrus, the adjacent frontal areas including the underlying white matter. However, more restricted lesions in the frontal operculum (Broca's area) produce only a transient deficit with delayed initiation of grammatically correct language. Transcortical motor aphasia with proximal limb paresis is observed in lesions of the territory of the left central artery involving the frontal operculum and the underlying white matter. Conduction aphasia is usually associated with bucco-lingual apraxia, slight right-sided facial weakness, and right hemisensory disturbances in relation to an infarct in the territory of the anterior parietal artery. Wernicke's aphasia is typically due to infarct in the territory of the posterior branches of the MCA or to lobar temporal hemorrhages and may also be found in lesions involving the posterior part of the basal ganglia. Isolated Wernicke's aphasia usually occurs in infarcts in the territory of the left temporal or temporo-occipital artery. Transcortical sensory aphasia (TSA) is found in lesions immediately posterior to Wernicke's area. However, transcortical aphasia variants may be observed with unilateral thalamic lesions involving the posterior or anterior nuclei complexes. Persisting global aphasia occurs in large perisylvian infarcts or extensive lesions of the basal ganglia and overlying insula. It can also develop without hemiparesis in double separate temporal and frontal strokes sparing the central region. Global aphasia is the most common type of aphasia in the acute phase of stroke, but it evolves over a few hours to a few days toward a more specific aphasia according to the stroke topography.

Hemineglect

Lesions in the frontal lobe, parietal lobe, and thalamus may produce hemineglect. It can be restricted to one sensory modality or involve all contralateral sensory modalities. Hemineglect occurs more commonly and is more severe with right hemisphere lesions, in which case it is often accompanied by denial of illness, dressing apraxia, constructional apraxia, and motor impersistence.

Dysarthria

Lesions in the lower motor cortex produce severe dysarthria characterized at onset by a severe mutism. Usually it is associated with dysprosody, buccofacial apraxia, and mild transient paresis predominantly affecting the hand and the lower part of the face. Right frontal operculum or putamen infarction may cause severe dysarthria and sometimes resemble cerebellar dysarthria. Interruption of the cerebello-cortical connections that regulate the modulation of speech is implicated. Dysarthria with characteristics similar to those found in parkinsonian patients can occur with bilateral thalamic infarcts sparing the internal capsule. This is probably related to involvement of the pallidal projections to the thalamic ventral nuclear group (30).

Rarely, cerebellar dysarthria is an isolated finding in infarcts in the territory of the medial branch of the superior cerebellar artery (SCA). This is not observed in patients with infarcts in the territory of the lateral branch of the posterior inferior cerebellar artery (PICA).

CONCLUSIONS

A broad spectrum of neurologic signs may be found in patients with stroke. The data provided by the history and a detailed examination may allow the clinician to make a topographic and etiologic diagnosis with high accuracy. The clinical evaluation is the basis for the choice and timing of investigations as well as for the selection of initial treatment.

ACKNOWLEDGMENT

Supported by a grant from the Fonds National Suisse de la Récherche Scientifique.

REFERENCES

1. Vingerhoets F, Bogousslavsky J. Respiratory dysfunction in stroke. *Clin Chest Med* 1994;15:729–737.
2. Cambier J, Viader F, Paquelin F, Poullot B, Pariser Ph. Dyspnée laryngée périodique au cours d'un syndrome bi-operculaire. *Rev Neurol (Paris)* 1983;139:531–533.
3. Labar DR, Mohr JP, Nichols FT, Tatemichi TK. Unilateral hyperhidrosis after cerebral infarction. *Neurology* 1988;38:1679–1682.
4. Korpelainen J, Sotaniemi K, Myllylä V. Ipsilateral hypodrosis in brain stem infarction. *Stroke* 1993;24:100–104.
5. Wayne Massey E, Davis JN. Decreased skin temperature contralateral to cerebral infarction: the cold stroke syndrome. *Neurology* 1989;39(suppl 1):184.
6. Besson G, Bogousslavsky J, Regli F. Posterior choroidal-artery infarct with homonymous horizontal sectoranopia. *Cerebrovasc Dis* 1991;1:117–120.
7. Frisén L. Quadruple sectoranopia and sectorial optic atrophy syndrome of the distal anterior choroidal artey. *J Neurol Neurosurg Psychiatry* 1979; 42:590–594.
8. Tijssen CC. Contralateral conjugate eye deviation in acute supratentorial lesions. *Stroke* 1994,25:1516–1519.
9. Bogousslavsky J, Regli F, Ghika J, Hungerbühler JP. Internuclear ophthalmoplegia, prenuclear paresis of contralateral superior rectus, and bilateral ptosis. *J Neurol* 1983;230:197–203.
10. Bogousslavsky J. Syndromes oculomoteurs résultant de lésions mésencéphaliques chez l'homme. *Rev Neurol (Paris)* 1989;145:546–559.
11. Kim JS, Kang JK, Lee SA, Lee MC. Isolated or predominant ocular motor nerve palsy as a manifestation of brain stem stroke. *Stroke* 1993; 24:581–586.

12. Dehaene I, Lammens M, Marchau M. Paretic ocular bobbing. A clinico-pathological study of two cases. *Neuro-ophthalmology* 1993;13: 143–146.

13. Halmagyi GM, Aw ST, Dehaene I, Curthoys IS, Todd MJ. Jerk-waveform see-saw nystagmus due to unilateral meso-diencephalic lesion. *Brain* 1994;117:789–803.

14. Marshall R, Sacco RL, Kreuger R, Odel JG, Mohr JP. Dissociated vertical nystagmus and internuclear ophthalmoplegia from a midbrain infarction. *Arch Neurol* 1991;48:1304–1305.

15. Munro NAR, Gaymard B, Rivaud S, Majdalani A, Pierrot-Deseilligny Ch. Upbeat nystagmus in a patient with a small medullary infarct. *J Neurol Neurosurg Psychiatry* 1993;56:1126–1128.

16. Freund HJ, Hummelsheim H. Lesions of premotor cortex in man. *Brain* 1985;108:697– 733.

17. Bogousslavsky J. Sémiologie des AVC ischémiques. Syndromes artériels ischémiques cérébraux. In: Bogousslavsky J, Bousser MG, Mas JL, eds. *Accidents vasculaires cérébraux.* Paris: Doin Editeurs. 1993: 111–137.

18. Besson G, Bogousslavsky J, Regli F, Maeder P. Acute pseudobulbar or suprabulbar palsy. *Arch Neurol* 1991;48:501–507.

19. Hopf H, Müller-Forell W, Hopf NJ. Localization of emotional and volitional facial paresis. *Neurology* 1992;42:1918–1923.

20. Bassetti C, Bogousslavsky J, Regli F. Sensory syndromes in parietal stroke. *Neurology* 1993;43:1942–1949.

21. Breuer AC, Cuervo H, Selkoe DJ. Hyperpathia and sensory level due to parietal lobe arteriovenous malformation. *Arch Neurol* 1981;38: 722–724.

22. Youl BD, Adams RW, Lance JW. Parietal sensory loss simulating a peripheral lesion, documented by somatosensory evoked potentials. *Neurology* 1991;41:152–154.

23. Martin R, Bogousslavsky J, Regli F. Pure sensory stroke heralding large hemispheric infarction. *Schweiz Arch Neurol Psychiat* 1992;143: 339–342.

24. Kim JS. Restricted acral sensory syndrome following minor stroke. Further observation with special reference to differential severity of symptoms among individual digits. *Stroke* 1994;25:2497–2502.

25. Kim JS. Trigeminal sensory symptoms due to midbrain lesions. *Eur Neurol* 1993;33:218–220.

26. Bogousslavsky J, Martin R, Moulin T. Homolateral ataxia and crural paresis: a syndrome of anterior cerebral artery territory infarction. *J Neurol Neurosurg Psychiatry* 1992;55:1146–1149.

27. Ghika J, Bogousslavsky J, Van Melle G, Regli F. Hyperkinetic motor behaviors contralateral to hemiplegia in acute stroke. *Eur Neurol* 1995; 35:27–32.

28. Masdeu JC, Gorelick PB. Thalamic astasia: inability to stand after unilateral thalamic lesions. *Ann Neurol* 1988;23:596–603.

29. Bogousslavsky J. Frontal stroke syndromes. *Eur Neurol* 1994;34: 306–315.

30. Ackermann H, Ziegler W, Petersen D. Dysarthria in bilateral thalamic infarction. *J Neurol* 1993;240:357–362.

Cerebrovascular Disease, edited by H. Hunt Batjer.
Lippincott-Raven Publishers, Philadelphia © 1997.

CHAPTER 15

Computed Tomography of Cerebrovascular Disease

Michael I. Ginsburg, David P. Chason, and Dianne B. Mendelsohn

Since the introduction of the EMI scanner in 1972, computed tomography (CT) has revolutionized imaging in medicine and for a decade was the mainstay for evaluation of the central nervous system (CNS). Its innovative collection of data and image production in part paved the way for magnetic resonance imaging (MRI), a technique that in many ways supplanted CT as the premier modality to image the brain and spine. However, CT remains a versatile and effective way to evaluate cerebrovascular disease. The ability of CT to measure subtle density differences gives this technique an edge when evaluating bony anatomy, acute hemorrhage, and the presence of mineralization. Moreover, CT is cost-effective, fast, and less motion-sensitive than MRI. Furthermore, CT can be used for patients with pacemakers, non-MRI-compatible aneurysm/vascular clips, and for those in whom monitoring is essential or in emergency situations. New helical scanning techniques enable CT to provide angiographic and three-dimensional (3D) surface rendering of the intra- and extracranial vasculature for the evaluation and diagnosis of vascular lesions. Lastly, CT can be coupled with xenon inhalation to evaluate cerebral blood flow.

The purpose of this chapter is to briefly describe and present an overview of how CT can be employed in the diagnosis of cerebrovascular disease.

INFARCTION/ISCHEMIA

Although MRI is more sensitive for the detection of ischemic changes in the first 12–24 hours after clinical presentation, CT is usually the initial study performed on patients who present with an acute neurologic deficit in many institutions. Furthermore, in this acute phase CT is useful for detecting associated hemorrhage and excluding a primary

intracerebral bleed or an underlying structural lesion that can clinically mimic an infarct (1).

Infarction may be the result of arterial (occlusive or non-occlusive) or venous occlusive disease. The distribution and appearance of the infarction that may result from these etiologies varies markedly and is highly dependent on the age of the lesion as well as the availability of collateral blood supply.

Following an acute cerebral infarction, CT is often unrevealing in the first 24 hours with only approximately 60% of CT scans demonstrating an abnormality (2). The earliest CT signs are subtle, ill-defined hypodensity of the affected region with loss of the normal gray–white matter distinction. Early edema results in subtle mass effect revealed by sulcal effacement (Fig. 1). Early infarcts typically do not enhance after intravenous contrast administration. Associated high density, representing thrombus, may be seen occasionally within the artery supplying the involved territory (Fig. 2). This is most frequently seen in the middle cerebral artery (MCA) and is referred to as the "dense MCA sign." It has also been described in the basilar artery (3). Taken alone, however, this sign is unreliable as arteries may be dense from atherosclerotic mineralization. Other early manifestations include obscuration of the lentiform nucleus and loss of the insular ribbon in cases of acute middle cerebral artery infarction (4–6).

Between 24 and 48 hours the ischemic parenchyma further decreases in attenuation and mass effect peaks between days 1–5 (3). This phenomenon is largely due to cytotoxic and vasogenic edema of both the gray and white matter. During this period, the lesion becomes better marginated.

The location of a lesion may provide an indication as to its etiology. Infarctions may reside in an end-artery distribution (Fig. 3) or involve multiple vascular regions (Fig. 4). Others, however, may occur in a border zone distribution that may be in a superficial or deep location (Fig. 5) (7,8).

The administration of intravenous contrast material for

M. I. Ginsburg, D. P. Chason, and D. B. Mendelsohn: Department of Radiology, University of Texas Southwestern Medical Center at Dallas, Dallas, TX 75235.

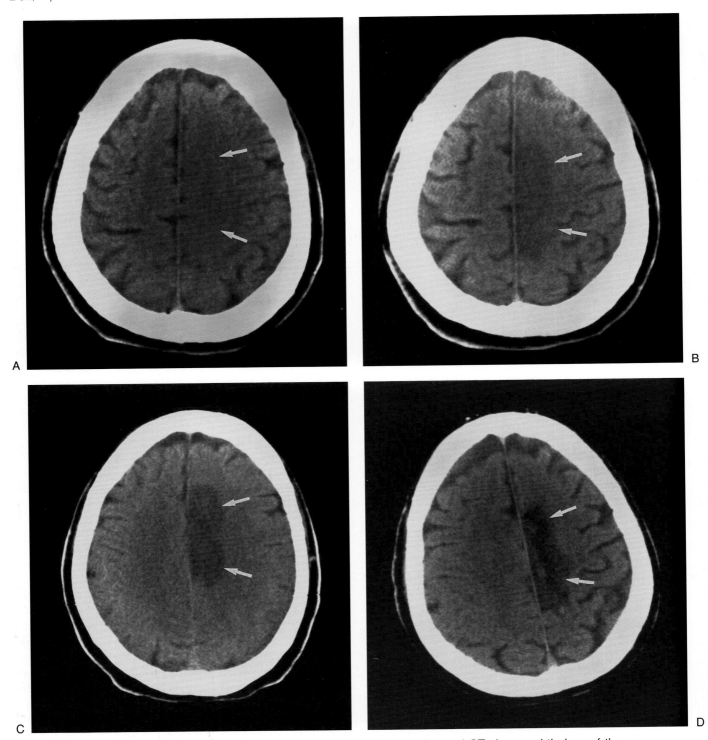

FIG. 1. Evolving anterior cerebral artery infarct. **A:** Initial nonenhanced CT shows subtle loss of the gray–white distinction in a parasagittal location *(arrows)* with early medial sulcal effacement consistent with acute infarction. **B:** Twelve hours later the region of infarction is lower in density and is better defined *(arrows)*. Follow-up scans at 3 days **(C)** and at 4 months **(D)** show progressive decrease in density of the infarcted region with volume loss and enlargement of the sulcal spaces at the convexity D, consistent with chronic infarction *(arrows)*.

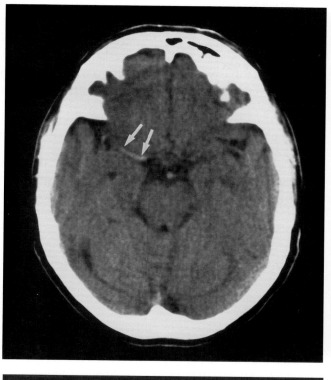

A

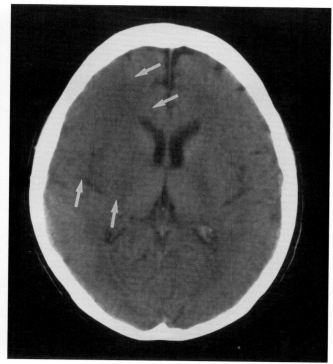

B

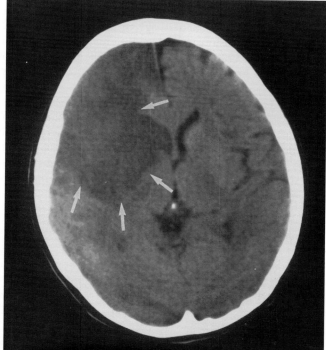

C

FIG. 2. Acute right middle cerebral artery (MCA) distribution infarct. **A:** Initial nonenhanced axial CT demonstrates the "hyperdense MCA sign" with high-density thrombus seen in the M1 segment of the middle cerebral artery *(arrows).* **B:** More cephalad image reveals low density, loss of the gray–white distinction, and sulcal effacement in the right MCA territory including the basal ganglia *(arrows).* **C:** One week later, the region of infarction has become lower in density, better defined, and demonstrates more mass effect *(arrows).*

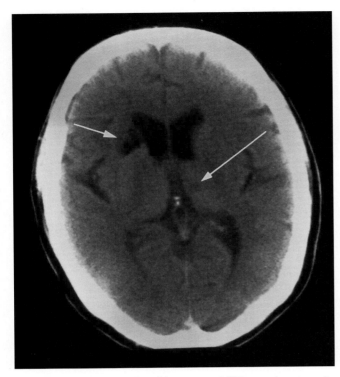

FIG. 3. Chronic infarction. Noncontrast CT reveals a remote infarct of the anterior inferior caudate head and the adjacent anterior limb of the internal capsule and putamen *(arrow)* in the distribution of the recurrent artery of Huebner. Note ex vacuo enlargement of the frontal horn and a lacunar infarct of the left thalamus *(long arrow)*.

detection of stroke is controversial (9). Unlike MRI, whereby intravascular, meningeal, and parenchymal enhancement may be seen, CT only reliably demonstrates the parenchymal form of enhancement (10). Parenchymal enhancement may have a gyriform, transcortical, wedge-shaped, or geographic appearance (9). The enhancement is maximal between 3 days and 3 weeks and should diminish by approximately 3 months (Fig. 6C, D) (11). Intravenous contrast material may be of particular value in demonstrating infarcts that have been obscured by the presence of the "fogging" effect (Fig. 6). Two to three weeks following the initial event, the region of infarction may change from its initial hypodensity on a nonenhanced study to a region of isodensity (12). A CT performed during this time could be misinterpreted as normal. Intravenous contrast administration, however, will establish the diagnosis with enhancement of the affected area. The precise mechanism of fogging on CT images is unknown. Some investigators have speculated that the CT attenuation returns to normal due to a decrease in edema that occurs during the reparative stage along with increasing attenuation secondary to the accumulation of proteinaceous material, lipid-laden macrophages, and from the diapedesis of red blood cells (13). This phenomenon of fogging has also been described by MRI (13).

Between 6 weeks and 3 months, a region of chronic infarc-

tion will further decrease in attenuation to become hypodense and well demarcated (Fig. 7). This transition is reflective of encephalomalacic change and may be associated with parenchymal volume loss and increasing prominence of adjacent cerebrospinal fluid (CSF) spaces and compensatory ventricular enlargement depending on the size and location of the infarct. Smaller peripheral or lacunar infarcts involving the basal ganglia, thalami, or brainstem, however, may not result in significant secondary changes and may only demonstrate low density.

Following chronic infarction there may be evidence of Wallerian degeneration. Though better demonstrated by MRI, low density and asymmetry of descending white matter tracts can be seen occasionally as decreased volume of the affected cerebral peduncle, pons, and medulla.

Hemorrhagic Transformation of Cerebral Infarction

The presence of hemorrhage on CT in a region of infarction is a critical factor in the management of acute stroke and affects the decision to initiate anticoagulant therapy. Hemorrhagic transformation within an infarcted area is more common in embolic-type infarcts due to reperfusion of the compromised arterial territory (Fig. 8) and with venous infarcts (14). Hemorrhagic transformation may be seen as small petechial-type hemorrhage or may be extensive and devastating, occasionally making differentiation from a primary intracerebral hematoma difficult. The latter, however, tends to be more spherical and well demarcated. Furthermore, a hypertensive hemorrhage is usually enveloped by normal brain.

CT may underdiagnose hemorrhagic transformation, particularly when lesions are small or when the hemorrhage is similar in density to brain parenchyma (15). Acute infarcts that initially enhance with high doses of contrast or on 3-hour postcontrast delayed imaging may be predictive of later hemorrhagic transformation (16).

Venous Infarction/Thrombosis

Venous infarction or cortical vein thrombosis may occur alone or in conjunction with venous sinus thrombosis, all of which may be suggested by CT scanning. Venous infarction/thrombosis may develop for a variety of reasons including hypercoagulability states (eg dehydration and oral contraceptives), pregnancy, paranasal sinus disease, sepsis, and neoplastic or infectious involvement of dural sinuses (17).

The CT findings in venous ischemia/thrombosis may be divided into the manifestations of infarction and the signs of intraluminal thrombosis. Venous, in contrast to arterial, infarctions are more often hemorrhagic and primarily affect the white matter rather than the cortex (1). Additional differentiating features are the lack of a specific arterial distribution and bilaterality (14). Patchy foci of edema and petechial hemorrhage may be seen. These infarcts are often parietal

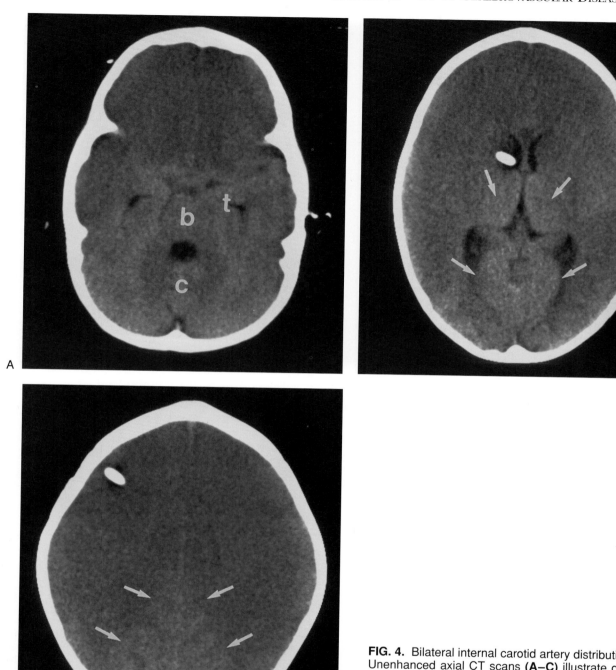

FIG. 4. Bilateral internal carotid artery distribution infarction. Unenhanced axial CT scans **(A–C)** illustrate diffuse loss of the gray–white distinction throughout the anterior and middle cerebral artery territories bilaterally. Sparing of the posterior circulation, including **(A)** the brainstem (b), cerebellum (c), and medial temporal lobes (t); and **(B)** the thalami and posterior cerebral artery (PCA) territory *(arrows)*; and **(C)** PCA territory *(arrows)*, is seen.

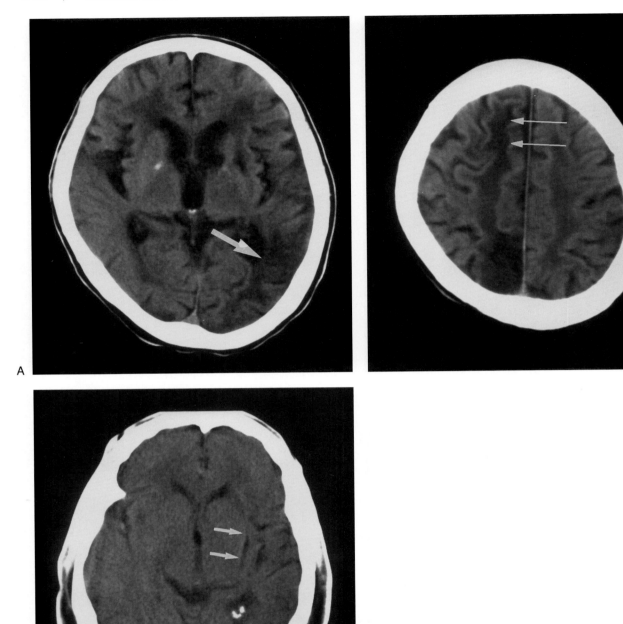

FIG. 5. Border zone infarction. Border zone infarction may occur in a superficial (leptomeningeal) location, eg, **A,** between the MCA and PCA distribution *(arrow)* or involve deeper penetrating branches, eg, **B,** between the ACA and MCA territories *(arrows).* **C:** Deep border zone infarction can occur between the lateral lenticulostriate and Sylvian branches of the MCA. This is seen lateral to the putamen and deep to the insula and is commonly mistaken for a deep MCA infarct (arrows).

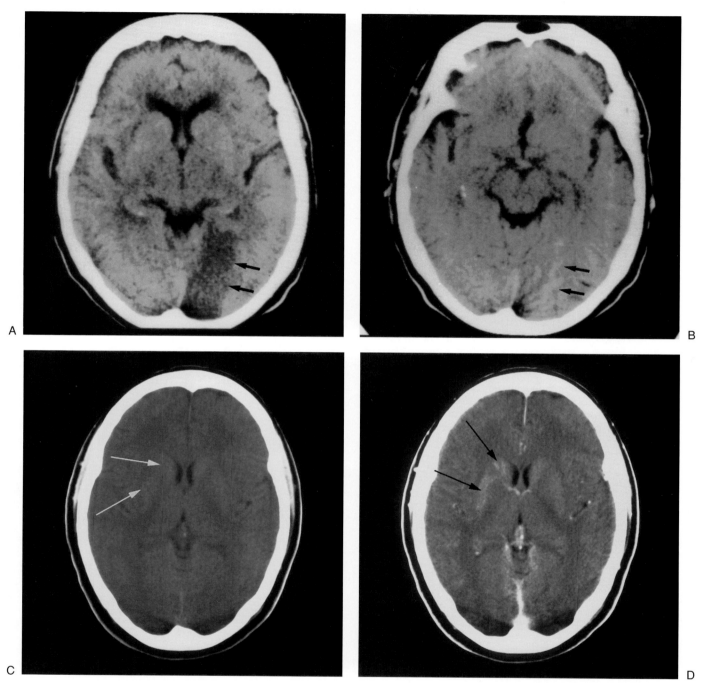

FIG. 6. "Fogging effect." **A:** Acute posterior cerebral artery distribution infarct is seen as a well-defined low-density region with loss of the gray–white junction *(arrow).* **B:** Two to three weeks later the region of infarction has become isodense giving a normal appearance *(arrow).* (Courtesy of Joseph Hise, M.D.). **C:** In a similar case, the right caudate head and putamen appear unremarkable on a noncontrast CT 2 weeks following infarction *(arrows).* The diagnosis can be made, however, following contrast infusion where there is geographic enhancement of the infarcted area **(D)** *(arrows).*

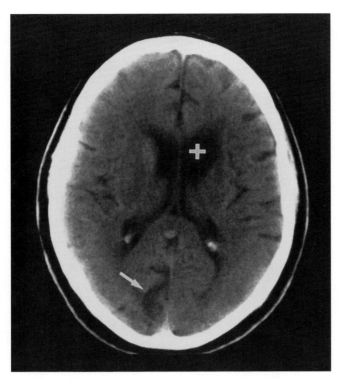

FIG. 7. Chronic infarction. Nonenhanced CT illustrates chronic infarction of the caudate head on the left with compensatory dilatation of the adjacent frontal horn (+) and in the right posterior cerebral artery distribution *(short arrow)*.

or parieto-occipital in location. CT may also demonstrate cerebral edema from venous engorgement resulting in small ventricles and sulcal effacement (18). Unusual findings such as hydrocephalus and small subdural hematomas or effusions have been described (19,20). The latter may be due to extravasated serum from bridging subdural veins.

Thrombosed cortical or deep cerebral veins may be visualized on CT as a linear region of increased density (cord sign) usually occurring with dural sinus thrombosis rather than in isolation (20). Of the dural sinuses, the superior sagittal sinus is the most commonly occluded followed by the transverse, sigmoid, and cavernous sinuses (1). Cortical and subcortical hemorrhage may be associated. On non-contrast CT, clot results in a triangular hyperdensity within the superior sagittal sinus when viewed in cross-section, referred to as the delta sign. When a contrast-enhanced CT is performed, the thrombus appears as a hypodense triangular filling defect surrounded by peripheral enhancement of the sinus dura, giving the appearance of an "empty delta" sign. Furthermore, collateral venous drainage may manifest as prominently enhancing cortical or medullary veins and result in a shaggy or thick-appearing tentorium (1).

NONTRAUMATIC INTRACRANIAL HEMORRHAGE

The list of possible etiologies leading to nontraumatic intracranial hemorrhage is lengthy. Initial CT scanning, how-

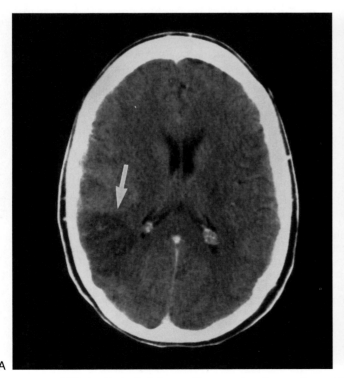

A

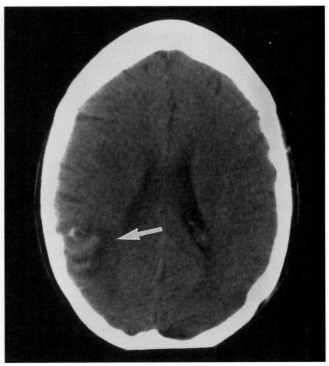

B

FIG. 8. Embolic infarct with secondary hemorrhage. Non-enhanced axial CT scans A and B demonstrate a peripheral wedge-shaped region of low density with loss of the gray–white junction (**A,** *arrow*) and high density hemorrhage (**B,** *arrow*).

ever, can often diagnose or suggest its etiology, direct early patient management, and guide further imaging studies. Clues to the underlying etiology may be provided by the anatomic compartment or location of the hemorrhage, as well as the presence or absence of mineralization, dilated vascular structures, and associated mass. The CT findings of the more common vascular processes leading to intracranial hemorrhage will be reviewed below.

Aneurysms

Approximately 85% of nontraumatic subarachnoid hemorrhage (SAH) is caused by rupture of an intracranial aneurysm (21). Most aneurysms arise from the circle of Willis and its branches. Approximately 30% of intracranial aneurysms arise from the anterior communicating artery, 25% from the posterior communicating artery, 15–20% from the middle cerebral bifurcation, 5% from the basilar apex, and 2% from the posterior inferior cerebellar artery (PICA). Aneurysms are multiple in 20–45% of patients (22–24).

Despite newly developed MRI imaging sequences capable of demonstrating acute subarachnoid blood, CT remains the modality of choice in most institutions for the initial detection of SAH (25,26).

The majority of patients who present with an acute ruptured aneurysm have SAH that is readily detected on CT by its high density relative to CSF (Fig. 9). There is a linear relationship between the CT density (Hounsfield units) of blood and the hematocrit and hemoglobin level (27). SAH in anemic states may be less conspicuous. Similarly, small volumes of SAH in a large cistern with hemodilution may be less conspicuous, particularly in the posterior fossa. Non-enhanced CT detects more than 90% of SAHs (28). After a week, 90% of subarachnoid blood has usually been cleared from the CSF and approximately only 50% of SAHs will then still be detectable by CT examination (29,30). Subarachnoid blood visualized on CT more than a week after the initial event may suggest rebleeding (29).

Sensitive locations for the CT detection of acute SAH are the cistern of the lamina terminalis and the interpeduncular cistern, as subarachnoid blood may layer in these regions with the patient in the supine position. Conversely, subarachnoid blood in the basal cisterns near the foramen magnum, close to bone of the posterior fossa, may be difficult to detect because of beam-hardening artifact.

When SAH is detected, CT may also aid in predicting the location of the offending aneurysm. The aneurysm may be located where the highest concentration of subarachnoid blood has accumulated. Associated parenchymal, ventricular, or subdural hemorrhage may also provide information in this regard.

Extension of hemorrhage into the anterior interhemispheric fissure, subcallosal and anterior cingulate gyri, septum pellucidum, or frontal horns is suggestive of a ruptured

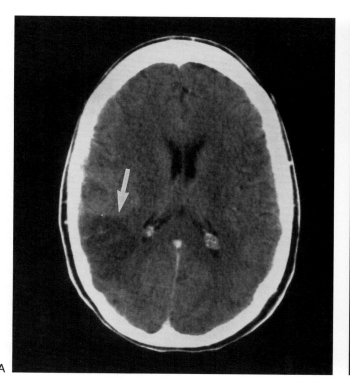
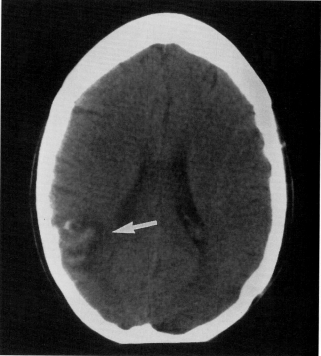

A
B

FIG. 9. Diffuse subarachnoid hemorrhage (SAH) in two patients following aneurysm rupture. **A:** Extensive SAH is present throughout the basal cisterns and Sylvian fissures. **B:** More peripheral SAH is seen with blood in the third and lateral ventricles. Example of the "zipper" sign of SAH is demonstrated (arrow).

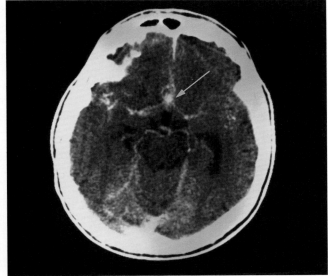

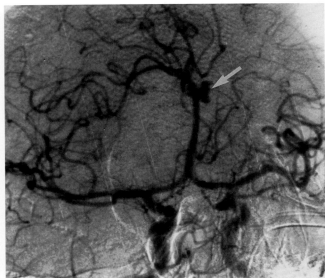

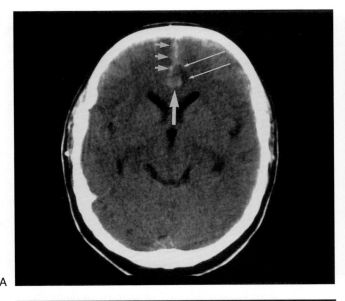

FIG. 10. Anterior cerebral artery aneurysms. **A:** Subarachnoid hemorrhage interdigitates into the pia-arachnoid space along the anterior interhemispheric fissure *(short arrows)* with a rounded density that abuts the genu of the corpus callosum *(arrow)*. Note the associated edema of the adjacent medial frontal lobe *(long arrows)*. **B:** An azygos pericallosal artery with a lobulated aneurysm *(arrow)*. **C:** Anterior communicating artery aneurysm in another patient is seen after contrast enhancement *(arrow)*.

anterior communicating artery aneurysm (Fig. 10). Subarachnoid blood within the anterior interhemispheric cistern interdigitates within the pia-arachnoid space giving a zipperlike appearance (Fig. 9B). Localized SAH in the peri-Sylvian and insular cistern is suggestive of a ruptured MCA aneurysm. Hemorrhage in the interpeduncular cistern is seen most conspicuously with basilar apex aneurysms but not exclusively as it may be associated with other aneurysms arising from the circle of Willis.

In approximately 15% of patients with SAH, no aneurysm is found on angiography (31). A large portion of these patients have a characteristic distribution of SAH in the basal cisterns referred to as "nonaneurysmal perimesencephalic hemorrhage" (31,32). Though a diagnosis of exclusion, blood is typically seen in the prepontine and interpeduncular cisterns without extension into the anterior interhemispheric fissure, lateral portion of the Sylvian cisterns or

the ventricular system (Fig. 11) (32). Interestingly, the patients in this subset of SAH usually have a less complicated clinical course and are less likely to have a rebleed (31,32).

The majority of aneurysms are not visualized by CT, even after infusion of contrast material. They are, however, occasionally seen as an incidental finding (Fig. 12). Those that are readily detectable are usually large, partially or completely thrombosed, or demonstrate peripheral calcification (Fig. 13) (33). Giant aneurysms may manifest as mass lesions with surrounding edema and peripheral enhancement, suggesting a reactive inflammatory process. Aside from the detection of subarachnoid hemorrhage, CT can also provide information useful in the initial management of an acute ruptured aneurysm, such as associated intraventricular or intraparenchymal hemorrhage, developing hydrocephalus or ischemic complications.

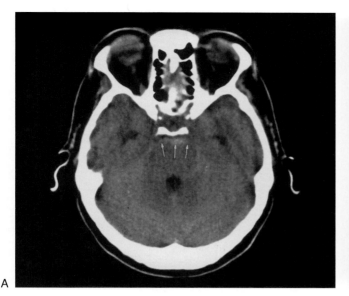
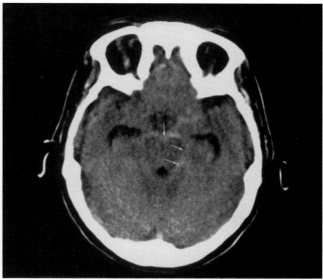

FIG. 11. Nonaneurysmal perimesencephalic hemorrhage. The typical distribution of blood includes the **(A)** prepontine *(arrows)* and **(B)** interpeduncular and ambient cisterns *(arrows)* with varying amounts in the proximal portions of the other basal cisterns.

Arteriovenous Malformation

The CT assessment for the presence of an arteriovenous malformation (AVM) can be difficult once hemorrhage has occurred. A large parenchymal hematoma, surrounding edema, mass effect, or hydrocephalus, may be present and obscure a small underlying AVM. In these cases, CT may only be capable of suggesting, and not demonstrating, the presence of the AVM.

The nonenhanced CT evaluation of a nonruptured AVM may be normal or may demonstrate enlarged feeding arteries or draining veins. The abnormal vessels, nidus, and affected brain may or may not be partially mineralized. Focal areas of hypodensity may be seen adjacent to the AVM, reflective of localized atrophy. Conversely, there may be mass effect secondary to the malformation from its nidus or feeding vessels (34,35).

Following contrast administration, there is often prominent enhancement of the nidus. The enhancement may also be serpiginous in nature, reflective of dilated vessels within the malformation. Individual feeding vessels and draining veins may be identified (Fig. 14). The presence of associated

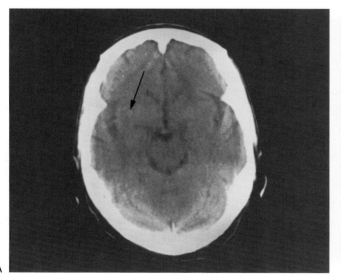
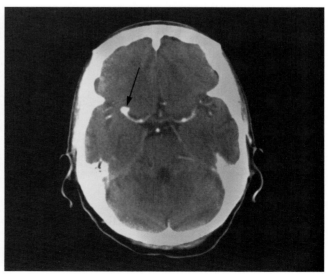

FIG. 12. Incidental aneurysm of the M1–M2 junction. **A:** Non-enhanced axial CT reveals a subtle rounded density adjacent to the Sylvian fissure *(arrow).* **B:** Following the administration of contrast the aneurysm is easily identified *(arrow).*

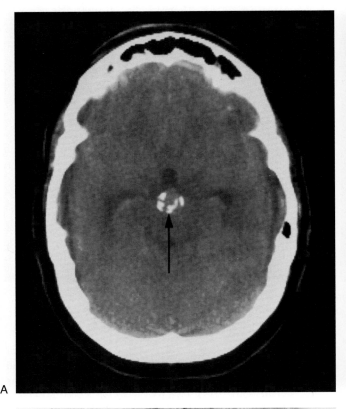

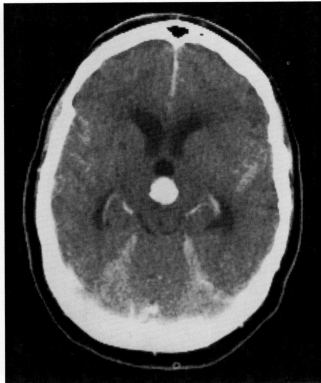

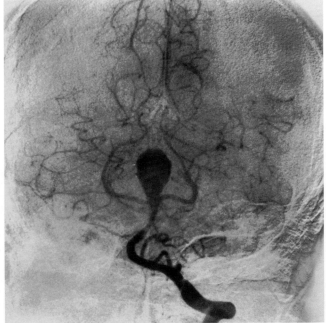

FIG. 13. Basilar tip aneurysm. **A:** Nonenhanced CT demonstrates a rounded density with peripheral mineralization impressing on the inferior third ventricle resulting in obstructive hydrocephalus *(arrow).* **B:** Dense enhancement is noted after injection of contrast. **C:** Angiogram confirms the diagnosis.

flow-related aneurysms should be sought as they predispose to hemorrhage but are seldom discovered by CT (36).

Dural Arteriovenous Malformation

Dural AVMs or dural arteriovenous (AV) fistulae (DAVFs) are arteriovenous malformations with a nidus lo-

cated within the dura. Feeding arteries are meningeal or dural and the draining structures include dural sinuses, cortical veins, or both. Dural AVFs are frequently, but not always, acquired lesions and account for 10–15% of intracranial AVMs (34). Most DAVFs are infratentorial and predominantly involve the sinuses along the base of the brain (37).

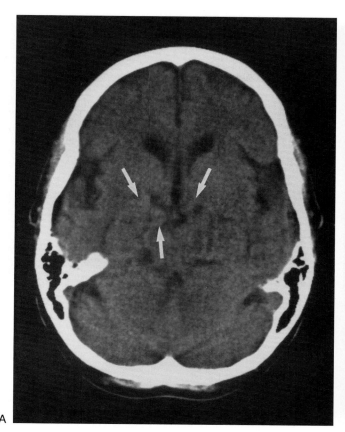
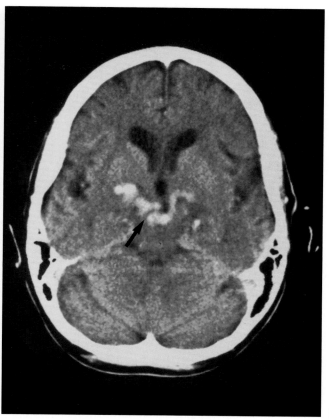

A

B

FIG. 14. Arteriovenous malformation. **A:** Noncontrast CT reveals several abnormally prominent feeding vessels in the interpeduncular cistern and proximal Sylvian fissures *(arrows)* much better illustrated with intravenous contrast **(B)** *(arrow).*

The CT examination in uncomplicated DAVF is usually non-revealing. Hemorrhage, which may be intraparenchymal or subdural, is the most common complication and may be related to sinus or venous occlusive disease (34). Venous infarction is the second most frequent complication and is probably due to venous congestion secondary to arterialization of cortical veins (34).

Venous Angioma

Venous angiomas are the most common vascular malformations seen at autopsy. They are felt to result from an accident of embryogenesis with resultant occlusion of normal medullary veins and compensatory enlargement of other medullary veins that converge toward enlarged transcerebral or transcerebellar veins (38,39). Such dilated vessels account for the stellate appearance on angiography. The most common CT manifestation of venous angioma is visualization of a linear enhancing transcerebral vein without associated parenchymal abnormality. A "caput Medusa" appearance can occasionally been seen similar to the angiographic finding (40). There is usually no evidence of edema or mass effect unless recent hemorrhage has occurred. There may be

a focus of increased attenuation in the adjacent brain on unenhanced CT (41).

Cavernous Angioma

Cavernous angiomas (cavernomas) are multilobulated sinusoidal vascular spaces lined by a single layer of epithelium and separated by fibrous septae without intervening neural tissue. They are characteristically well demarcated from adjacent parenchyma and can present with hemorrhage or seizure, often with a familial history.

On unenhanced CT, cavernomas frequently appear as oval or nodular areas of mild to moderately increased density related to the presence of calcification and/or hemosiderin (Fig. 15A). Up to one third of the lesions contain calcium (42). There is usually little or no enhancement seen after contrast is given and mass effect or edema is usually absent unless hemorrhage has occurred. If the lesion has bled, it may not be detectable; however, it may sometimes be demonstrated adjacent to the hematoma, as a small nodular enhancing lesion (43). Multiple lesions may occur in up to 33% of patients and are more common in the familial (73%) than the sporadic form (44). Lesion characterization and multiplicity are much better revealed by MRI (Fig. 15B).

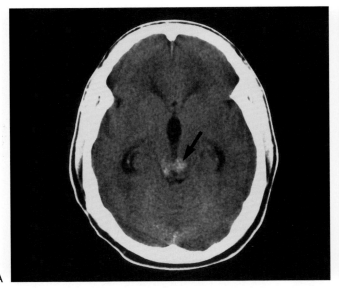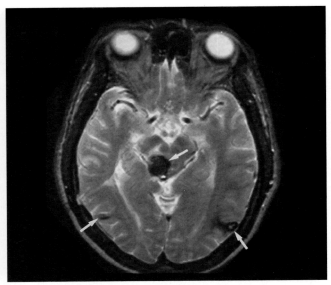

A   B

FIG. 15. Cavernous malformation of the midbrain. **A:** Non-contrast CT demonstrates a calcified lesion in the midbrain *(arrow)* adjacent to the aqueduct with mild hydrocephalus. **B:** Follow-up T2-weighted axial MRI better depicts the malformation and reveals surrounding edema as well as other smaller cavernomas not seen by CT *(arrows).*

Hypertensive Intracranial Hemorrhage

In adults, hypertension is one of the most common causes of nontraumatic intracranial hemorrhage. In the appropriate clinical setting, CT is extremely helpful in initially detecting the presence of a hypertensive hemorrhage and can often exclude other etiologies that may mimic the clinical presentation. Furthermore, CT can provide information about the size and location of the hematoma and evaluate for associated midline shift, intraventricular rupture, and the presence of hydrocephalus.

Hypertensive hemorrhage frequently occurs in territories supplied by perforating branches of the middle and posterior cerebral and basilar arteries. Approximately two thirds of the hemorrhages occur in the basal ganglia, followed by the thalamus (15–25%), pons (5–10%) and, cerebellum (2–5%) (1). Lobar hypertensive hemorrhages do occur but less frequently and may be difficult to differentiate from those caused by amyloid angiopathy or an underlying AVM.

On noncontrast CT, an acute hypertensive hemorrhage is easily identified as a large dense hematoma in a site listed above with associated mass effect and edema (Fig. 16). Intraventricular extension of hemorrhage and hydrocephalus may commonly occur as a result.

Hypertensive Encephalopathy

Hypertensive encephalopathy is a syndrome that can occur in normotensive patients who for numerous reasons may be afflicted with an acute and marked elevation of blood pressure or in those with accelerated malignant hypertension (46). Predisposing conditions include preeclampsia/eclampsia, renal failure, thrombotic thrombocytic purpura, hemolytic uremic syndrome, and systemic lupus erythematosus (45). Clinically, these patients present with severe headaches, drowsiness, vomiting, convulsions, focal neurologic signs, or coma (46,47). These encephalopathies are felt to result from a failure of cerebrovascular autoregulation leading to breakdown of the blood–brain barrier and consequent cerebral edema (45).

The CT findings in nongestational and gestational hypertensive encephalopathy are similar. Associated lesions include cortical and subcortical edema, particularly prominent at the gray–white junction with a predilection for the occipital lobes (Fig. 17) (46). Cortical and subcortical petechial hemorrhages and involvement of the basal ganglia and white matter may be seen. These changes of edema usually resolve following treatment.

Tumor Associated Intracranial Hemorrhage

Lesions commonly associated with hemorrhage include pituitary adenoma, malignant glial lesions, and metastatic lesions, especially from lung, kidney, choriocarcinoma, and melanoma. Factors that may induce tumoral hemorrhage include neovascularity, rapid tumor proliferation, vascular infiltration, and necrosis (48). Distinguishing benign from neoplastic hemorrhage is difficult. Tumors are generally more complex and heterogeneous in appearance and often exhibit nonhemorrhagic areas that enhance after contrast adminis-

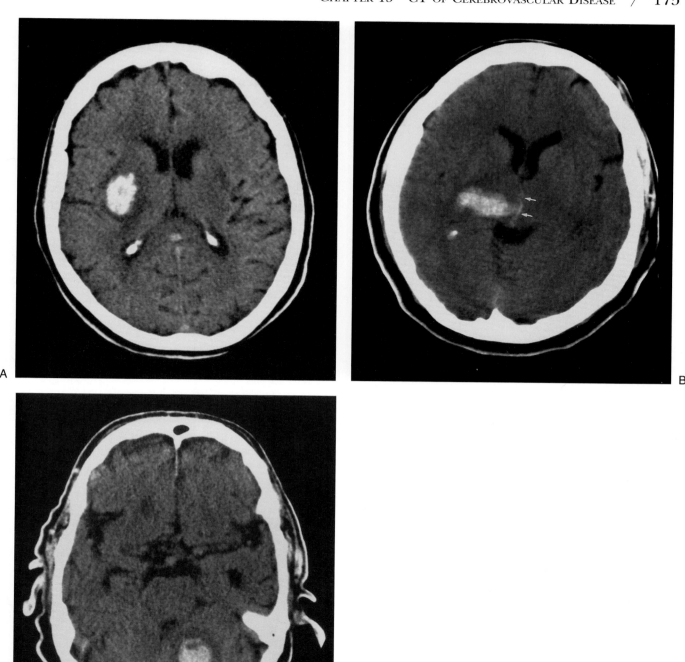

A

B

C

FIG. 16. Common locations of hypertensive hemorrhage. Basal ganglionic **(A)**, thalamic **(B)**, and cerebellar **(C)** hypertensive hemorrhages are seen with surrounding edema and mass effect on the adjacent ventricles. The thalamic hemorrhage has ruptured into the third ventricle *(arrows)* B. Lobar hemorrhages are much less common.

tration. Benign lesions, conversely, tend to follow an orderly evolution on sequential scans. Edema and mass effect characteristically resolve with benign lesions but persist with tumor (49). In patients with leukemia, hemorrhage may be caused by the abnormal neoplastic tissue or by a malignancy-induced coagulopathy (Fig. 18) (49).

CT ANGIOGRAPHY

In 1989, spiral CT was introduced as an advancement of the prior CT technology (50). Spiral CT is accomplished by the simultaneous advancement of the patient through the gantry at a constant rate during continuous rotation of the

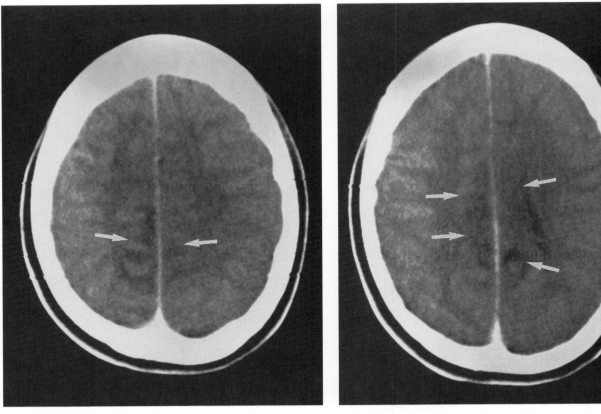

FIG. 17. Hypertensive encephalopathy. Axial-enhanced CT scans A and B of a patient with eclampsia demonstrate bilateral parasagittal subcortical edema/ischemic changes in an parietal distribution *(arrows).*

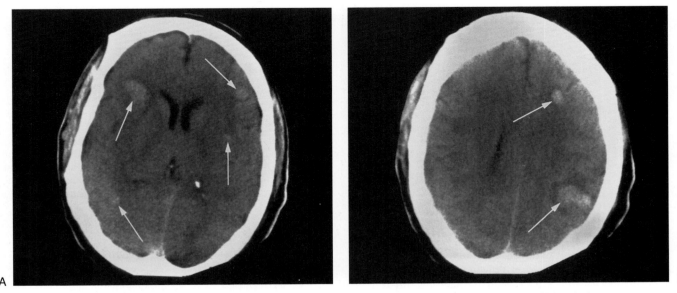

FIG. 18. Multiple intracranial hemorrhages in a patient with chronic myelocytic leukemia (CML) during an acute blastic crisis. Noncontrast CT (A and B) reveal numerous regions of hemorrhage and associated edema in the subcortical white matter of the cerebral hemispheres *(arrows).*

X-ray tube/detector unit (51). The X-ray source describes a spiral or helical path about the portion of the patient being scanned as opposed to traditional axial scanning. This results in the acquisition of a volume data set from which images can be generated in the standard transaxial plane or, alternatively, in multiplanar or three-dimensional views. This technological improvement has largely been afforded by the development of slip-ring gantry assemblies and larger heat capacity X-ray tubes that allow for continuous scanning (52).

CT angiography (CTA) is a relatively new technique that has emerged from this spiral technology. It is currently being used and studied as a method to assess the intra- and extracranial vasculature and shows promise in the noninvasive evaluation of cerebrovascular disease.

CTA is performed as a dynamic CT study during the intravenous bolus of a nonionic contrast agent with a scan time of up to 60 seconds depending on the region to be covered. From this spiral acquisition, variable-thickness transaxial

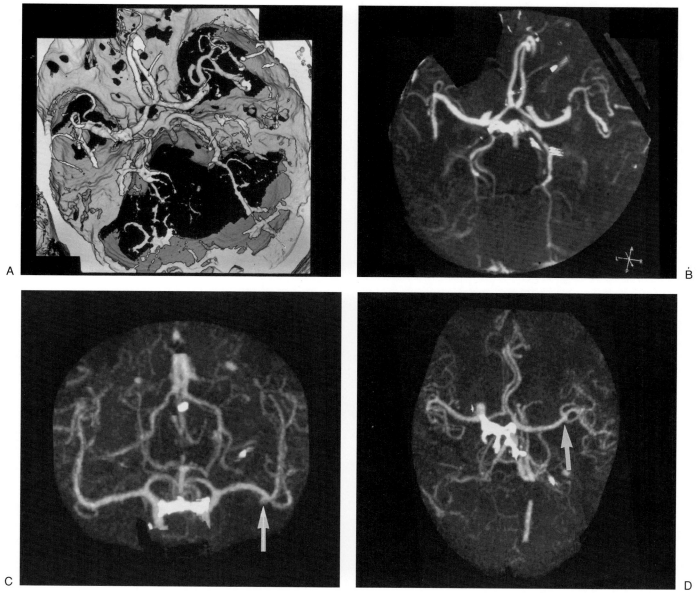

FIG. 19. CT angiography. **(A)** Three-dimensional, shaded-surface display (SSD) and **(B)** maximum intensity projection (MIP) images through the circle of Willis. The calvarium has been removed from the MIP image B, allowing for better visualization of the vessels when changing the frame of reference. **(C)** Towne's-like MIP projection through the circle of Willis reveals a questionable middle cerebral artery (MCA) bifurcation aneurysm *(arrow)*. **(D)** Rotation of the imaging volume, however, demonstrates this to be an overlapping branch of the MCA trifurcation *(arrow)*. Review of the source images would also prevent this misdiagnosis.

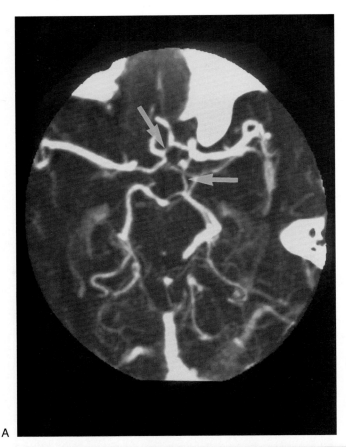

A

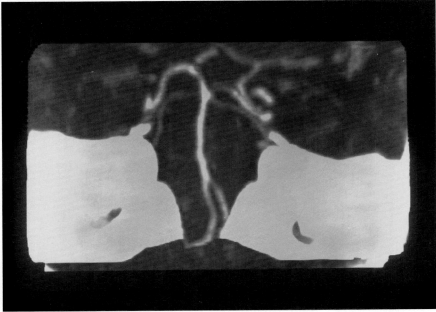

B

FIG. 20. "Target volume" maximum intensity projection CT angiography (CTA) (Picker International) allows for faster reconstruction of images because adjacent bone need not be removed to visualize vessels of interest, eg, the anterior and posterior communicating arteries *(arrows)* **(A)** and the posterior circulation **(B)**. Instead of viewing the entire spirally acquired volume, only "slabs" or rectangular boxes of interest are used to create the reconstructed images. This permits rapid evaluation and better demonstration of the vessels of clinical concern.

images can be reconstructed through the volume of interest scanned and may be viewed as source images. The image data are then transferred to a computer workstation where the data volume can be manipulated to produce three-dimensional images. These reconstructed images allow the data set or region of interest to be viewed from any angle.

Unlike MRA in which vascular imaging depends on flow dynamics, and velocity or duplex ultrasound, which depends on flow velocity, CTA depends only on the presence of con-

trast in the vessel at the time of imaging (53). Consequently, CTA can offer information not available by these other imaging techniques. This is particularly true when imaging a region where there is complex or turbulent flow, eg, in an aneurysm or region of stenosis.

CTA of the circle of Willis can be used to characterize the arterial anatomy quickly and accurately with various bone suppression techniques and reconstruction paradigms (Figs. 19 and 20). The information obtained can be useful in the

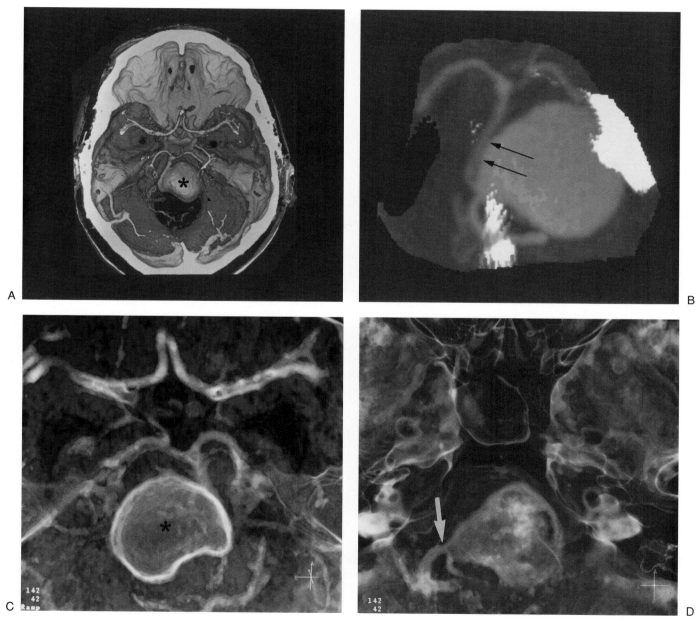

FIG. 21. CT angiography of giant aneurysm. **(A)** Shaded surface display CT angiography (SSD-CTA) shows a large vertebral artery confluence aneurysm (*) displacing the basilar artery. **(B)** Maximum intensity projection view with the bone removed better illustrates the separation of the giant aneurysm from the adjacent basilar artery (arrows). "Four-dimensional" (4-D) Angio (Picker International) (volume compositing) images through the posterior fossa **(C, D)** allow one to "look through" the dense aneurysm (*) to identify the aneurysm neck D *(arrows).*

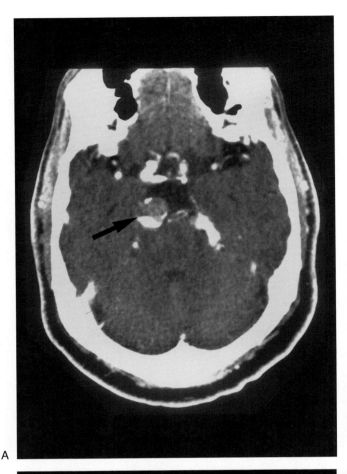

A

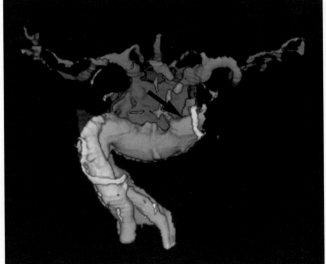

B

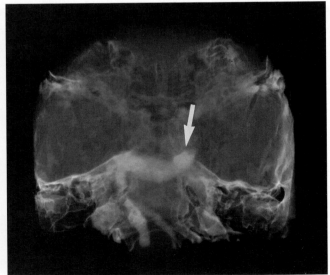

C

FIG. 22. CT angiography of basilar artery thrombosis. **(A)** Axial source image reveals thrombosis of a dolicoectatic basilar artery with contrast seen about the thrombus *(arrow)*. SSD-CTA **(B)** and 4-D Angio **(C)** reconstructions illustrate the occlusion in its entirety *(arrow)*.

evaluation of cerebral aneurysms, AVMs, moya-moya, vasospasm, and vascular occlusions or stenoses (Figs. 21 and 22) (53–56).

Furthermore, CTA of the neck has been used in the evaluation of carotid artery stenosis with success (57,58). In certain situations, MRA may overestimate the degree and length of stenosis when moderate to severe stenosis is present due to complex flow and intravoxel dephasing (Fig. 23) (59–63). Similarly, calcified plaque can lead to inaccurate assessment of the degree of stenosis by MRA and ultrasound but can usually be separated from the region of stenosis on CTA (53).

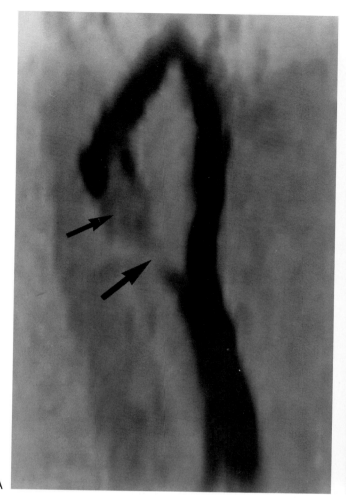

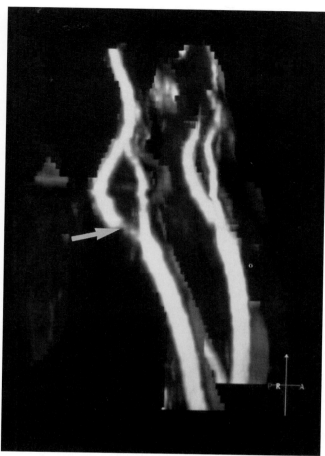

A   B

FIG. 23. MR and CT angiography of the carotid artery bifurcations. **A:** Phase contrast MRA demonstrates a tight stenosis at the origin of the internal carotid artery *(arrow)*. Clot or long segment stenosis versus dephasing artifact from turbulent flow is suggested just distally *(arrows)*. **B:** CTA MIP reconstruction of the carotid arteries shows only a focal segment of tight stenosis of the proximal internal carotid artery *(arrow)* without evidence of thrombus confirmed at surgery.

Lastly, CTA can be helpful in situations where MRI is contraindicated, when there are time constraints or when the patient is unstable.

XENON CEREBRAL BLOOD FLOW IMAGING

Xenon is a highly lipid-soluble noble gas ($Z = 54$) that freely diffuses across the blood–brain barrier. The stable xenon technique utilizes the Fick principle in order to calculate flow based on AV differences in concentrations of a freely diffusible inert indicator (64). The radiodensity of xenon allows its concentration within the brain to be determined directly by the CT scanner. In practice, cerebral blood flow (CBF) is determined indirectly by measuring the density (Hounsfield units) of a particular region before and after xenon administration. The technique is particularly accurate in quantifying low-blood-flow states.

Xenon CT CBF determination has proven to be useful in cases of brain death and acute stroke (65). Autoregulation, clinical challenge of reserve in occlusive vascular disease, and reserve testing in vasospasm are further useful applications. Xenon CBF testing has shown better correlation with clinical deficits and CT demonstrated infarction than has transcranial Doppler, which is insensitive to second-order vasospasm.

The main advantage of stable xenon CT is that it noninvasively provides relatively high-resolution quantitative local CBF information coupled to CT anatomy. CBF studies can be repeated at 20-minute intervals allowing for the evaluation of hemodynamic states as well as the response to therapeutic interventions (66).

CONCLUSION

CT is a rapid, cost-effective means by which to evaluate cerebrovascular disease. With the continued development of spiral CT, CTA has become a useful adjunct in the noninvasive assessment of the cerebral and extracranial vasculature. Despite the superior sensitivity of MRI, CT remains an important modality in the initial triage and follow-up of CNS pathology.

REFERENCES

1. Osborne AG. *Diagnostic Neuroradiology*. New York: CV Mosby, 1994.
2. Atlas S. *MRI of Brain and Spinal Cord*. New York: Raven Press, 1991; 420–435.
3. Schuier FJ, Hossmann KA. Experimental brain infarcts in cats II. Ischemic brain edema. *Stroke* 1980;11:593–601.
4. Pressman BD, Tourje EJ, Thomson JR. An early sign of ischemic infarction: increased density in a cerebral artery. *AJR* 1987;149(3): 583–586.
5. Tomura N, Vemura K, Inugami A, Fujita H, Higano S, Shishido F. Early CT finding in cerebral infarction: obscuration of the lentiform nucleus. *Radiology* 1988;168:463–467.
6. Truwit CL, Barkovich A, Gean-Marton A, Hibri N, Norman D. Loss of the insular ribbon: another early CT sign of acute MCA infarction. *Radiology* 1990;176:801–806.
7. Bories J, Derhy S, Chiras J. CT in hemispheric ischemic attacks. *Neuroradiology* 1985;27:468–483.
8. Valk J. *Computed Tomography and Cerebral Infarction*. New York: Raven Press, 1980.
9. Houser OW, Campbell JK, Baker HL Jr, Sundt TS Jr. Radiologic evaluation of ischemic cerebrovascular syndromes with emphasis on CT. *Radiol Clin North Am* 1982;20:123–142.
10. Bryan RN, Levy LM, Whitlow WD, Kilian JM, Preziosi TJ, Rosario JA. Diagnosis of acute cerebral infarction: comparison of MR and CT imaging. *AJNR* 1991;12:611–620.
11. Elster A. CT and MR imaging of stroke. *ASNR Core Curriculum Course in Neuroradiology* 1996.
12. Becker H, Desch H, Hacker H, Pencz A. CT fogging effect with ischemic cerebral infarcts. *Neuroradiology* 1979;18:185-192.
13. Asata R, Okumura R, Konishi J. Case report: "Fogging effect" in MR of cerebral infarct. *J Comput Assist Tomogr* 1991;15(1):160–162.
14. Secrist RD, Traynelis V, Schochet SS. MR imaging of acute cortical venous infarction: preliminary experience with an animal model. *Magn Res Imag* 1989;7:149–153.
15. Yagamuchi T. Clinical and neuroradiologic analysis of thrombotic and embolic cerebral infarctions. *Jap Circ J* 1984;48:50.
16. Hayman L, Evans RA, Bation FO, Hinck VC. Delayed high dose contrast CT: identifying patients at risk of hemorrhagic infarction. *AJR* 1981;136:1151.
17. Brant-Zawadzki M. *MRI of Central Nervous System*. New York: Raven Press, 1987;231–234.
18. Rao KC, Knipp HC, Wagner EJ. CT findings in cerebral sinus and venous thrombosis. *Radiology* 1981;140:391–398.
19. Zimmerman RD, Ernst RJ. Neuroimaging of cerebral venous thrombosis. *Neuroimag Clin North Am* 1992;2(3).
20. Buonanno FS, Moody DM, Ball MR, Laster DW. Computed cranial CT findings in cerebral sinovenous occlusion. *JCAT* 1978;2:281–290.
21. Bozzola FG, Borelich PB. Epidemiology of intracranial hemorrhage. *Neuroimag Clin North Am* 1992;2:1–10.
22. Inagawa T. Multiple intracranial aneurysms in elderly patients. *Acta Neurochir (Wien)* 1990;106:119–126.
23. Kassel NF, Torner JC, Haley EC, Jane JA, Adams HP, Kongable GI. The international comparative study on timing of aneurysm surgery. *J Neurosurg* 1990;73:18–47.
24. Wilson FM, Kaspam T, Holland IM. Multiple cerebral aneurysms: a reappraisal. *Neuroradiology* 1989;31:232–236.
25. Ogawa T, Inugami A, Shimosegawa E, et al. SAH evaluation with MRI. *Radiology* 1993;186:345–351.
26. Atlas SW. MRI is highly sensitive for acute SAH . . . Not! *Radiology* 1993;186:319–332.
27. New PFJ, Aronow S. Attenuation measurements of whole blood and blood fractions in CT. *Radiology* 1976;121:635.
28. Watanabe AT, Mackey K, Lufkin RB. Imaging diagnosis and temporal appearance of SAH. *Neuroimag Clin North Am* 1992;2:53.
29. Scotti G, Ethier R, Melancon D, Terbrugge K, Tchang S. CT in the evaluation of intracranial aneurysms and SAH. *Radiology* 1977;123: 85.
30. Silver AJ, Pederson ME, Ganti SR. CT of SAH due to ruptured aneurysm. *AJNR* 1981;2:13.
31. Rinkel TJE, Wijdicks EFM, Vermeulen M, et al. Nonaneurysmal perimesencephalic subarachnoid hemorrhage: CT and MR patterns that differ from aneurysmal rupture. *AJNR* 1991;12:829–834.
32. Tomsick TA. Aneurysm: CT, angiography, MR/MRA. *ASNR Core Curriculum in Neuroradiology* 1995;11–16.
33. Ramsey R. *Diagnostic Neuroradiology*, 3rd ed. Philadelphia: WB Saunders, 1993.
34. Hoang T, Hasso AN. Intracranial vascular malformations. *Neuroimag Clin North Am* 1994;4(4):823.
35. Atlas SW. Intracranial vascular malformations and aneurysms: current imaging applications. *Radiol Clin North Am* 1988;26:821–837.
36. Willinsky R, Lasjaunias P, Terbrugge K. Brain AVMs: analysis of angioarchitecture in relationship to hemorrhage. *J Neuroradiol* 1988; 15:225–237.
37. Chen J, Tsuruda JS, Halbach VV. Dural AVFs: results of screening MRA in 7 patients. *Radiology* 1992;183:265–271.
38. Scott JA, Augustyn GT, Gilmor RL, Mealey J, Olson EW. MRI of a venous angioma. *AJNR* 1985;6:284–286.
39. Rothfus WE, Albright AL, Casey KF, Latchaw RE, Roppolo HMN. Cerebellar venous angioma: "benign" entity. *AJNR* 1984;5:61–66.
40. Hyman RA, Black KS. Aneurysms and vascular malformations: topics in MRI. *J MRI* 1989;2:49–62.
41. Lotz PR, Quisling RG. CT of venous angiomas of the brain. *AJNR* 1983;4:1124–1126.
42. Rigamonti D. MR appearance of cavernomas. *J Neurosurg* 1987;67: 518–524.
43. Savoiardo M, Strada L, Passerini A. Intracranial cavernoma: neuroradiologic review in 36 operated cases. *AJNR* 1983;4:945–950.
44. Rigamonti D, Hadley MN, Drayer BP, et al. Cerebral cavernous malformations: incidence and familial occurrence. *N Engl J Med* 1988;319: 343–347.
45. Adams JH, Duchen LW. *Greenfield's Neuropathology*, 5th ed. New York: Oxford University Press, 1992.
46. Rail DL, Perkin GD. Computerized tomographic appearance of hypertensive encephalopathy. *Arch Neurol* 1980:37;310–311.
47. Leeds NE, Sawaya R, VanTassel P, Hayman LA. Intracranial hemorrhage in the oncologic patient. *Neuroimag Clin North Am* 1992;2: 119–136.
48. Schwartz RB, Jones KM, Kalina P, et al. Hypertensive encephalopathy: findings on CT, MR and SPECT I 14 cases. *AJR* 1992;159:379–383.
49. Atlas SW, Grossman RI, Gomori JM, et al. Hemorrhagic malignant intracranial neoplasms. *Radiology* 1987;164:71–77.
50. Heiken J, Brink JA, Vannier MW. Spiral (helical) CT. *Radiology* 1993; 189:647–656.
51. Kalender WA, Sissler W, Klotz E, Vock P. Spiral volumetric CT with single breath-hold technique, continuous transport and continuous scanner rotation. *Radiology* 1990;176:181–183.
52. Kalender WA, Polacin A, Marchal G, Baert AL. Current status and new perspectives in spiral CT. In: Felix R, Langer M, eds. *Advances in CT: II*. New York: Springer-Verlag, 1992;87–94.
53. Marks M. Spiral CT angiography of the cerebrovascular circulation. In: Fishman EK, eds. *Sprial CT: Principles, Techniques and Clinical Applications*. New York: Raven Press, 1995.
54. Dorsch NW, Young N, Kingston RJ, Compton JS. Early experience with spiral CT in the diagnosis of intracranial aneurysms. *Neurosurgery* 1995;36(1):230–238.
55. Aoki S, Sasaki Y, Machida T, Ohkubo T, Miniami M, Sasaki Y. Cerebral aneurysms: detection and delineation using 3D CT angiography. *AJNR* 1992;13:1115–1120.
56. Tsuchiya K, Makita K, Furui S. Moyamoya disease: diagnosis with three-dimensional CT angiography. *Neuroradiology* 1994;36:432–434.
57. Marks MP, Napel S, Jordan JE, Enzmann DR. Diagnosis of carotid artery disease: preliminary experience with maximum-intensity projection spiral CTA. *AJR* 1994;160:1267–1271.
58. Schwartz RB, Jones KM, Chernoff DM, et al. Common carotid bifurcations: evaluation with spiral CT. *Radiology* 1992;185:513–519.
59. Litt AW, Eidelman EM, Pinto RS, et al. Diagnosis of carotid artery stenosis: comparison of 2D FT time-of-flight MR angiography with contrast angiography in 50 patients. *AJNR* 1991;149:154.

60. Massaryk AM, Ross JS, DiCello MC, Modic MT, Paranandi L, Masaryk TJ. 3D FT MR angiography of the carotid bifurcations: potential and limitations as a screening examination. *Radiology* 1991;179:797–804.

61. Heiserman JE, Drayer BP, Fram EK, et al. Carotid artery stenosis: clinical efficacy of two-dimensional time-of-flight MR angiography. *Radiology* 1992;182:761–768.

62. Polak JF, Bajakian RL, O'Leary DH, Anderson MR, Donaldson MC, Jolesz FA. Detection of internal carotid artery stenosis: comparison of MR angiography, color Doppler sonography, and arteriography. *Radiology* 1992;182:35–40.

63. Huston J III, Lewis BD, Wiebers DO, Meyer FB, Riederer SJ, Weaver AL. Carotid artery: prospective blinded comparison of 2D TOF MRA with conventional angiography and duplex ultrasound. *Radiology* 1993;186:339–344.

64. Kety SS. The theory and applications of the exchange of an inert gas at the lungs and tissues. *Pharmacol Review* 1951;3:1–41.

65. Hughes RL. Cerebral blood flow determination within the first 8 hours of cerebral infarction using stable xenon-enhanced CT. *Stroke* 1989;20:754–760.

66. Johnson D. Stable xenon CT CBF imaging: rationale for and role in clinical decision making. *AJNR* 1991;12:201–213.

Cerebrovascular Disease, edited by H. Hunt Batjer.
Lippincott-Raven Publishers, Philadelphia © 1997.

CHAPTER 16

MRI of Cerebrovascular Disease: Capabilities and Limitations

Robert W. Androux, Eric J. Russell, and Joel R. Meyer

Advances in magnetic resonance imaging (MRI) technology have had a tremendous impact on our ability to evaluate and diagnose patients with cerebrovascular disorders. In this chapter we will discuss the role of magnetic resonance (MR) in the diagnosis of cerebral infarction, emphasizing widely available conventional MR applications. In addition, we will briefly discuss diffusion imaging, a new application that allows an earlier diagnosis of cerebral infarction than is possible with conventional techniques. Finally, we will discuss the role of MR imaging in the diagnosis of intracranial hemorrhage with emphasis on hemorrhage associated with neurovascular disorders. A simplified approach to the physical basis of the MR appearance of hemorrhage will also be presented, and we will explore specific disorders where an understanding of the appearance of associated hemorrhage permits a more precise diagnosis.

CEREBRAL INFARCTION

Cerebral ischemia is a dynamic process with multiple factors leading to tissue recovery or permanent damage (infarction). The clinical deficit associated with infarction depends upon its size and distribution (cortical and subcortical). The value of imaging for detection and characterization of cerebral infarction is limited but well established (1,2). Computed tomography (CT) is often negative in the first 24 hours following the acute onset of neurologic signs and symptoms (3). The improved soft tissue contrast afforded by MRI permits earlier detection of the subtle changes in tissue water content that accompany stroke, permitting an earlier diagnosis and clear delineation of the extent of tissue damage. The

R. W. Androux, E. J. Russell, and J. R. Meyer: Department of Radiology, Northwestern University Medical School, Chicago, Illinois 60611

purpose of this section is to review the sequential MRI appearance of cerebral infarction.

CORTICAL INFARCTION

The early MRI detection and characterization of cortical infarction depends on alteration of blood flow and the pathophysiologic response of brain tissue to ischemia. Cerebral oxygen depletion provokes anaerobic glycolysis, and the accumulation of intracellular sodium results in an increase in intracellular fluid (cytotoxic edema). These mechanisms develop rapidly within the first 30 minutes of the insult. Cytotoxic edema produces tissue swelling and mild mass effect. With prolonged ischemia, neuronal, glial, and capillary endothelial cell damage occurs, leading to blood–brain barrier (BBB) disruption with leakage of intravascular fluid into the extracellular space (vasogenic edema), where water is bound to macromolecules (4).

MR signal intensity alteration due to ischemic stroke is the result of altered blood flow, the combination of accumulated cytotoxic and vasogenic edema, and the presence or absence of hemorrhage. Cytotoxic edema results in swelling and subtle effacement of cortical sulci, a morphologic change that can occur without signal alteration on T2-weighted images due to the lack of binding of intracellular water to macromolecules. With the onset of vasogenic edema, bound water accumulates and there is a characteristic increase in T2 signal. The high signal of extracellular edema can be seen as early as 4–6 hours after ictus and is virtually always demonstrated at 24 hours (5–7).

Significant carotid stenosis or vascular occlusion may be detected by careful review of images made with conventional MR pulse sequences. In normals, fast-flowing blood does not experience the entire MR pulse sequence, resulting in low signal intensity referred to as high-velocity signal loss (flow void). High-grade stenosis or occlusion results in altered flow dynamics resulting in loss of this intravascular signal void, producing a relative increase in intensity resulting in homogeneous signal within the vessel lumen on T1-weighted scans. With less severe stenosis, a partial flow void pattern may be demonstrated within the affected vessel, characterized by increased intraluminal signal intensity at the periphery of a persistent central flow void, or mixed intensity related to turbulent flow (8,9). Increased peripheral intensity represents slow-moving protons that remain in the imaging plane during the entire MR pulse sequence and are thus available to emit a detectable signal. Intravascular signal beyond a proximal stenosis may also increase further with contrast injection (Fig. 1). Thrombosis may also be responsible for increased intravascular signal intensity distal to an occlusion (8,9).

Hemorrhagic infarction is defined as hemorrhage occurring in an infarct within the first 24 hours post-ictus. Hemorrhagic transformation refers to delayed appearance of hemorrhage after the first 24 hours post-ictus, usually due to reperfusion of an occluded artery by migration of an embolus distally. Hemorrhagic transformation occurs in up to 40% of ischemic strokes, most commonly between 48 hours and 2 weeks (10,11). The hemorrhagic component of an embolic infarct can be confined to gray matter or involve both gray and white matter (petechial hemorrhage). The MR characteristics of hemorrhagic infarction vary according to the age of the bleed (see next section). Mineralization of infarction can occur in the chronic stage, represented, in some cases, by high signal intensity seen on T1-weighted images related to hydration layer effect (Fig. 2).

Intravenous paramagnetic contrast media has been shown to be very useful for MRI characterization of cortical cerebral infarction (5,12,13). The time course for typical subacute parenchymal enhancement is similar to that described with contrast-enhanced CT (14). Two distinct patterns of enhancement, meningeal and intravascular, may be observed in the more acute stages of infarction. These patterns usually occur before the appearance of classic gyriform parenchymal enhancement; however, they may occur coincident with parenchymal enhancement.

The intravascular enhancement sign is most commonly observed during the first three days after stroke and is found in 75% of cortical infarctions (12). This sign frequently predates the signal intensity changes observed on noncontrast T2-weighted MR images and therefore may be the earliest

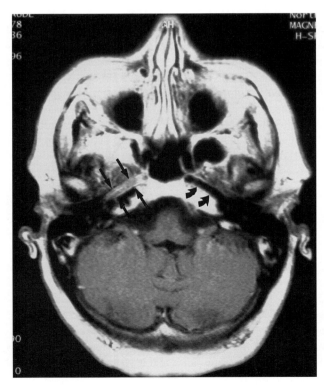

FIG. 1. Axial T1-enhanced scans through the skull base show homogeneous high signal intensity within the lumen of the right internal carotid artery *(arrows)*, representing slow flow–related enhancement beyond a proximal cervical internal carotid stenosis. Note the normal dark flow void in the contralateral left petrous carotid *(curved arrows)*.

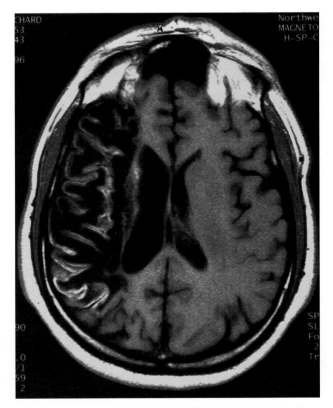

FIG. 2. A 60-year-old woman with left hemiparesis and new onset seizures. T1 noncontrast axial images demonstrate a large area of chronic infarction in the distribution of the right middle cerebral artery involving frontal and temporal cortex, as well as subcortical white matter and the basal ganglia. Surface (gyral) high signal intensity represents cortical mineralization.

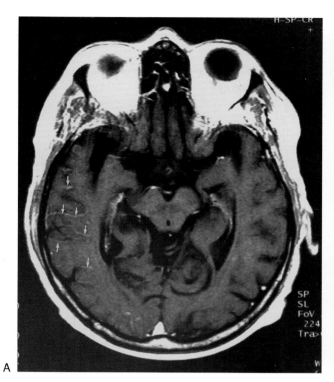

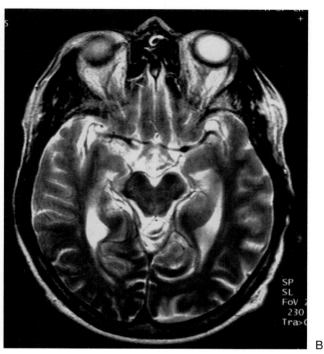

FIG. 3. Detection of acute infarction with contrast-enhanced MRI: Intravascular enhancement sign. **A:** Contrast-enhanced axial T1-weighted MR scan obtained a few hours after symptoms of a right middle cerebral artery (MCA) infarction reveals extensive intravascular enhancement within MCA branches in temporal sulci *(arrows)*. **B:** Axial T2-weighted MR scan demonstrates no signal abnormality within the right temporal lobe. T2-weighted scans are insensitive to cytotoxic edema seen early in ischemia.

positive MR finding in acute infarction (Fig. 3). Enhancement is due to slow flow within the arteries in the area of the acute infarct. With slow flow, contrast material remains in the imaging plane during the entire MR sequence, resulting in T1 shortening and increased signal intensity within the blood vessels. This sign may be seen within large vessels such as the internal carotid or vertebral arteries or within smaller intracranial branches such as M2 branches of the middle cerebral artery. It may also be seen within the proximal segment of distally occluded or narrowed arteries. In cases with complete proximal arterial occlusion, with enhancement may be due to slow retrograde collateral arterial flow beyond the occlusion. The intravascular enhancement sign can persist for 2 weeks but usually disappears in 5–7 days (6,12,13).

Meningeal enhancement may be detected in an area of cerebral infarction within the first 3 days post ictus. This sign is less constant than the intravascular enhancement sign and is observed in only 30% of cortical infarctions (12). The true incidence may be higher since it is demonstrated best on coronal images, which are not routinely acquired in the setting of acute stroke (Fig. 4). While there is no satisfactory explanation for the meningeal enhancement sign, this phenomenon has been attributed to collateral flow from the inner aspect of the dura toward leptomeningeal anastomoses and pial arteries. Irritation of the meninges by the adjacent in-

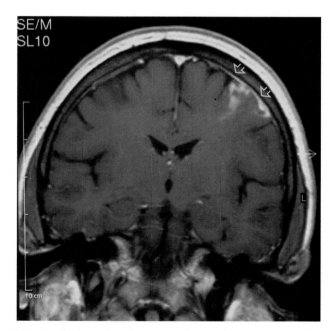

FIG. 4. Meningeal enhancement associated acute cortical infarct. Contrast-enhanced coronal T1-weighted MR scan shows pathologic gyriform parenchymal enhancement in a small zone within the distribution of the left middle cerebral artery. Note associated meningeal enhancement adjacent to the infarct *(small arrows)*.

jured brain is another speculative explanation. This type of enhancement is usually associated with large supratentorial cortical infarctions and is rarely seen with brainstem infarct (6,12,13,15,16).

Parenchymal (cortical) enhancement has the same gyral (surface) pattern and time course as that observed with enhanced CT. Most commonly seen 10–14 days postinfarction, it is present in nearly 100% of cases at some time during the first 2 months after the insult (Fig. 5) (6). Few infarcts will enhance after 6 weeks. Parenchymal enhancement can occur only when the BBB is disrupted and when there is sufficient inflow to allow delivery of contrast media to the injured tissue (17). Tissue perfusion during an acute ischemic event may be incomplete, depending on the presence or absence of collateral flow. In cases of arterial occlusion without collaterals, parenchymal enhancement cannot occur even in the presence of a disrupted BBB. In such cases, parenchymal enhancement is absent, whereas signal abnormalities on T2-weighted images may be extensive due to the presence of vasogenic edema. When tissue perfusion is partly preserved or restored, early parenchymal enhance-

ment can occur because contrast material can reach the ischemic tissue through collateral channels or recanalized proximal arteries. The T2 signal abnormality is often less extensive than that observed in complete occlusion due to a lesser ischemic insult. These two different patterns of parenchymal enhancement therefore reflect the underlying pathophysiology. Early parenchymal enhancement may also be seen in transient ischemic events that allow reperfusion after the insult, or in watershed infarctions, because of the dual nature of the blood supply that allows delivery of contrast agent from adjacent vascular territories.

BBB disruption alone does not explain the persistence of parenchymal enhancement for several weeks or months after the insult. Radiologic/pathologic correlation studies have shown that immature capillaries (neovascularity) within the damaged tissue are responsible for parenchymal enhancement during the later weeks following injury. This enhancement will progressively diminish as these capillaries are surrounded by new glial tissue and the effectiveness of the BBB is restored (18,19).

During the second week following infarction, the high signal intensity initially observed on T2-weighted images (related to edema) can diminish before the loss of brain tissue (encephalomalacia) produces a permanent zone of high intensity. During this brief time, the area of infarction may become isointense with adjacent normal brain, making the infarct hard to detect. This phenomenon is called the "fogging effect." The use of contrast media during this time period typically demonstrates gyriform enhancement, which facilitates localization of the infarction since both unenhanced proton density and T2-weighted images may be relatively normal (20).

Chronic infarcts, several weeks to years old, represent the end result of a destructive process. MR findings of chronic infarction reflect the effects of volume loss and glial scarring, so-called encephalomalacia. Mass effect will be absent. Instead, atrophy results in dilatation of adjacent sulci and ipsilateral ventricular enlargement. Contrast enhancement is not present because after 6–12 weeks the integrity of the BBB is reestablished. Ipsilateral brain stem atrophy can occur in the chronic stages due to secondary axonal (Wallerian) degeneration (Fig. 6) (21).

DIFFUSION-WEIGHTED IMAGING

MR is often normal within the first 6 hours after the initial ischemic injury because cytotoxic edema does not alter T1 or T2 relaxation times. Later on, conventional MRI is positive, but it may not identify the true extent of permanent tissue damage within the edematous area represented by the abnormal signal intensity seen on T2-weighted images.

These difficulties are addressed by MR pulse sequences, which are sensitive to the diffusion of water protons: diffusion-weighted imaging (DWI). Animal experimentation and several clinical investigations have shown that this technique

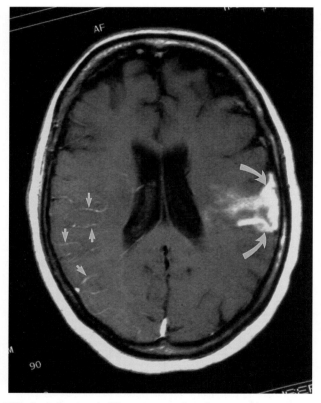

FIG. 5. Infarcts of different age, demonstrated by contrast-enhanced MR, in a patient with a sudden onset of left hemiparesis. Postinfusion axial T1-weighted MR scan shows abnormal intravascular enhancement in the distribution of the right middle cerebral artery *(arrows)*, related to slow arterial flow in an area of acute infarction. There is also classic gyral and subcortical white matter enhancement on the left *(curved arrows)*, consistent with subacute left hemispheric infarction.

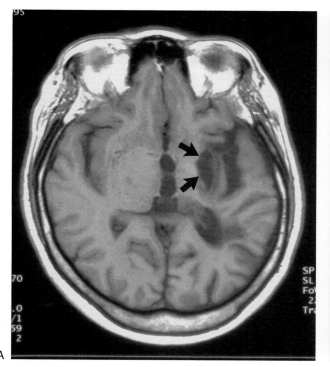

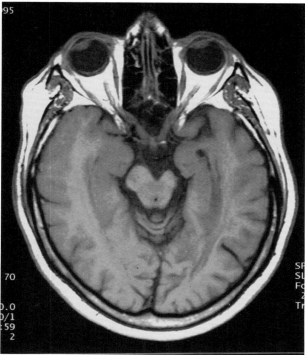

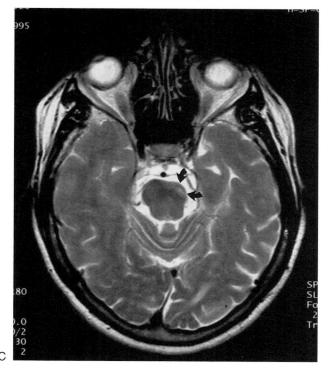

FIG. 6. Wallerian degeneration to postinfarction encephalomalacia within the left basal ganglia. **A:** Axial T1-weighted images show a lateral ganglionic infarct *(arrows)*, with ipsilateral atrial and Sylvian fissure enlargement. **B:** Lower axial T1-weighted MR scan shows asymmetric atrophy of the ipsilateral left cerebral peduncle due to secondary axonal (Wallerian) degeneration. **C:** Axial T2-weighted MR scan shows abnormal signal and volume loss within the left pons *(arrows)*, due to corticospinal tract degeneration.

is highly sensitive for the detection of impaired water diffusion associated with acute cerebral infarction (22–27). While similar MR pulse sequences have been available for years, new faster scanning techniques now permit DWI scanning in a practical amount of time. In fact, with echo planar scanning techniques, a whole-brain diffusion-weighted scan can be acquired in 15–20 seconds. The dramatic improvement in

examination speed will lead to the routine use of this technique, as an addition to the standard imaging protocol in stroke patients.

Diffusion-weighted images depict the random microscopic motion of water molecules that occurs in biological tissue. The length of the molecular displacement is proportionally expressed by an apparent diffusion coefficient

(ADC) (28). These normal transitional movements, which occur over a linear range of 10–20 μm, provoke spin dephasing effects in normal tissue, and as seen with flowing blood, this results in loss of local MR signal. The increase in intracellular water associated with dysfunction of the cell membrane's Na,K pump results in water entering the more restricted intracellular environment for water diffusion compared with the relatively unrestricted extracellular environment (29,30). Acute ischemic cerebral tissue with impaired diffusion related to cytotoxic edema (cell swelling) does not experience normal diffusion-related signal loss when exposed to diffusion gradients and therefore will demonstrate relatively increased signal intensity on DWI (low ADC). In the later stages of infarction, cellular necrosis results in a reduction in restricted diffusion, and the ADC increases, leading to a loss of the high signal intensity characteristic of acute ischemia. ADC is significantly reduced in the first hours to days, whereas ADC becomes high (and MR signal becomes normal or low) in all patients 1–2 weeks after the onset of the stroke (31). Because changes in ADC vary with the age of the infarct, DWI can differentiate between acute and chronic infarcts (Figs. 7 and 8).

Experimental models suggest that DWI can also depict the zone of reversible ischemia (periinfarct zone or ischemic penumbra) at the margins of the infarcted tissue. Return of normal low signal on DWI has been shown at the margin of the infarct after reperfusion of the ischemic penumbra zone (32). This area, where blood perfusion is initially reduced but not completely interrupted, may be a target for therapeutic intervention with thrombolytic and cytoprotective agents, such as cytocholine. There is considerable interest in the salvage of the ischemic penumbra in order to reduce the severity of permanent neurologic deficit. There is evidence that DWI can provide an earlier and more specific diagnosis of ischemia, leading to better management of this patient population within the first few hours after the ischemic event.

DEEP CEREBRAL (LACUNAR) AND CEREBELLAR ISCHEMIC INFARCTION

MR images are extremely sensitive for the detection of focal white matter diseases that produce cerebral edema or demyelination. Foci of abnormal white matter high signal intensity can be found in approximately 20–30% of clinically healthy elderly patients and are related to a wide variety of diseases that produce infarction, gliosis, and demyelination. Some of these bright spots represent dilatation of normal anatomic structures, the perivascular Virchow–Robin (VR) spaces. These consist of extensions of the subarachnoid space along cerebral perforating arteries. Differentiation between dilated VR spaces and ischemic infarction or gliosis can be made by anatomic location and MR signal intensity patterns: ischemic lesions tend to be higher in signal intensity than cerebrospinal fluid (CSF) on proton density (short TE, long TR) spin echo–weighted images, whereas VR spaces have signal intensity similar to CSF on all MR pulse sequences (Fig. 9) (33,34).

Whereas the intravascular and meningeal enhancement signs are very common in acute cortical infarction, they are uncommon in deep (subcortical) cerebral and brainstem infarctions. The majority of these infarctions are the result of occlusion of small penetrating arteries supplying the central portions of the telencephalon and diencephalon. These vessels arise from the proximal portions of the three major intracranial vessels: anterior cerebral artery (ACA), middle cerebral artery (MCA), posterior cerebral artery (PCA), and the associated communicating arteries that form the circle of Willis. These deep perforating arteries represent terminal territories and so their occlusion leads to a complete absence of blood flow perfusion within a very well-defined tissue territory. This explains the lack of the intravascular enhancement usually seen in cortical infarctions. The remote location of the infarction from the dura, and the small size of the majority of deep cerebral and brainstem infarcts, explains the lack of meningeal enhancement.

Several studies have shown that contrast infusion may produce parenchymal enhancement in deep subacute acute cerebral infarcts. This enhancement occurs in 50% of cases, usually before the end of the first week (35,36). Thus, contrast administration is very useful for detecting and dating acute/subacute deep infarcts, especially in patients with multiple chronic deep matter lesions that may obscure the presence of a newer lesion. Despite a relative lack of sensitivity in depicting very early deep cerebral infarcts, MR is still the best available study. The multiplanar imaging capabilities of MR and the absence of bone artifact make the vascular distribution of such lesions more apparent than with CT, particularly in the posterior fossa (37) (Fig. 10).

BORDER ZONE INFARCTIONS

Infarction that occurs at the interface of two arterial territories is referred to as border zone or watershed infarction. Border zone infarctions can occur between two superficial vascular distributions (ACA and MCA or MCA and PCA), or between superficial and deep arterial territories (ie, lenticulostriate and MCA). Typically a parasagittal area extending from the posterior frontal lobe to the parietal lobe delineates the border zone between the anterior and middle cerebral artery territories, whereas the area between the posterior parietal and occipital lobes represents the border zone between the posterior and middle cerebral artery distributions. Arterial pressure is lowest in border zones. These regions therefore receive the lowest relative cerebral blood flow and are therefore more susceptible to ischemia in situations of global hypoxia or systemic hypotension due to myocardial infarction, arrhythmia, tamponade, or other cause of congestive heart failure (38). The sequential MR appearance of these

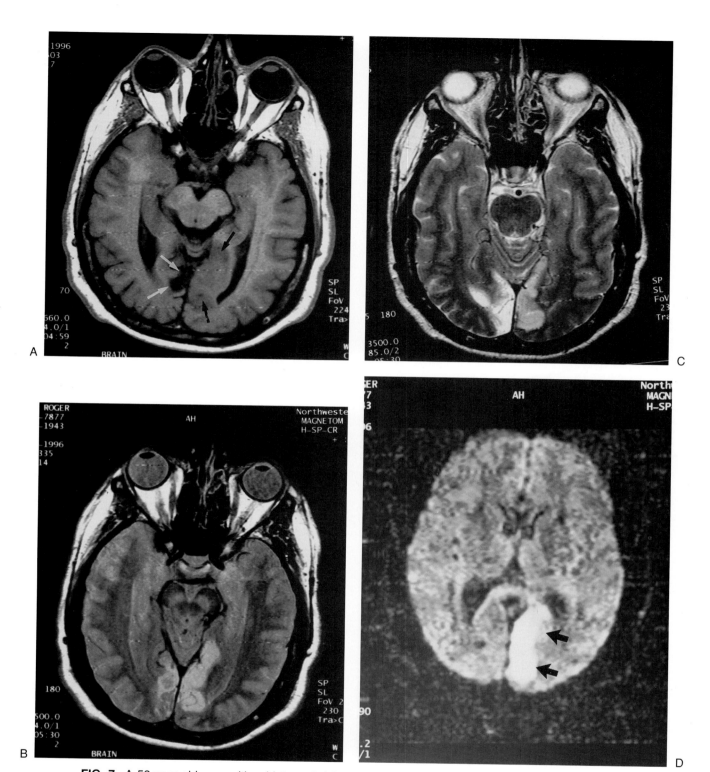

FIG. 7. A 53-year-old man with a history of right posterior cerebral artery infarct and a new onset of left-sided homonymous hemianopsia. **A:** Axial noncontrast T1-weighted scan shows prominence of the sulci in the area of an old right occipital lobe infarction *(white arrows),* and subtler more diffuse low intensity and sulcal effacement (gyral swelling) in the contralateral left medial occipital lobe *(black arrows).* **B,C:** Proton density (B) and T2-weighted (C) spin echo MR images show abnormally increased occipital lobe signal intensity bilaterally. The intensity of the old right-sided infarct closely resembles cerebrospinal fluid, since it represents cystic encephalomalacia, whereas the less marked left occipital high intensity is consistent with a more acute infarction. **D:** A diffusion-weighted MR image obtained in 15 seconds using an echo planar imaging technique demonstrates hyperintense signal (low ADC), only in the area of acute infarction on the left *(arrows).*

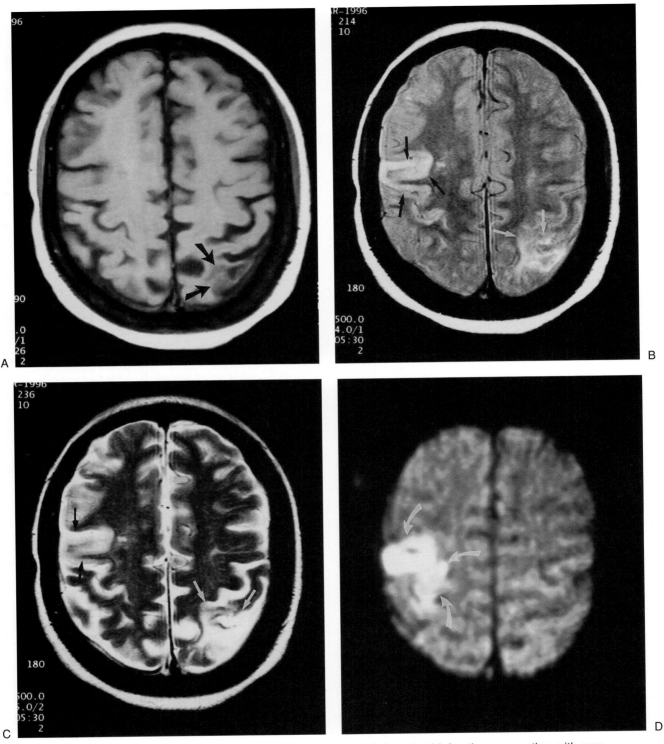

FIG. 8. A 75-year-old woman with a history of a chronic left parietal infarction, presenting with new onset of mental status change. **A–C:** Transverse-axial T1- (A), proton density (B), and T2- (C) weighted spin echo MR images were obtained within 2 days of the onset of symptoms. The T1-weighted scan (A) reveals focal atrophy and encephalomalacia in the left parietal region *(arrows)*, consistent with the known old infarct. The proton density and T2-weighted spin echo images (B, C) demonstrate abnormal high signal in the old left sided infarct *(white arrows, B, C)*, and also within the right posterior fronto-parietal gyrus in the area of the acute infarction *(black arrows, B, C)*. As is typical, the proton density image (B) is more revealing because the signal intensity from adjacent cerebrospinal fluid (CSF) is suppressed, permitting distinction of the superficial infarct from CSF. **D:** Diffusion-weighted image (DWI) demonstrates increased signal (low ADC) only within the right-sided lesion *(white arrows)*, confirming that this represents the acute infarct.

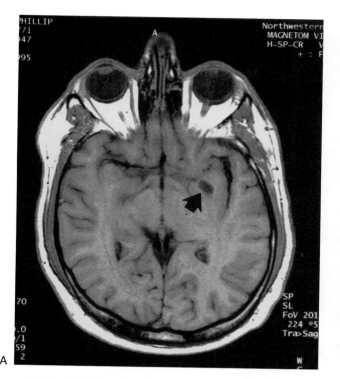

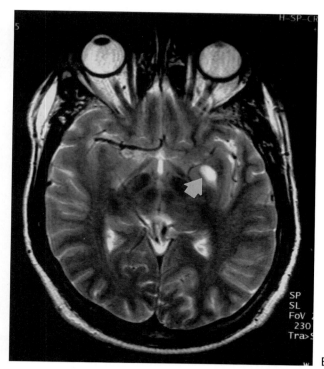

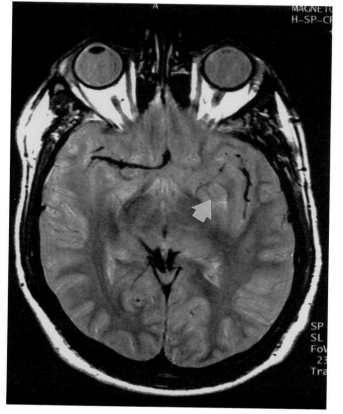

FIG. 9. Ganglionic region perivascular space dilatation resembling lacunar infarction. **A–C:** Axial T1-weighted (A), T2-weighted (B), and proton density weighted (C) MR scans show the typical MR pattern of perivascular space (Virchow–Robin space) dilatation and cyst formation. The intensity of this small rounded perivascular space *(arrows)* characteristically follows cerebrospinal fluid intensity on all MR pulse sequence. It seems to disappear on the proton density scan (C), since cerebrospinal fluid is isointense to brain with this sequence.

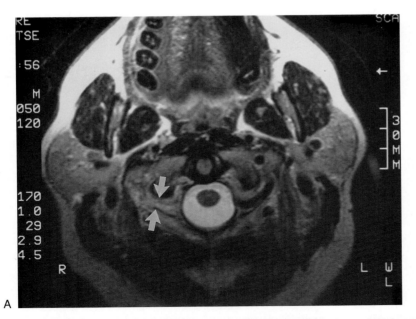

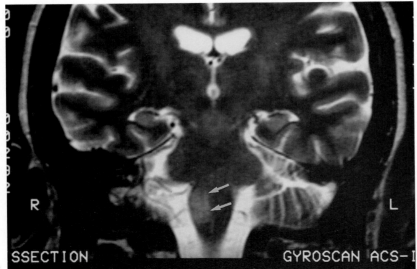

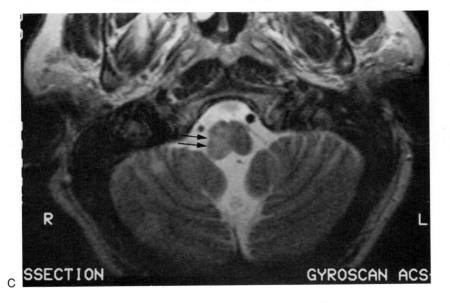

FIG. 10. Patient with a Wallenberg syndrome following right cervical vertebral artery dissection. **A:** Axial T2-weighted MR scan shows absence of flow void within the right vertebral artery at the level of the transverse foramen of the atlas *(arrows)*, due to proximal dissection. **B, C:** Coronal (B) and axial (C) T2-weighted MR scans show hyperintense signal *(arrows)*, within the right lateral medulla, corresponding to infarction in the brainstem distribution of the right posteroinferior cerebellar artery (PICA).

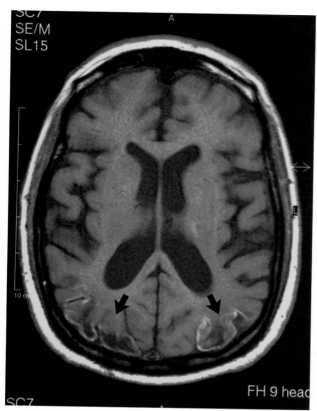

FIG. 11. Chronic watershed infarction with cortical hemorrhage. Noncontrast axial T1-weighted MR scan in a patient following an hypoxic-ischemic episode shows bilateral parieto-occipital low signal with peripheral hyperintensity representing watershed infarction, at the border zone between the middle and posterior cerebral artery territories *(arrows).*

infarcts depends on location, with a cortical pattern for the superficial type and a deep lacunar pattern for the subcortical type (Fig. 11).

INFARCTION RELATED TO VENOUS THROMBOSIS

Acute cerebral venous thrombosis may lead to a fatal outcome if the diagnosis is delayed. A large number of conditions can lead to cerebral venous thrombosis: coagulation disorders, dehydration, infection, trauma, neoplasm, hematologic disorders, and pregnancy (39). The superior sagittal sinus is most commonly occluded, followed by the transverse and cavernous sinuses (40). Clinical symptoms range from headaches to severe neurologic deficit and coma. The clinical picture of venous thrombosis is often nonspecific and depends on location, extent of thrombus, and the presence or absence of venous collaterals (41). Therefore, the diagnosis of venous thrombosis is often unsuspected before radiologic evaluation.

While CT is an excellent screening test, MR with MR venography (MRV) is more definitive for the detection of

intracranial venous thrombosis. Accurate diagnosis in the early phase is important because therapeutic interventions such as direct thrombolysis of clot may prevent permanent neurologic sequelae (41).

Because of the marked developmental variation of intracranial venous anatomy, detection of partial venous thrombosis can be difficult. Portions of the venous sinuses can be absent or hypoplastic and this must not be misinterpreted as thrombosis. There are two common anatomic variations. The first is hypoplasia or absence of the rostral portion of the superior sagittal sinus, anterior to the coronal suture. In this case, well-developed cortical veins can be demonstrated running parallel to the course of the hypoplastic or absent portion of the sinus. The second anatomic variation is hypoplasia or absence of one transverse sinus, usually the left. The deep venous system, especially the internal cerebral veins, basal vein of Rosenthal, and vein of Galen, are much more consistent in their anatomy.

MR with MRV can readily demonstrate venous thrombosis and its consequences on the brain parenchyma. Direct evidence of thrombosis may be seen as absence of the normal hypointense flow void within a dural venous sinus (Fig. 12A). The intensity of intraluminal blood clot will change with time. Acute thrombus is relatively isointense to brain on T1-weighted images. On T2-weighted images, isointensity changes to hypointensity over time as deoxyhemoglobin accumulates. At this time on T2-weighted scans, intraluminal signal may resemble the flow void of a patent sinus. Subacute clots have high signal on all pulse sequences when, T2 shortening is lost due to cell lysis, and T1 hyperintensity occurs due to the accumulation of methemoglobin. Contrast enhanced scans may also be helpful. A normal patent sinus will enhance homogeneously on postcontrast T1-weighted images. Absence of this normal enhancement can be seen in the occluded portion of the sinus. The use of contrast enhancement, however, can lead to confusion in distinguishing chronic thrombus, which may enhance directly from a normal patent sinus that enhances uniformly (Fig. 12B). The fact that chronic clot enhances, makes the distinction of clot from the adjacent normal patent sinus impossible with this technique. Thus, a false-negative diagnosis may occur in patients with chronic dural sinus occlusion using contrast-enhanced studies alone (42,43).

MRA with an inferior presaturation pulse to eliminate arterial signal (MR venography) can be very useful for distinguishing chronic sinus occlusion from normal patent sinus. Various MRA techniques are available, eg, time-of-flight (TOF) or phase contrast (PC) MR angiography. Because subacute clot has a short T1, and tissues with a short T1 are visible on TOF MRA, the distinction between the high signal of subacute clot and similar intensity produced by slow flow within the sinus cannot always be made with TOF MRA. PC MRA is considered the most accurate technique for distinguishing flow within a patent sinus from subacute thrombus because this technique employs subtraction, which elim-

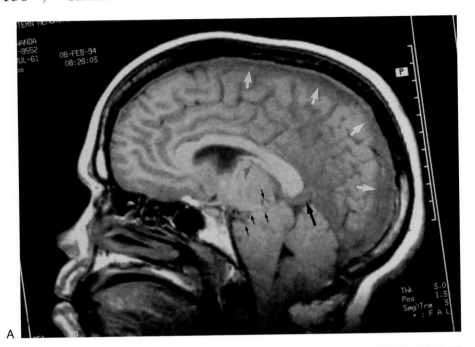

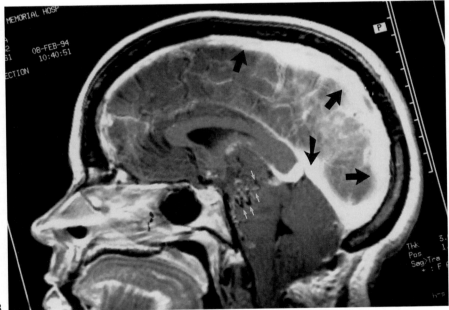

FIG. 12. Cerebral venous thrombosis in a 28-year-old woman. A: Noncontrast sagittal T1-weighted MR scan fails to reveal a normal hypointense flow void in the superior sagittal sinus *(white arrows)* and in the deep cerebral veins and Vein of Galen *(black arrow)*. The sinus is only slightly hypointense relative to gray matter. Collateral venous drainage, represented by signal voids along the brainstem *(small arrows)*, are also evident. B: Following contrast administration, a T1-weighted sagittal MR scan shows extensive abnormal enhancement within the superior sagittal sinus, the deep cerebral veins, the vein of Galen, and the straight sinus (note enhancement of chronic thrombus and dura, *arrows*). The collateral mesencephalic veins *(small arrows)* are visible.

inates high intensity clot from the image, leaving signal only related to flow (44).

The MR pattern of parenchymal ischemic damage due to venous thrombosis differs from that observed in cases of arterial ischemia. There are three patterns observed in venous infarction: brain swelling, hydrocephalus, and parenchymal hematoma. Brain swelling is characterized by cortical sulcal effacement, inconstantly accompanied by T2 signal abnormalities. When present, the signal intensity changes are less extensive than the overall mass effect. This abnormal signal may be reversible with treatment because it does not necessarily reflect infarction.

Ventricular enlargement probably occurs due to decreased venous drainage and constant or increased CSF production. Parenchymal hemorrhage is seen more frequently with venous infarction than with ischemic arterial infarction. Parenchymal and subarachnoid hemorrhage may occur when venous pressure exceeds the limit of the structural vascular wall. These infarcts tend to involve venous territories, which are quite different and anatomically less consistent than arterial territories. The abnormal arterial and parenchymal enhancement patterns observed in arterial occlusive infarction generally do not occur with venous infarction, reflecting an absence of BBB breakdown (39).

Deep cerebral venous infarction is a rare condition, representing only 6% of all venous occlusions. Bilateral signal intensity abnormalities within the basal ganglia and thalami may be the only imaging abnormality in some cases. This finding is not specific because it can be seen in other pathologic conditions such as glioma, germinoma, Wernicke's encephalopathy, carbon monoxide intoxication, and arterial infarction related to basilar artery occlusion (41,45).

VASCULITIS

The vasculitides are a group of uncommon central nervous system (CNS) pathologies characterized by inflammation and necrosis of blood vessel walls. There are infectious and noninfectious etiologies. Non-infectious causes include systemic lupus erythematous, polyarteritis nodosa, Wegener's granulomatosis, primary angiitis of the CNS (PACNS), and idiopathic granulomatous angiitis (IGANS) (46). Angiitis is also commonly associated with drug abuse (methamphetamine) and, recently, HIV infection.

MRI appears to be very sensitive for the detection of the parenchymal effects of vasculitis, which include cerebral infarction and parenchymal hemorrhage. Recent reports have demonstrated that vasculitis patients with positive angiography almost uniformly have abnormal MRI (47). If MRI demonstrates no abnormalities, the possibility of vasculitis is unlikely, and these patients may not need angiography. Conversely, if an MR study is abnormal, angiography should be performed to confirm the diagnosis. However, MR may be abnormal when angiography is negative, particularly in cases of IGANS. In such cases a meningeal biopsy may be required for diagnosis. MR should be the initial screening test for the evaluation of patients with suspected intracranial vasculitis (47,48).

MR abnormalities usually consist of punctate areas of abnormal high signal on T2-weighted images, most often found within the periventricular and subcortical white matter. Alternatively, frank cortical infarction may occur. While these findings are not specific, in the correct clinical context, they are highly suggestive of vasculitis. Contrast-enhanced studies can demonstrate linear or punctate enhancement in white matter, with or without abnormal signal on T2-weighted images (47). These areas of abnormal enhancement correspond to a combination of vascular and perivascular inflammatory changes.

Arteritis may also cause focal aneurysmal dilatation of cortical arteries (mycotic aneurysms), which may be associated with infectious subacute bacterial endocarditis (SBE). The slow turbulent flow within the areas of dilatation can be demonstrated by contrast-enhanced MR as focal intravascular enhancement. Resulting nodular sulcal lesions may resemble superficial cortical metastases (Fig.13) (49).

MRI OF HEMORRHAGE

Diagnostic imaging of nontraumatic intracranial hemorrhage is currently accomplished with noncontrast CT and/or MRI. CT offers several practical advantages relative to MRI. CT is fast, widely available, less expensive, and easier to interpret in the acute setting. On the other hand, MRI offers multiplanar imaging, more precise lesion localization, and improved tissue characterization, which often results in improved specificity regarding the etiology of hemorrhage. Although CT and MRI are clearly complementary, it is increasingly important for the practicing clinician to choose the most appropriate diagnostic test for specific clinical circumstances. Toward that end, this section will review the main factors responsible for the MR appearance of intraparenchymal hemorrhage. Unique considerations that affect the MR evaluation of subarachnoid hemorrhage and extraaxial hematomas will be discussed. Finally, select entities where the MR appearance of hemorrhage facilitates a more precise differential diagnosis will be presented.

Physical Factors

The appearance of intracranial hemorrhage on MRI is influenced by intrinsic factors such as age, location, and etiology of the hemorrhage, as well as extrinsic factors such as the strength of the magnetic field and the pulse sequence parameters utilized for imaging. For the purposes of this discussion, the appearance of hemorrhage will be examined in five time frames, hyperacute (12–24 hours), acute (12 hours to 3 days), early subacute (3 days to 1 week), late subacute (1 week to months), and chronic (months to years). A complete discussion of the physical basis for the appearance of intracranial hemorrhage on MRI is beyond the scope of this chapter. Interested readers are referred to excellent reviews by Bradley, Gomori, and Hayman (50–52). A simplified approach will be presented that requires review of two physical concepts: magnetic susceptibility and dipole–dipole interactions.

Magnetic susceptibility refers to the ability of tissues within a magnetic field to generate their own local magnetic field. When a substance generates a local magnetic field that augments the main magnetic field, it is termed *paramagnetic*. The number of unpaired electrons within the outer shell of atoms or molecules is responsible for the paramagnetic effect. The greater the number of unpaired electrons, the larger the effect. In the normal state, oxyhemoglobin, which is nonparamagnetic (diamagnetic), predominates within the afferent cerebral circulation. When oxyhemoglobin is isolated from an oxygen-rich environment, progressive changes occur that yield three paramagnetic products: deoxyhemoglobin, methemoglobin, and hemosiderin. The paramagnetic effects of these three hemoglobin byproducts are in large part responsible for the distinctive MR appearance of the various stages of intracranial hemorrhage, particularly at high field (1.5 T) (51).

Paramagnetic substances alter the local magnetic environment experienced by individual hydrogen nuclei in water. When placed within an external magnetic field (the MR

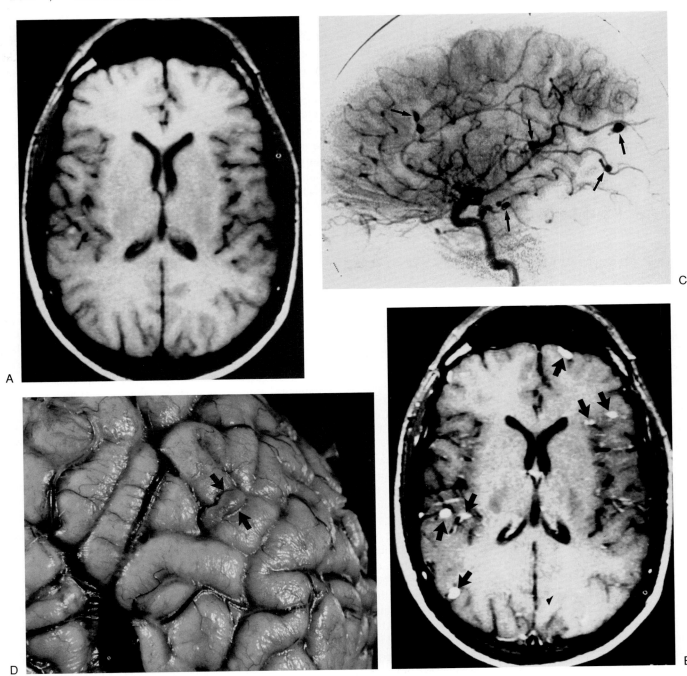

FIG. 13. Slow arterial flow resulting in intravascular enhancement in a case of mycotic aneurysm formation related to HIV infection and chronic methamphetamine abuse. **A,B:** Pre- (A) and post- (B) infusion T1-weighted MR scans show multiple bilateral peripheral areas of contrast enhancement, representing focal regions of arterial ectasia and mycotic aneurysm formation. Arterial structures may enhance when flow is sluggish, as in this case. **C:** Right internal carotid angiogram confirms the presence of focal arterial aneurysms *(arrows)*, corresponding to the areas of nodular sulcal enhancement seen in (B). **D:** Gross pathologic specimen shows focal dilatation of a frontal cortical artery *(arrow)*, also corresponding to the enhancement seen in (B). (From ref. 49.)

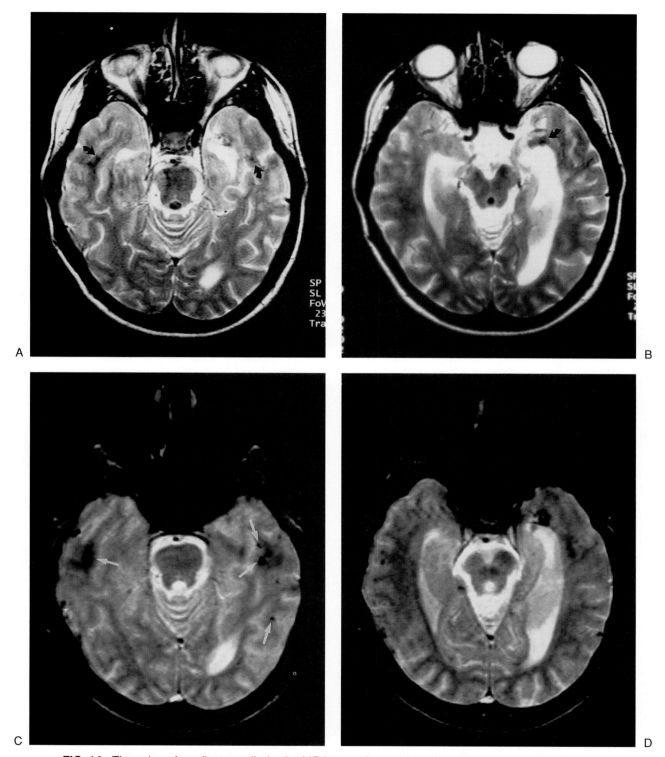

FIG. 14. The value of gradient-recalled echo MR images for the detection of hemorrhage, in a 26-year-old woman with a history of subacute/chronic head trauma and diffuse axonal (shearing) injury. **A, B:** Routine T2-weighted turbo-spin-echo MR images obtained through the temporal lobes at two adjacent levels reveal mild ventricular dilatation, and a few subtle areas of low signal intensity at the junction of gray and white matter (*arrows,* A, B). **C, D:** Gradient-recalled MR images at levels corresponding to those obtained in A and B better demonstrate multiple focal areas of magnetic susceptibility (low signal intensity related to T2* shortening) in areas of hemorrhage within the sites of axonal injuries *(white arrows)*. Gradient echo pulse sequences, which do not incorporate a 180° refocusing pulse, are more sensitive to tissues that create a local magnetic field, such as hemorrhage. The turbo-spin-echo pulse sequences in widespread use today are less sensitive to hemorrhage than the old standard spin echo sequences in use several years ago.

199

scanner) paramagnetic substances generate their own local magnetic field, which is additive with the externally applied field. This induces magnetic field inhomogeneity that affects MR relaxation processes, causing accelerated signal loss due to spin dephasing and loss of transverse coherence (enhanced T2 relaxation). This results in decreased signal intensity on T2-weighted images, with an effect roughly proportional to the square of the field strength of the MR scanner. Therefore, high-field MR scanners (1.5 T) are more sensitive for the detection of hemorrhage than low-field scanners (<1.0 T) (53). Furthermore, signal loss due to hemorrhage is exaggerated on $T2^*$ (parital flip angle) gradient-refocused echo se-

quences, which are highly sensitive to magnetic susceptibility effects due to the absence of a 180° refocusing pulse (Fig. 14). The T2 hypointensity from hemorrhage is less prominent on turbo or fast spin echo sequences, which employ multiple 180° refocusing pulses. For this reason, many centers include a $T2^*$ gradient echo sequence in imaging protocols tailored for the detection of intracranial hemorrhage (54).

Dipole–dipole interactions are responsible for the T1 shortening associated with the paramagnetic methemoglobin found in subacute hemorrhage, which results in increased signal intensity on T1-weighted images. This interaction is

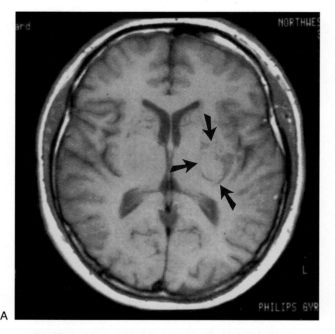

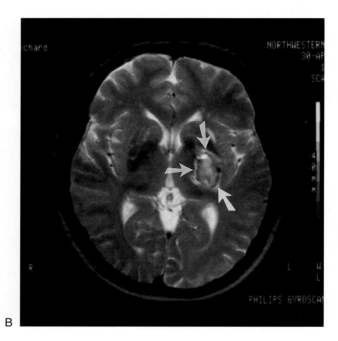

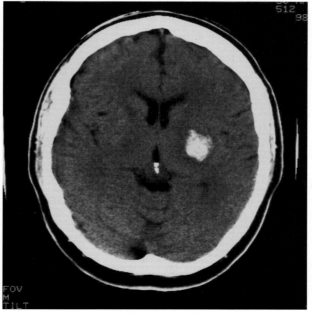

FIG. 15. Intracerebral hematoma in a 59-year-old man with left hemiplegia. **A, B:** Axial T1- (A) and T2- (B) weighted MR scans demonstrate a lesion located at the junction of the posterior limb of the left external capsule and lateral lentiform nucleus *(arrows)*. The signal characteristics (isointense to gray matter on T1- and hyperintense on T2-weighted MR images) are consistent hyperacute hematoma. A tumor would likely be hypointense on T1 images. Later on, deoxyhemoglobin accumulates within red cells, resulting in T2 hypointensity, and even later methemoglobin will accumulate, resulting in T1 hyperintensity. A faint hypointense ring at the periphery of the lesion is poorly defined. **C:** Noncontrast CT scan shows high attenuation within this left basal ganglionic acute hematoma.

proportional to the inverse of the distance between the hydrogen nucleus and methemoglobin to the sixth power. Although deoxyhemoglobin is also paramagnetic, the conformation of the hemoglobin molecule results in a relatively large distance between hydrogen nuclei and deoxyhemoglobin such that T1 shortening is not observed. Deoxyhemoglobin is referred to as a shielded paramagnetic substance.

Timing

Hyperacute Hemorrhage

Hyperacute hemorrhage refers to a collection of blood in which oxyhemoglobin predominates. This is rarely encountered in the clinical setting because several hours commonly elapses between the onset of hemorrhage and a patient being referred for MRI. A hyperacute hematoma may have a nonspecific appearance on MRI because oxyhemoglobin is not paramagnetic. Hyperacute hemorrhages can behave like other lesions with increased water content, and are typically iso- or low signal on T1-weighted images and high signal on T2-weighted images. With clot retraction in the hyperacute phase, the increased protein content of the hemorrhage will result in the lesion being iso- or hyperintense on T1-weighted images, which can facilitate differentiation from other mass lesions. Furthermore, a hypointense rim may be seen along the periphery of hyperacute hemorrhage, which may provide an additional clue to the diagnosis (55). Hyperacute hemorrhage, however, is more readily identified on CT, which remains the initial examination of choice for its evaluation (Fig. 15).

Acute Hemorrhage

In the acute setting, after the initial accumulation of blood within the brain parenchyma, there is clot retraction and resorption of serum. The hematoma becomes isolated from the normal cerebral circulation, and oxyhemoglobin rapidly deoxygenates to yield deoxyhemoglobin. The increased protein content of the retracted clot, which is responsible for the high attenuation noted on noncontrast CT, causes the hematoma to be slightly hyperintense relative to white matter on T1-weighted images. Unlike CT in the acute setting, which typically demonstrates high attenuation characteristics of acute hemorrhage, the MR appearance on T1-weighted images remains relatively nonspecific.

T2-weighted images demonstrate a marked decrease in signal intensity related to magnetic susceptibility effects. This is due to local field inhomogeneity related to paramagnetic deoxyhemoglobin within intact red blood cells. Gradient echo images will exaggerate this effect and are often useful for diagnosis of acute hemorrhage (Fig. 16).

Subacute Hemorrhage: Early

In the early subacute stage, oxidation of deoxyhemoglobin to methemoglobin occurs within intact red blood cells. Methemoglobin is paramagnetic, and the change in structure of hemoglobin associated with further oxidation promotes T1 shortening, which results in marked increased signal intensity on T1-weighted images. Typically this begins at the periphery of the clot and progresses inward, resulting initially in a bright rim on T1-weighted images. The differential diagnosis of lesions that demonstrate increased signal intensity on non-contrast T1-weighted images is relatively limited and deserves mention at this time. Fat, substances with elevated protein content (mucous or fluid within certain intracranial tumors, ie, craniopharyngioma), paramagnetic moieties such as melanin, free radicals (in the wall of parenchymal abscesses), and ions including calcium, manganese, and copper exhibit high signal intensity on T1-weighted images. Correlation with the clinical history, morphology, and location of the lesion, as well as appearance on other imaging sequences (ie, T2, fat suppression) typically allows differentiation of these from subacute hemorrhage.

On T2-weighted images, paramagnetic methemoglobin in intact red blood cells results in low signal intensity similar to that of deoxyhemoglobin. The combination of bright signal intensity on T1 and markedly decreased signal intensity on T2 is relatively specific for paramagnetic substances and, with the appropriate morphology, is highly suggestive of subacute hemorrhage (Fig. 17) (56).

Subacute Hemorrhage: Late

The late subacute stage is characterized by lysis of red cells. Concurrently, there is dilution of extracellular methemoglobin and breakdown of the proteinaceous clot. High signal intensity persists on T1-weighted images due to methemoglobin; however the loss of the red cell membrane and the decrease in protein content results in increased signal intensity on T2-weighted images. Bright signal intensity on T1 and T2 images is highly specific for hemorrhage. Furthermore, at the periphery of the hemorrhage, the early accumulation of hemosiderin and ferritin within macrophages produces a low signal intensity ring, most prominent on T2-weighted images.

Chronic Hemorrhage

The hallmark of chronic hemorrhage is low signal intensity on T2-weighted images due to accumulation of ferritin and hemosiderin in macrophages, the final breakdown products of hemoglobin. The resulting low intensity first appears at the margin of the lesion during the late subacute stage of hematoma evolution. With time, the rim thickens. Encephalomalacia (areas of low signal intensity) is the residuum of

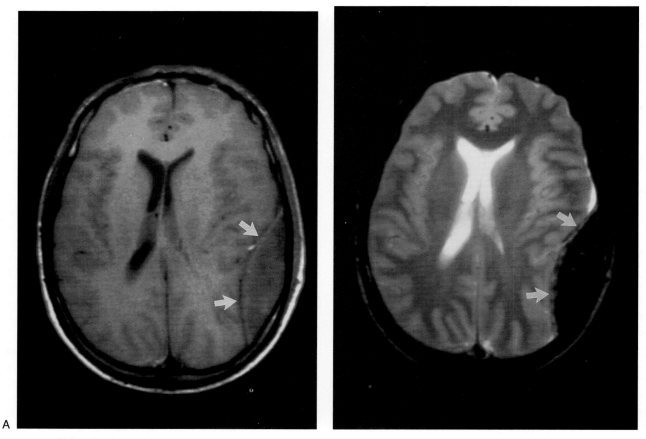

A   B

FIG. 16. A 32-year-old man with an acute epidural hematoma. **A, B:** MR scans obtained 6 hours posttrauma. Axial T1-weighted (A) and T2-weighted (B) scans demonstrate an extraaxial left frontoparietal lenticular-shaped clot, with signal intensity characteristics of acute blood. T1-weighted scans show isointensity (the lesion is too acute to contain oxidized hemoglobin—methemoglobin), whereas T2-weighted scans show marked hypointensity related to intracellular deoxyhemoglobin. The diagnosis is easily made by the anatomic configuration; the intensity characteristics are less important in this case.

an uncomplicated intraparenchymal hemorrhage. This appearance can persist indefinitely.

Subarachnoid and Extraaxial Hemorrhage

It is generally accepted that MRI is less sensitive than non-contrast CT for the diagnosis of acute subarachnoid hemorrhage. One important explanation for this observation is the exposure of red blood cells to the oxygen-rich environment of cerebral spinal fluid rather than the relatively oxygen-poor environment encountered by an intraparenchymal hematoma (57). Blood deoxygenates more slowly within the subarachnoid space than within the brain parenchyma, prolonging the time course for demonstrating the sequential MRI signal changes characteristic of hemorrhage (58). CSF pulsation artifacts, as well as the inhibition of clot retraction and the absence of hemoconcentration, are additional factors that make the diagnosis of acute subarachnoid hemorrhage difficult and less reliable on MRI.

Recently, investigators have applied FLAIR (fluid attenuation inversion recovery) MR pulse sequences for the diagnosis of subarachnoid hemorrhage. This technique involves the application of inversion prepulses that null the bright signal intensity from CSF, thereby yielding heavily T2-weighted images with dark CSF. Subarachnoid hemorrhage appears bright relative to nulled low-signal-intensity CSF. The appearance is not specific because meningitis, leptomeningeal metastatic disease, and fat within the subarachnoid space from a ruptured dermoid tumor may also produce this pattern. However, clinical history and attention to chemical shift artifact should facilitate the differential diagnosis. MRI can be used to confirm the diagnosis of subacute subarachnoid hemorrhage when CT findings have returned to normal. It may be helpful in determining which aneurysm bled in patients with multiple berry aneurysms, by showing localized perianeurysmal clot.

Similar considerations apply to the MR evaluation of subdural and epidural hematomas. Although these lesions follow an orderly progression between the five stages from

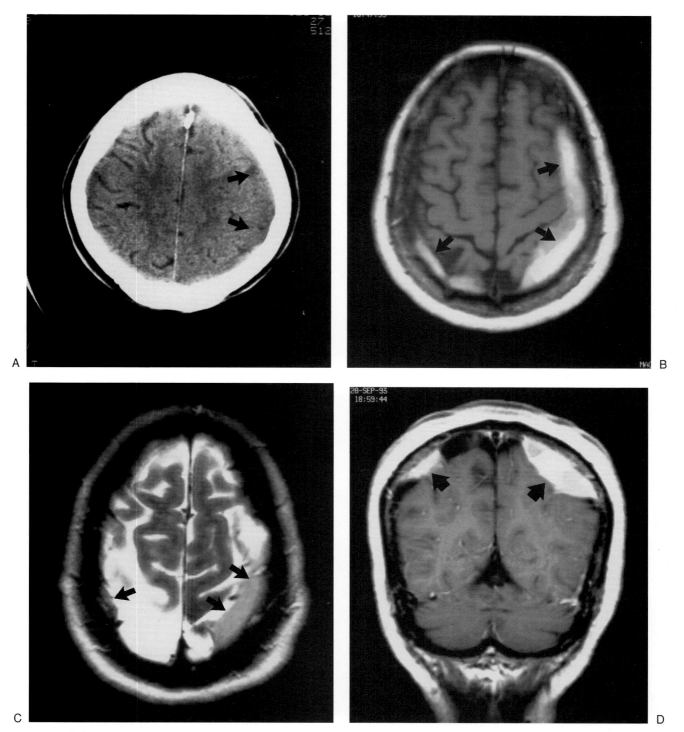

FIG. 17. Bilateral subacute subdural hematomas, relatively occult on CT, well demonstrated on MRI. **A:** Noncontrast CT scan suggests the presence of an isodense left subdural hematoma *(arrows)*. **B–D:** Axial T1- (B), T2- (C), and coronal T1- (D) weighted images demonstrate bilateral subdural hematomas *(arrows)*. The high intensity on T1-weighted images is related to T1 shortening due to accumulation of methemoglobin, and the low intensity on T2-weighted images is due to other blood products, which may include residual intracellular methemoglobin and accumulating ferritin and hemosiderin.

hyperacute to chronic, the progression is typically slower than that for intraparenchymal hemorrhage, due to the high vascularity of the dura, which results in high oxygen tension for extraaxial red blood cells. Nevertheless, the exquisite anatomic detail provided by MR readily detects extraaxial hemorrhage without attention to intensity patterns. MR is also extremely valuable in differentiating various causes of CT-documented low-attenuation extraaxial fluid collections. Chronic subdural hematomas can have a relatively nonspecific appearance on CT. Whereas MRI usually demonstrates slightly greater intensity than CSF on T1 and hyperintensity on proton density images. Subdural hygromas are typically isointense with CSF on all pulse sequences.

Select Disease Entities

The ability to characterize and diagnose different types of intracranial hemorrhage has proven invaluable for the diagnosis of a variety of cerebrovascular disorders. The remainder of this section will review several of these disorders (cervicocephalic dissection, giant aneurysm, vascular malformation, and intracranial vascular tumors) where an understanding of the varying appearances of hemorrhage on MR facilitates differential diagnosis.

Cervicocephalic Arterial Dissection

Cervicocephalic dissection is an underdiagnosed cause of stroke. Carotid or vertebral dissection may be spontaneous or posttraumatic in nature. Dissection may be associated with fibromuscular dysplasia, Marfan's syndrome, arteritis, atherosclerosis, chiropractic manipulations, and seemingly insignificant trauma. Clinically, patients with carotid dissection characteristically present with ipsilateral headache with or without neck pain, Horner's syndrome, and in some cases hemispheric symptoms in the distribution of the affected circulation. A high index of suspicion is necessary for diagnosis and early MRI is should be performed because of the potential for a good long-term prognosis with appropriate therapy.

MRI typically demonstrates subintimal hemorrhage (methemoglobin) within the wall of the affected vessel in the subacute phase. On T1-weighted images, the subintimal clot shows increased signal intensity adjacent to the compromised or occluded lumen (crescent sign) (Fig. 18) (59). Evaluation of the vessel in question with T1-weighted fat-suppressed sequences is recommended because high-signal-intensity fat around the vessel may obscure visualization of high-signal-intensity subintimal methemoglobin. Depending on the clinical circumstances, patients with an MR diagnosis of dissection may not require catheter angiography to confirm the diagnosis prior to initiating therapy. Catheter angiography is recommended if the presence of a pseudoaneurysm would affect clinical decision making, particularly when the dissection extends intracranially, where rupture could result catastrophic subarachnoid hemorrhage.

Giant Aneurysm

Giant aneurysms (diameter >2.5 cm) often present with symptoms of mass effect. Prior to the advent of MRI, they were frequently confused with other mass lesions, most commonly neoplasm, based on less than specific CT features.

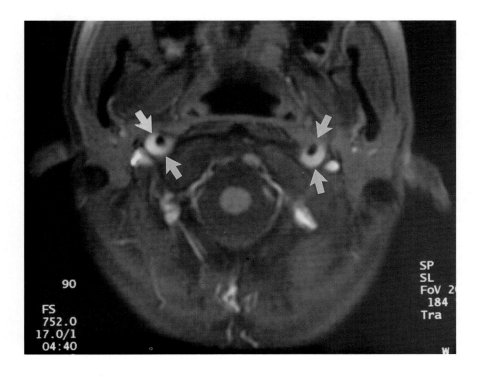

FIG. 18. Traumatic bilateral internal carotid artery dissection in a 35-year-old-woman with pain in both arms and neck following a bicycle accident. A noncontrast axial T1-weighted MR scan with fat suppression shows circumferential regions of high signal intensity blood (methemoglobin) around the lumen of the two internal carotid arteries (ICAs) near the skull base *(arrows)*. Note relative enlargement of both ICAs due to subadventitial extension of blood, a finding characteristic of dissection.

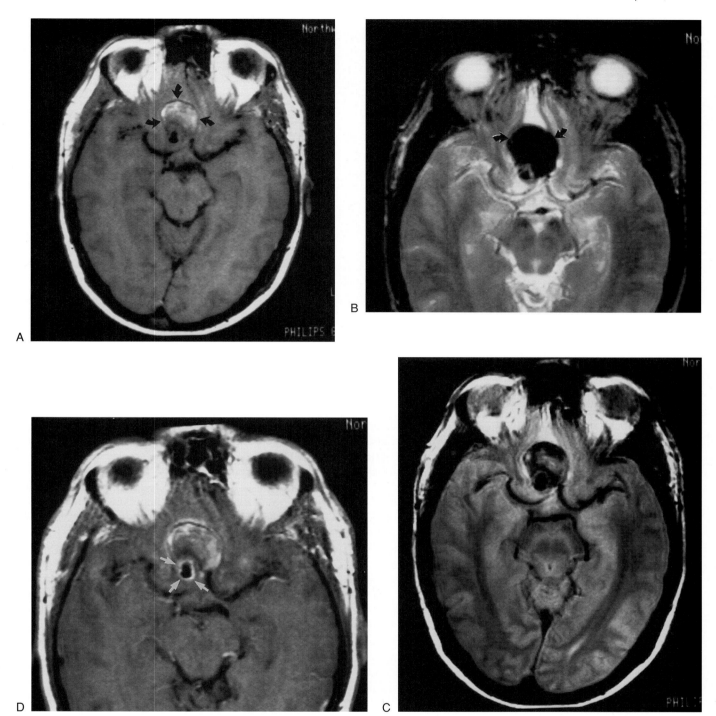

FIG. 19. Giant partially thrombosed internal carotid artery aneurysm. **A–C:** Axial T1- (A), T2- (B), and proton density (C) weighted MR scans demonstrate a mixed signal intensity mass with concentric laminated rings projecting above the planum sphenoidale. Asymmetric, peripheral, heterogeneous hyperintensity on T1- and proton weighted images and hypointensity on T2- *(black arrows)* indicate mural thrombus within the aneurysm, due to blood in various stages of evolution. **D:** The patent lumen of the aneurysm enhances peripherally after gadolinium administration *(arrows)*. The enhancement corresponds to slow flow in the periphery of the patent lumen.

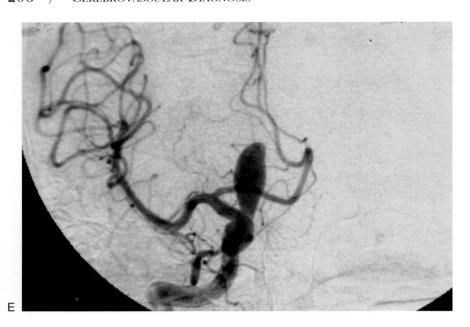

E

FIG. 19. *Continued.* **E:** Conventional carotid angiography confirms aneurysm luminal anatomy.

The sensitivity of MR to blood flow and aneurysmal thrombus result in a characteristic MR appearance of giant aneurysm. The need for preoperative catheter angiography of solid intracranial lesions to exclude the possibility of aneurysm is rarely necessary.

MR typically demonstrates low signal (flow void) within the parent vessel and patent lumen of the aneurysm. Because giant aneurysms are frequently partially thrombosed, MR shows a laminated appearance of blood products of various ages. The blood closest to the patent lumen is typically subacute methemoglobin, which is bright on both T1- and T2-weighted images. The blood products at the periphery of the lesion are more chronic (hemosiderin) and demonstrate low signal on T2-weighted images. Altered flow dynamics within the lumen of the aneurysm also contribute to this appearance. Phase contrast MRA may be more effective at distinguishing slow flow in a patent aneurysm lumen from laminated clot (Fig. 19). Giant aneurysms are also frequently associated with a low-signal-intensity rim, particularly when they are peripherally calcified (better detected on CT), and may be associated with parenchymal edema depending on their location. Artifact related to pulsation of blood flow seen along the phase encoding direction with MRI is an important clue to the diagnosis of giant aneurysm. Recognition of this constellation of findings allows confident differentiation of a solid neoplasm from aneurysm.

Arteriovenous Malformation

Initial imaging evaluation of pial arteriovenous malformations (AVMs) is typically accomplished with CT and MR. CT is most useful in the acute setting to detect intracranial hemorrhage. Additional findings that suggest the presence of an AVM on noncontrast CT include curvilinear calcification (20–30%), and serpiginous areas of high attenuation, which represent blood pool within dilated vessels. These enhance with contrast. AVMs that have not bled typically have very little if any associated mass effect and may be difficult to detect on CT without intravenous contrast material.

MRI adds additional specificity to CT in the acute setting and is the screening examination of choice in patients presenting with headaches, seizures, or cranial nerve palsy. MRI demonstrates serpiginous areas of flow void (low signal intensity), often associated with mixed signal intensity from slower flow. MRI also provides important prognostic information by demonstrating the size and location of the lesion as well as the presence of acute or prior hemorrhage. The capability of MRI to detect chronic blood products also permits recognition of small or thrombosed AVMs that are occult to CT (or catheter angiography). The detection of flow voids adjacent to or within an intraparenchymal hematoma suggests the diagnosis of AVM. These lesions may be further evaluated with MRA, although conventional angiography is required for therapeutic planning.

Other Vascular Malformations

Vascular malformations consisting of capillaries (capillary telangiectasias) and cavernous veins (cavernous malformations), and thrombosed AVMs may be occult to angiography. These lesions are best diagnosed on MRI but may be indistinguishable from one another.

Cavernous malformations (angiomas) are usually congenital abnormalities of cerebral vessels that affect 0.5–0.7% of the population. They can occur as isolated lesions or in a familial form where multiple lesions are the rule. Imaging features are related to the presence of blood products of varying ages within the lesion. The lesions are typically lob-

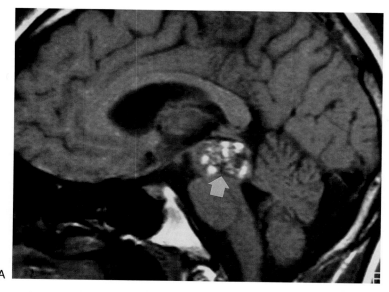

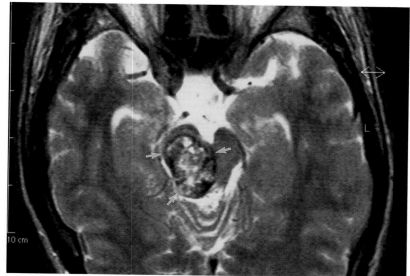

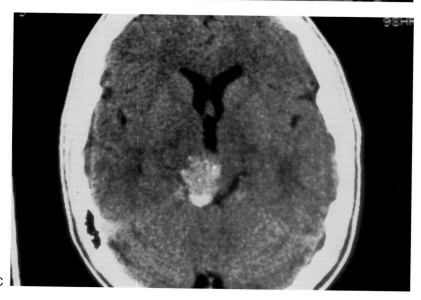

FIG. 20. Cavernous malformation (angioma) in 21-year-old woman with left arm numbness and tingling. **A, B:** Noncontrast T1 sagittal (A) and axial T2 (B) MR images demonstrate a popcorn-like intraaxial mass of mixed signal intensity, within the right midbrain (arrow). Focal areas of increased signal intensity are seen within the lesion on the T1-weighted image, and a rim of low signal intensity is seen around the lesion (arrows) on the T2-weighted image. This mixed signal corresponds to different stages of blood product degradation and is characteristic of cavernous malformation. **C:** Noncontrast CT scan demonstrates calcification within the lesion.

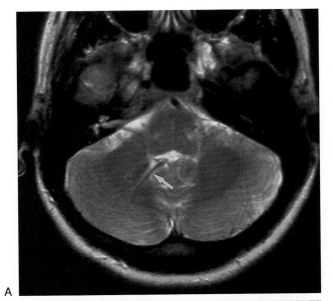

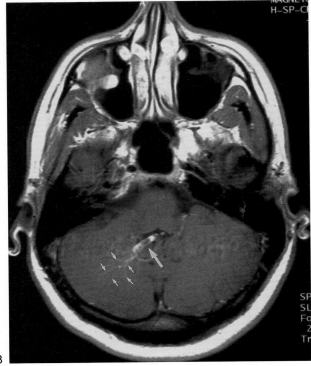

FIG. 21. Infratentorial venous malformation (angioma). **A, B:** T2-weighted precontrast (A) and T1-weighted postcontrast (B) MR scans show radially arranged dilated medullary veins *(small arrows, B)*, and a large central draining vein *(white arrow)*, typical of venous malformation. While often found incidentally, some lesions in the posterior fossa have been associated with hemorrhage.

ulated with a well-defined hypointense rim consisting of chronic blood breakdown products. Decreased signal intensity is often seen extending into the adjacent white matter, due to blood products that diffuse outside of the lesion. This is well-demonstrated on T2-weighted spin echo images, al-

though blooming of the low signal abnormality is better seen on T2*-weighted gradient echo images. Centrally, the lesions frequently show high signal intensity on T1- and T2-weighted images due to the presence of subacute methemoglobin. Rebleeding studies occurs frequently, leading to an ever-changing pattern of intralesional intensity (Fig. 20). Due to the increased sensitivity of T2* gradient echo images and the common occurrence of multiple cavernous angiomas, if a solitary OCVM is detected on conventional MRI, evaluation of the entire brain with a T2* gradient echo sequence is suggested.

Recent studies suggest that the familial form of cavernous malformation is a dynamic disease. New lesions have been documented in up to 29% of patients on follow-up MRI within a 5-year time frame (60). Surgery is recommended only for lesions that produce repetitive or progressive symptoms. High-resolution multiplanar MRI offers a significant advantage in localization of cavernous malformations, particularly in the posterior fossa and spinal cord. Identification of extension of the lesion to a pial surface facilitates surgical planning.

Capillary telangectasia is a common lesion, infrequently identified during life, and rarely symptomatic. Radiation-induced telangiectasias bleed frequently and can mimic multiple cavernous malformations on MRI. These lesions are due to ectatic thin-walled vessels surrounded by hemosiderin and gliosis, with minimal evidence of necrosis. They present with varying amounts of hemorrhage, occasionally frank parenchymal hematoma. A high frequency in children suggest that the developing brain may be more sensitive to radiation damage (61).

Venous malformations are composed of dilated, radially oriented, medullary veins that drain to cortical or ventricular veins (Fig. 21). They are common at autopsy but rarely symptomatic, frequently presenting as an incidental finding on MRI. Patients may rarely present with seizures, headaches, and hemorrhage (more common with cerebellar lesions). A high association with cavernous malformations (30–40%) likely accounts for many of the hemorrhagic venous angiomas reported in the literature, although hemorrhage may be associated with thrombosis of the central drainage vein (62). MRI with contrast is diagnostic and frequently obviates the need for catheter angiography. Postcontrast T1-weighted images demonstrate the radially oriented caput medusae appearance of dilated medullary veins converging toward a large draining central vein. Noncontrast images frequently demonstrate a linear flow void within the draining vein without evidence for edema or mass effect. MR venography can help confirm the diagnosis but is not necessary when conventional scans are diagnostic. The lesion is readily detected by angiography, which is rarely necessary for asymptomatic lesions.

REFERENCES

1. Bryan RN, Willcott MR, Schneiders NJ, et al. Nuclear magnetic resonance evaluation of stroke. *Radiology* 1983;149:189–192.

2. Zimmerman RA, Gill F, Goldberg HI, et al. MRI of sickle cell cerebral infarction. *Neuroradiology* 1987;29:232–235.

3. Inove Y, Takemota K, Miyamoto T, et al. Sequential computed tomography scans in acute cerebral infarction. *Radiology* 1980;135:655–662.

4. Bell BA, Branston NM: CBF and time thresholds for the formation of ischemic cerebral edema, and effect of reperfusion in baboons. *J Neurosurg* 1985;62:31–41.

5. Yuh WTC, Crain MR, Loes DJ, et al. MR imaging of cerebral ischemia: findings in the first 24 hours. *AJNR* 1991;12:621–629.

6. Crain MR, Yuh WTC, Greene GM, et al. Cerebral ischemia: evaluation with contrast-enhanced MR imaging. *AJR* 1991;157:575–583.

7. Bryan RN, Levy LM, Whitlow WD, et al. Diagnosis of acute cerebral infarction: comparison of CT and MR imaging. *AJNR* 1991;12:611–620.

8. Heinz RE, Yeates AE, Djang WT. Significant extracranial carotid stenosis: detection on routine cerebral images. *Radiology* 1989;170:843–848.

9. Russell EJ. Detection of significant extracranial carotid stenosis with routine cerebral MR imaging. *Radiology* 1989;170:623–624.

10. Hornig CR, Dorndorf W, Agnoli AL. Hemorrhagic cerebral infarction: a prospective study. *Stroke* 1986;17:179–185.

11. Hart RG, Easton JD. Hemorrhagic infarcts. *Stroke* 1986;17:586–589.

12. Elster AD. Magnetic resonance contrast enhancement in cerebral infarction. *Neuroimag Clin North Am* 1994;4:89–100.

13. Virapongse C, Brown E, Malat J. Brain ischemia. *Top Magn Reson Imag* 1989;2(1):63–75.

14. Weingarten K. Computed tomography of cerebral infarction. *Neuroimag Clin North Am* 1992;2(3):409–419.

15. Akiro S, Takahashi S, Soma Y, et al. Cerebral infarction: Early detection by means of contrast-enhanced cerebral arteries at MR imaging. *Radiology* 1991;178:433–439.

16. Mathews VM, Monsein LH, Pardo CA, Bryan RN. Histologic abnormalities associated with Gadolinium enhancement on MR in the initial hours of experimental cerebral infarction. *AJNR* 1994;15:573–579.

17. Gado MH, Phelps ME, Coleman RE. An extravascular component in contrast enhancement in cranial computed tomography. *Radiology* 1975;117:589–597.

18. Goldstein GW, Betz AL. Recent advances in understanding brain capillary function. *Ann Neurol* 1983;14:389–395.

19. Virapongse C, Mancuso A, Quisling R. Human brain imaging: Gd-DTPA-enhanced MR imaging. *Radiology* 1986;161:785–794.

20. Asato R, Okumara R, Konishi J. Fogging effect in MR of cerebral infarct. *J Comput Assist Tomogr* 1991;15:160–162.

21. Kuhn MJ, Mikulis DJ, Ayoub DM, et al. Wallerian degeneration after cerebral infarction: evaluation with sequential MR imaging. *Radiology* 1989;172:170–182.

22. Pierpaoli C, Righini A, Linfante I, et al. Histopathologic correlates of abnormal water diffusion in cerebral ischemia: diffusion-weighted MR imaging and light and electron microscopic study. *Radiology* 1993;189:439–448.

23. Maeda M, Itho S, Ide H, et al. Acute stroke in cats: comparison of dynamic susceptibility-contrast MR imaging with T2- and diffusion-weighted MR imaging. *Radiology* 1993;189:227–232.

24. Le Bihan D, Turner R, Douek P, Patronas N. Diffusion MR imaging: clinical application: *AJR* 1992;159:591–598.

25. Nomura Y, Sakuma H, Takeda K, et al. Diffusional anisotropy of the human brain assessed with diffusion-weighted MR: relation with normal brain development and aging. *AJNR* 1994;15:231–238.

26. Chien D, Buxton RB, Kwong KK, et al. MR diffusion imaging of the human brain. *J Comput Assist Tomogr* 1990;14:514–520.

27. Van Bruggen N, Cullen BM, King MD, et al. T2 and diffusion-weighted magnetic resonance imaging of a focal ischemic lesion in rat brain. *Stroke* 1992;23:576–582.

28. Einstein A. *Investigation on the Theory of the Brownian Movement.* New York: Dover, 1956.

29. Sevick RJ, Kucharczyk J, Mintorovitch J, et al. Diffusion-weighted MR imaging and T2 weighted MR imaging in acute cerebral ischemia: comparison and correlation with histopathology. *Acta Neurochir Suppl* 1990;51:110–122.

30. Sevick R, Kanda F, Mintorovitch J. Cytotoxic brain edema: assessment with diffusion-weighted MR imaging. *Radiology* 1992;185:687–690.

31. Spielman D, Butts K, de Crespigny A, Moseley M. Diffusion-weighted imaging of clinical stroke. *Int J Neuroradiol* 1995;1(1):44–55.

32. Minematsu K, Li L, Fisher M, et al. Diffusion-weighted magnetic resonance imaging: rapid and quantitative detection of focal brain ischemia. *Neurology* 1992;42:235–240.

33. Brafman BH, Zimmerman RA, Trojanowski JQ, et al. Brain MR: pathologic correlation with gross and histopathology 1. Lacunar infarction and Virchow–Robin spaces. *AJNR* 1988;9:621–628.

34. Hunt AL, Orrison WW, Yeo RA et al. Clinical significance of MRI white matter lesions in the elderly. *Neurology* 1989;39:1470–1474.

35. Elster A. MR contrast enhancement in brainstem and deep cerebral infarction. *AJR* 1991;158:173–178.

36. Regli L, Regli F, Maeder P, Bogousslavsky J. Magnetic resonance imaging with gadolinium contrast in small deep (lacunar) cerebral infarction. *Arch Neurol* 1993;50:175–180.

37. Cormier PJ, Long ER, Russell EJ. MR imaging of posterior fossa infarctions: vascular territories and clinical correlates. *Radiographics* 1992;2:1079–1096.

38. Adams JH. Patterns of cerebral infarction on their topography and pathogenesis. *Scott Med J* 1967;12:339–348.

39. Yuh WT, Simonson TM, Wang AM, Koci TM, Tali ET, Fisher DJ, Simon JH, Jinkins JR, Tsai F. Venous sinus occlusive diseae: MR findings. *AJNR* 1994;15:309–316.

40. Yasargil A, Damur M. Thrombosis of the cerebral veins and dural sinuse. In: Newton TH, Potts DG, eds. *Radiology of the Skull and Brain: Angiography,* vol 2, book 4. St Louis: CV Mosby, 1974:2375–2400.

41. Erbguth F, Brenner P, Schuierer G, et al. Diagnosis and treatment of deep cerebral vein thrombosis. *Neurosurg Rev* 1991;14:145–148.

42. Zimmerman RD, Ernst RJ. Neuroimaging of cerebrovenous thrombosis. *Neuroimag Clin North Am* 1992;2:463–485.

43. Dormont D, Sag K, Biondi A, Wechsler B, Marsault C. Gadolinium-enhanced MR of chronic dural sinus thrombosis. *AJNR* 1994;16:1347–1352.

44. Crosby DL, Turski PA, Davis WL. Magnetic resonance angiography and stroke. *Neuroimag Clin North Am* 1992;2:509–531.

45. Bell DA, Davis WL, Osborn AG, Harnsberger HR. Bithalamic hyperintensity on T2-weighted MR: vascular causes and evaluation with MR angiography. *AJNR* 1994;15:893–899.

46. Savage COS, Ng YC. The aetiology and pathogenesis of major systemic vasculitis. *Postgrad Med J* 1986;62:627.

47. Greenan TJ, Grossman RI, Goldberg HI. Cerebral vasculitis: MR imaging and angiographic correlation. *Radiology* 1992;182:65–72.

48. Harris KG, Tran DD, Sickels WJ, Cornell SH, Yuh WT. Diagnosing intracranial vasculitis: the roles of MR and angiography. *AJNR* 1994;15:317–330.

49. Lazar EB, Russell EJ, Cohen BA, Brody B, Levy RM. Contrast-enhanced MR of cerebral arteritis: Intravascular enhancement related to flow stasis within area of focal arterial ectasia. *AJNR* 1992;13:271–276.

50. Bradley WG Jr. Hemorrhage and hemorrhagic infections in the brain. *Neuroimag Clin North Am* 1994;4(4):707–732.

51. Gomori JM, Grossman RI: Mechanisms responsible for MR appearance and evaluation of intracranial hemorrhage. *Radiographics* 1988;8(3):427–440.

52. Hayman LA, Taber KH, Ford JJ, Bryan RN. Mechanisms of MR signal alteration by acute intracerebral blood: old concept and new theories. *AJNR* 1991;12(5):899–907.

53. Brooks RA, DiChiro G, Patonas N. MR imaging at different field strenghts: theory and applications. *J Comput Assist Tomogr* 1989;13:194–206.

54. Atlas SW, Mark AS, Grossman RI, Gomori JM. Intracranial hemorrhage gradient-echo MR imaging at 1.5 T: comparison with spin-echo imaging and clinical applications. *Radiology* 1988;168:803–807.

55. Thulborn KR, Brady TJ: Iron in magnetic resonance imaging of cerebral hemorrhage. *Magn Res Imag Q* 1989;5(1):23–28.

56. Gomori JM, Grossman RI, Hackney DB, et al. Variable appearance of subacute intracranial hematomas on high-field spin-echo MR. *AJNR* sman RI, Hackney DB, et al. Variable appearance of subacute intracranial hematomas on high-field spin-echo MR. *AJNR* 1987;8:1019–1026.

57. Grossman RI, Kemp SS, Yu-Ip C, et al. Importance of oxygenation in the appearance of acute subarachnoid hemorrhage on high field magnetic resonance imaging. *Acta Radiol* 1988;139:56–58.

58. Gomori JM, Grossman RI, Yu-Ip C, et al. NMR relaxation times of

blood: dependence on field strength, oxidation state, and cell integrity. *J Comput Assist Tomogr* 1987;11:684–690.

59. Goldberg HI, Grossman RI, Gomori JM, et al. MR diagnosis of cervical internal carotid artery dissecting hemorrhage. *Radiology* 1986;158:157–161.

60. Zambramski JM, Wascher TM, Spetzler RF, Johnson B, et al. The natural history of familial cavernous malformations: results of an ongoing study. *J Neurosurg* 1994;80(3):422–432.

61. Gaensler EHL, Dillon WP, Edwards MSB, Larson DA, Rosenau W, Wilson CB. Radiation-induced telangectasia in the brain simulates cryptic vascular malformations at MR imaging. *Radiology* 1994;193(3):629–636.

62. Field LR, Russell EJ. Spontaneous hemorrhage from a cerebral venous malformation related to thrombosis of the central draining vein: demonstration by serial MRI and conventional angiography. *AJNR* 1995;16:1885–1888.

Cerebrovascular Disease, edited by H. Hunt Batjer.
Lippincott-Raven Publishers, Philadelphia © 1997.

CHAPTER 17

Cerebral Angiography: Capabilities and Indications

Ralph G. Greenlee, Jr., Rance A. Boren, and Phillip D. Purdy

For decades following its introduction in 1952, cerebral angiography was the definitive neurodiagnostic procedure. The advent of computed tomography (CT) and magnetic resonance imaging (MRI) greatly reduced reliance on angiography, especially in the assessment of space-occupying lesions. The development of magnetic resonance angiography (MRA) and continued refinements in ultrasound technology have challenged angiography's role in the assessment of cerebrovascular disease. In addition, angiography is not without risk. This coupled with its relative expensiveness makes it unattractive to some doctors, many patients, and most third-party payers.

The primary goal of angiography is to define vascular anatomy and localize clinically relevant lesions. In general, angiography is indicated when the cause of a neurologic deficit cannot be determined clinically and when rational treatment decisions cannot be made on the basis of less invasive tests. Angiography is unsurpassed in visualizing the cerebral vasculature and allowing the clinician to interpret the significance of individual lesions within the context of the overall vascular anatomy. For example, smooth mid-grade stenosis of the internal carotid becomes less important if high-grade intracranial stenosis is detected. These "tandem lesions" are thought to be uncommon, but their presence may alter individual patient management. Angiography also allows visualization of collateral perfusion pathways. A patient with extensive collateralization may not require surgery or angioplasty, whereas a patient with a compromised vascular distribution and no collateral supply might require prompt and aggressive therapy.

The extent to which angiography is utilized varies widely among institutions and from physician to physician. Unfortunately, financial and political considerations have isolated the clinicians who care for patients with cerebrovascular disease from the radiologists who perform angiography. As a result, one group often has a poor appreciation of the technical limitations of the procedure whereas the other lacks insight into the clinical circumstances that warrant its use. In this chapter we discuss the strengths and weaknesses of angiography as well as the absolute and relative indications for its use. Special attention will be paid to a comparison between angiography and noninvasive imaging modalities, and suggestions for an appropriate mixture of the two will be offered. This chapter is intended to provide a rational model for the clinical use of angiography in the evaluation of ischemic and hemorrhagic cerebrovascular disease. The rapidly expanding field of endovascular therapy is beyond the scope of this chapter and is discussed elsewhere.

TECHNICAL CONSIDERATIONS

Early cerebral angiography was performed via direct carotid puncture or brachial artery injection. Frequently cross-compression was necessary to opacify the vessels of interest or to demonstrate collateral circulation. These techniques have been replaced by the percutaneous femoral approach using the Seldinger technique. With selective catheterization of individual vessels, cross-compression is seldom necessary except in cases of suspected aneurysm where the anterior communicating artery must be visualized. Digital subtraction technology has produced greater resolution with reduced dye loads. Current technology allows simultaneous filming in two planes and provides computerized images that are immediately available for review (1).

In our opinion a complete study for ischemic cerebrovascular disease includes an oblique view of the aortic arch and the origins of the great vessels, lateral and anteroposterior (AP) views of the common carotids and their branches, as well as of the intracranial anterior and posterior circulations.

R. G. Greenlee, Jr., R. A. Boren, and P. D. Purdy: Department of Neurology, University of Texas Southwestern Medical Center, Dallas, Texas 75235.

Under most circumstances only the dominant vertebral artery is injected. However, in cases of suspected aneurysm, both posterior internal carotid artery (PICA) origins should be demonstrated and all communicating vessels visualized. Selective internal carotid artery catheterization should be used to avoid overlap of the extracranial vessels and oblique views should be obtained as necessary.

The minimum laboratory evaluation prior to angiography includes studies of renal function and the coagulation pathways, as well as a hematologic profile. Screening labs obtained initially in our evaluation of suspected stroke patients include determination of serum creatinine, blood urea nitrogen (BUN), prothrombin time (PT), activated partial thromboplastin time (aPTT), and complete blood count (CBC). Informed consent is obtained from the patients by the angiographer. However, the reason for angiography and its risks and benefits are first discussed with the patient by the treating physician. The patient is typically made NPO or allowed only clear liquids prior to the procedure. When necessary, sedation during the procedure is accomplished with short-acting benzodiazepines.

COMPLICATIONS

The most common clinically relevant complications of angiography are nonneurologic and consist largely of hematomas confined to the site of arterial puncture. In a recent study of adverse events associated with cerebral angiography, a 6.9% incidence of hematomas was noted (2). Advancing age, size and number of catheters used, hypertension, and the presence of vascular disease increased the likelihood of hematoma formation. Careful attention to the puncture site, adequate compression after the procedure, and immobilization of the leg in the prone position for 6 hours help to prevent hematoma formation. If the patient requires heparinization for ischemic symptoms, it is preferable to start it several hours after the procedure. If a hematoma develops it can usually be managed by reapplying pressure, but if bleeding continues or distal blood supply is compromised, emergency surgery may be required. Thrombus formation at the puncture site may limit distal flow and is also treated surgically. Frequent monitoring of the pedal pulses should be routine after angiography. Occasionally, paresthesias in the distribution of the median cutaneous nerve of the thigh have been observed following angiography.

Systemic complications secondary to the administration of radiocontrast agents also occur following angiography. These agents may cause a frank allergic response or a more insidious compromise of renal function. Stroke patients are often hypertensive and diabetic, and they frequently have baseline impairment of their renal function. Diabetic nephropathy seems to place the patient at higher risk for subsequent worsening of renal function than does hypertensive nephropathy. The presumed mechanism is local ischemia secondary to decreased renal blood flow and the risk of renal insufficiency increases with the dye load. Solomon et al recently showed that hydration with 0.45% saline for 12 hours before and after angiography is superior to similar hydration with the addition of mannitol or furosemide in the prevention of renal complications (3).

Hypersensitivity reactions ranging from puritis or urticaria (2–3%) to cardiorespiratory collapse (0.01–0.005%) may occur without warning (1). A history of seafood allergy or prior allergic reaction to contrast media should prompt pretreatment with corticosteroids. Prior contrast reaction should not be viewed as an absolute contraindication to angiography because intravenous contrast is much more allergenic than intraarterial contrast. Mild hypersensitivity reactions may be treated with Benadryl (25–50 mg IM) whereas epinephrine (0.2–0.3 mg of 0.01% solution) may be given IV in severe cases. Vagally mediated episodes of hypertension or bradycardia respond to atropine in 0.4-mg boluses.

Recent prospective studies have demonstrated a 1–3% risk of neurologic injury with cerebral angiography. A set of interrelated variables has been repeatedly shown to predict these complications. These include advancing age, increased catheter size, duration of the procedure, increased contrast volume, and transient ischemic attack (TIA) or stroke as an indication for angiography. A variety of mechanisms can account for these neurologic events, and one or more may be operative in a given patient. The catheter tip may serve as a nidus for thrombus formation with emboli arising spontaneously or during contrast injection. Heparin-coated catheters and frequent flushing with heparinized saline can minimize this problem. Incidental contact between the guide wire and the vessel wall may raise an endothelial flap; local thrombus formation with embolization or dissection may then occur. In this instance, a brief course of anticoagulation may be warranted. Surgery is reserved for severe cases. Atherosclerotic plaques may be dislodged or disrupted during angiography with similar consequences. Contrast-induced activation of platelet aggregation is another possibility, but its clinical significance is unknown. Transient encephalopathy and cortical blindness are recognized complications of angiography and may be due to sluggish flow in the microcirculation or fluid shifts due to the osmotic load of the contrast agent dye. Minimizing the total contrast volume and utilizing nonionic contrast media may combat these problems.

In the largest study to date on the major complications of cerebral angiography, Mani et al demonstrated a 1.4% complication rate (2). Slightly over half (35 of 68, or 51%) of the complications were transient neurologic deficits lasting <48 hours. Three patients cleared completely over a slightly longer period. Two patients had a residual hemiparesis and one, a technically difficult case, died. Five patients (6%) required thrombectomy or embolectomy related to thrombosis at the groin. Five patients had hypotensive episodes that responded to conservative measures. Complications were nearly five times more likely at training institutions than at private hospitals. Permanent deficits, however, were identical in both private and academic settings (0.1%).

In skilled hands the overall complication rate remained <1%.

Dion et al prospectively analyzed 1002 patients undergoing cerebral angiography (4). These patients were examined serially by neurologists, so that preexisting conditions were likely to be noticed and postangiography deficits were unlikely to be missed. These authors demonstrated a 1.2% risk of transient neurologic deficit in the 24 hours following angiography and a 1.5% risk in the subsequent 48 hours. In the four patients (0.4%) who suffered permanent neurologic injury or death, the apparent cause was progression of the underlying illness rather than angiographic complications. Slightly over half of the transient neurologic deficits were noted in patients with TIA, and approximately two thirds of all deficits reproduced presenting complaints.

Headache is frequently reported during and immediately after angiography but is seldom considered a serious complication. Ramadan et al found a 33% incidence of postangiography headache (5). The headache was vascular in nature in almost every instance and unilateral in over half of the cases. Postangiography headache was over twice as likely to occur in patients with a history of prior recurrent headaches. These authors suggested that the pain is mediated by catheter- or contrast-induced release of vasoactive substances. Shuaib and Hochinski showed a comparable complication rate between migraineurs and nonmigraineurs (6).

It is clear from these and other studies that patients being evaluated for cerebrovascular disease fare poorly in relation to those undergoing angiography for evaluation of headache, tumor, or epilepsy. Many of the "changes" in these patients' clinical status may reflect progression of their underlying disease rather than actual complications of angiography. Some centers prefer to delay angiography (and endarterectomy) for up to 6 weeks to allow "stabilization." However, the results of the North American Symptomatic Carotid Endarterectomy Trial (NASCET) trial do not support this practice, and the trend now is toward early angiography and surgical intervention (7). Moreover, if thrombolytic therapy for acute stroke proves efficacious, early angiography in carefully selected patients will be imperative.

INDICATIONS

Carotid Occlusive Disease

Atherosclerotic plaques of the cervical carotid are well recognized as a major cause of ischemic infarction. The vast majority of such lesions occur in the proximal 3–4 cm of the internal carotid in the region of the carotid bulb, although the distal common carotid and proximal external carotid may be involved as well. For hemodynamic reasons, the majority of internal carotid plaques form on the posterior wall of the carotid bulb and are best visualized in the lateral projection. In recent controlled clinical trials, the carotid stenosis has been measured at it greatest, regardless of the plane, and the anteroposterior projection may demonstrate significant narrowing that is unappreciated in the lateral projection. For this reason both views are mandatory.

Well-designed clinical trials conclusively link the extent of carotid stenosis as measured by angiography to both the risk of ischemic stroke and benefit from endarterectomy (8,9). The European Carotid Surgery Trial (ECST) measured stenosis by comparing the smallest residual lumen with the expected width of the carotid bulb at that point. In NASCET, the stenosis was measured by comparing the smallest residual lumen with the width of the normal vessel distal to the bulb. Some authors suggest simplifying matters by measuring the residual lumen at its narrowest point without further calculations. The NASCET method has become preferred for a number of reasons:

1. It is based on the sound hemodynamic principle that stenosis is only significant when related to distal vessel caliber. In other words, since the carotid bulb is dilated with respect to the distal internal carotid artery, it can be partially filled with plaque without any effect on blood flow. It is only when the stenosis exceeds the width of the distal vessel that hemodynamic compromise occurs.
2. While still subjective, the NASCET method does not call for the degree of imagination required by the ECST method. Although normative values exist for the carotid bulb, it is difficult to measure something that "isn't there."
3. The majority of recent trials have utilized the NASCET method and confirmed its usefulness, thereby adding to its validity.

Clearly, any assessment based on hemodynamic principles alone ignores a number of factors related to the production of ischemic strokes. For example, a 50% stenosis by the ECST method suggests that a fair amount of potentially embologenic plaque is present, but this lesion would be graded as a 0% stenosis by the NASCET criteria. Bladin et al suggest a "carotid stenosis index" that uses the width of the common carotid artery to obtain a theoretical width for the carotid bulb (10). This method is probably more reproducible than the NASCET or ECST methods. The final resolution of these issues is of more than theoretical concern as it influences clinical decision making. The NASCET method, flaws included, has proven to be valid in the evaluation of patients with minor stroke and TIA, and is currently the preferred standard.

Although cerebral angiography has previously been considered a prerequisite for carotid endarterectomy, several recent reports challenge its necessity. Approximately half of the 30-day morbidity and mortality of endarterectomy on the ACAS trial was associated with angiography rather than the surgical procedure (11). This study showed a 93% concordance between duplex and angiographic estimation of stenosis, refuting the earlier suggestion from the NASCET data that ultrasound alone was an inadequate screening test.

In large part, this was due to the increased availability of color duplex sonography. Dawson et al prospectively evaluated the impact of angiography on treatment decisions in patients previously screened by duplex ultrasound (12). In 87 patients (93%), angiography confirmed the ultrasound findings. In six patients the need for confirmatory angiography was evident from the results of duplex scans. In only one patient (1%) was a significant intracranial stenosis detected by angiography. The authors concluded that technically adequate duplex scans were sufficient to select candidates for endarterectomy and to predict the need for preoperative angiography.

Although there is not a perfect correlation between the angiographic demonstration of ulceration and the pathologic specimen obtained at endarterectomy, angiography remains the gold standard for diagnosis of ulceration. In the NASCET study a plaque was classified as ulcerated if an ulcer niche was visible with or without the appearance of a double-contrast density. In NASCET, even patients treated surgically had a twofold increase in the risk for stroke or death at 2 years if angiographic ulceration was present.

A decade ago, O'Donnel et al showed carotid ultrasound to be superior to angiography in the detection of ulceration and intraplaque hemorrhage when both modalities were compared to pathologic specimens obtained in endarterectomy (13). This suggests that ultrasound evaluation of the extracranial carotid is a powerful diagnostic tool. To balance the highly persuasive arguments against the routine use of angiography prior to endarterectomy, several facts must be considered.

1. Only luminal reduction as measured by angiography has been validated by controlled clinical trials as a marker of benefit from endarterectomy.
2. Only the angiographic appearance of plaque ulceration has been shown to adversely affect outcome.
3. Rarely, but unpredictably, angiography reveals intracranial abnormalities that drastically alter treatment strategies.

A retrospective study showed no difference in perioperative morbidity in patients screened by ultrasound alone (14). These results, if supported by prospective clinical trials with long-term follow-up, may continue to minimize the need for conventional angiography in the evaluation of carotid stenosis. At present, angiography remains the standard by which other procedures are judged and the only method that has been validated in randomized studies.

Total occlusion of the internal carotid is generally felt to be a contraindication to endarterectomy due to propagation of the clot distally. In the setting of a documented acute occlusion (ie, a patient who has been recently studied noninvasively for TIA symptoms) emergency surgery with thrombectomy is an option. However, care must be taken not to confuse complete occlusion with high-grade stenosis. Often the vessel may collapse due to the low pressure beyond a tight stenosis, resulting in a mere trickle of blood distally.

In other cases contrast may flow retrograde into the cervical carotid via ophthalmic or other collaterals. In these instances angiography may be the only means of establishing patency, although contrast-enhanced CT may also be useful. Ultrasound is known to overestimate the degree of stenosis.

Clearly, the decision to use or defer angiography must be based on the relative skill of the ultrasonographers and angiographers at a given center; technically poor ultrasound may be dangerously misleading and ill-performed angiography may be harmful. A dialogue between the referring physician and radiologist is necessary to ensure proper use of diagnostic procedures. As financial considerations gain importance, the relative expense of angiography may further limit its use. The morbidity associated with the procedure always calls for careful patient selection.

Intracranial Occlusive Disease

Another prominent site of atheromatous plaque formation is the carotid siphon, and these plaques may lead to local occlusion or give rise to distal emboli. The appropriate therapy is unknown, but a recent retrospective study suggests that patients with symptomatic intracranial stenosis benefit from therapy with coumarin (15). Roeder et al found no appreciable effect of siphon disease on the outcome of endarterectomy in 2 years (16). In addition, it was noted that siphon plaques, when present, tended to be less severe than the carotid bulb lesions. The NASCET study included patients with siphon stenosis as long as the carotid stenosis was greater. The proximal portions of the large intracranial vessels are also affected by atheromatous disease. Distal tertiary and quaternary branches may also be involved. Typically, the atherosclerotic process produces irregularly spaced areas of focal stenosis, rather than the "beading" of fibromuscular dysplasia or the "sausage on the string" of cerebral vasculitis. Migraine and vasospasm following subarachnoid hemorrhage may also produce narrowing of the vessels at the base of the brain.

Transient Ischemic Attack

In our practice we use angiography more liberally in the evaluation of TIA than in completed stroke. The classic TIA of a few minutes duration often leaves no imaging or clinical clues as to its mechanism. In the absence of a clearly defined carotid or cardiac source, it seems prudent to evaluate the cerebral circulation as thoroughly as possible. Unsuspected arterial dissection or emboli from an unruptured berry aneurysm may present with transient symptoms and require dramatically different therapy. A mild, fluctuating hemiparesis may reflect impending basilar artery occlusion rather than lacunar infarction or cervical carotid stenosis. With so little to offer the patient once a stroke has occurred, the risk of angiography in skilled hands seems worthwhile to preserve a neurologically normal patient.

Lacunar Stroke

The idea that most small deep infarcts in the brainstem, basal ganglia, and subcortical white matter have a unique pathologic mechanism—lipohyalinosis—is now well accepted. When CT and MRI scanning reveals an appropriate lesion in a patient with one of the recognized lacunar syndromes the need for angiography is doubtful.

Studies of patients presenting with lacunar syndromes have reported variable prevalence of significant carotid stenosis. Hypertension, the presumed etiologic factor in the production of lipohyalinosis, is also recognized to promote large vessel atherosclerosis. Millikan has suggested that microembolism or atherosclerosis in the intracranial conductance vessels may give rise to lucunar infarctions (17). These vessels are best evaluated with angiography, but the clinical relevance of possible intracranial large vessel disease is unknown. Kappille et al found one case of intracranial (M1) occlusion in 45 patients with lacunar syndromes and corresponding small deep infarcts (18). We recommend that angiography be reserved for patients without obvious risk factors for microvascular disease in whom noninvasive screening reveals no cervical carotid stenosis.

Stroke in the Young Patient

Approximately 5% of patients with stroke are children or young adults. These patients differ from their elders in that hemorrhagic and ischemic infarction occur with fairly equal frequency. Cardiac disease, arterial dissection, migraine, and hematologic disorders are more frequent in young patients with stroke. We agree with Riela and Roach that patients with a clear cardiac lesion, hematologic disorder, or collagen vascular disease predisposing to stroke need not be subjected to angiography (19). However, if an intracranial vascular abnormality is suspected or the cause is unknown, angiography is indicated. Children and young adults are less likely to have widespread vascular disease, hypertension, or renal insufficiency, and therefore should tolerate angiography well. Some physicians are hesitant to expose children to invasive tests but we believe that children have the most to gain from a thorough workup and the most to lose from an incorrect diagnosis.

Dissection

Young and old patients alike may develop dissection of the cervical and (less often) intracranial vessels. This disease process is increasingly recognized as a cause of stroke in both populations. Often a history of neck trauma or torsion may be elicited. However, a large percentage of craniocervical dissections appear to be spontaneous. Dissection is a well-recognized complication of even the most careful angiography and is often clinically silent. The major differential diagnosis in this instance is arterial spasm induced by the presence of the catheter or contrast media. Although dissection can occur in otherwise normal arteries, it should prompt consideration of underlying vasculopathy.

The most frequent site of dissection in the cervical carotid is several centimeters distal to the bulb. The direction and degree of extension may vary widely. Subintimal extension of blood results in compression of the true lumen and a tapered, stenotic vessel is seen. Often a classic ''double-barrel'' lumen is observed. If the blood dissects between the media and adventitia a pseudoaneurysm results. The cervical carotid may also be affected at the level of the petrous bone where the transition to its fixed intracranial segment exposes it to shearing forces (20). The vertebral arteries are prone to dissection in their highly mobile upper cervical portion. Lesions here are more likely to be bilateral but are angiographically similar to dissections elsewhere.

Mullges and colleagues demonstrated that the diagnosis of carotid dissection could be made with noninvasive methods (21). The most compelling reason for angiography is to confirm the presence or absence of underlying vasculopathy or associated aneurysms (22). The authors suggest that angiography is most safely performed after a period of recuperation but no prospective studies using modern angiographic techniques indicate that a delay is of any clinical benefit. Currently, we anticoagulate patients with heparin when the diagnosis of dissection is made on clinical grounds and hemorrhage has been excluded. Angiography is then used as the first and only diagnostic procedure. If necessary, noninvasive methods can then be used to document regression of the lesion and to aid in determining the duration of therapy.

Moyamoya Disease

Moyamoya disease (idiopathic progressive anteriopathy) is characterized by gradual stenosis or occlusion of the intracranial carotid artery and its large branches. In addition to these findings, angiography demonstrates an extensive anastamotic network formed by dilated lenticulostriate and other basal perforating vessels. Leptomeningeal and other collateral vessels are also well developed (23). Ischemic strokes predominate early in the course of moyamoya disease, but patients may also present later with hemorrhage caused by rupture of the abnormal perforating vessels. The typical angiographic pattern can also be seen in other diseases that cause gradual occlusion of the proximal intracranial vasculature, including accelerated atherosclerosis secondary to radiation therapy or recurrent endothelial injury in sickle cell disease. Both processes may produce a pattern indistinguishable from moyamoya disease of the idiopathic or primary type.

Houkin et al argue persuasively that MRA is an ideal test for screening at-risk patients and for long-term follow-up of angiographically proven disease. They point out that early in the course of disease progression the enlarged anastomotic vessels may be absent or below the resolution of even catheter angiography (24). In the Western world there is little need for a widespread, noninvasive screening program for moyamoya disease. Because most cases in non-Oriental patients are due to secondary moyamoya disease, we prefer conventional angiography to thoroughly evaluate the intracranial vasculature.

Fibromuscular Dysplasia

Fibromuscular dysplasia (FMD) usually affects young to middle-aged women and is a well-recognized cause of ischemic stroke and TIA in this population. The angiographic appearance of this disease is one of alternating dilatation and constriction of the arterial lumen. The distinction should be made between this appearance and that of atheromatous disease or vasospasm in which focal stenosis without dilatation may occur. The midportion of the internal carotid artery is usually involved whereas the proximal and distal segments are spared. However, intracranial FMD has been reported. Aside from atheromatous disease, catheter spasm and granulomatous arteritis constitute the major differential diagnoses. Even when the diagnosis is made on the basis of noninvasive studies, angiography is still indicated due to the increased incidence of saccular aneurysms in patients with FMD (25). Just as in FMD of the renal arteries, angioplasty is a therapeutic option.

Cerebral Vasculitis

Central nervous system (CNS) vasculitis may present with headache, encephalopathy, seizures, or focal neurologic deficits. The causes range from isolated (primary) CNS angiitis, to a variety of connective tissue disorders (ie, lupus, Takayasu's), infection (syphilis), or drug use (cocaine, amphetamines). Such a varied clinical spectrum ensures that vasculitis often appears in the differential diagnosis of neurologically impaired patients. The gold standard for diagnosis of CNS vasculitis is meningeal biopsy, but many physicians are understandably hesitant to resort to this procedure prior to angiography. Harris et al reviewed the records of 92 patients with suspected CNS vasculitis. Angiography was considered diagnostic in 8 of 11 (72%) cases of biopsy-proven vasculitis whereas MRI was "abnormal" in all 9 cases of confirmed vasculitis in which it was performed. The authors were unable to discern any characteristic MRI pattern of abnormality associated with vasculitis but concluded that a normal MRI made the likelihood of abnormality on subsequent angiography "negligible" (26). They point out that the yield of angiography in this series was 6%. Stone et al compared the sensitivity of lumbar puncture (LP), CT, and MRI in patients with angiographic evidence of vasculitis in the appropriate clinical setting. The respective sensitivities were as follows: LP 53%, CT 65%, and MRI 75%. The greatest yield was obtained with a combination of LP and MRI with a sensitivity of 92% (27). Angiography should

also be considered in cases of suspected vasculitis to exclude unsuspected aneurysm formation and to aid biopsy planning.

Venous Thrombosis

Occlusive disease of the dural sinuses and intracerebral veins is a well-documented cause of stroke. However, even in the appropriate clinical setting it is often unrecognized. Predisposing conditions include inherited and acquired hypercoagulable states, the puerperal period, dehydration, trauma, and malignancy. The angiographic findings are those of filling defects or occlusion of veins or dural sinuses, enlarged venous collaterals, flow reversal in the veins, and prolonged contrast transit time.

With a high index of suspicion, the diagnosis of venous thrombosis may be made by CT; edema or infarction that fails to respect arterial territories is highly suggestive of venous occlusion. Contrast enhancement along the falx and tentorium as well as the "empty delta" sign are well-known markers of sinus thrombosis occlusion. However, up to 20% of CT scans may be normal. Yuh et al have thoroughly reviewed the MRI findings in sinus thrombosis and distinguished them from those of arterial disease (28). If a conservative therapeutic approach is planned, MRI with MRA is the test of choice. At our center, however, marked success with catheter-directed thrombolytic therapy has led us to consider all patients with confirmed or suspected venous disease as candidates for angiography (29). The unpredictable course of the disease and the potential severity of untreated cases has convinced us of the need for aggressive therapy of venous thrombosis, even in the presence of hemorrhagic infarction.

Infective Endocarditis

Despite the decrease in the incidence of rheumatic heart disease, infective endocarditis remains a significant medical problem. The majority of cases now occur in intravenous drug abusers and patients with artificial (mechanical or porcine) heart valves. A significant proportion (21%) of patients with infective endocarditis have neurologic complications. Subarachnoid hemorrhage from mycotic aneurysms occurs in 5–7% of patients. Brust et al followed the course of 28 mycotic aneurysms in 17 patients with endocarditis (30). Fifty percent of aneurysms followed with serial angiography remained unchanged during appropriate medical therapy. Twenty-five aneurysms were located on distal branches of the middle cerebral artery. Three others were located on the anterior communicating artery and remained unchanged despite therapy, raising the possibility that these were asymptomatic berry aneurysms unrelated to infection. In general, mycotic aneurysms are located in easily accessible areas and should be considered for surgical repair.

We agree with these authors that four-vessel cerebral angiography is indicated in all patients with infective endocarditis who present with neurologic complications or who develop them during treatment. In addition, all patients considered for long-term anticoagulation should have angiography regardless of their neurologic status. In medically stable patients with subarachnoid hemorrhage angiography should be undertaken as soon as possible. In patients with focal infarcts suggesting embolism, a waiting period of 48 hours may maximize the yield of the study because aneurysm formation may be delayed.

Headache

A variety of cerebrovascular, musculoskeletal, and psychogenic processes may result in headache. Few of these patients will require angiography if a careful history is obtained. The evaluation of aneurysmal subarachnoid hemorrhage, arterial dissection, and cerebral vasculitis are discussed under those headings. It is worth remembering that these disorders may be superimposed on preexisting headache syndromes and should be considered in the differential diagnosis of a patient with a change in headache character. Slivka and Philbrook suggest that patients with "thunderclap" headache who have normal CT scan and cerebrospinal fluid analysis do not need angiography (31). We consider this diagnosis one of exclusion and feel that angiography is indicated. Because of the morbidity of aneurysm rupture, we recommend angiography over any other modality in this clinical setting.

Aneurysms

The evaluation of intracranial aneurysms remains the domain of catheter angiography. Even the most vocal opponents of angiography recognize that the risk of the procedure pales in comparison to that of primary or recurrent subarachnoid hemorrhage: Approximately one third of patients die before hospitalization, and 20% die shortly thereafter. Another 20% are significantly disabled or neurologically devastated. When a diagnosis of intact or ruptured aneurysm is suggested, either by clinical history, radiographic findings, or spinal fluid analysis, four-vessel cerebral angiography is absolutely indicated if the patient is a candidate for surgical or endovascular therapy.

Estimates of the incidence of intracranial aneurysms vary. In a retrospective study, Atkinson excluded patients with intracranial or extracranial vascular disease, history compatible with subarachnoid hemorrhage, CT findings consistent with AVM, subarachnoid hemorrhage, or unruptured aneurysm. Eventually, 278 patients remained out of 9295 with "no bias" toward aneurysm formation, and a 1% incidence of asymptomatic aneurysm was noted (32). These data are of questionable clinical usefulness as most patients in whom the presence of an aneurysm is suggested by their clinical history have little in common with this highly selected group.

Autopsy data suggests a higher (6–7%) incidence of asymptomatic aneurysms, but these studies are skewed toward elderly patients. In addition, relatively healthy adults who suffer sudden death are likely candidates for autopsy and are perhaps overrepresented in some series. An intriguing study by Iwata et al revealed a 5.5% incidence of aneurysms in patients undergoing coronary angiography in Japan (33). Considering the greater incidence of subarachnoid hemorrhage in Japan (twofold), one arrives at an estimated incidence of 2–3% for Western patients.

Wiebers showed that unruptured aneurysms <10 mm in size were very unlikely to rupture (34). Proponents of MRA refer to this to justify the use of MRI and MRA in the evaluation of cerebrovascular diseases. This information has been called into question by observations that many ruptured aneurysms appear to be <10 mm in size. Schievink and his colleagues provided well-documented evidence of ruptured aneurysms less which were <10 mm. Postrupture (or postmortem) hemodynamic changes may account for this discrepancy (35).

Vasospasm of the cerebral vessels is a major factor contributing to morbidity associated with subarachnoid hemorrhage. Irregular narrowing of the intracranial vessels is most common at the base of the brain but may be more widespread. Eskesen reported that the diagnosis of vasospasm by angiography is highly subjective and the agreement between independent observations sometimes approached random chance (36). Vasospasm near an aneurysm may render it radiographically invisible. For this reason, repeat angiography may be warranted in patients with subarachnoid hemorrhage but no detectable aneurysm. Van Gijn reported a subset of patients with blood subarachnoid limited to the prepontine and perimesencephalic cisterns. The source of bleeding in these instances is probably venous rather than arterial, and repeat angiography may not be indicated in these patients (37).

Once the diagnosis of subarachnoid hemorrhage is made, regardless of the etiology, sequential transcranial Doppler has been shown to be a reliable test for vasospasm. In patients with subarachnoid hemorrhage who develop focal neurologic deficits and appropriate velocity changes on transcranial Doppler, angiography is indicated if angioplasty or papaverine injection is contemplated.

Arteriovenous Malformations

The classical AVM is composed of dilated serpiginous arteries and enlarged draining veins without an intervening capillary bed. In most instances this abnormal tangle of vessels includes no normal brain parenchyma. The corresponding angiographic appearance is one of single or multiple dilated arteries converging on a tangle of blood vessels drained by single or multiple veins. The absence of an intervening capillary bed and the rapid shunting of blood through the malformation leads to the simultaneous opacification of arterial and venous components. This appearance may mimic the "luxury perfusion" of ischemic infarction or the blush of a highly vascular tumor. Although approximately 98% of intravenous malformations are solitary, multiple malformations may be observed in Wyburn–Mason and Osler–Weber–Rendu syndromes.

The peak incidence of AVM rupture is between 20 and 40 years. These lesions are felt to rupture at approximately 2–4% per year and each rupture carries a 10–20% risk of death. Despite this, AVMs have a reputation as being relatively benign lesions in the neurologic literature. Marks et al determined the angiographic variables that were associated with an increased risk of hemorrhage (38). Some of these factors may be interrelated:

1. Deep venous drainage: There is a predisposition for stenosis in the vein of Galen that may result in increased incidence of hemorrhage.
2. Short feeding vessels: A shorter pedicle leading to the AVM results in a higher pressure head delivered to the nidus.
3. Intraventricular or periventricular location: It is presumed that loss of tamponade by the brain parenchyma may cause more extensive bleeding. In addition, a small amount of intraventricular blood may be more likely to cause clinical symptoms than a mild parenchymal bleed.
4. Associated aneurysms: In one series, almost 50% of hemorrhage associated with AVMs were found to be related to intracranial aneurysms.

Arteriovenous malformations are frequently diagnosed by CT scan in patients who present with subarachnoid hemorrhage or by MRI during the evaluation of patients with headache or seizure. Angiography remains an obligatory part of the workup of these patients and should be carried out in centers with the capability for superselective catheterization of the intracranial vessels.

Intracerebral Hemorrhage

Approximately 50% of parenchymal brain hemorrhages are associated with hypertension and are most common in the basal ganglia, thalamus, pons, and cerebellum. The remainder are associated cerebral amyloid angiopathy, vascular malformations, drug use, and pathologic or iatrogenic disturbance of the coagulation pathways. For patients who fit the clinical profile of hypertensive hemorrhage and have a characteristic hemorrhage on CT, angiography is unnecessary. However, in nonhypertensive patients or those with lobar hemorrhages, an argument can be made for angiography. Depending on the series, up to three quarters of patients with intracerebral hemorrhage related to cocaine use had an underlying vascular lesion ranging from necrotizing vasculitis to aneurysm and AVM. We typically delay angiography until the patient has clinically stabilized and the hematoma has resolved to maximize the yield of the study. In the series

of 72 patients with lobar intracerebral hemorrhage described by Wukai et al, 29 patients had negative angiography in the acute setting (39). However, 30% of these patients proved to have underlying vascular malformations at surgery. Presumably some of these malformations would have been visible on angiography performed after convalescence.

Brain Death

The President's Commission established stringent criteria for the determination of brain death. In the majority of instances these tests are conducted rapidly and without complication at the bedside. Confirmatory testing is warranted when craniofacial trauma compromises the evaluation of brainstem function, in possible organ donor cases when time is precious, or when specifically requested by the patient's family. Kricheff et al described the angiographic findings in 20 patients who met the clinical criteria for brain death and had isoelectric EEGs: In ten patients no filling of the intracranial vasculature was noted. Three patients demonstrated "static" filling of the proximal intracranial vessels but no contrast entered the venous system. Four other patients had reflux and retrograde filling via the circle of Willis but no venous contrast appeared. Two patients had markedly slowed circulation (ie, appearance of contrast in the venous system) in the posterior fossa and one had extravasation of contrast from the posterior cerebral artery on a common carotid artery injection (40). These data reveal variability in the angiographic findings in brain death and highlight the difficulty of reliance on ancillary tests. Due to expense, technical requirements, and the increased risks of hemodynamic instability, angiography has largely been replaced by cerebral perfusion scans with intravenous injection of technetium-90.

CONCLUSION

Cerebral angiography remains the gold standard in the diagnosis of cerebrovascular disorders. Because of the small but significant risk associated with the procedure, it must be used judiciously. We recommend angiography under the following circumstances:

1. As the primary diagnostic procedure in the evaluation of confirmed or suspected subarachnoid hemorrhage from ruptured saccular aneurysms.
2. As the primary diagnostic procedure in cases of suspected arterial dissection and in patients in whom intracranial atheromatous disease is likely.
3. As an integral part of the workup of arteriovenous malformations, both to define the feeding and drainage patterns and to locate associated aneurysms.
4. As an adjunct in the evaluation of intracerebral hemorrhage in atypical locations or in nonhypertensive patients.

5. In patients with infective endocarditis and neurologic symptoms or those in whom anticoagulation is considered.

6. As an adjunct to duplex ultrasonography in the evaluation of asymptomatic and symptomatic carotid stenosis.

7. As an adjunct in cases of suspected cerebral venous thrombosis, especially in cases where thrombolytic therapy is an option.

8. In any case where the cause of stroke remains obscure despite thorough noninvasive testing.

Caplan and Wolpert (41) wisely suggest an open dialogue between the angiographer and the clinician, but we feel strongly that the referring physician bears primary responsibility for ensuring that angiography is indicated and that the patient is an acceptable candidate for the procedure. The clinician must be available for personal or telephone consultation during the procedure and should be involved in the management of complications. We also feel that the complication rate of the individual angiographer should be a matter of record and that a major complication rate of <1% should be expected.

Clearly, we can expect the indications for cerebral angiography to change as technical advances in noninvasive imaging are made. Physician and patient bias will continue to affect the use of angiography. The decision to use angiography should be based on the clinical circumstance and the availability and sensitivity of non-invasive tests rather than on the possible risks of the procedure, which we feel are overstated.

REFERENCES

1. Osborn A. *Introduction to Cerebral Angiography*. New York: Harper and Row, 1980;1–22.
2. Mani R, Eisenberg E, et al. Complications of catheter cerebral arteriography: analysis of 5,000 procedures. I. Criteria and incidence. *AJR* 1978;131:861–865.
3. Solomon R, Werner C, et al. Effects of Saline, Mannitol, and Furosemide on acute decreases in renal function induced by radiocontrast agents. *N Engl J Med* 1994;1416–1420.
4. Dion J, Gates P, et al. Clinical events following neuroangiography: A prospective study. *Stroke* 1987;18:997–1004.
5. Ramadan N, Gilkey S, et al. Postangiography headache. *Headache* 1995;35:21.
6. Shuaib A, Hachinski V. Migraine and the risks from angiography. *Arch Neurol* 1988;45:911–912.
7. Gasecki AP, Ferguson GG, et al. Early endarterectomy after a nondisabling stroke: results for the North American Symptomatic Endarterectomy Trial. *J Vasc Surg* 1994;20:288–295.
8. North American Symptomatic Carotid Endarterectomy Trial Collaborators. Beneficial effect of carotid endarterectomy in symptomatic patients with high-grade carotid stenosis. *N Engl J Med* 1991;325:445–453.
9. European Carotid Surgery Trialists' Collaborative Group. MRC European Carotid Surgery Trial: Interim results for patients with severe (70–99%) with mild (0–29%) carotid stenosis. *Lancet* 1991;337:1235–1243.
10. Bladen CF, Alexander AV, et al. Carotid stenosis index: a new method of measuring internal carotid artery stenosis. *Stroke* 1995;26:230–234.
11. Executive Commitee for the Asymptomatic Carotid Atherosclerosis Study. Endarterectomy for asymptomatic carotid artery stenosis. *JAMA* 1995;273:1421–1428.
12. Dawson D, Zierler R, et al. The role of duplex scanning and arteriography before carotid endarterectomy: a prospective study. *J Vasc Surg* 1993;18:673–683.
13. O'Donnel T, Erdoes L, et al. Correlation of B-mode ultrasound imaging and arteriography with pathologic findings at carotid endarterectomy. *Arch Surg* 1985;120:443–449.
14. Cartier R, Cartier P, Fontaine A. Carotid endarterectomy without angiography: the reliability of Doppler ultrasonography and duplex scanning in preoperative assessment. *Can J Surg* 1993;36:411–421.
15. Chimowitz MI, Kokkinos J. The Warfarin-Aspirin Symptomatic Intracranial Disease Study. *Neurology* 1995;45:1488–1493.
16. Roederer G, Langlois Y, et al. Is siphon disease important in predicting outcome of carotid endarterectomy? *Arch Surg* 1983;118:1177–1181.
17. Millikan C, Futrell N. The fallacy of the lucunae hypothesis. *Stroke* 1991;21:1251–1257.
18. Kappelle L, Koudstaal P, et al. Carotid angiography in patients with lacunar infarction. *Stroke* 1988;19:1093–1096.
19. Riela A, Roach ES. Etiology of stroke in children. *J Child Neurol* 1993;8:201–220.
20. Ojemann RG, Fisher CM, Rich JC. Spontaneous dissecting aneurysms of the internal carotid artery. *Stroke* 1972;3:434–400.
21. Mullges W, Ringelstein E, Leibold M. Non-invasive diagnosis of internal carotid artery dissections. *JNNP* 1992;55:98–104.
22. Schievink W, Mokri B, Piepgras D. Angiographic frequency of saccular intracranial aneurysms in patients with spontaneous cervical artery dissection. *J Neurosurg* 1992;76:62–66.
23. Suzaki J, Takaku A. Cerebrovascular ''moyamoya'' disease showing abnormal net-like vessels in the base of the brain. *Arch Neurol* 1969;20:288–299.
24. Houkin K, Aoki T, et al. Diagnosis of moyamoya disease with magnetic resonance angiography. *Stroke* 1994;25:2159–64.
25. Sandok B, Houser O, et al. Fibromuscular dysplasia. *Arch Neurol* 1971;24:462–466.
26. Harris K, Tran D, et al. Diagnosing intracranial vasculitis: the roles of MR and angiography. *AJNR* 1994;15:317–330.
27. Stone J, Pomper M, et al. Sensitivities of noninvasive tests for central nervous system vasculitis: a comparison of lumbar puncture, computed tomography, and magnetic resonance imaging. *J Rheumatol* 1994;21:1277–1282.
28. Yuh W, Simonson T, et al. Venous sinus occlusion disease: MR findings. *AJNR* 1994;15:309–316.
29. Horowitz m, Purdy P, et al. Treatment of dural sinus thrombosis using selective catheterization and urokinase. *Ann Neurol* 1995;38:58–67.
30. Brust J, Dickinson P, et al. The diagnosis and treatment of cerebral mycotic aneurysms. *Am Neurol* 1990;27:238–46.
31. Slivka A, Philbrook B. Clinical and angiographic features of thunderclap headache. *Headache* 1995;35:1–6.
32. Atkinson J, Sundt T, et al. Angiographic frequency of anterior circulation intracranial aneurysms. *J Neurosurg* 1989;70:551–555.
33. Iwata K, Misu N, et al. Screening for unruptured asymptomatic intracranial aneurysms in patients undergoing coronary angiography. *J Neurosurg* 1991;75:52–55.
34. Wiebers DO, Whisnat JP, O'Fallon WM. The natural history on ruptured intracranial aneurysms. *N Engl J Med* 1981;304:696–1406.
35. Schievink W, Piepgras D, Wirth F. Rupture of previously documented small asymptomatic saccular intracranial aneurysms. *J Neurosurg* 1992;76:1019–1024.
36. Eskesen V, Kruse K, et al. Observer variability in assessment of angiographic vasospasm after aneurysmal subarachnoid hemorrhage. *Acta Neurochir* 1987;87:54–57.
37. Van Gign J, Van Donger KJ, et al. Perimesencephalic hemorrhage: a non-aneurysmal and benign form of subarachnoid hemorrhage. *Neurology* 1985;35:493–497.
38. Marks M, Lane B, et al. Hemorrhage in intracerebral arteriovenous malformations: angiographic determinants. *Radiology* 1990;176:807–813.
39. Wakai S, Kumakura N, Nagai M. Lobar intracerebral hemorrhage. *J Neurosurg* 1992;76:231–238.
40. Kricheff I, Pinto S, et al. Angiographic findings in brain death. *Ann NY Acad Sci* 1971;169:183.
41. Caplan L, Wolpert S. Angiography in patients with occlusive cerebrovascular disease: views of a stroke neurologist and neuroradiologist. *AJNR* 1991;12:593–601.

Cerebrovascular Disease, edited by H. Hunt Batjer.
Lippincott-Raven Publishers, Philadelphia © 1997.

CHAPTER 18

Magnetic Resonance Angiography of Cerebrovascular Disease

James L. Fleckenstein and John N. Oshinski

Technical refinements have propelled magnetic resonance angiography (MRA) into the forefront of the cerebrovascular disease diagnostic armamentarium. MRA offers clinicians not only the ability to define structural aspects of vascular pathology but the potential to study hemodynamic consequences of the disease. Although it is hoped that MRA might eventually obviate the need for the more invasive procedure of conventional X-ray angiography, there are multiple factors that ensure a limit to the reliance on MRA to comprehensively evaluate cerebrovascular disease.

An important limitation of MRA is that correct interpretation of these scans requires a good understanding of basic MR physics in order to avoid misdiagnoses. This is even more true than in the case of conventional MR image interpretation because that study generally ignores complex details inherent to the imaging of protons that are in motion, such as in flowing blood. Optimal MRA pulse sequence selections and interpretations rely heavily on knowing the strengths and weaknesses of the various sequences and the different kinds of data they make available. Hence, interpretation of MRA scans requires not only the same knowledge of pathophysiology, pathology, and anatomy that conventional X-ray angiography of cerebrovascular disease requires, but also an understanding of the relative strengths and limitations of different MRA techniques and how MRA images are formed.

Because these requirements cannot be ignored, this chapter will first review basic MR imaging principles with special emphasis on blood flow and flow-sensitive sequences. This will be followed by a brief review of current literature regarding clinical applications of MRA.

J. L. Fleckenstein: Algur H. Meadows Diagnostic Imaging Center, University of Texas Southwestern Medical Center, Dallas, Texas 75235.
J. N. Oshinski: Department of Radiology, Emory University School of Medicine, Atlanta, Georgia 30322.

BASICS OF MR PHYSICS

Detailed references on the generation of MR images are widely available (1). Briefly, the magnetic resonance effect dictates that when protons are placed in a static magnetic field, a statistically significant number of them will line up in the direction of the magnetic field. Taken as a group, these protons are said to have longitudinal magnetization, or magnetization aligned with the static magnetic field. The more protons aligned in a certain tissue, the larger the value of the magnetization. When a radiofrequency (rf) pulse is applied at the resonant frequency for protons, the protons will absorb the energy and the magnetization will be tipped away from alignment with the static magnetic field. This absorption of energy is referred to as excitation. The amount the magnetization is tipped from alignment with the static magnetic field is referred to as the flip angle (Fig. 1). If a flip angle of 90° is used, the tissue becomes saturated, meaning that no magnetization remains in the direction of the static magnetic field. When the rf pulse is terminated, the protons will begin to return to alignment with the static magnetic field, at a rate that is governed by the T1 of the tissue in which the protons reside. The return of the protons toward alignment with the static magnetic field is termed relaxation, and energy will be emitted in the form of a sine wave at the resonant frequency. This signal is referred to as the free induction decay (FID).

The FID signal is not usually used for generating an MR image because it tends to decay too rapidly. Instead, magnetic gradients, or rf pulses, are used to generate an MR signal at a somewhat later time. This signal is referred to as an echo. The vast majority of MRA techniques use magnetic field gradients to generate an echo, and the technique is aptly named a gradient echo sequence. Magnetic field gradients are also used to assign position-dependent phase and frequency values to the MR signal during the time between excitation and detection of the echo. The MR signals can

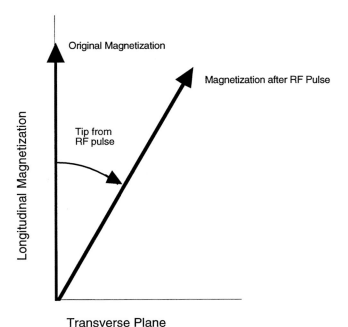

FIG. 1. Longitudinal magnetization. When tissue is placed in a static magnetic field, the protons line up to form longitudinal magnetization. A radiofrequency pulse at the resonant frequency of protons tips the magnetization from alignment with the static magnetic field. The relaxation of the magnetization back to alignment with the static magnetic field generates the MR signal.

then be spatially localized within an image. In most MR imaging, the magnitude of the MR signal is displayed as image intensity.

There are two major types of MRA techniques: time-of-flight (TOF) and phase contrast angiography (PCA). TOF techniques display the magnitude of the MR signal, and phase contrast techniques display the phase of the MR signal. Both of the techniques make images by maximizing signal from flowing blood and minimizing the signal from static tissue.

TIME-OF-FLIGHT MRA

TOF MRA relies on inflow of blood into an imaging slice. It maximizes the contrast between flowing blood and static tissue by retaining a high level of signal from flowing blood and suppressing signals from static tissue by using a series of rapidly applied rf pulses (2,3).

Understanding how contrast between flowing blood and static tissue is generated depends on understanding the magnetization of static tissue. Static tissue is subjected to a series of rapidly applied rf pulses. The series of rf pulses drives the magnetization of static tissue to a low level by exciting the tissue rapidly before it can recover toward alignment with the static magnetic field (Fig. 2). Note that after several rf pulses the magnetization from static tissue remains at a

low level, or nearly saturated. The low level of magnetization generates a very small MR signal. Inherent in the method is the assumption that the repetition time (TR) of the sequence is much shorter than the T1 of blood (1000 msec). This assumption is valid for all MRA techniques done on modern scanners.

Now let us examine magnetization of flowing blood. If blood is flowing rapidly through the imaging slice, it will exit the slice after receiving only one rf pulse (Fig. 3). Therefore, it will have a large longitudinal magnetization. The large value of longitudinal magnetization yields a larger MR signal. For maximum inflow contrast in an image, the blood must be flowing with sufficient velocity that it will exit the slice within one TR. Written in an equation form, the following relationship must be satisfied for maximum blood signal:

$$V > d/\text{TR} \tag{1}$$

where V = blood velocity (cm/sec), d = slice thickness (cm), and TR = repetition time (sec). In TOF imaging, it is best to have vessels where the blood is flowing through (perpendicular to) the slice in order to satisfy the above equation.

2D Time of Flight

Two-dimensional (2D) TOF is a technique that separately acquires each slice in a series of parallel slices. The advantage of 2D TOF is that it can provide a large area of coverage, and if the flow is perpendicular to the slice, good inflow contrast is maintained. However, there are also several disadvantages to 2D TOF imaging, including the need for fairly thick slices (about 3–4 mm) to obtain adequate MR signal. This slice thickness may be too large for detecting abnormalities in very small vessels. Thick slices cause vessels flowing through the slices at an oblique angle to have a "stair step" appearance in projection displays. This artifact can be reduced by using a slice overlap. Second, in 2D TOF, flow within the plane of the slice will not generate inflow contrast and vessels will not be visible. The in-plane flow will become saturated if it does not exit the slice within one TR. Lastly, 2D TOF has a fairly long echo time, which makes the technique susceptible to signal loss artifacts from the turbulent flow in stenoses. Because it can cover a large area, 2D TOF is often used in the carotid arteries to examine the entire carotid vasculature, and for examining venous flow (Fig. 4).

3D Time of Flight

In order to overcome some of the disadvantages of 2D TOF, a three-dimensional (3D) version TOF method was introduced (2). In the 3D TOF method, a large volume is excited with the rf pulse rather than a single slice. The volume is then divided into slices during image reconstruction.

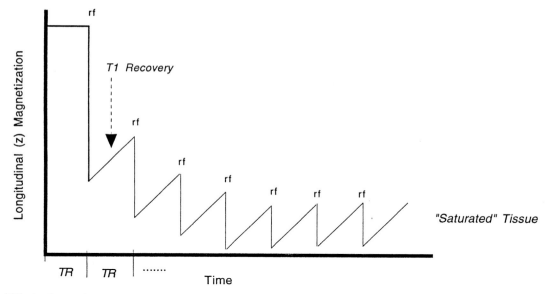

FIG. 2. Static tissue suppression. Tissue starts out with a substantial amount of longitudinal magnetization. When a radiofrequency (rf) pulse is applied to the tissue, longitudinal magnetization is driven to a lower value. If the rf pulses are applied rapidly, before T1 recovery can occur, the rf pulses will drive the longitudinal magnetization to a low level, or "saturate" the tissue.

Because of its larger excitation volume, the 3D method produces a larger signal-to-noise ratio (SNR). Because signal from the 3D method is greater, thinner slices and smaller pixels can be used. The advantages of 3D are, therefore, higher SNR, better resolution, enhanced ability to detect flow in multiple directions, and shorter echo times.

There are, however, disadvantages to the 3D method. Because slices are thinner, the scan cannot cover large areas. Also, it is more difficult to excite a larger volume properly and the slices near the edges of a 3D volumes will have poor image quality. Saturation of flowing blood can occur near the distal end of thick 3D volumes because the blood can receive several RF pulses before leaving the volume. The blood then becomes saturated in the same manner as the

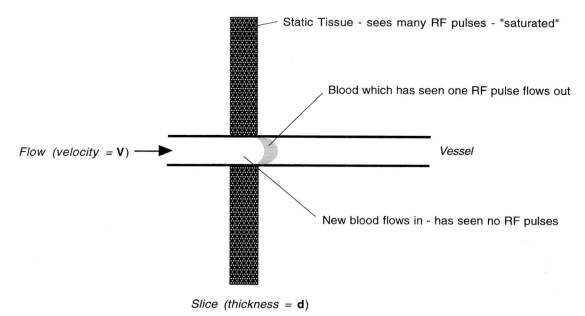

FIG. 3. Inflow effect. In time-of-flight (TOF) angiography, the signal from static tissue becomes saturated by the application of several rapidly applied rf pulses. The saturated tissue produces a small magnetic resonance (MR) signal. Blood that flows into the slice between successive rf pulse receives only a single rf pulse. The inflowing blood produces a large MR signal.

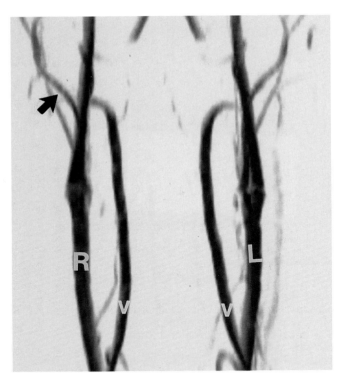

FIG. 4. Example of 2D time-of-flight (TOF). cervical carotid and vertebral arteries. Although each 2D TOF scan results in only one slice, a summation of all the slices allows for a large volume to be covered in a single scan. This coronal maximum intensity projection (MIP) image was produced from a series of transverse slices of the right (R) and left (L) carotid arteries. Note that vertebral arteries (v) are also included. Note also the stairstep artifact in oblique vessels *(arrow)*.

static tissue. In order to prevent saturation in 3D imaging, Eq. (1) must be satisfied where *d* is now the 3D volume thickness.

3D TOF is often used for imaging the circle of Willis because flow in several directions is present and high resolution is needed. 3D TOF is also used in imaging the carotid bulb, where multidirectional flow and signal loss from turbulent flow may be present.

3D Multislab Time of Flight

To overcome the problems of saturation and limited coverage in 3D TOF, a 3D multislab method was developed (4). 3D multislab uses multiple overlapping thin 3D volumes (called slabs) to create a single large image volume. The 3D multislab method eliminates most of the saturation and coverage problems seen in single volume 3D imaging, but it does introduce a new artifact called the ''Venetian blind'' artifact. This artifact appears as lines in the images where the individual 3D volumes overlap and is caused by variation in the saturation effect across the slab. In order to keep the effect of this artifact to a minimum, Eq. (1) must be satisfied

for each slab, where *d* is now the slab thickness. 3D multislab is used in the same locations as single-volume 3D imaging, such as the carotid bifurcation, the circle of Willis, and the posterior cerebral circulation, and locations where tortuous vessels are present (Fig. 5).

Presaturation

In order to image only arterial or venous flow, a presaturation slab may be applied to selectively eliminate signal from either flow direction. Presaturation slabs work by saturating the magnetization in a region with a 90° excitation before imaging begins. Blood that flows into the imaging slice from the region where a presaturation slab has been applied will not generate any signal because it has already been saturated. If a presaturation slab is positioned cranially with respect to the imaging slice, inferiorly directed blood flow, chiefly venous, will be eliminated from the image. If the slab is placed caudally with respect to the imaging slice, superiorly directed flow, primarily arterial, will be eliminated from the image (Fig. 6).

PHASE CONTRAST ANGIOGRAPHY

Phase contrast angiography (PCA) is fundamentally different from TOF angiography in that it relies on the phase of the MR signal (5). It requires two to four preliminary images to produce a final image and requires postprocessing where image subtraction is done. Unlike TOF imaging, PCA does not rely on the inflow effect; therefore saturation effects are not nearly as important. Static tissue suppression is accomplished with phase effects and image subtraction.

To form a phase contrast image illustrating flow in one direction, two images are made. One image is flow-compensated, which means that specialized gradients are applied during the sequence so that flow does not affect the phase of the MR signal. The second image is flow-sensitive, which means that the phase of the MR signal is affected by flow. These two-phase images are then subtracted to eliminate residual signal from static tissue and remove the effects of magnetic field inhomogeneities. The magnitude of the subtracted image is then used to form an image where only blood flowing in a single direction is visible.

To make the image show blood flowing in all three directions (left-to-right, cranial-to-caudal, anterior-to-posterior), image acquisitions and subtractions are somewhat more complex, but the bottom line is that a series of four images is required to produce the final image where flow in all directions is visible. In PCA, the signal intensity is related to the flow velocity through the velocity encoding value (V_{enc}), a parameter that must be set before the scan begins. The value of V_{enc} is usually set to about 75% of the peak systolic velocity expected in the image. Setting V_{enc} too high causes a lack of contrast between flowing blood and static tissue, and setting V_{enc} too low causes aliasing of high veloci-

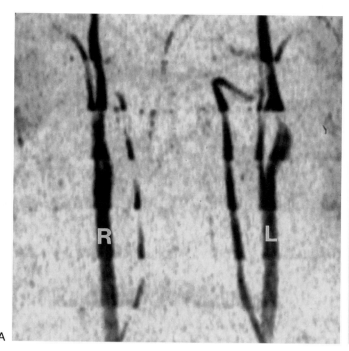
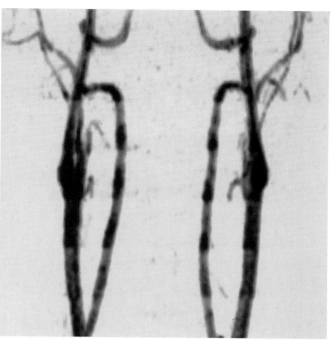

A   B

FIG. 5. Examples of 3D multislab time-of-flight (TOF). Cervical carotid and vertebral arteries. A coronal projection image of the right (R) and left (L) carotid bifurcations was acquired with a 3D multislab TOF technique. The image on the right shows a better example of the technique. The image on the left shows a more pronounced "Venetian blind" artifact.

ties, whereby high velocities actually appear as low signal intensity.

PCA can be implemented in either a 2D or a 3D method. 2D methods are usually thick-slice-localizing scans used to determine vessel location or to test values for the V_{enc}. As in TOF, 3D PCA has the advantages of higher SNR, better resolution, and shorter echo times. Note that the saturation problems associated with TOF methods are not present in PCA due to the different methodology used to suppress signal from static tissue.

The major advantage of PCA is that it is sensitive to flow in multiple directions and does not suffer from in-plane flow saturation effects. The disadvantages of PCA are that it involves longer scan times, has more stringent hardware requirements, is more sensitive to artifacts, and setting the V_{enc} value properly can be difficult.

The sensitivity of PCA to flow in multiple directions makes it a choice for imaging the carotid bulb and the cerebral vasculature. The sensitivity of PCA to in-plane flow make it a good choice for imaging long sections of vessels within a single plane as well as areas of tortuous slow flow (Fig. 7).

Quantitative Flow

Quantitative flow (QF) imaging is related to phase contrast angiography except that QF imaging yields an image whereby image intensity is directly proportional to the blood flow velocity in a single direction (6). Blood flowing in the positive direction will appear as bright pixels, blood flowing in the negative direction will appear as dark pixels, and static tissue will appear as midgray pixels. By using a region of interest (ROI) either the velocity or volume flow of blood through a vessel can be determined. QF will yield a curve of blood flow velocity (or volume) versus time (Fig. 8). The blood flow velocity curve produced from a QF scan can help set the V_{enc} value in PCA. In contrast to PCA, the V_{enc} value in QF scans should be set above the highest velocity expected; otherwise an artifact called phase wrap (phase aliasing) will occur. When velocities above the V_{enc} value are present in QF image, phase wrap causes the high-velocity values to "wrap around" and appear as negative velocities.

FLOW ARTIFACTS

The majority of artifacts in MRA are caused by hemodynamics. Blood flow in healthy vessels is organized and follows smooth streamlines. This type of smooth flow is referred to as laminar flow. Flow that is unorganized and chaotic in nature is referred to as turbulent flow. Turbulent flow can occur in the human body and is usually associated with disease. Turbulent flow affects MRA by causing intervoxel dephasing and signal loss distal to stenoses (7). The signal loss artifact can cause overestimation of stenosis severity or can cause a vessel to appear occluded. Normally, the signal loss artifact can be distinguished from occlusion

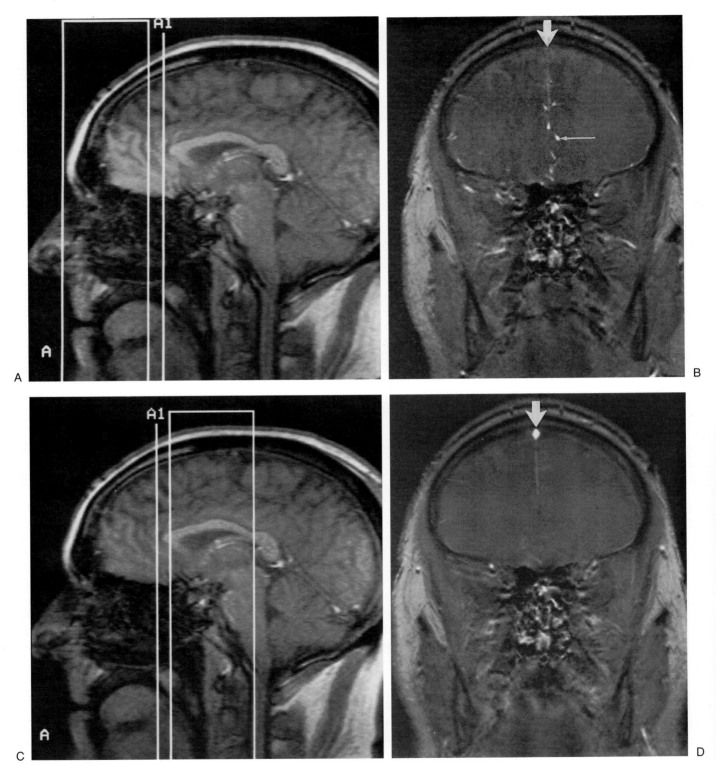

FIG. 6. Presaturation. **A:** Scout sagittal image shows a saturation band (box) anterior to the subsequently acquired slice (A1). **B:** The saturation box results in attenuation of signal within the posteriorly directed blood flow, eg, sagittal sinus *(arrowhead)*. Note that anteriorly directed flow within branches of the anterior cerebral artery show flow enhancement *(thin arrow)*. **C:** With the saturation band placed posterior to the slice (A1), anteriorly directed flow is suppressed while posteriorly projecting flow remains enhanced, as shown in D. **D:** Posteriorly directed flow within the sagittal sinus is enhanced *(arrowhead)*. Note that the anterior cerebral arteries fail to show flow-related enhancement.

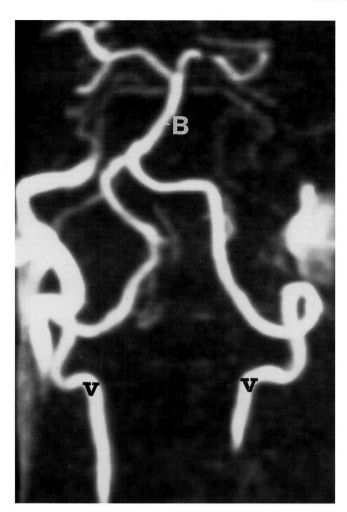

FIG. 7. Example of phase contrast angiography (PCA): verte-brobasilar system. A coronal maximum intensity projection (MIP) image produced from a sagittal 3D PCA scan of the vertebral (V) and basilar (B) arteries. The scan was acquired with flow sensitivity in all three directions. PCA scans are an excellent choice for imaging vessels that lie in the imaging plane or in which direction of blood flow varies.

by recognizing that the flow signal from the vessel reappears downstream of the signal loss artifact (Fig. 9).

A second artifact that appears in MRA is ghosting. Ghostings (or ghost vessels) are faint images of vessels that appear in ungated scans (8). The vessels appear in the phase-encoding direction within the image (Fig. 10). The ghost vessels are caused by the pulsatile nature of the flow. Since flow is not constant over the entire image acquisition but repeats over cardiac cycles, the differences in flow cause differences in phase of the MR signal. The scanner cannot differentiate between the phase used for spatial positioning and the phase acquired from the pulsatile flow. Ghosting can be eliminated by gating the acquisition to the cardiac cycle and imaging only during periods of more constant flow within the cardiac cycle.

ECG Triggering and Gating

Electrocardiographic (ECG) triggering and gating are techniques that are used to reduce artifacts due to pulsatile flow or to view flow dynamics over the cardiac cycle. ECG triggering is a technique whereby several images are acquired at different time points within the cardiac cycle. ECG gating is a technique that uses only a specified portion of the cardiac cycle for imaging. ECG triggering and ECG gating both will increase scan time when used with TOF or PCA. ECG triggering and gating are not always used in neuroimaging because cerebral flow is fairly constant over the cardiac cycle.

Cine Imaging

Cine imaging is a technique that uses cardiac triggering to acquire a series of images over the cardiac cycle (9). It is done to view flow dynamics over the cardiac cycle and is most often employed with gradient echo techniques. In standard cine imaging, one phase-encoding step is acquired per heart phase interval. A single image is acquired for each heart phase interval, which corresponds to a time in the cardiac cycle.

Fast (or turbo) cine imaging is a variation of cine imaging whereby several phase encoding steps are acquired per heart phase interval. With turbo cine imaging, scan time is decreased by the number of phase encoding steps acquired per heart phase interval. Cine and turbo cine imaging techniques can be implemented on TOF or PCA scans.

Gated Imaging

Gated imaging is a technique that acquires data only during a user-selectable portion of the cardiac cycle. In effect a "gate" is opened during the cardiac cycle where imaging is done. The imaging time is usually specified by setting a delay time after the QRS wave and setting a time period (gate window) in which to acquire data. Gated imaging is done to eliminate artifacts from pulsatile flow. The size of the data acquisition window governs the length of the scan. The larger the window, the shorter the scan. Unlike cine imaging, only a single image over the cardiac cycle is acquired.

DISPLAY TECHNIQUES

Most MRA scans consist of a large number of slices. Because examination of each individual slice can be very time consuming, several methods of image display have been devised to condense the image data. The most popular and widespread method of viewing MRA images is a maximum intensity projection (MIP) (12). MIP images are formed by first stacking up the individual slices to form an image vol-

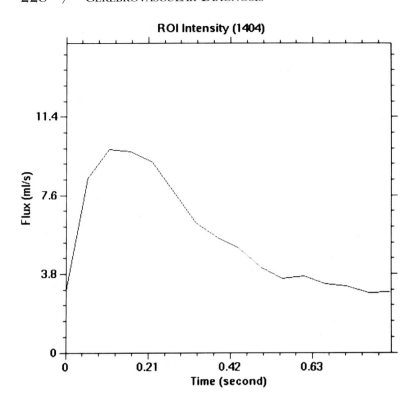

FIG. 8. Quantitative flow curve. The curve was obtained from a slice in the common carotid artery using 16 temporal images over the cardiac cycle. The curve shows flow (in ml/sec) on the vertical axis and time over the cardiac cycle (in msec) on the horizontal axis.

ume. A projection direction is then chosen. A computer algorithm then passes imaginary rays through the imaging volume from the projection direction onto a projection image. The maximum image intensity values encountered by the rays are recorded on the projection image. The projection image is referred to as an MIP image (Fig. 11). The main disadvantages of the MIP display are that overlapping vessels can cause confusion and signal from bright tissue, such as fat, can blur the image.

CLINICAL APPLICATIONS

Given the rapid evolution of MRA, conclusions regarding its clinical utility and impact on the practice of cerebrovascular neurology and neurosurgery is evolving. Early studies arguing for a potentially advantageous role of MRA are supported by more recent, larger studies.

Extracranial Arteries: Indications and Limitations

When a patient presents with symptoms of a transient ischemic attack or stroke, conventional arteriography is frequently performed to evaluate for potentially treatable causes of the event. Such a study usually includes aortography and selective catheterization of the common carotid arteries. MRA can noninvasively reveal evidence of flow and luminal dimensions, as well as the presence or absence of occlusion. Although the large body size of the chest renders

the aortic arch more difficult to study than vessels in the neck, anatomic detail is often sufficient to demonstrate the presence or absence of significant disease, particularly using phase contrast techniques that allow coverage over substantial volumes of tissue and can be optimized for imaging fast or turbulent flow (Fig. 12).

Imaging of the cervical carotid arteries takes advantage of the smaller volume of tissue that can be centrally located within a volume imaging coil, thus providing better SNR than imaging of the arch and proximal great vessels. Phase contrast and 2D TOF (Fig. 13) sequences can each evaluate arterial patency and the degree of stenosis, when present. Unfortunately, even when using optimal technique by current standards, MRA is limited in the evaluation of arterial stenoses.

Overestimating the degree of stenosis is an important and common problem both in intracranial and extracranial arterial diseases (10,11). Another well-documented limitation of MRA is in the false identification of a high-grade stenosis as an occlusion. This is particularly a problem when too many sections are included in the MIP image; lower intensity features of vessels may be lost, apparent vessel diameters reduced, and stenosis overestimated. In such cases, the individual sections that constitute the basis for the projection image are best evaluated singly, although targeted MIPs can also be helpful, ie, those in which only sections showing the lesion are included in the projection image.

Arterial dissection is another important area where MR techniques can noninvasively detect disease that traditionally requires conventional angiography. Routine MR imag-

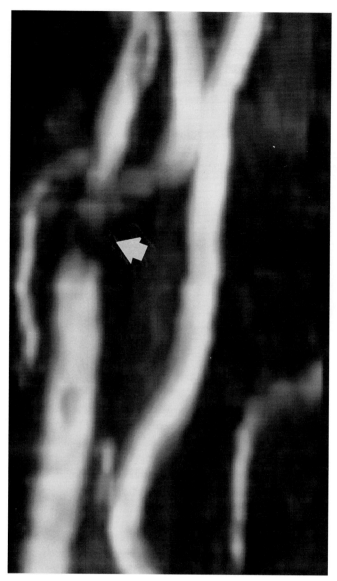

FIG. 9. Signal loss artifact in a time-of-flight image. Signal loss is caused by turbulent flow distal to stenoses. The signal loss makes it difficult to estimate the severity of stenoses and can cause a stenosis to appear as an occlusion.

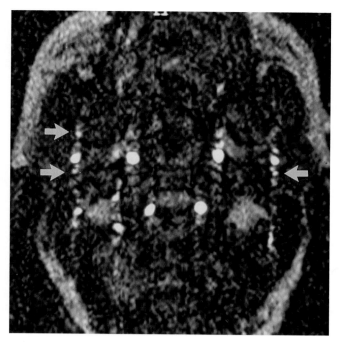

FIG. 10. Example of ghost vessels. Ghosting or ghost vessels are caused by the effects of pulsatile flow. Axial source image from 2D time-of-flight sequence shows ghost images in the phase encoding directions *(arrows)*. These may not be visible on maximum intensity projection (MIP) images, despite their conspicuous presence on source image.

ing can be helpful in identifying blood that is trapped in a subadventitial location, in which case it is recognized as a semilunar region of signal intensity increase. MRA may reveal slow or no flow, as well as apparent double lumens (12). As in conventional angiograms, abnormality of the luminal dimensions may be observed, appearing as an eccentric, tapered stenosis arising approximately 2 cm distal to the origin of the internal carotid artery. Such changes may be subtle, however, and close inspection of the individual (source) images that contribute to the overall projection angiogram is important. No large series has been reported to argue for one MR technique over another in this application.

Intracranial MRA in Stroke

When a major intracranial artery is occluded, MRA typically reveals lack of the expected flow-related enhancement, which is easily visualized (Fig. 15). Pitfalls exist, however, and include the fact that since the TOF sequences have short repetition and echo times, they are inherently T1-weighted and so substances that have short T1 times, such as subacute blood, may mimic flow. When the blood has a characteristic appearance, such as in a gyriform pattern of a hemorrhagic infarct (Fig. 14), this does not pose a diagnostic dilemma. However, when subacute thrombosis is present within the lumen of a vessel, it may appear identical to flowing blood and go unnoticed. For this reason, when subacute blood is anticipated, such as in sinus thrombosis or when an underlying lesion is being sought in a known parenchymal hematoma, phase contrast MRA sequences are most helpful because they are sensitive to differences in motion-dependent phase of protons and stationary blood will not be visible.

In stroke patients, MRA has been demonstrated to be sensitive in identifying stenoses and occlusions of intracranial arteries (13,14). In one report, occlusions or severe stenoses were observed in 16 of 34 cases of acute cerebral ischemia (13). Such MRA findings can be observed even before abnormalities develop on routine MRI (15). A larger study found posterior cerebral artery abnormalities in 84% of 70 patients with posterior circulation infarcts (14).

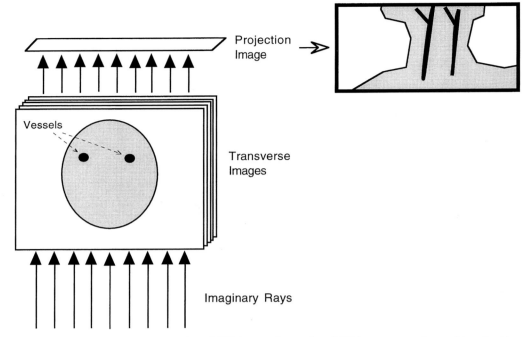

FIG. 11. Maximum intensity projection (MIP) image formation. MIP images are formed by stacking up a series of slices (usually axial) to form a volumetric dataset. A computer program then directs imaginary rays through the volumetric dataset and the maximum intensity value encountered by the ray is recorded on the projection image.

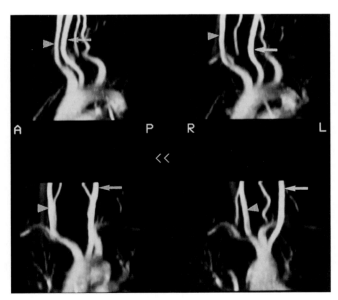

FIG. 12. Transient cerebral ischemia: aortic arch and proximal great vessel magnetic resonance angiography. Phase contrast MIP images of the arch and great vessels (20 axial increments) in this patient who presented with symptoms of transient cerebral ischemia. Note absence of significant stenoses of the takeoffs of the great vessels including the right common carotid artery *(arrowhead)* and the left common carotid artery *(arrow)*.

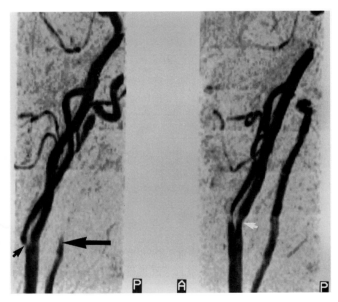

FIG. 13. Transient cerebral ischemia: cervical carotid arteries. Same patient as in Figure 12; maximum intensity projection (MIP) images from 2D time-of-flight sequences, filmed with inverted gray scale format (black on white background). On left is the right carotid artery showing high-grade stenosis at origin of external carotid artery *(small arrow)* but no significant stenosis of internal carotid artery. Note that the vertebral artery appears (but is not) occluded *(large arrow)*. It was excluded by the technologist from the MIP region of interest. On the right, the left internal carotid artery shows a 30% stenosis *(arrow)*.

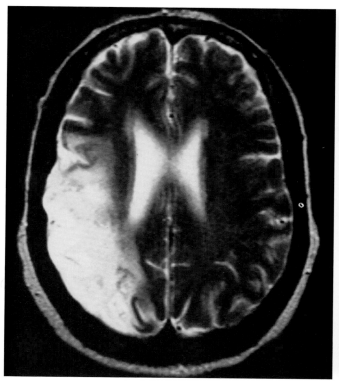

A

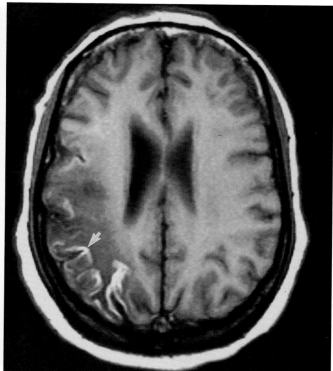

B

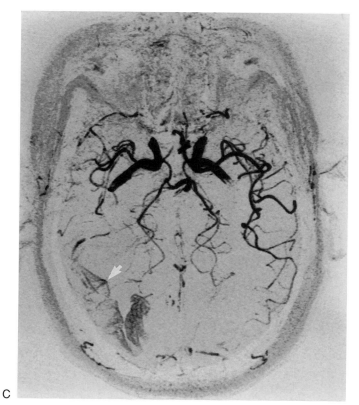

C

FIG. 14. Hemorrhage appearance on magnetic resonance angiography (MRA). **A:** T2-weighted image of the brain shows a large confluent area of edema-like change within the right parietal lobe, involving gray and white matter. **B:** T1-weighted image at the same level shows gyriform hyperintensity in the region, consistent with hemorrhagic transformation of cerebral infarct. **C:** 3D time-of-flight (TOF) MRA shows a paucity of vessels in the middle cerebral artery distribution on the right. Note that the T1 hyperintensity from the gyriform hemorrhagic change appears on the MRA image as if due to flow-related enhancement *(arrow)*. This is a common problem resulting from the short T1 time of methemoglobin and T1 weighting of TOF source images.

A study comparing digital subtraction arteriography to MR angiography found that MRA was 100% specific and 95% sensitive for detection of vessel occlusion (16). Accuracy of MRA in identifying stenoses was lower, however, at 86% specificity and sensitivity. Of course, these data do not consider the fact that angiography can identify vessels having much smaller calibers than those visible on MRA and so conclusions reached when major branches are evaluated can not be extrapolated to small vessel disease. Although the spatial resolution of MRA is inferior to conventional angiography in evaluating moyamoya, recent data argue that MRI and MRA are sufficiently sensitive (92%) to merit further investigation as an important tool in the evaluation of this disease (17,18).

Cerebral Arterial Anatomy: Normal, Variant, and Pathologic

In a 1995 study comparing computed tomographic angiography (CTA) to MRA, with conventional angiography as the gold standard, CTA and MRA were similarly sensitive to identification of the arterial anatomy of the circle of Willis (sensitivity 88.5% for CTA and 85.5% for MRA). While neither modality was significantly impaired in detecting anterior, middle, posterior, or anterior communicating arteries, only 59% of posterior communicating arteries were seen by CTA or MRA. However, it should be noted that only the MIP projection images were studied and smaller arteries are more difficult to see on projection images than on source images (19).

Despite imperfect accuracy for identifying normal arteries, displacements and elongations of intracranial arteries can be important clinical information easily provided by MRA (20). For example vascular loops compressing the fascial nerve root and causing hemifacial spasm has been well documented with MRA (21). Dilated, elongated arteries found in dolichoectasia of the basilar artery can also be readily defined, particularly with the inclusion of slow velocity encoding sensitivity of phase contrast MRA, or by the addition of intravenous gadolinium chelates to TOF sequences (20). Displacement of arteries by mass lesions is another application previously necessitating arteriography that may now be accomplished noninvasively (Fig. 15).

Aneurysms

Many studies have addressed the issue of cerebral aneurysms with MRI and MRA (Fig. 16). Most of these reported MRA to be quite sensitive, on the order of 86–92% (22–24). This accuracy has led to large screening programs, including one recently reported to have detected aneurysms in 37 of 400 asymptomatic members of families in which two or more cases of subarachnoid hemorrhage resulted from aneurysms (25). This success, however, must be viewed in the context of limitations that are also recognized. For example, while 30 of the 43 aneurysms were listed as very small (0–6 mm), the smallest aneurysm detected was actually 2.5 mm. The size limitation of MRA techniques was further emphasized in another important article (26).

In that study, the primary goal was to determine the effect

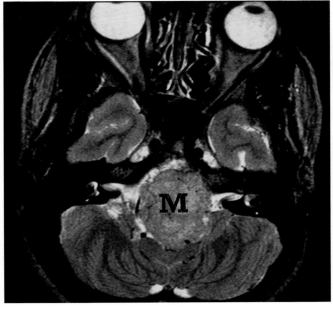

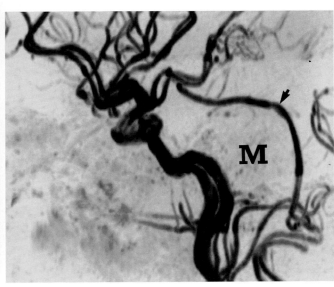

A

B

FIG. 15. MRA road mapping. This patient presented with a meningioma in the posterior fossa. **A:** Axial T2-weighted MRI shows the mass (M) anterior to the cerebellum in the midline. **B:** Phase contrast MRA shows posterior bowing and displacement of the basilar artery *(arrow)* by the mass. Small foci of signal within the mass are difficult to distinguish from background noise but may represent hypervascularity.

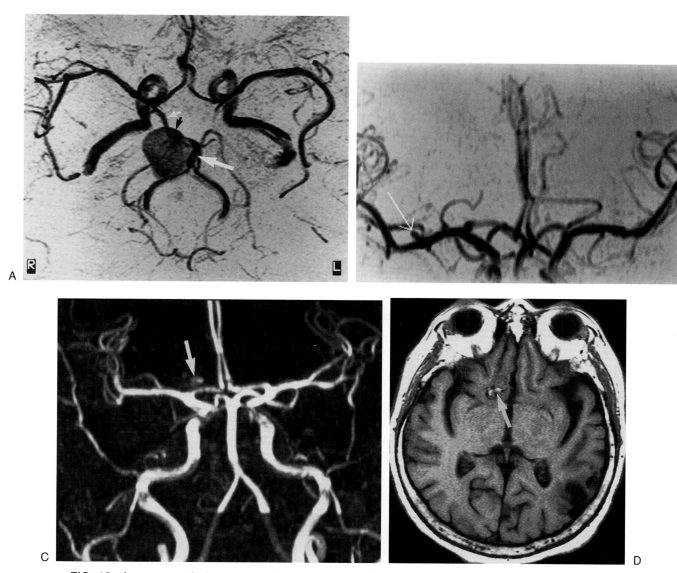

FIG. 16. Aneurysms. **A:** Large, saccular aneurysm originates from the right posterior cerebral artery *(black arrow)* in close proximity to the posterior communicating artery *(small white arrow)*. Note slight deviation of the basilar artery to the left *(arrow)*. **B:** Small, approximately 4-mm aneurysm of the right middle cerebral artery is noted *(arrow)*. **C:** Mimic of aneurysm, exemplified by focal rounded area of increased signal intensity near the right proximal anterior cerebral artery *(arrow)*. **D:** Axial T1-weighted image of the same patient as in C, without intravenous contrast, shows T1 shortening in a cavernoma near the anterior cerebral artery *(arrow)*. The short T1 of subacute blood is visible on time-of-flight MRA source images and can project, along with flow-related enhancement of the intracranial arteries, as it did in C.

of size on aneurysm detection. Interestingly, only 56% of all 27 aneurysms were identified using the most sensitive technique, 3D TOF. Importantly, that study included a relatively large number of aneurysms smaller than 5 mm. Of the 11 aneurysms measuring 5 mm or less, phase contrast MRA had a 0% sensitivity whereas the 3D TOF had a 9% sensitivity. Of the eight aneurysms not diagnosed, all but one were smaller than 5 mm; above 5 mm, the true positive rate was 94%. While sobering, that study required all three observers to detect an aneurysm. Also, patients' MRI studies

and the two MRA sequences that were performed were studied independently. It is likely that better results would have accompanied interpreting each patient's studies concurrently, as is done in clinical practice (27). In any case, the study was pivotal in elucidating the size of aneurysms at which the sensitivity of MR techniques can be expected to decay sharply.

Another important caveat in MRA of aneurysms relates to evaluation of giant aneurysms. This pitfall relates to difficulties in imaging slow or turbulent flow in larger aneurysms, particularly using phase contrast techniques (28). Turbulent flow in such a situation is frequently better imaged with phase contrast than TOF techniques. However, because phase contrast sequences are sensitive to operator-selected ranges of velocities, flow that falls below this range, such as may occur in large aneurysms, likely accounts for the occasional inability of phase contrast MRA to identify large aneurysms. This was documented in one case in which a giant aneurysm was visible only when the V_{enc} was reduced to 10 cm/sec (28). Unfortunately, use of such a low V_{enc} poses its own hazards, as signals from higher velocities will be aliased using such low V_{enc} values, thereby mimicking slow flows.

As a final caution, it should be restated that while MRA can be used to screen for aneurysms, a negative MRA in a setting of a subarachnoid hemorrhage is a well-established indication for catheter angiography. In fact, depending on the circumstances, subarachnoid hemorrhage is one indication in which catheter angiography should not be delayed by an MR study of any kind.

Arteriovenous Malformations

Arteriovenous malformations (AVMs) can be seen on routine MRI scans. These can provide information such as the size and location of the nidus, mass effect, regions of gliosis, and evidence of hemorrhage (29–31). The utility of gradient echo sequences to distinguish vessels from calcium or hemosiderin within the AVM was confirmed in one study in which thrombosis was correctly identified in the nidi of 8 of 8 patients in whom it was proven angiographically (29). Arteries feeding an AVM are best seen with 3D TOF MRA or PCA MRA. When it is important to determine venous anatomy noninvasively, 2D TOF MRA can be used effectively (20).

Limitations of MRA are again important to recognize. In the case of AVMs, similar to that of aneurysms, smaller lesions are less frequently visualized. In a study of 33 patients, sensitivity of MRA sequences were 100% and 95% for source and MIP images, respectively, when AVMs were greater than 1 cm in diameter (29). However, source and MIP sensitivities for detecting AVMs less than 1 cm were 50% and 27%, respectively. In addition to problems of detection, there is a problem in resolving the relevant vascular anatomy. Overlapping of arteries and veins is a common problem, particularly on MIP images due to the projection of many vessels in a limited volume of interest (Fig. 17). In such cases, the technique of presaturation, described above, can be used to selectively eliminate sources of flow-related enhancement.

MRA can aid not only in the detection of vascular malformations but in monitoring the response to therapy. For example, cardiac gated QF images were used to observe postembolization reductions of flow into AVMs by an average of 55% in embolized vessels and by 5% in nonembolized vessels (31). Interestingly, the study also suggested disturbed autoregulation in two patients in whom postembolization flow enhancement was observed in the contralateral hemispheres.

Veins and Sinuses

In 3D TOF MRA, slowly flowing venous blood tends to become saturated such that it loses signal. Because blood is less saturated in 2D TOF MRA, flow-related enhancement dominates over signal loss. Hence, 2D TOF MRA is the favored technique for identifying slowly flowing blood in veins and dural sinuses. Intravenous gadolinium chelates are frequently used to enhance venous flow–related signal enhancement, an example of which is in depicting venous angiomas (32).

As discussed above, presaturation slabs can be used to target spins in any given direction. For example, when flow in the sagittal sinus is desired to be evaluated, a saturation band is placed posterior to the slices so that anteriorly directed flow is suppressed (Fig. 6). This leaves posteriorly projected flow within patent sagittal sinuses and other posteriorly directed vessels to be enhanced. These techniques can be used to show cerebral venous and sinus thromboses, cerebral venous angiomas, and of veins draining from AVMs.

Assessment of patency of venous sinuses in the setting of dural based lesions such as meningiomas or in patients at increased risk for sinus thrombosis (eg, pregnant women) are common indications for these techniques. From the foregoing, one can see that inadvertent placement of a saturation band in the wrong location could produce nonvisualization of a sinus. This occurs routinely in the transverse sinuses when the sagittal sinus is studied using coronal MRA with presaturation. Usually, a presaturation band is placed posterior to the plane of acquisition (Fig. 6C). Visualization of posteriorly projecting flow results, as in the sagittal and straight sinuses and the vein of Labbé. Anteriorly projecting flow is removed, by design. A potential false-positive result is that since flow in the transverse sinus is directed anteriorly, it is saturated and not visible on MRA, thereby mimicking sinus occlusion. Cognizance of such technical factors is of obvious importance in correctly interpreting MRA images.

Another important limitation, a potential false-negative result, can occur when using MRA to assess clot within a dural sinus. If the clot is subacute and contains methemoglobin, it will appear hyperintense on T1-weighted images. Importantly, TOF images are heavily T1-weighted, and at this stage blood can easily be projected into the MIP image. This then gives the incorrect perception that flow is present within the sinus when in fact the sinus is occluded by subacute clot (18). Such a situation is obviated by the prudent selection of a phase contrast sequence, on which stationary tissue, including subacute clot, is invisible. This same principle dictates that when a subacute parenchymal hematoma is present and an underlying bleeding lesion is being sought, TOF sequences will be unhelpful because the hematoma will mimic

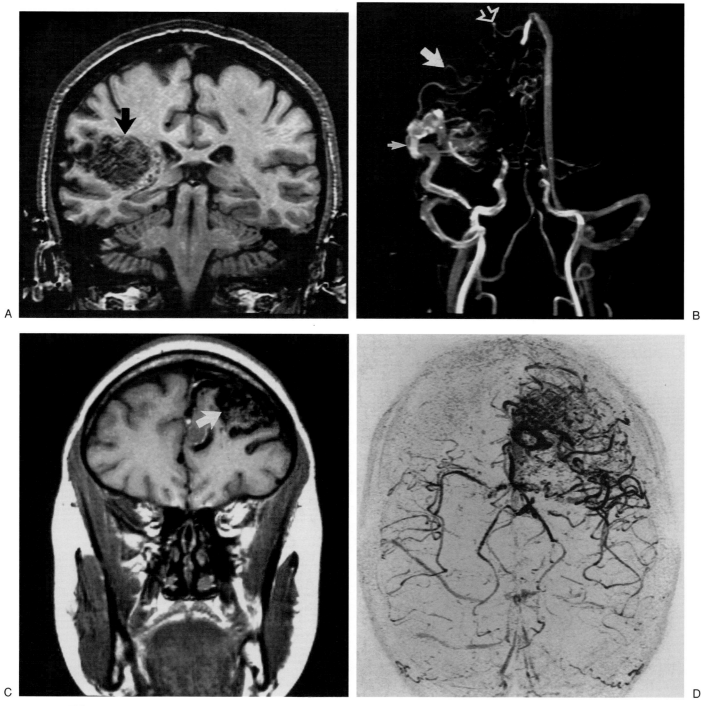

FIG. 17. Arteriovenous malformations: **A:** T1-weighted coronal image of a right opercular arteriovenous malformation *(arrowhead)* is characterized by mixed signal intensity and many tubular signal voids. **B:** Phase contrast magnetic resonance angiography (MRA) shows both and arterial anatomy. Note that the right cerebral hemisphere shows much more arterialization than the left, including flow from the anterior cerebral artery distribution *(open arrowhead)* and middle cerebral artery distribution *(closed arrowhead)*. Note superficial venous drainage into the right sigmoid sinus *(small arrow)*. The nidus is not well demonstrated on the MRA. **C:** In a second patient, coronal T1-weighted image through the frontal lobes shows multiple serpiginous signal voids characteristic for draining venous channels from an arteriovenous malformation. Also seen are smaller areas of signal dropout *(arrowhead)*, at least some of which represent the nidus. **D:** Axial 3D time-of-flight maximum intensity projection shows prominence of left middle and anterior cerebral artery branches in configuration that is typical for arteriovenous malformation.

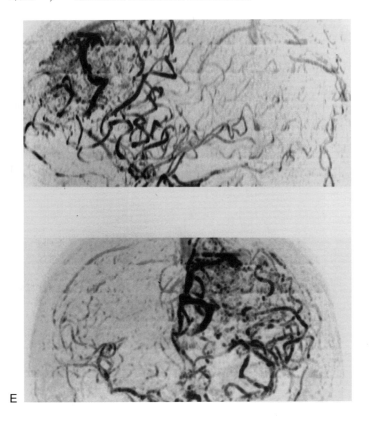

E

FIG. 17. *Continued.* **E:** Sagittal *(top)* and coronal *(bottom)* projections of the same case as D.

an aneurysm. Again, phase contrast MRA will not be similarly limited and will be able to probe the involved tissue for an underlying bleeding lesion.

CONCLUSIONS

In addition to the techniques discussed above, which have already been implemented in clinical practices, a host of newer technologies are emerging, which may become clinically important in the next several years, including functional MRI (33) and perfusion and diffusion techniques (34,35). Because these techniques are not currently widely available, their discussion exceeds the scope of this review and are discussed elsewhere (36).

MRA has dramatically enhanced the clinical assessment of patients with cerebrovascular disease by noninvasively characterizing intracranial and extracranial vascular pathologies. However, appropriate planning of the MRA examination is required to realize substantial benefit from this technology. Knowledge of the various 2D and 3D pulse sequences, their capabilities, and their limitations will continue to determine the extent by which MRA positively impacts patient management.

REFERENCES

1. Fullerton GD. Basic concepts for nuclear magnetic resonance imaging. *Magn Reson Imag* 1882;1:39–55.

2. Haacke EM, Masaryk TJ, Wielopolski PA, et al. Optimizing blood vessel contrast in fast three-dimensional MRI. *Magn Reson Med* 1990; 14:202–221.
3. Sheppard S. Basic concepts of magnetic resonance angiography. *Radiol Clin N Am* 1995;33:91–112.
4. Parker DL, Yuan C, Blatter DD. MR angiography by multiple thin slab 3D acquisition. *Magn Reson Med* 1991;17:434–451.
5. Dumoulin CL, Souza SP, Walker MF, Wagle W. Three-dimensional phase contrast angiography. *Magn Res Med* 1989;9:139–149.
6. Pettigrew RI, Daniels W, Galloway JR. Quantitative phase flow MR imaging in dogs by using standard sequences: comparison with in-vivo flow meter measurements. *AJR* 1987;148:411–414.
7. Oshinski JN, Ku DN, Pettigrew RI. Turbulent fluctuation velocity: the most significant determinant of signal loss in stenotic vessels. *Magn Res Med* 1995;33:193–199.
8. Nishumura DG, Jackson JI, Pauly JM. On the nature and reduction of the displacement artifact in flow imaging. *Magn Res Med* 1991;22: 481–492.
9. Siebert JE, Rosenbaum TL. Image presentation and postprocessing. In: Potchen EJ, Haacke EM, Siebert JE, Gottschalk A, eds. *Magnetic Resonance Angiography: Concepts and Applications.* St. Louis: CV Mosby, 1993;220–245.
10. Heisermann JE, Drayer BP, Fram EK, et al. Carotid artery stenosis; clinical efficacy of two-dimensional time-of-flight MR angiography. *Radiology* 1992;182:761–768.
11. Huston J III, Lewis BD, Weubers Dim, et al. Carotid artery: Prospective blinded comparison of two-dimensional time-of-flight MR angiography with conventional angiography and duplex US. *Radiology* 1993; 186:339–344.
12. Klufas RA, Hsu L, Barnes PD, Patel MR, Schwartz RB. Dissection of the carotid and vertebral arteries: imaging with MR angiography. *AJR* 1995;164:673–677.
13. Warach S, Li W, Ronthal M, Edelman RR. Acute cerebral ischemia: evaluation with dynamic contrast-enhanced MR imaging and MR angiography. *Radiology* 1992;182:41–47.
14. Bogousslavsky J, Regli F, Maeder P, Meuli R, Nader J. The etiology of posterior circulation infarcts: a prospective study using magnetic resonance imaging and magnetic resonance angiography. *Neurology* 1993;43:1528–1533.

15. Warch S, Chien D, Li W, Ronthal M, Edelman RR. Fast magnetic resonance diffusion-weighted imaging of acute human stroke. *Neurology* 1992;42:1717–1723.

16. Stock KW, Radue EW, Jacob AL, Bao XS, Steinbrich W. Intracranial arteries: prospective blinded comparative study of MR angiography and DSA in 50 patients. *Radiology* 1995;195:451–456.

17. Yamada I, Matsushima Y, Suzuki S. Moyamoya disease: diagnosis with three-dimensional time-of-flight MR angiography. *Radiology* 1992;184:773–778.

18. Yamada I, Suzuki S, Matsushima Y. Moyamoya disease: comparison of assessment with MR angiography and MR imaging versus conventional angiography. *Radiology* 1995;196:211–218.

19. Katz DA, Marks MP, Napel SA, Bracci PM, Roberts SL. Circle of Willis: evaluation with spiral CT angiography, MR angiography, and conventional angiography. *Radiology* 1995;195:445–449.

20. Baumgartner RW, Matle HP, Aaslid R. Transcranial color-coded duplex sonography, magnetic resonance angiography, and computed tomography angiography: methods, applications, advantages, and limitations. *J Clin Ultrasound* 1995;2:90–111.

21. Adler CH, Zimmerman RA, Savino PJ, Bernardi B, Bosley TM, Sergott RC. Hemifacial spasm: evaluation by magnetic resonance imaging and magnetic resonance tomographic angiography. *Ann Neurol* 1992;32:502–506.

22. Ross JS, Massaryk TJ, Modic MT, et al. Intracranial aneurysms: evaluation by MR angiography. *AJNR* 1990;11:449–456.

23. Schuierer G, Huk WJ, Laub G. Magnetic resonance angiography of intracranial aneurysms: comparison with intra-arterial digital subtraction angiography. *Neuroradiology* 1992;35:50–54.

24. Gouliamos A, Gotis E, Vlahos L, Samara C. Magnetic resonance angiography compared to intra-arterial digital subtraction angiography in patients with subarachnoid hemorrhage. *J Neuroradiol* 1992;35:46–49.

25. Ronkainen A, Puranen MI, Hernesniemi JA, et al. Intracranial aneurysms: MR angiographic screening in 400 asymptomatic individuals with increased familial risk. *Radiology* 1995;195:35–40.

26. Huston J III, Nichols DA, Luetmer PH, et al. Blinded prospective evaluation of sensitivity of MR angiography to known intracranial aneurysms: importance of aneurysm size. *AJNR* 1994;15:1607–1614.

27. Litt AW. MR angiography of intracranial aneurysms: proceed, but with caution. *AJNR* 1994;15:1615–1616.

28. Araki Y, Kohmura E, Tsukaguchi I. A pitfall in detection of intracranial unruptured aneurysms on three-dimensional phase-contrast MR angiography. *AJNR* 1994;15:1618–1623.

29. Mukherji SK, Quislin RG, Kubilis PS, Finn JP, Friedman WA. Intracranial arteriovenous malformations: quantitative analysis of magnitude contrast MR angiography versus gradient-echo MR imaging versus conventional angiography. *Radiology* 1995;196:187–193.

30. Edelman RR, Wentz KU, Mattle HP, et al. Intracerebral arteriovenous malformations: evaluation with selective MR angiography and venography. *Radiology* 1989;173:831–837.

31. Wasserman BA, Lin W, Tarr RW, Haacke EM, Müller E. Cerebral arteriovenous malformations: flow quantitation by means of two-dimensional cardiac-gated phase-contrast MR imaging. *Radiology* 1995;194:681–686.

32. Crecco M, Floris R, Vidiri A, et al. Venous angiomas: plain and contrast-enhanced MRI and MR angiography. *Neuroradiology* 1995;37:20–24.

33. Belliveau JW, Kennedy DN, McKinstry RC, et al. Functional mapping of the human visual cortex by magnetic resonance imaging. *Science* 1991;254:716–719.

34. Edelman RR, Mattle HP, Atkinson DJ. Cerebral blood flow: assessment with dynamic contrast-enhanced T-weighted MR imaging at 1.5 T. *Radiology* 1990;176:211–220.

35. De Crespigny AJ, Tsuura M, Moseley ME, Kucharczyk J. Perfusion/diffusion MRI of thromboembolic stroke. *J Magn Reson Imag* 1993;3:746–754.

36. Meairs S, Röther J, Neff W, Hennerici M. New and future developments in cerebrovascular ultrasound, magnetic resonance angiography, and related techniques. *J Clin Ultrasound* 1995;23:139–149.

ACKNOWLEDGMENTS

The authors thank Scott Sheppard, M.S. of Philips Medical Systems for his help in compiling and reviewing this chapter. Also, thanks are due to Barbra Lebron of Philips Medical Systems for facilitating use of some of the images shown here.

Cerebrovascular Disease, edited by H. Hunt Batjer.
Lippincott-Raven Publishers, Philadelphia © 1997.

CHAPTER 19

Positron Emission Tomography: Experimental and Clinical Applications

Colin P. Derdeyn and William J. Powers

Positron emission tomography (PET) uniquely provides accurate, quantitative, and repeatable in vivo measurements of regional cerebral hemodynamics and metabolism in humans. These measurements have both confirmed the presence of known cerebrovascular physiologic and pathologic mechanisms and yielded new information about hemodynamics and metabolism. In this chapter, we review the basic principles of PET in order to make apparent the advantages and limitations of this technique, discuss normal cerebral hemodynamics and metabolism, and review the knowledge of cerebrovascular pathophysiology gained with PET technique. PET has been used extensively to study two broad categories of cerebrovascular disease: the measurement of the effects of chronic hemodynamic compromise that may predispose to infarction and the pathophysiology of acute ischemic stroke. We discuss the use of PET in assessing the hemodynamic effects of arterial stenosis and occlusion and the clinical relevance of these measurements, and review the knowledge we have gained using PET to study the pathophysiology of acute ischemic stroke. We also discuss the use of PET in the study of aneurysmal subarachnoid hemorrhage and leukoariosis. The final section of this chapter covers future clinical and research applications of PET.

BASIC PRINCIPLES OF PET

PET relies on three major components to accurately measure physiologic processes in vivo: a radiotracer, a radiation detection system, and a mathematical model relating the physiologic process under study to the detected radiation. These three factors will be discussed in order to make apparent some of the assumptions, advantages, and limitations inherent in the study of cerebrovascular physiology using PET.

Radiotracers are radioactive molecules that are administered to the organism in very small quantities such that they do not affect the physiologic process under study. There are two general groups of radiotracers used for PET: radioisotopes of normal biological molecules, such as ^{11}C, ^{13}N, ^{15}O, and radioisotopes of nonbiological elements that are attached to organic molecules as radiolabels (^{18}F, ^{68}Ga, ^{75}Br). The half-lives of these positron-emitting radionuclides range from a few minutes to a few hours. These relatively short half-lives allow high administered radioactivity with less total radiation dose to the patient or subject as well as the ability to perform sequential studies. The limitation of a short half-life is that the radiotracer often has to be prepared very nearby or on site. The most commonly used radiotracers, ^{15}O, ^{11}C, and ^{18}F, require a linear accelerator or cyclotron for production. In addition, the synthesis of molecules incorporating a radiotracer is a specialized field of chemistry and requires great expertise. Synthesis must be achieved rapidly and with adequate purity for safe administration to human subjects (1).

The radiation detection system has historically been the barrier to the application of radiotracer methods to the quantitative in vivo study of human cerebrovascular pathophysiology. Ex vivo quantitative methods such as tissue autoradiography have been used in animal studies for decades. These methods expose a special film to the tissue slice. The intensity of the photographic image is proportional to the radioactivity in the slice. A major problem with the application of this concept to in vivo measurement is that of attenuation by surrounding tissue. Gamma rays (photons) emitted by radionuclides are absorbed to a variable extent by surrounding tissue, depending on several factors, including the photon

C. P. Derdeyn: Mallinckrodt Institute of Radiology, Washington University School of Medicine, St. Louis, Missouri 63119.

W. J. Powers: Division of Radiological Sciences, Mallinckrodt Institute of Radiology, Department of Neurology and Neurological Surgery (Neurology), Washington University School of Medicine, and the Lillian Strauss Institute of the Jewish Hospital of St. Louis, St. Louis, Missouri 63119.

energy, the tissue composition, and the pathlength of these photons. With conventional external detectors (Anger cameras), overlying structures are superimposed on those underneath. Major improvements have been made in detection systems for γ-emitting tracers with the development of single photon emission computed tomography (SPECT). Multiple two-dimensional slices permit three-dimensional visualization. However, quantitative data are difficult to generate with SPECT for two basic reasons. First, γ photons are variably attenuated by tissue; some may travel a long distance through tissue and reach the detector whereas another of the same energy and location may be absorbed by surrounding tissue. Second, the spatial resolution of external γ-ray detectors is distance dependent; as the distance between the source of γ rays and the external detector increases, the spatial resolution of detectors decreases (1). Most existing SPECT systems incorporate empiric or other corrections for attenuation and mathematical adjustments for distance-dependent resolution. Despite such limitations, these systems have been used extensively for the investigation of cerebral blood flow (CBF) and other physiologic variables.

The major advantage of PET over other external detection methods, including SPECT, derives from the use of positron-emitting radionuclides. These radionuclides decay by emission of a positron, a small particle with the same mass as an electron but the opposite charge. These particles travel a few millimeters within the tissue, losing energy, and interact with an electron. This interaction results in the annihilation of both positron and electron and the generation of two γ photons of equal energy but headed in opposite directions. A pair of detectors positioned on either side of the source of the annihilation photons will detect them simultaneously. Annihilation coincidence detection presents the solution to the problems of spatial resolution and attenuation experienced with SPECT. The spatial resolution of a pair of annihilation coincidence detectors is nearly uniform for most of the region found between detectors (1). The fraction of activity lost to attenuation can be measured and corrected for. For any pair of annihilation photons, the total distance and tissue composition traveled by both will be the same regardless of where the annihilation occurred. The attenuation fraction for a given path through an object will therefore be the same whether the annihilation to the object occurs internally or externally. The attenuation fraction for any detector pair can be measured before radiotracer administration using a source within the detector field but outside of the head.

A PET scanner consists of a large number of detector pairs connected by coincidence circuits. After the correction for attenuation, the data from the detector pairs is used to construct a series of projections, each representing the distribution of regional radioactivity viewed from a different angle. These projections are then combined by a computer to produce a two-dimensional reconstruction of the regional radioactivity within the combined field of view of all the detector pairs. Scanners with multiple rings of detectors are capable of generating several reconstructed slices of the im-

aged volume simultaneously, each depicting a different level of the brain and together providing a three-dimensional image. Newer scanners with more rings and more sophisticated software are capable of collecting data from coincidence circuits that employ detector pairs in many different slices. Less administered activity per scan is needed with this three-dimensional acquisition, allowing a greater number of scans to be performed on a given individual for a given total radiation dose.

A variety of technical factors have an impact on the ultimate accuracy of the reconstructed PET image as a quantitative measure of regional radioactivity (1–3). Most of these are beyond the scope of this chapter; however, one key concept should be discussed because ignorance of it can lead to errors in the interpretation of PET data. This is the effect of image resolution on the accuracy of measurement of regional radioactivity. In any external radiation detector system such as PET, detected radiation will be redistributed or smeared over a larger area (Fig. 1). The pattern of redistribution is approximately Gaussian for a point source of radiation, with the maximum measured value occurring at the original point. The resolution of the reconstructed image is described in terms of this point spread function and is usually given as the width of the point spread function at half its maximum amplitude. This is known as the full width, half maximum (FWHM) of a given detector system. The FWHM therefore describes the degree of smearing of radioactivity in a reconstructed image. The ability of a PET scanner to discriminate between two small adjacent structures or accurately measure the activity in a small region will depend on the FWHM of the system as well as the amount and distribution of activity within the region of interest and the surrounding areas. Because of the smearing or redistribution of detected radioactivity, any given region in the reconstructed image will not contain all of the activity actually within the region. Some of the activity will spill over into adjacent areas. Similarly, activity in the surrounding tissue or structures will also be redistributed into the region of interest. This phenomenon is known as the partial volume effect. An important consequence of this principle is that PET will always measure a gradual change in activity where an abrupt change actually exists, such as in an infarct or hemorrhage. Measurements made at the borders of such lesions will not be accurate.

Another consequence of the partial volume effect is that true gray and white matter measurements will be difficult to obtain. This is particularly true for cortical regions of interest, which will always contain both cortical gray and subcortical white matter. In addition, cortical areas adjacent to the subarachnoid space will also include cerebrospinal fluid (CSF) in the region of interest. This will result in a reduction in measured activity due to the low or absent radiotracer accumulation in the CSF. This becomes a problem in patients with hydrocephalus or cerebral atrophy.

The influence of the partial volume effect on the regional quantitation will depend on both the pattern of regional activity and the image resolution. Only when there is no activity

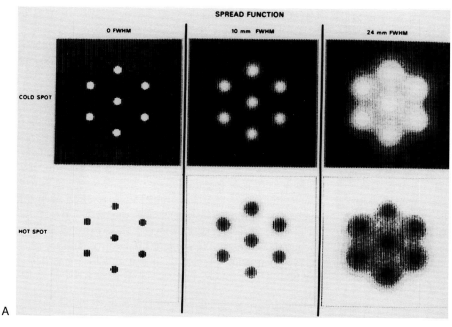

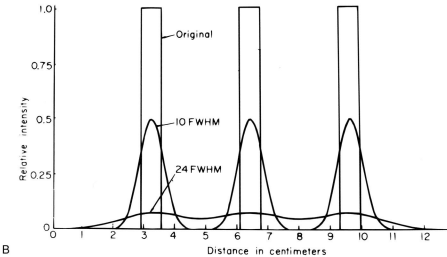

FIG. 1. The effect of differences in external detector resolution on the measurement of regional radioactivity from hexagonal arrays of cold spots (no radioactivity surrounded by radioactivity) and hot spots (radioactivity surrounded by no radioactivity) 8 mm in diameter with 32 mm center-to-center spacing. **A:** Simulated images from a system with perfect resolution (0 FWHM) *(left)* and those from two other systems with resolutions of 10 mm FWHM and 24 mm FWHM *(center and right,* respectively). **B:** Profiles of the relative intensity of radioactivity through the simulated images depicted in A. (From ref. 43.)

in surrounding areas can truly accurate PET measurements of regional radioactivity be made in the center of a homogeneous region with a diameter of at least twice the FWHM. If the surrounding tissue activity is greater than zero, the homogeneous region of interest must be made larger to achieve accurate quantitation at the center. The consequence of these considerations is that a region of interest of low activity surrounded by higher activity areas will be difficult to measure accurately. If small enough, it may not be detected at all.

The third requirement for PET measurement of cerebrovascular physiology is a mathematical model that quantitatively relates the externally measured tissue concentration of the positron-emitting radiotracer (PET counts) to the physiologic variable under study. The PET scanner simply measures the total counts in a volume of tissue. It falls on

the models to sort out how that measured activity reflects the physiologic parameter under study. These models must take into account a number of factors related to the tracer biomechanics and metabolism. These factors include the mode of tracer delivery to the tissue, the distribution and metabolism of the tracer within the tissue, the egress of the tracer and metabolites from the tissue, the recirculation of both the tracer and its labeled metabolites, and the amount of tracer and metabolites remaining in the blood. The model must be practically applicable given the constraints imposed by PET designs and the amount of radioactivity that can be safely administered to human subjects. Finally, the validity of all underlying assumptions and possible sources of error for each model when applied to the study of both normal physiology and disease states must be clearly understood. Ideally, each PET technique used in the study of cerebrovascular physiology should be rigorously validated by paired comparison to an accepted ''gold standard'' under the specific conditions for which it will be used. The specific discussion of the different models used to measure physiologic variables is beyond the scope of this chapter and the reader is referred to published comprehensive discussions and reviews (1–3).

A related issue of great importance in the analysis of PET data is that of statistics. PET counts measured during a study are statistical data and are subject to the same rules as other experimental data. Analysis of PET data must therefore employ statistically valid methods. For example, when comparing the data from several regions of interest, a correction for the potential error introduced by multiple comparisons must be used. The selection of proper control subjects and regions of interest is also crucial to accurate data analysis.

NORMAL CEREBRAL HEMODYNAMICS AND METABOLISM

The following sections will outline the important factors that affect cerebral blood flow and metabolism in normal and pathologic states. Many of these principles were proposed and proven in animals long before the advent of PET. Investigators using PET, however, have confirmed these mechanisms in living humans, discovering new information regarding cerebrovascular physiology and helping to synthesize our knowledge of cerebrovascular physiology. In this section, we will first define some commonly used terms and then review normal cerebrovascular hemodynamic mechanisms and metabolism.

Cerebral Blood Flow

Cerebral blood flow (CBF) is the volume of blood delivered to a defined mass of tissue per unit time, usually expressed in milliliters of blood per 100 grams of brain per minute [ml/(100 g min)]. Most PET laboratories use ^{15}O-labeled water to measure CBF. PET is capable of making highly accurate regional measurements of CBF within the limits of spatial resolution and the volume averaging phenomena as discussed above.

Cerebral Blood Volume

Cerebral blood volume (CBV) is the volume of blood within a defined mass of tissue and is generally expressed as milliliters of blood per 100 g of brain. Regional CBV measurements serve as an indicator of the degree of cerebrovascular vasodilatation. CBV can be measured by PET with trace amounts of either $C^{15}O$ or ^{11}CO. Both carbon monoxide tracers label the red blood cells. Blood volume is calculated using a correction factor for the difference between peripheral vessel and cerebral vessel hematocrit.

Cerebral Metabolism

PET employs $O^{15}O$ and independent measurements of CBF and CBV to measure the regional cerebral metabolic rate of oxygen (CMRO$_2$). The fraction of available oxygen extracted by the brain from the blood is the measurement actually made by PET (oxygen extraction fraction, or OEF). The quantitative value for the regional oxygen metabolism can then be calculated from an equation using rOEF, rCBF, and arterial oxygen content (CaO$_2$). The glucose analog ^{18}F-fluorodeoxyglucose (FDG) can be used to measure the regional cerebral metabolic rate of glucose (CMRGlu). CMRglu measurements are limited in pathologic conditions such as ischemia, however, because the ratio of tissue uptake of glucose and its analog, FDG, varies with the severity of ischemia. Recently, a practical method to measure glucose metabolism with 1-^{11}C- D-glucose and PET has been described (4).

Normal Cerebrovascular Physiology

Under normal resting conditions, whole-brain mean CBF of the adult human brain is 50 ml per 100 g per minute. Regional cerebral blood flow (rCBF) is determined by the ratio of regional cerebral perfusion pressure (rCPP) and regional cerebral vascular resistance (rCVR).

$$rCBF = \frac{rCPP}{rCVR}$$

Cerebral perfusion pressure is the difference between the arterial pressure forcing blood into the cerebral circulation and the venous back pressure. The venous back pressure is negligible under normal conditions, so the rCPP is generally equal to the systemic arterial pressure (CPP = MAP). Increased venous pressure would be found in pathologic conditions such as venous thrombosis and increased intracranial pressure (CPP = MAP − ICP).

Under normal conditions when rCPP is constant, any change in rCBF must be caused by a change in rCVR. rCVR is usually mediated by alterations in the diameter of small arteries or arterioles. An approximation of this relationship can be derived from this equation:

$$rCVR = \frac{Ln}{\pi r^4}$$

where L is vessel length, n is blood viscosity, and r is vessel radius (5).

This equation is not strictly true because blood is a non-Newtonian fluid and viscosity *(n)* changes with velocity. There is a direct correlation between rCBF and the intravascular regional cerebral blood volume (rCBV). rCBF and rCBV both will increase as vessels dilate and both decrease as vessels constrict. Examples include changes in rCBF produced by alterations in hematocrit in humans studied with PET (6).

In the resting brain with normal CPP, rCBF is also closely matched to the metabolic rate of the tissue. Gray matter areas with higher metabolic rate have higher rCBF and white matter areas with lower metabolic rates have lower rCBF. The ratio between rCBF and metabolism is nearly constant in all areas of the brain. Because of this resting balance between flow and metabolism, the extraction of oxygen and glucose from the blood shows little regional variation (7). The actual values for the regional oxygen extraction fraction (rOEF) and regional glucose extraction fraction vary from person to person and between measurements in the same individual. When increases in rCBF are generated by physiologic activation of neuronal tissue, this regional uniformity of rOEF is lost (8). OEF decreases while glucose extraction appears to remain relatively constant. This relative uncoupling of oxidative and glucose metabolism and the accompanying local increase in cerebral blood flow measured with neuronal activation are the basis for the use of neuroimaging as a means to map brain function.

HEMODYNAMIC EFFECTS OF ARTERIAL STENOSIS OR OCCLUSION

Measurements of rCBF, rCBV, and rOEF made with PET can accurately define in a given subject the presence and degree of hemodynamic impairment caused by arterial occlusive disease. Before discussing the assessment of hemodynamic stage, we will review the basic cerebrovascular responses to and hemodynamic and metabolic consequences of chronically reduced perfusion pressure.

Autoregulation

Cerebral perfusion pressure may be altered by any condition affecting either arterial inflow or venous back pressure. Reductions in systemic arterial pressure or increases in intracranial pressure transmitted through thin-walled veins will produce whole-brain reductions in CPP. Local arterial and venous occlusive disease can produce corresponding reductions in regional CPP.

Changes in rCPP have little effect on rCBF over a wide range of values (Fig. 2). This phenomenon is known as autoregulation and is mediated by changes in rCVR. This principle has been well demonstrated in animal preparations (6) but has been confirmed in humans with PET. An increase in rCPP will produce vasoconstriction of the pial arterioles, whereas a decrease in rCPP leads to vasodilatation. Similar changes in the intravascular volume have been measured in vivo in primates over a wide range of rCPP values (9). When rCPP falls, therefore, the rCBV/rCBF ratio is increased. The flow remains constant whereas the volume increases due to vasodilatation with a reduction in rCPP. There is evidence, however, that while an increased ratio is a more sensitive indicator of reduced perfusion pressure, it is less specific than increased rCBV alone because it can be elevated in situations that lead to reduction in flow with no change in

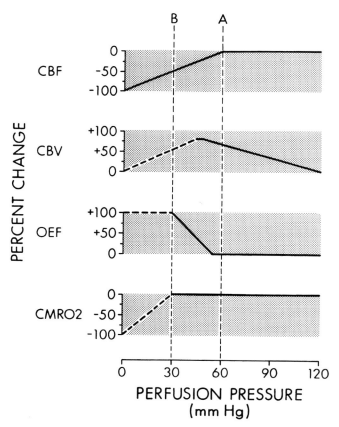

FIG. 2. Compensatory responses to reduced perfusion pressure. As cerebral perfusion pressure falls, cerebral blood flow (CBF) is initially maintained by the dilation of precapillary resistance vessels. As a result, both the cerebral blood volume (CBV) and the CBV/CBF ratio (not shown) increase. When vasodilatation can no longer compensate for the reduce perfusion pressure, cerebral autoregulation fails and blood flow begins to fall **(A)**. This occurs prior to maximal vasodilatation. As perfusion pressure continues to fall, CBV may decrease as vessels collapse, but the CBV/CBF ratio remains elevated. A progressive increase of the oxygen extraction fraction (OEF) now maintains cerebral oxygen metabolism (CMRO$_2$). Once this mechanism becomes maximal **(B)**, further declines in blood flow cause disruption of normal cellular metabolism and function. Dashed lines indicate conditions for which the data are inadequate to draw firm conclusions. (From ref. 6.)

perfusion pressure (10). The rCBV/rCBF ratio is mathematically equivalent to the mean transit time for red blood cells to pass through the cerebral circulation; an increased ratio indicates slowing of the cerebral circulation. Autoregulatory vasodilatation in response to reduction in rCPP impairs the ability of cerebral blood vessels to react to other vasoactive stimuli. Thus, while increases in PaCO$_2$ produce marked vasodilatation and increases in rCBF at normal rCPP, as rCPP is reduced this response is attenuated and then lost.

Beyond Autoregulation

When the capacity for compensatory vasodilatation has been exceeded, autoregulation fails. Further reductions in rCPP now produce decreases in rCBF. Direct measurements of arteriovenous oxygen differences have demonstrated the brain's capacity to increase OEF and maintain normal cerebral oxygen metabolism ($CMRO_2$) while the oxygen delivery diminishes due to decreasing CBF (6). If the perfusion pressure of the brain continues to fall, rCBF will progressively decline until the increase in rOEF is no longer adequate to supply the energy requirements of the brain (11). Clinical dysfunction now appears. This may be reversible if circulation is rapidly restored. Persistent or further declines in rCPP and rCBF can lead to permanent tissue damage. Sette et al. have postulated that reversible metabolic downregulation of $CMRO_2$ occurs when CBF is reduced to a point short of tissue damage as a compensatory phenomenon (11).

Once tissue damage has occurred, the normal mechanisms of cerebrovascular control may no longer operate, even when rCPP has returned to normal. Therefore, in some patients who have had transient ischemic attacks (TIAs) or mild ischemic strokes with subsequent normal carotid arteriograms, autoregulation or the normal cerebrovascular response to $PaCO_2$ may be abnormal for up to several weeks (6). The normal resting relationship between rCBF, rCBV, and rOEF is also lost in the first few weeks after infarction (6).

Thresholds for Permanent Cellular Damage

The lower limits of blood flow and oxygen metabolism for the maintenance of brain function have been documented with PET (12). Values of rCBF as low as 19 ml per 100 g per minute and $rCMRO_2$ of 60 μmol per 100 g per minute (1.3 ml per 100 g per minute) may occur without neurologic dysfunction. $CMRO_2$ below 60 μmol per 100 g per minute has been found only in infarcted tissue. CBF in infarcted tissue depends on the stage of reperfusion, but values below 12 ml per 100 g per minute have only been measured within infarcts (except in newborns) (13).

Hemodynamic Effect of Arterial Stenosis or Occlusion

Methods of Assessment of Hemodynamic Stage

The hemodynamic effect of arterial stenosis or occlusion depends on the adequacy of collateral circulation as well as on the degree of stenosis. An occluded carotid artery, for example, often has no measurable effect on the distal cerebral perfusion pressure because the collateral flow through the circle of Willis is adequate. Many imaging techniques, such as arteriography, magnetic resonance imaging (MR), computed tomography (CT) angiography, and Doppler ultrasound, can identify the presence of these collaterals. However, the actual contribution of collateral pathways to CBF and perfusion pressure can be accurately measured only with PET. In addition, measurement of CBF alone, by PET, SPECT, or xenon CT, is inadequate for the determination of the degree of hemodynamic compromise because the CBF may be maintained by vasodilatation when CPP falls, or the

CBF may be low because of reduced metabolic demand, as occurs with both stroke and deafferentation (Fig. 3).

Two basic strategies for defining the degree of hemodynamic compromise caused by arterial occlusive disease have emerged. Both are based on the known compensatory responses of the brain to reduction in CPP as discussed above. The first strategy involves resting measurements of rCBV and rCBF, sometimes in combination with rOEF (Fig. 4). When CPP is normal, all three will be normal. When rCPP is reduced, autoregulatory vasodilatation will cause an increase in rCBV. The rCBV/rCBF ratio will increase and the rOEF will remain normal. When autoregulation is no longer capable of maintaining an adequate blood flow to the brain, the fraction of oxygen extracted from the blood (OEF) will increase in order to maintain normal metabolism of oxygen. Baron and coworkers have called this stage of exceeded autoregulatory capacity "misery perfusion" (14).

The second strategy employs paired measurements of rCBF at rest and during some form of vasodilatory stimulus, such as with acetazolamide (Diamox), CO_2 inhalation, and even breath holding. Reduction of the normal increase in CBF seen in response to these stimuli is taken as evidence of preexisting autoregulatory vasodilatation, which would mute such an increase.

Arteriographic Correlation of Hemodynamic Stage

Studies of regional cerebral hemodynamics using PET have demonstrated no consistent relationship between the degree of carotid artery stenosis and the hemodynamic status of the ipsilateral hemisphere (15). In the setting of a high-grade stenosis or occlusion of the ipsilateral carotid artery, these studies have, however, confirmed a strong relationship between the hemodynamic stage and the pattern of collateral circulation as seen by intraarterial angiography. Reversal of ophthalmic artery flow has been consistently linked to an increased rCBV or rCBV/rCBF ratio. Pial collaterals have been correlated with increased rOEF. An intact circle of Willis, in contrast, has been associated with normal or abnormal hemodynamic stages. When the hemodynamic stage is abnormal, the contralateral carotid artery usually had >50% stenosis.

The concept of a hemodynamically significant arterial stenosis as it relates to the pathogenesis and treatment of cerebrovascular disease is therefore too simplistic. The status of the collateral circulation must be taken into account. This is a very important observation and one that is often overlooked. In other words, the presence of occlusion or high-grade stenosis may have no measurable affect on the distal cerebral perfusion pressure or blood flow.

Border Zone Hemodynamics

Infarction at arterial border zone regions is a well-recognized complication of global hypotension. Selective hemodynamic compromise at the arterial border zones has been

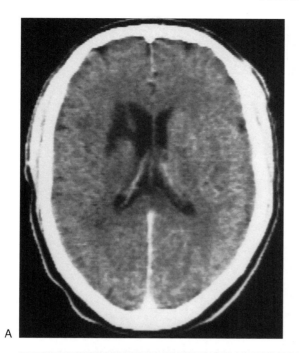

FIG. 3. CT scan from a 62-year-old man who had a left hemisphere stroke 2 months earlier (A). An infarct of the left (CT image reversed to match the PET scans) head of the caudate nucleus and the anterior limb of the internal capsule is present. The overlying cortex appears normal. Carotid arteriography demonstrated 99% stenosis of the origin of the left internal carotid artery and the patient underwent left carotid endarterectomy. In this and all subsequent figures, the right cerebral hemisphere is on the reader's right and the front of the head at the top of the image. (B) The preoperative PET study *(upper row)* shows matched reduction in cerebral blood flow (CBF) and cerebral metabolic rate of oxygen (CMRO₂) in the left frontal cortex which was normal on CT. This indicates that the reduction in CBF is not due to reduced flow through a stenotic carotid artery but rather is secondary to reduced metabolic demand from disruption of afferent and efferent pathways by the subcortical infarct. Following left carotid endarterectomy *(bottom row)*, there was no change in CBF *(left)* or CMRO₂ *(right)*, confirming the nonhemodynamic nature of the abnormalities. (From ref. 6.)

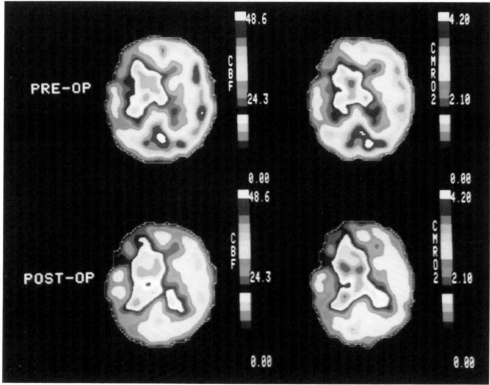

suspected as a cause of stroke in patients with carotid occlusion. Several PET studies have addressed this subject and varying results have been reported. However, when methodologic and statistical issues are carefully examined, selective hemodynamic compromise of the border zone regions in patients with chronic carotid occlusion has not been conclusively demonstrated (16).

Research and Clinical Applications of Hemodynamic Information

Measurement of cerebral hemodynamics can be used to (a) monitor the effects on the brain circulation of both medical and surgical therapy for cerebral ischemia and (b) define, within an otherwise clinically and angiographically homoge-

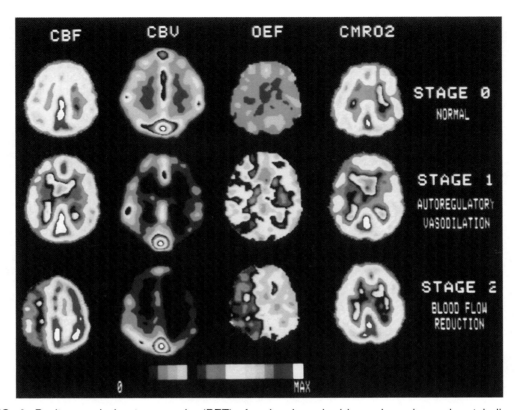

FIG. 4. Positron emission tomography (PET) of regional cerebral hemodynamics and metabolism in three patients with severe internal carotid artery disease. Each horizontal panel shows a single tomographic slice depicting a different physiologic measurement in the same patient. Each tomographic slice is scaled to its maximum value according to the color scale shown at the bottom, except for oxygen extraction fraction (OEF), for which the maximum is set at 1. *Top row:* Stage 0 or normal cerebral hemodynamics. PET studies of a 63-year-old woman with separate episodes of transient monocular blindness in the right eye and left arm weakness. Arteriography showed a 75% right internal carotid artery stenosis. Cerebral blood flow (CBF), cerebral blood volume (CBV), the CBV/CBF ratio (not shown), OEF, and the cerebral metabolic rate of oxygen metabolism ($CMRO_2$) are all normal. *Center row:* Stage 1 or autoregulatory vasodilatation. PET studies of a 64-year-old man with episodes of transient aphasia. Arteriography showed left internal carotid artery occlusion. CBV is elevated in the left hemisphere. Both CBF and $CMRO_2$ are slightly and proportionately reduced in the left frontal region as evidenced by uniform OEF throughout the brain. *Bottom row:* Stage 2 or blood flow reduction, also called misery perfusion. PET studies of a 56-year-old man who had transient episodes of right arm and leg weakness. Arteriography showed left internal carotid artery occlusion. Left hemisphere CBF is reduced relative to $CMRO_2$. CBV and OEF are both elevated in the left hemisphere. (From ref. 6.)

neous population, subgroups of patients who might respond differently to treatment.

To date, most of this work has been carried out in patients with carotid artery occlusion or high-grade stenosis undergoing superficial temporal artery to middle cerebral artery (STA-MCA) bypass surgery. Although this surgery was subsequently shown not to be of value in preventing stroke (17), preoperative and postoperative studies in these patients have provided valuable information about the circulatory physiology of the brain. Patients with focal preoperative reduction in rCBF and elevation in rOEF have often shown improvement after surgery (6). Perfusion pressure frequently does not return to normal in these patients, however, as the rCBV often remains elevated. PET has also been used to evaluate the efficacy of different revascularization techniques in other cerebrovascular disorders such as moya-moya and Takeyasu's arteritis.

In an analogous application of PET in assessing the hemodynamic effects of revascularization procedures discussed above, PET has also been used to evaluate the effects of different medical interventions on blood flow and metabolism. Yamauchi and coworkers assessed the effect of hemodilution on the cerebral circulation and metabolism in five patients with unilateral carotid artery occlusion and chronic stroke (18). No control subjects were used. They observed mild increases in blood flow and oxygen delivery (CBF × CaO_2) with no change in $CMRO_2$. Oxygen extraction fraction fell in the hemisphere contralateral to the occlusion. Hino and colleagues studied eight normal volunteers before and after hemodilution. They observed similar findings of slight augmentation of blood flow without change in $CMRO_2$ but with reduced oxygen delivery and increased OEF (19). Both of these studies showed an apparently paradoxical decrease in CBV accompanying the increase in CBF. No increase in arterial blood pressure occurred to suggest that the reduction in CBV was due to autoregulatory vasoconstriction. It may be explained by decreased viscosity producing decreased CVR with secondary compensatory vasoconstriction or because the same correction factor for the ratio of peripheral vessel to brain vessel hematocrit was used in all cases when in fact the ratio decreases as hematocrit decreases (19). PET has also been used to assess pharmacologic effects on the cerebral circulation, such as after the administration of adenosine (20).

The discussion of treatment implications of hemodynamic information is moot for carotid stenosis, as there is a proven benefit for surgical endarterectomy of high-grade lesions. However, these data suggest that the benefit seen with surgery in the endarterectomy trials may be due to removing the potentially embologenic atherosclerotic plaques rather than improving CBF distal to a lesion. The important issue, however, is whether or not this improvement in perfusion pressure translates into a reduction in stroke risk to the patient. The hypothesis that reduced perfusion pressure increases stroke risk has yet to be proven. If emboli are the most common cause of stroke in patients with reduced CPP, then revascularization will not be beneficial. The lack of benefit of STA–MCA bypass demonstrated in the extracranial/intracranial bypass trial, even in those patients with evidence of reduced CPP as evidenced by ophthalmic artery collaterals, lends support to the primacy of embolic causes. Further information is needed to identify the best therapy for patients with carotid artery or MCA occlusion.

To date, there is no clear answer as to whether or not reduced perfusion pressure (stages 1 and 2) is an independent risk factor for stroke. In a 2-year longitudinal PET study of 59 patients with primarily carotid occlusion, no relationship between abnormal hemodynamics (stages 1 and 2 combined) and subsequent stroke in medically treated patients was observed (21). In this study, only 14 patients had increased rOEF (stage 2), so that the significance of this most severely compromised population remains unknown.

Investigators using other modalities have presented conflicting data. Klieser and Widder reported a 3-year prospective study of 85 patients with carotid occlusion examined annually by transcranial Doppler before and after a CO_2 challenge (22). They observed a statistically significant increase in stroke occurrence in the patients with impaired CO_2 reactivity: 0/48 in patients with normal CO_2 reactivity, 5/23 (3 ipsilateral) in patients with impaired CO_2 reactivity, and 7/11 (5 ipsilateral and 3 of these occurring during drops in systemic arterial pressure) in patients with exhausted CO_2 reactivity. The increased risk of contralateral stroke in the patients with impaired or exhausted CO_2 reactivity suggests that these two groups were not matched with the normal

CO_2 reactivity group for other stroke risk factors and this may explain the differences observed.

Yonas and colleagues retrospectively reviewed their acetazolamide challenge xenon CT (Xe CT) CBF studies for symptomatic patients with high-grade stenosis or occlusion of the ipsilateral carotid artery (23). Sixty-eight patients met inclusion criteria and could be located for clinical follow-up. A higher rate of stroke occurrence was identified in the patients with the combination of impaired blood flow reactivity and CBF below 45 ml per 100 g of brain per minute. These criteria were set based on an analysis of patients in the study who had suffered a stroke and still need to be confirmed prospectively. In addition, some patients underwent revascularization procedures and dropped out of the study. A longitudinal, prospective study of the stroke risk of patients with carotid occlusion with measurement of cerebral hemodynamics and known risk factors is required to resolve the issue of whether hemodynamic factors are an independent risk factor. The evidence that measurement of hemodynamic stage yields any clinical information relevant to the care of individual patients is insufficient.

ACUTE ISCHEMIC STROKE

PET has provided us with unique information regarding the pathophysiologic mechanisms involved in the evolution of acute ischemic stroke. PET information has both confirmed and complemented data from experimental stroke models using more invasive methods of measurement. In this section, we will first briefly review the basics of the pathophysiology of acute ischemic stroke at a tissue and cellular level. Following this, we will discuss the relevant PET literature, including both animal and human studies of the time course of hemodynamic and metabolic events, the phenomenon of diaschisis, the possible prognostic value of PET data, and, finally, some recent data regarding possible mechanisms behind functional recovery after stroke.

Pathophysiology of Acute Ischemic Stroke

Ischemic stroke is produced by a reduction in blood flow to a region of the brain that is of sufficient duration and severity to cause infarction. Experimental and clinical data have shown that most stroke is due to embologenic cardiac disease or carotid artery atherosclerosis. Most intracerebral emboli resolve spontaneously but unfortunately not before permanent tissue damage in many patients. Transient ischemic attacks presumably occur when this lysis is rapid. True hemodynamic stroke from an acute reduction in CPP distal to a chronic large artery occlusion or stenosis is rare.

Studies with animal stroke models have provided a detailed description of the time course of changes in CBF and metabolism that occur during and after transient and permanent interruption of normal blood flow. When a vessel becomes occluded, a central core of severe ischemia is produced, surrounded by a zone with less reduction in blood flow in which perfusion is being maintained by collateral circulation. The adequacy of these collaterals will determine the size and severity of the ultimate infarction. The flow through the collateral vessels is dependent on CPP and reduction in systemic arterial pressure can lead to a substantial increase in the size and severity of the zone of ischemia. As long as blood flow is maintained above approximately 20 ml per 100 g per minute, no change in brain function or metabolism will occur. Below this level, however, normal brain electrical activity ceases and neurologic symptoms may appear. The energy supply becomes insufficient because of the inadequate supply of oxygen, preventing normal aerobic glycolysis. The high-energy phosphate stores of ATP and PCr (phosphocreatinine) become depleted. Anaerobic metabolism of the small amount of glucose remaining in the intracellular stores or from the diminished blood flow leads to a lactic acidosis. Once CBF has fallen to 10–12 ml per 100 g per minute, the integrity of cell membranes is lost and intracellular K⁻ leaks out of the cells while extracellular Ca leaks in. Cell death ultimately follows unless reperfusion occurs quickly.

Following reperfusion, the biochemical and ionic abnormalities resolve to a degree dependent on the severity of the initial ischemic insult. The acidosis of anaerobic glycolysis may be replaced by alkalosis. A biphasic evolution in CBF has been observed. First, a brief period of hyperperfusion occurs immediately after the arterial occlusion ceases. A prolonged period of depressed CBF, ie, below normal values, follows. During this period of postischemic hypoperfusion, metabolism may recover or even rise above normal levels. OEF consequently may increase as a result. Later, CBF may rise above normal whereas metabolism falls. These changes are typically observed over a period of several days. CBF eventually returns to a level that matches that of the reduced metabolic rate of the infarcted tissue.

PET Studies in Acute Ischemia

PET studies performed in the setting of acute ischemia (<24 or 48 hours) have demonstrated regions of both decreased and increased blood flow. The regions of decreased rCBF are thought to be due to persisting ischemia or postischemic hypoperfusion. Regions with increased rCBF are attributed to early postischemic hyperperfusion, caused by either clot lysis or collateral reperfusion. In acute ischemic stroke, focal reduction of rCBF is accompanied by a reduction in rCMRO$_2$. The rOEF is often elevated due to a greater reduction in rCBF than rCMRO$_2$ (6).

This initial period of increased OEF has been interpreted as reflecting a state of critical perfusion in still viable tissue during which a restoration of flow should restore both metabolism and function. The length of time that a group of neurons can survive a period of transient cerebral ischemia depends on both the severity and duration of ischemia. Other factors such as age, temperature, glucose availability, and

species also have an impact on the ability of a neuron to survive an ischemic insult. The pathophysiologic state of a group of neurons that are nonfunctional due to ischemia but salvageable on reperfusion has been called the ischemic penumbra. The increased OEF, however, is also consistent with changes in CBF and CMR that occur during postischemic hypoperfusion in animals. In one patient with persistently increased rOEF 4 days after acute stroke, Wise and coworkers raised the systemic blood pressure via angiotensin infusion (24). Flow to the infarcted region increased, rOEF fell, but rCMRO$_2$ remained unchanged and no neurologic improvement was observed. They were therefore unable to confirm an association between increased OEF and the ischemic penumbra.

Regional glucose metabolism has been difficult to measure during acute ischemic stroke due to limitations of the ¹⁸FDG method mentioned earlier. In one study of four patients studied within 48 hours of ischemia who had CBF <30 ml per 100 g per minute and thus were unlikely to have glucose metabolism limited by delivery of substrate, CMRO$_2$ was 35% of normal whereas CMRGlu was 81% of normal. The molar ratio of oxygen to glucose was 1.7 rather than the normal 5.5 (25). The evidence for the relatively increased glycolysis in the presence of adequate oxygen delivery has been attributed to glycolytic activity in neutrophils and macrophages.

The area of CBF and metabolism reduction associated with an infarction is often larger than the lesion seen on anatomic imaging studies such as MR. This surrounding zone has sometimes been interpreted as indicating the ischemic penumbra, especially because rCBF values of 15–20 ml per 100 g per minute have been measured in this area. The difficulty in making this assumption, however, is that these measurements can be attributed to the poor spatial resolution of PET methods and may not indicate a zone of reversible ischemic neuronal dysfunction (Figs. 5 and 6).

Studies performed in human subjects a few days to a week following infarction have shown mild increases in rCBF whereas the rate of oxygen metabolism remains low and unchanged. rOEF consequently is reduced below normal values. This increase in rCBF peaks at on 1–2 weeks and then declines. By 1 month CBF and CMRO$_2$ are decreased to the same degree, and OEF is either normal or slightly reduced (6).

Studies in animal models of acute ischemia have helped to better define the time course of early hemodynamic and metabolic events. Recently, Pappata et al showed in a baboon model of MCA occlusion that a zone of increased OEF first develops centrally and then moves progressively more peripherally over time (26). OEF was elevated in the MCA territory both at 1 hour and at 3 hours after occlusion. At 3 hours the rCMRO$_2$ had fallen in the central or deep MCA territory, consistent with infarction. In peripheral, cortical regions, however, CMRO$_2$ was only moderately reduced, suggesting possible viability. These peripheral regions usually go on to infarction within hours even without further

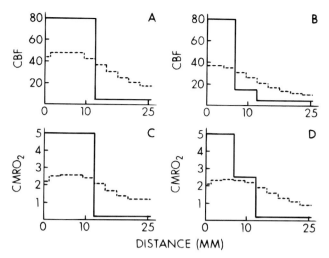

FIG. 5. Graphical representation of simulated PET measurements of cerebral blood flow (CBF) and cerebral metabolic rate of oxygen ($CMRO_2$) in ml per 100 g per minute. Solid lines represent the true values and dashed lines represent the values measure by PET. **A:** Cerebral infarct without penumbra. True CBF in normal brain surrounding the infarct is 80 and abruptly changes to a value of 5 within the infarct. **B:** Cerebral infarct with penumbra. True CBF in normal brain is 80, penumbral flow is 15, and infarct is 5. **C:** Cerebral infarct without penumbra demonstrates an abrupt decrease in true $CMRO_2$ from 5 (normal brain) to 0.2 (infarct). **D:** Cerebral infarct with penumbra demonstrates true $CMRO_2$ of 5 in normal brain, 2.5 in penumbra, and 0 in the infarct. Values measure by PET in the area surrounding the infarct are approximately the same whether or not there is a penumbra. (From ref. 44.)

reduction in CBF. This gradual movement of reduced oxygen metabolism from central to peripheral has been termed the dynamic penumbra by Heiss and coworkers, who have described this phenomenon in cats lasting up to 24 hours (27). Similar observations of potential viable periinfarct tissue that go on to infarction have also been made in humans. The authors referenced above have proposed a therapeutic window for the treatment of ischemia based on these studies. Whether these areas are salvageable, however, remains to be proven.

Investigators have also used PET to measure central benzodiazapine receptor binding sites after acute ischemia. Sette and coworkers measured ^{11}C-labeled flumazenil, an antagonist of central benzodiazepine receptors and ^{11}C-labeled PK 11195, a peripheral benzodiazepine receptor antagonist, as well as rCBF, rCBV, and rOEF in a baboon model of stroke (28). They demonstrated a delayed (20–40 days to maximal binding) increase of the uptake of the peripheral antagonist, likely reflecting glial and macrophage reaction. More importantly, they noted a marked early and prolonged reduction in the uptake of the central receptor antagonist, ^{11}C-flumazenil, within the area of infarction that was unchanged after day 2 postinfarction. This reduction was independent of time and perfusion and said to reflect neuronal damage.

Stroke Treatment

Similar to the use of PET to monitor the hemodynamic and metabolic effects of surgical revascularization and medical intervention in carotid occlusive disease, PET has also been used to assess the effect of medical therapy for acute

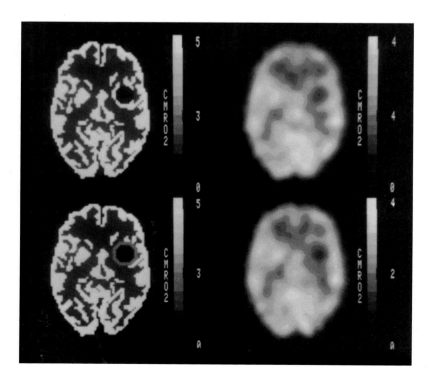

FIG. 6. Simulated PET images corresponding to $CMRO_2$ data shown in Fig. 5. *Left:* Digitized brain slices simulating true $CMRO_2$ values from a right Sylvan infarct without penumbra *(upper left)* and with penumbra *(lower left)*. *Right:* Simulated PET reconstructions of the digitized data show no obvious difference between infarct without penumbra *(upper right)* and with penumbra *(lower right)* except that the latter appears slightly larger. (From ref. 44.)

ischemic stroke. Hakim and colleagues studied the effect of nimodipine in 14 patients randomized to either intravenous nimodipine or carrier solution within 48 hours of acute ischemia (29). PET scans were obtained prior to randomization and 7 days later. They reported increased rCBF and rCMRO$_2$ within the infarct in the treatment group. However, the data analysis neither was corrected for the multiple comparisons nor was a conventional two-tailed probability used. It is unlikely that the observed increase in CMRO$_2$ is statistically valid.

Diaschisis

A common finding in PET studies of both acute and chronic stroke has been areas of reduced flow and metabolism at sites distant from the site of infarction (Fig. 3). The reduction in CBF and CMR are often but not always matched, ie, reduced to the same degree at these sites. This indicates that the cause of the reduced flow is not a limited supply but rather a reduction in metabolic demand due to reduced neuronal demand. The remote reductions in flow and metabolism generally occur in areas subserved by afferent or efferent pathways from the primary lesion. This phenomenon has been termed diaschisis. Diaschisis has been observed in the visual cortex with local reduction in CMRGlu after infarction involving the optic radiations (30). Similar findings have been reported in other cortical sites, particularly those overlying subcortical infarctions. Decreased metabolism of the ipsilateral thalamus after cortical or subcortical infarction has been reported as well as the converse condition of decreased cortical metabolism after ipsilateral thalamic infarction. Decreased flow and metabolism of the contralateral cerebral and cerebellar hemispheres have been observed after hemispheric cerebral infarction.

Clinical neurologic deficit correlating with these remote areas of decreased metabolism has been reported. Karbe and coworkers investigated 26 patients with aphasia after left MCA distribution infarction with PET, CT, and a language test battery including the Token test (31). Token test performance correlated with the degree of parietotemporal metabolism, regardless of infarct location. They concluded that infarcts of the basal ganglia or anterior MCA distribution disturb language comprehension via remote effects of parietotemporal metabolism (diaschisis). Similarly, neuropsychiatric abnormalities have also been reported after thalamic infarction (32).

Prognostic Value of PET

Some data suggest that PET scans may have prognostic value in acute stroke by allowing assessment of the hemodynamic and metabolic sequelae of ischemia that may have no clinical manifestations. In the acute setting, this information may be useful in identifying patients who would benefit from different therapies. Before PET can be used for this application, however, it must be shown to be yield useful prognostic information not discernible from clinical examination.

Marchal et al studied regional blood flow and oxygen metabolism in 18 patients with acute middle cerebral stroke between 5 and 18 hours after onset of symptoms and correlated their findings with neurologic outcome at 2 months (33). They could separate their patients into three groups based on the PET scan results. The first group had reduced blood flow and metabolism, suggesting irreversible damage. These patients had a poor outcome. The second group of patients demonstrated reduced flow and metabolism but to a lesser extent than the first group. This pattern was associated with a variable recovery of function. The third group showed increased perfusion and largely unchanged oxygen metabolism. This group had excellent return of function, suggesting early spontaneous reperfusion and collaterals that were able to maintain the minimum necessary flow during the period of occlusion. These patterns of blood flow and metabolism may be useful in designing therapeutic trials by screening out patients who would be unlikely to benefit from a specific therapy.

Recent data also suggest that PET may also help predict the long-term rehabilitation potential following infarction. DiPiero et al studied 10 patients with motor deficit with serial PET scans and found no predictive value of the CMRO$_2$ at the lesion site and the degree of recovery but found a correlation between CMRO$_2$ change and degree of recovery when PET scans were repeated 3 months later (34). Heiss et al performed a multivariate analysis of 76 stroke patients to assess predictors of social recovery and rehabilitation (35). They measured rCMRGlu several days following supratentorial infarction and assessed outcome at approximately 2 months. They found significant correlation with age, hypertension, and cardiac disease and poor recovery. In addition, reduced glucose metabolism in regions outside of the area of infarction also correlated with poor outcome but only for the hypertensive patients and this correlation was not strong ($r = 0.56$). Serrati et al found poor predictive value of the degree of contralateral cerebellar hypometabolism (diaschisis) measured 5–30 hours with recovery (36). However, patients without significant contralateral cerebellar hypometabolism (diaschisis) on acute PET scans all made a good neurologic recovery.

Mapping Functional Recovery

The mechanisms of recovery of function after infarction is poorly understood. Recently, however, researchers using PET techniques of functional brain mapping have begun to study brain recovery after stroke. An important implication of this line of inquiry includes the potential for identifying the optimal therapy for functional recovery. Researchers from the MRC cyclotron unit at Hammersmith Hospital have found that recovery of motor function after MCA distribution infarction was associated with either recovered or preserved tissue in the ipsilateral motor cortex or recruitment of tissue contralateral to the infarct (34). The contralateral activation observed in this study may have been due to mirror motion of the patient's other hand, which was not controlled for.

SUBARACHNOID HEMORRHAGE

The factors affecting cerebral oxygen metabolism and blood flow after aneurysmal subarachnoid hemorrhage are not completely defined. Several investigators have shown a depression of oxidative metabolism shortly after aneurysm rupture not related to vasospasm or ischemia (37,38). The reason for the primary reduction in $CMRO_2$ is not known but may be related to direct toxic effects of blood on cerebral metabolism.

Patients studied during periods of arteriographically confirmed vasospasm have yielded conflicting data. Most of these studies have demonstrated reduced CBF and $CMRO_2$ with increased CBV (38). These studies may be complicated by the inclusion of postoperative patients in whom brain retraction or other postoperative sequelae, such as hemodilution, may have changed the normal cerebrovascular and metabolic consequences of vasospasm. Carpenter and coworkers studying patients prior to surgery found reduced blood flow and normal $CMRO_2$ and CBV in regions without vasospasm (37). Regions with vasospasm demonstrated reduced blood flow and blood volume with increased OEF and no change in $CMRO_2$.

LEUKOARIOSIS

Leukoariosis refers to the white matter lucencies seen on CT and the high T2-weighted signal seen on MR. These imaging findings are nonspecific and reflect many different pathologies. The generally accepted hypothesis is that they are due to chronic ischemia, either ongoing or an old event. Most PET studies only look at large confluent areas. Two studies have specifically looked for evidence of ongoing ischemia. Yao and coworkers studied a group of patients with vascular dementia of the Binzwanger type and found reduced gray and white matter CBF and $CMRO_2$, but normal OEF (39). Meguro et al examined 21 patients with periventricular hyperintensities on MR and found similar results (40). De-Reuck and colleagues studied 30 patients and found reduced blood flow and $CMRO_2$ (41). rOEF was elevated in the frontal white matter. This may not be statistically valid due to the multiple comparisons employed in the analysis. In addition, these same investigators found similar data in ten patients after cardiac arrest in whom no ongoing ischemia should be occurring. Therefore, while leukoariosis may reflect the sequelae of ischemia, it does not appear to be due to ongoing chronic ischemia.

Conversely, in a study of 16 patients with carotid occlusive disease, Yamauchi et al found a correlation between regions of high T2 signal in white matter and hemispheric increases in OEF (42). These data suggest that leukoariosis in the setting of carotid occlusive disease may reflect hemodynamic compromise.

FUTURE CLINICAL APPLICATIONS

PET is well established as a unique research tool for the accurate measurement of regional cerebral metabolism and hemodynamics, both for animal models of ischemia and for clinical research in humans. Two basic principles must be satisfied in order for PET to find a clinical application, however. First, the data it provides must be unobtainable by other cheaper or less invasive means. Second, the data must be shown to have some impact on clinical decision making in terms of guiding therapy or establishing prognosis. Keeping these two criteria in mind, we will discuss future clinical and clinical research applications of PET. These applications can be separated into two topics: the prognostic value of cerebrovascular measurements and the use of these measurements as surrogate treatment endpoints to guide and evaluate therapy.

Establishing Prognosis

In patients with carotid occlusive disease, PET has been shown to provide an accurate and valid method for the in vivo assessment of cerebral hemodynamics in uninfarcted brain tissue. This information does not provide useful information in the clinical management of individual patients because the accurate knowledge of cerebral hemodynamics does not yet permit identification of a subgroup of patients at high risk for subsequent stroke. A longitudinal study of stroke risk in those with and without abnormal PET studies as well as a controlled trial of surgical versus medical treatment in those patients with PET evidence of reduced CPP are needed. Prognostic or therapeutic significance cannot be attributed to PET findings of hemodynamic compromise without good data. In fact, if emboli are the most common cause of stroke even in patients with reduced CPP, this entire line of reasoning may be incorrect. In summary, although PET can provide an accurate indication of the cerebral hemodynamic status in individual patients with cerebrovascular disease, the value of this information in improving patient care remains to be demonstrated.

If such value is demonstrated, PET must compared with other diagnostic tests such as SPECT, TCD, or Xenon-CT in order to determine which would be the most cost efficient means of predicting stroke risk and choosing therapy. While PET is clearly the most accurate technology, it is also the most expensive.

Recent data described in this chapter suggest that PET may provide useful prognostic information in both the acute and chronic stage of ischemic stroke. If PET can separate patients with salvageable tissue from those with completed infarction in the acute setting and this information is unobtainable by cheaper means, PET may find a valuable role in the triage of stroke patients in the intensive care unit (ICU) (33). The cost of a PET scan in this situation might be offset by the benefits of reducing the length of ICU stay. This is an extremely promising area of future research. Experimental treatment protocols of acute ischemic stroke would be improved significantly if they could target a population most likely to benefit. This is particularly true in thrombolysis trials where the incidence of complications such as hemorrhage and edema are significantly increased in patients with completed infarctions. The time required to make the necessary PET measurements may be an obstacle to routine clinical application. In acute stroke, where the time interval between the onset of ischemia and the institution of therapy is likely to have a direct bearing on outcome, the additional time necessary to perform PET may be critical. The data obtained would have to have crucial bearing on therapeutic decisions in order to justify the delay. Unless the treatment carried significant morbidity and mortality and the data derived from PET reduced these complications, PET may not be worthwhile.

Similar benefits could be seen in the rehabilitation setting, using PET or other functional imaging methods to identify subgroups of patients most likely to benefit from specific therapies. In summary, PET measurements in patients with acute or chronic ischemia have the potential to be of value in selecting candidates for both acute and chronic therapeutic interventions.

Use of Surrogate Physiologic Measurements

Currently, a great deal of research in cerebrovascular disease is devoted to the development of methods to improve cerebral oxygenation and blood flow in the immediate period following acute focal cerebral ischemia with the aim of salvaging reversible ischemic brain tissue before infarction. PET measurements of cerebral hemodynamics and metabolism may be useful in monitoring the consequences of these interventions. The accurate measurement of regional CBF and $CMRO_2$, currently possible only with PET, is indispensable for determining if therapeutic measures designed to improve oxygenation of ischemic tissue actually achieve that end. With such information, the rational adjustment of both intensity and duration of treatment can be carried out to ensure therapeutic benefit and reduce side effects. For example, in treating patients with ischemic vasospasm due to subarachnoid hemorrhage by volume expansion and induced hypertension, intravenous fluids and vasopressors could be adjusted to maintain CBF above 25–30 ml per 100 g per minute. Already infarcted areas with very low $CMRO_2$ could also be identified and futile attempts at further blood pressure elevation could be avoided. Similar monitoring and adjustment of other therapies aimed at improving blood flow and oxygen delivery could be possible.

This approach has considerable potential for drug development in terms of identifying therapeutic windows and dose. While these applications are exciting and represent a current avenue of clinical PET research, the routine clinical use of PET for these purposes is limited by three issues. It must be demonstrated that (a) PET measurements can accurately distinguish reversibly ischemic from infarcted tissue; (b) interventions designed to improve oxygenation of acutely ischemic cerebral tissue actually do so and can be applied in clinical settings to actually reduce morbidity and mortality; and (c) the use of PET monitoring provides benefit by improving safety, reducing costs, or increasing efficacy. While PET will play a major role in the clinical research necessary to establishing these data, until such studies are completed its application for individual patient care in this setting cannot be justified. These same criteria will apply to other imaging modalities, such as diffusion-weighted MR. Like PET, diffusion-weighted MR may be able to distinguish reversibly ischemic tissue from infarcted tissue. However, before it can be applied to routine patient care, its accuracy must be validated, and it must yield some benefit to the patient in terms of reducing mortality, morbidity, and cost.

CONCLUSION

Positron emission tomography provides unique, quantitative regional measurements of cerebral hemodynamics and metabolism in humans. These measurements have yielded important information regarding the pathophysiology of cerebrovascular disease. It is tempting to conclude that any test that provides accurate data related to the pathophysiology of the disease under consideration is clinically useful. PET remains primarily a research tool for two basic reasons. PET is expensive and physician-intensive and, most importantly, measurements of cerebral hemodynamics and metabolism have not yet been shown to provide clinically important information. The data provided by PET do not currently improve patient care by reducing either morbidity and mortality or expense. If the data PET can provide become necessary for making rational treatment decisions and the same information cannot be gathered with cheaper imaging modalities, then a clinical role for PET may be established. Until then PET will continue to play a significant role in clinical research into the pathophysiology and treatment of human cerebrovascular disease.

ACKNOWLEDGMENTS

Dr. Derdeyn is supported as the Siemens Medical Systems/Radiological Society of North America Research and Education Fund Fellow and by a training grant from the Charles S. Dana Foundation through the Dana Consortium on Neuroscience: Neuroimaging Leadership Training.

Dr. Powers is supported by a grant from the Charles S. Dana Foundation through the Dana Consortium on Neuroscience: Neuroimaging Leadership Training and NIH NINDS grants NS28947, NS06833, DK27085, and NS32568.

REFERENCES

1. Powers WJ, Raichle ME. Positron emission tomography and its application to the study of cerebrovascular disease in man. *Stroke* 1985;16:361–376.
2. Lammertsma AA, Frackowiak RSJ. Positron emission tomography. *CRC Crit Rev Biomed Eng* 1985;13:125–169.
3. Baron JC, Frackowiak RSJ, Herholz K, et al. Use of PET methods for measurement of cerebral energy metabolism and hemodynamics in cerebrovascular disease. *J Cereb Blood Flow Metab* 1989;9:723–742.
4. Powers WJ, Dagogo-Jack S, Markham J, Larson KB, Dence CS. Cerebral transport and metabolism of 1-^{11}C-D-glucose during stepped hypoglycemia. *Ann Neurol* 1995. In press.
5. Wood JH, Kee Jr DB. Hemorheology of the cerebral circulation in stroke. *Stroke* 1985;16:765–772.
6. Powers WJ. Cerebral hemodynamics in ischemic cerebrovascular disease. *Ann Neurol* 1991;29:231–240.
7. Baron JC, Rougemont D, Soussaline F, et al. Local interrelationships of cerebral oxygen consumption and glucose utilization in normal subjects and in ischemic stroke patients: a positron emission tomography study. *J Cereb Blood Flow Metab* 1984;4:140–149.
8. Fox PT, Raichle ME, Mintun MA, Dence C. Nonoxidative glucose consumption during focal physiologic neural activity. *Science* 1988;241:462–464.
9. Grubb RL Jr, Raichle ME, Phelps ME, Ratcheson RA. Effects of increased intracranial pressure on cerebral blood volume, blood flow and oxygen utilization in monkeys. *J Neurosurg* 1975;43:385–398.
10. Powers WJ. Is the ratio of cerebral blood volume to cerebral blood flow a reliable indicator of cerebral perfusion pressure? *J Cereb Blood Flow Metab* 1993;13 Suppl 1:S325.
11. Sette G, Baron JC, Mazoyer B, et al. Local brain haemodynamics and oxygen metabolism in cerebrovascular disease. *Brain* 1989;113:931–951.
12. Powers WJ, Grubb RL Jr, Darriet D, Raichle ME. Cerebral blood flow and cerebral metabolic rate of oxygen requirements for cerebral function and viability in humans. *J Cereb Blood Flow Metab* 1985;5:600–608.
13. Altman DI, Powers WJ, Perlman JM, et al. Cerebral blood requirement for brain viability in newborn infants is lower than in adults. *Ann Neurol* 1988;24:218–226.
14. Baron JC, Bousser MG, Rey A, Guillard A, Comar D, Castaigne P. Reversal of focal "misery-perfusion syndrome" by extra-intracranial arterial bypass in hemodynamic cerebral ischemia. *Stroke* 1981;12:454–459.
15. Powers WJ, Press GA, Grubb RL Jr, Gado M, Raichle ME. The effect of hemodynamically significant carotid artery disease on the hemodynamic status of the cerebral circulation. *Ann Intern Med* 1987;106:27–35.
16. Carpenter DA, Grubb RL Jr, Powers WJ. Border zone hemodynamics in cerebrovascular disease. *Neurology* 1990;40:1587–1592.
17. The EC/IC Bypass Group. Failure of extracranial–intracranial arterial bypass to reduce the risk of ischemic stroke. results of an international randomized trial. *N Engl J Med* 1985;313:1191–1200.
18. Yamauchi H, Fukuyama H, Ogawa M, Ouchi Y, Kimura J. Hemodilution improves cerebral hemodynamics in internal carotid artery occlusion. *Stroke* 1993;24:1885–1890.
19. Hino A, Ueda S, Mizukawa N, Imahori Y, Tenjin H. Effect of hemodilution on cerebral hemodynamics and oxygen metabolism. *Stroke* 1992;23:423–426.
20. Sollevi A, Ericson K, Eriksson L, Lindqvist C, Lagerkranser M, Stone-Elander S. Effect of adenosine on human cerebral blood flow as determined by positron emission tomography. *J Cereb Blood Flow Metab* 1987;7:673–678.
21. Powers WJ, Grubb Jr RL, Raichle ME. Clinical results of extracranial–intracranial bypass surgery in patients with hemodynamic cerebrovascular disease. *J Neurosurg* 1989;70:61–67.
22. Klieser B, Widder B. Course of carotid artery occlusions with impaired cerebrovascular reactivity. *Stroke* 1992;23:171–174
23. Yonas H, Smith HA, Durham SR, Pentheny SL, Johnson DW. Increased stroke risk predicted by compromised cerebral blood flow reactivity. *J Neurosurg* 1993;79:483–489.
24. Wise RJS, Bernardi S, Frackoiak RSJ, Legg NJ, Jones T. Serial observations on the pathophysiology of acute stroke. *Brain* 1983;106:197–222.
25. Wise RJS, Rhodes CG, Gibbs JM, et al. Disturbance of oxidative metabolism of glucose in recent human cerebral infarcts. *Ann Neurol* 1983;14:627–637.
26. Pappata S, Fiorelli M, Rommel T, et al. PET study of changes in local brain hemodynamics and oxygen metabolism after unilateral middle cerebral artery occlusion in baboons. *J Cereb Blood Flow Metab* 1993;13:416–424.
27. Heiss, W-D, Graf R, Wienhard K, et al. Dynamic penumbra demonstrated by sequential multitracer PET after middle cerebral artery occlusion in cats. *J Cereb Blood Flow Metab* 1994;14:892–902.
28. Sette G, Baron JC, Young AR, et al. In vivo mapping of brain benzodiazepine receptor changes by positron emission tomography after focal ischemia in the anesthetized baboon. *Stroke* 1993;24:2046–2058.
29. Hakim AM, Evans AC, Berger L, et al. The effect of nimodipine on the evolution of human cerebral infarction studied by PET. *J Cereb Blood Flow Metab* 1989;9:523–534.
30. Feeney DM, Baron JC. Diaschisis. *Stroke* 1986;17:817–830.
31. Karbe H, Herholz K, Szelies B, Pawlik G, Wienhard K, Heiss WD. Regional metabolic correlates of Token test results in cortical and subcortical left hemispheric infarction. *Neurology* 1989;39:1083–1088.
32. Pappata S, Mazoyer BM, Tran-Dinh S, Cambon H, Levasseur M, Baron JC. Effects of capsular or thalamic stroke on metabolism in the cortex and cerebellum. A positron tomography study. *Stroke* 1990;21:519–524.
33. Marchal G, Serrati C, Rioux P, et al. PET imaging of cerebral perfusion and oxygen consumption in acute ischemic stroke: relation to outcome. *Lancet* 1993;341:925–927.
34. DiPiero V, Chollet FM, MacCarthy P, Lenzi GL, Frackowiak RSJ. Motor recovery after acute ischemic stroke: a metabolic study. *J Neurol Neurosurg Pyschiatry* 1992;55:990–996.
35. Heiss W-D, Emunds H-G, Herholz K. Cerebral glucose metabolism as a predictor of rehabilitation after ischemic stroke. *Stroke* 1993;24:1784–1788.
36. Serrati C, Marchal G, Rioux P, et al. Contralateral cerebellar hypometabolism: a predictor for stroke outcome? *J Neurol Neurosurg Psychiatry* 1994;57:174–179.
37. Carpenter DA, Grubb RL Jr, Tempel LW, Powers WJ. Cerebral oxygen metabolism after aneurysmal subarachnoid hemorrhage. *J Cereb Blood Flow Metab* 1991;11:837–844.
38. Kawamura S, Sayama I, Yasui, Uemura K. Sequential changes in cerebral blood flow and metabolism in patients with subarachnoid haemorrhage. *Acta Neurochir* 1992;114:12–15.
39. Yao H, Sadoshima S, Kuwabara Y, Ichiya Y, Fujishima M. Cerebral blood flow and oxygen metabolism in patients with vascular dementia of the Binswinger type. *Stroke* 1990;21:1694–1699.
40. Meguro K, Hatazawa J, Yamaguchi T, et al. Cerebral circulation and oxygen metabolism associated with subclinical periventricular hyperintensity as shown by magnetic resonance imaging. *Ann Neurol* 1990;28:378–383.
41. De Reuck J, Decoo D, Strijckmans K, Lemahieu I. Does the severity of leukoariosis contribute to senile dementia? A comparative computerized and positron emission tomographic study. *Eur Neurol* 1992;23:199–205.
42. Yamauchi H, Fukuyama H, Yamaguchi S, Miyoshi T, Kimura J, Konishi J. High-intensity area in the deep white matter indicating hemodynamic compromise in internal carotid artery occlusive disease. *Arch Neurol* 1991;48:1067–1071.
43. Budinger TF, Derenzo SE, Guilberg GT, et al. Emission computer assisted tomography with single-photon and positron annihilation photon emitters. *J Comput Assist Tomogr* 1977;1:131–145.
44. Powers WJ, Mintun MA. The role of positron tomography in identification of the ischemic penumbra. In: Powers WJ, Raichle ME, eds. *Cerebrovascular diseases. Proceedings of the fifteenth research (Princeton) conference.* New York: Raven Press, 1987:273–281.

Cerebrovascular Disease, edited by H. Hunt Batjer.
Lippincott-Raven Publishers, Philadelphia © 1997.

CHAPTER **20**

Ultrasonic Evaluation of the Cervical Vasculature

Jesse Weinberger

The extracranial carotid artery is a frequent source of cerebral ischemia because atherosclerotic disease develops at the bifurcation of the internal and external carotid arteries (1). There are two primary mechanisms for production of cerebral ischemia from the extracranial carotid: emboli can arise from atheroma at the bifurcation and occlude distal intracranial arteries (2), or complete occlusion or high-grade stenosis of the internal carotid artery at the bifurcation can cause hemodynamic compromise resulting in cerebral infarction when collateral circulation is inadequate (3).

Patients with extracranial carotid artery disease may present with symptoms of transient cerebral ischemia (also termed transient ischemic attack, TIA) or irreversible cerebral infarction (CVA) (4) and can often be identified before the onset of cerebrovascular symptoms by auscultation of a vascular bruit in the neck (5). It has become important to recognize, categorize, and quantify atherosclerotic disease at the carotid artery bifurcation because both medical (6) and surgical (7,8) treatments have been developed for the prevention of stroke.

The extracranial carotid artery is the etiologic source of TIA in about 50% of patients (9), with other sources of cerebral ischemia such as cardioembolic phenomena or intracranial vascular disease accounting for the other half. Only 60% of patients with a cervical vascular bruit have identifiable extracranial carotid artery disease (5), and most do not have sufficient obstruction to warrant surgical intervention. Intraarterial contrast angiography is painful and carries about a 1% risk of complications in patients with cerebrovascular disease (10). Therefore, noninvasive sonographic methods have developed to image the extent of extracranial carotid artery disease with real-time B-mode scanning and to determine the degree of compromise of

blood flow by Doppler sonography. These techniques have been combined in the technique of duplex Doppler B-mode sonography to image the carotid bifurcation and determine blood flow in the corresponding regions of the artery. The addition of color flow Doppler sonography to the B-mode image has enhanced the accuracy of the ultrasound examination and made it easier to perform, resulting in widespread use of duplex Doppler sonography in screening patients for carotid artery disease.

DOPPLER SONOGRAPHIC TECHNIQUES

Doppler sonography employs high-frequency sound waves in the range of 2.0–10.0 MHz to measure the velocity of the red cells flowing through a blood vessel. Lower frequencies penetrate deeper into the underlying tissue; higher frequencies yield better resolution. The sound wave beam is passed through the artery underlying the skin and is reflected back from the red cells as they go by. The returning echo is detected by the Doppler instrument. The frequency of the echo is altered by the reflecting object (red cells) to a degree proportional to their velocity. The frequency shift is also dependent on the frequency of the emitted ultrasound beam and the angle at which the beam reflects off of the flowing particles (red cells). The frequency shift is related to the velocity of the red cells by the following equation:

$$fd = 2fd\ v \cos\theta\ (c - v \cos\theta)$$

where fd = frequency of the ultrasound beam, v = velocity of the flowing particles, c = sound propagation of the surrounding tissue, and θ is the angle of insonation (11).

The shift of frequency of the sound waves caused by the flow of blood is in the audible range. The Doppler instrument calculates the frequency shift of the incoming reflected sound wave from the original outgoing sound wave and produces a signal that can be heard by the examiner. The fre-

J. Weinberger: Department of Neurology, Mount Sinai School of Medicine, and Division of Neurology, North General Hospital, New York, New York 10029.

quency shift is displayed quantitatively on an analyzer by a fast Fourier transform that shows all of the frequency shifts being received or a mean of the frequency shifts. This results in a waveform with a peak in systole and runoff in diastole referred to as spectral analysis of Doppler frequency shifts. Because of Bernoulli's principle, the velocity of the red blood cells is proportionately increased and the resultant frequency shift is higher the smaller the area of the lumen through which the cells are passing (11). Thus, the degree of stenosis of an artery can be determined by the Doppler frequency shift compared to the frequency shift in a normal artery of the same size.

There are two basic types of Doppler sonography: continuous wave and pulsed. Continuous wave Doppler instruments emit an ultrasound beam constantly and the receiving transducer records all frequency shifts returning to the Doppler probe. If the cervical carotid artery is being auscultated and the sound wave beam passes through the internal and external carotids and jugular vein, all frequency shifts from these structures will be recorded and superimposed on spectral analysis of the Doppler frequencies. Pulsed Doppler instruments emit an ultrasound beam at a constant interval and receive the returning sound wave from a specified distance from the probe, which can be adjusted so that recordings of frequency shifts can be obtained from a distinct location in an individual artery. Pulsed Doppler instruments can distinguish the differences in laminar flow in a particular artery, demonstrating smooth higher velocity flow in the center of the stream and lower velocity, turbulent flow at the walls of the vessel. Continuous wave Doppler records all frequency shifts coming from the vessel from the center of lumen to the arterial walls (11).

Pulsed Doppler is commonly used in duplex systems with B-mode sonography because of its specificity. The artery is visualized with the B-mode scan and a cursor is placed within the segment from which signals are to be recorded. This sets the depth from which the pulsed Doppler instrument will receive the frequency shift signals. The disadvantage of a pulsed Doppler system is aliasing. When the frequencies reflected from the flowing particles are greater than twice the rate of emission of the pulsed Doppler signal, the recorded frequency shifts will be lower than the corresponding blood flow velocity would indicate and may even be negative. This causes underestimation or sometimes failure in detection of the highest velocity flows from the most severe stenoses. This can be obviated by increasing the pulse repetition frequency (PRF) to higher rates but can still be the source of false-negative results. With continuous wave Doppler, there is no aliasing of signal and the highest frequency shifts from the most stenotic vessels can be recorded accurately. Also, since continuous wave Doppler is recording all frequency shifts emanating from the artery, it can detect turbulent flow of the blood passing by a plaque on the wall of the artery, which disrupts laminar flow but does not increase the velocity of the red cells in the center of the lumen from which the pulsed Doppler recording would be obtained. Thus, pulsed Doppler is more specific than continuous wave Doppler, whereas continuous wave Doppler is more sensitive and can be used accurately by an experienced examiner to interpret the recorded sounds by auscultation as well as by reading the frequency shifts on spectral analysis (12).

Color flow Doppler records all of the frequencies reflected from an artery and displays them across the B-mode image. Flow toward the probe is recorded in red and flow away from the probe is recorded in blue, or these can be reversed. Frequency shifts above a set limit are coded in white or yellow so that areas of high-velocity flow from stenosis of the artery can be visualized. The pulsed Doppler cursor is then placed in the area of turbulence to record the spectral analysis of the Doppler frequency shifts in order to quantify the degree of stenosis.

The frequency shift information derived from spectral analysis can be used directly, but since the frequency shift recorded is dependent on the frequency of the emitted ultrasound beam, the frequency shift for a given degree of stenosis may vary among instruments. If the frequency of the emitted sound wave is known and the angle of insonation of the arterial lumen can be determined by lining up the pulsed Doppler cursor parallel to the direction of the artery, the actual velocity of the flowing red blood cells can be calculated by the Doppler equation. This provides a more reproducible method for determining the degree of stenosis of an artery independent of the particular Doppler equipment being used (11).

DOPPLER EXAMINATION OF THE CAROTID ARTERY BIFURCATION

The normal common, internal, and external carotid arteries have characteristic Doppler frequency shift patterns. The internal carotid artery is a low-resistance vessel, and the spectral pattern shows a rapid rise of flow velocity (frequency shift) in systole and a gradual decline in diastole, with flow continuing through diastole. With pulsed Doppler systems, there is a clear "window" where there are no frequency shifts below the envelope of flow signals recorded by the pulsed Doppler probe (Fig. 1A). The external carotid artery is a high-resistance vessel, with a shorter systolic waveform than the internal carotid and a precipitous decline of flow into diastole. There is little or no flow in the external carotid in diastole (Fig. 1B). The common carotid artery has a flow pattern intermediate between the internal and external carotid arteries, with more resistance to flow in both systole and diastole than the internal but less than the external (Fig. 1C). All three vessels in the bifurcation must be demonstrated before the examination is satisfactorily completed.

Stenosis of the carotid artery can be detected by changes in the spectral pattern of the Doppler frequency shifts or calculated velocities (15). In an internal carotid artery with mild to moderate stenosis of 0% to 15%, the systolic peak

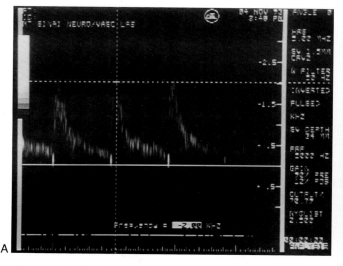

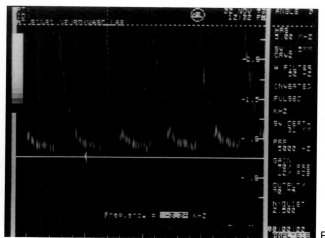

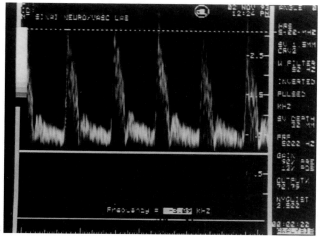

FIG. 1. The normal spectral analysis of a pulsed Doppler wave form from a color flow duplex instrument (ATL 9000 HDI, Seattle, WA) for the internal **(A)**, external **(B)**, and common **(C)** carotid arteries are shown. Note the smooth runoff in diastole in the internal carotid, the abrupt drop-off of systole in the external carotid, and the intermediate pattern in the common carotid.

frequencies will remain normal at about 2500 Hz for most Doppler instruments with 4- to 5-MHz probes but will show low frequencies filling in the normal "window" below the systolic waveform (Fig. 2B). This is referred to as spread of spectral frequencies. A moderate stenosis of 15–49% will cause progressive elevation of the systolic peak of the Doppler spectral pattern from 3000 Hz to 4000 Hz with spread of frequencies in systole (Fig. 2C). A moderately severe stenosis of 50–79% will cause elevation of the systolic peak of the Doppler spectral pattern from 4000 Hz to 5000 Hz and diastolic velocities may start to become elevated as well (Fig. 2D). With severe stenosis greater than 80%, the systolic peak will be elevated to 5000 Hz or greater, and there will be an increase in the end-diastolic frequency shifts to >2000 Hz (Fig. 2E). With pulsed Doppler instruments, aliasing may occur at the highest frequencies, with flow recorded below the baseline. The continuous wave Doppler frequency shifts for internal carotid arteries with no stenosis, moderate stenosis, and severe stenosis are shown in Fig. 3.

When there is severe stenosis, flow velocities in the internal carotid artery proximal to the stenosis may be in the normal range but will not have the typical low-resistance pattern of the normal internal carotid artery. Flow in the internal carotid distal to a severe stenosis may also be compromised, with normal velocities but a slow upsweep in systole and poor runoff in diastole. This can lead to false-negative readings if Doppler recordings are not made directly from the stenotic segment of the artery. The examiner must be careful not just to rely on the recorded frequency shifts but to be certain that the velocity waveform pattern in the internal carotid is normal before being satisfied that there is no stenosis in the internal carotid artery. Auscultation of high-frequency turbulence with the Doppler instrument that is not showing up on spectral analysis can help the examiner to realize that more accurate probe placement is necessary.

The velocity of blood flow may vary among individuals. Therefore, the flow velocities in the internal carotid artery are often compared to the flow velocities in the common carotid artery. If the systolic peak velocity or mean flow velocity is elevated in both the common and internal carotid arteries in a young individual or in a patient with exaggeration of the initial systolic peak by cardiac valve artifact (such

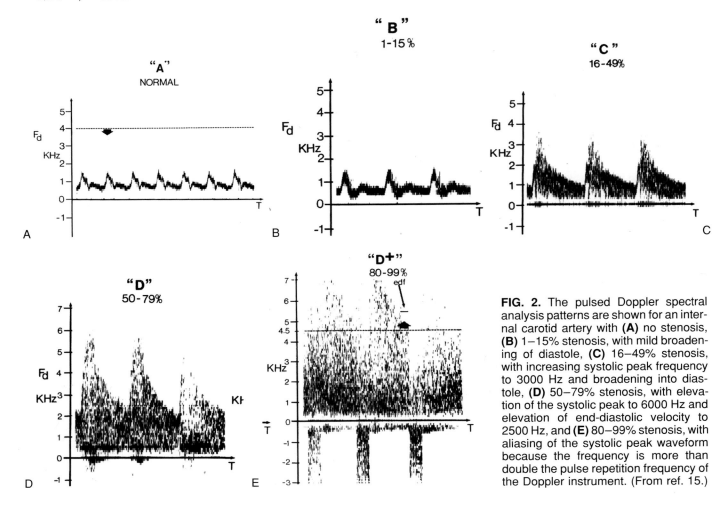

FIG. 2. The pulsed Doppler spectral analysis patterns are shown for an internal carotid artery with **(A)** no stenosis, **(B)** 1–15% stenosis, with mild broadening of diastole, **(C)** 16–49% stenosis, with increasing systolic peak frequency to 3000 Hz and broadening into diastole, **(D)** 50–79% stenosis, with elevation of the systolic peak to 6000 Hz and elevation of end-diastolic velocity to 2500 Hz, and **(E)** 80–99% stenosis, with aliasing of the systolic peak waveform because the frequency is more than double the pulse repetition frequency of the Doppler instrument. (From ref. 15.)

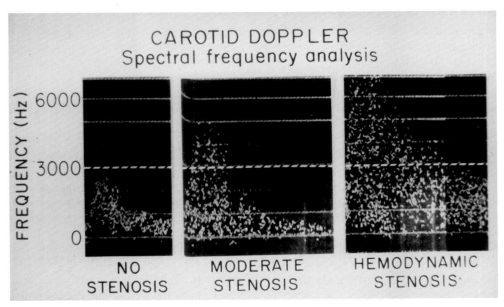

FIG. 3. Continuous wave Doppler spectral analysis patterns of an **(A)** normal, **(B)** moderately stenotic, and **(C)** severely stenotic internal carotid artery are shown.

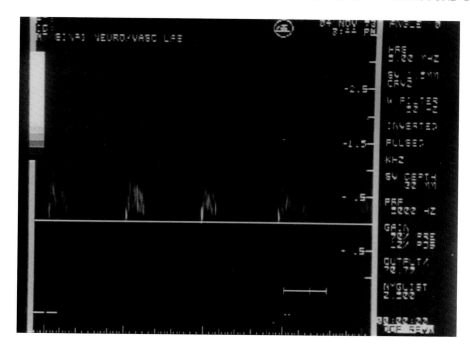

FIG. 4. The pulsed Doppler frequency pattern of a completely occluded internal carotid artery representing decreased flow in the remaining stump of the internal carotid artery.

as aortic stenosis or mitral regurgitation), the ratio of the flow velocities in the internal and common carotid arteries will remain normal. When the frequency shifts in the internal carotid artery are elevated by a stenosis, the internal carotid/ common carotid ratio will be elevated, particularly in a very severe stenosis where flow proximally in the common carotid artery is reduced. A ratio greater than 1.8 is considered to represent severe stenosis.

Complete occlusions of the internal carotid artery are difficult to diagnose. There may be no recording of the characteristic internal carotid artery signal. There will be to-and-fro flow with reduced velocities proximal to the lesion in the common carotid artery or internal carotid artery stump, with a short systole followed by a short wave of retrograde flow (Fig. 4). There may be a change in the flow pattern in the external carotid artery waveform that becomes more like the internal carotid artery, so that false-negative results can be obtained. If the internal carotid artery signal is not found without concomitant signs of proximal reduction in flow, a false-positive result can be obtained. Ancillary tests that assess distal flow such as pneumooculoplethysmography, supraorbital directional Doppler, or transcranial Doppler sonography may be helpful in confirming the diagnosis of complete occlusion by demonstrating a reduction in distal flow or perfusion pressure (13,14).

Real-Time B-Mode Ultrasonography

Real-time B-mode sonography is performed with a piezoelectric crystal that emits sound waves in the range of 2–10 MHz. As with Doppler sonography, lower frequencies are used to image deeper structures whereas higher fre-

quency probes provide greater resolution. The source can be a mechanical sector scanner or a phased array linear scanner. The mechanical sector scanner rotates to image tomographic planes of the vessel being insonated. The phased array device consists of individual ultrasound transducers that are configured in a linear arrangement and emit sound waves in a timed sequence to scan across the artery to give information in length and depth. The sound waves are reflected back from underlying structures and received by the transducer.

The intensity of the reflection is dependent on the density of the reflecting tissue. Liquids such as flowing blood are seen as black on the display monitor (television screen or oscilloscope). Calcium has high echodensity and is reflected as bright white. The walls of the artery are also echodense and are intermediate between calcium and blood (11). The intimal–medial wall thickness can be visualized and measured. The earliest atherosclerotic changes produce thickening of the intimal wall (16). Exophytic plaques extending into the arterial lumen can be visualized. When there is calcification of the plaque, there is anechoic shadowing of the arterial wall adjacent to the plaque (Fig. 5). The artery can be displayed in longitudinal or transverse views (Fig. 6).

B-mode sonography allows direct visualization of plaque morphology, constitution, and configuration that is not provided by conventional arteriography. Echolucent plaques contain recent hemorrhage and lipids in a liquid state (17). Identification of recent hemorrhage or intraluminal thrombus is important because symptomatic thromboembolic events from carotid atheroma are associated with recent hemorrhage (18–20). The degree of underlying lucency can be graded on a scale from type I through type IV (Fig. 7) (21). Clinical correlation with sonographic images has shown that echolucent plaques are associated with signifi-

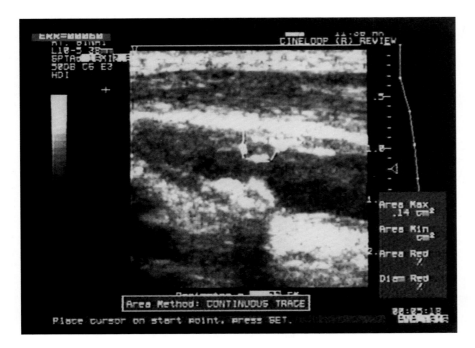

FIG. 5. A heterogeneous calcified plaque with acoustic shadowing of the wall beneath the plaque such that the wall of the artery is not reflected back to the ultrasound transducer and a void is seen underneath the plaque.

cantly more ipsilateral ischemic symptoms than echodense plaques regardless of the degree of stenosis (17). The degree of echolucency and heterogeneity of the plaque also has a predictive correlation with future thromboembolic ischemic events (22).

Plaque configuration also correlates with the degree of intraplaque hemorrhage and resultant symptomatic cerebral ischemic events. Plaques growing in a nodular configuration (Fig. 8) are homogeneous with higher echodensity, are usu-

ally simple fibrous plaques with calcification on histologic examination (23), and have the same frequency of ipsilateral ischemic symptoms as normal bifurcations (24). Plaques growing in a mural configuration along the wall of the bifurcation in a crescentic pattern, often with scalloped borders (Fig. 9), are heterogeneous, are associated with intraplaque hemorrhage and intraluminal thrombus (23), and are associated with a similar frequency of symptoms as arteries with high-grade stenosis of greater than 75% even when they are

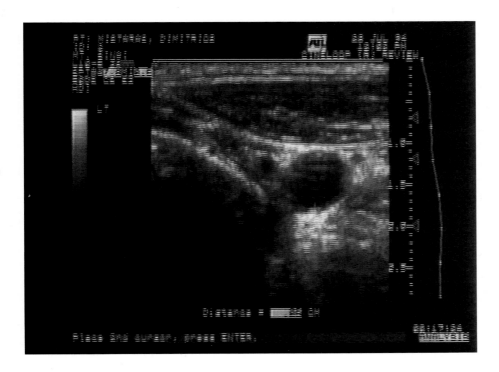

FIG. 6. A transverse view of the plaque seen in Fig. 5, showing soft echodensities of plaque in the upper half of the lumen. Transverse views help in calculating the percent stenosis of the internal carotid artery.

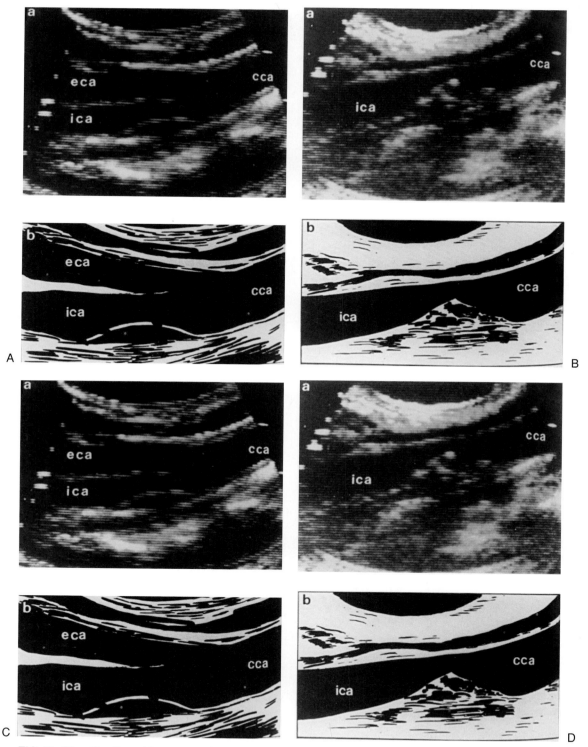

FIG. 7. Classification of heterogeneity of plaques, representing intraplaque thrombus. **A:** Type I, predominantly echolucent raised lesion with thin cap of echodensity, indicating a recent hemorrhage into the plaque. **B:** Type II, a heterogeneous lesion with mixed areas of echolucency, particularly near the luminal surface, indicating subacute hemorrhage with a moderate amount of thrombus. **C:** Type III, predominantly echogenic with small deep areas of lucency, indicating resolving thrombus. **D:** Type IV, uniformly echodense lesion without thrombus. (From ref. 21.)

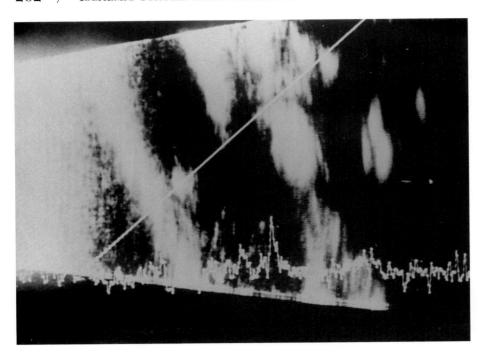

FIG. 8. A nodular plaque, indicating simple fibrous plaque, in the bifurcation near the origin of the internal carotid artery. (From ref. 24.)

not hemodynamically obstructive (24). When patients are followed over a 3-year period with carotid sonography and clinical evaluation, new events of ipsilateral cerebral ischemia are associated with plaque growth, particularly into a mural configuration suggesting recent hemorrhage into the plaque. The outcomes were independent of the degree of stenosis of the internal carotid (25). These findings correlate directly with the data on acute coronary occlusive disease with crescendo angina or myocardial infarction, in which

recent plaque hemorrhage is responsible for acute events rather than the degree of stenosis prior to the hemorrhage (26) and can be identified on angiography by the finding of crescentic plaque with scalloped borders (27).

Craters in plaques can also be identified (Fig. 10) but do not necessarily correlate with ulceration of the endothelial lining, which cannot definitely be ascertained by B-mode sonography (28). Craters may have importance in identifying a plaque that has recently produced a thromboembolism and

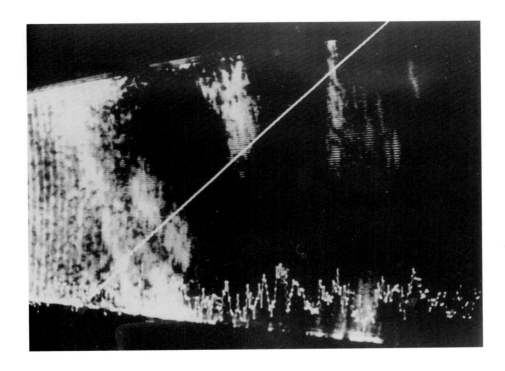

FIG. 9. A mural plaque with crescentic shape, scalloped borders, and heterogeneous lucencies, suggesting recent thrombus and embolization in a patient with ipsilateral transient ischemic attack. (From ref. 24.)

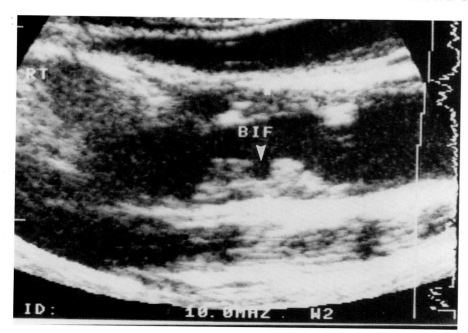

FIG. 10. A crater in a plaque that is otherwise homogeneous. Most of the plaque material has been extravasated, though the crater could conceal ulceration of the endothelium or be a nidus for further thrombus formation.

avulsed plaque material, in some cases to such an extent that the remaining plaque does not pose a source of recurrent embolization. However, blood flowing through the region of the crater may become exposed to tissue factor in the lipid core of the plaque, which can precipitate thrombus formation (29). The actual clinical relevance of craters requires further study. However, when symptoms of ipsilateral ischemia are correlated with histologic examination of plaques, recent plaque hemorrhage bore a significant relationship to thromboembolic events whereas plaque ulceration did not (18,19). Therefore, identification of plaque lucencies and heterogeneities by B-mode ultrasonography is clinically more relevant than identification of plaque craters.

Duplex Sonography

Estimation of the degree of stenosis of the internal carotid artery can be made by examination of the plaque and residual lumen on B-mode sonography (30). However, the image of the vessel is dependent on the angle of insonation of the probe, and changing probe position can alter the diameter of the visualized lumen. In very-high-grade stenosis, it is sometimes not possible to identify the lumen of the internal carotid at all. Soft thrombus overlying a plaque may not be visualized by B-mode sonography because the echodensity of the thrombus is similar to the echodensity of the blood.

Duplex sonography was developed to obtain Doppler frequency information in combination with B-mode sonography (31). The frequency shifts of the Doppler examination are directly proportional to the area of the residual lumen of the artery and are more accurate than B-mode sonography alone in determining the degree of stenosis in an obstructive lesion. The B-mode sonography localizes the region of the artery that is being insonated by the Doppler to help identify the part of the vessel from which the Doppler signal is originating. This is particularly advantageous in differentiating the internal carotid artery from the external carotid artery because branches of the external carotid can often be seen, whereas the internal carotid has no branches.

Traditional duplex sonography has proven to be very accurate in identifying carotid stenosis when compared to angiography. Blackshear et al. (32) reported an accuracy of over 95% in detecting lesions causing greater than 50% stenosis. Angiography was then necessary to delineate the spectrum of disease between 50% and 99%. Further categorization into mild, moderate, and severe degrees of stenosis can be obtained by duplex Doppler sonography with 68–82% accuracy and a 90% predictive value (33,34). Hunink et al. (35) reported that analysis of the initial systolic peak velocity of duplex Doppler signals correlated with angiographic stenosis of 70% or more by regression analysis ($p = 0.0006$).

The accuracy of traditional duplex sonography was impeded because samples of Doppler signals were taken from specific points along the artery, but the whole artery was not scanned. Therefore, the point of maximal stenosis might not be detected. This could be improved by employing continuous wave Doppler to scan across the whole artery and identify the region of greatest stenosis from which to sample, resulting in correlations with angiography of over 90% (36,37). However, continuous wave Doppler is difficult to employ and requires a great deal of experience by the examiner before reproducible results can be obtained. The addition of color flow duplex sonography has greatly enhanced the accuracy of the ultrasonographic evaluation of the carotid arteries.

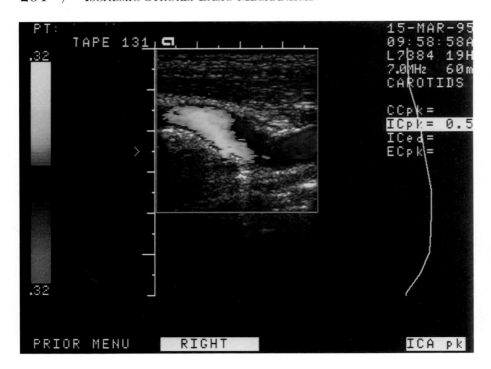

FIG. 11. Color flow imaging of the carotid sinus and internal carotid artery in red (bright). Note the normal flow reversal in blue (dark) and flow void in the curvature of the posterior wall of the carotid sinus. Plaque has a predilection to form in this region, possibly because of the low-velocity flow with a retrograde component. (Acuson, Mountain View, CA.)

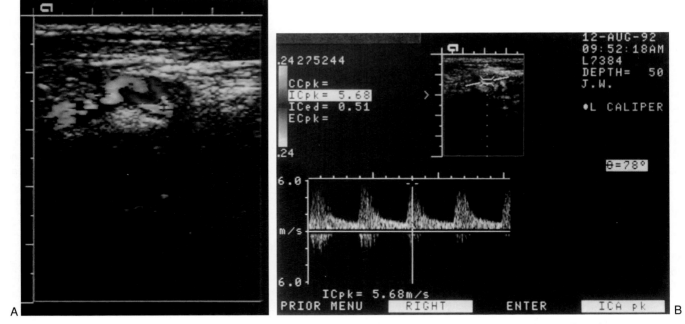

FIG. 12. High-grade stenosis of the internal carotid artery demonstrated by color flow duplex Doppler. **A:** The whole image is shown, with (bright) yellow indicating the region of turbulence overlying a large plaque. There is turbulent back flow below the plaque seen in blue (dark). **B:** Spectral analysis of pulsed Doppler sample taken from the region of turbulence seen at top. Velocity is increased to almost 6 m/sec (normal <1) and there is spread of frequencies. The backflow below the stenosis is also seen. Flow was reduced above the stenosis as well. This could have been misinterpreted as a complete occlusion of the internal carotid artery if the color image had not been available to indicate that flow was present distally, allowing placement of the pulsed Doppler probe in the correct position to measure the high-velocity Doppler shifts. Also note that to obtain the correct image and Doppler signal, the probe had to be lined up with the artery at an angle of 80° rather than 60°, causing some overestimation of the velocity. A high-grade stenosis was confirmed with angiography and surgery.

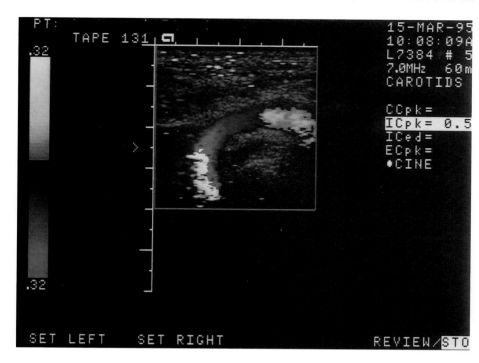

FIG. 13. Color flow imaging shows increased velocity in yellow (bright) in the distal internal as it curves medially from the bifurcation to course cephalad. This is a source of false-positive results indicating a stenosis because of increased velocities recorded on spectral analysis without stenosis.

Color Flow Duplex Sonography

Color flow Doppler imaging of the carotid bifurcation was developed so that Doppler signals in the entire artery could be represented visually (38). Flow toward the probe is imaged in either red or blue and flow away from the probe in the alternate color. A frequency shift value is set above which the image is recorded in yellow or white. This enhances the accuracy of the Doppler examination because spectral analysis is performed at the locations where turbulent flow is identified.

In the normal bifurcation, the posterior wall of the carotid sinus just opposite the origin of the external carotid artery often has a flow void or flow reversal (Fig. 11). This region of reduced flow is the site where most atheromata develop. In a stenotic vessel, the cursor representing the pulse wave Doppler probe is placed in the artery parallel to the direction of flow at the site of the turbulent flow marked in yellow. The spectral patterns are recorded to obtain quantitative analysis of the peak height and end-diastolic velocity of the waveform and to see the extent of spread of frequencies (Fig. 12). There are reports of greater accuracy in assessing the degree of internal carotid artery stenosis compared to angiography with color flow duplex Doppler than two-dimensional magnetic resonance angiography (MRA) (34,38), though three-dimensional MRA may provide greater accuracy than two-dimensional MRA (41).

Reproducibility of Doppler Sonography

Doppler sonography, even with the aid of color flow, is a user-dependent technique. There are several sources of error of which the examiner must be aware in order to obtain accurate results. Calcification in the arterial wall can change the tissue propagation of the ultrasound beam in the Doppler equation, causing false elevation of frequency shifts and spread of frequencies (11). Cardiac valve dysfunction can alter the systolic peak frequencies. Mitral regurgitation and aortic stenosis can elevate the initial systolic peak, causing exaggeration of the calculation of degree of stenosis. These valve artifacts can be detected by examination of the waveform on spectral analysis rather than just recording the numeric value of the frequency shift and by hearing characteristic sound patterns that cannot be interpreted through spectral analysis (42). Poor cardiac output, cardiac arrhythmias, or vasodilator medications that reduce the inotropic force of the heart can cause reduction in flow velocities and turbulence and thus cause underestimation of the degree of stenosis.

There are false-positive and false-negative results with complete occlusion of the internal carotid artery. Sometimes the internal carotid artery cannot be identified even though it is present. Sometimes no flow is detected in the internal carotid artery distal to the lesion with the Doppler instrument although the artery is still patent. These difficulties can usually be overcome with color flow imaging (43), which makes it easier to locate the internal carotid artery and can visualize flow in the internal carotid distal to a highly stenotic lesion. Also, when there is hemodynamic obstruction to flow in one carotid artery, frequency shifts may be exaggerated in the contralateral internal carotid artery, which is supplying a high volume of flow for collateral circulation. This can lead to overestimation of the degree of stenosis of the contralateral internal carotid.

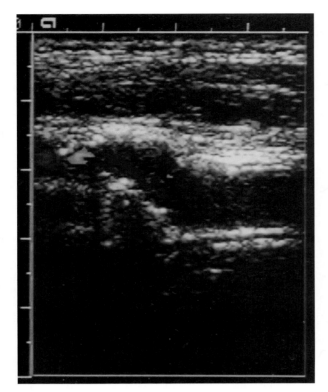

FIG. 14. Color flow imaging outlines a plaque near the origin of the internal carotid artery at the bifurcation and a plaque in the internal carotid artery distal to the bifurcation. Failure to continue the examination distally beyond the bifurcation can yield false-negative results and failure to identify a potential stenosis.

The most common source of error is not recording from the most appropriate angle of insonation. The relationship of Doppler frequency shifts and velocity of the flowing particles is dependent on the angle of insonation (11). The optimal angle for recording Doppler frequency shifts is 60°. It is necessary to line up the cursor of the pulsed Doppler so that it is directly parallel to the direction of flow in the artery while recording at an angle of 60° or just below 60°. The position of the sonographic probe on the neck may have to be altered in order to record Doppler flow patterns at an angle of about 60°. Failure to do so results in inaccurate measurements of Doppler frequency shifts or flow velocities.

The normal internal carotid artery curves medially to a varying degree after leaving the bifurcation and proceeding cephalad. When the curvature is extensive, frequency shifts in the distal cervical internal carotid are exaggerated, even with angle correction, resulting in false-positive readings suggestive of high-grade stenosis (Fig. 13). Plaque often forms in these regions of distal curvature of the internal carotid, producing even greater spurious elevations of frequency shifts. However, failure to carry the Doppler examination distal to the bifurcation may cause a stenosis or plaque in this region to be missed (Fig. 14). Examination of the B-mode image can usually aid in assessing the degree of stenosis more accurately when it can demonstrate that plaque is not causing narrowing of the lumen.

Some discrepancies arise between duplex Doppler sonography and intraarterial angiography when there is extensive atherosclerotic disease in the carotid sinus not involving the origin of the internal carotid artery. These lesions may not be detected on conventional arteriography, although in reality the normal dilatation of the carotid bulb will not be seen.

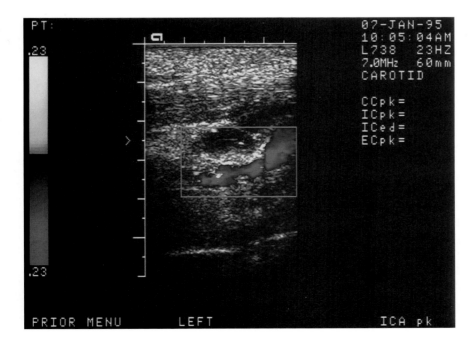

FIG. 15. A color flow image was obtained on a patient who developed mild contralateral hand weakness 1 day following carotid endarterectomy. A small lesion is seen in the distal internal carotid artery, probably representing a platelet plug.

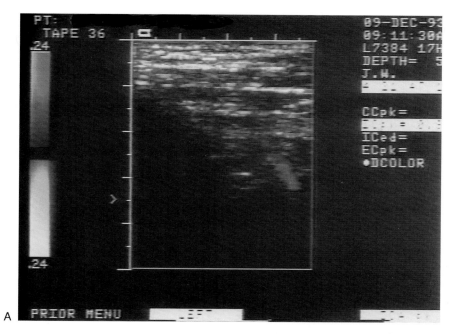

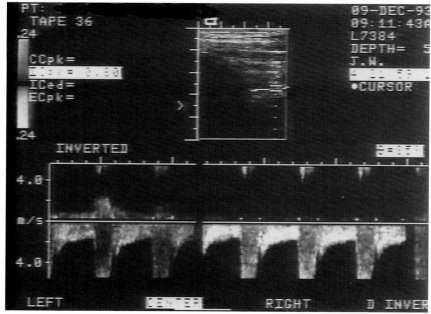

FIG. 16. The origin of the vertebral artery from the subclavian is shown with color flow imaging **(A)** and spectral analysis **(B)**. The large-volume flow in the subclavian is seen as retrograde whereas the smaller signal represents flow cephalad in the vertebral artery.

Sonography will visualize a large amount of plaque that can cause elevation of frequency shifts and be interpreted as a high-grade stenosis of the internal carotid artery. Usually when this occurs the systolic peak is elevated but there is little or no elevation of diastolic flow velocities. In this instance, duplex sonography is actually more sensitive than angiography in detecting severe atherosclerotic disease in the bifurcation. MRA is also sensitive to turbulent flow, and these lesions are often detected as flow voids and considered to be false-positive overestimations of the degree of stenosis. Occasionally MRA will not detect a high-grade stenosis that only involves a short segment of the internal carotid artery,

resulting in false-negative findings; these lesions are detected with ultrasonography. In instances when the MRA and duplex studies do not concur, intraarterial contrast angiography is necessary to quantify the degree of stenosis definitively.

CLINICAL APPLICATIONS OF CAROTID ULTRASONOGRAPHY

Duplex sonography can be employed as the primary screening test to identify carotid artery occlusive disease in patients with focal transient cerebral ischemic attacks or mild strokes, since most of these patients will not have significant carotid stenosis (7,9). Patients with transient monocular blindness or amaurosis fugax have an even lower proportion of significant lesions (44). If a stenosis of over 50% is identified, further imaging procedures such as MRA or contrast angiography are indicated to document whether a lesion more amenable to carotid endarterectomy than medical treatment is present. The combination of carotid duplex sonography and MRA has been found to be adequate for determining whether there is sufficient stenosis of greater than 70% (7) to warrant carotid endarterectomy in 87% of cases (45), avoiding the need for invasive procedures and hospitalizations in most instances.

Patients with asymptomatic carotid stenosis of greater than 60%, usually identified by presence of a carotid artery bruit, have also been shown to benefit from carotid endarterectomy to prevent stroke (8). These patients can be screened with duplex sonography because only 60% will be found to have any degree of stenosis (5), and those having greater than 60% stenosis can be readily identified by sonography (8). Previous studies have suggested that among patients with carotid artery bruit, the ones with progressive stenosis over time approaching 80% stenosis are at the highest risk for stroke (5). Duplex sonography is an effective and convenient technique for sequentially following patients with carotid artery stenosis to determine if there is significant

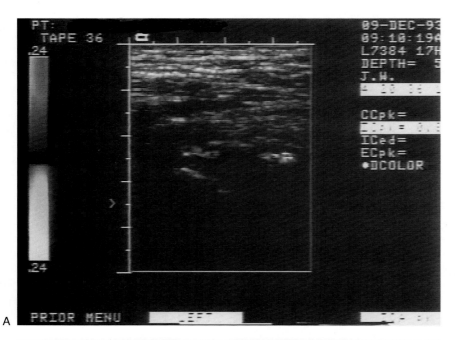

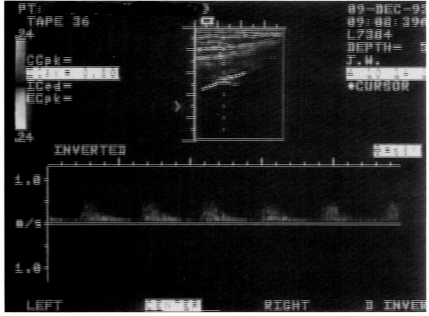

FIG. 17. The vertebral artery from C8 to C4 is imaged with color flow (A) and a sample for spectral analysis is measured with pulsed Doppler (B). Note the high resistance pattern with little runoff in diastole.

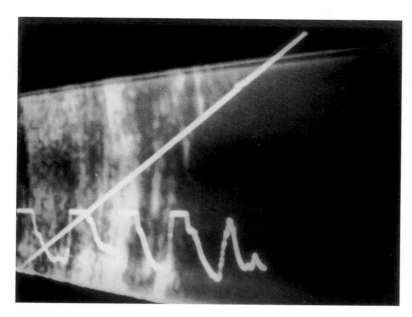

FIG. 18. A large heterogeneous plaque is seen in the proximal vertebral artery using analog mechanical sector scanning (High-Stoy SP100-B, Sonomed, Lake Success, NY) in a patient with an ipsilateral cerebellar stroke. Angiography showed a complete occlusion of the vertebral with retrograde filling and the distal lumen can still be seen above the plaque on the B-mode image.

progression. Duplex sonography is also useful in imaging the carotid bifurcation following endarterectomy to rule out recurrence of thrombus or stenosis (Fig. 15).

Not all patients with significant carotid artery stenosis present with a focal transient ischemic attack or a carotid artery bruit. Up to 20% of elderly patients with nonspecific symptoms such as lightheadedness, orthostatic visual disturbance, or evidence of vertebrobasilar insufficiency are found to have hemodynamically obstructive carotid artery lesions (46). Duplex sonography is an appropriate method for screening these patients to rule out occlusive carotid artery disease. Patients with other nonspecific symptoms suggestive of cerebral ischemia, such as transient global amnesia, can also be screened for carotid artery stenosis with duplex sonography (47).

DUPLEX SONOGRAPHY OF THE CERVICAL VERTEBRAL ARTERIES

The cervical vertebral arteries can be visualized with B-mode sonography by placing the probe over the transverse processes of the vertebrae. The vertebral artery can be followed from the origin at the subclavian artery to about C4 (Fig. 16), where it leaves the foramen transversarium to enter the cranium. Accuracy of 85% has been reported in identifying stenosis of the cervical vertebral artery by B-mode imag-

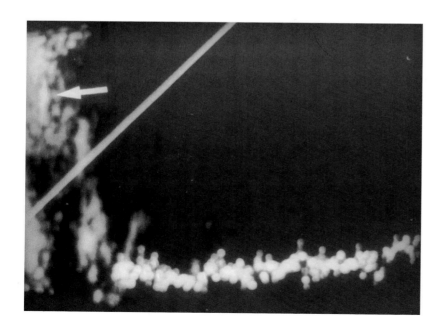

FIG. 19. A low-echodensity lesion, probably representing thrombus, is seen occluding the vertebral artery at about C6 in a patient who presented with a lateral medullary syndrome. Angiography confirmed a complete occlusion of the vertebral artery. (From ref. 48.)

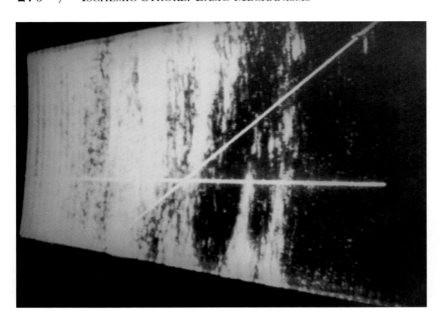

FIG. 20. Vertebral artery dissection demonstrating a true and false lumen with B-mode sonography. The false lumen is communicating with the true lumen and was probably a source of embolic thrombus which caused recurrent cerebellar and occipital lobe strokes in this patient. (From ref. 52.)

ing when compared to angiography (48). Reduction in flow in the vertebral artery can also be detected by Doppler analysis (49). Color flow imaging can aid in placement of the Doppler probe to obtain accurate recordings of direction and velocity of flow (Fig. 17). The distal cervical carotid artery can be insonated at C2 with a hand-held continuous wave Doppler probe, even though it is not visualized well in this region by duplex sonography (50).

Atherosclerotic plaques form mainly at the origin of the vertebral artery from the subclavian artery and occasionally at the transverse processes of the vertebral bones (Fig. 18) (51). Collateral circulation usually fills the vertebral artery distal to the plaques at the origin, but these lesions can be the source of emboli to distal vessels in the posterior circulation. Thrombus in the vertebral artery can also be identified (Fig. 19). Dissection of the wall of the vertebral artery can also be detected by B-mode sonography when it occurs between C8 and C4 (Fig. 20) (52). Dissections more commonly occur at the atlanto-occipital joint and can be detected by recordings of high frequencies at C2 with continuous wave Doppler. Lesions in the cervical vertebral artery are present in 28% of patients with definite symptoms of posterior circulation transient ischemic attacks and 44% of patients with vertebrobasilar territory stroke (48). Visualization of the cervical vertebral arteries with ultrasonography, particularly in conjunction with transcranial Doppler, is a useful screening test in evaluating patients with nonspecific symptoms such as vertigo and dizziness, to rule out vertebrobasilar insufficiency.

CONCLUSION

Duplex sonography of the cervical carotid and vertebral arteries is an accurate noninvasive procedure for evaluating the degree of obstruction to flow in the extracranial circulation when adequate quality control is employed, comparing ultrasonography to intraarterial contrast angiography. The information derived from duplex sonography can be used to determine whether to proceed with further imaging investigations. In most instances, however, when a satisfactory study is obtained it can be used to rule out significant occlusive disease without resorting to other modalities.

Duplex sonography provides complementary information to intraarterial contrast angiography in that it images the morphologic features of the plaque within the bifurcation rather than a silhouette of the wall of the vessel created by intraluminal contrast material. This provides a more accurate assessment of the extent of plaque burden within the bifurcation as well as the degree of plaque proliferation, which may be prognostic indicators in addition to the percentage stenosis of the internal carotid artery. In most instances, duplex sonography in combination with MRA can provide adequate imaging of the carotid bifurcation in preparation for surgery, avoiding the complications and inconveniences of intraarterial contrast angiography.

REFERENCES

1. Fisher CM, Gore I, Okabe N, White PD. Atherosclerosis of the carotid and vertebral arteries: extracranial and intracranial. *J Neuropathol Exp Neurol* 1965;24:455–476.
2. Moore WS, Hall AD. Importance of emboli from carotid bifurcation in pathogenesis of cerebral ischemic attacks. *Arch Surg* 1970;101: 708–711.
3. Sundt TM, Sharbrough FW, Piepgras DG, et al. Correlation of cerebral blood flow and electroencephalographic changes during carotid endarterectomy. *Mayo Clin Proc* 1981;56:533–543.
4. Fisher CM. Transient monocular blindness associated with hemiplegia. *Arch Ophthalmol* 1952;47:167–203.
5. Chambers BR, Norris JW. Outcome in patients with asymptomatic neck bruits. *N Engl J Med* 1986;315:860–869.

6. Canadian Cooperative Study Group. A randomized trial of aspirin and sulfinpyrazone in threatened stroke. *N Engl J Med* 1978;299:53–59.
7. North American Symptomatic Carotid Endarterectomy Trial Collaborators. Beneficial effect of carotid endarterectomy in symptomatic patients with high-grade carotid stenosis. *N Engl J Med* 1991;325:445–453.
8. Executive Committee for the Asymptomatic Carotid Atherosclerosis Study. Endarterectomy for asymptomatic carotid artery stenosis. *JAMA* 1995;273:1421–1428.
9. Fields WS, Maslenikov V, Meyer JS, et al. Joint study of extracranial arterial occlusion. V. Progress report of prognosis following surgery or nonsurgical treatment for transient cerebral ischemic attacks and cervical carotid artery lesions. *JAMA* 1970;211:1993–2003.
10. Faught E, Trader SD, Hanna GR. Cerebral complications of angiography for transient ischemia and stroke: prediction of risk. *Neurology* 1979;29:4–15.
11. Kremkau FW. Doppler principles. *Semin Roentgenol* 1992;27:6–16.
12. Barnes RW, Nix L, Rittgers SE. Audible interpretation of carotid Doppler signals: an improved technique to define carotid artery disease. *Arch Surg* 1981;116:1185–1189.
13. Weinberger J, Biscarra V. Noninvasive carotid artery testing in cerebrovascular disease. In: Weinberger J, ed. *Noninvasive imaging of cerebrovascular disease.* New York: Alan R Liss, 1989:17–25.
14. Ackerman RH, Candia MR. Identifying clinically relevant carotid disease. *Stroke* 1994;25:1–3.
15. Nicholls SC, Zierler E, Strandness DE Jr. Duplex scanning of the carotid arteries. In: Weinberger J, ed. *Noninvasive imaging of cerebrovascular disease.* New York: Alan R Liss, 1989:49–65.
16. Bond MG, Barnes RW, Riley WA, et al. High-resolution B-mode ultrasound scanning methods in the Atherosclerosis Risk in Communities (ARIC) cohort. *J Neuroimag* 1991;1:68–73.
17. Reilly LM, Lusby RJ, Hughes I, et al. Carotid plaque histology using real-time ultrasonography: clinical and therapeutic implications. *Am J Surg* 1983;146:188–193.
18. Imparato AM, Riles TS, Gorstein F. The carotid bifurcation plaque: pathologic findings associated with cerebral ischemia. *Stroke* 1977;10:238–245.
19. Imparato AM, Riles TS, Mintzer K, Baumann FG. The importance of hemorrhage in the relationship between gross morphologic characteristics and cerebral symptoms in 376 carotid artery plaques. *Ann Surg* 1983;197:195–203.
20. Lusby RJ, Ferrell LD, Ehrenfeld WK, et al. Carotid plaque hemorrhage: its role in production of cerebral ischemia. *Arch Surg* 1982;117:1479–1488.
21. Steffen CM, Gray-Weale AC, Byrne KE, Lusby RJ. Carotid artery atheroma: ultrasound appearance in symptomatic and asymptomatic vessels. *Aust NZ J Surg* 1989;59:529–534.
22. Langsfeld M, Gray-Weale AC, Lusby RJ. The role of plaque morphology and diameter reduction in the development of new symptoms in asymptomatic carotid arteries. *J Vasc Surg* 1989;9:548–557.
23. Weinberger J, Marks SJ, Gaul JJ, et al. Atherosclerotic plaque at the carotid artery bifurcation: correlation of ultrasonographic imaging with morphology. *J Ultrasound Med* 1987;6:363–366.
24. Weinberger J, Robbins A. Neurologic symptoms associated with nonobstructive plaque at carotid bifurcation: analysis by real-time B-mode ultrasonography. *Arch Neurol* 1983;40:489–492.
25. Weinberger J, Ramos L, Ambrose JA, Fuster V. Morphologic and dynamic changes of atherosclerotic plaque at the carotid artery bifurcation: sequential imaging by real time B-mode ultrasonography. *J Am Coll Cardiol* 1988;12:1515–1521.
26. Falk E. Unstable angina with fatal outcome: dynamic coronary thrombosis leading to infarction and/or sudden death. Autopsy evidence of recurrent mural thrombosis with peripheral embolization culminating in total vascular occlusion. *Circulation* 1985;71:699–708.
27. Ambrose JA, Winters SL, Arora RR, et al. Angiographic evolution of coronary artery morphology in unstable angina. *J Am Coll Cardiol* 1986;7:472–478.
28. Bluth EL, Kay D, Merritt CRB, et al. Sonographic characterization of carotid plaque: detection of hemorrhage. *Am J Neuroradiol* 1986;7:311–315.
29. Sakariassen KS, Barstad RM. Mechanisms of thromboembolism at arterial plaques. *Blood Coagul Fibrinolysis* 1993;4:615–625.
30. Ricotta JS, Bryan FA, Bond MG, et al. Multicenter validation study of real-time (B-mode) ultrasound, arteriography and pathologic examination. *J Vasc Surg* 1987;6:512–520.
31. Blackshear WM Jr, Phillips DJ, Thiele BL, et al. Detection of carotid occlusive disease by ultrasonic imaging and pulsed Doppler spectral analysis. *Surgery* 1979;86:698–703.
32. Blackshear WM Jr, Phillips DJ, Chikos PM, et al. Carotid artery velocity patterns in normal and stenotic vessels. *Stroke* 1979;11:67–71.
33. Lamb S, Murtagh R, Anderson J, et al. Pulsed Doppler ultrasonic arteriography and spectrum analysis for quantitating carotid occlusive disease. *J Cardiovasc Ultrason* 1985;4:105–112.
34. Mittl RL, Broderick M, Carpenter JP, et al. Blinded-reader comparison of magnetic resonance angiography and duplex ultrasonography for carotid artery bifurcation stenosis. *Stroke* 1994;25:4–10.
35. Hunink MGM, Polak JF, Borlan MM, O'Leary DH. Detection and quantification of carotid artery stenosis: efficacy of various Doppler velocity parameters. *AJR* 1993;160:619–625.
36. Hennerici M, Freund HJ. Efficacy of CW–Doppler and duplex system examinations for the evaluation of extracranial carotid disease. *J Clin Ultrasound* 1984;12:155–161.
37. Weinberger J, Biscarra V, Weitzner I, et al. Noninvasive carotid artery testing: role in the management of patients with transient ischemic attacks. *NY State J Med* 1981;81:1463–1468.
38. Erickson SJ, Mewissen MW, Foley WD, et al. Stenosis of the internal carotid artery: assessment using color Doppler imaging compared with angiography. *AJR* 1989;52:1299–1305.
39. Riles TS, Eidelman EM, Litt AW, et al. Comparison of magnetic resonance angiography, conventional angiography and duplex scanning. *Stroke* 1992;23:341–346.
40. Polak JF, Bajakian RL, O'Leary DH, et al. Detection of internal carotid artery stenosis: comparison of MR angiography, color Doppler sonography and arteriography. *Radiology* 1992;182:35–40.
41. Anderson CM, Saloner P, Lee RE, et al. Assessment of carotid artery stenosis by MR angiography: comparison with x-ray angiography and color-coded Doppler ultrasound. *Am J Neuroradiol* 1992;13:989–1003.
42. Weinberger J, Goldman M. Detection of mitral valve abnormalities by carotid Doppler flow study: implications for the management of patients with cerebrovascular disease. *Stroke* 1985;16:977–980.
43. Kiell SC, McPharlin M, Shepard AD, McManus MP. Efficacy of color flow Doppler in the diagnosis of carotid artery occlusion. *J Vasc Tech* 1993;17:81–86.
44. Gaul JJ, Marks SJ, Weinberger J. Visual disturbance and carotid artery disease. 500 symptomatic patients studied by non-invasive carotid artery testing including B-mode ultrasonography. *Stroke* 1986;17:393–398.
45. Polak JF, Kudina P, Donaldson MC, et al. Carotid endarterectomy: preoperative evaluation of candidates with combined Doppler sonography and MR angiography. *Radiology* 1993;186:333–338.
46. Weinberger J, Biscarra V, Weisberg MK. Hemodynamics of the carotid artery circulation in the elderly "dizzy" patient. *J Am Geriat Soc* 1981;29:402–406.
47. Feuer D, Weinberger J. Extracranial carotid artery in patients with transient global amnesia: evaluation by real-time B-mode ultrasonography with duplex Doppler flow. *Stroke* 1987;18:951–953.
48. Weinberger J. Noninvasive imaging of the cervical vertebral artery in the diagnosis of vertebrobasilar insufficiency. *J Stroke Cerebrovasc Dis* 1991;1:21–25.
49. Ringelstein EB, Zeumer H, Poeck K. Non-invasive diagnosis of intracranial lesions in the vertebrobasilar system: a comparison of Doppler sonographic and angiographic findings. *Stroke* 1985;16:848–854.
50. Ringelstein EB. Continuous-wave Doppler sonography of the extracranial brain-supplying arteries. In: Weinberger J, ed. *Noninvasive imaging of cerebrovascular disease.* New York: Alan R Liss, 1989:27–48.
51. Fisher CM. Occlusion of the vertebral arteries. *Arch Neurol* 1970;22:13–19.
52. Weinberger J, Rudolph S, Lidov M. Evidence for arterial embolization in dissecting aneurysm of the cervical vertebral artery. *J Stroke Cerebrovasc Dis* 1991;1:95–97.

Cerebrovascular Disease, edited by H. Hunt Batjer.
Lippincott-Raven Publishers, Philadelphia © 1997.

CHAPTER **21**

Transcranial Doppler Ultrasound in the Assessment of Stroke

Cole A. Giller and Camilo R. Gomez

The assessment of abnormalities of cerebral blood flow with ultrasound has been of clinical utility for several decades. Although originally restricted to the heart and great vessels, recent technological advances have allowed routine and convenient measurement of blood velocity in the intracranial vessels using transcranial Doppler (TCD) ultrasound (1,2). This chapter will focus on the explosion of applications of TCD to the assessment of stroke that have occurred over the past decade. Although these applications include the diagnosis of hemodynamically significant lesions, we believe that a major utility of TCD lies in its ability to serially assess the physiologic and clinical importance of such lesions when they have been diagnosed by other means.

BASIC ASPECTS OF TRANSCRANIAL DOPPLER ULTRASOUND

Description of the Technique

In 1982, Aaslid introduced the first practical ultrasonic device that could be used to obtain velocity measurements from the large intracranial vessels (3). Modern devices now allow direct insonation of blood velocity in the circle of Willis by simply holding an ultrasound probe to the head and setting the desired depth of insonation. The most commonly used areas of the skull allowing passage of the ultrasound beam are the ''temporal windows'' (just above the zygomatic arch), the ''orbital windows'' (through the superior orbital fissure), and the ''suboccipital window'' (posteriorly through the foramen magnum). By sequentially changing the depth of insonation and making small-angle adjustments of the probe, a skilled operator can obtain velocity signals from virtually the entire circle of Willis (4). Be-

C. A. Giller: Department of Neurosurgery and Radiology, The University of Texas Southwestern Medical School, Dallas, Texas 75235–8855

C. R. Gomez: Department of Neurology, University of Alabama at Birmingham, Birmingham, Alabama 35294

cause an image is not obtained, vessel localization is prone to error and is highly dependent on the skill of the operator. Newer technology allows a B-mode image of the intracranial contents to be obtained, with moving blood superimposed as a color image. These techniques provide striking images but may have less sensitivity to abnormal velocity changes than standard TCD (5).

Information Available from TCD Studies

The waveforms obtained from TCD contain much information but are commonly used to measure five quantities: mean velocity of blood flow, direction of blood flow, shape of the waveform, trends in mean velocity during various maneuvers, and presence of emboli.

Velocity

The systolic, diastolic, and mean velocities, continuously displayed by most devices, are derived from averages of the respective velocities within the sample volume of insonation over several heart beats (Fig. 1). The mean velocity appears to have more correlation to blood flow through the insonated vessel and has received most attention. It is crucial to make the distinction between velocity and flow. The flow through a vessel is given by the formula $Q = VA$, where Q = flow, V = velocity, and A = cross-sectional area. Since vessel caliber is not measured by TCD studies, any conclusions regarding blood flow derived from velocity measurements are based on the assumption that the diameter has remained constant. Conversely, any conclusions about vessel caliber depend on the assumption that flow has not changed. This represents an irrevocable limitation of TCD measurements that must be addressed in each clinical application.

Normal values of mean velocity have been summarized in several reviews (4) and are approximately 60, 50, and 40 cm/sec for the middle, anterior, and posterior/basilar cerebral

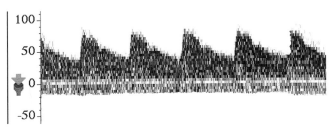

FIG. 1. Normal signal from middle cerebral artery. Mean velocity is about 50 cm/sec and pulsatility about 0.90.

arteries, respectively. These values are higher in children, decrease with age, and increase in the presence of anemia (6).

Direction of Blood Flow

The direction of blood flow through the insonated artery can be determined from the phase of the reflected ultrasound signal and is indicated by the convention of displaying signals corresponding to opposite direction above and below a zero line (Fig. 2). In this manner, blood flowing toward and away from the ultrasound probe can be easily distinguished.

Shape of the TCD Waveform

The contour of the velocity waveform is similar but not identical to that of blood pressure and is determined by multiple factors. These include the shape of the blood pressure waveform, vessel elasticity, wave reflections, and the peripheral hemodynamic resistance of the tissue bed. The dependence on distal resistance is put to use in clinical practice because a vasodilated tissue bed will produce a blunted, attenuated waveform (Fig. 2), whereas vasoconstriction of the arterioles produces a more "spiky" appearance (Fig. 3). Although various indices have been used to capture these concepts, the most popular is that of Gosling pulsatility, defined as the difference between systolic and diastolic velocities

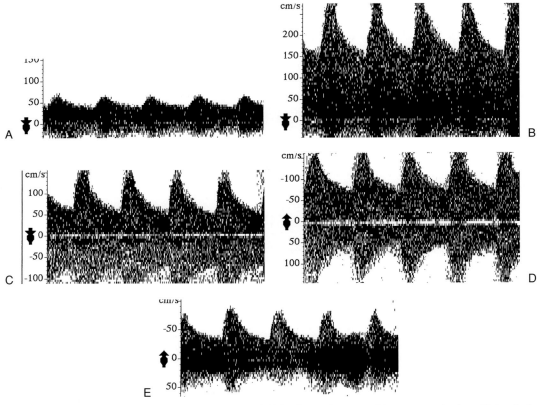

FIG. 2. A. Signal from middle cerebral artery (MCA) ipsilateral to carotid artery occlusion. Note diminished velocity and blunted pulsatility indicating proximal compromise as well as distal autoregulatory vasodilation. B. Signal from anterior cerebral artery (ACA) ipsilateral to carotid artery occlusion. Note high velocity due to high collateral flow and reversed flow direction (arrow points towards icon of probe). C. Signal from MCA contralateral to carotid artery occlusion. Note relatively normal velocity and evidence of orthograde flow in ACA (signal below zero line). D. Signal from ACA contralateral to carotid artery occlusion. Note high velocity due to demand for collateral flow and orthograde flow direction (arrow points away from icon). E. Signal from ophthalmic artery ipsilateral to carotid artery occlusion. Note reversal of flow direction and relatively low pulsatility indicating collateral flow from the extracranial to intracranial circulation.

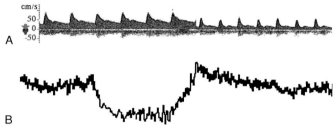

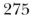

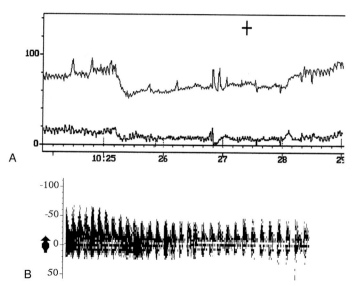

FIG. 3. A. Signals from middle cerebral artery (MCA) at baseline (left) and during hyperventilation (right). Note decrease in velocity and increase in pulsatility indicating vasoconstriction of the distal vasculature. B. Monitored velocity signals from MCA during hyperventilation. Total time is three minutes. Velocity falls from 50 cm/sec at baseline to 30 cm/sec during hyperventilation. Note the transient overshoot of velocity above baseline levels after hyperventilation suggesting a post-ischemic hyperemia.

FIG. 4. A. Simultaneous blood pressure (top signal) and posterior cerebral artery velocity (bottom signal) obtained during change in position accompanied by dizziness. The observed fall in blood pressure induced a similar fall in velocity suggesting orthostatic hypotension and perhaps an impairment in cerebral autoregulation as the source of symptoms. B. Signal from vertebral artery during head rotation evoking symptoms of dizziness. Note decrement of velocity suggesting proximal compromise.

divided by the mean velocity (4). Normal Gosling pulsatilities generally range between 0.8 and 1.0, are subject to tremendous variability, and are dependent on pulse rate. Nevertheless, a dramatically low pulsatility suggests proximal hemodynamic compromise or distal vasodilatation (Fig. 2), and side-to-side and serial comparisons can be useful in deriving the state of the tissue bed supplied by the insonated artery.

Velocity Trends During Maneuvers

TCD velocities can be obtained continuously over periods of time, and many devices that reliably fix the probe to the head are available for this purpose. The effects of such maneuvers as carotid occlusion (Figs. 4 and 5) or administration of medications can be assessed by examining the velocity trends during these maneuvers. Vascular reactivity to either CO_2 or blood pressure can also be assessed using TCD to examine velocity trends during alteration of CO_2 or blood pressure. Comparisons among velocity, blood pressure, intracranial pressure, and CO_2 allows an integrated interpretation of cerebral perfusion that would not otherwise be obtainable.

Emboli

It is now recognized that air and particulate emboli produce specific signals that can be identified within TCD waveforms as either intense vertical lines or globoid shapes when the gain is turned down (7,8) (Fig. 6). Identifying criteria include (a) short duration, (b) random occurrence within the pulse length, (b) higher acoustic intensity (>3 dB) above the background, and (d) a peculiar "plunking" or "clipping" sound (9). Nevertheless, there can be disagreement event among experienced operators in distinguishing emboli from artifact, and the promising strides in automatic detec-

tion and counting of emboli have not yet achieved the reliability needed for clinical use. Criteria to distinguish gaseous from particulate emboli are not firmly established, nor can the number of emboli be precisely counted when a large number occur in a "shower." The term HITS ("high-intensity transient signals") has been given to the signals produced by embolic particles in order to avoid the inherent clinical implication of the term "embolism." It has become clear, however, that HITS are rare in normal subjects and common in many clinical settings associated with cerebral embolism. Furthermore, the assumption that one embolus produces one stroke has proved to be false. Thresholds characterizing the number of embolic occurrence that are associa-

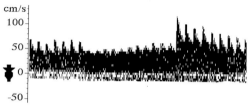

FIG. 5. Signals from middle cerebral artery during transient ipsilateral carotid artery occlusion. Velocity waveform becomes attenuated at onset of occlusion but velocity slowly rises after a few seconds, suggesting distal vasodilation due to autoregulation. Upon release of the occlusion, the velocity overshoots to levels above baseline as normal pressure is restored to this vasodilated tissue bed.

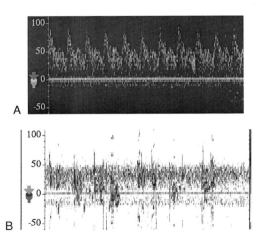

FIG. 6. A. HITS (high intensity transient signals) appearing as bright spots of color in TCD signal suggesting the occurrence of emboli. B. Signal suggesting showers of emboli during cardiac bypass. Note absence of systolic/diastolic signals while on bypass.

ated with neurologic deficit are emerging and will be addressed below.

Strengths and Advantages of TCD

The portability of TCD equipment and its noninvasive nature allow hemodynamic assessment of critically ill patients in difficult environments such as the operating room and the intensive care unit. Serial studies may be performed frequently, and monitoring may be used to assess the effect of almost any maneuver or therapeutic measure. The time resolution of continuous ultrasound signals allows a second-to-second assessment that cannot be obtained from any other modality. Finally, TCD remains the sole method to directly detect emboli in the cerebral circulation.

Limitations of TCD

Perhaps the most important limitation of TCD is the inability to distinguish velocity changes due to changes in flow from those due to changes in diameter. Comparison with flow measurements, angiography, and direct observation of vessel diameter (10–12) suggest that, in most cases, the error in middle cerebral artery (MCA) velocity produced by diameter changes is less than 15%. However, variations in diameter are less predictable for smaller and distal vessels, when severe changes in blood pressure occur, or when medications are given. In addition, cerebral blood flow and TCD velocity depend on a variety of factors that can also confound the interpretation. For example, velocity will increase at a hematocrit below 30 due to decreased viscosity (6) and will decrease with a low CO_2 or high intracranial pressure (1). Therefore, patients with various combinations of these parameters have TCD studies that can be difficult to interpret.

A proximal stenosis can also mask the velocity rise from a stenosis. A related difficulty is the distinction of a high velocity due to abnormal collateral flow through a vessel such as the anterior cerebral artery from that due to a focal stenosis. Finally, the absence of a signal from a defined artery does not always imply lack of perfusion because inability to insonate a vessel may be due to technical errors, obscuration by overlying bone such as the clinoid process, and confusion arising from the presence of retrograde flow through that arterial segment.

The dependence on operator skill and difficulty in transversing thick bone has also been mentioned and is at times insurmountable. Although successful insonation has been achieved in 97% of a relatively young European population (13), success rates in the elderly population range from 80% in white males to 30% in black females to 17% in Japanese females (14,15). This limitation therefore appears most pronounced in the very population of interest to the stroke physician.

TCD FOR DIAGNOSIS

Although TCD studies can theoretically be used in the diagnosis of almost any hemodynamic condition, in practice the availability of magnetic resonance imaging and angiography has limited TCD as a primary diagnostic tool. Nevertheless, there are a few settings in which the TCD study can provide a diagnosis that is not otherwise attainable.

Stenosis

A focal elevation in velocity that is at least twice that of baseline is highly suggestive of a focal stenosis. Diffuse velocity elevations over several centimeters or in several arteries are more difficult to interpret, but focal findings should provoke more definitive testing to determine appropriate treatment.

TCD studies of carotid siphon and MCA stenosis have compared well with angiography in several studies. Using a threshold of 65–80 cm/sec, sensitivity and specificity for siphon stenosis compared to angiography has been calculated at 73–86% and 95%, respectively (16,17). Using criteria of >80 cm/sec along with the requirement of a circumscribed length of velocity elevation and distal waveform dampening, sensitivity and specificity rates of 94% and 97% have been achieved for siphon stenosis and 86% and 99% for MCA stenosis (18). Similar agreements were found by Rorick et al., who noted an improvement in the correlations if attention was restricted to patients without a concomitant cervical carotid stenosis (19). It is clear that a focal elevation in carotid siphon or MCA velocities carries an excellent specificity and good sensitivity for stenosis. Confounding factors include a more proximal, flow-limiting stenosis and contralateral carotid occlusion with ipsilateral recruitment of collateral flow.

Stenosis in the other intracranial vessels has not been as well studied, but data are available for the posterior fossa. Thresholds for basilar artery velocity are generally >80 cm/sec, with sensitivity and specificity about 75% and 85%, respectively (19,20).

Finally, blunting of the TCD waveform carries a relatively high predictive value for proximal stenosis or occlusion. The blunting arises from the direct effect of the stenosis on the arterial pressure waveform as well as autoregulatory vasodilatation, which is induced by the associated ischemia. This latter process may preserve blood flow and velocity, and a severe blunting of the MCA waveform with normal velocity can be the earliest sign of proximal carotid artery occlusion (21). Kelley et al. found that a flow acceleration of <352 cm/sec in the MCA yielded a sensitivity of 82%, specificity of 73%, and positive predictive value of 79% for a proximal carotid stenosis of 70–100% diameter reduction (22). Furthermore, absence of either the ophthalmic artery or carotid siphon signal is a reliable indicator of proximal carotid occlusion or severe stenosis (specificity of 99.5% and 99%, respectively), although the sensitivity of this sign is quite low (23).

Vasospasm

Cerebral vasospasm is a common consequence of hemorrhagic stroke whenever there is significant subarachnoid hemorrhage (SAH) and so will be considered in this chapter. The metabolic products of hemoglobin produced after SAH apparently initiate a progressive narrowing of the large cerebral vessels that can limit blood flow and lead to clinical stroke. The causes of SAH include trauma and vasculitis, but vasospasm has been most studied following SAH due to aneurysmal rupture.

The utility of TCD for the diagnosis of vasospasm is largely due to the exquisite sensitivity of velocity to vessel narrowing. For example, a diameter decrease by only 30% (<1 mm in the case of the MCA) will double the TCD velocities if flow is assumed constant. For this reason, elevation of TCD velocity (Fig. 7) can be a more sensitive indica-

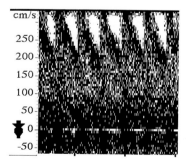

FIG. 7. Signals from narrowed segment of middle cerebral artery in a patient with vasospasm. Note the marked increase in velocity, sleep systolic upstroke, lack of dicrotic notching, spectral broadening and presence of low frequency bimodal signals typical of severe spasm.

tor of vasospasm than angiography and enjoys even further diagnostic importance because it can be frequently performed at the bedside.

Blood flow, as well as diameter, often varies during the complex changes following SAH, and velocity values that foretell hemodynamically significant spasm cannot be predicted from basic principles. However, empirical criteria are available that are surprisingly similar in various centers. For example, a mean MCA velocity of 120 cm/sec is generally interpreted as mild vasospasm, whereas a velocity of over 170 cm/sec generally suggests severe spasm (24,25). These criteria should be tailored to the individual patient. For example, an MCA velocity of 140 cm/sec may reflect severe spasm in an elderly patient for which the normal MCA velocity is low but may be normal in the presence of sickle cell anemia in which all velocities are high (26). Calculation of the ratio between MCA velocity and the cervical internal carotid artery (ICA) velocity has also been suggested as a method to distinguish between MCA spasm and hemispheric hyperemia (27,28). Mild spasm is suggested by a ratio of 3 and severe spasm by a ratio of greater than 6.

Protocols used for TCD evaluation of SAH reflect the natural history of vasospasm. Most centers obtain an initial study that is repeated daily until about 10 days after the hemorrhage. A decision to continue the studies is then based on the TCD exam and the neurologic status of the patient. Full studies are obtained to detect spasm in all vessels, and patients who are neurologically intact but have significant SAH seen on computed tomography (CT) are given special attention to evaluate early clinical consequences of spasm. The normal pattern shows a velocity elevation beginning 4 days following the hemorrhage and lasting about 2 weeks.

The sensitivity and specificity of TCD studies compared to angiography in detecting MCA vasospasm is quite high, ranging between 84–85% and 89–98%, respectively (25,27,28). In addition, the pattern of velocity elevation can be prognostic since a rapid elevation (50–70 cm/sec/day) carries a poor prognosis (29).

The use of TCD studies to follow various therapy for spasm is difficult because maneuvers that increase flow will increase velocity, as will worsening spasm. The use of the MCA/ICA ratio has not been completely successful in this setting, and unpredictable combinations of hyperemia due to dysautoregulation and spasm can produce high velocities. For example, persistent high velocity has been seen immediately following successful angioplasty for spasm, presumably due to hyperemia (30). Although a normal velocity following angioplasty is assurance against recurrence of spasm, these difficulties severely limit the utility of TCD to follow the therapy of spasm.

Serial TCD studies therefore, are of value in detecting arterial vasospasm following SAH, especially in the MCA. The lack of close correlation to clinical symptoms and outcome (31) is not surprising because it is the unpredictable recruitment of collateral supply and autoregulation and not simply vessel narrowing that determines tissue perfusion.

The clinical utility of these TCD studies lies in their ability to confirm the occurrence of spasm and serve as an early warning of significant vessel narrowing.

Intracranial Pressure

The appearance of high pulsatility throughout the cranium during a TCD study is suggestive of a significant rise in intracranial pressure (32). These changes may be seen either diffusely or limited to one hemisphere, and may be symptomatic. Other conditions that may produce these same changes include hyperventilation and the administration of vasoconstrictive agents such as pentothal.

Emboli

The consistent appearance of HITS during TCD examination is highly suggestive of the presence of an embolic source (Fig. 6). Emboli seen throughout the cranium suggest a cardiac or aortic source, and insonation of several sites along the arterial tree can often provide specific localization. There is no other modality available that provides primary diagnosis of the presence of emboli. An increasingly important example is the use of TCD to detect air emboli following intravenous injection of agitated saline for the detection of the presence of a patent foramen ovale (PFO). Although PFO can also be diagnosed with angiography and transesophageal echocardiography (TEE), TCD is less invasive and faster. Comparison of TCD to TEE has yielded sensitivities and specificities of 89–93% and 92–100% respectively (33,34), especially when augmented by the Valsalva maneuver. Itoh et al. (35) found TCD more sensitive than TEE, suggesting that TCD is the ideal tool for the diagnosis of PFO.

Hemodynamic Effects of Positional Maneuvers

The appearance of neurologic symptoms or vertigo during positional maneuvers such as head turning or standing may be due to orthostatic hypotension, stenosis induced by position, or otologic disease. The diagnosis of a hemodynamic source of these symptoms has been made in recent years by monitoring either the basilar, vertebral, or posterior cerebral arteries during these maneuvers. Simultaneous monitoring of blood pressure is helpful in distinguishing focal hemodynamic compromise from more global perfusion changes secondary to orthostatic hypotension (Fig. 4). In this setting, insonation of the vertebrobasilar system is difficult due to artifacts from angle changes and only dramatic changes can be reliably interpreted. On the other hand, changes seen in the posterior cerebral artery insonated through the temporal window are reliable and indicate hemodynamic change (36).

USE OF TCD IN THE PHYSIOLOGIC EVALUATION OF HEMODYNAMIC LESIONS

The information available from TCD studies is relevant to a wide variety of hemodynamic lesions and situations.

This section will touch on the major categories of such conditions, but similar considerations apply to virtually any pathologic state altering cerebral blood flow.

Assessment of Changes in Perfusion Due to Hemodynamic Lesions

Any decrease in cerebral blood velocity suggests a compromise of perfusion, especially if associated with a blunted pulsatility. The latter finding is due to either proximal vascular compromise or compensatory distal autoregulatory vasodilation (Fig. 2). Minor diminutions in velocity are common and probably not significant, whereas a drop to levels near zero suggests a critically low-level perfusion (Fig. 5). A rough rule of thumb for the threshold at which a drop in TCD velocity becomes significant is a drop of about 65–70%, with the evidence for this rule arising from several sources. A decrease in MCA velocity seen during transient manual compression of the cervical carotid artery in awake patients by more than 65% has been found to be associated with intolerance to a trial of balloon occlusion of the internal carotid artery (37). This association was based both on clinical tolerance and changes in SPECT studies. During carotid endarterectomy, clamping of the carotid artery produces a fall in the ipsilateral MCA velocity. A fall of this velocity by more than 65–70% has been associated with a stump pressure of less than 25 mm Hg, EEG changes, and poor outcome (38–42). Theoretical considerations are consistent with this same threshold as well. For example, the change between a normal cerebral blood flow of 50 cm^3/100 ml/min to that of the ischemic threshold of 20 is about 60%. Several investigators (38,43–45) found that an MCA velocity of <30% in the presence of ipsilateral carotid occlusion and stroke predicted poorer outcome and larger infarct on CT. Although there are many settings in which changes in velocity falls, the 65% threshold rule has only been confirmed in the studies of carotid occlusion above and must only be accepted as a rough estimation. In addition, diameter changes of the insonated vessels may occur to confound the interpretation of a velocity decrement as arising solely from impaired perfusion, as mentioned earlier.

Velocity decrements may be seen during changes in systemic blood pressure from a variety of causes, including arrhythmias and orthostatic hypotension. For example, during head-up tilt testing, a fall of greater than 65% in mean blood flow velocity is almost unequivocally associated with syncope (46). The intense sympathetic response induced by these changes may alter the diameter of the insonated vessel, but a profound fall of velocity suggests impairment of perfusion. A fall in the basilar or posterior cerebral artery during head turning has been used to implicate a hemodynamic cause of symptoms during evaluation of vertigo. The use of the 65% threshold has been mentioned previously when testing for tolerance to carotid occlusion or during carotid endarterectomy. Similarly, a fall in MCA velocity after endarterectomy has been associated with restenosis (47). The effects of an intracranial stenosis can be assessed by comparing the velocity distal to the stenosis with the contralateral comparable vessel, again using the 65% threshold. Decrements in velocity are also seen in the presence of increased intracranial pressure, although exact thresholds for clinical significance have not been determined. Finally, insonation of the vertebral or basilar arteries in the presence of subclavian steal often shows retrograde or altering flow in the vertebral artery but rarely in the basilar artery (48,49). These findings suggest alterations in perfusion pressure and are not tightly associated with symptoms.

The use of TCD to assess perfusion following acute stroke deserves special comment. As mentioned, a fall of MCA velocity to <30 cm/sec is associated with poor outcome. Other investigators have confirmed that early, persistent, and profound alteration in MCA velocity waveforms occurred frequently (70%) and predict poor outcome (50) and more profound CT changes (45,51). The combination of MCA velocity less than 40 cm/sec and an asymmetry index (defined as the difference between the right and left MCA velocities divided by their average) of more than 20% has been used to predict poor outcome from studies performed within 48 hours with a sensitivity of 67% and a specificity of 100% (52). Several authors have stressed the use of serial TCD studies to assess MCA reperfusion, which was noted to be common and predict a better outcome (50,51,53). The role of serial TCD studies to follow the effects of thrombolytic therapy is under investigation.

In addition to changes in velocity, changes in pulsatility also suggest alterations in perfusion. A lessened pulsatility with a blunted waveform scan arises from proximal compromise combined with distal autoregulatory vasodilatation. Although perfusion may be maintained in this setting, a blunted pulsatility combined with a lowered velocity strongly suggests compromise in perfusion with exhaustion of autoregulatory reserve (Fig. 2).

Although ischemia is commonly associated with vascular stenoses, successful treatment of a significant stenosis can lead to hyperemia and hemorrhagic stroke. For example, the chronic ischemia accompanying a severe carotid artery stenosis can lead to chronic vasodilatation and a loss of autoregulatory ability. An endarterectomy restores normal pressure to this vasodilated tissue bed, producing edema and hemorrhage. These changes are easily detected by measuring a rise in MCA velocities to above 120 cm/sec either immediately after the procedure or during serial studies over the subsequent several days (41). Treatment of this condition consists of rigid blood pressure control to normalize the MCA velocity on the affected side without producing a decrement on the unaffected side (41). Alternatively, one may surgically implant an adjustable clamp around the carotid artery and release it slowly over several days using the MCA velocities as guidance (54).

Assessment of Collateral Blood Supply

The patency of collateral channels can be reliably assessed with TCD, and abnormal patterns can suggest pathology such as proximal carotid compromise (55). Retrograde flow direction seen in the anterior cerebral artery suggests ipsilateral carotid artery compromise with collateral supply recruited from the contralateral side (Fig. 2). Detection of this condition is not straightforward because signals obtained from retrograde flow in the anterior cerebral artery (ACA) can mimic orthograde signals in the MCA. A clue to the presence of this phenomenon is the finding of two separate populations of MCA velocities, with the high velocity usually representing retrograde flow in the ipsilateral ACA. Similarly, increased velocity in the basilar artery suggests increased collateral flow across the posterior communicating arteries, whereas retrograde ophthalmic artery flow direction suggests extracranial to intracranial shunting.

TCD assessment of collateral flow has correlated well with angiography. Sensitivity, specificity, and positive predictive values for detecting flow across the anterior communicating artery in the presence of a unilateral carotid occlusion are about 94–95%, 100%, and 94%, respectively, and are 88–95% for collateral flow across the posterior communicating artery (13,56). Sensitivity and predictive value for collateral flow through the ophthalmic artery have been calculated as 100% and 80%, respectively (13). Furthermore, the appearance of these collateral patterns suggests profound hemodynamic changes because they are associated with more significant carotid lesions (57,58), and their absence has been associated with more profound MCA velocity changes during carotid endarterectomy (55). Finally, the ability of TCD to detect collateral channels has been found comparable or even superior to magnetic resonance angiography (59).

These collateral routes can be even more precisely tested by the use of transient manual carotid compression to induce flow direction reversal in the ACA and the ophthalmic artery as well as flow augmentation in the basilar or posterior cerebral arteries. Transient manual compression of the carotid artery has been safely used for this and other purposes in large series (60). However, the compression should be performed gently and arteries screened with duplex studies if significant atherosclerotic disease is suspected because there is at least one report of minor stroke following such a compression (61).

An important example of an abnormal collateral pattern is seen in subclavian steal. Reversal of flow direction in one vertebral artery is easily detected by TCD studies, although reversal of flow in the basilar artery is rare (62). Since intraarterial pressure differences vary during the cardiac cycle, it is not unusual to detect vertebral artery flow reversal only in diastole in producing a "reverberating" pattern.

An interesting example arises in the seeming paradoxical velocity elevation in the MCA contralateral to a carotid occlusion or an arteriovenous malformation (AVM). A potential explanation for this elevation is increased demand through leptomeningeal connections to the ipsilateral and anterior cerebral artery territory that is compromised due to steal from the AVM or collateral across the anterior communicating artery in the case of carotid occlusion.

These assessments of collateral channels require laborious insonation of multiple vessels. Furthermore, although the posterior communicating artery is occasionally identified by its relatively high pulsatility, it is rarely insonated directly. TCD imaging may allow insonation of several vessels simultaneously and may provide an easier assessment of collateral pathways (63).

Assessment of Intracranial Pressure

The hemodynamic resistance in the arterioles and pial vessels will increase dramatically with increased intracranial pressure, although hyperventilation or the administration of such agents such as pentothal can produce similar changes. The resulting TCD waveform is highly pulsatile and may at times be "reverberating" with alternating periods of flow toward and away from the probe (Fig. 8). In this case, the net flow in the insonated vessel is close to zero. As intracranial pressure rises, autoregulatory mechanisms that vasodilate the small vessels and oppose the increase in pulsatility are invoked. Thus, the appearance of a highly pulsatile signal indicates an advanced stage in which autoregulation has been overwhelmed (32). The TCD waveform is therefore unable to serve as a quantitative measure of intracranial pressure, although a trend of higher pulsatility toward a reverberating pattern indicates worsening of intracranial pressure.

Another interesting use of the waveform shape to evaluate subtle changes in hemodynamic resistance has been given by Ries et al. (64). Patients with Alzheimer's disease could be distinguished from those with multi-infarct dementia using a resistance index, suggesting that numerous small infarcts produce an elevated hemodynamic resistance not seen in Alzheimer's dementia.

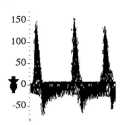

FIG. 8. Signal obtained from middle cerebral artery in a patient who is brain dead. The "reverberating" appearance of flow direction towards and away from the probe suggests little net forward flow.

Assessment of Vascular Reactivity

The measurement of vascular reactivity has attracted considerable attention, since impaired reactivity can be interpreted as concurrent vasodilatation due to the ischemic stimulus of a severe hemodynamic lesion. Measurements with external xenon detectors, stable xenon CT, and SPECT studies have been used to measure cerebral blood flow before and after vasodilating stimulation in an effort to quantitate this response. Although precise stratification of patient populations has been elusive, it is generally believed that a lack of response indicates significant small vessel vasodilatation and a significant hemodynamic lesion that may be worthy of aggressive therapy. This section discusses some of the efforts in this direction that have been made with TCD.

There are several major categories of physiologic response to vasodilatory stimulation that can be evaluated by TCD. Cerebral autoregulation is the ability of the vascular bed to maintain constant blood flow in the face of a change in blood pressure or appropriate blood flow in the face of changing metabolic demands. A large component of this response is mediated by the action of adenosine on the microcirculation, but there is also evidence that the larger vessels may respond to changes in blood pressure. A second and different vasodilatory stimulus, mediated by pH, is that produced by variation in partial pressure of carbon dioxide (pCO_2). The response to CO_2 can be dissociated from autoregulation, as seen in patients with head injury who commonly show impaired autoregulation but an intact response to pCO_2. Most of the response is due to reactivity of arterioles rather than that of the proximal circle of Willis. This explains the similarity in the magnitude of the response of both TCD velocity and cerebral blood flow as 3–5%/mm Hg, implicating the smaller vessels as the site of diameter change (65).

Many studies have addressed the role of CO_2 reactivity in assessing the hemodynamic state. Although vessels react to CO_2 by different mechanisms than autoregulation, it is reasoned that a vasodilatory response to CO_2 will be blunted in ischemic tissue in which autoregulatory mechanisms have already produced a vasodilatation. Ringelstein measured the velocity difference between hypercapnia induced by inhalation of 2–5% CO_2 and hypocapnia induced by hyperventilation, calculating an index expressed as a percentage of baseline (66). This index was 85% in normal subjects and was significantly decreased in the presence of unilateral or bilateral carotid occlusion. The association of a low reactivity with symptoms was significant, as was a level below 34% with low-flow infarct, ischemic ophthalmopathy, or TIAs of hemodynamic origin. Other authors have found association between low CO_2 reactivity and recent ischemic events (67), as well as correlation to velocity decrements of 60% during carotid endocarterectomy (68). A variant of the use of CO_2 is the administration of intravenous acetazolamide. This agent has identical action on cerebral blood flow as CO_2, and the intravenous administration of acetazolamide is well tolerated and more convenient than the use of inhaled CO_2. The response is not easily calibrated to dosage and a dose of 1000 mg is standard. Although one study showed that measurement of response to acetazolamide with TCD compares well to that derived from xenon-133 SPECT studies (69), another found a disagreement between the two modalities in 14 of 52 patients (70). Possible sources for this discovery included change induced by acetazolamide itself (vessel diameter or distribution of flow through vessel) and overestimation of high-flow status by SPECT (70,71). Association of reactivity to acetazolamide to hemodynamic states has nevertheless been noted. For example, one study found an association between high hemispheric difference in reactivity to carotid stenosis, occlusion, or ipsilateral TIAs (71).

A third type of vasodilatory stimulus involves the administration of vasoactive agents. Interpretation of the results upon the TCD velocity is difficult because the effect on large vessel diameter is essentially unknown. A fourth type of vasodilatory stimulus is seen in the use of the Valsalva maneuver, deep breathing and breath holding, and leg lifting. These also produce variations of blood pressure and velocity that can result in cerebral vasodilatation. Unfortunately, the invoked sympathetic response can be significant and has an unknown effect on the diameter of the insonated vessels. Finally, vascular activation by cognitive function or visual stimulation can be measured with TCD, although use in the clinical assessment of stroke is unexplored.

All of these stimuli have been used in combination with TCD to measure cerebral vasoreactivity. Stimuli that alter blood pressure must be used with caution, however, because both the agent used and the change in pressure itself may alter the diameter of the insonated artery. Aaslid and Lindegaard have employed pressure cuffs placed around both thighs to impose sudden drops in blood pressure (72). The slope of the calculated resistance using the recovering MCA velocity is then interpreted as autoregulatory ability. A subsequent study indicated that only minimal diameter changes were produced by this method (73). A simpler technique for altering local perfusion pressure relies on transient manual occlusion of the carotid artery (60). An observed overshoot of the velocity after the occlusion is released is interpreted as arising from autoregulatory vasodilatation occurring during the manual occlusion (Fig. 5). Another approach has utilized naturally occurring variations in blood pressure that can be dramatic in neurologically impaired patients. Comparison of the magnitude of the changes in TCD velocity to those of blood pressure yields an assessment of autoregulatory ability (74). Difficulties with these methods include dependence of natural variations to provide pressure changes at clinically meaningful frequencies and amplitudes, the unavailability of cerebral blood pressure, and the possibility of concomitant diameter changes of the insonated vessel. Other authors have used vasopressor agents or lower body negative pressure (75) or maneuvers to alter blood pressure, but the effects of these techniques on cerebral arterial diameter are largely unknown.

Assessment of Vessel Patency

The ability of TCD to assess patency of a vessel can be difficult because a signal may be absent due not only to vessel occlusion but to technical or anatomic factors. However, a diagnosis of vessel occlusion may be reliably determined if the same experienced operator detects the vessel in one study but not subsequently. TCD has been helpful in the assessment of patency of ECIC grafts, whereby the appearance of a signal of low pulsatility of intracranial characteristic confirms the flow of blood through the graft into the intracranial circulation. However, because the graft caliber will enlarge with time, quantitative assessment of flow through the lumen is impossible by TCD studies. TCD assessment of patency has also been used to follow the effects of thrombolytic therapy in settings where serial angiograms are otherwise contraindicated.

Assessment of Vessel Stenosis

The previous section addressed the effectiveness of TCD studies in diagnosing intracranial stenoses. This section will focus on the assessment of stenosis severity by TCD once the stenosis is known to exist. An unavoidable difficulty is the inability of velocity measurements to distinguish elevations arising from small diameter from those arising from high flow (30). Heuristic guidelines have nevertheless emerged and are useful in practice, and the availability of serial measurements adds to the utility of TCD in this setting (76). For example, the appearance of a focal increase in velocity is highly suggestive of stenosis of the insonated vessel with severity suggested by the finding of low velocity distal or proximal to the stenotic segment (Fig. 7). In addition, the large experience obtained from patients after subarachnoid hemorrhage has provided some empirical guidelines. Velocities in the MCA above 180 cm/sec generally indicate a clinically significant stenosis, whereas those below 120 cm/sec generally indicate a mild and insignificant stenosis. This is consistent with the theoretical fact that the velocity will double with only a 30% decrease in diameter if flow is otherwise constant.

These guidelines have been helpful in practice but have limitations. Stenoses of very severe magnitude may appear with normal velocity due to flow impediment, although the pulsatility would be blunted as autoregulation is triggered. Furthermore, the presence of a proximal tandem stenosis might result in decreased flow through the insonated stenosis and may confound interpretation.

Assessment of Emboli

Emboli are common during carotid endarterectomy (7,40) (Fig. 6), cardiac bypass (77,78), carotid angioplasty (79), and carotid atherosclerotic disease (80), and their ubiquity has been demonstrated since they were first noticed during underwater decompression. The appearance of one group of emboli signals (HITS) rarely leads to a clinical stroke, but large numbers of occurrences appear to be more ominous. The high embolic count has been associated with plaque ulceration in patients with carotid stenosis (81) and is more common in vessels that supply symptomatic tissue (82) or following a stroke (83). In patients who harbor prosthetic heart valves, HITS are more frequent in the presence of symptoms (84). Siebler et al. have shown that embolic counts greater than 2 per hour are highly associated with a history of recent symptoms (positive predictable value = 0.88) (80,83). Emboli were also seen in 9 of 10 carotid angioplasties, decreasing significantly after 1 month (79).

These data indicate that a high embolic count is associated with an increased risk for neurologic symptoms. Whether their occurrence represents an epiphenomenon rather than the critical event leading to the symptoms is not known. The threshold at which the number of emboli predicts neurologic compromise and mandates treatment is unknown, but patterns are emerging in specific settings. During cardiac bypass, emboli are almost always detectable (78), and Pugsley has found that identification of more than 1000 was associated with a 43% occurrence of neuropsychiatric worsening in contrast to a 9% chance in cases with fewer than 200 HITS (77). Patterns of emboli seen during carotid endocarterectomy have also been studied. The detection of more than 10 embolic signals while the carotid artery is being dissected is associated with MRI and CT changes suggestive of infarction, as well as a decrease in cognitive function (40,85,86). Embolic counts decrease at 1 and 12 weeks following endarterectomy (87), but persistent detection of emboli has been associated with occurrence of postoperative thrombi formation and neurologic deficits (86).

The use of emboli detection to diagnose PFOs has been mentioned and other applications are being considered. Although a decline in embolic counts would be anticipated following anticoagulation, reports are conflicting (88), and the exact relationship between observed counts and optimal anticoagulation has not been determined. Another promising application is the serial evaluation of intravascular thrombosis because thrombolysis can be detected by the reappearance of a normal velocity waveform and a decrease in the number of distal emboli (89).

There is emerging evidence that monitoring for emboli during procedures, or for 30–60 minutes during a screening TCD exam, can be helpful in assessing the significance of embolic disorders and embolic sources. The thresholds mentioned previously give rough guidelines for this assessment and will undoubtedly be refined in the near future. Systems designed to automatically count and detect emboli have been developed and may shortly be proven to have the reliability needed for clinical practice.

SUMMARY

TCD is a noninvasive, versatile diagnostic technique allowing assessment of hemodynamics and of embolic counts. The information can be conveniently obtained in a serial fashion at the bedside and in difficult hospital environments such as the intensive care unit or surgical suite. The major limitations of this method include the inability to distinguish changes in velocity from those of flow and the uncertainty of the significance of detected emboli. Nevertheless, clinically useful diagnoses and evaluations of lesions producing stroke are readily available with TCD that cannot be obtained otherwise.

REFERENCES

1. Newell D, Aaslid, R, ed. *Transcranial Doppler.* New York: Raven Press, 1992.
2. Babikian VL, Wechsler LR. *Transcranial Doppler Ultrasonography.* St Louis: Mosby, 1993.
3. Aaslid R, Markwalder TM, Nornes H. Noninvasive transcranial Doppler ultrasound recording of flow velocity in basal cerebral arteries. *J Neurosurg* 1982;57:769–774.
4. Ringelstein EB, Kahlscheuerer B, Niggemeyer E, Otis SM. Transcranial Doppler sonography: anatomical landmarks and normal velocity values. *Ultrasound Med Biol* 1990; 745–761.
5. Bogdahn U, Becker G, Winkler J, Greiner K, Perez J, Meurers B. Transcranial color-coded real-time sonography in adults. *Stroke* 1990; 21(2):1680–1688.
6. Brass LM, Pavlakis SG, DeVivo D, Piomelli S, Mohr JP. Transcranial Doppler measurements of the middle cerebral artery. Effect of hematocrit. *Stroke* 1988;19:1466–1469.
7. Spencer MP, Campbell, SD, Sealey JL, Lindenbergh J. Experiments on decompression bubbles in the circulation using ultrasonic and electromagnetic flowmeters. *J Occup Med* 1969;2:238–244.
8. Markus HS, Harrison MJ. Microembolic signal detection using ultrasound. *Stroke* 1995;26:1517–1519.
9. Russell D, Madden KP, Clark WM, Sandset PM, Zivin JA. Detection of arterial emboli using Doppler ultrasound in rabbits. *Stroke* 1991;22: 253–258.
10. Giller CA, Bowman G, Dyer H, Mootz L, Krippner W. Cerebral arterial diameters during changes in blood pressure and CO_2 during craniotomy. *Neurosurgery* 1993;32:737–742.
11. Huber P, Handa J. Effect of contrast material, hypercapnia, hyperventilation, hypertonic glucose and papaverine on the diameter of the cerebral arteries. *Invest Radiol* 1967;2:17–32.
12. Lindegaard KF, Lundar T, Wiberg J, Sjoberg P, Aaslid R, Nornes H. Variations in middle cerebral artery blood flow investigated with noninvasive transcranial blood velocity measurements. *Stroke* 1987; 18(6):1025–1030.
13. Grolimund P, Seiler RW, Aaslid R, Huber P, Zurbruegg H. Evaluation of cerebrovascular disease by combined extracranial and transcranial Doppler sonography. Experience in 1,039 patients. *Stroke* 1987;18: 1018–1024.
14. Halsey JH. Effect of emitted power on waveform intensity in transcranial Doppler. *Stroke* 1990;21:1573–1578.
15. Itoh T, Matsumoto M, Handa N, Maeda H, Hougaku H, Hashimoto H, Etani H, Tsukamoto Y, Kamada T. Rate of successful recording of blood flow signals in the middle cerebral artery using transcranial Doppler sonography. *Stroke* 1993;24:1192–1195.
16. Spencer MP, Whisler D. Transorbital Doppler diagnosis of intracranial arterial stenosis. *Stroke* 1986;17:916–921.
17. Babikian VL, Pochay V. Accuracy of transcranial Doppler in detecting carotid distribution—arterial stenoses. *Neurology* 1991;41(Suppl):122.
18. Lev-Pozo J, Ringelstein EB. Noninvasive detection of occlusive disease of the carotid siphon and middle cerebral artery. *Ann Neurol* 1990;28: 640–647.
19. Rorick MB, Nichols FT, Adams RJ. Transcranial Doppler correlation with angiography in detection of intracranial stenosis. *Stroke* 1994;25: 1931–1934.
20. Tettenborn B, Estol C, DeWitt D, Kraemer G, Pessin M, Caplan L. Accuracy of transcranial Doppler in the vertebrobasilar circulation. *J Neurol* 1990;237:159.

21. Giller CA, Mathews D, Purdy P, Kopitnik TA, Batjer HH, Samson DS. The transcranial Doppler appearance of acute carotid artery occlusion. *Ann Neurol* 1992;31:101–103.

22. Kelley RE, Namon RA, Mantelle LL, Chang JY. Sensitivity and specificity of transcranial Doppler ultrasonography in the detection of high-grade carotid stenosis. *Neurology* 1993;43:1187–1191.

23. Wilterdink JL, Feldmann E, Bragoni M. Brooks JM, Benavides JG. An absent ophthalmic artery or carotid siphon signal on transcranial Doppler confirms the presence of severe ipsilateral internal carotid artery disease. *J Neuroimag* 1994;4:196–199.

24. Aaslid R, Huber P, Nornes H. Evaluation of cerebrovascular spasm with transcranial Doppler ultrasound. *J Neurosurg* 1984;42:81–84.

25. Sloan MA, Haley ED, Kassell NF, Henry ML, Stewart SR, Beskin RR, Sevilla EA, Tomer JC. Sensitivity and specificity of transcranial Doppler ultrasonography in diagnosis of vasospasm following subarachnoid hemorrhage. *Neurology* 1989;39:1514–1518.

26. Adams R, McKie V, Nichols F, Carl E, Zhang DL, McKie K, Figueroa R, Litaker M, Thompson W, Hess D. The use of transcranial ultrasonography to predict stroke in sickle cell disease. *N Engl J Med* 1992; 326(9):605–610.

27. Lindegaard K, Nornes H, Bakke S, Sorteberg W, Nakstad P. Cerebral vasospasm after subarachnoid hemorrhage investigated by means of transcranial Doppler ultrasound. *Acta Neurol Chirurgica (Wien)* 1988; 42:81–84.

28. Lindegaard K, Nornes H, Bakke S, Sorteberg W, Nakstad P. Cerebral vasospasm diagnosis by means of angiography and blood velocity measurements. *Acta Neuro Chirurgica (Wien)* 1989;100:12–24.

29. Grosset DG, Straiton J, Trevou M, Bullock R. Prediction of symptomatic vasospasm after subarachnoid hemorrhage by rapidly increasing transcranial Doppler velocity and cerebral blood flow changes. *Stroke* 1992;23:674–679.

30. Giller CA, Purdy P, Giller A, Batjer HH, Kopitnik TA. Elevated transcranial Doppler ultrasound velocities following therapeutic arterial dilation. *Stroke* 1995;26:123–127.

31. Laumer R, Steinmeier R, Gonner F, Vogtman T, Priem R, Fahlbusch R. Cerebral hemodynamics in subarachnoid hemorrhage elevated by transcranial Doppler sonography. 1. Reliability of flow velocities in clinical management. *Neurosurgery* 1993;33:1–9.

32. Hassler W, Steinmetz H, Gawlowski J. Transcranial Doppler ultrasonography in raised intracranial pressure and in intracranial circulatory arrest. *J Neurosurg* 1988;68:745–751.

33. Job FP, Ringelstein EB, Grafen V, Flackskampf FA, Doherty C, Stockmann A, Hanrath P. Comparison of transcranial contrast Doppler sonography and trasesophageal contrast echocardiography for the detection of patent foramen ovale in young stroke patients. *Am J Cardiol* 1994;74:381–384.

34. Jauss M, Kaps M, Keberle M, Haberbosch W, Dorndorf W. A comparison of transesophageal echocardiography and transcranial Doppler sonography with contrast medium for detection of patent foramen ovale. *Stroke* 1994;25:1265–1267.

35. Itoh T, Matsumoto M, Handa N, Maeda H, Hougaku H. Paradoxical embolism as a cause of ischemic stroke of uncertain etiology. A transcranial Doppler sonographic study. *Stroke* 1994;25:771–775.

36. Sturzemegger M, Newell DW, Couville C, Byrd S, Schoonover K. Dynamic transcranial Doppler assessment of positional vertebrobasilar ischemia. *Stroke* 1994;25:1776–1783.

37. Giller CA, Mathews D, Walker B, Purdy P, Roseland A. Prediction of tolerance to carotid artery occlusion using transcranial Doppler ultrasound. *J Neurosurg* 1994;84:15–19.

38. Halsey JH. Prognosis of acute hemiplegia estimated by transcranial Doppler ultrasonography. *Stroke* 1988;19:648–649.

39. Halsey JH, McDowell HA, Gelmon S, Morawetz RB. Blood velocity in the middle cerebral artery and regional blood flow during carotid endarterectomy. *Stroke* 1989;20:53–58.

40. Jansen C, Ramos LMP, van Heesewijk JPM, Moll FL, van Gijn J, Ackerstaff RGA. Impact of microembolism and hemodynamic changes in the brain during carotid endarterectomy. *Stroke* 1994;25:992–997.

41. Jorgensen LG, Schroeder TV. Defective cerebrovascular autoregulation after carotid endarterectomy. *Eur J Vasc Surg* 1992;6:142–147.

42. Spencer MP, Thomas GI, Moehring MA. Relation between middle cerebral artery blood flow velocity and stump pressure during carotid endarterectomy. *Stroke* 1992;23:1439–1445.

43. Wechsler CR, Ropper AH, Kistler JP. Transcranial Doppler in cerebrovascular disease. *Stroke* 1986;17:905–912.

44. Hedera P, Traubner P, Bujdakova J. Short-term prognosis of stroke due to occlusion of internal carotid artery based on transcranial Doppler ultrasonography. *Stroke* 1992;23:1069–1072.

45. Kushner MJ, Zanette EM, Bastianello S, Mancini G, Sacchetti ML, Carolei A, Bozzao L. Transcranial Doppler in acute hemispheric brain infarction. *Neurology* 1991;41:109–113.

46. Gomez CR, Janosik DL, Lewis LM. Transcranial Doppler in the evaluation of global cerebral ischemia: syncope and cardiac arrest. In: Babikian VL, Wechsler LB, eds. *Transcranial Doppler Ultrasonography*. St. Louis: CV Mosby, 1993.

47. Laman DM, Voorwinde A, Davies G, Von Duijn H. Intraoperative internal carotid artery restenosis detected by transcranial Doppler monitoring. *Br J Surg* 1989;76:1315–1316.

48. Thomasson C, Aarli JA. Subclavian steal phenomenon. Clinical and hemodynamic aspects. *Acta Neurol Scand* 1994;90:241–244.

49. Hennerici M, Klemm C, Rautenberg W. The subclavian steal phenomenon: a common vascular disorder with rare neurologic deficits. *Neurology* 1988;38:669–673.

50. Alexandrov AV, Bladen CF, Norris JW. Intracranial blood flow velocities in acute ischemic stroke. *Stroke* 1994;25:1378–1383.

51. Ringelstein EB, Biniek R, Weiller C, Amelling B, Nolte PN, Thron A. Type and extent of hemispheric brain infarctions and clinical outcome in early and delayed middle cerebral artery recanalization. *Neurology* 1992;42:289–298.

52. Ni X-S, Horner S, Fazekas F, Niederkorn K. Serial transcranial Doppler sonography in ischemic strokes in middle cerebral artery territory. *J Neuroimag* 1994;4:232–236.

53. Zanette EM, Roberti C, Mancini G, Pozzilli C, Bragoni M. Toni D. Spontaneous middle cerebral artery reperfusion in ischemic stroke. A follow-up study with transcranial Doppler. *Stroke* 1995;26:430–433.

54. Smith RR, Burt T. Hyperperfusion after carotid endarterectomy managed by a removable clamp. *J Neuroimag* 1993;3:16–19.

55. Schneider PA, Ringelstein EB, Rossman ME, Dilly RB, Sobel DF, Otis SM, Bernstein EF. Importance of cerebral circulation pathways during carotid endarterectomy. *Stroke* 1988;19:1328–1334.

56. Muller M, Hermes M, Bruckmann H, Schimrick T. Transcranial Doppler ultrasound in the evaluation of collateral flood flow in patients with internal carotid artery occlusion: correlation with cerebral angiography. *Am J Neuroradiol* 1995;16:195–202.

57. Lindegaard K, Bakke SJ, Grolimund P, Aaslid R, Huber P, Nornes H. Carotid artery disease: assessment of intracranial hemodynamics in carotid artery disease by transcranial Doppler ultrasound. *J Neurosurg* 1985;63:890–898.

58. Schneider PA, Rossman ME, Bernstein EF, Tore S, Ringelstein B, Otis SM. Effect of internal carotid artery occlusion on intracranial hemodynamics. *Stroke* 1988;19:589–593.

59. Anzola GO, Gasparotti R, Magoni M, Prandini F. Transcranial Doppler sonography and magnetic resonance angiography in the assessment of collateral hemispheric flow in patients with carotid artery disease. *Stroke* 1995;26:214–217.

60. Giller CA. A bedside test for cerebral autoregulation using transcranial Doppler ultrasound. *Acta Neurochir* 1991;108:7–14.

61. Khaffaf N, Karnik, R, Winkler WB, Valentin A, Slany J. Embolic stroke by compression maneuver during transcranial Doppler sonography. *Stroke* 1994;25:1056–1057.

62. Otis SM, Ringelstein EB. Findings associated with extracranial occlusive disease. In: Newell DW, Aaslid R, eds. *Transcranial Doppler*. New York: Raven Press, 1992.

63. Martin PJ, Smith JL, Gaunt ME, Naylor AR. Assessment of intracranial primary collateral using transcranial color-coded real-time sonography. *J Neuroimag* 1995;5:199–205.

64. Ries F, Horn R, Hillekamp J, Honisch C, Konig M, Solymosi L. Differentiation of multi-infarct and Alzheimer demential by intracranial hemodynamic parameters. *Stroke* 1993;24:228–235.

65. Markwalder TM, Grolimund P, Seiler RW, Roth F, Aaslid R. Dependency of blood flow velocity in the middle cerebral artery on end-tidal carbon dioxide partial pressure: a transcranial ultrasound Doppler study. *J Cereb Blood Flow Metab* 1984;4:368–372.

66. Ringelstein EB, Sievers C, Ecker S, Schneider PA, Otis SM. Noninvasive assessment of CO_2-induced cerebral vasomotor response in normal individuals and patients with internal carotid artery occlusions. *Stroke* 1988;19:963–969.

67. Widder B. The Doppler CO_2 test to exclude patients not in need of

extracranial/intracranial bypass surgery. *J Neurol Neurosurg Psychiatry* 1989;52:38–42.

68. Thiel A, Zickman B, Stertmann WA, Wyderta T, Hempelmann G. Cerebrovascular carbon dioxide reactivity in carotid disease. Relation to intraoperative cerebral monitoring results in 100 carotid evaluations. *Anesthesiology* 1995;82:655–661.

69. Piepgras A, Schmiedek P, Leinsinger G, Haberl RL, Kirsch CM, Einhaupl KM. A simple test to assess cerebrovascular reserve capacity using transcranial Doppler sonography and acetazolamide. *Stroke* 1990; 21:1306–1311.

70. Dahl A, Russell D, Nyberg-Hansen R, Rootwelt K, Bakke SJ. Cerebral vasoreactivity in unilateral carotid artery disease. A comparison of blood flow velocity and regional cerebral blood flow measurements. *Stroke* 1994;25:621–626.

71. Dahl A, Russell D, Nyberg-Hansen R, Rootwelt K, Mowinckel P. Simultaneous assessment of vasoreactivity using transcranial Doppler ultrasound and cerebral blood flow in healthy subjects. *J Cereb Blood Flow Metab* 1994;14:974–981.

72. Aaslid R, Lindegaard KF, Sorteberg W, Nornes H. Cerebral autoregulation dynamics in humans. *Stroke* 1989;20:45–52.

73. Newell DW, Aaslid R, Lam A, Mayberg TS, Winn HR. Comparison of flow and velocity during dynamic autoregulation testing in humans. *Stroke* 1994;25:793–797.

74. Giller CA. The frequency-dependent behavior of cerebral autoregulation. *Neurosurgery* 1990;27:362–368.

75. Larsen FS, Olsen KS, Hansen BA, Paulson OB, Knudson GM. Transcranial Doppler is valid for determination of the lower limit of cerebral blood flow autoregulation. *Stroke* 1994;25:1985–1988.

76. Schwarz JJ, Babikian V, DeWitt LD, Sloan MA, Wechsler LR, Gomez CR, Pochay V, Baker E. Longitudinal monitoring of intracranial arterial stenoses with transcranial Doppler ultrasonography. *J Neuroimag* 1994; 4:182–187.

77. Pugsley W, Klinger L, Paschalis C, Treasure T, Harrison H, Newman S. The impact of microemboli during cardiopulmonary bypass on neuropsychological functioning. *Stroke* 1994;25:1393–1399.

78. Barbut D, Hinton RB, Szatrowski TP, Hartman GS, Bruefach M, Williams-Russo P, Charlson ME, Gold JP. Cerebral emboli detected during bypass surgery are associated with clamp removal. *Stroke* 1994;25: 2398–2402.

79. Markus HS, Clifton A, Buckenham T, Brown MM. Carotid angioplasty. Detection of embolic signals during and after the procedure. *Stroke* 1994;25:2403–2406.

80. Siebler M. Kleinschmidt A, Sitzer M, Steinmetz H, Freund HJ. Cerebral microembolism in symptomatic and asymptomatic high-grade internal carotid artery stenosis. *Neurology* 1994;44:615–618.

81. Valton L, Larrve V, Arrue P, Geraud G, Bes A. Asymptomatic cerebral embolic signals in patients with carotid stenosis. Correlation with appearance of plaque ulceration on angiography. *Stroke* 1995;26: 813–815.

82. Babikian VL, Hyde C, Pochay V, Winter MR. Clinical correlates of high-intensity transient signals detected on transcranial Doppler sonography in patients with cerebrovascular disease. *Stroke* 1994;25: 1570–1573.

83. Siebler M, Sitzer M, Rose G, Bendfeldt D, Steinmetz H. Silent cerebral embolism caused by neurologically symptomatic high-grade carotid stenosis: event rates before and after carotid endarterectomy. *Brain* 1993;116:1005–1015.

84. Braekken SK, Russell D, Brucher R, Svennevig J. Incidence and frequency of cerebral embolic signals in patients with a similar bileaflet mechanical heart valve. *Stroke* 1995;26:1225–1230.

85. Jansen C, Vriens EM, Eikelboom BC, Vermeulen FEE, Gijn J, Ackerstaff RGA. Carotid endarterectomy with transcranial Doppler and electroencephalographic monitoring: a prospective study in 130 operations. *Stroke* 1993;24:665–669.

86. Gaunt ME, Martin PJ, Smith, JL, Rimmer T, Cherryman G, Ratliff DA, Bell PR, Naylor AP. Clinical relevance of intraoperative embolization detection by transcranial Doppler ultrasonography during carotid endarterectomy: a prospective study on 100 patients. *Br J Surg* 1994;81: 1435–1439.

87. Van Zuilen EV, Moll FL, Vermeulen FEE, Mauser HW, van Gijn J, Ackerstaff RGA. Detection of of cerebral microemboli by means of transcranial Doppler monitoring before and after carotid endarterectomy. *Stroke* 1995;26:210–213.

88. Sturzemegger M, Beer JH, Rihs F. Monitoring combined antithrombotic treatments in patients with prosthetic heart valves using transcranial Doppler and coagulation markers. *Stroke* 1995;26:63–39.

89. Diehl RR, Sliwka U, Rautenberg W, Schwartz A. Evidence for embolization from a posterior cerebral artery thrombus by transcranial Doppler monitoring. *Stroke* 1993;24:606–608.

Cerebrovascular Disease, edited by H. Hunt Batjer.
Lippincott-Raven Publishers, Philadelphia © 1997.

CHAPTER 22

Invasive Cardiovascular Monitoring and Cerebrovascular Support

John B. Terry, Marek A. Mirski, and Daniel F. Hanley

The subspecialty of neurocritical care continues to rapidly expand and contribute to the care of patients with critical nervous system disease. This chapter, a presentation of a neurointensivist's approach to cerebrovascular disease, is divided into two main sections: (a) a review of noninvasive and invasive cardio- and cerebrovascular monitoring, which should provide some useful technical material and a short review of relevant physiology, and (b) a discussion of cerebrovascular support in specific neurologic disease states. Where it exists, relevant literature is cited. Where consensus has not been obtained regarding the most effective treatment approaches, the approach used in the Neurocritical Care Unit at the Johns Hopkins Hospital is outlined as a clinical reference point.

NONINVASIVE MONITORING

The basis of noninvasive assessment is the history and physical examination. A relatively extensive evaluation of a patient's current condition is possible with data derived from electrocardiography, blood pressure measurement, pulse oximetry, and capnography. The benefits of noninvasive monitoring are rapid availability of objective data and alarm capability and little or no risk to the patient. Also, after the initial capital investment, use of monitors is inexpensive (1). Noninvasive assessment technology continues to improve and in some situations rival invasive techniques. Although noninvasive methods exist for most organ systems, techniques for the cardiac and circulatory systems have been best implemented.

Electrocardiography

Electrocardiography (ECG) is one of the most well-entrenched, noninvasive monitoring techniques. Although vir-

tually every patient in an intensive care unit (ICU) undergoes continuous ECG monitoring, clinicians are unaware of over 75% of dysrhythmias and ischemic episodes detected (2–4). The patients are usually asymptomatic during these episodes, and neither past anginal history nor routine diagnostic testing characterizes their dysrhythmias or ischemic pattern.

Artifact created by electronic filtering of the ECG signal and the limited number of leads are problems with continuous ECG monitoring. If ECG changes on the monitor screen suggest an abnormality, a calibrated strip recording displays more accurate data. A 12-lead ECG may yield more accurate information; however, it may be altered by changes in patient position or lead placement. Also, the 12-lead ECG samples only a short amount of time with a significant chance of missing critical pathologic events. Preexisting cardiac abnormalities such as a left bundle branch block or left ventricular hypertrophy may obscure the diagnosis of ischemia because of repolarization changes in the baseline ST segment (1).

The optimal ECG lead system used in continuous ECG monitoring must be able to detect both ischemic changes and dysrhythmias (5). Ischemic changes are defined as ST segment depression or elevation of 1 mm beginning 60–80 milliseconds past the J point, lasting at least 60 seconds. T-wave changes alone are not diagnostic of ischemia or infarction and are remarkably common perioperatively with an incidence of 20% (6). The V5 lead has been shown to be the most sensitive for detecting acute ischemia regardless of the location of coronary artery pathology. The addition of lead V4 increases the sensitivity of detecting ischemia to ≥90% (7). The clarity of the displayed P waves in lead II facilitates the identification of dysrhythmias. Ideally leads II, V4, and V5 would be available for continuous monitoring. In a monitor with only three leads the use of a modified V5 lead may be useful (Fig. 1). The left arm lead is placed in the V5 position and the lead selector switch is set to lead I, resulting in a modified V5 lead. If a rhythm disturbance

J. B. Terry, M. A. Mirski, and D. F. Hanley: Department of Neurology, Neurosciences Critical Care Unit, Johns Hopkins Hospital, Baltimore, Maryland 21287.

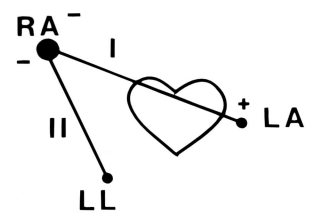

FIG. 1. With lead selector switch in the lead I position a modified V5 results. To evaluate a rhythm disturbance, lead II may be obtained without moving electrodes by changing the lead selector switch. (From ref. 34.)

occurs, the monitor may be switched to lead II without the need to move electrodes (1).

Poor-quality signal may be avoided by properly preparing the skin, using electrodes of a similar kind in similar positions, and keeping ECG cables away from other electrical equipment. Systems now available include computer-aided analysis of ECG data, which may increase detection and documentation of adverse cardiovascular events.

Neurogenic Cardiac Disease

The phenomenon of ECG changes associated with acute neurologic injury was first formally addressed 40 years ago by Byer et al. (8). He described four patients with stroke and one with hypertensive encephalopathy whose ECG was suggestive of acute myocardial infarction. At autopsy, however, the hearts of these patients were reportedly without signs of ischemic injury. Burch et al. (9) described peaked T waves, prolonged QT intervals, and U waves in patients with central nervous system (CNS) disease, predominantly subarachnoid hemorrhage (SAH). It is likely that this monograph spawned the term ''cerebral T waves.'' These electrocardiographic abnormalities were felt to be benign because pathologic evaluation of the patients' hearts at autopsy revealed no evidence of ischemic injury. The most common manifestation of neurogenic alteration of the ECG is T-wave and ST segment changes. However, large numbers of reports have described almost every type of electrocardiographic abnormality associated with acute neurologic illness. Interestingly, direct stimulation of Brodmann's area 13 in the orbitofrontal cortex has been shown to induce bradycardia (10). Also, the acute development of cardiac wall motion abnormalities after SAH without myocardial infarction has been reported (11).

Recent investigations using more advanced techniques have documented both the elevation of creatinine kinase MB fractions as well as pathologic changes in myocardium in patients who had neurogenic electrocardiographic changes.(12) Investigations using electron microscopy have revealed the presence of myofibrillar degeneration (coagulative myocytolysis and contraction band necrosis) in patients with SAH. Interestingly, this pathologic lesion differs from coagulation necrosis, the predominant lesion of myocardial infarction. Currently, the phenomenon is felt to result from high circulating levels of catechols that induce pathologic calcium influx in the myocardial cell via several biochemical cascades. These processes may account for some cases of sudden death early in the course of SAH. No treatment has been shown to be effective in humans but several pharmacologic methods to reduce catecholamine levels and calcium influx show promise in animal studies (12). Neurogenic ECG changes are a diagnosis of exclusion, however. Patients presenting with these changes should be initially evaluated for myocardial ischemia.

Oximetry and Capnometry

Hemoglobin Saturation Monitoring

Pulse oximetry utilizes the differential light absorption ratio of hemoglobin. Oxyhemoglobin absorbs more light at a wavelength of 990 nm and deoxyhemoglobin absorbs more light at a wavelength of 660 nm. Accordingly, a light source containing both wavelengths is positioned directly over a tissue capillary bed. The fingers, toes, or earlobe are most commonly used. Light passes through the tissue and is measured by a photodetector. The equipment measures the amount of light absorption at each wavelength and calculates the oxygen saturation. Only the light absorption characteristics that show a pulsatile variation are analyzed; this avoids artifact created by light absorption of venous blood and other tissues (1,5). The pulse oximetry measurements produce the most useful information in the range of hemoglobin saturations between 90% and 100%. For example, a change in PaO_2 of 120–100 does not cause a change in oximeter readings. The saturation values at each of these partial pressures of oxygen is virtually 100%. A decrease in PaO_2 from 100 to 60, however, causes the measured saturation to drop from 100% to 90%. At saturations <90% the accuracy of the measurements diminishes.

False monitoring information arises from several potential sources of artifact (1,5). Malposition of the sensor causes inaccurate saturation measurements. Excessive ambient light may interfere with readings. This may be avoided by placing the sensor on the palmar aspect of the hand, the plantar aspect of the foot, or the medial aspect of the earlobe. Covering the sensor also reduces ambient light. Nail polish, especially blue, green, or black, may cause inaccurate readings and should be removed. Motion of the sensor promotes equal absorption at both light wavelengths, resulting in an absorption ratio of 1:1. This ratio corresponds to a saturation of

85% and thus may cause artificially low saturation readings (5). Dependent positioning of the monitoring site enhances venous pulsations that may be erroneously detected as arterial pulsations; spuriously low saturation readings may result. Pulse oximetry cannot distinguish carboxyhemoglobin from oxyhemoglobin. Therefore it should not be used in patients with the possibility of CO exposure. Finally, monitoring may be difficult in patients with prominent peripheral vasoconstriction. A method of circumventing this problem is to induce vasodilatation by instilling lidocaine (1%) without epinephrine in the web space on either side of the digit used for monitoring. This may improve blood flow for a good-quality signal (1,5).

End-Tidal CO_2 Monitoring

Electronic capnometry also takes advantage of the specificity of absorption spectra. Light of a wavelength of 4.26 μm is directed through a stream of expired gas. The amount of light absorbed is measured by a photometer and is proportional to the concentration of CO_2. The highest concentration of CO_2 in the expired gas is expressed as a number (capnometry), and the changing concentrations over time are displayed as a waveform (capnography) (1,5).

A constant difference of approximately 5 mm Hg usually exists between end-expiratory CO_2 by capnometry and $PaCO_2$ by blood gas analysis. Once the relationship between these values is known, capnometry may provide continuous approximation of $PaCO_2$ values. This is especially desirable in patients who are being hyperventilated for treatment of increased intracranial pressure, both in confirming a therapeutic level of $PaCO_2$ initially and during weaning as the $PaCO_2$ is slowly normalized. With major changes in ventilation or lung perfusion the correlation between end-expiratory CO_2 and arterial CO_2 should be reevaluated.

Capnometry is also useful in confirming endotracheal (ET) tube position. Immediately after intubation the capnometer is attached to the ET tube. Detection of the presence of CO_2 during expiration on five consecutive respiratory cycles indicates that the ET tube is in the trachea. With intubation of the esophagus, CO_2 from the stomach may be initially detected but does not persist (1,5).

Blood Pressure

Manual Systems

The veracity of manual blood pressure (BP) readings obtained with the mercury sphygmomanometer depends on the accuracy of the equipment, appropriate BP cuff size, appropriate BP cuff deflation rate, and Korotkoff sound interpretation.

The ideal cuff is 20% wider than the diameter or 40% longer than the circumference of the limb being used. The length is twice as long as the width and the bladder covers at least 40% of the circumference of the limb. Cuffs that are too small give falsely elevated readings and those that are too large give falsely low readings (1).

The accuracy of ascertaining the pressure at which the appearance or disappearance of Korotkoff sounds occurs decreases with increased cuff deflation rates. The American Heart Association recommends that the cuff be deflated only 2–3 mm Hg between each heart beat. The systolic blood pressure is the pressure at which the Korotkoff sounds first appear (phase 1). Phase 1 sounds are characterized by a tapping quality. The diastolic pressure is the pressure at which the sounds completely disappear (phase 5). If they do not disappear, the point at which the sounds abruptly become muffled (phase 4) is used. A range of pressure occurring between Korotkoff sound phases 1 and 2 where the phase 1 sounds are transiently absent is termed the auscultatory gap. The range may span up to 50 mm Hg. This phenomenon occurs more frequently in hypertensive patients. If the cuff is not initially inflated above this pressure range, the blood pressure may be dramatically underestimated (1).

Auscultatory BP measurements can be misleading in patients with shock, with high total peripheral resistance, or on vasopressor drips. Invasive BP monitoring is recommended in these individuals.

Automated Systems

The three types of automated BP measurement systems commonly used are oscillometric, auscultatory, and arterial volume clamp. Oscillometric devices are the most common and provide automated, intermittent cycling of BP measurements with alarm capability. The cuff is automatically inflated. The pressure is decreased by steps, and the emergence and disappearance of minute arterial pressure oscillations is detected. These devices measure the mean arterial pressure (MAP) directly and calculate the systolic blood pressure (SBP) and diastolic blood pressure (DBP). The relationship among these pressure values is described by the equation $MAP = DBP - 1/3(SBP - DBP)$. The MAP values are the most accurate and remain so even if the machine fails to display the systolic or diastolic values. This type of automated BP monitoring is not altered by sensor positioning and will function on the arm, forearm, calf, or fingers with the proper sized cuff.

Auscultatory systems also provide automated, intermittent cycling of BP measurements and alarm capability. These devices detect Korotkoff sounds, determine systolic/diastolic blood pressure, and calculate MAP. They are very sensitive, however, to sensor placement and do not function well in nonstandard measurement sites such as the forearm or calf, where Korotkoff sounds may be less audible.

The third type of BP monitor utilizes the arterial volume clamp method (Finapres) and allows continuous BP readings. A finger cuff is used and the blood volume of the digit is determined by photoplethysmography. The instantaneous blood pressure in the digital arteries equals the cuff pressure needed to maintain a constant blood volume in the digit. This system is very sensitive to alterations in the peripheral circulation that may cause intermittent loss of sensitivity. This method may not function in individuals with prominent peripheral vasoconstriction (1).

INVASIVE MONITORING

Blood Pressure

Patient Selection

The use of an indwelling arterial catheter provides the opportunity for continuous BP monitoring, the obtaining of samples for arterial blood gas analysis, and calculation of cerebral perfusion pressure. Placement of an arterial line is indicated in cases that require close control of blood pressure. It is frequently useful in patients with stroke, cerebral aneurysm, arteriovenous malformation, increased intracranial pressure (ICP), head trauma, hypertensive encephalopathy, and carotid endarterectomy. Contraindications include the presence of a vascular prosthesis, local infection, or arterial occlusive disease with distal ischemia (1).

Accurate zeroing of the transducer is paramount for acquiring accurate data. The right midaxillary line is the point of reference most commonly used and corresponds to the level of the right heart (1). Movement of the transducer or the patient after zeroing may create inaccuracies in BP data. Generation of inaccurate data is an important complication of invasive BP monitoring and may lead to inappropriate therapy.

Complications of Arterial Lines

The most common complication of an arterial line is thrombosis. This occurs in 10% of 20-gauge catheters left in place for 3 days (13). Brachial arterial lines are associated with thrombosis rates as high as 41%. Large-bore catheters, hemodynamic instability, hypercoagulable states, preexisting atherosclerosis, and Raynaud's phenomenon increase the risk of thrombosis. The consequences of thrombosis range in severity from difficulty in withdrawing blood from the catheter to distal limb ischemia. Ischemia of the skin overlying the catheter has been reported and is attributed to occlusion of small perforating vessels. Use of small (20 gauge or less), Teflon-coated, nontapered catheters, pretreatment with aspirin, and stabilization of the limb in which the catheter is placed reduce the risk of thrombosis (13).

Significant bleeding is unusual during arterial line placement. However, femoral arterial line placement may result in delayed hematoma formation, often involving the retroperitoneum and producing a falling hematocrit. This occurs with frequency when the puncture site is proximal to the inguinal ligament. In patients with coagulation abnormali-

ties, femoral puncture should be performed distal to this ligament. Also, inadvertent disconnection of an arterial line may produce rapid blood loss. If the catheter site is not visible, significant amounts of blood may be lost before detection of the breach in the system. Appropriately defined low-pressure alarm parameters rapidly identify this situation.

Other potential complications of arterial catheter placement include infection (particularly *Staphylococcus* species) and peripheral nerve injury. Local vascular injury may result in formation of a pseudoaneurysm.

Finally, inadvertent injection of noxious substances, most commonly air or drugs, is another potential complication. Distal ischemia secondary to embolization or vasospasm may result. In these cases, intraarterial injection of lidocaine causes vasodilatation, increases perfusion, and may help to minimize injury (5). Arterial lines should remain inviolate, used only for pressure monitoring and arterial blood sampling. Pressure bags, tubing, and transducer systems should be sterile and bubble-free without access ports.

Arterial Waveform Analysis

Analysis of the arterial pressure waveform provides information on the fidelity of the BP data. Deviation from the normal waveform connotes suboptimal BP monitoring. The actual configuration of the waveform changes as blood moves distally in the arterial tree (Fig. 2). At the aortic root the elastic vessel wall absorbs kinetic energy from the ejected blood creating a broad and rounded systolic waveform. A cleft or incisura occurs at the end of the cardiac

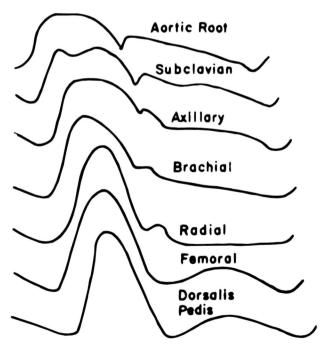

FIG. 2. Configuration of the arterial pressure waveform at several sites in the arterial tree. (From ref. 35.)

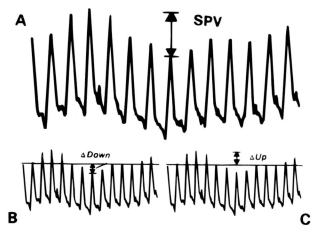

FIG. 3. The systolic pressure variation (SPV) is the difference between the maximal peak systolic and minimal peak systolic pressures during one respiratory cycle. The variable Δ down represents the difference between the peak systolic pressure at end expiration and the minimum peak systolic pressure. (From ref. 36.)

cycle and corresponds to the closing of the aortic valve. In general, the systolic wave increases in amplitude and decreases in length as it travels along the arterial tree. The incisura develops into a biphasic, dicrotic notch, most evident in the waveforms seen in the upper extremity, and disappears in those seen in the lower extremities (1,5). Retrograde, reflected pressure waves and differing arterial elasticity likely cause these changes.

The systolic pressure variation (SPV) is an aspect of the arterial pressure waveform analysis that may provide information on the volume status of the patient (Fig. 3). Increased venous return, left ventricular preload, and cardiac output occur during inspiration. During expiration these parameters decrease. This results in a sinusoidal variation in the peak systolic pressures generated during each respiratory cycle. This variation is termed the SPV. The magnitude of the change from the systolic peak pressure at end expiration to the minimum systolic peak pressure is referred to as the Δ down of the SPV. In hypovolemia, the extent of the SPV increases. More specifically, an increase in the Δ down in the presence of sinus rhythm and the absence of high inspiratory airway pressures, congestive heart failure, or pericardial tamponade is a sensitive marker of hypovolemia. In such circumstances, it may be more sensitive than the pulmonary artery wedge pressure in demonstrating decreased blood volume (1,5).

Measuring Cerebral Perfusion Pressure

In cerebrovascular disease, invasive BP monitoring may be used to evaluate and optimize cerebral perfusion pressure (CPP). The pressure of the blood entering the cerebral vasculature is the mean arterial pressure. The pressure of the blood exiting the cerebral vasculature is the central venous pres-

sure. The CPP equals the difference between these two pressures and may be expressed as MAP − CVP = CPP.

Usually the mean ICP exceeds the CVP, especially in the supine position, and it is substituted in the equation MAP − ICP = CPP. The target range of CPP for patients with cerebrovascular disease is 70–100 mm Hg. A CPP of 50–60 mm Hg may be tolerated in the special situation of induced hypotension under anesthesia to minimize blood loss during a surgical procedure such as aneurysm clipping. In laboratory studies using anesthetized animals with intact autoregulation, ischemia is not seen until the CPP falls below 40 mm Hg (12).

Autoregulation refers to the brain's ability to maintain cerebral blood flow (CBF) despite changes in MAP or CPP. This regulation occurs at the level of the cerebral arterioles. When the MAP falls, arteriolar dilatation occurs and more blood is allowed to enter the cerebral circulation. When the MAP rises, arteriolar constriction occurs allowing less blood to enter the cerebral circulation. Within a range of MAPs of 50–150 mm Hg the CBF of sedated, large mammals remains steady at approximately 50–60 cm³/100 g tissue/min. Below a MAP of 50 mm Hg, maximal arteriolar dilatation is present and autoregulation is lost. The CBF then becomes dependent on MAP in a linear fashion. At a MAP of greater than 150 mm Hg, arterioles are unable to maintain constriction against the pressure and their diameters increase. Again autoregulation breaks down and the CBF becomes dependent on the MAP. Additionally, in areas of brain injury autoregulation may be focally lost despite the MAP being in the normal range. In such a case, the CBF becomes dependent on the MAP in a linear relationship. In these situations the clinician may have the ability to maintain perfusion to the areas of injury by manipulating the MAP to maximize the CPP.

Pulmonary Artery Catheter

Use of a pulmonary artery (PA) catheter yields direct measurements of the pulmonary artery occlusion pressure and the cardiac output. Additional measurement of CVP and the calculation of the stroke volume, systemic vascular resistance, and various other hemodynamic parameters is also possible. In the context of neurologic dysfunction, the value of obtaining this full hemodynamic assessment is in the maximization of cerebral perfusion pressure. The most common neurologic or neurosurgical disorders where this catheter is utilized is in the treatment of cerebral vasospasm, conditions associated with increased ICP, or significant coexisting heart failure.

Furthermore, patients may require invasive monitoring of cardiac function as a means to effectively manage other complications of neurologic or neurosurgical disease such as "cardiac stun" following SAH or diabetes insipidus. Coexisting ischemic myocardium or cardiomyopathy makes this type of monitoring especially important.

PA Catheter Placement

Placement of a PA catheter should always be performed with ECG monitoring (preferably with an audible component) and where cardiac resuscitation drugs and a defibrillator are readily available. The catheter is placed in two steps. First, a vascular sheath is placed in the central venous vasculature. Then, under meticulously sterile conditions, the PA catheter is advanced through the sheath. As the catheter is advanced, pressure waveforms are used to infer the position of the tip (Fig. 4). The first waveform to be seen is that of the CVP or right atrial pressure (RAP).

The normal RAP waveform peaks and descents can be linked to physiologic events of the cardiac cycle. The first peak, termed the A wave, corresponds to atrial systole. A second smaller peak, termed the C wave, occurs with the closure of the tricuspid valve. During ventricular systole, conformational changes in the heart result in a decreased pressure in the right atrium creating the X descent. The V wave occurs as blood rushes back into the atrium during the end of the cardiac cycle. Finally, as the tricuspid valve opens prior to atrial systole, the atrial pressure trails off creating the Y descent (5).

As soon as the RAP waveform is identified, the balloon is inflated, which helps to carry the catheter along in the direction of blood flow (1,5). As the catheter passes into the right ventricle, large systolic pressure excursions appear and during ventricular diastole the pressure returns to close to zero. As the catheter passes into the pulmonary artery, the diastolic pressures become elevated and the systolic waveform develops an incisura that corresponds with the closing of the pulmonary valve. This waveform may be better seen if the catheter balloon is deflated. Once the pulmonary artery waveform is recognized, the balloon may be reinflated and advanced producing occlusion of a branch of the PA. This causes the ''wedge'' waveform to appear. This waveform is similar to the RAP waveform, although often the C wave is not visible. The wedge pressure is always read at end

expiration when the alveolar pressure is equal to atmospheric pressure (the zero reference pressure). In the patient on positive pressure ventilation the wedge waveform tracing is at its lowest point at end expiration. In a patient who is not mechanically ventilated, the wedge waveform is at its maximal at end expiration (1,5).

Changes in the morphology of the waveform components are seen in various rhythm disturbances as well as in valvular dysfunction. The effects of these pathologic states are well described in critical care texts (1,5).

PA Catheter Complications

The overall incidence of complications from PA catheter use has been estimated at 24%, with a 4.4% serious complication rate. The most common complications are rhythm disturbances. Atrial or ventricular dysrhythmias may occur. These are attributed to direct mechanical stimulation of the myocardium and usually resolve as the end of the catheter is moved out of the heart, either into the superior vena cava (SVC) or PA. Dysrhythmias may persist, however. The balloon of the catheter is inflated prior to entering the heart. This helps protect the endocardium from direct stimulation from the blunt tip of the catheter. Conduction defects, most commonly right bundle branch block, have been reported both during and after the procedure (5).

Pulmonary infarction is another complication and may occur from several etiologies. Thrombi may form around the catheter or in areas of denuded endothelium that were injured during placement. Also, even with the balloon deflated, the catheter tip may migrate and occlude small branches of the PA. Finally, if the balloon is allowed to stay inflated over long periods of time a large pulmonary infarction will result. Rupture of the pulmonary artery rarely occurs and has a high mortality. The incidence of rupture is 0.06–0.2% of all catheterizations (5). Other complications are balloon rupture and catheter-associated infection (5).

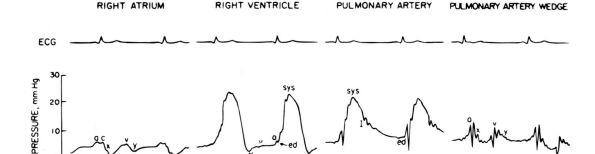

FIG. 4. Normal pressure waveforms of the right heart and pulmonary artery. sys, systolic; ed, end diastolic. (From ref. 37.)

Cardiovascular Physiology

The two important physiologic variables that may be directly measured with the PA catheter are the pulmonary artery occlusion pressure (PAOP) or the wedge pressure, and the cardiac output (CO). After placement of the catheter, the balloon at the tip may be inflated and "wedged" into position in a PA branch. This creates a stationary, continuous column of fluid between the left atrium and the pressure transducer of the PA catheter. Without flow in the column the pressures at each end equalize and the sensor reading represents the pressure in the left atrium (1). When the mitral valve is open, left atrial pressure equals left end-diastolic pressure. This value gives important information on the intravascular fluid volume of the patient.

Wedge Pressure Measurements

An implicit assumption in this measurement is that the column of blood between the catheter and left atrium is not obstructed. West has described three theoretical lung zones based on the pressure relationships between pulmonary arterial, pulmonary venous, and alveolar pressures (14). In zone 1, alveolar pressure exceeds both pulmonary arterial and venous pressures causing collapse of the vessels. In this region a continuous column of blood is impossible. In zone 2, the alveolar pressure is between the higher pulmonary arterial pressure and the lower pulmonary venous pressure. Under these conditions the blood column may be partially obstructed by the distended alveolus. In zone 3, the alveolar pressure is less than the arterial and venous pressures. The alveoli collapse, the vasculature remains patent, and the wedge pressure readings are accurate. Fortunately, the forces that create these zones also tend to direct the PA catheter to the desired zone 3 during placement. Other factors that affect the accuracy of the wedge pressure are changes in left ventricular compliance (such as seen in ischemic myocardium or in left heart failure) or valvular disease (1,5).

Thermodilution Measurements

Cardiac output, the second parameter directly measured, is most commonly determined by the thermodilution method. The PA catheter contains an electronic element (a thermistor) 4 cm proximal to its tip whose resistance varies with temperature. Cold saline is rapidly infused through the catheter's atrial port and passes through the heart and over the thermistor changing its resistance. These changes, the patient's body temperature, and the initial temperature of the injectate are used to calculate the cardiac output.

The information gained from the PA catheter is used to optimize cardiovascular hemodynamics and maximize CPP in the face of loss of autoregulation, increased ICP, vasospasm, or cerebrovascular stenosis. Since cerebral perfusion pressure is the difference between the MAP and the ICP,

increasing the MAP will lead to an increased CPP. The relationship between MAP, SVR, and CO is given by the following equation: $MAP = (SVR)(CO)/80 - CVP$. Therefore increasing the CO or SVR will increase the MAP. The cardiac output is the product of the heart rate and the stroke volume. Manipulation of the cardiac output may be achieved by altering either of these two factors. Extreme bradycardia or tachycardia decreases cardiac output and must be dealt with emergently. However, for patients with normal heart rates manipulation of the stroke volume is the most common strategy used to increase cardiac output.

Regulation of Cardiac Output

Starling first described the interrelation of factors that affect stroke volume: preload, afterload, and contractility (15). Preload corresponds to the length of the myocardial muscle cell immediately prior to contraction. It is affected by the intravascular fluid volume, the systemic driving pressure (MAP-RAP), systemic vascular resistance (SVR), and the atrial component of myocardial contraction. Increasing the preload increases the force of contraction of the myocardial cell and, in turn, the stroke volume until a critical muscle cell length is reached. Further stretching of the cell causes the force of contraction and stroke volume to decrease. The PA occlusion pressure approximates the left ventricular preload if certain conditions are met.

The true measure of left ventricular preload is the amount of stretch on the ventricular myocardium at the end of diastole. This is most closely approximated by the left ventricular end-diastolic volume (LVEDV). In practice this variable is extremely difficult to measure. Assuming normal left ventricular compliance, the left ventricular end-diastolic pressure (LVEDP) corresponds with the LVEDV relatively well. Furthermore, assuming that there is no mitral or aortic valve pathology, the LVEDP equals the left atrial pressure when the mitral valve is open. This relationship has been confirmed in patients in which a left atrial catheter and a PA catheter have been placed during cardiac surgery. Conditions such as mitral valve stenosis or aortic regurgitation create significant differences in the pressures of the left atrium and left ventricle and make the wedge pressure less meaningful (1,5).

Afterload corresponds to the force opposing muscle fiber shortening during contraction. This force is made up of various factors including the mass of blood in the aorta, blood viscosity, and SVR. The SVR is another factor besides CO that may be manipulated to augment the MAP. This is achieved pharmacologically.

Contractility is the amount of force that can be generated by the muscle cell during contraction at a given preload. Contractility is affected by endogenous catecholamine levels and also may be augmented by pharmacologic agents.

Many times patients who are critically ill are volume-depleted. In these patients the wedge is low, indicating that the left ventricular preload is low. This results in a suboptimal cardiac output. Initially, fluid expansion with crystalloids or colloids increases the preload and the cardiac output. In many cases all that is needed to maintain an adequate CPP is optimization of the cardiac output through fluid management. Continued fluid administration may result in the left ventricular myocardial cells being stretched beyond their critical length. When this occurs the cardiac output begins to decrease and the patient develops signs of fluid overload. This is the point at which volume expansion has been maximized. If the MAP is still inadequate, pressor support is added. Dopamine is usually the first pressor to be initiated. This drug acts by stimulating release of neuronal norepinephrine as well as by direct stimulation of autonomic receptors. The effects of dopamine vary qualitatively as well as quantitatively as the rate of infusion is increased. At rates of 0.5–2.0 μg/kg/min renal blood flow and urinary output is enhanced with little effect on heart rate or blood pressure. At these rates the enhanced urinary output may limit the effectiveness of other measures to increase the MAP. In the range of 2.0–5.0 μg/kg/min, cardiac contractility and cardiac output are increased with little effect on heart rate, blood pressure, or systemic vascular resistance. Doses of 5–10 μg/kg/min cause further increases in cardiac output as well as increases in blood pressure and tachycardia. Tachycardia may be dose limiting. At infusion rates of >10 μg/kg/min, a more pronounced effect on increasing mean arterial pressure is seen, resulting from both tachycardia and an increase in systemic vascular resistance (16).

If MAP requires further support despite maximal dopamine therapy, phenylephrine may be added. This drug increases the systemic vascular resistance. The pre- and postinfusion SVR may be calculated using data obtained with the PA catheter from the following equation:

$$SVR = MAP - CVP/CO \times 80.$$

Intracranial Pressure Monitoring

ICP monitoring techniques are divided between fluid-coupled systems with external transducers, such as intraventricular catheters (IVCs) and subarachnoid (SA) bolts, and fiberoptic systems that utilize a miniature pressure transducer within a catheter in the cranial vault (5).

Ventricular Catheter Method

The IVC, introduced in 1951, is a reliable and widely used technique. This device may be inserted in the ICU and is most commonly placed through the posterior aspect of the frontal lobe into the lateral ventricle of the nondominant hemisphere. The catheter is connected to a transducer and to an external drainage collection system via a three-way stopcock allowing for both ICP monitoring and CSF drainage. Infection is the most important complication of the IVC.

The risk of infection increases with time. Some studies have shown that between the 5th and 12th days of monitoring the infection risk rises from 8% to 40% (12). Although controversy exists over their usefulness, we use prophylactic antibiotics and sample the CSF every other day for laboratory evidence of infection. Other IVC complications are parenchymal brain injury or hemorrhage.

The IVC is generally considered the most accurate method of measuring ICP because it transduces pressure directly from the CSF in the lateral or third ventricles deep within the brain. All externally transduced ICP systems require an atmospheric pressure reference that should be zero-balanced to account for variations in patient head position. A commonly used anatomic reference point for adjusting the vertical position of the transducer is the external acoustic meatus (5). Several factors may create measurement inaccuracies. Air in the fluid coupling system will blunt the ICP recording. Clotted blood or other debris may obstruct the lumen of the catheter, or the ventricles may collapse around the catheter fenestrations.

Subarachnoid Bolt Method

The SA bolt technique for ICP monitoring was developed as an attempt to decrease the infection rate associated with ICP monitoring. Furthermore, in some cases small ventricular size makes IVC insertion unfeasible. Because the brain parenchyma is not punctured with this technique, there is a wider choice of insertion sites. The hollow, self-tapping bolt is inserted into a burr hole in the skull and the dura at the base of the bolt is perforated with a spinal needle to allow subarachnoid CSF to fill the bolt. Saline-filled pressure tubing is then connected to the bolt to establish communication to a transducer. Unlike the IVC, CSF drainage cannot be accomplished with this type of pressure-monitoring device. The infection rate is low for SA bolts (5).

The SA bolt usually provides a reliable ICP waveform and pressure reading but is susceptible to error if the dural perforations become plugged with blood or debris or if brain swelling obliterates communication with CSF. Flushing debris from the bolt with 0.2 ml of preservative-free (nonbacteriostatic) saline solution is one method to restore accurate ICP readings and does not cause dangerous ICP elevation in most circumstances. The SA bolt tends to underestimate the ICP, particularly when the ICP is high. The SA bolt is also less ideal than IVC monitoring in that it measures the local ICP at the surface of the hemisphere. It can be inaccurate if there is a pressure gradient between the left and right supratentorial compartments or the supratentorial and infratentorial compartments. This is an important phenomenon to consider, and if there is a discrepancy between the apparent ICP and the patient's clinical condition, emergency computed tomography (CT) scanning or treatment of elevated ICP may be warranted (5).

Miniaturized Pressure Transducer Method

Fiberoptic ICP monitors use miniature transducers coupled with fiberoptic cables to an external instrument. The transducer is incorporated into the end of a soft tube, which may be solid, or hollow for CSF drainage. Light is projected through an optic fiber to a miniature mirror in the catheter tip. The amount of light reflected to a collecting optic fiber depends on mechanical displacement of the mirror, which in turn is a function of ICP. Fiberoptic devices can be inserted in the lateral ventricle, brain parenchyma, subarachnoid space, or epidural space. If located on the brain surface, as in the SA bolt, infection rates are low (5).

The greatest advantage of fiberoptic catheters is that they lack fluid coupling for pressure transduction, which avoids the problems of waveform damping and artifacts from poor coupling. It also allows for a wide choice of insertion sites. Several disadvantages exist. The transducer cannot be recalibrated to zero once it has been inserted. The fiberoptic device has significant baseline drift after 5 days of use, which may necessitate replacement. Parenchymal fiberoptic pressure may consistently exceed IVC pressures by nearly 10 mm Hg. Finally, the fiberoptic system is not directly compatible with most ICU bedside monitoring systems and must be connected to a separate module for recording (5).

Clinical Utility of ICP Monitoring

In nontraumatic brain injury, the use of ICP monitoring has been studied most rigorously in subarachnoid hemorrhage. Early aggressive monitoring of intracranial hypertension and treatment of hydrocephalus has been shown to benefit patients with Hunt–Hess grade IV and V hemorrhages (5). Also, when patients enter the risk period for vasospasm, ICP monitoring allows titration of the CPP. Additionally, ICP reduction from external CSF drainage can reduce the amount of hypervolemic hypertensive therapy necessary to reverse ischemic deficits (5). The value of ICP monitoring in spontaneous intracerebral hemorrhage has not been rigorously evaluated, although in patients with hydrocephalus the placement of an IVC for CSF drainage is lifesaving. The use of ICP monitoring in large ischemic strokes has been evaluated in few studies. To date it has not been shown to be beneficial. As dural sinus thrombosis frequently results in increased ICP, it has been suggested that ICP monitoring in this disease process may have a beneficial effect on outcome (17).

This completes the discussion of the general aspects of cardio- and cerebrovascular monitoring and support. Specific disease states have unique monitoring and support issues. The following section addresses these issues.

SUBARACHNOID HEMORRHAGE

Of all the cerebrovascular diseases, the most specific information about perioperative and critical care management is known about aneurysmal subarachnoid hemorrhage (SAH). All potential SAH patients should have ECG and noninvasive BP monitoring initiated on arrival at the emergency room. Tachycardia is usually due to pain or anxiety and may be managed with relatively short-acting, reversible analgesics or sedatives. Bradycardia suggests increased ICP, and if it occurs the urgency of obtaining a CT scan is increased. The ECG may disclose the presence of dysrhythmias or signs of ischemia. If present, evaluation for cardiac ischemia should be undertaken. ECG changes are frequently present in SAH and may be ''neurogenic''; however, this is a diagnosis of exclusion. Blood pressure is usually elevated but should not be aggressively lowered. A MAP goal of <120 mm Hg can be achieved with small intravenous boluses of labetalol over a time period of 30–60 minutes. Once the patient is stable, if there is convincing history supporting an SAH, it is helpful to alert neurosurgery and neuroradiology of the possible diagnosis. Early and effective communication among physicians and surgeons greatly enhances the quality of care provided.

It takes hours to evaluate this type of patient. While the patient is in the CT scanner or angiography suite, focus tends to shift to completing the diagnostic maneuvers and the frequency of monitoring the patient's vital signs decreases. Accordingly, a member of the care team is assigned the duty of maintaining adequate, reversible sedation and BP control while closely following cardiorespiratory function.

Once the definitive diagnosis of aneurysmal SAH has been made, the patient is usually transferred to an ICU where more invasive monitoring procedures may be undertaken. Adequate anesthesia, analgesia, and sedation during these procedures must be given to prevent sympathetic responses and Valsalva maneuvers, which may cause arterial or intracranial hypertension or wide BP swings. We frequently use intravenous fentanyl 50–100 μg for sedation because it is short acting and readily reversible. Intravenous midazolam (1–2 mg) may be used in conjunction with or as an alternative to fentanyl. Adequate administration of lidocaine should be used at skin puncture sites. For central venous access, internal jugular cannulation is preferable because of the decreased risk of pneumothorax. In higher grade SAH (Hunt–Hess grade III or greater) an intraarterial line is often placed for continuous BP monitoring using the radial artery of the nondominant upper extremity or, if a hemiparesis is present, the paretic upper extremity. Subcutaneous infiltration of lidocaine around the artery prior to cannulation may help prevent spasm of the vessel if it is not entered on the initial attempt. Placement of an IVC is performed if the initial CT scan reveals severe hydrocephalus.

Two of the standard medications given to aneurysm patients have the potential to cause significant hypotension. Phenytoin is an effective anticonvulsant and may be loaded intravenously. The vehicle in which the drug is solubilized, propylene glycol, is vagotonic and may produce hypotension and bradycardia if given more quickly than 50 mg/min. The ECG and blood pressure should be monitored during administration. If noninvasive BP monitoring is used, frequent cycling (ie, every 1–2 minutes) should be used to evaluate for severe hypotension. The calcium channel blocker nimodipine also causes a decrease in blood pressure. The standard dose is 60 mg by mouth or nasogastric tube (NG) every 4 hours. If a patient's blood pressure is normal or low and concern of inducing hypotension exists, an initial test dose of 30 mg by mouth or via NG will demonstrate the patient's BP response to this agent. If problems with unacceptable hypotension (≥20 mm Hg drop in the MAP or increased neurologic symptoms with hypotension) occur, the drug may be given 30 mg every 2 hours or 15 mg every hour (12,18).

Vasospasm

Vasospasm of the large cerebral arteries occurs in 35% of patients with SAH. The mechanism of this phenomenon continues to perplex investigators, but it is thought to result from arterial irritation by breakdown products of whole blood in the subarachnoid space. The risk of vasospasm in any given patient is proportional to the amount of blood in the basal cisterns as seen on CT (12,18). The presence of a globular subarachnoid clot greater than 5 × 3 mm or a layer of blood ≥1 mm thick in the cerebral fissures carries a high risk for symptomatic vasospasm. Vasospasm usually occurs between the 3rd and 17th day after the initial bleed with a peak incidence of occurrence at 1 week.

Besides the amount of subarachnoid blood seen on CT, serial transcranial Doppler (TCD) examinations may help to predict which patients will develop vasospasm. TCD monitoring is also useful in following the temporal course of spasm and the response to treatment. A baseline study is obtained on the first or second postbleed day. On the third day, daily TCD examinations begin.

If the TCD velocities increase above 200 cm/sec or show a rapidly increasing trend, the asymptomatic patient is considered to be at extremely high risk for developing symptomatic vasospasm.

If the aneurysm is adequately clipped, the possibility of recurrent bleeding is reduced to almost zero. However, due to technical reasons the clip may not cover the entire neck of the aneurysm. If this occurs further bleeding may still occur, although the risk is significantly reduced. This is an important point to ascertain from the neurosurgeon as it also limits the aggressiveness with which circulatory manipulations may be used to treat vasospasm.

In a patient with low to moderate risk for vasospasm by CT criteria or normal TCD velocities, a goal is set to keep the patient's CVP between 8 and 12. If the CVP does not increase into the desired range, additional fluid boluses are given. Albumin administration or Florinef 0.1–0.2 mg po TID may also help increase the CVP. The patient is watched closely for signs of a decrease in level of consciousness or focal motor deficit, and the TCD velocities are followed. If the TCD velocities increase to ≥200 cm/sec treatment is

escalated. The patient's MAP is increased into the range of 100–120 mm Hg. This may require the use of pressors in addition to aggressive fluid administration. Dopamine is an excellent first-line pressor. Dobutamine is also effective. Echocardiographic evaluation of the ejection fraction, cardiac wall motion, and valvular function and placement of a pulmonary artery catheter in a patient with concomitant cardiovascular disease should be considered at this point. These help in determining the most advantageous way to support the blood pressure. If difficulty is encountered raising the pressure with the preceding measures, the addition of phenylephrine should be considered. A PA catheter is particularly helpful in titrating the dosage of this agent.

If focal neurologic signs or symptoms occur or if there is a decrease in the level of consciousness, the patient should be evaluated with head CT and angiography. The CT may be used to rule out hydrocephalus or hemorrhage or may suggest focal ischemia in a major arterial distribution. Angiography is used to quantitate the extent of vasospasm.

In patients with progressing neurologic signs despite maximal hypertensive therapy and evidence of significant cerebral edema on CT scan, the placement of an ICP monitoring device is considered. In these cases the IVC is the most useful type of monitor as it provides the ability to remove CSF and treat increased ICP as well as monitor the actual pressure. Once placed the monitor allows measurement of the CPP. This information helps to fine-tune hypertensive treatment and to guide CSF drainage.

ARTERIOVENOUS MALFORMATION

SAH arising from an arteriovenous malformation (AVM) poses fewer problems. Vasospasm is much less likely as the subarachnoid blood does not usually pool in the basal cisterns, and the risk of mortality from further hemorrhage is much less than that from aneurysmal SAH. Problems that may occur in the postoperative period consist of the development of hemorrhagic stroke and edema or obstructive hydrocephalus.

Continuous perioperative BP monitoring is indicated in all AVM patients. Hypertension is avoided both preoperatively and postoperatively. A well-known postoperative complication is the development of hemorrhagic stroke and malignant edema. Spetzler (19) posits that the high-volume AVM shunts blood from surrounding areas. Cerebral autoregulation causes a compensatory vasodilatation in these areas. When the AVM is treated, the shunt disappears and the full pressure of the MAP is brought to bear on unprotected capillaries, causing injury and associated edema formation and hemorrhage. This injury is readily seen on pathologic examination (19). Spetzler termed this proposed mechanism ''normal perfusion pressure breakthrough.'' More recently, this mechanism has been questioned (20). Some authors advocate perioperative antihypertensives to keep the MAP at 70–80 mm Hg (21). We prefer to use intermittent antihypertensive medications to keep the MAP at <90. Patients are monitored for 12–24 hours postoperatively unless complications mandate a longer period of monitoring. If hypertension is a consistent problem, an oral antihypertensive regimen is started in the ICU. Rarely, hemorrhagic stroke and edema have occurred up to 1 week after AVM resection.

Obstructive hydrocephalus is a potential complication in any case of subarachnoid hemorrhage regardless of etiology. Hydrocephalus occurs at any time and is heralded by the development of abulia or a decreased level of consciousness. The patient may complain of headache or nausea and may experience emesis. A CT scan of the head is obtained to evaluate ventricular size. If significant ventricular enlargement is present in a symptomatic patient an IVC is placed primarily for CSF drainage. In this situation ICP monitoring is used to guide management and weaning of the CSF diversion.

CAROTID ENDARTERECTOMY

Many carotid endarterectomy (CEA) procedures are followed by a benign postoperative course. However, postoperative complications may include carotid thrombosis, expanding neck hematoma, cerebrovascular emboli, cardiac ischemia, BP regulation anomalies, or bradycardia. Cardiovascular and cerebrovascular monitoring may be useful in detecting and treating these events.

McCory and Goldstein (22) found that the presence of two or more of the following risk factors was associated with a twofold increase in postoperative stroke, MI, or death: age >75 years, preoperative neurologic symptoms ipsilateral to the side of operation, severe hypertension, CEA performed prior to coronary artery bypass grafting, history of angina, evidence of internal carotid thrombus, and internal carotid artery stenosis close to the siphon. Sieber et al. (23) found that postoperative adverse events were best predicted by the preoperative presence of risk factors, which included heart or lung disease, neurologic symptoms, and angiographic evidence of complicated cerebrovascular disease. In CEA done under regional cervical block, intraoperative neurologic changes have strong predictability for postoperative adverse events (24).

Many postoperative complications occur in the immediate post-operative period, in the recovery room, or shortly after reaching the ICU. In the series of Sieber et al. of the 30 postoperative strokes reported, 23 occurred less than 10 hours after the procedure (14 of these occurred intraoperatively). Patients in whom a new deficit was noted early (ie, at emergence from anesthesia or on initial ICU evaluation) and who were emergently taken back to the operating room for exploration had significant improvement of their symptoms. Delay of even 1–2 hours resulted in permanent deficits (23). Thus, close attention to serial neurologic examinations by a seasoned examiner is an extremely important aspect of postoperative monitoring. The use of Doppler evaluation of extra- and intracranial blood flow as well as detection of emboli is a promising method of intra- and postoperative monitoring, although unproven by clinical trials at this time (23,25).

The majority of patients with cerebrovascular disease have coexistent cardiovascular disease. Myocardial infarction after CEA is the procedure's most common cause of mortality and may occur early in the postoperative period or may be delayed (25). The preoperative presence of unstable angina, congestive heart failure, or dysrhythmias increases the chances of postoperative adverse events and is a relative contraindication to the procedure. Although ECG changes unrelated to cardiac ischemia occur after bilateral and even unilateral CEA, most commonly changes indicate true cardiac ischemia (12). Accordingly, continuous postoperative ECG monitoring is indicated. ECG monitoring should continue for at least 12–24 hours and probably longer since postoperative MI may occur in a delayed manner (25). Postoperative hypertension has been reported to occur in 20–50% of cases. The significance of this phenomenon has been disputed. Predictive preoperative risk factors have not been described. Benzel and Hoppens (26) reported that 35% of the patients in their series developed postoperative hypertension requiring intravenous treatment. These investigators found that the occurrence of hypertension did not correlate significantly with other postoperative complications. Alternatively, Bernstein et al. (27) reported a case of fatal intracerebral hemorrhage occurring after endarterectomy. Despite the lack of postoperative hypertension, at autopsy the involved hemisphere had changes similar to those seen in malignant hypertension. These authors argued that this phenomenon was similar to the "normal perfusion pressure breakthrough" seen after embolization or resection of a large AVM reported by Spetzler and Wilson (19). Pre- and postoperative blood flow measurement or TCD examination may help to identify specific cases in which a high blood flow state is occurring. In these cases some investigators have recommended the MAP be maintained in the range of 95–105 for 2–3 days (25).

Hypotension is a well-known postoperative phenomenon that may occur in up to 40% of patients operated on under general anesthesia (12). Interestingly, it is uncommon in patients operated on under regional anesthesia. Hypotension is thought to occur as the carotid bodies experience increased BP resulting from correction of stenosis (25). Hypotension may produce inadequate cerebral perfusion pressure. Barnett et al. advocate maintaining the MAP in the 95–110 range (25). This may initially be achieved with volume expansion; however, these patients may require pressor support. Bradycardia may also occur and persist for up to 36 hours, necessitating treatment with atropine or chronotropic doses of dopamine (12).

For most patients continuous monitoring of blood pressure by noninvasive means is adequate. Patients at increased risk for adverse postoperative events or those requiring vasoactive drips should be monitored via an indwelling arterial line.

In patients with no postoperative complications, monitoring should continue for 12–24 hours after the procedure. Patients requiring intervention should be monitored for the duration of the intervention, which is usually less than 48 hours.

HYPERTENSIVE ENCEPHALOPATHY

The strict definition of hypertensive encephalopathy is the presence of cerebral symptoms (headache, delirium, generalized seizures, or cortical blindness) in a patient with severe hypertension (eg, diastolic blood pressure >130). Cerebral symptoms resolve with resolution of the hypertension, and no other metabolic or structural cause of symptoms should be present (28). Lateralizing signs may occur in this syndrome but are more commonly a result of hemorrhage or infarction and may not fully resolve. Any patient with an acute increase of blood pressure above 200/120 mm Hg or a MAP of >145 mm Hg may develop life-threatening complications within a short period of time (18). Persistent diastolic pressures exceeding 130 mm Hg are often associated with acute vascular damage. In practice, then, the clinical picture is frequently clouded by superimposed stroke. Uremia is often present as well (28).

Monitoring of blood pressure via an indwelling arterial line is recommended in this illness. Involvement of other organ systems (eg, pulmonary edema, renal failure, myocardial ischemia, aortic dissection, GI hemorrhage) may require placement of a central line or pulmonary artery catheter for better control of fluid and BP manipulations. As some patients with hypertensive encephalopathy have increased intracranial pressure, LP is not recommended unless intercurrent CNS infection is under consideration. As the hypertension is treated ICP decreases when autoregulation begins to function again. The mean arterial pressure should be followed and acutely brought down by only 10% in the first hour and an additional 10–15% over the next few hours (5). The initial clinical goal is to achieve a MAP that minimizes or stops progression of critical end-organ injury such as cardiac ischemia or acute renal failure. Longer range goals of therapy include the return of MAP to the upper limits of cerebral autoregulation over 12–36 hours and institution of an oral antihypertensive regimen. Close attention to monitoring for progressive neurologic, cardiac, or renal deterioration is important as the transition from acute control to long-term control of BP occurs. The BP range in which cerebral autoregulation functions normally for most individuals is a MAP between 50 and 150 mm Hg, systolic blood pressure below 170 mm Hg, and diastolic pressure below 110 mm Hg (18). In those with chronic hypertension this range is shifted to higher pressures.

In most cases nitroprusside is the best antihypertensive agent for initial treatment because of its ease of administration and fine control over titration. Although the theoretical possibility of this agent increasing ICP exists, it remains the agent of choice for patients with hypertensive emergency.

As the blood pressure decreases the ICP will decrease. Use of this agent mandates invasive BP monitoring and strongly argues for central venous monitoring. Other useful drugs are intravenous labetalol and esmolol.

Patients with aortic dissection present a special management problem. The most important aspect of treatment is to decrease the blood pressure at a rate that would normally be considered too rapid for other indications. For dissection pressure should be reduced to a systolic BP of 100–120 over 15–20 minutes. In these patients addition of a β blocker to nitroprusside helps to decrease the shear forces created by the blood ejected from the heart on the intima of the aorta (5).

Once the blood pressure is under control and the patient is stable, evaluation for secondary causes of hypertension should be undertaken.

STROKE

Cardiovascular monitoring in patients who have had a stroke is useful for two reasons. First, cerebrovascular disease commonly coexists with coronary artery disease. Stroke patients are more likely to die from cardiac dysfunction than from cerebral ischemia. Second, monitoring helps the physician to support cerebral perfusion pressure and to prevent the development of acute hypertensive cardiac or renal injury. ICP monitoring in stroke is of unconfirmed utility; however, it may be helpful in some situations.

An initial 12-lead ECG followed by continuous ECG monitoring is indicated, at least initially, in all stroke patients. Significant dysrhythmias occur in 5–10% of strokes (29), and myocardial infarction occurs in 2–3% of strokes (30). Although neurogenic ECG changes may be seen in stroke, myocardial ischemia must be ruled out in these situations.

Noninvasive BP monitoring is adequate in most cases. Typically, patients presenting with stroke have elevated blood pressures even if there is no history of hypertension (31). This is often attributed to a systemic response to cerebral ischemia. In areas of ischemia, vascular beds are maximally dilated without autoregulatory reserve. Blood flow in these areas is directly proportional to systemic blood pressure. Reduction of the blood pressure acutely entails the risk of decreasing the CPP and creating further ischemia.

Supratentorial Stroke

Appropriate treatment of blood pressure in each individual patient should be based on the blood pressure by history. Hypertension is not acutely detrimental to the stroke patient unless signs of acute end-organ injury (usually cardiac or renal) are present. Moreover, initial hypertension usually resolves over hours without treatment. Even in patients with parenchymal hemorrhage or hematoma, hypertension is well tolerated and has not been shown to significantly influence further hemorrhage. Hypotension on the other hand is detrimental. Hayashi et al. (32) examined the use of nifedipine, chlorpromazine, or reserpine in patients with increased intracranial pressure secondary to intracerebral hemorrhage. These workers found that decreasing the MAP using these drugs caused a similar or greater increase in the ICP and decrease in the CPP. In patients with ICP >40 mm Hg, a 20% decrease in MAP was associated with a 40% increase in ICP and a 40% decrease in the CPP.

Brott (33) suggests the following approach to treatment of hypertension in the patient with acute stroke. For DBP >140 on two readings 5 minutes apart begin sodium nitroprusside. For SBP >230 and/or DBP 121–140 on two readings 20 minutes apart treat with labetalol 20 mg iv q 10–20 minutes (labetalol is best avoided in patients with asthma, CHF, or cardiac conduction abnormalities due to its β-blocking actions). If SBP is 180–230 and/or DBP is 105–120 treatment should be deferred. If repeat BP in 1 hour remains elevated and the neurologic exam is unchanged, oral agents may be used. In acute stroke patients with SBP <180 and/or DBP <105 treatment is not indicated. Target BP ranges may be obtained over 6-12 hours. In patients with a history of hypertension the target is 160–170/90–100 or a MAP of 115–125; in patients without a history of hypertension the target is 140–150/85–95 or a MAP of 105–115.

The use of intracranial pressure monitoring in supratentorial stroke is of unconfirmed clinical utility. The theoretical advantage of this type of monitoring is the ability to directly measure and optimize the CPP.

Infratentorial Stroke

Infratentorial stroke monitoring is similar to that of supratentorial stroke. The most salient difference arises from the small size of the posterior fossa, approximately 250 cm^3. This volume leaves little margin for expansion of lesions before life-threatening complications of obstructive hydrocephalus or brainstem compression ensue.

Cardiovascular monitoring has greater importance in strokes in this location. The occurrence of hypertension is more uniformly associated with pontomedullary infarction. In this type of stroke, there is a higher likelihood of cardiorespiratory complications. Further, trends in vital signs may help in detecting increasing intracranial pressure or shifts in the contents of the posterior fossa. In these situations, the classic Cushing response of bradycardia, hypertension, and irregular respirations may be observed. More commonly, increased heart rate and blood pressure are seen. The additional use of serial neurologic exams as well as CT scanning enables the clinician to detect mass effect from progressive infarct edema, hematoma expansion, or hydrocephalus. Prompt placement of an IVC and/or surgical decompression of the posterior fossa is life saving. In this situation the utility of placement of an IVC is in the ability to drain CSF rather than measuring ICP.

SAGITTAL SINUS THROMBOSIS

The importance of cardiovascular monitoring in sagittal sinus thrombosis is similar to its importance in infratentorial stroke. Monitoring may give an indication of increasing ICP. There are no clearly defined recommendations for BP management in this disease. As intracranial pressure tends to be increased, the clinician must be cognizant of the need for an adequate CPP. Ideally, treatment would lead to acute relief of venous obstruction and a decrease in ICP. In the patient without coagulopathy, placement of an intracranial pressure-monitoring device enables the clinician to directly measure ICP and CPP. With this information the CPP may be maximized. The use of ICP monitoring is of unconfirmed benefit, although a report of its use in cases with favorable outcome exists (17).

REFERENCES

1. Civetta JM, Taylor RW, Kirby RR, eds. *Critical care*. 2nd ed. Philadelphia: JB Lippincott, 1992.
2. Shea MJ, Deanfield JE, Wilson R, et al. Transient ischemia in angina pectoris: frequent silent events with everyday activities. *Am J Cardiol* 1985;56:34E-38E.
3. Berger JJ, Donchin M, Morgan LS, et al. Perioperative changes in blood pressure and heart rate. *Anesth Analg* 1984;63:647-652.
4. Knight AA, Hollenberg M, London MJ, et al. Perioperative myocardial ischemia: importance of the preoperative ischemic pattern. *Anesthesiology* 1988;68:681-688.
5. Parrillo JE, Bone RC, eds. *Critical care medicine: principles of diagnosis and management*. St. Louis: Mosby, 1995.
6. Breslow MJ, Miller CF, Parker SD, et al. Changes in T-wave morphology following anesthesia and surgery: a common recovery-room phenomenon. *Anesthesiology* 1986;64:398-402.
7. Kubota I, Ikeda K, Ohyama T, et al. Body surface distributions of ST segment changes after exercise in effort angina pectoris without myocardial infarction. *Am Heart J* 1985;110:949-955.
8. Byer E, Ashman R, Toth LA. Electrocardiogram with large upright T wave and long QT intervals. *Am Heart J* 1947;33:796-801.
9. Burch GE, Myers R, Abildskov JA. A new electrocardiographic pattern observed in cerebrovascular accidents. *Circulation* 1954;9:719-726.
10. Fulton JF. *Functional localization in the frontal lobes*. London: Oxford University Press, 1949.
11. Pollick C, Cujec B, Parker S, Tator C. Left ventricular wall motion abnormalities in subarachnoid hemorrhage: an echocardiographic study. *J Am Coll Cardiol* 1988;12:600-605.
12. Ropper AH, ed. *Neurological and neurosurgical intensive care*. 3rd ed. New York: Raven Press, 1993.
13. Blitt CD, ed. *Monitoring in anesthesia and critical care medicine*. 2nd ed. New York: Churchill Livingstone, 1985.
14. West JB, Dollery CT, Naimark A. Distribution of blood flow in isolated lung: Relation to vascular and alveolar pressures. *J Appl Physiol* 1964;19:713.
15. Starling EH. The Linacre lecture on the law of the heart. Presented at Cambridge, 1915. London, Longmans, Green, 1918.
16. Chernow B, ed. *The pharmacologic approach to the critically ill patient*. Baltimore: Williams and Wilkins, 1994.
17. Hanley DF, Feldman E, Borel CO, Rosenbaum AE, Golberg AL. Treatment of sagittal sinus thrombosis associated with cerebral hemorrhage and intracranial hypertension. *Stroke* 1988;19:903-909.
18. Hacke W, Hanley DF, Einhäupl KM, et al, eds. *Neurocritical care*. New York: Springer-Verlag, 1994.
19. Spetzler RF, Wilson CB, Weinstein P, Mehdorn M, Townsend J, Telles D. Normal perfusion pressure breakthrough theory. *Clin Neurosurg* 1978;25:651-672.
20. Young WL, Kader A, Prohovnik I, et al. Pressure autoregulation is intact after arteriovenous malformation resection. *Neurosurgery* 1993;32:491-497.

21. Orlowski JP, Shiesley D, Vidt DG, et al. Labetalol to control blood pressure after cerebrovascular surgery. *Crit Care Med* 1988;16:765-768.

22. McCrory DC, Goldstein LB, Samsa GP. Predicting complications of carotid endarterectomy. *Stroke* 1993;24:1285-1291.

23. Sieber FE, Toung TJ, Diringer MN, Wang H, Long DM. Preoperative risks predict neurological outcome of carotid endarterectomy related stroke. *Neurosurgery* 1992;30:847-854.

24. Davies MJ, Mooney PH, Scott DA, Silbert BS, Cook RJ. Neurologic changes during carotid endarterectomy under cervical block predict a high risk of postoperative stroke. *Anesthesiology* 1993;78:829-833.

25. Barnett HJM, Stein BM, Mohr JP, Yatsu FM, eds. *Stroke pathophysiology, diagnosis, and management.* 2nd ed. New York: Churchill Livingstone, 1992.

26. Benzel EC, Hoppens KD. Factors associated with postoperative hypertension complicating carotid endarterectomy. *Acta Neurochir* 1991;112:8-12.

27. Bernstein M, Ross Fleming JF, Deck JHN. Cerebral hyperperfusion after carotid endarterectomy: a cause of cerebral hemorrhage. *Neurosurgery* 1984;15:50-56.

28. Healton EB, Brust JC, Feinfeld DA, Thomson GE. Hypertensive encephalopathy and the neurologic manifestations of malignant hypertension. *Neurology* 1982;32:127-132.

29. Rem JA, Hachinski VC. Value of cardiac monitoring and echocardiography in TIA and stroke patients. *Stroke* 1985;16:950-956.

30. Norris JW, Hachinski VC. Serum cardiac enzymes in stroke. *Stroke* 1979;10:548-553.

31. Britton M, Carlsson A, DeFaire U. Blood pressure course with acute stroke and matched controls. *Stroke* 1986;17:861-864.

32. Hayashi M, Kobayashi H, Kawano H, Handa Y, Hirose S. Treatment of systemic hypertension and intracranial hypertension in cases of brain hemorrhage. *Stroke* 1988;19:314-321.

33. Brott T, Reed RL. Intensive care for acute stroke in the community hospital setting: the first 24 hours. *Curr Conc Cerebrovasc Dis Stroke* 1989;24:1-5.

34. Gravenstein N, Good ML. Noninvasive assessment of cardiopulmonary function. In: Civetta JM, Taylor RW, Kirby RR, eds. *Critical Care.* 2nd ed. Philadelphia: JB Lippincott, 1992;298.

35. Bedford RF. Invasive blood pressure monitoring. In: Blitt CD, ed. *Monitoring in anesthesia and critical care.* New York: Churchill Livingstone, 1990;102.

36. Perel A, Segal E, Pizov R. Assessment of cardiovascular function by pressure waveform analysis. In: Vincent JL, ed. *Update in intensive care and emergency medicine.* New York: Springer-Verlag, 1989;542.

37. Grossman W, Barry WH. Cardiac catheterization. In: Braunwald E, ed. *Heart disease: a textbook of cardiovascular medicine.* Philadelphia: WB Saunders, 1988;250.

SECTION III
Ischemic Stroke

Stroke is one of the most common neurologic diseases that neurologists and neurosurgeons are challenged to treat. Fully 80% of strokes are due to brain ischemia while the remaining one-fifth are due to brain and subarachnoid hemorrhage. This portion of the book will deal with brain ischemia in its various garbs, always with the treating physician and surgeon in mind. The organization of the chapters in this section is unique among cerebrovascular textbooks and monographs; the focus remains consistently on treatment, disturbed physiology, and syndrome recognition.

The opening section of chapters (23–26) focuses on the basic physiology and pathophysiology of brain ischemia. Included is recent up-to-date information about biochemical changes at neuronal levels, and various natural (hypoperfusion, embolism, and reperfusion) and iatrogenic (anesthetic and surgical) stresses on normal and ischemic brain neuronal and white matter metabolism.

The next section (chapters 27–29) concentrates on the diagnosis and recognition of various clinical syndromes of brain ischemia. Symptoms and signs found in patients with ischemia, involving the various supratentorial branches of the internal carotid and basilar arteries, are presented, as well as a discussion of the findings in patients with brainstem and cerebellar ischemia and infarction. The special problems and situations encountered in patients with migraine and cardiac-origin brain embolism are also covered.

Various extracranial lesions and diseases have often been the focus of interventions by neurosurgeons, vascular surgeons, neurologists, and neuroradiologists. The section on extracranial occlusive vascular disease (chapters 30–37) considers the various disorders—atherostenosis, dissection, and trauma—that involve the carotid and vertebral arteries in the neck. Surgical treatment is emphasized, but alternative treatments such as angioplasty are also discussed. Data from recent randomized treatment trials are also included in many of the chapters.

Intracranial occlusive disease is a much less common cause of brain ischemia, and the pathology of the causative vascular lesions is more heterogeneous. A variety of different etiologies, including atherostenosis, inflammatory diseases, and venous occlusions, are discussed. Different surgical treatments, including intracranial angioplasty, embolectomy, bypass, and surgical decompressions of edematous space-taking brain, are reviewed. Medical therapy, especially anticoagulants, are also discussed in detail. Stroke prevention and rehabilitation are also included in this section (chapters 38–48) on intracranial disorders and their management.

Although the approaches in the various sections are comprehensive, the focus always remains targeted clearly to treatment. Information necessary for the surgeon and physician to eclectically choose the most appropriate treatment for their patients is always emphasized.

Louis R. Caplan, M.D.

Cerebrovascular Disease, edited by H. Hunt Batjer.
Lippincott-Raven Publishers, Philadelphia © 1997.

CHAPTER 23

Cerebral Ischemia: Insights from Animal Models of Focal Ischemia

R. Tyler Frizzell and H. Hunt Batjer

Stroke remains the leading cause of morbidity and ranks third as a cause of death in the United States. Cerebral ischemia is a potentially treatable condition, and data to support this statement are presented. This chapter reviews experimental studies that illustrate the pathophysiology associated with focal cerebral ischemia, a situation commonly encountered by neurologists and neurosurgeons. In this setting there is a dense central core of ischemia and a surrounding penumbral zone that contains cells at "risk" for stroke. Much evidence exists that penumbral tissue can be salvaged by therapy, lending insight into the pathophysiology of focal cerebral ischemia. We attempt to provide the reader with a basic understanding of the importance of cerebral blood flow (CBF), cerebral hemodynamics, brain temperature, and chemical modulators during focal cerebral ischemia and reperfusion (1). The final section describes the utilization of transgenic animals to assist in the "molecular dissection" of stroke.

EXPERIMENTAL STUDIES OF CEREBRAL ISCHEMIA

The depth and duration of ischemia affect the magnitude of stroke (Fig. 1). The "threshold concept" of CBF following acute ischemic stroke is the physiologic basis for revascularization attempts using surgical bypass or thrombolysis. It is apparent that revascularization in selected cases produces profound reversal of neurologic deficits. Early studies documenting the importance of the magnitude and duration of ischemia were performed by Sundt and colleagues (2). Using a squirrel monkey model of focal cerebral ischemia, these investigators established that infarction did not occur

R. T. Frizzell: Department of Neurological Surgery, University of Boise, Boise, Idaho 83702.

H. H. Batjer: Division of Neurosurgery, Northwestern University Medical School, Chicago, Illinois 60611.

immediately following the onset of cerebral ischemia but developed over a period of hours. Further studies established that potentially reversible effects (such as electroencephalogram changes) occurred at a CBF of approximately 18 ml/100 g/min in anesthetized patients undergoing carotid endarterectomy. Irreversible changes, characterized by an increase in extracellular K^+ concentration resulting from ionic pump failure, occurred when regional CBF fell below 10 ml/100 g/min. These studies involved the use of anesthesia, however, which modified the ischemic threshhold.

In 1981 Jones and colleagues, working in the Stroke Laboratory at Massachusetts General Hospital and Harvard Medical School, reported the tolerance of awake primates (with electrodes placed in the brain to assess CBF) to different periods of middle cerebral artery (MCA) occlusion (3). This method eliminated the effects of anesthetic agents on CBF that modified the results of earlier studies. They noted that the reduction of CBF below 23 ml/100 g/min resulted in reversible paralysis. Cerebral infarction occurred when CBF fell below 17–18 ml/100 g/min following permanent MCA occlusion and below 10–12 ml/100 g/min following 2–3 hours of MCA occlusion (Fig. 1). It is unlikely that similar experiments will be repeated given their expense and modern animal utilization guidelines.

Blood viscosity affects the magnitude of stroke (Fig. 2). Since it was recognized that the principles of fluid mechanics were applicable to the human circulatory condition, there has been interest in utilizing these laws to optimize cerebral blood flow. Poisseuille's law states that flow (F) through a vessel is proportional to the pressure (P) and the fourth power of the vessel radius (r^4) and inversely proportional to the vessel length (l) and the viscosity (vis) of the fluid:

$$F = k(\text{constant}) \times P \times r^4/l \times \text{vis}$$

It is obvious that blood flow increases as viscosity decreases but the experimental studies to demonstrate this are complex

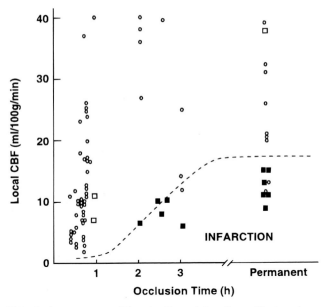

FIG. 1. Importance of the depth and duration of ischemia on the magnitude of stroke. The dashed line denotes an approximate infarction threshold and increases with time. Open boxes represent electrodes in normal tissue. Closed boxes represent electrodes located in infarcted tissue.

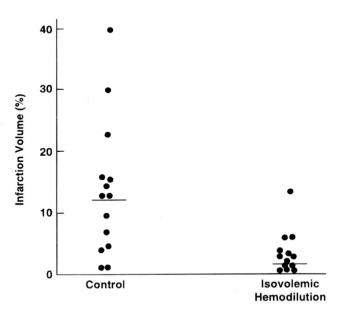

FIG. 2. Importance of a reduction of blood viscosity on stroke. Infarction averaged 12% in control animals and 2% in hemodiluted animals (low molecular weight dextran combined with blood withdrawal). Closed circles represent infarction volumes in control and isovolemic hemodiluted animals ($p < 0.05$).

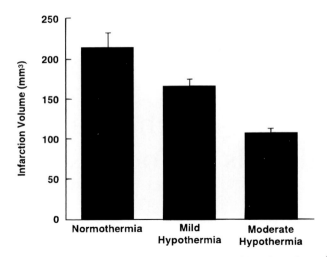

FIG. 3. Importance of mild hypothermia (33°C) and moderate hypothermia (28°C) on stroke following MCA occlusion in rats. Infarction volume following MCA occlusion averaged 214 ± 18 mm^3 in normothermic animals and was reduced to 166 ± 7 mm^3 in mildly hypothermic and 108 ± 6 mm^3 in moderately hypothermic animals ($p < 0.05$).

because concomitant hypervolemia makes it difficult to interpret the role of viscosity alone.

Korosue and colleagues, working in the laboratory of Dr. Roberto Heros, examined the effects of an isolated reduction in blood viscosity (using colloid solution in conjunction with repeated blood withdrawal) on the tolerance of dogs to 6 hours of internal carotid and MCA occlusion (4). Hemodilution was achieved 30 minutes after arterial occlusion, and blood viscosity was reduced to 16 seconds in the colloid-treated group and remained at 25 seconds in the control group. The hematocrit was 33% in the colloid-treated group and 41% in the control group. Central venous pressure remained constant in both groups. The infarction volume of the colloid-hemodiluted group (only 2% of the hemisphere) was significantly less than the infarction observed in the control group (12% of the hemisphere) (Fig. 2). Interestingly, reduction of the viscosity with crystalloid did not reduce cerebral infarction in this model. In fact, crystalloid infusion may have exacerbated cerebral edema by lowering the oncotic pressure.

Brain temperature affects the magnitude of stroke (Fig. 3). Although hypothermia has been regarded as a brain protectant for decades, its clinical utility has been limited by technical problems and impaired coagulation. Rosomoff reported almost 40 years ago that deep hypothermia (23°C) reduced ischemic damage after MCA occlusion in dogs (5). The mechanism by which hypothermia acts as a brain protectant likely involves more than just the reduction of the metabolic rate, and it is likely that decrements in excitatory amino acid release, brain edema, and the inactivation of the cascade involved in Ca^{2-} metabolism are important. In 1987 Busto and colleagues reported that a small reduction in brain temperature (2–3°C) is also neuroprotective (6), and subsequent studies have demonstrated that mild hypothermia decreases stroke in a focal model of ischemia.

Goto and colleagues studied the effects of both mild and moderate hypothermia on cerebral infarction in a reversible model of MCA occlusion in the rat (7). Temporalis muscle and rectal temperature were monitored in control animals (36°C), mild hypothermia animals (33°C in the temporalis muscle), and moderate hypothermia animals (28°C). All three groups of animals were subjected to 3 hours of MCA occlusion, and the total infarction volume was calculated and is shown in Fig. 3. Average infarct volume was 214 mm³ in the normothermia animals, 166 mm³ in the mild hypothermia animals, and 108 mm³ in the moderate hypothermia animals. Mild hypothermia appears to be efficacious, safe, and simple to employ.

• The glucose level affects the magnitude of stroke (Fig. 4). Myers and Yamaguchi fed a group of monkeys prior to the induction of cardiac arrest and serendipitously discovered that neurologic outcome following cardiac arrest was worse in the hyperglycemic animals (8). Subsequent studies in focal ischemia models showed that hyperglycemia increased blood viscosity and augmented lactate production through anaerobic glycolysis:

$$2\ \text{NAD}^+ \searrow 2\ \text{NADH}\quad 2\ \text{NADH} \searrow 2\ \text{NAD}^+$$
$$\text{GLUCOSE} \rightarrow 2\ \text{PYRUVATE} \rightarrow 2\ \text{LACTATE}$$
$$2\ \text{ADP} \nearrow 2\ \text{ATP}$$

Ischemia blocks the oxidation of pyruvate (along with the production of 36 ATP) via the citric acid cycle. Venables and associates later reported that hyperglycemia impaired water/ionic homeostasis during ischemia and exacerbated cerebral edema (9).

Nakai and colleagues performed an elegant study using triple-tracer autoradiography to define the role of hyperglycemia on CBF and pH in rats subjected to MCA occlusion (10). CBF was reduced more significantly in several brain regions in the ischemic hemisphere of the hyperglycemic rats compared to the normoglycemic rats. In addition, local tissue pH was markedly lower in the hyperglycemic animals during ischemia (Fig. 4). In the hyperglycemic animals, the threshold for a profound pH fall was only 63 ml/100 g/min compared to a threshold of 49 ml/100 g/min in the normoglycemic animals.

• Powerful mediators of inflammation affect the magnitude of stroke (Fig. 5). Reperfusion of cerebral tissue exacerbates tissue damage by the production of injurious cytokines and by the aggregation of leukocytes in the vasculature. Recent developments in the ability to modify leukocyte adhesion have increased our understanding of the role of leukocytes in stroke. Leukocytes are believed to play a role in the "no-

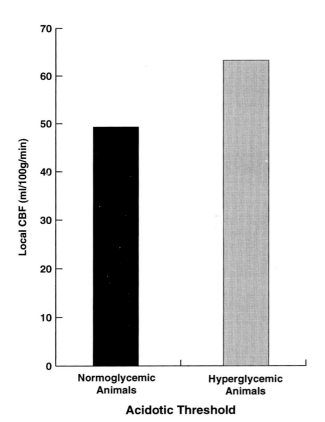

FIG. 4. Importance of hyperglycemia on lowering the threshold for tissue acidosis. The CBF must fall below 49 ml/100 g/min for a significant pH drop to occur in normoglycemic animals but only below 63 ml/100 g/min in hyperglycemic animals.

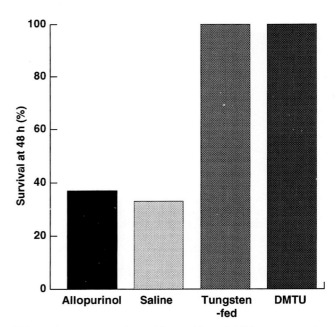

FIG. 5. Importance of xanthine oxidase inhibitors on stroke. Six-week tungsten-fed or DMTU-treated (a xanthine oxidase inhibitor given during reperfusion) gerbils demonstrated improved survival following carotid occlusion. Three of eight allopurinol-treated and three of nine saline-treated animals survived following carotid occlusion. In contrast, all tungsten-fed or DMTU-treated animals survived.

reflow'' phenomenon following cerebral ischemia by adhering to the endothelium and extravascular matrix via highly specific receptor–ligand interactions, leading to the release of free radicals and inflammatory cytokines. Of importance is that antibodies against these cellular adhesion molecules are available and intense studies are in progress in this area. For example, ICAM-1 (enlimomab) is a receptor expressed by cerebral endothelial cells, and .much interest has recently been devoted to the antagonism of leukocyte adherence to endothelial cells using ICAM-1 antibodies (11).

Antioxidants have been utilized in the treatment of human diseases ranging from cancer to aging. Almost 20 years ago Demopoulos, Flamm, and associates proposed that free radicals contribute to infarction (12). Cytotoxic oxygen species including superoxide, hydrogen peroxide, and hydroxyl radical are generated according to the equations:

$$Hypoxanthine + O_2 \rightarrow Xanthine + {}^{\cdot}O_2{}^- + H_2O_2$$

xanthine oxidase

$$Xanthine + O_2 \rightarrow Uric\ Acid + {}^{\cdot}O_2{}^- + H_2O_2$$

xanthine oxidase

$${}^{\cdot}O_2{}^- + Fe^{3+} \rightarrow O_2 + Fe^{2+}$$

$$H_2O_2 + Fe^{2+} \rightarrow OH^- + {}^{\cdot}OH + Fe^{3+}$$

$${}^{\cdot}O_2{}^- + H_2O_2 \rightarrow O_2 + OH^- + {}^{\cdot}OH$$

Antioxidants also play an important role in the limitation of free radical damage to the brain. Cells contain vitamins (including α-tocopherol and ascorbic acid) and enzymes (superoxide dismutase and catalase), which inactivate free radicals. These systems play an important role, particularly following ischemia when the amount of reduced compounds is increased.

The importance of antioxidants in the pathophysiology of stroke was demonstrated by Patt and colleagues in a study in which gerbils were fed a tungsten-rich diet for 6 weeks and then subjected to 3 hours of carotid artery occlusion (13). Sodium tungstate inactivates xanthine oxidase by preventing its biosynthesis in a process that involves the metal molybdenum. The 6-week tungsten-fed gerbils had lower brain xanthine oxidase activities (0 units) than the control animals (9 units). These animals also had lower brain H_2O_2 levels and brain edema following carotid artery ligation and reperfusion. Of particular importance was the finding that all tungsten-fed or DMTU-treated dimethylthiuvrea (a xanthine oxidase inhibitor that crosses the blood–brain barrier), gerbils survived carotid artery ligation whereas more than 60% of the control animals died (Fig. 5). Allopurinol (also a xanthine oxidase inhibitor) was found to be ineffective in improving survival, a result possibly related to its poor blood–brain transport ability.

The intracellular calcium level affects the magnitude of stroke (Fig. 6) An event widely implicated in the pathophysiology of ischemic brain damage is the presence of high concentrations of intracellular calcium (14). High levels of calcium activate a number of calcium-dependent enzymes, which results in neurotoxicity. Influx of calcium occurs primarily by voltage-sensitive as well as agonist channels and much experimental work has employed blockers of these channels in an attempt to reduce stroke. Efflux of calcium is due to an ATP-driven transporter and to electrogenic $3Na^+/Ca^{2+}$ exchange. Agonists interact with receptors coupled to phospholipase C, resulting in a rise in intracellular phosphorylated inositol compounds and diglycerides. The latter acti-

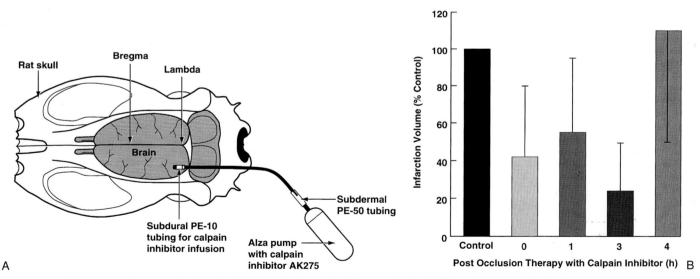

FIG. 6. A: "Supracortical perfusion" method to administer calpain inhibitors into the subdural space onto the ischemic cortex of rats. Polyethylene tubing is placed through a burr hole anterior to the lambdoid suture. **B:** The calpain inhibitor AK 275 reduced infarct size when administered at 0, 1, or 3 hours (p < 0.05) but not 4 hours (p = n.s.) after MCA occlusion in the rat. Stroke was reduced by 75% at 3 hours but no effect was observed when the infusion was delayed for 4 hours.

vates protein kinase C, which modulates mitochondrial membrane proteins. Calpains are recently recognized cytosolic neutral thiol proteases that degrade numerous cytoskeletal proteins and activate or degrade specified intracellular signal transducers such as protein kinases, phospholipases, and phosphatases. Calpains normally exist in the inactive state and become proteolytically active when high levels of intracellular calcium are present. Calpain inhibitors may therefore serve as a therapeutic tool to block the calcium-mediated cascade involved in cerebral ischemia.

The calpain inhibitor AK 275, a known inhibitor of the calcium cascade, was infused into the subdural space (parenteral formulations were not available) of rats by Bartus and colleagues (15). Anesthetized rats had a burr hole placed 5 mm from the midline at the lambdoid suture, and a polyethylene tube was placed subdurally and connected to a subcutaneously implanted pump (Fig. 6A). In order to prevent an excessive volume administration intracranially, a flow rate of only 4 μl/hr was utilized. Following MCA occlusion, 45% and 75% reductions in cerebral infarction were noted if AK 275 perfusion was initiated 1 and 3 hours postocclusion, but no effect was observed if AK 275 was not administered until 4 hours postocclusion (Fig. 6B). These studies strongly suggested that stroke can be minimized even 3 hours following the onset of ischemia.

Glutamate levels affect the magnitude of stroke (Fig. 7). It is now well established that the excitatory neurotransmitter glutamate plays an important role in ischemic neuronal injury (16). Glutamate is an agonist of NMDA (N-methyl-D-aspartate) and AMPA (amino-3-hydroxy-5-methyl-4-isoazoleproprionic acid) receptors. The NMDA channel in response to glutamate becomes permeable to Ca^{2+}, Na^+, K^+, and H^+, whereas the AMPA channels become permeable to Na^+, K^+, and H^+. The channels are normally blocked by Mg^{2+}. In response to glutamate stimulation, ischemic membranes become leaky secondary to ionic pump failure. NMDA as well as AMPA receptor antagonists are cerebroprotective in several models of ischemia and are believed to act by salvaging "penumbral" tissue.

New NMDA antagonists are potent protectants of the ischemic penumbral region. Takizawa and colleagues (17) infused the competitive NMDA antagonist CGS 19755 immediately following MCA occlusion in the rat. CGS-19755 has a low blood–brain permeability but is a potent NMDA antagonist. CGS 19755 improved CBF and corrected the pH decline in several cortical regions of the ischemic hemisphere but not the basal ganglia. Infusion of the NMDA antagonist reduced cortical infarction by approximately 50% in the treated group but had no effect on basal ganglia (a "core" region) infarction (Fig. 7). Hemodynamic parameters and temperature were similar in the two groups.

Nitric oxide (NO) is a potent cerebral vasodilator, although its role in stroke remains unclear (Fig. 8). NO, also called endothelium-derived relaxing factor, is an important determinant of CBF and acts via cyclic GMP:

$$\text{L-Arginine} \xrightarrow[\substack{\text{nitric oxide} \\ \text{synthetase}}]{} \text{NO} \rightarrow \begin{array}{l} \text{via activation of} \\ \text{GTP guanylate cyclase} \\ \searrow \\ \text{cGMP} \end{array}$$

NO has potential beneficial effects during ischemia including maintenance of CBF, inhibition of platelet aggregation, and antagonism of NMDA receptor actions. The detrimental effects of excessive NO production include a well-known cytotoxic effect and a potential role in NMDA-mediated brain injury. Studies on the role of NO during cerebral ischemia are ongoing, but it is clear that NO has a potential "double-edged sword" effect.

An elegant study by Zhang and associates showed a small therapeutic effect of nitric oxide in spontaneously hypertensive rats with MCA occlusion (18). In one group, the NO donor 3-morpholino-sydnonimine (SIN) was infused into the carotid artery for 60 minutes while papaverine (without NO donor capacity) was infused in a second group of rats. Phenylephrine was infused systemically in both groups to prevent hypotension (Fig. 8A). SIN but not papaverine increased the recovery of CBF and reduced the size of the infarct by 28% compared to papaverine (Fig. 8B).

The use of transgenic animals will better define the role of specific mediators in stroke (Fig. 9).

Transgenic animals are now being utilized to assist with the "molecular dissection" of stroke. Immediate early gene products and growth factors may play a role in the pathophysiology of stroke (19). How is a transgenic animal cre-

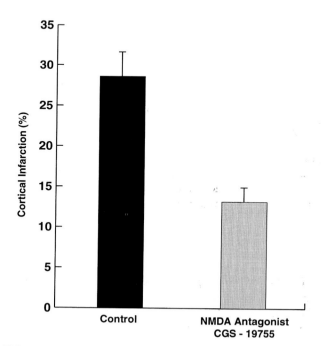

FIG. 7. Importance of NMDA antagonists in reducing infarction in the "penumbral region." The competitive NMDA antagonist CGS 19755 reduced cortical infarction by approximately 50% in MCA-occluded rats ($p = 0.05$). Basal ganglia infarction in the two groups was similar ($p = $ n.s.).

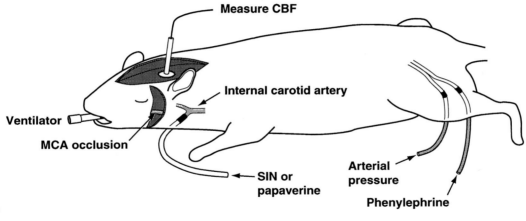

A

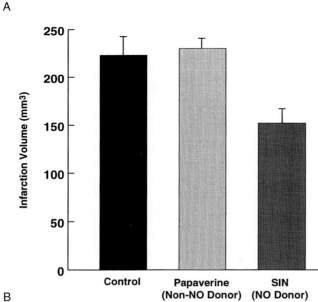

B

FIG. 8. A: Experimental protocol to assess the effect of nitric oxide (NO) during focal cerebral ischemia. An NO donor (SIN) or a non-NO donor (papaverine) was infused into the internal carotid artery of a rat in which the MCA had been occluded. Phenylephrine was infused peripherally as required to maintain baseline arterial pressure. B: The NO donor SIN reduced infarction from 223 ± 18 mm^3 to 152 ± 15 mm^3 ($p < 0.05$) whereas papaverine had no effect (p = n.s.).

ated? In the example of a p53 mutant mouse, a p53 targeting sequence containing a foreign piece of DNA (which prevents the p53 protein from being made) is placed into an embryonic stem cell using a process called electroporation (Fig. 9A). A genetic rearrangement termed homologous recombination transfers the target construct into the stem cell's DNA in a small number of stem cells. These stem cells are then microinjected into blastocysts and placed in pseudopregnant mice. The offspring are heterozygous (one copy) for the null mutation of the p53 gene. By mating the heterozygous animals, one fourth of the animals will have two copies of the null p53 gene.

This transgenic approach was utilized to assess the role of the p53 gene in stroke. p53, better known as a tumor suppressor gene, is involved in a series of steps requiring gene activation and protein synthesis for the cell to undergo its own destruction (20). Increased p53 expression has been observed in brain tissue after ischemia, and Crumrine and associates postulated that animals lacking p53 should have reduced infarction following MCA occlusion (21). Animals homozygous and heterozygous for a p53 null gene were sub-

jected to MCA occlusion, and both transgenic groups had a slight reduction in infarction compared to the control group (27% reduction in the heterozygous group and 15% reduction in the homozygous group) (Fig. 9B). The authors suggested that attenuated p53 expression may be protective after an ischemic event. We expect the application of this technology in dissecting the pathophysiology of stroke to become widespread in the 21st century.

SUMMARY

The aim of this chapter was to present animal studies of focal cerebral ischemia that offer insight into the horrors of human stroke. Animal models of stroke have long been criticized as irrelevant to the study of stroke in humans because little of this work has been applied to clinical medicine. We argue that the experimental work is often good and in some cases astonishing, and a major obstacle remains the lack of public education about stroke. The idea that stroke is a ''brain attack,'' as espoused by Camarata, Heros, and

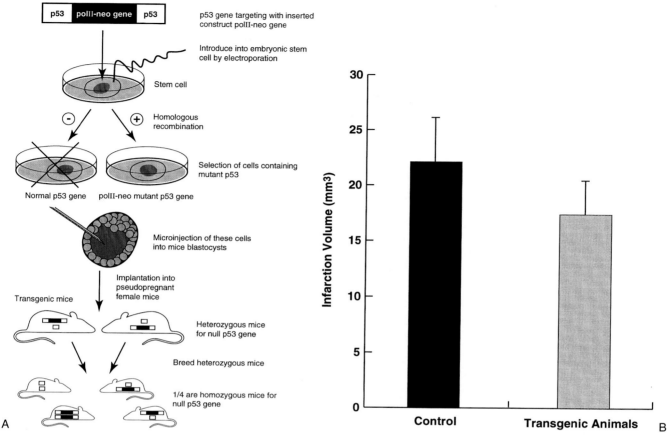

Transgenic Mice Deficient for the p53 Gene

FIG. 9. A: Transgenic mice deficient for the p53 gene "null p53 gene animals" are created using a p53 targeting construct that contains the polII-neo gene to prevent the production of the p53 protein. The targeting construct is introduced into the stem cells using electroporation. Homologous recombination occurs in some of the stem cells, and the cells containing the mutant p53 are selected. These cells are then microinjected into mice blastocysts and implanted into pseudopregnant females. Animals heterozygous for the null p53 gene are produced. Homozygous animals are obtained by breeding the heterozygous animals. **B:** Transgenic mice heterozygous or homozygous for a p53 null gene demonstrated a mild reduction in infarction following MCA occlusion. Infarction volume was 22.1 mm^3 in the wild-type animals and averaged 17.4 mm^3 in the transgenic animals ($p < 0.05$).

Latchaw (22), is a sound one and efforts should be made to continue both needed stroke basic research and public education.

REFERENCES

1. Siesjo BK. Pathophysiology and treatment of focal cerebral ischemia. 1. Pathophysiology. *J Neurosurg* 1992 :169–184.
2. Sundt TM, Grant WC, Garcia JH. Restoration of middle cerebral artery flow in experimental infarction. *J Neurosurg* 1969;31:311–322.
3. Jones TH, Morawetz RB, Crowell RM, Marcoux FW, FitzGibbon SJ, DeGirolami U, Ojemann RG. Thresholds of focal cerebral ischemia in awake monkeys. *J Neurosurg* 1981;54:773–782.
4. Korosue K, Heros RC, Ogilvy CS, Hyodo A, Tu Y-K, Graichen R. Comparison of crystalloids and colloids for hemodilution in a model of focal cerebral ischemia. *J Neurosurg* 1991;73:576–584.
5. Rosomoff HL. Hypothermia and cerebral vascular lesions. 1. Experimental interruption of the middle cerebral artery during hypothermia. *J Neurosurg* 1956;13:244–255.
6. Busto R, Dietrich WD, Globus MY-T, Valdes I, Scheinberg P, Ginsberg MD. Small differences in intraischemic brain temperature critically determine the extent of ischemic neuronal injury. *J Cereb Blood Flow Metab* 1987;7:729–738.
7. Goto Y, Kassell NF, Hiramatsu K, Soleau SW, Lee KS. Effects of intraischemic hypothermia on cerebral damage in a model of reversible focal ischemia. *Neurosurgery* 1993;32:980–985.
8. Myers RE, Yamaguchi S. Nervous system effects of cardiac arrest in monkeys. *Arch Neurol* 1977;34:65–74.
9. Venables GS, Miller SA, Gibson G, Hardy JA, Strong AJ. The effect of hyperglycaemia on changes during reperfusion following focal cerebral ischaemia in the cat. *J Neurol Neurosurg Psychiatry* 1985; 48:663–669.
10. Nakai H, Yamamoto YL, Diksic M, Worsley KJ, Takara E. Triple-tracer autoradiography demonstrates effect of hyperglycemia on cerebral blood flow, pH, and glucose utilization in cerebral ischemia of rats. *Stroke* 1988;19:764–772.
11. Kochanek PM, Hallenbeck JM. Polymorphonuclear leukocytes and monocytes/macrophages in the pathogenesis of cerebral ischemia and stroke. *Stroke* 1992;23:1367–1379.
12. Demopoulos H, Flamm E, Seligman M, et al. Molecular pathology of lipids in CNS membranes. In: Jobsis FF, ed. *Oxygen and physiological function.* Dallas: Professional Information Library, 1977:491–508.

13. Patt A, Harken AH, Burton LK, et al. Xanthine oxidase–derived hydrogen peroxide contributes to ischemia reperfusion–induced edema in gerbil brains. *J Clin Invest* 1988;81:1556–1562.

14. Siesjo BK. Pathophysiology and treatment of focal cerebral ischemia. 2. Mechanisms of damage and treatment. *J Neurosurg* 1992;77:337–354.

15. Bartus RT, Baker KL, Heiser AD, Sawyer SD, Dean RL, Elliott PJ, Straub JA. Postischemic administration of AK 275, a calpain inhibitor, provides substantial protection against focal ischemic brain damage. *J Cereb Blood Flow Metab* 1994;14:537–544.

16. Choi DW. Glutamate neurotoxicity and diseases of the nervous system. *Neuron* 1988;1:623–634.

17. Takizawa S, Hogan M, Hakim AM. The effects of a competitive NMDA receptor antagonist (CGS-19755) on cerebral blood flow and pH in focal ischemia. *J Cereb Blood Flow Metab* 1991;11:786–793.

18. Zhang F, White JG, Iadecola C. Nitric oxide donors increase blood flow and reduce brain damage in focal ischemia: evidence that nitric oxide is beneficial in the early stages of cerebral ischemia. *J Cereb Blood Flow Metab* 1994;14:217–226.

19. Kogure K, Kato H. Altered gene expression in cerebral ischemia. *Stroke* 1993;24:2121–2127.

20. Donehower LA, Harvey M, Slagle BL, McArthur MJ, Montgomery CA, Butel JS, Bradley A. Mice deficient for p53 are developmentally normal but susceptible to spontaneous tumors. *Nature* 1992;356:215–221.

21. Crumrine RC, Thomas AL, Morgan PF. Attenuation of p53 expression protects against focal ischemic damage in transgenic mice. *J Cereb Blood Flow Metab* 1994;14:887–891.

22. Camarata PJ, Heros RC, Latchaw RE. ''Brain attack'': the rationale for treating stroke as a medical emergency. *J Neurosurg* 1994;34:144–157.

Cerebrovascular Disease, edited by H. Hunt Batjer.
Lippincott-Raven Publishers, Philadelphia © 1997.

CHAPTER 24

Pathophysiology of White Matter Anoxic Injury

Bruce R. Ransom, Stephen G. Waxman and R. Fern

Ischemia of the mammalian central nervous system (CNS), including the secondary vascular embarrassment that frequently accompanies traumatic brain and spinal cord insults, damages both gray (GM) and white matter (WM). In fact, about 20% of ischemic strokes involve predominantly WM as a result of occlusion of small penetrating arteries that supply the deep parenchymal areas of the cerebral hemispheres (1). Ischemia in the form of delayed WM hypoperfusion also plays a prominent role in the response of the spinal cord to trauma (2); clinical deficits in spinal cord injury are in large part due to damage to WM, emphasizing the importance of understanding the pathophysiology of WM ischemia. The pathophysiology of anoxic injury is likely to be different in WM than in GM because WM contains no neuronal cell bodies or synapses but does contain myelinated axons, which have a unique, highly specialized structure (3). It follows that the strategies needed to confer protection against anoxic injury may also vary in these vastly different areas of the CNS.

In GM, it is now well established that anoxia results in extracellular accumulation of glutamate (4), which activates postsynaptic receptors, especially *N*-methyl-D-aspartate (NMDA) receptors, in an unrestrained fashion, causing increased intracellular $[Ca^{2+}]$ ($[Ca^{2+}]_i$) and neuronal damage (5). We have developed a highly quantitative model for studying the pathophysiology of anoxic injury in CNS white matter using the rat optic nerve, a WM tract (6,7). The nonsynaptic ionic mechanisms that are critical in the development of irreversible anoxic injury in WM are the focus of this chapter.

IRREVERSIBLE INJURY IN WM CAN BE QUANTITATIVELY STUDIED USING THE ISOLATED RAT OPTIC NERVE

The rat optic nerve has proven to be a highly reproducible model system for studying WM injury. The importance of

B. R. Ransom and R. Fern: Department of Neurology, University of Washington School of Medicine, Seattle, WA 98195.
S. G. Waxman: Department of Neurology, Yale University School of Medicine, New Haven, CT 06510.

this approach to our current understanding of how central axons are injured justifies a brief description of the experimental approach. Optic nerves from adult Long–Evans rats are dissected free and placed in a tissue slice chamber of interface design (6). Optic nerves from animals of this age have mature physiologic properties (8–10). Experiments were conducted at 37°C, and the nerves were perfused continuously with a physiologic saline containing 3 mM K^+ and 2 mM Ca^{2+} (6). The tissue is oxygenated in a 95% O_2–5% CO_2 atmosphere; anoxia is achieved by switching to a 95% N_2–5% CO_2 gas mixture, which results in a fall in chamber O_2 tension from 95% to zero in approximately 2.5 minutes (6).

Two broad categories of ischemic insult have been defined; the motivation for this subdivision is that the two types of insults produce different pathologic lesions (11). Global ischemia refers to complete cessation of blood flow to the brain with total deprivation of both oxygen and energy substrates; the equivalent clinical situation is cardiac arrest. Focal ischemia refers to a focal disturbance in cerebral blood flow, as with occlusion of a single intracranial vessel; under these circumstances some glucose can diffuse into the ischemic tissue from surrounding brain that is still normally perfused. It should be noted that our experiments are conducted in such a manner that they are more analogous to focal ischemia. After switching to anoxia, perfusion of the nerve with glucose-containing solution continues so the anoxic tissue has the same access to glucose as before.

The effects of anoxia on optic nerve function were assessed by measuring the compound action potential (CAP), using quantitative electrophysiologic techniques (12). Orthodromic stimulation and recording from optic nerves was accomplished using suction electrodes (Fig. 1A). The stimulus strength was set to 25% above the strength that elicited a maximum CAP. Area under the CAP was examined before and after experimental manipulations using a method that corrected for changes in recording electrode impedance (12); CAP amplitude is shown as percent of the control CAP integral. The extracellular currents generated by individual

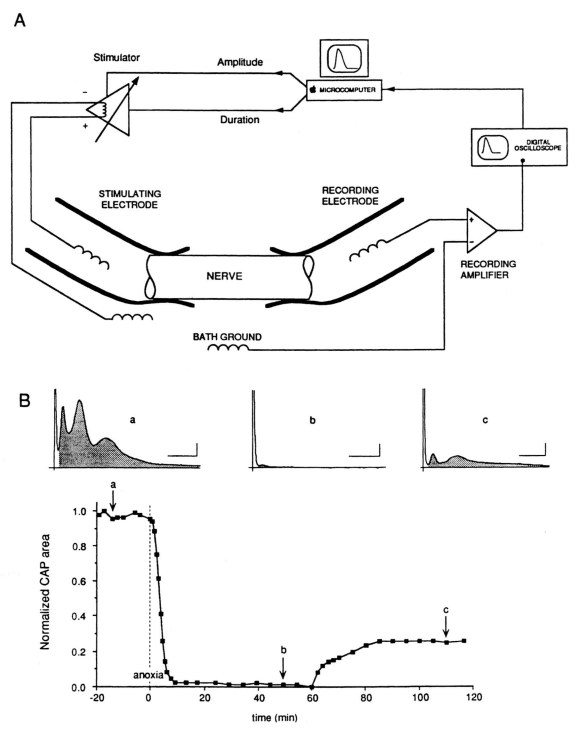

FIG. 1. A: Diagram of recording arrangement. The optic nerve is stimulated with a supramaximal voltage pulse via one suction electrode and the compound action potential (CAP) is recorded from the other end of the nerve with a second suction electrode. Signals are amplified, digitized, and transferred to a microcomputer for processing and storage. **B:** Effects of anoxia on white matter function. The function of the optic nerve was monitored as the area under the CAP (a–c); this is shown graphically as percentage of the control CAP integral. Anoxia was begun at time zero by switching from an atmosphere of 95% O_2/5% CO_2 to one with 95% N_2/5% CO_2. CAP area rapidly declined becoming virtually zero after 10 min of anoxia (residual area was mostly stimulus artifact). A standard 60 min period of anoxia was used for all experiments. After O_2 was reintroduced, CAP area gradually recovered to a mean of 28.5 $\pm$ 10.6 ($\pm$1 SD)% of control in perfusate containing 2.0 mM $[Ca^{2+}]$. For quantification, postanoxic CAP measurements were routinely made 60 min after the end of anoxia because recovery always reached a plateau by this time. Specimen records of the CAP under control (a), anoxic (b), and postanoxic (c) conditions are shown. Calibration marks are 1 msec and 1 mV. (Modified from ref. 6.)

axons sum to produce the CAP so that the CAP area reflects the number of axons that are capable of conducting action potentials (12,13).

The CAP rapidly diminished after the start of anoxia and virtually disappeared after 8–10 minutes (Fig. 1B); conceivably, the presence of hemoglobin in the capillaries of the freshly dissected nerves may have provided some O_2 to the axons and thereby prolonged function somewhat during anoxia (14). As shown in Fig. 1B, 60 minutes was the standard anoxic insult used in all experiments. During re-oxygenation, the CAP showed partial recovery and attained a plateau value within 1 hour (Fig. 1B) (6,15). The degree of functional recovery depended on duration of the anoxic period and was, in general, much greater in this WM structure than in GM (15–18). For example, 15 minutes of anoxia in the hippocampal brain slice preparation results in complete, irreversible loss of evoked synaptic activity (16,18), whereas the optic nerve exposed to a similar period of anoxia shows only a 10–15% loss of CAP following reoxygenation (Ransom and Davis, unpublished observations). The average CAP recovery from the standard 60 minutes of anoxia was approx. 35% (Fig. 1B) (6).

ANOXIA CAUSES RAPID INCREASES IN EXTRACELLULAR K^+ AND H^+ IN WM

The rapid changes in brain extracellular ion concentrations that occur with anoxia are important in understanding the pathophysiology of anoxic/ischemic brain injury (19). These changes convey information about the metabolic state of local brain tissue (20) and can have direct effects on neural behavior. Elevated $[K^+]_o$ depolarizes neuronal membranes, reducing and then blocking action potentials, causes uncontrolled transmitter release (4), reduces electrogenic glial uptake of neurotransmitters including the excitotoxin glutamate (21), induces cell swelling (22), and may affect cerebral blood flow (23). Extracellular acidosis can have direct toxic effects on both neuronal and glial membranes (24,25), may alter ion channel function (26), and blocks currents generated by activation of NMDA receptors (27,28).

Anoxia in WM causes rapid changes in the extracellular concentrations of K^+ and H^+ that are qualitatively similar to those seen in GM but smaller (19,25,28). In the optic nerve $[K^+]_o$ begins to increase within 3–4 minutes and reaches a final concentration averaging 14.0 mM. An acid shift in pH_o develops during anoxia with a time-course similar to the change in $[K^+]_o$. The average maximum acid shift in standard physiologic solution is 0.31 pH units (28). As in GM (25), the magnitude of the extracellular acid shift increases with higher levels of bath glucose concentration, and this is associated with smaller increases in $[K^+]_o$ and delayed loss of the CAP (28). In the presence of 20 mM glucose, compared to 10 mM, there is more substrate for anaerobic metabolism and presumably greater generation of lactic acid and ATP. The higher levels of ATP would act to slow the deterioration of ion gradients during anoxia accounting for the smaller increases in $[K^+]_o$ and delayed loss of the CAP (28).

In WM, glial cells have been shown to contribute directly to anoxia-induced changes in the concentration of extracellular ions, based on studies using optic nerves that contain only glial cells (as a result of retinal ablation and resultant loss of axons) (29). Technical reasons cause the ionic changes recorded in the "glial" nerve to be smaller and more variable than ionic changes in the intact nerve (29), so that the quantitative degree to which glial cells contribute to the ionic changes seen in normal WM is presently not known.

The extent to which extracellular ionic changes participate in the development of anoxic injury in WM is not known. Certainly these early changes predispose to some of the other ionic events that are critical for injury (see below). Increasing $[K^+]_o$ to 30 mM for 60 minutes under normoxic conditions is not harmful to the optic nerve (28), and preliminary experiments indicate that the optic nerve is also undamaged by 20 mM lactate buffered to a pH of 6.4. In contrast to the situation in GM (30), WM suffers less rather than more injury during anoxia in the presence of higher-than-usual glucose concentrations (28), in spite of the fact that the elevated bath glucose concentration causes a greater acid shift, which is believed to worsen outcome in anoxic GM (30–32).

EXTRACELLULAR CALCIUM IS NECESSARY FOR THE PRODUCTION OF IRREVERSIBLE ANOXIC INJURY IN WHITE MATTER

Experimental evidence indicates that extracellular Ca^{2+} is critical in the production of anoxic injury in WM (6). Test solutions with different concentrations of Ca^{2+} were applied for a period extending from 10 minutes before the onset of anoxia to 10 minutes after the end of anoxia (Fig. 2B, inset). As the $[Ca^{2+}]$ was decreased from 2 mM to zero, the degree of CAP recovery from anoxia gradually increased. If Ca^{2+} was entirely omitted from the perfusing fluid, the optic nerve displayed essentially complete recovery, as judged by the area under the CAP, even after 60 minutes of anoxia; the latencies of the CAP peaks, however, did not fully recover, suggesting that although most of the axons within the nerve are protected from anoxic injury by perfusion with zero $[Ca^{2+}]$, some axons conduct more slowly after anoxia. Exposure of the nerve to an increase in $[Ca^{2+}]$ (ie, 4 mM rather than 2 mM) during anoxia significantly worsened outcome (Fig. 2B). Other experiments indicate that the deleterious effects of Ca^{2+} accumulate slowly over the entire anoxic period (6).

Pyramidal tract responses can be recorded after 60-minute periods of anoxia in vivo (33). At first glance this observation seems to suggest that pyramidal tract axons in vivo can tolerate such periods of ischemia without any damage. The method used to obtain these results, however, does not allow

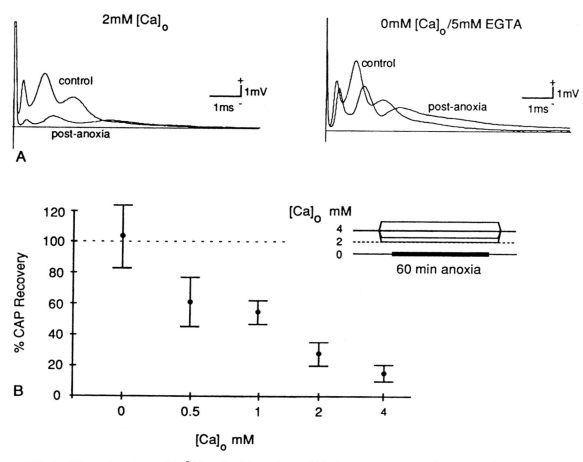

FIG. 2. Effect of perfusate $[Ca^{2+}]$ and calcium channel blockers on recovery of compound action potential (CAP) from 60 min of anoxia. **A:** CAPs before ("control") and 60 min after anoxia ("postanoxia") in 2.0 mM $[Ca^{2+}]$ or zero $[Ca^{2+}]$/5 mM EGTA are shown. CAP recovery from anoxia is enhanced in the zero $[Ca^{2+}]$ solution. **B:** Average (± 1 SD) percent recovery after a standard 60-min period of anoxia as a function of perfusate $[Ca^{2+}]$ during anoxia. Test solutions were begun 10 min before anoxia onset and continued until 10 min after the end of anoxia *(see inset)*. The percent recovery of the CAP gradually diminished as perfusate $[Ca^{2+}]$ increased from 0 to 4 mM. All points were significantly different from the normal $[Ca^{2+}]$ of 2 mM ($p < 0.005$). (Modified from Ref. 6).

quantitative evaluation of axonal function in the same way that it can be assessed under the conditions of our experiments on the optic nerve (12), and thus it is unclear if a real discrepancy exists between our in vitro observations on WM and those made in vivo. Assuming that there is less damage in vivo than in vitro, for the purposes of discussion, what could be the explanation for this? The argument has been offered that under in vivo circumstances the extracellular $[Ca^{2+}]$ falls to very low levels and in effect corresponds to the in vitro situation where bath Ca^{2+} is zero during anoxia (cf. Fig. 2). Were this the case, the degree of in vivo axonal injury following 60 minutes of anoxia might be expected to be very slight or nonexistent, as in the in vitro experiments. Although $[Ca^{2+}]_o$ falls to low levels in GM during anoxia both in vivo and in vitro (19), the situation in WM is less

clear. Further measurements of $[Ca^{2+}]_o$ in WM during anoxia should be carried out to resolve this question.

Although it is not directly shown by these experiments, extracellular Ca^{2+} probably acted as a source for inward Ca^{2+} flux into a cytoplasmic compartment. Because it is the axons that become dysfunctional during anoxia based on the loss of the CAP, a damaging increase in intraaxonal $[Ca^{2+}]$ seems likely. Some support for this view comes from observations in our laboratory on the ultrastructural correlates of anoxia in the optic nerve that indicate that 60 minutes of anoxia causes striking pathologic alteration within axons (34). Large empty spaces appear between axons and their ensheathing myelin, axoplasmic mitochondria are swollen and disrupted, and neurofilaments and microtubules disappear. Not all axons are so affected and the changes seem most prominent in large axons. Paranodal myelin retracts from the node and this may slow or abolish saltatory conduction. Some resolution of these anoxia-induced ultrastructural changes occur during the standard 60-minute recovery period, although neurofilament and microtubule damage persists. Particularly notable is a partial restitution in many fibers of the normal relationship between axon membrane and paranodal myelin, which might represent the ultrastructural substrate for some of the postanoxic recovery that is measured as a partial return of the CAP (see Fig. 1B). Interestingly, many of the cytoskeletal alterations seen after 60 minutes of anoxia are prevented by perfusion with zero $[Ca^{2+}]$ solution during anoxia (35). The destruction of the axonal cytoskeleton seen in our experiments on the optic nerve is similar to that induced by exposure of peripheral nerve axons to the calcium ionophore A23187 (36).

ANOXIA-INDUCED Ca^{2+} ENTRY IN WM IS MEDIATED BY THE Na^+–Ca^{2+} EXCHANGER AND BY Ca^{2+} CHANNELS

Experimental evidence reviewed above indicates that irreversible anoxic injury in WM, as in GM, depends on the presence of extracellular Ca^{2+}, which appears to serve as the source of inward Ca^{2+} flux into axons. How does this inward Ca^{2+} flux occur? At the outset it seemed likely that the mechanism would be different to that operating in GM where anoxia-mediated Ca^{2+} influx occurs predominantly via NMDA receptor channels and, to a lesser extent, by voltage-gated Ca^{2+} channels (5,37). Axons in the rat optic nerve do not appear to have glutamate receptors and, not surprisingly, optic nerve axons are not damaged by high concentrations of excitotoxins (15). Furthermore, the NMDA antagonist ketamine, at low concentrations that are relatively specific for blocking this receptor, had no protective effects on anoxia-induced injury in white matter. (At high concentrations ketamine is protective, but this effect is probably related to the drug's anesthetic-like actions on Na^+ channel permeability and not to NMDA receptor blockade [15].)

Recent evidence from our laboratory indicates that during anoxia Ca^{2+} influx occurs by way of reverse operation of the Na^+–Ca^{2+} exchanger, a ubiquitous membrane protein that normally operates to extrude cytoplasmic Ca^{2+} in exchange for Na^+ influx. This exchange mechanism does not consume ATP directly and is primarily driven by the transmembrane Na^+ gradient. The stoichiometry of this process, at least in some instances, is that three Na^+ ions exchange for each Ca^{2+} ion; this exchange ratio implies that the exchange process is electrogenic and, in fact, membrane current is generated by its operation (38). For this reason, the exchanger is also thermodynamically dependent on membrane potential (38,39), with membrane depolarization favoring reverse exchange (ie, Na^+ efflux and Ca^{2+} influx).

The disruption of cellular energy supply caused by anoxia in WM rapidly leads to an increase in $[K^+]_o$, resulting in axonal depolarization (28). This would also result in the activation of voltage-dependent Na^+ channels and an increase in intracellular Na^+ concentration ($[Na^+]_i$). Both membrane depolarization and the increase in $[Na^+]_i$ favor reverse operation of the Na^+–Ca^{2+} exchanger that would continue until a higher, steady-state intracellular $[Ca^{2+}]$ is reached. Modest increases in $[Na^+]_i$, coupled with membrane depolarization, can cause $[Ca^{2+}]_i$ to rise into the micromolar range (38,39). Procedures that would block the increase in $[Na^+]_i$ during anoxia should protect against irreversible injury according to the above scenario. In fact, reducing $[Na^+]_o$ during anoxia or adding tetrodotoxin (TTX) to block voltage-gated Na^+ channels results in dramatically improved CAP recovery (Fig. 3). Of particular interest is the observation that TTX significantly protects the nerve from anoxic damage at concentrations (eg, 10 nM) (see Fig. 3) that do not have much effect on the control CAP. Intracellular Na^+ appears to accumulate slowly during anoxia, suggesting the presence of persistently open Na^+ channels (40); one class of voltage-dependent Na^+ channels inactivates slowly or not at all (41), and such channels are candidates for mediating anoxia-induced increases in $[Na^+]_i$ in WM (40,42).

If reversal of Na^+–Ca^{2+} exchange mediates the damaging influx of Ca^{2+} during anoxia, then blocking the exchanger during anoxia could be expected to improve outcome. This hypothesis was tested using two different inhibitors of this transporter, bepridil and benzamil. Both drugs markedly improved post anoxic recovery (Fig. 4) (40). The amount of postanoxic CAP recovery seen following treatments that limit reverse operation of the Na^+–Ca^{2+} exchanger approaches the level of recovery seen when the nerve is bathed in zero Ca^{2+} solution during anoxia (compare Figs. 2B and 4). From a quantitative standpoint this suggests that reverse operation of the exchanger is playing a central role in mediating the damaging Ca^{2+} influx into axons during anoxia.

Voltage-gated calcium channels, however, are also involved in loading axons with Ca^{2+} during anoxia (Fig. 5). Recent work has shown that blockade of L-type or N-type Ca^{2+} channels partially protect anoxic axons from injury (40,43). Combined block of both L-type and N-type Ca^{2+} channels is just as protective as blocking the Na^+–Ca^{2+} exchanger (43). There are two possible explanations for this observation. Either an influx of Ca^{2+} via L-type and N-type Ca^{2+} channels is a prerequisite for reverse operation of the Na^+–Ca^{2+} exchanger, as has been reported (44), or Ca^{2+} influx via both Ca^{2+} channels and the Na^+–Ca^{2+} exchanger is required to overload the Ca^{2-} buffering capacity of CNS white matter. Calcium channels do not, however, support spike electrogenesis in optic nerve axons (8,43) and their role in normal axons has not been established.

THE IONIC MECHANISMS OF ANOXIC INJURY ARE DIFFERENT IN WM COMPARED TO GM

A schematic diagram of the events leading to anoxic injury in GM and WM is given in Fig. 6. This outline emphasizes

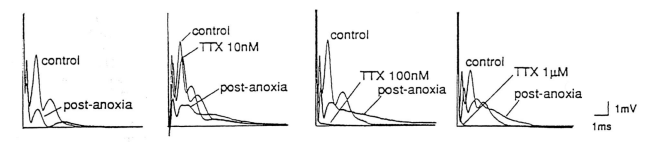

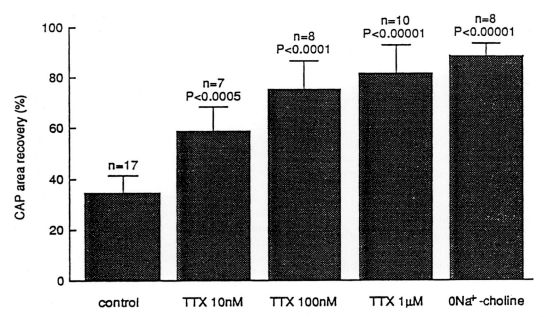

FIG. 3. The effects of zero-Na$^+$ solution or the Na$^+$ channel blocker tetrodotoxin on recovery of compound action potential (CAP) area following 60 min of anoxia. In normal artificial cerebrospinal fluid, CAP area recovered to 36.7 ± 7% of control. Recovery of CAP area was greatly improved in zero-Na$^+$ solution; pretreatment with zero-Na$^+$ (introduced 20 min before and maintained until 15 min after the anoxic insult) resulted in 88.0 ± 5% CAP area recovery. Nerves pretreated with tetrodotoxin (TTX) begun 15 min before and continued until 15 min after the 60-min anoxic period, showed significantly improved CAP recovery even at the lowest concentration used (10 nM). All *p* values show the comparison between the test condition and control. (Modified from Ref. 40).

the early ionic events that lead to an increase in [Ca^{2+}]$_i$ and ultimately to irreversible damage (45); it is presumed that the increase in [Ca^{2-}]$_i$ to some critical level activates additional biochemical reactions, including the formation of free radicals, activation of proteases, and appearance of nitric oxide, that are the ultimate cause of cell death (20,46).

Anoxia causes an increase in [K$^+$]$_o$ in both WM and GM; the increase is greater in GM (60–80 mM) than in WM (approx. 15 mM), although both occur shortly after anoxia onset (19,28). The anoxia-induced increase in [K$^+$]$_o$ correlates well with loss of function in WM, probably due to

depolarization of axons, but lags the loss of GM function, which has its onset within seconds of anoxic exposure and is associated with neuronal hyperpolarization rather than depolarization (47). The mechanism in GM responsible for this early hyperpolarization may be the opening of Ca^{2+}–dependent or ATP-sensitive K$^+$ channels (47); if this occurs in WM, it has little effect on the CAP. Once the massive increase in [K$^+$]$_o$ does occur in GM, it causes a spreading depression-like event (48) that is associated with massive release of glutamate and other transmitters (49). Glutamate activates both NMDA and non-NMDA receptors leading to

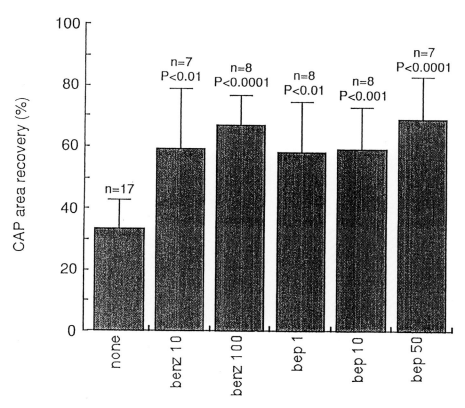

FIG. 4. Effects of blocking Na^+/Ca^{2+} exchange on recovery from 60 min of anoxia. Two different blockers of the Na^+/Ca^{2+} exchanger, bepridil (bep) and benzamil (benz), were applied individually, and at different concentrations, during the anoxic period. Both drugs significantly improved recovery as shown (the number of nerves tested with each drug ranged from 7 to 8). Bars represent standard deviations. (Modified from Ref. 40)

neuronal depolarization and Ca^{2+} influx. As indicated, voltage-gated Ca^{2+} channels also participate in mediating Ca^{2+} influx into GM. Release of intracellular stores of Ca^{2+} may be another means by which anoxia increases $[Ca^{2+}]_i$ in GM (50), and perhaps in WM as well. The anoxia-induced increase in $[Ca^{2+}]_i$ probably occurs very rapidly in GM neurons based on the response of neurons to high sustained applications of glutamate (50).

Anoxia probably also causes an increase in axonal $[Ca^{2-}]_i$, but the evidence for this in WM, although compelling, is admittedly indirect. It is clear, however, that the anoxia-induced (presumed) increase in $[Ca^{2+}]_i$ develops in part via a different mechanism and in a slower fashion in WM compared to GM. In WM, Ca^{2+} entry is by non-synaptic routes, namely reversal of the Na^+-Ca^{2+} exchanger and voltage-gated Ca^{2+} channels. The slowness of the Ca^{2-} loading process in WM is related to the fact that the $[Na^+]_i$ must increase before the exchanger runs in reverse, and this latter process appears to proceed gradually (40). It is entirely possible that this mechanism operates to increase cytosolic Ca^{2+} in GM as well, in addition to the mechanisms outlined above; in fact, this could be of major importance if the other modes of Ca^{2+} entry were blocked pharmacologically.

THE PATHOPHYSIOLOGY OF WM ANOXIC INJURY SUGGESTS THERAPEUTIC STRATEGIES

Advances in our understanding of the molecular and ionic mechanisms underlying anoxic/ischemic WM injury lead

naturally to insights about how to limit the consequences of such insults. For example, the demonstrated involvement of Na^+ and Ca^{2+} channels in leading to intracellular Ca^{2+} overload in WM suggests that blockade of these channels may be protective. Experimental studies have begun to test these expectations and should eventually lead to clinically useful approaches (50,52).

The specific Na^+ channel blockers TTX and saxitoxin, if applied before the anoxic insult, are strongly protective of WM function (40). Unfortunately, these drugs are not therapeutic candidates because they also block normal WM function. Local anesthetics and some antiepileptic and antiarrhythmic drugs are very effective blockers of Na^+ channels and can do this without greatly disrupting normal function. The tertiary anesthetics procaine and lidocaine, at 0.1 mM, significantly improve outcome following anoxia while producing only minimal reduction in the control CAP (53). The quaternary anesthetics, especially QX-314, are even better at protecting WM from anoxic damage without disrupting normal function. One factor that may favor enhanced Na^+ channel block during anoxia compared to normal conditions is greater Na^+ channel blocking action when the axons are depolarized, as would be the case during anoxia (53). QX-314 may be the best of this class of compound because it binds preferentially to non-inactivating Na^+ channels and these are likely to be most involved in the damaging Na^+ influx associated with anoxia (42).

The antiarrhythmic drugs tocainide, prajmaline, ajmaline, and disopyramide were strongly protective of WM anoxic

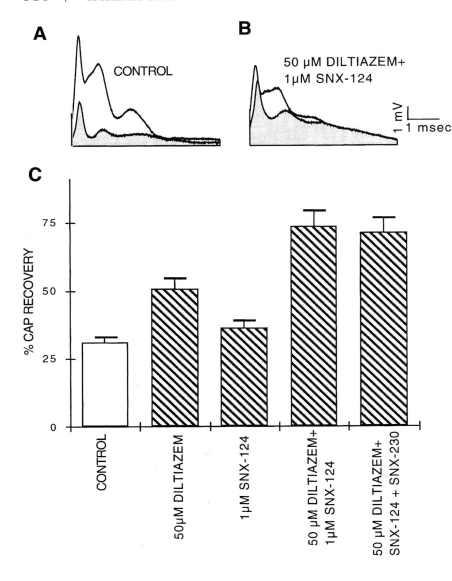

FIG. 5. Ca^{2+} channels contribute to anoxic injury of CNS white matter. **A:** Superimposed recordings of pre- and postanoxic compound action potentials (CAPs) recorded under control conditions. **B:** Examples of pre- and postanoxic CAPs showing the protective effect of perfusion with 50 μM diltiazem (which will block L-type Ca^{2+} channels) + 1 μm SNX-124 (which will block N-type Ca^{2+} channels). **C:** Mean CAP recovery under control conditions and in the presence of 50 μM diltiazem, 1 μM SNX-124, 50 μM diltiazem + 1 μM SNX-124, and 50 μM diltiazem + 1 μM SNX-124 + 1 μM SNX-230. CAP recovery during combined block of L-type and N-type Ca^{2+} channels was 73.6 ± 6.0%. (Modified from ref. 43.)

injury in the optic nerve model system (52). Moreover, the benefits were obtained without significant blockade of the normoxic CAP. This may be explained by the fact that these drugs produce a use-dependent type of Na$^+$ channel blockade; single action potentials are relatively unaffected, while the non-inactivating Na$^+$ channels, preferentially involved during anoxia, are readily blocked in the chronically open state caused by anoxic axonal depolarization (28). Procainamide was not protective (52).

Like the antiarrhythmic drugs, the antiepileptic compounds phenytoin and carbamazepine are use-dependent Na$^+$ channel blockers. Both drugs protect WM from anoxic injury, and do so at concentrations that have no effect on the control CAP (51). In fact, the drugs have maximal protective efficacy at concentrations that are lower than the normal unbound serum and cerebrospinal fluid levels that are found in patients under treatment for epilepsy.

The Na$^+$–Ca^{2+} exchanger is importantly involved in the Ca^{2+} loading phase of the anoxic sequence in WM (40). Depolarization and increased intracellular [Na$^+$] lead to reverse Na$^+$–Ca^{2+} exchange with Ca^{2+} influx. Blockers of Na$^+$–Ca^{2+} exchange are protective if they are applied before anoxia (40). Available blockers are not ideal, however, because they block both forward and reverse Na$^+$–Ca^{2+} exchange. Blockade of forward exchange, ie, Na$^+$-driven Ca^{2+} efflux, could seriously compromise cellular function, particularly after a period of intracellular Ca^{2+} loading, such as would occur during anoxia. Therefore, an agent most likely to be useful in the clinical setting of anoxia would block reverse Na$^+$–Ca^{2+} exchange selectively, leaving the forward, Ca^{2+}-exporting mode unaffected. Progress in understanding the molecular details of the Na$^+$–Ca^{2+} exchanger is well underway and it is conceivable that a selec-

Pathophysiology of Anoxic Injury: White Matter vs Gray Matter

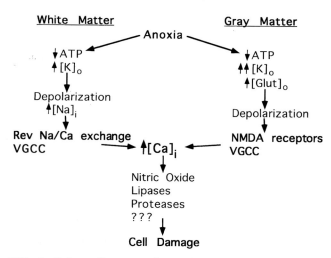

FIG. 6. Schematic comparison of the sequence of pathophysiologic events that characterize anoxic injury in gray matter (GM) and white matter (WM) of the mammalian CNS. The critical event in GM is the anoxia-induced unrestrained release of glutamate, and perhaps other transmitters, into the extracellular space leading to the activation of both NMDA receptors and, secondary to depolarization, voltage-dependent Ca^{2+} channels that mediate the influx of Ca^{2+} into neuronal cytoplasm. In WM, the critical event is the depolarization-induced activation of Na^+ channels (perhaps a subpopulation of non-inactivating Na^+ channels) leading to an increase in intracellular $[Na^+]$ followed by Ca^{2+} influx via reverse operation of the Na^+-Ca^{2+} exchanger (see text). In both GM and WM, the increase in cytosolic $[Ca^{2+}]$ activates a sequence of imprecisely defined biochemical events that lead to cell damage or death.

tive blocker of its reverse function might be engineered sometime in the future.

Ca^{2+} channels also mediate Ca^{2+} influx during anoxia in WM. In all, optic nerve axons appear to express three types of Ca^{2+} channel (43), but only the N and L types are involved in allowing Ca^{2+} entry during anoxia. Verapamil, diltiazem, and nifedipine, L-type Ca^{2+} channel blockers, were protective against anoxic injury. Blockade of N-type Ca^{2+} channels, with a specific synthetic ω-conotoxin, was also associated with improved outcome from the standard 60-minute period of anoxia.

Studies on the pathophysiology of WM anoxic damage are contributing to an overall improved understanding of the response of the CNS to injury. Moreover, the concept is emerging that the therapeutic strategies for protecting WM from anoxic injury must be tailored to the unique mechanisms leading to irreversible damage in this tissue. Our increasingly sophisticated understanding of the molecular nature of the Na^+-Ca^{2+} exchanger (54) and Na^+ and Ca^{2+}

channels will undoubtedly be of benefit in pursuing this central issue to a clinically useful end. An important challenge for the future is to extend our observations on the isolated rat optic nerve to WM in vivo, and ultimately it is in that setting that critical experiments must test our hypotheses about the mechanisms of anoxic injury in this tissue.

ACKNOWLEDGMENTS

This work was supported by NIH grant NS 15589 (BRR) and a Veterans Administration grant (SGW). R. F. was supported by a Blinded Veterans Association fellowship.

REFERENCES

1. Fisher CM. Capsular infarcts: the underlying vascular lesions. *Arch Neurol* 1979;36:65–73.
2. Young W. Blood flow, metabolic and neurophysiologic mechanisms in spinal cord injury. In: Becker D, Povlishock J, eds. *Central Nervous System Trauma Status Report 1985.* Washington, DC: NIH, NINCDS, 1985;463–473.
3. Black JA, Kocsis JD, Waxman SG. Ion channel organization of the myelinated fiber. *Trends Neurosci* 1990;13:48–54.
4. Benveniste H, Drejer J, Schousboe A, Diemer NH. Elevation of the extracellular concentrations of glutamate and aspartate in rat hippocampus during transient cerebral ischemia monitored by intracerebral microdialysis. *J Neurochem* 1984;43:1369–1374.
5. Choi D. Glutamate neurotoxicity and diseases of the nervous system. *Neuron* 1988;1:624–634.
6. Stys PK, Ransom BR, Waxman SG, Davis PK. The role of extracellular calcium in anoxic injury of mammalian central white matter. *Proc Natl Acad Sci USA* 1990;87:4212–4216.
7. Ransom BR, Waxman SG, Stys PK. Anoxic injury of central myelinated axons: Ionic mechanisms and pharmacology. In: Waxman SG, ed. *Molecular and Cellular Approaches to the Treatment of Neurological Disease.* New York: Raven Press, 1993;121–151.
8. Foster RE, Connors BW, Waxman SG. Rat optic nerve: electrophysiological, pharmacological and anatomical studies during development. *Dev Brain Res* 1982;3:371–386.
9. Connors BW, Ransom BR, Kunis DM, Gutnick MJ. Activity-dependent K accumulation in the developing rat optic nerve. *Science* 1982;216:1341–1343.
10. Ransom BR, Yamate CL, Connors BW. Activity-dependent shrinkage of extracellular space in rat optic nerve: A development study. *J Neurosci* 1985;5:532–535.
11. Ginsberg MD, Busto BS. Rodent models of cerebral ischemia. *Stroke* 1989;20:1627–1642.
12. Stys PK, Ransom BR, Waxman SG. Compound action potential of nerve recorded by suction electrode: a theoretical and experimental analysis. *Brain Res* 1991;546:18–32.
13. Buchthal F, Rosenfalck A. Evoked action potentials and conduction velocity in human sensory nerves. *Brain Res* 1966;3:1–122.
14. Kraus DW, Colacino JM. Extended oxygen delivery from the nerve hemoglobin of *Tellina alternata* (Bivalvia). *Science* 1986;232:90–92.
15. Ransom BR, Waxman SG, Davis PK. Anoxic injury of CNS white matter: protective effect of ketamine. *Neurology* 1990;40:1399–1403.
16. Kass IS, Lipton P. Mechanisms involved in irreversible anoxic damage to the in vitro rat hippocampal slice. *J Physiol (Lond)* 1982;332:459–472.
17. Smith M-L, Auer RN, Siesjo BK. The density and distribution of ischemic brain injury in the rat following two to ten minutes of forebrain ischemia. *Acta Neuropathol (Berl)* 1984;64:319–332.
18. Taylor MD, Mellert TK, Parmentier JL, Eddy LJ. Pharmalogical protection of reoxygenation damage to in vitro brain slice tissue. *Brain Res* 1985;347:268–273.
19. Hansen AJ. Effects of anoxia on ion distribution in the brain. *Physiol Rev* 1985;65:101–148.

20. Siesjo BK. Cell damage in the brain: a speculative synthesis. *J Cereb Blood Flow Metab* 1981;1:155–185.
21. Schwartz EA, Tachibana M. Electrophysiology of glutamate and sodium co-transport in a glial cell of the salamander retina. *J Physiol (Lond)* 1990;426:43–80.
22. Kimelberg HK, Ransom BR. Physiological and pathological aspects of astrocytic swelling. In: Federoff S, Vernadakis A, eds. *Astrocytes,* Vol. 3. Orlando: Academic Press, 1986, 1986;129–166.
23. Paulson OB, Newman EA. Does the release of potassium from astrocyte endfeet regulate cerebral blood flow? *Science* 1987;237:896–898.
24. Goldman SA, Pulsinelli WA, Clarke WY, Kraig RP, Plum F. The effects of extracellular acidosis on neurons and glia in vitro. *J Cereb Blood Flow Metab* 1989;9:471–477.
25. Kraig RP, Petito CK, Plum F, Pulsinelli WA. Hydrogen ions kill brain at concentrations reached in ischemia. *J Cereb Blood Flow Metab* 1987; 7:379–386.
26. Chesler M. The regulation and modulation of pH in the nervous system. (1990) *Prog Neurobiol* 1990;34:401–427.
27. Tang CM, Dichter M, Morad M. Modulation of the N-methyl-D-aspartate channel by extracellular H^+. *Proc Natl Acad Sci USA* 1990;87: 6445–6449.
28. Ransom BR, Walz W, Davis PK, Carlini WG. Anoxia-induced changes in extracellular K^+ and pH in mammalian central white matter. *J Cereb Blood Flow Metab* 1992;12:593–602.
29. Ransom BR, Philbin DM. Anoxia-induced extracellular ionic changes in CNS white matter: the role of glial cells. *Can J Physiol Pharmacol* 1992;70:181–189.
30. Pulsinelli WA, Waldman S, Rawlinson D, Plum F. Moderate hyperglycemia augments ischemic brain damage: a neuropathologic study in the rat. *Neurology* 1982;32:1239–1246.
31. Plum F. What causes infarction in ischemic brain? *Neurology* 1983; 33:222–233.
32. Giffard RG, Monyer H, Christine CW, Choi DW. Acidosis reduces NMDA receptor activation, glutamate neurotoxicity, and oxygen-glucose deprivation neuronal injury in cortical cultures. *Brain Res* 1990; 506:339–342.
33. Hossmann KA, Sato K. Recovery from neuronal function after prolonged cerebral ischemia. *Science* 1970;168:375–376.
34. Waxman SG, Black JA, Stys PK, Ransom BR. Ultrastructural concomitants of anoxic injury and early post-anoxic recovery in rat optic nerve. *Brain Res* 1992;574:105–119.
35. Waxman SG, Black JA, Ransom BR, Stys PK. Protection of the axonal cytoskeleton in anoxic optic nerve by decreased extracellular calcium. *Brain Res* 1993;614:137–145.
36. Schlaepfer WW. Structural alterations of peripheral nerve induced by the calcium ionophore A23817. *Brain Res* 1977;136:1–9.
37. Choi DW. Calcium-mediated neurotoxicity: relationship to specific channel types and role in ischemic damage. *Trends Neurosci* 1988;11: 465–469.
38. Lagnado L, Cervetto L, McNaughton PA. Ion transport by the Na–Ca exchange in isolated rod outer segments. *Proc Natl Acad Sci USA* 1988; 85:4548–4552.
39. Blaustein MP. Calcium transport and buffering in neurons. *Trends Neurosci* 1988;11(10):438–443.
40. Stys PK, Waxman SG, Ransom BR. Ionic mechanisms of anoxic injury in mammalian CNS white matter: role of Na^+ channels and Na^+–Ca^{2+} exchanger. *J Neurosci* 1992;12:430–439.
41. Stafstrom CE, Shwindt PC, Chubb MC, Crill WE. Properties of persistent sodium conductance and calcium conductance of layer V neurons from cat sensorimotor cortex. *J Neurophys* 1985;53:153–170.
42. Stys PK, Sontheimer H, Ransom BR, Waxman SG. Noninactivating, tetrodotoxin-sensitive Na^+ conductance in rat optic nerve axons. *Proc Natl Acad Sci USA* 1993;90:6976–6980.
43. Fern R, Ransom BR, Waxman SG. Voltage-gated calcium channels in CNS white matter: role in anoxic injury. *J Neurophysiol* 1995;74: 369–377.
44. DiPolo R, Beauge L. Regulation of Na–Ca exchange. An overview. *Ann NY Acad Sci* 1991;639:100–111.
45. Schanne FA, Kane AB, Young EE, Farber JL. Calcium-dependence of toxic cell death: a final common pathway. *Science* 1979;206: 700–702.
46. Siesjo BK, Wieloch T. Cerebral metabolism in ischemia: neurochemical basis for therapy. *Br J Anaesth* 1985;57:47–62.
47. Krnjevic K. Adenosine triphosphate-sensitive potassium channels in anoxia. *Stroke* 1990;21(suppl III): 190–193.
48. Somjen GG, Aitken PG, Balestrino M, Herreras O, Kawasaki K. Spreading depression-like depolarization and selective vulnerability of neurons; a brief review. *Stroke* 1990;21:III-179–III-183.
49. Globus MY-T, Busto R, Martinez E, Valdes I, Dietrich WD, Ginsberg MD. Comparative effect of transient global ischemia on extracellular levels of glutamate, glycine, and γ-aminobutyric acid in vulnerable and nonvulnerable brain regions in the rat. *J Neurochem* 1991;57:470–478.
50. Dubinsky JM, Rothman SM. Intracellular calcium concentrations during ''chemical hypoxia'' and excitotoxic neuronal injury. *J Neurosci* 1991;11:2545-2551.
51. Fern R, Ransom BR, Stys PK, Waxman SG. Pharmacological protection of CNS white matter during anoxia: actions of phenytoin, carbamazepine and diazepam. *J Pharmacol Exp Ther* 1993;266:1549–1555.
52. Stys PK. Protective effects of antiarrhythmic agents against anoxic injury in CNS white matter. *J Cereb Blood Flow Metab* 1995;15: 425–432.
53. Stys PK, Ransom BR, Waxman SG. Tertiary and quarternary local anesthetics protect CNS white matter from anoxic injury at concentrations that do not block excitability. *J Neurophysiol* 1992;67:236–240.
54. Reuter H. Ins and outs of Ca^{2+} transport. *Nature* 1991;349: 567–568.

Cerebrovascular Disease, edited by H. Hunt Batjer.
Lippincott-Raven Publishers, Philadelphia © 1997.

CHAPTER 25

Protection of the Brain from Ischemia

Ted M. Dawson and Valina L. Dawson

Ischemic neuronal injury occurs through mechanisms directly related to the initial ischemic event. The brain requires a continuous supply of oxygen and glucose to maintain normal function and viability. Loss of this supply for only a few minutes can trigger a cascade of events leading to further neuronal cell death through amplification of a variety of secondary pathologic processes set in motion by ischemia. These secondary pathways, which may significantly contribute to the overall neuronal injury, arise from derangements in normal metabolic and physiologic functions. Thus, both restoration of blood supply and control of these secondary processes limit ischemic neuronal damage and represent areas of active research. Though many such pathways have been proposed, the most extensively investigated mediators include glutamate, intracellular calcium, nitric oxide, and free radicals. This chapter will focus on emerging strategies for control of the secondary processes that accompany ischemia.

EXCITOTOXICITY

Olney coined the term ''excitotoxicity'' for the conditions that result from excessive activation of glutamate receptors leading to neuronal injury or death (1). Glutamate is the major excitatory neurotransmitter in the mammalian central nervous system (CNS) (2) (Fig. 1). It is released into the synapse following presynaptic depolarization and is inactivated by sodium-dependent reuptake. Glutamate receptors play a role in ischemic neuronal damage through their involvement in excitotoxicity. Glutamate acts postsynaptically at four major types of receptors. At least 20 separate genes encode the subunits of these receptors and many combinations of subunits and alternative splicing occur (3). The metabotropic glutamate receptor is linked to phosphatidylinositol turnover and possibly other second- messenger systems.

T. M. Dawson and V. L. Dawson: Departments of Neurology, Neuroscience, and Physiology, The Johns Hopkins University School of Medicine, Baltimore, Maryland 21287.

The other three receptors are ligand-gated cation channels named by their prototypic agonist. The α-amino-3-hydroxy-5-methyl-4-isoxazoleproprionate (AMPA) and kainate receptors are linked to a cation channel that normally passes sodium but little calcium under most conditions. The N-methyl-D-aspartate (NMDA) receptor is a cation channel that passes both calcium and sodium. Calcium that enters the cell through the NMDA receptor is capable of activating a variety of cellular enzymes including proteases, kinases, phospholipases, and nitric oxide synthase (NOS) (Fig. 1). Some variants of AMPA and kainate receptors are coupled to ion channels that are permeable to calcium (4). Furthermore, stimulation of any of the ionotropic glutamate receptors results in membrane depolarization and indirect activation of voltage-dependent calcium channels (5). Calcium influx can also trigger the mobilization of additional calcium from intracellular stores, which can contribute to excitotoxic damage (6).

Primary neurons grown in culture die when exposed to glutamate from excess excitation of glutamate receptors (7). Neuronal death through activation of non-NMDA receptors can occur rapidly over the course of several minutes, or cell death through activation of NMDA receptors may be delayed over the course of 24 hours. Although a number of neurons may die in the initial rapid phase, most neurons instead suffer a delayed cell death. The rapid phase of death is characterized by neuronal swelling that leads to osmotic lysis of the neurons and can be prevented by eliminating sodium or chloride, two ions responsible for the massive influx of water when glutamate-gated cation channels are open. Delayed cell death is primarily caused by NMDA receptor activation and in most cases is calcium-dependent (8). Delayed cell death is not dependent on acute neuronal swelling because blockade of the acute toxicity does not prevent the progression of delayed neurotoxicity. The elevation of intraneuronal calcium need not be prolonged to produce neuronal damage. Since glutamate levels rise in the central nervous system following ischemia, excitotoxic damage from activation of NMDA and non-NMDA receptors could enhance neuronal injury.

Ischemia

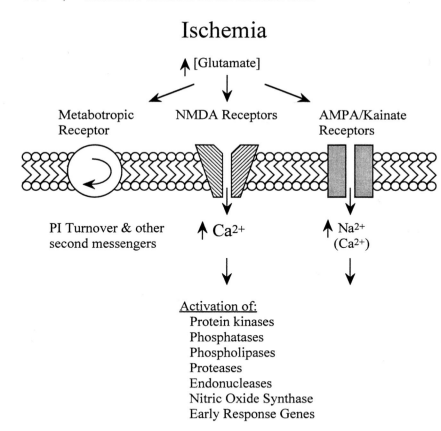

FIG. 1. Ischemic neuronal damage. Ischemia leads to an increase in extracellular glutamate, which acts at multiple postsynaptic receptors. Activation of AMPA/kainate (AMPA = α-amino-3-hydroxy-5-methyl-4-isoxazoleproprionate) receptors leads to sodium influx and depolarization of the neuron. A subset of AMPA/kainate receptors are able to flux calcium (Ca^{2-}) directly. Depolarization relieves the magnesium blockade of the NMDA receptor. Calcium directly fluxes through the NMDA receptor channel. Calcium then acts on many cellular processes to cause long-term changes or excitotoxicity.

Understanding the role of NMDA receptors in ischemic neuronal damage requires a discussion of the unusual pharmacologic properties of the NMDA receptor. It has an agonist binding site for glutamate and requires glycine as a co-agonist (9). Magnesium blocks the channel at normal resting membrane potential but is removed by depolarization (9). Thus, calcium enters only if the cell has recently been depolarized, so that this receptor may act as a molecular coincidence detector. A variety of pharmacologic agents interact with the NMDA receptor. The open channel is blocked by agents such as dizolcipine (MK 801), dextromethorphan, and ketamine (10). Competitive antagonists of glutamate and glycine also prevent channel opening. Polyamines such as spermine and spermidine increase channel opening probability and frequency at low concentration but block the channel at higher concentrations (11). Divalent cations such as magnesium have multiple effects on the NMDA receptor and a site for redox reagents has also been characterized (10). The noncompetitive antagonist ifenprodil may block the receptor directly or through antagonism of polyamine effects (12). Clinical drugs and drugs of abuse also act at the NMDA receptor. Dextromethorphan, ketamine, and the amantadine derivative memantine all block the ion channel of the NMDA receptor (10), and the new anticonvulsant felbamate may also act here. Phencyclidine (PCP) is a potent NMDA receptor blocker and is thought to exert its psychotomimetic effects through its action at the NMDA ion channel (10).

A variety of evidence implicates NMDA receptors and excitotoxicity in focal ischemia and non-NMDA receptors may play a more important role in global ischemia. Glutamate levels rise several fold in the brain following ischemia, beginning the cascade of excitotoxicity. The hippocampal formation, which has the highest levels of excitatory amino acid receptors, is easily damaged in cerebral ischemia (13). Blockade of either NMDA or non-NMDA receptors decreases the damage from ischemia in in vitro models of stroke (13). Antagonists at the glutamate, glycine, and channel sites of the NMDA receptor can lessen neuronal damage in animal models of focal ischemia and antagonists of non-NMDA receptors prevent neuronal damage in global ischemia (13,14). In addition, a variety of physiologic measures of secondary neuronal damage are blocked by NMDA receptor antagonists. Consistent with the concept of an excitotoxic cascade, NMDA receptor antagonists block the increase in excitatory amino acid release following focal ischemia (13,14). More importantly, the functional sequelae of ischemia are prevented in part by blockade of NMDA receptors. All of these results suggest an excitotoxic component to secondary neuronal damage following ischemia. Non-NMDA receptor antagonists are also neuroprotective in a variety of models and blockade of both NMDA and non-NMDA receptors provides additional protection.

With the wealth of animal data, human trials of glutamate receptor antagonists would seem a reasonable approach. At present, such studies are limited both by the timing of administration of potential protective agents and by side effects. The results from animal studies examining excitotoxic mechanisms in stroke emphasize the necessity of treating animals before the initial event or shortly following it. This obviously limits such therapies in clinical practice, though a few agents may be able to limit damage even when given hours after the initial insult (10,13). Because of the diversity of glutamatergic neurotransmission, total blockade of glutamate receptors causes a variety of side effects (10). The most important of these include coma and psychosis observed with MK 801, consistent with the similarity in mechanism between this agent and phencyclidine (PCP). Approaches to solving this problem include use of partial agonists at the various regulatory sites of the glutamate receptors, as well as development of more selective drugs for each site.

Newly discovered findings from molecular biological approaches elucidating the structure of NMDA receptors may help to direct the search for clinically useful NMDA receptor antagonists. The receptor is likely constructed of a key subunit (designated NMDA R1) that combines with a series of other subunits (designated NMDA R2A, 2B, 2C, and 2D) to create a functional ion channel (3,15). In the brain different combinations of these subunits likely associate to create subtypes of NMDA receptors. Each of these subunits conveys specific properties. By ligand binding assays the glycine site is localized to the NR 1 subunit, whereas stimulatory effects of polyamines and high-affinity inhibition by ifenprodil are mediated by the NR 2B subunit (16). Combinations of these subunits also have different physiologic properties and may confer differing susceptibilities to excitotoxicity on cells in culture (Anegawa NS, Lynch DR, and Pritchett D, personal communication). Each subunit also has a limited distribution within the brain. These differences raise the possibility that more selective agents that interact with only one subtype of receptor would allow selective targeting for specific therapeutic purposes. Thus development of agents to act at restricted sites in the brain or developing agents that block specific excitotoxic properties of each subtype may lessen the probability of significant side effects. Approaches aimed at investigating the characteristics of NMDA subtypes present an area for development of new agents to lessen damage in cerebral infarction.

INTRACELLULAR CALCIUM

The calcium-mediated effects of glutamate receptor activation leading to neuronal injury and death may involve a number of different pathways. Intracellular calcium is important for a number of physiologic processes, but excessive amounts may contribute to the overstimulation of normal processes, thus damaging neurons. Normally, intracellular calcium is tightly controlled in the range of 100 nM and is regulated by transport systems in the plasmalemma, the mitochondria, the nucleus, and the endoplasmic reticulum.

Ischemia rapidly affects cellular ion regulation through impairment of energy metabolism, plasma membrane integrity, ion translocation systems, and transmembrane signaling. Altered regulation of intracellular calcium plays a key role in processes leading to irreversible injury (17). Elevation of intraneuronal calcium levels activate a series of enzymes, including protein kinases, proteases, phospholipases, endonucleases, protein phosphatases, NOS, and the expression of several immediate-early genes (Fig. 1). Excessive activation of any of these enzymes could contribute to neuronal injury and a variety of studies have indicated that antagonists of these enzymes are protective in both in vivo and in vitro models of ischemia. Phospholipases can mediate much of the membrane damage that accompanies stroke and probably accounts for the mitochondrial swelling and the ultimate plasmalemmal decay that occurs in cell death (17). Calcium-activated proteases, such as calpains, appear to be capable of modifying the calcium-dependent ATPase in the plasma membrane as well as cytoskeletal components. Since much of the damage from excitotoxicity is mediated through intracellular calcium, attempts have been made to limit neuronal damage by blockade of calcium channels. In models of ischemia in tissue culture, dihydropyridine calcium channel antagonists protect neurons from death (13). Blockade of neuronal damage by calcium channel antagonists is potentiated by blockade of NMDA receptors. In addition, blockers of intracellular calcium release channels are also neuroprotective in in vitro models (6). Calcium channels blockers thus represent another possible method to decrease cytotoxic effects of intracellular calcium on neurons following ischemia. However, they may prove less efficacious for several reasons. Calcium channel antagonists have direct effects on blood vessels and they may have substantial side effects when given systemically. In addition, the source of calcium may affect its ability to cause toxicity. They may, however, serve as agents that add to the efficacy of glutamate receptor antagonists.

REACTIVE OXYGEN SPECIES

The inherent biochemical and physiologic characteristics of the brain, including high lipid concentrations and energy requirements, make it particularly susceptible to free radical–mediated insult. In ischemia, oxygen free radicals can be generated in excess of a cell's antioxidant capacity resulting in severe damage to cellular constituents including proteins, DNA, and lipids. The oxygen species that are typically linked to oxidative stress are superoxide anion, hydroxyl radical ($\cdot$OH), hydrogen peroxide (H_2O_2), nitric oxide ($NO\cdot$), and peroxynitrite (ONOO-). The collective term often used for these molecules is reactive oxygen species (ROS). Generation of these species from molecular oxygen is a normal aspect of mammalian respiration (18).

Ischemia results in the formation of ROS probably through activation of excitotoxic processes, in particular activation of the NMDA receptor. NMDA receptor-mediated stimulation of phospholipase A_2 and the subsequent release of arachidonic acid, prostaglandins, leukotrienes, thromboxanes, and platelet-activating factor leads to a variety of toxic events. Platelet-activating factor increases neuronal calcium levels, apparently by stimulating the release of glutamate. Arachidonic acid potentiates NMDA-evoked currents and inhibits reuptake of glutamate into astrocytes and neurons, further exacerbating the situation. Oxygen free radicals can be formed during arachidonic acid metabolism, leading to further phospholipase A_2 activation, which represents positive feedback. These processes can cause the neuron to digest itself by protein breakdown, free radical formation, and lipid peroxidation. Furthermore, arachidonic acid metabolites may exert untoward vascular effects on the affected area. In cerebral ischemia, tissue reperfusion increases this damage by providing additional free radicals in the form of superoxide anions. Under conditions of calcium elevation and energy failure, xanthine dehydrogenase is converted to xanthine oxidase, the activity of which results in $O_2^{\cdot-}$ formation. Elevations in intracellular calcium following NMDA receptor activation lead to the activation of neuronal NOS (nNOS) and formation of $NO^{\cdot}$ (19). Formation of $NO^{\cdot}$ in the presence of excess $O_2^{\cdot-}$ is likely to result in ONOO- formation and subsequent oxidation of intracellular components.

The chemical reactivity of ROS varies significantly. Perhaps the most potent and reactive species is the $^{\cdot}OH$. The $^{\cdot}OH$ reacts with almost all molecules in living cells (20). The estimated diffusion distance is 3 Å or one tenth the diameter of a typical protein (20). Consequently, where $^{\cdot}OH$ is formed is where the damage will occur. $^{\cdot}OH$ long has been implicated to be the primary toxic mediator of damage to proteins, carbohydrates, DNA, and lipids. However, there is a dissociation between the sources of $^{\cdot}OH$ generation and the proposed targets for toxic reaction. Although $^{\cdot}OH$ undoubtedly mediates some toxic events, it likely is not the only mediator of toxicity.

The superoxide anion $O_2^{\cdot-}$ is generated by multiple pathways and is often placed at the start of an oxidative stress cascade. The brain derives most of its energy exclusively from oxidative respiration through the mitochondrial electron transport chain. Mitochondria are located throughout the neuronal perikarya and its processes. During the production of ATP there is a small high-energy electron leak (1–3%) resulting in the generation of $O_2^{\cdot-}$ (21). $O_2^{\cdot-}$ is also produced by cells involved in the host immune response such as neutrophils, monocytes, macrophages/microglia, and in the brain in the response to neuronal injury. Extracellularly the diffusion limit of $O_2^{\cdot-}$ is estimated to be approximately 20 μm. Intracellularly, $O_2^{\cdot-}$ is constrained by membranes that it cannot cross.

It is likely that most of the $O_2^{\cdot-}$ generated in a cell undergoes superoxide dismutase (SOD)–catalyzed conversion to H_2O_2, which is diffusible within and between cells. In addition to the dismutation of $O_2^{\cdot-}$, H_2O_2 can be produced by the action of several oxidase enzymes including xanthine oxidase. H_2O_2 is effectively scavenged by glutathione peroxidase and catalase (22).

$NO^{\cdot}$ is synthesized on demand by the enzyme NOS from the essential amino acid L-arginine. Molecular cloning experiments have led to the identification of three NOS genes, neuronal NOS (nNOS), endothelial NOS (eNOS), and immunologic NOS (iNOS) that were named by the tissue from which they were first cloned. All three isoforms have been identified in numerous tissues. $NO^{\cdot}$ is small, diffusible, membrane-permeable, and reactive. It is rapidly being recognized as an important biological messenger molecule in the fields of immunology, cardiovascular pharmacology, toxicology, and neurobiology (19,23). In the nervous system, $NO^{\cdot}$ as a messenger molecule is changing the conventional concepts of neuronal communication. The biochemical reactions involving $NO^{\cdot}$ are not well characterized. $NO^{\cdot}$ can react with molecular oxygen (O_2) yielding nitrogen dioxide (NO_2) rapidly in the gas phase at high concentrations of reactants but in solution at physiologically relevant concentrations the $t_{1/2}$ is several hours, indicating that O_2 is not the primary biochemical target of $NO^{\cdot}$ (24).

Probably the most important oxidant involved in the genesis of neurotoxicity is peroxynitrite (ONOO-) (Fig. 2). ONOO- is formed from the reaction of $NO^{\cdot}$ with $O_2^{\cdot-}$ (25). In vitro the rate of this reaction is three times faster than the rate of reaction of the enzyme, superoxide dismutase (SOD), in catalyzing the dismutation of the $O_2^{\cdot-}$ to H_2O_2. Therefore, when present at appropriate concentrations, $NO^{\cdot}$ can effectively compete with SOD for $O_2^{\cdot-}$. Although a simple molecule, ONOO- is chemically complex. It has the activity of the $^{\cdot}OH$ and the $NO_2^{\cdot}$ although it does not readily decompose into these entities. ONOO- can also directly nitrate and hydroxylate aromatic rings on amino acid residues. It is also a potent oxidant that reacts readily with sulfhydryls, with zinc thiolate, lipids, proteins, and DNA (25,26).

Under normal physiologic conditions $NO^{\cdot}$ is predominantly a neuronal messenger molecule. However, when present in higher concentrations, $NO^{\cdot}$ can initiate a neurotoxic cascade (Fig. 3) (19). $NO^{\cdot}$ is formed following NMDA receptor activation, increases in intracellular calcium, and stimulation of nNOS. NMDA neurotoxicity is mediated in large part through this pathway. Treatment of cortical cultures with NOS inhibitors or removal of L-arginine from the media blocks NMDA neurotoxicity (27). Additionally, reduced hemoglobin, which binds $NO^{\cdot}$ and prevents it from reaching its target cells, completely prevents NMDA neurotoxicity. Blockade of NMDA neurotoxicity by NOS inhibitors is also observed in cultures of caudate-putamen and hippocampus. Additionally, cortical cultures from transgenic mice that lack neuronal NOS are relatively resistant to NMDA neurotoxicity (28). If $NO^{\cdot}$ is the mediator of NMDA neurotoxicity, then compounds that release $NO^{\cdot}$ directly should also be neurotoxic. Cortical cultures exposed to the $NO^{\cdot}$ donors, sodium nitroprusside (SNP), S-nitroso-N-acetylpenicillamine (SNAP), or 3-morpholino-sydnonimine-hydrochloride (SIN-1) exhibit a delayed neurotoxicity that follows the same time course as NMDA neurotoxicity (27).

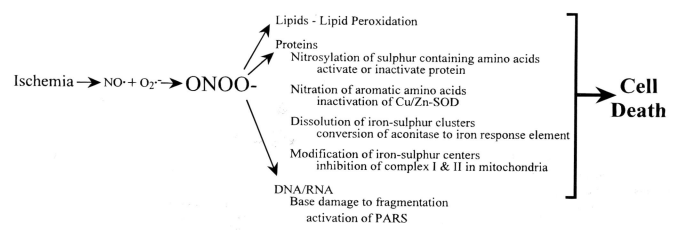

FIG. 2. ONOO- neurotoxicity. NO˙ and $O_2^{\cdot-}$ combine to form peroxynitrite. Both NO˙ and $O_2^{\cdot-}$ levels increase during ischemia and peroxynitrite is thought to be the major toxic moiety. Peroxynitrite is highly reactive and can damage a number of cellular processes leading to cell death.

The mechanism of NO˙ neurotoxicity likely involves the formation of ONOO- as neurotoxicity elicited by NO˙ donors is attenuated by the removal of $O_2^{\cdot-}$ by superoxide dismutase (27).

NOS catalytic activity can be inhibited at regulatory sites other than the catalytic site thus providing alternative strategies for protection against NO˙-mediated cell death. The flavoproteins, FAD and FMN, are critical for the necessary shuttling of electrons involved in the conversion of L-arginine to NO˙ and L-citrulline. The flavoprotein inhibitor diphenyleneiodonium is potently neuroprotective against NMDA neurotoxicity, although it is unlikely to be therapeutically useful. Calmodulin is an essential cofactor of NOS. Agents that inhibit or bind calmodulin such as calmidazolium or W7 decrease NOS catalytic activity and provide neuroprotection. Certain gangliosides also bind calmodulin. Gangliosides are neuroprotective in a variety of animal models possibly due in part to inhibition of NOS. Gangliosides inhibit NOS activity and the potency of NOS inhibition closely parallels their affinities for binding calmodulin and providing neuroprotection (29). Phosphorylation of NOS and the attendant reduction of its catalytic activity also provides another potential approach to neuroprotection. The immunosuppressants FK 506 and cyclosporin A bind small, soluble receptor proteins designated FK 506–binding proteins (FKBP) and cyclophilins, respectively. This complex binds to and inhibits the calcium-activated phosphatase, calcineurin. Inhibition of calcineurin prevents the dephosphorylation and activation of NOS; thus NOS remains in the inactive phosphorylated state (29). FK 506 is potently neuroprotective against NMDA neurotoxicity (30). The physiologic relevance of this observation was recently confirmed by the report that FK 506 is profoundly neuroprotective in a rat model of focal ischemia (31).

Most NOS inhibitors are not useful in the study of nNOS function in the CNS of intact animals. For instance, experiments with nonselective NOS inhibitors are confounded by inhibition of eNOS, which results in hypertension and alterations in cerebral blood flow. The lack of specificity of NOS inhibitors has confounded in vivo investigations of NO˙ particularly in the role of NO˙ in stroke. Following cerebrovascular infarction, release of excitatory amino acids in the extracellular space stimulates NMDA receptors, increasing NOS activity and NO˙ levels. Marked increases in NO˙ production in the brain occur during focal ischemia (32). Once formed, NO˙ can react with the $O_2^{\cdot-}$, levels of which are also increased during ischemia, to form ONOO-. If ONOO-is the toxin of physiologic importance, then one would expect that inhibiting accumulation of $O_2^{\cdot-}$, or decreasing production of NO˙, would be associated with decreased brain injury after focal ischemia. Consistent with this notion is the observation that in animals treated with SOD before focal ischemia and in transgenic mice that overexpress SOD, the

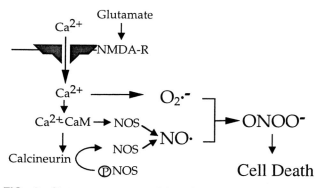

FIG. 3. Glutamate neurotoxicity. Glutamate activates the NMDA receptor allowing calcium (Ca^{2-}) to enter the cell. Calcium binds calmodulin (CaM) and activates nitric oxide synthase (NOS) and calcineurin. Calcineurin dephosphorylates NOS. NMDA receptor activation may activate other free radical–generating enzymes producing $O_2^{\cdot-}$. NO˙, and $O_2^{\cdot-}$ combine to form ONOO-, which leads to cell death.

infarct volume following focal ischemia is markedly attenuated (33). In a similar manner, NOS inhibitors reduce infarct volume following middle cerebral artery occlusion in mice, rats, and cats (19). Recent studies show that low doses of NOS inhibitors are neuroprotective whereas high doses are ineffective, suggesting that partial inhibition of neuronal NOS is sufficient to obtain an optimal neuroprotective effect (34). Exacerbation of injury occurs at high doses of NOS inhibitors through adverse vascular effects from inhibition of endothelial NOS, resulting in decreased regional cerebral blood flow and increased infarction volume. Further support for this hypothesis is the recent study in transgenic mice that lack nNOS. These mice have reduced infarct volumes compared to age-matched wild-type controls following focal permanent middle cerebral artery occlusion (35). When the nNOS null mice are treated with the NOS inhibitor, nitro-L-arginine methyl ester, the dilatation of the pial vessels is inhibited and stroke volume is increased. Thus, neuronally derived NO˙ plays an important role in mediating neuronal cell death following focal ischemia and endothelially derived NO˙ plays an important protective role by regulating and maintaining proper cerebral blood flow.

What are the cellular targets for NO˙ or ONOO- that result in neuronal cell death? Several investigations have determined that it is not activation of guanylyl cyclase (19). The toxic effects of NO˙-may occur through multiple mechanisms. One pathway that has been implicated is NO˙-damaged DNA and subsequent activation of the nuclear enzyme poly(ADP-ribose) synthetase (PARS) (Fig. 4) (36). Once activated, PARS catalyzes the attachment of ADP ribose units to nuclear proteins, such as histone and PARS itself (37). For every mole of ADP ribose transferred, 1 mole of NAD is consumed and four free energy equivalents of ATP are consumed to regenerate NAD. Thus, activation of PARS can rapidly deplete energy stores. Consistent with this possibility is that cortical cell cultures are protected from glutamate and NO˙ neurotoxicity by a series of PARS inhibitors

TABLE 1. *Protective strategies to limit neuronal damage from ischemia*

Site or mode of action	Drug class
Restoration of blood flow	Thrombolytic agents
Decrease glutamate release	Adenosine derivatives
	Sodium channel blockers
	Calcium channel blockers
Glutamate receptors	NMDA receptor antagonists
	NMDA-glycine binding site antagonists
	NMDA-polyamine binding site modulators
	non-NMDA antagonists
Downstream from glutamate receptors	Antioxidants
	Free radical scavengers
	Inhibitors of lipid peroxidation
	Nitric oxide synthase inhibitors
	Protease inhibitors
	Phosphatase inhibitors
	Growth factors
	Apoptosis inhibitors
	Phospholipase inhibitors
	Platelet-activating factor antagonists
	Cytokine antagonists
Miscellaneous	Hypothermia

NMDA, *N*-methyl-D-aspartate.

(36). The neuroprotective effects of these agents parallels their potency as PARS inhibitors.

CONCLUSIONS

Understanding the basic mechanisms of cell death in ischemia and related conditions is just beginning. It is likely that the importance of glutamatergic damage, NO˙-related damage, and free radical effects will vary in different models of stroke. Other potential therapeutic targets exist as well (Table 1). Side effects elicited by inhibition of these various

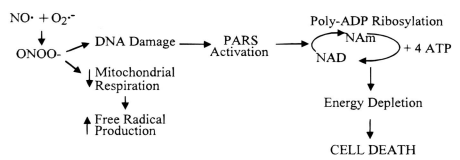

FIG. 4. PARS activation kills neurons. NO˙ and O_2^- combine to form ONOO- during ischemia. These free radicals then damage DNA and also inhibit mitochondrial function leading to more free radical formation. The damaged DNA activates poly(ADP-ribose) synthetase (PARS), which transfers ADP-ribose groups to nuclear proteins from NAD. NAD is resynthesized from nicotinamide (NAm), a reaction that consumes four high-energy equivalents of ATP. Poly(ADP-ribose) synthetase is highly promiscuous and adds numerous ADP-ribose groups to nuclear proteins consuming a very large amount of energy. NMDA-induced free radicals such as NO˙ activate a futile cycle of DNA damage followed by poly(ADP-ribose) synthetase activation, which depletes cells of their energy stores, ultimately leading to cell death.

pathways may limit the potential therapeutic value of these agents. However, blockade of these mechanisms represents an area with potential for novel clinical strategies in the near future.

ACKNOWLEDGMENTS

VLD is supported by grants from USPHS NS33142 and the American Heart Association. TMD is supported by grants from the USPHS NS01578, NS33277, and the Paul Beeson Physician Scholars in Aging Research Program and International Life Sciences Institute. TMD owns stock in and is entitled to royalties from Guilford Pharmaceuticals, Inc., which is developing technology related to the research described in this chapter. The stock has been placed in escrow and cannot be sold until a certain date as predetermined by The Johns Hopkins University.

REFERENCES

1. Olney JW. Neurotoxicity of excitatory amino acids. In: McGeer EG, Olney JW, McGeer Pl, eds. *Kainic acid as a tool in neurobiology.* New York: Raven Press, 1978:95–121.
2. Gasic GP, Hollmann M. Molecular neurobiology of glutamate receptors. *Annu Rev Physiol* 1992;54:507–536.
3. Nakanishi S. Molecular diversity of glutamate receptors and implications for brain function. *Science* 1992;258:597–603.
4. Hollmann M, Harley M, Heinemann S. Ca^{2-} permeability of KA-AMPA-gated glutamate receptor channels depends on subunit composition. *Science* 1991:252:851–853.
5. Siesjo BK. Calcium-mediated processes in neuronal degeneration. *Ann N Y Acad Sci* 1994;747:140–61.
6. Frandsen A. Schousboe A. Mobilization of dantrolene-sensitive intracellular calcium pools is involved in the cytotoxicity induced by quisqualate and N-methyl-D-aspartate but not by 2-amino-3-(3-hydroxy-5-methylisoxazol-4-yl)propionate and kainate in cultured cerebral cortical neurons. *Proc Natl Acad Sci USA* 1992;89:2590–2594.
7. Choi DW. Calcium mediated neurotoxicity: relationship to specific channel types and role in ischemic damage. *Trends Neurosci* 1988;7:357–368.
8. Choi DW. Glutamate neurotoxicity and diseases of the nervous system. *Neuron* 1988;1:623–634.
9. Collingridge GL, Lester RAJ. Excitatory amino acid receptors in the vertebrate central nervous system. *Pharmacol Rev* 1989;41:143– 210.
10. Lipton S, Rosenberg PA. Excitatory amino acids as a final common pathway for neurologic disorders. *N Engl J Med* 1994;330:613–622.
11. Rock DM, MacDonald RL. The polyamine spermine has multiple actions on N-methyl-D-aspartate receptor single-channel currents in cultured cortical neurons. *Mol Pharmacol* 1992; 41:83–88.
12. Reynolds IJ, Miller RJ. Ifenprodil is a novel type of N-methyl-D-aspartate receptor antagonist: interaction with polyamines. *Mol Pharmacol* 1989;36:758–765.
13. Choi DW. Cerebral hypoxia: some new approaches and unanswered questions. *J Neurosci* 1990;10:2493–2501.
14. Meldrum B, Garthwaite J. Excitatory amino acid neurotoxicity and neurodegenerative disease. *Trends Pharmacol Sci* 1990;11:379–387.
15. Monyer H, Sprengel R, Schoepfer R, Herb A, Higuchi M, Lomeli H, Burnashev N, Sakmann B, Seeburg PH. Heteromeric NMDA receptors: molecular and functional distinction of subtypes. *Science* 1992;256: 1217–1221.
16. Lynch DR, Anegawa NJ, Verdoorn T, Pritchett DB. N-methyl-d-aspartate receptors: different subunit requirement for binding of glutamate antagonists, glycine antagonists and channel blocking agents. *Mol Pharmacol* 1994;45:540–545.
17. Trump BF, Berezesky IK. Calcium-mediated cell injury and cell death. *FASEB J* 1995;9:219–228.
18. Chance B, Sies H, Boveris A. Hydroperoxide metabolism in mammalian organs. *Physiol Rev* 1992;59: 527–605.
19. Dawson TM, Snyder SH Gases as biological messengers: nitric oxide and carbon monoxide in the brain. *J Neurosci* 1994;14: 5147–5159.
20. Beckman JS. Peroxynitrite versus hydroxyl radical: the role of nitric oxide in superoxide-dependent cerebral injury. *Ann NY Acad Sci* 1994; 738:69–75.
21. Fridovich I. Superoxide dismutases. *Meth Enzymol* 1986;58:61–97.
22. Cohen G, Hochstein P. Glutathione peroxidase: the primary agent for the elimination of hydrogen peroxide in erythrocytes. *Biochemistry* 1963;2:1420–1428.
23. Moncada S, Higgs A The L-arginine-nitric oxide pathway. *N Engl J Med* 1993;329: 2002–2012.
24. Butler AR, Flitney FW and Williams DLH. NO, nitrosonium ions, nitroxide ions, nitrosothiols and iron-nitrosyls in biology: a chemists perspective. *Trends Pharmacol Sci* 1995;16: 18–22.
25. Radi R, Beckman JS, Bush KM, Freeman BA. Peroxynitrite induced membrane lipid peroxidation. The cytotoxic potential of superoxide and nitric oxide. *Arch Biochem Bhiophys* 1991;288: 481–487.
26. Dawson VL, Dawson TM. Free radicals and Neuronal Cell Death. *Cell Death and Differentiation* 1996;3:71–78.
27. Dawson VL, Dawson TM, Bartley DA, Uhl GR, Snyder SH. Mechanisms of nitric oxide mediated neurotoxicity in primary brain cultures. *J Neurosci* 1993;13:2651–2661.
28. Dawson VL, Kizushi VM, Huang PL, Snyder SH, Dawson TM. Resistance to Neurotoxicity in Cortical Cultures from Neuronal Nitric Oxide Synthase Deficient Mice. *J Neurosci* 1996;16:2479–2487.
29. Dawson TM, Hung K, Dawson VL, Steiner JP, Snyder SH. Neuroprotective effects of gangliosides may involve inhibition of nitric oxide synthase. *Ann Neurol* 1995;37: 115–118.
30. Dawson TM, Steiner JP, Dawson VL, Dinerman JL, Uhl GR, Snyder SH. Immunosuppressant, FK506 enhances phosphorylation of nitric oxide synthase and protects against glutamate neurotoxicity. *Proc Natl Acad Sci USA* 1993;90:9808–9812.
31. Sharkey J, Butcher SP. Immunophillins mediate the neuroprotective effects of FK506 in focal cerebral ischemia. *Nature* 1994;371:336–339.
32. Malinski T, Bailey F, Zhang ZG, Chopp M. Nitric oxide measured by a porphyrinic microsensor in rat brain after transient middle cerebral artery occlusion. *J Cereb Blood Flow Metab* 1993;13:355–358.
33. Kinouchi H, Epstein CJ, Mizue T. Attenuation of focal cerebral ischemic injury in transgenic mice overexpressing CuZn superoxide dismutase. *Proc Natl Acad Sci USA* 1991;88:11158–11162.
34. Carreau A, Duval D, Poignet H, Scatton B, Vige X, Nowicki J-P. Neuroprotective efficacy of N^{ω}-nitro-L-arginine after focal cerebral ischemia in the mouse and inhibition of cortical nitric oxide synthase. *Eur J Pharmacol* 1994;256:241–249.
35. Huang Z, Huang PL, Panahian N, Dalkara T, Fishman MC and Moskowtiz MA. Effects of cerebral ischemia in mice deficient in neuronal nitric oxide synthase. *Science* 1994;265:1883–1885.
36. Zhang J, Dawson VL, Dawson TM, Snyder SH. Nitric oxide activation of poly (ADP-ribose) synthetase in neurotoxicity. *Science* 1994;263: 687–689.
37. Lautier D, Lagueux J, Thibodeau J, Menard L, Poirier GG. Molecular and biochemical features of poly(ADP-ribose) metabolism. *Mol Cell Biochem* 1993;122:171–193.

Cerebrovascular Disease, edited by H. Hunt Batjer.
Lippincott-Raven Publishers, Philadelphia © 1997.

CHAPTER 26

Anesthetic Considerations for Carotid Endarterectomy

René Tempelhoff, Mary Ann Cheng, Shailendra Joshi, and William L. Young

Carotid endarterectomy (CEA) entails occlusion of the common, external, and internal carotid arteries and removal of atheromatous plaque from the arterial lumen. This plaque may serve as a source of emboli, resulting in transient or permanent ischemic syndromes. Less frequently, the plaque serves as a hindrance to adequate cerebral blood flow; more commonly, it limits the cerebrovascular reserve. Despite a major decrease in indications for this procedure in the mid-1980s, it has regained popularity for the treatment of patients with symptomatic and, more recently, asymptomatic disease (1).

There are a number of challenges in anesthetizing the CEA patient. The two primary perioperative complications of CEA are myocardial infarction and stroke, the occurrence of which may be influenced by anesthetic management. Myocardial infarction (MI) is the most frequent cause of perioperative and late death following CEA, occurring in 1–2% of cases (2). The frequency of perioperative stroke ranges from 2% to 6% (3). The incidence of perioperative stroke and MI in selected studies is shown in Tables 1–3 (4–6). Significantly, patients undergoing CEA are frequently in their sixth or seventh decade of life. These patients have comorbid disease processes and age-related changes in pharmacodynamics and pharmacokinetics.

This chapter will focus on some of the basic pathophysio-logic concepts involved in the genesis of cerebral damage and those aspects of anesthetic management that have an impact on the prevention of adverse neurologic outcomes.

CEREBRAL HEMODYNAMICS AND METABOLISM: A BRIEF REVIEW

Anesthesia for surgical procedures complicated by cerebral ischemia requires an understanding of cerebral pathophysiology with respect to ischemia. Cerebral perfusion during such procedures is influenced by preexisting cerebrovascular pathology in addition to the effects of anesthetic management and surgical manipulation of cerebral arterial inflow.

Cerebral Metabolism

The brain is an end-organ requiring about 15% of the cardiac output for its metabolic needs, including 20% of the total body oxygen consumption and 25% of the total body glucose requirement. This high global energy requirement for oxygen ($CMRO_2$), associated with a near-complete lack of reserve substrates, results in a complete dependence on a constant and adequate cerebral perfusion.

Arterial Supply of the Brain

The primary arterial supply to the brain consists of the anterior circulation, comprising the two carotid arteries and their derivations, and the posterior circulation, consisting of the two vertebral arteries that join to form the basilar artery.

Collateral arterial inflow channels are a cornerstone of cerebral-blood-flow compensation during ischemia (Fig. 1). The principal pathways are embodied in the circle of Willis. This hexagonal ring of vessels lies in the subarachnoid space,

R. T. Tempelhoff: Department of Anesthesiology and Neurological Surgery, Washington University School of Medicine, St. Louis, Missouri 63110.

M. A. Cheng: Department of Anesthesiology, Washington University School of Medicine, St. Louis, Missouri 63110.

S. Joshi: Department of Anesthesiology, College of Physicians and Surgeons of Columbia University, Columbia-Presbyterian Medical Center, New York, New York 10032.

W. L. Young: Departments of Anesthesiology, Neurological Surgery and Radiology, College of Physicians and Surgeons of Columbia University, Columbia-Presbyterian Medical Center, New York, New York 10032.

TABLE 1. *Risk groups for patients undergoing carotid endarterectomy*

Medical Risk Factors[a]
Angina
Myocardial infarction <6 months
Congestive heart failure
Severe hypertension
Chronic obstructive pulmonary disease
Obesity
Age >70

Neurologic Factors
Progressing neurologic deficit
Deficit of 24 hours' duration
Frequent daily TIA
Neurologic deficits by multiple cerebral infarctions

Angiographic Risk Factors
Occlusion of the opposite ICA
Stenosis of the ICA in the region of the siphon
Plaque extending >3 cm distally or 5 cm proximally
Bifurcation of the carotid at the level of C-2
Soft thrombus extending from an ulcerative lesion

[a] Diabetes and smoking were not part of this classification but were included in the North American Symptomatic Carotid Endarterectomy Trial (NASCET).

TABLE 2. *Risk groups for patients undergoing carotid Endarterectomy as defined by Sundt and colleagues*

Sundt Group	Medical	Neurologic	Angiographic
I	−	−	−
II	−	−	+
III	+	−	±
IV	±	+	±

(From ref. 4)

TABLE 3. *Reported rates of postoperative MI and stroke following carotid endarterectomy stratified according to the Sundt classification of risk factors[a]*

	Risk Group	n	MI	%	Stroke	%
Sundt et al.	I	129	0	0	1	0.8
(4)	II	56	0	0	1	1.8
	III	76	2	2.6	1	1.3
	IV	70	0	0	7	10
Modica et al.	I	23	0	0	1	4.3
(5)	II	18	0	0	0	0
	III	74	2	2.7	0	0
	IV	56	0	0	1	1.8
Sieber et al.	I	227	1	0.4	4	1.8
(6)[b]	II	61	0	0	6	9.8
	III	196	12	6.1	9	4.6
	IV	77	4	5.2	11	14.3

[a] In all three studies, the rate of MI was highest in risk group III. Stroke rate was highest in risk group IV in two of the three studies. The higher rate of stroke in risk group I found in Modica's study may be explained by the comparatively lower number since only symptomatic patients were included.

[b] This was a retrospective study of the variable over a specific number of preceding periods.

centered about the pituitary gland. In many patients, the circle of Willis is incomplete. The primary "collateral" pathways are the anterior communicating arteries, joining the two carotid circulations, and the posterior communicating arteries, joining the vertebral and carotid circulations bilaterally. Normally, there is probably no net flow through these communicating vessels. These channels are called into play if a pressure differential develops across their span.

When the normal arterial supply is compromised and remedy does not exist from the circle of Willis, other mechanisms may be activated. Adequate intraparenchymal collateral pathways are usually not present between major arterial territories. However, there exists the potential for pial-to-pial (leptomeningeal) communications that bridge "watershed" areas, represented by surface connections between surface branches of the anterior and middle cerebral arteries and the middle and posterior cerebral arteries. These pial-to-pial collaterals may compensate for reduced flow at the periphery of an arterial distribution; if the driving pressure is high enough, pial-to-pial channels may allow for complete retrograde filling of an adjacent arterial territory. However, if systemic pressure is globally reduced, these watershed areas, located farthest from the arterial input, become vulnerable to ischemic damage.

In addition, there exists the potential for communication between the external and internal carotid arteries, most commonly manifested as flow from the external carotid artery via facial pathways through the ophthalmic artery. Thus, retrograde flow may be provided to the circle of Willis. Other pathways that may develop between the intra- and extracranial systems are described elsewhere in this volume.

In summary, an elegant macrocirculatory arrangement is available for recruiting accessory inflow channels to the end-arterial perfusion territories of the brain in the event of acute interruption of a major arterial inflow channel. During normal circumstances, these channels lie dormant, becoming critical only when a pathologic stress is imposed on the circulation. In general, it is the circle of Willis that can be counted on to remedy an acute interruption of the proximal circulation, as during carotid cross-clamping; the other pathways described above are more applicable to the gradual compensation for chronic cerebral insufficiency.

Autoregulation

Cerebral blood flow (CBF) is maintained constant over varying perfusion pressures. This is achieved by regulation of cerebrovascular resistance. Autoregulatory vasomotion takes place primarily in the smaller arteries and arterioles (muscular or resistance vessels), and not the larger arteries that are visible on an angiogram (elastic or conductance vessels).

CBF to normal brain is maintained constant over the often-quoted range of 50–150 mm Hg. It is important to consider that these limits describe population mean values, and there

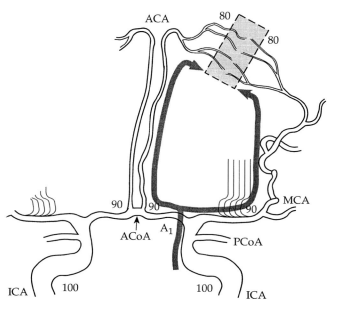

Figure 1 - Panel A

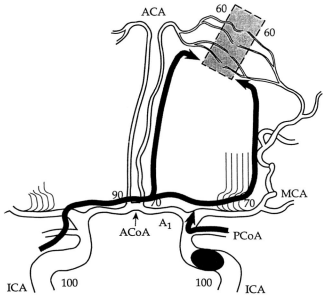

Figure 1 - Panel B

FIG. 1. Collateral pathways. The basic considerations for collateral flow disturbances are presented in the following series of panels. The principal collateral conduits are the anterior communicating artery (ACoA), which connects to the contralateral carotid circulation, and the posterior communicating artery (PCoA), which connects to the vertebrobasilar circulation. The shaded boxes refer to the "watershed" areas between the territories of the anterior cerebral artery (ACA) and middle cerebral artery (MCA) circulations. This is the equal pressure boundary between multiple sources of arterial input pressure and may shift according to changes in vascular anatomy. The *small black triangles* represent regions of hemodynamically significant stenosis in collateral pathways. The *thick gray lines* represent the general sources and direction of arterial flow. The *numbers* represent hypothetical mean arterial pressure (in mm Hg) that might be encountered in each scenario. The *black ovals* represent an obstruction to arterial flow as would be encountered with carotid cross-clamping or a postoperative arterial thrombosis. The arterial pressure values are illustrative only and other potential collateral pathways exist. The lenticulostriate arteries that arise from the first portion of the MCA are seen as multiple thin curved lines. **(A)** Normally, flow supplies the ACA and MCA via the ipsilateral carotid artery. Although they are both patent, no appreciable flow is delivered through the ACoA or PCoA. **(B)** With an occlusion of the internal carotid artery (ICA), pressure decreases in the distal territory, and flow now is recruited from the ACoA and PCoA conduits. The distal watershed remains in the same location, but pressure is reduced significantly. **(C)** With occlusion of the ICA and poor collateral pathways, eg, stenosis of both the ACoA and PCoA conduits, the distal watershed is now severely hypotensive and at risk for infarction. Although not shown in the figure, augmentation of systemic mean arterial pressure would improve the distal cerebral pressure by compensating for the pressure drop across the stenotic conduit pathways. (Adapted from ref. 66, with permission.)

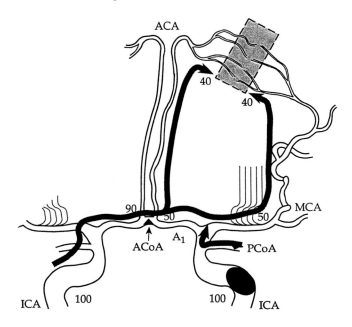

Figure 1 - Panel C

may be considerable variation among individuals. When either the upper or lower limit is exceeded, flow becomes pressure-passive. When mean arterial pressure (MAP) exceeds this range, disruption of the blood–brain barrier, vasogenic edema, and cerebral hemorrhage are possible. Reduction in CBF below the lower limit may lead to ischemia and infarction.

Patients with chronic systemic hypertension will compensate for their higher MAP by shifting the autoregulatory curve to the right. While this makes CBF pressure-dependent at a higher MAP, it protects the blood–brain barrier from disruption at the usual elevated level of systemic arterial pressure. It is not clear what happens to the autoregulatory curve in chronic cerebral hypotension in the setting of occlusive cerebrovascular disease.

One of the most striking differences between the systemic and cerebral circulations is the relative lack of humoral and autonomic influences on regulation of cerebrovascular tone. The systemic circulation is regulated to a large extent by sympathetic nervous activity, whereas autonomic factors do not appear to uniquely control the cerebral circulation. Autonomic influences, however, modify autoregulatory responses in several important ways.

At the lower limits of autoregulation, sympathetic activity will modify the autoregulatory response of CBF to a decrease in blood pressure. At equivalent blood pressures, CBF is lower during hemorrhagic hypotension than during pharmacologically induced hypotension (7). Thus, when reflex sympathetic constriction of larger cerebral arteries in response to hypotension is prevented by acute surgical sympathectomy or α-receptor blockade, CBF is better maintained. This explains in part why drug-induced hypotension during anesthesia is better tolerated than hypotension as a result of hemorrhagic shock.

Carbon Dioxide Reactivity

The most potent extrinsic physiologic determinant of CBF is $Paco_2$. In the physiologic range of 20–80 mm Hg, $Paco_2$ varies directly with CBF. Carbon dioxide reactivity is not significantly affected by clinical doses of anesthetic agents. However, ischemia and brain injury will attenuate carbon dioxide reactivity. Global or regional cerebral hypotension will diminish carbon dioxide reactivity. In severe hypotension, appropriate maximal vasodilation in an attempt to maintain flow in the normal range by autoregulatory relaxation of resistance arterioles will render carbon dioxide ineffective in causing additional vasomotion. This is the basis for using cerebrovascular responsiveness to inhaled carbon dioxide (or acetazolamide, which also acidifies interstitial fluid) as an index of "cerebrovascular reserve" in the assessment of ischemic cerebrovascular disease.

Temperature

Decreasing the temperature of the brain decreases its metabolic rate about 7%/°C. Between 17°C and 27°C, electrical activity of the brain will cease. Unlike pharmacologic suppression of electroencephalogram (EEG), however, decreasing temperature after electrical silence will further decrease cerebral metabolic activity.

Common Anesthetic Drugs

Inhalation Agents

The most commonly used inhaled anesthetics include nitrous oxide and the volatile agent isoflurane. There is evidence that nitrous oxide in humans is a potent cerebral vasodilator when administered alone. When used in addition to isoflurane, nitrous oxide increases CBF 39% under normocapnic conditions, but this increase in CBF is abolished with mild hypocapnia (8). Intracranial pressure is generally not a concern for carotid endarterectomy (CEA), and nitrous oxide has a long history of safety in this setting. However, some animal models have suggested nitrous oxide may have an unfavorable interaction with cerebral ischemia (9,10), but the clinical relevance of these data are unclear.

Although halothane had been the most commonly used neuroanesthetic in the past, it was eclipsed by the introduction of enflurane and isoflurane. Enflurane dropped out of favor in the neurosurgical setting when it was suggested that higher concentrations of enflurane could induce seizure activity when combined with hypocarbia (<30 mm Hg). The current volatile agent of choice since its introduction in 1981 is isoflurane. It depresses $CMRO_2$, while CBF is increased by cerebral vasodilatation. The increase in CBF can be attenuated by hyperventilation since carbon dioxide reactivity is not affected by volatile agents (11). In animal studies, isoflurane is a more potent metabolic depressant than halothane; some authors have advocated isoflurane as the best inhalation agent for CEA on this basis (12). In higher doses, isoflurane can be used to achieve burst suppression on the electroencephalogram. However, studies in CEA patients do not uniformly support a clinically significant difference between anesthetics in their cerebral metabolic depressant effects in the range employed in routine anesthesia (13).

Desflurane is a newly approved inhalational anesthetic and, like nitrous oxide, has a low blood-gas solubility and a resultant rapid onset and recovery (14). Desflurane is a potent airway irritant and may also cause direct sympathetic stimulation and give rise to tachycardia and hypertension. Sevoflurane is the newest of the inhalation agents approved in this country. It is characterized by rapid onset and offset, allowing a fast recovery from anesthesia similar to desflurane, although it is nonirritant to the airway. The clinical data regarding its use in anesthesiology are still sparse. Both sevoflurane and desflurane appear to share the same general effects on cerebral metabolism, dynamics, and electrophysiology as isoflurane (15,16).

Intravenous Agents

The classic intravenous anesthetic drug is thiopental sodium (Pentothal). It decreases $CMRO_2$ with a concomitant decrease in CBF. Pierce et al [17] demonstrated intact carbon dioxide reactivity even at the high doses of thiopental that induce an isoelectric EEG. At these dosages, hemodynamic stability may be jeopardized since thiopental is a myocardial depressant and a venodilator. If titrated carefully in a euvolemic patient, however, it is generally well tolerated [18]. Once the EEG is isoelectric, additional thiopental does not further decrease $CMRO_2$.

The intravenous agents etomidate and propofol have recently been studied as alternatives to thiopental for neuroanesthesia [19,20]. Both agents resemble thiopental in that they decrease both CBF and $CMRO_2$ in a dose-dependent fashion and have shorter effective half-lives than thiopental; burst suppression can be achieved with clinical doses of either agent.

Modica and Tempelhoff [21] demonstrated that etomidate titrated to burst suppression maintains hemodynamic stability while decreasing intracranial pressure (ICP) during endotracheal intubation. Prolonged etomidate infusion causes adrenocortical suppression, and this side effect should be weighed against the indications for its use, primarily impaired myocardial performance. Although unlikely, it is possible there is adrenocortical suppression even after a single dose. The clinical significance of such suppression after a single dose is not known. Prolonged use of an etomidate infusion also carries the risk of renal compromise due to its carrier agent propylene glycol.

The newest intravenous agent, propofol, has an extremely short effective half-life. Burst suppression is possible at clinically useful doses. Its main disadvantage is that it is a potent circulatory depressant, perhaps more so than thiopental. Therefore, any "protective" effects of the drug must be weighed against potential decreases in cerebral perfusion pressure (CPP) [20]. Because of the importance of maintaining CPP in patients at risk for cerebral ischemia, propofol should be used with caution, especially during the induction period.

The much-maligned ketamine has recently been of interest because of its N-methyl-D-aspartate antagonist property. Its ability to block these excitatory receptors has been shown to be protective during ischemia in animal models [22]. In humans, ketamine increases CBF and may minimally increase $CMRO_2$. In addition, clinically it has been shown to increase ICP in patients with and without intracranial pathology and has a marked proconvulsant effect. Although pretreatment with diazepam or thiopental may attenuate these untoward effects, there is little enthusiasm for its use in patients with intracerebral pathology or cerebrovascular disease.

Benzodiazepines are used as premedicants and as adjuncts to other anesthetics due to their favorable amnestic property. $CMRO_2$ is decreased with a concomitant decrease in CBF, while carbon dioxide reactivity is preserved. Benzodiazepines at clinical dosages do not cause burst suppression.

Narcotics, especially the synthetic opioids, are frequently used in the neurosurgical patient. However, their effects on cerebral hemodynamics are somewhat controversial. Narcotics, like nitrous oxide, are not used as sole anesthetic agents; hence their effects in the absence of a background anesthetic are difficult to evaluate. In studies with a vasodilator such as halothane, narcotics decrease CBF [23]. In the absence of any hypnotics, narcotics may increase CBF or ICP or have no effect [24]. A problem with many recent studies with the synthetic opioids has been that the systemic arterial pressure was not well controlled. It is possible that after drug administration the resulting increase in ICP was a result of an appropriate autoregulatory vasodilation. Narcotics do not affect carbon dioxide reactivity or pressure autoregulation. Synthetic opioids, such as fentanyl, may have a proconvulsant effect at very high doses [25]. In the CEA patient, however, narcotics are extremely useful adjuncts to minimize systemic cardiovascular changes that occur during induction and maintenance of anesthesia.

Muscle Relaxants

Muscle relaxants are ionized and therefore do not cross the blood–brain barrier and have no direct action on cerebral hemodynamics and metabolism. However, some of the newer agents such as atracurium besylate or mivacurium chloride can release histamine and increase CBF or lower MAP if administered too rapidly. The depolarizing agent succinylcholine chloride has been traditionally used for muscle relaxation during intubation of the trachea; it may indirectly increase CBF by activation of muscle spindles in the periphery. Vecuronium bromide is an intermediate-acting nondepolarizing agent that may also be used for intubation and maintenance of muscle relaxation in the presence of a normal airway. It is conspicuously devoid of systemic and cerebral effects. In the presence of a normal airway, it is an attractive choice as both an induction and maintenance relaxant.

Vasoactive Agents

Stimulation of central β-adrenergic receptors increases CBF and $CMRO_2$. However, intravascular catecholamines such as epinephrine and norepinephrine cannot gain access to these β receptors unless there is a disruption of the blood–brain barrier [26]. Similarly, α-adrenergic agonists such as phenylephrine and dopamine do not appear to change CBF in animals or humans, although there are some conflicting data [27]. Generally, phenylephrine is the drug of choice for temporary or short-term manipulation of systemic vascular resistance to increase MAP because of its lack of β-adrenergic chronotropic effects on the heart .

The classic antihypertensive drug used for neurosurgical

anesthesia has been sodium nitroprusside, primarily an arterial vasodilator. However, despite providing easy titration as an infusion for blood pressure control, nitroprusside has the side effect of increasing ICP and the possibility of cyanide toxicity. Nitroglycerin has been used as an infusion for its antihypertensive properties, but it also increases ICP, primarily by increasing venous capacitance. A major drawback to both these agents for controlling hypertension in the intraoperative setting is the potential for inadvertent hypotension.

Labetalol, a combined α- and β-adrenergic antagonist, and esmolol, a pure β-adrenergic antagonist, have both been used in the setting of cerebrovascular surgery and have minimal effects on CBF (28,29). Smooth blood pressure control is relatively easy compared with the short-acting nitrovasodilators. Calcium channel blocking drugs are an important group of antihypertensive and antianginal drugs used in CEA patients. These drugs may provide some degree of neuronal protection. Recently, the new generation calcium channel blocker nicardipine has been shown to reduce ischemic brain injury in cats (30). Nicardipine is short-acting and can be administered as an infusion.

PATHOPHYSIOLOGY OF CEREBRAL INJURY

Cerebral Ischemia

The neurons of the central nervous system are extremely sensitive to ischemic insult and cannot regenerate. During periods of decreased oxygen delivery, the brain's higher energy requirement in combination with a low metabolic reserve will cause the cessation of oxidative phosphorylation followed by ineffective anaerobic metabolism. This chain of events leads to a derangement of normal neuronal ion gradients involving potassium, sodium, and calcium and results in destabilization of cell membranes. At a CBF of approximately 15 ml/100 g/min, electrical activity of the brain stops, indicating cessation of synaptic transmission. In the absence of hypothermia or pharmacologic interventions, cell death will inevitably occur when CBF decreases to <6 ml/100 g/min. Depending on the degree and duration of the flow reduction, hypoperfusion will lead to either a state of penlucida (when tissue may regain function after flow normalization irrespective of time) or penumbra (when function will be salvaged only if flow is restored within a certain time frame). The development of infarction after a reduction in CBF depends both on the degree and the duration of the ischemic episode. (Clinically, it is almost never possible to determine exact degrees of CBF reductions, and one must work within a framework of relative changes in perfusion.)

Carotid surgery exposes the brain to two mutually interactive types of cerebral ischemia. The first is hemodynamic ischemia as a result of interruption or reduction in carotid flow during cross-clamping. The primary perioperative ischemic event is embolic, similar to the mechanism in transient ischemic attacks (TIA) or retinal lesions. However, hemodynamic and embolic ischemia are processes that are synergistic; reduced perfusion pressure will limit autoregulatory reserve to enhance collateral inflow to an area of focal ischemia.

The primary protection against focal or regional ischemia with acute cerebral hypotension is autoregulatory vasodilatation and decreased resistance. This adaptive decrease in resistance allows recruitment of collateral blood flow via the circle of Willis or other channels described above. Collateral failure may result either when pathways do not exist or when resistance vessels are already maximally vasodilated (see Fig. 1).

In an area of brain that is ischemic (relatively hypotensive), the resistance vessels will be maximally vasodilated. Therefore, pharmacologic vasodilation of surrounding normal vascular territories (either by carbon dioxide or drugs) may result in a "steal" syndrome. Flow may be diverted away from the ischemic area. Conversely, the vasoconstriction of normal tissue may produce a "Robin Hood" syndrome with possible shunting of flow to the ischemic region. Due to the paucity of convincing data in humans, the clinical significance of these syndromes is indeterminate at present.

Reperfusion Injury

Restoration of normal regional perfusion following an ischemic event can result in direct cellular injury or inappropriate vasoadaptive responses. The former is a continuation of the cascade of metabolic derangements that occur during ischemia and may involve free radicals. The latter is the poorly understood syndrome of "cerebral hyperperfusion" that occurs in the setting of carotid endarterectomy (31) and after treatment of cerebral arteriovenous malformations (32). It has been proposed that the chronic hypotension present in the vascular bed distal to a carotid stenosis renders that circulation, at least temporarily, unable to accommodate restoration of normal perfusion pressures after flow is established through the reconstructed carotid artery. Alternatively, the upper limit of autoregulation may be shifted to a lower perfusion pressure, and normal perfusion pressure after restoration of carotid blood flow may result in "circulatory breakthrough," vasogenic edema from disruption of the blood–brain barrier and cerebral hemorrhage. This phenomenon, poorly understood at the present time, is discussed further below.

ANESTHETIC MANAGEMENT

Preoperative Assessment

The patient with arteriosclerotic extracranial vascular disease frequently has associated peripheral and cardiac vasculopathy. Other comorbid processes are usually present as well, including chronic hypertension, diabetes, chronic pulmonary disease, and obesity.

Patients should be evaluated for symptoms related to the neurologic disease process, as well as coexisting systemic problems such as cardiovascular disease. The neurologic examination by the anesthesiologist should focus on the general level of consciousness and motor function. During the routine assessment of the airway, neck mobility should be related to any ischemic symptoms.

Frequently, these patients will have anticoagulant or antiplatelet therapy. Prior to surgery, coagulation studies should be obtained and corrected. A bleeding time or thromboelastogram may be considered for patients who have been on antiplatelet therapy. Preoperative oral anticoagulant therapy should be discontinued and, if necessary, replaced by heparin therapy. Patients with cardiac valvular pathology represent a separate entity, as the valvular pathology may be the cause of cerebral ischemic events. It is therefore of utmost importance to continue full anticoagulation until a few hours prior to surgery and restart it as soon as possible in the postoperative period.

It is important to document the preoperative blood pressure range tolerated by the patient. Adequate cerebral perfusion pressure (CPP) will likely be insured by maintaining intraoperative pressures within an individual patient's "normal" range. To avoid possible rebound hypertension, antihypertensive drugs should be continued until the morning of surgery. Importantly, uncontrolled systemic hypertension in the preoperative period is probably associated with an increased perioperative morbidity and mortality, and blood pressure should be under optimal medical control before elective surgery is undertaken.

Specific attention should be paid to the cardiac status of CEA patients for several reasons. Perioperative cardiovascular complications are a leading cause of mortality associated with CEA (4–6,33) (34)

Carotid artery disease is often a component of generalized arterial disease, frequently involving the coronary arteries. Concurrent ischemic heart disease may also require simultaneous or even prior surgical intervention. Carotid sinus manipulation or clamping is often associated with severe hypertension or bradycardia that poses a significant myocardial stress. Cerebral injury may manifest with perioperative cardiovascular changes.

Over 50% of CEA patients will have concurrent cardiac disease. This is evidenced by the patient profile seen in the North American Symptomatic Carotid Endarterectomy Trial (Table 4) (35). During the clinical evaluation of the patient, it is important to have a high index of suspicion regarding concurrent cardiovascular or systemic diseases. The cardiac risk factors associated with perioperative cardiac complications include a history of myocardial infarction, angina, congestive heart failure, and severe hypertension (4).

Routine cardiac assessment with 1-minute rest electrocardiography (ECG) has a very low sensitivity and specificity for detecting ischemia. A normal ECG offers little reassurance in such a population. Further, in the presence of left bundle branch block, ST-segment analysis may not be possible. Echocardiography is useful in quantifying ejection fraction and chamber volume. Identification of preexisting wall-motion abnormalities also helps in evaluating intraoperative changes seen with transesophageal echocardiography. It has been recommended that all patients for CEA should undergo coronary angiography (33). We recommend, however, that further cardiac evaluation be guided by the patient's symptoms and functional status.

Perioperative cardiovascular changes may also be due to cerebral injury. These manifestations range from asymptomatic ECG changes to arrhythmias, modifications in myocardial wall function, myofibril necrosis, myocardial infarction, or frank cardiopulmonary failure. Once a decision to undertake CEA has been made, the available time should be used for optimizing the patient. Control of blood pressure, congestive heart failure, and angina are important and have bearing on the short- and long-term outcome (36,37).

Patients with significant pulmonary disease should be assessed with pulmonary function tests, if indicated. Pulmonary function should be medically optimized prior to surgery and postoperative ventilation support should be arranged if appropriate.

Due to the adverse interaction of high serum glucose with cerebral ischemia, particular attention should be given to

TABLE 4. *NASCET patient profile[a]*

Concurrent medical condition	Randomized (%) (n = 1212)	Nonrandomized (%) (n = 1044)	Total (%) (n = 2256)
Hypertension	63	58	60
Past smoking	45	36	40
Current smoking	37	37	37
Angina	24	23	24
Previous MI	19	21	20
Diabetes	21	17	19
Claudication	14	17	15

[a] Data are from ref. 35. Randomized patients were randomly selected for either medical or surgical treatment, whereas the nonrandomized group, though eligible for carotid endarterectomy received medical or surgical treatment in a nonrandom fashion for a variety of reasons; the two groups are essentially comparable with regard to the baseline medical profile.

maintaining relative normoglycemia in the diabetic or patient with high-dose steroid therapy. Regarding preoperative insulin management, tight rather than loose control of serum glucose seems reasonable; it is probably not worth risking hypoglycemia in an anesthetized patient for any presumptive protective effect of lowering a mildly elevated glucose level.

Intraoperative Considerations

Monitoring

Standard monitors include blood pressure cuff, pulse oximetry, and ECG, including V5 monitoring for cardiac ischemia. Direct transduction of arterial blood pressure is recommended for beat-to-beat monitoring and, if indicated, for monitoring of respiratory gas exchange. The indications for central venous or pulmonary artery catheter placement in the CEA patient are the same as for any surgical patient. In general, monitoring of intravascular volume status is not as critical for CEA because there is relatively minimal blood loss and fluid shifts.

Hemodynamic Control

Patients undergoing CEA frequently have labile intraoperative blood pressure, which is often a challenge to control adequately, especially since the risk of inadvertent hypotension may have such grave consequences for the cerebral and coronary circulations. The genesis of this "dysautonomia" is probably multifactorial. Many patients are being treated for hypertension, and probably most are at least labile hypertensives by virtue of some underlying autonomic dysfunction or advanced age. The carotid sinus baroreceptors are located in the region of the carotid bifurcation. This region is involved in both the disease process and the surgical manipulation. The patient with a recent contralateral endarterectomy can be expected to have an especially labile intraoperative hemodynamic course, reflecting bilateral carotid sinus dysfunction. For this reason, as well as bilateral cranial nerve damage (see below), at least 6 weeks is recommended between staged bilateral endarterectomies (38).

As in any surgical procedure, it is prudent to relate any changes in blood pressure and heart rate to the events taking place on the operative field. Manipulation or traction of the baroreceptors may induce a variety of changes in blood pressure and heart rate. In the context of this autonomic lability, every change in blood pressure is not necessarily an indication of "light anesthesia." From a nociceptive perspective, the initial skin incision and dissection are the most stimulating portions of the procedure. If adequate anesthetic depth is achieved during that period, it is not unreasonable to manage the remainder of the case by treating blood pressure swings intraoperatively with vasoactive drugs rather than with changing the depth of anesthesia. This also serves to enhance the reliability of EEG monitoring.

Bradycardia deserves special mention in this context. Bradycardia during laryngoscopy may occur, especially in patients receiving β blockers or calcium channel antagonists. Manipulation of the carotid bifurcation may result in severe bradycardia or sinus arrest, especially during carotid cross-clamping. One should be prepared to administer atropine or, if necessary, isoproterenol, in this setting. However, most bouts of bradycardia will resolve if the surgeon is immediately informed and desists from the offending maneuver. The surgeon may attempt to attenuate these autonomic changes by injection of local anesthesia into the region of the bifurcation, but the effectiveness of this maneuver has never been rigorously demonstrated.

Use of a "pure" α-agonist such as phenylephrine as a vasopressor has the relative advantage of inducing a reflex reduction in heart rate. In patients with overt or covert coronary artery disease, this is probably a beneficial effect. One caveat is that extremely slow heart rates, eg, 40–50 bpm (at normotension), can make detection and treatment of significant carotid sinus manipulation more difficult and predispose to ventricular escape ectopy. Such low heart rates may be expected in patients treated with calcium channel blockers or β antagonists.

Myocardial ischemia should always be suspected when difficulty is encountered in maintaining adequate mean arterial pressure (MAP), especially in the setting of induced hypertension. Pump failure initiates a vicious cycle that further decreases MAP and increases central venous and hence cerebral venous pressure, leading to decreased net cerebral perfusion pressure (CPP).

Ventilation

The phenomena of cerebral steal and "Robin Hood" syndrome have been discussed earlier in this chapter. Most clinicians agree that the maintenance of normocapnia is desirable in patients undergoing CEA. However, there appears to be an improvement in collateral perfusion pressure in the presence of hypocapnia (38). Therefore, modest degrees of hypocapnia should be considered, especially in the treatment of an ongoing episode of cerebral ischemia. In patients with lung disease who retain carbon dioxide, mechanical ventilation should be managed by bearing in mind what is normal for an individual patient.

Blood and Fluid Management

Due to the balance between rheologic factors and the oxygen-carrying capacity of the blood, oxygen delivery to ischemic brain appears to be optimized when the hematocrit is in the range of 30–35%. Volume status is an important factor in the maintenance of an adequate cerebral perfusion and systemic cardiovascular stability. It is important to assess the preoperative volume status, especially in the elderly or patients who have been at bed rest for prolonged periods.

The combination of anesthetic-induced vasodilatation and some degree of myocardial depression with even a relative state of hypovolemia can produce catastrophic consequences on CPP. Therefore, it is important to optimize fluid status in the perioperative period. In patients with cardiac or renal failure, fluid administration is best assessed with pulmonary artery pressure monitoring. Hypoosmolar solutions such as 5% dextrose in water should be avoided in favor of isotonic electrolyte solutions. High plasma glucose is deleterious during cerebral ischemia (39). Tight control of perioperative plasma glucose levels seems advisable.

Choice of Anesthetic Technique

Although CEA is a common procedure, there is no general agreement as to what method of anesthetic is best for intraoperative management and monitoring of central nervous system (CNS) function. Direct monitoring of the neurologic status during surgery requires an awake cooperative patient and an effective regional block. Although the awake patient will allow effective neurologic monitoring, extenuating considerations (including long operative time, extensive surgical exposure, or high neck lesions) can be quite stressful for the patient. A state of agitation or confusion may ensue that may be difficult to discern from an ischemic event and may require administration of sedatives to a patient whose airway is unprotected and difficult to control. Furthermore, in the event of an acute ischemic process, the anesthesiologist is faced with a dramatic situation in which the patient requires emergency airway management under the drapes with the neck open.

Regional anesthesia for CEA is an attractive alternative in patients with risk factors for anesthesia and may offer better control of postoperative hypertension (40–42). Poorly controlled blood pressure in the perioperative period has been suggested to increase the incidence of neurologic deficits, myocardial infarction, and mortality. Evidence of the earlier return of blood pressure stability and shorter requirements for the use of vasopressors and vasodilators with regional anesthesia for CEA is readily found (43,44). A correlate of these findings is shorter stays in the intensive care unit and in the hospital overall (40,43–45). In addition, a higher incidence of perioperative myocardial infarction has been observed in those patients who had CEA with general anesthesia (44–46). These issues have not been resolved and are disputed by some authors (47,48).

Regional anesthesia may be accomplished by a deep and superficial cervical plexus block (49,50). The deep cervical plexus can be blocked with a single injection of 12–15 ml of 0.5% bupivacaine at C-4, although some recommend individual injections at the C2-4 nerve root levels. A fan of local anesthetic placed over the posterior margin of the middle third of the sternocleidomastoid muscle will enhance cutaneous anesthesia.

General anesthesia provides airway protection, allows for electrophysiologic monitoring, aggressive management of intraoperative ischemia with pharmacologic intervention, blood pressure augmentation, and control of respiratory gas exchange. However, this is at the cost of the requirement for indirect CNS monitoring and the possibility of delayed awakening. The supplementation of a light general anesthetic with a regional block may be a suitable compromise between the two techniques. A combined technique offers airway protection, an ability to perform electrophysiologic monitoring, a potential for decreasing the chance of delayed emergence, and the promise of better postoperative blood pressure control. There are no data available yet on the use of a combined technique.

Although the debate continues over the optimal type of anesthetic for CEA, a recent survey of 216 anesthesiologists in North America and Europe showed that about 85% use general anesthesia (51).

To Shunt or Not to Shunt

Much has been written about the advantages and disadvantages of intraoperative shunting during carotid cross-clamping. In some centers, the standard surgical approach is systematic shunting of every patient, regardless of the individual preoperative history or angiographic findings. Conversely, some surgeons never shunt. Most surgical teams prefer to use a bypass shunt either when there is preoperative evidence of impaired collateral circulation or when signs of cerebral ischemia develop intraoperatively.

Monitoring of CNS Status

There is no ideal way to perfectly monitor cerebral function during CEA; all methods have their advantages and disadvantages (38). There is a tendency to debunk or discredit methodologies because of less than perfect sensitivity and specificity for the prediction of postoperative stroke. This is a disingenuous approach to monitoring because the point of assessing intraoperative cerebral function is not to passively predict postoperative complications. Rather, it is to alert the operative team of a condition of compromised perfusion so that a proactive intervention can take place, for example, by insertion of a shunt or augmentation of systemic arterial pressure.

During awake surgery under regional block, the patient serves as his or her own CNS monitor, and some authors suggest that this may represent the best neurologic assessment available. It should be borne in mind, however, that the intraoperative "neurologic exam" generally consists primarily of a gross motor evaluation and that subtler degrees of neurocognitive or language function may be missed entirely.

For CNS monitoring during general anesthesia, a commonly used method to detect ischemia during carotid cross-clamping is EEG. Depending on the series and the methodology, ischemic EEG changes have been reported to occur in roughly 10–30% of cases. Ischemic changes in a standard 16-channel EEG correlate well with decreases in CBF. In one series, a critical blood flow of 15–17 ml/100 g/min was required to maintain a "normal" EEG tracing; discrete changes appeared at flows of 18–30 ml/100 g/min, and no EEG changes were recorded at a blood flow >30 ml/100 g/min (52,53). Classic 16-channel EEG monitoring of raw EEG is impractical in most centers (54). Computerized EEG (CEEG) is a practical alternative that processes the raw EEG signal through fast Fourier transformation. CEEG appears to be a reliable indicator of decreases in CBF.

Authors agree that patients with sustained ischemic EEG changes are likely to sustain new permanent postoperative deficits. In patients with preexisting cerebral infarction or abnormal EEG, both standard and CEEG monitoring are unreliable and complicated, and results are more controversial. However, new postoperative deficits occur at a rate of about 0.9% in the absence of EEG changes (55,56).

With all EEG monitoring, an important thing to bear in mind is that relatively stable levels of anesthesia are necessary to rationally interpret EEG changes as due to ischemia.

Stump pressure measured in the internal carotid artery (ICA) distal to the carotid cross-clamp has been used to monitor adequacy of cerebral circulation after clamping of the external and common carotid arteries. A stump pressure >60 mm Hg is usually considered a sign of adequate cerebral perfusion during cross-clamping of the carotid and appears to be a sensitive, but not specific, indicator for ischemic events (57). For example, if the angiogram demonstrates normal intracranial vessels, then a severe stump pressure reduction (ie, <20 mm Hg) is probably associated with inadequate CBF; but false negatives may occur (ie, normal stump pressure may be associated with inadequate CBF). Therefore, there is no consensus regarding a safe absolute level of stump pressure guaranteeing adequate collateral flow. Furthermore, the fact that stump pressure may be influenced by anesthetic agents has convinced most clinicians to use a combination of monitors rather than stump pressure alone. Some authors have recommended simultaneous measurement of jugular venous pressure to improve the accuracy of predicting true CPP.

Other types of electrophysiologic monitoring may be performed, such as somatosensory evoked potentials (SSEP). There is no clear advantage to the use of SSEP over EEG, and there is generally a requirement for more specialized personnel (38).

CBF measurement techniques, typically ^{133}Xe washout, have mostly been reserved for the experimental setting due to the requirement for use of radioisotopes, ultraspecialized equipment, and support staff. A relatively new technique that may be more readily available is transcranial Doppler (TCD) ultrasonography. TCD ultrasound measures blood flow velocities in the vessels of the circle of Willis (53). For monitoring during CEA, the middle cerebral artery (MCA) stem may be monitored via the temporal bone window. Since flow velocities are dependent on vessel diameter, TCD ultra-sound presumes a static diameter of the MCA stem. Absolute values vary from person to person, and relative trends are followed. Although results have been promising, the TCD probe is sometimes difficult to position over the temporal bone window, and it is often challenging to keep the proper position maintained during the course of surgery.

The greatest advantages of TCD ultrasonography are that it is relatively inexpensive, noninvasive, and nonradioactive and furnishes beat-to-beat (ie, continuous) information about the cerebral circulation. This is of use during occlusion of the carotid artery, and TCD may also give indication of shunt failure. An additional advantage of TCD monitoring is that it can also monitor the distal passage of particulate emboli.

Monitoring jugular venous oxygen saturation has also been proposed, but this technique suffers from the drawback that blood draining into each jugular vein is contaminated by venous outflow from the contralateral hemisphere. The recently developed instruments for assessing transcranial oxygen saturation using near-infrared spectroscopy are currently undergoing assessment. There are no convincing data that this method has more to offer than current means, but further inquiry is needed.

Induced Hypertension

A generally accepted method of preventing cerebral ischemia during carotid artery cross-clamping is the artificial maintenance of MAP at levels 20% higher than baseline by infusion of an α-adrenergic agonist (54). Such induced hypertension is of primary use in improving collateral perfusion pressure through the circle of Willis. During an ischemic episode, maintenance of a high perfusion pressure combined with optimal oxygen delivery may reduce neuronal death. Even small increases in CBF may shift a region from penumbra to penlucida or even restore normal function (55). Unfortunately, in a patient population already at risk for perioperative cardiac morbidity, induced hypertension may result in myocardial ischemia and a higher incidence of myocardial infarction when compared with the same patient population not submitted to induced hypertension (56). Caution must be used when elevating MAP in patients with preoperative cerebral infarction since this may worsen edema and transform a pale infarct into a hemorrhagic one (57). In an effort to minimize the risk–benefit ratio of an induced hypertension technique, some authors suggest limiting α-adrenergic agonist use to situations of impending cerebral ischemia defined by electrophysiologic criteria. The selective use of phenylephrine based on cerebral electrophysiology has been shown to decrease the rate of both myocardial and cerebral ischemia (58).

Pharmacologic Brain Protection

In order to delay triggering of the ischemic cascade during temporary cerebral vessel occlusion, pharmacologic protection has been proposed. As mentioned earlier, anesthetics may protect by decreasing cellular electrophysiologic or neurotransmitter function, as well as by decreasing metabolic rate. Because of the potential for cardiovascular depression, it is important that these agents are carefully titrated. Although EEG burst suppression is a convenient clinical endpoint, there is no good evidence that it correlates with maximum cerebral protection. For example, the two most frequently quoted papers used to support the position that there is a dose-dependent effect at those high concentrations did not control for brain temperature (59,60). It was not recognized at the time of these studies that minor temperature alterations were so critical in the outcome from an ischemic insult. In fact, recent animal model evidence indicates no advantage of burst suppression over a sedative dose, and in fact the protective effect versus awake was relatively small (D. S. Warner, oral personal communication, 1995, unpublished data). Burst suppression on the EEG may also interfere with monitoring of ischemic changes. If the burst-suppression ratio is fairly constant, however, EEG changes should still correlate with ischemia (61).

Thiopental is the classic cerebroprotective agent and must be administered cautiously to avoid cardiovascular depression and delayed awakening (62). To avoid these side effects, the use of either etomidate or propofol, which are both shorter-acting, has been proposed by some authors. Unfortunately, the evidence for protection by etomidate and propofol are not as compelling as that for barbiturates.

Temperature

Recent animal and human studies suggesting a protective effect with deliberate mild hypothermia in the range of 33–34°C has renewed interest for this type of cerebral protection (63,64). When used during anesthesia for craniotomy in otherwise healthy patients, deliberate mild hypothermia does not appear to have the problems associated with deep hypothermia, such as arrhythmias and myocardial ischemia, and coagulopathies appear limited (65). Deliberate mild hypothermia during CEA remains to be studied. There are several daunting problems for its application during CEA under general anesthesia. The cases are relatively short, decreasing time available for temperature manipulation. Even mild hypothermia may result in a delayed emergence and therefore delayed neurologic assessment. Compared with craniotomy patients, the population has a higher cardiac risk and is older; increased morbidity may not be offset by cerebral protective effects. Hypothermia cannot be used with regional anesthetic techniques.

Cerebral Hyperemia

The occurrence of postrepair cerebral hyperemia appears to be related to certain complications, including cerebral hemorrhage and severe brain swelling. These occurrences

are rare but often fatal complications of CEA. Also included in this category, but with a lower morbidity, are postendarterectomy headache (especially unilateral headache) and certain instances of seizures. Although patients with previous stroke may suffer intracranial hemorrhage after endarterectomy, it occurs in otherwise normal brain as well. Postendarterectomy intracerebral hemorrhage occurs in about 0.5–1.0% of cases. Poorly controlled blood pressure probably contributes to this complication.

Postoperative Concerns

The main postoperative concern remains the preservation of a stable CPP in a patient who will often exhibit labile blood pressure. Postoperative hypotension may be the result of a hyperfunctioning carotid sinus that is now exposed to a higher pressure secondary to plaque removal. On the other hand, patients with preoperative hypertension sometimes exhibit postoperative hypertension, although this mechanism is not well understood. Postoperative hemodynamic control is geared toward the maintenance of blood pressure in the range determined to be "normal" in the preoperative period. This is accomplished by either fluid therapy or vasoactive drugs.

Cranial nerve dysfunction can result from surgical trauma during neck dissection or retraction. Although usually minor and transient, occasionally problems will be encountered in the immediate recovery from anesthesia. Vocal cord malfunction, impaired gag reflex, or inability to handle secretions may result from glossopharyngeal or vagal nerve injury. Rarely, hypoglossal nerve injury results in tongue weakness that contributes to upper airway obstruction. The response to hypoxemia may be affected in patients having undergone bilateral carotid endarterectomies.

One special postoperative condition worthy of mention is the postoperative neck hematoma. Compression of the airway and respiratory embarrassment may result; with distortion of airway anatomy, tracheal intubation may be difficult. If there is suspicion of an enlarging mass, it is probably better to err on the side of caution and electively secure the airway. Swelling that compromises the airway may also impair carotid blood flow as well. A patient who returns to the operating room for neck swelling must have the airway secured in a conservative fashion. Awake direct laryngoscopy or fiberoptic intubation would be appropriate in this instance. When the patient has the airway secured and anesthesia is induced, one must also be prepared for rapid, uncontrollable blood loss. There may be a tamponade effect stemming flow from a ruptured or leaking arteriotomy. On opening of the skin or subcutaneous layers, exsanguination from the decompressed carotid artery may rapidly occur.

Future Considerations

Cerebral protection may depend on early blockade of the ischemic cascade. The more upstream the intervention is, the better will be chance of decreasing the effects of the cascade and providing some degree of neuronal protection. The new direction of research therefore is geared toward this goal. Barbiturates, electrophysiologic suppression, induced hypertension, and hypothermia may play a positive role in patient outcome if instituted before the triggering of the ischemic cascade. At the present time, anesthetic management that provides hemodynamic stability with optimal CPP is mandatory to minimize major complications referable to the coronary and cerebral circulation.

ACKNOWLEDGMENTS

David S. Warner, MD, for comments and suggestions.

REFERENCES

1. Executive Committee for the Asymptomatic Carotid Atherosclerosis Study. Endarterectomy for asymptomatic carotid stenosis. *JAMA* 1989; 273:1421–1428.
2. Towne JB, Weiss DG, Hobson RW II. First phase report of cooperative Veterans Administration asymptomatic carotid stenosis study: Operative morbidity and mortality. *J Vasc Surg* 1990;11:252–259.
3. Handelsman H. Carotid endarterectomy. AHCPR Health Technology Assessment Report—1990 (Number 5). US Dept of Health and Human Services publication PHS 91-3472 1990;1–13.
4. Sundt TM Jr, Sandok BA, Whisnant JP. Carotid endarterectomy: Complications and preoperative assessment of risk. *Mayo Clin Proc* 1975; 50:301–306.
5. Modica PA, Tempelhoff R, Rich KM, Grubb RL Jr. Computerized electroencephalographic monitoring and selective shunting: Influence on intraoperative administration of phenylephrine and myocardial infarction after general anesthesia for carotid endarterectomy. *Neurosurgery* 1992;30:842–846.
6. Sieber FE, Toung TJ, Diringer MN, Wang H, Long DM. Preoperative risks predict neurological outcome of carotid endarterectomy related stroke. *Neurosurgery* 1992;30:847–854.
7. Young WL, Ornstein E. Cerebral and spinal cord blood flow (review). In: Cottrell JE, Smith DS, eds. *Anesthesia and Neurosurgery*, 3rd ed. St. Louis, MO: Mosby-Year Book, 1994;17–57.
8. Hoffman WE, Charbel FT, Edelman G, Albrecht RF, Ausman JI. Nitrous oxide added to isoflurane increases brain artery blood flow and low frequency brain electrical activity. *J Neurosurg Anesthesiol* 1995; 7:82–88.
9. Hoffman WE, Baughman VL, Albrecht RF. Interaction of catecholamines and nitrous oxide ventilation during incomplete brain ischemia in rats. *Anesth Analg* 1993;77:908–912.
10. Hartung J, Cottrell JE. Nitrous oxide reduces thiopental-induced prolongation of survival in hypoxic and anoxic mice. *Anesth Analg* 1987; 66:47–52.
11. Scheller MS, Todd MM, Drummond JC. Isoflurane, halothane, and regional cerebral blood flow at various levels of $Paco_2$ in rabbits. *Anesthesiology* 1986;64:598–604.
12. Messick JM Jr, Casement B, Sharbrough FW, Milde LN, Michenfelder JD, Sundt TM Jr. Correlation of regional cerebral blood flow (rCBF) with EEG changes during isoflurane anesthesia for carotid endarterectomy: Critical rCBF. *Anesthesiology* 1987;66:344–349.
13. Young WL, Prohovnik I, Correll JW, Ornstein E, Matteo RS, Ostapkovich N. Cerebral blood flow and metabolism in patients undergoing anesthesia for carotid endarterectomy: A comparison of isoflurane, halothane, and fentanyl. *Anesth Analg* 1989;68:712–717.
14. Young WL. Effects of desflurane on the central nervous system. *Anesth Analg* 1992;75(suppl 4S):S32–S37.
15. Scheller MS, Tateishi A, Drummond JC, Zornow MH. The effects of sevoflurane on cerebral blood flow, cerebral metabolic rate for oxygen, intracranial pressure, and the electroencephalogram are similar to those of isoflurane in the rabbit. *Anesthesiology* 1988;68:548–551.
16. Koenig HM. What's up with the new volatile anesthetics, desflurane and sevoflurane, for neurosurgical patients (editorial). *J Neurosurg Anesthesiol* 1994;6:229–232.
17. Pierce EC, Lambertson CJ, Deutsch S, et al. Cerebral circulation and metabolism during thiopental anesthesia and hyperventilation in man. *J Clin Invest* 1962;41:1664–1671.
18. Stone JG, Young WL, Khambatta HJ, et al. Effect of massive intraoperative thiopental loading on cardiovascular hemodynamics and myocardial performance (case report). *J Neurosurg Anesthesiol* 1991;3: 132–135.
19. Batjer HH, Frankfurt AI, Purdy PD, Smith SS, Samson DS. Use of etomidate, temporary arterial occlusion, and intraoperative angiography in surgical treatment of large and giant cerebral aneurysms. *J Neurosurg* 1988;68:234–240.
20. Ravussin P, Tempelhoff R, Modica PA, Bayer-Berger M-M. Propofol vs. thiopental-isoflurane for neurosurgical anesthesia: Comparison of hemodynamics, CSF pressure, and recovery. *J Neurosurg Anesthesiol* 1991;3:85–95.
21. Modica PA, Tempelhoff R. Intracranial pressure during induction of anaesthesia and tracheal intubation with etomidate-induced EEG burst suppression. *Can J Anaesth* 1992;39:236–241.
22. Shapira Y, Lam AM, Artru AA, Eng C, Soltow L. Ketamine alters calcium and magnesium in brain tissue following experimental head trauma in rats. *J Cereb Blood Flow Metab* 1993;13:962–968.
23. Matsumiya N, Dohi S. Effects of intravenous or subarachnoid morphine on cerebral and spinal cord hemodynamics and antagonism with naloxone in dogs. *Anesthesiology* 1983;59:175–181.
24. Milde LN, Milde JH, Gallagher WJ. Effects of sufentanil on cerebral circulation and metabolism in dogs. *Anesth Analg* 1990;70:138–146.
25. Tempelhoff R, Modica PA, Bernardo KL, Edwards I. Fentanyl-induced electrocorticographic seizures in patients with complex partial epilepsy. *J Neurosurg* 1992;77:201–208.
26. Artru AA, Nugent M, Michenfelder JD. Anesthetics affect the cerebral metabolic response to circulatory catecholamines. *J Neurochem* 1981; 36:1941–1946.
27. Darby JM, Yonas H, Marks EC, Durham S, Snyder RW, Nemoto EM. Acute cerebral blood flow response to dopamine-induced hypertension after subarachnoid hemorrhage. *J Neurosurg* 1994;80:857–864.
28. Orlowski JP, Shiesley D, Vidt DG, Barnett GH, Little JR. Labetalol to control blood pressure after cerebrovascular surgery. *Crit Care Med* 1988;16:765–768.
29. Ornstein E, Young WL, Ostapkovich N, Matteo RS, Diaz J. Deliberate hypotension in patients with intracranial arteriovenous malformations: Esmolol compared with isoflurane and sodium nitroprusside. *Anesth Analg* 1991;72:639–644.
30. Kucharcyzk J, Chew W, Derugin N, et al. Nicardipine reduces ischemic brain injury. Magnetic resonance imaging/spectroscopy study in cats. *Stroke* 1989;20:268–274.
31. Schroeder T, Sillesen H, Sorensen O, Engell HC. Cerebral hyperperfusion following carotid endarterectomy. *J Neurosurg* 1987;66:824–829.
32. Young WL, Kader A, Ornstein E, et al. The Columbia University AVM Project: Cerebral hyperemia after AVM resection is related to "breakthrough" complications but not to feeding artery pressure. *Neurosurgery* 1996;38:1085–1095.
33. Hertzer NR, Lees CD. Fatal myocardial infarction following carotid endarterectomy. *Ann Surg* 1981;194:212–218.
34. Prough DS, Scuderi PE, Stullken EH, Davis CH Jr. Myocardial infarction following regional anaesthesia for carotid endarterectomy. *Can Anaesth Soc J* 1984;31:192–196.
35. North American Symptomatic Carotid Endarterectomy Trial (NASCET) Steering Committee. North American Symptomatic Carotid Endarterectomy Trial: Methods, patient characteristics, and progress. *Stroke* 1991;22:711–720.
36. Rihal CS, Gersh BJ, Whisnant JP, et al. Influence of coronary artery disease on morbidity and mortality after carotid endarterectomy: A population based study in Olmsted County, Minnesota (1970–1988). *J Am Coll Cardiol* 1992;19:1254–1260.
37. Riles TS, Kopelman I, Imparato AM. Myocardial infarction following carotid endarterectomy: A review of 683 operations. *Surgery* 1979;85: 249–252.
38. Loftus CM, Quest DO. Technical issues in carotid artery surgery 1995. *Neurosurgery* 1995;36:629–647.
39. Lanier WL, Stangland KJ, Scheithauer BW, Milde JH, Michenfelder JD. The effects of dextrose infusion and head position on neurologic

outcome after complete cerebral ischemia in primates: Examination of a model. *Anesthesiology* 1987;66:39–48.

40. Corson JD, Chang BB, Leopold PW, et al. Perioperative hypertension in patients undergoing carotid endarterectomy: shorter duration under regional block anesthesia. *Circulation* 1986;74:I1–4.

41. Shifrin EG, Gertel M, Anner H, Olshwang D, Levy P. Local anesthesia in carotid endarterectomy: An alternative method. *Isr J Med Sci* 1985; 21:511–513.

42. Stullken E, Prough D, Balestrieri F, Davis C, Sixx E. Anesthesia for carotid surgery: Does regional anesthesia reduce the risk of postoperative hypertension? (abstract). *Anesthesiology* 1984;61:A320.

43. Corson JD, Chang BB, Shah DM, Leather RP, DeLeo BM, Karmody AM. The influence of anesthetic choice on carotid endarterectomy outcome. *Arch Surg* 1987;122:807–812.

44. Gabelman CG, Gann DS, Ashworth CJ Jr, Carney WI. One hundred consecutive carotid reconstructions: Local versus general anesthesia. *Am J Surg* 1983;145:477–482.

45. Muskett A, McGreevy J, Miller M. Detailed comparison of regional and general anesthesia for carotid endarterectomy. *Am J Surg* 1986; 152:691–694.

46. Lee KS, Davis CH, McWhorter JM. Low morbidity and mortality of carotid endarterectomy performed with regional anesthesia. *J Neurosurg* 1988;69:483–487.

47. Palmer MM. Comparison of regional and general anesthesia for carotid endarterectomy. *Am J Surg* 1989;157:329–330.

48. Forssell C, Takolander R, Bergquist D, Johansson A, Persson NH. Local versus general anesthesia in carotid surgery: A prospective, randomised study. *Eur J Vasc Surg* 1989;3:503–509.

49. Scott DB. *Techniques of Regional Anesthesia*. New York: Appleton & Lange, 1989:74–76.

50. Winnie AP, Ramamurthy S, Durrani Z, Radonjic R. Interscalene cervical plexus block: A single-injection technique. *Anesth Analg* 1975;54: 370–375.

51. Cheng MA, Theard MA, Tempelhoff R. Anesthetic technique for carotid endarterectomy: The reality (abstract). *J Neurosurg Anesthesiol* 1995; 1995;7:312.

52. Sharbrough FW, Messick JM, Sundt TM. Correlation of continuous electroencephalograms with cerebral blood flow measurements during carotid endarterectomy. *Stroke* 1973;4:674–683.

53. Sundt TM, Sharbrough FW, Piepgras DG, Kearns TP, Messick JM, O'Fallon WM. Correlation of cerebral flood flow and electroencephalo-graphic changes during carotid endarterectomy. *Mayo Clin Proc* 1981; 56:533–543.

54. Chiappa KH, Burke SR, Young RR. Results of electroencephalographic monitoring during 367 carotid endarterectomies: Use of a dedicated minicomputer. *Stroke* 1979;10:381–388.

55. Tempelhoff R, Modica PA, Grubb RL Jr, Rich KM, Holtmann B. Selective shunting during carotid endarterectomy based on two-channel computerized electroencephalographic/compressed spectral array analysis. *Neurosurgery* 1989;24:339–344.

56. Modica PA, Tempelhoff R. A comparison of computerized EEG with internal carotid artery stump pressure for detection of ischemia during carotid endarterectomy. *J Neurosurg Anesthesiol* 1989;1:211–218.

57. Halsey JH, McDowell HA, Gelmon S, Morawetz RB. Blood velocity in the middle cerebral artery and regional cerebral blood flow during carotid endarterectomy. *Stroke* 1989;20:53–58.

58. Boysen G, Engell HC, Henriksen H. The effect of induced hypertension on internal carotid artery pressure and regional cerebral blood flow during temporary carotid clamping for endarterectomy. *Neurology* 1972;22:1133–1144.

59. Hoff JT, Smith AL, Hankinson HL, Nielsen SL. Barbiturate protection from cerebral infarction in primates. *Stroke* 1975;6:28–33.

60. Corkill G, Sivalingam S, Reitan JA, Gilroy BA, Helphrey MG. Dose dependency of the post-insult protective effect of pentobarbital in the canine experimental stroke model. *Stroke* 1978;9:10–12.

61. Young WL, Solomon RA, Pedley TA, et al. Direct cortical EEG monitoring during temporary vascular occlusion for cerebral aneurysm surgery. *Anesthesiology* 1989;71:794–799.

62. Young WL, Cole DJ. Deliberate hypertension: Rationale and application for augmenting cerebral blood flow. *Probl Anesth* 1993;7: 140–153.

63. Sano T, Drummond JC, Patel PM, Grafe MR, Watson JC, Cole DJ. A comparison of the cerebral protective effects of isoflurane and mild hypothermia in a model of incomplete forebrain ischemia in the rat. *Anesthesiology* 1992;76:221–228.

64. Marion DW, Obrist WD, Carlier PM, Penrod LE, Darby JM. The use of moderate therapeutic hypothermia for patients with severe head injuries: A preliminary report. *J Neurosurg* 1993;79:354–362.

65. Baker KZ, Young WL, Stone JG, Kader A, Baker CJ, Solomon RA. Deliberate mild intraoperative hypothermia for craniotomy. *Anesthesiology* 1994;81:361–367.

66. Young WL: Clinical Neuroscience Lectures. Munster, IN, Cathenart Publishing, 1996 in press.

Cerebrovascular Disease, edited by H. Hunt Batjer.
Lippincott-Raven Publishers, Philadelphia © 1997.

CHAPTER 27

Supratentorial Ischemic Syndromes

D. Hal Unwin

Localization of the lesion has long been considered the quintessence of neurology as a medical specialty. The delineation of many of these functions has been a result of lesions induced by cerebrovascular disease. Broca's description of the verbal output of language in the frontal lobes, as well as many additional brain functions such as calculation, reading, praxis, and object recognition, were associated with specific brain areas based on clinical observation and pathologic verification of the site of brain damage (1).

As a result of modern imaging techniques, great progress has been made in defining the anatomical localization of higher cortical functions. With the advent of acute, early interventional therapies in ischemic cerebrovascular disease, localization of specific syndromes might enhance early patient selection even before imaging modalities show any abnormality. This chapter highlights certain syndromes of the supratentorial region that can be reliably related to a specific arterial distribution. Syndromes resulting from proximal carotid artery occlusion are only discussed briefly as they are covered elsewhere in this volume.

INTERNAL CAROTID ARTERY

Carotid Ischemic Syndromes

Most carotid ischemic symptoms relate to its distal supply of the middle and anterior cerebral arteries (to be covered later in the chapter). Infarction of the watershed zone between the middle and anterior cerebral arteries leads to proximal greater than distal weakness and sensory loss of the contralateral arm, variable lower extremity weakness, and sparing of the face and hand. In the dominant hemisphere, a transcortical aphasia may also occur (see below). Infarction of the watershed zone between the middle and posterior cerebral arteries may cause a contralateral hemianopic or quadrantanopic field defect and a transcortical aphasia or hemi-inattention, depending on hemispheric dominance (2).

There are two syndromes associated with carotid ischemia that warrant mention. An unusual brief, involuntary, coarse, irregular, wavering movement or tremble involving the arm and hand alone, or arm, hand, and leg together has been described in severe carotid occlusive disease (3). The movements are without electroencephalographic changes and are felt to represent generalized hemispheric ischemia. Limb-shaking transient ischemic attacks (TIAs) have also been seen in moyamoya disease. Recognition of this uncommon form of transient ischemic attack is important in the early recognition and treatment of carotid occlusive disease.

The presence of a partial Horner's syndrome (meiosis and ptosis) accompanied by hemispheric symptoms should alert the examiner to the possibility of carotid disease. Since the sympathetic fibers to the pupil travel in the internal carotid sheath, involvement of the vasa nervorum due to severe carotid atherosclerosis and/or occlusion can lead to a partial Horner's syndrome.

Ophthalmic Artery

Transient monocular blindness, or amaurosis fugax, is one of the most important syndromes pointing to carotid artery disease. The patient usually experiences a dimming or blackening of vision, frequently described as a shade coming down from above. Some patients report that their vision may gray out. Most report a total loss of vision. The episodes typically last from seconds to several minutes and are due to decreased blood flow to the retina, either from embolization from proximal sources or from occlusion of the carotid or ophthalmic arteries. There most often follows a gradual return of vision. A relatively rare syndrome described as bright light amaurosis occurs in patients who experience visual loss only when exposed to bright light. The mechanism is believed to be related to neuronal ischemia brought on when retinal activity exceeds the available oxygen delivery in the presence of severe carotid occlusive disease (4,5).

D. H. Unwin: Department of Neurology, University of Texas Southwestern Medical School, Dallas, Texas 75235.

TABLE 1. *Risk of stroke at 2 years with presenting symptom of amaurosis fugax, 70–99% carotid stenosis*

Stenosis (%)	Risk of stroke at 2 years (%)
95	28.9
85	17.8
75	11.2

Data from ref. 6 and 7.

Patients frequently will not volunteer that amaurosis fugax has occurred because the episodes tend to be brief, infrequent over time, and without sequelae. Though the symptom of amaurosis rarely results in permanent visual loss, its importance as a risk factor for ischemic stroke cannot be stressed enough. Data from the North American Symptomatic Carotid Endarterectomy Trial (NASCET) shows a 17% risk of ipsilateral stroke at 2 years for patients with amaurosis fugax and the presence of >70% carotid stenosis. The risk increases with increasing stenosis (Table 1) (6,7). Though usually associated with carotid or intrinsic ophthalmic arterial disease, amaurosis can be caused by a cardiac embolus, a source that should be excluded if evaluation of the carotid-ophthalmic system is unrevealing.

Anterior Choroidal Artery

The anterior choroidal artery is the third intracranial branch of the internal carotid artery after the ophthalmic and posterior communicating arteries. It supplies the choroid plexus of the lateral ventricle after it enters the temporal lobe through the choroidal fissure. More importantly, however, is the supply to the lateral geniculate body, globus pallidus, and the posterior limb of the internal capsule. Anterior choroidal artery infarcts usually result in a contralateral dense hemiparesis affecting the face, arm, and leg; contralateral hemisensory loss; and, if the lateral geniculate is involved, a contralateral hemianopsia with sparing of an arc-shaped portion within the central region of the hemianopic field (8).

ANTERIOR CEREBRAL ARTERY

Recurrent Artery of Heubner

The recurrent artery of Heubner is the major branch of the A-1 segment of the anterior cerebral artery. In most people, there are actually two or more recurrent perforating arteries that are grouped as the recurrent artery of Heubner. The artery reliably supplies the medial portion of the head of the caudate and the anterior limb of the internal capsule. Infarction as a consequence of occlusion of this artery is due to intrinsic arterial disease, although embolization from proximal sources must also be considered (9). Infarction may lead to mild weakness in the contralateral limb commonly accompanied by dysarthria. While restlessness and hyperactivity can be seen, abulic patients who are apathetic and have

inertia of movement are more frequently documented with occlusion in this arterial distribution. Hemichorea contralateral to caudate infarction has also been described (10).

Anterior Cerebral Artery

Infarction in the distribution of the anterior cerebral artery (ACA) produces contralateral weakness of the leg and shoulder. Cortical sensory deficit with poor touch localization and extinction with bilateral stimuli are frequent accompaniments, distinguishing anterior cerebral artery infarction from the easily confused disorders of the cervical spine. The presence of apraxia of the left arm only can also be a significant clue to anterior cerebral artery territory infarction. In this instance, infarction of the anterior corpus callosum or adjacent white matter disrupts the pathways for praxis from the left frontal region to the right hemisphere. As the former region is intact, praxis of the right upper extremity is normal. Transcortical motor and sensory aphasia with the unusual ability to repeat phrases while both spontaneous speech and comprehension are impaired has been described with isolated anterior cerebral territory infarction (11). Abulia, apathy, and incontinence can occur following unilateral anterior cerebral artery infarction, although these are most commonly seen with bilateral lesions.

MIDDLE CEREBRAL ARTERY

The clinical result of occlusion of a middle cerebral artery (MCA) is greatly influenced by whether the thrombus is proximal to the lateral lenticulostriate arteries, or distal to them, resulting in what are commonly called branch occlusion syndromes. Branch occlusion syndromes can be defined in terms of involvement of superior or inferior divisions of the MCA as well as their lateralization to the left or right hemisphere.

In either hemisphere, the most prominent feature of proximal (M-1) MCA occlusion is contralateral spastic hemiplegia. More distal occlusion, at the M-2 origins, for example, causes a characteristic hemiparesis affecting the face and arm more severely than the leg. With ischemia of superior division occlusion, contralateral conjugate gaze palsy occurs due to infarction of the frontal eye fields, which control saccadic eye movements, and initially results in the conjugate deviation of the eyes toward the side of the infarct. Since subcortical brain-stem structures are intact, gaze to the side contralateral to the stroke can be accomplished with Doll's eye maneuver or by provoking voluntary smooth pursuit movements. Visual field abnormalities are also commonly seen in MCA occlusion. Both proximal and superior division occlusions are associated with a contralateral homonymous hemianopsia, frequently associated with visual neglect toward the hemianopic field. Inferior division occlusion is associated with the oft described "pie-in-the-sky" visual deficit, a contralateral superior homonymous quadrantanopsia. This defect occurs due to disruption of Meyer's

TABLE 2. *Aphasia*

Condition	Expression	Comprehension	Repetition
Broca's	−	+	−
Wernicke's	+	−	−
Conduction	+	+	−
Global	−	−	−
Transcortical motor	−	+	+
Transcortical sensory	+	−	+
Mixed transcortical	−	−	+

loop, which contains the inferior retinal fibers and loops into the posterior temporal lobe prior to traveling to the calcarine cortex.

LANGUAGE-DOMINANT (USUALLY LEFT) HEMISPHERE LESIONS

Language is one of the most reliable features that aids in cortical localization of supratentorial ischemic syndromes (12). Motor aphasia, or Broca's aphasia, is due to infarction in the region of the frontal operculum of the dominant hemisphere, which is supplied by the anterior or superior branch of the MCA. The patient's speech is characterized by the ability to think the words but an inability to articulate them. Acutely, patients are frequently mute. As the aphasia improves, the patient's speech becomes halting and telegraphic, with articles frequently omitted. In addition, the speech may contain word substitutions of a semantic (eg, breen for brick) or phonemic (breen for green) nature and patients are unable to repeat what is said to them. A more distal watershed region infarction causes similar symptoms, except repetition is preserved. This is then called a transcortical motor aphasia (Table 2). Isolated Broca's aphasia is frequently due to an embolus.

Wernicke's or receptive aphasia results when the superior temporal gyrus of the dominant hemisphere is infarcted due to occlusion of the posterior or inferior branch of the MCA. These patients are frequently seen as "confused" and may be agitated. They may be able to follow some simple, one-step, usually midline commands (eg, stick out your tongue, close your eyes) but frequently have difficulty with more laterally placed (eg, show two fingers) or complex two-step commands. Speech is fluent with neologisms and paraphasic errors. Similar to Broca's aphasia, patients with a Wernicke's aphasia cannot repeat. Wernicke's aphasia frequently resolves completely.

There are a variety of more limited language defects associated with dominant MCA branch occlusions that may be overlooked if not specifically sought in the clinical evaluation. Conduction aphasia occurs due to posterior MCA branch occlusions with involvement of the arcuate fasciculus. These patients are fluent and have normal comprehension, but repetition is significantly impaired. Alexia with agraphia occurs due to involvement of speech areas in the dominant hemisphere. With involvement of Wernicke's and Broca's areas, patients are both unable to read and unable to write. Pure word deafness is an extremely rare ischemic syndrome due to infarction in the region of the superior temporal gyrus whereby patients are able to speak but spoken words uttered by others have no meaning for them. These patients may be able to spell the word aloud and via that mechanism are able to understand.

Large proximal MCA occlusions frequently lead to a global aphasia with impairment in all spheres of language. The aphasia typically improves with evolution into a classic Broca's aphasia.

Praxis is a Greek term meaning "to do" and when present means that a patient has the ability to understand a command and the motor power to perform it (13). A motor act initiated to spoken command begins in the language dominant parietal lobe, traveling to the dominant prefrontal region and across the corpus callosum to the contralateral prefrontal region. Lesions of the superior division of the MCA are most commonly associated with apraxia. If the occlusion is in the dominant hemisphere, the patient often will be apractic in both upper extremities. If the infarct occurs in the nondominant hemisphere, the patient will be apractic in the left upper extremity only. Oral-buccal apraxia is due to a lesion in the dominant hemisphere whereby the patient who may not be aphasic has great difficulty in positioning the mouth and coordinating the complex movements of the palate and mouth when trying to speak. These patients frequently sound as if they are speaking "baby talk." With inferior division lesions of the non-dominant hemisphere, constructional apraxia and difficulty with maps, shapes, and so forth may occur. Apraxia is frequently grouped into either ideomotor, ideational, or limb kinetic (Table 3).

NON-DOMINANT (USUALLY RIGHT) HEMISPHERE LESIONS

Proximal or superior branch MCA occlusion in the non-dominant hemisphere is associated with a profound neglect

TABLE 3. *Apraxia*

Type	Features	Localization
Ideomotor	Inability to carry out learned motor pattern to command	Dominant parietal lobe if bilateral. Nondominant frontal lobe if unilateral
Ideational	Inability to sequence and plan complex motor acts	Dominant parietal lobe
Limb-kinetic	Lack of skill and dexterity of learned motor movements	Contralateral premotor cortex

TABLE 4. *Aprosodia*

Condition	Expression	Comprehension	Repetition
Motor aprosodia	−	+	−
Sensory aprosodia	+	−	−
Conduction aprosodia	+	+	−
Global aprosodia	−	−	−

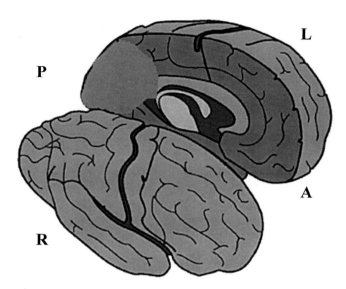

FIG. 1. Location of ischemic lesion causing alexia without agraphia.

of the left side of space. In addition, these patients frequently have an impersistence to tasks if the frontal lobe is involved. Confusion and delirium are frequently noted with lesions of the right temporal lobe, an area subserved by the inferior division (14).

Prosody is the emotional content of speech, with motor, sensory, and conduction aprosodias having been described (15). Similar to the dominant hemisphere lesions of speech, mirror image infarction of the nondominant hemisphere leads to corresponding aprosodias (Table 4).

POSTERIOR CEREBRAL ARTERY

Proximal Posterior Cerebral Arteries

The posterior cerebral artery (PCA) arises from the basilar artery in the majority of patients but in the persistent fetal arrangement can arise from the carotid system. Infarction of the proximal segment of the PCA can lead to specific deficits involving the thalamus as outlined in Table 5. Infarction of the more distal posterior choroidal artery can lead to a contralateral field cut due to infarction of the lateral geniculate body. The paramedian diencephalic syndrome is due to bilateral infarction of the thalamus and is characterized by the triad of hypersomnolent apathy, an amnesic syndrome, and impaired (frequently downward) vertical gaze (17).

Infarction of the distal region of the PCA causes a defect in the corresponding contralateral and contra-altitudinal visual field. Divided vertically by the sagittal sulcus and horizontally about the calcarine fissure, the occipital lobes and hence the visual fields can be divided into quadrants. Macular vision is located posteriorly along the calcarine fissure and may be spared in occipital lobe infarctions due to collateral blood supply from the MCA. Visual field deficits from PCA occlusion are similar to those of MCA occlusion. However, unlike hemianopic defects in MCA disease, most patients are aware of the deficit.

Palinopsia, which may occur with occipital lobe infarction, is the persistence of a visual image after the image has disappeared. The image may also return later and persist for a short time.

Infarction of the proximal dominant PCA leads to a unique syndrome of alexia without agraphia (Fig. 1). With printed words presented in the left visual field, the information is unable to access the language centers in the left hemisphere due to infarction of the splenium of the corpus callosum. Because language centers are intact, the patient is able to write normally but unable to read what has just been written.

TABLE 5. *Thalamic infarction syndromes*

Artery	Origin	Symptoms
Ventrolateral	P-2 segment of PCA	Contralateral numbness and tingling Pain (less common) Delayed Dejerine–Roussy syndrome Mild contralateral weakness
Tuberothalamic	Posterior communicating artery	Dysphasia in left-sided infarcts, hemineglect, and impaired visuospatial processing in right-sided infarcts Minor and transient contralateral motor signs
Posterior choroidal	P-2 segment of PCA	Partial hemianopia
Paramedian	P-1 segment of PCA	Transient loss of consciousness or somnolence Unilateral infarcts similar to tuberothalamic symptoms Confusion, amnesia, confabulation if bilateral (thalamic dementia)

From ref. 16.

TABLE 6. *Posterior cerebral artery syndromes*

Syndrome	Features	Location
Prosopagnosia	Inability to recognize familiar faces	Bilateral (or right) occipital lesions
Anton's	Denial of blindness with confabulation	Bilateral occipital lesions
Gerstmann's	Acalculia	Dominant angular gyrus
	Agraphia	
	Right/left disorientation	
	Finger agnosia	

Similarly, color agnosia may also be present whereby the patient is unable to name the color of an object presented in the left visual field.

Infarction in the region of the angular gyrus of the dominant hemisphere results in Gerstmann's syndrome. The syndrome can be seen in dominant inferior division MCA cortical infarction or dominant PCA infarction of deep white matter in the inferior parietal lobule (2). This is classically represented by four major components: (a) finger agnosia (the inability to name either the examiner's fingers or the patient's own fingers), (b) acalculia, (c) right–left disorientation, and (d) agraphia, though most patients will manifest only two or three of the components (Table 6).

Infarction of the right (or both right and left) PCA territory may lead to prosopagnosia (the inability to recognize familiar faces). When presented with a picture of a familiar person, perhaps even a member of their own family, these patients are unable to name or recognize the person pictured.

Bilateral occipital lobe infarction, usually due to distal basilar occlusion, leads to cortical blindness, though rarely the patient may be left with tunnel vision because of sparing of the macular areas due to the collateral blood supply from the anterior circulation. These patients may not recognize that they are blind (Anton's syndrome). Balint's syndrome may also occur in which the patient is unable to view the entire visual field at once, has poor hand–eye coordination, and gaze apraxia. These patients usually cannot read a paragraph because they omit words or lines while reading (18). Bilateral temporal lobe infarction may lead to an amnestic syndrome indistinguishable from Korsakoff's psychosis.

A unilateral dominant PCA territory infarction may cause a transcortical sensory aphasia, in which the patient is unable to understand but can repeat normally.

CONCLUSION

The importance of recognition of supratentorial ischemic syndromes lies not so much in the features of the specific syndromes, though they are intellectually interesting, but perhaps in the etiology and pathophysiology of the syndrome when due to cerebrovascular disease. Bogousslavsky stressed that the thalamic perforator syndromes could be due to embolus or aneurysm (15). Similarly, the presence of an isolated Wernicke's aphasia would lead one to a search for an embolic source, whether cardiac, carotid, or proximal MCA, and thus allow for appropriate therapy.

REFERENCES

1. Benson DF. The history of behavioral neurology. *Neurol Clin* 1993; 11(1):1–8.
2. Gavrilescu T, Kase CS. Clinical stroke syndromes: clinical–anatomical correlations. *Cerebrovasc Brain Metab Rev* 1995;7(3):218–239.
3. Baquis GD, Pessin MS, Scott RM. Limb shaking—a carotid TIA. *Stroke* 1985;16(3):444–448.
4. Furlan AJ, Whisnant JP, Kearns TP. Unilateral visual loss in bright light. *Arch Neurol* 1979;36:675–676.
5. Wiebers DO, Swanson JW, Cascino TL, Whisnant JP. Bilateral loss of vision in bright light. *Stroke* 1989;20:554–558.
6. North American Symptomatic Carotid Endarterectomy Trial Collaborators. Beneficial effect of carotid endarterectomy in symptomatic patients with high-grade carotid stenosis. *N Engl J Med* 1991;325(7): 445–453.
7. Streifler JY, Eliasziw M, Benavente OR, et al. The risk of stroke in patients with first-ever retinal vs hemispheric transient ischemic attacks and high-grade carotid stenosis. *Arch Neurol* 1995;52:246–249.
8. Helgason C, Caplan LR, Goodwin V, et al. Anterior choroidal territory infarction: case reports and review. *Arch Neurol* 1986;43:681–686.
9. Caplan LR, Schmahmann JD, Case CS, et al. Caudate infarcts. *Arch Neurol* 1990;47:133–143.
10. Saris S. Chorea casused by caudate infarction. *Arch Neurol* 1983;40: 590–591.
11. Ross ED. Left medial parietal lobe and receptive language functions: mixed transcortical aphasia after left anterior cerebral artery infarction. *Neurology* 1980;30:144–151.
12. Geschwind N. Aphasia. *N Engl J Med* 1971;284(12):654–656.
13. Geschwind N. Disconnexion syndromes in animals and man. *Brain* 1965;88:585–644.
14. Mesulam MM, Waxman SG, Geschwind N, and Sabin TD. Acute confusional states with right middle cerebral artery infarctions. *J Neurol Neurosurg Psychiatry* 1976;39:84–89.
15. Ross ED. The aprosodias. *Arch Neurol* 1981;38:561–569.
16. Bogousslavsky J, Regli F, Uske A. Thalamic infarcts: clinical syndromes, etiology, and prognosis. *Neurology* 1988;38:837–848.
17. Meissner I, Sapir S, Kokmen E, Stein SD. The paramedian diencephalic syndrome: a dynamic phenomenon. *Stroke* 1987;18:380–385.
18. Caplan LR. "Top of the basilar" syndrome. *Neurology* 1980;30:72–79.

Cerebrovascular Disease, edited by H. Hunt Batjer.
Lippincott-Raven Publishers, Philadelphia © 1997.

CHAPTER 28

Infratentorial Ischemic Syndromes

Lee H. Schwamm and Seth P. Finklestein

NORMAL VASCULAR ANATOMY OF THE POSTERIOR FOSSA

The vascular supply to the brainstem and cerebellum consists of the paired vertebral arteries (VAs) and the basilar artery (BA). These arteries course along the anterior aspect of the brainstem, and their perforating end-arterioles are the only blood supply to the substance of this region (Fig. 1A, B). At all levels of the medulla, pons, and midbrain, the large vessels lie on the outer surface of a cyclindrical structure. The pattern of penetrating arteries is maintained throughout, with the ventromedial brainstem supplied by paramedian branches, the ventrolateral brainstem by short circumferential branches, and the dorsolateral brainstem and cerebellum by long circumferential branches (Fig. 2). In addition, there is a great degree of variability in the site of vessel origins, vessel-specific vascular territories, side-to-side dominance, and in the arrangement of collateral channels. The least variable anastomotic design is found in the circle of Willis, connecting the anterior (carotid) and posterior (vertebrobasilar) circulations at the base of the brain (1) (Figs. 3, 22, 24). The details of the normal anatomy of the posterior fossa are outlined below.

Vertebral Arteries

The left and right VAs commonly arise from the subclavian arteries, although the right VA may also arise from the right brachiocephalic trunk and the left may arise directly from the aortic arch (Fig. 4). The VAs are of equal size in a quarter of normal patients and the left VA is dominant in about half (2). Total blood flow to the intracranial VAs (ICVAs) is approximately 15% of total cerebral blood flow. This disparity reflects the different perfusion requirements of the brainstem, which is predominantly white matter, vs.

L. H. Schwamm and S. P. Finkelstein: Stroke Service, Department of Neurology, Massachusetts General Hospital and Harvard Medical School, Boston, Massachusetts 02114.

the cerebral cortex, which is predominantly gray matter, with the former requiring approximately 20 ml/100 g/min and the latter requiring 100 ml/100 g/min, respectively. The VAs can be divided into four segments: the *prevertebral* segment (arch origin to C6), the *cervical* segment (transverse foramina of C6 to C2), the *atlantic* segment (posterior atlas to atlanto-occipital membrane), and, after entering the cranium via the foramen magnum and piercing the dura, the *intracranial* or *subarachnoid* segment (anterolateral medulla to vertebrobasilar junction) (3) (Fig. 5). The cervical segment gives rise to small perforating branches to muscle and contributes to the anterior and posterior spinal arteries. The intracranial segment gives rise to paramedian arteries, short circumferential arteries, long cirumferential arteries known as posterior inferior cerebellar arteries (PICAs), as well as the anterior spinal arteries (ASAs) (4). This segment may contain several sites of persistent fetal anastomoses between the carotid and vertebral systems, including the trigeminal, hypoglossal, and acoustic arteries (2). The average ICVA diameter is between 3.2 and 3.5 mm, and the majority of the small brainstem perforators originate within 7 mm of the vertebrobasilar junction (Fig. 6). Normally, reduction in flow in a single VA does not produce symptoms of basilar territory ischemia, assuming that flow through the contralateral VA compensates for the loss. Congenital variations may occur in which one VA terminates as the ipsilateral PICA whereas the other is continuous with the BA, or one VA may be atretic or stenosed while the other supplies both PICAs and the BA. In both these instances, the VA is said to be "basilarized" because hemodynamic compromise in this vessel may now be indistinguishable from flow reductions in the BA itself (Fig. 28).

The *paramedian* arteries (Figs. 2 and 8) of the proximal ICVA and ASAs supply the following medial medullary structures: pyramidal tract, medial inferior olive, medial lemniscus, medial longitudinal fasciculus (MLF), and the hypoglossal (XII) nucleus and emerging XII nerve fibers.

The *short circumferential* (Figs. 2 and 9) branches of the ICVA supply the lateral medulla, with some overlap at the

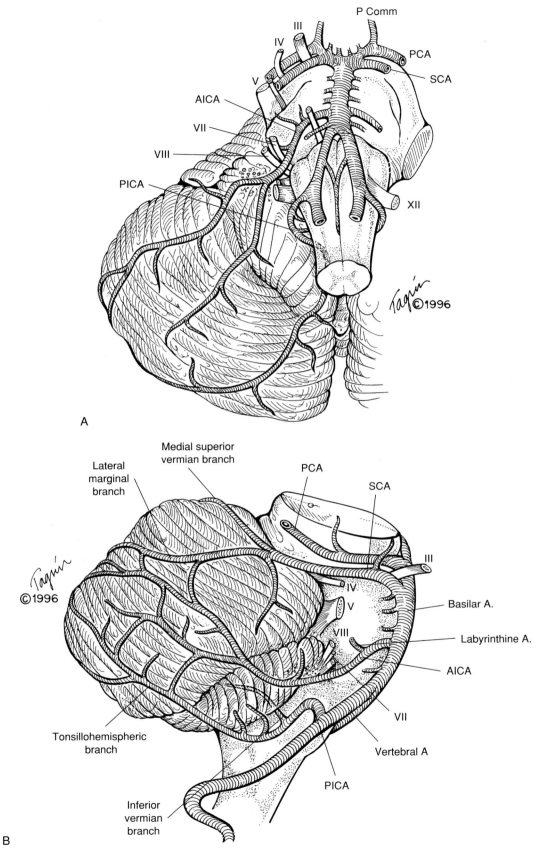

FIG. 1. A: Anteroposterior view of the posterior fossa and its vascular supply. **B:** Lateral view of the posterior fossa and its vascular supply.

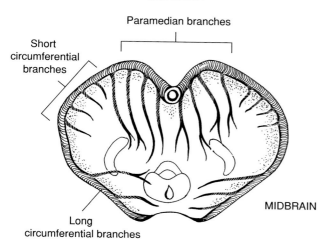

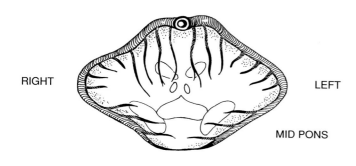

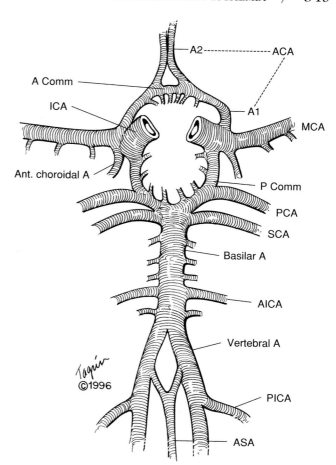

FIG. 3. Circle of Willis.

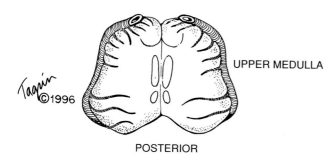

FIG. 2. Axial sections of the brainstem at three levels, illustrating the pattern of penetrating vessels.

dorsolateral border with the PICA. This territory contains the spinothalamic tract, spinal tract and nucleus of V, descending sympathetic fibers, lateral inferior olive, nucleus and tractus solitarius, the cuneate and gracile nuclei, inferior cerebellar peduncle (restiform body, ICP), the nucleus ambiguus (contributions to IX, X, XI), and the exiting fibers of the vagus nerve (X).

The most caudal of the long circumferential arteries is the *posterior inferior cerebellar* artery (PICA) (Figs. 1B and 25), which usually arises from the ICVA at the level of the

olive but can also arise from the atlantic segment of the VA, directly from the BA, or from a common trunk with the anterior inferior cerebellar artery (AICA). The four segments of the PICA are the *anterior medullary, lateral medullary, posterior medullary,* and *supratonsilar.* The first three segments give rise to perforating bulbar branches to the lateral and posterior medulla en route to the inferior cerebellum. The supratonsilar segment comprises an inferior vermian branch and a tonsillohemispheric branch, which supply cerebellum and overlying occipital lobe. If the PICA diameter is small, its territory may be supplied by the adjacent ipsilateral AICA or the contralateral PICA. End-to-end anastomoses commonly exist between the cerebellar hemispheric branches of the PICA and the ipsilateral AICA or contralateral PICA (5). This extensive collateral flow may allow the brain to tolerate occlusive VA lesions that occur between PICA and AICA better than those lesions proximal to the PICA origin.

Basilar Artery

The BA begins at the junction of the VAs, and gives off 5–10 paramedian vessels, 5–7 short circumferential vessels,

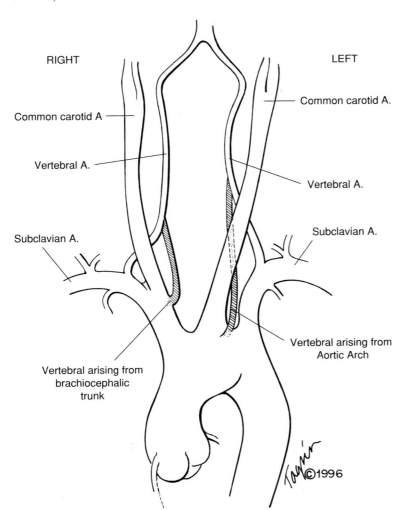

RIGHT

LEFT

Common carotid A

Common carotid A.

Vertebral A.

Vertebral A.

Subclavian A.

Subclavian A.

Vertebral arising from
Aortic Arch

Vertebral arising from
brachiocephalic
trunk

©1996

FIG. 4. Relationship of the vertebral arteries to the aotic arch. Shaded vessels indicate common congenital variations.

and 2 long circumferential vessels (AICA and SCA) before it terminates as the bifurcation of the posterior cerebral arteries (PCAs) in the interpeduncular cistern, above the level of the oculomotor nuclei. At the level of the midbrain, the paramedian perforators and short circumferential arteries arise from the distal tip of the basilar, the proximal portions of the PCA and the *posterior communicating* artery (PComm) (Fig. 2). Occlusion of these vessels may produce the ''top of the basilar'' syndrome, a constellation of vertical gaze palsy, abnormal convergence, skew deviation, corectopia, behavioral disturbances, and hallucinations (Figs. 16 and 18) (6). In 10–20% of individuals, the proximal segment of the PCA (mesencephalic artery) is atretic and one PCA arises from the carotid system via the PComm (unilateral fetal PCA) (Fig. 24). In this instance, the paramedian perforating arteries that usually originate from the mesencephalic segment of the PCA now arise from the basilar tip. In 5–10% of individuals, both PCAs arise from the carotid system (bilateral fetal PCAs) (2,7). The average proximal BA diameter is 4.5 mm and the vertebrobasilar junction may occur any-

where from 2 mm below to 7 mm above the pontomedullary junction (4).

The *paramedian* arteries (Figs. 2, 10, 12, 14) originate on the posterior surface of the BA, enter the pons a few millimeters lateral to midline and travel in an anteroposterior plane. They supply the structures of the medial basis pontis and ventral tegmentum, including the corticobulbar tract (CBT), corticospinal tract (CST), pontine nuclei, MLF, medial lemniscus, and pontine reticular formation.

The *short circumferential* arteries (Figs. 2, 11, 13, 15) arise from the lateral wall of the BA and travel laterally over the surface of the pons for 1 cm before entering to supply the lateral two thirds of the pons, middle cerebellar peduncle (brachium pontis, MCP), and superior cerebellar peduncle (brachium conjunctivum, dentatorubrothalamic tract, SCP). The pontine structures include pontine nuclei, lateral CST, lateral medial lemniscus, and trigeminal (V) and facial (VII) nuclei.

The *anterior inferior cerebellar* artery (AICA) (Figs. 1B and 11) arises from the lateral wall of the lower third of the

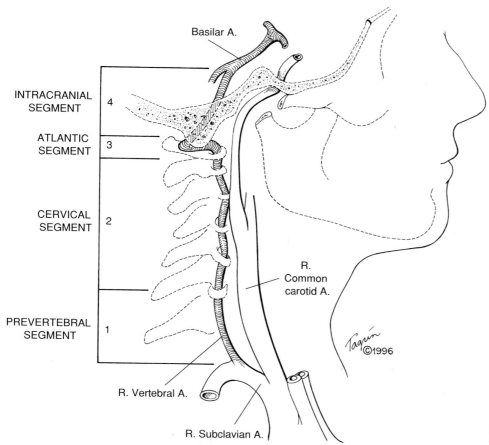

INTRACRANIAL SEGMENT 4

ATLANTIC SEGMENT 3

CERVICAL SEGMENT 2

PREVERTEBRAL SEGMENT 1

Basilar A.

R. Common carotid A.

R. Vertebral A.

R. Subclavian A.

©1996

FIG. 5. Anatomic segments of the vertebral artery.

BA, passes ventrally across the inferior pons, and gives off penetrating arteries en route to the cerebellum. It is the most caudal long circumferential artery of the pons and supplies the emerging facial nerve (VII), trigeminal nerve (V) root, vestibular and cochlear nuclei and acoustic nerve (VIII), and the spinothalamic tract. When the AICA reaches the internal auditory meatus, it gives rise to the labyrinthine artery, which traverses the internal auditory canal (IAC), with the facial and vestibulocochlear nerves to supply the cochlea and labyrinth. Alternatively, the labyrinthine artery may arise as a branch directly off the BA. Distal to the IAC, the AICA then courses over the anterior inferior cerebellum, supplying the MCP and adjacent cerebellum.

The *superior cerebellar* artery (SCA) (Fig. 1b, 15, 31) is the most rostral long circumferential artery of the pons, arising from the distal BA just inferior to the PCA bifurcation. The SCA passes below the oculomotor nerve (III) and past the cerebral peduncle, giving off perforating branches into the upper pons and low midbrain on its way to the superior cerebellum. The SCA then divides into two main branches, the *lateral marginal* and the *medial superior vermian,* which freely anastomose with one another and with the other cerebellar arteries. The lateral marginal branch supplies the SCP,

MCP, dentate nucleus, and anterolateral superior cerebellum. The medial superior vermian branch merges with the inferior vermian branch of the PICA to supply the dentate nucleus, inferior colliculus, and posteromedial superior cerebellum.

The *posterior cerebral* artery (PCA) (Figs. 1B and 2) arises as the terminal bifurcation of the BA and passes above the oculomotor nucleus and around the cerebral peduncle on its way to thalamic nuclei and the occipital lobe. The proximal PCA is divided into the peduncular, ambient, and quadrigeminal segments according to the cistern it traverses. The *peduncular* segment (mesencephalic artery or basilar communicating artery) gives rise to dense paramedian perforating arteries that supply the red nucleus, substantia nigra, medial aspect of the cerebral peduncle, oculomotor and trochlear (IV) nuclei and nerves, periaqueductal gray and reticular formation, decussation of the SCP, MLF, and medial lemniscus. The *ambient* segment gives rise to the *thalamoperforating* arteries, which supply the hypothalamus, subthalamus, and midline and medial thalamic nuclei. Included within the complex of *thalamoperforating* arteries is the *posterior thalamosubthalamic paramedian* artery (artery of Percheron), which can also arise as a single midline vessel from the proximal peduncular

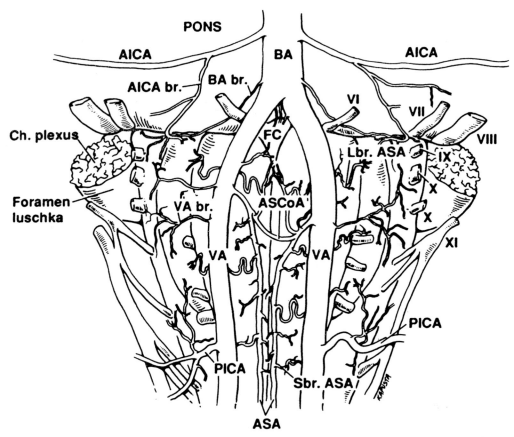

FIG. 6. Schematic drawing of the proximal intracranial part of the vertebrobasilar system. The branches to the anterior aspect of the medulla oblongata are shown. ASA, anterior spinal artery; ASCoA, anterior spinal communicating artery; br, branch; ch. Plexus, choroid plexus; FC, foramen caecum; Lbr, long branch; Sbr, short branch. (Reprinted from Neurological Research by permission of Forefront Publishing.)

segment and bifurcate to supply bilateral thalamic and hypothalamic structures. More distal are the *thalamogeniculate* arteries, which supply the medial and lateral geniculate nuclei and central and posterior thalamus, and the *posterior choroidal* arteries, which supply the pulvinar, and medial dorsal and lateral geniculate thalamic nuclei. Additional supply to the cerebral peduncle arises from perforators off the PComm. The *quadrigeminal* segment gives rise to perforating arteries, which supply the lateral cerebral peduncle and lateral pontine and midbrain tegmentum.

PATHOLOGIC PROCESSES AFFECTING ARTERIES

Atherosclerosis and Thrombosis

Atherosclerosis typically affects vessels greater than 500 μm in diameter and is found in characteristic locations in the posterior circulation. It consists of the intimal accumulation of extracellular lipids and necrotic cellular debris with resultant fibromuscular proliferation. As the lesions progress the lumen narrows, hemodynamic flow is compromised, and a nidus for in situ thrombosis develops (Figs. 19 and 20). Though seen less commonly in the posterior circulation vessels than in the carotid arteries, necrosis, ulceration, and rupture of the atherosclerotic plaque into the intraluminal surface may cause acute thrombo-occlusion or distal embolization of atheromatous debris or thrombus (5). When atherosclerosis involves a segment of vessel wall, which includes the osteum of a smaller penetrating branch artery, it may produce infarction that simulates occlusive small branch vessel disease (8).

Atherosclerotic disease in the posterior circulation vessels reflects the same pathophysiologic process as in the carotid circulation, with the proximal ICVA mirroring the proximal extracranial internal carotid artery. Thrombosis of the ICVA also produces anterograde or retrograde propogation of clot to the level of the nearest inflowing branch vessel. (This is a rare occurrence in the extracranial VA due perhaps to its tortuous course or multilevel collateral anastomoses.) Ischemic symptoms in both of these vascular territories arise from hemodynamically significant stenoses or distal embolization, and collateral circulation may blunt the effects of proximal stenoses. The contralateral ICVA often provides collateral flow, as evidenced by the finding that many proximal ICVA occlusions are silent. In addition, the cerebellar anastomoses between PICA and AICA provide further potential collateral channels and may explain why ICVA occlusions proximal to the PICA are more symptomatic than those that occur between PICA and AICA.

The distribution of cerebral atherosclerotic lesions varies with race and gender. Caucasian men tend to develop stenosis at the VA origins, the distal ICVA, and the proximal and distal ends of the BA (Figs. 7 and 23). Postmenopausal Caucasian women, and black and Asian men and women are more prone to intracranial rather than extracranial disease, with preferential involvement of the mid-basilar, distal ICVA and the origins of the PICA, SCA, and PCA (2,9).

Lipohyalinosis

Segmental fibrinoid arterial degeneration of small penetrating cerebral arteries (75–300 μm) of the cerebral circulation is the pathophysiology underlying lacunar infarction (10,11). It is most often a complication of longstanding systolic hypertension or diabetes. Neuropathologically the distinctions between vessel intima, media and adventitia are lost and these tissue layers are replaced by a brightly eosinophilic material. This arterial pathology leads to secondary aneurysmal dilatation, periarterial hemorrhage, or occlusive thrombosis with subsequent ischemia to the distal territory. Since this process affects end-arterioles there is typically no collateral circulation and ischemic infarction ensues. Lacunar infarction is most common in the pons and thalamus, but may also occur in the midbrain and medulla (Fig. 14). In the brainstem, lacunae occur most often in the medial basal seg-

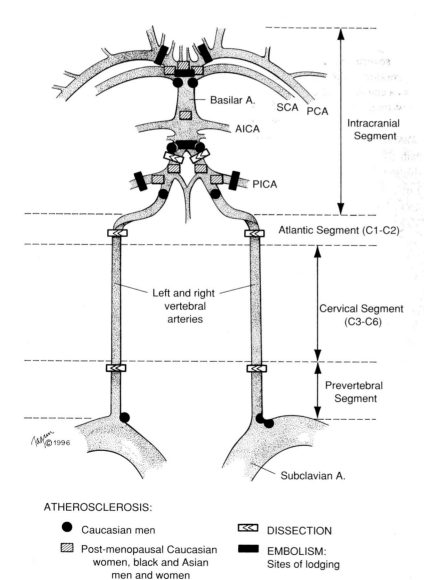

ATHEROSCLEROSIS:

● Caucasian men

▨ Post-menopausal Caucasian women, black and Asian men and women

◩ DISSECTION

▬ EMBOLISM: Sites of lodging

FIG. 7. Sites of predilection for atherosclerosis, dissection, and embolism arrest.

ments, in the territory of the paramedian penetrating arterioles (2,12).

Dissection

Arterial dissection of one or both extracranial VAs may occur spontaneously or in the setting of minimal trauma. Chiropractic neck manipulation and activities involving rapid neck rotation have been reported to cause intimal injury to the extracranial VA (13,14). Rotational force is maximal at the C1–C2 junction in the atlantic segment and in the distal prevertebral segment of the VA (Figs. 5 and 7). Vascular injury at these sites may be due to in situ thrombosis without true dissection, dissection and thrombosis with or without hemodynamic compromise, or dissection with thrombosis and distal embolization (Case examples 3 and 4). Magnetic resonance imaging can be useful in noninvasive diagnosis of arterial dissection by detecting diminished flow signal in the affected vessel and associated ischemic brain lesions (Fig. 25). Occasionally, T1 hyperintensity (seen best on axial sections) due to subintimal methemoglobin deposition can be appreciated. In patients with severe cervical spondylosis, mechanical osteophytic compression of the VA during head rotation has been postulated as a cause of vertebrobasilar insufficiency, but there are few data to support this hypothesis.

The most common symptom of extracranial vertebral dissection is the sudden onset of severe pain in the posterior neck, often with radiation to the occiput. Ischemic symptoms generally localize to the lateral medulla or cerebellum and may occur simultaneously with, or at some delay from, the onset of the head and neck pain (15). ICVA and BA dissections are much rarer and often present with subarachnoid hemorrhage. The risk of rupture into the interstitium is greater in intracranial vessels because they have a thinner subintima than extracranial vessels and no external elastic lamina to help contain hemorrhage within the vessel wall. Conditions that predispose to dissection include fibromuscular dysplasia, cystic medial necrosis and some heritable collagen vascular disorders (16).

Embolism From Other Sites

In the posterior circulation emboli arising from the heart or proximal arteries frequently lodge in the distal ICVA, distal BA, PICA, SCA, or PCA (Fig. 7). An embolus capable of passing through the distal ICVA will not be arrested until it reaches the top of the BA unless preexisting atherosclerosis has narrowed the lumen of the more proximal BA (Fig. 23). Emboli may arise in any part of the left-sided circulatory system, including the pulmonary veins, left atrium, left ventricle, and mitral or aortic valves. Additionally, the aorta, subclavian, or vertebral arteries may be the source of cholesterol or thrombotic artery-to-artery emboli (17,18). Approximately 40% of posterior circulation emboli arise from cardiac or intraarterial sources (9). Left ventricular mural thrombus may occur in severe myocardial failure with or without left ventricular aneurysm and after acute anterior wall infarction. Any procedure that involves passage of a catheter into the proximal aorta can damage the arterial wall and liberate cholesterol or platelet debris (Case example 2). Tumors of the left atrium may present as sources of embolic material. Valvular disease in the mitral or aortic position may produce emboli, consisting of infectious, thrombtic, immune complex, or atheromatous particles. Right-sided circulation disease may generate cerebrovascular emboli if a right-to-left shunt exists (eg, patent foramen ovale or pulmonary arteriovenous malformation). Acute right heart strain such as occurs in left ventricular failure or pulmonary embolism may raise right ventricular end-diastolic pressures sufficiently to open a patent foramen ovale that was functionally occluded at normal intracardiac pressures. Lipid from long bone fractures and thrombus from limb and pelvic veins are other potential sources of embolic material.

Arteritis

Partial focal inflammation of the arterial wall can lead to aneurysmal dilatation and rupture, and circumferential inflammation can lead to progressive stenosis and in situ thrombosis. Although rare, arteritis may affect the subclavian and vertebral arteries and, to an even lesser degree, the intracranial posterior circulation branch vessels. Arteritis can involve the vessel wall directly or indirectly via inflammation of the vaso vasorum, causing ischemic injury to the arterial wall. Takayasu's arteritis and giant cell arteritis demonstrate a type IV (granulomatous) hypersensitivity reaction that may affect the subclavian and vertebral origins. When the proximal left subclavian artery occludes, collateral blood supply to the distal subclavian develops via retrograde flow down the vertebral and basilar arteries. In this setting, vigorous exercise of the limb may cause some symptoms of lower brainstem ischemia, *subclavian steal,* such as lightheadedness, dizziness, or vertigo. Rarely, if ever, does it produce such focal brainstem ischemic signs as hemiparesis, sensory disturbance, cranial nerve dysfunction, or nystagmus, and thus it is almost never confused with atherosclerotic or embolic disease of the vertebral or basilar arteries. Behçets disease demonstrates either a type III (immune complex) or type IV (granulomatous) hypersensitivity reaction and may give rise to ischemia in the brainstem. Infectious arteritis (syphilitic or tuberculous) involves the arteries of the rostral brainstem and when untreated can lead to progressive infarction (19).

GENERAL PRINCIPLES OF BRAINSTEM ISCHEMIA

Localization of ischemic symptoms within the vertebrobasilar system can be a daunting task, especially for the clinician who does not routinely encounter these syndromes. The clinical syndrome and anatomy of BA disease has been well described by many authors (2,3,6,9,20–33). It consists of the abrupt onset of altered consciousness and bilateral motor and cranial nerve signs, the severity of which may wax and wane in the first few hours. The constellation of ''confusion,'' vertigo, pupillary and extraocular movement abnormalities, dysarthria, hemiplegia, ataxia, and bilateral extensor plantar responses should convince the clinician of disease in the BA (Case examples 1 and 2).

In their landmark paper in 1948, Kubik and Adams reported clinicopathologic correlation in 18 cases of BA occlusion (29). They noted frequent disturbances of consciousness (18 of 18), hemiplegia (18 of 18), pupillary abnormalities (15 of 18), and dysarthria (13 of 18). Dizziness (7 of 18), headache (4 of 18), paresthesias (4 of 11), and unilateral abducens palsy (2 of 18) were less common and observed only in BA thrombotic occlusion. Oculomotor palsy was found more frequently in embolism. This reflects the tendency of emboli to lodge at the uppermost BA (at the level of the paramedian artery supply to the oculomotor nuclear complex) and thrombosis to occur in the mid-BA at the level of the pons. The examination of the eyes often provides the clue for localization within the brainstem. Lesions confined to the pons interrupt descending sympathetic fibers and horizontal gaze centers but spare the pupillary reflex arc and vertical gaze centers, whereas midbrain lesions tend to spare the former and interrupt the latter. Thus pontine pupils are miotic, equal, and reactive, but midbrain pupils are irregular and poorly reactive to light. Pupil size and contour depend on the relative balance of sympathetic and parasympathetic inputs and the integrity of the Edinger–Westphal nucleus.

Early clinical recognition of BA ischemia becomes increasingly important as novel therapies for acute stroke continue to emerge. Although the reduced metabolic requirements of white matter tracts may render them less vulnerable to periods of decreased cerebral perfusion, the success of intraarterial or intravenous thrombolysis in posterior circulation ischemia still depends on rapid recognition and treatment.

Occlusion of branches of the VA or BA may produce focal infarction within the brainstem or cerebellum. Some general principles apply: As noted above, infarction of the medial brainstem generally occurs following occlusion of short paramedian branches from the BA. Infarction of the lateral brainstem occurs following occlusion of the long or short circumferential branches of the VA or BA. Hallmark clinical features of infarction of the medial brainstem include contralateral weakness (through involvement of the corticospinal tract), contralateral loss of vibration and position sense (through involvement of the medial lemniscus), ataxia (through involvement of cerebellar tracts), and dysfunction of cranial nerves VI and III (through involvement of their nuclei). Hallmark features of infarction of the lateral brainstem include ipsilateral ataxia (through involvement of the cerebellar tracts), contralateral loss of pain and temperature

sensation (through involvement of the spinothalamic tract), facial pain and numbness (through involvement of the nucleus and tract of V), nystagmus and vertigo (through involvement of the vestibular nuclei), and Horner's syndrome (through involvement of sympathetic pathways). Weakness, loss of position and vibration sense, and IIIrd nerve dysfunction can also occur in some lateral brainstem syndromes. When brainstem infarction fails to produce hemiparesis, the diagnosis of stroke is sometimes missed. In these cases, the clinician must be alert to other findings, such as the acute onset of ataxia, vertigo, nystagmus, diplopia, loss of pain and temperature sensation, Horner's syndrome, or facial pain to make the correct diagnosis.

Described below are specific clinical syndromes resulting from infarction of the brainstem, with representative axial sections from ten levels of the brainstem. To facilitate comparison with actual case material, the axial sections are displayed in the same orientation as conventional radiologic images. These sections contain the important anatomic structures useful in clinical localization; however, actual strokes rarely respect these arbitrary borders. The figures depict common deficits associated with the shaded areas of infarction, and all lesions are drawn on the right half of the brainstem. The tables list the clinical symptoms and signs associated with injury to each anatomic structure; for additional clarity, the items in bold-face are also depicted in the illustrated figures. Common eponyms are listed at the bottom of each table with their cardinal symptoms listed in parentheses. The glossary (see p. 356) lists all abbreviations used in the axial sections, figures, and tables.

ISCHEMIC SYNDROMES OF THE POSTERIOR CIRCULATION

Medulla

Lesions of the Medial Upper Medulla (Fig. 8) (Table 1)

Occlusion of the VA or ASA may cause a unilateral or bilateral medial medullary infarction. This is a relatively uncommon lesion that produces ipsilateral tongue weakness, contralateral hemiparesis sparing the face, and contralateral decreased position and vibration (dorsal column) sense. A bilateral vascular insult may cause a quadriparesis. If the lesion is more caudal in the medulla, it may involve the motor fibers to the arm after they have decussated, producing ipsilateral arm and contralateral leg weakness.

Lesions of the Lateral Upper Medulla (Figs. 9, 28–30) (Table 2)

The lateral medullary syndrome of Wallenberg is a common form of brainstem stroke. Since this is one of the brainstem syndromes that spares the corticospinal tracts and hemiparesis does not occur, this diagnosis of stroke is sometimes

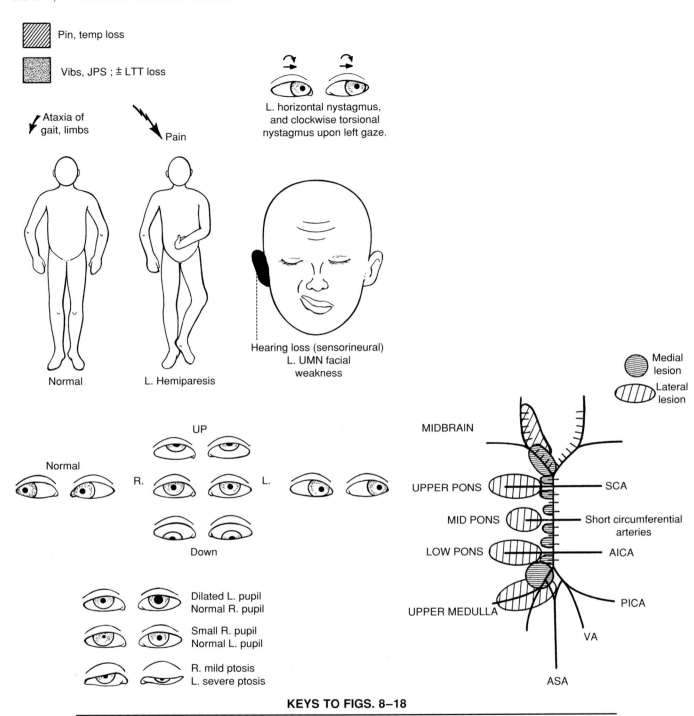

Pin, temp loss

Vibs, JPS ; ± LTT loss

Ataxia of gait, limbs

Pain

L. horizontal nystagmus, and clockwise torsional nystagmus upon left gaze.

Normal

L. Hemiparesis

Hearing loss (sensorineural) L. UMN facial weakness

UP

Normal

R.   L.

Down

Dilated L. pupil
Normal R. pupil

Small R. pupil
Normal L. pupil

R. mild ptosis
L. severe ptosis

Medial lesion

Lateral lesion

MIDBRAIN

UPPER PONS — SCA

MID PONS — Short circumferential arteries

LOW PONS — AICA

UPPER MEDULLA — PICA

VA

ASA

KEYS TO FIGS. 8–18

Glossary

a., artery; AICA., anterior inferior cerebellar artery; BA., basilar artery; C., contralateral; CBT., cortico-bulbar tract; CST., corticospinal tract; DMN., dorsal motor nucleus of X; F-P., frontopontine fibers; I., ipsilateral; I-XII., Cranial nerves I-XII; ICP., inferior cerebellar peduncle; inf., inferior; INO., internuclear ophthalmoplegia; IO., inferior oblique; IR., inferior rectus; L., left; LMN., lower motor neuron; LR., lateral rectus; MCP., middle cerebellar peduncle; MGB., medial geniculate body; ML., medial lemniscus; MLF., medial longitudinal fasiculus; MR., medial rectus; n., nerve; N., non-lateralizing; nucl., nucleus; PAG., periaqueductal grey matter; PCA., posterior cerebral artery; PComm., posterior communicating artery; PICA., posterior inferior cerebellar artery; P-T-OP., parieto-temporo-occipitopontine fibers; R., right; SCA., Superior cerebellar artery; SCP., superior cerebellar peduncle; SN., substantial nigra; SO., superior oblique; SR., superior rectus; ST., spinothalamic tract; subnucl., subnucleus; sup., superior; UMN., upper motor neuron; VA., vertebral artery.

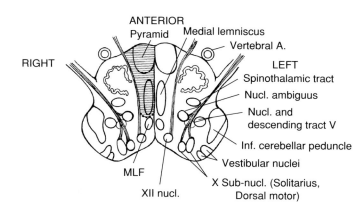

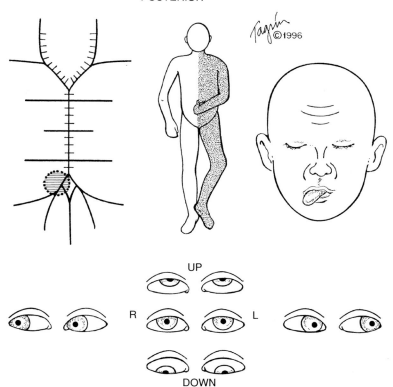

FIG. 8. Occlusion of the vertebral or anterior spinal artery causing infarction of the medial upper medulla.

TABLE 1. *Lesions of the medial upper medulla*

Neuroanatomy	Clinical manifestations
XIIth nerve	(a) I: **tongue weakness, deviating toward the lesion when protruded**
Corticospinal tract	(b) C: **weakness arm and leg**
Medial lemniscus	(c) C: **decreased vibration, proprioception ± light touch**

Eponyms: Dejerine anterior bulbar (a, b, c).

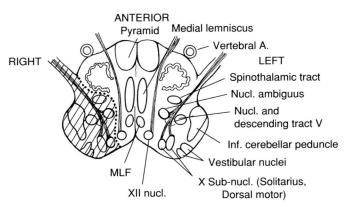

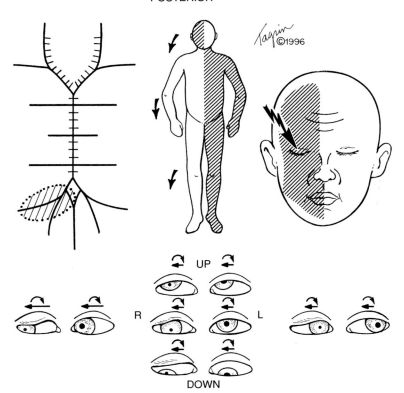

FIG. 9. Occlusion of the vertebral or posterior inferior cerebellar artery causing infarction of the lateral upper medulla.

TABLE 2. *Lesions of the lateral upper medulla*

Neuroanatomy	Clinical manifestations
Vth nucl.	(a) I: **periorbital ± facial pain**
Descending tract of Vth nucl.	(b) I: **facial numbness**
ICP ± cerebellar tracts	(c) I: **ataxia of limbs and gait,** hypermetric saccades toward side of lesion
Vestibular nuclei	(d) I: **horizontal nystagmus** (fast phase), **tonic gaze deviation**
	(e) C: **torisional nystagmus** (fast phase)
	(f) N: diplopia, vertigo, nausea, vomiting
Descending sympathetics	(g) I: **Horner's syndrome**
Nucl. ambiguus, Xth nerve	(h) I: hoarseness, dysphagia, decreased gag
Nucl. and tractus solitarius	(i) I: decreased taste
Spinothalamic tract	(j) C: **body numbness**
Uncertain localization	(k) N: hiccups

Eponyms: Wallenberg (a–k), Cestan–Chenais (c, g, h, j).
ICP, inferior cerebellar peduncle.

missed. Lateral medullary infarction is due to occlusion of the VA (75% of cases) or PICA (15% of cases). It is sometimes accompanied by cerebellar infarction, which may result in life-threatening brain swelling in the posterior fossa (7). When PICA occlusion occurs, it is most often due to emboli arising from the proximal VA or the heart (2,34).

The classic syndrome consists of dysequilibrium, crossed sensory loss, and Horner's syndrome (see below). Patients complain of sudden onset of vertigo, nausea, vomiting, hoarseness, dysphagia, often with hiccups and diplopia. They have ipsilateral periorbital or facial pain within a field of numbness, and contralateral body numbness. Nystagmus and visual disturbances are common but often unrecognized. However, due to differences in the vascular supply and territory of infarction among individuals, the clinical presentation can be quite variable and the only firm clue may be the facial pain characteristic of injury to the spinal tract of V (35).

The nucleus of the spinal tract of V sends afferent fibers for facial sensation to the thalamus in a somatotopic array, with the mandibular (V3) representation most rostrally and the ophthalmic (V1) representation descending caudally into the cervical spine. Afferent sensory fibers leaving the spinal nucleus of V cross to the ventral trigeminothalamic tract and shift laterally as they ascend into the pons, coming to lie adjacent to the lateral spinothalamic tract. If the lateral medullary lesion extends rostrally enough into the low pons, these crossing fibers may be interrupted, adding contralateral perioral or mandibular division numbness to the contralateral body numbness caused by spinothalamic involvement. Occasionally, the nucleus of the spinal tract of V is organized in an alternative somatotopic array, in a medial-to-lateral plane, and lesions produce an onion skin pattern of facial numbness (24).

The complete Horner's syndrome includes ipsilateral ptosis, miosis, and anhidrosis (asymmetric sweating over the whole face). This occurs when autonomic sympathetic fibers are injured proximal to the origin of the external carotid artery. If the injury is distal to this site, sweating over the face is unaffected. Pharmacologic testing of the pupil assists in localizing the level at which the sympathetic outflow has been interrupted. In a preganglionic or central Horner's such as occurs in lateral medullary infarction, the miotic pupil will dilate to a 1% hydroxyamphetamine solution but not to a drop of 10% cocaine solution. This is because hydroxyamphetamine causes the release of presynaptic norepinephrine (NE), which then acts appropriately on the normal postganglionic neuron. Cocaine is an indirect sympathomimetic that blocks reuptake of NE, and since the injured preganglionic neuron is incapable of releasing NE, there is no effect on the pupil.

The ptosis that occurs in Horner's syndrome is mild because approximately 30% of levator palpebrae action (upper eyelid elevation) is innervated by sympathetic fibers compared with 70% by the IIIrd nerve (30). Lower lid contraction is due to Mueller's muscle, which is innervated by sympathetic fibers only.

Lateral medullary infarction often produces visual disturbances, such as tilt of the visual environment, skew deviation with ipsilateral hypometria (skew deviation of Hertwig–Magendie), tonic conjugate gaze deviation increasing with eye closure, and downbeat monocular nystagmus upon gaze toward the affected side (23,36,37).

Pons

Lesions of the Medial Lower Pons (Fig. 10) (Table 3)

Occlusion of the proximal paramedian BA branch vessels produces infarction in the medial lower pons. Contralateral hemiparesis and ipsilateral VIth nerve or conjugate gaze palsy are the hallmark clinical features. The hemiparesis is due to involvement of the uncrossed corticospinal and corticobulbar tracts and the gaze palsy is due to involvement of the VI nucleus ± the horizontal gaze center. When the lesion extends laterally, involvement of the VIIth nucleus or nerve produces peripheral (ie, lower motor neuron) facial weakness involving the forehead. Central (ie, corticobulbar tract) facial weakness spares the forehead, owing to the bilateral descending cortical motor input to each frontalis.

The horizontal gaze center (parapontine reticular formation) receives input from the contralateral frontal eye fields and generates a conjugate horizontal saccade to the ipsilateral side. Because neurons of the horizontal gaze center are intermingled so closely with those of the VIth nucleus, many authors believe that it is impossible to have a pure horizontal gaze center lesion that preserves ipsilateral abduction. However, since a chronic VIth nerve palsy produces medial deviation of the eye (esotropia) due to the unopposed action of the ipsilateral medial rectus, a chronic abducens palsy may be detected in the presence of an acute horizontal gaze palsy (23).

If the lesion involves the MLF and the horizontal gaze center, all voluntary horizontal eye movements except abduction of the contralateral eye are lost. When each eye is assigned one point for full horizontal gaze, this lesion causes loss of one-and-a-half eye movements, and thus the descriptive term "one-and-a-half syndrome" (40).

The "locked-in syndrome" results from bilateral infarction of the corticospinal tracts, corticobulbar tracts, and the exiting VIth nerve fibers. This produces quadriparesis with spared vertical eye movements, volitional blinking, and awareness, due to the ventral location of the infarction. This syndrome is caused by occlusion of paramedian BA perforators, usually in the setting of BA main trunk thrombosis. When horizontal gaze is fully abolished, attempts at horizontal gaze may produce ocular bobbing, ie, a rapid downbeat jerk of the eyes followed by a slow return to primary position (31,40).

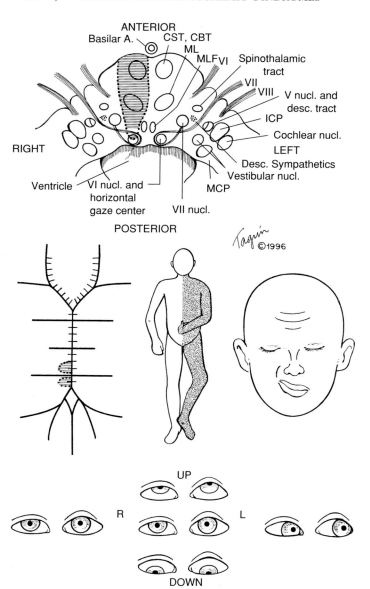

FIG. 10. Occlusion of the proximal paramedian basilar artery branch vessels causing infarction of the medial lower pons.

TABLE 3. *Lesions of the medial lower pons*

Neuroanatomy	Clinical manifestations
Horizontal gaze center	(a) I: **slow or absent saccades**
MCP ± cerebellar tracts	(b) I: ataxia of limbs and gait
VIth nerve	(c) I: **weakness of abduction**
VIIth nucl. or nerve	(d) I: peripheral facial palsy
CST ± CBT	(e) C: **weakness of arm and leg ± face**
Medial lemniscus	(f) C: **decreased vibration, proprioception, ± light touch**
MLF	(g) I: INO

Eponyms: Millard–Gubler (c, d, e), Foville (a, d, e ± c), Raymond (c, e), Fisher one-and-a-half (a, g). MCP, middle cerebellar peduncle; CST, corticospinal tract; CBT, corticobulbar tract; MLF, medial lemniscus and pontine reticular formation; INO, internuclear ophthalmoplegia.

Lesions of the Lateral Lower Pons (Fig. 11) (Table 4)

Occlusion of the AICA may produce infarction of the lateral lower pons or cerebellum. The combination of ipsilateral deafness or tinnitus with facial weakness and numbness and ipsilateral ataxia (due to involvement of nerves VIII, VII, and V, and cerebellar tracts) is the clinical signature. Nystagmus and "crossed sensory loss" to pain and temperature also occur. The unilateral syndrome is almost always a consequence of AICA occlusion at its origin from the BA and occurs primarily in patients with hypertension or diabetes. A bilateral syndrome, a large area of infarction, or the presence of brainstem signs referable to another BA branch vessel should raise the concern for impending basilar thrombosis (20,38).

Lesions of the Medial Midpons (Fig. 12) (Table 5)

Isolated occlusion of the paramedian mid-BA branches may produce internuclear ophthalmoplegia (INO), ipsilateral ataxia, and contralateral weakness with decreased dorsal column sensation. Infarction at this level may also represent a more diffuse BA thrombotic infarction. INO describes an eye movement abnormality reflecting injury to the internuclear connections (via the MLF) between the contralateral VIth and ipsilateral IIIrd nuclei that are essential in maintaining conjugate gaze. Attempts at conjugate horizontal gaze to the contralateral side produce slowed or absent adduction) of the ipsilateral eye and nystagmus of the contralateral abducting eye that beats in the direction of gaze. Convergence testing helps distinguish an INO from a partial IIIrd nerve palsy, since in an INO the ipsilateral eye can still adduct to convergence (32).

Lesions of the Lateral Midpons (Fig. 13) (Table 6)

Occlusion of short circumferential mid-BA branch vessels produces infarction in the lateral midpons. When infarction involves the main Vth motor and sensory nuclei, it produces weakness in the muscles of mastication and decreased facial vibratory and proprioceptive sensation, respectively. It is usually accompanied by the ipsilateral ataxia, ipsilateral Horner's syndrome, and contralateral body numbness (crossed sensory loss) that characterize the lateral pontomedullary syndromes. When due to BA branch disease alone, the medial and lateral syndromes remain distinct. When the BA trunk is diseased, infarction usually occurs in both the medial and lateral territories.

Lesions of the Medial Upper Pons (Figs. 14 and 21) (Table 7)

Occlusion of the paramedian distal BA branches is often due to lipohyalinosis and produces small infarcts ("la-

cunae") in the medial upper pons (8,10–12). Lacunar clinical syndromes due to infarction in this region include the following: In ataxic hemiparesis the corticospinal and adjacent pontocerebellar projections are injured, producing a contralateral ataxia and hemiparesis. Pure motor hemiparesis and dysarthria–clumsy hand syndrome affect only descending corticospinal and corticobulbar fibers. Occasionally, a seemingly "pure" motor hemiparesis is the earliest sign of impending BA thrombosis, and the evidence for bilateral multilevel brainstem ischemia is subtle (39).

Lesions in the paramedian pontine territory including the central tegmental tract may occasionally produce palatal myoclonus, although this localization remains uncertain. A lesion that extends rostrally and dorsally may produce a pontomesencephalic syndrome with ipsilateral ataxia, IIIrd nuclear palsy, INO, and disorder of vertical gaze (Nothnagel's syndrome).

Lesions of the Lateral Upper Pons (Fig. 15, 31) (Table 8)

Occlusion of the SCA may produce infarction from the lateral upper pons into the dorsal midbrain. Decreased vibration and position sense is caused by injury to the medial lemniscus, which is ascending superolaterally toward the thalamus at this level. Because the medial lemniscus is organized with the leg most lateral, the leg tends to be more severely affected. This is usually accompanied by the ipsilateral ataxia, ipsilateral Horner's, and contralateral body numbness to pain and temperature, which typify the lateral pontomedullary syndromes. Notably lacking are ipsilateral facial sensory changes because the afferent fibers from the spinal nucleus of V have already crossed. However, if the lesion extends quite far lateral, it may interrupt the contralateral afferent trigeminothalamic fibers that have already crossed producing contralateral facial anesthesia (24).

Midbrain

Lesions of the Medial Midbrain (Fig. 16) (Table 9)

Occlusion of paramedian terminal BA or proximal PCA branches produces infarction of the medial midbrain. Proximal PCA trunk occlusions cause lateral midbrain, mesial temporal, and occipital infarction if flow through the ipsilateral PComm is compromised. Lesions at this level are characterized by contralateral hemiparesis accompanied by abnormalities of vertical gaze, pupillary function, and oculomotor activity. The finding of hemiparesis with a IIIrd nerve palsy is specific to the medial midbrain.

Whereas lesions at the pontomedullary junction produce vertical nystagmus, lesions in the mesencephalon produce disorders of vertical gaze. While most medial midbrain lesions impair both up- and downgaze, a more caudal lesion of the rostral interstitial nucleus of the MLF may spare up-

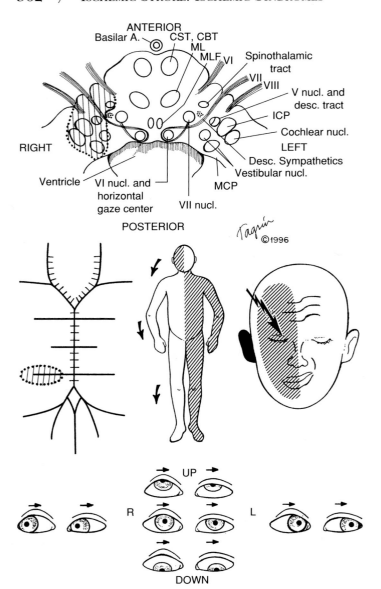

FIG. 11. Occlusion of the anterior inferior cerebellar artery causing infarction of the lateral lower pons.

TABLE 4. *Lesions of the lateral lower pons*

Neuroanatomy	Clinical manifestations
Vestibular nucl. or nerve	(a) N: vertical or **horizontal nystagmus**, vertigo, nausea, vomiting
Cochlear nucl., auditory nerve,	(b) I: **sensorineural deafness**, tinnitus
Horizontal gaze center	(c) I: slow or absent saccades
MCP ± cerebellar tracts	(d) I: **ataxia of limbs and gait**
VIIth nucl. or nerve	(e) I: **peripheral facial palsy**
Vth nucl.	(f) I: **periorbital ± facial pain**
Descending tract of Vth nucl.	(g) I: **facial numbness**
Descending sympathetics	(h) I: Horner's syndrome
Spinothalamic tract	(i) C: **Body numbness**

MCP, middle cerebellar peduncle.

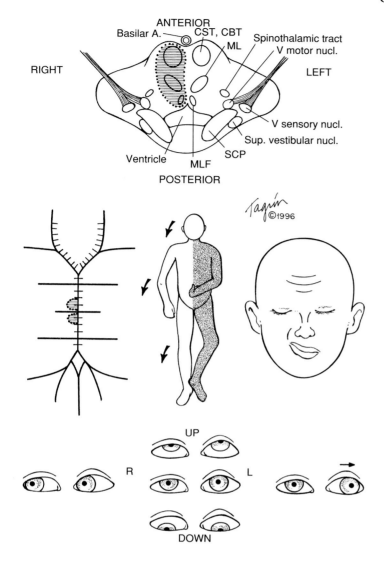

FIG. 12. Occlusion of the paramedian midbasilar artery branch vessels causing infarction of the medial mid-pons.

gaze and cause an isolated downgaze palsy. Diplopia results when the eyes become dysconjugate in the vertical plane. Even when the patient denies double vision, persistent closure of one eye may suggest diplopia and, by implication, disease of the mesencephalon.

The Edinger–Westphal (EW) nucleus in the medial midbrain subserves pupillary constriction for both the light and near reflexes. The phenomenon of light–near dissociation refers to pupillary constriction to convergence but not to light. This reflects a greater proportion of fibers (approximately 30:1) innervating the EW nucleus devoted to constriction in response to convergence compared to that in response to light. Pupillary size and shape are controlled by tonic influences of the autonomic nervous system. Descending parasympathetic fibers synapse on the EW nucleus, and then travel to the ciliary ganglion and body via the superficial surface of the IIIrd nerve. Pupillary dilatation may reflect dysfunction of the IIIrd nerve due to aneurysmal compres-

TABLE 5. *Lesions of the medial mid pons*

Neuroanatomy	Clinical manifestations
MCP ± cerebellar tracts	(a) I: **ataxia of limbs and gait**
MLF	(b) I: **INO**
CST ± CBT	(c) C: **weakness of arm and leg ± face**
Medial lemniscus	(d) C: **decreased body vibration, proprioception, ± light touch**

Eponyms: Raymond-Cestan (a, c ± d, spinothalamic). Abbreviations as in Table 3.

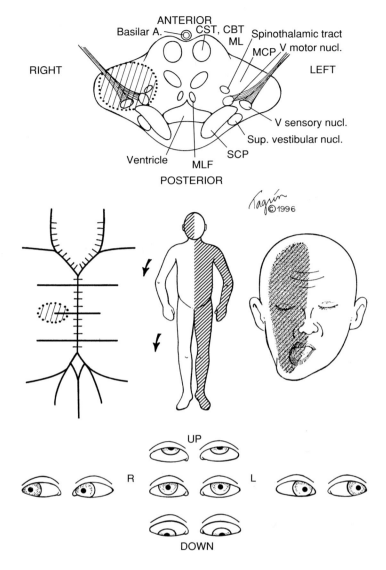

FIG. 13. Occlusion of short circumferential midbasilar artery branch vessels causing infarction of the lateral midpons.

sion or increased intracranial pressure rather than midbrain infarction. Interruption of parasympathetic fibers alone produces 7- to 10-mm diameter pupils; additional involvement of sympathetic fibers may reduce the diameter to 4–6 mm (40). Pharmacologic testing of the mydriatic (dilated) non-

reactive pupil with various concentrations of a miotic agent can be useful in distinguishing benign from life-threatening etiologies.

In the tonic dilated pupil (Adie's), a benign longstanding mydriasis is present, presumably due to denervation hyper-

TABLE 6. *Lesions of the lateral mid pons*

Neuroanatomy	Clinical manifestations
MCP ± cerebellar tracts	(a) I: **ataxia of limbs and gait**
Vth motor nucl. or nerve	(b) I: asymmetric jaw jerk and **chin deviates to side of lesion with jaw opening**
Vth sensory nucl.	(c) I: **decreased facial vibration, proprioception, ± light touch**
Vth sensory nerve	(d) I: **facial numbness,** weak corneal reflex
Descending sympathetics	(e) I: Horner's syndrome
Spinothalamic tract	(f) C: **body numbness**

MCP, middle cerebellar peduncle.

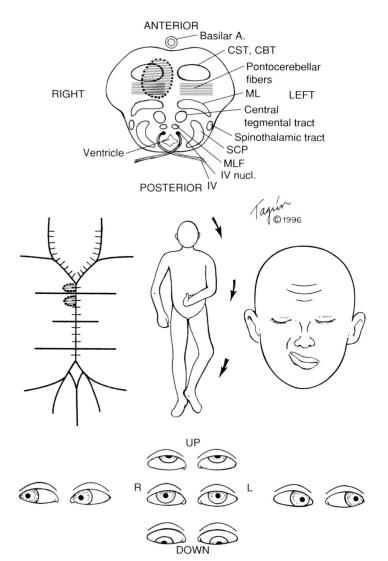

FIG. 14. Occlusion of the paramedian distal basilar artery branch vessels causing infarction of the medial upper pons.

sensitivity of the pupillary constrictors. A dilute (0.1%) pilocarpine solution will constrict this pupil but is not potent enough to constrict normally innervated or midbrain pupils. By contrast, 1% pilocarpine solution will constrict a pupil that is dilated because of IIIrd nerve or nucleus dysfunction (midbrain disease) but is not potent enough to overcome the mydriatic effects of inadvertent pharmacologic instillation or direct iris injury. The levator palpebrae and pupillary constrictors are innervated bilaterally by their respective IIIrd subnuclei, the obliques and inferior rectus muscles by the ipsilateral subnuclei, and the superior rectus muscle by the contralateral subnucleus (Fig. 17). Therefore, a IIIrd nuclear

TABLE 7. *Lesions of the medial upper pons*

Neuroanatomy	Clinical manifestations
MCP or SCP	(a) I: ataxia of limbs and gait
MLF	(b) I: INO
CST ± CBT	(c) C: **weakness of arm and leg ± face**
Medial lemniscus	(d) C: decreased body vibration, proprioception ± light touch
Pontocerebellar fibers	(e) C: **ataxia of limbs and gait**

Eponyms: ataxic-hemiparesis (c, e), pure motor hemiparesis (c), dysarthria–clumsy hand (c), Nothnagel (a, d, + nucl. III lesion).
SCP, superior cerebellar peduncle. All other abbreviations as in Table 3.

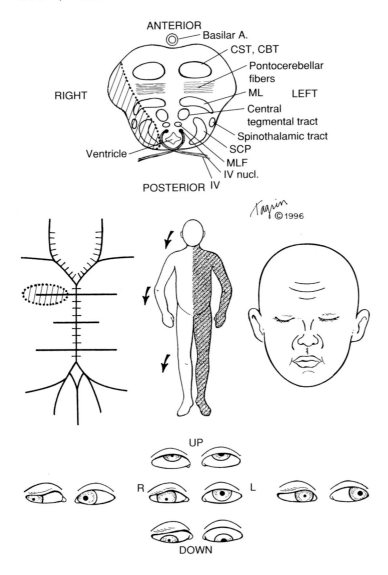

FIG. 15. Occlusion of superior cerebellar artery causing infarction of the lateral upper pons.

lesion always produces a mild contralateral ptosis in addition to the severe ipsilateral ptosis and involves the contralateral but not ipsilateral superior rectus. A peripheral IIIrd nerve lesion never involves the contralateral eye.

A corectopic pupil is one that is irregular and eccentrically placed within the iris. Both corectopia and skew suggest brainstem disease but are poorly localizing signs. A

''pseudo-sixth'' palsy is an apparent slowing of abduction during refixation, caused by excessive convergence tone. It is often bilateral and may be accompanied by convergence-retraction nystagmus. The constellation of vertical gaze palsy, abnormal convergence, skew deviation, corectopia, behavioral disturbances, and hallucinations strongly suggests a ''top-of-the-basilar'' syndrome (6).

TABLE 8. *Lesions of the lateral upper pons*

Neuroanatomy	Clinical manifestations
MCP or SCP	(a) I: **ataxia of limbs and gait**
Superior vestibular nucl.	(b) I: horizontal nystagmus, vertigo, nausea, vomiting
Descending sympathetics	(c) I: **Horner's syndrome**
Spinothalamic tract	(d) C: **body numbness**
Medial lemniscus	(e) C: **decreased body vibration, proprioception, ± light touch**

MCP, middle cerebellar peduncle; SCP, superior cerebellar peduncle.

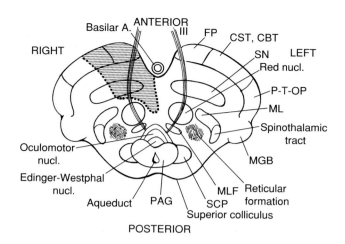

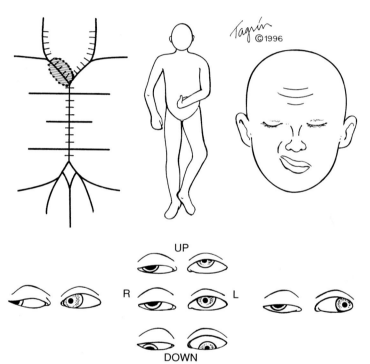

FIG. 16. Occlusion of the paramedian terminal basilar or proximal posterior cerebral artery branches causing infarction of the medial midbrain.

TABLE 9. *Lesions of the medial midbrain*

Neuroanatomy	Clinical manifestations
IIIrd nerve	(a) I: **dilated pupil, ptosis, exohypotropia with preserved abduction, intortion**
IIIrd nucl.	(b) I: dilated pupil, ptosis, exohypotropia with preserved abduction, intortion
	C: hypotropia, mild ptosis
MLF below IIIrd nucl.	(c) I: INO
Red nucl. or SCP	(d) C: hemiataxia ± hemichorea, tremor
Cerebral peduncle:	(e) C: **weakness of arm and leg ± face**
→CST ± CBT	
→frontopontine fibers	(f) I: slow or absent saccades
Rostral interstitial MLF	(g) N: vertical gaze palsy, tonic downgaze
Edinger–Westphal nucl.	(h) N: light-near dissociation
Uncertain localization	(i) N: skew deviation and corectopia
Reticular formation	(j) N: confusion, disturbance of consciousness

Eponyms: Weber (a, e), Claude (a, d).

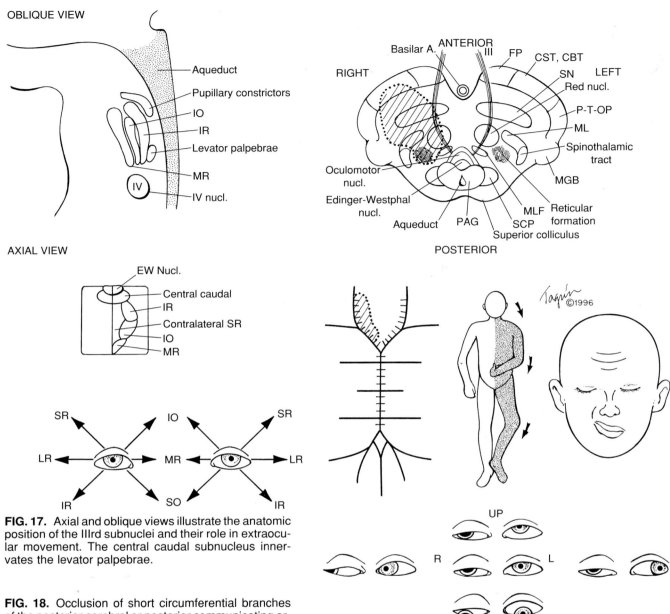

FIG. 17. Axial and oblique views illustrate the anatomic position of the IIIrd subnuclei and their role in extraocular movement. The central caudal subnucleus innervates the levator palpebrae.

FIG. 18. Occlusion of short circumferential branches of the posterior cerebral or posterior communicating artery causing lateral midbrain infarction.

TABLE 10. *Lesions of the lateral midbrain*

Neuroanatomy	Clinical manifestations
IIIrd nerve	(a) I: **dilated pupil, ptosis, exohypotropia with preserved abduction, intortion**
Descending sympathetics	(b) I: Horner's syndrome
Spinothalamic tract	(c) C: body numbness
Red nucl. or SCP	(d) C: **hemiataxia** ± hemichorea, tremor
Medial lemniscus	(e) C: **decreased body vibration, proprioception, ± light touch**
Cerebral peduncle	(f) C: **weakness of arm and leg ± face**
Uncertain localization	(g) skew deviation and corectopia
Reticular formation	(h) confusion, disturbance of consciousness

Eponyms: Benedikt (a, d, f), Claude (a, d), Chiary-Foix-Nicolesco (d, e, f).
SCP, superior cerebellar peduncle.

Lesions of the Lateral Midbrain (Fig. 18) (Table 10)

Occlusion of short circumferential branches of the PCA or PComm results in lateral midbrain infarction. Clinical symptoms include an ipsilateral IIIrd nerve paresis, a contralateral hemiparesis and ataxia, and a contralateral sensory loss to position and vibration sense as well as to pain and temperature. Peduncular hallucinations are vivid and well-formed illusions that are recognized by the patient as unreal. They may be associated with bizarre and inappropriate verbal responses and behavior. They are thought to be due to deafferentation of the lateral geniculate nucleus or lesions of the reticular formation (41,42). Interruption of crossed cerebellar fibers from red nucleus or SCP produces the contralateral ataxia or tremor, and involvement of the subthalamic nucleus may produce hyperkinetic movements (eg, hemiballismus).

Cerebellar Infarction

The cerebellum is supplied predominantly by the SCA, with contributions from the AICA and PICA. Because these arteries also supply the brainstem, it is often difficult to determine whether a clinical sign is caused by brainstem or cerebellar dysfunction. Isolated cerebellar infarction classically occurs in the PICA territory and presents with prominent dizziness, vertigo, and nausea. The unsteadiness, nystagmus, and ipsilateral dysmetria that suggest cerebellar localization may be overlooked at the onset if not specifically examined.

Due to the restricted space of the posterior fossa, acute cerebellar disease is often a life-threatening condition. The increase in infratentorial pressure is poorly tolerated. Whereas supratentorial herniation syndromes demonstrate a rostral-to-caudal progression of brainstem signs and metabolic encephalopathies demonstrate diffuse, patchy brainstem signs, the posterior fossa herniation syndromes affect discrete levels of the brainstem. Midline cerebellar lesions may produce isolated truncal ataxia, which can sometimes be recognized with the patient seated but most often requires that the patient be standing or walking. If gait and balance are not tested, a midline lesion will not be appreciated until further cerebellar or brainstem signs emerge due to ongoing brain swelling. Lateral hemispheric lesions produce symptoms ipsilateral to the lesion. Patients complain of limb incoordination and demonstrate ataxia with falling toward the side of lesion, dysmetria (overshoot) on appendicular testing, dysdiadokinesia (inaccuracy) of rapid alternating movements, intention tremor (tremor amplitude increases as target is approached), and nystagmus (often bilateral but worse when looking toward side of the lesion). Speech may be dysarthric (slurred) or explosive.

Patients with large infarctions may develop nausea, vomiting, headache, decreasing alertness, and symptoms of pontine compression over the next 12–96 hours. Suboccipital decompression is a life-saving procedure when medical management fails to reduce the increasing posterior fossa pressure (31,43).

CASE EXAMPLES

Case 1: Basilar Artery Thrombosis

A 45-year-old man presented with sudden onset of quadriparesis, ophthalmoparesis, dysarthria, and decreased alertness while singing in church. He was treated with intraarterial thrombolysis within hours but sustained paramedian pontine infarction despite successful vascular recanalization (Figs. 19–21).

Case 2: Basilar Artery Embolus

A 61-year-old man developed the sudden onset of quadriparesis, ophthalmoparesis, multiple cranial nerve palsies, and coma during cardiac catheterization. He died despite aggressive medical therapy (Figs. 22 and 23).

Case 3: Vertebral Artery Dissection and Lateral Medullary Infarction

A 28-year-old man developed sudden left facial numbness, left limb and gait ataxia, right body numbness, dizziness, and dysphagia. Transfemoral angiography demon-

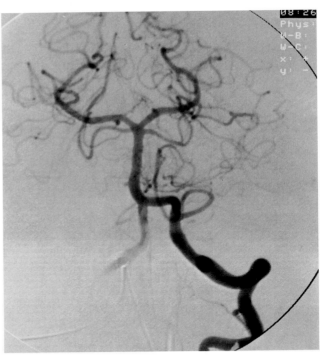

FIG. 20. Repeat injection after 1.25 million units of urokinase demonstrates lysis of thrombus and restored patency to the basilar artery and its long circumferential branches. (Courtesy of Dr. Insup Choi.)

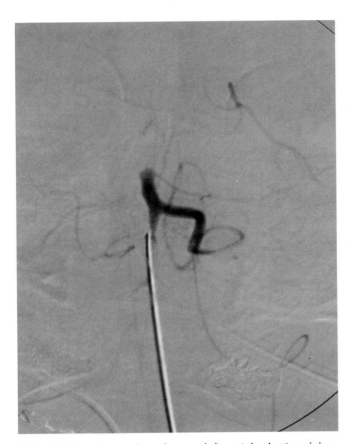

FIG. 19. Transfemoral angiogram left vertebral artery injection demonstrates reflux into right vertebral artery and occlusion of the midbasilar artery. (Courtesy of Dr. Insup Choi.)

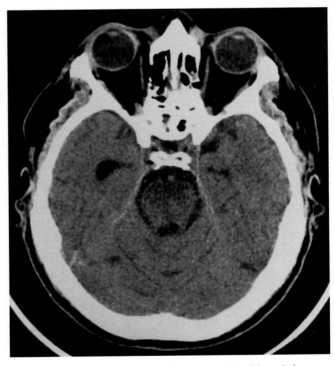

FIG. 21. Axial plain computed tomograph of head demonstrates bilateral infarction of the tectum of the upper pons in the territory of the paramedian penetrating vessels.

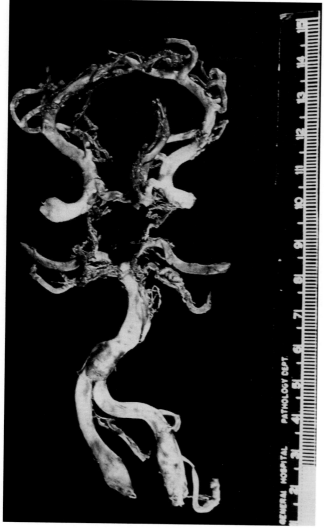

FIG. 22. Autopsy specimen of circle of Willis and its major contributing vessels. Note the atherosclerosis of the proximal basilar artery.

strated focal stenosis of the prevertebral segment of the left VA consistent with dissection (Figs. 24–26).

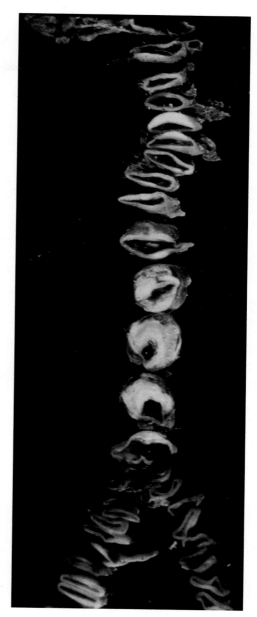

FIG. 23. Serial axial sections through the vertebral and basilar arteries demonstrates eccentric narrowing of the basilar artery lumen by atherosclerosis.

Case 4: Vertebral Artery Dissection and Brainstem and Cerebellar Infarction

A 26-year-old man presented with severe occipital headache followed by right-sided cerebellar ataxia and diplopia 12 hours after vigorously hyperextending his neck to drink several shots of tequilla. MR angiography revealed a right vertebral dissection (Fig. 27).

Case 5: Intracranial Vertebral Artery Occlusion and Lateral Medullary Infarction

A 57-year-old man developed left-sided facial pain and numbness, limb and gait ataxia, Horner's syndrome, dimin-

ished gag; right-sided body numbness; and nausea, vomiting, dizziness, and hoarseness. Transfemoral angiography demonstrated occlusion of the distal left VA and PICA (Figs. 28–30).

Case 6: Superior Cerebellar Infarction

A 58-year-old black female with a history of hypertension and diabetes presented with the sudden onset of nausea, vomiting, vertigo, and left-sided ataxia (Fig. 31).

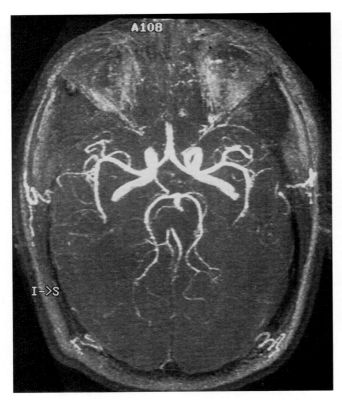

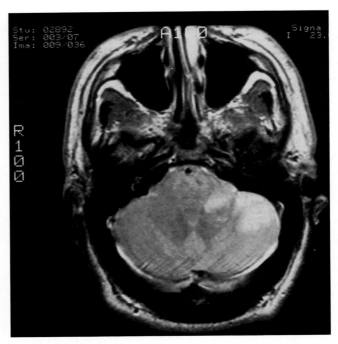

FIG. 24. Magnetic resonance three-dimensional time-of-flight angiography of the circle of Willis. Note the absent left posterior communicating artery.

FIG. 25. Magnetic resonance T2-weighted axial image demonstrates left lateral cerebellar infarction in the posterior inferior cerebellar artery (PICA) territory.

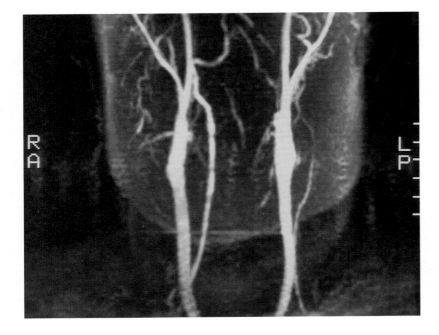

FIG. 26. Magnetic resonance coronal SPGR angiography demonstrates a prominent ascending cervical branch vessel arising from the left subclavian artery and reconstituting the left vertebral artery.

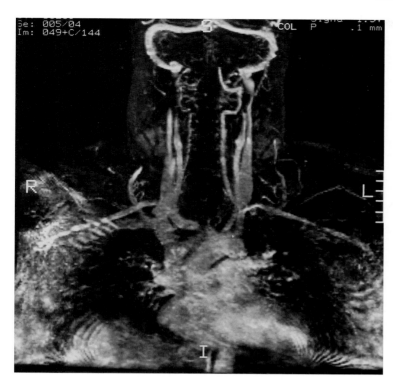

FIG. 27. Magnetic resonance coronal three-dimensional time-of-flight gadolinium-enhanced angiography of the great vessels demonstrates diminished signal in the right vertebral artery.

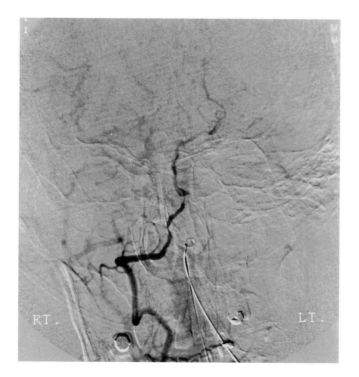

FIG. 28. Transfemoral angiogram right subclavian artery injection demonstrates distal stenosis of the right vertebral artery and no evidence of flow in the distal left vertebral artery.

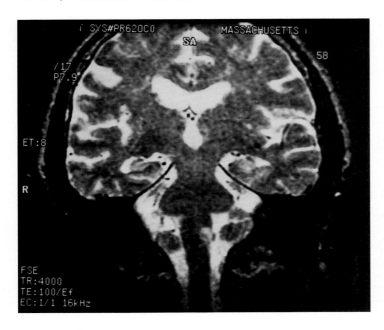

FIG. 29. Magnetic resonance T2-weighted coronal image demonstrates left lateral medullary infarction.

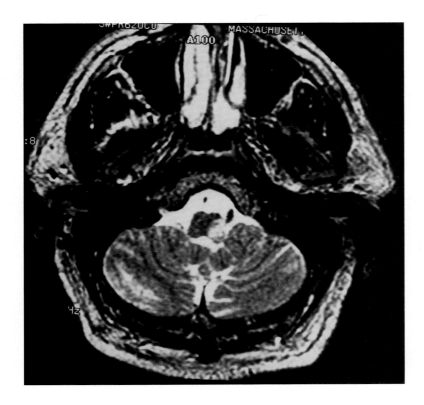

FIG. 30. Magnetic resonance T2-weighted axial image demonstrates left lateral medullary infarction.

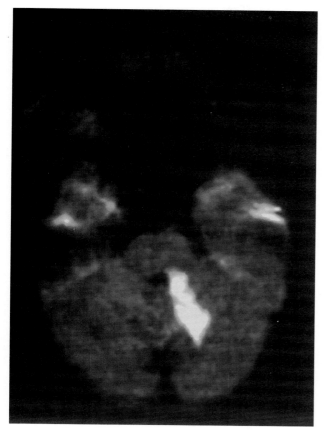

FIG. 31. Magnetic resonance diffusion-weighted image demonstrates infarction of the superior cerebellum and SCP in the territory of the SCA. (Courtesy of Drs. A. Gregory Sorensen and R. Gilberto González.)

REFERENCES

1. Fisher CM. The circle of Willis anatomical variations. *Vasc Dis* 1965; 2:99–105.
2. Caplan LR. Vertebrobasilar occlusive disease. In: Barnett HJM, Mohr JP, Stein BM, Yatsu FM, eds. *Stroke: Pathophysiology, Diagnosis, and Management.* 2nd ed. New York: Churchill Livingstone, 1992.
3. Netter FH. *Nervous System: Anatomy and Physiology (Part I).* West Caldwell, NJ: CIBA Pharmaceutical Co., 1986.
4. Akar ZC, Dujovny M, Slavin KV, Gomez-Tortosa E, Ausman JI. Microsurgical anatomy of the intracranial part of the vertebral artery. *Neurol Res* 1994;16:171–180.
5. Adams RD, Sidman RL. *Introduction to Neuropathology.* New York: McGraw-Hill, 1968.
6. Caplan LR. "Top of the basilar" syndrome. *Neurology* 1980;30:72–79.
7. Kistler JP, Ropper AH, Martin JB. Cerebrovascular diseases. In: Braunwald E, Isselbacher KJ, Petersdorf RG, Wilson JD, Martin JB, Fauci AS, eds. *Harrison's Principles of Internal Medicine.* 11th ed. New York: McGraw-Hill, 1987.
8. Fisher CM, Caplan LR. Basilar artery branch occlusion: A cause of pontine infarction. *Neurology* 1971;21:900–905.
9. Caplan LR. Vertebrobasilar ischemic stroke. In: Fisher M, ed. *Clinical Atlas of Cerebrovascular Disorders.* Boston: Mosby–Year Book, 1994.
10. Fisher CM. Lacunes: small, deep cerebral infarcts. *Neurology* 1965; 15:774–784.
11. Fisher CM. Lacunar infarcts—a review. *Cerebrovasc Dis* 1991;1: 311–320.
12. Fisher CM. Ataxic hemiparesis. *Arch Neurol* 1978;35:126–128.
13. Biller J. Cervicocephalic arterial dissections: a ten-year experience. *Arch Neurol* 1986;43:1234–1238.
14. Frisoni GB, Anzola GP. Vertebrobasilar ischemia after neck motion. *Stroke* 1991;22:1452–1460.
15. Fisher CM, Ojemann RG, Roberson GH. Spontaneous dissection of cervico-cerebral arteries. *Can J Neurol Sci* 1978;5(1):9–18.
16. Mettinger KL, Ericson K. Fibromuscular dysplasia and the brain: observations on angiographic, clinical and genetic characteristics. *Stroke* 1982;13(1):46–58.
17. Koroshetz WJ, Ropper AH. Artery-to-artery embolism causing stroke in the posterior circulation. *Neurology* 1987;37:292–296.
18. George B, Laurian C. Vertebro-basilar ischemia with thrombosis of the vertebral artery: report of two cases with embolism. *J Neurol Neurosurg Psychiatry* 1982.
19. Parums DV. The arteritides. *Histopathology* 1994;25:1–20.
20. Adams RD. Occlusion of the anterior inferior cerebellar artery. *Arch Neurol Psychiatry* 1943;49:765–770.
21. Adams RD, Victor M. *Principles of Neurology.* New York: McGraw-Hill, 1993.
22. Barnett HJ. Cerebral ischemia and infarction. In: Wyngaarden JB, Smith LH, eds. *Cecil's Textbook of Medicine.* 18th ed. Philadelphia: WB Saunders, 1988.
23. Bogousslavsky J, Meienberg O. Eye-movement disorders in brain-stem and cerebellar stroke. *Arch Neurol* 1987;44:141–148.
24. Brazis PW, Masdeu JC, Biller J. *Localization in Clinical Neurology.* 2nd ed. Boston: Little, Brown, 1990.
25. Brust JC. Cerebral Infarction. In: Rowland LP, ed. *Merritt's Textbook of Neurology.* 8th ed. Philadelphia: Williams and Wilkins, 1989; 246–256.
26. Caplan LR. *Stroke: A Clinical Approach.* Boston: Butterworth-Heinemann, 1993.
27. DeArmond SJ, Fusco MM, Dewey MM. *Structure of the Human Brain.* New York: Oxford University Press, 1989.
28. Gilman S, Newman SW. *Manter and Gatz's Essentials of Clinical Neuroanatomy and Neurophysiology.* 7th ed. Philadelphia: FA Davis, 1987.
29. Kubik CS, Adams RD. Occlusion of the basilar artery—a clinical and pathological study. *Brain* 1946;69(2):73–121.
30. Lindsay KW, Bone I, Callander R. *Neurology and Neurosurgery Illustrated.* 2nd ed. London: Churchill Livingstone, 1991.
31. Plum F, Posner JB. *The Diagnosis of Stupor and Coma.* 3rd ed. Philadelphia: FA Davis, 1982.
32. Rowland LP. Clinical syndromes of the brainstem. In: Kandel ER, Schwartz JH, eds. *Principles of Neural Science.* 2nd ed. New York: Elsevier, 1985.
33. Wolf JK, ed. *The Classical Brainstem Syndromes: Translations of the Original Papers with Notes on the Evolution of Clinical Neuroanatomy.* Springfield: Charles C Thomas, 1971.
34. Caplan LR, et al. Embolism from vertebral artery origin occlusive disease. *Neurology* 1992;42:1505–1512.
35. Currier RD, Giles CL, DeJong RN. Some comments on Wallenberg's lateral medullary syndrome. *Neurology* 1961;11:778–791.
36. Ropper AH. Illusion of tilting of the visual environment: report of five cases. *J Clin Neuro-ophthalmol* 1983;3:147–151.
37. Silfverskiöld BP. Skew deviation in Wallenberg's syndrome. *Acta Neurol Scand* 1965;41:381–386.
38. Amarenco P, Rosengart A, DeWitt LD, Pessin MS, Caplan LR. Anterior inferior cerebellar artery territory infarcts: mechanisms and clinical features. *Arch Neurol* 1993;50:154–161.
39. Fisher CM. The "herald hemiparesis" of basilar artery occlusion. *Arch Neurol* 1988;45:1301–1303.
40. Fisher CM. Some neuro-ophthalmological observations. *J Neurol Neurosurg Pschiatry* 1967;30:383–392.
41. Bogousslavsky J, Maeder P, Regli F, Meuli R. Pure midbrain infarction: clinical syndromes, MRI, and etiologic patterns. *Neurology* 1994;44: 2032–2040.
42. Segarra JM. Cerebral vascular disease and behavior: I. the syndrome of the mesencephalic artery (basilar artery bifurcation). *Arch Neurol* 1970;22:408–418.
43. Lehrich JR, Winkler GF, Ojemann RG. Cerebellar infarction with brain stem compression. Diagnosis and surgical treatment. *Arch Neurol* 1970; 22(6):490–498.

Cerebrovascular Disease, edited by H. Hunt Batjer.
Lippincott-Raven Publishers, Philadelphia © 1997.

CHAPTER 29

Cardiac Sources of Embolism: Diagnosis, Management, and Prevention

R. Michael Poole and Marc I. Chimowitz

Cardioembolism is responsible for approximately 15–20% of ischemic strokes. Therefore, in the United States, about 65,000 strokes are caused by cardioembolism annually. Cardioembolism is more prevalent in younger patients (23–36% of ischemic strokes in patients younger than 45 years), primarily because of the lower incidence of atherosclerotic disease in this age group. These statistics are only approximate estimates of the prevalence of cardioembolic stroke, since establishing the diagnosis of cardioembolism is often difficult. Reasons for this difficulty include the lack of well defined diagnostic criteria for cardioembolism, the coexistence of atherosclerotic cerebrovascular disease in some patients with cardiac sources of embolism (eg, nonvalvular atrial fibrillation), and, until recently, the lack of sensitive cardiac imaging modalities for detecting cardiac sources of embolism.

A list of cardiac abnormalities that have been associated with cardioembolism is shown in Table 1. Some of these abnormalities are associated with a high risk of cardioembolism, whereas the risk associated with other abnormalities either is low or remains to be established. Of the high risk sources, atrial fibrillation, mural thrombi related to acute myocardial infarction, prosthetic heart valves, and cardiomyopathy are the most common. While endocarditis and cardiac myxomas are less common, they are very high risk lesions for cardioembolism when present.

DIAGNOSIS

Certain features of the history, cardiac and neurologic examinations, and brain imaging findings can suggest a diagnosis of cardioembolism. A maximal neurologic deficit at onset and a history of heart disease or systemic embolism are important clues in the history. On examination of the heart of a patient with an ischemic stroke, finding an irregularly irregular pulse (atrial fibrillation), a middiastolic murmur (mitral stenosis), or a newly diagnosed regurgitant murmur in a patient with fever (endocarditis) raises the suspicion of cardioembolism. Certain neurologic syndromes favor diagnosis of an embolic mechanism (from the heart or a proximal arterial source such as the aortic arch or carotid artery). These include isolated Wernicke's or Broca's aphasia, top-of-the-basilar syndromes, and an isolated hemianopia from occipital infarction. On brain imaging, a wedge-shaped cortical infarction should suggest an embolic mechanism. Multiple infarcts in different vascular territories should always suggest a proximal source of embolism from the heart or aortic arch.

Although many cardiac abnormalities that predispose to embolism can be diagnosed on the basis of a careful bedside cardiac evaluation (eg, atrial fibrillation, mitral stenosis), other abnormalities (eg, intermittent atrial fibrillation or sick sinus syndrome, left atrial spontaneous contrast, atrial septal aneurysm, patent foramen ovale, and aortic atherosclerosis) can only be detected with electrocardiography (ECG) or echocardiography.

Electrocardiography

Standard 12-lead ECG provides helpful diagnostic information about certain cardiac abnormalities that are associated with cardioembolism. Abnormalities of cardiac rhythm such as atrial fibrillation and sick sinus syndrome, both of which are important causes of cardioembolism, are diagnosed primarily with ECG. ECG continues to play an important role in the diagnosis of myocardial infarction and cardiomyopathy, although the latter is more commonly identified with echocardiography.

R. M. Poole: Department of Neurology, University of Rochester School of Medicine and Dentistry, Rochester, New York 14621.
Marc I. Chimowitz: Department of Neurology, Emory University School of Medicine, Atlanta, Georgia 30322.

TABLE 1. *Potential sources of cardioembolism*

High Risk Sources
Atrial fibrillation
Mural thrombus associated with acute MI
Prosthetic heart valve
Dilated cardiomyopathy
Bacterial endocarditis
Rheumatic mitral stenosis
Ascending aorta atheroma ≥4 mm in size
Intracardiac thrombus
Left atrial spontaneous echo contrast (invariably occurs with
   atrial fibrillation or mitral stenosis)
Left ventricular aneurysm or large area of dyskinesia
Nonbacterial endocarditis (eg, Libman–Sacks, marantic)
Cardiac myxoma or other tumors

Lower Risk Sources
Sick sinus syndrome
Calcific aortic stenosis
Patent foramen ovale or atrial septal defect
Atrial septal aneurysm
Mitral annulus calcification
Ventricular septal defect
Mitral valve prolapse

Ambulatory ECG monitoring can provide important information about occult arrhythmias in stroke patients. In a prospective study of 184 patients with transient ischemic attack (TIA) or stroke, 12 patients (6.5%) whose history, bedside cardiac evaluation, and baseline ECG did not suggest an arrhythmia were found to have important arrhythmias on Holter or 48-hour automatic arrhythmia monitoring (1). Six patients had atrial fibrillation, four had Mobitz type II second-degree atrioventricular block, and one each had third-degree heart block and sick sinus syndrome. This study suggests a rationale for performing continuous cardiac monitoring in patients with stroke of undetermined cause in whom there is no clinical or baseline ECG evidence of cardiac arrhythmia.

Transthoracic and Transesophageal Echocardiography

Although other modalities such as ultrafast cardiac computed tomography (CT) and cardiac magnetic resonance imaging (MRI) are available in some centers, echocardiography is the cardiac imaging procedure of choice for the evaluation of potential cardiac sources of embolism. Each of the two commonly used echocardiographic methods, transthoracic echocardiography (TTE) and transesophageal echocardiography (TEE), has advantages and disadvantages.

TTE is performed by placing an ultrasound probe on the chest wall and interrogating heart structures through the intervening tissue, utilizing the spaces between or under the ribs. The more anterior structures of the heart, namely the ventricles, are most accurately imaged. TTE easily assesses atrial and ventricular dimensions, wall-motion abnormalities, stenotic or regurgitant valvular lesions, and pericardial

disease. It is a relatively insensitive method for imaging the left atrium and left atrial appendage and therefore is insensitive for detecting thrombus or spontaneous echo contrast in these locations. TTE has been the mainstay of cardiac imaging for patients with potential sources of cardioembolism because it is widely available, relatively inexpensive, and noninvasive.

TEE is accomplished with an ultrasound probe on the tip of a flexible endoscope that is inserted into the esophagus and positioned behind the left atrium. In this location, the esophagus is immediately adjacent to the left atrium; ultrasonic waves pass into posterior cardiac structures without having to traverse bone, lung, or other more anterior regions of the heart or mediastinum. For these reasons, TEE is superior to TTE for imaging the left atrium and left atrial appendage, the interatrial septum, certain portions of the left ventricle, and the atrial surfaces of the mitral and tricuspid valves. It also provides excellent images of the descending aorta, immediately posterior and to the left of the esophagus at the level of the left atrium. TEE yields better images of the cardiac chambers and the valvular structures than TTE. Although sedation is necessary for esophageal intubation, TEE is safe and usually well tolerated by patients.

Several studies have compared the accuracy of TTE and TEE for detecting certain cardiac abnormalities. TEE is superior to TTE for identifying left atrial thrombi, while TTE may be superior for identifying ventricular thrombi because of the higher sensitivity of TTE for detecting apical thrombi (2). TTE is nearly as sensitive as TEE for the diagnosis of intracardiac tumors. In one study, TTE and TEE both correctly diagnosed 13 left and two right atrial myxomas (3); however, TEE was slightly better at identifying the tumor attachment site. In another study, TTE detected eight of nine left atrial tumors and three of four right atrial tumors that were found on TEE (4).

In patients with bacterial endocarditis, echocardiography can help to identify patients who are at risk for systemic embolization because of valvular vegetations. A review of 28 studies of echocardiography in patients with endocarditis showed that the detection rate for vegetations was 64% for TTE and 88% for TEE (5). TEE is also more accurate than TTE for the detection of valvular abscesses. In patients with prosthetic valves TEE, is superior for identifying valvular abnormalities. In one recent study in which prosthetic valve pathology was confirmed at surgery or autopsy, TEE was superior to TTE in identifying endocarditis, thrombi, or morphologic abnormalities such as valve leaflet thickening or restricted motion (6). TEE is also more sensitive than TTE for the detection of left atrial spontaneous echo contrast, patent foramen ovale, and interatrial septal aneurysms (see below).

TEE AND STROKE RISK ASSOCIATED WITH CARDIAC ABNORMALITIES

The use of TEE over the past decade has led to a better understanding of the association between certain cardiac abnormalities and stroke risk. These abnormalities include mitral valve prolapse, patent foramen ovale, atrial septal aneurysm, aortic atheromatous disease, and spontaneous echo contrast.

Mitral Valve Prolapse

Mitral valve prolapse (MVP) is a relatively common cardiac abnormality, occurring in approximately 4% of the general population. MVP is associated with a midsystolic click and late systolic murmur on cardiac examination. Clinically unsuspected MVP is often discovered during echocardiography performed for other reasons. Several studies have shown a significantly higher frequency of MVP in young patients with stroke compared with age- and sex-matched controls without stroke; however, it is not clear that MVP is the underlying cause of stroke in these patients. The risk of stroke in patients with MVP is low overall, but some studies have suggested that certain patients with MVP are at increased risk of embolism. In one prospective study, complications such as endocarditis, sudden death, and cerebral embolism occurred more frequently in MVP patients with redundant valve leaflets (7). Other retrospective studies have shown that patients with redundant and thickened mitral valve leaflets have a higher risk of endocarditis but a similar risk of stroke when compared with MVP patients without these characteristics. A recent population-based study showed that older patients (average age 71 years) with echocardiographically diagnosed MVP and stroke usually had other important stroke risk factors and most had other potential stroke mechanisms (8).

Patent Foramen Ovale

Patent foramen ovale (PFO) is a common cardiac abnormality, present in up to 27% of patients in some autopsy series. The prevalence of PFO declines with age, whereas the size of the interatrial defect increases with age. PFO is identified during echocardiographic studies when microbubbles cross from the right atrium into the left atrium following intravenous injection of agitated saline contrast. There is no agreed-on echocardiographic standard for the diagnosis of PFO. Some echocardiographers consider PFO to be present when two or more microbubbles are seen in the left atrium within three cardiac cycles of contrast appearance in the right atrium. Others are less strict, accepting either a smaller number of microbubbles or allowing a longer period of time for contrast to cross the atrial septum. Having the patient cough or perform a Valsalva maneuver as the contrast appears in the right atrium increases right-to-left shunting and improves the detection rate of PFO.

Several studies have shown that TEE is superior to TTE in identifying PFO (9). Recent studies have also documented the accuracy of transcranial Doppler (TCD) ultrasound for detection of right-to-left cardiac shunts (10). Occasionally, it may be difficult to document an interatrial shunt by contrast-enhanced TEE, and PFO is recognized by the appearance of left-to-right jets on color-flow Doppler.

Paradoxical embolism through a PFO has been recognized for many years and has been presumed to be the mechanism of stroke in patients with PFO when no other cause has been identified. Several studies have shown that patients with cryptogenic stroke have a significantly higher frequency of PFO than age-matched patients with another unequivocal cause of stroke (eg, carotid stenosis) (11). The results of these studies suggest a possible etiologic link between PFO and stroke; however, some authors doubt that paradoxical embolism is the underlying mechanism of stroke in the majority of patients with PFO (12). They cite the improbability of paradoxical embolism occurring in the absence of associated pulmonary embolism or associated venous thrombosis, as well as the rare occurrence of systemic or cerebral embolism in patients with thrombophlebitis despite the high frequency of PFO in the general population.

Certain echocardiographic characteristics of PFO may help to stratify risk for cardioembolism. Some studies of patients with stroke and PFO have shown that the size of PFO and the number of microbubbles traversing the septum within four cardiac cycles are significantly greater in patients with cryptogenic stroke compared with patients with another cause of stroke (13). The finding of >20 microbubbles in the left atrium within four cardiac cycles has been associated with abnormal morphology of the foramen ovale, including hypermobility, discontinuity of the septum, and distention.

Atrial Septal Aneurysm

Atrial septal aneurysm (ASA) is a local bulging of the septum primum through the fossa ovalis into the right atrium, the left atrium, or both. ASA, present in 1% of a large adult autopsy series (14), is most reliably detected in vivo by TEE. Echocardiographers must distinguish ASA from other intraatrial structures and interatrial septal abnormalities. Occasionally, it is confused with atrial myxoma; the eustachian valve (valve of the inferior vena cava) and its extension, the Chiari network; the thebesian valve (valve of the coronary sinus); or bulging of the entire atrial septum. ASA is associated with other cardiac abnormalities including mitral and tricuspid valve prolapse and right-to-left shunt through a PFO.

ASA has been associated with an increased risk of cardioembolism. Postulated mechanisms include embolization from thrombi formed near or within the aneurysm and paradoxical embolism through a coexistent PFO. In one retrospective study, the relative risk of stroke in patients with coexistent ASA and PFO was 33.3 compared with patients with neither of these abnormalities (15); however, the true risk is probably substantially lower.

Aortic Atheromatous Disease

Strictly speaking, strokes resulting from emboli from aortic arch atheromatous disease are not considered cardioembolic. Nevertheless, this subtype of stroke is included in this discussion because TEE has played a central role in establishing the association between aortic atheromatous disease and stroke in the elderly. Although aortic atherosclerosis is a common autopsy finding in patients with vascular risk factors, a causal relationship between aortic arch disease and stroke had not been established until recently. An autopsy study showed that ulcerated plaques in the aortic arch are much more common in patients with cryptogenic stroke than in patients with an unequivocal cause of stroke or in patients with neurologic diseases other than stroke (16). This association was present even after controlling for age, heart weight (an indirect estimate of the presence of hypertension), and carotid artery stenosis.

TEE provides excellent cross-sectional images of the aorta from the level of the transverse arch to the more distal portions of the descending thoracic aorta and is a sensitive method for detecting atheromatous changes. However, portions of the aorta proximal to the origin of the innominate artery must be evaluated to be most useful in the evaluation of stroke patients. Several factors make TEE examination of this portion of the aorta difficult: (a) The interposition of the trachea and mainstem bronchi between the esophagus and the proximal aorta partially obscures the view of the proximal aorta; (b) to view the proximal aorta, the transducer must be positioned at a level of the esophagus that is more likely to provoke gagging; (c) the aorta is usually examined at the end of the TEE study when the patient is often anxious for the procedure to end; and (d) to obtain detailed views of the aortic wall, the operator must remember to change the transducer frequency to a higher setting (7 MHz).

Several studies have documented an association between aortic plaque seen on TEE and stroke risk. In a prospective case-control study of TEE of the aorta in patients older than 60 years with ischemic stroke, Amarenco and coworkers (17) demonstrated an independent association between atherosclerotic plaque in the aorta and the risk of ischemic stroke. The relative risk of ischemic stroke in the group with plaques ≥ 4 mm was 9.1 (95% confidence interval [CI], 3.3–25.2; $p < 0.001$). Aortic plaques with a mobile component were associated with a relative risk of 14 among patients with ischemic strokes of uncertain cause. There was no association between the presence of plaques ≥ 4 mm and extracranial internal carotid stenosis or atrial fibrillation. Hypertension, diabetes, cigarette smoking, history of myocardial infarction, and hypercholesterolemia were more frequent in patients than controls, although there was no difference in the rates of atrial fibrillation or peripheral vascular disease.

Another recent case-control study using TEE showed that complex proximal aortic atheromas are a risk factor for stroke independent of vascular risk factors (18). The investigators demonstrated a significant association between the severity of aortic atheroma and the severity of carotid stenosis determined either by duplex scanning or angiography, suggesting that proximal aortic atheroma may be a marker for extracranial cerebrovascular disease in some patients. The presence of carotid disease was not a reliable predictor of aortic atheroma in this study, however. Recent studies have also shown that the aortic arch is a major source of embolism during coronary artery bypass surgery when the aorta is cross-clamped or cannulated.

Spontaneous Echo Contrast

Spontaneous echo contrast (SEC) is a dynamic smoke-like signal that is detected on TEE in patients with stasis of blood in one or more of the cardiac chambers. SEC is most commonly seen in the left atrium but can also be seen in the left ventricle, the aorta, and occasionally in the right atrium and right ventricle. The most common conditions associated with the formation of left atrial SEC are atrial fibrillation and mitral stenosis. Studies in dogs indicate that SEC represents intracardiac erythrocyte or platelet microaggregates, suggesting that SEC may be a precursor of thrombus. SEC has also been associated with elevated fibrinogen levels and elevated serum viscosity in patients with acute stroke.

Several studies have shown an association between the presence of left atrial SEC and previous stroke or peripheral embolism. One study of patients with atrial fibrillation or mitral stenosis showed that left atrial SEC was associated with previous stroke independently of traditional vascular risk factors (19). The presence of left atrial SEC may be useful for stratifying cardioembolic risk in patients with nonvalvular atrial fibrillation. A retrospective study showed that six of 12 patients with nonvalvular atrial fibrillation and left atrial SEC had previous stroke or peripheral embolism, compared with only one of 28 patients (4%) with nonvalvular atrial fibrillation who did not have left atrial SEC (relative risk 27.0; 95% CI, 2.7–267.8; $p < 0.001$) (19). In a prospective study of 272 patients with nonvalvular atrial fibrillation who underwent TEE, the rate of stroke, TIA, or systemic embolism was 12% per year in 161 patients with SEC compared with 3% per year in 111 patients without SEC ($p = 0.002$). Mortality rates during a mean follow-up of 17.5 months were 16% in patients with SEC compared with 10% in patients without SEC ($p = 0.025$) (20).

PREVENTION OF CARDIOEMBOLIC STROKE

Once a cardioembolic source is identified, the physician needs to start antithrombotic therapy to prevent embolism. The choice between anticoagulation and antiplatelet therapy depends on a number of factors, including recent history of TIA or stroke, severity of stroke, the specific cardiac abnormality, and whether any contraindications to the use of anti-coagulation are present (eg, marked ataxia, alcoholism).

Anticoagulation and Acute Cardioembolic Stroke

The decision to use heparin for anticoagulation in the setting of an acute cardioembolic stroke is particularly vexing. On the one hand, there is concern that hemorrhagic transformation of an ischemic infarct, which is particularly common after cardioembolic stroke (up to 68% in some MRI series), may be more severe in patients given heparin. On the other hand, there is the risk of early recurrent cardioembolism, which may be as high as 12% in the first 2 weeks after a cardioembolic stroke. In the only randomized study of patients (n = 45) with acute cardioembolic stroke that compared immediate anticoagulation with no anticoagulation, there was a trend toward reduction of early recurrent embolism and no bleeding complications in patients randomized to anticoagulation (21). Pooled data from six studies of patients with cardioembolic stroke (two prospective, four retrospective) show that three of 147 patients (2%) who received early anticoagulation had recurrent stroke within 21 days, compared with 49 of 280 (17.5%) who received delayed or no anticoagulation (22). Since the risk of symptomatic brain hemorrhage in patients treated with early anticoagulation is relatively low (1–4%), the available data favor early anticoagulation with heparin (without a bolus) in the setting of acute cardioembolic stroke, unless the patient has infectious endocarditis, a large infarction, or severe hypertension or the initial brain CT shows areas of hemorrhagic transformation. In those circumstances, aspirin is the alternative treatment to prevent recurrent cardioembolism.

In the setting of stroke related to infectious endocarditis, anticoagulation is usually not recommended because valvular vegetations are not platelet-fibrin thrombi and can break off regardless of anticoagulation and the risk of intracranial bleeding may be particularly high when cerebral emboli are septic. Since fewer than 3% of patients with infectious endocarditis have cerebral emboli after infection is controlled, appropriate antibiotic therapy is critical to prevent recurrent embolism (23). Patients with recurrent emboli despite antibiotics who have vegetations >10 mm on TEE should be considered for cardiac surgery. Patients with mechanical valves and infectious endocarditis who have not had cerebral embolism should be continued on anticoagulation. If cerebral embolism occurs in these patients, Pruit (23) has suggested stopping anticoagulation for 48 hours because of the high risk of cerebral hemorrhage.

Antithrombotic Therapy After Recovery from Cardioembolic TIA or Stroke

It is generally accepted that warfarin is the long-term therapy of choice for stroke prevention in patients who have recovered from a TIA or stroke caused by one of the following high-risk cardiac abnormalities: mitral stenosis, atrial fibrillation, intracardiac clot or left atrial spontaneous echo contrast, prosthetic valve, dilated cardiomyopathy, and a large area of left ventricular dyskinesia, particularly if a mural thrombus is present. The dose of warfarin is usually adjusted to maintain the international normalized ratio (INR) for the prothrombin time between 2.0 and 3.0, except in patients with mechanical prosthetic heart valves, for whom the target INR is usually 3.0–4.0.

One recent study suggests that the addition of aspirin to warfarin in patients with a prosthetic valve significantly reduces their risk of major systemic embolism or vascular death (24). In this double-blind randomized study of patients with a prosthetic valve (mechanical valve or a tissue valve if associated with a history of atrial fibrillation or thromboembolism), 186 patients were assigned to aspirin (100 mg/d) plus warfarin and 184 to placebo plus warfarin. The target INR was 3.0–4.5. During a mean follow-up of 2.5 years, there were 13 vascular deaths (11 cardiac, two ischemic stroke) in the placebo group and two in the aspirin group. There were 13 major embolic events in the placebo group and five in the aspirin group. There were three fatal intracranial hemorrhages in each group, but there were five nonfatal intracranial hemorrhages in four patients, all in the aspirin group. Analysis of the composite endpoint of major embolism, nonfatal intracranial hemorrhage, fatal hemorrhage, and vascular death showed 12 in the aspirin group (3.9% per year) vs. 28 in the placebo group (9.9% per year; p = 0.005) (24). The results of this study suggest that combined aspirin and warfarin may be the preferred treatment for certain patients with prosthetic valves, but studies with longer follow-up are needed to determine if the benefits of aspirin over 2.5 years can be extended to lifetime follow-up. If a patient with a prosthetic valve has a cardioembolic event while taking warfarin alone, antiplatelet therapy (aspirin 100–325 mg/d or dipyridamole 300–400 mg/d) should be added to the treatment regimen if the INR was therapeutic at the time of the event.

The choice of antithrombotic therapy in patients with a TIA or stroke who have a lower-risk cardioembolic source (eg, patent foramen ovale, atrial septal aneurysm without a right-to-left shunt, mitral valve prolapse, mitral annular calcification) is empiric. Long-term warfarin is frequently used in this setting; however, there are no data indicating that aspirin is less effective. In patients with patent foramen ovale (PFO) who have recurrent TIA or stroke despite adequate anticoagulation, surgical closure of the interatrial septal defect should be considered. There are reports, however, of patients having recurrent TIA or stroke despite successful closure of the septal defect (25). These reports suggest that the mechanism of cerebral ischemia in these patients may be unrelated to the PFO. Aspirin is usually the treatment of choice in patients with mitral valve prolapse (because of the low risk of recurrent embolism) and in patients with mitral annular calcification, whose emboli are usually calcific and not related to intracardiac thrombus.

Antithrombotic Therapy in Patients with a High-Risk Cardioembolic Source and No History of TIA or Stroke

The two most important causes of cardioembolic stroke in the United States are atrial fibrillation (AF) and acute myocardial infarction (MI). AF accounts for almost 50% of cardiogenic emboli, and acute MI accounts for 15%. The incidence of ischemic stroke during hospitalization in patients with acute MI is approximately 1%. Recent studies have indicated that the use of thrombolytic agents in these patients has reduced the incidence of cardioembolic stroke after MI, but the higher incidence of intracranial hemorrhage related to thrombolysis offsets this benefit. The usual mechanism of ischemic stroke after MI is embolism of a mural thrombus. These thrombi occur in up to 30% of patients with an anterior-wall transmural MI and only rarely in patients with inferior-wall MI. Factors that have been associated with mural thrombus formation in patients with anterior-wall infarction are an ejection fraction $\leq$35% and apical dyskinesia or aneurysm. Mobility of thrombus has been associated with increased embolic risk. A recent metaanalysis of seven studies indicates that the odds ratio of anticoagulation vs. no anticoagulation in preventing embolization in patients with acute anterior-wall MI was 0.14 (95% CI, 0.04–0.52), whereas evidence for a similar benefit of antiplatelet therapy was lacking (26).

It has long been recognized that patients with AF associated with mitral stenosis should be treated with long-term warfarin because of the extremely high rate of thromboembolism associated with this condition (the relative risk of stroke in these patients is 17 times that of age-matched controls in sinus rhythm). Although patients with nonvalvular AF are also at a higher risk of stroke than age-matched controls in sinus rhythm (relative risk, 5.6), the efficacy of antithrombotic therapy in these patients has only recently been established.

Over the past 5 years, seven multicenter studies on the efficacy of warfarin or aspirin for stroke prevention in patients with nonvalvular AF have been completed (27–29). Six of these studies enrolled mainly patients without preceding neurologic events (27,29), while one study restricted enrollment to patients with TIA or minor stroke (28). Other inclusion and exclusion criteria for these trials were similar, although two of the trials did not include patients with intermittent AF. All seven trials had a warfarin arm, and four trials had an aspirin arm. The dose of aspirin was 75 mg/d in one study, 300 mg/d in another, and 325 mg/d in two other studies. Aspirin was administered in a double-blind fashion in three of the studies. Warfarin was administered in a double-blind fashion in two of the studies, none of which had an aspirin arm. Three studies used prothrombin time ratios to monitor the intensity of anticoagulation, three studies used INR values, and one study used prothrombin time ratios initially and later switched to INR values.

In the first five trials, warfarin consistently reduced the frequency of thromboembolic events by 37–86% compared with control patients (most of whom received placebo; the remainder received aspirin). Analysis of pooled data from these five trials showed an annual stroke rate of 4.5% for the control group and 1.4% for the warfarin group (risk reduction of 68%; 95% CI, 50–79%) (27). Warfarin reduced the risk of stroke by 84% (95% CI, 55–95%) in women compared with 60% (95% CI, 35–76%) in men. The efficacy of warfarin was evident in all subgroups except in patients younger than 65 years who had no vascular risk factors (ie, those with lone AF). In this subgroup, the annual stroke rate was 1% in patients treated with either warfarin or placebo (27). The primary concern when using warfarin is the risk of major systemic or intracranial hemorrhage. Pooled data from the first five studies show that the annual rate of major hemorrhage (intracranial hemorrhage, bleeding requiring hospitalization, transfusion of 2 units of blood) was 1.0% for the control group and 1.3% for the warfarin group (27).

In the three trials that have included a comparison between aspirin and placebo, the efficacy of aspirin has been less consistent than that of warfarin. The risk reduction with aspirin compared with placebo has varied between 18% (95% CI, 60–58%) in the Copenhagen study (in which patients received aspirin 75 mg/d) to 44% (95% CI, 7–66%) in the Stroke Prevention in Atrial Fibrillation study (in which patients received aspirin 325 mg/d) (27).

While the results of studies that compared warfarin with placebo and aspirin with placebo suggest a higher reduction in the risk of thromboembolism in patients taking warfarin, studies that have directly compared the efficacy and safety of warfarin with aspirin have produced discordant results. In the Copenhagen study, the major hemorrhage rates in patients treated with warfarin or aspirin were <1% per year, and the thromboembolic rates were 2.0% per year in the warfarin group and 5.5% per year in the aspirin group (27). In the European Atrial Fibrillation Trial (EAFT) study, the major hemorrhage rates were 2.8% per year in the warfarin group and 0.9% per year in the aspirin group, and the rates of stroke were 4% per year in the warfarin group and 10% per year in the aspirin group (28). In the Stroke Prevention in Atrial Fibrillation (SPAF) II study, however, warfarin was associated with only a 0.8% lower rate of thromboembolism than patients treated with aspirin but was associated with a higher rate of major hemorrhage than aspirin, especially in patients older than 75 years (29). These studies are not directly comparable because the dose of aspirin was smaller in the Copenhagen study, the intensity of anticoagulation was highest in SPAF II, there were substantially more patients older than 75 in SPAF II, and only the EAFT study restricted enrollment to patients with a history of TIA or minor stroke.

Given the results of these trials, which antithrombotic therapy should be prescribed for patients with nonvalvular AF? For patients younger than 65 with lone AF, the data from these trials show that aspirin therapy is probably sufficient. The most effective dose of aspirin has not been established, but most of the trials used 300–325 mg/d. For high-risk patients younger than 65 (ie, patients with a history of hypertension, diabetes, congestive heart failure, or TIA or stroke) and all patients 65–75 years old, warfarin therapy, with a target INR of 2.0–3.0, appears warranted based on the weight of the evidence. In patients older than 75, warfarin should probably only be used in patients at high risk of thromboembolism (ie, those with previous TIA or stroke, left atrial spontaneous echo contrast or thrombus on TEE, or congestive heart failure) because of the higher risk of major hemorrhagic complications in this age group. Further research is needed to develop safer antithrombotic therapy in older patients. One approach that is currently under investigation in patients with nonvalvular AF is low-intensity anticoagulation with warfarin (target INR 1.2–1.5) combined with aspirin.

Ideally, when patients present with recent onset AF for the first time, consideration should be given to pharmacologic or electric cardioversion to achieve sinus rhythm. Maintenance of sinus rhythm would then obviate the need for long-term anticoagulation. TEE has assumed an important role in the selection of patients for electric cardioversion because detection of atrial thrombi mandates postponement of cardioversion. The absence of atrial thrombi on TEE, however, does not obviate the need for short-term anticoagulation (at the time of cardioversion and for 4 weeks thereafter), since stroke can occasionally occur within 2 hours to 7 days after electric cardioversion in patients with no evidence of atrial thrombus on TEE (30).

REFERENCES

1. Rem JA, Hachinski VC, Boughner DR, Barnett HJM. Value of cardiac monitoring and echocardiography in TIA and stroke patients. *Stroke* 1985;16:950–956.
2. Pearson AC, Labovitz AJ, Tatineni S, Gomez CR. Superiority of transesophageal echocardiography in detecting cardiac source of embolism in patients with cerebral ischemia of uncertain etiology. *J Am Coll Cardiol* 1991;17:66–72.
3. Múgge A, Daniel WG, Haverich A, Lichtlen PR. Diagnosis of noninfective cardiac mass lesions by two-dimensional echocardiography. *Circulation* 1991;83:70–78.
4. Reeder GS, Khandheria BK, Seward JB, Tajik AJ. Transesophageal echocardiography and cardiac masses. *Mayo Clin Proc* 1991;66:1101–1109.
5. Múgge A. Echocardiographic detection of cardiac valve vegetations and prognostic implications. *Infect Dis Clin North Am* 1993;7:877–898.
6. Daniel WG, Múgge A, Grote J, et al. Comparison of transthoracic and transesophageal echocardiography for detection of abnormalities of prosthetic and bioprosthetic valves in the mitral and aortic positions. *Am J Cardiol* 1993;71:210–215.
7. Nishimura RA, McGoon MD, Shub C, Miller FA Jr, Ilstrup DM, Tajik AJ. Echocardiographically documented mitral-valve prolapse. Long-term follow-up of 237 patients. *N Engl J Med* 1985;313:1305–1309.
8. Petty GW, Orencia AJ, Khandheria BK, Whisnant JP. A population based study of stroke in the setting of mitral valve prolapse: Risk factors and infarct subtype classification. *Mayo Clin Proc* 1994;69:632–634.
9. Nemec JJ, Marwick TH, Lorig RJ, et al. Comparison of transcranial Doppler ultrasound and transesophageal contrast echocardiography in the detection of interatrial right-to-left shunts. *Am J Cardiol* 1991;68:1498–1502.
10. Chimowitz MI, Nemec JJ, Marwick TH, Lorig RJ, Furlan AJ, Salcedo EE. Transcranial Doppler ultrasound identifies patients with right-to-left cardiac or pulmonary shunts. *Neurology* 1991;41:1902–1904.
11. Di Tullio M, Sacco RL, Gopal A, Mohr JP, Homma S. Patent foramen ovale as a risk factor for cryptogenic stroke. *Ann Intern Med* 1992;117:461–465.
12. Falk RH. PFO or UFO? The role of a patent foramen ovale in cryptogenic stroke (editorial). *Am Heart J* 1991;121:1264–1266.
13. Homma S, Di Tullio MR, Sacco RL, Mihalatos D, Li Mandri G, Mohr JP. Characteristics of patent foramen ovale associated with cryptogenic stroke. A biplane transesophageal echocardiographic study. *Stroke* 1994;25:582–586.
14. Silver MD, Dorsey JS. Aneurysms of the septum primum in adults. *Arch Pathol Lab Med* 1978;102:62–65.
15. Pearson AC, Nagelhout D, Castello R, Gomez CR, Labovitz AJ. Atrial septal aneurysm and stroke: A transesophageal echocardiographic study. *J Am Coll Cardiol* 1991;18:1223–1229.
16. Amarenco P, Duyckaerts C, Tzourio C, Henin D, Bousser MG, Hauw JJ. The prevalence of ulcerated plaques in the aortic arch in patients with stroke. *N Engl J Med* 1992;326:221–225.
17. Amarenco P, Cohen A, Tzourio C, Bertrand B, et al. Atherosclerotic disease of the aortic arch and the risk of ischemic stroke. *N Engl J Med* 1994;331:1474–1479.
18. Jones EF, Kalman JM, Calafiore P, Tonkin AM, Donnan GA. Proximal aortic atheroma. An independent risk factor for cerebral ischemia. *Stroke* 1995;26:218–224.
19. Chimowitz MI, DeGeorgia MA, Poole RM, Hepner A, Armstrong WM. Left atrial spontaneous echo contrast is highly associated with previous stroke in patients with atrial fibrillation or mitral stenosis. *Stroke* 1993;24:1015–1019.
20. Leung DY, Black IW, Cranney GB, Hopkins AP, Walsh WF. Prognostic implications of spontaneous echo contrast in nonvalvular atrial fibrillation. *J Am Coll Cardiol* 1994;24:755–762.
21. Cerebral Embolism Study Group. Immediate anticoagulation of embolic stroke: A randomized trial. *Stroke* 1983;14:668–676.
22. Pessin MS, Estol CJ, Lafranchise F, Caplan LR. Safety of anticoagulation after hemorrhagic infarction. *Neurology* 1993;43:1298–1303.
23. Pruit AA. Neurologic complications of infective endocarditis: A review of an evolving disease and its management issues in the 1990s. *Neurologist* 1995;1:20–34.
24. Turpie AG, Gent M, Laupacis A, et al. A comparison of aspirin with placebo in patients treated with warfarin after heart-valve replacement. *N Engl J Med* 1993;329:524–529.
25. Zhu WX, Khandheria BK, Warnes CA, Seward JB, Danielson GK. Closure of patent foramen ovale for cryptogenic stroke in young patients: Long-term follow-up (abstract). *Circulation* 1992;86:I-147.
26. Vaitkus PT, Barnathan ES. Embolic potential, prevention and management of mural thrombus complicating anterior myocardial infarction: A meta-analysis. *J Am Coll Cardiol* 1993;22:1004–1009.
27. Atrial Fibrillation Investigators. Risk factors for stroke and efficacy of antithrombotic therapy in atrial fibrillation. Analysis of pooled data from five randomized controlled studies. *Arch Intern Med* 1994;154:1449–1457.
28. European Atrial Fibrillation Trial (EAFT) Study Group. Secondary prevention in non-rheumatic atrial fibrillation after transient ischemic attack or minor stroke. *Lancet* 1993;342:1266–1262.
29. Stroke Prevention in Atrial Fibrillation Investigators. Warfarin versus aspirin for prevention of thromboembolism in atrial fibrillation: Stroke Prevention in Atrial Fibrillation II Study. *Lancet* 1994;343:687–691.
30. Black IW, Fatkin D, Sagar KB, et al. Exclusion of atrial thrombus by transesophageal echocardiography does not preclude embolism after cardioversion of atrial fibrillation. A multicenter study. *Circulation* 1994;89:2509–2513.

Cerebrovascular Disease, edited by H. Hunt Batjer.
Lippincott-Raven Publishers, Philadelphia © 1997.

CHAPTER 30

Cervicocephalic Carotid and Vertebral Artery Dissection: Management

Constantino Takis and Jeffrey L. Saver

First reported in 1915, cervicocephalic arterial dissections are now recognized as a major cause of brain ischemia. Dissections transpire when blood erupts into the wall of a vessel, producing an intramural hematoma. When the dissection plane is located in the subintima or inner media, the intramural hemorrhage bulges inward, narrowing the vessel lumen. When located in the outer media or subadventitia, the intramural hematoma produces an arterial dilatation (dissecting aneurysm) (Fig. 1). With surprising frequency, dissections of the cervicocerebral vasculature occur without provocation or in association with trivial arterial trauma. Dissections are also a natural consequence of major penetrating or nonpenetrating trauma to the head and neck.

ETIOPATHOGENESIS

The pathogenesis of spontaneous cervicocephalic arterial dissections is still incompletely understood. Some authors suggest that an endothelial tear is the initial event, permitting blood from the lumen to infiltrate into the arterial wall, and others favor an intramedial hematoma as the primary insult, secondarily rupturing into the true lumen. It is likely that both mechanisms occur. In some autopsied cases an intimal tear is demonstrated near the proximal margin of the dissection; in others no communication between false and true lumens can be detected. Cerebral ischemia may ensue from (a) low-flow hemodynamic failure due to stenosis or occlusion of the lumen at the level of the dissection, or (b) artery-to-artery embolism occurring when endothelial disruption exposes highly thrombogenic material within the vessel wall. Most investigators suspect

that distal thromboembolism occurs somewhat more frequently than low-flow perfusion failure. The plane of dissection likely depends on systemic blood pressure, vessel location, and presence and site of underlying vasculopathy. The dissection plane is most commonly in the media and subadventitia in extracranial carotid, extracranial vertebral, and intracranial vertebral artery dissections, and most commonly subintimal in intracranial carotid, basilar, and middle cerebral artery dissections.

While most spontaneous cervicocephalic dissections occur in healthy subjects, underlying congenital arteriopathies do account for a substantial proportion of patients. Fibromuscular dysplasia is present in about 15%, and associations have also been noted with cystic medial necrosis, Marfan's syndrome, Ehlers–Danlos syndrome type IV, and α_1-antitrypsin deficiency (1,2). Several causes of acquired vasculopathy have also been linked with dissection in case series, including hypertension, migraine, oral contraceptives, atherosclerosis, temporal arteritis and other vasculitides, tortuous arterial coiling, and moyamoya syndrome (1–3). It is likely that many healthy-appearing individuals suffering dissection actually harbor a subtle and unrecognized predisposing congenital or acquired vasculopathy (1,2,4). Pathologic specimens frequently demonstrate disorganization of the media and internal elastic lamina, although dissection in microscopically normal arteries is well documented.

As minor trauma or intense physical activity precedes spontaneous cervicocerebral dissections in 20–25% of reported cases, the traditional dichotomy between traumatic and unprovoked dissections is best discarded, recognizing instead a spectrum of predisposing mechanical insults. Particular activities that have been implicated in association with cervicocerebral dissection include head turning while leading a parade, yoga, ceiling painting, sneezing, coughing, sexual concourse, a wide variety of sporting maneuvers, tonic-clonic seizures, chiropractic manipulation, and vigorous nose blowing (1,2).

C. Takis: New England Medical Center, Boston, Massachusetts 02111.
J. L. Saver: UCLA Stroke Center, Reed Neurologic Research Center, Los Angeles, California 90095.

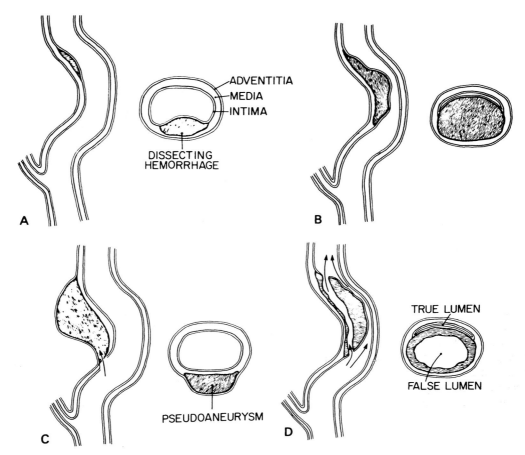

FIG. 1. Lateral and cross-sectional views of differing planes of dissection. **A:** Subintimal dissection, distending vessel wall inward. **B:** More extensive subintimal hemorrhage, almost fully occluding arterial lumen. **C:** Subadventitial hemorrhage, causing outward protrusion of vessel wall (dissecting aneurysm). **D:** False lumen channel established when intramural hemorrhage communicates at proximal and distal ends with true lumen. (From ref. 33.)

CLINICAL FEATURES

The clinical features, course, and management of cervico-cephalic dissections differ with the arterial segment involved, warranting separate consideration.

EXTRACRANIAL INTERNAL CAROTID ARTERY DISSECTION

The cervical internal carotid artery (ICA) is the most frequently encountered site of cervicocephalic dissection, representing >70% of cases in the literature. In a population-based registry, cervical carotid dissections accounted for 2.5% of all first ischemic strokes, and in several registries they account for 10–25% of ischemic stroke in young adults (5). The average annual incidence among persons 20 years and older is 3.5 per 100,000 (6). Cervical ICA dissection is predominantly a disease of midadulthood, with 70% of patients between the ages of 35 and 50, and a mean age of 44 years. Males and females are equally affected.

The classic mode of clinical presentation of cervical ICA dissection consists of the triad of unilateral neck or head pain, ipsilateral oculosympathetic paresis, and focal cerebral ischemic symptoms (2,5,7). Clinical manifestations may be quite variable, however, and patients not infrequently present with only one or two of these symptoms, or with ipsilateral lower cranial nerve palsies (8,9). The clinical features of 626 cases collected from the literature are presented in Table 1.

Transient ischemic attacks appear in one third of patients, producing symptoms typical of anterior intracranial circulation ischemia. Transient monocular blindness constitutes approximately one third of all transient ischemic episodes (2). Infarcts have been reported in 70% of cases, with preceding TIAs in only a minority. Infarct severity varies widely. Cervical ICA dissections are fatal in about 5%, severely disabling in about 25%, and produce no or mild residual deficits in about 70% (Table 4).

Headache, neck pain, or facial pain often precedes the onset of ischemic symptoms by a few hours or days. Among reported cases, cervicocephalic pain was the inaugural symp-

TABLE 1. *Clinical features of cervical ICA dissection*

No. cases	626
Mean age (years)	44
Sex	
Male	52%
Female	47%
Laterality	
Unilateral	86%
Left	60%
Right	40%
Bilateral	14%
Major presenting complaint	
Asymptomatic bruit	2%
Neck or head pain	21%
Pulsatile tinnitus alone	2%
TIA	30%
Stroke	46%
Symptoms present at diagnosis	
Neck pain	20%
Headache	64%
Neck or head pain	66%
Tinnitus or subjective bruit	26%
Signs present at diagnosis	
Horner's syndrome	32%
Cervical bruit	18%
Lingual paresis	6%
Associated conditions	
Oral contraceptives	35%
Tobacco	29%
Hypertension	28%
Migraine	22%
Fibromuscular displasia	16%

ICA, internal carotid artery; TIA, transient ischemic attack.

tom in one fifth of patients and reported at some time in the clinical course in two thirds. Pain is homolateral to the dissection in about four fifths of patients, more often affects the head than face or neck, and generally lasts for several days (median 5 days) (10). The headache is severe in the majority, and may be throbbing, but is more often steady. Rarely, positive visual phenomena are observed.

A partial Horner's syndrome may also be a heralding or accompanying finding. Direct pressure on the sympathetic fibers of the internal carotid plexus produces an oculosympathetic paresis with miosis and ptosis, while sparing of the external carotid plexus subserving sweating of the face accounts for the absence of anhidrosis. A partial Horner's deficit is evident in one third of patients. Pulsatile tinnitus and subjective bruits are conspicuous complaints in about one quarter of patients.

Palsies of one or more cranial nerves are a less common but well-documented complication of cervical ICA dissection (8,9). Cranial nerve XII is most frequently affected, producing lingual paresis, followed by nerves IX, X, XI, and V. The lower cranial nerves are most often compromised by local compression from an outwardly expanding subadventitial dissection that causes the carotid wall to encroach on the upper cervical parapharyngeal space (Fig. 2). Ipsilateral tongue paresis, throat numbness, facial dysesthesia, dysgeu-

sia, and dysarthria, dysphagia, and dysphonia may result. Rarely, oculomotor cranial nerves are involved, generally when the dissection extends intracranially into the cavernous sinus. Nerve ischemia due to a compromised blood supply may also sometimes occur.

Combinations of these clinical features, which are uncommon in atherothrombotic stroke, appear in three quarters of patients with cervical ICA dissection, facilitating clinical detection. Prominent head or neck pain accompanying cerebral ischemia should always suggest dissection as a potential diagnosis. A particularly high index of suspicion is required in patients presenting with local signs alone, including new head or neck pain, oculosympathetic paresis, or both, to permit diagnosis before cerebral ischemia occurs. In the series of Biousse et al, 43% of patients with inaugural local signs experienced ensuing cerebral or retinal infarction, after a mean delay of 6 days (11).

History taking in patients with cervical internal carotid dissection reveals preceding minor neck torsion or trauma in almost one fourth. Cervical rotation or extension can juxtapose the distal extracranial carotid artery and the transverse processes of the upper cervical vertebra, precipitating dissection in the vulnerable individual (Fig. 3). The frequent location of the hematoma in the posterior wall of the distal extracranial portion of the cervical ICA supports the role of mechanical injury (1). However, in the substantial number of patients with dissection beginning below the C1-2 vertebral level, direct bony injury seems improbable. Dissections ordinarily spare the carotid bifurcation, beginning 2 or more cm distal to the origin of the internal carotid artery and extending variable distances rostrally. Tears generally terminate before or at the level of the entrance of the artery into the petrous canal, where bony support prevents further upward extension except in rare circumstances.

Hypertension is reported in one third of patients. Oral contraceptives, which may provoke medial and intimal proliferation, are taken by one third of women suffering cervical ICA dissections. A history of migraine is present in one fifth of patients. At least one case-controlled study found migraine and anticonception treatment to constitute independent risk factors for extracranial ICA dissection (12). Most prominent among the arteriopathies associated with ICA dissection is fibromuscular dysplasia, present in <1% of the general population but 15% of cases, with a female preponderance. Ehlers–Danlos disease, Marfan's syndrome, arterial coiling, and atheromatous plaques have occasionally been implicated. Familial occurrence of cervical ICA dissection has been reported.

The diagnosis of extracranial ICA dissection depends on a consonant clinical picture and characteristic neuroimaging findings. Noninvasive studies with magnetic resonance imaging (MRI) and ultrasound supplement, and with increasing frequency supplant, conventional arteriography. Five typical angiographic appearances have been delineated: (a) irregular, extended narrowing of the distal ICA, resulting in a string sign if severe, the most common pattern; (b) a gradually tapering

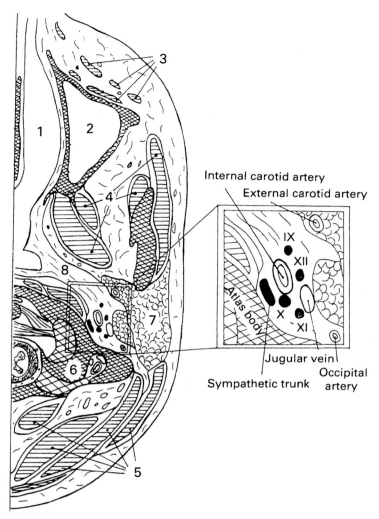

FIG. 2. Anatomic basis of lower cranial nerve palsies with extracranial carotid artery dissection. Illustration displays the close relationship between the internal carotid artery and cranial nerves IX, X, XI, and XII at the level of the first cervical vertebral body (atlas). (From ref. 8.)

occlusion starting distal to the carotid sinus, the least specific finding but present in one fifth of cases; (c) intimal flaps evident near the proximal margin of a smooth or scalloped narrowing extending only a few centimeters; (d) an extraluminal pouch (dissecting aneurysm), usually occurring distally, near the base of the skull; and (e) accompanying findings of intracranial embolic occlusions, fibromuscular dysplasia, or tortuosity (Fig. 4) (2,7). Rarely, dissections are visualized originating in the common carotid artery or extending distally to involve the intracranial anterior circulation.

MRI possesses several advantages over conventional arteriography (8,13,14). It clearly depicts the vessel wall and surrounding structures as well as the lumen, allowing direct visualization of the intramural hematoma. MRI avoids the minor risks of arteriographic catheterization. The pathognomonic MRI finding of dissection is an eccentrically narrowed lumen with adjacent semilunar-shaped increased signal (crescent sign), representing the extravasated blood

within the vessel wall (Fig. 5A). Other, less specific findings are (a) an increased signal from the entire vessel, (b) poor or absent visualization of the vessel, and (c) significant compromise of the vessel lumen by adjoining abnormal increased signal tissue (13). These findings are best observed on axial, high cervical T1-weighted and proton density images, which afford excellent contrast between vessel wall, lumen, and surrounding cervical structures. Magnetic resonance angiography (MRA) may increase the yield of MR studies, displaying the same features of dissection as conventional angiography noninvasively (Fig. 5B). Taking conventional arteriography as a gold standard, one study found that MRI had a sensitivity of 84% and a specificity of 99% for the diagnosis of carotid dissection, and MRA a sensitivity of 95% and a specificity of 99% (14). Several case reports have described conventional angiogram-negative, MRI-positive dissections, which may arise when intramural hematoma fails to compromise the arterial lumen.

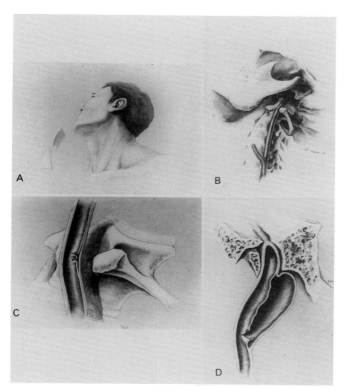

FIG. 3. Mechanism of mechanical injury to carotid artery during neck movement. **A:** Simultaneous neck hyperextension and rotation, surface view. **B:** Simultaneous neck hyperextension and rotation, bone and vessel view. **C:** Impingement of artery on vertebra produces intimal tear. **D:** Extravasation of blood into vessel wall through intimal tear. (From ref. 34.)

Carotid duplex, high extracranial Doppler, and transcranial Doppler sonography may also be useful in the evaluation of patients with ICA dissections (15–18). Standard carotid duplex studies interrogate the carotid bifurcation proximal to the level of most dissections and therefore only rarely provide imaging evidence of dissection directly, such as a tapering luminal stenosis or double lumen (Fig. 6). Carotid duplex will often demonstrate consequences of more distal carotid stenosis, however, including reduced flow, absent flow, or, most commonly, high-resistance flow with a bidirectional signal component. Retromandibular placement of the probe allows insonation of the distal portion of the extracranial carotid artery and may demonstrate increased velocities reflecting high extracranial carotid stenosis. Transcranial Doppler delineates effects of carotid pathology on the intracranial circulation, including reduced velocities, collateral flow patterns, and distal emboli. Multimodal ultrasound studies demonstrate up to 95% sensitivity for carotid dissection and are particularly helpful for serial monitoring of lesion evolution (18). Lack of specificity of findings and inability to identify dissecting aneurysms are limitations.

The proper management of extracranial internal carotid artery dissections remains controversial. Recognition of the strong tendency to natural improvement in the vessel wall has swung support to initial medical rather than surgical management. Anticoagulation and/or antiplatelet agents are often advocated, though unsupported by controlled clinical trials (1,2,5,7,17). The use of antithrombotics may appear counterintuitive in a disease defined by bleeding into the arterial wall, but early angiograms suggest that distal embolization of thrombotic fragments from the dissection site and in situ thrombus propagation are the most common causes of neurologic worsening rather than extension of intramural hemorrhage. We favor initial anticoagulation with heparin followed by warfarin in patients who have no contraindication to anticoagulation, and initial antiplatelet therapy in the remainder.

The time frame of recovery of the vessel wall determines the duration of therapy. Among 439 cases collected from large series, 86% percent of stenoses due to extracranial carotid dissection, 46% percent of occlusions, and 43% percent of aneurysms improved or returned to normal on follow-up imaging. Serial ultrasound studies demonstrate that the median time to resolution of carotid dissections is 6–7 weeks, most vessels recover by 3 months, and arteries failing to reconstitute a normal lumen by 6 months are unlikely to improve subsequently (5,17). We continue anticoagulation until the dissection has largely healed. Serial ultrasound is an option to follow the time course of vessel recovery closely in an individual patient. At 3 months (or earlier if ultrasound has normalized) a follow-up MRI/MRA or conventional angiogram is obtained to evaluate lumen recovery and screen for the formation of a persistent dissecting aneurysm. If the artery is normal, antithrombotic therapy is discontinued. If mild luminal abnormalities persist, platelet antiaggregants are employed. When hemodynamically significant stenosis or dissecting aneurysm persist, anticoagulation is continued for 3 additional months and repeat imaging obtained. Late strokes, defined as infarctions occurring after discharge from the initial hospitalization, are infrequent in extracranial ICA dissections. Among 388 cases with follow-up (average 3.5 years) information, fewer than 2% experienced late cerebral infarction, and most of these occurred in the first year.

We reserve surgery for patients with cranial nerve compression due to expanding dissecting aneurysms or with cerebral ischemic episodes despite medical therapy. Aneurysmal resection and carotid reconstruction is the most common surgical strategy (19). Cervical-to-intracranial ICA bypass procedures may occasionally be employed for poorly accessible aneurysms of the very distal ICA. Carotid ligation or balloon occlusion is safe and simple in individuals with good collateral circulation but likely increases the risk of cerebral ischemia and perhaps intracranial aneurysms later in life.

The risk of recurrent dissection in the initially dissected artery is low; the risk of subsequent dissection of a different cervicephalic vessel slightly higher. In a Mayo Clinic series of 200 extracranial cervicocephalic arterial dissections, patients experienced recurrent dissection at a rate of 2% in the first month, and 1% per year thereafter. All dissections

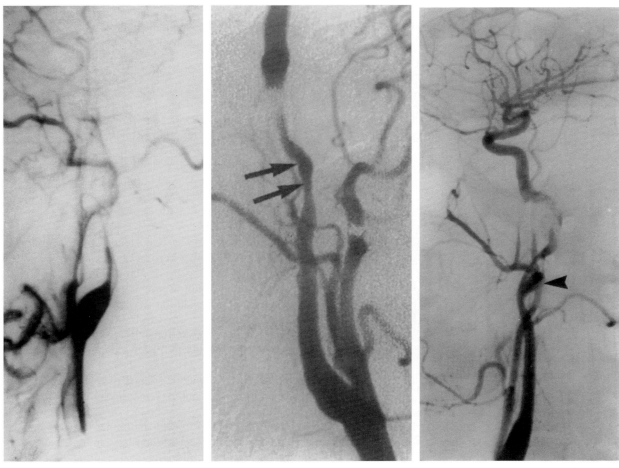

FIG. 4. Spectrum of arteriographic appearances of extracranial internal carotid artery dissection. **A:** Long, tapering occlusion beginning distal to the bulb. **B:** Extended irregular scalloping of the distal ICA *(arrows)*, with reconstitution of normal caliber on entry to the petrous canal. **C:** Dissecting aneurysm *(arrowhead)*. (Part A from ref. 35; parts B and C from ref. 14.)

occurred in cervicocephalic or renal arteries not previously involved by dissection. Younger age was the only independent risk factor for recurrence (20). In a collaborative European study of 105 patients, the rate of recurrent dissection also approximated 1% per year over 10 years (21). All patients in this study with recurrence had underlying arteriopathies, either Ehlers–Danlos syndrome or fibromuscular dysplasia. It seems prudent to recommend that survivors of dissection avoid activities that predispose to abrupt cervical rotation or extension. Vigorous control of hypertension and discontinuation of estrogen-containing compounds also are reasonable steps.

EXTRACRANIAL VERTEBRAL ARTERY DISSECTION

The extracranial vertebral artery is the second most common site of cervicocerebral arterial dissection, accounting for 15% of cases in the literature. It occurs most commonly in young to mid-adulthood, with a mean age of onset of 38

years among reported cases. However, an ascertainment bias favoring younger patients is likely, as in older individuals angiography is less frequently performed in ischemia of the posterior circulation compared with the anterior circulation, and the coexistence of atherosclerotic disease limits diagnostic certainty. A modest female preponderance is noted.

The characteristic clinical presentation of vertebral artery dissection is abrupt onset of neck pain or headache, and simultaneous or delayed onset of focal ischemic symptoms (Table 2) (1–3,22–24). Cervicocranial pain is reported in three fourths of patients and headache, when present, tends to be occipital. Cerebral ischemia is almost invariable among reported cases, with infarction in over 70% and transient symptoms in about 30%. Cases producing headache alone likely often go unrecognized. Cerebral ischemia usually occurs after an interval, with almost 90% of strokes delayed in onset. The most common stroke syndromes are (a) a lateral medullary infarct, partial or complete, observed in 35% of cases, and (b) cerebellar infarction. Pontine, midbrain, and posterior cerebral artery territory infarcts are much less often

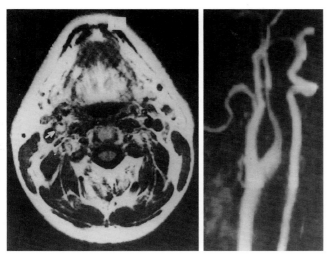

FIG. 5. Magnetic resonance studies of extracranial internal carotid artery (ICA) dissection. **A:** Distal cervical axial T2-weighted image shows hyperintense intramural hemorrhage (crescent sign) with eccentrically located residual vessel lumen flow void *(arrow)*. **B:** Magnetic resonance angiogram in the same patient displays extended narrowing of the ICA beginning distal to the bulb (string sign). (From ref. 17.)

TABLE 2. *Clinical features of extracranial vertebral artery dissection*

No. of cases	131
Mean age (years)	38
Sex	
Male	37%
Female	63%
Laterality	
Bilateral	35%
Unilateral	65%
Left	55%
Right	45%
Symptoms and signs	
Neck pain	51%
Headache	56%
Neck or head pain	75%
TIA	32%
Stroke	72%
At onset	13%
Delayed	87%
After TIA	13%
Lateral medullary syndrome	34%
Preceding minor mechanical insult	53%
Neck rotation	72%
Minor trauma	15%
Associated conditions	
Hypertension	28%
Oral contraceptives	28%
Fibromuscular dysplasia	18%
Migraine	17%

TIA, transient ischemic attack.

encountered. The unique dependence of the posterior inferior cerebellar artery on a single extracranial vertebral artery accounts for its vulnerability. The anatomy of the posterior circulation also contributes to the relatively high prevalence of bilateral dissections in the literature, approximately one third of cases. Unilateral vertebral artery dissections, especially if proximal, may not produce ischemia, due to preserved flow through the contralateral vertebral artery, and the dissection may elude detection.

Similar risk factors have been implicated in extracranial vertebral artery dissections as in extracranial carotid artery

dissection (1–3,22–24). Hypertension is present in more than a quarter, migraine in almost one fifth of patients, and among women oral contraceptive use occurs in more than one quarter. Structural arteriopathies clearly underlie some extracranial vertebral artery dissections, with fibromuscular dysplasia accounting for almost one fifth of cases in large series.

Minor trauma is a common precipitating event, present in more than half of cases. A wide array of mildly traumatic activities have been noted, including ceiling painting and trampoline exercises, but chiropractic manipulation looms as a particularly frequent offender. Underlying degenerative or inflammatory arteriopathies are more common in patients without any history of trauma, whereas mild neck torsion or trauma has been found to precipitate dissection in histologically normal arteries.

The third anatomic segment of the vertebral artery (V3) from its exit through the transverse foramen of C2 to its entry into the dura, is the most favored site for dissection, affected in approximately one half of cases (3,22–25). The first and third segments of the vertebral artery are more mobile than the foraminal V2 and intracranial V4 segments, which are fixed by bony attachments. Rotation and hyperextension of the neck stretch the artery maximally within the V3 segment (1,24,26). Chiropractic and minor neck torsion traumas are almost always associated with dissections at the V3 level (23). V3 is also the most common site of dissection

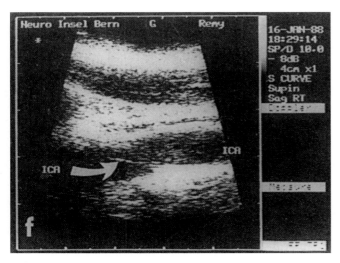

FIG. 6. B-mode high cervical ultrasound demonstrating intimal flap *(arrow)* from extracranial internal carotid artery dissection. (From ref. 36.)

among patients without any elicitable history of trauma, suggesting that mechanical features play a role in individuals with apparent wholly spontaneous dissections, with or without underlying arteriopathies.

Diagnosis of extracranial vertebral artery dissection rests on a compatible clinical picture and characteristic imaging findings. MRI and ultrasound are less sensitive at detecting vertebral dissection than carotid dissection, mandating more frequent conventional angiographic investigation. In one small series, MRI detected vertebral artery dissection with a sensitivity of 60% and specificity of 98% and MRA with a sensitivity of 20% and specificity of 100%, compared with standard angiography (14). The smaller size and broad variation in caliber of vertebral arteries make their imaging on MR more vulnerable to technical artifact. Similarly, transcranial Doppler ultrasound can demonstrate vertebral artery stenosis due to dissection and its intracranial consequences, but not invariably, hampered by the greater tortuosity and anatomic variability of the vertebral artery.

On conventional angiography, dissections of the vertebral artery exhibit the same set of patterns as carotid dissections. The most frequent angiographic finding is an irregularly tapering stenosis, present in almost three quarters of cases (Table 3). Findings of double lumen or intimal flap are more specific but are uncommon.

Data to guide therapy of extracranial vertebral artery dissection rest on an even less secure base of nonrandomized case series than that of extracranial carotid artery dissection. Most natural history studies suggest a broadly similar time course of vessel recovery within 3 months, low incidence of late cerebral ischemia, and low incidence of recurrent dissection. We therefore follow a parallel treatment strategy of (a) early anticoagulation in patients without contraindication and (b) a follow-up imaging study 3 months later with continued anticoagulation if severe luminal compromise and irregularity or dissecting aneurysm persists, antiplatelet therapy for mild luminal abnormalities, and discontinuation of antithrombotics when the vessel appears normal. In the minority of patients whose dissection extends intracranially, computed tomography and lumbar puncture to rule out subarachnoid hemorrhage, which would preclude anticoagulation, are mandatory. The prognosis for patients with extracranial vertebral dissection tends to be favorable. Approximately 80% have normal outcome or mild residual deficits, vs. 70% for extracranial internal carotid dissection (Table 4).

TABLE 3. *Angiographic findings in extracranial vertebral artery dissection*

Irregular stenosis	73%
Occlusion	29%
Aneurysm	14%
Dissection origin in V3 segment	50%
Bilateral vertebral dissection	35%
Vertebral and internal carotid dissection	18%

TABLE 4. *Outcome of cervical artery dissection*

Outcome	ICA	VA
Normal or mild deficit	71%	83%
Major, disabling deficit	25%	9%
Death	5%	8%

ICA, internal carotid artery; VA, vertebral artery.

INTRACRANIAL CAROTID SYSTEM DISSECTION

Intracranial carotid system dissection is an infrequently reported disease entity. Its true incidence is unknown because specific angiographic and noninvasive imaging features are lacking. Consequently, many nonfatal cases are likely unrecognized, and postmortem diagnosed cases dominate the literature. In a review of 59 reported cases, the mean age of onset was 30 years, younger than for extracranial cervicocephalic dissections, and a slight male preponderance was noted (27).

The majority of affected patients are healthy, without evident risk factors or arteriopathy. Hypertension, migraine, oral contraceptives, alcohol, and recreational drug use have been reported sporadically. Vasculopathies implicated in isolated cases include fibromuscular dysplasia, cystic medial necrosis, moyamoya syndrome, atherosclerosis, polyarteritis nodosa, and meningovascular syphilis. About one quarter of patients have a history of antecedent minor trauma, intense physical activity, or a surgical intervention.

Associated pain and sudden focal neurologic deficits are the characteristic clinical features, present in over 80% of cases. The headache is often severe, may exhibit a migrainous character, and is commonly localized to ipsilateral periorbital or frontotemporal regions. Focal cerebral ischemia usually appears within minutes or hours of onset of pain, only rarely after delays of days to weeks. Neurologic deficits are most often profound from inception, although infrequently TIAs or a stuttering progression are seen. Seizures or syncope can be the initial symptom, and 50% of patients have early alterations of consciousness. Horner's syndrome is seen only rarely, in contrast to extracranial carotid dissection. Subarachnoid hemorrhage, arising when subadventitial hematomas erupt through the external wall of the vessel, is observed in 20% of cases.

Neuroimaging is often nonspecific. Computed tomography may disclose brain infarction, subarachnoid hemorrhage, or both. Angiography only rarely shows pathognomonic findings of double lumen and intimal flap. The concurrence of subarachnoid bleeding, intracranial arterial stenosis, and an aneurysm originating at a non-bifurcation location is also highly suggestive, but uncommon. Most often arterial occlusion or stenosis is visualized. These only occasionally suggest dissection, if they exhibit the appearance of an extended, tight stenosis (string sign), irregular scalloping (pearl and string sign), or a wavy ribbon pattern. Follow-up angiographic studies may support the diagnosis in retrospect, by demonstrating rapid resolution of luminal narrowing, uncommon with atherosclerotic disease, or by showing the development of a dissecting aneurysm.

The usual site of dissection is the intracranial internal carotid artery or the middle cerebral artery trunk, affected in 78% of cases. The anterior cerebral artery and branches of the middle cerebral artery are involved infrequently. Restricted mobility of the distal intracranial internal carotid artery and middle cerebral artery stem may render them more vulnerable to shear forces during acceleration–deceleration head movements. Intracranial extension of an extracranial dissection is rare, and bilateral or multivessel dissections are less frequent in the intracranial than extracranial circulation. The usual plane of intracranial anterior circulation dissection is subintimal, with subadventitial dissections that predispose to subarachnoid hemorrhage in about one fifth of cases. Intracranial arteries lack well-developed external elastic membranes, and their muscularis and adventitial layers are only two thirds as thick as extracranial arteries, rendering them more vulnerable to rupture.

The prognosis appears to be poor. Fatal outcome was observed in 72% of reported cases, and moderate to severe neurologic deficits were present in 50% of the survivors, though dependence on autopsy diagnosis likely distorts the true natural history (27). No therapy has clearly been proven effective. Vigorous regulation of blood pressure and bed rest are likely to be beneficial. Anticoagulation to prevent artery-to-artery embolism and local thrombus propagation has been proposed on analogy to extracranial carotid dissection, but is of uncertain benefit and should certainly be avoided when subarachnoid hemorrhage is present. A variety of surgical procedures have been performed in individual cases with successful outcome either due to or despite the intervention, including ligation of the carotid artery, arteriotomy, and extracranial–intracranial bypass.

INTRACRANIAL VERTEBRAL ARTERY DISSECTION

Intracranial posterior circulation dissection is uncommon, roughly equal in incidence to intracranial anterior circulation dissection. All together, intracranial dissections account for roughly 10% of cervicocerebral dissections. In isolated intracranial vertebral artery dissection, mean age tends to be the late 40s, slightly older than in dissection at other sites, and a slight male preponderance is noted. A relatively younger mean age (late 30s) is noted among patients with intracranial vertebral artery dissections that extend to involve the basilar artery (2,28–30).

Hypertension has been noted in one third of cases, but oral contraceptive use has rarely been reported. Structural alterations in the vessel wall have been noted in a minority of cases, including fibromuscular dysplasia, cystic medial degeneration, subtle defects in the internal elastic lamina, and atherosclerosis. Antecedent cervical manipulation, physical exertion, and minor head trauma have been present infre-

quently. Both mechanical and histologic factors likely explain the usual site of origin of dissection, just distal to the foramen magnum near the origin of the posterior inferior cerebellar artery. Here the artery may be compressed during head maneuvers, the media and adventitia diminish in size and elastic components, and the external elastic lamina terminates.

The clinical picture departs sharply from carotid or extracranial vertebral artery dissection. More than half of patients present with subarachnoid hemorrhage (2,28–30). One third present with cerebral ischemia, and one tenth with both. Patients with subarachnoid hemorrhage sometimes have prodromal headaches, but more often massive hemorrhage accompanied by headache is present at onset. Patients with subarachnoid bleeding tend to have dissections in the subadventitial plane that are confined to the intracranial vertebral artery and often develop aneurysmal dilatation. Patients with cerebral ischemia generally exhibit headache and simultaneous or delayed brainstem symptoms. Lateral medullary infarction is most common, and extension to bilateral pontine infarction not infrequent. Patients with ischemic deficits tend to have dissections in the subintimal plane that may extend to the basilar artery. Rarely, an outwardly expanding dissecting aneurysm can present as a mass lesion, compressing lower cranial nerves, the brainstem, and/or the cerebellum.

Noninvasive imaging with MRI may demonstrate a crescent sign of high signal within the vessel wall representing intramural hematoma. Transcranial Doppler may detect luminal stenosis if present. Angiography is most helpful, though only rarely will it show definite findings of double lumen or intimal flap. Indirect angiographic signs of dissection such as string sign, string and pearl sign, and wavy ribbon sign may be present. Aneurysmal dilatation of the vertebral artery is often demonstrated. Angiographic distinction from a saccular aneurysm of the posterior inferior cerebellar artery may be difficult, though the irregular contour and early appearance of nearby vessel narrowing should suggest dissection rather than vasospasm. Often dissection is recognized only as an unexpected finding at surgery for presumed saccular aneurysm. Serial angiographic studies in patients without subarachnoid hemorrhage demonstrate resolution or stabilization of the lesions over 2–6 months (30).

In patients presenting with subarachnoid hemorrhage, optimal treatment is surgical, as rebleeding appears to occur in about one fourth of patients. The fusiform dissection precludes clipping of an aneurysmal neck. If the affected vessel is the nondominant vertebral artery, clip occlusion or trapping procedures are often recommended. For dissection in a dominant vertebral artery, wrapping has been advocated, although systematic reports of its effectiveness are sparse. Test balloon occlusion of an apparent dominant vertebral artery followed by permanent clipping if well tolerated has been successful in several series. Permanent endovascular occlusion with platinum coils, silicone balloons, or other detachable agents has shown promise in small series and is especially useful for less surgically accessible dissecting

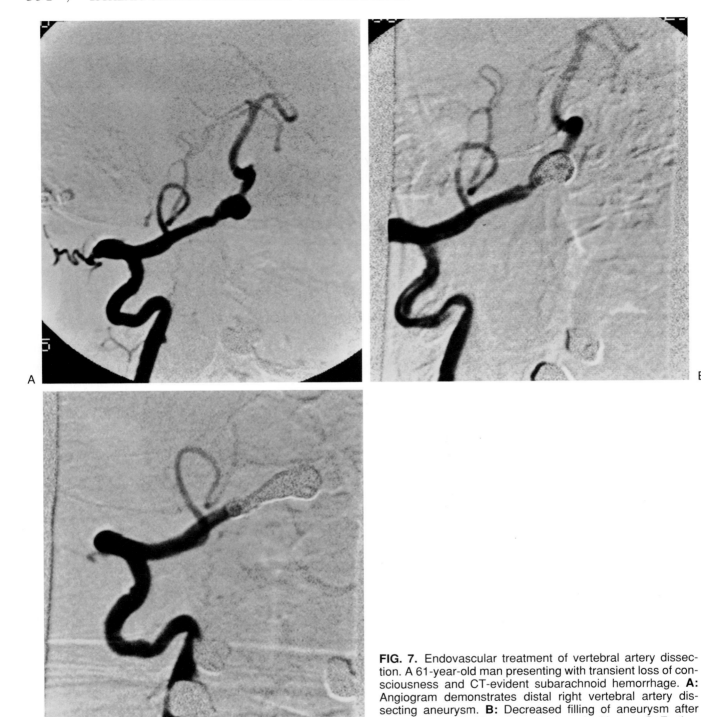

FIG. 7. Endovascular treatment of vertebral artery dissection. A 61-year-old man presenting with transient loss of consciousness and CT-evident subarachnoid hemorrhage. **A:** Angiogram demonstrates distal right vertebral artery dissecting aneurysm. **B:** Decreased filling of aneurysm after Guglielmi detachable coils were deposited in sac. **C:** Further placement of coils in aneurysm and artery isolates the aneurysm from the circulation.

aneurysms distal to the posterior inferior cerebellar artery (Fig. 7) (31). Delayed vasospasm may develop following dissection-related subarachnoid hemorrhage and is managed in the customary manner.

In patients presenting with ischemia and without subarachnoid hemorrhage, management is controversial. Bed rest, quiet environment, and treatment of severe elevations in blood pressure to reduce the chance of delayed subarachnoid hemorrhage may be the best initial course. Anecdotal reports of bleeding into the subarachnoid space following initiation of anticoagulation suggest that heparin is probably best avoided in most cases.

BASILAR ARTERY DISSECTION

Primary dissection of the basilar artery is a rare and apparently grave disease. Approximately 30 cases have been reported (2,32). Mean age is younger, about 35 years, and the sexes are equally affected. Hypertension is present in more than one third, and among the vasculopathies reported are defects in the internal elastic lamina and homocystinuria. The plane of dissection is usually subintimal, although subadventitial and transmural eruptions producing subarachnoid hemorrhage and dissecting aneurysm have been observed. Abrupt onset of severe brainstem ischemia leading rapidly to coma is the typical course. Almost 90% of the cases in the literature had a fatal outcome. No treatment is of demonstrated benefit. Data on antithrombotics for cases without subarachnoid hemorrhage are lacking.

REFERENCES

1. Hart RG, Easton JD. Dissections of cervical and cerebral arteries. *Neurol Clin* 1983;1:155–182.
2. Saver JL, Easton JD, Hart RG. Dissections and trauma of cervicocerebral arteries. In: Baranett JHM, Mohr JP, Stein BM, Yatsu FM, eds. *Stroke: Pathophysiology, Diagnosis, and Management.* 2nd ed. New York: Churchill Livingstone, 1992:671–688.
3. Mokri B, Houser OW, Sandok BA, Piepgras DG. Spontaneous dissections of the vertebral arteries. *Neurology* 1988;38:880–885.
4. Schievink WI, Mokri B, Michels V, Piepgras DG. Familial association of intracranial aneurysms and cervical artery dissections. *Stroke* 1991; 22:1426–1430.
5. Bogousslavsky J, Despland PA, Regli F. Spontaneous carotid dissection with acute stroke. *Arch Neurol* 1987;44:137–140.
6. Schievink WI, Mokri B, Whisnant JP. Internal carotid artery dissection in a community: Rochester, Minnesota, 1987–1992. *Stroke* 1993;24:1678–1680.
7. Fisher CM, Ojemann RG, Roberson GH. Spontaneous dissection of cervico-cerebral arteries. *Can J Neurol Sci* 1978;5:9–19.
8. Sturzenegger M, Huber P. Cranial nerve palsies in spontaneous carotid artery dissection. *J Neurol Neurosurg Psychiatry* 1993:56:1191–1199.
9. Mokri B, Schievink WI, Olsen KD, Piepgras DG. Spontaneous dissection of the cervical internal carotid artery: presentation with lower cranial nerve palsies. *Arch Otolaryngol Head Neck Surg* 1992;118:431–435.
10. Biousse V, D'Anglejan-Chatillon J, Massiou H, Bousser M-G. Head pain in non-traumatic carotid artery dissection: a series of 65 patients. *Cephalalgia* 1994;14:33–36.
11. Biousse V, D'Anglejan-Chatillon J, Touboul P-J, Amarenco P, Bousser M-G. Time course of symptoms in extracranial carotid artery dissections. *Stroke* 1995;26:235–239.
12. D'Anglejan-Chatillon J, Ribeiro V, Mas JL, Youl BD, Bousser M-G. Migraine. A risk factor for dissection of cervical arteries. *Headache* 1989;29:560–561.
13. Sue DE, Brant-Zawadski MN, Chance J. Dissection of cranial arteries in the neck: correlation of MRI and anteriography. *Neuroradiology* 1992;34:273–278.
14. Levy C, Laissy JP, Raveau V, Amarenco P, Servois V, Bousser M-G, Tubiana JM. Carotid and vertebral dissections: three dimensional time-of-flight MR angiography and MR imaging versus conventional angiography. *Radiology* 1994;190:97–103.
15. Early TF, Gregory RT, Wheeler JR, Snyder SO, Gayle RG, Parent N, Sorrell K. Spontaneous carotid dissection: duplex scanning in diagnosis and management. *J Vasc Surg* 1991;14:391–397.
16. Mullges W, Ringelstein EB, Leibold M. Non-invasive diagnosis of internal carotid artery dissections. *J Neurol Neurosurg Psychiatry* 1992; 55:98–104.
17. Steinke W, Rautenberg W, Schwartz A, Hennerici M. Noninvasive monitoring of internal carotid artery dissection. *Stroke* 1994;25:998–1005.
18. Sturzenegger M, Mattle HP, Rivoir A, Baumgartner RW. Ultrasound findings in carotid artery dissection: analysis of 43 patients. *Neurology* 1995;45:691–698.
19. Schievink WI, Piepgras DG, McCaffrey TV, Mokri B. Surgical treatment of extracranial internal carotid artery dissecting aneurysms. *Neurosurgery* 1994;35:809–816.
20. Schievink WI, Mokri B, O'Fallon WM. Recurrent spontaneous cervical-artery dissection. *N Engl J Med* 1994;330:393–397.
21. Leys D, Moulin T, Stojkovic T, Begey S, Chavot D, DONALD Investigators. Follow-up of patients with history of cervical artery dissection. *Cerebrovasc Dis* 1995;5:43–49.
22. Hart RG. Vertebral artery dissection. *Neurology* 1988;38:987–989.
23. Hinse P, Thie A, Lachenmayer L. Dissection of the extracranial vertebral artery: report of four cases and review of the literature. *J Neurol Neurosurg Psychiatry* 1991;54:863–869.
24. Josien E. Extracranial vertebral artery dissection: nine cases. *J Neurol* 1992;239:327–330.
25. Friedman DP, Flanders AE. Unusual dissection of the proximal vertebral artery: description of three cases. *AJNR* 1992;13:283–286.
26. Sherman DG, Hart RG, Easton JD. Abrupt change in head position and cerebral infarction. *Stroke* 1981;12:2–6.
27. Bassetti C, Bogousslavsky J, Eskenasy-Cottier AC, Janzer RC, Regli F. Spontaneous intracranial dissection in the anterior circulation. *Cerebrovasc Dis* 1994;4:170–174.
28. Caplan LR, Baquis GD, Pessin MS, D'Alton J, Adelman LS, DeWitt LD, Ho K, Izukawa D, Kwan ES. Dissection of the intracranial vertebral artery. *Neurology* 1988;38:868–877.
29. Sasaki O, Ogawa H, Koike T, Koizumi T, Tanaka R. A clinicopathological study of dissecting aneurysms of the intracranial cerebral artery. *J Neurosurg* 1991;75:874–882.
30. Kitanaka C, Tanaki JI, Kuwahara M, Teraoka A, Sasaki T, Takakura K. Nonsurgical treatment of unruptured intracranial vertebral artery dissection with serial follow-up angiography. *J Neurosurg* 1994;80:667–674.
31. Halbach VV, Higashida RT, Dowd CF, Fraser KM, Smith TP, Teitelbaum GP, Wilson CB, Hieshima GB. Endovascular treatment of vertebral artery dissections and pseudoaneurysms. *J Neurosurg* 1993;79:183–191.
32. Bogousslavsky J. Dissections of the cerebral arteries: clinical effects. *Curr Opin Neurol Neurosurg* 1988;1:63–68.
33. Friedman WA, Day AL, Quisling RG, et al. Cervical carotid dissecting aneurysms. *Neurosurgery* 1980;7:207–214.
34. Stringer WL, Kelly DL. Traumatic dissection of the extra cranial internal carotid artery. *Neurosurgery* 1980;6:123–130.
35. Cohen M, Biller J, Saver JL. Advances in the management of carotid disease. *Current Prob Cardiol* 1994;8:473–532.
36. Sturzenegger M. Ultrasound findings in spontaneous carotid artery dissection. *Arch Neurol* 1991;48:1057–1063.

Cerebrovascular Disease, edited by H. Hunt Batjer.
Lippincott-Raven Publishers, Philadelphia © 1997.

CHAPTER 31

Clinical Trials in Carotid Endarterectomy

Marc R. Mayberg

Clinical trials have become an important component of current medical practice. This trend is due to a variety of factors, including the widespread acceptance of design for multicenter studies, increasing public awareness regarding health care decision-making, the role of clinical trials in determining reimbursement policies, and a consensus in the medical community that any treatment administered should be proven effective according to rigorous scientific criteria. More recently, emphasis has been placed on the requirement to document the efficacy of surgical procedures by clinical trials.

The effect of clinical trials on clinical practice has been especially notable in the field of cerebrovascular surgery and carotid endarterectomy in particular. The publication of a single clinical trial regarding extracranial-to-intracranial (EC-IC) bypass surgery markedly changed the indications for a previously common neurosurgical operation (1). In addition, the widespread recognition of this trial and its consequences were responsible in part for the inception of several subsequent studies designed to test the efficacy of another cerebrovascular procedure, carotid endarterectomy.

Extensive data have been published from retrospective studies in cerebrovascular disease; the focus of this chapter on prospective randomized trials does not discount the validity of these prior studies. Nevertheless, as discussed below, prospective randomized trials have several distinct scientific advantages in demonstrating causality, or the cause-and-effect relationship between treatment (eg, surgery) and outcome (eg, stroke or perioperative death). Retrospective analyses, on the other hand, are subject to a number of factors that may bias the interpretation of data. Prospective randomized trials have become one standard by which surgical procedures are judged and from which practice guidelines and reimbursement schedules are derived, thus ultimately determining their application in clinical practice.

As clinical trials in cerebrovascular disease assume a greater role in clinical practice, it becomes imperative for the practicing physician to become familiar with the general methodology of clinical research and to critically examine the methodology of individual trials. This chapter will describe the basic elements of clinical trial design as they apply to clinical studies of carotid endarterectomy.

BASIC METHODOLOGY OF CLINICAL TRIALS

The design of clinical trials determines in large part their validity, their applicability to broader populations, and ultimately the clinical usefulness of the data. A successful trial should be designed to provide internal validity, or conclusions that are not due to erroneous observations. External validity, on the other hand, describes the relationship of observations in the study sample to broader populations. To accomplish this, the clinical trial should be constructed to minimize random error (due to chance occurrences) and systematic error (due to bias of some type). In addition, the study must pose a research question that is novel, relevant to clinical practice, feasible, ethical, and important. Failure to encompass one or more of these criteria can seriously limit the extent to which findings from a clinical trial may be applied to clinical decision-making.

Population Studies: Incidence and Prevalence

Cross-sectional studies measure a set of variables in a given population at one point in time. They are usually derived from general populations or data banks. Prevalence reflects the number of patients with a disease at one point in time divided by the total number of patients. Although prevalence provides important demographic information, population studies provide less evidence for causality between any variable and outcome. For example, the prevalence of myocardial infarction is high in patients with carotid stenosis; nevertheless, it is unlikely that carotid stenosis is the cause of heart attack or that carotid endarterectomy will effectively prevent it. By following patients over time, popu-

M. R. Mayberg: Department of Neurological Surgery, University of Washington, Seattle, Washington 98195.

TABLE 1. *Comparison of clinical trial methodologies*

| Feature | Cohort | | Cross-sectional (population) |
	Retrospective	Prospective	
Simplicity	Yes	No	No
Duration	Short	Longer	Longer
Patient selection	Uncontrolled	Controlled	Population
Bias	Potential	Less	Less
Causality	No	Yes	No
Cost	Low	High	+/−
Ethical concerns	No	Yes	No

lation trials determine disease incidence, or the number of new cases over a period of time divided by the total number of individuals. In summary, cross-sectional studies provide important information about the frequency of certain disease variables in a given population. In contrast, cohort studies can infer causality, measure predictive variables, examine several outcomes over time, and determine the relative risk reduction provided by a specific therapy (Table 1).

Cohort Studies

External validity for any clinical trial is determined in large part by the parameters used to define the population being studied. Inclusion criteria are those parameters that describe the predictive variables to be studied, such as carotid stenosis and transient ischemic attacks as risk factors for subsequent cerebral infarction. Exclusion criteria, on the other hand, define those variables that might otherwise confound the analysis, such as atrial fibrillation in patients with carotid stenosis. These criteria together define a cohort or subset of patients who are followed over a given interval to analyze the influence of specific risk factors or describe the natural history of the condition being studied. A careful balance between inclusionary and exclusionary criteria is essential to define a cohort that is selective for a specific condition and relatively uniform, yet large enough to provide adequate sample size (see below) and general enough to be applicable to larger populations. Care must be taken to insure that the study population is not biased by undefined selection crite-

ria. For example, the EC-IC Bypass Trial (1) was criticized for including only a portion of all qualified patients at participating centers (2–4). In that study, referral bias may have produced a subset of patients with a stroke risk that was different from that of the general population. To assess this issue, most subsequent clinical trials in cerebrovascular surgery have incorporated follow-up of nonrandomized qualified patients to insure against this potential deficit.

Collection of Data: Specificity and Sensitivity

The means by which data are collected in any clinical trial contributes to its accuracy and validity. The precision of observations is defined as the consistency of repeated measurements, which are affected by random errors from the observer, variability in the subject, and the inherent inaccuracy of instruments used to gather data. Precision can be enhanced by several methods, including training the observer, blinding the observer to the treatment group and standardizing the data collection instrument (ie, a questionnaire in most clinical trials). The sensitivity of any instrument or test is defined as the number of positive observations divided by the total number of true positive occurrences; conversely, specificity is defined as the number of negative observations divided by the total number of true negative occurrences (Table 2). Variables can be continuous (eg, serum glucose), discrete (eg, number of prior transient ischemic attacks [TIAs]), or categorical (eg, stroke). The

TABLE 2. *Determining specificity and sensitivity*

| | | Experimental observation | | |
		Present	Absent	Total
Actual occurrence	Present	A (True positive)	B (Falst negative)	A + B
	Absent	C (False positive	D (True negative)	C + D

$$Sensitivity = \frac{A}{A + B}$$

$$Specificity = \frac{D}{C + D}$$

precision of categorical variables can be enhanced by using preestablished scales (eg, stroke disability ratings).

Types of Cohort Trials

Retrospective cohort trials identify a group of patients and analyze the presence or absence of potential predictive variables at a prior time. For example, Sundt (5) and others (6) used retrospective analysis to define perioperative risk factors in patients undergoing carotid endarterectomy. The advantages of retrospective trials are their relative simplicity, short duration, and low cost (see Table 1). The major disadvantages are uncontrolled patient selection, potential bias in determining predictors, and the lack of evidence for sequential cause-and-effect. Although data from retrospective trials may be compared with that derived from other trials or cross-sectional studies, any conclusions are weakened by potential or unrecognized differences in populations studied. Prospective cohort trials, on the other hand, define in advance one or more predictive variables (or treatments) in a given population and measure outcome (endpoints) over time. By reducing bias and controlling subject selection, true causality between treatment and outcome can be inferred with a much greater level of confidence compared with retrospective trials. The disadvantages of prospective trials include their complexity, duration, cost, and potential ethical concerns. The validity of prospective trials can be further enhanced by randomization, stratification, and blinding. Randomization reduces bias from confounding variables by ensuring treatment groups are comparable in every regard. In most contemporary studies, treatment group is assigned by computer-generated or random number lists. Although certain variables may be analyzed retrospectively in prospective trials, additional validity can be obtained by prospective stratification of subgroups (eg, TIA vs. amaurosis fugax vs. completed stroke) in which separate randomization occurs for each group. Blinding of the observer to the treatment arm (single-blind) or both patient and observer (double-blind) can reduce bias from unintended treatment or inaccurate outcome determination. In certain settings (eg, surgical procedures), blinding is impossible.

The validity of the final analysis in prospective trials is enhanced by maximizing the follow-up of patients. Considerable effort must be made to follow as many patients as possible for the entire duration of the trial and to minimize cross-over from one treatment group to another. Intent-to-treat analysis follows outcome in all randomized patients regardless of whether they receive the intended treatment. This technique minimizes variability from unexpected occurrences such as cross-over between groups but can produce seemingly inaccurate outcome determinations (eg, a patient randomized to carotid endarterectomy who has a stroke prior to surgery).

Statistical Analysis

In any experiment, the null hypothesis predicts that there will be no association between the predictive variable (or treatment) and outcome. Statistical measures of outcome analyze the possibility that any observed association might have occurred by chance (α or p value). A one-tailed analysis assumes the association occurs in only one direction (eg, fewer strokes after carotid endarterectomy), whereas a two-tailed analysis assumes the association might occur in either direction (eg, either fewer or more strokes after carotid endarterectomy). Type I errors occur when a positive association is falsely demonstrated. Type II errors occur when a falsely negative association is shown. The likelihood of type I or type II errors is determined by (1) the magnitude of the difference in expected outcome between groups and (2) the sample size. Fewer patients are necessary to demonstrate a valid association when endpoints are much more frequent in one group compared with the other. Statistical power is defined as the value [1 − the percentage likelihood of a type II error]. In most clinical trials, a p value of 0.5 (ie, <5% chance of type I error) and a statistical power of 0.9 (ie, a <10% chance of type II error) are used to calculate sample size in the design of the study. These values are arbitrary. Calculation of sample size prior to design of the study is critical for preventing either type of error and thereby producing misleading results. However, in many cases the incidence of the particular outcome being studied is not known before the study, and sample size estimates must be based on limited data. For example, if perioperative morbidity and mortality from carotid endarterectomy are estimated at 5%, with a subsequent 1% annual stroke risk at five years, a total of 10% of surgical patients would experience an endpoint (stroke). If the annual stroke rate in unoperated patients is constant at 4%, total strokes at five years would equal 20% (Fig. 1). In this case, the absolute risk reduction is 10%, and the relative risk reduction is 50%. Based on these figures, approximately 600 patients would be required to demonstrate a statistically significant difference between groups at $p = 0.5$ and power = 0.9. However, assuming a 6% stroke rate in the nonsurgical group (total strokes, 30%) would produce an absolute risk reduction of 20% and a relative risk reduction of 67% and would require a sample size of only 350 patients to demonstrate a difference with the same degree of confidence (7).

Data Monitoring and Interim Analysis

At the time of inception, most major prospective cohort trials are designed to include endpoint and data-monitoring committees. Both committees are usually composed of individuals not associated with the trial. The endpoint committee independently and blindly reviews every clinical incident that has been designated as an endpoint to assure the accuracy of the designation. The data-monitoring committee re-

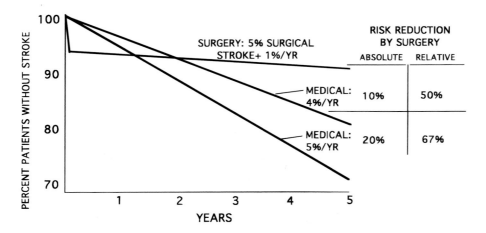

FIG. 1. Schematic representation of estimated stroke rates used to calculate sample size for a prospective study of carotid endarterectomy. In each case, a perioperative stroke and death rate of 5% and subsequent annual stroke rate of 1% are used for the surgical group. If the annual stroke rate in the nonsurgical group is 4%, at five years there will be a 10% absolute reduction and a 50% relative reduction in strokes for surgery patients. Assuming an annual 6% stroke rate for nonsurgical patients provides a 20% absolute reduction and a 67% relative reduction in stroke for surgery at five years.

views the accuracy of all data collected, monitors adverse events, and oversees interim analyses. At the study inception, a protocol is written for statistical outcome analysis at defined intervals during the trial (eg, every six months). Stop rules are defined so that the trial can be halted if the difference in outcome between groups reaches a certain level of significance (usually $p < 0.01$) prior to the end of the trial. Stop rules insure that additional patients will not be subjected to the less favorable treatment. Five of seven major trials for carotid endarterectomy have been prematurely discontinued by data-monitoring committees (see below).

PROSPECTIVE RANDOMIZED TRIALS FOR CAROTID ENDARTERECTOMY

Early Trials

Three randomized trials for carotid endarterectomy were published before 1990. The Joint Study of Extracranial Arterial Occlusion (8) involved 24 centers in the United States. From 1962 to 1968, 316 patients with TIA and angiographic carotid stenosis were randomized to surgical or nonsurgical therapy. At a mean follow-up of 42 months, stroke occurred in 19 of 167 surgical patients (11%) compared with 18 of 145 nonsurgical patients (12%). In the endarterectomy group, the majority of strokes (13/19) occurred in the perioperative period, with a relatively low subsequent stroke rate of approximately 1.5% per year. This study was flawed by a number of significant methodologic errors, including limited sample size, lack of follow-up for eligible nonrandomized patients, variability in stroke diagnosis, and inconsistency of adjunctive therapies. In 1984, Shaw et al (9) published a limited trial involving 41 symptomatic patients in Great Britain. This trial was terminated due to an excessive perioperative stroke rate (25%). A limited randomized trial for asymptomatic stenosis involving only 29 patients was inconclusive (10). In summary, perhaps the only meaningful data from early prospective randomized trials for carotid endar-

terectomy concerned the relatively low (1–2% annual) risk of subsequent stroke in those patients surviving surgery. Due to serious methodologic flaws, other data regarding comparison between surgical and nonsurgical therapy in these studies were of limited value.

Current Trials for Carotid Endarterectomy

In late 1984, coincident with the release of results from the EC-IC bypass trial (1), a series of articles appeared expressing the need for prospective randomized trials to determine the efficacy of carotid endarterectomy in preventing stroke (11–14). These studies were based on several premises. First, the frequency of carotid endarterectomy in North America at that time was increasing to levels approximating 100,000 cases annually (13). Second, considerable individual variations existed in perioperative morbidity and mortality after carotid endarterectomy, with total complication rates in the range of 1–20% (15). Third, the natural history of untreated carotid stenosis was not well defined, with annual stroke incidence for asymptomatic stenosis estimated at 1–4% (16) and for symptomatic stenosis at 4–10% (14). Fourth, wide geographic variations in the frequency of carotid endarterectomy existed within the United States (17) and between countries (14). Fifth, depending on the definition, indications for carotid endarterectomy varied widely with as few as 35% of operations being performed for "appropriate" reasons (18). Sixth, prior randomized trials for carotid endarterectomy were flawed (see above) and did not provide a scientific basis for determining the efficacy of the operation. Finally, the EC-IC bypass trial demonstrated the feasibility of large-scale, multicenter prospective randomized trials for cerebrovascular disease (1).

These expressions of concern about carotid endarterectomy precipitated several trends that profoundly affected clinical practice in cerebrovascular surgery. Policy statements regarding these indications for carotid endarterectomy were issued by several organizations, including the American Neurological Association (19), the American Heart Association (20), and various ad hoc committees (21,22). In addition, there was a marked (approximately 35%) reduction in the number of endarterectomies performed in the United States (23). Finally, a number of prospective, randomized trials for carotid endarterectomy were undertaken.

By 1990, seven carotid endarterectomy trials were in planning or in progress (Tables 3 and 4). Four trials randomized patients with asymptomatic carotid stenosis: the Veterans Administration Asymptomatic Stenosis Trial (VAAST), the Carotid Artery Stenosis Asymptomatic Narrowing Operation Versus Aspirin (CASANOVA), the Asymptomatic Carotid Atherosclerosis Study (ACAS), and the Mayo Asymptomatic Carotid Endarterectomy (MACE). Three trials dealt with symptomatic patients: the European Carotid Surgery Trial (ECST), the North American Symptomatic Carotid Endarterectomy Trial (NASCET), and the Veterans Administration Symptomatic Stenosis Trial (VASST). All seven studies were prospective, randomized, nonblinded, multicenter trials. Although these studies had certain features in common, some important differences in study design affect the generalizability of each trial to wider populations and complicate intertrial comparisons (24).

TRIALS FOR ASYMPTOMATIC CAROTID STENOSIS

Comparison of Study Design (Table 3)

VAAST was funded by the Veterans Administration (VA) Cooperative Studies Program. A cohort of 444 patients was entered into the trial by 1988 and completed follow-up in 1991. CASANOVA was funded by the Federal Republic of Germany and entered 400 patients by 1988. ACAS was funded by the National Institute of Neurological Disorders and Stroke (NINDS) and randomized 1662 patients by 1993.

MACE was funded by NINDS and had an estimated sample size of 900 patients (25). Follow-up was planned to be five years for VAAST and ACAS, three years for CASANOVA and two years for MACE. All four trials set an α-level of 0.05. ACAS and VAAST screened participating centers for perioperative morbidity and mortality <3%, and VAAST pretrained ultrasonographers to ensure diagnostic accuracy. Anesthesia and surgical technique were not standardized among centers for any trial.

Patients could not have symptoms of cerebral ischemia ipsilateral to carotid stenosis in any of the four trials, although contralateral symptoms were permitted in ACAS and VAAST. Criteria for carotid stenosis among trials were comparable at 60% for ACAS and 50% for the other trials. VAAST required angiographic documentation for all patients, whereas ACAS required angiography only in surgical patients and CASANOVA and MACE used noninvasive assessment only. ACAS and CASANOVA patients were drawn from general populations at multiple centers; MACE randomized only Mayo Clinic patients, and VAAST included only men from participating VA medical centers. CASANOVA employed a complicated randomization procedure for patients with bilateral carotid stenosis in which one or both carotid arteries could be operated (see below).

Exclusion criteria were relatively consistent among the four asymptomatic trials. In general, patients who would otherwise not be considered for surgery were excluded according to a variety of neurologic, cardiovascular and general medical (eg, renal failure, diabetes, etc) criteria. Confounding neurologic (eg, seizures, dementia, etc) and cardiac (eg, atrial fibrillation, severe valvular disease) conditions that might affect evaluation of stroke outcome were generally grounds for exclusion. All asymptomatic trials applied best medical management including risk factor reduction and aspirin therapy to both medical and surgical groups, with

TABLE 3. *Prospective randomized trials for carotid endarterectomy: asymptomatic stenosis*

Trial	Principal investigator	Stenosis criteria (%)	Aspirin	CT	Follow-up (yr)	Sample size (Actual)	Primary endpoints	Completion date
VAAST	R. R. Hobson	>50 (all angio)	1300 mg/d	No	5 (mean = 4)	500 (444)	TIA or stroke in distribution of randomized artery; death <30 days after randomization	1992
CASANOVA	H. C. Dienes H. Homann	50–90 (noninvasive)	1000 mg/d + dipyridamole 225 mg/d	Yes	3	400 (410)	TIA, stroke or death	1991
ACAS	J. Toole	>60 (angio-surgery only)	325 mg/d	Yes	5 (mean = 2.7)	1500 (1662)	TIA or stroke in distribution of randomized artery; death <30 days after randomization*	1995
MACE	D. Wiebers	>50 (noninvasive)	80 mg/d (nonsurgical group only)	Option	2	900	TIA, RIND, stroke, or death	Terminated

* TIA was later removed as an endpoint.

the exception of MACE, in which the surgery group did not receive aspirin. The aspirin dose varied among trials. Computed tomography (CT) scans were required in ACAS and CASANOVA and optional in MACE.

Results from Asymptomatic Trials

The MACE trial was stopped shortly after initiation due to increased frequency of a secondary endpoint (myocardial infarction) in the surgical group, who were not receiving aspirin (24).

The CASANOVA study randomized patients with asymptomatic carotid stenosis (>50% but <90%) to either immediate carotid endarterectomy (n = 206) or no immediate surgery, including some patients who underwent delayed surgery after developing ischemic symptoms, progressive severe stenosis, bilateral stenosis, or contralateral stenosis (n = 204) (26). At three-year follow-up, using death or new stroke as endpoints, there was no difference in outcome between the immediate surgery group and the other group of patients (10.7% vs. 11.3%). However, nearly half of the patients in the no-immediate-surgery group eventually did have an endarterectomy for one of the reasons stated above. The unusual study design for this trial considerably lessens its statistical validity.

The VAAST study randomized patients with asymptomatic carotid stenosis (>50%) to operative (n = 211) or nonoperative therapy (n = 233) (27–29). At a mean follow-up of four years, the combined incidence of ipsilateral neurologic ischemic events (TIA and stroke) was reduced in the surgical group (8%) in contrast to the medical group (20.6%) ($p < 0.001$) (Fig. 2). However, the sample size was not sufficiently large enough to provide statistical power to show a difference in stroke alone. The ipsilateral stroke rate in the

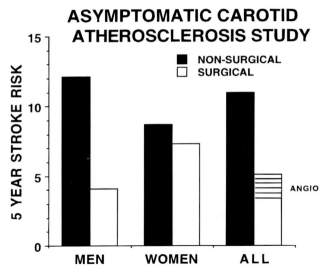

FIG. 3. Comparison of five-year stroke risk for various subgroups of medical and surgical patients in the Asymptomatic Carotid Atherosclerosis Study (ACAS) trial.

surgical group was 4.7% (including perioperative strokes) in contrast to 9.4% in the medical group ($p = 0.056$). However, when perioperative mortality (1.9%) was added to the surgical stroke rate, the difference between the two groups was not statistically significant.

The ACAS trial substantiated the hypothesis that carotid endarterectomy may prevent stroke in certain patients with asymptomatic carotid stenosis (30). Among 1662 individuals randomized with high-grade carotid stenosis (>60% diameter reduction by ultrasound and/or angiography), there was a projected overall 53% relative risk reduction in ipsilateral stroke over five years (mean follow-up, 2.7 years) in patients receiving carotid endarterectomy (5.1%) compared with unoperated patients (11.0%) (Fig. 3). Although 9% of patients were not treated according to their randomization status, the stroke risk reduction was comparable for analysis by intent-to-treat or actual treatment. The stroke risk reduction was more prominent in men and was apparently independent of degree of stenosis or contralateral carotid artery disease. A substantial portion of the surgical risk was attributable to angiography (1.2% stroke rate), and the initial risk for surgery plus angiography was offset by a constant risk of stroke at approximately 2.2% per year in the nonsurgical group. The surgical benefit was apparent by ten months and was statistically significant at three years.

Asymptomatic Trials—Summary

Data from the ACAS and VAAST trials provide strong evidence that the risk of ipsilateral stroke can be lessened by endarterectomy in selected asymptomatic patients with >50–60% carotid stenosis. Several important caveats

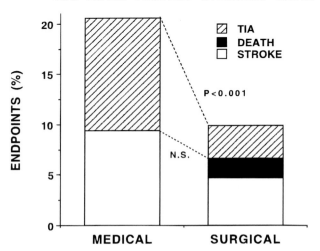

FIG. 2. Comparison of endpoints for medical and surgical groups in the Veterans Affairs Cooperative Studies Program Asymptomatic Stenosis Trial (VAAST) (N.S., not significant).

TRIALS FOR ASYMPTOMATIC STENOSIS

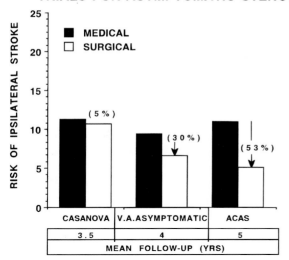

FIG. 4. Comparison of stroke risk in medical vs. surgical patients for three major asymptomatic stenosis trials (relative risk reduction in parentheses).

should be noted, however. In both studies, patients, surgeons, and institutions were selected for low surgical risk. Women were not studied in the VA trial, and the surgical benefit for women was less prominent in ACAS. Nonwhites represented only 5% of patients studied in the ACAS trial. In both studies, medically treated asymptomatic carotid stenosis was associated with a relatively low annual rate of ipsilateral stroke (approximately 2% per year) compared with that observed for symptomatic high-grade stenosis (>10% per year) (Fig. 4). On this basis, 19 endarterectomies in patients with asymptomatic stenosis would be necessary to prevent one stroke, compared with five to six procedures required to prevent one stroke in symptomatic patients (see below). Physicians should carefully evaluate patients with asymptomatic stenosis in terms of surgical risk and life expectancy to determine those individuals who will benefit from carotid endarterectomy.

TRIALS FOR SYMPTOMATIC CAROTID STENOSIS

Comparison of Study Design (Table 4)

The ECST was funded by multiple sources and estimated a sample size of 400 patients. NASCET was funded by NINDS and projected a sample size of 3000. VASST estimated a sample size of 500 but was terminated after entering 192 patients (see below). Follow-up was intended to be five years for ECST and NASCET and three years for VASST; all three trials were terminated early. NASCET and VASST followed eligible nonrandomized patients outside of the study. All three studies determined sample size based on α = 0.05 and power = 0.9. NASCET and VASST screened participating centers for surgical morbidity and mortality of <6%. Anesthesia and surgical technique were not standardized among centers for any trial.

Inclusion criteria were relatively standard among the symptomatic trials and included transient cerebral or retinal ischemia or minor completed stroke within 120 days of randomization in the distribution of a stenotic carotid artery. ECST and NASCET entered men and women from general referral populations at multiple centers, whereas VASST enrolled only men at VA centers. Angiography was mandatory in all three trials, although entry criteria varied: 0–99% diameter reduction in ECST, 30–99% in NASCET, and 50–99% in VASST. All three studies randomized by center according to various stratification schemes, although ECST randomized 60% of patients to surgery. As in the asymptomatic trials, exclusionary criteria were relatively standard for NASCET and VASST and attempted to exclude patients who would not otherwise be candidates for surgery. ECST, on the other hand, employed undefined (discretionary) guidelines for patient exclusion. Among symptomatic trials, only VASST defined best medical management as risk reduction plus aspirin 325 mg/d; ECST and NASCET allowed discretionary administration of aspirin or other medications. CT scans were required in all studies at entry and at endpoint occurrence.

Primary endpoints in all three trials were defined as clini-

TABLE 4. *Prospective trials for carotid endarterectomy: symptomatic stenosis*

Trial	Principal investigator	Stenosis criteria (%)	Aspirin	CT	Follow-up (yr)	Projected sample size (Actual)	Primary endpoints	Completion date
ECST	C. Warlow	0–99 (all angio)	Discretion	Yes	5 (mean = 2.7) (mean = 3)	400 (<30% = 374) (>70% = 395)	Ipsilateral stroke	1991
NASCET	H. J. M. Barnett	30–99 (all angio)	Discretion	Yes	5 (mean = 2)	3000 (>70% = 659)	Ipsilateral stroke; stroke-related death; death <30 days after randomization	1991 (<70%) 1996 (30–69%)
VAAST	M. Mayberg S. E. Wilson F. Yatsu	50–99 (all angio)	325 mg/d	Yes	3 (mean = 1)	500 (192)	Ipsilateral stroke or crescendo TIA; death <30 days	1991

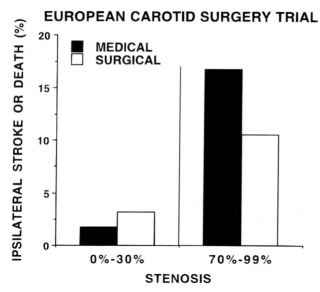

FIG. 5. Risk of ipsilateral stroke or death in medical vs. surgical patients in low-grade and high-grade stenosis categories for the European Carotid Surgery Trial (ECST).

cal infarction ipsilateral to the randomized carotid artery; ECST and VASST also included death within 30 days of randomization. VASST included crescendo TIAs in the appropriate vascular distribution as a primary endpoint. Secondary endpoints for all studies included death from causes other than stroke, stroke in other vascular distributions, or myocardial infarction.

Results from Symptomatic Trials

The ECST enrolled patients with mild (<30%), moderate (30–69%), or severe (70–99%) carotid stenosis, who were

then randomized to surgical or nonsurgical treatment (31). Interim analysis of 2200 patients (mean follow-up, 2.7 years) led to premature termination of the trial for mild and severe stenosis groups. For mild stenosis, among 374 randomized patients there was no significant difference in ipsilateral stroke between the surgical and nonsurgical groups. There were more treatment failures in the surgery group, which was attributed to the 2.3% risk of death or disabling stroke during the first 30 days after surgery. For severe stenosis, however, surgery was shown to be beneficial in preventing stroke. There was a 7.5% risk of ipsilateral stroke or death within 30 days of surgery. At three years of follow-up, there was an additional 2.8% risk of stroke in the surgery group (total, 10.3%), compared with 16.8% in the nonsurgery group ($p < 0.0001$) (Fig. 5). More important, the risk of death or ipsilateral disabling stroke was reduced from 11% in the nonsurgery group to 6% in the surgery group. Entry of patients with moderate stenosis (30–69%) continues in this trial.

The NASCET prematurely stopped randomizing patients with carotid stenosis >70% due to the overwhelming stroke risk reduction observed in the surgical group (32). A total of 659 patients in this category of stenosis were randomized to surgical (n = 331) or nonsurgical (n = 328) therapy. At a mean follow-up of 24 months, ipsilateral stroke was noted in 26% of nonsurgical patients, compared with 9% of patients with endarterectomy (Fig. 6), for an overall risk reduction of 17% (relative risk reduction, 71%). The benefit for surgical patients was highly significant ($p < 0.001$) for a variety of outcomes, including stroke in any territory, major strokes, and major stroke or death from any cause. A perioperative morbidity and mortality of 5.8% was rapidly surpassed in the nonsurgical group, such that surgical benefit was apparent by three months. In addition, the protective

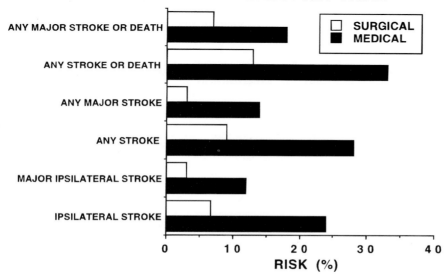

FIG. 6. Analysis of stroke risk for various endpoint analyses in medical and surgical patients for the North American Symptomatic Carotid Endarterectomy Trial (NASCET).

effect of surgery was durable over time, with few strokes noted in the endarterectomy group beyond the perioperative period. Functional disability (assessed by a standardized disability scale) was significantly less in the surgery group over time ($p < 0.001$) (33). Multivariate analysis demonstrated that surgical benefit was independent of a variety of concurrent demographic variables such as age, sex, or risk factors for stroke. There was a direct correlation between surgical benefit and the degree of angiographic stenosis. NASCET continues to randomize symptomatic patients with carotid stenosis of 30–69%; the benefit of carotid endarterectomy in this group of patients remains indeterminate.

Enrollment in the VASST was discontinued in February 1991 based on preliminary data consistent with the NASCET findings. Subsequent analysis demonstrated a statistically significant reduction in ipsilateral stroke or crescendo TIA for patients with carotid stenosis >50% (34). A total of 193 men aged 35–82 years (mean, 64.2 years) were randomized to surgical (n = 91) or nonsurgical (n = 98) treatment. The complication rate of cerebral angiography was low, with no permanent residual deficits and transient complications in 5% (2% local vascular; 2% transient neurologic, 1% minor allergic). Two thirds of randomized patients demonstrated angiographic internal carotid artery stenosis >70%. Duplex ultrasound examination was performed in 152 patients who subsequently underwent cerebral angiography. There was poor accuracy in the lower ranges of stenoses, especially underestimating the degree of stenosis between 30% and 49%. Non-endpoint complications of surgery were relatively infrequent, including respiratory insufficiency requiring extended intensive care monitoring (5%), minor-to-moderate wound hematoma (5%), cranial nerve deficit (5%), myocardial infarction (2%), and pulmonary embolism (1%).

At a mean follow-up of 11.9 months, there was a significant reduction in stroke or crescendo TIA in patients receiving carotid endarterectomy (7.7%), compared with nonsurgical patients (19.4%), representing a risk reduction of 11.7% (relative risk reduction, 60%; $p = 0.028$) (Fig. 7). Among subgroups, the benefit of surgery was most prominent in TIA patients compared with transient monocular blindness (TMB) or stroke, although these differences were not statistically significant. The benefit for surgery was apparent as early as two months after randomization and persisted over the entire period of follow-up. The efficacy of carotid endarterectomy was durable with only one ipsilateral stroke beyond the 30-day perioperative period. Discounting one preoperative stroke, a perioperative morbidity of 2.2% and mortality of 3.3% (total, 5.5%) was achieved over multiple centers among relatively high-risk patients.

Conclusions from Symptomatic Stenosis Trials

The NASCET, ECST and VASST trials unequivocally showed that carotid endarterectomy reduced stroke risk compared to medical therapy in patients with high-grade (>70%)

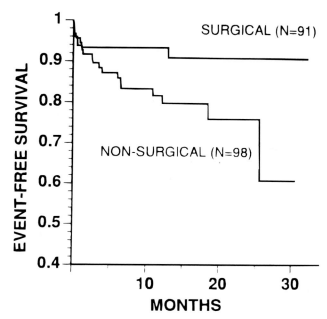

FIG. 7. Kaplan–Meier analysis of ipsilateral cerebral ischemic endpoints in VASST.

symptomatic carotid stenosis. However, these data should also be viewed critically when patients for surgery are being selected. First, a major determinant for surgical benefit in all three studies was the low surgical complication rate observed. This underscores the fact that this procedure should be done only by surgeons with experience in the operation and low morbidity for endarterectomy. Second, the patients in these studies were carefully selected to include a highly specific cohort within well defined clinical parameters. In a nonselected population, the benefit of surgery in reducing stroke risk is less predictable. Finally, although the benefit of carotid endarterectomy in patients with severe carotid stenosis is clear, the fate of symptomatic patients with moderate carotid stenosis has not been resolved. NASCET and ECST continue to randomize patients with 30–69% stenosis.

On the other hand, several features common to the symptomatic stenosis trials can be generalized to broader medical populations. First, carotid endarterectomy provided a profound protection against subsequent ipsilateral stroke or crescendo TIA in patients with high-grade symptomatic stenosis. The stroke risk reduction was realized early after surgery, persisted over extended periods of time, and was independent of other risk factors (Fig. 8). Second, stroke in the nonsurgical group considerably exceeded those reported from prior prospective and retrospective studies. Symptomatic patients receiving aspirin in prior prospective multicenter trials had annual stroke rates in the range of 3–7% (4,9,11), compared with rates between 15% and 20% in unoperated patients from NASCET and VASST. Third, the inaccuracy of carotid duplex ultrasonography noted in both NASCET and VASST (see below) suggests that symptomatic patients with intermediate degrees of stenosis by duplex

TRIALS FOR SYMPTOMATIC STENOSIS

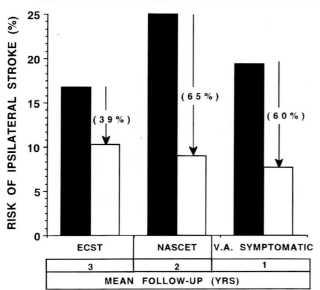

FIG. 8. Comparison of ipsilateral stroke rates in three major trials for carotid endarterectomy in patients with symptomatic carotid stenosis (relative risk reduction in parentheses).

ultrasound should have definitive assessment by angiography prior to determination of therapy.

SUBSEQUENT ANALYSES OF DATA FROM ENDARTERECTOMY TRIALS

Following publication of the three major trials for symptomatic carotid stenosis, a number of post hoc analyses have been performed. These reports provide additional data regarding accuracy of diagnostic measures for carotid stenosis and specific clinical factors that increase stroke risk in patients with symptomatic carotid stenosis.

Accuracy of Diagnostic Measures

Angiograms from the NASCET trial were examined by three groups of observers to test the accuracy of subjective assessments of stenosis (mild, moderate, severe, or occluded) against measured stenosis. Using a 70% stenosis cut-point, the sensitivity among groups was 84–95% and specificity was 78–88% (38). Bruits were a relatively poor predictor of high-grade stenosis in NASCET patients, with a sensitivity of 63% and a specificity of 61% (38). Similarly, ulcers documented at surgery were poorly detected by angiography (sensitivity, 46%; specificity, 74%) (39). Two studies examined the accuracy of noninvasive testing with Doppler ultrasound compared with angiography. In NASCET, for a 70% stenosis cut-point, the specificity was 60% and the sensitivity was 88% (40). In VASST, duplex ultrasound sensitivity compared with angiography varied from 24% in the 30–49% range to 71% for 50–79% stenosis and 91% for occlusion. Using a cut-point of 50% stenosis, duplex sensitivity was 90% and specificity was 76%; the degree of stenosis was underestimated in nearly half of patients with moderate (30–49%) stenosis (41). A metaanalysis showed that duplex, Doppler, and magnetic resonance angiography have equivalent sensitivity (82–86%) and specificity (89–94%) for detecting high-grade carotid stenosis (42). These data are in contradistinction to single-center retrospective analyses that show much greater accuracy for duplex ultrasound and point out the important differences observed in retrospective compared with prospective studies (43). More important, they substantiate the concept that decisions regarding patient management should not be based solely on noninvasive assessment of carotid stenosis.

Other Risk Factors for Stroke

Subgroup analysis for ECST and VASST was limited by relatively small patient samples. For NASCET, however, a number of factors were identified in nonsurgical patients that contributed to stroke risk. Angiographic ulceration nearly doubled the stroke risk for patients with high-grade (>70%) stenosis (44). These data must be interpreted in light of the poor accuracy of angiography for detecting ulcers (see above) (39). Hemispheric ischemia (stroke or TIA) portended a stroke risk three times higher than that observed for amaurosis fugax (45). Although increased age was associated with higher stroke risk, surgery provided benefit independent of age. Contralateral carotid occlusion was a strong risk factor for stroke; contralateral stenosis was not (45). Evidence of prior asymptomatic stroke by CT scan also increased stroke risk (45). Carotid endarterectomy was uniformly beneficial in reducing stroke risk independent of these associated risk factors. A retrospective metaanalysis of surgical risk at 12 academic medical centers identified the following factors as significant; ipsilateral carotid occlusion or siphon stenosis, intraluminal thrombus, or age (increased myocardial infarction but not stroke) (6). On the other hand, degree of carotid stenosis or ulcers, symptom type, sex, race, cardiac history, contralateral stenosis were not associated with increased surgical risk. Timing of surgery in patients with completed stroke in NASCET did not affect surgical risk (46). In combination, these data may allow the determination of stroke risk and surgical risk profiles based on demographic, symptomatic, and diagnostic criteria, which will identify cohorts most likely to benefit from carotid endarterectomy.

GUIDELINES FOR CAROTID ENDARTERECTOMY

At various times, guidelines for carotid endarterectomy have been developed; these reports have attempted to distill existing data into practical documents intended to facilitate clinical decisions. Whether by consensus or scientific analy-

TABLE 5. *AHA Consensus guidelines on carotid endarterectomy*

Asymptomatic stenosis					
Ipsilateral carotid stenosis	Contralateral stenosis	Ulcer	Surgical risk (%)		
			<3	3–5	5–10
>75%	No	—	A[a]	U[a]	N
>75%	Yes	—	A[a]	A[a]	N
>75%	—	Yes	A[a]	U[a]	N
<50%	—	Yes	U	U	N
Dissection	—	—	N	N	N

Symptomatic Stenosis			
Ipsilateral carotid stenosis	Symptom	Surgical risk (%)	
		<6	6–10
>70%	TIA, mild stroke	P	P
>50%	TIA, mild stroke	A	U
>70%	Progressive stroke	A	U
<50%	TIA, mild stroke	U	U
>75%	Global ischemia	U	U
Dissection	TIA on heparin	U	U
Acute occlusion	Mild stroke	U	U
<50%	Evolving or moderate stroke	N	N
<50%	TIA, mild stroke	U	N
<50%	Global ischemia	U	N

Key: A, acceptable; U, uncertain; N, proven not beneficial; P, proven beneficial.
[a] ACAS data change the recommendation.

sis, these guidelines are necessarily limited by the quality of the data, the inherent generalization of unique clinical situations, and the subsequent emergence of new data. In this regard, initial guidelines for carotid endarterectomy (19–22), were superseded by contemporary guidelines after the symptomatic stenosis trials (47–49). These guidelines in turn were published prior to ACAS and do not incorporate important new data concerning treatment of asymptomatic stenosis.

In 1993, an ad hoc committee of the American Heart Associate (AHA) established guidelines for carotid endarterectomy based on committee consensus or a modified Delphi procedure. These guidelines (summarized in Table 5) describe indications for endarterectomy in a variety of clinical situations.

Ad hoc committees of the AHA for management of TIA based guidelines for endarterectomy on review and grading of published reports according to predetermined criteria (48). For patients with single or multiple TIAs and ipsilateral carotid stenosis >70%, endarterectomy was recommended only for recurrent TIAs in patients on antiplatelet therapy (grade C data). Similarly, carotid endarterectomy was recommended for patients with an ulcer on angiography and no other source of emboli. Similar guidelines for the management of patients with acute stroke did not reach a conclusion regarding emergent carotid endarterectomy after stroke due to insufficient data (47).

SUMMARY

It has been stated that "if carotid endarterectomy was a drug its efficacy would require scrutiny and licensure . . . .

by the Food and Drug Administration" (14). Although this contention has widespread proponents, surgical procedures are in fact not drugs and cannot necessarily be studied according to the same criteria. Clinical decision-making in surgery is a multifactorial process involving both subjective and objective evaluations. A variety of factors can otherwise interfere with the best clinical trial design, including referral patterns, fiscal concerns, and local variations in treatment. Most important, there remains the profound ethical concern regarding withholding previously accepted therapy from one group of patients in a randomized trial of a surgical procedure. Nevertheless, the clinical trial has become the means by which existing and new surgical procedures may be judged in the near future, and the results of such trials may dictate surgical practice to some extent. For these reasons, it is important that surgeons become familiar with the methodology of clinical trials and examine these studies in a critical light.

REFERENCES

1. The ECIC Bypass Study Group. Failure of extracranial–intracranial arterial bypass to reduce the risk of ischemic stroke: Results of an international randomized trial. *N Engl J Med* 1985;313:1191–1200.
2. Day AL, Rhoton AL Jr, Little JR. The extracranial–intracranial bypass study. *Surg Neurol* 1986;22:222–226.
3. Langfitt T, Goldring S, Zervas N. The extracranial–intracranial bypass study. A report of the committee appointed by the American Association of Neurologic Surgeons to examine the study. *N Engl J Med* 1987;316:817–820.
4. Sundt TM Jr. Was the international randomized trial of extracranial–intracranial arterial bypass representative of the population at risk? *N Engl J Med* 1987;316:814–816.

5. Sundt TM Jr, Sandok BA, Whisnant JP. Carotid endarterectomy: Complications and preoperative assessment of risk. *Mayo Clin Proc* 1975; 50:301–306.
6. Goldstein LB, McCrory DC, Landsman PB, et al. Multicenter review of preoperative risk factors for carotid endarterectomy in patients with ipsilateral symptoms. *Stroke* 1994;25:1116–1121.
7. Taylor DW, Sackett DL, Haynes RB. Sample size for randomized trial in stroke prevention. How many patients do we need? *Stroke* 1984;15: 968–971.
8. Fields WS, Maslenikov V, Meyer JS, et al. Joint study of extracranial arterial occlusion, V: Progress report of prognosis following surgery or nonsurgical treatment for transient cerebral ischemic attacks and cervical carotid artery lesions. *JAMA* 1970;211:1993–2003.
9. Shaw DA, Venables GS, Cartilidge NEF, et al. Carotid endarterectomy in patients with transient cerebral ischemia. *J Neurol Sci* 1984;64: 45–53.
10. Clagett PG, Youkey JR, Brigham RA, et al. Asymptomatic cervical bruit and abnormal ocular pneumoplethysmography: A prospective study comparing two approaches to management. *Surgery* 1984;96: 823–830.
11. Awad IA, Spetzler RF. Extracranial–intracranial bypass surgery: A critical analysis in light of the international cooperative study. *Neurosurgery* 1986;19:655–664.
12. Barnett HJM, Plum F, Walton JN. Carotid endarterectomy—An expression of concern. *Stroke* 1984;15:941–943.
13. Dyken ML, Pokras R. The performance of endarterectomy for disease of the extracranial arteries of the head. *Stroke* 1984;15:948–950.
14. Warlow C. Carotid endarterectomy: Does it work? *Stroke* 1984;15: 1068–1076.
15. West H, Burton R, Roon AJ, et al. Comparative risk of operation and expectant management for carotid artery disease. *Stroke* 1979;10: 117–121.
16. Hertzer NR. Presidential address: Carotid endarterectomy—A crisis in confidence. *J Vasc Surg* 1988;7:611–619.
17. Leape LL, Park RE, Solomon DH, et al. Relation between surgeon's practice volumes and geographic variation in the rate of carotid endarterectomy. *N Engl J Med* 1989;321:653–657.
18. Winslow CM, Solomon DH, Chassin MR, et al. The appropriateness of carotid endarterectomy. *N Engl J Med* 1988;318:721–727.
19. Whisnant JP, Fisher L, Robertson JT, et al. Does carotid endarterectomy decrease stroke and death in patients with transient ischemic attacks? *Ann Neurol* 1987;22:72–76.
20. Beebe HG, Clagett GP, DeWeese JA, et al. Assessing risk associated with carotid endarterectomy. *Circulation* 1989;79:472–473.
21. Callow AD, Caplan LR, Correll JW, et al. Carotid endarterectomy: What is its current status? *Am J Med* 1988;85:835–838.
22. Cebul RD, Whisnant JP. Indications for carotid endarterectomy. *Ann Intern Med* 1989;111:675–677.
23. Pokras R, Dyken ML. Dramatic changes in the performance of endarterectomy for diseases of the extracranial arteries of the head. *Stroke* 1988;19:1289–1290.
24. Wiebers DO. Effectiveness of carotid endarterectomy for asymptomatic carotid stenosis: Design of a clinical trial. *Mayo Clin Proc* 1989;64: 897–904.
25. Howard VJ, Toole JF, Grizzle J, et al. Comparison of multicenter study designs for investigation of the efficacy of carotid endarterectomy. *Stroke* 1992;23:583–593.
26. CASANOVA Study Group. Carotid surgery versus medical therapy in asymptomatic carotid stenosis. *Stroke* 1991;22:1229–1235.
27. Hobson R, Weiss D, Fields W, et al. Efficacy of carotid endarterectomy for asymptomatic carotid stenosis. *N Engl J Med* 1993;328:221–227.
28. Towne JB, Weiss DG, Hobson RW. First phase report of cooperative Veterans Administration asymptomatic carotid stenosis study—Operative morbidity and mortality. *J Vasc Surg* 1990;11:252–259.
29. Veterans Administration Cooperative Study. Role of carotid endarterectomy in asymptomatic carotid stenosis. *Stroke* 1986;17:534–539.
30. The Asymptomatic Carotid Atherosclerosis Study Group. Endarterectomy for asymptomatic carotid artery stenosis. *JAMA* 1995, in press.
31. European Carotid Surgery Trialists Collaborative Group. European carotid surgery trial: Interim results for symptomatic patients with severe (70–99%) or with mild (0–29%) carotid stenosis. *Lancet* 1991;337: 1235–1243.
32. North American Symptomatic Carotid Endarterectomy Trial Collaborators. Beneficial effect of carotid endarterectomy in symptomatic patients with high-grade stenosis. *N Engl J Med* 1991;325:445–453.
33. Haynes RB, Taylor DW, Sackett DL, Thorpe K, Ferguson GG, Barnett HJ. Prevention of functional impairment by endarterectomy for symptomatic high-grade carotid stenosis. North American Symptomatic Carotid Endarterectomy Trial Collaborators. *JAMA* 1994;271:1256–1259.
34. Mayberg MR, Wilson SE, Yatsu F, et al. Carotid endarterectomy and prevention of cerebral ischemia from symptomatic carotid stenosis. *JAMA* 1991;266:3289–3294.
35. Barnett HJM. A randomized trial of aspirin and sulfinpyrazone in threatened stroke. *N Engl J Med* 1978;299:53–59.
36. Bousser MG, Eschwege E, Hagvenau M, et al. "AICLA" controlled trial of aspirin and dipyridamole in the secondary prevention of atherothrombotic cerebral ischemia. *Stroke* 1983;14:5–14.
37. Candelise L, Landi G, et al. A randomized trial of aspirin and sulfinpyrazone in patients with TIA. *Stroke* 1982;13:175–179.
38. Sauvé JS, Thorpe KE, Sackett DL, et al. Can bruits distinguish high-grade from moderate symptomatic carotid stenosis? The North American Symptomatic Carotid Endarterectomy Trial. *Ann Intern Med* 1994; 120:633–637.
39. Streifler JY, Eliasziw M, Fow AJ, et al. Angiographic detection of carotid plaque ulceration. Comparison with surgical observations in a multicenter study. North American Symptomatic Carotid Endarterectomy Trial. *Stroke* 1994;25:1130–1132.
40. Haynes RB, Taylor DW, Sackett DL, Fox A, Rankin R, Barnett H. Poor performance of Doppler in detecting high-grade carotid stenosis. *Clin Res* 1992;40:184A.
41. Srinivasan J, Weiss D, Mayberg MR. Duplex accuracy compared to angiography in the Veterans Affairs cooperative studies trial for symptomatic carotid stenosis. *Neurosurgery* 1995;36:648–655.
42. Blakeley DD, Oddone EZ, Hasselblad V, Simel DL, Matchar DB. Noninvasive carotid artery testing. A meta-analytic review. *Ann Intern Med* 1995;122:360–367.
43. Hames TK, Ratliff DA, Humphries KN, Gazzard VM, Birch SJ, Chant AD. The accuracy of duplex scanning in the evaluation of early carotid disease. *Ultrasound Med Biol* 1985;11:819–825.
44. Eliasziw M, Streifler JY, Fox AJ, Hachinski VC, Ferguson GG, Barnett HJ. Significance of plaque ulceration in symptomatic patients with high-grade carotid stenosis. North American Symptomatic Carotid Endarterectomy Trial. *Stroke* 1994;25:304–308.
45. Barnett HJM. Status report on the North American symptomatic carotid surgery trial. *J Mal Vasc* 1993;18:202–208.
46. Gasecki AP, Ferguson GG, Eliasziw M, et al. Early endarterectomy for severe carotid artery stenosis after a nondisabling stroke: Results from the North American Symptomatic Carotid Endarterectomy Trial. *J Vasc Surg* 1994;20:288–295.
47. Adams HP Jr, Brott GH, Crowell RM, et al. Guidelines for the management of patients with acute ischemic stroke. *Circulation* 1994;90: 1588–1601.
48. Feinberg WM, Albers GW, Barnett HJM, et al. Guidelines for the management of transient ischemic attacks. *Stroke* 1994;25:1320–1335.
49. Moore WS, Barnett HJ, Beebe HG, et al. Guidelines for carotid endarterectomy. A multidisciplinary consensus statement from the ad hoc committee, American Heart Association. *Stroke* 1995;26:188–201.

Cerebrovascular Disease, edited by H. Hunt Batjer.
Lippincott-Raven Publishers, Philadelphia © 1997.

CHAPTER 32

Carotid Endarterectomy: The Asymptomatic Carotid Artery

Christopher M. Loftus

Carotid circulation disease can be divided into both asymptomatic and symptomatic forms. Asymptomatic carotid disease includes patients with asymptomatic carotid bruits and those with symptoms referable to one carotid territory with radiographic demonstration of clinically silent contralateral carotid stenosis or ulceration; it also includes patients who are found to have auscultatory or radiographic evidence of carotid pathology, while being prepared for major surgical procedures, most commonly coronary or peripheral vascular surgery. I also include in the asymptomatic category patients with silent Hollenhorst plaques in the retina, silent cerebral infarcts, and high-grade asymptomatic stenoses that are seen to be progressing on serial evaluations. Symptomatic carotid disease encompasses a spectrum of presentations from transient ischemic attacks (TIAs) to stroke in evolution and persistent strokes; it also includes acute or subacute carotid occlusion, as well as the so-called "stump" syndromes. Symptomatic carotid disease or operative technique will not be further addressed in this chapter.

Both asymptomatic and symptomatic carotid disease have been the subject of considerable debate in years past, and the literature dealing with surgical indications was confusing and often contradictory. It is gratifying to see that various cooperative trials have now given firm answers for both problems and that surgery has been upheld as the cornerstone of therapy in patients with carotid stenosis.

SCIENTIFIC FOUNDATION OF ASYMPTOMATIC CAROTID SURGERY

The propriety of performing surgery for asymptomatic carotid stenosis has been evaluated with retrospective and prospective studies and finally and most recently with randomized trials. In an attempt to answer this question definitively, several populations of patients have been studied: those with (a) bruit or stenosis identified through screening procedures (in both historical and randomized trials), (b) asymptomatic disease contralateral to a symptomatic carotid, and (c) carotid disease identified while being evaluated preoperatively for other types of surgery. Unfortunately, the data for each of these groups are conflicting in many ways, and this chapter examines each type of study in some detail. I should also mention here, however, that the Asymptomatic Carotid Atherosclerosis Study (ACAS) trial data are now available and show a surgical benefit for all groups of asymptomatic patients with stenosis ≥60% (1). This study will be discussed in greater detail later in this chapter, but because of its importance references to it throughout the text are unavoidable.

ASYMPTOMATIC BRUIT

Carotid bruits are heard in 3–4% of the asymptomatic population over 45 years of age in the United States and are present in 10–23% of patients in referral populations with symptomatic atherosclerosis in other arterial distributions. The presence of such bruits on routine examination invariably poses a series of questions to both the patient and the primary physician. Is the patient at risk for stroke based on this finding? Should further evaluation, such as duplex ultrasonography or arteriography, be performed? What medical treatments should be proposed?

Historically, two major studies have advocated surgery for asymptomatic carotid bruits (2,3). Both studies followed a group of unoperated patients with asymptomatic bruits and reported higher rates of neurologic sequelae, with stroke rates of 15–17%, as compared with operated controls. These data were used to justify the propriety of surgery in such cases. Nei-

Modified in part from Loftus CM: *Carotid Endarterectomy: Principles and Techniques.* St. Louis, MO: Quality Medical Publishing, 1995. Reprinted with permission.

C. M. Loftus: Department of Surgery (Neurosurgery), The University of Iowa College of Medicine, Iowa City, Iowa 52242.

ther of these reports, however, documented the relationship of the neurologic events to the territory of the carotid bruit (eg, whether the stroke was ipsilateral or contralateral to the carotid with the bruit), nor was it reported whether the patients who later had strokes had experienced a warning TIA before that event (which would have justified prophylactic endarterectomy in most centers). These questions were addressed, however, in several population studies (4,5). The first of these, in Evans County, Georgia, identified and followed carotid bruits in 72 patients, ten of whom went on to have subsequent strokes. The incidence of stroke was clearly higher in the bruit group (13.9% vs. 3.4% in the nonbruit population), and strokes were more common in men with bruits than in women with the same findings (27.8% vs. 9.3%, respectively). Three of these strokes occurred on the side of the auscultated midcarotid bruit (at least one was preceded by a warning TIA), but seven were in other vascular distributions. These authors did not feel that their data justified workup of the asymptomatic bruit beyond modification of risk factors (4). In the second study, 171 patients in the Framingham cohort were identified as having carotid bruits and followed for 8 years. Twenty-one patients in this group had subsequent neurologic events, but most of these events were in other territories. In the territory of the carotid bruit, six patients had TIAs followed by stroke and two had TIAs only. Most events were either in other cerebrovascular territories or were etiologically related to noncarotid factors, such as aneurysms, lacunar infarcts, or emboli following myocardial infarction (5).

Both the Evans County and the Framingham studies confirmed that patients with asymptomatic bruit are at increased risk for cerebrovascular and/or cardiac problems. Neither group felt their data could provide justification for prophylactic surgery for the asymptomatic bruit alone.

Asymptomatic patients have been followed prospectively to evaluate their risk of stroke. Chambers and Norris (6) followed 500 asymptomatic bruit patients prospectively with serial noninvasive studies. Carotid-circulation ischemic events, mostly TIAs, were seen in 31 patients during follow-up. The incidence of unwarned stroke was 1% at 1 year for all patients and 3% in the severe-stenosis category. Although the authors did recommend following these bruit patients with duplex scans, they did not feel prophylactic endarterectomy was warranted (6). Hennerici et al (7) followed 339 patients with serial Doppler ultrasound examinations; all patients had ≥50% stenosis at admission to the trial. In their group overall, the risk of stroke without premonitory TIAs was a low 0.4%. However, significant progression of disease was noted in 36% of the patients during the follow-up interval (median, 29 months), and indeed such rapid progression of disease was the only predictor of negative cerebrovascular prognosis that they could identify, suggesting that a high-risk subgroup might exist.

CRITICAL STENOSIS

A subset of the asymptomatic bruit/stenosis population was felt by many neurovascular surgeons to represent a high-

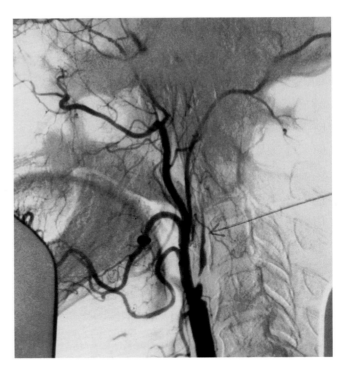

FIG. 1. Lateral angiogram of a 99% carotid stenosis with the string sign distal to the obstruction. This type of lesion would be considered an indication for surgery by any criteria. (From ref. 75, with permission.)

risk group for acute carotid occlusion with neurologic catastrophe. These patients included two groups. The first group consisted of those who had an initial stenosis ≥80% documented by noninvasive studies, angiography (Fig. 1), or magnetic resonance angiography (MRA). The other group involved patients with lesser degrees of stenosis who were followed with serial examinations and stenosis then progressed to ≥80%. The optimal management of these ''critical'' high-grade asymptomatic stenoses was greatly debated. Hemodynamic studies have indicated that critical reductions in cerebral blood flow may not be reached until 75–84% diameter stenosis has occurred, indicating that stenosis must be of a very high grade to be significant (8). Ojemann et al (9) believed that a 2-mm residual angiographic lumen represented a 70% narrowing and that carotid reconstruction was justified. Roederer et al (10) studied prospectively 167 asymptomatic bruit patients who were followed with duplex scans at 6 month to 1 year intervals. Smoking, diabetes mellitus, and age >65 years were identified as major risk factors for progression of silent stenosis. Ten patients suffered subsequent neurologic events (all ipsilateral to the carotid bruit), and 90% of these were in patients who had a ≥80% stenosis. The authors felt that this high degree of correlation between progression of stenosis and the onset of clinical events justified serial scanning to monitor the progression of carotid stenosis and that lesions ≥80% should be reconstructed. Moneta et al (11) studied 129 asymptomatic high-grade (80–99%) stenosis patients, 56 of whom underwent endarterectomy and 73 were followed. One perioperative stroke (1.8%) occurred, and there were nine strokes, all unwarned (five from carotid occlusion), in the unoperated group. Their data provided convincing evidence that surgery may be protective in these high-grade stenosis patients. Based on these reports, many surgeons felt justified in correcting such severe but otherwise asymptomatic lesions.

As mentioned earlier, however, Chambers and Norris (6) reported that in asymptomatic patients with stenosis of all degrees, the risk of cardiac ischemia was higher than that of stroke. In their series, although the risk of cerebral ischemic events was highest in patients with severe carotid artery stenosis, in most instances these patients did not have strokes without some sort of warning event, and even those who progressed to complete occlusion while being observed had a relatively benign outcome. Bogousslavsky et al (12) had likewise followed 38 patients with asymptomatic stenosis ≥90% for a mean period of 48 months. This patient group with severe stenosis had a 1.7% annual rate of unwarned stroke, sufficiently low that the authors could not justify prophylactic endarterectomy. Most recently, Norris et al (13) followed 696 patients for a mean of 41 months with noninvasive studies. While the combined TIA/stroke rate for patients with >75% stenosis was a significant 10.5%; the ipsilateral stroke rate (without warning TIA) was 2.5% for patients with >75% stenosis and 1.1% for those with <75% stenosis. These data reemphasized the need for surgical action in symptomatic high-grade stenosis patients but did not identify a high-risk asymptomatic subgroup (13). Many reviews of this subject recommended medical management of the patient with asymptomatic carotid bruit or stenosis with antiplatelet-aggregating therapy and attention to contributing risk factors, such as hypertension, with surgical intervention deferred until such time as frank TIAs develop (14–17). Others, like Moneta et al (11), felt justified in prophylactically reconstructing lesions causing ≥75–80% stenosis. In my opinion, ACAS has essentially resolved this conflict in favor of surgery.

SILENT CEREBRAL INFARCTION

There had been some evidence to suggest that silent small cerebral infarction, which may be seen on computed tomography (CT), may justify carotid endarterectomy in otherwise asymptomatic patients. Norris and Zhu (18) compared CT scans with carotid Doppler sonograms in patients identified to have asymptomatic carotid stenosis. They reported ipsilateral small (<15 mm) silent infarcts in 10% of mild (35–50%), 17% of moderate (50–75%) and 30% of severe (>75%) stenosis patients. They concluded that silent cerebral infarction may be an indication for ipsilateral carotid endarterectomy, particularly in severe stenosis. In light of the ACAS trial data now available, I agree that such lesions should be reconstructed if ≥60% stenosis exists, and I feel

that the gray area will now be the management of patients with <60% stenosis and silent cerebral ipsilateral infarction.

COOPERATIVE TRIALS

The continuing controversy over asymptomatic carotid disease spawned several large clinical trials. There have been four major completed prospective, randomized trials comparing medical and surgical therapies in patients with asymptomatic internal carotid artery stenosis: the Carotid Artery Stenosis with Asymptomatic Narrowing Operation Versus Aspirin (CASANOVA) study, the Mayo Asymptomatic Carotid Endarterectomy (MACE) trial, the Veterans Administration Cooperative Trial on Asymptomatic Carotid Stenosis (VA CSP 167) and the Asymptomatic Carotid Atherosclerosis Study (ACAS). There is also one European trial, the Asymptomatic Carotid Surgery Trial (ACST), which is continuing patient entry. The results of these trials are tabulated in Table 1. The first installment of the final answers to the asymptomatic question became available just before the time of this writing, with the release of the ACAS trial data mentioned above (1) to the coinvestigators. Unlike symptomatic carotid disease, where all three cooperative trials came to essentially the same conclusion (that surgery was justified), the asymptomatic trials have yielded somewhat conflicting results.

The first of these trials to be completed was the German CASANOVA study of 410 patients. This trial did not show any surgical benefit in reducing morbidity and mortality for patients with asymptomatic internal carotid artery stenosis of <90%. Medical treatment in this study consisted of aspirin and dipyridamole. No recommendations were made for patients with higher (>90%) grades of stenosis, since such patients unfortunately were excluded from this trial (19,20). The MACE study, published in 1992, was interrupted after only 71 patients had been randomized because an excess of patients in the surgical group suffered myocardial infarction (21). No surgical benefit could be demonstrated in this small study. If anything, findings from this trial pointed to the benefit of prophylactic aspirin in preventing myocardial infarction in patients having carotid endarterectomy (21). The VA CSP 167 trial randomized 444 male patients in 1987. Patients in the medical arm of this study received aspirin 325 mg twice daily. Findings from this trial showed that carotid endarterectomy reduced the overall incidence of ipsilateral neurologic events (TIAs included) for patients with asymptomatic internal carotid artery stenosis ≥50%. However, this trial found no significant effect from carotid endarterectomy on the combined incidence of stroke and death, and thus no surgical benefit was conferred for these endpoints (22). Whereas some argued that the VA trial provided justification for surgery on asymptomatic lesions, many others felt that the demonstrated reduction of only TIAs, without an impact on stroke or death, was not sufficient justification for prophylactic endarterectomy, since the onset of TIAs in

TABLE 1. *Randomized trials of asymptomatic carotid stenosis*

Trial	Patients (no.)	Entry criteria	Medical treatment	Follow-up period	Endpoint	Results
Carotid Artery Stenosis with Asymptomatic narrowing: Operation versus Aspirin (CASANOVA)	410	50–90% linear stenosis by angiography	Aspirin 330 mg/d + dipyridamole 75 mg/d	Minimum 36 mo (median 41.8–42.9 mo)	Ischemic neurologic deficit lasting >24 hrs; death	No surgical benefit for <90%; ≥90% not evaluated
Mayo Asymptomatic Carotid Endarterectomy Trial (MACE)	71	>50% linear stenosis on IV DSA or >75% cross-sectional area stenosis by duplex echocardiography	Aspirin 80 mg/d in medical arm; aspirin discouraged in surgical patients	Mean 23.6 mo when trial stopped	TIA, stroke, death	Trial stopped due to high rate of MI in surgical arm; No surgical benefit
Veterans Affairs Cooperative Study on Asymptomatic Carotid Stenosis (VA CSP 167)	444	>50% linear stenosis by biplanar arteriogram	Aspirin 650 mg twice daily in both medical and surgical arms	Mean 47.9 mo	TIA, stroke, death	Surgical benefit for prevention of TIA only, not for stroke or death
Asymptomatic Carotid Artery Stenosis Trial (ACAS)	1662	Hemodynamically significant stenosis (≥60%) by Doppler, OPG-Gee, or arteriogram (all surgical patients had arteriogram preop)	Aspirin 325 mg/d	Median 2.7 yr, trial stopped when surgical benefit demonstrated	Stroke or death within 30 days (surgical) or 42 days (medical), ipsilateral stroke thereafter	Surgical benefit for all patients with ≥60% stenosis
Asymptomatic Carotid Stenosis Trial (ACST)	approx. 600	"Tight" carotid stenosis (no minimum specified)	?	NA	?	Ongoing

previously asymptomatic patients would customarily trigger carotid reconstruction, especially in patients with high-grade stenosis (23).

The largest of these asymptomatic trials, the ACAS, reached a stopping rule on September 16, 1994, and the data were released to the coinvestigators. The ACAS trial involved 1662 patients at 39 centers. All patients had ≥60% stenosis of the carotid artery and were randomized into either the medical arm in which they received aspirin 325 mg/d or the surgical arm in which aspirin was also given. The primary endpoints in the ACAS study were stroke or death during the 30-day perioperative period and, thereafter, stroke ipsilateral to the carotid under study. ACAS showed a 55% relative risk reduction conferred by surgery, and it will be used as justification for performing prophylactic carotid artery reconstruction in any patient identified to have ≥60% stenosis (1). In my opinion, the plethora of conflicting historical studies and even the discordant results of the smaller randomized trials are overshadowed by the definitive results of ACAS, a beautifully designed and scrupulously documented cooperative trial.

CONTRALATERAL CAROTID STENOSIS

Patients with symptomatic carotid stenosis who undergo angiography and surgery very often are found to have disease in the contralateral extracranial carotid system as well. Some small number of these patients will have bilateral TIAs and will require bilateral (staged, in our hands—never concurrent) carotid endarterectomy. For those patients who have only unilateral symptoms, the question is often raised by the patient and or the referring physician as to what treatment is required for the asymptomatic side. A number of clinical studies, primarily retrospective, have been performed with the aim of ascertaining the risks of long-term neurologic sequelae in such patients with contralateral carotid stenosis managed nonoperatively. The critical point, much as in the follow-up of asymptomatic bruits, was to determine what percentage of these patients progressed to frank stroke in the appropriate carotid distribution without warning TIAs.

Most of the studies of this problem have specified 50% stenosis of the contralateral carotid as the criterion for significant disease (24–28), and most study designs have followed the contralateral asymptomatic side without surgery to see if and when TIAs and/or unwarned stroke would develop in that territory. In three of these reports, no patients followed with contralateral asymptomatic lesions developed a stroke without warning TIAs (26–28). In two other reports, a few patients did develop unwarned strokes, but the incidence was invariably <3%, and thus less than the accepted risk of surgical morbidity and mortality (24,25). A single study included all patients with contralateral stenosis (1–99%) and reported the incidence of direct stroke in unoperated patients to be 3%. The authors recommended prophylactic surgery on this basis and concluded that the percentage stenosis did not correlate with the risk of neurologic sequelae (29). Aside from this one group's findings, however, no authors in these small series could demonstrate that prophylactic surgery for contralateral lesions of >50% stenosis had any protective effect in the absence of clinical symptoms referable to that lesion.

This subject has most recently been evaluated by the investigators of the European Carotid Surgery Trialists (ECST) Cooperative Group. The investigators in this trial of symptomatic stenosis have kept records on the contralateral carotid in the 2295 randomized patients in their study, making this the largest series of this type. Their three-year Kaplan–Meier risk of stroke referable to the contralateral artery was 2.1%, and they did not feel surgery or screening examinations were justifiable based on these data (30). Even for their asymptomatic group with 70–99% stenosis, the 3-year risk only increased to 5.7%. Once again, the ACAS data supersede nonrandomized data such as this, no matter how large the population.

Until the release of the ACAS findings, my policy for lesions of this kind had been one of expectant observation with annual duplex ultrasonography, with consideration of surgery for lesions that progressed to ≥80% under observation. The ACAS data now available will lead to a modification of this position, and I will reconstruct contralateral stenoses of ≥60%, although still with staged procedures whenever possible. When second-side carotid procedures are indicated, I am careful to evaluate the cervical nerves preoperatively, lest an occult vocal cord paresis be converted to a disabling bilateral one.

CAROTID RISKS IN NONCAROTID PREOPERATIVE PATIENTS

Since carotid surgery has become routine and the consequences of carotid embolization or occlusion have become well recognized, considerable interest has been generated in the proper management of preoperative patients who are found to have auscultatory or radiographic evidence of otherwise silent carotid artery disease. There were a number of studies performed to address this problem, with nearly unequivocal conclusions. Once again, however, the ACAS data will change this picture significantly.

One early group performed prophylactic endarterectomies in 34 surgical patients and was able to demonstrate low morbidity and good long-term survival following the procedure (31). It was not clear, however, that their patients were at increased risk for cerebrovascular events, and thus whether these prophylactic procedures, albeit safe in their hands, were necessary. This point was soon resolved by a series of retrospective studies of surgical patients identified to have asymptomatic bruits but followed without carotid surgery

(32–35). These studies established the incidence of asymptomatic bruits in random preoperative patients to be near 15%. Although they documented a perioperative stroke rate of about 1% in their patient groups, none of these investigators could find a correlation between presence or location of carotid bruits and risk of perioperative stroke. More recent investigations have prospectively examined asymptomatic bruit patients with noninvasive carotid studies in an attempt to correlate percentage stenosis with risk of perioperative stroke (36–40). Although some of their reports documented higher perioperative mortality in the carotid stenosis groups, these deaths were primarily attributable to an increased risk of myocardial infarction, and once again no correlation between bruit or stenosis and perioperative stroke risk could be demonstrated (36,37). In one recent prospective study of preoperative patients with asymptomatic bruits only, the incidence of bruits in this group was 14%, and all strokes (0.7% of patients) were found in patients having coronary bypass surgery (41). The concept that the increased risk of perioperative stroke in coronary bypass patients arises from femoral arterial cannulation (and consequent retrograde aortic flow during bypass) rather than incidental carotid disease with carotid embolization and/or hypoperfusion has been supported by a Canadian study that found femoral cannulation to be the only statistically significant common denominator among a group of bypass patients with embolic stroke (42). Furlan and Craciun (43) have studied patients undergoing coronary bypass surgery who had angiographically documented asymptomatic stenosis >50% and showed that stroke risk was not increased in patients with either <90% stenosis or total internal carotid artery occlusion. There was an insufficient number of patients in the 90–99% group to allow statistical conclusions.

On the basis of these older studies, then, there was no strong evidence to support prophylactic endarterectomy in preoperative patients with either asymptomatic bruit or stenosis detected by noninvasive carotid studies. The ACAS data will change this policy. It will be my practice to recommend duplex ultrasound and/or angiographic study of preoperative patients found to have bruits or carotid stenosis, and carotid reconstruction will be advised in those patients found to have ≥60% stenosis. Whether carotid endarterectomy should precede the primary surgical procedure is unclear at present, as will be discussed later.

HOLLENHORST PLAQUE

In 1961, Hollenhorst (44) described 31 patients with orange-yellow or copper-colored plaques observed ophthalmoscopically at bifurcations of the retinal arterioles. Twenty-seven of these patients had occlusive disease in the carotid tree and four in the vertebral basilar tree. He also described five patients who underwent carotid endarterectomy and subsequently were found to have showers of these plaques in the retina. Hollenhorst felt that these plaques represented cholesterol emboli from the extracranial circulation and that their presence should warrant aggressive investigation of the cardiovascular and cerebrovascular system for surgically correctable disease. The atheromatous nature of this embolic material was confirmed in a case report by David et al (45) in 1963.

It is important to distinguish symptomatic retinal plaques from asymptomatic ones. Multiple authors have reported plaques associated with either amaurosis fugax or retinal artery occlusion with visual field deficits (46–48), and I have little doubt that these represent symptomatic carotid lesions. Russell (47,48) classifies these refractile, cholesterol-containing flakes as his third type of retinal emboli and points out that they customarily disappear from the retina within a few weeks, with or without leaving a permanent field deficit. Once again these symptomatic lesions certainly deserve active investigation for carotid-origin embolization.

In 1973, Hollenhorst's group (49) reported on 208 consecutive patients observed to have retinal cholesterol emboli who had been followed for at least 6 years. This group was mixed and many in the group had visual symptoms associated with this condition. This group of patients had significantly decreased survival compared with a heterogeneous comparison group, with a survival rate 13% less than expected in the first year of observation and increasing to 80% less than expected by the eighth year. The cause of death in many of these patients was related to diffuse vascular disease, with myocardial infarction being the greatest factor. Hollenhorst (49) once again concluded on the basis of these data that these plaques warrant aggressive cardiac and cerebrovascular investigation.

Patients with truly asymptomatic retinal cholesterol emboli represent a much more unusual and smaller group. Very little evidence is available as to the natural history and prognosis of these patients. Bruno et al (50) recently studied 70 consecutive men with asymptomatic retinal cholesterol emboli and compared them with a control group of 21 randomly selected subjects without retinal emboli. Patients in their study group had a significantly higher prevalence of hypertension and smoking history than did the control group. The prevalence of carotid stenosis ≥50% ipsilateral to the embolus was only 13%, however; and this was not significantly different from that in control subjects. However, carotid stenosis ≥50% on either side was more common in patients with asymptomatic retinal cholesterol emboli. According to Bruno et al's data, asymptomatic retinal cholesterol emboli did indicate a higher prevalence of systemic vascular disease and ischemic heart disease, similar to that reported by Pfaffenbach and Hollenhorst (49). Their data, however, did not support the concept that asymptomatic retinal cholesterol emboli are the harbingers of cerebrovascular events or of the presence of an unstable carotid atherosclerotic plaque. In this regard, it should be noted that asymptomatic retinal cholesterol emboli were not considered entry criteria for the North American Symptomatic Carotid Endarterectomy Trial (NASCET).

What, then, can be said about the presence of Hollenhorst plaques? Certainly any identifiable retinal lesion with visual symptoms must be considered a symptomatic carotid event until proven otherwise and warrants full investigation. I have performed carotid endarterectomy on many patients whose initial presentation was visual loss from central retinal artery occlusion by an embolic plug. The significance of asymptomatic lesions in the retina is confusing and not well studied at present. Available data would indicate that these do not represent a high-risk group, but it had been my inclination to investigate these patients actively even on the few occasions when absolutely no visual symptoms could be elicited. Of course, I now recommend carotid endarterectomy for any such patients found to have ≥60% stenosis.

CLINICAL APPROACH TO THE ASYMPTOMATIC CAROTID PATIENT

Patients present to the cerebrovascular surgeon in a number of different ways. Asymptomatic patients are customarily elective and seen in the office or clinic and are most often sent by primary care physicians for a surgical opinion, as well as surgical treatment. They may or may not have had noninvasive carotid studies performed, but most likely will not yet have undergone angiography.

My diagnostic plan for asymptomatic patients differs from that for patients with neurologic symptoms. In the absence of symptoms, I proceed first with noninvasive scanning (duplex ultrasonography) to ascertain the degree of stenosis present, whereas in symptomatic patients I usually go directly to angiography. The quality of the noninvasive laboratory is crucial at this step, and I prefer to use a validated and standardized laboratory with which I am familiar. If the stenosis is found to be ≥60%, I proceed with a rapid workup with the aim of performing surgery as soon as possible. It is my preference to have formal and complete angiography in every case including selective injection of both carotids and both vertebral arteries. Attention to intracranial cross-filling is also important, and I insist on biplane cervical angiography in every case so that the relationship of the external and internal carotid arteries can be determined. When digital angiography is performed (as is common in my center now), I ask that the arterial image be superimposed on a bone image so that I can ascertain the height of the carotid bulb in relationship to the cervical spine, the angle of the mandible, and the hyoid bone.

There is at present a considerable degree of interest in operating on patients based on magnetic resonance angiography alone. This has not been my practice as yet, but clearly, as the technology develops, it may become more prevalent. I have not operated on patients on the basis of duplex scanning alone and do not imagine I will do so in the future.

Patients who are seen for consideration of carotid surgery are customarily on aspirin or some form of anticoagulation, but if not, they are started on aspirin at the time of first visit.

I do not stop preoperative antiplatelet therapy in preparation for surgery.

The remainder of the preoperative evaluation is uneventful. A careful neurologic examination is performed, and a history is carefully obtained to be certain that neurologic symptoms have not been overlooked. Any history of cardiac disease warrants a cardiology consultation, and patients who are smokers are advised to cease smoking as much as possible in advance of the surgical procedure.

SPECIAL SURGICAL CONSIDERATIONS

Recurrent Carotid Stenosis

There is a small but finite incidence of recurrent carotid stenosis following primary carotid endarterectomy. Most authors quote a symptomatic recurrence rate of approximately 4–5%, and in one study of noninvasive follow-up after carotid surgery, a 4.8% recurrence rate of symptomatic carotid restenosis was documented with an additional 6.6% silent restenosis rate (51). Piepgras et al (52) have quoted somewhat lower figures with their use of patch graft repair: 1% symptomatic restenosis, with a 4–5% total at 2-year follow-up).

Aside from technical inadequacies, it has been difficult to identify risk factors associated with recurrent carotid stenosis. However, continuation of smoking habits after endarterectomy proved to be a significant risk factor in one study, whereas hypertension, diabetes mellitus, family history, lipid values, aspirin use, and coronary disease were not found to be significant risk factors by this group (53).

Reoperation for carotid stenosis is a technically difficult procedure. It is associated with significantly higher risks than primary endarterectomy, and Piepgras et al (52) documented a 10.5% risk of complications—four times their customary figure. In our institution, the possibility of reoperation for carotid stenosis is entertained in patients who present with angiographically proven disease and classic neurologic symptoms referable to the appropriate artery. Until the ACAS data were released, I had been unwilling to assume this surgical risk in asymptomatic patients and therefore had not routinely followed patients with noninvasive studies beyond the first year if they remained clinically stable. Others with great experience in this field, however, do feel that changing bruits or rapidly progressive stenoses justify surgical intervention (52). It is still unclear to me whether the clear surgical benefits shown by ACAS for primary cases can be extrapolated to recommend reconstruction for asymptomatic recurrent disease. Although I have begun to follow my patients for longer periods with duplex ultrasound, it's unclear whether the higher risk of reoperation should be assumed in the absence of symptoms.

Concurrent Coronary and Carotid Disease

It is well established that patients with extracranial carotid artery disease have a higher than normal incidence of coronary disease, as well as other peripheral vascular problems. Indeed, the risk of perioperative myocardial infarction exceeds the risk of perioperative stroke in many clinical series of carotid endarterectomy. Several major questions arise in treatment planning for concurrent coronary and carotid disease. First, what is the risk of coronary revascularization in a patient with a high-grade asymptomatic stenosis or bruit? Second, in patients with symptomatic carotid disease, what is the appropriate workup of the coronary circulation? And third, if surgical carotid artery and coronary artery disease are identified in the same patient, what is the appropriate surgical management: (a) staged carotid surgery followed by coronary revascularization, (b) a combined procedure, or (c) a "reverse staged" coronary revascularization followed by delayed carotid endarterectomy?

The first of these questions regarding asymptomatic bruit in symptomatic coronary patients was dealt with earlier in this chapter. Based on the ACAS and NASCET data (and noting the current paradox concerning significant percentage stenosis between the two studies until the moderate-grade NASCET data are analyzed), I would now recommend carotid endarterectomy for patients with ≥60% asymptomatic stenosis or ≥70% symptomatic stenosis prior to coronary revascularization whenever possible.

The second question regarding appropriate workup of coronary disease in symptomatic carotid artery patients is a more difficult one. In this situation, workup is customarily guided by the patient's history and symptoms. It has been my practice to obtain cardiology consultation in any patient with a history of angina, known heart disease, or abnormal resting ECG. The workup proceeds with a thallium stress test with exercise or dipyridamole; if there is any evidence of myocardial ischemia, coronary angiography is performed (54,55).

When the results of cardiac evaluation indicate the need for coronary revascularization, the question becomes one of timing of the surgical procedures. Our preference is to do staged procedures whenever possible. With careful hemodynamic monitoring and good anesthetic technique, I am routinely able to perform safe unilateral carotid endarterectomies prior to coronary revascularization. An occasional patient with severe unstable angina may require a combined procedure, but this entails a significantly higher surgical risk and I attempt staged procedures whenever possible (54,56). Most series dealing with reverse-staged coronary/carotid procedures (ie, coronary artery revascularization first with delayed carotid endarterectomy) discuss these in the context of asymptomatic carotid disease. Clearly, the answer to this is not known at present. While my old position was that asymptomatic disease did not need to be reconstructed, I would now prefer to treat ≥60% stenosis with staged carotid reconstruction followed by coronary revascularization, just as in a symptomatic carotid patient.

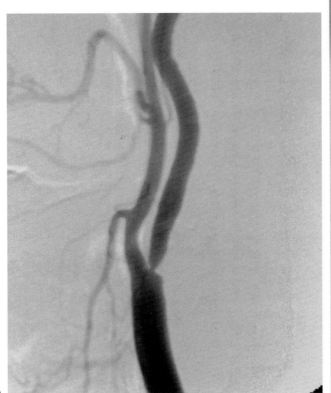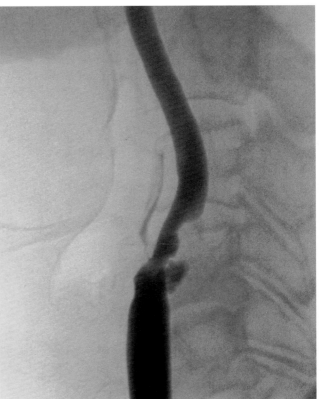

A   B

FIG. 2. Lateral digital angiographic views of the right **(A)** and left **(B)** cervical carotid arteries. The patient was asymptomatic. The right carotid showed a 90% linear stenosis and met the ACAS criteria for surgery, and a right carotid endarterectomy was performed without incident. The left carotid (to my mind) represents a far more dangerous lesion, with deep and irregular ulcerations over a long segment of the carotid bulb. In an asymptomatic patient, however, this 50% lesion has not been proven to benefit from surgery. I elected to perform a left carotid endarterectomy as a staged procedure in this patient, but I must emphasize that the scientific basis for this, as outlined in the text, is not well established.

In conclusion, then, any patient with cardiac symptoms prior to carotid endarterectomy should have an aggressive workup. If procedures in both circulations are indicated, staged procedures are preferable for symptomatic patients, unless the coronary circulation disease makes anesthesia for carotid endarterectomy an untenable proposition. In such case, a combined procedure may be acceptable. The role of reverse-staged procedures for asymptomatic carotid stenosis discovered in patients awaiting coronary revascularization is unclear, but in my mind reverse staging may prove to be a reasonable approach. There are at present no good data to suggest that asymptomatic stenosis increases the risk of stroke during coronary artery bypass grafting, but the ACAS data do indicate that ≥60% carotid lesions should be reconstructed. A reverse-staged approach to this problem, which I previously avoided, may now be appropriate. ACAS subgroup analyses will hopefully address this problem further.

Bilateral Carotid Endarterectomy

Bilateral asymptomatic lesions of ≥60% are routinely seen. Whereas my old policy was one of observation in such

cases, I have begun recommending staged carotid endarterectomy for such patients, staged 6 weeks apart wherever possible (Fig. 2). The surgeon's question then becomes which procedure should be performed first. In symptomatic cases, of course, or in cases where there is one symptomatic and one silent carotid (both ≥60%), it has been my preference to operate first on the side with the most recent or crescendo TIAs. In cases of bilateral silent disease, I prefer to operate first on the side with the higher-grade or preocclusive lesion, with the idea that reconstruction of the opposite carotid first would lead to thrombosis of a 99% lesion once collateral circulation was increased.

Bilateral carotid endarterectomy runs the risk not only of extreme swings of blood pressure from concurrent denervation of both carotid sinuses (57) but also of bilateral cranial nerve injury. For this reason, when bilateral carotid endarterectomy is required in my patients, I stage these procedures 6 weeks apart and have the patient examined by an otolaryngologist to ensure that no occult cranial nerve or vocal cord dysfunction is present prior to the second procedure. Unilateral nerve dysfunction in the cervical region is troublesome, but a bilateral one can be disabling. On several occasions, I have deferred second-side surgery and maintained the patient on medical therapy when an occult vocal cord paralysis was diagnosed.

Postoperative Considerations

Following carotid endarterectomy, the patient is awakened in the operating theater and does not leave the room until a screening neurologic examination has been performed. The superficial temporal artery (STA) pulse, which was checked preoperatively, is palpated again on the operative side. I anticipate that all carotid patients will be neurologically intact at the conclusion of the procedure. I examine them carefully for grip strength, function of the hypoglossal nerve, and function of the marginal mandibular branch of the facial nerve (by asking them to smile). In patients who are neurologically unstable preoperatively or who have had a preexistent stroke, it is not uncommon to find some decreased grip strength for the first several hours after surgery. This is most commonly a transient phenomenon that occasionally responds to a slight increase of blood pressure and almost always resolves spontaneously. However, the process of waiting for this to resolve is a nerve-racking one for the surgeon. I take comfort in the fact that we have tested the artery intraoperatively with Doppler imaging after the repair and immediately before closing the neck. In patients who were normal preoperatively and who awaken with a new postoperative deficit, however, or in stroke patients who do not appear to be making steady progress over the first several hours, I proceed immediately to the angiographic suite to confirm patency of the vessel. If there is any question of inadequate technical repair or a postoperative occlusion, I return to surgery for reexploration of the wound.

I have not adopted the policy of exploring the wound without radiographic confirmation of technical error in patients who awaken with a neurologic deficit. It has been my feeling that the patient is better served by obtaining a good snapshot of the anatomy and areas of technical difficulty before reexploring the vessel. In fact, most patients who have angiography do not have an identifiable technical error and go on to make a reasonable recovery from what is assumed to be a transient ischemic deficit. My overall perioperative stroke rate in patients including all classes of preoperative risk has been (gratifyingly) <2%.

I monitor all patients in the recovery room for an hour or so and then transfer them to the intensive care unit (ICU) for overnight observation before returning them to the dedicated stroke unit. My reasons for ICU management of the patients are primarily for control of blood pressure and prevention of the risk of myocardial infarction. After transfer to the floor the following day, the Hemovac is removed and the patient is mobilized. Customarily, the hospital stay lasts 2–3 days beyond this. As the wound is customarily closed with subcuticular stitches, there is no need for suture removal.

My long-term follow-up of carotid patients involves a visit at 6 weeks and another at 3 months. Although previously I did not routinely perform a postoperative duplex ultrasound examination in normal patients (because of my policy of only operating on symptomatic recurrent carotid disease), I have begun to follow these patients with prospective duplex scans since the ACAS results have been available. Patients are also maintained on aspirin 325 mg/d for the rest of their lives.

Complications

It is generally recognized that patients with cerebrovascular disease severe enough to warrant carotid artery surgery often have serious associated medical conditions and that the surgical morbidity and mortality risks in such patients are directly related to the degree of these complicating systemic factors. Several authors (58,59) have demonstrated that perioperative risks of 1% in patients without associated medical or angiographic risk factors increase to at least 7% in individuals with such predisposing medical conditions as angina pectoris, recent myocardial infarction, congestive heart failure, severe hypertension, chronic obstructive pulmonary disease, or obesity. Nonetheless, patients with classic carotid symptoms who are consequently at high risk for embolic stroke may still benefit from surgical therapy, and all precautions must be taken to avoid aggravation of underlying disease.

The complications of carotid endarterectomy can be divided into three major groups: (a) perioperative, medical, and anesthetic nonneurologic events, (b) vascular events in the territory of the operated carotid, and (c) local wound problems.

The major perioperative complication of carotid surgery is myocardial infarction, with an incidence of 1–4% in carotid procedures (60–63). As Sundt et al (58) have demonstrated, the risk of carotid surgery is markedly increased in patients with strong histories of cardiac disease. In addition, Yeager et al (63) demonstrated that diabetes mellitus was a significant risk factor for perioperative myocardial infarction in their series of 249 procedures, and Riles et al (61) showed that the use of vasopressors in carotid endarterectomy patients was associated with a fourfold rise (2.0% to 8.1%) in the incidence of postoperative myocardial infarction.

Complications referable to the vascular territory of the operated carotid artery include devastating embolic, ischemic, and/or hemorrhagic strokes and, rarely, postoperative TIAs. Postoperative stroke rates, although generally decreasing with advances in surgical and anesthetic skills, vary from Sundt's figure (58) of 0.6% for embolic stroke to a rate of 14.5% in one community hospital series (64). It is generally accepted that embolic stroke rates can be reduced by the gentlest possible dissection of the carotid and that thrombosis of the operated carotid is often a reflection of technical error, whether from dissection of a distal intimal flap or stenosis in the arteriotomy suture line (59). Postoperative hypotension, the consequence of carotid baroreceptor dysfunction (65,66), has been shown to be associated with an increased incidence of complications (65,67) and may contribute to ischemic neurologic deficits. The etiology of the commonly observed postoperative hypertension and its effect on hemorrhagic stroke is less well understood (65). There is good evidence, however, that clinically elevated preoperative blood pressure is the major contributory factor in this problem, and in one study the incidences of both postoperative neurologic deficit and operative death were significantly increased in the patient group manifesting postoperative hypertension (68). Hemorrhagic complications after endarterectomy are probably multifactorial. Hyperperfusion related to revascularization of a severe stenosis and systemic hypertension play a predominant role (69). The use of anticoagulants or perhaps antiplatelet-aggregating medications can be implicated in some cases, and they should be used with recognition of the increase in risk. Postoperative TIAs are disturbing in that they may represent acute carotid occlusion requiring surgical intervention. Nonocclusive TIAs, however, have been successfully managed with anticoagulation (58).

As mentioned, I manage any postoperative neurologic deficit, including TIA alone, with immediate angiography (Fig. 3). In my experience, lesser measures, such as duplex scanning, are inadequate for definitive surgical decision-making in these cases, where quick judgments and emergent surgery may be required.

Problems related to the wound constitute the final group of carotid surgical complications. Injuries to local cranial nerves, including the marginal mandibular, hypoglossal, superior laryngeal, and recurrent laryngeal nerves, are among the most common of these complications, and in one prospective series such injury was found in 12.5% of patients (70). The majority of these injuries were subclinical or mild and resolved spontaneously; in addition they were attributed to retraction rather than transection injury. The incidence of hemorrhage from the carotid suture line is low—much <1% in two major series (58,62)—despite the use of intraoperative anticoagulants (71). Such hemorrhage can, however, be catastrophic with tracheal obstruction and can lead to false aneurysm formation (72). Wound infections, usually staphylococcal, have occasionally been reported and rarely may contribute to the genesis of a false aneurysm (73).

CONCLUSIONS

Previously, it was very difficult for me to sort out the complexities of historical and nonrandomized trials and to determine which, if any, asymptomatic patients required surgery. At the risk of seeming oversimplified, this problem has essentially been solved. I recommend surgery to any asymptomatic patient with linear carotid stenosis ≥60%.

There are still problems with this approach. It assumes that I have ignored the data from CASANOVA, MACE, VA

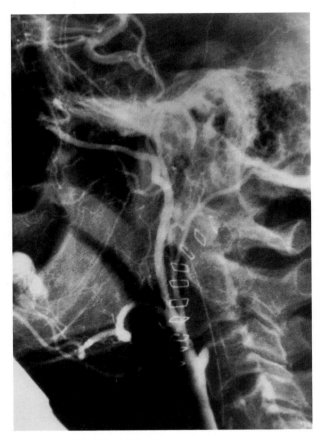

FIG. 3. Lateral projection of a common carotid arteriogram. This patient developed left-arm weakness in the recovery room following uneventful (but shunted) carotid endarterectomy. Immediate formal angiography showed an internal carotid artery occlusion with a patent external carotid artery and retrograde flow into the cavernous and petrous carotid artery. The patient was taken directly to surgery to reestablish flow with a saphenous vein patch angioplasty; there was a full neurologic recovery. (From ref. 75, with permission.)

CSP 167, and the countless nonrandomized trials that could not show a surgical benefit. This is essentially what I have done, putting my trust in ACAS, which I feel is the largest and most scientifically valid trial.

For the present, there are still paradoxes that are not easily resolved (74,75). Although I have not discussed symptomatic carotid trials in this chapter, the reader must understand that so far (with the exception of the small VA CSP 309), no benefit from surgery has been demonstrated by randomized trials except for ≥70% stenosis. This puts me in the unusual position of recommending surgery for asymptomatic stenosis of 60% in some patients, while I either treat the contralateral symptomatic 60% stenosis with aspirin or randomize it potentially into the medical arm of NASCET! There is and will continue to be much room for debate among neurologists and neurosurgeons regarding the indications for carotid reconstruction. In my opinion, however, the ACAS data will stand the test of time, just as the EC-IC bypass data have done, and will reshape practice patterns for carotid endarterectomy in much the same fashion.

REFERENCES

1. Asymptomatic Carotid Atherosclerosis (ACAS) Study Group. Endarterectomy for asymptomatic carotid artery stenosis. *JAMA* 1995;273:1421–1428.
2. Cooperman M, Martin EW, Evans WE. Significance of asymptomatic carotid bruits. *Arch Surg* 1978;113:1339–1340.
3. Thompson JE, Patman RD, Talkington CM. Asymptomatic carotid bruit. Long-term outcome of patients having endarterectomy compared with unoperated controls. *Ann Surg* 1978;188:308–315.
4. Heyman A, Wilkinson WE, Heyden S, et al. Risk of stroke in asymptomatic persons with cervical arterial bruits. A population study in Evans County, Georgia. *N Engl J Med* 1980;302:838–841.
5. Wolf PA, Kannel WB, Sorlie P. Asymptomatic carotid bruit and risk of stroke. The Framingham study. *JAMA* 1981;245:1442–1445.
6. Chambers BR, Norris JW. Outcome in patients with asymptomatic neck bruits. *N Engl J Med* 1986;315:860–865.
7. Hennerici M, Hulsbomer HB, Hefter H, Lammerts D, Rautenberg W. Natural history of asymptomatic extracranial artery disease. *Brain* 1987;110:777–791.
8. Archie JP, Feldtman RW. Critical stenosis of the internal carotid artery. *Surgery* 1981;1:67–72.
9. Ojemann RG, Crowell RM, Roberson GH, Fisher CM. Surgical treatment of extracranial carotid occlusive disease. *Clin Neurosurg* 1975;22:214–263.
10. Roederer GO, Langlois YE, Jager KA, et al. The natural history of carotid artery disease in asymptomatic patients with cervical bruits. *Stroke* 1984;15:605–613.
11. Moneta GL, Taylor DC, Nicholls SC, et al. Operative versus nonoperative management of asymptomatic high-grade internal carotid artery stenosis: improved results with endarterectomy. *Stroke* 1987;18:1005–1010.
12. Bogousslavsky J, Despland PA, Regli F. Asymptomatic tight stenosis of the internal carotid artery: Long-term prognosis. *Neurology* 1986;36:861–863.
13. Norris JW, Zhu CZ, Bornstein NM, et al. Vascular risks of asymptomatic carotid stenosis. *Stroke* 1991;22:1485–1490.
14. Corman LC. The preoperative patient with an asymptomatic carotid bruit. *Med Clin North Am* 1979;63:1335–1340.
15. Fields WS. The asymptomatic carotid bruit—operate or not? *Stroke* 1978;9:269–271.
16. Mohr JP. Asymptomatic carotid artery disease. Stroke 1982;13:431–433.
17. Yatsu FM, Hart RG. Asymptomatic carotid bruit and stenosis: A reappraisal. *Stroke* 14:301–304, 1983
18. Norris JW, Zhu CZ. Silent stroke and carotid stenosis. *Stroke* 1992;23:483–485.
19. CASANOVA Study Group. Carotid surgery versus medical therapy in asymptomatic carotid stenosis. *Stroke* 1991;222:1229–1235.
20. Diener HC, Hamann H, Schafer H, et al. Carotid surgery versus medical therapy in asymptomatic carotid stenosis. *Neurology* 1990;40(suppl 1):415.
21. Mayo Asymptomatic Carotid Endarterectomy Study Group. Results of a randomized controlled trial of carotid endarterectomy for asymptomatic carotid stenosis. *Mayo Clin Proc* 1992;67:513–518.
22. Hobson RW, Weiss DG, Fields WS, et al. Efficacy of carotid endarterectomy for asymptomatic carotid stenosis. *N Engl J Med* 1993;328:221–227.
23. Barnett HJM, Haines SJ. Carotid endarterectomy for asymptomatic carotid stenosis. *N Engl J Med* 1993;328:276–279.
24. Durward QJ, Ferguson GG, Barr HWK. The natural history of asymptomatic carotid bifurcation plaques. *Stroke* 1982;13:459–464.
25. Humphries AW, Young JR, Santilli PH, et al. Unoperated asymptomatic significant internal carotid artery stenosis: A review of 182 cases. *Surgery* 1976;80:695–698.
26. Johnson N, Burnham SJ, Flanigan DP, et al. Carotid endarterectomy: A follow-up study of the contralateral non-operated carotid artery. *Ann Surg* 1978;188:748–752.
27. Levin SM, Sondheimer FK. Stenosis of the contralateral asymptomatic carotid artery—to operate or not? *J Vasc Surg* 1973;7:3–13.
28. Levin SM, Sondheimer FK, Levin JM. The contralateral diseased but asymptomatic carotid artery: To operate or not? *Am J Surg* 1980;140:203–205.
29. Podore PC, DeWeese JA, May AG, et al. Asymptomatic contralateral carotid artery stenosis: A five-year follow-up study following carotid endarterectomy. *Surgery* 1980;88:748–752.
30. European Carotid Surgery Trialists Collaborative Group. Risk of stroke in the distribution of an asymptomatic carotid artery. *Lancet* 1995;345:209–12.
31. Lefrak EA, Guinn GA. Prophylactic carotid artery surgery in patients requiring a second operation. *South Med J* 1974;67:185–189.
32. Carney WI, Stewart WB, DePinto DJ, et al. Carotid bruit as a risk factor in aortoiliac reconstruction. *Surgery* 1977;81:567–570.
33. Evans WE, Cooperman M. The significance of asymptomatic unilateral carotid bruits in preoperative patients. *Surgery* 1978;83:521–522.
34. Treiman RL, Foran RF, Cohen JL, et al. Carotid bruit. A follow-up report on its significance in patients undergoing an abdominal aortic operation. *Arch Surg* 1979;114:1138–1140.
35. Treiman RL, Foran RF, Shore EH, et al. Carotid bruit. Significance in patients undergoing an abdominal aortic operation. *Arch Surg* 1973;106:803–805.
36. Barnes RW, Liebman PR, Marszalek PB, et al. The natural history of asymptomatic carotid disease in patients undergoing cardiovascular surgery. *Surgery* 1981;90:1075–1083.
37. Barnes RW, Marszalek PB. Asymptomatic carotid disease in the cardiovascular surgical patient: Is prophylactic endarterectomy necessary? *Stroke* 1981;12:497–500.
38. Breslau PJ, Fell G, Ivey TD, et al. Carotid arterial disease in patients undergoing coronary bypass operations. *J Thorac Cardiovasc Surg* 1981;82:765–767.
39. Gerraty RP, Gates PC, Doyle JC. Carotid stenosis and perioperative stroke risk in symptomatic and asymptomatic patients undergoing vascular or coronary surgery. *Stroke* 1993;24:1115–1118.
40. Turnipseed WD, Berkoff HA, Belzer FO. Postoperative stroke in cardiac and peripheral vascular disease. *Ann Surg* 1980;192:365–368.
41. Ropper AH, Wechsler LR, Wilson LS. Carotid bruit and risk of stroke in elective surgery. *N Engl J Med* 1982;307:1388–1390.
42. Martin WRW, Hashimoto SA. Stroke in coronary bypass surgery. *Can J Neurol Sci* 1982;9:21–26.
43. Furlan AJ, Craciun AR. Risk of stroke during coronary artery bypass graft surgery in patients with internal carotid artery disease documented by angiography. *Stroke* 1985;16:797–799.
44. Hollenhorst RW. Significance of bright plaques in the retinal arterioles. *JAMA* 1961;178:123–129.
45. David NJ, Klintworth GK, Friedberg SJ, et al. Fatal atheromatous cerebral embolism associated with bright plaques in the retinal arterioles: Report of a case. *Neurology* 1963;13:708–713.
46. Balla JI, Howat ML, Walton JN. Cholesterol emboli in retinal arteries. *J Neurol Neurosurg Psychiatry* 1964;27:144–148.
47. Russell RW. Atheromatous retinal embolism. *Lancet* 1963;2:1354–1356.
48. Russell RW. The source of retinal emboli. *Lancet* 1968;2:789–792.
49. Pfaffenbach DD, Hollenhorst RW. Morbidity and survivorship of patients with embolic cholesterol crystals in the ocular fundus. *Am J Ophthalmol* 1973;75:66–72.
50. Bruno A, Russell PW, Jones WL, et al. Concomitants of asymptomatic retinal cholesterol emboli. *Stroke* 1992;23:900–902.
51. Salvian A, Baker JD, Machleder HI, et al. Cause and noninvasive detection of restenosis after endarterectomy. *Am J Surg* 1983;146:29–34.
52. Piepgras DG, Sundt TM, Marsh WR, et al. Recurrent carotid stenosis: Results and complications of 57 operations. In: Sundt TM (ed): *Occlusive Cerebrovascular Disease: Diagnosis and Surgical Management.* Philadelphia: WB Saunders, 1987:286–297.
53. Clagett GP, Rich NM, McDonald PT, et al. Etiologic factors for recurrent carotid artery stenosis. *Surgery* 1983;2:313–318.
54. Graor RA, Hertzer NR. Management of coexistent carotid artery and coronary artery disease. Current concepts of cerebrovascular disease and stroke 1988;23:19–23.
55. Jones RH, Loftus CM, Sheldon WC, et al. Concomitant carotid and coronary disease. *Patient Care* 1992;15:49–66.
56. Cosgrove DM, Hertzer NR, Loop FD. Surgical management of syn-

chronous carotid and coronary artery disease. *J Vasc Surg* 1986;3: 690–692.

57. Wade JG, Larson CP, Hickey RF, et al. Effect of carotid endarterectomy on carotid chemoreceptor and baroreceptor function in man. *N Engl J Med* 1970;282:823–829.

58. Sundt TM, Sandok BA, Whisnant JP. Carotid endarterectomy. Complications and preoperative assessment of risk. *Mayo Clin Proc* 1975;50: 301–306.

59. Thompson JE. Complications of carotid endarterectomy and their prevention. *World J Surg* 1979;3:155–165.

60. Matsumoto GH, Cossman D, Callow AD. Hazards and safeguards during carotid endarterectomy. Technical considerations. *Am J Surg* 1977; 133:458–462.

61. Riles TS, Kopelman I, Imparato AM. Myocardial infarction following carotid endarterectomy: A review of 683 operations. *Surgery* 1979; 859:249–252.

62. Wylie EJ, Ehrenfeld WK. *Extracranial Occlusive Cerebrovascular Disease: Diagnosis and Management.* Philadelphia: WB Saunders, 1970.

63. Yeager RA, Moneta GL, McConnell DB, et al. Analysis of risk factors for myocardial infarction following carotid endarterectomy. *Arch Surg* 1989;124:1142–1145.

64. Easton JD, Sherman DG. Stroke and mortality rate in carotid endarterectomy: 228 consecutive operations. *Stroke* 1977;8:565–568.

65. Bove EL, Fry WJ, Gross WS, et al. Hypotension and hypertension as consequences of baroreceptor dysfunction following carotid endarterectomy. *Surgery* 1979;85:633–637.

66. Tarlov E, Schmidek H, Scott RM, et al. Reflex hypotension following carotid endarterectomy: mechanism and management. *J Neurosurg* 1973;39:323–327.

67. Ranson JHC, Imparato AM, Clauss RH, et al. Factors in the mortality and morbidity associated with surgical treatment of cerebrovascular insufficiency. *Circulation* 1969;269(suppl 1):39–40.

68. Towne JB, Bernhard VM. The relationship of postoperative hypertension to complications following carotid endarterectomy. *Surgery* 1980; 88:575–580.

69. Solomon RA, Loftus CM, Quest DO, et al. Incidence and etiology of intracerebral hemorrhage following carotid endarterectomy. *J Neurosurg* 1986;64:29–34.

70. Hertzer NR, Feldman BJ, Tucker HM. A prospective study of the incidence of injury to the cranial nerves during carotid endarterectomy. *Surg Gynecol Obstet* 1980;151:781–784.

71. Dunsker SB. Complications of carotid endarterectomy. *Clin Neurosurg* 1976;23:336–341.

72. Ehrenfeld WK, Hays RJ. False aneurysm after carotid endarterectomy. *Arch Surg* 1972;104:288–291.

73. Smith RB, Perdue GD, Collier RH, et al. Post-operative false aneurysms of the carotid artery. *Am Surg* 1970;36:335–341.

74. Loftus CM, Hopkins LN. Paradoxical indications for carotid endarterectomy. *Neurosurgery* 1995;36:99–100.

75. Loftus CM. *Carotid Endarterectomy: Principles and Technique.* St. Louis, MO, Quality Medical Publishing, 1995.

Cerebrovascular Disease, edited by H. Hunt Batjer.
Lippincott-Raven Publishers, Philadelphia © 1997.

CHAPTER 33

Carotid Endarterectomy: Technical Considerations

Julian E. Bailes

CONTROVERSIES IN CAROTID ENDARTERECTOMY

Few procedures in modern medicine have been as carefully scrutinized and highly debated as carotid endarterectomy. Spurred by stroke prevalence and high medical and societal costs of caring for victims and survivors of stroke, there has been an evolution in the consideration regarding and techniques related to carotid endarterectomy. Although we are still debating its efficacy in certain situations (eg, moderate stenosis), this procedure has been deemed beneficial for many groups of patients.

The procedure of carotid endarterectomy has often been considered as merely a method of increasing ipsilateral cerebral blood flow and of removing angiographically visualized stenoses. Our current knowledge has progressed to allow detailed analysis of the entire cerebrovascular supply, beginning at the aortic arch and continuing through to the cerebral microcirculation. In conjunction with the neuroradiologic investigation, we are able to individualize treatment according to the clinical manifestations of each patient's embolic or hemodynamic phenomena. The past few years has seen tremendous advances in areas such as magnetic resonance angiography, transcranial Doppler (TCD) ultrasound, critical care medicine, cardiology, anesthesiology, and other areas. These have added greatly to our ability to successfully accomplish carotid endarterectomy in order to improve the natural history of the untreated disease (Fig. 1).

Carotid endarterectomy has undergone an evolution in indications, preoperative patient assessment, intraoperative technique, anesthetic management, and postoperative patient care. The North American Symptomatic Carotid Endarerectomy Trial (NASCET) study, published in 1991, demon-

J. E. Bailes: Department of Neurosurgery, Medical College of Pennsylvania and Hahnemann University, and Allegheny General Hospital, Pittsburgh, PA 15212.

strated that patients with symptomatic, >70% stenosis benefited from surgical intervention. The absolute risk reduction for surgery compared with the best medical therapy was 17%, with a relative risk reduction of 65% for ipsilateral stroke and stroke death (1). Two additional contemporaneous trials, the European Collaborative Group (2) and the Veteran's Administration report by Mayberg et al (3), corroborated the success of endarterectomy for symptomatic stenosis.

The defining of benefited populations notwithstanding, there still are many areas of carotid endarterectomy that are controversial. Technical issues have centered around the avoidance of cerebral ischemia. Although historically it was felt that the period of carotid cross-clamping was of paramount importance, newer evidence shows that this is usually well tolerated and that other technical factors may be predominant in outcome. All aspects of the surgical protocol for carotid endarterectomy must be carefully considered and justified. The protocol described herein, based on certain modern principles of neurologic surgery such as the use of the operating microscope, intraoperative monitoring of cerebral function, pharmacologic protection, and avoidance of routine use of carotid shunts, has yielded favorable outcomes in patients undergoing endarterectomy (4). This chapter will describe the techniques of microsurgical carotid endarterectomy and thromboendarterectomy, but it will also focus on the controversies of the procedure. The major complications and their avoidance will be addressed.

Tandem Carotid Lesions

The complete assessment of the cerebrovascular circulation begins with angiographic visualization of the aortic arch. In such an evaluation it is important to visualize the origins of the carotid and vertebral arteries. Patients with cerebral ischemic symptoms may have atherosclerotic stenosis, ulcerative lesions, or occlusion of the origin of these great vessels. The full consideration of the cerebrovascular

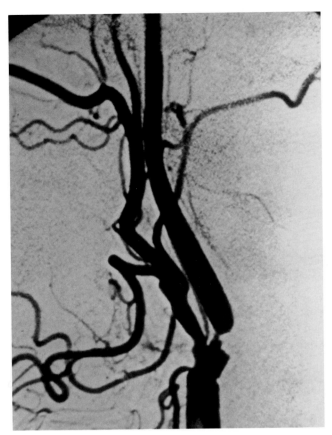

FIG. 1. Serial Doppler examinations disclosed that this asymptomatic patient had progressive stenosis of the internal carotid artery as confirmed by this angiogram. Successful endarterectomy was performed.

supply and an understanding of the patient's symptomatology is not possible without such a comprehensive evaluation. When tandem lesions exist, they usually involve the cervical carotid bifurcation along with abnormalities in the cavernous portion of the internal carotid artery (ICA). However, carotid bifurcation lesions may also exist in tandem with stenosis of the origin of the common carotid artery.

In patients with tandem carotid bifurcation and carotid siphon lesions, the former are usually responsible for cerebral ischemic symptoms. Cerebral infarction, which often occurs in the middle cerebral artery (MCA) territory, is more likely to be of thromboembolic than hemodynamic origin. The characteristics of atheromatous plaques at the ICA origin are more likely to provide a substrate for atheromatous debris, thrombus, or platelet aggregate material for embolization than plaques in the carotid siphon (Fig. 2). Removal of an ICA origin lesion should eliminate a symptomatic embolic source. In addition, studies using oculoplethysmography have shown that cervical carotid bifurcation and carotid siphon stenoses may have an additive affect in hemodynamic terms. Considering cerebral blood flow, carotid origin lesions have been shown to have a greater detrimental impact than carotid siphon lesions.

It has been shown that carotid endarterectomy can be successfully performed in patients with coexistent carotid siphon lesions without an apparent increased risk of morbidity and mortality. Day et al. reported two patients with severe preoperative carotid siphon stenosis that resolved following carotid endarterectomy. Their experience emphasizes that tandem lesions are not a contraindication to carotid endarterectomy and that the carotid siphon stenosis may be a reversible phenomenon (5). Repeat angiography or magnetic resonance angiography may be obtained to ascertain the status of the carotid siphon lesion. Carotid siphon tandem stenosis can be caused by embolization, reactive arterial spasm, anterograde flow disturbance, or a combination of factors. Alcock demonstrated a similar phenomenon with occlusive lesions of the MCA (6). Little et al. had a similar experience in two patients with resolving carotid siphon lesions that they termed pseudotandem stenosis. They postulated that laminar flow through the poststenotic carotid segment beyond the cervical bifurcation may produce the appearance of marked diminution in arterial caliber, secondary to either a reduced amount of contrast medium or actual slow contrast flow (7). Collateral flow of a substantial nature through either the anterior cerebral artery or posterior communication artery likewise could displace or dilute a column of contrast medium.

It appears, therefore, most patients with tandem carotid lesions are probably symptomatic from the cervical bifurcation atheromatous plaque. It is believed that carotid endarterectomy in patients with tandem lesions can be safely performed without significant increase in the incidence of cerebral ischemic symptoms or in the stroke rate following carotid endarterectomy. It has also been suggested that there is potential for an additive effect. In addition, carotid siphon stenosis is a predictor of future coronary disease and indicates widespread systemic atherosclerotic changes.

Cerebral Protection

Many technical facets of carotid endarterectomy are aimed at providing a good outcome by protecting cerebral tissue either directly or indirectly. Intraoperatively, the threshold for tolerance of cerebral ischemia is increased by pharmacologic agents; the most common are barbiturates. Barbiturates are used widely in cerebrovascular surgery, during both carotid endarterectomy and periods of temporary cerebral arterial occlusion, particularly in aneurysm surgery.

The mechanism of action of barbiturates providing cerebral protection is believed to be a reversible, dose-dependent depression of cerebral blood flow and, ultimately, of the cerebral metabolic rate (8,9). When the electroencephalogram (EEG) reaches an isoelectric state, barbiturates have reduced cerebral blood flow and the cerebral metabolic rate of oxygen by about 50%. This protective effect is more prominent in the nonischemic portions of the brain (8, 10–12). Vasoconstriction of the normal portions of the brain

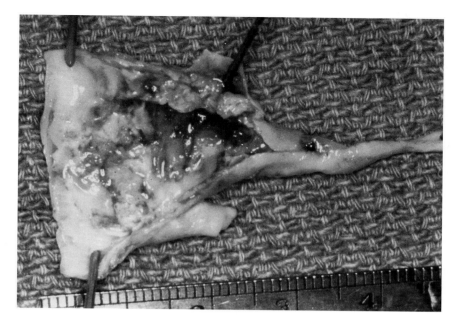

FIG. 2. An operative specimen shows a complex, ulcerated lesion with platelet thrombotic material beginning to accumulate.

occurs and is thought to improve cerebral blood flow to the ischemic areas (13). Barbiturates may also decrease the rate of edema formation. By reducing cerebral blood flow and cerebral blood volume, barbiturates also decrease the intracranial pressure. Barbiturates may also serve as free radical scavengers and reduce the production of free fatty acids from damaged cells (14,15). The exact mechanism of barbiturate cerebral protection in the setting of arterial occlusion is probably multifactorial and incompletely understood. It is clear, however, that these agents can modify or prevent cerebral damage secondary to focal ischemia (8,16). Laboratory experience with a primate model has demonstrated that prior administration of barbiturates provides dramatic cerebral protection for as long as 6 hours of MCA occlusion (8,12, 17). This degree of cerebral protection far surpasses that provided by other general anesthetic agents. Barbiturates administered after the onset of cerebral ischemia are not believed to provide protection and may in fact be deleterious, especially in the presence of a permanent vascular occlusion (10,18).

Barbiturate use has disadvantages including intraoperative hypotension, myocardial depression, and a prolonged postoperative wake-up period in some patients. The use of vasopressor agents and intravenous volume expansion has led to intraoperative hypotension not being a problem. In patients with severe myocardial dysfunction, the anesthesiologist may be concerned that the cardiovascular effects of barbiturates could be detrimental or significantly adversely affect function. In such cases, we have used etomidate with excellent results. Etomidate is a short-acting intravenous anesthetic agent that induces a reversible, dose-dependent reduction in the cerebral metabolic rate. The EEG effects of etomidate are similar to the characteristics of barbiturates: isoelectric EEG pattern associated with about a 50% de-

crease in the cerebral metabolic rate of oxygen. The cardiovascular depressive affects of etomidate are likely insignificant (19). We have used this drug safely and efficaciously during carotid endarterectomy, as others have for temporary cerebral arterial occlusion (20). We find that the addition of barbiturate therapy for cerebral protection provides an opportunity for the surgeon to perform a precise and relaxed endarterectomy, including the time needed for complicated arterial reconstruction. In our series, the administration of barbiturates was both feasible and safe (4).

Carotid Patch Graft

Materials that have been used for carotid patch angioplasty are saphenous vein, Dacron, or polytetrafluoroethylene. Autogenous saphenous vein has been the preferred material because of its ease in handling; its relatively antithrombotic properties; and its size, tensile strength, and resistance to infection. Proponents of vein patch carotid angioplasty propose that this technique enlarges the endarterectomized segment and restores normal contour to the carotid bulb. Immediate postoperative and subsequent flow disturbances are thereby minimized. It is also thought to prevent or minimize intimal hyperplasia (21,22). The saphenous vein interposition graft contains viable endothelium that may reduce thrombogenicity compared to the otherwise denuded surface present following conventional endarterectomy (23).

Routine use of saphenous vein patch grafts has been advocated during carotid endarterectomy to reduce the incidence of postoperative restenosis, which has ranged from 1% to 49% in reported series (24–27). Sundt regularly employed saphenous vein interposition grafts with excellent success (9,23). He believed that the vein angioplasty enlarged the endarterectomized segment and improved the blood flow in this region of the carotid bifurcation. It has been postulated that the saphenous vein interposition graft reorients the configuration of the bifurcation. Consequently, the ICA becomes the primary extension of the common carotid artery, improving the rheologic characteristics at the operative site (23).

A saphenous vein interposition graft may be most beneficial in the immediate postoperative period, when the potential for thrombosis is highest. Little et al compared early postoperative intravenous digital subtraction angiograms of 70 cases of carotid endarterectomies with primary closure to 50 patients who underwent saphenous vein interposition graft endarterectomy. By postoperative angiography, the ICA was consistently larger and the incidence of postoperative thrombosis at the operative site was less in the 50 patients treated with saphenous vein interposition graft endarterectomy. In the conventional endarterectomy group, four patients had ICA occlusions; two patients had internal, external, and common carotid artery occlusions; and nine patients had various degrees of ICA stenosis. No patients with saphenous vein interposition graft had postoperative occlusion and only two had stenosis. In the conventional endarterectomy patients with postoperative occlusions who underwent reexplorations, thrombosis was revealed in the angiographically nonvisualized arteries, but no obvious causes were found. Overall, of the six patients in the conventional endarterectomy group, three had cerebral infarctions that were the main cause of postoperative morbidity. With no occlusions present in the saphenous vein interposition graft endarterectomy patients, the difference was statistically significant and led the authors to recommend the routine use of saphenous vein interposition graft. In this study, the surgical microscope was not used and heparinization was neutralized at the end of the procedure (28).

Other authors have reported similar encouraging benefits from the routine use of a saphenous vein interposition graft, believing that it prevents early thrombosis and late recurrent stenosis (23–25,29,30). However, Rosenthal et al retrospectively studied 1000 consecutive patients who underwent endarterectomy. The patients were divided into four equal groups: 250 patients had a conventional endarterectomy closure, 250 had an expanded polytetrafluoroethylene patch, 250 had a Dacron patch, and 250 had saphenous vein interposition graft. Postoperative patency was documented by B-mode ultrasonography. The difference in the incidence of early or late postoperative stroke and restenosis was not statistically significant among the various methods of arterial closure. The authors recommended saphenous vein interposition graft angioplasty for patients with small arteries and for habitual smokers (36).

By contrast, Hans reported a series of 90 carotid endarterectomies using saphenous vein interposition graft. He performed arteriography at both intermediate (21 months) and late (55 months) follow-up periods. He documented recurrent stenosis in three patients and carotid occlusion in five patients at the intermediate follow-up and recurrent stenosis

in an additional three patients at the late follow-up. He thus concluded that saphenous vein interposition graft did not uniformly prevent either early or late postoperative carotid stenosis (21).

Studies have supported both primary suture closure for endarterectomy or saphenous vein interposition graft. The consensus suggests that specific groups of patients may benefit most from saphenous vein interposition grafts: patients undergoing reoperation for postoperative recurrent carotid stenosis, patients with an unusually small ICA (primarily women), patients who have had cervical radiation treatments, patients who are habitual heavy smokers, and patients whose external arterial walls hold sutures poorly.

A saphenous vein interposition graft does, however, have disadvantages. It increases operative and carotid cross-clamp time because two suture lines are required. Postoperatively, the angioplasty segment can balloon, slowing blood flow or causing eddy currents. Such a blood flow pathway can predispose the patient to the formation of mural thrombi and pseudoaneurysms. Vital lower extremity veins, which may later be needed for other arterial reconstruction (eg, coronary artery bypass) procedures, are often utilized and thus sacrificed. The most dreaded complication of saphenous vein interposition graft angioplasty is rupture of the vein patch, which has been reported in 0.4–4.0% of patients. This catastrophic event most often occurs in the first few days after the procedure. Its incidence is increased with hypertension. The associated morbidity and mortality rates, which are high, follow hemorrhagic shock, cerebral ischemia, or airway compression (29,32–34).

Our experience suggests that the routine use of saphenous vein interposition graft is unnecessary for microsurgical carotid endarterectomy (4,15). Although not regularly performed in our patients, postoperative angiography has demonstrated a slight enlargement, not a narrowing, of the endarterectomized segment. Our low symptomatic early stroke rate of 1% suggests that postoperative patency rates are excellent. It is doubtful that these rates could be improved by saphenous vein interposition graft or synthetic graft angioplasty (4). We do recommend saphenous vein interposition graft in operations for recurrent carotid stenosis and in extraordinary circumstances such as after cervical radiation for malignancy.

Intraoperative Carotid Shunt

An area of great discordance is the indication for placement of a carotid artery shunt during the period of carotid cross-clamping. Many surgeons have believed that the cerebral ischemia induced during the period of carotid cross-clamping is the primary reason for the morbidity associated with the procedure of carotid endarterectomy. Others believe that embolic rather than hemodynamic events cause most cerebral ischemic episodes during carotid endarterectomy. Many surgeons have reported excellent results with the use of intraluminal shunting, believing that the hemodynamic intolerance to carotid cross-clamping is very common (35, 36).

Various criteria have been used during carotid endarterectomy to help determine the need for shunt placement. Sundt et al measured intraoperative regional cerebral blood flow using extracranial detection of intraarterially injected xenon-133. Their protocol employed shunt insertion for all patients with occlusion flow of <18 ml/100 g/min. They concluded that with intraoperative carotid occlusion the critical regional cerebral blood flow is approximately 15 ml/100 g/min. Blood flow <10 ml/100 g/min during occlusion, which was seen in 8% of their patients, always produced rapid changes in the EEG pattern (23). Intraoperative measurement of CES stump pressures has also been used as an indication for shunting, with significant ischemia believed to occur with a mean blood pressure of <25 mm Hg (37).

The use of intraoperative temporary carotid shunting does have risk (Fig. 3). Many believe that a shunt can produce more problems than benefits. An intraluminal shunt has several major drawbacks. First, the shunt may allow the embolization of atherosclerotic debris, thrombotic material, or air into the distal cerebral circulation. This phenomenon is often unrecognized by the surgeon until it is detected by changes in the EEG or by a signal change on TCD. At that point, sometimes little can be done to stop further embolization by this route or to reverse the damaging cerebral effects. It also often undoubtedly occurs without detection. Second, when inserted into either the common carotid artery or the distal ICA, the shunt can injure the intimal surface of these vessels. Such an injury can lead to postoperative thrombosis at the operative site. Finally, the presence of a shunt severely limits the surgeon's ability to expose and dissect the atheroma, especially the distal portion. The creation of an intimal flap or the inability to recognize and repair the intima or to re-move all of the atherosclerotic debris can contribute to a poor technical outcome. This is true even when the surgical microscope, with its improved visualization, is utilized. Furthermore, significant periods of ischemia can occur when the shunt is placed and after it is withdrawn, before the arteriotomy closure is completed and carotid cross-clamping is removed. Instances of shunt occlusion and improper placement leading to potential upper extremity ischemia have also occurred (38,39).

Ott et al conducted a prospective study of 240 patients to determine the effectiveness of carotid endarterectomy performed without shunting. The incidence of perioperative stroke was 1.3% and the mortality rate was 0.64%, the latter caused by myocardial infarction in two patients. The incidence of permanent neurologic deficit compared favorably with other published series, regardless of whether shunting was used. Furthermore, none of their 102 patients who had either partial or complete occlusion of the contralateral ICA experienced a postoperative stroke (33).

Bland and Lazar reported a series of 280 consecutive carotid endarterectomies performed without using EEG monitoring or an intraluminal shunt. A third of their patients had contralateral stenosis or ICA occlusion. They believed that adequate cerebral protection was provided by general anesthesia and moderate induced hypertension. Their carotid occlusion time, however, was an average of only 10 minutes. They reported no operative mortality, no strokes in the immediate postoperative period, and only three (1.1%) strokes during the first postoperative month. They concluded that intraluminal shunts and intraoperative monitoring such as EEG and carotid stump pressures are unnecessary, reinforcing the concept that most intraoperative strokes during carotid endarterectomy are embolic in origin (41). In 282 consecutive carotid endarterectomies, Ferguson et al reported that intraoperative stroke occurred in four (1.4%) patients,

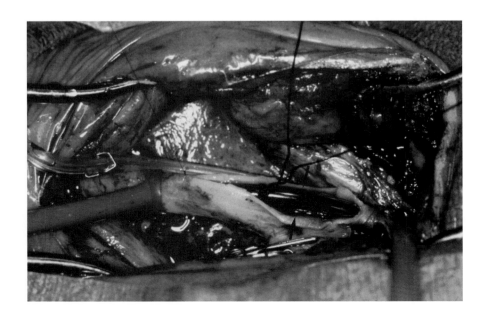

FIG. 3. An intraluminal (Sundt) shunt *(arrow)* provides ipsilateral hemispheric blood supply during endarterectomy but was inserted only following asymmetry developing on EEG. It is always best to complete at least the distal plaque removal prior to shunt insertion; otherwise the poor visualization may compromise the technical results.

all of whom were in a small subgroup with major EEG changes and a mean carotid stump pressure of <25 mm Hg. They concluded that this subgroup of patients is at high risk for hemodynamic stroke and could benefit from shunting (42).

Halsey reported a multicenter, retrospective study of 1495 carotid endarterectomy patients in which EEG, regional cerebral blood flow, and TCD were used to determine the ischemic threshold during the period of carotid cross-clamping. The routine use of carotid shunting offered no benefit in neurologic outcome, and he concluded that intraoperative monitoring (TCD <40% of baseline flow velocities) could be used to determine the need for selective shunt placement (35). Sandmann and colleagues (31) conducted a multicenter, randomized, prospective study in 503 patients to assess the need for or benefit of routine carotid shunting during endarterectomy. Their overall stroke rate was 4.0%, with the incidence of perioperative stroke not differing significantly between patients who were routinely shunted (4.2%) and those whose endarterectomy was performed without a shunt (3.3%).

Carotid shunting is an answer to only one problem associated with carotid endarterectomy, ie, cerebral hemodynamic insufficiency. Many other factors, eg, technical, embolic, thrombotic, anesthetic, systemic, and the surgeon's experience, play a major role along with global cerebral blood flow (31). It is believed that a small subpopulation of carotid endarterectomy patients exists in whom temporary carotid artery occlusion will cause hemispheric hypoperfusion that will result in cerebral infarction, which is correctable by shunt placement. Many patients, however, will respond to moderate induced hypertension, which increases collateral flow. We use a major change in EEG and, more recently, in TCD (mean ipsilateral MCA velocity reduced to less than one third of the preocclusion value) as indications for selective carotid intraluminal shunting (5) if there is no response to induced hypertension (Fig. 4). A recent series by Jansen et al claimed that TCD may be more sensitive than EEG in detecting subcortical ischemia and embolic phenomena (43).

Since instituting this criterion, about 7% of our patients have required intraoperative shunts. None of these patients has experienced a permanent cerebrovascular accident postoperatively. EEG monitoring should be used, and it predicts postoperative deficits (26,44) more accurately than TCD criteria alone, especially when cerebroprotective agents are circulated.

Operating Microscope

The operating microscope, which has revolutionized neurologic surgery with its unparalleled lighting, visualization, and wide range of magnification, is the cornerstone of microsurgical carotid endarterectomy. The size of the operating field can be varied by as much as 12 times that of ordinary operating surgical loupes. The ability to zoom to higher magnification to inspect fine details and to retreat to low degrees of magnification for portions of the procedure, such as tying sutures, makes this flexible instrument a mainstay in our surgical protocol. In addition, the operating microscope provides excellent illumination, even in the depths of a wound and in the intraluminal area of the carotid artery. The operating microscope is usually employed once the gross portion of the atheromatous plaque and intraluminal thrombotic material has been removed. If difficult, ulcerated, or indistinct plaques, the microscope can facilitate dissection in the correct plane. Remaining portions of the atheromatous material are best removed under higher power. The view is unequaled and the luminal surface can be assessed in detail (Fig. 5).

Findlay and Lougheed described their technique and results in 60 consecutive patients with symptomatic carotid stenosis who underwent microsurgical carotid endarterectomy. Only one (1.7%) patient suffered a perioperative stroke after common carotid artery occlusion, without an obvious cause. With an average follow-up of 18 months, no patient experienced a postoperative hemorrhagic or ischemic stroke. They believed that using the surgical microscope helped to minimize difficulties with the surgical technique (45). The benefits of the surgical microscope in the performance of carotid endarterectomy have also been emphasized by other neurosurgeons (44,46–48). A previously reported series from the Barrow Neurologic Institute included 200 consecutive endarterectomies performed in 180 patients using a defined protocol of microsurgical endarterectomy. Barbiturate protection was used during carotid cross-clamping, the period of potential focal cerebral ischemia. The protocol also included preoperative antiplatelet therapy, barbiturate anesthesia, routine avoidance of an internal shunt, and strict postoperative control of blood pressure. On the fifth postoperative day, one patient died from a hypertensive cerebral hemorrhage and two patients suffered postoperative cerebrovascular accidents. The combined permanent morbidity and mortality rate was 1.5% (48). Results of our larger series have upheld our opinion that using the operative microscope greatly improves the technical result and ultimate clinical outcome of carotid endarterectomy (4). The utility of the operating microscope and its ability to improve the manipulation of the diseased artery is highlighted when one realizes that embolic events and technical errors are probably the two leading causes of neurologic morbidity with carotid endarterectomy.

Technical failures were found in the series of Rosenthal et al in two thirds of the postoperative strokes. The causes were intimal flaps, lateral carotid tears, or carotid clamp injury. The remaining strokes were caused by embolic occlusion of intracranial vessels (36). Moore described three patients who developed postoperative neurologic deficits from thromboembolic propagation that originated from an external carotid artery intimal flap. Thrombotic material accumulated in the external carotid artery and passed through the ICA into the cerebral distribution. This report emphasizes

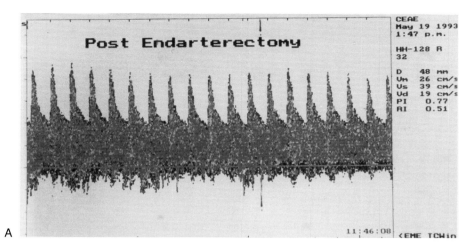

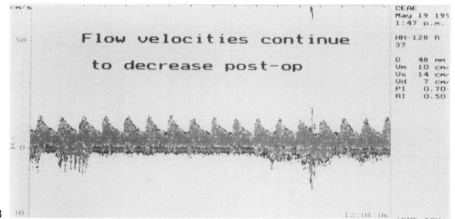

FIG. 4. Transcranial Doppler spectrum illustrating **(A)** a normal postendarterectomy flow initially after completion of the procedure. In the recovery room, the patient **(B)** had continued diminishment in flow velocities that were indicative of an acute thrombus at the operative site.

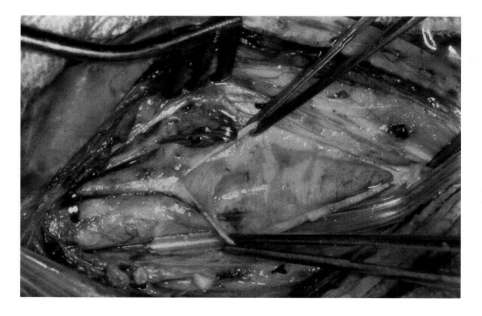

FIG. 5. Luminal view of the carotid artery following plaque resection, as seen through the operating microscope. With magnification and lighting superior to other methods, the intimal surface is inspected for remaining plaque material, intimal flaps of the distal internal carotid artery, or proximal origin of the external carotid artery on an improper dissection plane into the arterial wall.

the potential of interaction between the external carotid circulation and the intracranial circulation (49).

Magnification and illumination provided by the operating microscope improves the ability to inspect the luminal surface of both the external and internal carotid arteries. Blaisdell reported that after routine utilization of intraoperative angiography, approximately 25% of the endarterectomized carotid arteries demonstrated a significant technical abnormality that would not have been noted without angiography. They believed that correction of these deficits at the time of the angiography resulted in a 100% late patency rate in their endarterectomy series (50).

OPERATIVE ANATOMY AND EXPOSURE FOR CAROTID ENDARTERECTOMY

For carotid endarterectomy, the patient is positioned supine with the head turned slightly to the contralateral side. A towel roll may be placed in the interscapular area to permit cervical extension and to improve deep exposure. Care must be taken during the surgical prep to minimize the likelihood of mechanical dislodgement of atheromatous or thrombotic debris.

The surgical incision begins about 2 finger widths above the clavicle and sternal notch along the anterior border of the sternocleidomastoid muscle and proceeds superiorly until it approaches the angle of the mandible (Fig. 6). Further cephalad exposure is attained by gently curving the incision posteriorly toward the mastoid tip. Directing the incision away from the side of the cheek improves cosmesis and avoids injury to the branches of the facial nerve.

Operative planning is facilitated by review of the angiogram to ascertain the location of the carotid bifurcation as well as the level and extent of the carotid lesion, which are noted in relation to the cervical vertebral bodies and mandibular angle. When the bifurcation is unusually high or low, the incision should be adjusted accordingly. A submandibular incision 1 cm below and parallel to the lower mandibular margin and a zigzag incision along the anterior border of the sternocleidomastoid muscle are alternatives that can also improve cosmesis. These incisions, however, require developing wide skin flaps and do not offer as good exposure, particularly proximally on the common carotid. The incision along the anterior edge of the sternocleidomastoid is preferred and gives fully acceptable cosmetic results, especially with subcuticular suture closure.

The dissection next proceeds through the subcutaneous tissues and platysma along the medial border of the sternocleidomastoid. Hemostasis from the skin incision down to the carotid artery must be complete and meticulous because heparinization is not reversed at the end of the procedure. Oozing commonly occurs from the dermis following heparinization. The loose areolar tissue, which adheres the sternocleidomastoid to the strap muscles overlying the trachea, is dissected. A deep, self-retaining retractor or retaining sutures

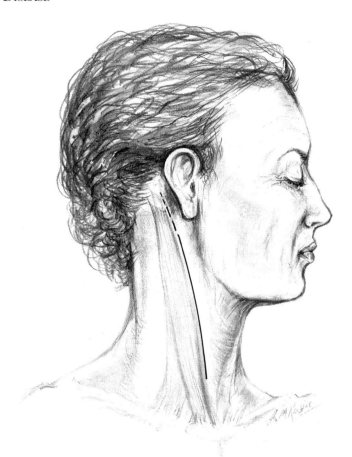

FIG. 6. The standard incision for carotid endarterectomy begins along the medial border of the sternocleidomastoid approximately 1 in. above the clavicle and proceeds superiorly as judged by the angiographic appearance and location of the lesion. For an unusually high bifurcation or lesion, the incision may be extended behind the ear for cosmesis and to avoid the facial nerve *(dotted line)*.

are placed to expose the carotid sheath. The common carotid artery pulse can serve as a guide to the proper dissection plane.

Several nerves are in the vicinity of the exposure, superficial to the sternocleidomastoid muscle. The great auricular nerve crosses obliquely over the sternocleidomastoid toward the posterior auricular region and mandibular angle. The lesser occipital nerve courses across the posterior sternocleidomastoid attachment to the occipital and mastoid regions. The spinal accessory nerve runs on the posterior aspect of the sternocleidomastoid across the posterior triangle to innervate the trapezius muscle. A cervical branch of the facial nerve runs deep to the platysma. By maintaining the dissection in the correct plane, these nerves will not typically be encountered or injured during the endarterectomy. Often, however, the transverse cervical nerve, which crosses the midbelly of the sternocleidomastoid, is transected. This often results in transient numbness in the anterior neck. Regeneration, however, typically occurs and the numbness disappears by 6 months. It is important to avoid placing a self-retaining retractor in a deep plane medially due to the likelihood of nerve injury.

As the dissection proceeds posteriorly lymph nodes are often present. These are best handled by medial dissection and lateral deflection. In the upper end of the incision, the parotid gland may be recognized by its lobulated architecture and pale color compared with subcutaneous adipose tissue. The carotid sheath is opened with sharp dissection and careful bipolar coagulation of any small vessels within the fibrous sheath. The common carotid artery, located in the proximal region of the dissection posteromedial to the internal jugular vein, is exposed first. The vagus nerve usually is situated dorsal to the vessels within the carotid sheath. The internal jugular vein must be mobilized, which often requires dividing medial venous tributaries, the largest of which is usually the common facial vein located near the carotid bifurcation. Access to the carotid bifurcation and ICA is best facilitated by reflecting the internal jugular laterally.

The proximal extent of the exposure is usually the omohyoid muscle. This muscle may be divided partially or completely to attain adequate access to the common carotid; however, this is rarely necessary. Occasionally, as the dissection proceeds cephalad, the ansa cervicalis is encountered. It is composed of an inferior division, which originates from the ventral rami of the second and third cervical nerves, and a superior division, which descends from the hypoglossal nerve and connects with the inferior division after the latter courses over the internal jugular vein. Dividing the descending limb of the ansa gives improved access to the carotid artery. This maneuver also will shift the hypoglossal nerve medially and slightly superiorly away from the carotid bifurcation, but is not performed unless necessary. The carotid bifurcation is most often located at the level of the thyroid cartilage. In about 20% of the cases, however, it bifurcates between the thyroid cartilage and the hyoid bone. Rarely, the bifurcation is below the thyroid cartilage; or the common carotid artery is absent, and the internal and external carotid arteries originate directly from the aortic arch or the innominate artery. These details are discernible on the preoperative angiogram and should be considered during the preoperative planning stage.

The common carotid artery typically possesses no branches, although the superior thyroid artery often may originate within 2 cm proximal to the carotid bifurcation. When the superior thyroid artery is dissected for temporary clipping, its posterior aspect—a location where the superior laryngeal nerve may be injured—should be avoided. The carotid body is ovoid, usually <5 mm, and is situated immediately dorsal to the carotid bifurcation. Its chemoreceptor elements form a portion of the visceral afferent system innervated by the vagus nerve.

The routine injection of local anesthetic into the carotid body to avoid reflexive bradycardia and hypotension is often advocated. However, experience has shown that a carotid body injection does not significantly affect the patient's cardiovascular response, and consequently this technique is not ordinarily employed. If, however, the anesthesiologist notes any hemodynamically significant changes during dissection or handling of this area, the physiologic effects may be blocked temporarily with an injection of 1% lidocaine.

The distal ICA must be dissected, usually 3–5 cm distal to the bifurcation, depending on the extent of the carotid plaque. This distal exposure is readily gained by dissecting laterally and superiorly to the hypoglossal nerve. Leaving the areolar connective tissue attached on the medial side will tend to pull the hypoglossal nerve somewhat medially and superiorly as desired. Occasionally, distal exposure is improved by careful placement of retraction sutures in the medial connective tissue or perineurium of the hypoglossal nerve or by dividing or incising the digastric muscle.

Often an external carotid branch to the sternocleidomastoid muscle, accompanied by a vein, will be encountered and must be divided. Rarely, this structure, together with the twelfth nerve, has been the source of carotid compression, the so-called "carotid sling." More complex maneuvers for distal exposure, such as osteotomy of the mandibular ramus, are not ordinarily necessary. Careful and deliberate dissection along the distal ICA, working lateral to the hypoglossal nerve, ordinarily provides adequate cephalad exposure. The adventitial layer, which must be included within the arteriotomy closure, should be avoided. Small venous tributaries of the internal jugular vein, which are often encountered in this area, can readily be handled by bipolar coagulation or suture ligation. The external carotid artery is dissected for about 2 cm beyond the bifurcation. Exposure is necessary only to guarantee vascular control and sufficient space for temporary clipping.

Once the exposure is completed, the carotid artery is inspected for the extent of the plaque. The plaque is usually yellow tinged compared with the gray walls of a healthy carotid artery. The step-off transition zone at the distal end of the lesion can be gently palpated with a moistened gloved finger. This intraoperative judgment is combined with the preoperative angiographic data to confirm plaque location, placement of the arteriotomy, and adequacy of proximal and distal dissection and thus vascular control.

At this junction in the procedure, the patient undergoes full systemic heparinization by an anesthesiologist who administers 100 IU/kg intravenously or, alternatively, a standard adult dose of 5000 IU. Cerebral protection is attained by placing the patient in 15- to 30-second electroencephalographic burst suppression, usually with bolus doses of thiopental (150–250 mg). Patients with considerable myocardial dysfunction receive an intravenous bolus loading dose of etomidate (0.4–0.5 mg/kg) and then 0.1 mg/kg to maintain burst suppression. During infusion of these agents, and particularly during carotid cross-clamping when a moderate degree of hypertension is desired to optimize collateral cerebral blood flow, blood pressure must be controlled carefully.

Phenylephrine infusion may be required to maintain systemic blood pressure in the desired range.

With stable blood pressure and the EEG, the distal ICA is occluded with a temporary aneurysm clip. This initial maneuver prevents any cerebral embolization of plaque or thrombotic material as the vessels are occluded. The proximal common carotid artery is immediately occluded with a 45° angled DeBakey vascular clamp, tightened only enough to prevent hemorrhage. The external carotid and superior thyroid arteries are closed using temporary aneurysm clips. For ultimate proximal vascular control, a vascular loop with a rubber tubing occluder (Rummell tourniquet) can be placed proximal to the DeBakey clamp. When encircling tapes are placed for occlusion, the vessel should be dissected from its underlying soft tissue only where the tape is to be passed. Otherwise, troublesome oozing can occur from the relatively inaccessible back wall, especially once heparinization is performed.

Using the angiographic data to judge the proximal extent of the lesion, the common carotid artery is incised, usually about 2 cm proximal to the carotid bifurcation (Fig. 7). The incision must completely penetrate through the plaque and proceed into the carotid lumen, extending about 5 mm in length. Otherwise, the muscularis layer may contract and, together with the adventitial layer, occlude the incision. An angled Pott's scissors is used to extend the arteriotomy cephalad into the ICA until the distal extent of the atherosclerotic plaque is passed. Care must be taken to extend the arteriotomy down the center axis of the ICA. The closure will be more difficult if the arteriotomy veers either medially into the region of the bifurcation or laterally on the vessel. Especially in tightly stenotic carotid arteries, it is important that the lower blade of the scissors seek and follow the remaining luminal channel. The surgeon should learn and appreciate a proprioceptive feel with the bottom blade of the Pott's scissors.

The endarterectomy is performed using two microsurgical dissectors, which are used to find the cleavage plane between the atherosclerotic plaque and the arterial wall (Fig. 8). However, the characteristics of these lesions vary. They usually begin in the distal common carotid artery, are thickest in the anterolateral position of the carotid sinus, and thin distally after considerable involvement at the ICA origin. Typically, the atherosclerotic plaque is first separated from the arterial wall in the common carotid artery using the dissectors to pass along the back or dorsal wall of the artery. The plaque is incised at its proximal end and lifted superiorly as the plaque–media interface is dissected in a distal direction into the ICA (Fig. 9). The back wall must not be injured nor should the media be dissected through the adventitial layer, which can be identified by its pinkish coloration.

The external carotid plaque is removed by an eversion technique that circumferentially dissected the plaque off the artery. Simultaneously, the external carotid artery is grasped with forceps and pulled away from the atheroma. Removal of this external carotid plaque can be assisted by briefly opening the temporary clip, allowing the tail of the lesion to be removed. This is often required when a calcified portion of the plaque involves the proximal external carotid artery. If required to remove residual plaque or a potential intimal plaque, a separate external carotid incision and endarterectomy should be performed.

The critical portion of plaque removal is that portion within the distal ICA. This provides the leading edge of the plaque–vessel interface, which may lead to formation of an intimal flap and postoperative thrombosis. Gentle elevation and traction of the plaque will often cause it to break with an even contour or a feathering effect at the distal ICA transition

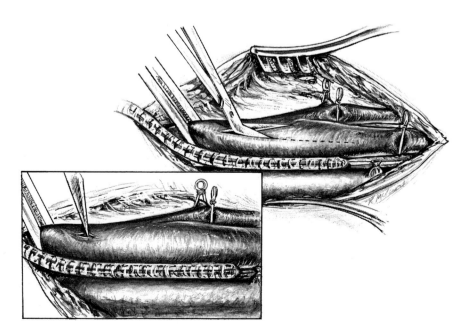

FIG. 7. After the vessels have been prepared, a vascular clamp occludes the common carotid artery and temporary aneurysm clips occlude the superior thyroid, external and internal carotid arteries. A 5-mm incision is made with an 11-blade scalpel in the common carotid artery. The arteriotomy is then extended distally into the internal carotid artery to a point beyond the plaque using angled Pott's scissors. If the arteriotomy extends too far laterally or deviates medially into the bifurcation, difficulty in closing may result.

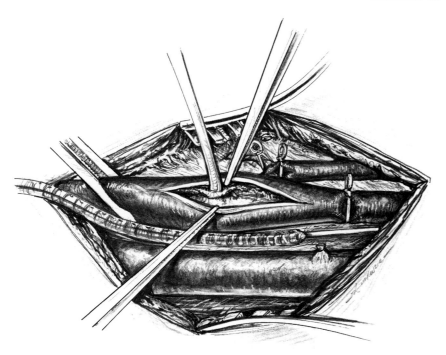

FIG. 8. Inspection is performed to visualize the correct dissection plane between the atherosclerotic plaque and the intimal surface. In difficult or indistinct lesions, this process is aided by the surgical microscope.

zone. This maneuver not only removes the remainder of the hemodynamically offending lesion but also prevents an intimal flap from developing. Often, the final cleavage of the plaque can be optimized by combining traction and eversion of the plaque as the back wall of the vessel is pushed away (Fig. 10). Transecting the plaque proximal to the end of the arteriotomy makes closure easier and avoids stenosis

of the vessel. When the vessel wall is handled, the layers of the wall should not be separated. Rather, the walls should be held together only at the edges with little pressure, using only wide-grip vascular forceps. Fine sutures also should not be picked up or pinched between the jaws of the forceps because this may cause the suture to crimp and weaken.

The operating microscope is now positioned to allow the

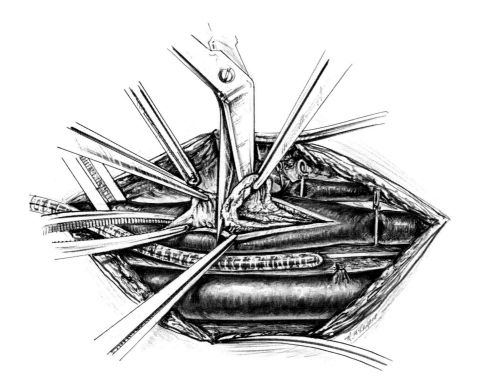

FIG. 9. The plaque is best handled by transecting it at the proximal (common carotid) end and reflecting it superiorly as dissection proceeds.

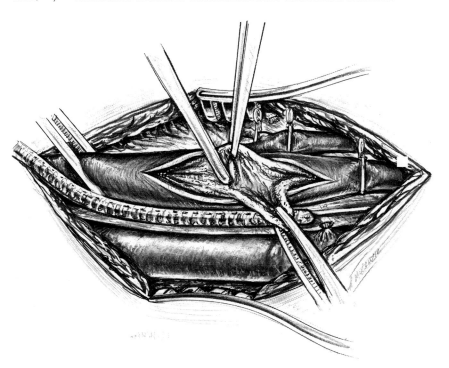

FIG. 10. The dissection is carried out meticulously using Penfield or other neurosurgical dissections. Attention must be directed to avoid creating an irregularity or intimal flap as the plaque is removed from the external carotid artery origin.

surgeon and assistant to have unimpeded binocular vision. The internal surface of the carotid artery is carefully inspected. Remaining atheromatous debris is removed, usually by circumferentially stripping it from the intimal surface. Continuous heparinized saline (1000 IU/L) irrigation of the luminal surface is performed. Small fragments of plaque filaments are likewise removed. The arterial surface is inspected proximally but especially distally, where thrombosis-causing intimal flaps are usually located (Fig. 11). Rarely, there is an abrupt transition zone in the distal ICA,

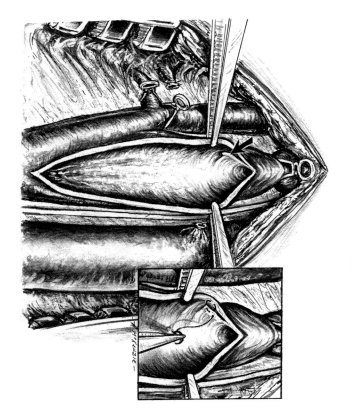

FIG. 11. Following plaque removal, careful inspection through the microscope is performed to exclude the creation of an initial flap. The best technical result is obtained by gently pulling the internal carotid plaque with constant tension while dissection at the plaque–intima interface is carried out. This usually results in a feathered transition zone. Any significant intimal flap *(arrow)* should be secured with 8-0 nylon tacking sutures.

or, if the intima adheres loosely to the media, interrupted 8-0 monofilament (nylon) tacking sutures should be placed. The luminal surface is inspected in detail using the superior lighting and magnification afforded by the operating microscope (see Fig. 5).

Shunting is not performed routinely and is reserved for patients who experience major EEG changes that cannot be reversed by inducing moderate hypertension (vide infra). Both internal (eg, Sundt) and external (eg, Javid) shunts have been used successfully. Recent experience over the last several years has shown that only 6% of our patients have required shunting (4).

Closure

Beginning distally, the arteriotomy is closed with a continuous 6-0 monofilament (Prolene) suture to below the bifurcation. Another 6-0 monofilament is used starting proximally on the common carotid artery, and the two joined. Alternatively, a single 6-0 suture may be used to close from distal to proximal, which is an easier and preferred method. When the arteriotomy is almost complete and prior to tying the two sutures, back-bleeding of the internal and external carotid arteries is accomplished by briefly opening the temporary aneurysm clips. The quality and extent of the back bleeding from the ICA is important. Poor or no flow often indicates thrombosis at or distal to the operative site. This requires immediate reexploration and is usually caused by an unrecognized or insufficiently repaired intimal flap. Al-

ternatively, a suture grabbing both the anterior and posterior walls of the artery may be responsible. The superior vision afforded by the operating microscope, however, has made this technical mistake exceedingly rare. In our experience, it occurs significantly <1% of the time. Failure to restore acceptable back-flow once the sutures are removed implies distal ICA thrombosis and may necessitate balloon catheter or suction thrombectomy, intraoperative angiography, or intraarterial thrombolysis.

The common carotid clamp is also opened momentarily to permit any thrombotic or atheromatous material to be expelled through the open lumen. The superior thyroid artery clip is removed permanently. Consequently, the slow, continuous back-bleeding pushes trapped air out through the arteriotomy opening or through the small spaces between the sutures. All microsutures must be handled delicately, and crimping must be avoided. Multiple throws are required to hold the knot of this suture (Fig. 12). Including only 1 or 2 mm of the cut edge of the artery permits only small bites with each suture to avoid kinking of the vessel (Fig. 13). Postoperative angiographic evaluation has shown that there is consistently no ICA stenosis with the microsurgical closure (Fig. 14).

Following arteriotomy closure, the vessels are opened in a specific order (Fig. 15). The external carotid artery is opened first. The common carotid clamp is opened temporarily to permit atheromatous debris, thrombotic material, or air to wash up the external carotid artery distribution and away from the hemispheric or retinal blood supply. Next, the ICA clip is released momentarily to allow any debris accumulated

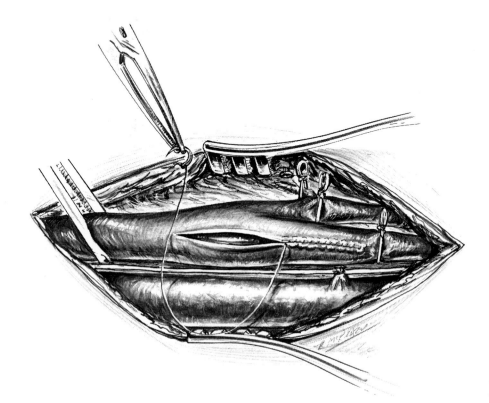

FIG. 12. Closure is easiest and most efficiently effected by running a 6-0 prolene suture from distally to proximally. The routine use of two sutures or patch grafts is not necessary with the microsurgical technique.

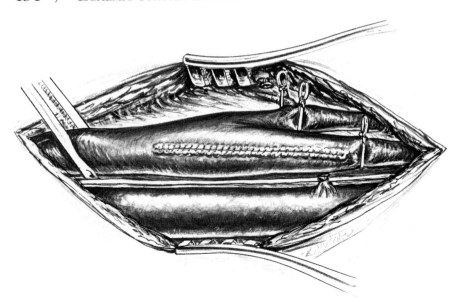

FIG. 13. The microsurgical closure includes just the edge of the vessel, causing no narrowing and markedly reducing the incidence of subsequent carotid restenosis.

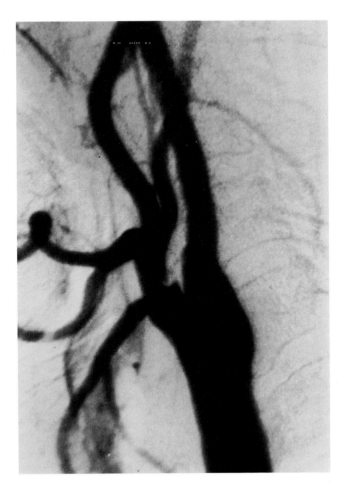

FIG. 14. Postoperative carotid angiogram following microsurgical endarterectomy demonstrates relief of the stenotic lesion without iatrogenic narrowing.

between the endarterectomy site and the distal ICA clip to travel by retrograde flow into the external carotid system. The first maneuver with opening both the external and common carotid arteries is repeated. The common carotid clamp is then permanently removed, finally restoring anterograde flow through the ICA.

The arteriotomy suture line should be hemostatic except for slight oozing through needle holes or between sutures. Any source of pumping blood or area that does not immediately stop is closed with single, interrupted 6-0 monofilament sutures. Surgicel may be placed as a monolayer over the arteriotomy. Complete hemostasis is attained, and a topical hemostatic agent (Avitene) may be applied to the wound after copious irrigation with a topical antibiotic solution. The blood pressure is brought to or very near normal to avoid hypertension-induced intracerebral hemorrhage in a dysautoregulated cerebral hemisphere. The systemic heparinization is not reversed. The wound is closed in two layers with absorbable sutures and sterile strips are used for the skin.

In the recovery room and during the patient's first overnight stay, blood pressure must be strictly controlled to avoid hypertension. Hypertension can lead to intracerebral hemorrhage, especially following the reopening of tightly stenotic lesions. In these patients, it is believed that the ipsilateral cerebral hemisphere is likely to have faulty autoregulation. Conversely, hypotension can promote thrombosis at the operative site and should be avoided. Aspirin (650 mg) is administered rectally in the recovery room and then orally each day for an indefinite period. Routine antibiotics are administered for 24 hours.

Invasive cardiac or other monitoring is performed postoperatively as indicated. Many patients who receive intraoperative barbiturates for cerebral protection may experience postoperative respiratory depression, neurologic depression, or both. Usually these effects diminish rapidly. Even when pa-

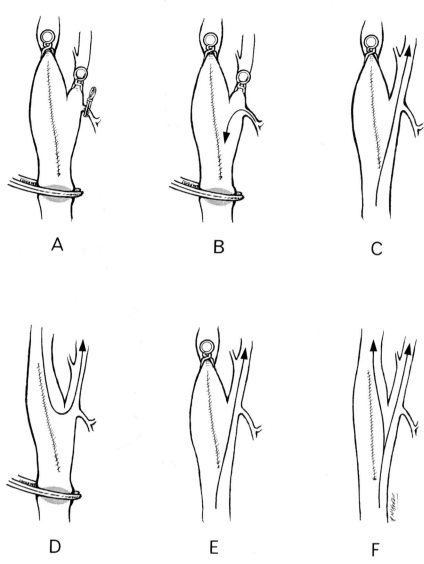

A   B   C

D   E   F

FIG. 15. Following arteriotomy completion, deocclusion is best accomplished by the following method. **A:** Careful attention is paid so that the suture line is not handled with forceps and any bipolar coagulation of adventitial bleeding points does not occur near the sutures. **B:** The temporary aneurysm clip on the superior thyroid artery has been previously removed just prior to arteriotomy closure, which causes a constant, low-volume blood backflow through the arteriotomy site. This helps to maintain a full column of fluid and to expel air bubbles. **C:** The external carotid artery is opened to allow any trapped thrombotic or atherosclerotic debris as well as air bubbles caused by retrograde flow to be at least partially removed through the arteriotomy. In addition, this retrograde flow will often reveal any sources of significant leaks in the arteriotomy closure. With the internal carotid artery still occluded by a temporary aneurysm clip, the vascular clamp on the common carotid artery is opened, allowing a few moments for blood and any proximal debris to flow out through the external carotid system. **D:** With the proximal common carotid artery again temporarily occluded, the clip on the distal internal carotid artery is released, allowing any debris distal to the internal carotid clip to travel back into the external carotid artery by retrograde flow. **E:** The maneuver in C is then briefly repeated. **F:** All clips are removed and the common carotid artery is opened, establishing antegrade internal carotid artery flow. Transcranial Doppler monitoring has shown in our experience that embolization into the cerebral circulation is markedly diminished or eliminated by use of these maneuvers.

tients are deeply pharmacologically obtunded, brainstem reflexes are intact and meaningful movement or a withdrawal pattern to painful stimuli can be seen. Consequently, a basic examination can ordinarily detect focal or localizing findings even at this stage. In the occasional patient who is initially deeply sedated upon arrival at the recovery room, EEG or TCD monitoring may be continued until a neurologic examination becomes possible. Of all the methods of postoperative monitoring, TCD gives the earliest warning of impending carotid occlusion by showing a marked decline in ipsilateral flow velocities. Often, TCD findings significantly precede other methods of detection, even the clinical neurologic examination, especially in a patient just emerging from a general anesthetic.

Postoperative Care

The postoperative treatment of patients with carotid endarterectomy follows the guidelines for routine postoperative care, but several important aspects are given special consideration. Careful cardiac monitoring and assessment of the patient's cardiac clinical status are stressed in the immediate postoperative period.

In the past, patients were usually maintained in the intensive care unit (ICU) for at least 24 hours after endarterectomy. Recent advances have shown that routine ICU admissions may not be necessary in many patients. Having patients maintain their oral medications, especially cardiac and hypertensive agents the night prior to surgery and the morning of surgery (with a sip of water), seems to provide much more stable blood pressure postoperatively. Other maneuvers, such as optimizing medical conditions preoperatively and utilizing regional anesthesia, appear to increase the number of patients who do not require postoperative ICU care and reduces the overall length of the hospital stay (51). Invasive monitoring (eg, arterial blood pressure lines, Swan–Ganz catheters, central venous pressure catheters, saturation monitors) are utilized as indicated in selected patients. Patients who have received significant doses of intraoperative barbiturate (usually >1 g of thiopental) are subject to postoperative respiratory depression. This effect usually resolves in several hours. An occasional patient may require intubation and ventilation overnight and often are managed by consulting with specialists in intensive care medicine. Although deep vein thrombosis prophylaxis therapy (subcutaneous heparin) is considered safe for use in the postoperative period, we only use it to treat patients considered to be at high risk.

Patients are mobilized early in the postoperative period and allowed out of bed on the first postoperative day if their general and cardiac conditions permit. If patients are otherwise stable, they are transferred from the intensive care unit to a regular care bed on the first postoperative day. Postoperative antiplatelet therapy is continued indefinitely (650 mg aspirin daily), and the patient is allowed a general diet and full ambulatory activity.

During the next 2 days, blood pressure must be monitored closely, particularly as patients become fully ambulatory. Postoperative hypertension, even if mild, should be considered for aggressive treatment. Early postoperative hypertension, especially in patients with preoperative tight carotid stenotic lesions, may predispose patients to postoperative intracerebral hemorrhage. Symptoms such as severe ipsilateral headache, facial pain, or seizures may also herald a cerebral hyperperfusion syndrome and possible intracerebral hemorrhage. During these first postoperative days, the wound is carefully inspected for any evidence of hematoma or infection. If there are no complicating or extenuating events, the patient is usually discharged on the second or third postoperative day and followed closely as an outpatient.

CAROTID THROMBOENDARTERECTOMY

Occlusion of the ICA has often been considered to have an uncertain clinical course and natural history. Although most occlusions of the ICA are discovered incidentally and are apparently asymptomatic, those patients with associated signs and symptoms of stroke or transient ischemic attacks (TIAs) may benefit from aggressive medical and surgical management. Operative treatment is sometimes recommended for patients with acute blockages but no major neurologic deficits. In such patients, ICA occlusions can potentially be opened successfully with minimal morbidity and mortality. Patients with a chronic occlusion may have symptoms resulting from embolization from the proximal segment (stump) of the ICA.

The natural history of ICA occlusion has varied and was not clearly elucidated by some of the earlier literature. In several retrospective series, the incidence of subsequent stroke or TIAs after complete ICA occlusion varied between 0 and 23% (52–54). Prospective series, which may be a more sensitive indicator when minor syndromes are considered, have found between 7% and 54% incidence of subsequent stroke, with a mean of 23.6% (55–57). In about two thirds of the patients, the strokes occurred ipsilateral to the carotid occlusion and in one third strokes were located in a contralateral distribution. Fields and Lemak (56) followed 359 patients with ICA occlusion for a mean period of 44 months. New strokes occurred in 25% of the patients and 64% of the strokes were ipsilateral to the occluded ICA. Furlan et al reported a 3% annual stroke rate following angiographically proven ICA occlusion; one third occurred on the contralateral side (53). Various other studies have shown a wide variation in the incidence of ischemia ipsilateral to an occluded ICA, ranging from 5% to 10% annual rate for stroke and approximately twice that for TIAs (55,58). Cardiac deaths are more likely to occur in the follow-up period (59).

With regard to surgical management, Meyer et al (60) described their experience with 34 patients treated with carotid thromboendarterectomy for acute ICA occlusion. All of these patients except one experienced changes in their level of consciousness and major neurologic deficits that began while they were hospitalized. Nine (26.5%) patients returned to normal, four patients (11.8%) were left hemiplegic, and seven (20.6%) died. Walters et al (61) performed emergency carotid endarterectomies in 64 patients, 16 of whom had presumed acute, complete occlusion, with some of which proved later to have pseudoocclusions. Blood flow through the ICA was reestablished in all cases. Postoperatively, 14 patients were unchanged or improved, 1 patient's neurologic status deteriorated, and 1 patient died from cardiopulmonary arrest on the 24th postoperative day.

Results with surgical thromboendarterectomy for ICA occlusion in patients who presented early and without profound deficits have been reported. This category of patients was the one most likely to benefit from surgery. Hugenholtz and Elgie (62) excluded patients with drowsiness, major neurologic deficits, and tandem lesions distal to the ICA occlusion. With these criteria, they reduced the surgical morbidity rate to 10% and the surgical mortality rate to 0% in a group of 35 patients. Using similar selection criteria in 47 patients, Hafner and Tew (59) achieved surgical mortality and neurologic morbidity rates of 0%. Kusunoki et al (63) studied two groups of patients: those with neurologic, medical, and angiographic risk factors and those without. The latter group of 14 patients had no operative mortality. Clearly, case series that excluded patients with severe neurologic deficits demonstrate that restoring blood flow in the ICA is beneficial. Despite the identification of a subgroup of patients expected to benefit from restoring blood flow through the ICA and the publication of two clinical series showing favorable surgical morbidity and mortality rates in this group, a recent poll indicated that, according to expert opinion, ICA occlusion was a contraindication to ICA surgery. In fact, after reviewing 1000 carotid endarterectomies, the responders categorized the 60 endarterectomies (6%) performed for complete ICA occlusion as inappropriate (64).

The optimal treatment of carotid occlusion, especially surgical intervention, is controversial. The controversy partially reflects the difficulties in defining the population best suited for surgical intervention and in performing prospective studies to determine the outcome of different treatment groups. There does appear to be a subgroup of patients who fare well if they can be diagnosed and treated expeditiously before significant cerebral infarction occurs. As experience with intraarterial thrombolytic therapy occurs, it is anticipated that some patients with acute ICA occlusions may benefit from such treatment. If restoration of anterograde blood flow is successful, carotid bifurcation and ICA origin angioplasty by balloon or stent techniques may be a temporizing or preferred treatment. Protection against distal propagation of thrombotic material is of obvious and paramount importance.

Technique

In patients who are candidates for thromboendarterectomy, a standard carotid endarterectomy longitudinal incision is made along the medial border of the sternocleidomastoid muscle, through the platysma muscle and cervical fascia, to expose the carotid sheath. After the carotid artery is isolated above and below the level of the bifurcation, the vessel is inspected to determine its size and external appearance. If the ICA is small, thin, and fibrotic, no attempt is made to reopen it and surgery is directed to performing a stumpectomy if otherwise indicated. Before cross-clamping the common carotid artery, thiopental sodium (145–250 mg) is administered intravenously to achieve 15- to 30-second burst suppression on the electroencephalogram (15). Dissection is then completed to expose the common, internal, and external carotid arteries. Care is used to avoid manipulating the occluded ICA.

Next a small arteriotomy is made on the lateral ICA beyond the obvious atheromatous disease. At this point, one of three phenomena occur: (a) The clot spontaneously expresses itself with good backflow. (b) The clot does not spontaneously exit and backflow is not observed. A small amount of clot exits and is followed by poor backflow (Fig. 16). In the first instance, standard cross-clamping of the vessels is performed followed by an endarterectomy. In the case of the latter two events, a no. 2 French Fogarty catheter with a 0.2-ml balloon is passed up the ICA with very gentle pressure to near (10–12 cm) the carotid siphon. The balloon is inflated with saline and gently withdrawn. In cases of acute or subacute thrombosis, especially where collateral flow has kept the distal ICA patent, it is often possible to remove the clot. Brisk bleeding from the distal ICA is then immediately encountered. After good retrograde flow is established, the distal ICA along with the common carotid artery should be rapidly occluded. The endarterectomy is then completed in the standard fashion by extension of the arteriotomy into the common carotid artery. Shunting is not recommended unless indicated by a major EEG change as described in the stan-

dard endarterectomy protocol. If the ICA could not be reopened with passing the catheter approximately three times, it is safest to discontinue the effort.

When the ICA cannot be reopened or is atretic upon inspection as described earlier, if indicated a proximal remnant angioplasty (stumpectomy) and an external carotid endarterectomy are performed. Proximal remnant angioplasty is performed by closing the ICA flush at its origin with a large vascular clip, dissecting along the posterior wall of the ICA, and transecting it from the distal portion. These maneuvers avoid angulation as flowing blood passes into the external carotid artery. This maneuver may reduce the propensity for stagnated blood, eddy currents, and embolic material to form in the area of the ICA origin.

In 1992, we reported our experience with 42 patients with symptomatic carotid occlusion (65). Clinical presentations included focal TIAs in 68%, amaurosis fugax in 28%, new fixed deficits in 28%, and stroke in evolution in 9% of patients. Forty-six operations were performed on the 42 patients, including 24 (52%) successful ICA reopenings, 9 (20%) stumpectomies with concomitant external carotid endarterectomies, and 4 (9%) of the latter who ultimately required extracranial-intracranial bypass for persistent ischemic symptoms. Three (7%) patients experienced transient surgical morbidity, one (2%) patient's hemiparesis worsened with restoration of antegrade blood flow, and there were no deaths.

Long-term arterial patency was assessed in 17 (73%) of the 24 patients. Carotid Doppler ultrasound studies were performed a mean of 28 months after surgery. In 15 (88%) of these patients, the ICAs were widely patent. Of the other two, one had more than 70% stenosis and one had reocclusion.

Three patients were lost to follow-up, which for the remaining 39 patients was an average of 40 months after their last operation. Five (13%) patients died, two of cancer and three of myocardial infarction. Four (10%) patients experienced neurologic events: TIAs in two and vertebrobasilar insufficiency in two. Six (15%) patients had new myocardial infarctions of new-onset angina. The outcome for patients with successful restoration of ICA flow as not significantly different from that of patients who were treated until asymptomatic with the alternative surgical strategies described. No patient had a subsequent stroke during the follow-up period, and the rates for neurologic transient events (TIAs and vertebrobasilar insufficiency) for both groups were comparable with the expected natural history for completed stroke in nonsurgically treated patients.

These data further strengthen the conclusion that a subgroup of patients chosen primarily from their presenting neurologic examination will have low surgical morbidity and mortality rates from restoration of ICA flow. The issue of timing of surgery remains unclear. The precise timing between ICA occlusion and attempted restoration of flow is known in few series. These include postangiographic or postsurgical occlusions that represent a pathophysiology other than spontaneous occlusion associated with atheroscle-

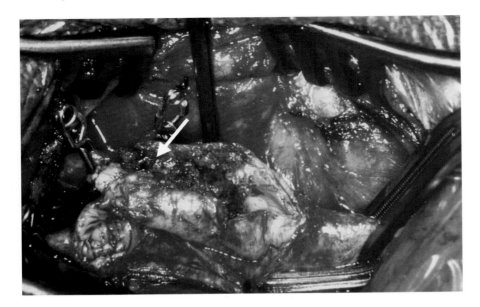

FIG. 16. Following the arteriotomy, no backflow resulted from this thrombotic material *(arrow)*, which extended several centimeters distally.

rotic disease. The impression of those reporting such series is that the earlier surgery is performed, the better patients fare.

The literature concerning thromboendarterectomy of spontaneously occluded symptomatic ICAs consistently demonstrates a subgroup of patients who have successful restoration of flow with little morbidity and mortality. This subgroup is best defined as those without severe neurologic deficits, a decreased level of consciousness, or intracerebral hemorrhage. Clinical experience with such patients at our institution and others shows a low surgical morbidity and mortality rate associated with carefully performed thromboendarterectomy of the ICA. During long-term follow-up review, the vessels remained patent and the patients had fewer strokes than would be anticipated from natural history data. Our patients followed a prospectively designed diagnostic, anesthetic, and surgical protocol. Their evaluation and treatment were interdisciplinary. The data, however, were collected retrospectively and no simultaneous control group was available for comparison. This experience cannot definitively establish the efficacy of surgical management for ICA occlusion. However, based on the available data, we currently recommend surgery for patients with acute symptomatic ICA occlusion who do not have a major neurologic deficit or hemorrhage on CT scan.

The natural history of carotid occlusion has been ill defined, and its treatment is controversial. Even when presenting initially in an asymptomatic fashion, probably as many as one fifth of patients may suffer a cerebral infarction ipsilateral to the occluded carotid artery within 3 years. This likelihood suggests that initially asymptomatic ICA occlusion may not be as benign or stable as originally believed. The determination that an occlusion of the ICA is of recent onset is not always made with certainty. Patients with a documented ICA occlusion that is symptomatic are not uncommon and often pose difficulty in terms of being able to dis-

cern optimal treatment. ICA occlusion may present with either acute, transient, or evolving cerebral ischemic symptoms.

Emergency carotid thromboendarterectomy for patients with acute ICA occlusion has often been considered contraindicated. This attitude is due to the perceived high incidence of neurologic morbidity and mortality, the fact that it was thought that blood flow must be restored in the first few hours after the occlusion, and because of the previously perceived lack of definite benefit.

As our microsurgical technique, anesthesia methods, and perioperative management through the years have improved, we have improved our ability to reopen these occluded arteries with minimum neurologic morbidity and no operative mortality. We have also been able to achieve a higher patency rate in recent years by developing our current protocol of operating on patients with acute, symptomatic carotid occlusions who have not experienced a decreased level of consciousness, hemiplegia, or aphasia. This approach is viable in appropriately selected patients.

COMPLICATIONS OF CAROTID ENDARTERECTOMY

Although carotid endarterectomy is proven to be efficacious treatment, as with any surgical procedure it has inherent characteristic risks. For intervention upon the arterial vasculature, if properly performed, it carries exceeding low risks. In contrast to often and traditionally held beliefs, the actual risk of temporary carotid occlusion (ie, carotid cross-clamping) is low. This is especially true if carotid occlusion is performed under the controlled environment of the operating theater, with full compliment of cerebral monitoring, and the protective elements of general anesthesia and metabolic suppressive agents.

Embolization

It is now felt that the major risk of carotid endarterectomy is not the result of temporary ischemia during the period of carotid cross-clamping. Rather, other phenomena account for the neurologic morbidity of this procedure. Embolization of thrombotic material, portions of atherosclerotic plaque material or air particles have all been reported. With transcranial Doppler monitoring, emboli (usually gaseous) have been detected in one third of cases

The risk of intraoperative embolic events occurs primarily during three phases of carotid endarterectomy. In addition, care should be exercised by the nurse preparing the surgical field with antiseptic solution scrubbing because shearing of thrombotic material can occur from fragile plaque lesions. During the operation, the dissection of vessels in preparation for endarterectomy may cause embolization of particulate matter. This is the time of highest risk both due to the necessary handling and manipulation of the carotid artery and the presence of the plaque and associated thrombotic material. Another occasion of high risk of distal embolization, also confirmed in our experience by intraoperative TCD recording, is during vessel reopening following arteriotomy closure. Usually, however, this consists of gaseous emboli due to incomplete evacuation of intraluminal air. This can be minimized or eliminated by meticulous attention to proper surgical technique. It is paramount for the surgeon to always attempt to establish a full column of fluid intraluminally prior to clamp release. This is accomplished by back-bleeding via an open superior thyroid artery, or in cases of inadequate back-flow, filling the intraluminal carotid artery with heparinized saline solution.

The use of intraluminal carotid shunts has been controversial, and it has been further complicated by a lack of scientific and surgical confirmatory data. Although some have advocated routine employment of intraluminal carotid shunts, they have actually been required in only 6% of our cases (4). Among several drawbacks, shunts are responsible for the highest incidence of cerebral embolization.

Carotid Artery Thrombosis

Operative site carotid thrombosis can occur in the absence of technical errors and can cause ischemic complications. The thrombogenic nature of the fresh luminal surface after endarterectomy makes it susceptible to mural thrombosis and/or subsequent embolization. Removal of the atherosclerotic plaque exposes the underlying media and occasionally portions of the adventitial layer. When flow is restored, platelets actively adhere to the underlying collagen (66). A pseudoendothelial monolayer of platelets, which is thought to be nonthrombogenic, forms (33,67,68). The adhering platelets release vasoactive substances including adenosine diphosphate and thromboxane A2, both potent platelet aggregators. Factor XII is activated by the exposed collagen and also initiates the hemostatic cascade that forms a fibrin clot. Platelet factor III, released by the activated platelets, dissipates in the activation of the intrinsic coagulation system (69,70,71). The combination of aggregated platelets, fibrin, and red blood cells constitutes a thrombus at the operative site. This thrombus can fragment with distal embolization. The size of the clot can also continue to increase locally until the vessel is occluded. There can also be propagation of thrombus distally. Before carotid cross-clamping, heparin is routinely administered to prevent intravascular thrombosis and thromboembolism of areas of stasis caused by the carotid occlusion (72–74). With a half-life of only 90 minutes, it appears that superior results are obtained if heparinization is not neutralized because the platelet monolayer can form to protect the exposed elements in the media (69). Some authors have recommended the routine use of postoperative heparin infusion. Such a regimen, however, has the potential to cause postoperative hematomas at the operative site and is probably unnecessary, except in special circumstances where there is unusual potential for postoperative vessel occlusion.

Aspirin interferes with normal platelet function by inhibiting the formation of thromboxane A2 in ADP-induced platelet aggregation (66). Findlay et al reported a series in which a combination of aspirin and dipyridamole or a placebo was administered perioperatively to patients undergoing carotid endarterectomy. Autologous indium-3-labeled platelets were injected postoperatively, and platelet collection and deposition were measured at the endarterectomy site. The degree of platelet aggregation and accumulation in the treatment group was significantly reduced compared with the placebo group. Two patients in the control group had postoperative strokes. In one of these patients, a thick, white, mural thrombus, indicative of a platelet clot, was found upon reexploration. None of the patients had a postoperative wound hematoma. They recommended aspirin at a dosage of 300 mg every 8 hours and dipyridamole 75 mg every 8 hours (75). The cyclooxygenase system is inhibited by aspirin. Dipyridamole interferes with the platelet phosphodiesterase system, elevating the cyclic adenosine monophosphate levels in a synergistic fashion. We have utilized aspirin alone with excellent results. Ercius et al showed that in canines a single dose of aspirin (10 mg/kg) resulted in the formation of the platelet monolayer, which inhibited thrombus formation at the endarterectomy site. In contrast, doses in the range of 0.5 mg/kg were ineffective (68).

The incidence of recurrent carotid artery stenosis after an endarterectomy may be lessened by antiplatelet treatment. Degranulated platelets release smooth muscle and fibroblast mitogens with subsequent migration of these elements to the underlying neointima. Exaggerated or exuberant growth of layers of this neointima may be the origin of recurrent stenosis. This growth is termed neointimal hyperplasia or fibromuscular hyperplasia (34,73,76). A recent report suggests that aspirin plus dipyridamole was ineffective in reducing the incidence of carotid restenosis when evaluated at 1-year

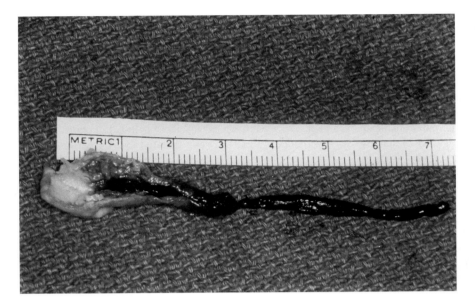

FIG. 17. This thrombus was successfully removed and arteriograde flow restored using a thrombectomy balloon catheter.

follow-up (77). Hansen et al likewise noted no difference between treatment with low doses of aspirin (75 mg daily) and a placebo 1-year after carotid endarterectomy. Two months after surgery, 39% of the patients had recurrent carotid artery stenosis of 30% or greater; it also recurred in 42% of patients 6 months after surgery. More than 50% stenosis was seen in 9% of patients and 2% had occlusion at the 6-month follow-up (78). Bischoff et al compared antiplatelet therapy with anticoagulation in 328 patients who underwent carotid endarterectomy with a subgroup of patients treated without medication and found no statistically significant difference between the two groups. There was also no difference in their cause of death or in the incidence of intracerebral hemorrhage. They concluded that long-term antiaggregant and anticoagulant therapy did not affect the rate of complications or survival after carotid endarterectomy; however, survival was increased in the treated group because the incidence of postoperative myocardial infarction was reduced (79). We advocate aspirin administered about a week before surgery and extended indefinitely throughout the postoperative period. As mentioned, aspirin is also administered to the patient rectally in the recovery room immediately after the procedure.

Intracerebral Hemorrhage

Although infrequent in occurrence, intracerebral hemorrhage is a potentially devastating complication of carotid endarterectomy (80–83). Postoperative intracerebral hemorrhage, which usually occurs several days after the operation, has been the source of significant morbidity and mortality in series where operative techniques have otherwise demonstrated excellent outcomes. The incidence of postoperative intracerebral hemorrhage is thought to be <1%. In our series,

intracerebral hematoma caused one postoperative morbidity and one death, which was the only neurologically related death in the series (4). Bruetman et al reported that intracerebral hemorrhage complicated 6 of 900 (0.67%) endarterectomies (81). Spetzler et al in 1986 reported a 0.5% incidence of postoperative intracerebral hematoma, in one case leading to death (15). Solomon et al described 8 patients out of 1930 carotid endarterectomies (0.41%) who sustained a postoperative intracerebral hemorrhage (8). Postoperative intracerebral hemorrhage was thought to occur only in patients with preexisting cerebrovascular accidents in which reperfusion of cerebral blood flow to that region could cause hemorrhage into or adjacent to the infarcted zone. In their 1978 review, Caplan et al described 17 reported cases, all of whom had preoperative stroke. Two of these patients had severe unilateral carotid stenosis and underwent carotid endarterectomy 4 and 5 weeks after cerebral infarction (82). However, most patients with postoperative intracerebral hemorrhage have a profile of a recent antecedent brain infarct and preoperative hypertension. Postoperative intracerebral hemorrhage usually occurs in the first few days after surgery and is associated with systemic hypertension. In reported series, these hemorrhages occurred an average of 3 days after surgery and were ipsilateral to the carotid endarterectomy in >90% of cases (20,74,82).

Hypertension often accompanies carotid endarterectomy. Lehv et al found that mean systolic blood pressure was elevated >15 mm Hg in 15 of 27 (55%) of patients undergoing unilateral carotid endarterectomy. Seven of these patients developed neurologic complications and one died. In a third of these hypertensive patients, blood pressure was extremely elevated, ie, 195–250 mm Hg systolic and 105–130 mm Hg diastolic. They believed that postoperative hypertension occurred after the normal carotid sinus reflex was interrupted and therefore was common after bilateral carotid procedures (51). The absence of other systemic (eg, retinal, renal, or cardiac) signs of hypertension in some patients suggested that preoperative occult or asymptomatic hypertension did not exist and that a new onset of postoperative hypertension can cause capillary breakdown and hemorrhage (82). Besides recent cerebral infarction and hypertension, TIAs and anticoagulation have been regarded as steps contributing to postoperative hemorrhage.

In addition to the risk caused by uncontrolled postoperative hypertension, Sundt documented that postoperative cerebral blood flow increased to the cerebral hemisphere ipsilateral to carotid endarterectomy despite the absence of systemic hypertension (26). It has been suggested that cerebral hyperperfusion may be symptomatic in certain patients causing severe headache, facial pain, orbital pain, and paroxysmal lateralizing epileptiform discharges (PLEDs) (72,73, 84,85). Brick and colleagues reported a case of a patient who 8 days after endarterectomy developed acute confusion, agitation, and headaches. His workup disclosed that he had PLEDs and severe angiographic cerebral vasoconstriction. These symptoms subsided in 1 week, did not recur, and were thought to be secondary to impaired cerebral autoregulation (86). Both focal and generalized seizures have been described in patients with negative CT scans after carotid endarterectomy (70). Akers et al (87) found that somnolence, clinical depression, and psychiatric disturbances were present in their postoperative endarterectomy patients. These features were characteristic of patients who had high-grade stenoses corrected and who were believed to be secondary to a cerebral hyperperfusion syndrome. These phenomena tended to be self-limited within an 8-week period. TCD ultrasonography has been shown to be an effective, accurate, and noninvasive method to document and follow such patients with suspected hyperperfusion until it resolves (80).

Solomon and his colleagues reported that of eight patients with postoperative intracerebral hemorrhage after carotid endarterectomy, six had no evidence of a previous cerebral infarction in the area of the subsequent hemorrhage. Most hemorrhages occurred within the first 5 days of surgery and were not associated with postoperative hypertension. It was believed that a cerebral hyperperfusion syndrome existed in these patients in areas where severe, chronic ICA stenosis had paralyzed autoregulation of cerebral blood flow (8). This state is reminiscent of, and perhaps has a mechanism similar to that underlying, normal perfusion pressure breakthrough after an arteriovenous malformation (AVM) has been resected. In this circumstance, a cerebral blood flow steal causes chronic ischemia in the area surrounding the AVM. The surrounding vessels are in a chronic state of maximal dilatation and have lost the capacity for autoregulation. When the AVM is removed, the surrounding cerebral tissue is unable to react with normal vasoconstriction to a normal perfusion pressure. In certain cases, cerebral hemorrhage or edema can result.

Myocardial Infarction

In series of microsurgical carotid endarterectomy, myocardial infarction is one of the commonest complications and certainly the greatest systemic complication of the procedure. It occurred in approximately 3% of patients in our series (4). Undoubtedly, this is due to the frequent concomitant presence of coronary and carotid artery atherosclerosis. In addition, the systemic or coronary operative stresses of carotid endarterectomy and general anesthesia are significant.

The reported incidence of perioperative myocardial infarction with carotid endarterectomy is 2–3%. Myocardial infarction has been reported to be the most common complication, reported to account for up to 50% of late deaths (4). This is due to the natural progression of the coronary atherosclerotic process. Various cardiac syndromes are seen including activation of previously stable angina, onset of unstable angina, and development of acute intraoperative or immediate postoperative myocardial infarction. Myocardial oxygen demand, probably altered by increased catecholamine production, may exceed oxygen delivery. Intraoperative or postoperative hypertension, increased intravascular volume, and tachycardia may exacerbate this situation. In addition, if intraoperative barbiturates are utilized for cerebral protection, myocardial suppression may occur. Patients with aortic and mitral valve insufficiency seem especially vulnerable to the above scenario and may suffer congestive failure with or without myocardial infarction.

Careful preoperative screenings for critical coronary perfusion and myocardial function at rest and in response to stress are necessary to minimize morbidity. Strict attention to intraoperative hemodynamic parameters and their response to anesthetic manipulation is required. Immediate postoperative hemodynamic and cardiac monitoring is useful in minimizing the possibility of perioperative cardiac morbidity.

CONCLUSION

Carotid endarterectomy has evolved, both in indications and technique, remarkably over the recent years. Defined by the recent clinical trials for both symptomatic and asymptomatic populations, the procedure is now supported by firm data and more sophisticated methods. Improvements have also accrued in the cardiac, medical, and anesthetic management of these patients. Attention meticulously paid to technical details and participation by qualified nursing and other support personnel contribute heavily to an excellent outcome. No other procedure in medicine highlights, as does carotid endarterectomy, the importance of minimizing operative morbidity and mortality if the natural history of the disease process is to be exceeded. The principles of surgery, including the microsurgical technique described herein, have provided minimal morbidity and no mortality for carotid endarterectomy. Current studies are underway to continue to define the patient population most likely to benefit from this procedure, including those patients with moderate (30–60%) degrees of carotid stenosis, and the role of future developments in endovascular techniques.

ACKNOWLEDGMENTS

The author thanks Barbara Berry and Cathie Campbell for assistance with manuscript preparation. Randy McKenzie provided the artwork, which accurately depicts the issues involved in the procedure.

REFERENCES

1. NASCET Collaborators: Beneficial effect of carotid endarterectomy in symptomatic patients with high-grade carotid stenosis. *N Engl J Med* 1991;325:445–453.
2. European Carotid Surgery Trialists Collaborative Group. MRC European carotid surgery tiral: interim results for symptomatic patients with severe (70–99%) or with mild (0–29%) carotid stenosis. *Lancet* 1991;337:1235–1243.
3. Mayberg MR, Wilson SE, Yatsu F, et al. Carotid endarterectomy and prevention of cerebral ischemia in symptomatic carotid stenosis. *JAMA* 1991; 226:3289–3294.
4. Bailes JE, Spetzler RF (eds). *Microsurgical Carotid Endarterectomy.* New York: Lippincott-Raven, 1996.
5. Day, AL, Rhoton, AL, Quisling RG. Resolving siphon stenosis following endarterectomy. *Stroke* 1980;11:278–281.
6. Alcock, JM. Occlusion of the middle cerebral artery: serial angiography as a guide to conservative therapy. *J Neurosurg* 1967;27:353–357.
7. Little JR, Sawhny B, Weinstein M. Pseudo-tandem stenosis of the internal carotid artery. *Neurosurgery* 1980;7:574–577.
8. Solomon RA, Loftus CM, Quest DO, et al. Incidence and etiology of intracerebral hemorrhage following carotid endarterectomy. *J Neurosurg* 1986;64:29–34.
9. Sundt TM Jr., Anderson RE, Michenfelder JD. Intracellular redox states under halothane and barbiturate anesthesia in normal, ischemic, and anoxic monkey brain. *Ann Neurol* 1979;5:575–579.
10. Selman WR, Spetzler RF, Roski RA, et al. Barbiturate coma in focal cerebral ischemia: relationship of protection to timing of therapy. *J Neurosurg* 1982;56:685–690.
11. Shiu GK, Nemoto EM. Barbiturate attenuation of brain free fatty acid liberation during global ischemia. *J Neurochem* 1981;37:1448–1456.
12. Sundt TM, Sharbrough FW, Piepgras DG, et al. Correlation of cerebral blood flow and electroencephalographic changes during carotid endarterectomy. *Mayo Clin Proc* 1981;56:533–543.
13. Feustel PJ, Ingvar MC, Severinghaus JW. Cerebral oxygen availability and blood flow during middle cerebral artery occlusion: effects of pentobarbital. *Stroke* 1981;12:858–863.
14. Demopoulos HB, Flamm ES, Seligman ML, et al. Antioxidant effects of barbiturates in model membranes undergoing free radical damage. *Acta Neurol Scand* (Suppl) 1977;64:152–153.
15. Spetzler RF, Martin N, Hadley MN, et al. Microsurgical endarterectomy under barbiturate protection: a prospective study. *J Neurosurg* 1986;65:63–73.
16. Moseley JI, Laurent JP, Molinari GF. Barbiturate attenuation of the clinical course and pathological lesions in primate stroke model. *Neurology* 1975;25:870–874.
17. Nehls D, Todd M, Spetzler RF, et al. A comparison of the cerebral protective effects of isoflurane and barbiturates during temporary focal ischemia in primates. *Anesthesiology* 1987;66:453–464.
18. Corkill G, Chikovani OK, McLeish I, et al. Timing of pentobarbital administration for brain protection in experimental stroke. *Surg Neurol* 1976;5:147–149.
19. Milde LN, Milde JH, Michenfelder JD. Cerebral functional, metabolic, and hemodynamic effects of etomidate in dogs. *Anesthesiology* 1985;63:371–377.
20. Batjer HH, Frankfurt AI, Purdy PD, et al. Use of etomidate, temporary arterial occlusion, and intraoperative angiography in surgical treatment of large and giant cerebral aneurysms. *J Neurosurg* 1988;68:234–240.
21. Hans SS. Late follow-up of carotid endarterectomy with venous patch angioplasty. *Am J Surg* 1991;162:50–54.
22. Van Dammer H, Grenade T, Creemers E, et al. Blowout of carotid venous patch angioplasty. *Ann Vasc Surg* 1991;5:542–544.
23. Sundt TM, Whisnant JP, Houser OW, et al. Prospective study of the effectiveness and durability of carotid endarterectomy. *Mayo Clin Proc* 1990;65:625–635.
24. Deriu GP, Ballotta E, Bonavina L, et al. The rationale for patch-graft angioplasty after carotid endarterectomy: early and long-term follow-up. *Stroke* 1984;15:972–979.
25. Hertzer NR, Beven EG, O Hara PJ, et al. A prospective study of vein patch angioplasty during carotid endarterectomy. Three-year results for 801 patients and 917 operations. *Ann Surg* 1987;206:628–635.
26. Sundt TM Jr, Sandok BA, Whisnant JP. Carotid endarterectomy: complications and preoperative assessment of risk. *Mayo Clin Proc* 1975;50:301–306.
27. Thompson JE, Austin DJ, Patman RD. Carotid endarterectomy for cerebrovascular insufficiency: long-term results in 592 patients followed up to thirteen years. *Ann Surg* 1970;172:663–679.
28. Little JR, Bryerton BS, Furlan AJ. Saphenous vein patch grafts in carotid endarterectomy. *J Neurosurg* 1984;61:743–747.
29. O Hara PJ, Hertzer NR, Krajewski LP, et al. Saphenous vein patch rupture after carotid endarterectomy. *J Vasc Surg* 1992;15:504–509.
30. Thomas M, Otis SM, Rush M, et al. Recurrent carotid artery stenosis following endarterectomy. *Ann Surg* 1984;20:74–79.
31. Sandmann W, Kolvenback R, Willeke F. Risks and benefits of shunting in carotid endarterectomy (Letter). *Stroke* 1993;24:1098.
32. Javid H, Ostermiller WE, Hangesh JW, et al: Natural history of carotid bifurcation atheroma. *Surgery* 1970;67:80–83.
33. Ott DA, Colley DA, Chapa L, et al. Carotid endarterectomy without temporary intraluminal shunt. *Ann Surg* 1980; 191:708–14.
34. Waring PH, Kraftson DA. Another complication of carotid artery shunting during endarterectomy (letter). *Anesthesiology* 1990;72:1099.
35. Halsey JH. Risks and benefits of shunting in carotid endarterectomy. *Stroke* 1992;23:1583–1587.
36. Rosenthal D, Archie JJP, Garcia-Rinaldi R, et al. Carotid patch angioplasty: immediate and long-term results. *J Vasc Surg* 1990;12:326–333.
37. Hunter GC, Sieffert G, Malone JM, et al. The accuracy of carotid back pressure as an index for shunt requirements: a reappraisal. *Stroke* 1981;13:319–326.
38. Gumerlock MK, Neuwelt EA. Carotid endarterectomy: to shunt or not to shunt. *Stroke* 1988;19-1485–1490.
39. Winslow CM, Solomon DH, Chassin MR, et al. The appropriateness of carotid endarterectomy. *N Engl J Med* 1988;318:721–727.
40. Plecha FR, Pories WJ. Intraoperative angiography in the immediate assessment of arterial reconstruction. *Arch Surg* 1972; 105:902–907.
41. Bland JE, Lazar ML. Carotid endarterectomy without shunt. *Neurosurgery* 1981;8:153–157.
42. Ferguson GG, Blume WT, Farras JK. Carotid endarterectomy: an evaluation of results in 282 consecutive cases in relationship to intraoperative monitoring. Abstract 54, Program of Annual Meeting of the American Association of Neurologic Surgeons, Atlanta, April 23, 1985.
43. Jansen C, Vriens EM, Eikelboom BC, et al. Carotid endarterectomy with transcranial Doppler and electorencephalographic monitoring. A prospective study in 130 operations. *Stroke* 1993;24:665–669.
44. Giannotta L, Dicks RE, Kindt GW. Carotid endarterectomy: technical improvements. *Neurosurgery* 1980;7:309–312.
45. Findlay JM, Lougheed WM. Carotid microendarterectomy. *Neurosurgery* 1993;32:792–798.
46. Barrow KL, Mizuno J. Carotid endarterectomy: technical aspects and perioperative management. In: Awad IA, ed. *Cerebrovascular Occlusive Disease and Brain Ischemia.* Chicago: American Association of Neurological Surgeons, 1992;162–185
47. Pessin MS, Paris W, Prager RJ, et al. Auscultation of cervical and ocular bruits in extracranial occlusive carotid disease. *Stroke* 1983; 14:246
48. Sundt TM Jr, *Occlusive Cerebrovascular Disease: Diagnosis and Surgical Management.* Philadelphia: WB Saunders, 1987.
49. Moore WS, Martello JY, Quinones-Baldrich WJ, et al. Etiologic importance of the intimal flap of the external carotid artery in the development of postcarotid endarterectomy stroke. *Stroke* 1990;21:1497–1502.

50. Blaisdell FW, Lim R, Hall AD. Technical result of carotid endarterectomy: arteriographic assessment. *Am J Surg* 1962;114:239–246.

51. Lehv MS, Salzman EW, Silen W. Hypertension complicating carotid endarterectomy. *Stroke* 1970;1:307–313.

52. Dyken ML, Klatte E, Kolar OJ, et al. Complete occlusion of common or internal carotid arteries. Clinical significance. *Arch Neurol* 1974; 30:343–346.

53. Furlan AJ, Whisnant JP, Baker HL. Long-term prognosis after carotid artery occlusion. *Neurology* 1980;30-986–988.

54. Gurdjian FS, Lindner DW, Hardy WG, et al. Completed stroke due to occlusive cerebrovascular disease. *Neurology* 1961;11:724–732.

55. Cote R, Barnett HJM, Taylor DW. Internal carotid occlusion: a prospective study. *Stroke* 1983;14:898–902.

56. Fields WS, Lemark NA. Joint study of extracranial arterial occlusion. X. Internal carotid artery occlusion. *JAMA* 1976;235:2734–2738.

57. Wiebers DO, Whisnant JP, Sandok BA, O Fallon WM. Prospective comparison of a cohort with asymptomatic carotid bruit and a population-based cohort without carotid bruit. *Stroke* 1990; 21:984–988.

58. Hennerici M, Hulsbomer H-B, Rautenberg W, et al. Spontaneous history of asymptomatic internal carotid occlusion. *Stroke* 1986;17: 718–722.

59. Hafner CD, Tew JM. Surgical management of the totally occluded internal carotid artery: a ten-year study. *Surgery* 1981;89:710–717.

60. Meyer FB, Sundt TM Jr, Piepgras DG, et al. Emergency carotid endarterectomy for patients with acute carotid occlusion and profound neurological deficits. *Ann Surg* 1986;203:82–89.

61. Walters BB, Ojemann RG, Henos RC. Emergency carotid endarterectomy. *J Neurosurg* 1987;66:817–823.

62. Hugenholtz H. Elgie RG. Carotid thromboendarterectomy: a reappraisal. Criteria for patient selection. *J Neurosurg* 1980;53:776–783.

63. Kusunoki T, Towed DW, Tator CH, et al. Thromboendarterectomy for total occlusion of the internal carotid artery: a reappraisal of risks, success rate and potential benefits. *Stroke* 1978;9:34–38.

64. Wylie EJ, Hein MF, Adams JE. Intracranial hemorrhage following surgical revascularization for treatment of acute strokes. *J Neurosurg* 1964;21:212–215.

65. McCormick PW, Spetzler RF, Bailes JE, et al. Thromboendarterectomy of the symptomatic occluded internal carotid artery. *J Neurosurg* 1992; 76:752–758.

66. Bailes JE, Quigley MR, Kwaan HC, et al. The effects of intravenous prostacyclin in a model of microsurgical thrombosis. *Microsurgery* 1988;9:2–9.

67. Baumgartner HR, Haduenschild C. Adhesion of platelets to subendothelium. *Ann NY Acad Sci* 1972;201:22–36.

68. Ercius MS, Chandler WF, Ford JW, et al. Early versus delayed heparin reversal after carotid endarterectomy in the dog. A scanning electron microscopy study. *J Neurosurg* 1983;58:708–713.

69. Dirrenberger RA, Sundt TM Jr. Carotid endarterectomy: temporal profile of the healing process and effects of anticoagulation therapy. *J Neurosurg* 1978;48:201–219.

70. Kieburtz K, Ricotta JJ, Moxley RT. Seizures following carotid endarterectomy. *Arch Neurol* 1990;568–570.

71. Mustard JF, Jorgenson L, Hovig T, et al. Role of platelets in thrombosis. *Thromb Diath Haemorrh* 1966;21(Suppl):131–158.

72. Dolan JG Mushlin AI. Hypertension, vascular headaches, and seizures after carotid endarterectomy. Case report and therapeutic considerations. *Arch Intern Med* 1984;144:1489–1491.

73. Metke MP, Lie JT, Fuster V. Reduction of intimal thickening in canine coronary bypass vein grafts with dipridamole and aspirin. *Am J Cardiol* 1979;43:1144–1148.

74. Zierler R, Bandyk DF, Thiele BL, et al. Carotid artery stenosis following endarterectomy. *Arch Surg* 1982;117:1408–1412.

75. Findlay JM, Lougheed WM, Gentill F, et al. Effect of perioperative platelet inhibition on postcarotid endarterectomy mural thrombus formation. *J Neurosurg* 1985;63:693–698.

76. Thompson JE, Pataman RD, Talkington CM. Asymptomatic carotid bruit: long-term outcome of patients having endarterectomy compared with unoperated controls. *Ann Surg* 1978; 188:308–16.

77. Harker LA, Bernstein EF, Dilley RB, et al. Failure of aspirin plus dipyridamole to prevent restonosis after carotid endarterectomy. *Ann Intern Med* 1992;116:731–736.

78. Hansen F, Lindblad B, Persson NH, et al. Can recurrent stenosis after carotid endarterectomy be prevented by low-dose acetylsalicylic acid? A double-blind, randomized and placebo-controlled study. *Eur J Vasc Surg* 1993;7:380–385.

79. Bischoff G, Pratschner T, Kail M, et al. Anticoagulants, antiaggregants or nothing following carotid endarterectomy? *Eur J Vasc Surg* 1993; 7:364–369.

80. Bernstein M, Fleming JFR, Deck JHN. Cerebral hyperperfusion after carotid endarterectomy: a cause of cerebral hemorrhage. *Neurosurgery* 1984;15:50–56.

81. Bruetman ME, Fields WS, Crawford ES, et al. Cerebral hemorrhage in carotid artery surgery. *Arch Neurol* 1963;9:458–467.

82. Caplan LR, Skillman J, Ojemann R, et al. Intracerebral hemorrhage following carotid endarterectomy: a hypertensive complication? *Stroke* 1978;9:457–460.

83. Tempelhoff R, Modica PA, Grubb RL, et al. Selective shunting during carotid endarterectomy based on two-channel computerized electroencephalographic/compressed spectral array analysis. *Neurosurgery* 1989;24:339–344.

84. Leviton A, Caplan L, Salzman E. Severe headache after carotid endarterectomy. *Headache* 1975;15:207–210.

85. Messert B, Black JA. Cluster headache, hemicrania, and other head pains: morbidity of carotid endarterectomy. *Stroke* 1978;9:559–562.

86. Brick JF, Dunker RO, Gutierreg AR. Cerebral vasoconstriction as a complication of carotid endarterectomy. *J Neurosurg* 1990;73: 151–153.

87. Akers DL, Brinker MR, Engelhadt TC, et al. Postoperative somnolence in patients after carotid endarterectomy. *Surgery* 1990;107:684–687.

88. Sundt TM Jr. The ischemic tolerance of neural tissue and the need for monitoring and selective shunting during carotid endarterectomy. *Stroke* 1983;14:93–98.

89. Allen GS, Preziosi TJ. Carotid endarterectomy: a prospective study of its efficacy and safety. *Medicine* 1981;60:298–309.

90. Quinones-Baldrich WJ, Moore WS. Intraoperative monitoring and use of the interanl shunt during carotid endarterectomy. *Int Surg* 1984;69: 207–213.

Cerebrovascular Disease, edited by H. Hunt Batjer.
Lippincott-Raven Publishers, Philadelphia © 1997.

CHAPTER 34

Extracranial Carotid and Vertebral Artery Stenosis: The Future of Angioplasty

Robert D. G. Ferguson, John G. Ferguson, and Laurance I. Lee

The focus of this chapter is the state of the science in cerebral percutaneous transluminal angioplasty (CPTA) of the extracranial carotid and vertebral arteries—and its future directions. CPTA refers to high-pressure dilation of vaso-occlusive, atherosclerotic target lesions in cerebral arteries, using nonelastomer balloons. Despite more than a decade of clinical research, the clinical effectiveness of CPTA is unclear. However, recently published prospective angiographic outcome and safety data justify the evaluation of CPTA in prospective, multidisciplinary, externally monitored cooperative studies.

RATIONALE FOR CPTA IN CAROTID AND VERTEBRAL DISEASE

There are two mechanisms by which an atherosclerotic plaque can reduce blood flow and cause cerebral infarction: (a) atheroocclusion, that is, encroachment of the plaque, with or without associated thrombus, on the arterial lumen; and (b) artery-to-artery embolus, or liberation of plaque fragments and/or thrombi that narrow or occlude distal elements of the arterial tree (1). Consequently, there are two main reasons for proposing CPTA: (a) to reduce the risk of hemodynamic (low-flow) stroke by increasing the cross-sectional area of the target artery, thereby increasing flow reserve; and (b) to favorably alter perilesional rheology and restore endothelial function at the target site. Achieving these goals may prevent cerebral ischemia and infarction in patients who are at risk for stroke due to large-vessel thrombotic occlusion, hemodynamic instability, or plaque-derived thromboembolism.

There are no reliable morphologic data on the mechanism of successful human cerebral angioplasty. The consequences of CPTA may be similar to those described for lesions that have similar morphology and pathophysiology (2,3); that is, endothelial denudation with cracking and splitting of the plaque, along with stretching of the adjacent media and adventitia, leading to aneurysmal dilatation of the target segment and an attendant increase in cross-sectional area (4). There is a need for pathologic, intravascular ultrasound, and angioscopy studies to expedite refinement of CPTA by correlating technical parameters with mechanical effects.

HISTORY OF CPTA IN HUMANS

Kerber and colleagues (5) performed the first human carotid artery dilatations in 1980, demonstrating that atherosclerotic lesions of the common carotid artery could be dilated without necessarily provoking symptomatic atherothromboembolism. Later that year, Mullan et al (6) reported the first human internal carotid artery dilation. Angioplasty of this nonatherosclerotic, web-like lesion resulted in immediate disappearance of the patient's complaint of a pulsating noise in the ear and a vibration (thrill) in the neck.

There have been several case series that included patients with extracranial carotid and vertebral target lesions. They demonstrated the technical feasibility of performing cerebral angioplasty for treatment of structural occlusive disease in some patients (7–10). However, no definitive, comparative clinical CPTA study has been published, and the long-term angiographic results are unknown. Therefore, the therapeutic role of cerebral angioplasty needs to be defined before widespread implementation is justifiable.

STATE OF CPTA RESEARCH

Before a review of the state of CPTA research, it is necessary to clarify the problems in calibrating angioplasty results.

All authors: Memphis Vascular Research Foundation, Memphis, Tennessee 38103

Heretofore, the referral pathway leading to cerebral angioplasty has been biased against CPTA. The typical angioplasty patient was a poor surgical candidate because of comorbidity and anesthetic risk. In addition, a significant proportion of CPTA patients were referred after failed endarterectomy, which was performed in the as yet unsubstantiated hope of reducing operative risk for coronary artery bypass surgery or neurosurgery.

Retrospective Case Reports and Case Series

Retrospective case reports and case series represent the bulk of the published CPTA literature. Taken as a whole, this body of work has serious limitations that go beyond the inferential limitations of the case-report design. The limitations—weakness of the research paradigm, defective implementation of the research design, and questionable ethics in the reporting of study results—preclude a reliable synthesis of the data even for descriptive purposes; pooling results for a systematic overview is particularly unrealistic, even with techniques proposed for combining observational studies (11).

Even exemplary case reports and case series cannot establish the clinical effectiveness of extracranial carotid and vertebral angioplasty. The case series is a relatively weak clinical research paradigm that does not meet evidentiary standards for establishing cause and effects. It is an imprecise design that is highly susceptible to multiple forms of bias in: patient selection, management, measurement, and follow-up, as well as in the reporting of study results. Moreover, investigators have, in general, failed to acknowledge these limitations, and they have done a poor job of identifying, preventing, and discussing the potential biases that may have distorted their results.

CPTA case series have a plethora of implementation problems. In general, they lack standardization, a well defined basis for patient inclusion and exclusion, quantification of patients' baseline risk for adverse events, objective diagnostic criteria, procedures to ensure consistent interpretation of diagnostic procedures, objective methods for quantifying angiographic and clinical results, systematic follow-up and event surveillance, descriptive summaries of pertinent results, external monitoring, an adequate description of censoring, angiographic quantification of target restenosis, and discussion of the impact that potential biases may have had on study results. In addition, many authors draw inferences from their results that go well beyond the descriptive nature of the study design. As a result, it is difficult to characterize the referral pathway, to define sample characteristics, and to estimate risk for significant adverse events in follow-up. Consequently, there is typically no identifiable target population and no basis for comparison with therapeutic alternatives.

In addition to the aforementioned shortcomings, some investigators who reported early cerebral angioplasty studies did not adhere to widely accepted reporting standards (12–14). Contrary to customary editorial policy (15), some authors submitted for publication reports that were substantively indistinguishable and involved essentially the same cases. Occasionally, this practice eluded detection by journal reviewers, resulting in duplicate publication (16–19). In addition, some investigators lumped their data with large unreferenced external data sets, rendering their results inscrutable (20). The tendency for investigators to report CPTA results in journals that do not reserve the right to audit raw data has done little to mitigate the negative impact of these actions on critics' perceptions. Rightly or wrongly, the conduct of a few investigators has prompted deprecation of early cerebral angioplasty research and undermined the credibility of CPTA research in general.

Despite their inferential limitations concerning the clinical effectiveness of CPTA, retrospective reports initiated and perpetuated interest in CPTA. Kerber et al's (5) and Mullan et al's (6) reports were milestones in the emergence of human carotid and internal carotid CPTA. They demonstrated that dilatation of the carotid artery could be performed without necessarily provoking symptomatic cerebral embolization. Concerned by the theoretical risk of procedure-related cerebral embolism, Latchaw proposed a mechanical cerebral protection paradigm (Val d'Ysère Working Group on Interventional Neuroradiology, 1983) that was modified and implemented by Theron et al (21). Along the way, investigators demonstrated the technical feasibility of CPTA in individual patients as well as efficacy with regard to assorted surrogate endpoints, such as postdilatation increase in translesional blood flow (22) and regional cerebral blood flow (23).

Prospective Studies

There are at least two ongoing prospective, protocol-based studies. The Carotid and Vertebral Artery Transluminal Angioplasty Study (CAVATAS) is attempting to compare surgery with angioplasty for treatment of carotid and vertebral occlusive lesions (M. Brown, oral personal communication, 1994). The largest prospective experience to date comes from the North American Cerebral Percutaneous Transluminal Angioplasty Register (NACPTAR) (24). These studies have different goals and reflect philosophic variance regarding the state of CPTA research (see discussion of the future of CPTA below). CAVATAS includes a multicenter, randomized comparison of carotid angioplasty and endarterectomy; the results are unpublished.

NACPTAR is a prospective, multicenter, protocol-based pilot study that was designed (a) to provide relatively precise estimates of immediate angiographic success, angiographic restenosis, and clinical outcomes in nonsurgical patients undergoing CPTA for symptomatic intracranial and extracranial cerebrovascular disease; and (b) to determine the advisability of, and formulate a tractable hypothesis for, a randomized controlled trial comparing CPTA with therapeutic alternatives, as well as developing the infrastructure, institutional ties, and logistics needed to ensure its success. Phase 1 of NACPTAR ended in January 1995. Published NACPTAR results provide preliminary evidence concerning the immediate angiographic success and clinical complications (24), restenosis rate (25), and predictors of angiographic success (26) in CPTA for symptomatic, intracranial and/or extracranial cerebrovascular disease. The NACPTAR design, data management, and analysis were developed and implemented by a clinical epidemiologist. The study protocol stipulated mandatory inclusion/exclusion criteria and diagnostic procedures, and it proposed standardized treatment, measurement, and follow-up procedures. The primary outcome, angiographic effectiveness, was a self-controlled analysis. A coordinating center was established to administer the project. Coordinating center personnel included a dedicated data entry clerk, a dedicated programmer, and an experienced study coordinator. Data validation procedures and a computerized database were developed along with precoded case-report forms to maximize data integrity. Site visits were conducted when the completion of case reports lagged behind schedule. Although data on the extracranial carotid and vertebral lesion subsets will not be available until publication of the final study results, preliminary NACPTAR reports constitute the only large-scale, prospective CPTA experience so far.

Interim angiographic results and neurologic complications were presented at the 66th Scientific Sessions of the American Heart Association (AHA) in 1993. There were 113 angioplasties in 102 symptomatic nonsurgical patients. The average pre-CPTA stenosis was 80%. The average stenosis immediately postangioplasty was 30%, yielding a mean difference of 50% (95% confidence interval [CI], 47–53%). This corresponds to an immediate angiographic success rate of 88% (95% CI, 81–92%), when success is defined as >20% reduction in baseline stenosis and <50% residual stenosis. Major complications included death in two of 113 angioplasties and stroke in an additional eight angioplasties, resulting in a combined major complication rate of 8.8% (24).

Preliminary NACPTAR data concerning the rate of restenosis in 44 lesions with angiographic follow-up at a mean of 260 days were presented at the AHA 20th International Joint Conference on Stroke and the Cerebral Circulation in 1995 (25). The mean pre-CPTA stenosis was 83%, and the mean difference pre-CPTA vs. post-CPTA was 49%. Restenosis was defined as angiographically documented narrowing >50%. Of the 37 lesions that were ≤50% after the initial dilatation, restenosis occurred in eight (22%; 95% CI, 10–38%). Of the patients who had restenosis, five of eight (63%) were symptomatic at the time of follow-up. Cox proportional hazards modeling revealed that symptoms and the degree of pre-CPTA stenosis were independent predictors of angiographic restenosis in follow-up. This self-controlled angiographic substudy, which is the largest angiographic follow-up evaluation so far, suggests that restenosis may be a significant problem after successful CPTA. However, the small proportion of the total sample who consented to repeat angiography raises the possibility of selection bias; that is, symptomatic patients may be more likely to consent to repeat angiography than their asymptomatic counterparts.

Preliminary NACPTAR results also suggest that the success of CPTA in a given patient may depend on target lesion characteristics (26). Data presented at the 1995 American Academy of Neurology meeting suggested that vertebral location and calcification are independent predictors of immediate angiographic success; that is, the adjusted odds of failure in a logistic regression model with immediate angiographic success as the dependent variable were 4.0 times greater in vertebral vs. nonvertebral target arteries and 4.1 times greater in calcified vs. noncalcified target lesions.

Definitive interpretation of these data must await publication of the final NACPTAR results. However, it is reasonable to conclude tentatively that in selected patients CPTA can effect a marked change in the degree of stenosis of target lesions, with a complication rate like that seen in the angioplasty of other vessels at the same stage in technical development (27).

Adjuncts to CPTA

The list of adjunctive pharmaceutical agents and medical devices that have an impact on CPTA study design is large and growing rapidly. There is no proof that any of these has a positive cost–benefit ratio when used in conjunction with CPTA. Analogy to percutaneous transluminal coronary angioplasty (PTCA) suggests that stenting might be the most promising adjunctive approach. Randomized trials have produced compelling evidence that coronary stenting produces better initial results and a lower rate of restenosis than angioplasty alone (28,29). In the hands of some operators, stent implantation is successful in up to 95% of cases (30,31). These results suggest that primary stenting may be of value in the cerebral circulation as well. In addition, stenting may reduce the risk of embolism following CPTA, and it is a potential form of vascular rescue for CPTA-induced occlusion due to intimal dissection or intraplaque hemorrhage. Preliminary reports from the Memphis Vascular Research Foundation and the University of Alabama at Birmingham (G. S. Roubin, oral personal communication, 1995) of the combined use of CPTA and stents suggest better initial technical results with stenting, ie, a larger postprocedure lumen, which is widely regarded as the most important determinant of long-term patency. We are of the opinion that primary stenting warrants further study in this context.

CURRENT INDICATIONS

Nonbrachiocephalic CPTA should only be attempted by multidisciplinary teams with formal training in the anatomy, pathophysiology, prognosis, and treatment of occlusive cerebrovascular disease with CPTA devices. Until definitive therapeutic studies are published and accepted by the medical community, nonbrachiocephalic CPTA should be performed under the auspices of an internal review board–approved investigational protocol except under extraordinary circumstances.

COSTS

There are no reliable estimates of the relative cost of CPTA and surgery for lesions that are amenable to both therapeutic approaches. Both procedures appear to be susceptible to restenosis (25,32); however, the relative frequency and clinical significance of restenosis for both procedures remain to be elucidated. Thus, it remains to be seen whether the theoretical fiscal advantages of CPTA related to the elimination of general anesthesia, blood-type screen, and transfusion, as well as shorter stays in the recovery room, intensive care unit, and hospital, will make CPTA more affordable than surgery.

THE FUTURE OF CPTA: ENSURING A FAIR AND SCIENTIFIC INQUIRY

"Prejudice: a disease characterized by hardening of the categories."—*William A. Ward*

These words succinctly capture the rigid, unreasonable, preconceived convictions that impede progress in carotid angioplasty research. Some elements of the neuroscience community appear to think that the recent level-1 evidence (33) for the clinical effectiveness of carotid endarterectomy (34–36) justifies a moratorium on the use of CPTA in general and carotid angioplasty in particular. However, the existence of effective therapy does not preclude the advent of more effective and acceptable alternatives. Moreover, CPTA is tractable in some lesions that are surgically inaccessible, such as those in the high-cervical, prepetrous, and cavernous internal carotid arteries. In addition, CPTA and surgery may be complementary in some instances; that is, CPTA may be useful after failed carotid endarterectomy. A variegated strategy is needed to optimize the secondary prevention of atherosclerotic cerebrovascular disease. Our efforts to expand the preventive armamentarium should include an authoritative and dispassionate evaluation of CPTA.

Progress in CPTA research does not mean that endarterectomy can be replaced by angioplasty. The success of CPTA does not portend the end of surgical therapy, just as surgery for coronary and peripheral vascular disease thrives despite the advent of angioplasty. Between 1979 and 1989, the adoption of angioplasty for peripheral vascular disease of the lower extremities was associated with an increase in the use of peripheral bypass surgery; the rate more than doubled from 32 to 65 per 100,000 (37). Between 1981 and 1986 in the National Hospital Discharge Survey, the rate of coronary artery bypass graft (CABG) procedures increased 36% from 69.9 to 95.3 per 100,000 (38); and between 1981 and 1989 the rate of CABG in Ontario, Canada, increased 31% from 50.3 to 66.0 per 100,000 (39).

The future of cerebral angioplasty depends on creating a network of multidisciplinary neurointerventional teams committed to and cognizant of the tremendous demands that reliable clinical research entails, and on organizing a cadre of disinterested clinicians and methodologists who will ensure the scientific rigor of future CPTA studies by providing external oversight. This implies the close cooperation of subspecialties that have traditionally viewed one another with suspicion. Participants and their societies must subordinate their interests and differences to patient welfare and use the research paradigm to foster interdisciplinary cooperation. The orderly implementation of CPTA, if and when it is proven to be of therapeutic value, can be modeled on the team approach used in scientific inquiry.

Efficient large-scale CPTA evaluation requires the collaboration of several medical subspecialties: neurology, neurosurgery, cardiovascular medicine, cardiovascular surgery, and radiology, including interventional radiology and neuroradiology. Properly trained operators may designate any one of these as their primary specialty; that is, CPTA is the prerogative of the appropriately trained and proficient operator who maintains an adequate caseload, regardless of his or her subspecialty. In addition, close collaboration with a team of clinical epidemiologists, statisticians, and data management personnel is the sine qua non of definitive modern CPTA research.

The disparate study designs mentioned earlier bespeak the controversy surrounding the optimal approach to CPTA validation. Phase III randomized controlled trial proponents believe that the state of the science is evolved enough and stable enough to conduct a multicenter study to compare CPTA and carotid endarterectomy (40). We disagree. First, we are not convinced that the state of the science establishes the theoretical clinical equipoise that is necessary to justify randomization in this context. Second, techniques and technology are evolving so rapidly that the results of an ostensibly definitive study run a genuine risk of being irrelevant (eg, the pending release of endovascular devices, in particular endoluminal stents, that may improve the success rate and decrease the adverse outcome rate associated with CPTA). Third, a test of angioplasty vs. endarterectomy would be unfair at this time because of the relative technical maturity of endarterectomy and because of the scarcity of accomplished CPTA operators.

Despite the controversy concerning the specifics of optimal study design, adequately controlled studies are a precondition to proving the clinical effectiveness of CPTA for the prevention of stroke and death in patients with external carotid and vertebral disease. The reasons for this are several: (a) the majority of patients with transient ischemic attacks (TIAs) do not suffer permanent dysfunction in follow-up

(41,34); (b) there is significant variability in the risk for subsequent stroke among patients who suffer a TIA (42); (c) some risk factors for stroke are unknown; and (d) a significant proportion of strokes and deaths that occur in follow-up are due to extraneous factors such as hemorrhage, lacunar infarction, cardiogenic embolism, and myocardial infarction (43,44).

SUMMARY

We are still in the early stages of the clinical evaluation of CPTA. There are no definitive reports concerning the long-term clinical and angiographic results of this procedure. Angioplasty techniques and technology are evolving rapidly. Although preliminary prospective results are encouraging, CPTA's therapeutic role remains unclear. Rigorous controlled studies are needed to establish this role; however, interdisciplinary cooperation, networked multidisciplinary research teams, technological stabilization, and additional basic research are needed before a meaningful comparison of CPTA and therapeutic alternatives, in stroke prevention for extracranial carotid and vertebral cerebrovascular disease, is practicable.

REFERENCES

1. Classification of cerebrovascular diseases III. *Stroke* 1990;21:637–676.
2. Gomez CR. Carotid plaque morphology and the risk for stroke. *Stroke* 1990;21:148–151.
3. Fuster V, Badimon L, Badimon JJ, Chesebro JH. The pathogenesis of coronary artery disease and the acute coronary syndromes. *N Engl J Med* 1992;326:242–250.
4. Landau C, Lange Ra, Hillis LD. Percutaneous transluminal angioplasty. *N Engl J Med* 1994;330:981–993.
5. Kerber CW, Lange RA, Hillis LD. Percutaneous transluminal angioplasty. *N Engl J Med* 1994;330:981–993.
6. Mullan S, Duda EE, Patro NAS. Some examples of balloon technology in neurosurgery. *J Neurosurg* 1980;52:321–329.
7. Tsai FY, Matovich V, Hieshima G, et al. Percutaneous angioplasty of the carotid artery. *Am J Neuroradiol* 1986;7:349–358.
8. Becker G, Katzen B, Dake M. Noncoronary angioplasty. *Radiology* 1989;170:921–940.
9. Theron J. Angioplasty of brachiocephalic vessels. In: Vinuela F, Halbach VV, Dion JE, eds. *Interventional Neuroradiology: Endovascular Therapy in the Central Nervous System.* New York: Raven Press, 1992; 167–180.
10. Munari LM, Belloni G, Perretti A, Ghia HF, Moschini L, Porta M. Carotid percutaneous angioplasty. *Neurol Res* 1992;14(suppl): 156–158.
11. Fleiss JL, Gross AJ. Meta-analysis in epidemiology, with special reference to studies of the association between exposure to environmental tobacco smoke and lung cancer: A critique. *J Clin Epidemiol* 1991;44: 127–139.
12. Broad WJ. The publishing game: Getting more for less. *Science* 1981; 211:1137–1139.
13. Huth EJ. Irresponsible authorship and wasteful publication. *Ann Intern Med* 1986;104:257–259.
14. Angell M, Relman AS. Redundant publication. *N Engl J Med* 1989; 320:1212–1213.
15. International Committee of Medical Journal Editors. Uniform requirements for manuscripts submitted to biomedical journals. *Can Med Assoc J* 1994;150:147–154.
16. Freitag G, Freitag J, Koch RD, Wagemann W. Percutaneous angioplasty of carotid artery stenosis. *Neuroradiology* 1986;28:126–127.
17. Freitag G, Freitag J, Koch RD, et al. Transluminal angioplasty for the treatment of carotid artery stenosis. *Vasa* 1987;16:67–71.
18. Higashida RT, Hieshima GB, Tsai FY, Halbach W, Norman D, Newton TH. Transluminal angioplasty of the vertebral and basilar artery. *Am J Neuroradiol* 1987;8:745–749.
19. Higashida RT, Tsai FY, Halbach W, et al. Transluminal angioplasty for atherosclerotic disease of the vertebral and basilar arteries. *J Neurosurg* 1993;78:192–198.
20. Kachel R, Basch ST, Heerklotz, I, Grossman K, Endler S. Percutaneous transluminal angioplasty (PTA) of supra-aortic arteries especially in the internal carotid artery. *Neuroradiology* 1991;33:191–194.
21. Theron J, Courtheoux P, Alachkar F, Maiza D. New triple coaxial catheter system for carotid angioplasty with cerebral protection. *Am J Neuroradiol* 1990;11:869–874.
22. Courtheoux P, Tournade A, Theron J, et al. Transcutaneous angioplasty of a vertebral artery atheromatous ostial stricture. *Neuroradiology* 1985;27:259–264.
23. Purdy PD, Devous MD Sr, Unwin DH, Giller CA, Batjer HH. Angioplasty of an atherosclerotic middle cerebral artery associated with improvement in regional blood flow. *Am J Neuroradiol* 1990;11:878–880.
24. Ferguson R, Ferguson J, Schwarten D, et al. Immediate angiographic results and in-hospital central nervous system complications of cerebral percutaneous transluminal angioplasty. *Circulation* 1993;88(suppl): 1–393.
25. The NACPTAR Investigators: Ferguson R, Schwarten D, Purdy P, et al. Restenosis following cerebral percutaneous transluminal angioplasty. Presented at the Forty-sixth Annual Meeting of the American Academy of Neurology in Seattle; May 1995.
26. The NACPTAR Investigators. Vascular determinants of successful cerebral percutaneous transluminal angioplasty. Presented at the Forty-sixth Annual Meeting of the American Academy of Neurology in Seattle; May 1995.
27. Detre K, Holubkov R, Kelsey S, et al. Percutaneous transluminal coronary angioplasty in 1985–1986 and 1977–1981. The National Heart, Lung and Blood Institute Registry. *N Engl J Med* 1988;318:265–270.
28. Serruys PW, de Jaegere P, Kiemeneij F, et al. A comparison of balloon-expandable stent implantation with balloon angioplasty in patients with coronary artery disease. Benestent Study Group. *N Engl J Med* 1994; 331:489–495.
29. Fischman DL, Leon MB, Baim DS, et al. A randomized comparison of coronary-stent placement and balloon angioplasty in the treatment of coronary artery disease. Stent Restenosis Study Investigators. *N Engl J Med* 1994;331:496–501.
30. Haude M, Erbel R, Hafner G, et al. Multicenter results after coronary implantation of balloon-expandable Plamaz–Shatz stents. *Z Kardiol* 1993;82:77–86.
31. George BS, Voorhes WD III, Roubin GS, et al. Multicenter investigation of coronary stenting to treat acute or threatened closure after percutaneous transluminal angioplasty: Clinical and angiographic outcome. *J Am Coll Cardiol* 1993;22:135–143.
32. Hunter GC, Palmaz JC, Hayashi HH, Raviola CA, Vogt PJ, Guernsey JM. The etiology of symptoms in patients with recurrent carotid stenosis. *Arch Surg* 1987;122:311–315.
33. Sacket DL. Rules of evidence and clinical recommendations on the use of antithrombotic agents. *Chest* 1986;89(suppl):2S–3S.
34. North American Symptomatic Carotid Endarterectomy Trial Collaborators. Beneficial effect of carotid endarterectomy in symptomatic patients with high-grade carotid stenosis. *N Engl J Med* 1991;325: 445–453.
35. Investigators of the Asymptomatic Carotid Atherosclerosis Study (ACAS). Clinical advisory on carotid endarterectomy for patients with asymptomatic carotid artery stenosis. National Institute of Neurological Disorders and Stroke Clinical Alert, September 30, 1994.
36. European Carotid Surgery Trialists Collaborative Group. MRC European carotid surgery trial: Interim results for symptomatic patients with severe (70–99%) or with mild (1–29%) carotid stenosis. *Lancet* 1991; 337:1235–1243.
37. Tunis SR, Bass EB Steinberg EP. The use of angioplasty, bypass surgery, and amputation in the management of peripheral vascular disease. *N Engl J Med* 1991;325:556–562.

38. Feinlieb M, Havlik RJ, Gillum RF, Pokras R, McCarthy E, Moien M. Coronary heart disease and related procedures. National Hospital Discharge Survey data. *Circulation* 1989;70(suppl I):I-13–I-18.

39. Ugnat AM, Naylor CD. Trends in coronary artery bypass grafting in Ontario from 1981 to 1989. *Can Med Assoc J* 1993;148:569–575.

40. Brown MM. Balloon angioplasty for cerebrovascular disease. *Neurol Res* 1992;14:159–163.

41. Hankey GJ, Slattery JM, Warlow CP. The prognosis of hospital-re-ferred transient ischemic attacks. *J Neurol Neurosurg Psychiatry* 1991; 54:793–802.

42. Robinson JG, Leon AS. The prevention of cardiovascular disease: Emphasis on secondary prevention. *Med Clin North Am* 1994;78:69–98.

43. Choi DW. Selective vulnerability of the brain: New insights into the pathophysiology of stroke. *Ann Intern Med* 1989;110:992–1000.

44. Sirna S, Biller J, Skorton DJ, Seabold JE. Cardiac evaluation of the patient with stroke. *Stroke* 1990;21:14–23.

Cerebrovascular Disease, edited by H. Hunt Batjer.
Lippincott-Raven Publishers, Philadelphia © 1997.

CHAPTER 35

Surgical Management of Vertebral Artery Lesions

Fernando G. Diaz, Thomas Cummings, Harvey Wilner, and Vickie Gordon

GENERAL BACKGROUND

The syndrome of vertebrobasilar ischemia has been a source of controversy since Kubik and Adams (1) described thrombosis of the basilar artery. Millikan described the syndrome that is now agreed to represent ischemic disease of the brainstem (2). Multiple diagnostic techniques have been used in the evaluation of patients with vertebrobasilar insufficiency, including angiography, Doppler ultrasound, transcranial Doppler, computed tomography (CT), magnetic resonance imaging (MRI) and MR angiography, and positron emission tomography (PET) scanning. Cerebral angiography remains the gold standard in the anatomic determination of occlusive lesions of the posterior circulation. Numerous medical approaches have been used with variable degrees of success. Millikan et al (2,3) recommended anticoagulation to treat patients suspected clinically of having basilar artery thrombosis and found a 50% decrease in the incidence of brainstem infarction in symptomatic patients. No angiographic correlation was undertaken in these patients. Surgical approaches to the vertebrobasilar circulation have included intracranial and extracranial procedures, but there has been no agreement among neurologists and neurosurgeons about the potential benefit of any surgical procedure used to treat patients with ischemia of the posterior circulation.

An overview of the clinical and pathologic characteristics of patients with lesions of the vertebral artery (VA) will be presented along with a discussion of the surgical alternatives available for lesions in the vertebral artery.

F. G. Diaz, T. Cummings and V. Gordon: Department of Neurological Surgery, Wayne State University, School of Medicine, Detroit, Michigan 48201.

H. Wilner: Department of Radiology, Wayne State University, School of Medicine, Detroit, Michigan 48201.

PERTINENT NEUROLOGIC AND VASCULAR ANATOMY AND VARIATIONS

The vertebrobasilar system is formed by the confluence of the VAs, which arise from the subclavian artery on the left and from the brachycephalic artery on the right. The VAs have four distinct anatomic portions: (a) first or proximal portion, extending from the origin of the VA to the foramen transversarium of C-6; (b) second or intraosseous portion, consisting of the VA section that traverses the foramina transversaria of C-6 through C-1; (c) third or atlantal portion, extending from the exit of the VA at the C-1 foramen to its entry into the dura through the atlanto-occipital membrane; and (d) fourth or intradural portion, extending from the point of entry, through the dura, to the point of convergence with the opposite VA to form the basilar artery (4) (Fig. 1).

The vertebrobasilar junction is located at the level of the mid-pons. The basilar artery then extends from the midpons to the upper midbrain where it bifurcates, giving rise to the two posterior cerebral arteries. The main arteries arising from the vertebrobasilar system are the posterior inferior cerebellar artery from the VAs, the anterior inferior cerebellar artery from the midportion of the basilar artery, and the superior cerebellar arteries from the distal basilar artery prior to its termination. Although these three arterial pairs are the main arteries originating from the vertebrobasilar system, numerous short and intermediate circumferential arteries, as well as perforators, originate directly from the basilar and vertebral arteries (1,5). The entire brainstem, cerebellum, and occipital lobes and part of the temporal lobes are irrigated by the vertebrobasilar circulation.

The carotid circulation connects with the vertebrobasilar circulation at the level of the posterior cerebral arteries normally through the posterior communicating arteries. The posterior cerebral arteries develop embryologically from the internal carotid arteries through the posterior communicating

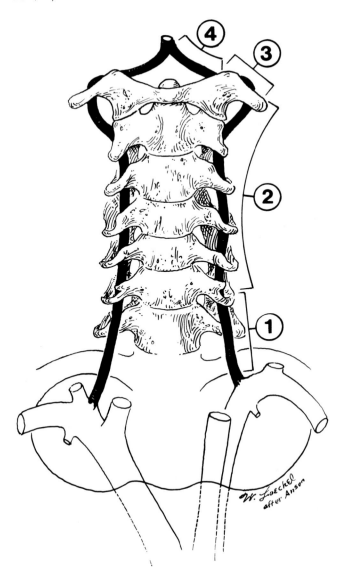

FIG. 1. Anatomic portions of the vertebral artery. 1: Origin to foramen transversarium of C-6; 2: Intraosseous portion within foramina transversaria of C-6 to C-1; 3: Horizontal portion from exit at C-1 foramen to dural entry; 4: Intradural portion from entry through the dura to the origin of the basilar artery.

artery, the otic artery connecting the intrapetrous carotid artery to the midportion of the basilar artery, the hypoglossal artery connecting the extracranial internal carotid artery to the intracranial VA, and the proatlantal artery connecting the extracranial internal carotid artery to the extracranial VA at the C-2 level (8). The trigeminal artery is purely subarachnoid and easy to identify intracranially. The otic artery is partly intrapetrous, coursing through the Vidian canal, to become subarachnoid and join the midportion of the basilar artery. The hypoglossal artery is extracranial in origin and gains access to the intracranial cavity through the hypoglossal canal. The proatlantal artery is purely extracranial.

The extracranial VA is surrounded by an extensive venous plexus that extends from the third portion of the artery, follows the artery in and throughout the second portion as it travels through the foramina transversaria, and drains into the vertebral vein at the level of the sixth or seventh transverse process, to drain into the subclavian vein.

PATHOLOGIC FEATURES

Vertebrobasilar circulation may be affected by a variety of pathologic processes of which arteriosclerosis is the most important (4,7,8). In a large group of autopsies, Schwartz and Mitchell (7) described arteriosclerotic plaques at the origin of the VA as the most common site of abnormality. The second most common site was the second portion of the VA, in the foramina transversaria. It is uncertain as to why the intraosseous portion of the VA is a site of deposition of arteriosclerotic material. It is possible that the segmental damping effect of the pulsatile expansion of the artery may contribute to the deposition of lipids in the wall. Third in frequency is the vertebrobasilar junction, probably resulting from the flow turbulence that develops as the two VAs come together to form the basilar artery. Arteriosclerotic lesions at other levels are less frequent and include the point of entry of the VA through the dura, and the mid- and distal basilar artery (1,2,6,7,10). The frequency of atherosclerosis in the VA varies and generally occurs less often than in the carotid artery (8).

Other pathologic conditions of the vertebrobasilar system include spontaneous VA dissections with the formation of pseudoaneurysms and complete occlusion. Spontaneous dissection is frequently observed in association with fibromuscular hyperplasia of the VAs (2,4). Fibromuscular changes have been observed in the first three portions of the VA but have not been reported in the fourth portion. Spontaneous dissections observed in association with fibromuscular disease have occurred mostly in the distal second and third portions of the VA (2,4).

Direct trauma to the VA by penetrating wounds or severe cervical spine fracture dislocations can result in occlusion, dissecting pseudoaneurysms, or arteriovenous fistula of the VA (11). Traumatic occlusion or dissection of the VAs, which may extend into the basilar artery, have been reported after chiropractic manipulation of the neck (11). The effect

arteries. These primitive posterior cerebral arteries join with the basilar artery at the P-1 or proximal portion of the posterior cerebral arteries. After the embryonic development is completed, the carotid origin of the posterior cerebral artery regresses and becomes the posterior communicating artery. In most cases the P-1 portion of the posterior cerebral artery then enlarges to form the proximal portion of the artery; it remains incompletely developed or atrophies in 25% of patients. Communication with the anterior circulation through the posterior communicating artery is functional in only 65% of individuals (5,6). Four normal embryologic arterial connections may persist after birth in some individuals. These arteries are the trigeminal artery connecting the intracavernous portion of the carotid artery to the tip of the basilar

of trauma to the VAs induced by chiropractic manipulation is not necessarily age-dependent or related to pre-existing pathology. The mechanism proposed for the disruption of the VA during chiropractic manipulation relates to *the areas of fixation of the artery at the level of the foramina transversaria* and the sudden traction inflicted by the manipulation. Since the artery is tethered at two fixed points within its intraosseous course, the sudden stretch of the artery between these two points causes it to tear and allows for a traumatic dissection and occlusion of the artery.

External encroachment on the VA from osteophytic spurs arising from the cervical vertebrae may compress the second portion of the VA and produce symptoms of vertebrobasilar insufficiency, generally associated with dynamic changes in position of the cervical spine (12,13). These changes are most frequently seen in individuals with severe spondylitic and osteoarthritic spurs and are frequently missed when arteriography is performed in neutral position. For the result to be positive the angiogram must be performed with the head turned in the direction known to induce the symptoms.

Ligamentous bands from the anterior scalene muscle compressing the VA at C-6 (13) can also cause vertebrobasilar insufficiency. In patients with osteophytic spurs compressing the second portion of the VA and in patients with ligamentous bands compressing the artery as it enters the C-6 foramen, it is frequently possible to precipitate the symptoms by rotation of the neck. In these patients, a dynamic angiogram is frequently positive, revealing the exact level of the occlusion.

The subclavian steal syndrome is a clinical entity that results from the occlusion of the subclavian artery, associated with symptoms of vertebrobasilar insufficiency, provoked by active use of the left arm (14,15). The increased demand for blood triggered by activity coupled with occlusion of the subclavian artery prior to the origin of the left VA result in the shunting of blood into the left subclavian artery through many muscular collaterals and reversal of the flow in the left VA. The left VA will carry flow from the intracranial circulation to the left arm. The flow reversal is generally well tolerated until the demand for blood flow in the left arm increases, diverting more arterial flow from the cerebral circulation and causing partial ischemia of the brainstem.

Most emboli in the vertebrobasilar territory originate from sources other than the VA itself, including the cardiac valves or areas of previous myocardial infarction; atrial thrombi; atrial myxomas; arteriosclerotic plaques of the aorta, subclavian or innominate arteries; and pathologic emboli of systemic origin (4).

CLINICAL PRESENTATION

The syndrome of vertebrobasilar insufficiency is characterized by intermittent episodes of neurologic dysfunction. The symptoms are usually repetitive but can be progressive or occur as a single, sudden, severe event with complete and permanent neurologic dysfunction. The syndrome of vertebrobasilar insufficiency (16) consists of at least two of the following symptoms: (a) motor or sensory deficits or both occurring bilaterally in the same attack; (b) ataxia of gait; (c) diplopia; (d) dysarthria; (e) dysmetria; or (f) bilateral homonymous hemianopsia. Additional symptoms compatible with this syndrome are vertigo, tinnitus, multiple cranial nerve involvement usually contralateral to the major sensory deficit, and motor involvement of the extremities. Dizziness by itself, syncope, drop attacks, and transient global amnesia do not form part of the syndrome of vertebrobasilar insufficiency. If any of these symptoms occur alone, other causes besides vertebrobasilar insufficiency should be considered (4,16). No study correlates the angiographic findings in patients with vertebrobasilar insufficiency and any specific combination of symptoms.

The differential diagnosis of vertebrobasilar disease should exclude cardiac problems such as dysrhythmias, myocardial insufficiency, and emboli. Emboli of cardiac origin may arise from an old myocardial infarction, valvular disease, or subacute bacterial endocarditis. Any potential hematologic problem associated with the development of hypercoagulability, including thrombocytosis, sickle cell disease, or macroglobulinemias, should be ruled out. Women who smoke, are taking contraceptives, and present with events of basilar migraine may develop symptoms that mimic vertebrobasilar ischemia. Bleeding disorders with intraparenchymal hemorrhages could result in the development of sudden neurologic dysfunction in the vertebrobasilar distribution. The abrupt onset of symptoms in these patients and the severity of the clinical picture would be comparable only to thrombosis of the basilar artery with complete loss of function of the brainstem.

Other processes that may resemble vertebrobasilar insufficiency include demyelinating disease, usually occurring in younger individuals, and intracranial neoplasms, such as cerebellopontine angle region tumors or intraaxial tumors of the cerebellum. In some cases, Meniere's syndrome mimics vertebrobasilar insufficiency and therefore must be excluded.

Routine laboratory examinations include a complete differential blood count with a blood smear and complete coagulation profile, a metabolic battery, a 12-lead electrocardiogram, and Holter monitoring for 24 or 36 hours. A CT scan will exclude most intracranial sources of nonvascular structural pathology (4). With the recent introduction of PET scanning, the metabolic function of the brainstem or cerebellum can be determined, although its application to the study of vertebrobasilar ischemic disease has been limited. MRI has rapidly improved the diagnostic capabilities and image resolution in patients evaluated for vertebrobasilar insufficiency (Fig. 2).

Selective cerebral angiography is the definitive diagnostic tool to establish the nature of the vascular involvement in the patient with vertebrobasilar insufficiency (5,6,17); the

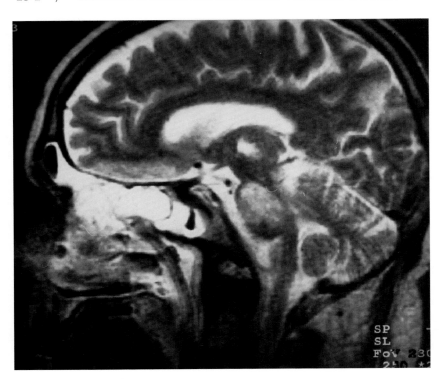

FIG. 2. Sagittal T2 MRI of 65-year-old woman admitted to the hospital with sudden onset of coma, quadriparesis, bilateral ophthalmoplegia, and tachypnea. Scan shows extensive area of brain edema within the substance of the pons compatible with a pontine infarction.

currently acceptable overall mortality rate is 0.6% with major complications under 1% (5). The recent introduction of intraarterial digital cerebral angiography and nonionic contrast agents has made cerebral angiography even safer. Digital angiography requires lower doses of contrast to obtain excellent diagnostic images and reduces the contrast load required in patients with serious renal or cardiac problems.

Two exciting vascular imaging techniques are now in progress: CT and MR angiography. For CT angiography the patient is studied in a helical CT instrument that produces instantaneous real-time three-dimensional reconstruction of the intracranial vessels. MR angiography produces two-dimensional images that resemble a conventional angiogram but does not require the administration of contrast material. As the diagnostic accuracy and precision of CT and MR angiography increases, they will become the ideal diagnostic tools for evaluation of the cerebral circulation (Fig. 3).

MEDICAL TREATMENT

The medical management of patients with vertebrobasilar insufficiency has made little progress in the last 40 years. Millikan et al (3) introduced systemic anticoagulation in the 1950s and observed a decline in mortality rate from 43% in an untreated group of patients to 24% in a group of patients treated with heparin. Angiography was not performed, other major causes of symptoms were not ruled out, and patients were not randomized to treatment groups. All patients were assumed to have impending basilar occlusion before the

treatment started but no definitive clinical study was performed to document this conclusion. Whisnant et al (16) reported a decreased incidence of brainstem stroke from 35% to 15% within 4 years in patients with symptoms of vertebrobasilar ischemia who received oral anticoagulants. Treatment and control groups were chosen, but most patients had not undergone angiography and were not randomized to the treatment groups.

Other forms of treatment, such as antiplatelet agents, are used to treat patients with vertebrobasilar disease, but the effectiveness in averting strokes cannot be reliably predicted in an individual patient. In patients with angiographically confirmed impending basilar artery occlusion caused by a local thrombus or from a systemic embolus, some have used systemic or locally infused streptokinase and urokinase. The hemorrhagic complications of these drugs administered systemically and their limited efficacy have been enough to discourage their use. The local application of streptokinase met with some success and led to the introduction of tissue plasminogen activator (TPA). The cost of TPA has been a major limiting factor in its use. Comparative studies that evaluated the difference between TPA and streptokinase in cardiac patients have not shown a significant benefit of one over the other for intravascular clot lysis.

Strict blood pressure control should be discouraged in patients with angiographically demonstrated, hemodynamically significant lesions of the vertebrobasilar tree. In cases with severe lesions, a significant drop in blood pressure could acutely alter the perfusion to the ischemic brain and create a watershed area of ischemia (4,18). Hypertension in these patients could reflect ischemia of the brainstem.

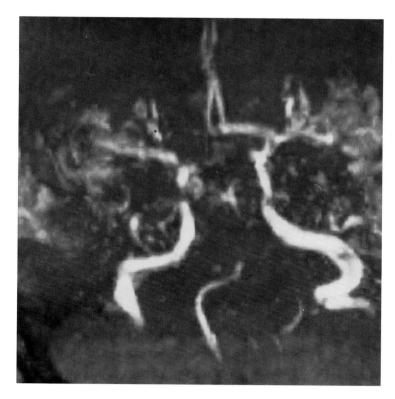

FIG. 3. MR angiogram of 65-year-old woman admitted with a pontine infarct showing left vertebral artery occlusion, occlusion of the basilar artery origin, and congenital absence of A-1 segment on the right.

SURGICAL PRINCIPLES AND STRATEGIES

Surgery for patients with vertebrobasilar insufficiency has been controversial since Crawford et al (17) reported the surgical approach to lesions of the extracranial VA in 1958. Initial surgical procedures (18–20), including endarterectomy of the VA origin through the VA wall or through the subclavian artery (19), were poorly received. These procedures were associated with many complications, including occlusion of the VA, postoperative hematomas, phrenic nerve paresis, lymphoceles, chyle fistulae, and others. It was not until the early 1970s that Edwards and Wright (20) reported a successful series of proximal extracranial VA reconstructions for the treatment of patients with vertebrobasilar insufficiency.

Transposition

Several procedures are currently used to treat extracranial VA lesions. The most common is the transposition of the VA from its origin to a new location, generally the ipsilateral common carotid artery (15,18,20). The VA is exposed through a supraclavicular incision placed 2 cm above the clavicle and just across the midline. The prevertebral fascia is approached by dissecting the space medial to the sterno-cleidomastoid muscle, exposing the common carotid artery, the jugular vein, and the vagus nerve. The sympathetic ganglia and their branches are found immediately beneath the prevertebral fascia, directly over the anterior scalene muscle.

The ascending pharyngeal artery and the posterior cervical arteries are frequently in the operative field adjacent to the cervical sympathetic plexus. The VA can be found as it travels from its origin to the foramen transversarium of C-6, lateral to the longus coli muscle, medial to the anterior scalene muscle, and deep to the vertebral vein and sympathetic chain.

Care must be taken to identify the thoracic duct as it enters the angle formed by the confluence of the jugular and subclavian veins. The lymphatic duct generally is formed by three or four small branches that enter the venous angle from a deep to a more superficial location. When dissecting the VA origin, the lymphatics are generally clearly visible under magnification. The lymphatics are larger on the left than on the right side but should and can be identified on either side and transfixion ligated to prevent the ultimate development of a chyle fistula or a chyle cyst. Lymphatics do not coagulate well and must be ligated to prevent a leak from occurring. Once the lymphatics are ligated, they can be transected to expose the origin of the VA.

When exposing the VA on the right side, it is important to pay special attention to the retraction exerted on the trachea and esophagus. The recurrent laryngeal nerve is located in the tracheo-esophageal groove after it loops around the subclavian artery to return to the larynx. On the left side, the recurrent laryngeal nerve is more lax because it loops around the aortic arch, and as a result the trachea can be retracted with more freedom. Extreme retraction of the recurrent laryngeal nerve will result in paresis of the ipsilateral vocal cord, in most cases a temporary condition but permanent in a small percentage.

Sufficient length of VA may be gained for an anastomosis by dissecting the entire VA from its origin to the foramen transversarium. The VA is located directly below the vertebral vein, and often it is necessary to coagulate and transect the vein to expose the artery. Coagulation of the vein may be difficult because it forms a plexus that surrounds the artery as it exits from the foramen transversarium. Coagulation of the vein can be difficult since the vein is sometimes densely adherent to the artery. Careful separation of the vein is required before the vein can be coagulated. The VA is transected after it has been ligated at its origin and temporarily clipped at the foramen transversarium. A fish mouth stoma is prepared on the free end of the VA, and the common carotid artery is then clamped proximally and distally. A fenestration is made on the lateral wall of the carotid artery and an end-to-side anastomosis is completed under magnification between the vertebral and the common carotid arteries (Fig. 4).

Transposition of the subclavian artery to the common carotid artery has been performed for patients with subclavian steal syndrome secondary to subclavian artery occlusion (20). This procedure is preferable to vertebral-to-carotid transposition in patients who have intermittent claudication of the upper extremity. Other angioplastic procedures of the VA origin include balloon angioplasty of the origin, vertebral endarterectomy, patch graft of the VA origin with removal of the atherosclerotic plaque, or angioplastic reconstruction that widens and shortens the VA in cases of poststenotic ectasia of the VA (Fig. 5) (19).

Direct Grafting

Saphenous vein grafts and prosthetic grafts have been placed from the subclavian artery to the VA or from the common carotid artery to the VA distal to the area of stenosis (21,22). The VA is exposed in the manner described for the vertebral-to-carotid transposition. A saphenous vein graft is then obtained from the lower portion of the leg. The greater saphenous vein may be found immediately posterior to the medial malleolus, superficial to the medial malleolar ligament. The graft is obtained in a conventional manner, and care should be taken to cauterize or ligate side branches without damaging the vein wall. It is also important not to strip the vein clean of all periadventitial tissue because this could damage the vasa vasorum and result in endothelial necrosis. When the dissection is complete, the vein should be gently distended with warm heparinized blood or saline using a pressure-regulated balloon with no more than 200–300 mm of water pressure. The vein is then stored in cold heparinized blood or saline until it is used. The distal portion of the vein must be identified so that the anastomosis is performed respecting the direction of the valves.

In patients where the graft will be placed from the carotid

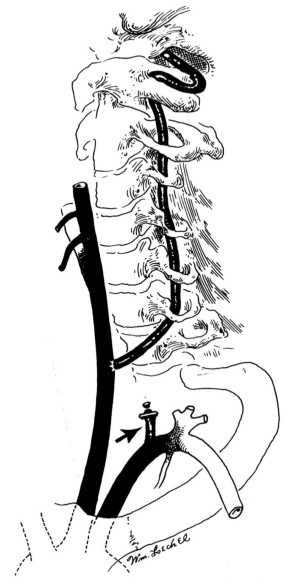

FIG. 4. Vertebral-to-carotid artery transposition. The vertebral artery is identified at its origin from the subclavian artery, transected, and anastomosed end-to-side to the common carotid artery.

to the VA, the carotid has been exposed during the initial dissection. In patients where it is decided to perform the anastomosis of the graft from the subclavian artery, it is necessary to disinsert the two heads of the sternocleidomastoid muscle to expose the length of the subclavian artery. The VA is then temporarily occluded at the transverse foramen and ligated at the origin. The proximal end is transected, a fish mouth stoma made, and an end-to-end anastomosis is completed with the vein graft. The proximal anastomosis is then performed on either the carotid artery or the subclavian artery in a manner similar to that described for the vertebral-to-carotid transposition. Special care must be taken to back

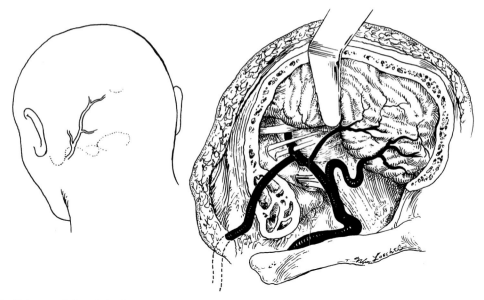

FIG. 5. Extracranial vertebral artery endarterectomy. The third portion of the vertebral artery is exposed via a suboccipital approach, the artery is isolated between temporary clips, an arteriotomy is made, and the arteriosclerotic plaque is removed. The arteriotomy is closed with a running suture.

bleed the anastomosis before closing the last suture to allow air and possible thrombi to exit the artery.

Balloon angioplasties have been performed successfully at the origin of the vertebral and in the subclavian artery proximal to the origin of the VA, but the recurrence rate is nearly 35% within the first 6 months postangioplasty.

Decompression

Decompressive procedures have been used to treat lesions in the second portion of the VA. Fibrous bands originating from the anterior scalene muscle can be released at the level of entry of the VA into the C-6 foramen (18,19,23). Decompressive osteotomies of the foramina transversia can be performed at single or multiple levels throughout the course of the VA from C-6 to C-1 foramina via an anterior or lateral route (12,13). When the foramina are enlarged for decompression, it is necessary to remove the periosteum that surrounds the VA because the areas of constriction could persist if the periosteum is not removed. In some patients it is not possible to remove all areas of stenosis in the second portion of the VA. In this situation it is possible to perform a high vertebral-to-carotid transposition to the external or the internal carotid artery.

Vascular Reconstruction

Vascular reconstruction using a long saphenous vein graft or a prosthetic from the subclavian or common carotid artery to the VA distal to the point of stenosis has been reported for patients with arteriosclerotic areas of stenosis in the second

portion of the VA (23,24). Anastomosis of a branch or the trunk of the external carotid artery to the second portion of the VA has also been reported (25). To accomplish this procedure, the anterior surfaces of one or two of the foramina above the level of stenosis are exposed through an anterior incision placed along the sternocleidomastoid muscle. The common carotid and the bifurcation are dissected in the usual manner and retracted laterally to expose the deep cervical fascia. The transverse processes are identified and the longus coli muscle is dissected from the anterior surface of the transverse process. The anterior and lateral walls of the transverse processes are removed and the periosteum adjacent to the VA canal is resected. It is generally necessary to remove two or three foramina to expose enough length of the VA.

When the VA is free, several alternatives may be used to deal with the problem. Whenever possible, the plaque may be dissected out by either inverting the VA and gradually separating the plaque until it feathers out or by a longitudinal arteriotomy and dissecting the plaque in a conventional manner. Either maneuver would leave a length of VA sufficient to then perform a transposition to the carotid bifurcation. If it is not possible to resect the plaque or mobilize enough VA to obtain a transposition, then it would be necessary to perform either a saphenous vein graft from the carotid artery or an anastomosis of one of the major branches of the external carotid artery to the second portion of the VA.

For arteriosclerotic lesions in the first or second foraminal level of the VA, it is sometimes possible to perform an anastomosis of the occipital artery or a saphenous vein graft to the third portion of the VA. The VA is exposed through an anterolateral incision that extends from the anterior border of the sternocleidomastoid muscle below the angle of the jaw to the highest point of the mastoid bone along the path of the external occipital artery. The mastoid attachment of the sternocleidomastoid muscle is transected and the posterior portion of the digastric disinserted to expose the occipital artery. The superior and inferior oblique muscles are transected at the level of the lateral mass of C-1 as the VA exits from the foramen. The VA is freed of the surrounding vertebral venous plexus and dissected from the foramen transversarium of C-1 to its entrance into the skull at the atlanto-occipital membrane. If the segment of VA dissected is not enough for the anastomosis, the atlanto-occipital membrane and dura mater may be opened to expose the fourth portion of the VA. Temporary clips are applied at the most proximal and distal ends of the VA, a longitudinal arteriotomy is performed, and an end-to-side anastomosis is completed with the occipital artery or a saphenous vein graft.

Endarterectomy

Vertebral endarterectomies have been performed in patients with highly stenotic areas in the third and fourth portions of the VA, usually associated with contralateral or high-grade stenosis or VA occlusion (9,10). The VA is approached through a suboccipital craniotomy performed with the patient lying in a three-quarter prone position. A midline or paramedian approach is performed and extended laterally until the VA is exposed and dissected from its exit at the first transverse process to its entry into the atlanto-occipital membrane. The VA is surrounded by a venous plexus that must be carefully dissected, cauterized, and transected. When dissection is completed, the dura is opened from the midline in the direction of the VA entry. The perimedullary portion of the VA is dissected to expose the origin of the posterior inferior cerebellar artery (PICA). If a vertebral endarterectomy is required, the artery can be clipped proximally at C-1 and distally prior to the PICA. A longitudinal arteriotomy is made, and the plaque is dissected under the microscope. After the plaque is removed, the arteriotomy is closed with running 6-0 or 7-0 polypropylene sutures. During the occlusion period, patients receive an intravenous bolus of 250 mg of thiopental, 100 mg of lidocaine (Xylocaine), and 5000 units of heparin.

Sundt (34) attempted balloon dilatation of the distal VA under direct observation but noted significant problems following the angioplasty, including VA dissections, thrombosis, and perforation. Sundt abandoned the use of intracranial vertebral angioplasties following this dismal experience. The results for endarterectomy were initially promising, but further experience revealed many complications, including brainstem infarctions like those found by Sundt during balloon angioplasties. Neither endarterectomy nor angioplasty of the distal VA is now recommended, although the introduction of newer endovascular angioplastic techniques may soon change this difficult treatment area.

Extracranial–Intracranial Bypass

For bilateral occlusion or high-grade stenosis of the distal VA, various forms of extracranial–intracranial anastomoses have been described. The occipital artery (OA) may be anastomosed to the postmedullary portion of the PICA (26–29). With the patient in the lateral position, the occipital artery is dissected from the level of the mastoid process to the inion. A lateral suboccipital craniectomy is performed and the postmedullary portion of PICA dissected free from the area of the lateral medulla. This portion of PICA is generally free of any branches to the brainstem and can be temporarily clamped for an anastomosis. The OA is clamped proximally, the distal end is cleaned of periadventitial tissue, and a fish mouth end is fashioned on its most distal portion. A longitudinal arteriotomy is performed on the segment of PICA that has been dissected and clamped, and an end-to-side anastomosis is completed from the occipital artery to PICA (Fig. 6).

For occlusive lesions of the vertebrobasilar junction, an anastomosis of the occipital artery to the second portion of the AICA (30) may be performed. The procedure is essentially the same as the one described for OA–PICA anastomosis in terms of the position, dissection of the OA, and suboccipital craniectomy, but the dissection of the AICA is performed on the anterior surface of the cerebellum just lateral to the foramen of Luschka. The rostral and caudal branches of the AICA may be found at that level, and usually there are no branches to the brainstem or the cerebellum at that point. The largest of the two branches is dissected and isolated, and an anastomosis of the occipital artery to AICA may then be completed in the manner described for the OA–PICA anastomosis.

The superficial temporal to superior cerebellar artery anastomosis (STA–SCA) has been used for mid- and distal basilar artery stenosis but has also been applied for more proximal lesions (31–33). With the patient in the supine position and the ipsilateral shoulder elevated, the head is placed flat on the table and rotated to the opposite side. The largest branch of the superficial temporal artery is dissected and a craniotomy is placed centered on the ear, with its inferior margin level with the floor of the middle fossa. The temporal lobe is elevated, preserving the posterior temporal lobe veins draining into the transverse sinus. The tentorial edge is identified and the tentorium is incised from the tentorial incisura behind the point of penetration of the IV cranial nerve toward the lateral cranial wall. The two tentorial flaps are elevated and fixed to the dural base, exposing the ambient cistern, the cerebral peduncles, the IVth cranial nerve, and the superior cerebellar arteries. The largest of the two SCA branches is dissected as it nears the anterior border of the cerebellum where there are no branches to the brainstem. The distal end of the STA is then prepared in the manner described for the OA anastomosis, taking care to leave enough length to allow the STA to reach the level of the cerebral peduncles. This usually requires 12–15 cm of

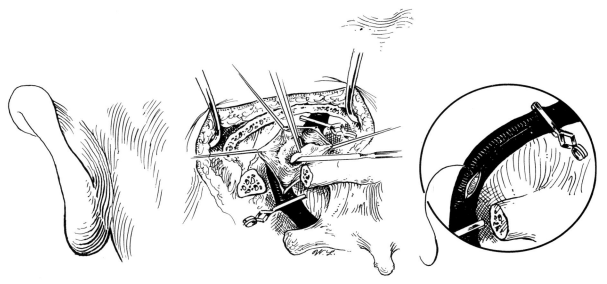

FIG. 6. Occipital to posterior inferior cerebellar artery (PICA) anastomoses. The occipital artery is dissected from its bed and through a suboccipital craniectomy anastomosed to the lateral medullary segment of PICA.

STA to complete the anastomosis without tension. Temporary clips are applied on the SCA, a longitudinal arteriotomy is completed, and an end-to-side anastomosis is performed from the STA to the SCA (Fig. 7).

The STA may also be anastomosed to the PCA (32). The procedure is essentially the same as the one described for the STA–SCA anastomosis, but it requires more retraction of the temporal lobe because the PCA lies somewhat higher than the superior cerebellar artery and enters the posterior interhemispheric fissure soon after it passes the posterolat-

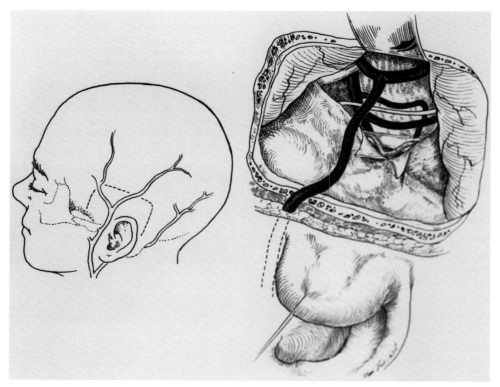

FIG. 7. Superficial temporal to posterior cerebral artery anastomosis. The superficial artery is dissected from its bed and through a subtemporal craniotomy anastomosed to the perimesencephalic portion of the superior cerebellar artery.

eral margin of the cerebral peduncle. The STA–PCA anastomosis is more risky because it requires temporary occlusion of the arterial supply to the visual cortex. The saphenous vein may be grafted from the extracranial carotid artery to the posterior cerebral artery (32) or to the superior cerebellar artery (32,33). The vein graft is obtained from the lower leg and care should be taken that the graft is oriented properly when the anastomoses are completed. The vein graft must be handled carefully because these grafts have a greater tendency to become occluded than the artery-to-artery grafts.

The surgical approaches described in this chapter have been designed to treat patients with symptoms suggestive of vertebrobasilar insufficiency, who have failed best available medical therapy and have a specific arterial lesion demonstrated by selective cerebral angiography compatible with their clinical picture. However, no attempt has been made to assign patients to a randomized controlled study.

COMPLICATIONS AND THEIR MANAGEMENT

The surgical results have been encouraging for patients who had an extracranial reconstructive procedure of the VA, with neurologic morbidity of 2% and mortality of 1% (35). The intracranial reconstructive procedures, including angioplasties of the fourth portion of the VA and all types of extracranial-to-intracranial anastomoses have had a greater number of complications (36). The highest number of complications were observed in patients who had unstable neurologic syndromes with signs of progressing ischemia or stroke in evolution.

OVERVIEW

Because patients with vertebrobasilar insufficiency may have symptoms arising from many areas, it is necessary to establish an accurate diagnosis before a treatment modality is chosen. Differential diagnostic possibilities include vascular and nonvascular causes that should be excluded before treatment is begun. The natural history of patients with vertebrobasilar insufficiency and arteriosclerotic lesions of the vertebrobasilar tree has not been studied well. Currently available information indicates that the stroke risk for untreated patients symptomatic for vertebrobasilar ischemia is 35% within 4 years after the onset of symptoms (16). The risk of stroke decreased by 50% in symptomatic patients treated with anticoagulants (16), although there was no angiographic proof that these patients had significant arterial lesions compatible with their symptomatology. The reported surgical morbidity for patients with angiographically proven, significant vertebrobasilar lesions is 5% and surgical mortality is 3% (22,31). Because to date there is no controlled study comparing best medical to best surgical treatment, each patient decision must be individualized. It is intuitively reasonable to treat patients medically first. If medical therapy fails,

surgery may then be justified in these otherwise untreatable patients.

REFERENCES

1. Kubick CS, Adams RD. Occlusion of the basilar artery. A clinical and pathological study. *Brain* 1946;69:73–121.
2. Millikan CH, Seikert RG. Studies in cerebrovascular disease. I. The syndrome of intermittent insufficiency of the basilar arterial system. *Mayo Clin Proc* 1965;3:61–68.
3. Millikan CH, Siekert RG, Shick RM. Studies in cerebrovascular disease. III. The use of anticoagulant drugs in the treatment of insufficiency or thrombosis within the basilar arterial system. *Proc Staff Meet Mayo Clin* 1955;30:116–126.
4. Sahs AL, Hartmann EC. Fundamentals of stroke care. DHEW Publ. (HRA) 76-14016. US Department of Health, Education and Welfare, Washington, D.C., 1976.
5. Caplan LR, Rosenbaum AE. Role of cerebral angiography and vertebrobasilar occlusive disease. *J Neurol Neurosurg Psychiatry* 1975;38:601–612.
6. Hass WK, Fields WB, North RR, Kricheff I, Chase NE, Bauer RB. Joint study of extracranial arterial occlusion. II. Arteriography, techniques, sites and complications. *JAMA* 1968;203:96–196.
7. Schwartz CJ, Mitchell JPA. Atheroma of the carotid and VA systems. *Br Med J* 1961;2:1057–1063.
8. Cerebral angiography. In: Taveras JM, Wood EH, eds. *Diagnostic Neuroradiology*. Baltimore: Williams and Wilkins, 1976;543–986.
9. Allen GS, Cohen RJ, Preziosi TJ. Microsurgical endarterectomy of the intracranial vertebral artery for vertebrobasilar transient ischemic attacks. *Neurosurgery* 1981;8:56–59.
10. Ausman JI, Diaz FG, Pearce JE, de los Reyes RA, Leuchter W, Mehta B, Petal S. Endarterectomy of the vertebral artery from C2 to posterior inferior cerebellar artery intracranially. *Surg Neurol* 1982;18:400–404.
11. Rosenwasser R, Delgado T, Buckheit W. Cerebrovascular complications of closed neck and head trauma. Injuries to the carotid artery. *Surg Rounds* 1983;12:56–65.
12. Hardin C. Vertebral artery insufficiency produced by cervical osteoarthritic spurs. *Arch Surg (Chicago)* 1965;90:629–633.
13. Sheehan S, Bauer R, Meyer JS. Vertebral artery compression in cervical spondylosis. *Neurology* 1960;70:968–986.
14. Fisher DM. A new vascular syndrome. The subclavian steal. *N Engl J Med* 1961;265:912–913.
15. Bohmfalk GL, Storey JL, Brown WE, Marlin AE. Subclavian steal syndrome. 1 and 2. *J Neurosurg* 1979;51:628–643.
16. Whisnant JP, Cartlidge NEF, Elvebach LR. Carotid and vertebrobasilar transient ischemic attacks. Effects of anticoagulants, hypertension, and cardiac disorders on survival and stroke occurrence. A population study. *Ann Neurol* 1978;3:107–115.
17. Crawford ES, DeBakey ME, Fields WS. Roentgenographic diagnosis and surgical treatment of basilar artery insufficiency. *JAMA* 1958;166:509.
18. Diaz FG, Ausman JI, Shrontz C, de los Reyes RA, Boulos R, Patel S, Pearce J. Combined reconstruction of the vertebral and carotid artery in one single procedure. *Neurosurgery* 1983;12:629–635.
19. Imparato AM. Surgery for extracranial cerebrovascular insufficiency. In: Ransohoff, ed. *Modern Techniques in Surgery. vol 14. Neurosurgery*. Futura: New York, 1979;1–38.
20. Edwards WH, Wright R. A new surgical technique for relief for subclavian stenosis. *Hosp Pract* 1972;7:78–87.
21. Berguer R, Bauer RB. Vertebral artery reconstruction. A successful technique in selecting patients. *Ann Surg* 1981;193:441–447.
22. Diaz FG, Ausman JI, de los Reyes RA, Boulos R, Patel S, Mehta B. Surgical correction of lesions affecting the vertebral artery. *Surg Forum* 1982;33:495–497.
23. Corkill G, French BN, Michas C, Cobb CA, Mims TJ. External carotid–vertebral artery anastomosis for a vertebrobasilar insufficiency. *Surg Neurol* 1977;7:109–115.
24. Clark K, Perry MO. Carotid vertebral anastomosis. An alternate for repair of the subclavian steal syndrome. *Ann Surg* 1966;163:414–406.
25. Pritz MB, Chandler WF, Kindt GW. Vertebral artery disease. Radiologic evaluation, medical management, and microsurgical treatment. *Neurosurgery* 1981;9:524–530.

26. Ausman JI, Nicoloff DM, Chou SN. Posterior fossa revascularization. Anastomosis of vertebral artery to PICA with interposition radial artery graft. *Surg Neurol* 9:281–286 (1978).

27. Kodadad G. Occipital artery–posterior inferior cerebellar artery anastomosis. *Surg Neurol* 1976;5:225–227.

28. Roski RA, Spetzler RF, Hopkins LN. Occipital artery to posterior inferior cerebellar artery bypass for vertebrobasilar ischemia. *Neurosurgery* 1982;10:44–49.

29. Ausman JI, Lee MC, Klassen AL, Seljeskog EL, Chou SN. Stroke. What's new? Cerebral revascularization. *Min Med* 1976;59:223–227.

30. Ausman JI, Diaz FG, de los Reyes RA, Pak H, Patel S, Boulos R. Anastomosis of the occipital artery to anterior inferior cerebellar artery for vertebrobasilar junction stenosis. *Surg Neurol* 1981;16:69–102.

31. Ausman JI, Diaz FG, de los Reyes RAN, Shrontz C, Pearce J, Dujovny M. Microsurgical techniques on cerebral revascularization. *Henry Ford Hosp Med J* 1983;31:3–15.

32. Sundt TM Jr, Whisnant JP, Piepgras DG, Campbell J, Holman CB. Intracranial bypass grafts for vertebrobasilar ischemia. *Mayo Clin Proc* 1978;53:12–18.

33. Sundt TM Jr, Whisnant JP, Piepgras DG, Campbell JK. Interposition saphenous vein grafts for advanced occlusive disease and large aneurysms in the posterior circulation. *J Neurosurg* 1982;56:205–215.

34. Sundt TM. Transluminal angioplasties for basilar artery stenosis. *Mayo Clin Proc* 1981;55:673–680.

35. Diaz FG, Ausman JI. Surgical therapy in vascular brainstem diseases. In: Hoffenberth B, Brunes GG, Sitzer G, Wegger HD, eds. *Vascular Brainstem Disease*. Basel: Karger, 1990;270–281.

36. Ausman JI, Diaz FG, Vacca DF, Sadasivan B. Superficial temporal artery and occipital artery bypass pedicles to superior, anterior inferior and posterior inferior cerebellar arteries for vertebrobasilar insufficiency. *J Neurosurg* 1990;72:554–558.

Cerebrovascular Disease, edited by H. Hunt Batjer.
Lippincott-Raven Publishers, Philadelphia © 1997.

CHAPTER 36

Extracranial Carotid Artery Injuries

Charles W. Wyble and Bruce L. Gewertz

This chapter will review the evolution of treatments for carotid artery trauma and then focus on current management of these life threatening vascular injuries. The discussion will address the specific diagnostic tests that allow selective nonoperative management of some patients with blunt and penetrating neck wounds. Finally, we will consider the critical decisions involved in revascularization in the presence of neurologic deficits.

HISTORY

The first documented carotid artery ligation for trauma was performed by Ambrose Pare in 1522 (1). Unfortunately, the French soldier undergoing the procedure developed aphasia and left-sided hemiplegia. A later account with a more successful outcome was documented in 1803 by Garrison; Mr. Fleming ligated the common carotid artery of a suicidal sailor aboard the H.M.S. Tonnant. He commented that "there was but one step to take with any prospect of success, mainly to cut down upon and tie the carotid artery below the wound"(2).

Remarkably, ligation remained the accepted mode of treatment for injuries of the carotid artery through World War I (3), although Sir Frederic Treves wrote in 1887, "I think the ligature of main arteries for arrest of bleeding in distant parts is often somewhat blindly advised and possibly too frequently carried out"(4). Utilizing this method, American surgeons reported mortalities from penetrating neck injuries of 15% in the Civil War (5), 18% in the Spanish-American War, and 11% in World War I (6). In the latter conflict, carotid ligation in American and British combatants was associated with a mortality of 44% (1); furthermore, those patients surviving had a 30% incidence of neurologic deficits (1,3).

During World War II and the Korean conflict, the mortality from such wounds decreased sharply. This was attributed to more expeditious performance of tracheostomy, early ex-

ploration, and the development of successful vascular surgical techniques (7). Ligation was discouraged and emphasis placed on prompt, mandatory exploration of all wounds penetrating the platysma (8,9). The best reports documented mortalities of less than 10%. These salutary results were undoubtedly influenced by the general improvements in care, including more attentive monitoring during anesthesia, antibiotics (10), and the aggressive management of shock (11). Paradoxically, mortality in the Vietnam conflict rose to 15% (12). This is usually attributed to the larger-caliber high-velocity injuries that were encountered. Nonetheless, taken together, the improved results in recent military experiences reaffirmed the fundamental principles that early exploration is essential and, whenever possible, primary repair is the most desirable management.

Despite knowledge gained from combat, outcomes for civilian carotid injuries during the 1950s and 1960s were surprisingly poor, with mortality rates as high as 11% (5). The trend was reversed only when young surgeons with military experience returned to their communities convinced of the utility of early mandatory exploration. Typical of these early civilian reports, Fogelman and Stewart (7) in 1956 demonstrated 6% mortality with early neck exploration as opposed to 35% mortality when surgery was delayed more than 6 hours.

As others followed these recommendations, the predictable yet undesirable consequence was a high incidence of negative explorations. For example, Ashworth et al (10) reported a 46% negative exploration rate, and Roon and Christensen (13) a 43% negative rate. A desire to maintain improved outcomes without undue utilization of resources prompted the most current trend in management of penetrating neck wounds—selective exploration, which will be discussed later in detail.

MECHANISMS OF INJURY

Although cervical neck trauma constitutes only 5–10% of all arterial trauma, morbidity and mortality of these inju-

C. W. Wyble and B. L. Gewertz: Department of Surgery, University of Chicago, Chicago, Illinois 60637

ries is significant (2). The most common cause of extracranial carotid artery injury is penetrating trauma, which accounts for roughly 90–95% of serious injuries. In most urban series, stab wounds and gunshots are equally represented. In addition to direct lacerations, the tragic increased use of high-velocity firearms adds the possibility of indirect "blast" injury when bullet paths are close to vascular structures.

Overall, blood vessels are injured in about 50% of penetrating wounds (14); major artery involvement is noted in approximately half of these. Most frequently injured is the common carotid artery followed by the subclavian artery (2,14). As would be predicted from its proximity, the most commonly injured venous structure is the internal jugular vein. In addition to the expected risk of massive hemorrhage, venous injuries may also be associated with potentially fatal air embolism.

Blunt carotid trauma is much less common (3–5% of injuries) but is being diagnosed more frequently due to expanded use of duplex ultrasonography and arteriography (2,15,16). Vessels can be injured directly by impact or indirectly by stretching and torsion. A final but relatively uncommon cause of vessel injury is iatrogenic injury related to the introduction of venous catheters or trauma from endoscopy or intubation.

Vascular injuries are often associated with damage to the trachea and larynx (10%), esophagus and pharynx (7%), and spinal cord and brachial plexus (2%) (17–22). As in all vascular injuries, late complications of untreated arterial trauma include false aneurysms, thrombotic occlusion, arteriovenous fistulas, and distal embolization (Fig. 1).

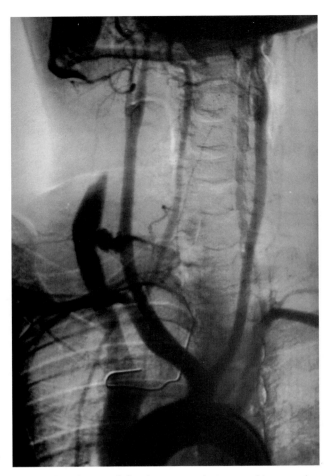

FIG. 1. Arteriogram following a gunshot wound in zone I reveals large arteriovenous fistula between the carotid artery and jugular vein.

PENETRATING INJURIES

Because of the benign appearance of a small entry wound, the initial evaluation of a patient with a penetrating cervical injury is often inaccurate (13). Unfortunately, the potential for sudden bleeding, airway compromise, and neurologic catastrophe demands swift and definitive management (5).

To aid in categorization and decision-making, the neck has been divided into three anatomic zones based on topographic landmarks. Original and still accepted work by Saletta et al (23) defined zone I as the area inferior to the sternal notch and zone III as the area above the angle of the mandible. The most commonly injured region, zone II, represents the region between the two. The neck can be further viewed as comprising anterior and posterior triangles, divided by the sternocleidomastoid muscle. In general, penetrating injuries to zone I carry the highest mortality (14).

Vascular Injury

Obvious indications of clinically important vascular injury include active bleeding, pulsatile or expanding hematoma, asymmetry of extremity blood pressure, and presence of a bruit. Systemic findings are common. In one series of 129 patients suffering penetrating neck injuries, Brown et al (17) observed that 25% were hypotensive on admission. Other related signs and symptoms include transient or permanent central neurologic deficits, especially involving the middle cerebral artery distribution, Horner's syndrome, and brachial plexus injuries. Overall, 10–45% of patients with carotid arterial injury have associated central nervous system damage (24).

Despite the frequency of such multiple organ involvement, which would be expected to increase the ease of diagnosis, the literature is replete with reports of misleading physical examinations in patients with serious injuries. Ashworth et al (10) noted that 33% of 41 patients with documented injuries were asymptomatic and without clinical signs. Bishara et al (25) reported that 23% of patients who had positive surgical explorations had injuries unsuspected on clinical grounds. While many of these injuries might not have resulted in serious complications if left untreated (eg, minor venous or lymphatic disruptions), it is generally accepted that substantial morbidity and mortality can result

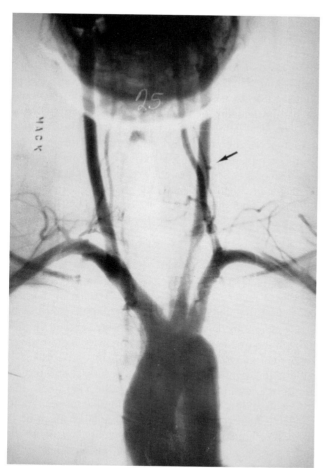

FIG. 2. Stab wound of the neck resulted in this minor irregularity on the lateral wall of the common carotid artery. On exploration, the vessel was found to be nearly transected.

from underestimating the serious nature of cervical injuries (13).

Arteriography is likely the single most valuable tool in the diagnosis and treatment of cervical trauma. The two most common signs of injury—intimal defects and extravasation of contrast medium—are usually apparent if multiple projections and selective injections are used (Figs. 2 and 3). It is noteworthy that in one large series, one half of the errors in diagnosis (5 in 244 cases) were attributed to incomplete single-view angiograms (26). Another frequent lapse in evaluation is underestimating the variability of a bullet's path and focusing the study on too limited an area.

Diagnostic algorithms for penetrating wounds are often referenced to the site of entry. In zone I injuries, most recommend arch aortography with complete visualization of the brachiocephalic vessels; optimal evaluation of zone III injuries should include arteriographic assessment of both carotid and vertebral arteries, the basilar artery, and intracranial vessels. The use of arteriography in unequivocal zone II injuries is less essential, especially if exploration is routinely performed. For example, Rivers et al (27) studied 61 patients

with 65 injuries distributed equally in all zones and found that no significant injuries were detected by arteriography in patients without physical findings.

Central Nervous System Complications

Neurologic complications remain dominant factors in mortality and long-term morbidity in patients with neck trauma (28). For example, Flint et al (29) found that 35% of patients with carotid artery injuries had neurologic deficits, while Richardson et al (4) demonstrated a 20% incidence in 133 patients. Although the classic neurologic presentation of carotid injury is profound cerebral ischemia with lateralizing deficits such as aphasia and hemiplegia, trauma may also directly involve the spinal cord, cranial nerves, and brachial plexus, as well as the phrenic and recurrent laryngeal nerves. Such associated injuries occur in as many as 20% of patients with penetrating carotid artery injuries (2).

It is essential but often difficult to perform a proper neuro-

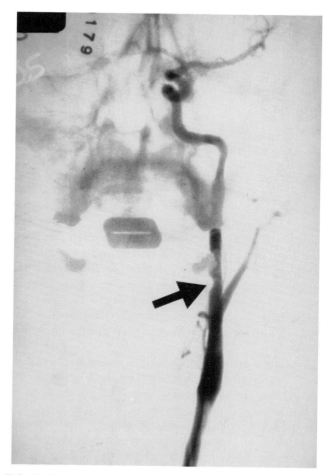

FIG. 3. Arteriogram following a gunshot wound at base of the skull reveals an intimal defect. Exploration demonstrated extensive blast injury to the base of the skull. The patient required extracranial–intracranial bypass to maintain flow in the middle cerebral artery distribution.

logic examination following major neck injury. Even after stabilization of airway and blood volume, acutely injured patients may be combative or unable to participate appropriately. The most critical initial evaluation—serial determinations of the level of consciousness—may be seriously compromised by drug and alcohol intoxication or hypotension. When closed head injury is a possibility and precise neurologic assessment is not possible, computed tomography (CT) is most helpful and should be obtained, if at all possible.

Associated Respiratory System Injuries

Major upper respiratory tract injuries are usually recognized on the initial physical examination due to the rapid occurrence of crepitus or subcutaneous emphysema. Bubbling of air through the wound is common, and palpation may reveal the instability of a fractured larynx (30). Symptoms may include respiratory distress, hoarseness, stridor, odynophagia, hemoptysis, and dyspnea. The presence, if not the nature, of injury can usually be confirmed with radiographic studies. Anteroposterior and lateral neck views may demonstrate a displaced trachea, narrowed airway, subcutaneous emphysema, cervical fractures, or projectile fragments. In cooperative or stable patients, direct visualization is more definitive. Meyer et al (31), using direct laryngoscopy combined with flexible tracheobronchoscopy, documented 100% accuracy in the diagnosis of tracheal and laryngeal injures.

Pharyngoesophageal Injuries

While esophageal trauma occurs in conjunction with extracranial carotid artery injury in only 7% of cases, these associated injuries account for considerable delayed morbidity and mortality (17–22). The most disastrous outcomes usually follow a missed esophageal leak that leads too quickly to abscess formation and fatal mediastinitis (31). Many have shown that early diagnosis and treatment is of paramount importance. Sankaran and colleagues (32) reported 107 patients undergoing operation for esophageal injuries. Only two of 98 undergoing early exploration died, whereas death occurred in four of nine undergoing delayed operation.

Indications of alimentary tract injuries are similar to those seen in respiratory tract trauma. In fact, tracheal and esophageal injuries are so commonly associated that the presence of one should redouble diagnostic efforts for the other. In addition to odynophagia and neck pain, physical examination may reveal crepitus. Radiographic markers include retropharyngeal air or pneumomediastinum.

Since pharyngeal or esophageal injuries may be difficult to detect even during surgical exploration, many authors recommend routine esophagograms and esophagoscopy to locate the exact site of injury. However, false-negative results of esophagography are high, in the range of 5–52% (6,33), while esophagoscopy misses 10–60% of injuries (6,34). A metaanalysis revealed that esophagograms detected 83% of injuries (31,33–37), whereas endoscopy located only 50% (31,33,34,36). Some argue that accuracy of esophagography may be improved if barium is used rather than water-soluble contrast (38). As an added benefit, Wood et al (37) notes that barium staining of the tissue makes identification of the esophageal defect more expeditious during exploration, without increasing infectious complications. Irrespective of the precise reliability of these tests, it is clear that endoscopy, in particular, is dependent on the experience of the examiner and that more than one modality should be employed to minimize missed injuries.

BLUNT INJURIES

Verneuil in 1872 was the first to report that cervical artery injury may result from nonpenetrating trauma of the head and neck (39). In the modern era, blunt trauma to the carotid vessels represents only 3–5% of all reported carotid injuries, although the true incidence of these often asymptomatic lesions is not known (15,40,41).

While the severity of blunt trauma necessary to injure the carotid arteries may be surprisingly mild (39), more than 50% of the cases in most reports follow high-speed motor vehicle accidents (15). The presumptive mechanism of injury is acceleration–deceleration, which also results in disruptions of the aortic isthmus or other brachiocephalic vessels. Other less common mechanisms may include direct blows, hyperextension of the neck, intraoral trauma, or basilar skull fractures (16). Irrespective of the specific mechanism, injuries range from localized intimal tears to extensive distal dissections and total or partial arterial disruptions (Fig. 4). In the former circumstance, platelet aggregation on the exposed subintimal connective tissue can cause thrombosis of the vessel or embolization to distal arteries (39).

In contrast to penetrating trauma, the distal internal carotid artery or bifurcation is involved in nearly all cases (2). Krajewski and Hertzer's review (15) found the bifurcation was involved in about half of patients, while the internal carotid artery was the site of injury slightly less frequently (38%). Predictably, blunt carotid injuries are frequently associated with direct central nervous system trauma; as an example, Yamada et al (42) reported that a full 75% of patients with blunt trauma to the carotid artery also had head trauma.

Physical diagnosis is difficult because symptoms and findings often appear at a time distant from the injury. In fact, only 10% of patients with nonpenetrating carotid trauma present with focal neurologic symptoms (15), and more than 50% manifest neurologic symptoms more than 24 hours after injury (2,16). When symptoms develop they include loss of consciousness, aphasia, hemiparesis, and Horner's syndrome.

While the most accurate test for the diagnosis of blunt carotid artery injuries is unquestionably selective arteriogra-

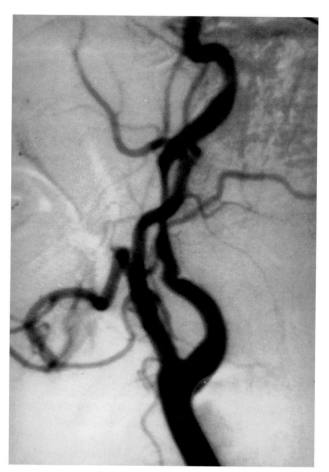

FIG. 4. Patient involved in a high-speed motor vehicle accident presented with sudden loss of speech and right-sided movement 48 hours after injury. Arteriogram reveals dissection of the distal left internal carotid artery. The patient was treated with anticoagulation. Repeat arteriogram at 1 month demonstrated no progression of narrowing.

phy (41,43), recent reports support the use of ultrasonography as a screening procedure (44). In one recent series of 14 patients evaluated for possible blunt carotid injuries, Davis et al (41) noted no false-negative and no false-positive scans. Nonetheless, in major acceleration–deceleration injuries, arteriography offers the distinct advantage of defining the integrity of the other brachiocephalic vessels. Furthermore, a positive ultrasound must be followed by a complete four-vessel arteriogram to fully define the extent of the injury and assess the collateral cerebral circulation prior to any operative intervention.

Limited injuries can be repaired by thrombectomy with intimal tacking; more severely injured vessels may require bypass grafting. In some instances, direct surgical correction is not possible because of the extension of lesions to the skull base. An alternative treatment for very distal disruption or pseudoaneurysm is planned ligation proximal to the pathology. Ligation is best performed with neurologic monitoring, either continuous electroencephalography or assessment of the conscious patient. At least 75% of patients with patent contralateral carotid arteries and vertebrobasilar vessels will tolerate ligation without deficit, if anticoagulated in the perioperative period. Posttraumatic dissections without extravasation can be treated with chronic anticoagulation much like the "spontaneous" dissections associated with fibromuscular dysplasia. Finally, newer interventional techniques such as intravascular stenting may have a role in selected lesions not presenting with embolization.

MANAGEMENT OF PENETRATING INJURIES

Successful management depends on early injury recognition, aggressive resuscitation, and an expedient systematic approach (29). Often immediate endotracheal tube intubation is required and must not be delayed. Maneuvers that assist in this procedure include suctioning secretions, removal of dentures, tongue traction, and placement of an oral airway. If concern exists for a cervical spine or cord injury, care must be taken to avoid hyperextension of the neck during visualization of the larynx. If the surgeon is unable to successfully secure the airway, alternatives include nasotracheal intubation or cricothyroidotomy. The surgeon must also be wary of possible late obstruction secondary to an expanding hematoma .

As previously discussed, most vascular injuries in zone II can be controlled by direct pressure. Importantly, "blind" clamping of neck structures is not productive and may cause inadvertent nerve injury or complicate primary vascular repair at the time of exploration (11). For the same reasons, probing of the wound is not justified.

The choice of incision depends on the mechanism of injury and the information available at the time of surgery. Regardless of these specific considerations, a wide area including both sides of the neck and chest should be prepared along with at least one thigh for possible vein graft harvest (9). The standard incision extends a variable distance from the mastoid process along the anterior border of the sternocleidomastoid muscle toward the sternum. If needed, the incision can be extended into a median sternotomy (to allow proximal control of the great vessels) or combined with a left lateral thoracotomy (to expose the left subclavian origin). Alternatively, the clavicle can be removed, affording access to the entire subclavian vessel.

Exposure at the base of the skull for repair of or bypass to the distal internal carotid artery is facilitated by anterior subluxation of the jaw. This can be performed atraumatically after the induction of general anesthesia; the position is maintained by dental wiring or circummandibular wires in edentulous patients.

If primary repair of the injury is not possible, the optimum conduit for bypass or patching is saphenous vein. Prosthetic grafts can be used if veins are not satisfactory in size or if associated injuries mandate an extremely rapid repair; however, their use in contaminated fields is clearly undesirable.

Regardless of the conduit, completion arteriography is recommended when grafting is performed. Alternatives include intraoperative duplex scanning or Doppler ultrasound to verify adequate reconstruction.

In rare instances in which the extracranial carotid artery cannot be reconstructed and ipsilateral ischemia is a concern, extracranial–intracranial arterial bypass can provide necessary collateral circulation. The procedure involves the construction of an end-to-end anastomosis between a branch of the external carotid artery or vein graft and a large cortical branch of the middle cerebral artery (45).

Issues Involving "Selective" Management of Penetrating Injuries

All surgeons agree that hemodynamically unstable patients with penetrating cervical injuries require urgent operation to obtain hemostasis. Neck exploration in these patients can be expected to reveal major injury in the vast majority of cases (35). However, more precise evaluations are appropriate in the stable patient, and in those without serious injury exploration may be avoided entirely. Besides limiting the number of negative neck explorations, so-called "selective" management may be justified by apparent cost containment. It must be cautioned that nonoperative management should not be considered less rigorous than mandatory exploration. In fact, observation requires more time and effort than routine exploration. Patients must be examined frequently, and ancillary studies must be obtained rapidly and repeatedly.

The controversy involving selective vs. mandatory exploration is focused on zone II injuries. Most agree that zone I and III injuries should be fully evaluated with arteriography and other studies prior to a decision to undertake operation. The advocates of routine exploration contend that (a) delayed treatment of a missed injury is associated with significant morbidity and mortality, especially in esophageal injuries; (b) physical examination and radiologic contrast studies are not uniformly reliable; (c) observation requires more manpower; (d) negative neck exploration is rarely accompanied by significant morbidity; and (e) hospital stay is not prolonged by a negative exploration (28,46).

Those favoring selective exploration argue that (a) the incidence of negative exploration among patients routinely explored is unacceptably high (40–60%); (b) the morbidity of a negative exploration is greater than that of observation alone; (c) selective observation is less expensive than routine operation (28,46); and (d) most morbidity occurs because injuries are missed despite formal neck exploration (34).

In view of the wide range of possible diagnostic tests (including arteriography, laryngoscopy, bronchoscopy, esophagoscopy, esophagograms, CT, duplex scan, and magnetic resonance imaging), it is understandable that some have questioned the cost savings associated with a selective approach to simple neck wounds. For example, Weigelt et al (36) in 1987 found that a negative exploration at a county

hospital cost $2,850, while a selective approach including arteriography, esophagography, and 1-day hospitalization was $2,670. Furthermore, the latter figure did not include additional fees for bronchoscopy and rigid esophagoscopy. Dunbar et al (47) found no significant difference in length of hospital stay between patients observed (2.6 days) and patients who had a negative neck exploration (3.0 days).

Allowing the vagaries of hospital-cost allocations, resolving the substantive issues of this controversy is not easy. Most reviews of the morbidity of neck exploration are presented by experienced high-volume trauma surgeons and demonstrate low perioperative risk, commensurate with that of anesthesia alone (48). Jones et al (49) reported 103 negative explorations with no deaths and only one wound infection. Similarly, Markey et al (46) noted no morbidity or mortality in 69 patients whose neck explorations were negative.

Even if neck exploration is not associated with untoward risk, perhaps the most compelling argument for preoperative studies is the fact that mandatory operation does not eliminate missed visceral injuries. Review of both historical and recent published series reveals numerous reports of major injuries that have been missed at exploration; predictably these errors were associated with considerable morbidity (24,50) and mortality (7,33,35).

The safety of a selective approach depends on the fact that delaying operation 6–12 hours for diagnostic studies does not substantially increase complications even in patients with injury. This is supported by numerous studies. For example, Stein and Seaward (50) selectively managed 200 patients with only one complication and no mortality. They avoided surgical procedures in 133 patients (67%) and found significant visceral injury in 61 of 67 patients explored. Campbell and Robbs (51), in a prospective study of 108 patients treated with a selective approach, found that they missed no serious injuries and performed only 26 operations. Dunbar and colleagues (47) noted no complications in 12 nonoperated patients with negative findings on arteriography and esophagograms. Ayuyao et al (52) observed 69 patients, none of whom required subsequent operative intervention. Narrod and Moore (34) confirmed the safety of selective exploration in a prospective study of 77 patients, while reducing the incidence of unnecessary neck explorations to 10%. These studies and many others suggest that careful clinical evaluation can reduce the number of unnecessary operations (6,8,11,28,33,35,37,53–61). However, diagnostic studies must be obtained immediately and any uncertainty must be resolved by operation.

Management of Neurologic Deficit

The question of how to treat carotid injuries associated with neurologic deficits is a remaining area of uncertainty. In the past, most recommended ligation of an injured and occluded carotid in the presence of a significant ipsilateral neurologic deficit. This approach was driven by the fear that revascularization increases the risk of hemorrhagic cerebral infarction (62). More recently, the tendency has been to revascularize irrespective of the presenting neurologic status. This evolution in management is based on two main assumptions: (a) the primary cause for progression of neurologic deficits is not cerebral hemorrhage but cerebral edema, which can be modified by judicious clinical care; and (b) the prognosis of patients presenting with major deficits or coma is so poor that the only rational hope for recovery is restoration of flow.

Ledgerwood et al (21) were among the first to refute the inevitability of intracerebral hemorrhage after revascularization of ischemic brain following traumatic carotid occlusion. They reported 36 patients suffering carotid artery injuries between 1972 and 1978. Nine patients presented with stroke or coma. While three of these patients died after revascularization procedures, all autopsies revealed cerebral edema and "bland" infarcts unassociated with hemorrhage.

In a literature review by Unger et al (40) of 186 patients with major preoperative neurologic deficits treated between 1952 and 1979, 34% improved after reconstruction compared with only 14% after ligation. In a classic collective review of 233 cases, Liekweg and Greenfield (24) documented 63 patients with carotid injuries and abnormal preoperative neurologic examinations. Forty-nine patients underwent revascularization procedures, while 14 were treated by ligation. The majority (59%) of those treated by ligation either deteriorated or died. Conversely, 67% of those in whom blood flow was restored either improved (47%) or were unchanged (20%). Further statistical evaluation revealed even greater improvement with revascularization if patients in coma were excluded from analysis; of those 34 with major deficits other than coma, 22 patients demonstrated improvement after revascularization. These authors concluded that all noncomatose patients with neurologic deficits should undergo primary vascular repair. They also recommended vascular reconstruction for patients in coma if antegrade flow can be documented in the carotid artery, although they acknowledged that no treatment appears to significantly effect the overall poor prognosis.

Additional support for revascularization is offered by Brown et al (17), who retrospectively reviewed 129 patients between 1947 and 1981. In their series, 16 patients were admitted in coma, nine of whom underwent reconstructive surgery. In this group, six patients had complete neurologic resolution of symptoms, while three patients died. The mortality of those revascularized (33%) was less than that associated with ligation (five of seven, or 71%). In another small series of four patients with preoperative severe neurologic deficits, Jebara et al (20) reported that three of three patients undergoing revascularization improved, while the one patient whose carotid artery was ligated had a persistent neurologic deficit.

In summary, while it is clear that comatose patients with carotid injuries have a grave prognosis regardless of management, there is evidence to support surgical repair in all cases with antegrade blood flow, as surgery offers the only possible chance for improvement. Ligation should be limited to those few distal injuries at the skull base in which revascularization is technically impossible and to severely comatose patients without either antegrade blood flow or retrograde flow after thrombectomy.

REFERENCES

1. Rubio PA, Reul GJ, Beall AC, Jordan GL, DeBakey ME. Acute carotid artery injury: 25 years' experience. *J Trauma* 1974;14:967–973.
2. Pearce WH, Whitehill TA. Carotid and vertebral arterial injuries. *Surg Clin North Am* 1988;68:705–723.
3. Karlin RM, Marks C. Extracranial carotid artery injury: Current surgical management. *Am J Surg* 1983;146:225–227.
4. Richardson R, Obeid FN, Richardson JD, et al. Neurologic consequences of cerebrovascular injury. *J Trauma* 1992;32:755–760.
5. Asensio JA, Valenziano CP, Falcone RE, Grosh JD. Management of penetrating neck injuries. *Surg Clin North Am* 1991;71:267–296.
6. Sheely CH, Mattox KL, Reul GJ, Beall AC, DeBakey ME. Current concepts in the management of penetrating neck trauma. *J Trauma* 1975;15:895–900.
7. Fogelman MJ, Stewart RD. Penetrating wounds of the neck. *Am J Surg* 1956;91:581–593.
8. Belinkie SA, Russell JC, DaSilva J, Becker DR. Management of penetrating neck injuries. *J Trauma* 1983;23:235–237.
9. Blass DC, James EC, Reed RJ, Fedde CW, Watne AL. Penetrating wounds of the neck and upper thorax. *J Trauma* 1978;18:2–7.
10. Ashworth C, Williams LF, Byrne JJ. Penetrating wounds of the neck: Re-emphasis of the need for prompt exploration. *Am J Surg* 1971;121:387–391.
11. Stroud WH, Yarbrough DR. Penetrating neck wounds. *Am J Surg* 1980;140:323–326.
12. Thal ER. Injury to the neck. In: Mattox KL, Moore EE, Feliciano DV, eds. *Trauma.* Norwalk, CT: Appleton & Lange, 1988;301–313.
13. Roon AJ, Christensen N. Evaluation and treatment of penetrating cervical injuries. *J Trauma* 1979;19:391–397.
14. Carducci B, Lowe RA, Dalsey W. Penetrating neck trauma: Consensus and controversies. *Ann Emerg Med* 1986;15:208–215.
15. Krajewski LP, Hertzer NR. Blunt carotid artery trauma: Report of two cases and review of the literature. *Ann Surg* 1980;191:341–346.
16. Fakhry SM, Jaques PF, Proctor HJ. Cervical vessel injury after blunt trauma. *J Vasc Surg* 1988;8:501–508.
17. Brown MF, Graham JM, Feliciano DV, Mattox KL, Beall AC, DeBakey ME. Carotid artery injuries. *Am J Surg* 1982;144:748–753.
18. Fabian TC, George SM, Croce MA, Mangiante EC, Voeller GR, Kudsk KA. Carotid artery trauma: Management based on mechanism of injury. *J Trauma* 1990;30:953–963.
19. George SM, Croce MA, Fabian TC, et al. Cervicothoracic arterial injuries: Recommendations for diagnosis and management. *World J Surg* 1991;15:134–140.
20. Jebara VA, Tabet GS, Ashoush R, et al. Penetrating carotid injuries—A wartime experience. *J Vasc Surg* 1991;14:117–120.
21. Ledgerwood AM, Mullins RJ, Lucas CE. Primary repair vs ligation for carotid artery injuries. *Arch Surg* 1980;115:488–493.
22. Timberlake GA, Rice JC, Kerstein MD, Rush DS, McSwain NE. Penetrating injury to the carotid artery: A reappraisal of management. *Am Surg* 1989;55:154–157.
23. Saletta JD, Folk FA, Freeark RJ. Trauma to the neck region. *Surg Clin North Am* 1973;53:73–85.
24. Liekweg WG, Greenfield LJ. Management of penetrating carotid arterial injury. *Ann Surg* 1978;188:587–592.
25. Bishara RA, Pasch AR, Douglas DD, Schuler JJ, Lim LT, Flanigan DP. The necessity of mandatory exploration of penetrating zone II neck injuries. *Surgery* 1986;100:655–660.
26. Sclafani SJA, Cooper R, Shaftan GW, Goldstein AS, Glanz S, Gordon DH. Arterial trauma: Diagnostic and therapeutic angiography. *Radiology* 1986;161:165–172.
27. Rivers SP, Patel Y, Delany HM, Veith FJ. Limited role of arteriography in penetrating neck trauma. *J Vasc Surg* 1988;8:112–116.

28. Golueke PJ, Goldstein AS, Sclafani SJA, Mitchell WG, Shaftan GW. Routine versus selective exploration of penetrating neck injuries: A randomized prospective study. *J Trauma* 1984;24:1010–1014.

29. Flint LM, Snyder WH, Perry MO, Shires GT. Management of major vascular injuries in the base of the neck: An 11-year experience with 146 cases. *Arch Surg* 1973;106:407–413.

30. Blass DC, James EC, Reed RJ, Fedde CW, Watne AL. Penetrating wounds of the neck and upper thorax. *J Trauma* 1978;18:2–7.

31. Meyer JP, Barrett JA, Schuler JJ, Flanigan DP. Mandatory vs selective exploration for penetrating neck trauma: A prospective assessment. *Arch Surg* 1987;122:592–597.

32. Sankaran S, Walt A. Penetrating wounds of the neck: Principles and some controversies. *Surg Clin North Am* 1977;57:139–150.

33. Obeid FN, Haddad GS, Horst HM, Bivins BA. A critical reappraisal of a mandatory exploration policy for penetrating wounds of the neck. *Surg Gynecol Obstet* 1985;160:517–522.

34. Narrod JA, Moore EE. Selective management of penetrating neck injuries: A prospective study. *Arch Surg* 1984;119:574–578.

35. Jurkovich GJ, Zingarelli W, Wallace J, Curreri PW. Penetrating neck trauma: Diagnostic studies in the asymptomatic patient. *J Trauma* 1985;25:819–822.

36. Weigelt JA, Thal ER, Snyder WH, Fry RE, Meier DE, Kilman WJ. Diagnosis of penetrating cervical esophageal injuries. *Am J Surg* 1987;154:619–622.

37. Wood J, Fabian TC, Mangiante EC. Penetrating neck injuries: Recommendations for selective management. *J Trauma* 1989;29:602–605.

38. Popovsky J. Perforation of the esophagus from gunshot wounds. *J Trauma* 1984;24:337–339.

39. Cornacchia LG, Abitbol JJ, Heller J, Schneiderman G, Garfin S, Marshall LF. Blunt injuries to the extracranial cerebral vessels associated with spine fractures. *Spine* 1991;16:S506–S510.

40. Unger SW, Tucker WS, Mrdeza MA, Wellons HA, Chandler JG. Carotid arterial trauma. *Surgery* 1980;87:477–487.

41. Davis JW, Holbrook TL, Hoyt DB, Mackersie RC, Field TO, Shackford SR. Blunt carotid artery dissection: Incidence, associated injuries, screening, and treatment. *J Trauma* 1990;30:1514–1517.

42. Yamada S, Kindt GW, Youmans JR. Carotid artery occlusion due to penetrating injury. *J Trauma* 1967;7:333–342.

43. Fry RE, Fry WJ. Extracranial carotid artery injuries. *Surgery* 1980;88:581–587.

44. Bashour TT, Crew JP, Dean M. Ultrasonic imaging of common carotid artery dissections. *J Clin Ultrasound* 1985;13:210–211.

45. Gewertz BL, Samson DS, Ditmore QM, Bone GE. Management of penetrating injuries of the internal carotid artery at the base of the skull utilizing extracranial-intracranial bypass. *J Trauma* 1980;20:365–369.

46. Markey JC, Hines JL, Nance FC. Penetrating neck wounds: A review of 218 cases. *Am Surg* 1975;41:77–83.

47. Dunbar LL, Adkins RB, Waterhouse G. Penetrating injuries to the neck: Selective management. *Am Surg* 1984;50:198–204.

48. McInnis WD, Cruz AB, Aust JB. Penetrating injuries to the neck: Pitfalls in management. *Am J Surg* 1975;130:416–420.

49. Jones RF, Terrell JC, Salyer KE. Penetrating wounds of the neck: An analysis of 274 cases. *J Trauma* 1967;7:228–237.

50. Stein A, Seaward PD. Penetrating wounds of the neck. *J Trauma* 1967;7:238–247.

51. Campbell FC, Robbs JV. Penetrating injuries of the neck: A prospective study of 108 patients. *Br J Surg* 1980;67:582–586.

52. Ayuyao AM, Kaledzi YL, Parsa MH, Freeman HP. Penetrating neck wounds: Mandatory versus selective exploration. *Ann Surg* 1985;202:563–567.

53. DeLa Cruz A, Chandler JR. Management of penetrating wounds of the neck. *Surg Gynecol Obstet* 1973;137:458–460.

54. Lundy LJ, Mandal AK, Lou MA, Alexander JL. Experience in selective operations in the management of penetrating wounds of the neck. *Surg Gynecol Obstet* 1978;147:845–848.

55. Mansour MA, Moore EE, Moore FA, Whitehill TA. Validating the selective management of penetrating neck wounds. *Am J Surg* 1991;162:517–521.

56. Massac E, Siram SM, Leffall LD. Penetrating neck wounds. *Am J Surg* 1983;145:263–265.

57. Meinke AH, Bivins BA, Sachatello CR. Selective management of gunshot wounds to the neck: Report of a series and review of the literature. *Am J Surg* 1979;138:314–319.

58. Merion RM, Harness JK, Ramsburgh SR, Thompson NW. Selective management of penetrating neck trauma: Cost implications. *Arch Surg* 1981;116:691–696.

59. Rao PM, Bhatti MFK, Gaudino J, et al. Penetrating injuries of the neck: Criteria for exploration. *J Trauma* 1983;23:47–49.

60. Roden DM, Pomerantz RA. Penetrating injuries to the neck: A safe, selective approach to management. *Am Surg* 1993;59:750–753.

61. Shirkey AL, Beall AC, DeBakey ME. Surgical management of penetrating wounds of the neck. *Arch Surg* 1963;86:955–963.

62. Wylie EJ, Hein MF, Adams JE. Intracranial hemorrhage following surgical revascularization for treatment of acute stroke. *J Neurosurg* 1964;21:212–215.

Cerebrovascular Disease, edited by H. Hunt Batjer.
Lippincott-Raven Publishers, Philadelphia © 1997.

CHAPTER 37

Vertebral Artery Trauma

R. James Valentine and G. Patrick Clagett

Vertebral artery injuries were once considered to be highly lethal. Early surgeons recognized injured vertebral arteries at the time of neck exploration, when the unwary were confronted with exsanguinating hemorrhage on entry into the posterior cervical tissues. Treatment was generally inadequate and consisted of proximal ligation or packing; more controlled exclusion of the injured segment was rarely feasible. Early mortality rates exceeded 80%, due most often to difficulty with vertebral artery exposure (1).

The first reported case of successful vertebral artery ligation is credited to Maisonneuve in 1853 (2), but outcomes were not significantly improved for more than 120 years. The decrease in mortality of vertebral artery injuries is generally ascribed to the institution of routine arteriography in patients with cervical injuries. Routine arteriography resulted in a sharp increase in the number of vertebral artery injuries that were diagnosed, especially in asymptomatic patients (2,3). Although early recognition and directed surgical treatment of vertebral artery injuries may have resulted in a decreased risk of exsanguination, it has been argued that reduced mortality rates of vertebral artery injuries are due largely to increased diagnosis of benign injuries (3,4).

Modern advances in endovascular techniques have afforded the opportunity to treat vertebral artery injuries without operation in many cases. Mortality rates are gratifyingly low, even in patients who are hemodynamically unstable. As a result, the respect for vertebral artery injuries has changed dramatically. In fact, some authors have advocated disregarding these injuries completely in asymptomatic individuals (5–7). However, the available evidence would suggest that vertebral artery injuries can be safely observed without intervention only in rare circumstances.

PERTINENT NEUROLOGIC AND VASCULAR ANATOMY AND VARIATIONS

The vertebral arteries are located beneath the posterior cervical fascia in the deep tissues of the dorsal neck (Fig.

R. J. Valentine and G. P. Clagett: Division Vascular Surgery, Department of Surgery, The University of Texas South Western Medical Center, Dallas, Texas 75235.

1). Although this location confers some protection from injury, it also renders surgical exposure more difficult. In the proximal third, the vertebral arteries course from their origins at the subclavian arteries to enter the transverse processes of C-6. The distal two thirds of the extracranial vertebral arteries are surrounded by the bony canal formed by the transverse processes of C1-6. After entering the cranium through the foramen magnum, the vertebral arteries converge to form the basilar artery. Approximately 15% of patients have a hypoplastic vertebral artery, more commonly on the right side (8). An aberrant vertebral confluence exists in 5% of patients: the vertebral artery terminates as a posteroinferior cerebellar artery on the right in 3.1% and on the left in 1.8% (8).

A useful classification of vertebral anatomy has been proposed by Berger (9). The V1 segment is the extraosseous portion that lies within the delta-shaped groove formed by the longus coli muscle medially and the anterior scalene muscle laterally. These muscles converge at a prominence on the C-6 transverse process known as the carotid or Chassaignac's tubercle. The V1 segment terminates at the transverse process of C-6 in 88% of humans, at C-5 in 7%, and at C-7 in 5% (10). In the V2 segment, the vertebral arteries course through the anterior portions of the transverse processes from C-6 to C-2. The roots of the cervical nerves occupy the posterior portions. The V3 segment begins at the top of the C-2 transverse process and ends at the base of the skull. In this segment, there is more space for access to the vertebral artery between C-1 and C-2 than in any other interspace due to the decreased bulk of the local bony architecture. The V4 segment is the intracranial portion that begins at the atlantooccipital membrane and terminates at the basilar artery.

ETIOLOGY AND CLINICAL FEATURES

Vertebral artery injuries are relatively rare, accounting for approximately 10% of all cervical vascular injuries (11,12). The vast majority of vertebral artery injuries are due to pene-

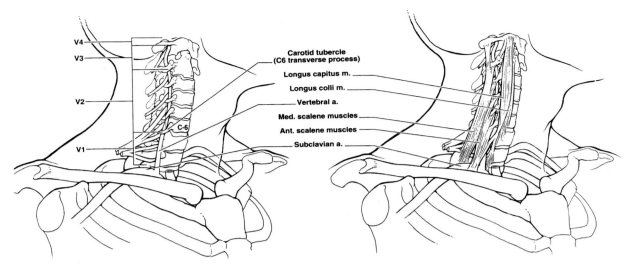

FIG. 1. The vertebral artery usually enters the transverse process of C-6 and courses through the upper transverse processes to enter the skull through the foramen magnum.

trating trauma, usually gunshot wounds. Most penetrating vertebral injuries present as zone II trauma, situated between the angle of the mandible and the clavicular heads (3), although the site of arterial injury is almost evenly distributed between segments V1, V2, and V3 (4). The anatomic location of the vertebral artery places it in close proximity to a number of other vascular, neural, and osseous structures. Associated injuries are frequent among patients sustaining penetrating vertebral artery trauma (Table 1).

Blunt vertebral artery injuries are associated with rotational or hyperextension forces or direct blows to the vessel (13). Most reported injuries have occurred during motor vehicle accidents (13). Blunt vertebral artery injuries have been associated with severe cervical injuries such as atlantooccipital dislocation (14) but have also been reported following

minor trauma such as chiropractic manipulation (15–17), minor head injury (18), neck flexion during paroxysmal coughing (19), Yoga exercises (20), and swimming (21).

Since the vertebral arteries represent a paired blood supply to the brain, the majority of patients who sustain vertebral artery trauma do not manifest central nervous system symptoms. In a series of 23 patients with vertebral artery injuries, Golueke et al (3) reported only one patient with transient vertebrobasilar ischemia that was not explainable by direct missile injury. None of the 43 patients with vertebral artery injuries reported by Reid and Weigelt (4) had neurologic sequelae attributable to vertebrobasilar ischemia. Approximately three fourths of patients with penetrating vertebral artery injuries present without any clinical findings suggestive of an arterial injury other than the penetrating neck wound or a stable hematoma (4). Blunt vertebral injuries rarely present with acute symptoms (22). However, delayed symptoms of midbrain ischemia and cerebellar infarction have been reported in patients with unrecognized vertebral injuries as late as 7 weeks after the initial traumatic episode (17,18,22,23). Since the natural history of unrepaired vertebral artery injuries is unknown, most authors favor intervention at the time of diagnosis.

Patients who sustain injuries in the most distal portion of the vertebral artery may experience interruption of the blood supply to the cerebellum and medulla via the posteroinferior cerebellar artery (3) (Fig. 2). This may lead to cerebellar or medullary infarction. Wallenberg's syndrome has been described in a patient with left lateral medullary infarction due to distal vertebral artery injury (17).

TABLE 1. *Associated injuries in penetrating vertebral artery trauma*

Injury	Number (%)
Arterial	
Carotid	20 (18)
Subclavian	5 (4.5)
Venous	
Internal jugular	10 (9)
Subclavian	2 (1.8)
Thoracic duct	2 (1.8)
Neural	
Spinal cord	14 (12.6)
Nerve root	3 (2.7)
Osseous	
Cervical spine	20 (18)
Mandible	9 (8)
Pharyngoesophageal	12 (10.8)
Total	97 (87.3)

(From data on 111 patients reported in refs. 3,4,34,41).

DIAGNOSIS

Prior to the routine use of arteriography, vertebral artery injuries were diagnosed at the time of cervical exploration, usually on the basis of major hemorrhage that was not controlled by carotid artery occlusion. As a consequence of the liberal use of arteriography, vertebral artery injuries have been diagnosed with increasing frequency. After the initiation of routine arteriography in patients with penetrating neck wounds at their institution in 1973, Meier et al (2) reported an increase in the proportion of diagnosed vertebral artery injuries from 3% of all cervical vascular injuries between 1957 and 1973 to 19.4% of such injuries during the years 1978–1980. Arteriography has become the gold standard for diagnosis of vertebral artery injuries, and many authors base their therapeutic decisions on the arteriographic appearance of the injured segment. In addition, arteriography is necessary to evaluate the collateral circulation in patients with vertebral artery injuries. Some authors feel that routine angiographic assessment of the vertebral arterial system overemphasizes injuries that would have gone unnoticed, suggesting that the natural history of these lesions is benign (5,6,24). However, most would argue that avoiding arteriography is tantamount to deliberate neglect of potentially serious injuries (2–4,25). The abundant literature on serious late sequelae lends credence to this argument.

TABLE 2. *Indications for arteriography in patients with possible vertebral artery Injuries*

Penetrating zone I or zone III cervical injuries
Selected zone II penetrating injuries with wounding path proximate to vertebral artery
Blunt trauma with cervical hematoma
Vertebral fracture that crosses transverse foramen
Posterior fossa ischemia
Patients with altered neurologic exam and
    Basilar skull fracture
    Significant external cervical trauma
    Focal neurological defect incongruent with CT findings

The indications for arteriography to exclude vertebral artery injury are listed in Table 2. Although some authors have challenged the value of routine arteriography in penetrating neck trauma (5,6,26), others have demonstrated that noninvasive criteria such as physical examination and mechanism of injury are not sufficiently accurate to exclude vascular injury in these patients (27,28). Therefore, most authors continue to favor the liberal use of arteriography following cervical trauma (2–4,5,26,28). Technical considerations are extremely important. The majority of patients should undergo four-vessel angiography, beginning with an arch aortogram. Arteriography can occasionally be limited to one side of the neck in patients with stab wounds that are clearly localized to one side of the cervical midline. If no injuries are identified at the origins of the great vessels, selective angiography should be performed with individual catheterization of both subclavian and common carotid arteries. If a vertebral artery injury is identified, selective catheterization of the contralateral vertebral artery should be performed with visualization of the entire vertebrobasilar system. Whenever possible, at least two views should be obtained of each artery.

The most common angiographic finding in an injured vertebral artery is occlusion (3,4) (Fig. 3). Other findings include pseudoaneurysms, arteriovenous fistulas, intimal disruption, dissections, and arterial spasm. Although arteriography accurately identifies the site of injury, the specific angiographic diagnosis can be unreliable (Fig. 4). Reid and Weigelt (4) found that the specific angiographic diagnosis was confirmed in only 50% of their patients who came to operation. Nine arteries thought to have been occluded proved at operation to be disrupted.

SURGICAL PRINCIPLES AND STRATEGIES

Surgical ligation has represented conventional treatment of a vertebral artery injury. Observation without intervention may be acceptable in the occasional asymptomatic patient with a minor vertebral artery injury detected on arteriogram, such as intimal disruption, dissection, or spasm (5,29,30) (Fig. 5). The need for anticoagulation in these patients remains controversial. Some authors have advocated observation alone in asymptomatic patients with occluded vertebral

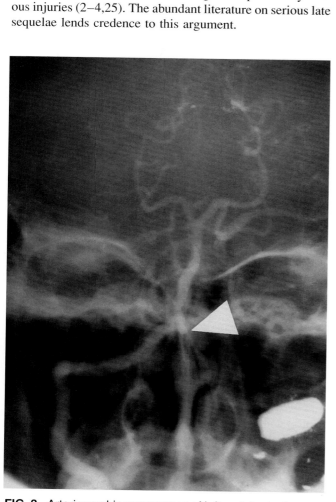

FIG. 2. Arteriographic appearance of left vertebral artery occlusion to the level of the basilar artery *(arrow)*. The patient had sustained a gunshot wound to the posterosuperior neck and was asymptomatic.

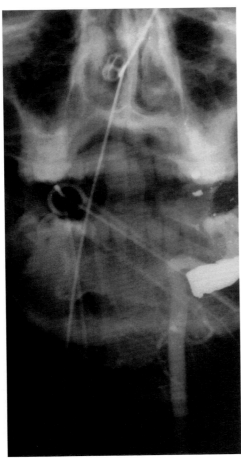

FIG. 3. Arteriogram demonstrating vertebral artery occlusion in the V3 segment due to penetrating trauma.

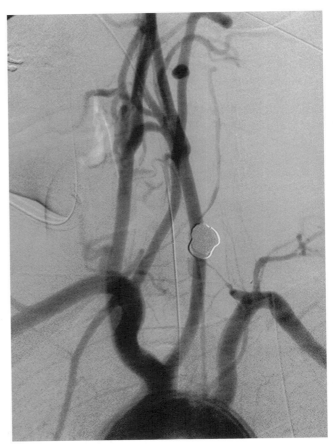

FIG. 4. Arteriographic appearance of a left vertebral artery injury associated with a low-velocity gunshot wound to the base of the neck. The injury was felt to be a proximal dissection associated with distal arterial spasm. However, on exploration, the artery proved to be transected just distal to its subclavian artery origin.

arteries, provided collateral circulation is adequate (5,6). However, others have reported that arteriographic appearances may be misleading in that supposed occlusions turned out to be complete arterial disruptions in a significant proportion of patients who underwent operative intervention (4,31). Although the natural history of untreated vertebral artery injuries remains unknown, most authors advocate intervention for patients with occlusions, extravasation injuries, arteriovenous fistulas, and pseudoaneurysms (32–36) (Fig. 6).

Modern advances in endovascular technology have led to the ability to embolize injured vertebral arteries with occlusive devices. Several types of occluding devices have been employed, including absorbable gelatin sponge, steel coils, silk suture, and detachable balloons (35–40). Although there are few reports of complications with this technique, tissue adhesives, coils, and silk suture carry the potential for midbrain infarction from microembolism prior to arterial occlusion. Detachable balloons are theoretically more appealing since complete arterial occlusion is immediate, but these devices are not currently approved for use by the Food and Drug Administration. Most interventionalists currently use coils (36,39).

Endovascular occlusion is convenient because it can be performed at the time of the diagnostic arteriogram without the need for general anesthesia. The technique is particularly attractive in unstable patients and in those with vertebral artery injuries that are difficult to expose, such as injuries in the V2 or V4 segments. Most authors recommend embolic occlusion both proximal and distal to the injured area. Although proximal occlusion is relatively easy, distal control is often difficult. This can be accomplished in patent arteries by traversing a guidewire across the injured area, then advancing a catheter can over the guidewire into the distal segment (3). It may occasionally be necessary to obtain distal control with a catheter passed via the contralateral vertebral artery, but this technique requires considerable experience and skill (40).

Operative intervention for vertebral artery injuries usually involves ligation. However, arterial repair may be necessary in patients with inadequate collateral circulation. Preoperative four-vessel arteriography is indicated in all patients with vertebral artery injuries in order to study the collateral circulation.

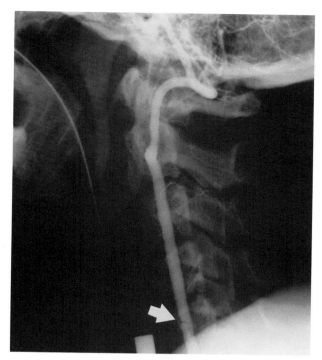

FIG. 5. Arteriographic appearance of intimal disruption in a vertebral artery *(arrow)*.

SURGICAL EXPOSURE

Exposure of the V1 segment is most easily accomplished through a supraclavicular incision, but it can also be exposed

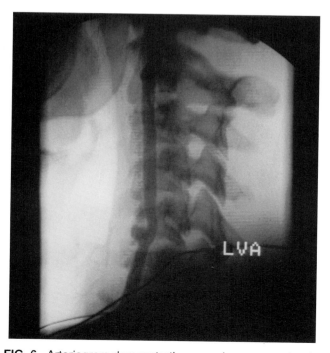

FIG. 6. Arteriogram demonstrating pseudoaneurysm involving the V2 segment of the left vertebral artery.

using the anterior cervical approach as described below. The supraclavicular incision is made approximately 1 cm above and parallel to the clavicle (Fig. 7). The lateral border of the sternocleidomastoid muscle can be mobilized and retracted medially, or the clavicular head of the sternocleidomastoid can be divided to enhance medial exposure. After the omohyoid muscle is divided, the carotid sheath is retracted medially with the sternocleidomastoid muscle. The scalene fat pad is mobilized on its medial border to expose the underlying anterior scalene muscle. On the left side, the thoracic duct should be ligated and divided near its termination into the confluence of the internal jugular and subclavian veins. The vertebral artery is identified by retracting the anterior scalene muscle laterally, with care to avoid injury to the phrenic nerve. The V1 segment can be exposed from its origin at the subclavian artery to the point where the artery dips under the longus coli muscle to enter the transverse process of C-6.

The V2 segment is exposed using an anterior cervical approach. The vertical incision is made along the anterior border of the sternocleidomastoid muscle, which is retracted laterally. After division of the omohyoid muscle, the carotid sheath and its contents are carefully mobilized and retracted medially. The underlying scalene fat pad is mobilized along its medial border and retracted laterally to expose the anterior scalene muscle. The V1 segment is exposed by retracting the medial border of the anterior scalene muscle laterally. The interosseous (V2) vertebral artery is exposed by mobilizing the carotid sheath, pharynx, and larynx. Medial retraction of these structures as far as possible exposes the retropharyngeal space. The anterior spinal ligament is incised vertically over the vertebral column for the length of the incision. The prevertebral fascia, longus coli, and longus capitis muscles are bluntly separated from the vertebral bodies and transverse processes using a periosteal elevator. The vertebral artery lies directly behind the bone forming the anterior border of each transverse process (Fig. 8). The artery is most safely exposed within the bony canal, since multiple venous tributaries surround the artery between the transverse processes. The bony canal is opened by removing the bone forming the anterior border.

The V3 segment is simpler to expose than the V2 segment, and it may often prove to be a better site for distal control after proximal ligation in the V1 segment. The V3 segment is best exposed in the space between the C1-2 transverse processes by extending the anterior cervical incision cephalad to the mastoid process (Fig. 9). Detachment of the sternocleidomastoid muscle origin greatly enhances exposure. The spinal accessory nerve should be mobilized and retracted anteriorly. The prevertebral fascia is incised beginning at the tip of the C-1 process, staying parallel to the spinal accessory nerve. The levator scapulae and splenius cervicis muscles should be divided as close to the transverse process of C-1 as possible, with care to preserve the anterior ramus of the C-2 nerve root. Division of the muscle fibers exposes the

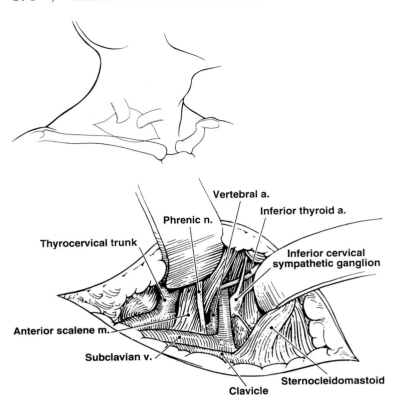

FIG. 7. Supraclavicular approach to the V1 segment of the vertebral artery.

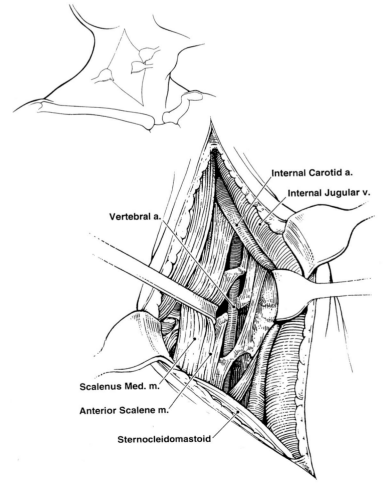

FIG. 8. Direct exposure of the V2 segment of the vertebral artery is most safely performed by unroofing the anterior borders of the transverse processes. Dissection between the transverse processes should be avoided due to the multiple venous tributaries that surround the artery in these areas.

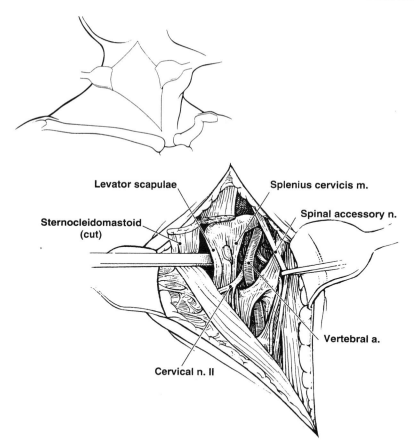

Levator scapulae

Splenius cervicis m.

Spinal accessory n.

Sternocleidomastoid
(cut)

Vertebral a.

Cervical n. II

FIG. 9. Distal control of vertebral artery injuries may be preferable in the V3 segment, which is simpler to expose than the V2 segment.

underlying C1-2 interspace. A 2-cm segment of the vertebral artery is accessible in this interspace.

COMPLICATIONS

Complications following surgical ligation or transluminal embolization of vertebral artery injuries are relatively rare. Based on autopsy studies, it has been estimated that midbrain necrosis follows occlusion of the left vertebral artery in 3.1% of patients and the right vertebral artery in 1.8% (2,8), which parallels the incidence of anomalous arteries in these locations. The vast majority of patients who are treated for vertebral artery injuries do well. Modern mortality rates for isolated vertebral artery injuries range from 6% (25) to 18% (33), with an average of 10% (3,4,11,13). Mortality rates for combined vertebral and carotid injuries are significantly higher, reported at 44% (28) to 50% (25). Up to 75% of the deaths are due to complications of associated trauma, especially central nervous system missile injury (3,4). The majority of the remaining deaths in cases of isolated vertebral artery injury are due to exsanguinating vertebral artery hemorrhage.

OVERVIEW

The number of diagnosed vertebral artery injuries has increased as a result of the routine use of arteriography in patients with cervical injuries. The majority of patients with vertebral trauma do not manifest symptoms of acute posterior circulation deficit. Although some authors consider vertebral artery injuries to be benign, anecdotal reports would suggest that serious late sequelae can result from untreated or unrecognized injuries. As a result, most authorities would recommend treatment of these injuries at the time of diagnosis.

Modern treatment options of vertebral artery injuries consist of surgical ligation, endoluminal occlusion via catheter, or selective observation. In rare cases of inadequate collateral circulation, surgical repair of an injured vertebral artery may be necessary. In most instances, ligation is appropriate but may be difficult in the V2 (interosseous) segment. Endoluminal occlusion can be performed at the time of diagnostic arteriography without the need for general anesthesia. Selective observation may be appropriate for patients with vertebral artery dissections or spasm.

The majority of patients do well after treatment of vertebral artery injuries. Mortality rates in modern series average 10%; in most cases deaths are due to associated injuries rather than to the vertebral artery injury per se.

REFERENCES

1. Matas R. Traumatisms and traumatic aneurysms of the vertebral artery and their surgical treatment, with a report of a cured case. *Ann Surg* 1893;18:477–521.

2. Meier DE, Brink BE, Fry WJ. Vertebral artery trauma. Acute recognition and treatment. *Arch Surg* 1981;116:236–239.
3. Golueke P, Sclafani S, Phillips T, et al. Vertebral artery injury: Diagnosis and management. *J Trauma* 1987;27:856–864.
4. Reid JDS, Weigelt JA. Forty-three cases of vertebral artery trauma. *J Trauma* 1988;28:1007–1012.
5. Menawat SS, Dennis JW, Laneve LM, Frykberg ER. Are arteriograms necessary in penetrating zone II neck injuries? *J Vasc Surg* 1992;16:397–401.
6. Jurkovich GJ, Zingarelli W, Wallace J, Curreri PW. Penetrating neck trauma: Diagnostic studies in the asymptomatic patient. *J Trauma* 1985;25:819–822.
7. Quencer RM. Angiography in penetrating neck injuries [editorial]. *AJR* 1986;147:1000–1001.
8. Thomas GI, Anderson KN, Hain RF, Merendino KA. The significance of anomalous vertebro-basilar artery communications in operations on the heart and great vessels. *Surgery* 1959;46:747–757.
9. Berger R. Surgical access to the vertebral artery. *Semin Vasc Surg* 1989;2:197–201.
10. Cavdar S, Arisan E. Variations in the extracranial origin of the human vertebral artery. *Acta Anat* 1989;135:236–238.
11. Feliciano DV, Bitondo CG, Mattox KL, et al. Civilian trauma in the 1980s: A 1-year experience with 456 vascular and cardiac injuries. *Ann Surg* 1984;199:717–724.
12. Hall RL, Anderson CA, Bickerstaff LK. Isolated vertebral artery injuries. *Contemp Surg* 1986;29:57–62.
13. Dragon R, Saranchak H, Lakin P, Strauch G. Blunt injuries to the carotid and vertebral arteries. *Am J Surg* 1981;141:497–500.
14. Lee C, Woodring JH, Walsh JW. Carotid and vertebral artery injury in survivors of atlanto-occipital dislocation: Case reports and literature review. *J Trauma* 1991;31:402–407.
15. Pratt-Thomas HR, Berger KE. Cerebellar and spinal injuries after chiropractic manipulation. *JAMA* 1947;133:600–603.
16. Davidson KC, Weiford EC, Dixon GD. Traumatic vertebral artery pseudoaneurysm following chiropractic manipulation. *Neuroradiology* 1975;115:651–652.
17. Schellhas KP, Latchaw RE, Wendling LR, Gold LHA. Vertebrobasilar injuries following cervical manipulation. *JAMA* 1980;244:1450–1453.
18. Auer RN, Krcek J, Butt JC. Delayed symptoms and death after minor head trauma with occult vertebral artery injury. *J Neurol Neurosurg Psychiatry* 1994;57:500–502.
19. Herr RD, Call G, Banks D. Vertebral artery dissection from neck flexion during paroxysmal coughing. *Ann Emerg Med* 1992;21:116–119.
20. Heros RC. Cerebellar infarction from traumatic occlusion of a vertebral artery. *J Neurosurg* 1979;51:111–113.
21. Tramo MJ, Hainline B, Petito F, et al. Vertebral artery injury and cerebellar stroke while swimming: Case report. *Stroke* 1985;16:1039–1042.
22. Davis JM, Zimmerman RA. Injury of the carotid and vertebral arteries. *Neuroradiology* 1983;25:55–69.
23. Amaral JF, Grigoriev VE, Dorfman GS, Carney WI. Vertebral artery pseudoaneurysm: A rare complication of subclavian artery catheterization. *Arch Surg* 1990;125:546–547.
24. Swan KG. In discussion: Golueke P, Sclafani S, Phillips T, et al. Vertebral artery injury: Diagnosis and management. *J Trauma* 1987;27:856–864.
25. Landreneau RJ, Weigelt JA, Megison SM, et al. Combined carotid-vertebral arterial trauma. *Arch Surg* 1991;126:301–304.
26. Rivers SP, Patel Y, Delany HM, Veith FJ. Limited role of arteriography in penetrating neck trauma. *J Vasc Surg* 1988;8:112–116.
27. Sclafani SJA, Cavaliere G, Atweh N, et al. The role of angiography in penetrating neck trauma. *J Trauma* 1991;31:557–563.
28. Rao PM, Ivatury RR, Sharma P, et al. Cervical vascular injuries: A trauma center experience. *Surgery* 1993;114:527–531.
29. Stain SC, Yellin AE, Weaver FA, Pentecost MJ. Selective management of nonocclusive arterial injuries. *Arch Surg* 1989;124:1136–1141.
30. Fakhry SM, Jaques PF, Proctor HJ. Cervical vessel injury after blunt trauma. *J Vasc Surg* 1988;8:501–508.
31. Snyder WH III, Thal ER, Bridges RA, et al. The validity of normal arteriography in penetrating trauma. *Arch Surg* 1978;113:424–428.
32. Asensio JA, Valenziano CP, Falcone RE, Grosh JD. Management of penetrating neck injuries. *Surg Clin North Am* 1991;71:267–296.
33. Pearce WH, Whitehill TA. Carotid and vertebral artery injuries. *Surg Clin North Am* 1988;68:705–722.
34. Blickenstaff KL, Weaver FA, Yellin AE, et al. Trends in management of traumatic vertebral artery injuries. *Am J Surg* 1989;158:101–105.
35. Halbach VV, Higashida RT, Hieshima GB. Treatment of vertebral arteriovenous fistulas. *AJR* 1988;150:405–412.
36. Halbach VV, Higashida RT, Dowd CF, et al. Endovascular treatment of vertebral artery dissections and pseudoaneurysms. *J Neurosurg* 1993;79:183–191.
37. Bergsjordet B, Strother CM, Crummy AB, Levin AB. Vertebral artery embolization for control of massive hemorrhage. *Am J Neuroradiol* 1984;5:201–203.
38. Ben-Menachem Y, Fields WS, Cadavid G, et al. Vertebral artery trauma: Transcatheter embolization. *Am J Neuroradiol* 1987;8:501–507.
39. Higashida RT, Halbach VV, Tsai FY, et al. Interventional neurovascular treatment of traumatic carotid and vertebral artery lesions: Results in 234 cases. *Am J Neuroradiol* 1989;153:577–582.
40. Miller RE, Hieshima GB, Gianotta SL, et al. Acute traumatic vertebral arteriovenous fistula: Balloon occlusion with the use of a contralateral approach. *Neurosurgery* 1984;14:225–229.
41. Hatzitheofilou C, Demetriades D, Melissas J, et al. Surgical approaches to vertebral artery injuries. *Br J Surg* 1988;75:234–237.

Cerebrovascular Disease, edited by H. Hunt Batjer.
Lippincott-Raven Publishers, Philadelphia © 1997.

CHAPTER 38

Middle Cerebral Artery Stenosis

Jeffrey I. Greenstein, Souvik Sen, and Shwe Z. Tun

Middle cerebral artery (MCA) stenosis is a relatively uncommon disorder (1,2) that has not been studied as extensively as either extra- or intracranial internal carotid artery (ICA) disease. Most studies have been retrospective and have included only small numbers of individuals. MCA stenosis is seen less frequently than MCA occlusion from either embolism or atherosclerotic occlusion. In most published series, MCA stenosis has not been adequately differentiated from MCA occlusion. To complicate matters, it is also difficult at times to differentiate between complete and partial occlusions and between embolic disease with recanalization and stenosis. Furthermore, the site of MCA stenosis has often not been adequately defined, and it is unclear as to which clinical presentations correspond with either proximal or distal MCA disease in many series (3).

ANATOMY OF THE MIDDLE CEREBRAL ARTERY

The MCA is the largest and most complex of the cerebral arteries. It supplies most of the convex surface of the cerebral hemispheres (4–10) including the lateral aspect of the frontal and parietal lobes, the superior temporal lobe, the outer segment of the globus pallidus, the putamen, much of the caudate nucleus, the internal capsule (with the exception of the lowest parts of the anterior and posterior limbs), and the adjacent corona radiata. The average length of the MCA is 1.6 cm (range 0.5–3.0 cm), with diameters ranging from 0.3 to 0.5 cm (5).

The MCA arises as the larger of two terminal branches of the ICA just lateral to the optic chiasm, at the medial end of the Sylvian fissure. Here it lies below the anterior perforated substance and posterior to the division of the olfactory tract into the olfactory striae. The MCA runs laterally from its origin, lying below the anterior perforated substance

and parallel but posterior to the sphenoid ridge. Within the Sylvian fissure, it divides and turns sharply to reach the surface of the insula. At the periphery of the insula, the MCA branches pass to the medial surfaces of the frontal, temporal, and parietal opercula and then project superiorly to supply the cortical surfaces of the frontal, parietal, and occipital convexities, and inferiorly to supply the temporal convexity. Anastomoses of the terminal branches of the MCA with those of the anterior and posterior cerebral arteries occur over the convexities.

In most cases (54%), the MCA stem gives rise to the lenticulostriate branches. These vessels arise from the first 12–15 mm of the stem and penetrate the substance of the brain to supply the lentiform and caudate nuclei and the internal capsule (6). Less frequently, these vessels arise after the MCA has divided (25.6%) or from one of the MCA branches (20.3%) (6). While as many as 20 lenticulostriate branches may be found, there are usually about 3–6 medial and 3–6 lateral vessels. The lenticulostriate vessels branch at right angles to the upper surface of the horizontal portion of the MCA and then course superiorly and posteriorly in a gentle convex curve to penetrate the anterior perforated substance laterally. The medial lenticulostriate vessels are usually smaller than the lateral vessels. These vessels are essentially end arteries because they do not anastomose with each other and only rarely do they anastomose with vessels originating from the cortical surface.

The medial lenticulostriate arteries supply the outer segment of the globus pallidus and part of the internal capsule; whereas the lateral lenticulostriate arteries supply the putamen, the claustrum and external capsule, much of the caudate nucleus, and the superior half of the internal capsule and adjacent corona radiata. One of the lateral lenticulostriate arteries is slightly larger than the others and this is the vessel most likely to rupture causing hypertensive ganglionic cerebral hemorrhage.

Beyond the lenticulostriate vessels, the MCA most commonly bifurcates (78% of vessels), but less often it will form a trifurcation (12%) or continue without branches (10%),

J. I. Greenstein, S. Sen, and S. Z. Tun: Department of Neurology, Temple University School of Medicine, Philadelphia, Pennsylvania 19140.

with the convexity vessels arising directly from this artery. The convexity of the cerebral hemispheres is usually supplied by 12 branches of the MCA.

When the MCA bifurcates, the orbitofrontal, prefrontal, and central (Rolandic) branches originate from the upper trunk; and the temporal polar, anterior, and middle temporal branches arise from the lower trunk. The anterior parietal branch usually originates from the upper trunk, whereas the temporo-occipital branch tends to arise from the lower trunk. The posterior temporal artery almost always arises from the lower division of the bifurcation, whereas the posterior parietal and angular branches have an almost equal chance of originating from either division.

When the MCA trifurcates, the orbitofrontal, prefrontal, and precentral branches originate from the upper division; the central, anterior parietal, and angular branches from the middle division; and the temporal polar, anterior, and middle temporal branches from the inferior division. The posterior temporal, temporo-occipital, precentral, and superior temporal branches may arise variably from either the middle or the inferior trunks.

The smallest and shortest MCA branches supply the frontal lobe. The largest MCA branch is usually the central branch. Fewer branches supply the more posterior portions of the MCA territory. Of these the temporo-occipital artery is usually large and it follows the cortical surface for a long distance. These features made this vessel the preferred artery for extracranial–intracranial anastomoses in surgical treatment of occlusive ICA and MCA disease (11).

The terminal twigs of the cortical MCA branches end in a narrow network of anastomotic vessels with the terminal anterior and posterior cerebral arteries. These vessels are usually 200–400 μm in diameter and are therefore too small to form effective collaterals between arterial territories. In addition, anastomoses between contiguous branches of the MCA are also either too sparse or too small to provide good collaterals.

Anomalies of the MCA are infrequent, occurring in less than 3% of cases (5,6). Duplication of the MCA is most commonly seen. Here the MCA arises from the ICA and an accessory MCA originates either from the anterior cerebral artery or, less commonly, from the ICA. Both vessels supply the same territory as normal MCA vessels.

The MCA differs histologically from extracranial vessels of comparable size. The internal elastic lamina is thicker and more finely fenestrated, the adventitia is thinner with little elastic tissue, and there are fewer perivascular supporting structures. In addition, there are no vasa vasorum. The potential role that these variations play in the pathogenesis of MCA stenosis in general, and in atherosclerotic disease of this vessel in particular, have not been explored.

Apart from a conventional anatomic approach, the MCA can also be characterized using radiographic anatomy. This approach is used to describe the angiographic appearances of the vessel. The MCA is divided into four segments (M1 to M4) based on major landmarks. The M1, or sphenoidal, segment starts at the origin of the MCA and extends laterally to the Sylvian fissure. The M1 segment is divided into two parts. The first, which accounts for most of its length, includes the MCA stem, from which the lenticulostriate vessels arise. The second part includes the MCA bifurcation and the branch vessels to their entry into the Sylvian fissure. The M2, or insular, segment originates at the genu of the MCA where the trunks pass over the limen insulae and it terminates at the circular sulcus of the insula. This segment includes the trunks that lie within and supply the insula. The M3, or opercular, segment begins at the circular sulcus of the insula and ends at the surface of the Sylvian fissure. The M4, or cortical, segment includes the named cortical branches and begins at the surface of the Sylvian fissure, extending over the cortical surface of the cerebral hemisphere.

ETIOLOGY OF MCA STENOSIS

A number of conditions are associated with MCA stenosis including atherosclerosis, moyamoya disease, spontaneous or post-traumatic MCA dissection, fibromuscular dysplasia, postirradiation angiopathy, and arteritis, including that associated with oral contraceptive or amphetamine use (12–16). The vast majority of cases of MCA stenosis in the literature are associated with atherosclerosis and these cases will form the subject of the rest of this chapter. Other causes are considered in other chapters.

EPIDEMIOLOGY OF MCA STENOSIS

MCA stenosis is an uncommon atherosclerotic cerebrovascular lesion. It was seen in 7.6% of 4748 individuals where the intracranial circulation was studied pathologically in the Joint Study of Extracranial Occlusions (1) and it ranks after ICA bifurcation and basilar artery atherosclerosis in frequency of occurrence in the cerebral blood supply at autopsy (17). In a number of clinical studies of MCA ischemic disease, markedly variable numbers of stenotic lesions (2–58%) have been found to be responsible for the development of symptoms (18–23).

Intracranial MCA occlusive disease is found with increased frequency in African, African-American (24–29), Japanese, and Chinese subjects (30–34), and MCA stenosis has been found more frequently in individuals from these ethnic groups compared to Caucasians (3,14,15,30,31,35). The highest risk for MCA stenosis appears to exist in Asian subjects, followed by African-American and then Caucasian individuals (3). A relative female preponderance has been demonstrated in a number of studies (14,15,36,37), but this finding was not confirmed in other series (19) including the extracranial–intracranial (EC/IC) bypass series, which is the largest documented group of MCA stenosis patients (3). MCA stenosis patients tend to be younger than those with extracranial atherosclerotic disease (3,14,15,19). Hypertension (3,14,36,37), smoking (3), and to a lesser extent diabetes (14,36,37) are risk factors. However, the presence of MCA stenosis does not correlate with hypercholesterolemia or either coronary or peripheral vascular disease (3,14,15). No information is available regarding different lipid component or lipoprotein levels and their possible relationship to MCA stenosis.

PATHOLOGY OF MCA STENOSIS

Although a vast body of data exists on the pathology and pathogenesis of atherosclerosis in general, there are no published studies on MCA stenosis in particular. It has been presumed that both recanalization of the MCA after embolization and atherosclerotic lesions of the vessel are similar to those found elsewhere, but this assumption should not be made lightly because of the epidemiologic differences between intra- and extracranial atherosclerotic disease discussed above.

Stenotic lesions of the MCA occur most frequently in the proximal stem, then in the superior trunk, and much less often in either the inferior trunk or the distal branches of the vessel (2,14,19,38). The majority of stenoses are less than 7 mm in length (2,19). In general, hemorrhage, ulceration, and calcification are found much less frequently in intracranial plaques compared with extracranial atherosclerotic plaques (39), and this situation would appear to be the case from the literature on MCA stenosis though no definitive data for all of these possibilities have been presented. The epidemiologic differences between MCA atherosclerotic stenosis and extracranial atherosclerotic disease may reflect an underlying pathogenetic process that has structural and functional differences in the generation of the atheromatous lesion at this site (40). Of interest in this regard is the finding of a deletion polymorphism in the angiotensin converting enzyme in African-American individuals at risk for stroke (41). This may play a role in the pathogenesis of hypertension in affected individuals. In addition, a study of restriction fragment length polymorphisms in the apoprotein A-I-C-III gene cluster found the frequency of a Sac I polymorphism to be significantly higher in African-American than in Caucasian American subjects (42). This polymorphism seemed to identify African-American individuals at risk for atherosclerotic cerebrovascular disease in the absence of elevated cholesterol or low-density lipoprotein, with or without reduced high-density lipoprotein levels.

Once established, MCA stenosis may lead to the development of ischemia presenting as either transient ischemic attacks (TIAs) or strokes by either reducing perfusion pressure distally or producing thrombosis with or without distal embolization (16,43). Artery-to-artery embolism of fibrin-platelet thrombi formed at the site of MCA atherosclerotic stenosis has been documented both at autopsy (44) and during bypass surgery (45), and this is clearly one cause of MCA territory ischemia.

CLINICAL PRESENTATION OF MCA STENOSIS

The clinical presentation of MCA stenosis is similar to that of ICA stenosis except that monocular blindness does not occur with MCA stenosis. Conversely, it may not be possible to distinguish clinically between ICA and MCA stenosis if blindness is not part of the clinical presentation.

MCA stenosis may present as either a TIA or a stroke (which may occur with or without an antecedent TIA) (2,3,14,16,19). TIAs occur less frequently with MCA stenosis than with ICA stenosis (14). Strokes occur less frequently in MCA stenosis compared with MCA occlusion (3). Most series of MCA stenosis have also noted that both TIAs and stroke reflect left more frequently than right MCA disease (2,3,14,19,46).

The clinical features of TIA are appropriate to the location of the luminal narrowing in all cases of MCA stenosis (3) and they occur in 20–71% of symptomatic patients (3,14,19). The number of TIAs prior to presentation is variable (3,14), but they tend to be multiple (2,3,14). In the medically treated group of 185 patients in the EC/IC bypass study TIAs were more common in the severely stenotic group of 116 individuals who had >70% luminal narrowing (mean = 8.1), compared with the 71 individuals in the moderately stenotic group, who had <70% luminal narrowing (mean = 4.4). The TIAs also lasted twice as long in the severe group (138 vs. 77 minutes). The majority of TIAs (86%) were stereotyped rather than variable in their clinical manifestations and 55% of TIAs were not followed by the development of stroke, compared with MCA occlusion where only 24% of TIAs do not progress to stroke. Unilateral weakness with a speech disorder (dysarthria or dysphasia) was the most common clinical abnormality found in the EC/IC bypass study (3). The degree of weakness tended to be more severe in the arm than the leg and least in the face. Isolated limb or hand weakness or combinations of weakness such as hand, tongue, and mouth weakness have been noted less commonly (3,19). Dysphasia occurred in half of the dominant hemisphere TIAs, whereas dysarthria was uncommon in the cases reported by Corston et al (19). They also found that pure sensory symptoms were present in only nondominant TIAs. Strokes occurred in 72% of subjects with moderate and 63% of subjects with severe MCA stenosis in the EC/IC bypass study (3). Preceding TIAs were noted in 28% and 40% of these cases, respectively. The majority of strokes in both MCA stenosis patient groups were maximal at the onset of symptoms. Smoothly progressive, stepwise, and fluctuating onsets were seen less frequently, although these presentations have been documented more commonly in smaller series (14,16). Headache occurred in 15%, and impaired levels of consciousness were noted in 14% of patients. Focal seizures developed in 2% of cases. Contralateral weakness of the face, arm, and leg with dysarthria or dysphasia were the most common clinical signs, with pure motor or sensory signs, or isolated dysphasia, presenting less commonly.

DIAGNOSTIC INVESTIGATIONS FOR MCA STENOSIS

The diagnostic evaluation of MCA stenosis includes non-invasive and invasive studies of the vessel lumen such as transcranial Doppler ultrasonography, magnetic resonance (MR) or spiral computed tomography (CT), and conventional cerebral angiography. In addition, both CT and MR imaging of the brain are useful to determine the presence of cerebral ischemia or infarction in the MCA territory. Single photon emission computed tomography (SPECT) and positron emission tomography (PET) imaging have not been used to evaluate MCA stenosis in reported series.

Transcranial Doppler Ultrasonography

Transcranial Doppler ultrasonography (TCD) is used in the non-invasive investigation of the intracranial vessels. It has been evaluated in a number of series of MCA stenosis (47–50) and has been found to be highly reliable for both the detection and exclusion of high-grade stenosis of the vessel (49). In a series of 133 patients with acute stroke studied with TCD and selective angiography, TCD was found to be 86% sensitive and 99% specific in the diagnosis of MCA stenosis (49). The diagnostic reliability of TCD is improved if multiple parameters of abnormal flow related to MCA stenosis are used (51).

The most common finding in MCA stenosis is an increase in the mean flow velocity above 80 cm/sec (Fig. 1). The flow change must be restricted to one or two insonation depths (5–10 mm) in order to determine that a circumscribed stenosis exists. The flow velocity distal to the stenosis should be damped. Side-to-side differences in mean flow velocity of 30 cm/sec are also helpful in the diagnosis of stenosis. Additional Doppler findings indicative of circumscribed

flow disturbance due to stenosis include spectral broadening with an increase in low-frequency components either during systole or during the whole cardiac cycle and arterial wall covibrations (51).

Rorick et al (50) studied 65 patients with acute cerebral ischemia using both an MCA mean flow velocity >80 cm/sec on TCD and cerebral angiography to evaluate MCA stenosis. When patients with high-grade stenosis of the cervical ICA were excluded, TCD using velocity criteria alone was found to be effective in screening of the M1 segment for stenosis. However, combining other Doppler criteria with another technique, such as MR angiography, would probably increase the diagnostic accuracy of noninvasive testing further.

The diagnostic accuracy of TCD also depends on operator skill and the absence of tortuous or anomalous vessels. In addition, the evaluation of the MCA may be limited technically by poor acoustic windows due to increased temporal bone thickness. This limitation is seen more frequently in African-American women (52), who are more susceptible to MCA stenosis.

Magnetic Resonance Angiography

Magnetic resonance angiography (MRA) has been used more recently in the evaluation of patients with intracranial occlusive vascular disease. Conventional spin-echo imaging has been used as well as two- and three-dimensional time-of-flight (TOF) MRA (53,54). In severe MCA stenosis, the spin-echo images may reveal absent or decreased flow voids in the MCA stem or Sylvian fissure (55). However, this finding does not satisfactorily distinguish between stenosis and occlusion (Fig. 2). In addition, abnormal flow may not be apparent in mild stenosis. Discontinuity of flow and narrowing of the vessel lumen are demonstrable in both two- and three-dimensional TOF angiograms (55). The degree of

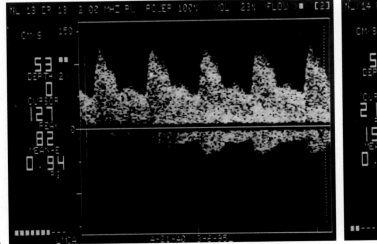
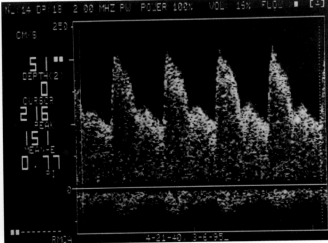

FIG. 1. Transcranial Doppler ultrasonography of middle cerebral artery (MCA) stenosis. **A:** Normal velocity in left MCA. **B:** Increased velocity in stenotic right MCA.

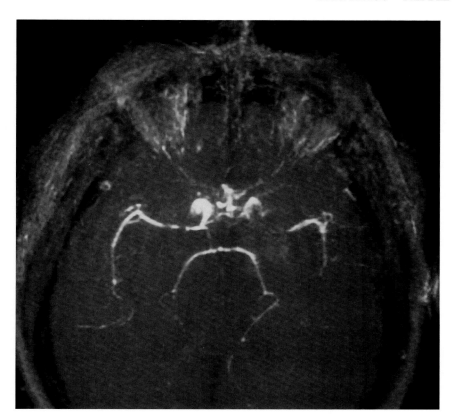

FIG. 2. Three-dimensional time-of-flight magnetic resonance angiogram demonstrating left middle cerebral artery stenosis. Discontinuity of flow is present in the main stem.

stenosis tends to be overestimated on two-dimensional TOF angiography because of flow-induced intravoxel dephasing through the area of stenosis. Conversely, three-dimensional TOF angiography may not detect slow distal flow because of insufficient spin saturation, suggesting total occlusion rather than stenosis. In spite of some technical limitations, MRA is a valuable noninvasive modality that can complement MR imaging in the assessment of MCA stenosis. MRA may also be of potential use in the noninvasive monitoring of selective vessel thrombolysis.

Spiral CT Angiography

Spiral CT angiography is a new modality that allows for rapid acquisition of blood vessel images following intravenous contrast injection. This technique was used to evaluate ten stroke patients with a diagnosis of MCA stenosis or occlusion by transcranial Doppler studies (56). All seven MCA stenoses were visualized with spiral CT angiography and the findings corresponded with the TCD localizations. Although this technique does not provide more information than TCD, it may be a useful extension of acute CT imaging studies when MCA stenosis or occlusion are suspected. Further studies are required to fully validate this modality and to determine whether quantitation of stenotic lesions is possible.

Cerebral Angiography

In spite of the slightly increased risk of mortality and morbidity, cerebral angiography still remains the standard for complete evaluation of stenosis of the MCA.

The most common site of angiographically defined stenosis is the proximal MCA (Fig. 3). Hinton et al (2) found the MCA stem involved in 13 of 16 patients. The origin of the vessel was involved in 5 of 13, the lenticulostriate segments in 4 of 13, and the distal stem in 4 of 13. The superior division of the MCA was involved in the remaining 3 patients. Caplan et al (14) also found the MCA stem involved more frequently, in 8 of 11 subjects, with the superior division involved in the other individuals. Similar findings were noted by Corston et al (19), with 12 of 14 stenoses found in the MCA stem. Distal branches of the MCA appear to be involved only rarely (19).

The length of artery involved varies considerably, with ranges from 0.8 to 25 mm reported in different series (2,3,14,19). In the EC/IC study (3), the length of stenosis was found to be slightly greater in severe compared with moderate MCA stenosis (6.8 mm vs. 5 mm on average, respectively). The degree of stenosis has likewise been variable, with stenoses from 33% to 85% of the vessel diameter being reported in these studies. In addition, the maximal length of the stenosis was greater in severe compared with moderate stenosis in the EC/IC study (2.9 mm compared

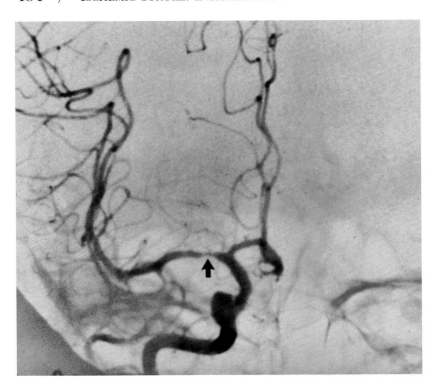

FIG. 3. Middle cerebral artery angiogram demonstrating stenosis in the main stem.

with 2 mm). Ulcerated stenoses were found in 2% of cases that could be evaluated (3).

CT and MR Imaging

The appearances of the brain may be normal unless significant ischemia or infarction results from MCA stenosis. In this instance, deep subcortical and ganglionic as well as wedge-shaped cortical hypodensities have been noted on CT images (3,14). Insufficient data are available on MR images. In our experience, the MR findings are similar to those on CT imaging (Fig. 4). It is to be expected that the MR imaging will detect ischemic change to a greater extent than CT, particularly soon after the occurrence of symptoms.

TREATMENT

A variety of different medical therapies have been used to treat MCA stenosis including acetylsalicylic acid, warfarin, and heparin. However, no rigorously designed and controlled studies are available. The effect of ticlopidine in the prevention of stroke due to MCA stenosis is unknown. The largest randomized controlled treatment trial of MCA stenosis was the EC/IC bypass study (3), which compared medical and surgical treatment, and which will be reviewed below. In the absence of definitive data, the best approach to the treatment of MCA stenosis is to use the guidelines for the treatment of occlusive cerebrovascular disease in general.

Hinton et al (2) treated 11 of 16 patients with TIAs secondary to MCA stenosis initially with heparin followed by war-

farin. One patient was started on warfarin from the beginning. Two other patients were treated with aspirin. All of these patients remained asymptomatic when followed for 4 months to 6 years. With long-term follow-up they noted a decrease in the degree of stenosis in two warfarin-treated patients. However, progression of stenosis was noted in another warfarin-treated patient.

Caplan et al (14) treated 16 of 24 patients with heparin and warfarin. Superior temporal artery-MCA bypass surgery was performed on two patients (one occlusion and one stenosis) for progressive disease despite appropriate anticoagulation. Antiplatelet agents were used in two patients. No clear outcome data are available for stenosis patients alone in this study.

Corston et al (19) primarily treated patients with ongoing warfarin therapy (10 of 21), but aspirin was also used (4 of 21). One patient each was treated with either dipyramidole or short-term intravenous heparin. No comment was made on the effect of therapy in these patients.

EC/IC bypass surgery was extensively investigated as a potential therapeutic modality for symptomatic ICA and MCA middle disease from 1967 when it was first described (57) until an international randomized trial was completed in 1985 (EC/IC Bypass Study Group). The EC/IC bypass study (3) was designed to determine whether anastomosis of the superficial temporal and middle cerebral arteries reduced the rate of stroke and stroke-related death in patients with symptomatic internal and middle cerebral artery disease. It was the largest study of its kind to be conducted, including 1377 patients, of whom 109 had severe MCA stenosis. Patients were randomized to either a surgical or non-

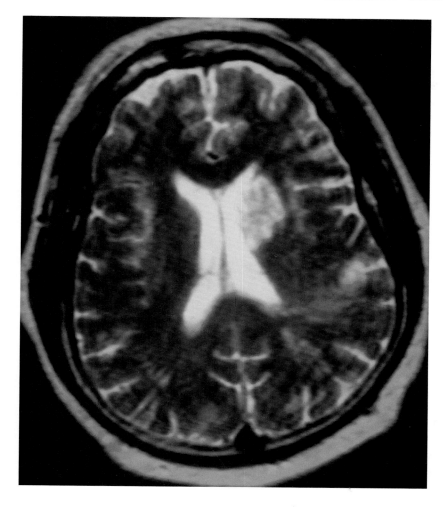

FIG. 4. Ganglionic and subcortical infarctions on MRI of patient with middle cerebral artery stenosis demonstrated in Fig. 2.

surgical group. Both groups were treated with 325 mg acetyl-salicylic acid four times per day. Not only did this study fail to confirm that the surgical procedure was effective in preventing cerebral ischemic events in both the whole patient group and the MCA stenosis group in particular, but both fatal and nonfatal strokes occurred earlier and more frequently in the surgically treated individuals in general and in the group of severe MCA stenosis patients in particular. The findings of this study differ from those of a case series of 47 patients treated surgically for MCA stenosis where outcome was assessed by comparison with a historical control group (58). The large patient number and randomization of the EC/IC bypass study supports the conclusion that this procedure is not effective. The poor outcome of EC/IC bypass in severe MCA stenosis may possibly be the result of subsequent thrombosis of the stenotic vessel (28–31, 43,59–62). This possibility is supported by a 14% rate of postoperative MCA occlusion seen in follow-up angiograms in the EC/IC study.

PROGNOSIS OF MCA STENOSIS

There are no natural history studies available to evaluate the effects of MCA stenosis without therapeutic interven-

tion. In general, the published series have been small, potentially limiting the extent to which one can draw definitive conclusions. However, comparisons between treatment groups and with MCA occlusion can be made to form the basis for the assessment of newer therapies in the future.

From early studies comparing unselected patients with MCA occlusion and stenosis, it appeared that MCA stenosis patients had a better long-term prognosis. For example, Lascelles and Burrows found that only 25% of patients with MCA occlusion recovered from their neurologic deficits (20). Kaste and Waltimo (46) found a 5% mortality rate in a study of long-term prognosis for MCA occlusion in 78 patients evaluated at postmortem or by angiography. This was lower than the mortality rate for acute embolic and ischemic cerebral infarction in general, probably because of the relatively younger age of their subjects and because the infarcts were smaller and less often associated with severe edema. They also found that 43% of MCA occlusion patients returned to work, that 27% required assistance, and that 1% were permanently disabled. Over a 30.3-month mean follow-up period strokes were more commonly a cause of death than cardiovascular disease.

An early study of prognosis in MCA stenosis was that

of Hinton et al (2). Sixteen patients with angiographically proven, medically treated MCA stenosis were followed for 1 month to 6 years. Fifteen of these patients had experienced TIAs and 11 developed cerebral infarction. One patient was neurologically intact but died of pulmonary embolism after a month. Fourteen of the patients treated with either warfarin or aspirin had an asymptomatic course following their initial presentation. Thirteen had no further neurologic events and one had recurrent TIAs for 2 years and none for the following 4 years.

Corston et al (19) investigated the outcome in 21 patients with angiographically demonstrated MCA stenoses. Patients were followed for a mean of 6 years and 10 months (range 3 months to 25 years). Ten patients died in this period. Three of the four who died of stroke had recurrent disease on the side of their stenosis. Two patients died of myocardial infarction and the others of unrelated causes. Strokes occurred more commonly in patients with either proximal or hemodynamically significant stenoses.

The largest body of data with regard to the prognosis of patients with MCA stenosis and occlusion comes from the EC/IC bypass study (3). Here 352 patients with either MCA stenosis or occlusion were treated with acetylsalicylic acid 325 mg four times daily and followed for 42 months. Cerebrovascular events were comparable in both the stenosis and occlusion groups (42% and 39%, respectively). Within this grouping, TIAs were slightly more common than stroke in the MCA stenosis patients. The death rate was comparable in the two patient groups as well. In the MCA occlusion group the total stroke rate was 10.1% per patient-year and the ipsilateral stroke rate 7.1% per patient-year, compared with rates of 9.5% and 7.8%, respectively, in the MCA stenosis group. Race, sex , age, smoking, hypertension, and diabetes did not significantly influence the occurrence of cerebrovascular events subsequent to patient entry into the study. TIAs during the follow-up period were significantly more common in moderate compared with severe MCA stenosis. Strokes were also more common in moderate stenosis, but not significantly so. Of the MCA stenosis survivors, 51% had abnormal neurologic examinations. Fifteen percent of these individuals were severely disabled, but 65.35% returned to their previous occupations. No differences were apparent between the severe and moderate stenosis groups. Compared with other studies, stroke occurred more frequently in follow-up in the MCA stenosis patients in this study. However, there was a lower death rate than in other studies.

REFERENCES

1. Hass WK, Fields WS, Norht RR, Kricheff II, Chase NE, Bauer RB. Joint study of extracranial arterial occlusion. II Arteriography, techniques, sites and complications. *JAMA* 1968;203:159–968.
2. Hinton RC, Mohr JP, Ackerman RH, Adair LB, Fisher CM. Symptomatic middle cerebral artery stenosis. *Ann Neurol* 1978;5:152–157.
3. Bogousslavsky J, Barnett HJM, Fox AJ, Hachinski VC, Taylor W for the EC/IC Bypass Study Group. Atherosclerotic disease of the middle cerebral artery. *Stroke* 1986;17:1112–1120.
4. Herman LH, Ostrowski AZ, Gurdjian ES. Perforating branches of the middle cerebral artery. *Arch Neurol* 1963; 8:32–34.
5. Jain KK. Some observations on the anatomy of the middle cerebral artery. *Can J Surg* 1964;7:134–139.
6. Crompton MR. The pathology of ruptured middle cerebral aneurysms with special reference to the differences between the sexes. *Lancet* 1962;2:421–425.
7. Kaplan HA, Rabiner AM, Browder J. Anatomical study of the blood vessels of the brain: the perforating arteries of the base of the forebrain. *Trans Am Neurol Assoc* 1954;79:38–40.
8. Kaplan HA. Arteries of the brain: an anatomic study. *Acta Radiol* 1956; 46:364–370.
9. Shellshear JL. The basal arteries of the forebrain and their functional significance. *J Anat* 1920–1;55:27–35.
10. Alexander L. The vascular supply of the strio-pallidum. *Res Publ Assoc Nerv Ment Dis* 1942;21:77–132.
11. EC/IC bypass study group. Failure of extracranial–intracranial arterial bypass to reduce the risk of ischemic stroke. *N Engl J Med* 1985;313:1191–1200.
12. Toole JF. Middle cerebral artery stenosis: a neglected problem? *Surg Neurol* 1987;27:44–46.
13. Kudo M, Lee JCK. Fibromuscular dysplasia of middle cerebral and renal arteries. *Acta Pathol Jpn 1985;* 35:775–780.
14. Caplan L, Babikian V, Helgason C, Hier DB, DeWitt D, Patel D, Stein R. Occlusive disease of the middle cerebral artery. *Neurology* 1985;35:975–982.
15. Caplan LR, Gorelick PB, Hier DB. Race, sex and occlusive cerebrovascular disease: a review. *Stroke* 1986;17:648–655.
16. Feldmeyer JJ, Merendaz C, Regli F. Symptomatic stenoses of the middle cerebral artery. *Rev Neurol* 1983;139:725–736.
17. Baker AB, Iannone A. Cerebrovascular disease. I. The large arteries of the circle of Willis. *Neurology* 1959;9:321–332.
18. Allcock JM. Occlusion of the middle cerebral artery: serial angiography as guide to conservative therapy. *J Neurosurg* 1967;27:353–363.
19. Corston RN, Kendall BE, Marshall J. Prognosis in middle cerebral artery stenosis. *Stroke* 1984;15:237–241.
20. Lascelles RG, Burrows EH. Occlusion of the middle cerebral artery. *Brain* 1965;88: 85–96.
21. Lhermitte F, Gautier JC, Derouesne C. Nature of occlusions of the middle cerebral artery. *Neurology* 1970;20:82–88.
22. Sinderman F, Dichgans J, Bergleiter R. Occlusion of the middle cerebral artery and its branches. Angiographic and clinical correlates. *Brain* 1969;92:607–620.
23. Silverstein A, Hollin S. Internal carotid versus middle cerebral artery occlusions. *Arch Neurol* 1965;12:468–471.
24. Gorelick P, Caplan LR, Hier D, Parker S, Patel D. Racial differences in the distribution of anterior circulation occlusive disease. *Neurology* 1984;34:54–59.
25. Heyden S, Heyman A, Goree J. Nonembolic occlusion of the middle cerebral and carotid arteries: a comparison of predisposing factors. *Stroke* 1970;1:363–369.
26. Heyman A, Fields WS, Keating RD. Joint study of extracranial arterial occlusion. VI. Racial differences in hospitalized patients with ischemic stroke. *JAMA* 1972;222:285–289.
27. Russo L. Jr. Carotid system transient ischemic attacks: clinical, racial and angiographic correlations. *Stroke* 1981;12:470–473.
28. Solberg LA, McGarry PA. Cerebral atherosclerosis in Negroes and Caucasians. *Atherosclerosis* 1972;16:141–154.
29. Bauer R, Sheehan S, Wechsler N, Meyer J. Arteriographic study of sites, incidence and treatment of arteriosclerotic cerebrovascular lesions. *Neurology* 1962;12: 698–711.
30. Brust R. Patterns of cerebrovascular disease in Japanese and other sub-population groups in Hawaii: an angiographical study. *Stroke* 1975;6:539–542.
31. Feldmann E, Daneault N, Kwan E, Ho KJ, Pessin MS, Langenberg P, Caplan LR. Chinese–white differences in the distribution of occlusive cerebrovascular disease. *Neurology* 1990;40:1541–1545.
32. Gould SE, Hayashi T, Tashiro T, Tanimura A, Nakashima T, Shohoji T, Ashley FW. Coronary heart disease and stroke. Atherosclerosis in Japanese men in Hiroshima, Japan and Honolulu, Hawaii. *Arch Pathol* 1972;93:98–102.
33. Kieffer S, Takeya Y, Resch J, Amplaz K. Racial differences in cerebro-

vascular disease: angiographic evaluation of Japanese and American populations. *Amer J Radiol* 1967; 101:94–99.

34. Resch JA, Okabe, N, Loewenson RB, Kimoto K, Katsuli S, Baker AB. Pattern of vessel involvement in cerebral atherosclerosis. A comparative study between a Japanese and Minnesota population. *J Atheroscler Res* 1969;9:239–250.

35. Nishimaru K, McHenry L, Toole J. Cerebral angiographic and clinical differences in carotid system transient ischemic attacks between American Caucasians and Japanese patients. *Stroke* 1984;15:56–59.

36. Kunitz S, Gross C, Heyman A, Kase C, Mohr J, Price T, Wolf P. The pilot stroke data bank: definition, design, and data. *Stroke* 1984;15:740–746.

37. Shinar D, Gross C, Mohr J, et al. Interobserver variability in the assessment of neurologic history and examination in the Stroke Data Bank. *Arch Neurol* 1985;42:557–565.

38. Kawase T, Mizukami M, Tazawa T, Araki G. The significance of lenticulostriate arteries in transient ischemic attack: neurological and regional cerebral blood flow studies. *No To Shinkei* 1979;31:1033–1040.

39. Moosy J. Cerebral infarcts and the lesions of intracranial and extracranial atherosclerosis. *Arch Neurol* 1966;14:124–128.

40. Nichols FT. Atherosclerosis. In: Fisher M, ed. *Stroke Therapy*. Boston: Butterworth-Heinemann, 1995;171–205.

41. Yatsu FM, Alam SS, Shan Q, Alam R. Insertion/deletion polymorphism in the angiotensin converting enzyme (ACE) gene: possible marker to identify stroke-prone individuals. *Stroke* 1995;26:29.

42. Kasturi R, Yatsu FM, Alam R, Rogers S. Restriction fragment length polymorphism of the apoprotein A-I-C-III gene cluster in control and stroke-prone white and black subjects: racial differences. *Stroke* 1992;23:1257–1264.

43. Furlan AJ, Little JR, Dohn DF. Arterial occlusion following anastomosis of the superficial temporal artery to middle cerebral artery. *Stroke* 1980;11:91–95.

44. Masuda J, Ogata J, Yutani C, Miyashita T, Yamaguchi T. Artery-to-artery embolism from a thrombus formed in stenotic middle cerebral artery. Report of an autopsy case. *Stroke* 1987;18:680–684.

45. Adams HP, Gross CE. Embolism distal to stenosis of the middle cerebral artery. *Stroke* 1981;12:228–229.

46. Kaste M, Waltimo O. Prognosis of patients with middle cerebral artery occlusion. *Stroke* 1976;7:482–485.

47. Hennerici M, Rautenberg W, Schwartz A. Transcranial Doppler ultrasound for the assessment of intracranial arterial flow velocity. 2. Evaluation of intracranial arterial disease. *Surg Neurol* 1987;27:523–532.

48. Lindegaard K-F, Bakke SJ, Aaslid R, Nornes H. Doppler diagnosis of intracranial artery occlusive disorders. *J Neurol Neurosurg Psychiat* 1986;49:510–518.

49. Ley-Pozo J, Ringelstein EB. Noninvasive detection of occlusive disease of the carotid siphon and middle cerebral artery. *Ann Neurol* 1990;28:640–647.

50. Rorick MB, Nichols FT, Adams RJ. Transcranial Doppler correlation with angiography in detection of intracranial stenosis. *Stroke* 1994;25:1931–1934.

51. von Reutern G-M, von Budingen. *Ultrasound Diagnosis of Cerebrovascular Disease*. New York: Thieme, 1993.

52. Halsey JH. Effect of emitted power on waveform intensity in transcranial Doppler. *Stroke* 1990;21:1573–1578.

53. Patrux B, Laissy JP, Jouini S, Kawiecki W, Coty P, Thiebot J. Magnetic resonance angiography (MRA) of the circle of Willis: a prospective comparison with conventional angiography in 54 subjects. *Neuroradiology* 1994;36:193–197.

54. Heiserman JE, Drayer BP, Keller PJ, Fram EK. Intracranial vascular stenosis and occlusion: evaluation with three-dimensional time-of-flight MR angiography. *Radiology* 1992;185:667–673.

55. Fujita N, Hirabuki N, Fujii K, Hashimoto T, Miura T, Sato T, Kozuka T. MR imaging of middle cerebral artery stenosis and occlusion: value of MR angiography. *Amer J Neuroradiol* 1994;15:335–341.

56. Wong KS, Liang EY, Lam WWM, Huang YN, Kay R. Spiral computed tomography angiography in the assessment of middle cerebral artery occlusive disease. *J Neurol Neurosurg Psychiat* 1995;59:537–539.

57. Yasargil MG, ed. *Microsurgery Applied to Neuro-surgery*. Stuttgart: Thieme Verlag, 1969.

58. Andrews BT, Chater NL, Weinstein PR. Extracranial-intracranial arterial bypass for middle cerebral artery stenosis and occlusion. *J Neurosurg* 1985; 62:831–838.

59. Chater NL, Weinstein PR. Progression of middle cerebral artery stenosis to occlusion without symptoms following superficial temporal artery bypass: case report. In: Fein JM, Reichman OH, eds. *Microvascular Anastomoses for Cerebral Ischemia*. New York; Springer-Verlag, 1974;269–271.

60. Gumerlock MK, Ono H, Neuwelt EA. Can a patent extracranial–intracranial bypass provoke the conversion of an intracranial stenosis to a symptomatic occlusion? *Neurosurgery* 1983;12:391–400.

61. Nakagawa Y, Tsuru M, Mabuchi S, Echizenya K, Satoh M, Kashiwaba T. EC-IC bypass surgery for the middle cerebral artery stenosis: outcomes and postoperative angiography. In: Spetzler RF, Carter LP, Selman WR, Martin NA, eds. *Cerebral Revascularization for Stroke*. New York: Thieme-Stratton, 1985;449–457.

62. Awad I, Furlan AJ, Little JR. Changes in intracranial stenotic lesions after extracranial–intracranial bypass surgery. *J Neurosurg* 1984;60:771–776.

Cerebrovascular Disease, edited by H. Hunt Batjer.
Lippincott-Raven Publishers, Philadelphia © 1997.

CHAPTER 39

Moyamoya Disease and Cerebral Ischemia

Bhuwan P. Garg, Askiel Bruno, and José Biller

Moyamoya disease is a chronic, noninflammatory, occlusive vasculopathy of unknown etiology. While it has been most commonly noted in Japan, it does occur in North America and is seen in both children and adults, especially women in their first or fourth decade of life. Moyamoya is a Japanese word that means "something hazy like a puff of cigarette smoke drifting in the air." Suzuki and Takaku (1) coined this term in 1969 for the peculiar angiographic pattern of an abnormal wisp-like network of vessels at the base of the brain seen in patients with the disorder.

Takeuchi and Shimizu reported the first angiograms of this disease at the 1955 meeting of the Japan Neurosurgical Society (2). They described the abnormality as carotid artery stenosis in a subsequent case report in 1957 (3). Suzuki and colleagues reported six cases in 1963 and proposed that this constituted a new disease (1). The first case outside Japan was reported by Weidner and colleagues (4) in 1965. Subsequently, Krayenbühl and Gerlach each recorded a case of moyamoya, and Leeds and Abbott reported two children of Japanese parentage with the disease (1,5). In Japan, further reports of this condition were forthcoming from Nishimoto and Takeuchi (6) and Fukuyama et al (7). By 1966, Kudo managed to collect 146 Japanese cases. Suzuki and Takaku (1) reported 20 cases in 1969 and named this peculiar disease the cerebral moyamoya disease.

EPIDEMIOLOGY

Moyamoya disease is common in Japan but has been reported all over the world. It is not a rare cause of childhood strokes, although incidence or prevalence studies are not available. In Japan, a mean incidence of 0.1 cases per 100,000 people per year has been found (2). Women are affected more than men at a reported ratio of 3:2 in a Japanese series (8). This difference in the sexes is most evident in children, with a ratio of 2.5:1 as compared with adults

in whom the ratio has varied from 1:1 to 1.40:1 (2). Moyamoya disease occurs in children and adults with a bimodal age distribution. There are peaks in the first and fourth decades of life. Half of patients are younger than 10 years (9). Onset of symptoms in children often occurs before 5 years of age, though diagnosis may not be made till later.

CLINICAL CHARACTERISTICS

The disorder may cause transient ischemic attacks (TIAs), headache, seizures, cerebral infarction, or intracranial hemorrhage with corresponding clinical symptoms. Clinical presentation in children is different from that in adults. In children, the disease most often causes TIAs or ischemic strokes that may alternate sides. Repeated strokes are not uncommon. Ischemic strokes are often multiple, affecting predominantly the carotid circulation. Infarctions are often encountered in "watershed" territories between the anterior, middle, and posterior cerebral arteries in the basal ganglia, as well as in the centrum semiovale. TIAs with brief episodes of sensorimotor, visual, or speech deficit—otherwise uncommon in childhood—occur often in childhood moyamoya disease and may be the presenting symptom. Ischemic symptoms in children may be precipitated by crying, blowing (eg, playing wind instruments or cooling a drink), and hyperventilation. Hot weather has been reported to worsen the symptoms (10). Alteration of mental status occurs, although loss of consciousness is rare. Motor and speech disturbance are present in more than half of these children, and seizures and mental deficits are common. Headache and sensory disturbances are not uncommon, and visual and psychic abnormalities have been reported. Involuntary movements have been reported to occur in 3–6% of patients and may be the presenting symptom (11). Seizures may be a presenting symptom in some children (12). Eighty percent of moyamoya patients with epilepsy are younger than 10 years (13).

Some patients present with symptoms of posterior cerebral hemisphere or global ischemia. Vertigo, dysphagia, sudden disturbance of consciousness, scintillating scotoma, cor-

B. P. Garg, A. Bruno, and J. Biller: Department of Neurology, Indiana University Medical Center, Indianapolis, Indiana 46202.

tical blindness, visual-field deficits, and other visual disturbances may be present (1,14). Visual-field deficits as a sign of occipital lobe ischemia were present in 11% of cases in one study (15). Intracranial hemorrhage is a rare event in childhood moyamoya disease. Delay in development and later mental retardation of varying severity occur (16,17).

In adults, the most common symptoms are hemorrhagic and due to subarachnoid, subependymal, intraparenchymal, or intraventricular hemorrhage. Headache, disturbed consciousness, and sensorimotor abnormalities are associated with this presentation. Speech and visual disturbances may also occur.

A history of repeated infections above the neck is frequently found. Suzuki reported that 74% of juvenile cases of moyamoya disease had sinusitis, otitis media, or other inflammation above the neck. Tonsillitis was present in 65% of juvenile cases and 40% of adults (2). Yamaguchi et al (18) found that 63.5% of moyamoya patients had an infection of some type, the majority of which were above the neck. Head trauma has been reported in 8–9.4% of cases (2,18). The significance of these observations in the etiology and pathogenesis of moyamoya disease is not clear but these observations may point to an abnormal immune-mediated mechanism.

DIFFERENTIAL DIAGNOSIS

A Japanese research committee on the spontaneous occlusion of the circle of Willis (cerebrovascular moyamoya disease) proposed the following guidelines for the diagnosis: (a) stenosis involving the region of the internal carotid artery bifurcation and the proximal portions of the anterior cerebral and middle cerebral arteries; (b) dilated basal collateral arteries, usually the lenticulostriate and thalamoperforate arteries; and (c) bilateral abnormalities (13). Occasionally, these abnormalities are found in association with other conditions, some of which may cause moyamoya disease and others may simply be associated with it (Table 1).

Care should be taken to distinguish the rich collateral circulation of idiopathic moyamoya disease from that which may be associated with specific causes of vascular occlusions, such as emboli, basilar inflammatory conditions, space-occupying masses with slow compression of the large vessels, and radiation of the optic chiasm and hypothalamic gliomas. The committee recommended that if any of these conditions is present, the angiographic abnormality should be termed *moyamoya syndrome* rather than moyamoya disease. In addition, the moyamoya angiographic pattern is sometimes found on one side only, and none of the above associations is present. The committee recommended that such cases be termed *probable* moyamoya disease. Diagnostic difficulties may arise in the presence of basal ganglia arteriovenous malformation, glioblastoma, or other tumors with rich vascularity at the base of the brain; sometimes

TABLE 1. *Conditions associated with moyamoya disease*

Down's syndrome
Neurofibromatosis
Tuberous sclerosis
Basilar meningitis
Tuberculous meningitis
Leptospirosis
Fibromuscular dysplasia
Vasculitis
Periarteritis nodosa
Sickle cell disease
Brain tumors
Radiation-induced arteritis
Fanconi's anemia
Type 1 glycogenosis
Renal artery stenosis
Homocystinuria
Retinitis pigmentosa
Pseudoxanthoma elasticum
Myopathy
Factor XII deficiency
Oral contraceptives?
Trauma
Sneddon's syndrome
Neonatal anoxia
Encephalotrigeminel angiomatosis
Alagille syndrome
Congenital heart disease
Hypertension

diagnosis may be difficult when bilateral hypoplasia of the carotid arteries is present (19–29).

NEUROIMAGING INVESTIGATIONS

Diagnosis of moyamoya disease is based on a distinct arteriographic appearance. The characteristic arteriogram shows progressive, bilateral stenosis of the distal internal carotid arteries extending to the proximal anterior and middle cerebral arteries, often with involvement of the circle of Willis, and development of an extensive collateral network at the base of the brain. Intracranial aneurysms can occur with this disorder. Magnetic resonance angiography (MRA) is emerging as a potential noninvasive tool to evaluate these patients. Positron emission tomography (PET) and single-photon emission computed tomography (SPECT) are valuable research techniques used to study cerebral blood flow and metabolism in this disease.

Cerebral CT

Computed tomography (CT) usually shows evidence of cerebral ischemia. Multiple focal ischemic lesions are commonly seen; a lesion representing a large area of ischemia may sometimes be present. Blush of enlarged vessels on contrast-enhanced CT scan has been reported but is not a common finding (30). In cases of intracranial hemorrhage, evidence of subarachnoid, intraventricular, or intraparenchymal blood may be present with a mass effect and shift of midline structures. Cerebral atrophy has been reported in up to 50–60% of cases.

Cerebral MRI

Magnetic resonance imaging (MRI) shows findings similar to those seen on CT. Lesions consistent with ischemia are scattered in the carotid artery distribution, though sometimes the posterior cerebral artery territory is also involved. Lesions are usually bilateral, even though the patient may only have unilateral symptoms (Fig. 1). There is a preponderance of lesions in the centrum semiovale. Another area where these lesions predominate is the watershed zone between the anterior, middle, and posterior cerebral arteries and the terminal territory of the brain supplied by the penetrating branches of the anterior and middle cerebral arteries (31). Occipital lobe lesions are present in patients with posterior cerebral artery occlusion. Thalamic lesions are rare in patients who have involvement of the vertebrobasilar system.

Additionally, MRI also shows the enlarged vessels in the basal ganglia region that correspond to the moyamoya vessels seen on the angiograms and only rarely seen on CT. These vessels are represented on MRI as dark, punctate areas

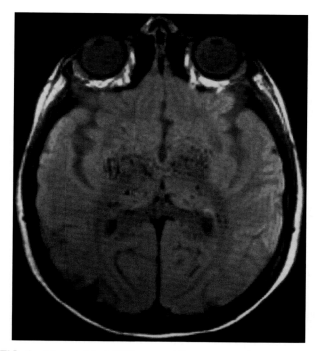

FIG. 2. T1-weighted MRI scan of the same patient as in Fig. 1 shows dilated lenticulostriate (moyamoya) vessels as "flow voids" in the basal ganglia region (TR 2400, TE 25).

of "flow void," best seen on T1-weighted images (Fig. 2). MRA is a recent advance in the imaging modalities available to the clinician for the study of cerebrovascular disorders. Large-to-medium size intracranial and extracranial vessels can be studied by this technique. Recent studies have shown the cerebral vascular pattern in good enough resolution that the more invasive study, angiography, may become unnecessary for the diagnosis of moyamoya disease in the future (Figs. 3 and 4). As yet, however, this study does not show the collateral circulation for which cerebral angiography is essential.

Cerebral Angiography

At present, cerebral angiography is considered the diagnostic study of choice. It not only defines the extent of the disease but also demonstrates the collateral vessels and adequacy of the compensatory circulation. The typical angiographic findings are in the vessels at the base of the brain (Figs. 5 and 6). The earliest angiographic finding is stenosis of the supraclinoid portion of the internal carotid arteries. Later, with disease progression, there is involvement of the proximal portions of the anterior and middle cerebral arteries and the circle of Willis; the posterior circulation is involved less often. The condition is usually bilateral, though asymmetric involvement is often seen. Progressive narrowing and subsequent occlusion of these cerebral vessels leads to collateral blood flow through the arteries supplying the basal ganglia, thalamus, hypothalamus, and mesencephalon. The

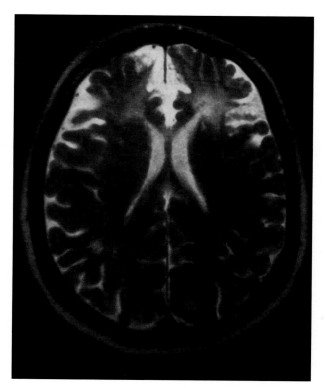

FIG. 1. T2-weighted MRI scan of a 9-year-old girl with moyamoya disease shows bilateral cerebral infarcts in the frontal lobes with atrophy (TR 5586, TE 90).

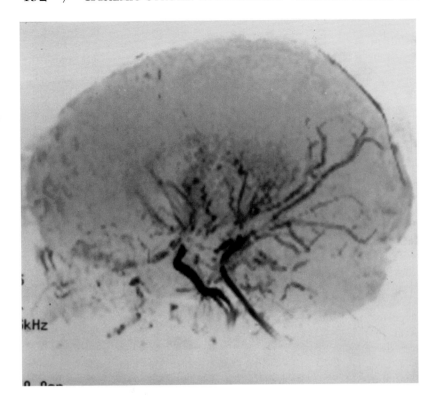

FIG. 3. MRA shows hypertrophied and tortuous lenticulostriate (moyamoya) vessels in a 2-year-old girl with moyamoya disease.

lenticulostriate arteries, Heubner's artery, and anterior choroidal and posterior communicating arteries dilate to help establish this collateral circulation. These dilated vessels give the appearance of a hazy puff of smoke on angiography. The external carotid artery initially becomes involved in this process through the anastomoses formed by the ophthalmic artery. Anterior and posterior ethmoidal arteries, the external

carotid artery, and the ophthalmic artery form a net-like collateral anastomosis in the orbit that communicates with the basal moyamoya vessels distal to the carotid stenosis. Suzuki and Kodoma (8) have termed this *ethmoidal moyamoya*. In children, this type of collateralization appears to correlate with the severity of the disease. This is not the case in adults and may reflect their diminished capacity to form collateral

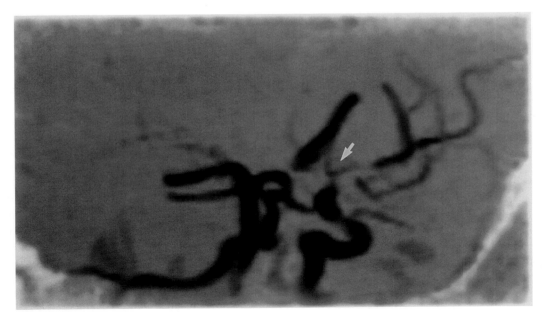

FIG. 4. MRA of a 35-year-old woman shows stenosis of the distal internal carotid artery and proximal segments of the anterior and middle cerebral arteries *(arrow)*.

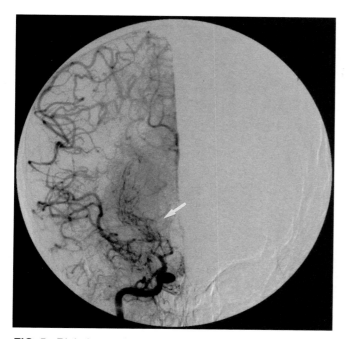

FIG. 5. Right internal carotid artery angiogram (anteroposterior view) of the same patient as in Fig. 4 shows a narrowed distal internal carotid artery and proximal segment of the middle cerebral artery. Dilated moyamoya vessels are seen *(arrow)*, and the anterior cerebral artery fills retrogradely through leptomeningeal collaterals.

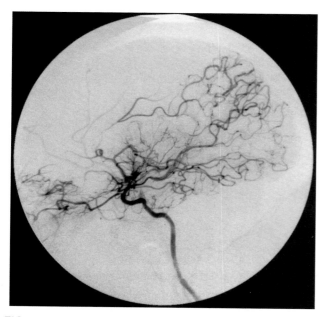

FIG. 6. Right internal carotid artery angiogram (lateral view) shows dilated lenticulostriate vessels and no antegrade flow in the anterior and middle cerebral arteries. The posterior cerebral artery fills from the internal carotid artery through the posterior communicating artery. There is retrograde filling of the anterior cerebral artery through leptomeningeal collateral from the posterior cerebral artery.

circulation. This differential correlation also occurs in the formation of the vault type of transdural collaterals that are derived from the middle meningeal and superficial temporal arteries. Angiography demonstrates these additional dural and leptomeningeal collateral vessels (32).

In patients who show involvement of the vertebrobasilar system, the quadrigeminal segment of the posterior cerebral artery is the earliest affected site. The proximal segment of the posterior cerebral artery and sometimes the distal portion of the basilar artery may become involved with further disease progression. Later in the course of the disease, the posterior cerebral arteries may become occluded. As a result of this occlusive process, posterior basal moyamoya develops, marked by dilated branches of the posterior choroidal arteries, thalamogeniculate arteries, and other thalamoperforate arteries. These may have anastomotic connections with the medullary vessels in the parietal subcortex. The leptomeningeal collateral anastomoses, which are usually the most prominent, have a tendency to decrease with the development of posterior cerebral artery stenosis (33). As the disease progresses, the cerebral perfusion finally becomes totally dependent on the collaterals from the extracranial arteries (34).

The angiographic findings in adults are somewhat different from those described above in children. The moyamoya vessels may be minimal or absent. There may be saccular defects and pseudoaneurysms, the latter especially in the small arteries in the ventricular wall and sometimes in the moyamoya vessels (35). Saccular aneurysms are often located at the basilar artery bifurcation (36). Cerebral dissecting aneurysms have also been reported (37). Hemorrhage as a presentation in adults is often due to rupture of subependymal or basilar bifurcation aneurysms (32).

Suzuki and Takaku (1) have divided the progression of moyamoya disease into six stages. In stage 1, there is only stenosis of the terminal, supraclinoid segment of the carotid arteries. Stage 2 is characterized by beginning basal moyamoya collateral vessels. The main cerebral arteries are dilated at this stage of the disease. Intensification of the moyamoya pattern in the basal ganglia region is associated with poor filling of the anterior and middle cerebral arteries in stage 3. There is progressive disappearance of the basal collateral network and minimization of the moyamoya pattern in stage 4. Narrowing and poor filling of the posterior cerebral arteries are often seen at this stage. The anterior and middle cerebral arteries are hardly visible in stage 5, as the transdural collateral and anastomotic vessels from the posterior cerebral arteries become more prominent. The basal moyamoya pattern continues to be further reduced during this stage. The final stage (stage 6) of disease progression is characterized by total obliteration of the main cerebral arteries and disappearance of the basal moyamoya. Cerebral blood flow is now exclusively supplied by the external carotid arteries via various transdural anastomoses.

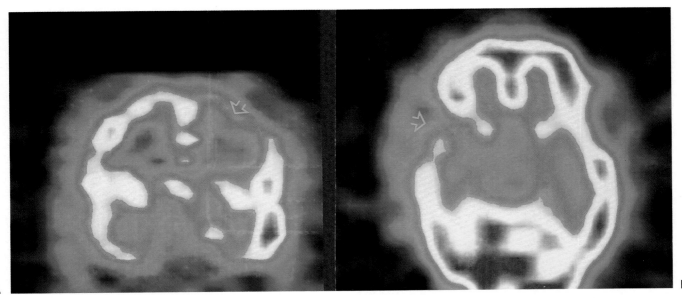

FIG. 7. Tc-99m HMPAO SPECT scans of the same patient as in Fig. 4 show decreased cerebral blood flow *(arrows)* in the left parietal region (coronal image) **(A)** and the right temporal region (axial image) **(B).**

Cerebral Blood Flow Studies

There is reduction in cerebral blood flow in moyamoya disease. This reduction is uneven and shows an anteroposterior gradient. Regional cerebral blood flow (rCBF) studies using xenon Xe 133 (^{133}Xe) inhalation SPECT technique have shown a striking bilateral frontooccipital blood flow gradient in young adults with moyamoya disease, with frontal hypoperfusion and occipital hyperemia in all patients studied (38). Technetium Tc 99m HMPAO SPECT may show perfusion defects corresponding to areas of ischemia (Fig. 7). Tc-99m DTPA HSA SPECT has been used to study the vasodilatory capacity of cerebral vessels to acetazolamide injection in moyamoya disease. The study showed that areas of diminished capacity could be demonstrated and cerebral infarction subsequently occurred in the same area (39). These observations suggest that this technique may identify cerebral areas at high risk for ischemic strokes. These or other similar techniques may become useful in selecting patients who would benefit from surgical intervention as compared with conservative therapy.

PET scan studies of rCBF showed a 20% decrease in the frontal and parietal region, with sparing of the occipital lobes in children with moyamoya compared with controls, although this did not reach statistical significance. However, a significant increase in the regional oxygen extraction fraction (rOEF) in the regions with low rCBF, especially the frontal and parietal regions, was found in children but not in adults (40). This observation indicates insufficient blood flow for the oxygen demand, which has been called "misery perfusion." Regional cerebral blood volume (rCBV) was significantly increased in the cerebral cortices and striatum of pediatric patients only. The regional transit time (rTT), calculated as rCBV/rCBF, was prolonged in the cerebral hemispheres of both adults and children. This correlates with dilated blood vessels seen in this condition. Regional cerebral metabolic rate for oxygen (rCMRO$_2$) was not decreased in either children or adults (40). A later study in children showed similar findings (41). The increased rOEF in children may be the reason why transient ischemic attacks (TIAs) are a common symptom in this age group compared with adults (40,41).

Cerebral blood flow autoregulation response to changes in blood pressure changes and carbon dioxide tension in the blood is reported to be impaired. The investigators found that the response to hypercapnia and low blood pressure (vasodilation) was impaired more than the response to hypocapnia and hypertension (vasoconstriction) (42,43).

Electroencephalogram

The electroencephalogram (EEG) may show a distinctive pattern following hyperventilation and has been termed the *rebuild-up phenomenon.* This consists of a return of high-voltage slow waves 20–60 seconds after cessation of hyperventilation (44). Although the mechanism responsible for this is unknown, the following sequence of events may occur. The vascular constriction after initiation of hyperventilation results in the typical pattern of high-voltage slow waves as seen in any individual. Recovery from this pattern occurs with gradual dilation of the cortical vessels after cessation of hyperventilation. It is postulated that the moyamoya vessels at the base of the brain are abnormal and are not as reactive to lowered carbon dioxide as the cortical vessels. Hence, when the cortical vessels dilate during the recovery phase following hyperventilation, there is a steal of blood from the deeper brain structures to the dilated cortical vessels with resultant ischemia—and thus a second phase of diffuse slow waves, the rebuild phenomenon. This EEG picture has not been seen in other conditions and therefore has been proposed as a useful screening test.

Pattern-reversal visual evoked potentials have been found to be useful in detecting occipital lobe abnormalities in patients with posterior cerebral artery occlusion (45).

LABORATORY INVESTIGATIONS

Routine hematology, biochemistry, and serology laboratory investigations are not revealing. Other appropriate laboratory investigations may be required for the associated conditions listed in Table 1. Patients should also be investigated for the usual stroke risk factors of young adults and children and appropriate measures taken. There is, however, no correlation of moyamoya disease with the presence of hypertension, hyperlipidemia, or other usual risk factors for stroke. Some of the more common investigations are listed in Table 2.

ETIOLOGY

Some patients with moyamoya disease have had neonatal anoxia, trauma, infections at the base of the brain, radiation

TABLE 2. *Selected investigations in children and young adults with ischemic stroke*

Complete blood count with differential, platelet count, and peripheral smear
Prothrombin time, partial thomboplastin time
Erythrocyte sedimentation rate
Blood glucose, serum electrolytes, blood chemistries
Total cholesterol, triglycerides, lipoprotein fractionation
Serologic tests for syphilis (VDRL, FTA-ABS)
Drug screen
Urine and blood amino acid and organic acids
Blood lactate and pyruvate
Plasma AT-III activity, protein C, and S levels
Antinuclear antibodies (ANA)
Rheumatoid factor
Lupus anticoagulant
Anticardiolipin antibodies
Pregnancy test (in women of childbearing age)
Urinalysis with microscopic evaluation
Chest roentgenogram
Electrocardiogram
M-mode and two-dimensional echocardiography
Contrast and transesophageal echocardiography in some cases
Duplex ultrasonography of the carotid arteries
Transcranial Doppler ultrasonography
Cranial CT
Brain MRI and MRA (in most instances)
Cerebral angiography (in most instances)

therapy, neurofibromatosis, tuberous sclerosis, brain tumors, fibromuscular dysplasia, cerebral dissecting and saccular aneurysms, sickle cell anemia, Fanconi's anemia, factor XII deficiency, type I glycogenosis, renal artery stenosis, and Down's syndrome. Etiologic factors in patients demonstrating the radiologic picture of moyamoya disease are diverse. Table 1 lists some of the conditions associated with this disease. It seems that any condition that causes a slow progressive narrowing and occlusion of basal cerebral vessels can result in a radiologic picture of resembling moyamoya disease. There is, however, an idiopathic variety in which genetic factors have been postulated. Investigations in 13 children and ten adults with angiographically proven moyamoya disease revealed an association with HLA antigens Aw24, Bw46 and Bw54, with relative risks of 3.83, 6.50 and 3.58, respectively (46). An increase in HLA-B40 antigen in children younger than 10 years was found in one study (47). HLA-B54 (20) was increased in patients older than 11 years of age in the same study. Autoantibody against double-stranded DNA showed higher than normal binding in the serum in four of 18 patients. Antivessel antibody was not detected in any of 23 patients. Natural T-cell toxic autoantibody was demonstrable by fluorescence-activated cell-sorter technique analysis in five of these 23 patients (46). Moyamoya disease type of phenomenon was also found to be associated with anti–Ro/SS-A and anti–La/SS-B antibodies in an adult black woman who had no risk factors for atherosclerosis and no signs of systemic lupus erythematosus or Sjögren's syndrome (48). These results suggest an underlying immunologic disturbance as the pathogenetic mechanism of moyamoya disease.

The role of infections, especially tonsillitis, pharyngitis, and other infections in the head and neck area, remains to be elucidated. Some authors have speculated that moyamoya disease may be a type of childhood vasculitis such as Kawasaki's syndrome that preferentially affects the carotid circulation (10). There is at present inadequate information to support such a hypothesis.

Moyamoya disease is characterized by a tendency for the formation of extensive collateral vessels. This tendency is most striking in the childhood form of the disease, and a role for basic fibroblast growth factor has been postulated (49). The recent finding of the presence of increased amounts of basic fibroblast growth factor and its receptor in the smooth muscle of the superficial temporal artery of moyamoya disease patients is provocative. It has been suggested that these smooth muscle cells with abundant basic fibroblast growth factor may stimulate themselves via an autocrine mechanism and migrate to and thicken the intima of patients with moyamoya disease (50).

Genetics

The role of genetic factors in moyamoya disease is not clear. Affected siblings have been reported in both Japanese and Caucasian families. We have seen two sisters with this disease. A mother–child pair and an uncle–nephew pair have also been reported (2). An incidence of 7% was found in the Japanese cases. This condition has also been reported in monovular twins (51). These reports point to a role for yet unknown and probably multifactorial genetic factors in this disease (52).

PATHOLOGY

Pathologic alterations are confined to the cerebral vasculature, with stenosis and occlusion of the distal internal carotid arteries and the proximal portions of the anterior and middle cerebral arteries. The vessel caliber is decreased. There is fibrocellular thickening of the intima. The internal elastic lamina is preserved all around the vessel wall but infolded and wavy and often duplicated. The media is usually attenuated. Inflammatory changes are absent. There is no atheroma, calcium, or lipid deposit. Complement components or immunoglobulins cannot be demonstrated. A number of small- and medium-sized arteries enter the base of the brain and form the moyamoya network of vessels. They also participate in the anastomoses with other vessels in the brain. Brain hemorrhage in the basal ganglia, thalamus, hypothalamus, and midbrain may be present in adults. Pseudoaneurysms have been described, and pathologic examination has shown their wall to be composed of concentric layers of fibrin and red blood cells. Saccular aneurysms have also been reported. Small arteries near the ventricular wall have a tendency to rupture. Recent and old cerebral infarcts may be present (53,54).

PATHOPHYSIOLOGY

Clinically and pathologically, moyamoya disease is progressive, with narrowing and eventual occlusion of the major cerebral vessels supplying the brain. The cerebral blood flow is maintained by collateral circulation from the external carotid arteries and the vertebral arteries. The symptoms in this disease are due to either cerebral ischemia or hemorrhage. Initial symptoms of TIA are common in children, although they also occur in adults. These events represent transient cerebral ischemia most likely due to the hemodynamic changes that precede vascular occlusion. This is supported by the blood flow studies cited earlier that show a decrease in the cerebral blood flow, especially in the carotid circulation. The increased regional oxygen extraction fraction (rOEF) in children suggests that they are at risk for more severe ischemia than adults and correlates with the observation that TIAs are more common in children than in adults. It probably also reflects the severity of the disease and more rapid progression in children.

Increased regional cerebral blood volume (rCBV) reflects the well developed network of basal moyamoya vessels characteristic of this disease. The role of collateral vessels on the brain surface to this increase in rCBV is not known. The rCBV very likely also reflects the compensatory vasodilation of these and other cerebral vessels in response to cerebral ischemia. The prolongation of regional transit time (rTT) demonstrated on PET studies supports this interpretation.

TREATMENT

Medical treatment of moyamoya disease with aspirin, steroids, vasodilators, mannitol, low molecular weight dextran, and antibiotics has been attempted but has proved to be ineffective (2). Calcium channel blocking drugs have been more successful in increasing the cerebral blood flow in moyamoya disease. Increased opacification of collateral vessels following intravenous verapamil infusion during cerebral angiography was noted in a 7-year-old girl with moyamoya disease who had presented with muteness and progressive right-sided weakness. She had previously had superficial temporal artery–middle cerebral artery (STA-MCA) bypass surgery. The clinical improvement associated with verapamil use in this girl was attributed to drug-induced vasodilation with reversal of cerebral ischemia. Similar clinical effect was present in another 3-year-old child with moyamoya disease (55). Nimodipine was also shown to be beneficial in a 40-year-old woman with moyamoya disease (56). Nicardipine was successfully used in two patients who remained symptomatic following surgery (57). However, the use of calcium channel blocking drugs has been recent and limited to only a few patients. More experience is required before their role in the medical therapy of moyamoya disease can be established. Medical therapy has otherwise largely been unsuccessful. As a result, surgical approaches have been advocated with the aim of increasing the cerebral blood supply (Table 3).

Surgical treatment of cerebrovascular disease has a long history. German and Taffel (58) in 1939 described the procedure of encephalomyosynangiosis (EMS). Kredel (59) was the first to attempt this procedure in man in 1942. Henschen and colleagues (60) revived the procedure in 1950, only to abandon it when postoperative angiograms consistently failed to show collateral flow through the graft. The follow-

TABLE 3. *Surgical procedures for the treatment of moyamoya disease*

Perivascular sympathectomy
Superior cervical sympathetic ganglionectomy
Superficial temporal artery–middle cerebral artery (STA-MCA) anastomosis
Superficial temporal artery–arterior cerebral artery (STA-ACA) anastomosis
Encephalomyosynangiosis (EMS)
Encephalomyoarteriosynangiosis (EMAS)
Encephaloduroarteriosynangiosis (EDAS)
Omental transposition
Gracilis-muscle transplantation

ing year Fisher (61), while discussing atherosclerotic strokes, suggested the possibility of a bypass from the extracranial to intracranial circulation (EC-IC bypass) to treat the underlying occlusive cerebrovascular disease. Technical difficulties in anastomosing small-caliber vessels hindered further progress till 1961 when Jacobson and Suarez (62) described the microsurgical technique to anastomose 2-mm-diameter vessels. Yasargil performed the first EC-IC bypass by anastomosing the superficial temporal artery to a distal cortical branch of the middle cerebral artery (STA-MCA bypass) in 1972 for the treatment of moyamoya disease (63).

The small caliber of the blood vessels in children has encouraged the development of other surgical procedures for this disease. Spetzler et al (64) reported the development of an impressive number of collaterals from the STA to the cortex and MCA distribution in a patient in whom he had found no satisfactory recipient vessel for STA-MCA bypass and had sutured the STA to the cortical arachnoid. Matsushima and colleagues (65–67) in 1981 described a procedure called encephaloduroarteriosynangiosis (EDAS). This procedure and its variations are now used mostly in children, while STA-MCA bypass is usually performed in adults as the initial surgical treatment.

The choice of surgical procedure depends on the age of the patient and availability of suitable donor and recipient arteries. Bilateral procedures are essential except perhaps in those rare cases in which the condition is unilateral. Postoperative angiograms after a suitable interval and close clinical follow-up are important. In some patients, adequate collateral revascularization does not seem to occur. In these patients, alternate procedures may need to be performed, especially if the disease continues to progress. Omental transplantation, though infrequently performed for revascularization of MCA territory, may be more useful in the territories of the anterior cerebral and posterior cerebral arteries. Recently, gracilis muscle transplantation has been used for similar purposes (77). Anastomosis of the STA to the anterior cerebral artery (ACA) (STA-ACA bypass) has also been used in some cases (68). The surgery, however, dose not prevent progressive carotid artery stenosis, although in successful cases TIAs and strokes, as well as further clinical progression, cease (67,69,70).

Perivascular Sympathectomy

Suzuki and colleagues (71) attempted to treat moyamoya disease by performing bilateral cervical perivascular sympathectomy. To this procedure, they added either unilateral or bilateral superior cervical ganglionectomy in some children. Despite initial encouraging results, they concluded that this procedure could slow the progress of moyamoya disease for short period only. This procedure is now rarely, if ever, performed for moyamoya disease.

STA-MCA Bypass

The STA-MCA bypass is most effective for TIAs, reversible ischemic neurologic deficits, and perhaps for minor or moderate neurologic symptoms (72). The STA is anastomosed to either the MCA or one of its main branches to augment the cerebral blood flow. Both side-to-side and end-to-side types of anastomosis are used. The angiographically demonstrated patency rate of this anastomosis is quite high. The procedure is technically difficult, especially in young children, due to the small caliber of both the STA and the MCA. Selection of appropriate recipient vessel is important, and several methods have been suggested. In some children, this procedure may not be feasible.

EMS and EDAS

These procedures are similar in that they avoid direct vessel-to-vessel anastomosis and are thus nonanastomotic EC-IC bypass procedures. The goal in these procedures is to increase cerebral vascularization and cerebral blood flow. Advantage is taken of the propensity of the brain, especially in this disease, to form collateral vessels from a readily available source.

In EMS, the temporalis muscle along with its blood supply is placed on the exposed cerebral cortex. This graft may or may not be sutured to the dural margins, and some surgeons open the arachnoid, while others do not. Focal seizures, wound infections, and chronic subdural hematoma are potential complications.

EDAS involves the placement of intact STA with a strip of attached galea on the cerebral arachnoid. Either the anterior or the posterior branch of the STA may be used. Sometimes the occipital artery may be used instead for this purpose. A variation of this operation involves opening the dura and the arachnoid and securing the transposition of the transplanted artery directly onto the cortex (69).

Omental Transposition

Omental transplantation for revascularization of ischemic heart had been done in 1936 by O'Shaughnessy (73). Goldsmith et al (74) in 1973 proposed the use of omental transposition to the brain surface for revascularization of the ischemic brain. The procedure has been done infrequently in moyamoya disease (75,76). It may find some use in revascularization in the anterior and posterior cerebral artery territories (76). It may also be used in cases where other surgical procedures have failed to stop disease progression. There may be theoretical concerns in the use of omentum, especially with regards to fibroblast proliferation and possible increased risk of epileptogenesis.

Gracilis Muscle Transplantation

Gracilis muscle transplantation is another technique that has been used to revascularize the territories supplied by the anterior and posterior cerebral arteries. Six children, aged 3–13 years, have been reported in whom this procedure was used. The gracilis muscle transplantation was in the territory of the anterior cerebral artery in three patients and in that of the posterior cerebral artery in the other three patients. The TIAs disappeared completely in five of the six patients and were markedly reduced in the remaining patient (77).

Considerations During and After Surgery

It has been pointed out above that ischemic symptoms in moyamoya disease can be precipitated by hyperventilation. It is therefore important to avoid hypocapnia during surgery. The choice of anesthetic agent should be made with this consideration. It should also be recognized that the brain in moyamoya disease is in a state of chronic ischemia, which is further aggravated by hypotension. Careful attention must be paid to prevent lowering of blood pressure during surgery and in the postoperative period.

PROGNOSIS

The natural history of moyamoya disease is not clearly understood. There are only a few reports of long-term follow up of patients with this disease, with or without surgical intervention (78–81). There is suggestion that the untreated condition may burn out (10). In one series, TIAs were most common in the first 4 years of the disease and decreased thereafter. Follow-up revealed no sequelae in 19%, occasional TIA or headache in 33%, mild intellectual and/or motor impairment in 26%, special school or care by parents/institution in teenage years in 11%, total 24-hour care in 7%, and death in 3% of patients (78). Poor prognosis was correlated with early onset, repeated TIAs followed by residual neurologic deficit, dominant-hemisphere or bilateral lesions, hypertension, and widespread lesions on angiography (78,79). Unfavorable outcome has also been reported in patients with repetitive ischemic attacks in the posterior cerebral artery territory (76).

EC-IC bypass surgery has been reported to increase cerebral blood flow and improve cognitive function, with an increase in IQ, especially the performance IQ (80,82). The frequency of TIAs, strokes and cerebral hemorrhage decreases following EC-IC bypass (81,83). Despite these observations, it is not yet clear whether surgery is superior to medical management in patients with moyamoya disease. A 5-year follow-up study of 628 patients by Yonekawa (83) showed that although the outcome seemed more favorable for the surgically treated patients compared with the conservatively treated patients, it did not reach statistical significance. It was noted that 70–80% of these patients had a rather benign natural history. This suggests that there is a need to define the criteria for patient selection for surgical treatment in moyamoya disease.

REFERENCES

1. Suzuki J, Takaku A. Cerebrovascular moyamoya disease showing abnormal net-like vessels in base of brain. *Arch Neurol* 1969;20:288–299.
2. Suzuki J. *Moyamoya Disease.* Springer-Verlag, Tokyo, 1986.
3. Takeuchi K, Shimizu K. Hypoplasia of the bilateral internal carotid arteries. *Brain Nerve (Tokyo)* 1957;9:37–43.
4. Weidner W, Hanagee W. Markham CH. Intracranial collateral circulation via leptomeningeal and rete mirabile anastomoses. *Neurology* 1965;15:39–47.
5. Leeds NE, Abbott KH. Collateral circulation in cerebrovascular disease in childhood via rete mirabile and perforating branches of anterior choroidal and posterior cerebral arteries. *Radiology* 1965;85:628–634.
6. Nishimoto A, Takeuchi S. Abnormal cerebrovascular network related to the internal carotid arteries. *J Neurosurg* 1968;29:255–260.
7. Fukuyama T, Suzuki Y. Segawa M. Acute recurrent transient hemiplegia in children with special reference to cases with telangiectasis-like vascularity at the base of brain. *Brain Nerve (Tokyo)* 1965;17:757–760.
8. Suzuki J, Kodama N. Moyamoya disease—A review. *Stroke* 1983;14:104–109.
9. Aicardi J. *Diseases of the Nervous System in Childhood.* London: Mac-Keith Press, 1992. Clinics in Developmental Medicine, No. 115/118.
10. Chaudhuri KR, Edwards R. Adult moyamoya disease. *BMJ* 1993;307:852–854.
11. Watanabe K, Negoro T, Maehara M, Takahaski I, Nomura K, Miura K. Moyamoya disease presenting with chorea. *Pediatr Neurol* 1990;6:40–42.
12. Schoenberg BS, Mellinger JF, Schoenberg DG, Barringer FS. Moyamoya disease presenting as a seizure disorder. *Arch Neurol* 1977;34:511–512.
13. Yonekawa Y, Handa H, Okuno T. Moyamoya disease: Diagnosis, treatment and recent achievement. In: Barnett HJM, Stein BM, Mohr JP, Yatsu FM, eds. *Stroke.* New York: Churchill Livingstone, 1986:805–829.
14. Miyamoto S, Kikuchi H, Karasawa J, Nagata I, Ihara I. Study of the posterior circulation in moyamoya disease. Part 2: Visual disturbances and surgical treatment. *J Neurosurg* 1986;65:454–460.
15. Miyamoto S, Kikuchi S, Karasawa J, Nagata I, Ikota T. Study on the vertebrobasilar system in moyamoya disease. *Brain Nerve (Tokyo)* 1984;36:491–499.
16. Gordon N, Isler W. Childhood moyamoya disease. *Dev Med Child Neurol* 1991;31:98–107.
17. Maki Y, Enomoto T. Moyamoya disease. *Childs Nerv Syst* 1988;4:204–212.
18. Yamaguchi T, Tashiro M, Minematsu K, Kitamura K. Summary of Japanese survey of occlusion of the circle of Willis. In: *Reports by the Research Committee on Spontaneous Occlusion of the Circle of Willis.* Tokyo: Japanese Ministry of Health and Welfare, 1980:13–22.
19. Pearson E, Lenn NJ, Cail WS. Moyamoya and other causes of stroke in patients with Down syndrome. *Pediatr Neurol* 1985;1:174–179.
20. Tsuji N, Kuriyama T, Iwamoto M. Moyamoya disease associated with craniopharyngioma. *Surg Neurol* 1984;21:588–592.
21. Rajakulasingam K, Cerullo LJ, Raimondi AJ. Childhood moyamoya syndrome: Postradiation pathogenesis. *Child's Brain* 1979;5:467–475.
22. Ellison PH, Largent JA, Popp AJ. Moyamoya disease associated with renal artery stenosis. *Arch Neurol* 1981;38:467.
23. Kapusta L, Daniels O, Renier WO. Moyamoya syndrome and primary pulmonary hypertension in childhood. *Neuropediatrics* 1990;21:162–163.
24. Coakham HB, Duchen LW, Scaraville F. Moyamoya disease: Clinical and pathological report of a case with associated myopathy. *J Neurol Neurosurg Psychiatry* 1979;42:289–297.
25. Cohen N, Berant M, Simon J. Moyamoya and Fanconi's anemia. *Pediatrics* 1980;65:804–805.
26. Fernandez-Alvarez E, Pineda M, Royo C, Manzanares R. Moyamoya disease caused by cranial trauma. *Brain Dev* 1979;1:133–138.
27. Scott IA, Boyle RS. Sneddon's syndrome. *Aust N Z J Med* 1986;16:799–802.
28. Ho C, Baraitser M. Neurological complications in one of a sib pair with aplasia cutis congenita. *Clin Dysmorphol* 1992;1:235–238.
29. Huang CY. Neurology in Asia. In: Bradley WG, Daroff RB, Fenichel GM, Marsden CD, eds. *Neurology in Clinical Practice.* Boston: Butterworth-Heinemann, 1991;1909–1910.
30. Takahashi M, Miyauchi T, Kowada M. Computed tomography of moyamoya disease: Demonstration of occluded arteries and collateral vessels as important diagnostic signs. *Radiology* 1980;134:561–676.

31. Bruno A, Yuh WTC, Biller J, Adams Jr HP, Cornell SH. Magnetic resonance imaging with cerebral infarction due to moyamoya. *Arch Neurol* 1988;45:303–306.

32. Huber P. *Krayenbuhl/Yasargil Cerebral Angiography.* New York: Georg-Thieme Verlag, 1982.

33. Satoh S, Shibuya H, Matsushima Y, Suzuki S. Analysis of the angiographic findings in cases of childhood moyamoya disease. *Neuroradiology* 1988;30:111–119.

34. Miyamoto S, Kikuchi H, Karasawa J, Nagata I, Ikota T, Takeuchi S. Study of the posterior circulation in moyamoya disease. *J Neurosurg* 1984;61:1032–1037.

35. Konishi Y, Kadowaki C, Hara M, Takeuchi K. Aneurysms associated with moyamoya disease. *Neurosurgery* 1985;16:484–491.

36. Adams HP, Kassell NF, Wisoff HS, Drake CG. Intracranial saccular aneurysm and moyamoya disease. *Stroke* 1979;10:174–179.

37. Yamashita M, Tanaka K, Matsuo T, Yokoyama K, Fujii T, Sakamoto H. Cerebral dissecting aneurysms in patients with moyamoya disease. *J Neurosurg* 1983;58:120–125.

38. Bruno A, Adams HP Jr, Biller J, Rezai K, Cornell S, Aschenbrener CA. Cerebral infarction due to moyamoya disease in young adults. *Stroke* 1988;19:826–833.

39. Inoue Y, Momose T, Machida K, Honda N, Tsutsumi K. Cerebral vasodilatory capacity mapping using Technetium-99m-DTPA-HSA SPECT and acetazolamide in moyamoya disease. *J Nucl Med* 1993; 34:1984–1986.

40. Kuwabara Y, Ichiya Y, Otsuka M, et al. Cerebral hemodynamic change in the child and the adult with moyamoya disease. *Stroke* 1990;21: 272–277.

41. Ikezaki K, Matsushima T, Kuwabara Y, Suzuki SO, Nomura T, Fukui M. Cerebral circulation and oxygen metabolism in childhood moyamoya disease: A perioperative positron emission tomographic study. *J Neurosurg* 1994;843–850.

42. Ogawa A, Yoshimoto T, Suzuki J, Sakurai Y. Cerebral blood flow in moyamoya disease. Part I: Correlation with age and regional distribution. *Acta Neurochir (Wien)* 1990;105:30–34.

43. Ogawa A, Nakamura N, Toshimoto T, Suzuki J. Cerebral blood flow in moyamoya disease. Part 2: Autoregulation and CO_2 response. *Acta Neurochir (Wien)* 1990;105:107–111.

44. Kodama N, Aoki Y, Hiraga H, Wada T, Suzuki J. Electroencephalographic findings in children with moyamoya disease. *Arch Neurol* 1979; 36:16–19.

45. Tashima-Kurita S, Matsuchima T, Kato M, Morioka T, Kuwabara Y, Hasuo K, Fukui M. Moyamoya disease. *Arch Neurol* 1989;46:550–553.

46. Kitahara T, Okumura K, Semba A, Yamaura A, Makino H. Genetic and immunologic analysis on moyamoya. *J Neurol Neurosurg Psychiatry* 1982;45:1048–1052.

47. Sekiguchi S, Kobagashik, Hatton M. HLA antigen in spontaneous occlusion of the circle of Willis. In: Gotoh F, ed. *Annual Report (1979) of the Research Committee on Spontaneous Occlusion of the Circle of Willis.* Tokyo: Japanese Ministry of Health and Welfare, 1979;76.

48. Provost TT, Moses H, Morris, EL, et al. Cerebral vasculopathy associated with collateralization resembling moyamoya phenomenon and with ANTI-Ro/SS-A and ANTI-La/SS-B antibodies. *Arthritis Rheum* 1991;34:1052–1055.

49. Hoshimaru M, Takahashi JA, Kikichi H, Nagata I, Hatanaka M. Possible roses of basic fibroblast growth factor in the pathogenesis of moyamoya disease: An immunohistochemical study. *J Neurosurg* 1991;75: 267–270.

50. Suzuki H, Hoshimaru M, Takahashi M, et al. Immunohistochemical reactions for fibroblast growth factor receptor in arteries of patients with moyamoya disease. *Neurosurgery* 1994;35:20–25.

51. Yamada H, Nakamura S, Kageyama N. Moyamoya disease in monovular twins: A case report. *J Neurosurg* 1980;53:109.

52. Kitahara T, Ariga N, Yamaura A, Makino H, Maki Y. Familial occurrence of moyamoya disease: Report of three Japanese families. *J Neurol Neurosurg Psychiatry* 1979;42:208–214.

53. Adams JH, ed. *Greenfield's Neuropathology,* 5th ed. New York: Oxford University Press, 1992.

54. Yamashita M, Oka K, Tanaka K. Histopathology of the brain vascular network in moyamoya disease. *Stroke* 1983;14:50–58.

55. McLean MJ, Gebarski SS, Van der Spak AF, Goldstein GW. Response of moyamoya disease to verapamil. *Lancet* 1985;i:163–164.

56. Spittler JF, Smektala K. Pharmacotherapy in moyamoya disease. *Hokkaido J Med Sci.* 1990;65:235–240.

57. Hosain SA, Hughes JT, Forem SL, Wisoff J, Fish I. Use of a calcium channel blocker (nicardipine HCl) in the treatment of childhood moyamoya disease. *J Child Neurol* 1994;9:378–380.

58. German WJ, Taffel M. Surgical production of collateral intracranial circulation. *Proc Soc Exp Biol Med* 1939w°:349–353.

59. Kredel FE. Collateral cerebral circulation by muscle graft. Technique of operation with report of 3 cases. *South Surg* 1942;10:235–244.

60. Henschen C. Cited by Onesti ST, Solomon RA, Quest DO. Cerebral revascularization: A review. *Neurosurgery* 1989;25:618–629.

61. Fisher CM. Occlusion of the internal carotid artery. *Arch Neurol Psychiatry* 1951;65:346–377.

62. Jacobson JH, Suarez E. Microsurgery in anastomosis of small vessels. *Surg Forum* 1960;11:243–245.

63. Krayenbuhl HA. The moyamoya syndrome and the neurosurgeon. *Surg Neurol* 1975;4:353–360.

64. Spetzler RF, Roski RA, Kopaniky DR. Alternative superficial temporal artery to middle cerebral artery revascularization procedure. *Neurosurgery* 1980;7:484–487.

65. Matsushima Y, Fukai N, Tanaka K, et al. A new surgical treatment of moyamoya in children: A preliminary report. *Surg Neurol* 1981; 15:313–320.

66. Matsushima Y, Inaba Y. Moyamoya disease in children and its surgical treatment. *Childs Brain* 1984;11:155–170.

67. Matsushima T, Fujiwara S, Nagata S, et al. Surgical treatment for paediatric patients with moyamoya disease by indirect revascularization procedures (EDAS, EMS, EMAS). *Acta Neurochir (Wien)* 1989;98: 135–140.

68. Ishii R, Koike T, Takeuchi S, Ohsugi S, Tanaka R, Konno K. Anastomosis of the superficial temporal artery to the distal anterior cerebral artery with interposed cephalic vein graft. *J Neurosug* 1983;58: 425–429.

69. Scott RM. Surgical treatment of moyamoya syndrome in children. *Concepts Pediatr Neurosurg* 1985;6:198–212.

70. Eller TW, Pasternak JF. Revascularization for moyamoya disease: Five year follow-up. *Surg Neurol* 1987;28:463–467.

71. Suzuki J, Takaku A, Kodama N, Sato S. An attempt to treat cerebrovascular moyamoya disease in children. *Childs Brain* 1975;1:193–206.

72. Karasawa J, Kikuchi H, Furuse S, Kawamura J, Sakaki T. Treatment of moyamoya disease with STA-MCA anastomosis. *J Neurosurg* 1978; 49:679–688.

73. O'Shaughnessy L. An experimental method of providing a collateral circulation for the heart. *Br J Surg* 1936;23:665–670.

74. Goldsmith HS, Chen W-F, Duckett SW. Brain vascularization by intact omentum. *Arch Surg* 1973;106:695–698.

75. Karasawa J, Kikuchi H, Kawamura J, Sakai T. Intracranial transplantation of the omentum for cerebrovascular moyamoya disease: A twoyear follow-up study. *Surg Neurol* 1980;14:444–449.

76. Karasawa J, Touho H, Ohnishi H, Miyamoto S, Kikuchi H. Cerebral revascularization using omental transplantation for childhood moyamoya disease. *J Neurosurg* 1993;79:192–196.

77. Touho H, Karasawa J, Ohnishi H. Cerebral revascularization using gracilis muscle transplantation for childhood moyamoya disease. *Surg Neurol* 1995;43:191–198.

78. Kurokawa T, Tomita S, Ueda K, et al. Prognosis of occlusive disease of the circle of Willis (moyamoya disease) in children. *Pediatr Neurol* 1985;1:274–277.

79. Maki Y, Nakada Y, Nose T, Yoshii. Clinical and radioisotopic follow-up study of moyamoya. *Childs Brain* 1976;2:257–271.

80. Ishii R, Takeuchi S, Ibayashi K, Tanaka R. Intelligence in children with moyamoya disease: Evaluation after surgical treatments with special reference to changes in cerebral blood flow. *Stroke* 1984;15:873–877.

81. Karasawa J, Touho H, Ohniski H, Miyamoto S, Kikuchi H. Long-term follow-up study after extracranial-intracranial bypass surgery for anterior circulation ischemia in childhood moyamoya disease. *J Neurosurg* 1992;77:84–89.

82. Suzuki R, Matsushima Y, Takada Y, Nariai T, Wakabayashi S, Tone O. Changes in cerebral hemodynamics following encephalo-duro-arteriosynangiosis (EDAS) in young patients with moyamoya disease. *Surg Neurol* 1989;31:343–349.

83. Yonekawa Y. Summary report of the research committee on spontaneous occlusion of the circle of Willis (moyamoya disease) (1988–1992). In: Yonekawa Y, ed. *1992 Annual Report of the Research Committee on Spontaneous Occlusion of the Circle of Willis (Moyamoya Disease).* Tokyo: Japanese Ministry of Health and Welfare, 1992:1–11.

Cerebrovascular Disease, edited by H. Hunt Batjer.
Lippincott-Raven Publishers, Philadelphia © 1997.

CHAPTER 40

Inflammatory Arteritis and Stroke

Robin L. Brey and Patricia M. Moore

Inflammation of the blood vessel wall, often resulting in compromise of blood flow and subsequent ischemia, is the central feature of the diverse group of diseases that make up the arteritides. Any size, location, and type of blood vessel may be involved. The immunogenic processes resulting in vessel wall inflammation are numerous but can be broadly categorized into the following: (a) immune complex–mediated, (b) antibody-associated, and (c) cell-mediated. In human diseases, the hypersensitivity vasculitides that are characterized by predominant involvement of the cutaneous venules and leukocytoclasis are often immune complex–mediated [1]. Two syndromes, Kawasaki's syndrome [2] and Wegener's granulomatosis [3], are associated with autoantibodies that may have a pathogenic role in vessel inflammation. Cell-mediated processes occur in numerous other disorders and are most frequently identified when the histologic picture is primarily mononuclear or lymphocytic. Isolated angiitis of the central nervous system (CNS) is a likely example of this [4].

Clinical manifestations of vasculitic damage in the nervous system can be quite variable. Stroke can occur during the stage of acute inflammation due to focal ischemia induced by the vasculitic process. In more chronic vasculitic conditions, stroke may be due to sustained ischemia induced by fibrotic narrowing of the cerebral vasculature. Other neurologic manifestations such as headache and mental status changes may be due to more diffuse CNS injury. Although global ischemia may play a role in these other manifestations, they may be due to direct toxic effects of cytokines and other soluble mediators of inflammation on nervous system tissue [5]. In most vasculitic syndromes, there is systemic involvement, although neurologic manifestations can be the heralding feature [4,6]. Vasculitis can also be isolated to the central or peripheral nervous system [6]. The pathogenesis of neither isolated nor secondary nervous vasculitis is well understood and is likely to involve multiple factors.

ROLE OF ENDOTHELIAL CELLS AND ADHESION MOLECULES

The interaction of endothelial cells and leukocytes via adhesion molecules is likely to be the initial event in most vasculitic disorders (Table 1). A decade of studies of the dynamic interaction of leukocytes and the endothelium provides information on the accumulation of inflammatory cells in and around the vessel wall. Much of the work utilizes endothelium of the systemic vasculature as antigen-presenting cells. Some of these studies may also be applicable to vascular inflammation within the central and peripheral nervous systems.

Adhesion molecules belong to a multiple receptor–ligand system consisting of three families of related proteins: (a) the selectins, (b) the integrins, and (c) the immunoglobulin superfamily [1,3,7]. The initial leukocyte attachment occurs when selectins on the endothelial surface bind to carbohydrate moieties on the leukocyte surface. Selectins support the adhesion of neutrophils, some T lymphocytes, and monocytes. Selectins are expressed only by endothelial cells, with little constitutive expression. Thus, immediately after an inflammatory stimulus, leukocytes are loosely adherent to endothelium in the vicinity of the stimulus. Involvement of specific types of leukocytes depends on the nature of the inflammatory stimulus. Chemokines that are displayed on or released from the endothelium further attract specific leukocytes and increase integrin adhesiveness. Other molecules also participate. Platelet-activating factor, a biologically active phospholipid, is coexpressed with P-selectin at the time of endothelial activation and appears to upregulate integrin expression on the leukocyte surface [8]. Firmer adhesiveness occurs when intercellular adhesion molecule 1 (ICAM-1) is upregulated and interacts with loosely bound leukocytes. ICAM-1 is a transmembrane protein and member of the immunoglobulin superfamily, and supports the adhesion of all

R. L. Brey: Division of Neurology, University of Texas Health Science Center, San Antonio, Texas 78284.

P. M. Moore: Department of Neurology, Wayne State University, Detroit, Michigan 48201.

TABLE 1. *Adhesion molecule–leukocyte interactions*

Adhesion molecule/ligand	Cell types expressing adhesion molecule	Factors increasing constitutive expression	Cells interacting with adhesion molecule
E-selectin/sialyated glycoprotein	Endothelial cells	TNF-α, IL-1 atherogenic lipids, hyperglycemia	Neutrophils, T-lymphocytes, monocytes
ICAM-1/LFA-1 (CD11a/CD18b)	Endothelial cells, glial cells, smooth muscle cells in atheroma	IFN-γ, IL-1, TNF-α, atherogenic lipids, hyperglycemia	All leukocytes
VCAM-1/VLA-4	Endothelial cells, macrophages, smooth muscle cells in atheroma	TNF-α, IL-1, IL-4, atherogenic lipids, hyperglycemia	Lymphocytes, monocytes

Key: ICAM-1, intercellular adhesion molecule 1; LGA-1, lymphocyte function–associated antigen 1; VCAM-1, vascular cell adhesion molecule 1; VLA-4, very late antigen 4; TNF-α, tumor necrosis factor alpha; IL-1, interleukin-1; INF-γ, interferon gamma; IL-4, interleukin-4.

leukocytes. It is also expressed in endothelial cells and smooth muscle cells in human atherosclerotic lesions. After interaction with ICAM-1, the firmly adherent leukocytes can then traverse the vessel wall. Lymphocytes and monocytes soon follow, usually beginning to arrive in the lesion about 4 hours after the initial inflammatory stimulus (9). This change from a predominantly neutrophil to a predominantly mononuclear cell infiltrate corresponds to a change in endothelial CAM expression. Vascular cell adhesion molecule 1 (VCAM-1) is also a transmembrane protein and member of the immunoglobulin superfamily, and supports the adhesion of monocytes and lymphocytes, but not neutrophils. VCAM-1 is expressed by macrophages, endothelial cells, and atherosclerotic lesions. Selectin expression diminishes about 4–6 hours after an acute inflammatory stimulus; however, ICAM-1 and VCAM-1 expression is increasing at this time, accounting for the change in the type of leukocyte attracted to the inflammatory lesion (8). Tissue injury depends on the location and number of fully activated leukocytes recruited to the lesion.

Endothelial cells also release cytokines and are important in the regulation of chemotaxis, vessel wall permeability, and molecular and cellular transport across the endothelial barrier, in addition to the direction of lymphocyte trafficking (10,11). Endothelial cells can present antigen to T cells in association with class II molecules and be induced to express Fc and complement receptors. In addition, endothelial cells themselves may be a target for cytotoxic T cells in the setting of certain infections.

SPECIAL IMMUNOLOGIC FEATURES OF THE CENTRAL NERVOUS SYSTEM

Brain endothelial cells differ markedly from other endothelial cells immunologically and morphologically (Table 2). Cerebrovascular endothelial cells together with astrocytes and pericytes form the blood–brain barrier. Under normal circumstances the blood–brain barrier blocks the entrance of large numbers of most immune effector cells into the CNS (10). Activated T lymphocytes enter the CNS under normal conditions for immunologic surveillance (9,11); however, if they do not encounter a specific CNS antigen, they do not remain. If the blood–brain barrier is already altered (eg, by proinflammatory cytokines), immune effector cells and soluble mediators of inflammation could enter the CNS freely (10). Even without a grossly disrupted blood–brain barrier, an increased influx of leukocytes into the brain can also occur if brain endothelial CAM expression is upregulated. Once present within the CNS, these effector cells can initiate a cascade of events that can result in an extension of tissue injury. Cytokines secreted by activated T lymphocytes and macrophages can upregulate the expression of major histocompatibility complex (MHC) class I molecules—tumor necrosis factor alpha (TNF-α) acting synergistically with interferon gamma (IFN-γ)—and MHC class II molecules (IFN-γ) on brain endothelial cells, microglial cells, and astrocytes (12). This MHC up-regulation, particularly of MHC class II, probably plays a crucial role in initiating and perpetuating a CNS-directed immune response. Finally, some of the cytokines secreted by lymphocytes and macrophages during an immune response—interleukin-1 (IL-1), IFN-γ, and TNF-α)—can be directly toxic to CNS tissue (5).

In the nervous system, much of our information on leukocyte–endothelial interactions comes not from the study of vasculitides but rather from the study of other disorders such as multiple sclerosis and experimental allergic encephalomyelitis (EAE). The constitutive expression of brain endothelial CAMs appears to be lower than in systemic endothelium (7). Some recent work has suggested that the degree of constitutive expression may be a susceptibility factor for developing some inflammatory and autoimmune nervous system diseases. For example, some murine strains found to be resistant to the development of EAE have no constitutive expression of brain endothelial CAMs, suggesting that the degree of constitutive expression may well be a susceptibility factor (13). Further, Raine and colleagues (14) have shown that ICAM-1 is upregulated on brain endothelial cells in the initial stages of demyelination. Interestingly, the expression of ICAM-1 on brain endothelium in this study had a dose and

TABLE 2. *Immunologic properties of brain and aortic endothelium*

Properties	Brain endothelium	Aortic endothelium
Major Histocompatibility (MHC) Expression		
MHC class expression	High	High
Effects of TNF-α and IFN-γ on MHC class I expression	Enhanced	Enhanced
MHC class II expression	Absent	Absent
Effects of INF-γ	Markedly increased expression	Mildly increased expression
Leukocyte Adhesion		
Leukocyte adhesion	Low	High
Effects of TNF-α and IFN-γ on leukocyte adhesion	High	No increase
Dependence on Ca^{++}/Mg^{++}	Present	Present
Enhancement by mitogens	High	No increase

Key: TNF-α, tumor necrosis factor alpha; INF-γ, interferon gamma.

time dependence on the presence of proinflammatory cytokines but, once expressed, could not be reversed, even when these cytokines were removed. This suggests a mechanism whereby, in some cases, chronic ischemic tissue injury could persist long after the acute inflammatory disorder is quiescent. Cannella and Raine (15) demonstrated an upregulated expression of ICAM-1 and VCAM-1 in the brains of patients with a variety of inflammatory and noninflammatory nervous system diseases. These investigators could not find a pattern of expression specific for any of them. This suggests that dysregulation of CAM expression in the CNS may be a key feature in CNS injury mediated by a number of different disease processes.

VASCULAR ENDOTHELIUM AND NORMAL HEMOSTASIS

In addition to the accumulation of cells, several other physiologic processes contribute to tissue ischemia in the vasculitic syndromes. Of these, the most important clinically are the changes in coagulation and hemostasis. Vascular endothelium is a highly active metabolic and endocrine organ with key roles in normal hemostasis (3). Situation-appropriate coagulation occurs locally in response to vascular injury through a complex interaction of coagulation factors, platelets, and the endothelial surface. It is highly regulated by the major natural anticoagulant systems: proteins C and S, antithrombin III, and fibrinolysis. Further aggregation of already adherent platelets is limited by local secretion of prostacyclin by neighboring endothelial cells (reviewed in ref. 3). The homeostatic balance in some patients appears to be perturbed by a variety of factors such as hypertriglyceridemia or vascular endothelial damage with subsequent increased expression of tissue factor. Angiotensin-converting enzyme that can activate the vasoconstrictor angiotensin II and inactivate the vasodilator bradykinin and is present on the endothelial surface. Also present are receptors and carrier proteins that play a role in the activation and metabolism of coagulation proteins and other vasoactive substances. In addition, to maintain blood fluidity, endothelial cells synthesize important substances, such as fibronectin, heparin-like substances, cytokines, tissue plasminogen–activating factor, growth factors, prostacyclin, endothelin-1, and others.

The normal anticoagulant properties of endothelial cells may be altered by the vasculitic process, resulting in thrombosis, as well as stroke if the injured vessel is in the brain. Coagulation products, such as thrombin, upregulate some members of the selectin family, potentially leading to the attachment of neutrophils in the area of thrombosis (16). This process can then lead to further ischemia in a cycle of thrombotic and inflammatory damage. In addition, the release of endothelin by activated endothelial cells may add to tissue injury by causing vasoconstriction, as well as thrombosis. Notably, corticosteroids, which diminish cytokine expression and inflammation, may also have a deleterious effect in vascular inflammation. Corticosteroids interfere with the metabolism of arachidonic acid by inhibiting phospholipase A$_2$ leading to decreased production of prostacyclin, thromboxane, and leukotrienes (17). Thus, clot lysis is inhibited, platelet aggregation is favored, and the secretion of vasodilating substances is inhibited. The net effect therefore could be both thrombosis and vasoconstriction. The use of both aspirin and calcium channel blockers has been suggested as a way to counteract this potential adverse corticosteroid effect (18).

NERVOUS SYSTEM INVOLVEMENT IN SYSTEMIC VASCULITIS (TABLE 3)

Polyarteritis Nodosa

Polyarteritis nodosa is the most common of the necrotizing vasculitides and involves the CNS in 20–40% of patients and the peripheral nervous system (PNS) in up to 50% (18,19). PNS involvement can include the classic mononeuropathy multiplex, polyneuropathies, plexopathies, radiculopathies, cutaneous neuropathies, and an ascending quadraparesis from extensive mononeuropathies (20,21). CNS

TABLE 3. *Prominent clinical features of the vasculitides and major organ involvement*

Vasculitic syndrome	Clinical features	Major organ involvement
Polyarteritis nodosa	Peripheral neuropathy, hematuria, visceral involvement, hepatitis B antigenemia in 30% of patients	Kidneys, skin, PNS gastrointestinal system
Churg-Strauss	Asthma, eosinophilia, peripheral neuropathy	Lungs, skin, PNS, CNS
Wegener's granulomatosis	Upper and lower respiratory tract involvement, glomerulo-nephritis, cranial neuropathies, presence of antineutro-phil cytoplasmic antibodies	Upper respiratory tract, lungs, kidneys, cranial nerves, PNA
Connective tissue diseases	SLE: any organ can be involved; when stroke occurs, it is usually related to a vasculopathy and not vascular inflammation in the brain Other: Any organ can be involved; although NS is involved less often than SLE, vasculitis is more likely to be present	Any organ
Giant-cell arteritis	New onset headaches in older person, jaw claudication, tender temporal arteries, high sedimentation rate, vis-ual loss, posterior circulation strokes, encephalopathy	Extracranial and posterior circulation vasculature
Takayasu's arteritis	Ischemic symptoms from aortic arch involvement (syn-cope, transient ischemic attacks, stroke)	Aorta and branches
Vasculitis due to infection/drugs	Any organ can be involved, including isolated CNS in-volvement	Any organ
Isolated CNS vasculitis	Global CNS dysfunction (headache, encephalopathy) and focal ischemia (stroke, cranial neuropathy, myelop-athy)	CNS

Key: PNS, peripheral nervous system; CNS, central nervous system; NS, nervous system; SLE, systemic lupus erythematosus.

abnormalities usually develop after the disease is established and include encephalopathies, seizures, subacute memory loss, stroke, and subarachnoid hemorrhage.

There are no serologic markers of disease, although the systemic inflammation is often reflected nonspecifically in anemia, leukocytosis, thrombocytosis, C-reactive proteins, and an elevated erythrocyte sedimentation rate (18). Hepatitis B antigenemia and immune complexes are found in about 30% of patients (22). Abdominal angiography can demonstrate vasculitic involvement of renal, hepatic, and visceral blood vessels. The diagnosis of polyarteritis nodosa is determined on the basis of evidence of systemic inflammation, angiographic evidence of enteric vascular disease, and histologic evidence of vasculitis (often seen in a peripheral nerve) (20,21).

Churg–Strauss Syndrome

Churg–Strauss syndrome, also known as allergic angiitis and granulomatosis, is a rare condition with prominent involvement of the pulmonary system. Prominent eosinophilic infiltration of blood vessels is seen. The disease is often heralded by an increasingly severe asthma in patients with a history of atopy (23). Asthma may precede the development of eosinophilia and systemic vasculitis by 2–20 years. PNS involvement frequently occurs early in the disease course in 50% of patients, whereas CNS involvement is unusual except late in the course in untreated patients (1,18,21,23).

Wegener's Granulomatosis

Wegener's granulomatosis affects the upper and lower respiratory tract and is accompanied by glomerulonephritis. Presenting symptoms reflect systemic inflammation and focal pulmonary or upper airway involvement. The characteristic histologic picture, necrotizing granulomatous angiitis, is most frequently detected in the lung (1,18,23). Recent studies suggest that the incidence of neurologic abnormalities may be declining with earlier and more aggressive therapy. Neurologic abnormalities occur either by proximity of a neurologic structure to a necrotizing process or by ischemia or hemorrhage from the inflammatory vascular disease. Thus, the prominent cranial neuropathies reflect erosion of the bony structures at the base of the skull by contiguous extension from sinus granulomas. Hearing loss, proptosis, and trigeminal and facial paresis are prominent features. Hypothalamic or pituitary abnormalities also appear to develop by this mechanism. The PNS is predominantly affected by this small-vessel vasculitic syndrome, but the CNS parenchyma is sometimes involved as well. Encephalopathies, seizures, and focal sensory or motor changes can be seen (1,25). Neurodiagnostic studies are often needed to differentiate compressive cranial nerve lesions from lesions resulting from ischemia.

Antineutrophil cytoplasmic antibodies are strongly associated with Wegener's granulomatosis and can be helpful diagnostically (1,3). The relationship of the titer to disease activity or the disease pathogenesis is uncertain. Diagnosis depends on the clinical features, histologic abnormalities, and exclusion of infection as a cause of chronic respiratory tract inflammation.

Vasculitis with Connective Tissue Diseases

Both CNS and PNS vasculitis may complicate connective tissue diseases. These are a group of systemic inflammatory disorders including systemic lupus erythematosus (SLE), Sjögren's syndrome, mixed connective tissue disease, rheumatoid arthritis, progressive systemic sclerosis, and dermatomyositis/polymyositis, which are characterized by the central involvement of joints, muscles, connective tissues, and the vascular system. Typically, a constellation of organ-system involvement, histopathologic features, and serologic abnormalities renders each disease distinctive. In some disorders, such as SLE, neurologic abnormalities are frequent; in others, such as progressive systemic sclerosis, they are unusual (1,18,21).

The immunopathogenesis of the neurologic abnormalities in SLE comprises several potential mechanisms, including autoantibody-mediated changes in neuronal cell surfaces, cytokine-influenced alterations in neuronal function, immune complex–mediated inflammation, and neurovascular disorders (1). Neurovascular disorders themselves result from several processes and illustrate the range of biologic responses to chronic and acute immune stimulus, as well as differences in the nervous system and systemic vasculature. Stroke occurs in SLE, although it remains difficult to distinguish ischemia from direct immune-mediated changes clinically. Among the histologic, hematologic, and serologic correlates of stroke are abnormalities in both the blood vessel walls and the coagulation system. Degenerative rather than inflammatory changes in CNS blood vessels characterize the vasculopathy associated with SLE, resulting in the loss of elasticity and normal contractile function of the vessel wall (1) (Fig. 1). Platelet thrombi have been described diffusely

in the arterioles of postmortem brains from patients with SLE, and CNS hemorrhage has been associated with both thrombocytopenia and qualitative platelet function abnormalities. Finally, antiphospholipid antibodies have been associated with both arterial and venous thrombosis in patients with SLE. Interestingly, when arterial thrombosis occurs the brain is most commonly affected (26).

In the other connective tissue diseases, neurologic abnormalities occur less frequently than in SLE, but when they do occur, inflammation of the blood vessels is more likely to be present. Recent studies of Sjögren's syndrome suggest that inflammatory vascular disease may play a role in the neuropsychiatric features of the disease (27). Neurologic abnormalities appear far less frequently in rheumatoid arthritis and progressive systemic sclerosis, but histologic studies reveal that vasculitis is often present (18). Polymyositis and dermatomyositis alone rarely seem to affect the nervous system.

Temporal Arteritis

Temporal arteritis is an acute inflammatory disease characterized by a systemic panarteritis primarily affecting vessels of the extracranial vasculature (1,18). Rarely, intracranial vessels can be involved, with particular predilection for the vessels of the posterior circulation (28). Classic histologic features seen in temporal artery biopsy specimens include giant cells in a granulomatous inflammation of the intima–media junction (28). Fragmentation of the internal elastic lamellae is typical but not pathognomonic and may occur in normal elderly patients. In almost all of the symptomatic patients with an abnormal temporal artery biopsy, the histologic features are different. In these cases, a mixed-cell inflammatory infiltrate that is predominantly mononu-

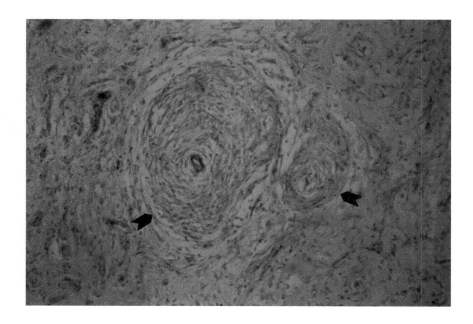

FIG. 1. A cortical vessel shows the typical layered, "onion skin" pattern of vasculopathy associated with systemic lupus erythematosus (hematoxylin-eosin, ×40).

clear with some neutrophils and eosinophils but without giant cells occurs (reviewed in ref. 1).

Clinically, a new-onset headache in a patient older than 50 years should alert the physician to the diagnosis. Tender or nodular temporal arteries and jaw claudication are useful features that are often observed. An elevated erythrocyte sedimentation rate is present in over 90% of patients. Visual loss, cranial neuropathies, and posterior circulation strokes are the most feared neurologic manifestations (1,18). In a small percentage of patients, peripheral neuropathies and encephalopathy are also reported. Because the neurologic manifestations are often preventable, an aggressive approach to obtaining the diagnosis is essential. Temporal artery biopsy usually establishes the diagnosis if a sufficient length of temporal artery is obtained (28). Occasionally, several discontinuous portions of artery are needed because the characteristic lesions are not always contiguous. Committing an elderly patient to a long course of corticosteroid therapy without a definitive tissue diagnosis remains problematic.

Polymyalgia rheumatica is a syndrome characterized by proximal muscle weakness and myalgias. Polymyalgia rheumatica may be one of the many clinical features associated with temporal arteritis. It should be distinguished from temporal arteritis, however, because a much lower dose of corticosteroids is usually required to treat polymyalgia rheumatica compared with that needed for temporal arteritis (1).

Takayasu's Arteritis

Takayasu's arteritis affects the aorta and its large branches by an initially inflammatory and later occlusive process. The disease, first described in young Asian women, is now recognized worldwide. The absence of pulses in at least one extremity in more than 90% of patients explains why Takayasu's arteritis is also called the pulseless disease (1). Neurologic abnormalities occur most often in the vasoocclusive phase, which is often complicated by hypertension. Visual changes are prominent as are syncope, transient ischemic attacks, and stroke (29).

Histologic features of early disease, including granulomatous changes in the media and adventitia of the aorta and its branches, are succeeded by intimal hyperplasia, medial degeneration, and adventitial fibrosis in the sclerotic stage (29). The time between stages of this disease varies widely. Diagnosis is usually suspected in a patient younger than 50 years whose complaint is limb claudication. On examination, the absence of one or more pulses, a systolic blood pressure difference >10 mm Hg between arms, and the presence of a bruit over the aorta or subclavian arteries should prompt a complete angiographic evaluation of the aorta and its branches for a firm diagnosis (1).

VASCULITIS RELATED TO INFECTION AND DRUGS

Infection-Associated Vasculitis

Vasculitis can occur in the setting of many infections, both systemic and those involving the CNS directly (30) (Fig. 2). These include tuberculosis and other infections with a variety of bacteria, fungi (coccidioidomycosis, cryptococcosis, and histoplasmosis), and viruses, including varicella zoster, cytomegalovirus, and human immunodeficiency virus 1 (HIV-1) (31). The clinical presentation usually includes prominent mental status changes and a stroke-like onset. In many cases, the vasculitic complications are unanticipated and associated with a delay in diagnosis and therapeutic intervention.

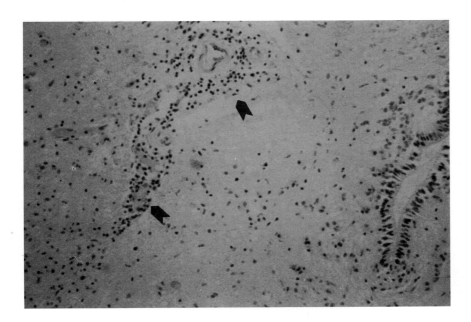

FIG. 2. The spinal cord at the level of T-10 from a patient with disseminated herpes zoster infection at the time of death from other causes (hematoxylin-eosin).

Infection-associated vasculitis results from several pathophysiologic mechanisms that ultimately damage vascular endothelium (reviewed in ref. 1). Clinical manifestations can result from involvement of any organ, including vasculitis isolated to the nervous system. Vascular endothelial cells can be infected directly (eg, equine virus) or can be damaged by microbial toxins (eg, *Mycoplasma gallisepticum*). Soluble immune complexes that damage endothelium occur in infections with hepatitis B, lymphocytic choriomeningitis, and cytomegalovirus. A prominent cell-mediated process resulting in vascular endothelial injury occurs from infections with *Neisseria* organisms and herpes zoster.

Drug-Associated Vasculitis

Vasculitis has been reported in association with a number of recreational and over-the-counter drugs (32,33). This association has been best documented with amphetamine abuse but has also been reported in patients using cocaine, heroin, phenylpropanolamine, ephedrine, and pseudoephedrine. A multiorgan-system necrotizing vasculitis resembling polyarteritis nodosa has been reported in patients using amphetamine alone or in conjunction with other drugs (33). In patients using cocaine alone, small-vessel cerebral vasculitis and endomyocardial hypersensitivity vasculitis have both been reported. Thus, there are at least two major pathologic profiles associated with drug-induced vasculitis: (a) a necrotizing vasculitis involving medium and small arteries and arterioles and (b) a nonnecrotizing, hypersensitivity vasculitis involving small arteries, arterioles, capillaries, and veins (32).

There also appear to be two major clinical patterns of involvement (32). Patients with skin involvement only tended to improve spontaneously with withdrawal of the offending drug, whereas many patients with systemic and CNS involvement at diagnosis die due to vasculitic complications.

Many of the drugs that have been reported in association with vasculitis have been associated with cerebral ischemia and hemorrhage without vasculitis as well. The pathophysiology of drug-related cerebral ischemia is likely to be complex and due to the interaction of multiple factors (33). With the increased use of recreational drugs in the past decade, most notably cocaine, the frequency of this complication is likely to increase. Vasculitis should be considered in the differential of any patient presenting with cerebral ischemia and a history of recent recreational drug use. The utility of steroids in treating drug-associated vasculitis is uncertain.

ISOLATED CNS VASCULITIS

Vasculitis isolated to the CNS is unusual but may occur in several settings, including infections, drugs, and neoplasia. A disorder currently called *isolated angiitis of the CNS* is an idiopathic process that has been recognized with increasing frequency in the past decade (6), possibly because

treatment methods are so effective. This disorder overlaps with granulomatous angiitis of the CNS and primary angiitis of the CNS, and the term used often depends on the author's criteria for diagnosis. When the disease is diagnosed on the basis of angiography alone, vasculitis may not be present histologically. It is therefore difficult to interpret therapeutic effects in series that include such patients with histologic confirmation of vasculitis. We suggest that in order to diagnose isolated angiitis of the CNS in patients with recurrent or persistent neurologic symptoms, systemic inflammation, infection, vasoconstriction syndromes, and neoplasia must be excluded, and both a four-vessel cerebral angiogram and a brain biopsy are needed.

Clinically, patients with isolated angiitis of the CNS present with or develop numerous neurologic abnormalities. Most frequently identified is a pattern of new-onset headaches, encephalopathy, and multifocal motor or sensory signs. However, the disease can present with seizures, subarachnoid hemorrhage, visual loss, cranial neuropathies, myelopathies, or a single stroke (4). Most patients are in their fourth to sixth decade, but patients have been reported ranging from 4 to 72 years of age. Blood studies are of little value in screening for this disease, as the erythrocyte sedimentation rate is almost invariably normal and autoantibodies and immune complexes are not present. The electroencephalogram is abnormal in 50–75% of patients, but the changes are nonspecific, usually consisting of diffuse slowing. Cerebrospinal fluid abnormalities occur in about half of the carefully diagnosed patients. These changes are most often a mild elevation in protein concentration, although occasionally a mild pleocytosis (<20 lymphocytes/mm^3) is present (4,34). Increased intracranial pressure is rare.

Angiography and biopsy are the mainstays of diagnosis. Angiographic abnormalities, present in 85–90% of patients, often suggest the disease. These include segmental narrowing (beading), abrupt termination of vessels, prolonged circulation time, collateral formation, and neovascularization. Brain biopsy is important in establishing the diagnosis and excluding alternate causes of clinical and angiographic features. This is important because fungal infections and neoplasia may be indistinguishable from isolated angiitis of the CNS both clinically and angiographically. The diagnostic sensitivity of combined meningeal/cortical biopsy is about 75% (34). Typical pathologic abnormalities include segmental inflammation of small arteries and arterioles, intimal proliferation and fibrosis with sparing of the media, and multinucleate giant Langerhan's cells.

The treatment for isolated CNS angiitis depends on identifying any possible causes. Infections, toxins, and neoplasia require specific therapy. Patients with a single well defined clinical event and one abnormal angiogram may be observed without specific treatment or with steroids alone because many of these patients have spontaneous remissions. Clinically, this less aggressive disorder differs from true isolated CNS angiitis in several ways: (a) the majority of patients are young women with sudden headache and focal sensory or motor deficits; (b) cerebrospinal fluid is normal; and (c) cerebral angiogram is usually abnormal and may suggest segmental vasoconstriction rather than vasculitis (34). In patients with recurrent or severe disease, however, a brain biopsy should be performed. If the diagnosis of isolated angiitis of the CNS is established, a combination of cyclophosphamide and corticosteroids has proved effective.

TREATMENT FOR THE VASCULITIC SYNDROMES

There are no prospective, randomized, controlled trials of therapy in vasculitis involving the CNS or PNS; however, some guidance is available (1,18,21,34,35). Many patients with systemic or isolated CNS vasculitis are treated initially with the combination of cyclophosphamide and corticosteroids (18,35). Treatment should be initiated with oral cyclophosphamide 2 mg/kg/d in combination with prednisone 1.5 mg/kg/d. Prednisone is given as a single daily dose every morning for 2–4 weeks. Cyclophosphamide is generally maintained for a least 1 year.

A trial of corticosteroids alone or a shorter course of cyclophosphamide may be indicated in some patients with isolated PNS vasculitis. In addition, patients with the benign form of isolated CNS vasculitis likewise appear to have a better prognosis and can be treated with corticosteroids alone (34).

REFERENCES

1. Moore PM. Neurological manifestations of vasculitis: Update on immunopathologic mechanisms and clinical features. *Ann Neurol* 1995; 37(suppl 1):S131–S141.
2. Leung DYM, Geha RS, Newburger JW, et al. Two monokines, interleukin-1 and tumor necrosis factor, render cultured vascular endothelial cells susceptible to lysis by antibodies circulating during Kawasaki syndrome. *J Exp Med* 1986;164:1958–1972.
3. Savage COS, Cooke SP. The role of the endothelium in systemic vasculitis. *J Autoimmun* 1993;6:237–249.
4. Moore PM. Diagnosis and management of isolated angiitis of the central nervous system. *Neurology* 1989;39:167–173.
5. Ellison MD, Merchant RE. Appearance of cytokine-associated central nervous system myelin damage coincides temporally with serum tumor necrosis factor induction after recombinant interleukin-2 infusion in rats. *J Neuroimmunol* 1991;33:245–251.
6. Alhalabi M, Moore PM. Serial angiography in isolated angiitis of the central nervous system. *Neurology* 1994;44:1221–1226.
7. Springer TA. Adhesion receptors of the immune system. *Nature* 1990; 346:425–434.
8. Springer TA. Traffic signals for lymphocyte recirculation and leukocyte emigration: The multistep paradigm. *Cell* 1994;76:301–314.
9. Bevilacqua MP, Pober JS, Mendrick DL, et al. Identification of an inducible endothelial-leukocyte adhesion molecule. *Proc Natl Acad Sci U S A* 1987;84:9238–9242.
10. Male D. Immunology of brain endothelium and the blood brain barrier.

In: MWB Bradbury, ed. *Physiology and Pharmacology of the Blood Brain Barrier.* Berlin: Springer-Verlag, 1992:397–415.
11. Hickey WF. Migration of hematogenous cells through the blood-brain barrier and the initiation of CNS inflammation. *Brain Pathol* 1991;1: 97–105.
12. Engelhardt B, Conley FK, Butcher EC. Cell adhesion molecules on vessels during inflammation in the mouse central nervous system. *J Neuroimmunol* 1994;51:199–208.
13. Dopp JM, Breneman SM, Olschowka JA. Expression of ICAM-1, VCAM-1, L-selectin, and leukosialin in the mouse central nervous system during the induction and remission stages of experimental allergic encephalitis. *J Neuroimmunol* 1994;54:129–144.
14. Raine CS, Cannella B, Duijvestijn AM, Cross AH. Homing to the central nervous system vasculature by antigen-specific lymphocytes, II: Lymphocyte/endothelial cell adhesion during the initial stages of autoimmune demyelination. *Lab Invest* 1990;63:476–489.
15. Cannella B, Raine CS. The adhesion molecule and cytokine profile of multiple sclerosis lesions. *Ann Neurol* 1995;37:424–435.
16. Lasky LA. Selectins: Interpreters of cell-specific carbohydrate information during inflammation. *Science* 1992;258:964–969.
17. Conn DT. Update on systemic necrotizing vasculitis. *Mayo Clin Proc* 1989;64:535–543.
18. Kissel JT, Rammohan KW. Pathogenesis and therapy of nervous system vasculitis. *Clin Neuropharmacol* 1991;14:28–48.
19. Travers RL, Allison DJ, Brettle RP, Hughes GRV. Polyarteritis nodosa. A clinical and angiographic analysis of 17 cases. *Semin Arthritis Rheum* 1979;8:184–189.
20. Kissel JT, Slivka AP, Warmolts JR, Mendell JR. The clinical spectrum of necrotizing angiopathy of the peripheral nervous system. *Ann Neurol* 1985;18:251–257.
21. Moore PM, Fauci AS. Neurologic manifestations of systemic vasculitis. A retrospective and prospective study of the clinicopathologic features and responses to therapy in 25 patients. *Am J Med Sci* 1981;71: 517–524.
22. Duffy J, Lidsky MD, Sharp JT, et al. Polyarthritis, polyarteritis and hepatitis B. *Medicine (Baltimore)* 1976;55:19–37.
23. Lanham JG, Elkon KB, Pusey CD, Hughes GRV. Systemic vasculitis with asthma and eosinophilia: A clinical approach to the Churg-Strauss syndrome. *Medicine (Baltimore)* 1984;63:65–81.
24. Hoffman GS, Kerr GS, Leavitt RY, et al. Wegener's granulomatosis: An analysis of 158 patients. *Ann Intern Med* 1992;116:488–498.
25. Nishino H, Rubino FA, DeRemee RA, et al. Neurological involvement in Wegener's granulomatosis: An analysis of 34 consecutive cases at Mayo Clinic. *Ann Neurol* 1993;33:4–9.
26. Brey RL. Gharavi AE, Lockshin MD. Neurologic complications of antiphospholipid antibodies. *Rheum Dis Clin North Am* 1993;19: 833–850.
27. Olney RK. Neuropathies in connective tissue disease. *Muscle Nerve* 1992;15:531–542.
28. Gibb W, Urry PA, Lees AJ. Giant cell arteritis with spinal cord infarction and basilar artery thrombosis. *J Neurol Psychiatry* 1985;48: 945–948.
29. Shelhamer JH, Volkman DJ, Parillo JE et al. Takayasu's arteritis and its therapy. *Ann Intern Med* 1985;103:121–126.
30. Williams PL, Johnson R, Pappagianis D, et al. Vasculitis and encephalitis complications associated with *Coccidioides immitis* infection of the central nervous system in humans: Report of 10 cases and review. *Clin Infect Dis* 1992;14:673–682.
31. Calabrese LH. Vasculitis and infection with the human immunodeficiency virus. *Rheum Dis Clin North Am* 1991;17:131–147.
32. Morrow PL, McQuillen JB. Cerebral vasculitis associated with cocaine use. *J Forensic Sci* 1993;38:732–738.
33. Fredericks RK, Lefkowitz DS, Challa VR, Troost BT. Cerebral vasculitis associated with cocaine abuse. *Stroke* 1991;22:1437–1439.
34. Calabrese LH, Furlan AJ, Gragg LA, Ropos TJ. Primary angiitis of the central nervous system: Diagnostic criteria and clinical approach. *Cleve Clin J Med* 1992;59:293–306.
35. Brey RL, Barohn RJ, Tami JA. Neuroimmunology: Clinical and therapeutic approach. *Neurologist* 1996;2:25–52.

Cerebrovascular Disease, edited by H. Hunt Batjer.
Lippincott-Raven Publishers, Philadelphia © 1997.

CHAPTER 41

Critical Management of Acute Ischemic Stroke: Triage and Diagnosis

Camilo R. Gomez and Marc D. Malkoff

Stroke continues to be the third leading cause of death as well as a primary cause of disability in our country (1). Despite these impressive statistics, only recently did the medical community begin to systematically emphasize the importance of managing acute stroke patients as aggressively as possible in an attempt to improve outcome and facilitate the development of useful treatment algorithms (2, 3). The population of victims of acute ischemic stroke is anything but homogeneous, and the care of patients with basilar artery occlusion is substantially different from that of patients with occlusion of a second-order cortical cerebral artery. Indeed, the former are likely to have more severe neurologic deficits, increased morbidity, and higher mortality—characteristics that make them candidates for more intensive care services. A fundamental step in the emergent management of patients with acute ischemic stroke is the accurate diagnosis of their condition, identifying and differentiating it from other disorders capable of causing acute focal neurologic deficit. Clinicians also face the challenge of determining the level of care each stroke patient requires; this depends on (a) the type of vascular occlusion suffered; (b) its known natural history; (c) the treatment strategies applicable to the situation; (d) the therapeutic window; and (e) the resources available (both human and technical).

The need for rapid evaluation and diagnosis of patients with acute ischemic stroke cannot be overemphasized because there is a close association between the results of the initial assessment and appropriate delivery of emergent management (2). In fact, in clinical practice it is often necessary to undertake the evaluation of stroke patients while treatment strategies are being planned or implemented (2). This chapter summarizes the most important considerations in the initial assessment and diagnosis of patients with acute ischemic stroke and describes how the diagnostic steps affect the treatment of patients. We will begin by outlining the objectives of the initial assessment and follow with a description of methodologic issues related to the emergency evaluation of patients with acute ischemic stroke.

OBJECTIVES OF THE INITIAL ASSESSMENT

The majority of patients with acute ischemic stroke are initially assessed in emergency departments by physicians whose priorities are the management of the patients, both immediately and in the days that follow. This is illustrated by the questions found in Fig. 1, which are variations of those used in the much larger task of diagnosing etiopathogenic ischemic stroke subtypes (4) and includes the following:

Does the patient have a stroke?
Is it an ischemic stroke?
What vascular territory has been compromised (or which vessel has been occluded)?
What is the risk of death or significant neurologic disability?
What is the likelihood of neurologic deterioration?

Notice that, in the emergency setting, early diagnostic priorities do not necessarily include a precise etiopathogenic definition of the stroke. In general, issues of causation (ie, etiology) and mechanism (ie, pathogenesis) assist in the early treatment only when obvious risk factors are uncovered. However, treatment does not need to be delayed while trying to define the type and cause of acute ischemic stroke. Conversely, etiopathogenic diagnosis has an indisputable impact on the choice of secondary stroke prevention strategies (4).

The evaluation of ischemic stroke patients in the emergency setting requires separating these individuals from pa-

C. R. Gomez: Comprehensive Stroke Center and Department of Neurology, The University of Alabama at Birmingham, Birmingham, AL 35294

M. D. Malkoff: Department of Neurology, Indiana State University, Indianapolis, Indiana, 46202

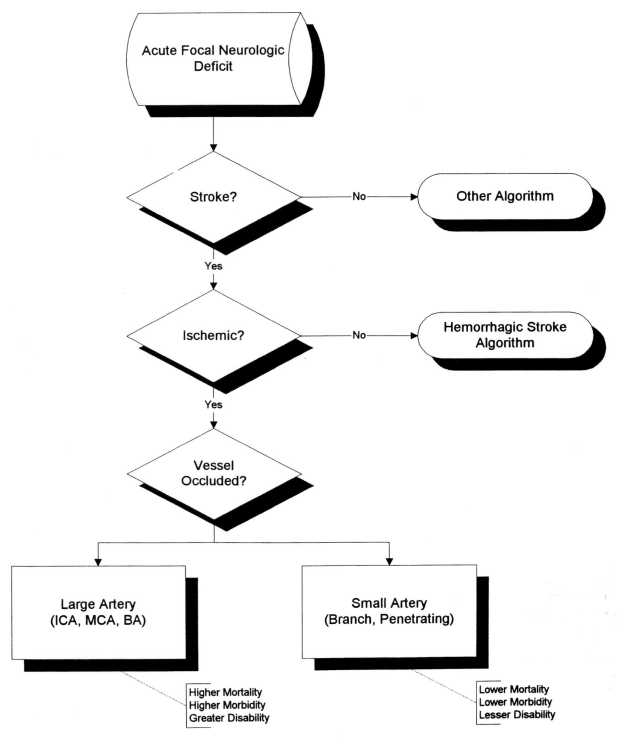

FIG. 1. Most important diagnostic questions in the emergency evaluation of patients with acute ischemic stroke. ICA, internal carotid artery; MCA, middle cerebral artery; BA, basilar artery.

tients whose acute focal neurologic deficit is not related to stroke (see Fig. 1). To this end, the initial diagnosis is based on three major factors: clinical data (symptoms and signs), temporal profile, and risk factors. In most cases, this information is readily available from the patient or the family, and it should be sufficient to allow a presumptive diagnosis of acute ischemic stroke. The result of this step guides the choice of further diagnostic testing as well as the implementation of preliminary management strategies. It is important to note that each of the three factors carries significant weight in the decision making process. In fact, there may be instances in which the clinical data are nonspecific and the temporal profile is equivocal, but the presence of strong risk factors alone will force a consideration of the patient as a stroke victim until proven otherwise. Furthermore, for experienced neurologists and neurosurgeons, assessment of these factors will also provide some suspicion about the vascular territory compromised and, often, the mechanism and cause of the stroke. For example, a patient who presents with the sudden onset of an isolated congruous homonymous hemianopia and who harbors a prosthetic heart valve is very likely to have suffered a cardiogenic embolism to one of his or her posterior cerebral arteries.

Once it has been determined that the patient has suffered a stroke, it is possible to address a second important issue: is it ischemic or hemorrhagic? In the past, it was thought that astute clinicians could easily make this differentiation at the bedside simply by considering certain aspects of the syndrome of presentation, particularly headache, impairment of consciousness, or degree of neurologic deficit. The introduction of computed tomography (CT) in the early 1980s, which makes it relatively easy to distinguish between ischemic and hemorrhagic strokes, showed how inaccurate such a method of differentiation was. In fact, we would like to emphasize the importance of imaging (particularly CT) in the early evaluation of patients with acute ischemic stroke.

Finally, instead of the traditional neurologic localization diagnostic strategy, it is necessary to go one step further and estimate which vascular territory is compromised. This task requires a certain amount of skill and familiarity with the clinical manifestations of occlusion of specific cerebral arteries. In addition, it requires knowledge of the prognostic and therapeutic implications of the specific vascular syndromes. We cannot overemphasize this point because we find it to be of extreme importance when making moment-to-moment decisions about the use of intensive care measures, the management of fluid therapy and hemodynamics, the use of antithrombotic and thrombolytic agents, considerations of emergency revascularization procedures, and the likelihood of survival. In general, occlusion of the large cerebral arteries, particularly the basilar, internal carotid, and middle cerebral arteries, carries with it a greater potential for disability as well as a higher morbidity and mortality. In contrast, occlusion of smaller arteries, either cortical or white matter (ie, penetrating) branches, is associated with generally better outcomes. This diagnostic dichotomy must not lead the reader to think that patients with small cerebral arterial occlusion should be given less attention than those with larger artery occlusion. Instead, it is introduced as a practical (though perhaps not perfect) method for quickly creating awareness among members of the treating team of the important issues that will highlight the treatment of the patient.

IMPORTANCE OF A SPECIFIC TRIAGE APPROACH

One of the most important and difficult tasks in emergency and critical care medicine is the efficient assessment and management of patients who present with rapidly evolving or potentially devastating disorders, including those with ischemic stroke. In the past, delays in the management of ischemic stroke have occurred because of a series of assumptions, such as (a) there is no treatment available; (b) because there is no treatment, there is no reason to hurry; and (c) the emergency personnel should be capable of handling the situation. These assumptions, which are incorrect, have done nothing but create obstacles for the delivery of basic, rational care to victims of stroke. It is important to emphasize that the fact that no drug available specifically reverses the effects of acute cerebral ischemia does not mean that there is no treatment, and unless we approach stroke patients with the same zeal that we approach other life-threatening emergencies (eg, cardiac arrest), we will never be able to prove that any strategy is effective because we will not be maximizing its potential. As with any other neurologic emergency, the evaluation and treatment of patients with acute ischemic stroke are guided by two important objectives: the preservation of life and the preservation of neurologic function (5). To this effect, the initial assessment is geared towards making the decisions noted above (see Fig. 1) and choosing the best diagnostic and therapeutic courses to follow.

Traditionally, the clinical evaluation of neurologic patients is taught as a one-to-one exercise, where one clinician usually concentrates all of his or her senses on identifying the ailment of one individual patient and in taking the necessary steps for further diagnostic and therapeutic measures. It is not unusual, however, for several patients to be present in an emergency facility concurrently, and the challenge of providing care simultaneously for a variety of diverse conditions becomes readily apparent. Part of the art of successfully completing the task of caring for patients in this type of environment is dependent on the ability to triage multiple patients, making the delivery of care to follow the most streamlined, efficient, and effective pattern. *Triage,* a term derived from the French "to sort," refers to the medical screening of patients to determine their priority for treatment. Although the experience of triage is inherent to certain specialties (eg, emergency medicine, trauma surgery), it has not been given proper emphasis in neurology. Indeed, the neurologic assessment is based on the acquisition of detailed clinical histories and the performance of almost obsessively precise neurologic examinations. This is followed by the traditional exercise of neurologic localization and, later, the generation of a differential diagnosis. The obvious problem with this approach when caring for victims of acute ischemic stroke is that as time elapses an increasing number of neurons in the ischemic penumbra are likely to become permanently damaged (6–8). Thus it is less likely that therapeutic measures will have a beneficial impact, and there will then be a larger area of infarction and a greater risk for loss of life or neurologic function. Consequently, a more pragmatic, priority-oriented approach to the initial assessment of stroke patients must be designed and widely disseminated. The one we use, based on a rapid definition of the issues noted earlier, provides such an alternative. Its application takes into consideration the most important diagnostic and therapeutic issues and can be carried out in a period of approximately 15–30 minutes.

STEP-BY-STEP IMPLEMENTATION OF ACUTE ISCHEMIC STROKE DIAGNOSIS

In order to better explain the tasks required in the rapid assessment and diagnosis of patients with ischemic stroke, we find it useful to divide the steps according to the ideal time it should take to carry them out. The concepts outlined below are derived from the clinical care protocol instituted at the University of Alabama, Birmingham (UAB) Hospital by the Vascular/Critical Care Neurology team. Although certainly not perfect, and some of them perhaps controversial, these steps have been successfully utilized to deliver what we view as optimal care for patients with acute ischemic stroke. In this chapter we will emphasize the diagnostic aspects of our protocol, although it is impossible to describe these without referring to the therapeutic steps, which are administered concurrently and constitute the Code Stroke system used in our institution (2).

Time: 0–15 Minutes (Arrival to Imaging)

The first step upon arrival of the patient with acute ischemic stroke is a rapid history and physical examination. Table 1 lists the most important issues to inquire of the patient and/or a family member. It is important to estimate the time of onset (ETO) of the stroke as precisely as possible. In patients whose deficit was found upon awakening, the time that they went to sleep or the last time that they were observed to be normal should be considered the ETO. The history of present illness should focus on the major deficit caused by the stroke, its functional effect, its temporal profile, concurrent symptoms (both systemic and neurologic), and whether the deficit is worsening or improving. Allergies, medications, and other medical problems should then be investigated. Prior cerebrovascular or cardiovascular events should be identified, as well as any treatment they may have

TABLE 1. *Important issues for patient history*

1. Age, sex, race of patient
2. Estimated time of onset (ETO)
3. Deficit (neurologic signs and symptoms)
4. Concurrent systemic symptoms
5. Temporal profile
6. Risk factor
    Cerebrovascular
    Others
7. Allergies
8. Medications
9. Other pertinent information
    Illicit Drug Use
    Chiropractic Manipulation
    Trauma to Head or Neck
    Previous Thrombotic Events

required. In addition, it is important to ask specific questions, for example, about the use of illicit drugs or over-the-counter medications, history of chiropractic cervical manipulation, and history of trauma to head and neck structures.

The physical examination should be quick and relevant and include both systemic and neurologic components. The most important aspects of the examination can and should be carried out while interviewing the patient. More specifically, the clinician should train himself or herself to look, listen, and feel. For example, while obtaining the history, one should observe the patient's appearance and as well as the pattern and content of speech. This method allows rapid identification of patients with severe hemiparesis, neglect, hemianopsia, aphasia, or dysarthria. Also, it allows the categorization of patients with concurrent heart failure or chronic obstructive pulmonary disease (COPD) since breathing difficulties and jugular venous distension would be easily identified. Auscultation of the neck vessels, the heart, the lungs, and the abdomen can be carried out in rapid sequence.

When it comes to the bedside assessment of neurologic function, the exam does not need to be comprehensive but rather relevant (Fig. 2). The most important neurologic functions that require emergency bedside testing are those that (a) create the bulk of the functional deficit; (b) are capable of leading to long-term disability; and (c) may respond to rapid intervention. They include consciousness, language, vision and eye movements, body-spatial perception, and motor function (both strength and coordination). It is possible to evaluate these clinically in just a few minutes, leaving assessment of other functions, such as two-point discrimination, for examination at a later time. It is our practice not to test gait at this time since this requires the patient to be upright (see below). In patients who are unconscious, assessment of the Glasgow coma score is not only useful but practical. At the end of the initial assessment, clinicians should be able to answer the questions posed in Fig. 1, at least presumptively.

As noted earlier, it is impossible to consider early triage and diagnosis of ischemic stroke independently of treatment. Ideally, general measures designed to optimize the chances

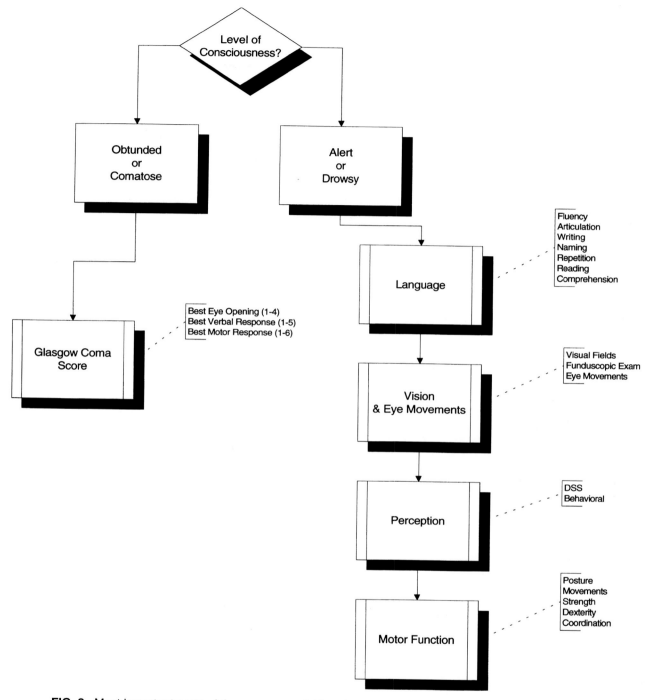

FIG. 2. Most important parts of the emergency (abbreviated and relevant) neurologic exam of patients with acute ischemic stroke. DSS, double simultaneous stimulation.

of recovering the function of neurons rendered ischemic but not irreversibly damaged (ie, the ischemic penumbra) can be implemented while the history and physical are being carried out. Some of these measures can be decided a priori, incorporated into a standing protocol and implemented automatically by nursing personnel upon the arrival of patients with acute ischemic stroke.

At the UAB Hospital, we have established a protocol that includes the following components: (a) patients are placed flat in bed and kept in that position until stable; (b) supplemental oxygen is administered by whatever method is appropriate for the clinical situation (with a target $SaO_2 = 100\%$), (c) a fluid bolus of 10–15 cm^3/kg of isotonic crystalloid is rapidly administered, followed by a continuous infusion at a rate of 80–125 cm³/hr, and (d) the patient is asked to chew on a 325-mg aspirin tablet (if unable to do so, a nasogastric tube is placed and water-soluble aspirin given through it). Although we recognize that these measures may be viewed by some as unfounded, unnecessary, or even useless, they are based on principles learned by managing ischemic events in a variety of clinical scenarios and their rationale stems from the pathogenesis of the ictus. Their effectiveness is difficult to measure, and they are not intended as a cure of the ischemic process but rather as the means of optimizing the cerebral circulatory environment. Theoretically, this will then facilitate flow restoration by whatever means are chosen later.

While all of the steps noted above are taking place,

blood should be drawn and sent to the laboratory for measurement of important variables (Table 2). In general, complete blood count, serum electrolytes, and basic coagulation studies should be obtained in all patients at this time. The remaining tests can usually wait until later. Also, an electrocardiogram can be obtained during this period; its review might uncover cardiac disorders that could be either the cause or the consequence of the cerebral ischemic process (Fig. 3). It is important to identify patients with concomitant acute cardiac disorders (eg, myocardial ischemia) because this may influence the type and level of care they will receive. Once all of these steps are carried out, the evaluation process can escalate to the next interval: imaging.

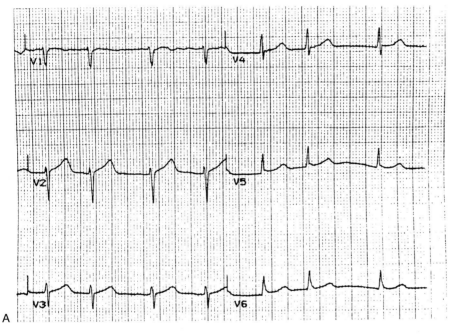

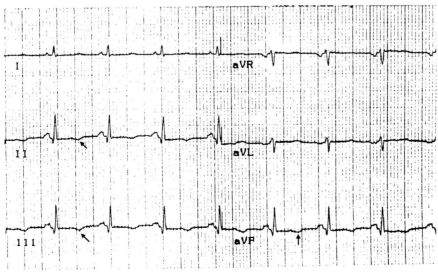

FIG. 3. A: Electrocardiogram of a patient presenting with a clinical syndrome consistent with acute brain embolism. The presence of atrial fibrillation with variable ventricular response is obvious and was found to be the cause of the stroke. B: Electrocardiogram of a patient who had evidence of acute myocardial ischemia after she had suffered a cerebral infarction. Note the inverted T waves (arrows) in leads II, III, and atrioventricular fibrillation, consistent with concurrent inferior myocardial ischemia.

TABLE 2. *Laboratory tests*

Hemoglobin/hematocrit
White blood cell count
Platelet count
Prothrombin time (PT)
Partial thromboplastin time (PTT)
Serum electrolytes
BUN and creatinine
Erythrocyte sedimentation rate (ESR)
FTA-abs or MHA-TP in serum
Additional studies:
  Antithrombin III
  Protein C
  Protein S
  Anticardiolipin antibodies
  Vitamin B$_{12}$
  Drug screening
  Cardiac enzymes

Time: 16–30 Minutes (Imaging to Admission)

The single most important diagnostic step in the critical management of acute ischemic stroke involves imaging of the brain. The following aspects of this topic require discussion: (a) choice of imaging, (b) expectations, (c) findings, and (d) impact on treatment. In order to be useful in the setting of acute ischemic stroke, the imaging modality utilized must be fast and informative, and to this end CT is the ideal technique because it is capable of providing information about ischemic as well as hemorrhagic processes potentially responsible for the clinical situation (9,10). In addition, it allows the identification of numerous conditions that may mimic acute ischemic stroke. CT scanning can be performed in a matter of minutes, and there are almost no restrictions in terms of a person's undergoing the procedure. Intravenous contrast administration is usually not required for proper evaluation of acute stroke patients. An alternative is the use of magnetic resonance imaging (MRI). Although clearly superior to CT in the demonstration of ischemic lesions, there are logistical problems in using it in the acute setting at this time (10,11). The test requires considerably longer scanning times; patients need to remain still for longer periods and it is impossible to properly monitor critically ill patients. Also, its capability for detecting small amounts of hemorrhage during the acute stage is not as good as with CT (10). Nevertheless, further research in MRI promises to bring to us the practical application of related techniques in the evaluation of acute ischemic stroke. Among these, diffusion MRI, perfusion MRI, and magnetic resonance spectroscopy (MRS) may allow the future characterization of the ischemic penumbra (12–15).

The findings in early CT of patients with acute ischemic stroke go hand in hand with the expectations of the clinician. It must be clear that if imaged early (ie, <6 hours after onset) most patients with acute ischemic stroke will display normal CT scans (9,10). This should not be a source of disappointment. On the contrary, the longer the brain tissue can be

preserved without any evidence of permanent damage, the better the chances that any treatment may help the patient. As time elapses, however, the likelihood of CT displaying the infarcted tissue becomes greater. The differentiation between a normal CT scan and one that already shows signs of infarctions has recently gained increased importance in lieu of the results of clinical trials that assessed the efficacy of thrombolytic agents in the treatment of acute ischemic stroke (16,17).

When the CT is not normal, it is possible to categorize the findings as (a) demonstrative of the acute ischemic stroke; (b) evidence of other previous ischemic insults; (c) consistent with cerebrovascular abnormalities related to the stroke; (d) diagnostic of processes other than ischemic stroke (new or old), or (e) a combination of the above. The clinical implications of each of these are different and, therefore, further discussion of each of them is warranted. Disclosure of a process other than acute ischemic stroke requires that alternative diagnostic and treatment algorithms be applied, some very different than those used in the management of acute brain ischemia (Fig. 4). Demonstration of the acute ischemic stroke not only confirms the diagnosis but helps to reach etiopathogenic and prognostic conclusions. For ex-

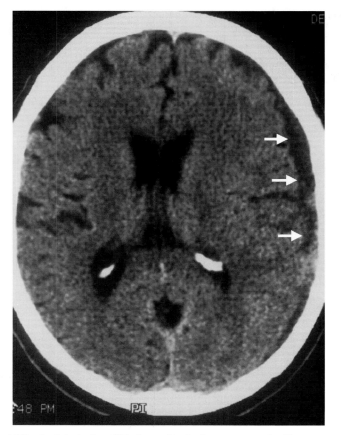

FIG. 4. Admission CT of a patient who presented with acute onset of speech arrest and weakness of the right hand. The images show a left subacute/chronic subdural hematoma *(arrows)*.

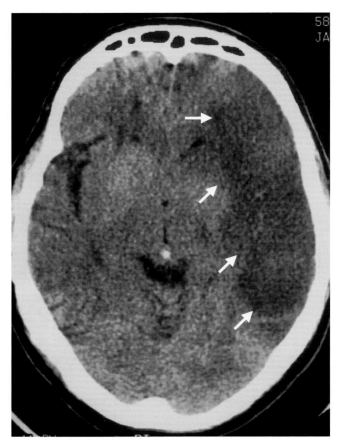

FIG. 5. Admission CT of a patient who presented with acute onset of right hemiplegia, right gaze palsy, right homonymous hemianopia, and global aphasia. The images are consistent with infarction of the left middle cerebral artery territory (arrows). The patient eventually died.

ample, finding an area of hypodensity involving the territory of a cortical branch will point the diagnostic search in the direction of a source of embolism. Furthermore, infarction of the territory of the middle cerebral artery implies increased chances of neurologic worsening over the first 96–100 hours of treatment due to edema and increased intracranial pressure (Fig. 5). These predictions help to determine the level of care the patient will require over the next few days.

The third possible finding in CT is that of old ischemic lesions. Their importance is that they may implicate an underlying etiopathogenic process. For example, patients with acute ischemic stroke whose CT scans show old lesions in multiple vascular territories should be suspected of having either a cardiogenic or aortogenic source of embolism (Fig. 6). Finally, there are patients whose admission CT scans, although not completely normal, do not show the acute ischemic lesion or an alternative explanation for the patient's deficit. Instead, they show subtle signs of cerebrovascular pathology. Perhaps the sign most referred to in the literature is the hyperdense middle cerebral artery, curiously associated with occlusion of that vessel (18,19). Hyperdensity of

other vessels, such as the basilar artery, has also been reported (20). More often, however, the CT findings to which we refer are more subtle and include calcification and dolichoectasia of the brain blood vessels, both suggestive of underlying atherosclerosis (Fig. 7). In the future, the introduction of spiral CT scanning may allow imaging of the cerebral blood vessels immediately following imaging of the brain (21).

Time: 31–60 Minutes (Admission to Treatment)

Once the initial imaging of the brain is completed, the clinician should be in a position to decide what therapeutic course to follow, depending on some of the variables noted in the introduction of the chapter. As such, the approach to the management of a patient with infarction secondary to occlusion of a small penetrating artery (eg, lacunar infarction) will be radically different from that of a patient with a middle cerebral artery stem occlusion. Furthermore, each of these could be further subdivided based upon the interval between the ETO and the time of admission (ie, therapeutic window). Additionally, not every hospital harbors the technology and human resources necessary to implement certain treatment protocols (eg, intraarterial thrombolysis). The tests that remain at the disposal of the clinician should at this point be used tactically in order to gain the most useful information as rapidly as possible while avoiding delays in the treatment protocol. A discussion of the role these tests play in the early diagnosis of acute ischemic stroke follows.

MAGNETIC RESONANCE IMAGING

We discussed earlier the potential disadvantages of MRI as the initial imaging modality in the management of acute ischemic stroke. Nevertheless, its clear advantages is that it allows visualizations of ischemic lesions earlier than CT, as well as identifying abnormalities that may never be uncovered by CT. (Fig. 8) (22–24). In addition, with the appropriate software, it is possible to concurrently perform magnetic resonance angiography (MRA) as an additional diagnostic procedure (Fig. 9) (11). Using spin echo (for MRI) and phase contrast (for MRA) sequences, it is thus feasible to acquire highly detailed images of the brain and its blood vessels in 35–45 minutes. The utility of MRI in the diagnosis of acute ischemic stroke is based on its role in (a) confirming the location and extent of ischemic damage; (b) identifying previous ischemic lesions that carry certain etiopathogenic implications (see above); and (c) identifying occlusion or high-grade stenosis of major cerebral arteries using MRA (22–26). Nevertheless, MRI is not a perfectly practical diagnostic technique, and several other disadvantages must be pointed out. These include the difficulty in imaging confused or combative patients, the inability to image patients who harbor pacemakers or certain other implanted metallic devices, the impossibility of properly monitoring unstable pa-

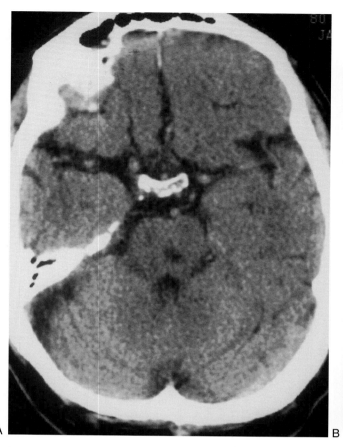

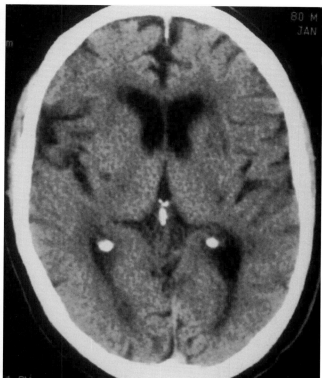

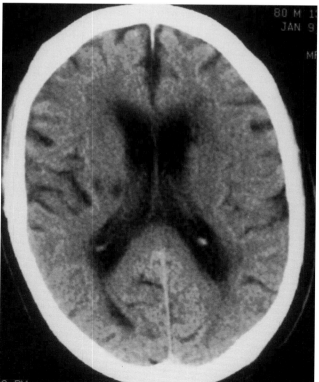

FIG. 6. Admission CT of a patient who presented with hemiparesis involving mostly the right leg. The images are consistent with infarctions of multiple vascular territories. He was found to have severe aortic atherosclerotic plaques with mobile elements.

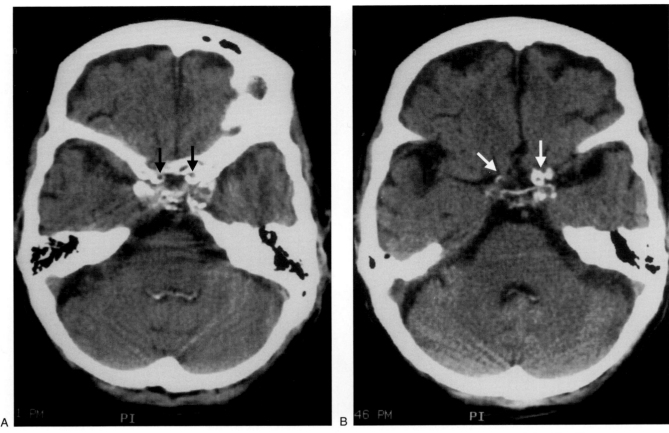

FIG. 7. Admission CT of a patient who presented with right hemiparesis and dysarthria. Significant calcification of the carotid arteries is obvious *(arrows)*, implying atherosclerosis with possible dolichoectasia or stenosis. This was later confirmed.

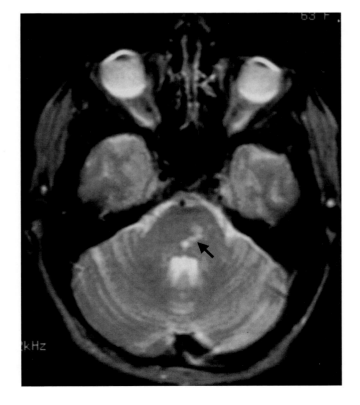

FIG. 8. Early T2-weighted MRI of a patient with a small pontine infarction *(arrow)*. These infarcts are usually not seen upon admission CT.

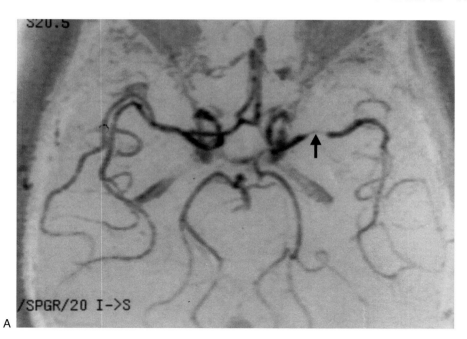

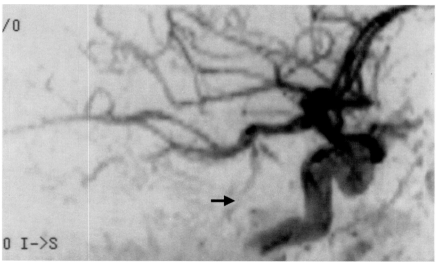

FIG. 9. Two important MRA patterns of vascular abnormality found in patients with acute stroke. Focal stenosis of an intracranial blood vessel (**A**, *arrow*) and decreased flow in an entire vascular territory (**B**, *arrow*).

tients, and the impracticality of repeating the test over the course of minutes or hours to follow the progression of the ischemic process.

The MRI findings in patients with acute ischemic stroke may be seen earlier than 6 hours (Table 3). Subtle swelling of the gyri, hyperintensity of blood vessels, and loss of flow void are the most prominent. During this period, hemor-

rhagic changes are difficult to detect. After the first 6 hours, progressively increased signal intensity in the infarcted tissue is obvious in T2-weighted imaging. Even at this time, it may be difficult to detect hemorrhagic changes.

NEUROVASCULAR ULTRASOUND

At this time, the two main ultrasonic techniques useful in the diagnosis of neurologic patients are color Doppler/duplex and transcranial Doppler (TCD). Their primary purpose is to assess the patency of the cerebral arteries while detecting hemodynamic derangements that lead to impairment of cerebral blood flow. From this point of view, both tests (one most useful in the extracranial and the other in the intracranial circulations) allow identification of occluded vessels

TABLE 3. *Magnetic resonance imaging findings*

Less than 6 hr	More than 6 hr
Gyral swelling	Hyperintensity in T2-weighted images
Hyperintense vessels	
Absent flow voids	Some swelling
Hemorrhage difficult to detect	Hemorrhage difficult to detect

and of vessels at risk for occlusion. The clear advantages of these tests are that they are simple, noninvasive, and provide moment-to-moment information about the status of the cerebral vasculature. Their disadvantages include the inability to assess all vessels of the brain circulation and their inherent operator dependency. The ability of color Doppler/duplex to characterize carotid atherosclerotic plagues is very high, having well over 90% of sensitivity and specificity when compared with angiography (27,28). The sensitivity and specificity of TCD in the detection of intracranial stenosis varies between 75–99%, depending on which vessel is being studied (29–36). The utility of either of these techniques during the first hour of acute ischemic stroke management depends upon how treatment will be implemented. It is our experience that the findings are most helpful when highly specific questions are being asked. For example, in a patient who presents with a clinical syndrome suggestive of ischemia of either the internal carotid or the middle cerebral artery territory, the signs and symptoms alone may not allow distinction of which the two vessels is compromised. Ultrasonic assessment in this instance may be very useful since the findings may help prepare the interventionist for the catheterization or they may allow follow-up of the effects of treatment.

CATHETERIZATION AND ANGIOGRAPHY

This is an invasive procedure whose main purpose is to study the cerebral blood vessels. It is the most definitive test available to diagnose cerebrovascular pathologic processes. It is, however, invasive and carries a small but definite risk (37). In our opinion, its use in the context of acute ischemic stroke should be reserved for patients in whom (a) the angiographic findings will have a direct impact upon the therapy administered or (b) catheterization is the method by which the intended treatment is to be delivered (eg, intra-arterial thrombolysis) (38,39). The angiographic findings largely depend on the process being investigated and include (a) occlusion (Fig. 10); (b) arterial stenosis from atherosclerosis (Fig. 11) or from other vascular pathology (eg, dissection), (c) changes in collateral patterns, or (d) normal vasculature. After a decision to perform this test is made, the procedure should not be delayed unnecessarily because its yield decreases progressively with time after the acute vascular occlusion has occurred (40).

TIME: BEYOND THE FIRST HOUR

After the first battery of tests (both clinical and ancillary) has been completed and some decisions about treatment have been made, it is possible to focus on other aspects of the etiopathogenic diagnosis of the patient. As discussed elsewhere (4), the tests available to clinicians caring for patients with ischemic stroke are geared toward assessment of one of three categories of etiopathogenic processes: cerebrovascular, cardiac, or hematologic/systemic. It is clear that the utilization of diagnostic procedures aiming at uncovering

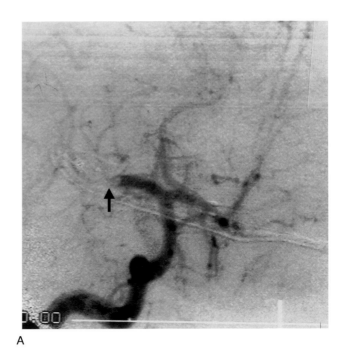

A

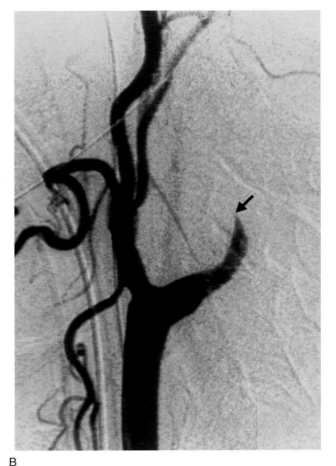

B

FIG. 10. A: Anteroposterior angiographic image of a patient with acute right middle cerebral artery cardiogenic embolic occlusion *(arrow).* **B:** Angiographic images of a patient with acute internal carotid artery occlusion *(arrow).*

by experienced individuals. However, this task requires a clear understanding of the diagnostic priorities and a vision of the impact that the results of the evaluation will have on the treatment of the patient. The diagnosis of acute ischemic stroke begins upon the patient's arrival at the emergency facility and ends when specific strategies for secondary stroke prevention are implemented.

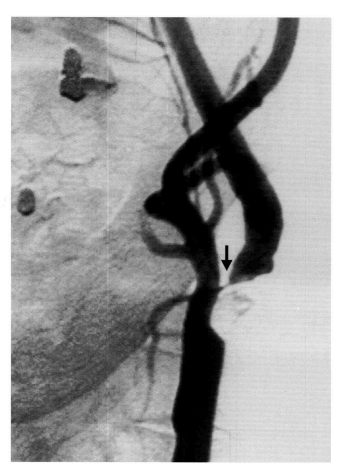

FIG. 11. Angiographic image of a patient with an acute cortical brain infarction ipsilateral to a severely stenotic internal carotid artery *(arrow)*.

processes in any of these categories is largely governed by both early presumptive diagnostic assessment and opportunity. For example, in some instances, the ultrasonic tests will be more readily accessible than MRI procedures. In others, echocardiography will have preference simply because of a clinical history suggestive of cardiogenic brain embolism. Finally, in a few cases, patients will be transported from the CT scanner to the catheterization laboratory for diagnostic angiography and endovascular intervention. It is important to note that all that will be altered is the order of the tests. We would like to emphasize our position that in order for strategies for secondary stroke prevention to be effective, all possible risk factors and causes of stroke must be explored. In our experience, this can be accomplished in a matter of 48–72 hours, leaving plenty of time to institute preventive protocols.

CONCLUSIONS

In summary, the triage and emergency diagnosis of acute ischemic stroke can be carried out in short periods of time

REFERENCES

1. American Heart Association. *Heart and Stroke Facts: 1994 Statistical Supplement.* Dallas: American Heart Association, 1993.
2. Gomez CR, Malkoff MD, Sauer CM, Tulyapronchote R, Burch CM, Banet GA. Code stroke: an attempt to shorten in-hospital therapeutic delays. *Stroke* 1994;25:1920–1923.
3. Camarata PJ, Heros RC, Latchaw RE. Brain attack: the rationale for treating stroke as a medical emergency. *Neurosurgery* 1994;34:144–157.
4. Gomez CR. Diagnostic evaluation of patients with cerebral ischemic events. In: Adams HP, ed. *Handbook of Cerebrovascular Disease.* New York: Marcel Dekker, 1993.
5. Gomez CR. Triage and stabilization of neurological patients. In: Malkoff MD, Gomez CR, eds. *Manual of Emergency and Critical Care Neurology.* In press.
6. Astrup J, Siesjo B, Symon L. [Editorial] Thresholds in cerebral ischemia—the ischemic penumbra. *Stroke* 1981;12:723–725.
7. Hossmann K-A. Viability threshold and the penumbra of focal ischemia. *Ann Neurol* 1994;36:557–565.
8. Ginsberg MD, Pulsinelli WA. Editorial: The ischemic penumbra, injury thresholds, and the therapeutic window for acute stroke. *Ann Neurol* 1994;36:553–554.
9. Adams HP, Brott TG, Crowell RM, et al. Guidelines for the management of acute ischemic stroke: a statement for healthcare professionals from a special writing group of the stroke council, American Heart Association. *Stroke* 1994;225:1901–1914.
10. Bryan RN, Levy LM, Whitlow WD, et al. Diagnosis of acute cerebral infarction: comparison of CT and MR imaging. *AJNR* 1991;12:611–620.
11. Yuh WTC, Crain MR. Magnetic resonance imaging of acute cerebral ischemia. *Neuroimag Clin North Am* 1992;2:421–439.
12. Moseley ME, De Crespigney A, Chew WM. Diffusion/perfusion magnetic resonance imaging. *Neuroimag Clin North Am* 1992;2:693–718.
13. van Gelderen P, de Vleeschouwer MHM, Des-Pres D, et al. Water diffusion and acute stroke. *Mag Reson Med* 1994;31:154–163.
14. Moseley ME, Cohen Y, Mintorovitch J, et al. Early detection of regional cerebral ischemia in cats: comparison of diffusion- and T2-weighted MRI and spectroscopy. *Mag Reson Med* 1990;14:330–346.
15. LeBihan D, Turner R, Douek P, et al. Diffusion MR imaging: clinical applications. *AJR* 1992;159:591–599.
16. Marler JR. Tissue plasminogen activator for acute ischemic stroke. *N Engl J Med* 1995;333:1581–1587.
17. Hacke W, Kaste M, Fieschi C, Lesaffre E, von Kummer R, Boysen G, et al. Intravenous thrombolysis with recombitant tissue plasminogen activator for acute hemispheric stroke. *JAMA* 1995;274:1017–1025.
18. Bastianello S, Pierallini A, Colonnese C, et al. Hyperdense middle cerebral artery sign. *Neuroradiology* 1991;33:207–211.
19. Rauch RA, Bazan C III, Larsson EM, et al. Hyperdense middle cerebral arteries identified on CT as a false sign of vascular occlusion. *AJNR* 1993;14:669–673.
20. Ehsan T, Haya G, Malkoff MD, Selhorst JB, Martin D, Manepalli A. Hyperdense basilar artery: an early computed tomography sign of thrombosis. *J Neuroimag* 1994;4:200–205.
21. Link J, Brossman J, Grabener M, Mueller-Huelsbeck S, Steffans JC, Brinkmann G, et al. Spiral CT angiography and selective digital subtraction angiography of internal carotid artery stenosis. *AJNR* 1996;17:89–94.
22. Yuh WT, Crain MR, Loes DJ, et al. MR imaging of cerebral ischemia: finding in the first 24 hours. *AJNR* 1991;12:621–629.
23. Truwit CL, Kucharczyk J. Reversible cerebral ischemia: magnetic resonance appearance and pathophysiology. *Neuroimag Clin* North Am 1992;2:557–595.

24. Shimosegawa E, Inugami A, Okudera T, et al. Embolic cerebral infarction: MR findings in the first 3 hours after onset. *AJR* 1993;160: 1077–1082.

25. Biller J, Yuh WTC, Mitchel GW, et al. Early diagnosis of basilar artery occlusions using magnetic resonance imaging. *Stroke* 1988;19: 297–306.

26. Katz BH, Quencer RM, Kaplan JO, et al. MR imaging of intracranial carotid occlusion. *AJNR* 1989;10:345–350.

27. Bluth EI, Wetzner SM, Stavros AT, et al. Carotid duplex sonography: a multicenter recommendation for standardized imaging and Doppler criteria. *RadioGraphics* 1988;8:487–506.

28. Moneta GL, Edwards JM, Chitwood RW, et al. Correlation of NASCET angiographic definition of 70% to 99% internal carotid artery stenosis with duplex scanning. *J Vasc Surg* 1993;17:152–159.

29. Spencer MP, Whisler D. Transorbital Doppler diagnosis of intracranial arterial stenosis. *Stroke* 1986;17:916–921.

30. Babikian VL, Pochay V. Accuracy of transcranial Doppler in detecting carotid distribution–arterial stenoses. *Neurology* 1991;41(suppl):122.

31. Lev-Pozo J, Ringelstein EB. Noninvasive detection of occlusive disease of the carotid siphon and middle cerebral artery. *Ann Neurol* 1990;28: 640–647.

32. Rorick MD, Nichols FT, Adams RJ. Transcranial Doppler correlation with angiography in detection of intracranial stenosis. *Stroke* 1994;25: 1931–1934.

33. Tettenborn B, Estol C, DeWitt D, Kraemer G, Pessin M, Caplan L. Accuracy of transcranial Doppler in the vertebrobasilar circulation. *J Neurol* 1990;237:159.

34. Giller CA, Mathews D, Purdy P, Kopitnik TA, Batjer HH, Samson DS. The transcranial Doppler appearance of acute carotid artery occlusion. *Ann Neurol* 1992;31:101–103.

35. Kelley RE, Namon RA, Mantelle LL, Chang JY. Sensitivity and specificity of transcranial Doppler ultrasonography in the detection of high-grade carotid stenosis. *Neurology* 1993;43:1187–1191.

36. Wilterdink JL, Feldmann E, Bragoni M, Brooks JM, Benavides JG. An absent ophthalmic artery or carotid siphon signal on transcranial Doppler confirms the presence of severe ipsilateral internal carotid artery disease. *J Neuroimag* 1994;4:196–199.

37. Heiserman JE, Dean BL, Hodak JA, Flom RFA, Bird CR, Drayer BP, et al. Neurologic complications of cerebral angiography. *AJNR* 1994; 15:1401.

38. Ferguson RDG, Ferguson JG. Cerebral intraarterial fibrinolysis at the crossroads: is a phase III trial advisable at this time? *AJNR* 1994;15: 1201.

39. Tsai FY, Berberian B, Matovich V, Lavin M, Alfieri K. Percutaneous transluminal angioplasty adjunct to thrombolysis for acute middle cerebral artery rethrombosis. *AJNR* 1994;15:1823.

40. Bozzao L, Fantozzi LM, Bastianello S, et al. Ischemic supratentorial stroke: angiographic findings in patients examined in the very early phase. *J Neurol* 1989;236:340–342.

Cerebrovascular Disease, edited by H. Hunt Batjer.
Lippincott-Raven Publishers, Philadelphia © 1997.

CHAPTER **42**

Critical Management of Acute Stroke: Medical and Surgical Therapy

Werner Hacke, Thorsten Steiner, and Stefan Schwab

While the incidence of cerebrovascular disease has decreased in the last two decades, it is still the third leading cause of mortality in first- and second-world countries (1). Reduction of mortality and improvement of outcome are therefore major goals for neurocritical care. Neurocritical care of stroke focuses on the management of acute stroke–related problems and the treatment of secondary complications (2,3). There is a great variety of clinical settings during the initial phase of critical care. In some situations, the physician initially will assess the patient's most important clinical findings: heart rate and blood pressure. Patients with large strokes at this time may already need intensive therapy. Increasing impairment or loss of consciousness and/or breathing, risk of aspiration, excessively elevated blood pressure, high intracranial pressure (ICP), and cardiac problems may require urgent intervention. Patients with extensive vertebrobasilar territory infarction, seizure activity, or massive intracranial or subarachnoid hemorrhage are usually unconscious and have a particular risk of aspiration. They may require immediate airway management, as do patients with severe hypoxemia and hypercarbia.

GENERAL THERAPY

Management of Respiratory Complications

Although respiratory problems in the first hours of an acute stroke are rare, pulmonary complications constitute a major cause of morbidity and mortality in intensive care unit (ICU) patients with cerebrovascular disease (4,5). Insufficient breathing, loss of protective reflexes with consecutive aspiration, or neurogenic pulmonary edema may lead to secondary hypoxia that can worsen stroke. Maintaining adequate ventilation and oxygenation is an important prerequisite for preservation of metabolic turnover in the marginal zone of an ischemic stroke, the so-called penumbra. Oxygen saturation should be measured at least transcutaneously in the emergency room.

Several specific problems are linked to intubation and mechanical ventilation of the stroke patient. The patient might have a full stomach; laryngoscopy and intubation often lead to a substantial hemodynamic response, which can be deleterious in case of severe carotid artery stenosis. Furthermore, some drugs may worsen increased ICP. As short-acting sedatives, we prefer thiopental (3–5 mg/kg), etomidate (0.3–0.5 mg/kg), and propofol (0.1–0.2 mg/kg/min) because they have only minimal cardiodepressive effects. These three drugs blunt the ICP response. This effect is most pronounced with thiopental (6–9). The depolarizing neuromuscular blocking agent succinylcholine (1.2 mg/kg) is also considered one of the above mentioned substances. For further analgesia and sedation, the combination of opioids and benzodiazepines that have additional ICP-lowering effects is widely accepted (eg, fentanyl 0.05 mg/ml and midazolam 1.8 mg/ml via separated infusion pumps) (10,11). Initial orotracheal intubation is preferred to nasotracheal intubation because of the high incidence of paranasal sinusitis (12).

Most intubated stroke patients require ongoing ventilatory support. Anesthesia reduces cerebral blood volume, arterial blood pressure, and central venous pressure (13). However, inhalational agents such as halothane, trichloroethylene, and methoxyflurane considerably increase ICP. Nitrous oxide has only minimal effect on ICP.

Often in intensive care of ischemic stroke, there must be a compromise of medical and neurologic benefits. Thus, positive end-expiratory pressure (PEEP) ventilation is frequently essential to prevent lung injuries such as pneumonia, pulmonary or neurogenic edema, and adult respiratory distress syndrome (ARDS), which leads to hypoxia and hypercapnia. It is important to know that PEEP ventilation may

---

W. Hacke, T. Steiner, S. Schwab: Department of Neurology, University of Heidelberg, Heidelberg, Germany D69120

TABLE 1. *Indication for endotracheal intubation*

Po_2 <50–60 mm Hg
Pco_2 >50–60 mm Hg
Vital capacity <500–800 ml
Signs of respiratory distress
Tachypnea >30 breaths/min
Dyspnea
Self PEEP with expiratory grunting
Use of accessory muscles
Respiratory acidosis
Comatose state
Risk for aspiration
Loss of maintenance of stable airway

TABLE 3. *Indications for tracheotomy*

Coma for >14 d
Bronchial toilet/protection
Laryngeal obstruction
Prolonged weaning

increase ICP (14). In general, early intubation and vigorous chest physical therapy can help prevent pulmonary complications and help improve the outcome of patients with cerebrovascular diseases. Table 1 shows the indications for endotracheal intubation and Table 2 shows the appropriate initial ventilator settings.

Neurogenic Pulmonary Edema

Neurogenic pulmonary edema (NPE) is a rare but often unrecognized complication. It can develop rapidly after subarachnoid hemorrhage and epileptic seizures and in pandysautonomia. The edema consists of protein-rich alveolar fluid. The pathophysiologic mechanisms have not been clarified until now. Contributing factors are left atrial hypertension, systemic hypertension, and increased sympathetic activity, which may be pharmacologically induced (eg, by catecholamines) (15,16). The goal of treatment is the lowering of hydrostatic pulmonary vascular pressure by decreasing pulmonary and peripheral vascular resistance, inotropic support, and mild reduction of blood volume. Therapy of NPE consists of mechanical ventilation with controlled hyperventilation ($Paco_2$, 30–35 mm Hg), low PPE (5 cm H_2O), and a targeted Pao_2 >80 mm Hg, followed by dobutamine and furosemide. For sufficient therapy control, a pulmonary artery catheter is often needed.

Tracheotomy

The development of high-volume, low-pressure cuffs has markedly decreased the risk for tracheal stenosis. However, prolonged orotracheal or nasotracheal intubation may cause

TABLE 2. *Initial ventilator setting*

IMV or CMV mode
Tidal volume: 12 ml/kg
Respiratory rate: Pco_2 <40 mm Hg (8–12 breaths/min)
Fio_2 = 1.0
I:E = 1:2–3
Inspiratory flow: 30 L/min

laryngeal damage and phonation disability, sores, and pansinusitis with consecutive impairment of auditory function. Though the need for tracheotomy in long-term ventilated patients is clear, the appropriate time for this procedure is still controversial (Table 3). Early tracheostomy assists mobilization and further rehabilitative measurements. From our experience, the risk of major complication after tracheotomy is low, although there are reports with an incidence up to 5% (17). We recommend tracheostomy 2–3 weeks after orotracheal intubation (18,19).

Antihypertensive Therapy and Metabolic Problems

Many patients with cerebrovascular diseases initially present with hypertensive blood pressure. Recently, there has been an extensive discussion about when to treat hypertension (20,21).

Systemic blood pressure, ICP, and cerebral perfusion pressure (CPP) are firmly linked. CPP is defined as the difference between midarterial blood pressure (MABP) and ICP:

$$CPP = MABP - ICP \ [mm \ Hg]$$

Normal ICP values in adults range up to 15 mm Hg. In children younger than 5 years, normal values are slightly than in adults. ICP can rise from 50 to 80 mm Hg during pressing maneuvers or coughing. Under physiologic circumstances, CPP is 80 mm Hg or higher. The threshold for secondary ischemia is <60 mm Hg (22). Raised blood pressure leads to an elevation of CPP as long as ICP is stable. CPP and cerebral blood flow (CBF) are physiologically connected by the Bayliss effect: A rise of CPP leads to a decrease of vessel diameter. Through this effect, CBF remains constant within a blood pressure range of 60–180 mm Hg. In stroke patients with hypertensive RR-recordings during the first hours, blood pressure should therefore not be lowered below a systolic pressure of 180 mm Hg. The previously hypertensive patient has adapted to an even higher regulatory range. In these patients, the risk of reaching the ischemic tolerance level while treating hypertension is higher. For these reasons, we restrict treatment of hypertension in acute settings and follow the therapeutic approach shown in Table 4 for acute hypertension in ischemic stroke (23). In the United States, the regimen of Brott is widely used (Table 5) (24).

Sodium nitroprusside and hydralazine are cerebral vasodilators that increase CBF and ICP and impair autoregulation. Angiotensin-converting enzyme (ACE) inhibitors should be avoided because they often cause extensive activation of the

TABLE 4. *Regimen for therapy of acute hypertension in ischemic stroke*

Clinical condition	Therapeutic action
Systolic BP <220, diastolic BP <120 mm Hg	Do not treat
Diastolic BP >120 mm Hg, systolic BP slightly increased on repeated measures 15 min apart	Nitroglycerine 5 mg IV or 10 mg PO
Systolic BP >220 mm Hg, or diastolic BP 110–120 or both on repeated measures	Nifedipine 10 mg PO, clonidine 0.075 mg SC, or urapidil 12.5 mg IV

(From ref. 23, with permission)
[a] Caution: Nifedipine may cause an overly rapid decline of blood pressure.

renin system (25). Antiadrenergic agents such as clonidine or short-acting β blockers such as labetalol (continuous 2 mg/min IV in the United States only) are favored.

Neurogenic Heart Disease

Neurogenic heart disease is a phenomenon that has been observed after acute lesions of the central nervous system like SAH, head trauma, and epileptic seizures. It presents with arrhythmias, repolarization disturbances, and increased cardiac enzyme levels (26). In the electrocardiographic (ECG) findings, large inverted T waves, large U waves, and prolonged QT intervals, seen predominantly in the anterolateral and inferolateral leads, are symptomatic. Autopsy findings of neurogenic heart disease reveal myofibrillar degeneration, also known as coagulative myocytolysis. It is easy to distinguish from coagulation necrosis, which is the cardinal finding in myocardial infarction (27). As in neurogenic pulmonary edema, an increased sympathetic drive with elevated catecholamine levels leads to Ca^{++} channel activation with eventual cell death and leakage of cardiac enzymes into the serum. For prevention and treatment, the administration of benzodiazepines, barbiturates, β blockers, calcium channel

TABLE 5. *Antihypertensive treatment in acute ischemic stroke*

Clinical condition	Therapeutic action
Systolic BP 180–230 mm Hg and/or diastolic BP <120 mm Hg	Do not treat
Diastolic BP >140 mm Hg, systolic BP slightly increased on repeated measures 5 min apart	Sodium nitroprusside 2 mg/kgBW/min, double dose after 3–5 min
Systolic BP >230 mm Hg, diastolic BP 120–140 mm Hg, or both on repeated measures 20 min apart	Labetalol 10 mg IV to be repeated if needed to max. 160 mg Nifedipine 10 mg PO

blockers, and free radical scavengers (which intervene in the above described cascade) may be favorable, especially when given early in the clinical course. Use of β blockers (eg, propranolol) has been shown to improve the hyperdynamic state in head-injured patients, most likely because neurogenic heart disease is caused mainly by sympathetic overdrive.

Fluid and Electrolyte Balance

A central venous catheter is essential for treatment of acute stroke patients and provides direct information about the intravascular volume. This is a safe route for administration of fluids, parenteral nutrition, and medication. The safest approach is via a cubital vein. If multilumen catheters become necessary, the subclavian or internal jugular vein approach is recommended. Even in patients with elevated ICP, internal jugular vein catheters can be inserted, as it has been shown that neither impediment of central venous drainage nor increase in ICP occurs (28,29). However, cerebral venous and dural sinus anatomy is highly variable. Bilateral jugular vein drainage should therefore be proven (eg, by Doppler ultrasound) before insertion of a catheter. The Queckenstedt maneuver is recommended if lumbar puncture will be performed or if an ICP-monitoring device has already been applied.

Sodium

Both hyper- and hyponatremia are commonly seen electrolyte disturbances in critically ill patients with ischemic stroke. Sodium is the major osmotic anion in the extracellular fluid. Changes in serum osmolality are therefore reflected in sodium concentration. Neurons are vulnerable to rapid changes of the osmotic gradient. Pharmacologic correction of sodium level should be performed cautiously.

Hypernatremia is most commonly due to application of osmotic diuretics. If osmotic agents are given, the above described relationship does not exist. Therefore, serum osmolality (therapeutic range: 300–320 mmol/l), in addition to sodium levels, should be monitored closely in those patients.

Hyponatremia may be due to an increase in body water, as in inappropriate secretion of antidiuretic hormone (SIADH) or to renal and gastrointestinal sodium loss. Fluid restriction and in some cases hypertonic saline infusion are the treatment of choice for SIADH. The rapid correction of hyponatremia should be avoided because it can precipitate central pontine demyelinization (30). Correction of serum sodium should not exceed 1–2 mval/h (31).

Potassium

Administration of diuretics, osmotic agents, and antibiotics cause hypokalemia. At least daily monitoring of potassium levels is necessary and approximately 20–60 mEq/l are needed in addition to parenteral nutrition.

Glucose Metabolism

Hyperglycemia is frequently seen after acute stroke due to stress and increased catecholamine serum levels. Administration of epinephrine may lead to an additional resistance to insulin. Elevated blood glucose levels increase infarct size, both experimentally and clinically (32,33). Therefore, glucose levels >200 mg/dl should be treated by subcutaneous injection or continuous IV administration of insulin. Glucose levels should be monitored to avoid hypoglycemia. In stroke patients, parenteral nutrition should not contain >40 g/d glucose.

Prophylaxis of Deep Venous Thrombosis

In all critically ill patients, prevention of pulmonary embolism is of great importance. Prophylaxis with subcutaneous low-dose heparin (10,000 IU every 12 hours) is recommended. Elastic or pneumatic compressive stockings decrease the risk of pulmonary embolism (34). In deep vein thrombosis, anticoagulation and, if possible, thrombolysis should be initiated.

THERAPY OF ELEVATED ICP AND EDEMA FORMATION

Brain edema with subsequent rise of ICP is the most dangerous complication of any acute brain damage. Cerebral blood flow (CBF) is reduced by compression of adjacent local brain tissue, and secondary neuronal damage may result. Potent analgesia and sedation is necessary, since coughing or elevated intraabdominal pressure increases ICP. Procedures such as endotracheal suction, turning the patient, and central venous catheterization have been shown to raise ICP considerably. The patient should be maintained in an upright position of approximately 30° (35). Body temperature should be maintained at normal because fever increases CBF and raises ICP. In addition, animal experiments have shown that hypothermia reduces infarct volume (36). Antipyretics should be used early, and a cooling blanket may help to decrease body temperature. For treatment of elevated ICP in hemispheric infarctions, we suggest a stepwise therapy escalation depending on development of both clinical and monitored findings (Table 6).

TABLE 6. *Stepwise escalation therapy for elevated intracranial pressure (ICP) in hemispheric Infarction[a]*

Therapy	Clinical condition and ancillary findings
Step 1: Baseline therapy: All cases of suspected elevated ICP	
1. Elevated body positioning 2. Glycerol 10%, 4 × 125 or 250 ml/24 h	Clinical findings: Spontaneous breathing, stable level of consciousness (awake or drowsy), normal or stable brainstem reflexes: pupil isocoria, corneal reflex normal Ancillary finding: CCT: Normal or early signs of infarction
Step 2: ICP crisis: Clinical signs of further increasing ICP	
1. Intubation (if not already necessary) and 2. Controlled hyperventilation (Pco₂ 28–35 mm Hg) *If no clinical reaction* 3. Mannitol 20%, 100 ml, up to 4–6 × 100 ml/d *If no clinical reaction* 4. Thiopental IV or bolus application of 0.25–0.5 g up to 1 g/10 kgBW/d, monitoring by EEG to burst-suppression pattern *If no clinical reaction* 5. Tromethamine, 3 mmol/h, pH <7,55, base excess < +10 mEq	Clinical findings: Increasing breathing insufficiency, vomiting, singultus, impairment of consciousness; if already intubated, decreasing brainstem function: anisocoria with/without sluggish or no reaction to light (perhaps after intermittent miosis); tachycardia Ancillary finding CCT: Increasing brain tissue edema with signs of midline and/or pineal gland shift, beginning tentorial or uncal herniation with/without brainstem compression (see Fig. 1) ICP monitoring: Elevated ICP (instructive only if correlating with clinical signs) TCD: Wave pattern of elevated ICP BAEP: Normal or early signs of brainstem compression (increasing interpeak latencies especially of late components)
Step 3: Surgical intervention: No reaction to treatment in step 2, only right hemispheric massive cerebral infarction	
Hemicraniectomy with application of ICP monitoring device Continued extended pharmacologic treatment as described under step 2 until improvement of CPP and ICP	Clinical findings: Worsening of the above mentioned findings despite step 2 therapy (see Fig. 2)

Key: CCT, cranial computed tomography; TCD, transcranial Doppler ultrasonography; BAEP, brainstem acoustic evoked potentials; CPP, cerebral perfusion pressure.
[a] See text for further information on dosage and application.

For proper management, an ICP-monitoring device is desirable, although it is used in fewer than 10% of stroke patients treated in our ICU (see below). Monitoring helps diagnose increasing ICP early, monitor effectiveness of therapy, and recognize iatrogenic errors that elevate ICP, such as excessive free water administration.

Osmotic Agents

Low-molecular-weight hypertonic solutions such as glycerol, mannitol, and sorbitol are frequently used to reduce brain water content. All of these compounds produce an osmolar gradient between blood and brain and thereby draw water from brain tissue into the plasma.

Glycerol can be administered orally or via a nasogastric tube (3–4 × 50 ml as a 50% glycerol solution) since enteral application has been proven to be more effective (37,38). If there are any reasons to avoid enteral applications, glycerol can be given IV. Depending on body weight, we infuse 125 ml or 250 ml of a 10% glycerol solution over 1 hour four times daily. Glycerol has a slow effect on ICP, which is lowered within 20–30 minutes after administration. It is metabolized by glycolysis within the brain tissue and is cleared by the kidney. Volume overload, hemolysis, and electrolyte disturbances are frequent problems encountered with glycerol-based osmotherapy (38–40). With glycerol treatment, glucose solution can be reduced. For example, 1000 ml of 10% glycerol solution and 500 ml glucose 40% contain 325 g carbohydrates, a sufficient carbohydrate intake for a patient weighing 70 kg. Renal function and central venous pressure must be watched carefully in patients with underlying cardiac disease.

Mannitol 20% (0.25–0.5 g/kg every 4 hours) is infused in severe cases of cytotoxic edema or in emergency situations (eg, decompensated ICP with dilated pupil). A serum osmolarity of 310–320 mOsm/l is desired. Mannitol is renally cleared and acts as an osmotic diuretic. Electrolyte disturbance, renal dysfunction, and hypovolemia are known complications. It should not be given for more than 3 days, since increasing tissue levels prevent or even reverse the osmotic drive, leading to a marked rebound phenomenon (41).

Loop diuretics decrease ICP by removing water from the edematous brain. However, the use of diuretics alone to control raised ICP has not been tested. Combined with osmotic agents these may be helpful.

Hyperventilation

Hyperventilation-induced hypercapnia leads to reduction of ICP by vasoconstriction of cerebral blood vessels due to serum and cerebrospinal fluid (CSF) alkalosis (42). Vasoconstriction lowers cerebral blood volume (CBV) without influencing CBF. An acute reduction of arterial CO_2 of 5–10 mm Hg to Pco_2 values of 28–33 mm Hg lowers ICP by 25–30% in most patients (43). Hypocarbia can be achieved by raising the ventilation rate by a constant tidal volume. Unfortunately, the effect of hyperventilation is limited. Through the compensation of CSF alkalosis, it may become less effective and sometimes may be followed by a rebound phenomenon if normal ventilation is resumed too rapidly (44). Currently, many ICU physicians are reluctant to use hyperventilation or prophylactic agents.

High-Dose Barbiturate Therapy

Short-acting barbiturates such as thiopental lead to a prompt and significant decrease of ICP mediated by a reduction of CBV and CBF (45). Barbiturates are free radical scavengers and may protect brain tissue against secondary damage. The ICP-lowering effect starts during (slow) application and lasts 15–20 minutes. Its use is restricted to acute ICP crisis. Complications of high doses of barbiturates, including hypotension, depression of cardiac contractility with reactive tachycardia, and predisposition to infections, limit its routine use. Thiopental acts as a respiratory depressant and has no muscle-relaxant effect (46). The watery thiopental sodium is a highly alkalotic solution with a pH 10.0. It is responsible for tissue and vessel damage and is incompatible with many drugs used in critical care (eg, benzodiazepines, fentanyl, and catecholamines). Administration of thiopental therefore requires a second independent central venous catheter. For exact hemodynamic monitoring, a Swan–Ganz catheter may be necessary.

The ICP-lowering effect can be monitored clinically (eg, pupil diameter, form, and reaction to light) and, if available, by an ICP-monitoring device or electroencephalography (EEG). An EEG is recorded with superficial adhesive skull electrodes during the injection of barbiturates. The administration of barbiturate is stopped when a burst-suppression pattern is reached. Beyond this electrophysiologic pattern, no further reduction of cerebral metabolism can be achieved (47).

It is still under discussion whether multiple boli or continuous administration is more effective. The effect of thiopental decreases after multiple boli applications and continuous IV infusion of thiopental is probably as effective as bolus dosage (7).

We prefer the multiple boli administration (250–500 mg bolus injections) of thiopental over a central venous catheter up to a maximum daily dosage of 0.1 g/kg. Advantages of multiple boli applications include better control of this highly lipophilic drug and reduction of total dose. Consequently, side effects are decreased since boli are only repeated if clinically necessary.

THAM Buffer

Tris(hydroxymethyl)aminomethane (THAM or tromethamine) induces vasoconstriction and decreases ICP after IV administration. The mode of action is not clearly understood. THAM increases the capacity of CSF to buffer pH changes and neutralize acidosis-mediated vasodilation. THAM (60 mmol/100 ml in 5% dextrose) may be infused over 45 minutes as a test dose. ICP should fall by 10–15 mm Hg. A central venous line should be used for continuous IV infusion (3 mmol/h), since it causes severe tissue necrosis. Hourly blood gas analyses are performed to ensure that base excess does not exceed +6 mEq and pH is ≤7.55. In high doses, THAM can impair ventilation. Since THAM is nephrotoxic, we use it only in cases in which all other conservative therapies have failed (48).

ICU MONITORING OF THE CRITICALLY ILL PATIENT

For all ICU patients, on-line monitoring of blood pressure, cardiac performance (ECG, Swan–Ganz catheter), and breathing is established. Continuous monitoring of blood pressure and arterial blood gases is achieved via an arterial line, preferably at the radial artery. A central venous catheter is needed in all patients. Pulmonary artery catheterization may sometimes become necessary for monitoring of cardiac output and fluid therapy.

Neurologic Monitoring

ICP Monitoring

Monitoring ICP helps provide the physician with data for rational treatment management (Table 7). The location of ICP-monitoring devices can be epidural, subdural, intraparenchymal, or intraventricular. ICP can be obtained fluid-coupled (ventricular catheter, subarachnoid bolt) or nonfluid-coupled (fiberoptic, pneumatic devices). However, neither system is completely satisfactory. The main disadvantages are unreliable measurements, drift of measurements, and the risk of infections. We favor the use of pneumatic devices for epidural (Fig. 1) and intraparenchymal ICP monitoring. They are easy to handle and allow at least the observation of individual changes. The application route of parenchymal devices is nearly the same as in ventricular catheters. The rate of epidural and subdural bleeding complications in ventricular catheters is 0.33–1%. Aschoffe (49) found a cumulative infection rate of 5.2% in 5056 ven-

tricular catheters (in 54 studies). The probability of infections is 0% on the first day and rises with the duration of implantation. The risk of infection is highly dependent on the quality of hygiene. The risk of bleeding and infections in epidural catheters is <1%.

Electrophysiologic Monitoring

Median nerve somatosensory evoked potential (MSEP) with both spinal and cortical leads, brainstem auditory evoked potential (BAEP), and, less frequently, visual evoked and middle latency acoustic potentials may be monitored in the ICU even under analgesia/sedation. BAEP and MSEP are part of the decision-making for aggressive treatment in cases of basilar artery thrombosis, space-occupying cerebellar lesions, and severe hemispheric strokes. Cerebellar infarction alterations of the BAEP and MSEP are indications for neurosurgical intervention, even in awake patients (50). On the other hand, missing contralateral cortical MSEP in patients with hemispheric infarction or intracranial hemorrhage support the decision toward less or no specific treatment. From our recently presented data, we concluded that patients with massive cerebral infarction and normal BAEP before surgery have a significantly lower mortality than those with uni- or bilateral preoperative BAEP changes (51).

EEG monitoring is rarely performed in acute stroke patients because extended pharmacologic therapy interferes with its specificity. However, EEG can be useful for monitoring of patients in barbiturate-induced coma. Spectral features and measures of period and amplitude may give further information.

Other Monitoring Methods

Magnetic resonance imaging (MRI) and cranial computed tomography (CCT) are necessary in most patients with acute cerebrovascular disease. Patients with space-occupying lesions often require daily scans during the first days. However, it should be kept in mind that flat position on the CCT or MRI gantry can be hazardous for patients with elevated ICP.

Transcranial Doppler ultrasonography (TCD) with uni- or bilateral on-line monitoring of the middle cerebral artery (MCA) trunk at an insonation depth of 45–55 mm can be useful for the assessment of cerebral blood flow. Especially

TABLE 7. *Comparison ICP-monitoring devices*

ICP monitor	Advantage	Disadvantage
Ventricular catheter	Drainage and exact measures	Major surgery, high infection rate
Subarachnoid bolt	Low infection rate, noninvasive	Often no exact monitoring possible, obstruction of device
Pneumatic device	Accurate measures	Expensive, dislocation possible
Fiberoptic device	Accurate measures, subdural, intraparenchymal, and intraventricular location	No further calibration possible, breakage risk, expensive

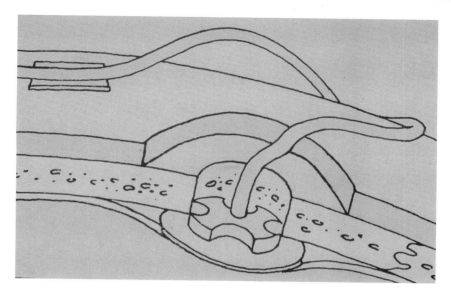

FIG. 1. Pneumatic epidural device for monitoring intracranial pressure. (Courtesy of A. Spiegelberg, Hamburg, Germany.)

after thrombolysis, the time window of recanalization can be obtained. Wave-pattern analysis with respect to ICP can be done (52).

Cerebral oxygen consumption can be monitored using a jugular bulb catheter or near-infrared laser spectroscopy. However, both methods still need validation in larger patient series (53,54).

ICU MANAGEMENT OF ACUTE ISCHEMIC STROKE

Results of the ECASS trial suggest that the first steps are being taken toward causative treatment strategies for acute ischemic stroke. However, it must be taken into account that ECASS strategies were proven to be beneficial for a selected and predefined subgroup of stroke patients (55). From the distant point of view, the intensive care of stroke patients might only be concerned with respiratory, cardiac, and nursing complications. Some stroke subtypes always require immediate neurocritical care treatment, such as acute basilar artery thrombosis, acute proximal MCA occlusion, and space-occupying cerebellar infarctions. For the future, acute arterial recanalization to restore blood flow to ischemic brain, neuroprotection, and improvement of emergency and intensive care management are major goals. The identification of patients who need ICU management requires the early identification of stroke subtype. This is indicated by the emergency examination (level of consciousness, pupillary reaction, oculocephalic response, and corneal reflex), additional tests (CCT, TCD), and the diagnosis of concomitant disease (eg, atrial fibrillation) (Table 8).

Acute MCA Territory Stroke

Clinically, most patients present with severe hemiparesis or hemiplegia. In the first hours after onset of symptoms, the level of consciousness is normal or only slightly depressed. Forced conjugate eye deviation often implies a large infarct. Hemiplegia, forced eye deviation, and decreased level of consciousness often indicate a poor outcome.

The diagnosis of acute intracranial internal carotid artery (ICA) or MCA occlusion is made either by ultrasound or angiography. CCT scan will reveal early signs of infarction within the first 2–3 hours (56). The dense MCA artery sign is present in 50% of acute ICA/MCA occlusions. Other signs such as effacement of the cortical sulci, compression of the insular cistern, loss of internal capsule definition, and focal loss of white/gray-matter contrast may be observed.

Intravenous or local thrombolysis may be performed following controlled, randomized protocols within a 6-hour margin after onset of symptoms. The use of full-dose heparin is discussed controversially (57–61). A beneficial effect of early full-dose heparin has never been shown prospectively, and it is not clear whether the risk of parenchymal hemorrhage outbalances the avoidance of recurrent emboli. The rationale for early anticoagulation is the prevention of local thrombus propagation and recurrent embolism, as in atrial fibrillation. Anticoagulation with full-dose heparin is often used in Europe immediately after the diagnosis has been confirmed. In North America, anticoagulation is often postponed for 48–72 hours if infarcts are present. Heparin is probably not indicated in lacunar stroke. Within the first 24 hours, formation of cerebral edema becomes a serious

TABLE 8. *Indications for ICU treatment of acute cerebral ischemia*

Progressing symptoms, crescendo TIA
Fluctuating, hemodynamically induced infarction
Embolic intracranial ICA/MCA occlusion
Endocarditis with septic cerebral emboli
Arterial dissection plus embolism
Thrombolytic or proposed hypervolemic therapy

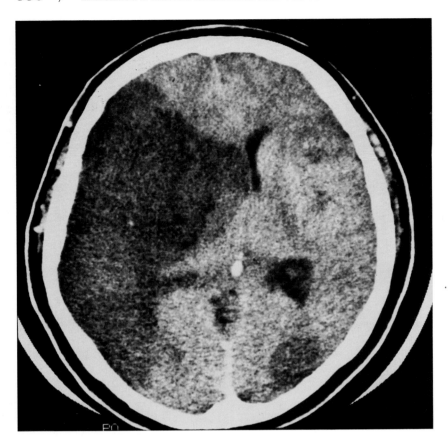

FIG. 2. CCT scan shows massive cerebral infarction, with midline and pineal gland shift.

complication of large MCA infarcts. It is necessary to monitor patients' alertness, pupillary reaction, and neurologic status very carefully. Serial CCT scans may show increasing edema formation, and functional deterioration may be monitored electrophysiologically.

Decompressive Surgery in Hemispheric Infarction

Edema formation may be life threatening, especially in younger patients. If early CCT scan reveals signs of a large MCA infarction and neurovascular diagnostics shows either a combined ICA/MCA or MCA trunk occlusion, we favor early surgical intervention (Figs. 2 and 3). In all other cases, surgical treatment is only discussed after failure of maximal conservative antiedematous therapy as described above (62). Our prospective data show a favorable long-term outcome after hemicraniectomy in patients with right hemispheric infarctions (63). Surgery was performed in 32 patients. The mean Barthel index was 60 points, and mortality was reduced to 40%. Nevertheless, until a large prospective study shows its superiority over conservative treatment, hemicraniectomy is still confined to desperate cases. It is very important to recognize the failure of conservative therapy early, which may be difficult in sedated and intubated patients. We determine the time point for decompressive surgery by a combination of clinical observation (ipsilateral dilated pupil

or decerebrate posture, both reversible with osmotherapy), ICP and repeated electrophysiologic data, and CCT monitoring of the space-occupying effect of brain edema insofar as the clinical condition allows transportation of patient. During the acute phase, additional ongoing monitoring includes daily BAEP and MSEP (64,65).

Acute Basilar Artery Occlusion

Patients with acute basilar artery occlusion are generally treated in an ICU. Diagnosis is made by clinical signs and confirmed with either Doppler ultrasound or angiography. In case of impaired consciousness, immediate endotracheal intubation and analgesia/sedation are necessary. Patients who are already comatose on admission with lost cortical SSEP have a poor prognosis despite acute treatment. From our experience with these patients, further interventional procedures or therapy have no additional benefit.

Patients with favorable predictors of outcome (eg, young age, presumed embolic occlusion, only slightly impaired consciousness) will profit from local thrombolysis (66). After initial analgesia/sedation and intubation, these patients receive intraarterial urokinase 1,000,000 IU/h. Successful thrombolysis can be especially expected with embolic-origin thrombus, good collateral blood flow, and lack of underlying arteriosclerotic vasculopathy (67). Full-dose heparin is

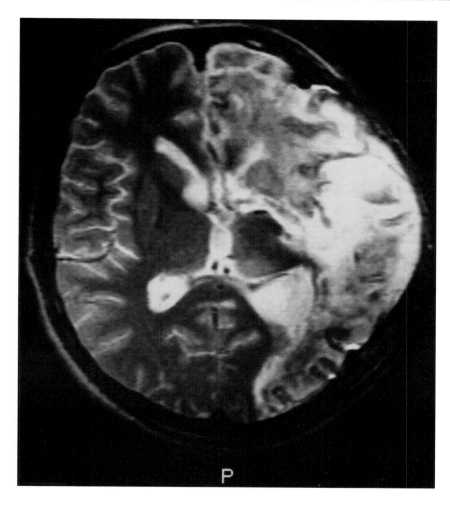

FIG. 3. MRI scan shows hemicraniectomy after extended infarction of the MCA.

started immediately after thrombolysis. Repeated CCT scans are performed after angiography to detect intracerebral hemorrhage and extension of ischemic infarction.

Cerebellar Infarction

Cerebellar infarction due to occlusion of vertebral or basilar artery branches in general has a good clinical outcome even without aggressive treatment. However, patients with large cerebellar infarcts are at particular risk for periischemic edema with occlusive hydrocephalus and brainstem compression with increased pressure in the posterior fossa. Even if these patients initially present with only mild clinical signs, they can rapidly deteriorate with further impairment of consciousness, oculomotor dysfunction and, if untreated, coma. Close clinical monitoring and often repeated CCT scans to estimate the grade of obstructive hydrocephalus are essential (Fig. 4). In comatose patients, decompressive surgery of the posterior fossa, with or without removal of infarcted cerebellar tissue, is significantly superior to ventriculostomy (68–70). As stated above, we do not use this approach in patients with additional basilar artery thrombo-

sis and large brainstem infarcts. We routinely use MSEP and BAEP to further inform decision-making in these patients. Patients with normal BAEP and SSEP are treated with osmotherapeutics. Prolonged interpeak latencies in BAEP and altered amplitudes in SSEP indicate decompressive surgery, and ventriculostomy should be performed if CCT shows signs of hydrocephalus.

Hypertensive-Hypervolemic Therapy in Progressive Stroke

Hypertensive-hypervolemic therapy has been widely advocated for treating vasospasm after subarachnoid hemorrhage. This therapeutic concept has been adopted for the treatment of progressive stroke due to hemodynamic failure of the blood supply. We use this strategy in patients with severe hemodynamic stenosis and reversible neurologic symptoms. It is induced by plasma expanders, with the aim of a central venous pressure of 8 mm Hg and arterial hypertension with systolic blood pressure values up to 180 mm Hg. The additional use of sympathomimetics may be mandatory. The benefit of hypertensive-hypervolemic therapy has not

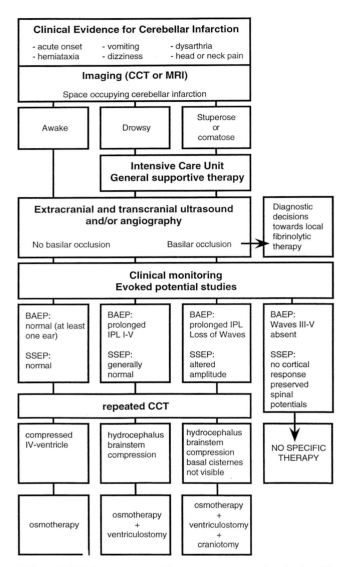

FIG. 4. Heidelberg protocol for management of patients with cerebellar stroke.

TABLE 9. *Hypertensive hypervolemic therapy*

High volume colloidal infusion (hetastarch, 500–1500 ml)
Ringer's solution (5000–10,000 ml)
Hemoglobin solution if necessary
Dopamine/dobutamine (10–30 mg/kg/min)

TABLE 10. *Required controls for hypertensive hypervolemic therapy*

Physical examination: edema
Laboratory studies including osmolarity of urine and serum
Mean arterial BP ≥ systolic BP: 160–180 mm Hg
Central venous pressure ≥ 10–12 mm Hg
Fluid status and weight control ≥ hematocrit: 33–38%
Daily chest x-ray
Wedge pressure (Swan–Ganz catheter) <20 mm Hg

been proven by randomized studies. However, our clinical data show a lower frequency of permanent ischemic deficits in patients with severe hemodynamic carotid stenosis treated with this method. The complications of this therapy are pulmonary and cerebral edema, cardiac dysregulation due to volume overload, and myocardial infarction (Tables 9 and 10).

REFERENCES

1. Homer D, Whisnant JP, Schoenberg BS. Trends in the incidence rates of stroke. *Ann Neurol* 1987;22:245–251.
2. Brott T, Fieschi C, Hackle W. General therapy of acute ischemic stroke. In: Hacke W, ed. *Neurocritical Care.* Berlin: Springer-Verlag, 1994: 552–577.
3. McMahon SM, Heyman A. The mechanism of breathing and stabilization of ventilation in patients with unilateral cerebral infarction. *Stroke* 1974;5:518–527.
4. Bounds JV, Wiebers DO, Whisnant JP, Okazaki H. Mechanisms and timing of deaths from cerebral infarction. *Stroke* 1981;19:1119–1124.
5. Burtin P, Bollaert P, Feldmann L, et al. Prognosis of stroke patients undergoing mechanical ventilation. *Intensive Care Med* 1994;20: 32–36.
6. Chesnut RM, Marshall LF. Management of head injury. Treatment of abnormal intracranial pressure. *Neurosurg Clin N Am* 1991:2:267–284.
7. Metz S, Slogoff S. Thiopental sodium by single bolus dose compared to infusion for cerebral protection during cardiopulmonary bypass. *J Clin Anesth* 1990:2:226–231.
8. Modica PA, Tempelhoff R. Intracranial pressure during induction of anaesthesia and tracheal intubation with etomidate-induced EEG burst suppression. *Can J Anaesth* 1992;39:236–241.
9. Pinaud M, Leslausque JN, Chetanneau A et al. Effects of propofol on cerebral hemodynamics and metabolism in patients with brain trauma. *Anesthesiology* 1990;73:404–409.
10. Kalkman CJ, Drummond JC, Ribberink AA, Patel PM, Sano T, Bickford RG. Effects of propofol, etomidate, midazolam, and fentanyl on motor evoked responses to transcranial electrical or magnetic stimulation in humans. *Anesthesiology* 1992;76:502–509.
11. Schulte-am-Esch J, Kochs E. Midazolam and flumazenil in neuroanaesthesia. *Acta Anaesthesiol Scand Suppl* 1990;92:96–102.
12. Arens JF, Le Jeune FE, Webre DR. Maxillary sinusitis, a complication of nasotracheal intubation. *Anesthesiology* 1981;40:415.
13. Kofke WA, Dong ML, Bloom M, Policare R, Janosky J, Sekhar L. Transcranial Doppler ultrasonography with induction of anesthesia for neurosurgery. *J Neurosurg Anesthesiol* 1994:6:89–87.
14. Aidinis SJ, Lafferty J, Shapiro HM. Intracranial response to PEEP. *Anesthesiology* 1976;45:275–286.
15. Ell SR. Neurogenic pulmonary edema. A review of the literature and a perspective. *Invest Radiol* 1992;26:499–506.
16. Malik AB. Mechanisms of neurogenic pulmonary edema. *Circ Res* 1985;57:1–18.
17. Heffner JE, Miller S, Sahn SA. Tracheostomy in the intensive care unit. Parts 1 and 2. *Chest* 1986;90:269–274.
18. Incze F. Certain aspects of continuous ventilation. *Orv Hetil* 1993;134: 2421–2426.
19. Stauffer JL, Olson DE, Petty TL. Complications and consequences of endotracheal intubation and tracheostomy. *Am J Med* 1981;70:65–76.
20. Powers WJ. Acute hypertension after stroke: The scientific basis for treatment decisions. *Neurology* 1993;43:461–467.
21. Spence J, del Maestro R. Hypertension in acute ischemic strokes: Treatment. *Arch Neurol* 1985;42:1000–1002.
22. Hartmann A, Stingele R, Schnitzer M. General treatment strategies for elevated intracerebral pressure. In: Hacke W, ed. *Neurocritical Care.* Berlin: Springer-Verlag, 1994:101–115.
23. Hacke W, del Zoppo GJ, Furlan A, von Kummer R. Ischemic stroke. In: Hanley DF, ed. *Principles and Practices in Neurocritical Care.* Baltimore, MD: Williams and Wilkins, 1996 in press.
24. Brott T, MacCarthey E. Antihypertensive therapy in stroke. In: Fischer M, ed. *Medical Therapy of Acute Stroke.* New York: Marcel Decker, 1989:117–143.

25. Strandgaard S, Paulsen O. Regulation of cerebral blood flow in health and disease. *J Cardiovasc Pharmacol* 1992;19:89–93.

26. Samuels MA. Cardiopulmonary aspects of acute neurologic disease. In: Ropper AH, ed. *Neurologic and Neurosurgical Intensive Care.* New York: Raven Press, 1993:103–120.

27. Kreiger D, Patel SV. Acute autonomic instability. In: Hacke W, ed. *Neurocritical Care.* Berlin: Springer-Verlag, 1994:353–365.

28. Garcia EG, Wijdicks EFM, Younge BR. Neurologic complications associated with internal jugular vein cannulation in critically ill patients: A prospective study. *Neurology* 1994;44:951–952.

29. Goetting MG, Preston G. Jugular bulb catherization does not increase intracranial pressure. *Intensive Care Med* 1991;17:195–198.

30. Sterns RH, Riggs JE, Schochet S. Osmotic demyelinization syndrome following correction of hyponatremia. *N Engl J Med* 1986:314:1535–1542.

31. Ayus JC, Krothapalli RK, Arieff AI. Changing concepts in treatment of severe symptomatic hyponatremia. *Am J Med* 1985;78:897–902.

32. Toni D, Sacchetti M, Argentino C, et al. Does hyperglycemia play a role in the outcome of acute ischaemic stroke patients? *J Neurol* 1992;239:382–386.

33. Wagner K, Kleinholz M, de Courten-Myers G, Myers R. Hyperglycemic versus normoglycemic stroke: Topography of brain metabolites, intracellular pH, and infarct size. *J Cereb Blood Flow Metab* 1992;12:213–222.

34. Scurr JH, Coleridge-Smith PD, Hasty JH. Regimen for improved effectiveness of intermittent pneumatic compression in deep venous thrombosis prophylaxis. *Surgery* 1987;102:817–820.

35. Feldmann Z, Kanter MJ, Robertson CS, et al. Effect of head elevation on intracranial pressure, cerebral perfusion pressure, and cerebral blood flow in head-injured patients. *J Neurosurg* 1992;76:207–211.

36. Ginsberg M, Sternau L, Globus M, et al. Therapeutic modulation of brain temperature: Relevance to ischemic brain injury. *Cerebrovasc Brain Metab Rev* 1992;4:189–225.

37. Nau R, Dreyhaupt T, Kolenda H, Prange H. Low blood-to-cerebrospinal fluid passage of sorbitol after intravenous infusion. *Stroke* 1992;23:1276–1279.

38. Bayer A, Pathy M, Newcombe R. Double-blind randomised trial of intravenous glycerol in acute stroke. *Lancet* 1987;1(8530):405–408.

39. Frank M, Nahata M, Hilty M. Glycerol: A review of its pharmacology, pharmacokinetics, adverse reactions, and clinical use. *Pharmacotherapy* 1981;1:147–160.

40. Yu YL, Kumana CR, Lauder IJ, et al. Treatment of acute cerebral hemorrhage with intravenous glycerol: A double-blind, placebo-controlled, randomized trial. *Stroke* 1992;23:967–971.

41. Kaufmann AM, Cardoso ER. Aggravation of vasogenic edema by multiple-dose mannitol. *J Neurosurg* 1992;77:584–589.

42. Grant R, Codon B, Patterson J, et al. Changes in cranial CSF volume during hypercapnia and hypocapnia. *J Neurol Neurosurg Psychiatry* 1989;52:218–222.

43. Marshall LF, Smith RW, Shapiro HM. The outcome of aggressive treatment in severe head injuries, part I: The significance of intracranial pressure monitoring. *J Neurosurg* 1979;50:20–30.

44. Muizelaar JP, Marmarou A, Ward JD, et al. Adverse effects of prolonged hyperventilation in patients with severe head injury: A randomized clinical trial. *J Neurosurg* 1991;75:731–739.

45. Eisenberg HM, Frankowski RF, Contant CF, et al. High dose barbiturate control of elevated intracranial pressure in patients with severe head injury. *J Neurosurg* 1988;69:15–23.

46. Estler. *Pharmakologie und Toxikologie.* Stuttgart: Schattauer Verlagsgesellschaft mbH, 1995.

47. Winer J, Rosenwasser R, Jimenez F. Electroencephalographic activity and serum and cerebrospinal fluid pentobarbital levels in determining the therapeutic endpoint during barbiturate coma. *Neurosurgery* 1991;29:739–742.

48. Wolf A, Levi L, Marmorou A, et al. Effect of THAM upon outcome in severe head injury: A randomized prospective clinical trial. *J Neurosurg* 1993;78:54–59.

49. Aschoff A. *In-vitro-Testung von Hydrozephalus-Ventilen. Habilitationsschrift zur Erlangung der Venia Legendi.* Heidelberg: Ruprecht-Karls-Universität, 1994.

50. Krieger D, Adams H, Rieke K, Schwarz S, Forsting M, Hacke W. Prospective evaluation of the prognostic significance of evoked potentials in acute basilar occlusion. *Crit Care Med* 1992;21:1169–1174.

51. Steiner T, Krieger D, Jauss M, Pilling P, Schwab S, Hacke W. Hemicraniectomy for massive cerebral infarction: Presurgical prognostic factors. *Stroke* 1995;26:172.

52. Klingelhöfer J. *Zur Physiologie und Pathophysiologie der zerebralen Hämodynamik: Neue Aspekte bei Untersuchungen mit der transkraniellen Dopplersographie. Habilitationsschrift zur Erlangung der Venia legendi.* Göttingen: Georg-August-Universität zu Göttingen, 1988.

53. McCornick PW, Stewart M, Goetting M, Balakrishnan G. Regional cerebrovascular oxygen saturation measured by optical spectroscopy in humans. *Stroke* 1991;34:596–602.

54. Stocchetti N, Paparella A, Bridelli F, et al. Cerebral venous oxygen saturation studied with bilateral samples in the internal jugular veins. *Neurosurgery* 1994;34:38–44.

55. Hacke W, Kaste M, Fieschi C, for the ECASS Study Group. The efficacy of IV-rtPA in acute ischemic stroke: First results of the ECASS trial. *Stroke* 1995;26:167.

56. von Kummer R, Meyding-Lamadé U, Michael F, et al. Sensitivity and prognostic value of early CT in occlusion of the middle cerebral artery trunk. *Am J Neuroradiol* 1994;15:9–15.

57. Eston CJ, Pessin MS. Anticoagulation. Is there still a role in atherothrombotic stroke? *Stroke* 1990;21:820–823.

58. Koller RL. Recurrent embolic cerebral infarction and anticoagulation. *Neurology* 1982;32:283–285.

59. Miller V, Hart R. Heparin anticoagulation in acute brain ischemia. *Stroke* 1988;19:403–406.

60. Phillips S. An alternative view of heparin anticoagulation in acute focal brain ischemia. *Stroke* 1989;20:295–298.

61. Scheinberg P. Heparin anticoagulation. *Stroke* 1989;20:173–174.

62. Delashaw JB, Broaddus WC, Kassell NF, et al. Treatment of right hemispheric cerebral infarction by hemicraniectomy. *Stroke* 1990;21:874–881.

63. Rieke K, Krieger D, von Kummer R, Aschoff A, Hacke W. Decompressive surgery in space occupying hemispheric infarction. *Crit Care Med* 1995;73:1576–1587.

64. Hacke W. Neuromonitoring. *J Neurol* 1985;232:125–132.

65. Nagao S, Kuyama H, Honma Y, et al. Prediction and evaluation of brainstem function by auditory brainstem responses in patients with uncal herniation. *Surg Neurol* 1987;27:81–86.

66. Hacke W, Zeumer J, Ferbert A, Brückmann H, del Zoppo G. Intra-arterial thrombolytic therapy improves outcome in patients with acute vertebrobasilar occlusive disease. *Stroke* 1988;19:1216–1222.

67. Del Zoppo GJ, Poeck K, Pessin MS. Recombinant tissue plasminogen activator in acute thrombotic and embolic stroke. *Ann Neurol* 1992;32:78–86.

68. Chen HJ, Lee TC, Wei CP. Treatment of cerebellar infarction by decompressive suboccipital craniectomy. *Stroke* 1992;23:957–961.

69. Heros R. Surgical treatment of cerebellar infarction. *Stroke* 1992;23:937–938.

70. Rieke K, Krieger D, Adams HP, Aschoff A, Meyding-Lamadé U, Hacke W. Therapeutic strategies in space-occupying cerebellar infarction based on clinical, neuroradiological, and neurophysiological data. *Cerebrovasc Dis* 1993;3:45–55.

71. Awad I, Carter P, Spetzler R, Medina M, Williams F. Clinical vasospasm after subarachnoid hemorrhage: Response to hypervolemic hemodilution and arterial hypertension. *Stroke* 1987;18:365–37.

Cerebrovascular Disease, edited by H. Hunt Batjer.
Lippincott-Raven Publishers, Philadelphia © 1997.

CHAPTER 43

Thrombolytic Therapy for Cerebral Infarction

Thomas Brott, Rashmi Kothari, and Joseph Broderick

Thrombolytic therapy has been in use for cerebral infarction since 1958. In the era before computed tomography (CT), seven case series were published describing thrombolytic therapy in 249 patients with ischemic stroke (1–7). Therapy involved an assortment of agents, including fibrinolysin (plasmin), streptokinase, and urokinase. Thrombolytic treatment was almost always administered more than 6 hours after symptom onset and often up to several days afterward. Because CT was unavailable, these early thrombolytic investigators could not exclude patients with small spontaneous intracerebral hematoma masquerading as cerebral infarction. In addition, neurologic deterioration due to hemorrhage after the initiation of thrombolytic therapy could not be definitively identified except at autopsy.

During this pre-CT period, two randomized trials evaluated small numbers of patients with ischemic stroke (3,4). These trials were interpreted to be negative because of poor patient outcomes, including intracerebral hemorrhage. Because of limited therapeutic success and a high rate of complications, enthusiasm for thrombolytic therapy waned.

During the 1980s, thrombolytic therapy was developed as treatment for acute myocardial infarction (MI), acute pulmonary embolism, and peripheral arterial disease (8–14). With acute MI, early studies investigated intraarterial, as well as intravenous, administration of thrombolytic agents (12–17). Possible advantages with regard to clot lysis for intraarterial delivery were overshadowed by much more rapid treatment with intravenous administration. By the late 1980s, intravenous treatment of patients with acute MI with either streptokinase or tissue plasminogen activator (t-PA) was demonstrated to improve patient survival and cardiac function compared with treatment with placebo (12,13,18–20).

Parallel to the successful development of thrombolytic therapy for acute MI, CT imaging became widely available throughout the United States. Therapeutic trials of other agents for ischemic cerebral stroke were also carried out during this time, and these trials emphasized earlier and earlier treatment as the decade progressed (21,22). By the end of the 1980s, multiple case series of thrombolytic therapy for stroke had been published (23–30). Several pilot protocols, preludes to larger randomized trials, emphasized dose finding, clot lysis, and methods for assessing neurologic outcome (31–35).

Experimental studies of thrombolytic therapy in the setting of acute focal cerebral ischemia in animal models were also accomplished. These studies suggested that thrombolytic agents, if administered within 30–60 minutes of the onset of ischemia, could lyse clots, decrease cerebral infarction size, and improve neurologic outcome (36–45).

FREQUENCY AND LOCATION OF ARTERIAL THROMBI IN ACUTE STROKE

How often are thrombi present in the setting of acute cerebral infarction? A partial answer can be provided by studies of patients with acute stroke that included very early cerebral arteriography. The largest and most detailed of such studies is the dose-finding trial of intravenously administered t-PA (duteplase) carried out by the Acute Stroke Study Group (ASSG) (35,46,47). This multicenter study included patients who were thought to have sustained a large-vessel thrombotic or embolic stroke. Patient evaluation, including cerebral arteriography, had to be completed so that a patient could be treated with IV t-PA within 8 hours of symptom onset. Cerebral arteriography was performed in 139 patients. Arterial occlusion appropriate to the patients' symptoms was present in 81% of these patients (47). In another study, Fieschi et al (48) reported 80 patients with acute ischemic stroke who were examined with cerebral arteriography within 6 hours of symptom onset. Sixty-one patients (76%) had an appropriately located arterial occlusion. Because both of these studies included only patients who presented very early after symptom onset and the ASSG trial of t-PA by

T. Brott and J. Broderick: Department of Neurology, University of Cincinnati Medical Center, Cincinnati, Ohio 45267.

R. Kothari: Department of Emergency Medicine, University of Cincinnati Medical Center, Cincinnati, Ohio 45267.

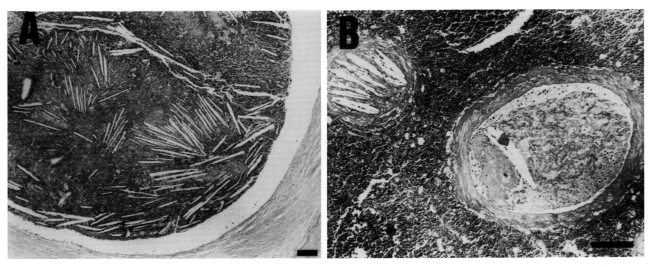

FIG. 1. Heterogeneous atheromatous emboli occlude the right middle cerebral artery trunk **(A)** and (in a second patient) two right temporal leptomeningeal arteries **(B)**. Cholesterol crystals are prominent in the largest embolus **(A)** and in the smallest embolus (bars = 100 μm). (From ref. 49, with permission.)

definition did not include patients thought to have small-vessel disease, these arteriographic results may not be representative of all ischemic strokes in the population.

The arteriographic data from these reports are also instructive concerning the sites of acute arterial occlusion. In the ASSG t-PA trial, 23 of 93 patients (25%) completing the study had occlusion of the extracranial internal carotid artery (ICA); 12 of these patients had tandem ipsilateral middle cerebral artery (MCA) occlusions, and in 11 others, the anatomy of the MCA ipsilateral to the extracranial occlusion was not visualized (47). Thirty-three of the 93 patients (35%) had occlusion of the MCA stem, and an additional 29 patients (31%) had occlusions of MCA branches. Thus, not only were thrombi frequent in this study, but the thrombi most commonly involved large vessels. The findings of the Fieschi et al (48) study were similar. Among the 61 patients with occlusions, 19 (31%) had extracranial ICA occlusions, 20 (33%) had intracranial occlusions associated with ICA plaque, and 18 (30%) had isolated occlusions of the MCA or its branches.

Unfortunately, cerebral arteriography does not provide answers with regard to the composition or age of the thrombi identified. Postmortem examination of thrombi is limited. As illustrated in Figure 1, acute thrombi are not only heterogeneous with regard to location but also with regard to composition. The characteristics of thrombi are likely to be important with regard to their susceptibility to disruption by either thrombolytic agents or mechanical means (50).

THROMBOLYTIC AGENTS

The thrombolytic agents currently under investigation as treatment for stroke are streptokinase, urokinase, prourokinase, and recombinant t-PA. Streptokinase is an indirect-acting plasminogen activator that is derived via chemical purification from a streptococcal bacterial filtrate. Streptokinase is generally infused over 30–60 minutes, has a half-life of approximately 20 minutes, results in a lytic state, and costs approximately $300 per treatment (51). In studies with patients with myocardial infarction, the incidence of hypotension requiring direct treatment was approximately 7%. Allergic reactions occur in approximately 4% of patients. Urokinase is a direct-acting plasminogen activator that may be obtained via purified human urine or cultured embryonic or transformed renal cells, or by recombinant DNA technology (52,53). For stroke, urokinase has been administered almost exclusively via the intraarterial route. Urokinase has a half-life of approximately 15 minutes and costs approximately $2,000 per treatment (51). The action of urokinase is enhanced in the presence of fibrin. The likelihood of a lytic state following urokinase treatment is related to the drug dose. Prourokinase (also known as single-chain urokinase plasminogen activator), obtained through recombinant DNA technology, is the precursor of urokinase and has much higher fibrin specificity than urokinase. In animal models, prourokinase induces thrombolysis more effectively than urokinase and is much less likely to induce a lytic state. Tissue plasminogen activator (t-PA) is the most important endogenous plasminogen activator. Recombinant t-PA (rt-PA) is obtained through recombinant DNA technology and may be synthesized in a single- or double-chain form (54). The most widely used form of rt-PA is the single-chain form (alteplase). For cerebral infarction, rt-PA is generally infused over 60 minutes, has a serum half-life of 5–8 minutes, and costs approximately $2,300 per treatment (51). In common with prourokinase, the activity of rt-PA is greatly increased in the presence of fibrin.

The rationale for these agents is that their administration

results in the activation of plasminogen to plasmin, which then results in thrombolysis. The plasminogen activators may be inhibited by plasminogen activator inhibitors (PAI), particularly PAI-1. Plasmin is inhibited by α_2-antiplasmin (55).

Intravenous Therapy

Clot Lysis and Recanalization

Each of the thrombolytic agents under investigation has been demonstrated to result in clot lysis. Given that t-PA is the most important endogenous plasminogen activator, it likely plays an important role in spontaneous recanalization. Spontaneous clot lysis has long been recognized and may occur in up to 40–70% of patients with stroke (48,56,57). Fieschi et al (48) reported serial transcranial Doppler ultrasound (TCD) examinations in 15 patients with MCA occlusion. Spontaneous recanalization occurred in 11 patients—in four of these within 24 hours. The other seven patients showed evidence of recanalization by TCD within one week. Importantly, there was no significant clinical improvement associated with arterial recanalization. Serial studies of arterial occlusions have also been done on the placebo patients evaluated in the randomized trials of rt-PA reported by Mori, Yamaguchi, and their colleagues (34,58). In these two studies, pretreatment and posttreatment angiograms were performed on a total of 58 patients. Spontaneous recanalization occurred between the time of the pretreatment angiogram and the time of the posttreatment angiogram (60 minutes) in only four patients (7%) (34,58).

With regard to clot lysis, three of four studies have reported recanalization rates in patients treated with IV rt-PA within 6 hours after symptom onset (33,34,58); one study reported recanalization within 8 hours (47). In the ASSG rt-PA trial, the recanalization rate for all 93 patients receiving active treatment was 34% (47). In the three smaller studies of von Kummer, Mori, and Yamaguchi, a total of 106 patients received treatment within 6 hours, and the combined recanalization rate was approximately 30% (33,34,58). Smaller clots were more likely to be recanalized. In the ASSG rt-PA trial, recanalization was accomplished in 2 (9%) of 23 patients with extracranial carotid artery occlusion, 12 (26%) of 46 patients with MCA stem occlusions, and 14 (44%) of 32 patients with occlusions of MCA divisions or branches (46). In the study by Mori et al (34), only one of the 10 patients with occlusion of the ICA had recanalization. In contrast, recanalization was achieved with IV rt-PA in 9 (69%) of 13 patients with occlusion of the MCA or its branches. Clot lysis is also time-dependent. Among 22 patients treated by von Kummer and colleagues (33) with IV rt-PA 100 mg after baseline angiography, complete recanalization was immediately obtained in only one of 21 patients. Repeat angiography at 24 hours demonstrated recanalization in 10 (45%) of 22 patients. Clot lysis can also be accomplished for occlusion of the basilar artery. Huemer et al (59) reported 16 patients treated with IV rt-PA 100 mg over 3 hours. Recanalization, assessed by angiography in two patients and by TCD in 14 patients, was accomplished in 10 (63%) of these patients.

In summary, intravenous thrombolytic therapy, if administered very early, can achieve arterial recanalization in 30–60% of cases. However, clot lysis rates for stroke are considerably lower than the rates (60–80%) achieved with thrombolytic therapy for acute myocardial infarction.

Neurologic Outcome

Intravenous thrombolytic therapy can lyse occlusive thrombi in the setting of acute stroke. However, does thrombolytic therapy improve neurologic outcome? In the National Institutes of Health (NIH) dose-finding safety study of rt-PA for stroke, 74 patients were treated, under a dose-escalation design, within 90 minutes of symptom onset (32). Major neurologic improvement occurred in 22 patients (30%) at 2 hours from the initiation of treatment and in 34 (46%) at 24 hours. In the small randomized trials of Mori, Yamaguchi, Haley, and their colleagues, a total of 156 patients were treated with either IV rt-PA or placebo (34,58,60). In each of these three trials, a treatment advantage was demonstrated for the rt-PA patients. However, benefits were often transient, and patient group numbers were small. Fortunately, the results addressing neurologic outcome in larger randomized controlled trials are becoming available (Tables 1 and 2).

The Multicenter Acute Stroke Trial—Europe (MAST-E) is a double-blind, randomized study of streptokinase compared with placebo in patients with hemispheric stroke who could be randomized and treated within 6 hours of stroke onset. Patients were treated with IV streptokinase 1.5 million IU or placebo given over 60 minutes. The target number of patients was 600, but MAST-E was terminated upon recommendation from the Data Monitoring and Safety Committee following the evaluation of 270 patients (61). The 10-day mortality in the 137 patients receiving streptokinase was 35% compared with 18% in the patients treated with placebo ($p = 0.001$) (see Table 1). The symptomatic hemorrhage rate was 18% in the streptokinase patients and 3% in the placebo patients ($p = 0.001$).

The Multicenter Acute Stroke Trial—Italy (MAST-I) is a randomized trial, with a factorial design, comparing treatment among four groups (62). Patients with acute carotid or vertebrobasilar stroke who could be treated within 6 hours were randomized to receive either IV streptokinase 1.5 million IU over 60 minutes, aspirin 300 mg/d for 10 days, IV streptokinase and aspirin, or control (standard treatment—no placebo). MAST-I was suspended following recommendation of the Safety and Monitoring Committee because of the increased risk of adverse events in the

TABLE 1. *Randomized trials of streptokinase (SK)*

Trial[a]	Time to treatment (hr)	Patients (no.)	Treatment group	Mortality (%)	Intracerebral hematoma (%)
Australian Streptokinase (ASK) (64,65)	<4	228	SK + 100 mg aspirin vs.	43*	NA
			100 mg aspirin	22*	NA
Multicenter Acute Stroke Trial—Europe (MAST-E) (61)	≤6	270	SK vs.	35*	18*
			placebo	18	3
Multicenter Acute Stroke-Trial—Italy (MAST-I) (63)	≤3	616	SK + 300 mg aspirin vs. SK vs. 300 mg aspirin vs. standard therapy	31	4

* $p \leq 0.001$; NA = not available.
[a] All studies terminated prior to completion due to increased mortality in treatment groups.

streptokinase group (63). Details from this study are not yet available.

The Australian Streptokinase Trial (ASK) is a double-blind, randomized, placebo-controlled trial of patients with ischemic stroke who could be randomized and treated within 4 hours of symptom onset (64). Patients were treated with IV streptokinase 1.5 million IU plus 325 mg aspirin or intravenous placebo and aspirin over 60 minutes. ASK was also suspended upon recommendation by the Safety and Monitoring Committee following analysis of 228 patients who had been treated between 3 and 4 hours after stroke onset. The recommendation was made because of increased mortality and symptomatic hemorrhage in the streptokinase patients. Death occurred in 46 (43%) of the 106 patients treated with streptokinase compared with 27 (22%) of the 122 patients treated with placebo, with an odds ratio of 2.65 favoring mortality in the streptokinase patients ($p < 0.001$) (see Table 1) (65).

Preliminary results from the three suspended streptokinase trials raise several issues. First, while pilot safety studies were carried out prior to beginning the randomized trials, dose-escalation and dose-finding studies were not performed. Rather, a 1.5 million unit dose of streptokinase was studied in small numbers of patients. This dose is identical to that used in the setting of acute myocardial infarction, which results in a lytic state. While a lytic state may be well tolerated by patients with myocardial infarction who have no known cerebral vascular disease, it may not be well tolerated by the more elderly stroke patients with acute focal cerebral injury. In contrast, two dose-finding, dose-escalation trials of IV rt-PA preceded the larger randomized trials of rt-PA. The doses ultimately selected for the subsequent randomized trials of rt-PA were approximately 60–75% of the total dose used in the treatment of acute myocardial infarction. Perhaps a lower dose of streptokinase (eg, 0.9–1.2 million IU) would have been better tolerated by stroke patients without sacrificing efficacy. Safety in the streptokinase trials may also have been significantly better if earlier treatment had been required. The two dose-finding, dose-escalation trials of IV rt-PA indicated a statistically significant relationship of later treatment with the occurrence of thrombolysis-related intracerebral bleeding. Finally, detailed analysis of the results of MAST-E, MAST-I, and ASK may reveal subgroups of patients for whom potential benefit is suggested, as well as subgroups of patients for whom excess risk is concentrated. Unfortunately, further development of streptokinase as intravenous therapy for acute ischemic stroke is unlikely because of the negative findings from these studies.

Three large multicenter, randomized, controlled trials of rt-PA for acute ischemic stroke have been in progress in Europe and the United States for the last five years. The

TABLE 2. *Preliminary results of European Cooperative Acute Stroke Study (ECASS)*

	Intent-to-treat population (n = 611)		Target population (n = 511)	
	t-PA	Placebo	t-PA	Placebo
30-Day mortality (%)	18	13	15	12
Parenchymal hematoma (%)	20	6	19	7
Rankin 0–1 at 3 mo (%)	37	28	41	29

* $p < 0.01$.

results of the European Cooperative Acute Stroke Study (ECASS) have recently been reported (66–68). In this trial, patients aged 18–80 years with a clinical diagnosis of moderate to severe hemispheric stroke were eligible for randomization if they could be evaluated and treated within 6 hours of symptom onset. Coma, hemiplegia with fixed eye deviation, global aphasia, vertebrobasilar stroke, or CT-scan hypodensity in more than one third of the middle cerebral artery territory were grounds for exclusion. Patients were then treated with IV rt-PA 1.1 mg/kg or placebo over 60 minutes. Prospectively, the ECASS intent-to-treat population sample size was planned for 600, while the fully evaluable population was planned for 480; the investigators anticipated that up to 20% of the patients would not be fully evaluable under the conditions of the protocol. Actual study enrollment was 620 patients. The preplanned evaluable group, which the ECASS investigators have now termed the "target population," comprised 511 patients. The reasons for exclusion from the target population were abnormalities on the CT scans in 66 patients (mainly major early infarct signs), prohibited therapy (eg, heparin in less than 24 hours) in 13 patients, deviation from the 90 (± 14)-day time window for follow-up or lost follow-up in 19 patients, and a variety of reasons (eg, randomized but not treated) in 11 others.

In the intent-to-treat population, neurologic outcome was not improved in patients treated with rt-PA (67). At three months, the median Barthel index, the median Rankin scale, and mortality were not significantly different in the two groups. Death associated with hemorrhage occurred in 19 of the rt-PA–treated patients and in seven of the placebo patients. In the target population, two primary endpoints indicated better outcome in the rt-PA–treated patients. First, the median modified Rankin scale score in the rt-PA patients was 2 and that for the placebo patients was 3. (A Rankin of 0 or 1 signifies a normal or a very good recovery; a Rankin of 2, 3, or 4 signifies a modest deficit; a Rankin of 5 signifies poor recovery, and a Rankin of 6 signifies death.) Of the rt-PA–treated patients in the target population, 41% had a 3-month modified Rankin score of 1 or 0 compared to 29% of the placebo-treated patients ($p < 0.01$) (see Table 2). Mortality was not different in the two target population groups. Death associated with hemorrhage occurred in 10 patients treated with rt-PA as compared with seven treated with placebo (NS). Overall, the total parenchymal hematoma rate in the target population was 19% for rt-PA and 7% for placebo.

The preliminary ECASS results have sparked considerable controversy. Skeptics point out that the real-world population is the intent-to-treat population. For that group, no efficacy or suggestion of efficacy was identified. Optimists point out that proper patient selection is necessary for adequate evaluation of a given therapy. Methods for proper selection have already improved since the beginning of the ECASS trial. They argue that 71 of the 109 patients excluded from the target population showed CT-scan evidence of an already established major cerebral infarction or were ran-

domized but not treated. Such patients would not be expected to benefit from thrombolysis, and therefore attention to the positive results in the target population is warranted. Furthermore, they state that subsequent analysis of the results may identify subgroups of patients for whom benefit is likely, as well as subgroups of patients for whom the risk of intracranial bleeding is excessive. Finally, rt-PA treatment was initiated after 4 hours from symptom onset for the majority of the ECASS patients. If all patients had been treated within 3 hours, perhaps outcomes for the rt-PA–treated patients could have been improved.

The second relatively large trial for which recruitment has been completed is the National Institute of Neurological Disorders and Stroke (NINDS) rt-PA stroke trial (68). This is a double-blind, randomized trial comparing patients with acute ischemic cerebral infarction randomized to receive IV rt-PA 0.9 mg/kg or placebo over 60 minutes. Treatment is required within 3 hours; for approximately 50% of the patients, treatment was required within 90 minutes. No heparin was allowed for the first 24 hours. For the first part of the trial (approximately half of the patients treated), the primary endpoint was a decrease (improvement) of ≥4 points on the NIH Stroke Scale score at 24 hours or resolution of the neurologic deficit at 24 hours from symptom onset. For the second part of the trial, the primary endpoint was a consistent and persuasive difference in the proportion of rt-PA–treated patients compared with the placebo-treated patients at 90 days, with a Barthel index ≥95, a Rankin score ≤1, a Glasgow Outcome Scale of 1, and an NIH Stroke Scale score ≤1. Six hundred and twenty-three patients were entered into this trial.

Safety

The major risk of intravenous thrombolytic therapy for stroke is intracranial hemorrhage. Intracranial bleeding associated with thrombolytic therapy may vary in severity from a petechial hemorrhagic change within infarcted tissue to frank hematoma with mass effect, herniation, and death (47) (Fig. 2). Among the 84 patients evaluated in the three smaller randomized studies, six (7%) parenchymal hematomas were reported with treatment with rt-PA (58–60). Overall, the symptomatic hemorrhage rate has been in the 4–10% range. In the larger MAST-E trial, the symptomatic hemorrhage rate in the streptokinase-treated patients was 18% vs. 3% in the placebo-treated patients (see Table 1). The breakdown of hemorrhage by treatment group or by whether or not the hemorrhage was symptomatic has not yet been reported for either the MAST-I trial or the ASK trial. In the ECASS trial of rt-PA, parenchymal hematoma occurred in 20% of the rt-PA–treated patients compared with 6% of the placebo-treated patients (see Table 2), and hemorrhagic infarction occurred in 23% of those given rt-PA compared with 30% of those given placebo (62). The breakdown of hemorrhagic infarction and parenchymatous hematoma into symptomatic

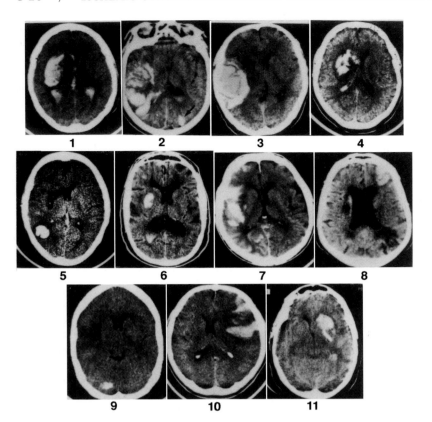

FIG. 2. CT scans from 11 patients with intracerebral hematoma following IV rt-PA administration for ischemic stroke. Differentiation between hematoma and hemorrhagic infarction may be difficult. (From ref. 47, with permission.)

and asymptomatic has not yet been reported for the ECASS patients.

Given the frequency of intracranial hemorrhage with thrombolytic therapy and an associated case mortality of 20–50%, identification of risk factors for such hemorrhage becomes important. In the ASSG rt-PA trial, in which 11 of the 93 treated patients had parenchymal hematomas, the only risk factor identified was time-to-treatment (see Fig. 2) (46). Hematoma occurred in 5 (8%) of 61 patients treated before or at 6 hours compared with 6 (19%) of 32 patients treated after 6 hours. In the NIH rt-PA pilot trial, patients treated with rt-PA at 90–180 minutes from symptom onset tended to have a higher risk than those treated in less than 90 minutes (31). Two other risk factors emerged in analysis of the patients treated in the NIH study. Higher doses of rt-PA were associated with a greater risk of posttreatment hemorrhage; in addition, those with hemorrhage had a statistically significantly higher initial diastolic blood pressure (mean, 104 ± 10 mm Hg) than those without (86 ± 14 mm Hg). Results from the three streptokinase trials and the two large rt-PA trials may identify additional risk factors.

Other adverse events potentially associated with thrombolytic therapy for stroke include cerebral reperfusion injury, arterial reocclusion, secondary embolization, and systemic hemorrhage. Potential for reperfusion injury has been demonstrated experimentally and suggested in humans (69–70). In the larger intravenous and intraarterial trials, the frequency of reperfusion injury and even its occurrence after

thrombolytic recanalization has not been established. However, none of the trials was designed to detect reperfusion injury. To do so would be difficult and would require serial neurologic assessments, arteriography pre- and posttreatment, and serial brain imaging with CT or magnetic resonance imaging.

Arterial reocclusion, another complication that is difficult to document, requires initial identification of an occlusion, subsequent documentation of thrombolysis, and later documentation of reocclusion. In the setting of acute myocardial infarction, reocclusion rates after thrombolytic recanalization have been approximately 10–20% (51). In this instance, the acute thrombus is characteristically superimposed on a complex underlying atherosclerotic plaque. In contrast, in cerebral infarction, the site of occlusion is not usually the site of a complex atherosclerotic plaque. Rather, the site of a blockage is usually an intracranial vessel occluded by an embolus that originated from a proximal plaque in an extracranial vessel, the aortic arch, or the heart. Hopefully, when an acute thrombus is lysed in an intracranial vessel, the absence of an underlying complex plaque provides less of a nidus for local rethrombosis and reocclusion. Von Kummer (33) and colleagues evaluated 40 patients who were studied at baseline angiographically, received rt-PA 100 mg over 90 minutes, had angiography repeated immediately on completion of the rt-PA infusion, and were reassessed at 24 hours with either transcranial Doppler ultrasound (n = 34) or a third angiogram (n = 9). Reocclusion was observed at 24 hours in one (7%) of the 14 patients who showed recanalization immediately on termination of the rt-PA infusion. (The rate of recanalization was 50% at 24 hours.)

Embolic complications could occur in the setting of thrombolytic therapy if, for example, the patient had a preexisting thrombus proximal to the brain (eg, left ventricle) that became fragmented at the time of thrombolytic therapy for ischemic infarction. Such secondary embolization has been reported in one patient (71). Finally, systemic complications have been infrequent in the setting of intravenous thrombolytic therapy for stroke. Pericardial tamponade, retroperitoneal hematoma, and gastrointestinal bleeding have been reported, but in no study has the rate of significant systemic bleeding exceeded 5% (32). Systemic bleeding complications have not yet been reported for the three large controlled trials of streptokinase or for the ECASS rt-PA trial.

Intraarterial Therapy

Because of the relatively low recanalization rates reported with intravenous therapy, interest in intraarterial thrombolytic therapy has increased over the past decade. The recanalization rates after intravenous thrombolytic therapy appear to be particularly low for large-vessel occlusions such as those involving the internal carotid artery and the middle cerebral artery stem (33,47). Intraarterial therapy has been investigated with streptokinase, urokinase, prourokinase, and rt-PA (71–77). Earlier studies reported on regional intraarterial administration. More recent studies report the results of local intraarterial treatment via the use of superselective microcatheters (Table 3). With this method, the patient is first studied by cerebral arteriography carried out through the transfemoral technique (Fig. 3). When the thrombus is located, the microcatheter is introduced, placed at the site of the clot, then used to penetrate the clot so that the terminus of the clot can be identified. Then the microcatheter is withdrawn either into the clot or immediately proximal to the clot, and drug is delivered. Infusion times vary from minutes to several hours. Clot penetration by this technique results in some mechanical disruption of the thrombus and very high concentrations of lytic drug at the site of the clot.

Clot Lysis and Recanalization

Clot lysis rates have been approximately 40–50% for streptokinase, 50–100% for urokinase, and 80–100% for rt-PA (71–74,78–82). Patient numbers are too small to draw conclusions regarding the efficacy of one drug compared with another. Zeumer et al (71) have the largest experience and opportunity to treat patients with either local intraarterial urokinase or local intraarterial rt-PA. In 19 patients treated within 6 hours with local intraarterial urokinase, the lysis rate was 100%. In 20 patients treated with local intraarterial rt-PA for vertebrobasilar occlusions, the lysis rate was 100%. In 20 patients treated with local intraarterial rt-PA for carotid distribution occlusions, the lysis rate was 90%. These investigators were unable to appreciate any significant differences in the rate or speed of clot lysis between urokinase and rt-PA.

The time required for recanalization with local thrombolysis has been considerably longer than anticipated. An analysis of the different time intervals required for local intraarterial therapy has not been published. However, at our center and others, evaluation and transport from the emergency

TABLE 3. *Intraarterial thrombolytic therapy series[a]*

Study	Patients (no.)	Agent	Onset to treatment (hr)	Treatment to recanalization (hr)[b]	Partial (P) or complete (C) recanalization (no./%)	Symptomatic hematoma (no./%)
Zeumer et al. (71)	40	t-PA	<6	1.5	19 (48)C 19 (48)P	0
	19	UK	<6	1.5	14 (74)C 5 (26)P	0
Ezura and Kagawa (72)	11	UK	7.7	2.8	1 (9)C 6 (55)P	0
Barnwell et al. (81)	13	UK plus mechanical clot disruption	12	2	7 (54)C 3 (23)P	0
Higashida et al. (82)	27	UK	NA	NA	37 of 45 vessels (82) C or P	3 (11)
Hiramoto et al. (78)[c]	60	UK	NA	NA	32 (53) C or P	1 (2)
Sasaki et al. (79)	44	t-PA or UK	4.6	NA	23 (52)C 14 (32)P	1 (2)
	18	UK intracarotid	4.3	NA	0 C 2 (11)P	0
Lamonte et al. (80)	11	UK	<8	NA	NA	0

Key: t-PA, tissue plasminogen activator; UK, urokinase; NA, not available.
[a] Studies with n >10 published 1991 or later.
[b] Time interval from admission to treatment.
[c] Retrospective study.

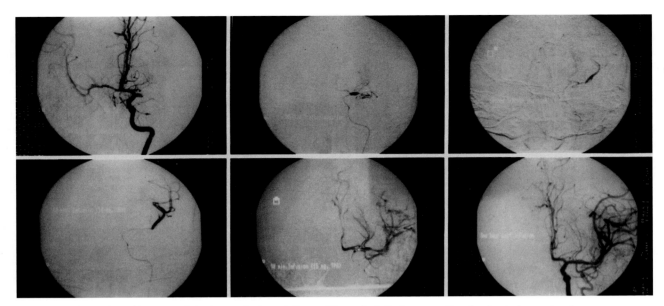

FIG. 3. Local intraarterial microcatheter–delivered thrombolytic therapy. Cerebral arteriography demonstrates occlusion of the right middle cerebral artery stem **(A)** in a 27-year-old man with acute onset of aphasia and right hemiplegia in the setting of rheumatic heart disease. A Tracker-18 microcatheter was introduced into **(B)** and through **(C)** the thrombus. IV rt-PA 15 mg were administered into the clot over 90 minutes, beginning 6 hours after symptom onset. Partial recanalization was present at 60 minutes **(D)** and 90 minutes. Recanalization was complete by 60 minutes postinfusion **(E)**. The patient's deficits improved slowly. At 6 weeks, he had modest aphasia and right hemiparesis but was able to walk. (Courtesy of M. Gaskill, MD, and R. Cornelius, MD, University of Cincinnati Medical Center, Ohio.)

medicine department to radiology and preparation of the patient take approximately 30 minutes. The cerebral angiogram and subsequent positioning of the microcatheter and initiation of local intraarterial therapy require 45–90 minutes. Thus, the time required from patient arrival at the hospital to initiation of treatment is 90–120 minutes (71). Added to this 1–3-hour period is the time to lysis once the infusion has begun (see Table 3). The Zeumer group (71) reported a median recanalization time of 60 minutes in stroke patients treated with urokinase and 120 minutes in the those treated with rt-PA. They attributed the longer recanalization times in the rt-PA group to the higher frequency of occlusions of the carotid siphon, the M1 segment of the middle cerebral artery, and the A1 segment of the anterior cerebral artery rather than to any differences in lytic potency between urokinase and rt-PA. The 3–4-hour period from patient arrival to recanalization is vexing.

"Plasminogen steal" has been suggested as one reason for the delay in clot lysis (83). When a therapeutic plasminogen activator is administered locally via the intraarterial route, the very high local concentrations of activator produce a profound local plasminemia and concomitant depletion of fibrinogen and plasminogen in the blood adjacent to the clot. This fluid-phase disequilibrium results in leaching of clot-bound plasminogen into the plasminogen-depleted adjacent fluid phase. Plasminogen steal and resulting diminution in clot lysis have been confirmed in vitro. For patients with stroke, Zeumer has suggested that simultaneous local delivery of a plasminogen activator plus plasminogen might be useful.

Another reason for delayed lysis with intraarterial therapy could be the use of radiologic contrast agents during the interventional procedure. The contrast agent is present briefly at high concentrations at the clot surface following each contrast injection. The three contrast agents most widely used are nonionic and generally given in hyperosmolar solution. Each has been shown in vitro to inhibit thrombolysis (84). Diatrizoate and iohexol have been shown in vivo to alter fibrin structure, making it more resistant to lysis (85).

Neurologic Outcome

Improved neurologic outcome has not been clearly established after anatomically successful thrombolysis with intraarterial thrombolytic therapy. In the largest series reported, 8 (24%) of 33 patients with carotid territory stroke died; 15 (45%) survived with either moderate or severe neurologic deficit (71). Among the 28 patients treated for vertebrobasilar stroke, 10 patients (36%) died within the first week. Of the ten patients who were alive at 3 months, seven had a minimal or mild deficit. In a second relatively large series, Higashida and colleagues (82) reported treatment of 27 patients with acute occlusion of a major intracerebral artery. All were treated with local intraarterial urokinase, and 18 patients (67%) demonstrated improvement. The majority of patients had some residual deficit immediately after treatment. However, the improvements from the baseline neurologic evaluation are difficult to attribute with certainty to the urokinase therapy. In randomized trials of other agents investigated for stroke, postbaseline improvement occurs in both the treatment and the placebo groups. As case series do not allow comparisons between active-treatment and placebo patients, conclusions regarding outcome cannot be made.

Safety

Complications of intraarterial therapy for stroke include intracerebral hemorrhage, arterial intracranial embolization, subarachnoid hemorrhage, arterial perforation, secondary embolization, hemorrhagic infarction, groin hematoma, and retroperitoneal hematoma (71,74,77,79,82,86). Most reports are small case series and therefore suffer from potential publication bias, particularly with regard to complications. Reported intracranial hemorrhage rates are frequently difficult to evaluate. In many of these small series, safety CT scans were not routinely performed at fixed times posttreatment (with or without patient deterioration). In addition, angiographic dye used during treatment can mimic hemorrhage on subsequent CT scans. In the largest series, no massive intracerebral hemorrhage occurred among the 59 patients treated; secondary asymptomatic hemorrhagic infarction occurred in eight patients (71). In the series of 27 patients treated by Higashida and colleagues (82), intracerebral hemorrhage occurred in three patients (11%), all of whom died. One cannot infer from these two larger series and other smaller series that local intraarterial therapy is safer than intravenous thrombolytic therapy.

NEW APPROACHES

In contrast to urokinase, which is relatively nonselective, prourokinase has a fibrin-dependent mode of action similar to rt-PA. However, unlike rt-PA, prourokinase is not activated by direct fibrin binding. Rather, prourokinase preferentially activates fibrin-bound glu-plasminogen. The plasmin thus formed can locally activate more prourokinase. Such activation can be relatively localized to sites of active clot. Clinically, prourokinase is currently being evaluated in multiple centers as part of a local intraarterial investigational protocol. Initially, the protocol involved evaluation of patients with acute middle cerebral artery territory stroke. Patients for whom intraarterial therapy could be initiated within 6 hours from time of symptom onset were randomized to receive prourokinase or placebo. Both patient groups underwent cerebral angiography. If an arterial occlusion was identified as appropriate to the patient's symptoms, a superselective catheter was positioned in the proximal one third of the thrombus. Then the patient was given the prourokinase or

placebo over 120 minutes. Patients were evaluated with the NIH Stroke Scale, CT scan, cerebral arteriography, and a disability outcome assessment over the 3-month period of the study. The cerebral angiography was carried out at baseline, 60 minutes into the infusion, and following the termination of the infusion at 120 minutes. Results from the trial have not been reported. The protocol is currently being modified.

Combined intravenous and intraarterial thrombolytic therapy is also under investigation. In a multicenter pilot trial designed to evaluate safety and potential efficacy, patients with acute ischemic stroke who can be treated within 3 hours are randomized to receive IV rt-PA 0.6 mg/kg or placebo over 30 minutes. Cerebral arteriography is then carried out in all patients. If the cerebral angiogram localizes an occlusion appropriate to the patient's symptoms, the patient receives intraarterial rt-PA. All patients with clot receive active treatment intraarterially whether or not they initially receive intravenous rt-PA or placebo. Before the start of the rt-PA infusion, the clot is penetrated, and rt-PA 1 mg is given distally. The catheter is retracted into the thrombus, another 1 mg bolus of rt-PA is administered, and then rt-PA is administered by infusion into the clot at a rate of 10 mg/h for up to 2 hours. Cerebral angiography is carried out on a local basis every 15 minutes during the infusion to assess clot lysis. Patients are evaluated at baseline and over the subsequent 90 days.

In addition to these larger multicenter efforts, neurointerventional techniques have been evolving at the single-institution level. Barnwell and colleagues (81) have reported distal clot lysis following penetration of a proximal occlusion of the internal carotid artery. Thrombolysis has been reported in association with local angioplasty (87,88) and for treatment of thrombotic complications of endarterectomy (89,90). High-dose local intraarterial therapy has been reported in the setting of acute vertebrobasilar occlusion (91).

COLLATERAL BLOOD SUPPLY AND RECANALIZATION

Studies of thrombolytic therapy that have required cerebral angiography have confirmed a longstanding supposition that collateral circulation is an important determinant of cerebral infarction. Von Kummer and colleagues (92), after recently analyzing their own patients and those reported by others, concluded that the state of collateral circulation was a more important determinant of outcome than accomplishing (or not accomplishing) arterial recanalization. The patient with acute occlusion of the middle cerebral artery stem with poor collaterals may be destined for a large cerebral infarction, even if arterial recanalization were to be accomplished very early, perhaps even within 90–120 minutes. The same patient with good collaterals would have the potential for beneficial arterial recanalization for 6 hours or longer. Ringelstein and colleagues (93) have stated that ''perhaps the extent of the leptomeningeal blood supply defines the temporal width of the therapeutic window.'' In the patient with good collaterals, drugs that provide neuronal protection may complement treatments based on arterial recanalization. Thrombolysis combined with neuronal protection has already shown promise in the laboratory and will likely be applied in clinical trials within the next decade.

SELECTED NEW THROMBOLYTIC AGENTS

A variety of new tissue plasminogen activators has been synthesized. TNK-rt-PA is an example of these agents. It has a 14-fold higher fibrin specificity than endogenous rt-PA, an eightfold slower clearance, and an 80-fold higher resistance to the principle inhibitor of endogenous rt-PA, PAI-1 (94). In a rabbit venous-shunt model, TNK-rt-PA achieved 50% lysis in one third the time required by endogenous rt-PA (94). It is now under investigation in patients with acute myocardial infarction. BM 06.022 is another recombinant plasminogen activator that has a threefold lower plasma clearance and a fivefold higher lytic potency in vitro than endogenous rt-PA (95,96). In preliminary studies carried out in patients with acute myocardial infarction, those treated with BM 06.022 had a trend toward a higher patency rate at 90 minutes and a lower 30-day mortality (96) compared with those treated with endogenous rt-PA. For stroke, an intravenous dose-finding BM 06.022 trial is about to begin in Europe.

A number of biological agents with antithrombotic or thrombolytic activity has generated interest in patients with stroke, including ancrod, hirudin, and recently Desmodus salivary plasminogen activator (DSPA) (an enzyme discovered in the saliva of the vampire bat, *Desmodus rotundus*) (97–99). DSPA is more dependent on fibrin cofactor than endogenous rt-PA. In a dog coronary thrombosis model, DSPA was found to be superior to rt-PA with regard to clot lysis and reocclusion (98). DSPA had a half-life of 195 minutes compared with that of 5 minutes for endogenous rt-PA.

Clearly, improved thrombolytic agents are needed for use in treatment of stroke. With myocardial infarction, the current agents offer good to excellent lysis rates and a high degree of safety. Patient outcomes, including mortality, are improved. With stroke, lysis rates are too low with intravenous therapy and too long with local intraarterial therapy. Complication rates are also high. Whether or not an agent can be developed that combines increased lytic potency without increased risk for bleeding remains to be established.

CONCLUSIONS

The time to recanalize an occluded vessel and the adequacy of collateral blood supply prior to recanalization are the key factors determining the success of thrombolytic therapy. Major questions regarding thrombolytic therapy for stroke remain unresolved. Efficacy has not been established for either intravenous or local intraarterial therapy. The best agent for intravenous or local intraarterial therapy has not yet been established. Intravenous streptokinase in high doses is unsafe when used in stroke patients beyond three hours after symptom onset. Potential theoretical advantages of pro-urokinase or any of the newer plasminogen activators under development must be established in clinical trials. The best route of delivery for thrombolytic agents administered for stroke has not been determined. The advantages of early treatment afforded by intravenous thrombolytic therapy won out in the setting of acute myocardial infarction; intraarterial therapy has been largely abandoned. With stroke, recanalization rates are low following intravenous therapy. For intraarterial therapy, the delays in treatment delivery and arterial recanalization are formidable, and the availability of neurointerventional teams is extremely limited. If intraarterial therapy is shown to be effective and to improve patient outcome, then expanded availability of neurointerventional capabilities could be accomplished. Such availability has already been accomplished for treatment of myocardial infarction. An optimal dose regimen has not been established for any of the agents, for either the intravenous or local intraarterial delivery strategy.

Which stroke patients are most likely to respond to thrombolytic therapy? Critics of the inclusive symptom-based intravenous trials have objected to lumping the various stroke subtypes rather than attempting to tease out those with the arterial occlusions most likely to benefit from thrombolysis. An alternative view is that our knowledge is rudimentary concerning which patients are most likely to benefit from thrombolytic therapy. For example, the patients thought during the 1980s to be ideal for thrombolytic therapy—those with large-vessel acute thrombi—may have clots too large for lysis with intravenous drugs. The patients thought previously to be poor candidates for thrombolysis, such as those with small clots or even lacunar syndromes, may benefit.

A fundamental problem with thrombolytic therapy for stroke continues to be the occurrence of treatment-related intracerebral hemorrhage. For intravenous thrombolytic therapy, analysis of the results from the randomized trials should allow clarification of which patients are at greatest risk and perhaps which patients should not receive thrombolytic therapy.

REFERENCES

1. Clarke RL, Clifton E. The treatment of cerebrovascular thromboses and embolism with fibrinolytic agents. *Am J Cardiol* 1960;6:546–551.
2. Herndon RM, Meyer JS, Johnson JF. Fibrinolysin therapy in thrombotic diseases of the nervous system. *J Mich State Med Soc* 1960;59: 1684–1692.
3. Meyer JS, Gilroy J, Barnhart MI, Johnson JF. Anticoagulants plus streptokinase therapy in progressive stroke. *JAMA* 1964;189:373.
4. Meyer JS, Gilroy J, Barnhart MI, Johnson JF. Therapeutic thrombolysis in cerebral thromboembolism. *Neurology* 1963;13:927–937.
5. Fletcher AP, Alkjersig N, Lewis M, et al. A pilot study of urokinase therapy in cerebral infarction. *Stroke* 1976;7:135–142.

6. Fears R. Biochemical pharmacology and therapeutic aspects of thrombolytic agents. *Pharmacol Rev* 1990;42:202–222.

7. Larcan A, Laprevote-Heully MC, Lambert H, et al. Indications des thrombolytiques au cours des accidents vasculaires cerebraux thrombosants traites par ailleurs par O.H.B. (2ATA). *Therapie* 1977;32: 259–270.

8. Sherry S. Thrombolytic therapy for noncoronary diseases. *Ann Emerg Med* 1991;20:396–404.

9. Levine MN. Bolus, front-loaded, and accelerated thrombolytic infusions for myocardial infarction and pulmonary embolism. *Chest* 1991; 99:128S–134S.

10. A Cooperative Study. Urokinase-streptokinase embolism trial. Phase 2 results. *JAMA* 1974;229:1606–1613.

11. Sharma GVRK, Burleson V, Sasahara A. Effect of thrombolytic therapy on pulmonary-capillary blood volume in patients with pulmonary embolism. *N Engl J Med* 1980;303:842–845.

12. Verstraete M, Bleifeld W, Brower RW, et al. Double-blind randomized trial of intravenous tissue-type plasminogen activator versus placebo in acute myocardial infarction. *Lancet* 1985;2:965–969.

13. Verstraete M, Bernard R, Bory M, et al. Randomized trial of intravenous recombinant tissue-type plasminogen activator versus intravenous streptokinase in acute myocardial infarction. *Lancet* 1985;1:842–847.

14. The TIMI Study Group. The thrombolysis in myocardial infarction (TIMI) trial: Phase I findings. *N Engl J Med* 1985;312:932–936.

15. Yusuf S, Collins R, Peto R, et al. Intravenous and intracoronary fibrinolytic therapy in acute myocardial infarction: Overview of results on mortality, reinfarction and side-effects from 33 randomized controlled trials. *Eur Heart J* 1985;6:556–585.

16. Khaja F, Walton J, Brymer J, et al. Intracoronary fibrinolytic therapy in acute myocardial infarction. *N Engl J Med* 1983;308:1305–1311.

17. Collen D, Topol E, Tiefenbrunn A, et al. Coronary thrombolysis with recombinant human tissue-type plasminogen activator: A prospective, randomized, placebo-controlled trial. *Circulation* 1984;70:1012–1017.

18. Gruppo Italiano per Lo Studio Della Streptochinasi Nell Infarto Miocardico (GISSI). Effectiveness of intravenous thrombolytic treatment in acute myocardial infarction. *Lancet* 1986;1:397–401.

19. Chesebro JH, Knatterud G, Roberts R, et al. Thrombolysis in myocardial infarction (TIMI) trial, phase I: A comparison between intravenous tissue plasminogen activator and intravenous streptokinase. *Circulation* 1987;76:142–154.

20. Wilcox RG, Von Der Lippe G, Olsson CG, Jensen G, Skene AM, Hampton JR. Trial of tissue plasminogen activator for mortality reduction in acute myocardial infarction. *Lancet* 1988;2:525–530.

21. Adams HP, Olinger CP, Barsan WG, et al. A dose-escalation study of large doses of naloxone for treatment of patients with acute cerebral ischemia. *Stroke* 1986;17:404–409.

22. Gelmers H, Gorter K, DeWeerdt CJ, Wiezer HJA. A controlled trial of nimodipine in acute ischemic stroke. *N Engl J Med* 1988;318:208–207.

23. Zeumer H, Freitag HJ, Grzyska V, et al. Interventional neuroradiology: Local intra-arterial fibrinolysis in acute vertebrobasilar thromboembolic disease. *Am J Neuroradiol* 1983;4:401–404.

24. Henze T, Boerr A, Tebbe U, et al. Lysis of basilar artery occlusion with tissue plasminogen activator (letter). *Lancet* 1987;2:1391.

25. Jafar JJ, Tan WS, Crowell RM. Tissue plasminogen activator thrombolysis of a middle cerebral artery embolus in a patient with an arteriovenous malformation. *J Neurosurg* 1991;74:808–812.

26. Kaufman HH, Lind TA, Clark DS. Non-penetrating trauma to the carotid artery with secondary thrombosis and embolism: Treatment by thrombolysin. *Acta Neurochir (Wien)* 1977;37:219–244.

27. Nenci GG, Gresele P, Taramelli M, Agnelli G Signorini E. Thrombolytic therapy for thromboembolism of vertebrobasilar artery. *Angiology* 1983;34:361–571.

28. Zeumer H, Hacke W, Kolmann HL, Poeck K. Lokale fibrinolysetherapie bei basilaris-thrombose. *Deutsche Med Wochenschr* 1982;107: 728–731.

29. Zeumer H, Ferbert A, Ringelstein EB. Local intra-arterial fibrinolytic therapy in inaccessible internal carotid occlusion. *Neuroradiology* 1984;26:315–317.

30. Jungreis CA, Wechsler LR, Horton JA. Intracranial thrombolysis via a catheter embedded in the clot. *Stroke* 1989;20:1578–1580.

31. Haley EC Jr, Levy DE, Brott TG, et al. Urgent therapy for stroke. Part II. Pilot study of tissue plasminogen activator administered 91–180 minutes from onset. *Stroke* 1992;23:641–645.

32. Brott TG, Haley EC Jr, Levy DE, et al. Urgent therapy for stroke. Part

I. Pilot study of tissue plasminogen activator administered within 90 minutes. *Stroke* 1992;23:632–640.

33. von Kummer R, Forsting M, Hacke W, Sartor K. Recanalization, infarct volume, cerebral hemorrhage, and clinical outcome after intravenous recombinant tissue plasminogen activator and heparin in acute carotid territory stroke. In: del Zoppo GJ, Mori E, Hacke W, eds. *Thrombolytic Therapy in Acute Ischemic Stroke II.* Berlin Heidelberg: Springer-Verlag, 1993:53–58.

34. Mori E, Yoneda Y, Tabuchi M, et al. Intravenous recombinant tissue plasminogen activator in acute carotid artery territory stroke. *Neurology* 1992;42:976–982.

35. del Zoppo GJ, Poeck K, Pessin MS, et al. Recombinant tissue plasminogen activator in acute thrombotic and embolic stroke. *Ann Neurol* 1992; 32:78–86.

36. Centeno RS, Hackney DB, Rothrock JR. Streptokinase clot lysis in acute occlusions of the cranial circulation: Study in rabbits. *Am J Neuroradiol* 1985;6:589–594.

37. Zivin JA, Lyden PD, DeGirolami U, et al. Tissue plasminogen activator reduction of neurologic damage after experimental embolic stroke. *Arch Neurol* 1988;45:387–391.

38. DeLey G, Weyne J, Demeester G, et al. Experimental thromboembolic stroke studied by positron emission tomography: Immediate versus delayed reperfusion by fibrinolysis. *J Cereb Blood Flow Metab* 1988; 8:539–545.

39. Clark WM, Madden KP, Zivin JA, Lyden PD, Sasse KC. Intracerebral hemorrhage: tPA versus streptokinase thrombolytic therapy. *Neurology* 1989;39(suppl 1):183.

40. Hirschberg M, Hofferberth B. Thrombolytic therapy with urokinase and pro-urokinase in a canine model of acute stroke. *Neurology* 1987; 37(suppl 1):132.

41. Hirschberg M, Korves M, Koc I, Hofferberth B, Wiesmann W. Untersuchungen zur Thrombolyse zerebraler Thrombembolien mittels urokinase an einem Tiermodell. *Schweiz Med Wochenschr* 1987;117: 1811–1813.

42. Zivin JA, Fisher M, DeGirolami U, Hemenway CC, Stashak JA. Tissue plasminogen activator reduces neurological damage after cerebral embolism. *Science* 1985;330:1289–1292.

43. del Zoppo GJ, Copeland BR, Waltz TA, Zyroff J, Plow EF, Harker LA. The beneficial effect of intracarotid urokinase on acute stroke in a baboon model. *Stroke* 1986;17:638–643.

44. Slivka A, Pulsinelli W. Hemorrhagic complications of thrombolytic therapy in experimental stroke. *Stroke* 1987;18:1148–1156.

45. Dujovny M, Vasquez M, Diaz FG, Ausman JI, Mirchandani HG, Berman SK. Anatomical basis for lenticulostriate microvascular surgery. *Stroke* 1987;18:292.

46. Alberts MJ for the rt-PA Acute Stroke Study Group. A safety and efficacy study of intravenous rt-PA in patients with acute stroke. In: del Zoppo GJ, Mori E, Hacke W, eds. *Thrombolytic Therapy in Acute Ischemic Stroke II.* Berlin Heidelberg: Springer-Verlag, 1993:45–52.

47. Wolpert SM, Bruckmann H, Greenlee R, Wechsler L, Pessin MS, del-Zoppo GJ for the rt-PA Acute Stroke Study Group. Neuroradiologic evaluation of patients with acute stroke treated with recombinant tissue plasminogen activator. *Am J Neuroradiol* 1993;14:3–13.

48. Fieschi C, Argentino C, Lenzi GL, Sacchetti ML, Toni D, Bozzao L. Clinical and instrumental evaluation of patients with ischemic stroke within the first six hours. *J Neuro Sci* 1989;92:311–322.

49. Masuda J, Yutani C, Ogata J, Kuriyama Y, Yamaguchi T. Atheromatous embolism in the brain: A clinicopathologic analysis of 15 autopsy cases. *Neurology* 1994;44:1231–1237.

50. Jang IK, Gold HK, Ziskind AA, et al. Differential sensitivity of erythrocyte-rich and platelet-rich arterial thrombi to lysis with recombinant tissue-type plasminogen activator. *Circulation* 1989;79:920–928.

51. Marder VJ, Hirsh J, Bell WR. Rationale and practical basis of thrombolytic therapy. In: Colman RW, Hirsh J, Marder VJ, Salzman EW, eds. *Hemostasis and Thrombosis: Basic Principles and Clinical Practice,* 3rd ed. Philadelphia: J.B. Lippincott, 1994:1514–1541.

52. Bernik MB, Kwaan HC. Plasminogen activator activity in cultures from human tissues. An immunological and histochemical study. *J Clin Invest* 1969;48:1740–1753.

53. White WF, Barlow GH, Mozen MM. The isolation and characterization of plasminogen activators (urokinase) from human urine. *Biochemistry* 1966;5:2160–2169.

54. Loscalzo J, Braunwald E. Tissue plasminogen activator. *N Engl J Med* 1988;319:925–931.

55. Hirsh, J, Salzman EW, Marder VJ, Colman RW. Overview of the thrombolytic process and its therapy. In: Colman RW, Hirsh J, Marder VJ, Salzman EW, eds. *Hemostasis and Thrombosis: Basic Principles and Clinical Practice*, 3rd ed. Philadelphia: J.B. Lippincott, 1994: 1151–1163.

56. Jorgensen HS, Sperling B, Nakayama H, Raaschou HO, Olsen TS. Spontaneous reperfusion of cerebral infarcts in patients with acute stroke. *Arch Neurol* 1994;51:865–873.

57. Irino T, Taneda M, Minami T. Angiographic manifestations in postrecanalized cerebral infarction. *Neurology* 1977;27:471–475.

58. Yamaguchi T, Hayakawa T, Kikuchi H for the Japanese Thrombolysis Study Group. Intravenous tissue plasminogen activator ameliorates the outcome of hyperacute embolic stroke. *Cerebrovasc Dis* 1993;3:269.

59. Huemer M, Niederwieser V, Ladurner G. Thrombolytic treatment for acute occlusion of the basilar artery. *J Neurol Neurosurg Psychiatry* 1995;58:227–228.

60. Haley EC Jr, Brott TG, Sheppard GL, et al for the tPA Bridging Study Group. Pilot randomized trial of tissue plasminogen activator in acute ischemic stroke. *Stroke* 1993;24:1000–1004.

61. Hommel M, Boissel JP, Comu C, et al for the MAST Study Group. Termination of trial of streptokinase in severe acute ischaemic stroke. *Lancet* 1994;315:57.

62. The MAST-I Collaborative Group. Thrombolytic and antithrombotic therapy in acute ischemic stroke. Multicenter acute stroke trial—Italy (MAST-I). In: del Zoppo GJ, Mori E, Hacke W, eds. *Thrombolytic Therapy in Acute Ischemic Stroke II*. Berlin Heidelberg: Springer-Verlag, 1993:86–94.

63. Roncagliona C. Multicenter Acute Stroke Trial—Italy (MAST-I): Poster presentation at 20th International Joint Conference on Stroke and Cerebral Circulation; February, 1995. *Stroke* 1995;26:163.

64. Donnan GA, Davis SM, Chambers BR, et al. Australian streptokinase trial (ASK). In: del Zoppo GJ, Mori E, Hacke W, eds. *Thrombolytic Therapy in Acute Ischemic Stroke II*. Berlin Heidelberg: Springer-Verlag, 1993:80–85.

65. Shahar E, McGovern P. Trials of streptokinase in severe acute ischaemic stroke. *Lancet* 1995;345:578–579.

66. Hacke W, Kaste M, Fieschi C for the ECASS Study Group. The efficacy of IV rt-PA in acute ischemic stroke: First results of the ECASS trial. *Stroke* 1995;26:167.

67. Kaste M, Hacke W, Fieschi C for the ECASS Study Group. ECASS: Safety data from the pilot study and the first 160 randomized patients. *Stroke* 1994;25:256.

68. Tilley BC for the NINDS tPA Stroke Trial Investigators. A Demming approach to recruiting: The National Institute of Neurological Diseases and Stroke (NINDS) tPA stroke trial experience. In: del Zoppo GJ, Mori E, Hacke W, eds. *Thrombolytic Therapy in Acute Ischemic Stroke II*. Berlin, Heidelberg: Springer-Verlag, 1993:282–284.

69. Davies SW, Ranjadayalan K, Wickens DG, Dormandy TL, Timmis AD. Lipid peroxidation associated with successful thrombolysis. *Lancet* 1990;335:741–743.

70. Koudstaal PJ, Stibbe J, Vermeulen M. Fatal ischaemic brain oedema after early thrombolysis with tissue plasminogen activator in acute stroke. *BMJ* 1988;297:1571–1574.

71. Zeumer H, Freitag HJ, Zanella F, Thie A, Arning C. Local intra-arterial fibrinolytic therapy in patients with stroke: Urokinase versus recombinant tissue plasminogen activator (rt-PA). *Neuroradiology* 1993;35: 159–162.

72. Ezura M, Kagawa S. Selective and superselective infusion of urokinase for embolic stroke. *Surg Neurol* 1992;38:353–358.

73. Wong MC, Htoo A. A pilot study of early angiography and intra-arterial streptokinase for acute ischemic stroke. *Neurology* 1993;43:A263.

74. Hacke W, Zeumer H, Ferbert A, Bruckmann H, del Zoppo GJ. Intra-arterial thrombolytic therapy improves outcome in patients with acute vertebrobasilar occlusive disease. *Stroke* 1988;19:1216–1222.

75. Casto L, Moschini L, Camerlingo M, et al. Local intra-arterial thrombolysis for acute stroke in the carotid artery territories. *Acta Neurol Scand* 1992;86:308–311.

76. Fletcher AP, Alkjaersig N, Lewis M, et al. A pilot study of urokinase therapy in cerebral infarction. *Stroke* 1976;7:135–142.

77. Mori E, Tabuchi M, Yoshida T, Yamadori A. Intracarotid urokinase with thromboembolic occlusion of the middle cerebral artery. *Stroke* 1988;19:802–812.

78. Hiramoto M, Yoshimizu N, Satoh K, Takamatsu S. Intra-arterial urokinase therapy in thromboembolic stroke. *Stroke* 1994;25:268.

79. Sasaki O, Takeuchi S, Koike T, Koizumi T, Tanaka R. Fibrinolytic therapy for acute embolic stroke: Intravenous, intracarotid, and intra-arterial local approaches. *Neurosurgery* 1995;36:246–253.

80. LaMonte MP, Hurst RW, Raps EC, et al. Selective intra-arterial thrombolysis for acute cerebral ischemia: A case-control comparison. *Neurology* 1995;45(suppl 4):A469.

81. Barnwell SL, Clark WM, Nguyen TT, O Neill OR, Wynn ML, Coull BM. Safety and efficacy of delayed intra-arterial urokinase therapy with mechanical clot disruption for thromboembolic stroke. *Am J Neuroradiol* 1994;15:1817–1822.

82. Higashida RT, Halbach VV, Barnwell SL, Dowd CF, Hieshima GB. Thrombolytic therapy for acute stroke. *J Endovasc Surg* 1994;1:4–15.

83. Torr SR, Nachowiak DA, Fujii S, Sobel BE. Plasminogen steal and clot lysis. *J Am Coll Cardiol* 1992;19:1085–1090.

84. Dehmer GJ, Gresalfi N, Daly D, Oberhardt B, Tate D. Impairment of fibrinolysis by streptokinase, urokinase and recombinant tissue-type plasminogen activator in the presence of radiographic contrast agents. *J Am Coll Cardiol* 1995;25:1069–1075.

85. Granger CB, Gabriel DA, Reese NS, et al. Fibrin modification by ionic and nonionic contrast media during cardiac catheterization. *Am J Cardiol* 1992;69:821–822.

86. Courtheoux P, Theron J, Derlon JM, Alachkar F, Casasco A. In situ fibrinolysis in supra-aortic main vessels. A preliminary study. *J Neuroradiol* 1986;13:111–124.

87. Tsai FY, Berberian B, Matovich V, Lavin M, Alfieri K. Percutaneous transluminal angioplasty adjunct to thrombolysis for acute middle cerebral artery rethrombosis. *Am J Neuroradiol* 1994;15:1823–1829.

88. Troughton AH, Morgan RA, Paxton RM, Wells IP. External carotid angioplasty in the treatment of developing stroke. *Br J Radiol* 1992; 65:825–827.

89. Morgan MK, Grinnell V, Little N, Day MJ Jr. Successful treatment of an acute thrombosis of an intracranial vertebral artery endarterectomy with urokinase. *Neurosurgery* 1994;35:978–981.

90. Barr J, Horowitz M, Mathis J, Sclabassi R, Yonas H. Intraoperative urokinase infusion for embolic stroke during carotid endarterectomy. *Neurosurgery* 1995;36:606–611.

91. Mayer TE, Bruckmann H, Mull M, Thron A. High dose local intra-arterial fibrinolytic therapy improves the outcome in acute vertebrobasilar occlusion. In: Huckman MS, ed. *Proceedings of the 33rd Annual Meeting of the American Society of Neuroradiology*. Published by American Society of Neuroradiology, Chicago, 1995:69.

92. von Kummer R, Holle R, Rosin L, Forsting M, Hacke W. Does arterial recanalization improve outcome in carotid territory stroke? *Stroke* 1995;26:581–587.

93. Ringelstein EB, Biniek R, Weiller C, Ammeling B, Nolte PN, Thron A. Type and extent of hemispheric brain infarctions and clinical outcome in early and delayed middle cerebral artery recanalization. *Neurology* 1992;42:289–298.

94. Paoni NF, Keyt BA, Refino CJ, et al. A slow clearing, fibrin-specific, PAI-1 resistant variant of tPA (T103N, KHRqR 296-299 AAAA). *Thromb Haemost* 1993;70:307–312.

95. Vermeer F, Bar F, Windeler J, Schenkel W. Saruplase, a new fibrin specific thrombolytic agent: Final results of the PASS study (1698 patients). *Circulation* 1993;88:I292.

96. Martin U, Sponer G, Strein K. Evaluation of thrombolytic and systemic effects of the novel recombinant plasminogen activator BM 06.022 compared with alteplase, anistreplase, streptokinase and urokinase in a canine model of coronary artery thrombosis. *J Am Coll Cardiol* 1992; 19:433–440.

97. Olinger CP, Brott TG, Barsan WG, et al. Use of Ancrod in acute or progressing ischemic cerebral infarction. *Ann Emerg Med* 1988;17: 1208–1209.

98. Witt W, Maass B, Baldus B, Hildebrand M, Donner P, Schleuning WD. Coronary thrombolysis with Desmodus salivary plasminogen activator in dogs. *Circulation* 1994;90:421–426.

99. Neuhaus KL, Essen R, Tebbe U, et al. Safety observations from the pilot phase of the randomized r-Hirudin for improvement of thrombolysis (HITT-III) study. A study of the Arbeitsgemeinschaft Leitender Kardiologischer Krankenhausarzte (ALKK). *Circulation* 1994;90: 1638–1642.

Cerebrovascular Disease, edited by H. Hunt Batjer.
Lippincott-Raven Publishers, Philadelphia © 1997.

CHAPTER 44

Intracranial Angioplasty: Current Use, Limitations, Future Implications

Cameron G. McDougall, Randall T. Higashida, Van V. Halbach, Christopher F. Dowd, Donald W. Larsen, and Grant B. Hieshima

This chapter reviews recent experience with intracranial percutaneous transluminal angioplasty (PTA). The discussion comprises two parts: firstly, PTA treatment of occlusive cerebrovascular disease and secondly, of vasospasm after subarachnoid hemorrhage.

ANGIOPLASTY FOR OCCLUSIVE CEREBROVASCULAR DISEASE

PTA for symptomatic cerebrovascular lesions is being performed with increasing frequency in highly selected cases. The initial techniques of transluminal angioplasty were first reported in 1964 by Dotter and Judkins (1). Since then, studies have shown that angioplasty can increase blood flow in the renal, femoral, iliac, distal peripheral, and coronary arteries, as well as in the aorta (2–6). In the early 1980s, the initial reports describing PTA for brachiocephalic vessels were published (7–11). Sundt et al (12) described the direct operative exposure of the vertebral artery at the C-1 level followed by insertion of a balloon coronary angioplasty catheter and dilation of a basilar artery stenosis. The study of PTA for cerebral vessels has lagged behind that for other vessels because of technical problems, including difficulty of access to the affected areas and the potential complication of stroke secondary to the embolization of debris from the angioplasty site. Intracranial PTA is inherently more difficult than peripheral angioplasty because of the smaller size and greater tortuosity of the vessels being treated, as well as the presence of critical perforating blood vessels. Although cerebral PTA is still under investigation, preliminary reports by Theron, Tsai, Higashida, and others (13–16) have demonstrated the safety, efficacy, and long-term success that angio-

plasty may provide in alleviating or preventing further symptoms of cerebral ischemia and stroke. Currently, prospective multicenter studies of the efficacy and safety of cerebral PTA are underway in North America and Europe (17).

Patients are being treated by PTA techniques for critically significant, symptomatic stenosis of the innominate, subclavian, vertebral, basilar, and internal and external carotid arteries. During the past several years, the more distal lesions involving the intracranial internal carotid, distal vertebral, and basilar arteries have been treated due to improvements in microballoon and guidewire technology. Other key reasons for the extension of angioplasty techniques include high-resolution radiographic imaging, proper neurologic monitoring, and careful patient selection. Rapid diagnosis and the start of appropriate therapy are critical in patients with cerebral ischemia in order to reduce injury of brain tissue. Just as the use of thrombolysis, angioplasty, and surgery to revascularize ischemic myocardium in patients with heart attacks has evolved in the past decade, so too must the use of similar rapid treatment for cerebral ischemia caused by "brain attacks." Education of the general population about the signs and symptoms of an acute stroke, transient cerebral ischemia, and acute cerebral hemorrhage is required, so that patients will recognize these problems and seek immediate treatment. Intervening before irreversible damage to brain tissue occurs will optimize the benefits of revascularization therapy.

Indications for Angioplasty

PTA is currently indicated in symptomatic patients with >70% stenosis of the intracranial arteries (internal carotid, anterior and middle cerebral, vertebral, and basilar) who are unresponsive to medical therapy and not considered surgical candidates. The vast majority of these patients will have

All authors: Department of Radiology, University of California, San Francisco Medical Center, San Francisco, California 94143.

stenoses due to atherosclerosis. Other pathologic entities may include acute arterial dissections, postradiation stenosis, arteritis, and fibromuscular dysplasia. These patients should have signs and symptoms of stroke or have experienced reversible neurologic deficits attributable to thromboemboli or cerebral ischemia. Patients whose signs and symptoms are stable and not progressing should initially be treated by standard medical therapies. These patients should have maximal medical therapy including administration of antiplatelet medications, control of blood pressure, and systemic anticoagulation—with angioplasty being considered only if they fail to respond to conventional medical therapies (18,19). Conversely, patients with stroke in evolution, crescendo cerebral ischemia, and acute arterial occlusion require more emergent therapeutic measures.

PTA Technique

The initial diagnostic evaluation should include computed tomography (CT) or magnetic resonance imaging (MRI) of the brain to determine whether the signs and symptoms are due to ischemia or to a completed stroke, the extent of brain injury, the vessels involved, and the presence or absence of recent cerebral hemorrhage (20,21). In appropriate cases, cerebral angiography is required to determine the degree of vascular stenosis and the presence of intraluminal thrombus, as well as to assess distal perfusion, occlusion of distal branches, and collateral blood flow. Rapid-sequence digital subtraction angiography is used to qualitatively assess blood flow distal to the stenosis before and after treatment. Other ancillary imaging studies may include nuclear medicine perfusion blood flow studies, Doppler ultrasound imaging, MR angiography (MRA), and three-dimensional CT of the cervical vessels.

PTA is usually performed via a transfemoral arterial approach, with mild sedation of the patient and local anesthesia at the puncture site. After angiographic documentation of a critical stenosis >70%, patients should be fully anticoagulated. A soft-tipped guidewire is then navigated across the zone of stenosis and advanced into the distal arterial segment. The proper balloon diameter is then selected for angioplasty (Fig. 1). In general, we choose a PTA balloon that matches the normal luminal diameter of the vessel just proximal or distal to the stenosis. To avoid rupture or damage of the vessels, the vessel size must be determined with corrected magnification using high-resolution angiography.

The balloon should have a minimum-rated burst pressure of 6–8 atm. While extracranial lesions, such as those of the innominate artery, may require a balloon as large as 8–12 mm in diameter, much smaller balloons, 2.0–5.0 mm in diameter, are required for intracranial vessels.

Once the balloon is guided over the wire and across the lesion, it is inflated to the maximum-rated burst pressure for 10–30 seconds. Dilatation of the lesion should be detected as the "waist" of the balloon expands. Long periods of inflation should be avoided to prevent further ischemia in already compromised vascular territories. Some vessels require more than one dilatation, and in cases in which significant opening is not achieved, a larger balloon diameter, up to a maximum of 120% of the normal luminal diameter may be required.

Patients presenting with symptoms of focal acute cerebral ischemia who are found to have a documented stenosis with intraluminal thrombus are now being treated with a combination of intraarterial thrombolysis and angioplasty of the underlying lesion (22). A microcatheter is navigated into the intraluminal thrombus and boluses of urokinase 25,000–50,000 IU are infused every 5–10 minutes to a maxi-

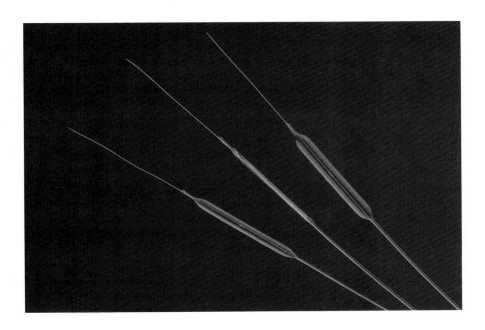

FIG. 1. Angioplasty balloons used for treating atherosclerotic lesions. These balloons are available in sizes ranging from 2.0 to 8.0 mm in diameter when inflated. The balloons are introduced over soft guidewires. (Courtesy of Cordis Endovascular Systems Inc., Miami Lakes, Florida, USA.)

mum dose of 2 million IU over 2–4 hours (23). If an underlying stenosis is identified, angioplasty may be performed to prevent reocclusion. These patients must be treated within a few hours of the onset of symptoms to minimize the amount of irreversible ischemic neuronal death and to reduce the risk of hemorrhagic transformation due to reperfusion of infarcted brain (24).

After the angioplasty procedure, patients should be monitored in a neurologic observation unit for at least 24 hours. If there is angiographic evidence that patency has improved to >60–70% without significant arterial dissection or thromboemboli, patients may be discharged on antiplatelet medications (eg, aspirin or dipyridamole) for a minimum of 6 months. If residual stenosis >50% is present or if significant arterial dissection or thromboemboli are present, then systemic anticoagulation should be maintained and follow-up angiography performed at 4–6 weeks to reassess the treated site.

Clinical and radiographic follow-up is performed at 1–3 and 6–12 months to assess long-term results of the angioplasty procedure. Radiographic assessment includes angiography and may include combinations of CT, MRI, MRA, and/or Doppler ultrasound.

Effect of Angioplasty

The mechanism for dilatation of intracranial vessels with atherosclerosis is similar to that of other lesions treated with this technique. The balloon mechanically dilates and fractures the hard plaque, compressing it against the intima and media (25,26). After PTA, the angiogram often shows vessel irregularity, subintimal hemorrhage, and fissuring of the plaque. Histologic examination frequently shows desquamation of the superficial plaque elements and dehiscence of the intima and media. Over time, platelets are deposited in the area of the traumatized vessel, and a new layer of endothelium develops. Eventually, there is further healing with retraction of the intimal flaps. With the formation of neointima, this usually results in a more even and regular surface, a finding often noted when follow-up angiography is performed 3–12 months after the procedure.

Representative Cases

Vertebrobasilar Stenosis

A 58-year-old professor of nursing with hypertension presented with new-onset vertigo, slurred speech, and right-arm ataxia. She was subsequently found to have an infarct of the right cerebellar peduncle. Investigations revealed a complete occlusion of the left vertebral artery as well as a high-grade stenosis of the right vertebrobasilar junction (Fig. 2A,B). She was initially treated with anticoagulation, but because of the severity of the stenosis and lack of adequate collateral supply, it was felt that angioplasty was a reasonable treatment for this individual. A 2.5-mm Stealth balloon (Target Therapeutics, Fremont, CA) was used to treat the high-grade stenosis, resulting in a dramatic improvement in posterior fossa circulation (Fig. 2C,D). The patient's in-hospital course was uncomplicated, and she was discharged home on oral anticoagulants 4 days after the treatment. At 6-month follow-up, the presenting symptoms had largely resolved, and no further ischemic events had occurred.

Vertebral and Basilar Stenosis

A 63-year-old man presented with several episodes of posterior fossa ischemia, and MRI revealed two small cerebellar infarcts on the right, as well as a pontine infarct on the left. Angiography revealed tandem stenoses involving the distal left vertebral artery and the proximal basilar artery (Fig. 3A,B). The right vertebral artery ended as the posteroinferior cerebellar artery. He was initially treated with intravenous anticoagulation, but on two occasions attempts to convert his intravenous anticoagulant medications to oral therapy resulted in worsening of his symptoms (dysarthria, diplopia, altered mental status, and vertigo). Fortunately, his symptoms improved upon resumption of intravenous heparin therapy. The patient was transferred emergently for angioplasty, but because of a severely tortuous vertebral artery, catheterization of the intracranial vertebral artery was not possible. Ultimately, repeated attempts resulted in dissection, but not occlusion, of the left vertebral artery. Subsequently, surgical exposure of the origin of the left vertebral artery was carried out, and a large loop of this vessel was resected. After this, access could be obtained to the vertebral artery, but only through a left axillary approach. Successful angioplasty was then achieved using a 3-mm Stealth balloon (Fig. 3C,D). The patient ultimately did well, suffering no new neurologic events as a result of treatment and at the time of discharge had only mild residual diplopia and right-arm drift. Follow-up angiography 3 months after the procedure revealed continued patency of the treated lesions, with no recurrent stenosis.

Internal Carotid Artery Stenosis

A hypertensive 81-year-old woman presented with a series of sudden events over a period of 3 days, resulting in a stepwise worsening of speech and right-arm weakness. In retrospect, her family had noted a prior episode of aphasia and right-arm weakness 2 months earlier, but she had made a near-complete recovery from that episode. On examination, she was found to have a marked, predominantly expressive aphasia and a marked paresis, but not plegia of the right arm. CT scan showed a small area of infarction of indeterminate age in the left frontal lobe. This was felt to be consistent with the history of an earlier stroke. No areas of hemorrhage were seen. Subsequent angiography revealed a severe stenosis of the petrous portion of the left internal

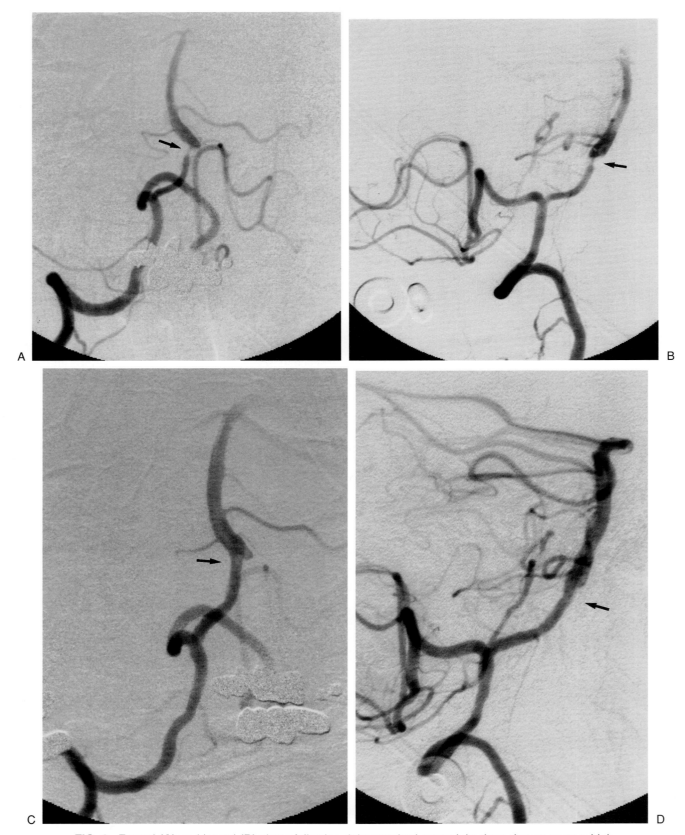

FIG. 2. Frontal **(A)** and lateral **(B)** views following right vertebral artery injections demonstrate a high-grade stenosis at the vertebrobasilar junction *(arrows)*. One-centimeter metallic markers are used to estimate the size of arteries to be treated. The left vertebral artery was occluded at its origin. Postangioplasty, images in the frontal **(C)** and lateral **(D)** projections demonstrate a marked improvement in posterior fossa perfusion with no significant residual stenosis at the angioplasty site *(arrows)*.

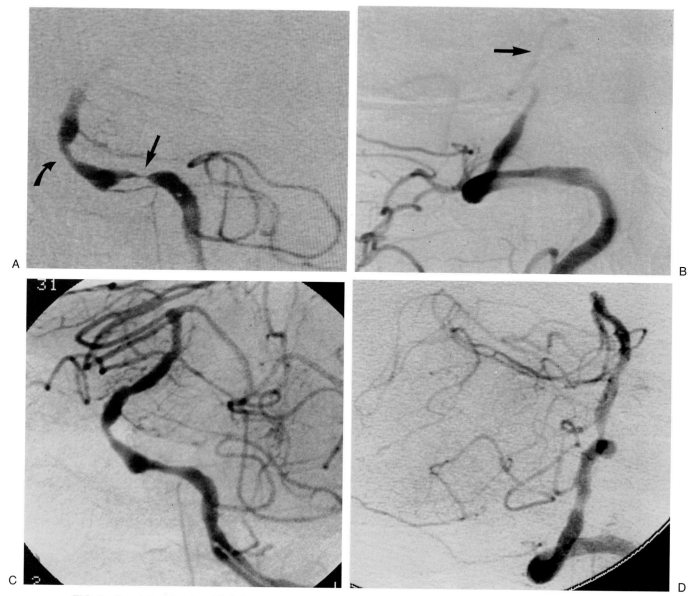

FIG. 3. Frontal projection **(A)** following a left vertebral artery injection shows tandem intracranial stenoses involving the vertebral artery *(straight arrow)* and the vertebrobasilar junction *(curved arrow)*. There is poor flow of contrast distally, with failure to opacify the distal basilar artery. The stenoses are not well seen on the lateral projection **(B)**; however, a trace of opacification of the distal basilar artery can bee seen *(arrow)*. After angioplasty of the more proximal (vertebral) lesion *(arrow)*, the posterior fossa perfusion is much improved. Frontal **(C)** and lateral **(D)** projections.

carotid artery (Fig. 4A,B). Because of the clear history of a rapidly deteriorating neurologic state, angioplasty of this lesion was carried out. The procedure was done using a 0.014-inch guidewire to cross the lesion and a Stealth balloon system. The balloon measured 4 mm in diameter and 20 mm in length. An excellent angiographic result was obtained (Fig. 4C,D). The patient was maintained on anticoagulants following the procedure, with a plan to taper and discontinue the anticoagulants after 24–48 hours. Unfortunately, several hours after the angioplasty she suffered a left temporal lobe hemorrhage that ultimately resulted in her death.

Vertebral Artery Stenosis

A 58-year-old man presented with several brief episodes of mild vertigo followed by two episodes of severe vertigo, diplopia , and right-sided weakness. Past history was significant for coronary artery stenosis treated on two occasions by angioplasty. After MRI evaluation at an outside institution failed to show any cerebral infarction or hemorrhage, he was started on anticoagulant therapy. Approximately 2 weeks later, while still on anticoagulant therapy, he experienced a further transient episode of vertigo, diplopia, and

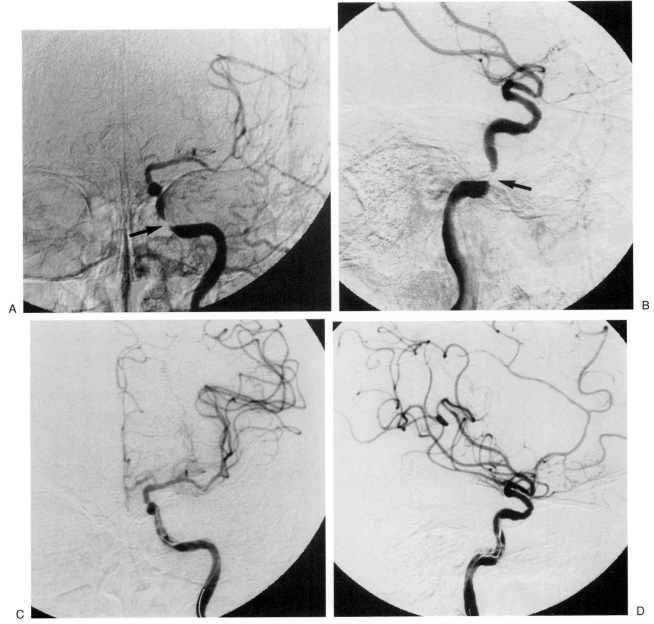

FIG. 4. Left internal carotid artery injections in the frontal **(A)** and lateral **(B)** projections show pin-hole stenosis of the petrous portion of the internal carotid artery *(arrows)*. Poor distal perfusion is apparent. After angioplasty, frontal **(C)** and lateral **(D)** views demonstrate marked improvement both in the caliber of the previously stenosed segment and in the distal intracranial circulation. These postangioplasty images were obtained after deflation of the angioplasty balloon but before its removal.

on this occasion, left-sided weakness. CT scan at this time again showed no evidence of infarction or hemorrhage. Angiography was then carried out, revealing a high-grade stenosis of the left vertebral artery (Fig. 5A,B). It was also found that the right vertebral artery terminated in the posteroinferior cerebellar artery, with no connection to the basilar artery. Angioplasty was carried out first using a 2.5-mm balloon, but as the stenosis did not appear to open adequately, a 3-mm balloon was then used. An excellent angio-

graphic result was achieved (Fig. 5C,D), with no further transient ischemic attacks to date.

Experience to Date

PTA for hemodynamically significant stenosis of the extracranial and intracranial cerebral circulation has been reported by numerous investigators in North America, Europe,

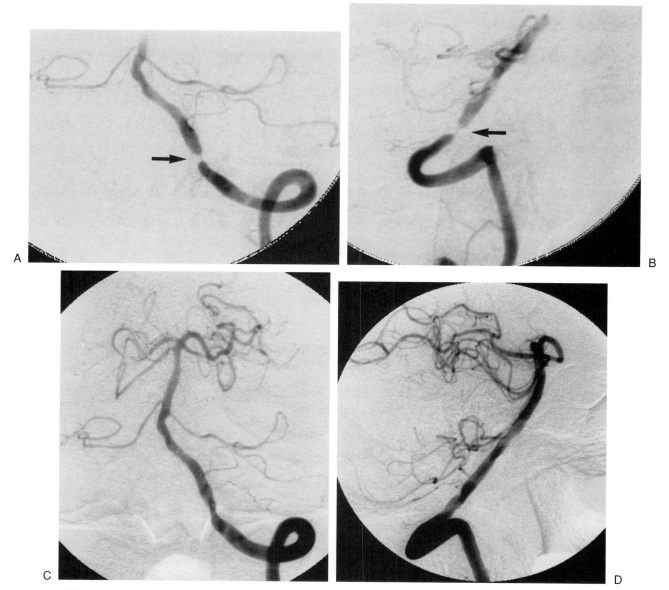

FIG. 5. Frontal **(A)** and lateral **(B)** views of a left vertebral artery injection show a high-grade stenosis *(arrows)* with poor filling distally. Post angioplasty frontal **(C)** and lateral **(D)** views show markedly improved flow through the area of former stenosis.

and Japan. The vast majority of these procedures have involved the extracranial circulation. Theron (13) in 1992 reported findings in 267 patients in whom brachiocephalic angioplasty was used successfully to treat stenosis of the carotid, innominate, subclavian, and vertebral arteries. The overall complication rate, including embolic stroke in three patients, was 5.3%. No deaths were reported. Ferguson et al (17) have reported preliminary results from the North American Cerebral PTA Register (NACPTAR). This was a multicenter study to determine the efficacy, safety, and clinical results of balloon angioplasty in patients with transient ischemic attacks. One hundred thirteen angioplasty procedures were done in 102 patients. Two patients died, eight

had strokes, and four had transient ischemia, for a total event rate of 14%.

Complications associated with angioplasty can include perforation, spasm, dissection, and occlusion of the treated vessel or thromboembolic events and occlusion of adjacent vessels. This may result in a worsening of the patient's signs and symptoms due to temporary occlusion during balloon inflation, or stroke and death. In the middle cerebral, distal vertebral, and basilar artery territories in particular, the potential complication rate is much higher because of the many perforating arteries leading to critical vascular territories of the cerebral cortex, brainstem, and upper cervical spinal cord. As softer, more compliant angioplasty balloons are developed specifically for use in intracranial vessels, the morbidity associated with these factors should decrease and the overall outcome improve.

Higashida et al (27) have reported the results of angioplasty in 325 cases treated since 1981. Patients ranged in age from 9 to 78 years. The underlying pathology was atherosclerosis in 95% of the cases and cerebral arteritis, fibromuscular dysplasia, acute arterial dissection, or intimal hyperplasia in the remaining 5%. Of these cases, 292 (90%) involved the extracranial cerebral circulation, with the remaining 33 cases involving intracranial stenoses.

Nine patients presented with an acute thromboembolic occlusion and were treated with a combination of intraarterial thrombolysis using urokinase followed by PTA of the underlying stenosis. This included the internal carotid artery in two cases, the middle cerebral artery in three cases, and the distal vertebral or basilar artery in four cases. Three patients had release of small thrombus emboli distally, resulting in small cortical strokes; however, their overall neurologic condition after clot lysis and angioplasty was greatly improved.

Three patients had iatrogenic arterial dissections at the time of the initial angioplasty, with acute occlusion or extravasation of contrast. The sites involved included the subclavian, internal carotid, and vertebral arteries. These patients were treated with intravascular stenting to avoid the need for emergency surgical intervention. No complications resulted from these three procedures.

Complications related to the procedure included 17 (5%) acute strokes. Eleven of these strokes were thromboembolic due to fragmentation of plaque, and six were caused by vessel rupture, dissection, or acute vessel closure. Four patients with stroke died as the result of cerebral infarction and edema. Of the four deaths, three involved either the distal vertebral or basilar artery region, and one involved the middle cerebral artery. All four of these patients had failed maximal medical treatment including antiplatelet and systemic anticoagulation therapy.

Twenty-three patients (7%) had symptoms of cerebral ischemia during or within 24 hours after the procedure. These patients were treated with continued systemic anticoagulation, volume expansion, and or antispasmodic agents, with resolution of symptoms. Follow-up has ranged from 6 months to 7 years. In 24 cases (7%), follow-up radiologic studies demonstrated restenosis at the angioplasty site.

Of the 292 patients in whom the extracranial cerebral circulation was involved, transient cerebral ischemic symptoms during the procedure occurred in 16 (5%) cases, restenosis in 21 (7%), and stroke in seven (2%). By comparison, PTA of the intracranial vessels accounted for only 33 of the 325 cases but resulted in ten cases of stroke. This results in a stroke rate of 30.3% if only the intracranial cases are considered. Four of these stroke complications ultimately resulted in death (12%). In addition, seven cases (21%) of transient cerebral ischemia and three cases (9%) of restenosis were observed.

The reported overall stoke and death rate of 6.4% compares favorably with that of other reported series. The much higher complication rate for the treatment of intracranial vessels must be carefully considered before such treatment is undertaken.

More recently, two other series have been reported (28,29). Clark et al (28) have reported a series of 17 patients with 22 intracranial atheromatous lesions treated by PTA. A good angiographic and clinical response was reported in 14 (82%) of the patients. One patient had no response to angioplasty, one had an increase in the degree of stenosis, and a third had a complete occlusion of the treated vessel. Two patients (12%) suffered a stroke, and with a mean clinical follow-up of 12 months, one patient had experienced recurrent transient ischemic attacks. Follow-up angiography at 3–10 months postprocedure was available for eight of the patients. Touho (29) reported a series of 19 patients with anterior circulation stenoses at or distal to the C-5 segment of the internal carotid artery. Angioplasty could not be carried out for technical reasons in six patients but was technically successful in 13 of the 19 (68%). Clinical improvement was noted in seven of the 13, but restenosis at follow-up angiography was seen in five of the 13 treated patients. Transient complications were reported in three patients, but no permanent neurologic worsening was seen. While these stroke rates are lower than that reported by Higashida et al (27), the risk remains sufficiently high that intracranial angioplasty can only be considered in the face of failure of more conservative measures.

Summary

The use of angioplasty for the treatment of intracranial lesions continues to evolve. Recent technological advances in imaging quality, as well as in catheter and balloon systems, have expanded the range of lesions that can be considered for treatment. Undoubtedly, further technical refinements will continue to improve both the safety and efficacy of these treatments. Combining angioplasty techniques with thrombolysis and intravascular stenting may soon yield significant advances in the management of acute, as well as chronic, occlusive cerebrovascular diseases.

To be successful, intervention in the acute phase will require considerable education of the general public, as well as health care professionals. The early recognition of symptoms of cerebrovascular disease, coupled with rapid assessment and treatment, has tremendous potential to lessen the enormous impact of this group of diseases on our society. The importance of abandoning the currently widespread nihilistic approach to stoke in favor of an early, aggressive, but individualized and appropriate response cannot be overstated.

For the present time, however, the many pitfalls involved in intracranial angioplasty limit its applicability to those patients who have failed maximal medical therapies and do not have viable surgical options for cerebral revascularization. The difficulties of access, arterial dissection, and thromboembolic complications, as well as the presence of critical perforating branches, are but a few of the problems that for the time being will continue to restrict the use of intracranial angioplasty. Much work remains not only to improve the safety and efficacy of intracranial angioplasty but to continue to define the appropriate role for angioplasty in the management of occlusive cerebrovascular disease.

ANGIOPLASTY FOR VASOSPASM AFTER SUBARACHNOID HEMORRHAGE

The use of intracranial angioplasty in post–subarachnoid hemorrhage treatment was first described by Zubkov et al (30) in 1984. First reports of experience with this technique in North America were published in 1986 by Hieshima et al (31), and further reports followed in 1989 by Barnwell, Higashida, Newell and their colleagues (32–34). Since then softer balloons have been developed, and the use of angioplasty for recalcitrant vasospasm has become widely accepted (35,36).

Indications for Angioplasty

Angioplasty is indicated for the treatment of symptomatic vasospasm that is not responsive to maximal medical therapies. A relative contraindication is acute cerebral infarction in the territories to be treated; however, successful treatment has been reported in patients with prolonged neurologic deterioration (>24 hours) or stroke (32).

In recent years, the management of vasospasm has evolved considerably. Many centers have moved to early definitive aneurysm treatment whenever possible. Once the aneurysm is secured, vasospasm may be treated with various combinations of ''triple H'' therapy, including hydration, hemodilution, and hypertensive therapies. Calcium channel antagonists, specifically nimodipine, have also become a standard adjunctive therapy. Unfortunately, despite these treatments, some patients will suffer neurologic deterioration as a result of vasospasm.

Technique of Angioplasty

When vasospasm is suspected as a cause of neurologic deterioration in a clinical setting, thorough but rapid evaluation and institution of treatment is essential. Other possible causes of neurologic deterioration must be considered and excluded. CT scan should be carried out to ensure that cerebral infarction has not occurred, as well as to rule out intracranial hemorrhage, hydrocephalus, and other causes of delayed neurologic deterioration. Transcranial Doppler ultrasonography (TCD) may be useful in the evaluation of vasospasm but should not delay angiographic assessment when clinical suspicion is strong (37). TCD may in fact be misleading, especially if baseline Doppler studies are not available for comparison. Unquestionably, angiography re-

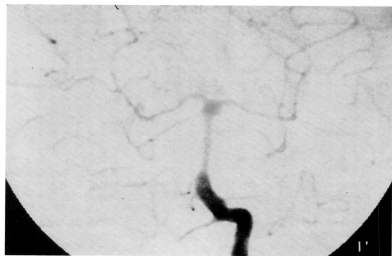
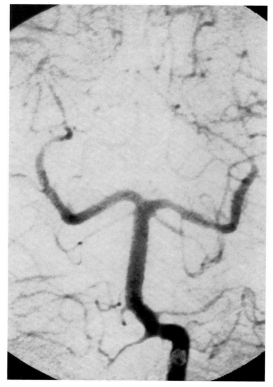

A

B

FIG. 6. A 76-year-old woman suffered two subarachnoid hemorrhages from a posterior fossa dural arteriovenous fistula. The fistula was cured by endovascular treatment, but she later became comatose and was found to have severe stenosis of the basilar artery. The vasospasm **(A)** was treated by angioplasty **(B)**, resulting in her regaining consciousness within hours of the treatment.

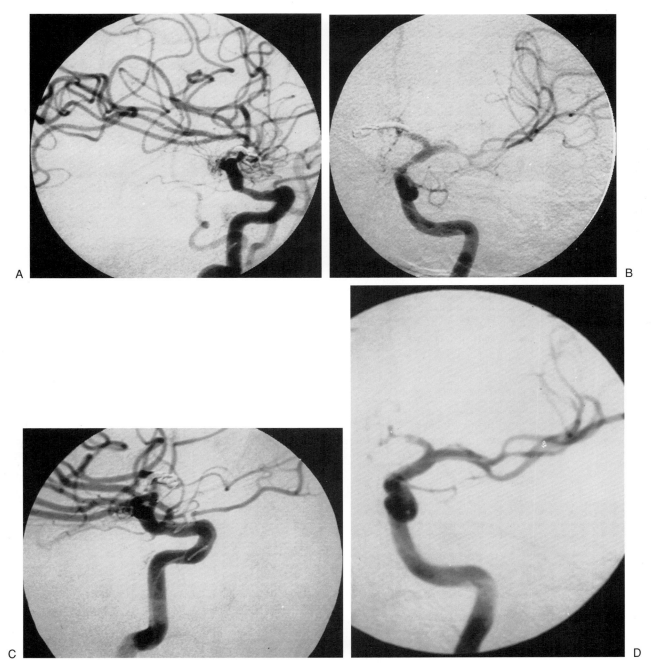

FIG. 7. A 47-year-old man with subarachnoid hemorrhage from an anterior communicating artery aneurysm was treated successfully by clipping of the aneurysm, but he went on to develop a right hemiparesis. Angiography showed vasospasm of the supraclinoid segment of the left internal carotid artery (**A**, *lateral view*), as well as vasospasm of the distal M1 and M2 segments of the left middle cerebral artery (**B**, *frontal view*). Angioplasty of the internal carotid artery (**C**) and of the M1 segment of the middle cerebral artery resulted in improvement of the hemiparesis. The M2 segment spasm was treated by intraarterial infusion of papaverine (**D**).

mains the gold-standard method of evaluation at the current time.

Only after the exclusion of other causes of neurologic deterioration and the failure of less invasive treatments (such as triple H) should angioplasty be considered. At this point,

if the symptoms have been present for less than 6 hours and angiographic studies confirm severe vasospasm in a vascular territory that corresponds to the clinical findings, angioplasty should be carried out. If more than 6 hours since the onset of symptoms has elapsed, the risk of causing a reperfusion hemorrhage into freshly infarcted tissue must be weighed against the potential benefits of angioplasty.

In the majority of cases, baseline angiography will be available. Comparison with these studies can be particularly useful in evaluating interval changes and differentiating between spastic and hypoplastic vessels. Angiographic evaluation is carried out before angioplasty, beginning with the territories considered most severely affected. After the selection of appropriate vessels to be treated, angioplasty is performed using a soft, compliant silicone balloon developed specifically for the treatment of vasospasm (Interventional Therapeutics, San Francisco, CA). This balloon is softer than that used for the angioplasty of atherosclerotic disease and is inflated using much lower inflation pressures. Inflation pressures are typically 0.5–2.0 atm. Silicone is used because of its softness and ability to conform to the shape of the artery lumen without exerting excessive pressure on the vessel wall.

The balloon is introduced through a larger transfemoral guide catheter and advanced from the cervical vessels intracranially, with gentle balloon inflation and deflation to flow-direct it to the appropriate locations. High-resolution digital subtraction angiography is required, as well as road-mapping capabilities. As spastic segments are encountered, the balloon is inflated more fully to treat the affected segment (Fig. 6). The balloon is then advanced to the next area to be treated, working sequentially from proximal to distal. Frequently, the predominant flow is to the middle cerebral artery and away from the anterior cerebral artery. Flow-directing the balloon to the A1 segment of the anterior cerebral artery is often not possible because of middle cerebral artery dominance. In this situation, as well as for the treatment of other territories where access is a problem, intraarterial papaverine has been used to treat vasospasm (38,39) (Fig. 7). While this has been a useful technique, the effect of papaverine does not appear to be as lasting as angioplasty, and retreatment within 24 hours has been necessary in some instances.

Effect of Angioplasty

It is unclear why angioplasty for vasospasm is successful not only in reversing vasospasm but also in preventing it from recurring in the majority of cases. The mechanism of action is thought to be different from that of angioplasty for atherosclerosis. Histologic examination in animal studies has shown minimal disruption of the intima and media when a soft, compliant balloon and low balloon-inflation pressures were used (40,41). The somewhat irregular surface seen frequently after angioplasty for atherosclerosis is generally not seen after angioplasty for vasospasm. Honma et al (42) described postmortem findings in two patients who died 5 days after angioplasty. Findings included disruption of the endothelial layer, stretching and disruption of the smooth muscle cells in the media, and changes in the extracellular matrix,

specifically the types III and V collagen laid down following subarachnoid hemorrhage.

Experience to Date

Zubkov et al (30), in their pioneering article of 1984, reported the treatment of 33 patients involving 105 vessels. A good outcome was reported in most cases. Mayberg et al (43) reported 21 cases of acute spasm treated by angioplasty, with 15 (71%) showing clinical improvement after therapy. Takahashi et al (44) found good to excellent neurologic improvement, defined as an improvement of two neurologic grades on the Hunt and Hess neurologic scale, in 15 (68%) of 22 treated patients. Higashida et al (45) reported that 19 (68%) of 28 patients showed clinical improvement with angioplasty. By combining angioplasty with papaverine infusion, Kaku et al (39) found a clinical improvement in eight of ten treated patients.

Complications related to angioplasty for vasospasm include vessel rupture, stroke, and reperfusion hemorrhages. Death has been reported from vessel perforation when angioplasty was carried out adjacent to a recently clipped aneurysm (46).

Summary

At present, angioplasty is a useful technique for the treatment of refractory vasospasm following subarachnoid hemorrhage. While angioplasty is of major benefit for the majority of such patients, treatment is often limited by problems of access, particularly access to the anterior cerebral arteries and the more distal territories of both the middle and anterior cerebral arteries. This problem of access is partly overcome through the use of intraarterial papaverine, and it is anticipated that further refinements in catheter and balloon technology will allow easier access to all major vascular territories. Finally, it is hoped that continued progress in understanding the pathophysiology of vasospasm will lead to the development of less invasive methods for the prevention and treatment of cerebral vasospasm following subarachnoid hemorrhage.

REFERENCES

1. Dotter CT, Judkins MP. Transluminal treatment of arteriosclerotic obstruction: Description of a new technic and a preliminary report of its application. *Circulation* 1964;30:654–670.
2. Becker GJ, Katzen BT, Dake MD. Non-coronary angioplasty. *Radiology* 1989;170:921–940.
3. Gallino A, Mahler F, Probst P, Nachbur B. Percutaneous transluminal angioplasty of arteries of the lower limbs: 5-year follow up. *Circulation* 1984;70:619–623.
4. Miller SW. Percutaneous transluminal angioplasty of the coronary arteries. In: Athanasoulis CA, Pfister RC, Greene GE, Roberson GH, eds. *Interventional Radiology.* Philadelphia: W.B. Saunders, 1982: 322–325.
5. Klinge J, Mali WP, Puijlaert CB, Geyskes GG, Becking WB, Feldberg

MA. Percutaneous transluminal renal angioplasty: Initial and long-term results. *Radiology* 1989;171:501–506.

6. Athanasoulis CA. Bowel ischemia: Management with intra-arterial papaverine infusion and transluminal angioplasty. In: Athanasoulis CA, Pfister RC, Greene GE, Roberson GH, eds. *Interventional Radiology.* Philadelphia: W.B. Saunders, 1982:334–342.

7. Bockenheimer SA, Mathias K. Percutaneous transluminal angioplasty in arteriosclerotic internal carotid artery stenosis. *Am J Neuroradiol* 1983;4:791–792.

8. Tsai FY, Matovich V, Hieshima G, et al. Percutaneous transluminal angioplasty of the carotid artery. *Am J Neuroradiol* 1986;7:349–358.

9. Motarjeme A, Keifer JW, Zuska AJ. Percutaneous transluminal angioplasty of the brachiocephalic arteries. *AJR* 1982;138:457–462.

10. Courtheoux P, Tournade A, Theron J, et al. Transcutaneous angioplasty of vertebral artery atheromatous ostial stricture. *Neuroradiology* 1985;27:259–264.

11. Hodgins GW, Dutton JW. Subclavian and carotid angioplasty for Takayasu's arteritis. *Can Assoc Radiol J* 1982;33:205–207.

12. Sundt TM, Smith HC, Campbell JK, Vlietstra RE, Cucchiara RF, Stanson AW. Transluminal angioplasty for basilar artery stenosis. *Mayo Clin Proc* 1980;55:673–680.

13. Theron J. Angioplasty of brachiocephalic vessels. In: Vinuela V, Halbach VV, Dion JE, eds. *Interventional Neuroradiology: Endovascular Therapy of the Central Nervous System.* New York: Raven, 1992:167–180.

14. Tsai FY, Hieshima GB, Higashida RT. Percutaneous transluminal angioplasty for the treatment of stroke. In: Fisher M, ed. *Medical Therapy of Acute Stroke.* New York: Marcel Decker, 1989:203–239.

15. Higashida RT, Tsai FY, Halbach VV, et al. Transluminal angioplasty for atherosclerotic disease of the vertebral and basilar arteries. *J Neurosurg* 1993;78:192–198.

16. Higashida RT, Halbach VV, Tsai FY, Dowd CF, Hieshima GB. Interventional neurovascular techniques for cerebral revascularization in the treatment of stroke. *AJR* 1994;163:793–800.

17. Ferguson R, Ferguson J, Schwarten D, et al. Immediate angiographic results and in-hospital central nervous system complications of cerebral percutaneous transluminal angioplasty (CPTA) (abstract). *Circulation* 1993;88:393.

18. Dyken ML. Anticoagulation and platelet anti-aggregating therapy in stroke and threatened stroke: Symposium on cerebrovascular disease. *Neurol Clin* 1983;1:223–242.

19. Weksler BB, Lewin ML. Anticoagulation in cerebral ischemia. *Stroke* 1983;14:658–663.

20. Wall SD, Brant-Zawadzki M, Jeffrey RB, Barnes B. High-frequency CT findings within 24 hours after cerebral infarction. *AJR* 1983;138:307–311.

21. Yuh WTC, Crain MR, Loes DJ, Greene GM, Ryals TJ, Sato Y. MR imaging of cerebral ischemia: Findings in the first 24 hours. *Am J Neuroradiol* 1991;12:621–629.

22. Tsai FY, Berberian B, Matovich V, Lavin M, Alfieri K. Percutaneous transluminal angioplasty adjunct to thrombolysis for acute middle cerebral artery rethrombosis. *Am J Neuroradiol* 1994;15:1823–1829.

23. Higashida RT, Halbach VV, Barnwell SL, Dowd CF, Hieshima GB. Thrombolytic therapy in acute stroke. *J Endovasc Surg* 1994;1:4–15.

24. Molinari GF. Pathogenesis of secondary brain hemorrhage after ischemia: Lessons from animal models . . . and a few from man too. In: del Zoppo GJ, Mori E, Hacke W, eds. *Thrombolytic Therapy in Acute Ischemic Stroke III.* New York: Springer-Verlag, 1993:29–36.

25. Castaneda-Zuniga WR, Formanek A, Tadavarthy M, et al. The mechanism of balloon angioplasty. *Radiology* 1980;135:565–571.

26. Block PC, Baughman KL, Pastenak RC, Fallon JT. Transluminal angioplasty: Correlation of morphologic and angiographic findings in an experimental model. *Circulation* 1980;61:778–785.

27. Higashida RT, Tsai FY, Halbach VV, et al. Angioplasty for the brachiocephalic and intracranial arteries. In: Proceeding of the 10th annual Endovascular Neurosurgical Society of Japan 1994:1–9.

28. Clark WM, Barnwell SL, Nesbit G, O'Neill OR, Wynn M, Coull BM. Safety and efficacy of percutaneous transluminal angioplasty for intracranial atherosclerotic stenosis. *Stroke* 1995;26:1200–1204.

29. Touho H. Percutaneous transluminal angioplasty in the treatment of atherosclerotic disease of the anterior cerebral circulation and hemodynamic evaluation. *J Neurosurg* 1995;82:953–960.

30. Zubkov YN, Nikiforov BM, Shustin VA. Balloon catheter technique for dilatation of constricted cerebral arteries after aneurysmal SAH. *Acta Neurochir (Wien)* 1984;70:665–679.

31. Hieshima GB, Higashida RT, Wapenski J, Halbach VV, Cahan L, Benston JR. Balloon embolization of a large distal basilar artery aneurysm. Case report. *J Neurosurg* 1986;65:413–416.

32. Barnwell SL, Higashida RT, Halbach VV, Dowd CF, Wilson CB, Hieshima GB. Transluminal angioplasty of intracerebral vessels for cerebral arterial spasm: Reversal of neurological deficits after delayed treatment. *Neurosurgery* 1989;25:424–429.

33. Higashida RT, Halbach VV, Cahan LD, et al. Transluminal angioplasty for treatment of intracranial arterial vasospasm. *J Neurosurg* 1989;71:648–653.

34. Newell DW, Eskridge JM, Mayberg MR. Angioplasty for the treatment of symptomatic vasospasm following subarachnoid hemorrhage. *J Neurosurg* 1989;71:654–660.

35. Higashida RT, Halbach VV, Dormandy B, Bell J, Brant-Zawadzki M, Hieshima GB. New microballoon device for transluminal angioplasty of intracranial arterial vasospasm. *Am J Neuroradiol* 1990;11:233–238.

36. Terada T, Nakamura Y, Yoshida N, et al. Percutaneous transluminal angioplasty for the M2 portion vasospasm following SAH: Development of the new microballoon and report of cases. *Surg Neurol* 1993;39:13–17.

37. Hurst RW, Schnee C, Raps EC, Farber R, Flamm ES. Role of transcranial Doppler in neuroradiological treatment of intracranial vasospasm. *Stroke* 1993;24:299–303.

38. Kassel NF, Helm G, Simmons N, Phillips CD, Cail WS. Treatment of cerebral vasospasm with intra-arterial papaverine. *J Neurosurg* 1992;77:848–852.

39. Kaku Y, Yonekawa Y, Tsukahara T, Kazekawa K. Superselective intra-arterial infusion of papaverine for the treatment of cerebral vasospasm after subarachnoid hemorrhage. *J Neurosurg* 1992;77:842–847.

40. Yamamoto Y, Smith RR, Bernake DH. Mechanism of action of balloon angioplasty in cerebral vasospasm. *Neurosurgery* 1992;30:1–5.

41. Kobayashi H, Ide H, Aradachi H, Arai Y, Handa Y, Kubota T. Histological studies of intracranial vessels in primates following transluminal angioplasty for vasospasm. *J Neurosurg* 1993;78:481–486.

42. Honma Y, Fujiwara T, Irie K, Ohkawa M, Nagao S. Morphological changes in human cerebral arteries after percutaneous transluminal angioplasty for vasospasm caused by subarachnoid hemorrhage. *Neurosurgery* 1995;36:1073–1081.

43. Mayberg M, Eskridge J, Newell D, Winn HR. Angioplasty for symptomatic vasospasm. In: Sano K, Takakura K, Kassell NF, Sasaki T, eds. *Cerebral Vasospasm: Proceedings of the IVth International Conference on Cerebral Vasospasm.* Tokyo: University of Tokyo Press, 1990:433–436.

44. Takahashi A, Yoshimoto T, Mizoi K, Sugawara T, Fujii Y. Transluminal balloon angioplasty for vasospasm after subarachnoid hemorrhage. In: Sano K, Takakura K, Kassell NF, Sasaki T, eds. *Cerebral Vasospasm: Proceedings of the IVth International Conference on Cerebral Vasospasm.* Tokyo: University of Tokyo Press, 1990:429–432.

45. Higashida RT, Halbach VV, Tsai FY, Dowd CF, Hieshima GB. Intravascular balloon dilatation for intracranial arterial vasospasm: Patient selection, technique, and clinical results. *Neurosurg Rev* 1992;15:89–95.

46. Linskey ME, Horton JA, Rao GR, Yonas H. Fatal rupture of the intracranial carotid artery during transluminal angioplasty for vasospasm induced by subarachnoid hemorrhage. Case report. *J Neurosurg* 1991;74:985–990.

Cerebrovascular Disease, edited by H. Hunt Batjer.
Lippincott-Raven Publishers, Philadelphia © 1997.

CHAPTER 45

Acute and Chronic Venous Sinus Thrombosis

Michael B. Horowitz, Ralph G. Greenlee, Jr., and Phillip D. Purdy

HISTORICAL PERSPECTIVE

Intracranial dural venous thrombosis is a poorly understood condition, and its etiology, incidence, natural history, treatment, and outcome are debated among clinicians caring for neurologic diseases. One fact that is not questioned, however, is that the disease process is unpredictable in terms of course and outcome and has the potential for creating devastating consequences. The advent of magnetic resonance imaging (MRI) and the capacity to selectively deliver thrombolytic agents have opened a new chapter in the diagnosis and treatment of this difficult clinical entity.

Possibly the earliest recorded observations of dural sinus thrombosis were made by Hippocrates who noted apoplexy in association with pregnancy and childbirth (1). Gowers (2) attributes the first description of dural sinus thrombosis to Ribes, who in 1825 ministered to a 45-year-old man with widespread malignancy, headache, seizures, and delirium. The postmortem examination of this patient revealed superior sagittal sinus (SSS), left transverse sinus (TS), and cortical vein thromboses. In 1888, Gowers (2) himself described aseptic dural sinus thrombosis in a cachectic patient, and in 1915 Holmes and Sargent (3) described posttraumatic thrombosis of the SSS. In 1936, Lhermitte et al (4) made the association between pediatric congenital heart disease and sinus thrombosis. In the 1940s, Martin and Sheehan (5) related thrombosis to the puerperal period. Based on these and other cases, the characterization of cerebral venous thrombosis as a rare and possibly fatal disease characterized by headache, papilledema, seizures, and focal neurologic

M. B. Horowitz: Department of Neurological Surgery and Department of Radiology, Division of Neuroradiology, The University of Texas Southwestern Medical Center at Dallas, Texas 75235.

R. G. Greenlee Jr.: Department of Neurology, The University of Texas Southwestern Medical Center at Dallas, Texas 75235.

P. D. Purdy: Department of Radiology, Division of Neuroradiology, Department of Neurology, and Department of Neurological Surgery, The University of Texas Southwestern Medical Center at Dallas, Texas 75235.

deficits began to evolve. During the period 1942–1990, approximately 203 cases of intracranial venous thrombosis were reported (6).

The finding of hemorrhagic infarction in pathologic material recovered from patients who died secondary to venous sinus thrombosis led to the widely accepted principle that anticoagulants could be dangerous in treating such cases. As will be shown, this view has been modified as our experience has broadened.

INCIDENCE AND DEMOGRAPHICS

Despite increasing ease of diagnosis, the true incidence of intracerebral venous thrombosis is unknown because many cases continue to go unrecognized. Ehlers and Courville (7) reported 16 cases of SSS thrombosis in 12,500 autopsies. According to Kalbag and Woolf (8), cerebral venous thrombosis was the principle cause of death in only 21.7 persons per year in England and Wales from 1952 to 1961. The female-to-male ratio is 1.29:1. While men of all ages are affected evenly, 61% of cases in women occur between the ages of 20–35 years, coinciding with the peak incidence of pregnancy, as well as the use of oral contraceptives (9).

ANATOMY AND PATHOPHYSIOLOGY

The cerebral sinuses are large, valveless, incompletely septated, venous structures, triangular in cross-section, with a plexus of adjacent venous channels that act as collateral pathways for drainage in the event of thrombosis. Cerebral veins, as well as calvarial emissary veins, discharge into the sinuses, and the latter may, in pathologic conditions, provide for extracranial drainage. Sinus variations are common. Located over the convexity in the midline, the SSS is the largest of the dural sinuses. The SSS rostral to the coronal suture may be functionally absent in 6% of specimens. In such cases, drainage occurs via cerebral veins. Such a situation should not be confused with pathologic occlusion. The inferior sagittal sinus lies within the inferior margin of the falx cerebri. It joins the vein of Galen to enter the straight sinus (SS). The SS courses to its confluence with the SSS to form the torcular Herophili, which in turn divides into the TS (lateral) and the less constant occipital sinus (more constant in children). Asymmetry of the TS is common with the right TS draining the SSS and the left TS draining the SS. The right TS provides the dominant drainage in 50–80% of cases. Agenesis or atresia of one of the TSs occurs in up to 5% of the cases and, again, should not be mistaken for dural sinus occlusion (10). The TS runs inferiorly to join the sigmoid sinus (SgS), which continues into the jugular bulb. The SgS runs within the inner aspect of the mastoid process and is susceptible to thrombosis secondary to infectious processes such as mastoiditis and otitis media, which involve the sinus via emissary veins.

The cavernous sinus (CS) is a multiseptated, dural-lined collection of venous channels through which the internal carotid artery and the sixth cranial nerve run. Cranial nerves III, IV, and V (divisions 1 and 2) are contained within the dural walls. Located on either side of the pituitary fossa, the CS receives drainage from superior and inferior ophthalmic veins, superior petrosal sinus, and the pterygoid plexus (through the foramen of ovale). Each CS communicates with the other across the midline via the circular or intercavernous sinus that surrounds the hypophysis. Communication with the TS/SgS and the jugular bulb occurs via the superior petrosal sinus and inferior petrosal sinus, respectively. Because of its connection with the deep facial veins via the pterygoid plexus and the ophthalmic veins, the CS may become thrombosed as a consequence of sphenoid and ethmoid sinus infections.

Cortical veins can be divided into superficial and deep systems. The largest of the superficial veins are the veins of Trolard and Labbé and the superficial middle cerebral vein (the anastomotic veins). The middle cerebral vein runs along the sylvian fissure. Trolard's vein is located over the parietal lobe, while Labbé's vein drains the posterior temporal region. Each vessel's diameter is variable, with the size of one often inversely related to the size of the other.

The organization and presence of veins of the superficial cortex are highly variable, making the angiographic diagnosis of isolated cortical vein thrombosis problematic. In contrast, the deep cerebral venous system that drains the deep white matter, thalamus, brainstem, ventricles, and basal ganglia is more constant. These vessels include the septal, anterior caudate, thalamostriate, internal cerebral, direct lateral, inferior ventricular, and medial atrial veins, the basal vein of Rosenthal, and Galen's vein.

In the case of venous sinus thrombosis, the SSS is the most commonly occluded dural sinus followed by the TS, SgS, and CS (10). Cortical vein thrombosis is rarely diagnosed in the absence of dural sinus thrombosis. From a pathophysiologic standpoint, sinus thrombosis can be conceived as a multistep process.

TABLE 1. *Conditions associated with cerebral venous thrombosis*

Infectious

Sinusitis, mastoiditis, dental infections, facial infections, meningitis, encephalitis

Noninfectious

Pregnancy, puerperium, circulating antiphospholipid antibodies, lupus anticoagulants, oral contraceptives, malignancies, dehydration, jugular vein cannulation, sickle cell disease, surgical trauma, congenital and acquired heart disease

Idiopathic

CLINICAL PATHOPHYSIOLOGY

Intracranial venous thrombosis is frequently associated with certain predisposing factors and conditions, a partial list of which is outlined in Table 1 (1,6,9,11–14). Such conditions may be divided into infectious and noninfectious categories.

Before the antibiotic era, infection was associated with the vast majority of cases, with frequent spread from the mastoids and other sinuses via the diploic veins. Today, such infectious cases reside primarily within the immunocompromised and diabetic populations.

Noninfectious etiologies now constitute the majority of thrombosis cases. In adults, disorders of coagulation are particularly important. These conditions are especially common during pregnancy and in the second and third weeks after delivery. In the case of the latter, propensity toward thrombosis may be due to elevated plasma fibrinogen, as well as factors VII, VIII, IX, and X (15,16). Other states that promote thrombosis include antithrombin-III, protein-C, and protein-S deficiencies. Activated protein C inhibits the activity of factors V and VIII, while at the same time stimulating fibrinolysis. Protein S increases the activity of protein C 10,000-fold. Levels of both of these proteins have been found to be deficient in the puerperium but may be congenitally low as well (17–19). In addition to the above, lupus anticoagulants and antiphospholipid antibodies have been associated with enhanced thrombosis (20) and should be investigated in every patient presenting with thrombosis of unknown etiology.

While cerebral vein thrombosis may present with a wide spectrum of signs and symptoms, headache is the most prominent presenting symptom in almost all series. A common presentation includes headache, focal neurologic deficits, seizures, and reduction in the level of consciousness. Many of the abnormalities may be related to increased intracranial pressure due to decreased cerebrospinal fluid absorption secondary to venous hypertension. Others can be attributed to intracranial venous hemorrhage (9,11,13). Ameri and Bousser (9) emphasize that the mode of presentation of symptoms is highly variable. In their series of 110 patients, only 28%

presented with acute illnesses, with symptoms developing over 48 hours; 42% presented with symptoms between 48 hours and 30 days. When the presentation is acute, focal signs are more frequent and the etiologic basis of sinus thrombosis is more often infectious or obstetric, whereas chronic onset was notable for the absence of focal signs and was associated with neoplastic or immune-related illnesses. This slow onset frequently mimics the syndrome of benign intracranial hypertension. Thus, cerebral venous thrombosis must be excluded by either MRI or angiography whenever benign intracranial hypertension is a diagnostic consideration. Finally, an often forgotten complication of sinus thrombosis is pulmonary embolism, 23 cases of which were reported in the literature between 1942 and 1990 (6).

DIAGNOSTIC INVESTIGATIONS

When signs and symptoms suggest sinus thrombosis, investigation should be directed first toward confirming the diagnosis and then toward the underlying predisposing factor or factors. Radionuclide studies and electroencephalography (EEG) are of historical interest and will not be covered. The cornerstones of diagnosis are the findings on computed tomography (CT), cerebral angiography, and MRI. Because CT images of the brain may be normal in 10–20% of cases, MRI and cerebral angiography must be pursued when sinus thrombosis is suspected (9). Until MRI results are universally validated, however, cerebral angiography remains the gold standard against which all other technologies should be compared.

Angiographic findings include partial or complete nonopacification of venous sinuses and veins, dilated cortical collateral veins with a corkscrew appearance, increased cerebral circulation transit time, and reversal of flow away from the obstructed sinus or vein (9,10). In the process of interpreting angiographic images, one must be aware of a number of pitfalls. Often the anterior SSS is normally absent, replaced by two superior cerebral veins that join behind the coronal suture. Absent opacification of the anterior SSS alone therefore is insufficient in and of itself to make the diagnosis of sinus thrombosis (9). The same statement can be made about the TS and SgS, which may normally fail to be visualized during cerebral angiography (21). Careful attention to technique must be observed, with visualization of the entire venous phase in both anterior and lateral projections. Oblique projections may help in the delineation of parasagittal sinuses and veins.

Although CT images of the brain may be normal in 10–20% of cases of venous thrombosis, common findings include hemorrhagic venous infarcts, nonhemorrhagic infarcts, small ventricles, intense contrast enhancement of the falx and tentorium, a cord sign representing thrombosed veins, a dense-triangle sign representing fresh thrombus in the posterior SSS, and an empty-delta sign secondary to enhancement of collateral veins in the SSS wall surrounding

a nonenhancing thrombus. Ventricles are frequently small and white matter may be edematous.

MRI represents a noninvasive means of assessing the presence of thrombosed sinuses and veins, as well as possibly determining thrombus age by analyzing its T1- and T2-weighted signal intensities (9). The advantage of MRI is its ability to demonstrate blood flow and parenchymal processes. In acute stages, there is an absence of "flow void" and thrombus appears hyperintense on T1-weighted images and hypointense on T2-weighted images. With the appearance of methemoglobin, the absence of flow persists and the thrombus becomes hyperintense on both T1- and T2-weighted images.

NATURAL HISTORY

An important clinical point concerning cerebral venous thrombosis is that the clinical course and prognosis are variable and unpredictable. Some feel that the rate of thrombus formation, presence or absence of coma, focal symptoms, hemorrhagic infarct, and age of presentation (infants and elderly doing worse) are useful prognosticators. While the mortality rate has been reported to approach 70%, more recent reviews estimate the range to be 5–30% (9). There is little information concerning prognosis for functional recovery after cerebral venous thrombosis. Eighty-three percent of 35 cases reported in the literature since 1980 survived (22). Only 15–25% of afflicted patients have any sequelae (9). Information concerning the outcome in the pediatric population is equally scant. Taha et al (23) reported a series of five patients with traumatic SgS thrombosis, all of whom had normal neurologic examinations 6 months after their initial symptoms. Four patients had complete resolution of the sinus obstruction. With SgS thrombosis, however, venous drainage can occur across a patent torcular and into the contralateral sinus system.

MANAGEMENT STRATEGIES

The management of intracerebral venous sinus thrombosis is varied. Controlled, randomized studies are difficult to perform in view of the rarity of symptomatic cases and the multiple etiologies, both of which make adequate randomization nearly impossible. Some physicians espouse a course of watchful waiting in view of the benign nature and uneventful recovery made by the majority of patients. Interventions are reserved for individuals who worsen while being observed (9,23,24). Medical management of these patients includes cerebral dehydrating agents (1,14), steroids (9,24,25), acetazolamide, cerebrospinal fluid drainage, barbiturates, decompressive craniectomy (14), sinus thrombectomy (24,25), heparin/warfarin (1,25–31), urokinase (11,25,32–36), and tissue plasminogen activator (t-PA) (37).

Stansfield (26) was the first to use heparin in a puerperal woman with focal neurologic deficits secondary to venous

TABLE 2.

Case	Sex	Age (yr)	Symptom duration	Physical and neurologic status	Heparin	Occlusion site	Treatment duration (hr)	Total dose (IU)
1	M	26	3 d	Diffuse headache, somnolent, left homonomous hemianopsia	Yes	SS, SSS, ICV, VG, BVR, bilateral TS	36	~3,380,000
2	F	27	<2 d	Headache, nausea, vomiting, neck pain	Yes	SSS, bilateral TS, VG, SS, left JB	72	~4,500,00
3	F	65	2 wk	Decline in mentation, dysarthria, right hemiparesis	Yes	SSS	48	~3,280,00
4	F	36	2 mo	Right orbital swelling, blurred vision, right eye pain, pulmonary embolus, cardiac failure	Yes	SSS, bilateral TS, deep venous system	48	~4,000,00
5	M	38	5 d	Headache, right hemiparesis, seizures	Yes	SSS, right TS	17	~2,600,00
6	M	35	<1 h	Hemiparesis, altered mental status	Yes	TS	12	~2,400,00
7	M	35	32 d	Seizure, change in mental status	Yes	TS, SSS	42	~3,600,00
8	M	32	2 wk (?)	Seizure, papilledema, bilateral cranial nerve VI palsies	Yes	SSS	48	~4,590,00
9	F	6 wks	0–5 d (?)	Seizures	Yes	VG, ICV, SS, SSS, TS	~84	~1,500,00
10	F	12	3 mo (?)	Headache, papilledema, chorea	Yes	SSS, SS, ICV, VG, TS	72	~4,320,00
11	F	43	2 d	Headache, left cranial nerve VI paresis, papilledema	Yes	SSS, right TS	~48	~2,750,00
12	F	27	~1.5 mo	Headache, bilateral papilledema	Yes	SSS, TS	~70	~7,000,00
13	F	22	2 wk	Headache, nausea, vomiting, blurred vision, atrophic papilledema, confusion	Yes	Posterior 2/3 SSS, torcula, right/left TS, right sigmoid sinus, partial left sigmoid sinus	~72	~5,800,00

Key: SS, straight sinus; SSS, superior sagittal sinus; ICV, internal cerebral veins; VG, vein of Galen; BVR, basal vein of Rosenthal; TS, transverse sinus; SLE, systemic lupus erythematosus; JB, jugular vein.

Treatment group

Urokinase bolus dose (IU)	Infusion/hr	Clinical outcome	Radiographic outcome	Complications	Presumed etiology	Pretreatment intraparenchymal hemorrhage/infarct	Warfarin at discharge
250,000	80,000	Excellent	All sinuses patent, deep venous system patent	None	Dehydration	Bilateral occipital lobe 1 cm hemorrhages	Yes
250,000–500,000	100,000	Excellent (slight residual headache)	All sinuses patent, residual occlusion left JB	None	Oral contraceptives	No	Yes
400,000	60,000	Excellent	Sinus patent	None	Malignancy	Biparietal hemorrhages	Yes
?	?	Death secondary to pulmonary emboli	No change from pretreatment	Hematuria, groin hematomas, death	Malignancy, protein C deficiency, antiphospholipid antibody syndrome	No	Yes
?	100,000	Excellent	Sinuses patent	Transient worsening of exam after initial improvement	Dehydration, mastoiditis	No	Yes
?	200,000	Excellent	Sinuses patent	Groin hematoma	Iatrogenic-balloon migration in interventional therapy case	No	Yes
250,000	80,000	Excellent	Sinuses patent	Bilateral groin hematomas	Unknown	No	Yes
250,000	80,000	Good; residual visual loss	Sinuses patent	None	Unknown (febrile illness?)	Right occipital lobe hemorrhage	Yes
50,000	10,000–20,000	? Follow-up period inadequate	Sinuses almost completely patent	None	Dehydration	Thalamic hemorrhage	Yes
500,000	60,000	Excellent; headache resolved	Good; anterograde drainage in sinuses reestablished	Retroperitoneal hematoma, blood transfusion	SLE	Right temperal lobe infarct	Yes
250,000	80,000	Good; cranial nerve VI paresis improved but not resolved	Good; SSS opened, TS remained occluded	? Bacteremia due to sheath	Ulcerative colitis, oral contraceptives, tooth abscess	No	Yes
250,000	80,000–100,000	Excellent; headache resolved	Good; anterograde from SSS to left TS reestablished, small residual clot SSS, torcula, right TS	Small groin hematoma	Sinusitis	No	Yes
250,000	80,000	Excellent; headache resolved, returned to neurologic baseline, papilledema minimally improved 1 wk posttherapy, visual fields restricted	Sinuses patent, right sigmoid sinus still with moderate thrombus	None	Medroxy-progesterone acetate injections	Right parietooccipital venous infarct	Yes

thrombosis. She recovered within 4 days of beginning therapy. Bousser et al (28) managed 38 patients with cerebral sinus thrombosis. Twenty-three patients were treated with heparin, none of whom died, 19 patients making a complete recovery. While this report answers no questions about heparin therapy vs. nonheparin therapy, it does point out the relative safety of using the former in a small group of patients. Einhaupl et al (31) performed the only randomized, blinded study of adjusted-dose heparin in 20 patients with venous sinus thrombosis. At 3 months after therapy, 80% of the heparin-treated patients were normal, with the remainder showing slight deficits. Only 10% of the nonheparinized patients were normal at 3 months, 60% had neurologic deficits, and 30% were dead. The author went on to a retrospective study involving 102 patients with thrombosis, 43 of whom had intracranial hemorrhage. Twenty-seven of the 43 were treated with heparin. Four of these patients (15%) died, and 14 (52%) had a normal recovery. The 16 remaining patients were treated without heparin, nine of whom (56%) died and three had a normal recovery (31). The authors concluded from this study that treatment with heparin was not only beneficial but also safe, even in the face of intracranial hemorrhage.

Other practitioners have advocated the use of fibrinolytic agents, with the goal of rapid clearance of thrombus from the venous system. In 1971, Vines and Davis (11) used urokinase and heparin in the treatment of four patients with sinus thrombosis, all of whom improved. In 1988, Scott et al (33) catheterized the SSS via a frontal burr hole and infused urokinase over an 8-hour period. The patient, who was initially decerebrate, had only a mild dysphasia 4 weeks after therapy. In 1989, Higashida et al (35) reported treatment of TS thrombotic occlusion in a newborn child with seizures by direct SSS puncture and instillation of urokinase 12,000 IU over a 12-hour period. The thrombus cleared, and the child remained neurologically normal 3 years later. Nevertheless, the safety and efficacy of urokinase therapy have not been established in pediatric patients. There are case reports of urokinase infusions to treat thrombosed catheters or right atrial thrombi in infants. The dosage has ranged between 2,000 and 8,800 IU/kg/h (38–43). Bolus doses of 5,000–10,000 IU have been used (42,43), as well as low-dose infusions of 70–500 IU/kg/h (42). There are also published reports of urokinase for treatment of arterial occlusions. Strife et al (43) used it in neonates to treat four cases of central thrombosis via umbilical artery catheterization of the abdominal aorta. The urokinase dose used was a loading bolus of 4,400 IU/kg followed by 4,000–20,000 IU/kg/h maintenance dose. The duration of therapy for these neonates was 3–9 days.

In 1990, Persson and Lilja (25) performed an open thrombectomy and instilled urokinase into the SSS. Despite formation of a small cerebellar hematoma, the patient gradually improved, although never to baseline. In 1991, Barnwell et al (32) reported the treatment of three patients with transjugular catheterization and instillation of urokinase, and Tsai et al

(34) reported five additional cases from the same institution in 1992. Seven of the eight patients in these two studies had excellent neurologic recoveries, and none had complications related to the therapy. Additionally, Smith et al (36) described similar results in seven patients in 1994, two of whom had previously been reported by Barnwell (32) (Dowd, personal communication). All patients in this last study did well. In total, we found 13 cases in the English literature of transjugular cerebral venous sinus catheterization and urokinase instillation.

Our series of 13 patients treated with transfemoral transvenous urokinase infusions directly into the cerebral dural sinuses demonstrates the efficacy that can be achieved using present catheter technology (Table 2). Twelve of the 13 individuals reported had significant radiographic improvement (reestablished venous sinus drainage) or complete resolution of their thrombus along with rapid neurologic improvements. One failure was in a patient with at least a 2-month history of sinus thrombosis and protein-C deficiency. We can only speculate that the clot was organized to the extent that it was resistant to urokinase's thrombolytic properties. This concept is supported by a number of studies concerning thrombolysis for deep venous and pulmonary thrombosis and lower-extremity arterial occlusions. Genton and Wolf (44) noted that emboli estimated to be less than 72 hours old responded well to fibrinolysis, while lesions older than 2 weeks responded less well. Lesions at 6 weeks showed no appreciable change after therapy. Amery et al (45) confirmed these findings in patients with lower-extremity arterial occlusions. The frequency of thrombus clearing was significantly higher in patients treated within 72 hours than in those treated later (68% vs. 7%). The urokinase—pulmonary embolism trial also showed an advantage for acute treatment (46). While venous and arterial thrombi are most susceptible to thrombolytic therapy early in their course, Duckert et al (47) did achieve patency in one of seven (14%) of patients treated 22–56 days after the onset of deep venous thrombosis symptoms.

In addition to demonstrating the effectiveness of selective fibrinolytic therapy, this series also suggests that the techniques described here are safe even in individuals with hemorrhagic and nonhemorrhagic venous infarcts. No significant complications from therapy, especially those of intracerebral hemorrhage, pulmonary embolism, and vessel damage were seen in our 13 patients despite the apparent risks.

PATIENT SELECTION AND THROMBOLYTIC TECHNIQUE

Thirteen patients (five males, eight females), ages 6 weeks to 65 years, presented with venous sinus thrombosis involving the SSS and at least one TS (see Table 2). After adequate patient preparation, a 6-French sheath was placed into a femoral vein, and another was inserted into the contralateral femoral artery using a single wall puncture needle and the

Seldinger technique. The artery and vein in a single leg were not catheterized because of the risk of creating an arteriovenous fistula when the sheaths were removed. Whenever possible, the right femoral vein was used because it would be closer to the interventionalist during microcatheter manipulations. A 5-French angiographic catheter and guidewire were then used to perform a complete cerebral angiogram, with imaging carried out into the late venous phase. Once the diagnosis of sinus thrombosis was made, the catheter was removed. A catheter and wire were then advanced via the femoral vein through the right atrium and into the superior vena cava. The decision of which internal jugular vein (IJV) to catheterize was made depending on the location of the sinus thrombosis. (Given a choice, the right IJV is generally the easier of the two to locate and negotiate.) Having entered the IJV, the catheter was placed at the C-1 level. A microcatheter (in all cases, either a Tracker-18 or Fast Tracker-18 catheter system, Target Therapeutics, Fremont, CA, or a Transit catheter, Cordis Corporation, Miami Lakes, FL, was used) was advanced coaxially over a guidewire through the jugular bulb and into the appropriate sinus or sinuses. The catheter and wire sometimes made several loops and turns as it passed through and around the thrombus. Advancement sometimes required many back and forth rotary motions of the wire as clot was macerated by the wire tip. During the advancement, we generally instilled urokinase in 50,000 IU aliquots approximately every 15 minutes to bathe the thrombus as we traversed its length. A total dose of 250,000–500,000 IU was given during a single sitting. The catheter was eventually positioned near the distal end of the thrombus, with careful attention not to leave it at a point where the urokinase would drain preferentially through venous collaterals. The system was then secured to the patient's thigh with an occlusive dressing, and the patient was returned to the intensive care unit (ICU) with a continuous urokinase infusion through the microcatheter at 60,000–100,000 IU/h.

Approximately 18–24 hours later, the patient was returned to the angiography suite where a repeat venogram was performed. If the sinuses appeared patent, a single common carotid arteriogram was obtained to visualize the arteriovenous relationship and transit time. When thrombolysis was not adequate, additional boluses were administered, the catheter was repositioned, and the patient was continued on the urokinase infusion. Follow-up venograms and arteriograms were obtained at 24-hour intervals until the desired effect was achieved. Once the infusions were completed, the catheters were removed. The patient remained on heparin and was eventually converted to warfarin. Anticoagulant therapy was continued for 3–6 months.

SELECTED CASE REPORTS

Case One

A 26-year-old right-handed man presented 72 hours after the onset of diffuse headache and gradually increasing som-

nolence. He had a history of working outdoors in extreme heat over the previous days and may have become dehydrated. Neurologic examination demonstrated the above findings plus a partial left homonomous hemianopsia. A head CT scan revealed density in the SS, SSS, torcular, TS, internal cerebral veins (ICV), and vein of Galen, as well as a cord sign in the left ambient cistern consistent with the location of the basal vein of Rosenthal. A 1-cm diameter hemorrhagic venous infarct was visible in the cortical and subcortical occipital lobes bilaterally (Fig. 1). Cerebral MRI demonstrated subacute thrombus in the venous sinuses and an abnormal signal in the left centrum semiovale and occipital lobes. A diagnosis of venous sinus thrombosis was made. The patient was referred for cerebral angiography, which confirmed the above findings (Fig. 2). After systemic heparinization, transfemoral catheterization of the right IJV was achieved, and a Fast Tracker-18 catheter was placed coaxially and advanced into the anterior SSS with minimal difficulty. Venograms obtained during the catheter positioning revealed diffuse thrombus within the right jugular bulb, right TS, and SSS. The left TS was not opacified. Retrograde venous flow was seen from the anterior SSS into dilated cortical veins. A bolus dose of urokinase 250,000 IU in 50,000 IU aliquots administered every 5–10 minutes was infused into the anterior SSS with minimal effect on thrombus appearance. The patient was returned to the ICU with the microcatheter in the SSS just anterior to the coronal suture. Urokinase was infused over the next 18 hours at a rate of 80,000 IU/h. The following day, repeat interval angiography demonstrated near-complete clearing of the SSS and right TS, although small filling defects representing a residual clot remained. We were unable to pass the catheter across the torcular to assess the left TS. Catheterization of the left IJV and placement of the catheter into the torcular revealed extensive thrombus within the left TS, SgS and left IJV. An additional 250,000 IU of urokinase were administered in boluses of 50,000 IU each, and the patient was infused over the next 18 hours with 80,000 IU/h. Follow-up venography and angiography 18 hours later revealed patency of the venous sinuses with decreased collateral drainage (Fig. 3). Follow-up cerebral CT demonstrated resolution of the occipital hemorrhage and small infarcts in the deep left parietal white matter. Within 48 hours of treatment, the patient's headaches had almost completely resolved, and visual fields were grossly normal to confrontational testing. He was discharged on warfarin. Coagulation studies investigating hypercoagulability were all within normal limits.

Case Two

A 27-year-old woman with a history of tobacco and oral contraceptive use presented with less than 24 hours of headache, nausea, vomiting, and neck pain. Cerebral CT and MRI studies revealed hyperdensity within the SSS, SS, and VG. No hemorrhages or infarcts were visible. Systemic heparin-

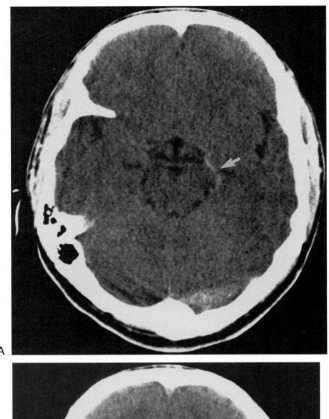

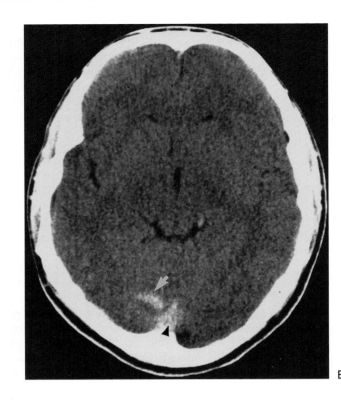

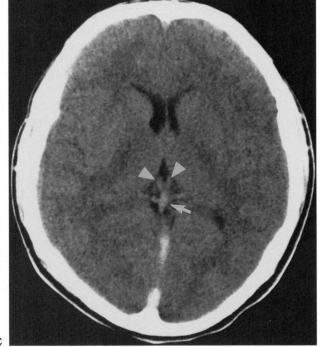

FIG. 1. CT scan **(A)** reveals thrombus in the left basal vein of Rosenthal *(arrow)*. **(B)** Intraparenchymal hemorrhage is present in the occipital lobe *(arrow)*, and thrombus is within the SSS *(arrowhead)*. **(C)** Thrombus is also apparent within the internal cerebral veins *(arrowheads)* and Galen's vein *(arrow)*.

ization was instituted. A cerebral angiogram and transvenous catheterization were performed (as described in case 1), revealing SSS and bilateral TS thrombosis. Over the next 72 hours, three venograms were performed. Bolus urokinase injections of 250,000–500,000 IU were made during each procedure, and the patient remained on a continuous infusion of 100,000 IU/h in the ICU. After 3 days, near-complete resolution of the thrombosis was achieved, except for residual occlusion of the left jugular bulb, which was compensated for by significant posterior fossa venous collateralization. The patient's nausea and vomiting abated and her headaches improved, although they never completely resolved even at 3-month follow-up. Warfarin was discontinued after 3 months.

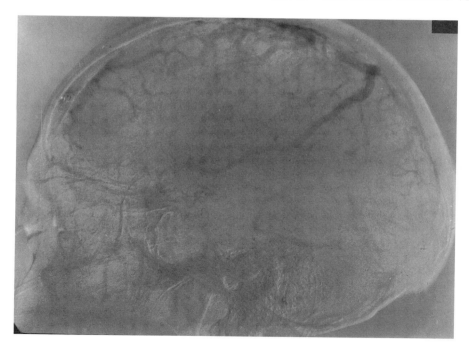

FIG. 2. In this lateral venous-phase carotid arteriogram, note absence of opacification of SSS, TS, and SgS.

Case Three

A 65-year-old woman presented with a 2-week history of a gradually declining level of consciousness along with progressive dysarthria, right-sided weakness, and right facial paresis. Prior to therapy, the patient was stuporous with right lower-extremity plegia and severe right upper-extremity paresis. Cerebral CT revealed biparietal hemorrhages, parietal edema, and sulcal effacement. Hyperdensity was seen in the torcular and SSS. Angiography confirmed the above and in addition demonstrated slow arterial flow and dilated cortical veins. A Tracker catheter was placed into the SSS, and a 400,000 IU urokinase bolus was infused over 40 minutes. A 48-hour infusion at 60,000 IU/h was carried out. The patient improved markedly over the next 12 hours such that she was alert and oriented with good right lower and upper extremity

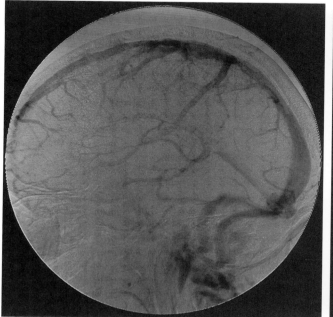

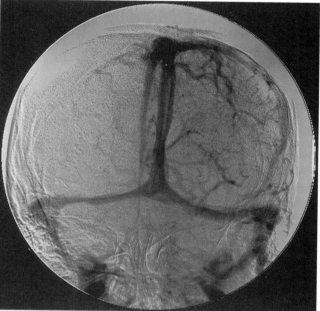

A   B

FIG. 3. Lateral **(A)** and anteroposterior **(B)** views of a venous-phase carotid arteriogram following urokinase infusion show that all sinuses are patent.

movement. Repeat angiography at 48 hours demonstrated near-complete thrombus resolution with only small filling defects remaining. The patient was converted from heparin to warfarin and at the time of discharge was ambulating with the assistance of a walker, had minimal right-handed weakness, and was capable of independent living. The patient returned 6 months later with an angiographically documented pulmonary embolus. Routine workup for a hypercoagulable state was negative (antithrombin III, proteins C and S, urine homocystine, and anticardiolipin/antiphospholipid antibody). An occult colon malignancy was discovered shortly afterward.

Case Four

A 32-year-old black man with a history of a febrile illness 3 weeks before admission to our institution presented with a single tonic-clonic seizure, bilateral papilledema with flame hemorrhages, and mild bilateral sixth nerve palsies. A cerebral CT scan revealed a small right occipital lobe parenchymal hemorrhage, while MRI demonstrated increased signal within the SSS suggestive of venous sinus thrombosis. Cerebral angiography confirmed the diagnosis (Fig. 4). Utilizing a transfemoral transvenous approach, a Tracker-18 catheter was advanced into the SSS, and urokinase 250,000 IU was infused over 60 minutes (50,000 IU every 12 minutes) with immediate lysis of clot surrounding the catheter tip. The catheter was left in position in the SSS, and 80,000 IU/h were infused over the next 48 hours. The patient had interval angiography at 24 hours, at which time an additional 500,000 IU was infused into the SSS and TS. At 48 hours after initiation of

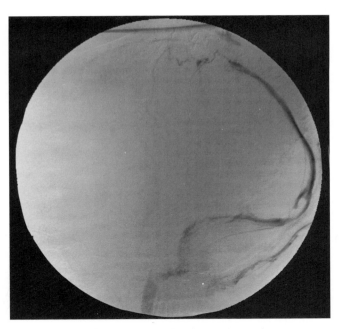

FIG. 5. Lateral venogram via Tracker catheter demonstrates recanalization of the venous sinuses following urokinase therapy.

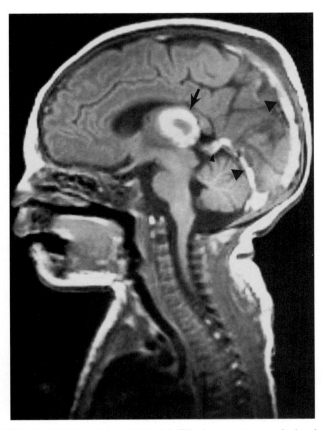

FIG. 6. Midline T1-weighted MRI demonstrates thalamic hemorrhage *(large arrow)* and thrombus in the SSS, SS *(large arrow head)*, vein of Galen *(small arrow head)*, and torcular.

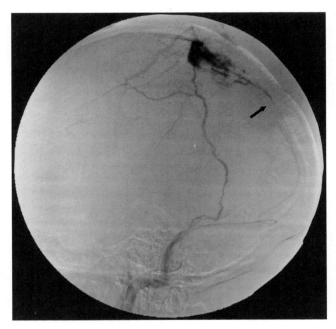

FIG. 4. Lateral venogram via Tracker catheter in the posterior SSS *(arrow)* shows nonopacification of the SSS and TS.

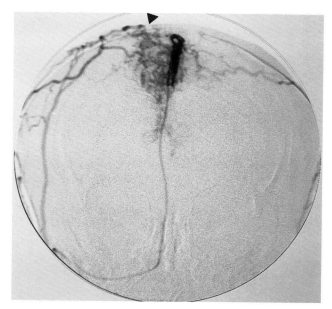

FIG. 7. Anteroposterior venogram reveals poor opacification of the SSS with transosseous drainage *(arrowheads).*

therapy, all venous sinuses were widely patent (Fig. 5). A follow-up CT scan at 48 hours showed resolution of the hemorrhage. A coagulopathy study revealed normal protein C and S levels. Antiphospholipid antibodies were also within normal limits. The patient was discharged on warfarin 7.5 mg/d.

Case Five

A 6-week-old girl was admitted, suffering from dehydration and malnutrition. On the fifth hospital day, she experi-

enced two focal seizures localized to the left hemisphere. Cerebral CT revealed a right thalamic hemorrhage, and thrombus within the VG, ICV, SS, SSS, and TS. The anterior fontanelle was tense. MRI confirmed the above findings (Fig. 6), and transfemoral transvenous selective catheterization and thrombolysis was initiated. A 3-French left common femoral sheath was placed, with the tip of the sheath in the inferior vena cava. This was exchanged for a 5-French sheath. A Tracker-18 catheter was advanced coaxially into the mid-SSS. A venogram confirmed the presence of complete thrombosis with venous collaterals via both cortical and scalp veins (Fig. 7). An infusion of urokinase 50,000 IU was delivered within 1 hour. Follow-up venography demonstrated little improvement, and the patient was transferred to the ICU with the Tracker catheter in place infusing urokinase 10,000 IU/h. The following day a venogram demonstrated minimal improvement. The infusion was increased to 20,000 IU/h. This rate was maintained for the next 72 hours, and subsequent venograms revealed gradual thrombolysis of the SSS, TS, and SgS (Fig. 8). Normal venous drainage was restored, and abnormal venous collateral flow disappeared. A follow-up MRI obtained 3 days after the termination of therapy showed patency of the SSS, left TS, left SgS, and SS, along with residual clot in the ICV and VG (Fig. 9). Multiple CT scans were obtained during the thrombolysis procedure, and there was no enlargement of the right thalamic hemorrhage (Fig. 10).

CONCLUSION

The management of cerebral venous sinus thrombosis is controversial. This series does not establish which patients

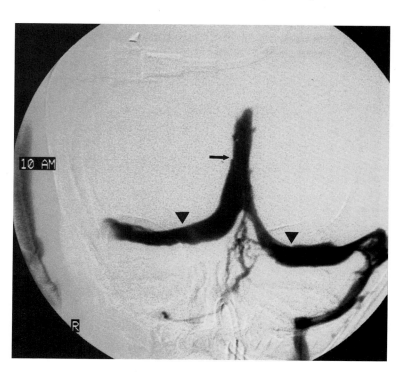

FIG. 8. Anteroposterior venogram following urokinase therapy demonstrates patent SSS *(arrow)* and TS *(arrowheads).*

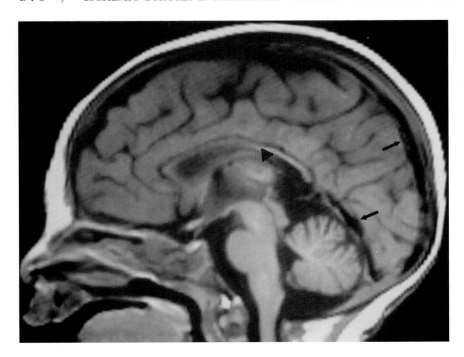

FIG. 9. Sagittal MRI scan 3 days after therapy shows no progression of thalamic hemorrhage *(arrowhead)* and patency of the dural venous sinuses *(arrows)*.

warrant intervention and which can be followed conservatively with expectant care or systemic heparinization. Because of our favorable experience with dural sinus urokinase infusions, we tend to favor aggressive interventional management because it is impossible to predict which patients will succumb to the ravages of venous infarction. Unlike heparin therapy, which inhibits thrombus progression while the body lyses the clot in a natural fashion, thrombolytic therapy hastens clot dissolution, thus opening venous channels in a more timely fashion. Though outcome improvement with urokinase has not been definitively shown, we believe rapid restoration of venous outflow by clot dissolution should be to the patient's benefit.

ACKNOWLEDGMENTS

This series was initially accepted in March 1995 for publication in the *Annals of Neurology* and entitled "Treatment of cerebral dural sinus thrombosis using selective catheterization and urokinase infusion." Many thanks to Robert A. Fishman, MD, Editor, *Annals of Neurology*, for permitting its publication in textbook format.

Thanks to Leslie Mihal for her help in preparing this manuscipt; to Bill Perkins, MD, Mike Graber, MD, and Preston Harrison, MD, for patient referal; to Carol Zimmerman, MD, for ophthalmologic management; and to George Carstens, MD, Hal Unwin, MD, Joe Hise, MD, Tom Kopitnik, MD, Hunt Batjer, MD, Nancy Rollins, MD, and Duke Samson, MD, for assistance in patient management.

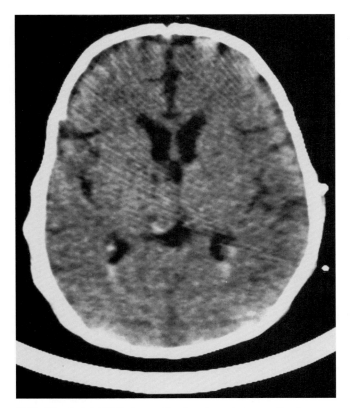

FIG. 10. Axial CT 3 days after treatment shows the hemorrhage has completely resolved.

REFERENCES

1. Carrol JD, Leak D, Lee HA. Cerebral thrombophlebitis in pregnancy and the puerperium. *Q J Med, New Series XXXV* 1966;139:347–367.

2. Gowers WR. *Manual of Diseases of the Nervous System*, ed 2. London: Churchill, 1888:416.

3. Holmes G, Sargent P. Injuries of the superior longitudinal sinus. *BMJ* 1915;2:493–498.

4. Lhermitte J, Lereboullet J, Kaplan B. Ramollissement hemorragipare d'origine nerveuse chez un enfant, atteint de malformations cardiaques. *Rev Neurol (Paris)* 1936;65:305.

5. Martin JP, Sheehan HL. Primary thrombosis of cerebral veins (following childbirth). *BMJ* 1941;1:349.

6. Diaz JM, Schiffman JS, Urban ES, Maccario M. Superior sagittal sinus thrombosis and pulmonary embolism: A syndrome rediscovered. *Acta Neurol Scand* 1992;86:390–396.

7. Ehlers H, Courville CB. Thrombosis of internal cerebral veins in infancy and childhood. Review of the literature and report of five cases. *J Pediatr* 1936;8:600–623.

8. Kalbag RM, Woolf AL. *Cerebral Venous Thrombosis*. London: University Press, 1967.

9. Ameri A, Bousser MG. Cerebral venous thrombosis. In: Barnett HJM, Hachinski VC, eds. *Cerebral Ischemia: Treatment and Prevention*. *Neurol Clin* 1992;10:87–111.

10. Osborne A. *Diagnostic Neuroradiology*. St. Louis, MO: Mosby, 1994.

11. Vines FS, Davis DO. Clinical-radiological correlation in cerebral venous occlusive disease. *Radiology* 1971;98:9–22.

12. Barnett HJM, Hyland HH. Non-infective intracranial venous thrombosis. *Brain* 1953;76:36–49.

13. Atkinson EA, Fairburn B, Heathfield KWG. Intracranial venous thrombosis as a complication of oral contraception. *Lancet* 1970;914–918.

14. Shende MC, Lourie H. Sagittal sinus thrombosis related to oral contraceptives. *J Neurosurg* 1970;33:714–717.

15. Estanol B, Rodriguez A. Intracranial venous thrombosis in young women. *Stroke* 1979;10:680.

16. Strauss HS, Diamond LK. Elevation of factor VIII during pregnancy in normal persons and in a patient with von Willebrand's disease. *N Engl J Med* 1963;269:1251.

17. Marlar RA, Kleiss AJ, Griffin JH. Protein C: Inactivation of factors V and VIII in plasma. *Ann N Y Acad Med* 1981;370:303.

18. Roos AI, Pascuzzi RM, Kuharik M. Prior intracranial venous thrombosis associated with dysfunctional protein C and deficiency of protein S. *Obstet Gynecol* 1990;76:492.

19. Cros D, Loup PC, Beltran G, Gum G. Superior sagittal sinus thrombosis in a patient with protein S deficiency. *Stroke* 1990;21:633–635.

20. Levin SR. Cerebral venous thrombosis with lupus anticoagulants. Report of 2 cases. *Stroke* 1987;18:801–804.

21. Hacker H. Normal supratentorial veins and dural sinuses. In: Newton TH, Potts DG, eds. *Radiology of the Skull and Brain*. St Louis, MO: CV Mosby, 1974.

22. Fincher RME, Swift TR. Case Report: Improvement in sagittal sinus thrombosis by MRI. *Am J Med Sci* 1991;301:262–264.

23. Taha JM, Crone KR, Berger TS, Becket WW, Prenger EC. Sigmoid sinus thrombosis after closed head injury in children. *Neurosurgery* 1993;32:541–546.

24. Estanol B, Rodriguez A, Conte G, Aleman JM, Loyo M, Pizzuto J. Intracranial venous thrombosis in young women. *Stroke* 1979;10:680–684.

25. Perrson L, Lilja A. Extensive dural sinus thrombosis treated by surgical removal and local streptokinase infusion. *Neurosurgery* 1990;26:117–121.

26. Stansfield FR. Puerperal cerebral thrombophlebitis treated by heparin. *BMJ* 1942;436–438.

27. Brown JIM, Coyne TJ, Hurlbert RJ, Fehlings MG, Ter Brugge KG. Deep cerebral venous system thrombosis: Case report. *Neurosurgery* 1993;33:911–913.

28. Bousser MG, Chiras J, Borias J, Castaigne P. Cerebral venous thrombosis. A review of 38 cases. *Stroke* 1985;16:199–213.

29. Gettelfinger DM, Kokmen E. Superior sagittal sinus thrombosis. *Arch Neurol* 1977;34:2–6.

30. Fairburn B. Intracranial venous thrombosis complicating oral contraception: Treatment by anticoagulant drugs. *BMJ* 1973;2:647.

31. Einhaupl KM, Villringer A, Meister W, et al. Heparin treatment in sinus venous thrombosis. *Lancet* 1991;338:597–600.

32. Barnwell SL, Higashida RT, Halbach VV, Dowd CF, Hieshema GB. Direct endovascular thrombolytic therapy for dural sinus thrombosis. *Neurosurgery* 1991;28:135–142.

33. Scott JA, Pascuzzi RM, Hall PV, Becker GJ. Treatment of dural sinus thrombosis with local urokinase infusion. *J Neurosurg* 1988;68:284–287.

34. Tsai FY, Higashida RT, Matovich V, Alferi K. Acute thrombosis of the intracranial dural sinus: Direct thrombolytic therapy. *Am J Neuroradiol* 1992;13:1137–1141.

35. Higashida RT, Helmer E, Halbach VV, Hieshema GB. Direct thrombolytic therapy for superior sagittal sinus thrombosis. *Am J Neuroradiol* 1989;10:S4–S6.

36. Smith TP, Higashida FT, Barnwell SL, et al. Treatment of dural sinus thrombosis by urokinase infusion. *Am J Neuroradiol* 1994;15:801–807.

37. Alexander LF, Yamamoto Y, Ayoubi S, Al-Mefty O, Smith R. Efficacy of tissue plasminogen activator in the lysis of thrombosis of the cerebral venous sinus. *Neurosurgery* 1990;26:559–564.

38. Pongiglione G, Marasini M, Ribaldone D, Silvestri G, Tuo P, Cantoni-Garello L. Right atrial thrombosis in two premature infants: Successful treatment with urokinase and heparin. *Eur Heart J* 1986;7:1086–1089.

39. Zureikat GY, Martin GR, Silverman NH, Newth CJL. Urokinase therapy for a catheter-related right atrial thrombus and pulmonary embolism in a 2-month old infant. *Pediatr Pulmonol* 1986;2:303–306.

40. Delaplane D, Scott JP, Riggs TW, Silverman BL, Hunt CE. Urokinase therapy for a catheter related right atrial thrombus. *J Pediatr* 1982;100:149–152.

41. Winthrop AL, Wesson DE. Urokinase in the treatment of occluded central venous catheters in children. *J Pediatr Surg* 1984;19:536–538.

42. Ragnall HA, Gomperts E, Atkinson JB. Continuous infusion of low dose urokinase in the treatment of central venous catheter thrombosis in infants and children. *Pediatrics* 1989;83:963–966.

43. Strife JL, Ball WS, Towbin R, Keller MS, Dillon T. Arterial occlusions in neonates: Use of fibrinolytic therapy. *Radiology* 1988;166:395–400.

44. Genton E, Wolf PS. Urokinase therapy in pulmonary thromboembolism. *Am Heart J* 1968;76:628.

45. Amery A, Deloof W, Vermylen J, Verstraete M. Outcome of recent thromboembolic occlusion of limb arteries treated with streptokinase. *BMJ* 1970;4:639–644.

46. *Urokinase–Pulmonary Embolism Trial*. A National Cooperative Study. *Circulation* 1973;47(4): Suppl 2:1–108.

47. Duckert F, Muller G, Nyman D. Treatment of deep venous thrombosis with streptokinase. *BMJ* 1975;1:479–481.

Cerebrovascular Disease, edited by H. Hunt Batjer.
Lippincott-Raven Publishers, Philadelphia © 1997.

CHAPTER 46

A Paradigm for the Use of Antiplatelet Agents in Stroke Prevention

Cathy M. Helgason and Larry D. Brace

This chapter addresses the use of antiplatelet therapy for the treatment of cerebrovascular disease, in particular for prevention of ischemic stroke. The biologic and clinical response to antiplatelet agents may differ for a person with a history of ischemic stroke compared with one without previous vascular occlusion. Antiplatelet therapy is prescribed when there is reason to believe that it will address a pathogenic mechanism for vascular occlusion or stroke that will respond to or be prevented by its use. The use of antiplatelet therapy to prevent stroke is therefore based on full knowledge of the patient's potential for vascular occlusion. The latter may originate from any number of etiologies existing alone or in concert in the same individual. A pure identification of those instances where antiplatelet agents are likely to be effective for recurrent stroke prevention may be difficult, and combined anticoagulant–antiplatelet therapy may be appropriate in some persons to prevent vascular occlusion.

RESPONSE TO ANTIPLATELET AGENTS IN PRIMARY VS. SECONDARY STROKE PREVENTION

This discussion of stroke prevention will focus on secondary stroke. Not much is known about the efficacy of antiplatelet therapy for primary stroke prevention. The distinction may be an important one; it is conceivable that a patient who has already had an ischemic event will have a different baseline thrombotic state and respond in a different fashion to therapeutic maneuvers. Patients who have had a stroke, including those with more than one potential etiology, may have hyperactive platelets (1). It is not unreasonable to think

that these patients may need a different dosage or type of antiplatelet therapy than those who have never had an ischemic event and may not have hyperactive platelets. Plasma factors may also contribute to ischemic events, and patients who have had a previous stroke may be more likely to have a hypercoagulable state (2). In a recent study done at our center, nearly 30% of patients had protein-S deficiency at repeated measurement months beyond the acute phase of the stroke (2). This is new information and may indicate that a hypercoagulable state is often a concomitant contributor to the final event of vascular occlusion in the ischemic stroke patient. The hypercoagulable state may be genetically determined or have other precipitants. There is no evidence that it excludes the potential presence of cardiac or vascular disease, which may also contribute to increased stroke risk or occurrence. Likewise, the presence of cardiac or vascular disease does not exclude the concomitant existence of the hypercoagulable state. The contribution of the presence of protein-S deficiency or any other hypercoagulable state to platelet hyperactivity is not known at present. Theoretically, an increased amount of thrombin formation will cause platelet hyperactivity as thrombin is a very (if not the most) potent stimulant of platelet aggregation.

In common with patients who have already had a stroke, individuals without previous vascular ischemia vary fairly widely in response to a fixed dose of aspirin (3,4). It is not known whether these patients have the potential for developing a need for an increased aspirin dosage over time, as shown in our study of patients with previous stroke (5). It is also not known whether an individual's response to a particular dose of aspirin fluctuates over time (5). These questions may be raised regarding the use of other antiplatelet agents for stroke prophylaxis.

At present, it appears that the potential side effects of the main alternative to aspirin, ticlopidine (Ticlid), are too serious (leukopenia, irreversible thrombocytopenia) to merit its use as a prophylactic agent in the same way as aspirin (6),

C. M. Helgason: Department of Neurology, University of Illinois at Chicago, Illinois 60612.

L. D. Brace: Department of Pathology, College of Medicine, University of Illinois at Chicago, Illinois 60612.

particularly for those without a previous history of vascular occlusion. Fish oil, eicosapentaenoic acid (EPA), garlic, alcohol, and other natural products may inhibit platelet aggregation and have a role in stroke prophylaxis. However, the long-term efficacy of these substances has not been proven, and it is unclear, although doubtful, whether these agents would put people at an increased risk for intracranial hemorrhage, as was suggested for aspirin use in the primary prevention of myocardial ischemia (7).

DIAGNOSIS OF STROKE SUBTYPE BY DEDUCTION RATHER THAN INDUCTION AND PARADIGM FOR THERAPEUTIC DECISIONS FOR RECURRENT STROKE PREVENTION (8)

The distinction between risk factor, etiology, and mechanism is of paramount importance when stroke diagnosis and treatment options are concerned. Risk factors and systemic disease may lead to vascular, cardiac, or hypercoagulable states that in turn lead to vascular occlusion or decreased perfusion. In this context, a *risk factor* is a clearly defined condition or characteristic that has been epidemiologically related to an increased incidence of stroke. Cerebral ischemia may occur in association with a wide variety of conditions. *Etiology* is defined as the cause of stroke. It is the pathology and vehicle by which the risk factors lead to the mechanisms. The *mechanisms* of stroke are the physiologic and biologic processes by which the disease progresses or occurs. The use of any therapy or measure to prevent the occurrence of cerebral infarction will need to be specific for the particular risks, etiology, and mechanisms of stroke.

Stroke caused by ischemia is the common endpoint of thrombosis, embolism, and decreased perfusion. These are the three mechanisms by which the etiologies of cerebral ischemia become manifest in the signs and symptoms of stroke. The etiologies of stroke are those cardiac, hematologic, or vascular conditions that lead to the formation of thrombosis, embolism, or decreased perfusion. The risk factors for stroke may relate to the etiologies (causes) or mechanisms in a causative or other manner.

Antiplatelet agents used prophylactically for primary or recurrent stroke address a mechanism of stroke by preventing thrombosis or thromboembolism. The fact that the patient may develop thrombosis or thromboembolism is based on detailed knowledge of the patient's risk factors and potential etiologies for stroke. Again, the latter involves the diagnosis of cardiac, hematologic, or vascular conditions, as well as risk factors, such as a particular systemic disease, known to contribute to the occurrence of thrombosis and thromboembolism. Antiplatelet agents are not considered, in general, to play a role in preventing stroke due to decreased perfusion, although their position in this instance has not been defined. They may play a role in the treatment of acute stroke, although their mode of action in this setting may not be limited to this mechanism.

Since most ischemic strokes are considered to be caused by thrombosis or thromboembolism, antiplatelet agents have been assumed to be applicable to a wide variety of patients. This consideration exists separately from the fact that a patient with previous stroke has a high likelihood of harboring hyperactive platelets (1). Although the use of any therapeutic agent is tailored toward a particular pathogenic mechanism, not all strokes are due to thromboembolism, and a therapeutic agent targeted to prevent thromboembolism is unlikely to be effective prophylaxis. For example, antiplatelet agents may not be useful for intracranial hemorrhage and vascular occlusion due to cholesterol, calcium, or infective embolization. Furthermore, antiplatelet agents may not be effective for the prevention of all types of thrombi. Red thrombi and fibrin plugs are two thrombi for which anticoagulant agents are likely to be more useful than antiplatelet agents. A thorough and extensive investigation of the patient's blood, heart, and vessels to determine the potential etiology of stroke is unlikely to be undertaken prior to a first stroke. This has also been true for those over a particular age or who are considered to be at increased risk. Therefore, the discussion of the use of antiplatelet therapy in relation to potential etiologies and mechanisms of stroke has been centered on prevention of recurrent stroke, because patients who have had an event are those likely to have undergone the investigations necessary to identify conditions likely to cause future problems. In addition, these are the patients likely to have hyperactive platelets. Diagnostic investigations are performed to enable the clinician to choose the treatment best suited for that particular individual. Even if one has decided that the patient has hyperactive platelets because he or she has had an ischemic stroke and is therefore in need of antiplatelet therapy, failure to investigate the patient for conditions likely to respond to other therapeutic measures will lead to incomplete diagnosis, as well as inadequate therapy.

Most stroke patients are investigated for the risk factors, etiology, and mechanism of stroke with the hope that the disease process can be ameliorated and additional morbidity and mortality prevented. We believe the proper way to do this is to investigate each patient for risk characteristics, systemic disease, hypercoagulable state, cardiac source for embolism, and arterial disease. These entities clearly are not mutually exclusive. In fact, the conditions that give rise to one may make the presence of others more likely. It is not the purpose of this discussion to digress into the topic of determination of stroke causes. However, for antiplatelet therapy to be effective for the prevention of thrombosis or thromboembolism, it is necessary to identify the etiologies and mechanisms likely to be responsive to antiplatelet agents.

Red Thrombus vs. White Thrombus

Several questions surround the use of antiplatelet agents for the prevention of stroke recurrence. Why is antiplatelet therapy expected to prevent thrombosis and thromboembolism? When or under what circumstances will antiplatelet therapy be of benefit? Is it possible that all patients with previous cerebral ischemia, whether of transient or permanent symptomatology, will benefit from platelet inhibition?

The use of antiplatelet therapy is currently defined by the white clot–red clot paradigm (9). If the clinician can determine that a particular patient is at risk for formation of white thrombi, antiplatelet therapy can rationally be chosen for prevention of such an occurrence. White thrombi are platelet and fibrin rich and form in fast-moving arterial streams where the endothelium of the artery has been damaged (eg, in an atherosclerotic artery) (10). Platelet adhesion to the arterial endothelium or underlying subendothelial structures and platelet activation and aggregation are considered to be the main events that lead to white-clot formation (11). An antiplatelet agent might be expected to inhibit platelet adhesion, activation, or aggregation. However, each of the known antiplatelet agents inhibits one or the other process to a greater or lesser degree and the mechanisms by which it does so may differ from those of other agents used to achieve the same effect. The determination of clinicopathologic circumstances under which antiplatelet therapy will be effective for prevention of thromboembolism is currently under study.

Endothelial damage or reduced endothelial function are considered essential for the occurrence of arterial thrombosis. Atherosclerotic arterial disease is the most studied circumstance in which endothelial damage leads to platelet- and fibrin-rich arterial thrombi. However, the arterial endothelium may also be damaged or dysfunctional in association with infectious processes, such as syphilis or arterial vasculitis. The endothelium of coronary arteries and, conceivably, veins may also be damaged in these or other pathologic states. The use of antiplatelet therapy to prevent thrombosis in these settings is not well studied, but theoretically it is likely to be beneficial (12).

Platelet hyperaggregability or hyperactivity has been described and is considered to be a prothrombotic state. It is not entirely understood how hyperactivity of platelets directly causes vascular occlusion. However, the participation of platelets in the atherosclerotic process has been extensively studied. Platelets participate in normal vascular repair processes through the release from alpha granules of stimulatory substances such as platelet-derived growth factor (PDGF). PDGF and other mitogens stimulate smooth muscle cell proliferation and migration into the damaged area. These substances also stimulate lipid metabolism and accumulation in macrophages that have attached and become entrapped in the tissues at the site of damage. With time, the injury heals with minimal or no narrowing of the arterial lumen. However, if repeated injury occurs at the same site, the lumen will progressively narrow, lipid-laden macrophages (foam cells) will accumulate, and atherosclerotic plaque will develop (13,14). The process is accelerated in the presence of hyperactive platelets or hyperlipidemia (15–17). When

platelets are hyperaggregable or hyperactive, it is likely that factors that otherwise may not have been critical in vascular occlusion will suddenly become lethal in this regard, as when the endothelium of the heart or cerebral vasculature is damaged.

Red thrombi are rich in red blood cells and fibrin, although they contain all formed cellular elements. Their formation occurs preferentially under conditions of stasis, such as those encountered in a dilated cardiac chamber or in vessels with low shear rates such as veins or tightly stenosed large arteries adjacent to the stenosis (18). While platelets are present in these thrombi, the role of coagulation factors and natural fibrinolytic processes are generally considered to be more important. The role that antiplatelet therapy might play in preventing formation of this type of thrombus is unclear. As a result, anticoagulant therapy is typically used to prevent red-clot formation. The role of anticoagulant therapy is understandable when the primary risk for thrombotic occlusion is stasis. However, when the patient has a hypercoagulable state (eg, anticardiolipin antibodies or deficiency of proteins C or S, antithrombin III, or activated protein C) and stasis is not the major risk for thrombosis, the use of anticoagulant therapy to prevent red-clot formation seems nonetheless justified. The role of platelets in thrombus formation associated with deficiencies of the fibrinolytic system proteins is unclear.

Role of Platelet Hyperactivity in the Thrombotic Process and Stroke

The presence of platelet hyperaggregability has been described in patients with the antiphospholipid syndrome (19). It would appear that the use of anticoagulants at doses sufficient for intensive effect are required to prevent thrombi in patients with this syndrome (20). The addition of antiplatelet agents in antiphospholipid syndrome patients with platelet hyperaggregability may be justified, although no large randomized studies have been designed to address this issue. Platelet hyperaggregability is present in many patients with atherosclerotic disease (21,22), has been described in patients with diabetes mellitus (23), and has been emphasized as an important contributor to vascular occlusive disease in diabetics. While it is unclear whether all diabetics should be tested for platelet aggregability and placed on antiplatelet therapy for primary prevention of stroke or other vascular occlusion, it seems reasonable for all diabetics who have had an event and demonstrate platelet hyperactivity to be placed on this therapy for prevention of recurrence. In our institution, the presence of platelet hyperaggregability in patients with lower-limb occlusive disease is used as an indication to add an antiplatelet agent to the treatment regimen for these patients.

The presence of deficient proteins C or S or antithrombin III may demand anticoagulation when stasis is an important issue, as in prevention of deep venous thrombosis. However, if the arterial wall is damaged or small-vessel occlusion is to be prevented, it may well be that antiplatelet agents have a role in the prevention of vascular occlusion. Antiplatelet therapy may be particularly valuable in an older population or those with hypertension, diabetes, vasculitis, and the like, where arteries are diseased and the endothelium damaged. For patients who have an underlying hypercoagulable state, combined anticoagulation–antiplatelet therapy would seem more comprehensive. For instance, deficiency of proteins C or S or antithrombin III may not become significant for the arterial tree until arterial vessels become diseased. At such time, the patient may be considered to be in double jeopardy, and the chance for stroke, myocardial infarction, or peripheral vascular occlusion may be increased many times (24). Finally, it is possible (even probable) for patients to harbor more than one condition that, in combination with other conditions, predispose to both red- and white-thrombus formation. Such an example would be a patient who has atherosclerosis, has had a myocardial infarction, and has dilated ischemic cardiomyopathy. Furthermore, the presence of a white clot may in itself predispose to red-clot formation and vice versa. It follows that there may well be a group of patients in whom combination therapy will provide the best therapeutic and prophylactic effect.

Combined Anticoagulant–Antiplatelet Therapy and Aspirin Resistance

The safety of combined warfarin–aspirin therapy has been shown in patients with cardiac disease (25). On the other hand, to our knowledge, no studies have ever been performed comparing the efficacy of combination antiplatelet–anticoagulant therapy with monotherapy with agents of each class for the prevention of thrombosis. We have shown that in a cohort of patients taking warfarin for primary stroke prevention in the Stroke Prevention in Atrial Fibrillation (SPAF I) study at our center, nearly one third of patients receiving warfarin had hyperaggregable platelets (26). This was also the case for patients taking warfarin for recurrent stroke prevention who did not have nonvalvular atrial fibrillation (27). The addition of aspirin to the antithrombotic regimen eliminated the hyperaggregability in some patients who took aspirin 325 mg. Others required aspirin 650 mg, and even at this dosage some were unable to achieve inhibition of platelet hyperaggregability (27). The presence of platelet hyperactivity has been shown to exist in many patients who have had a stroke and not just in those with diabetes or antiphospholipid syndrome. These patients may harbor various etiologies of stroke (1,27).

The potential risk, etiology, and mechanism of stroke in a given person is defined by the extent of the investigation. Frequently, multiple concomitant conditions are discovered in the same individual. It is of paramount importance to note that the site and size, as well as the clinical severity of the cerebral infarct, do not define the risk, etiology, or mechanism of the infarct. A lacunar, or any other sized infarct,

may have a cardiac or arterial source of embolism, or it may be associated with hypercoagulability. The mere definition of infarction by neuroimaging does not reveal information as to its cause. For preventing recurrence or for other purposes, a full investigation of the patient is mandated to determine the appropriate therapy as indicated by diagnosis of risk, etiology, and mechanism. Classifications of stroke subtypes that ignore this fact preclude the above paradigm for therapeutic decision in the setting of stroke.

Platelet hyperactivity may be eliminated by antiplatelet therapy. The dose required for this purpose may vary from individual to individual. If a patient is resistant to a particular therapy, combined therapy (two antiplatelet agents or antiplatelet–anticoagulant therapy) may be justified (28). Because platelet hyperactivity is common in patients in the chronic phase of stroke, it may be that the use of antiplatelet agents in these patients is justified regardless of what else is found.

Normal individuals, as well as patients with previous stroke, may require an individualized dosage of aspirin to achieve antiplatelet effect (29). The efficacy of dosing the antiplatelet agent according to the desired antiplatelet effect has not been studied on a large scale when recurrent stroke prevention has been the endpoint. However, Grotemeyer and colleagues (30), using a "platelet reactivity test," showed that when aspirin effect was not achieved after stroke, individuals were more likely to have a recurrent cerebral ischemic event than those who had full aspirin inhibition of platelet reactivity. Similarly, we have shown that some individuals who at one time had full aspirin effect as judged by inhibition of platelet aggregation had recurrent stroke at a time when the same dose of aspirin appeared to be inadequate to maintain its prior antiaggregant effect (5). Others required increasing dosage of aspirin in order to regain the full antiplatelet aggregation effect of aspirin. Still others had a fluctuating effect of aspirin without dosage change. Some individuals had become resistant to aspirin effect in spite of increase in dosage up to 1300 mg. The importance of monitoring the antithrombotic effect of aspirin or any other antiplatelet agent is not appreciated at present but certainly has been suggested by these studies.

Ticlopidine has not been studied with respect to its antiplatelet effect to the same extent as aspirin (31). However, aspirin and ticlopidine appear to inhibit platelet function by different mechanisms. The inhibitory action of aspirin through its irreversible inhibition of platelet cyclooxygenase is well known. On the other hand, ticlopidine appears to inhibit platelet function through an adenosine diphosphate (ADP)–dependent mechanism, although the details of this mechanism have not been completely elucidated. Thus, ticlopidine may be expected to inhibit the ADP-induced platelet response in a more pronounced fashion than aspirin, while epinephrine (Epi), arachidonic acid (AA), and collagen responses are only mildly affected. On the other hand, aspirin has marked inhibitory action on Epi-, collagen-, and AA-induced aggregation but only mild effects on ADP-induced platelet aggregation. Combined antiplatelet therapy with agents possessing different mechanisms of action should produce effects that are at least additive if not synergistic (32).

The maximum ticlopidine effect on platelet aggregation is at present undefined. Based on our observations, we suggest that a 50% decrease in the response to 5 μmol/l ADP–induced aggregation could define the maximum ticlopidine response, although further data are required to support this suggestion. Several of our patients have in fact exhibited a decreased response to ADP by 90%.

There have been no studies to date that have attempted to determine whether different individuals require a different dosage of ticlopidine in order to achieve the same degree of platelet inhibition. Once the antiplatelet effect is achieved, it is not known if a constant dose will maintain that effect over time. We have studied the inhibition of platelet aggregation in a few individuals taking ticlopidine for recurrent stroke prevention. One of these patients has been on combined warfarin–ticlopidine therapy and has developed platelet hyperactivity according to the platelet-aggregation test. Other individuals have maintained an antiplatelet effect on combined aspirin–ticlopidine therapy. In other instances, the therapy has been a combination of ticlopidine at a lower-than-usual dosage—125 mg (half a tablet) twice a day—and enteric-coated aspirin 325 mg/d. It may be that the combination of the two antiplatelet agents at low doses will give additional antiplatelet effect to that of either given alone. Again, this may only be true for some individuals. Others may need a full dose of both to achieve the same effect. Furthermore, the side effects of each, but particularly those of ticlopidine, may be fewer or less severe when given at a lower dose. This is true for the diarrhea associated with ticlopidine. The efficacy of this combination therapy for recurrent stroke prevention has not been studied, nor has the need for individualized dosing and repeated measurements for maintenance of effect over time.

One additional effect of ticlopidine is that it may be expected to reduce shear-induced platelet aggregation that is dependent on ADP but not on products of cyclooxygenase activity. The effect of ticlopidine on shear-induced platelet aggregation may be another way to measure its biologic effect (32). While aspirin is not expected to inhibit shear-induced platelet aggregation, it has been shown to do so in high doses (33,34). One explanation for this observation is that any process that activates platelets, in this instance shear stress, ultimately causes release of arachidonic acid from membrane phospholipids. The free arachidonic acid is rapidly metabolized by cyclooxygenase to intermediate prostaglandins, which are then converted to thromboxane. Thromboxane promotes the platelet-release reaction and platelet aggregation. If cyclooxygenase is inhibited, then shear-induced aggregation would not be reinforced by thromboxane formation. Therefore, it is conceivable that one might also use the effect of high-dose aspirin on shear-induced platelet aggregation as another marker of its biologic activity.

Antiplatelet Effect of Aspirin: Prostacyclin and Bleeding Time

Aspirin is believed to exert its antithrombotic effect through inhibition of platelet aggregation. This effect can be measured for the individual patient, and the test can be performed repeatedly over time in order to judge the maintained efficacy of a given dosage of a medication. As mentioned previously, a large randomized study has not yet been done to show whether dosage adjustment based on monitored antiplatelet effect is clinically important.

Criticism of measuring inhibition of platelet aggregation has come from those who believe that no matter what the antiplatelet effect of a given dosage of aspirin, no conclusion about antithrombotic efficacy can be made if the inhibition of prostacyclin is not measured concomitantly. This argument is based on the fact that prostacyclin production, like thromboxane production, depends on functional cyclooxygenase. Since prostacyclin is a potent inhibitor of platelet aggregation and has vasodilatory effects, inhibition of endothelial cell prostacyclin production would theoretically be detrimental. However, another potent inhibitor of platelet aggregation, nitric oxide, also promotes vasodilatation, and its production is not commonly considered to be affected by aspirin. Nitric oxide is also produced by the endothelium, although the interdependence and relative importance of nitric oxide compared with prostacyclin is not yet clear. Feinberg and colleagues suggested that in spite of inhibition of prostacyclin, vasodilatation was inhibited in an ex vivo heart perfusion model where vasoconstrictors and aspirin were in the perfusing fluid (35). These authors suggested that in this model the production of nitric oxide (or other vasodilators) was stimulated by aspirin. If this is correct, the relative importance of prostacyclin production may be less than that previously thought.

Another possibility is that inhibition of prostacyclin metabolism in the endothelium of systemic arteries is not inhibited by aspirin. Some preparations of aspirin are absorbed into the portal circulation and may well have exerted its effect on cyclooxygenase (platelet and endothelial) prior to leaving the portal circulation (36), in which case aspirin would not be presented to the systemic circulation. If this argument applies to the enteric-coated aspirin used in our study, the importance of inhibition of prostacyclin production would be minimal. It may also be that diseased arteries are incapable of producing prostacyclin or nitric oxide in effective concentrations. Under these circumstances, the antithrombotic effect of the antiplatelet agent would be of paramount importance in the prevention of thrombosis, and the potential inhibition of prostacyclin production would be of questionable significance (37). Finally, no one has shown that the inhibition of prostacyclin production by aspirin contributes to thrombosis, and it may be that inhibition of thromboxane production overrides the importance of diminished prostacyclin production. The nagging issue of the prothrombotic potential of aspirin in relation to its usage to prevent vascular occlusion needs to be clarified since it has given rise to a wide variety of dosing schemes for aspirin. Some believe that aspirin 80 mg/d will inhibit platelet function but not endothelial cell prostacyclin production. Some use aspirin 325 mg every other day, believing that the time between doses allows endothelial cell recovery of prostacyclin production, while retaining antiplatelet effect. Finally, others use aspirin 325–1300 mg/d, believing that the most important benefit from aspirin treatment is the inhibition of platelet function by diminished platelet thromboxane production. It is not clear that the effects achieved by a given dose of aspirin can be predicted; the data show that the doses needed to achieve certain biologic effects vary and that some people are aspirin resistant, and this may be dependent on characteristics particular to the individual (eg, weight, absorption, genetic susceptibility of the platelet and vascular endothelium to aspirin, concomitant disease states, concomitant medications).

Platelet aggregation inhibition is one test that is available to measure the biologic effect of aspirin. The bleeding time test has been cited by some as the preferred test to measure aspirin efficacy. Bleeding time is primarily a measure of platelet adhesion, and adhesion is not affected to a significant degree by aspirin. It is only to the degree that platelet aggregation, which is affected by aspirin, participates in hemostasis after platelet adhesion that aspirin's effect may be expressed. Even in experienced hands, bleeding time is a crude measurement. While it is true that most individuals respond to aspirin with an increase in bleeding time, the variation from person to person is wide. In some individuals, there is a large increase in bleeding time (the so-called aspirin responders), while in others only a minor increase or no change is seen (aspirin nonresponders). Finally, for some patients residual scar formation at the incision site is a significant problem. In our opinion, bleeding time is an inadequate measurement of aspirin efficacy or effect.

Aspirin and Acute Stroke

While antiplatelet agents are typically used in the prevention of recurrent stroke, they may have a role in the treatment of the acute event. Platelet activation from products released by ischemic tissue plays a role in reperfusion injury, and aspirin or ticlopidine may be useful during this phase of the acute event. Aspirin can be given intravenously, but ticlopidine is not available for parenteral administration. When ticlopidine is given orally, it may take days for the antiplatelet effect to be expressed (6,31,38). The efficacy of combined antiplatelet–anticoagulant effect for the treatment of acute stroke has not been studied.

At this time, heparin remains the standard treatment for thrombotic/thromboembolic stroke. However, in some patients heparin induces the formation of antibodies to platelet factor 4 expressed on the platelet surface. The antibody will only bind in the presence of heparin, but once bound to the platelet surface, it causes platelets to be eliminated by the reticuloendothelial system. These patients have the syndrome of heparin-induced thrombocytopenia (HIT). Some patients with HIT develop arterial and venous thrombi due to in vivo platelet aggregation. Heparin-dependent antibody-induced platelet aggregation is dependent on thromboxane formation, and aspirin prevents platelet aggregation in this circumstance (39,40). Patients receiving both heparin and aspirin may develop HIT, but in our experience such patients have not developed thrombi and their platelet count falls more gradually than in the patient with HIT who is not on aspirin. For patients who develop HIT while on heparin and aspirin, thrombocytopenia develops progressively over 4–6 days; for those who develop HIT on heparin only, thrombocytopenia develops rapidly over 1–2 days. It is not known what the effect of ticlopidine would be in these circumstances. Heparin can also cause platelet aggregation by mechanisms that do not involve antibody formation and are aspirin sensitive. For these reasons, it has become our practice to strongly consider the use of aspirin–heparin combination therapy whenever heparin is used for the treatment of acute stroke.

Aspirin and Stroke Etiology

The most commonly used antiplatelet agent is aspirin. The considerations discussed above for the use of aspirin therapy may require a major shift in paradigm by which its use is chosen.

Large randomized trials of aspirin have focused on prevention of ischemic stroke as a disease, not the common endpoint of multiple etiologies. Choice of dosage has focused on intrinsic properties of the drug itself and not on patient response to or need for a particular dosage based on stroke pathogenesis. The etiologies and mechanisms of ischemic stroke may be broadly investigated in the individual patient by examination of the blood, heart, and vessels. Blood tests define the presence or absence of systemic disease or hypercoagulable states associated with stroke; cardiac examination is performed to define arrhythmia, alteration of flow, or morphologic details commonly accompanied by thromboembolism; and examination of the extra- and intracranial vasculature helps define vascular morphologic irregularities and/or stenosis consistent with endothelial damage or alterations of flow that can lead to thrombosis. The treating physician can then logically decide whether antiplatelet, anticoagulant, combination antiplatelet–anticoagulant, or another therapeutic modality (carotid endarterectomy) is indicated for the prevention of ischemic stroke in that patient. For the present, this choice almost always includes the use of appropriate antithrombotic therapy because the majority of ischemic strokes are thought to be caused by vascular occlusion by thrombosis or thromboembolism. Situations of decreased perfusion are difficult to predict, but causes include decreased cardiac output due to dilated cardiomyopathy and decreased cerebral blood flow through tight arterial stenoses. If it is determined that a state of decreased perfusion exists, one may also include antithrombotic therapy as part of the therapeutic regimen, since these states are also predictive of thrombosis and cerebral embolism. Vascular occlusion may also occur by means of embolism of nonthrombotic matter, such as infectious material, cholesterol, fat, air, or calcium. Antithrombotic therapy probably would not be solely effective in such cases. Clinically, it may be impossible to distinguish these events from thrombotic occlusion, unless the embolus is somehow visualized, as may be the case in the ocular fundus (Hollenhorst plaque). With further refinements, Doppler and other ultrasound imaging techniques may be able to define embolus composition.

For the etiologies of ischemic stroke that can be identified, very little data are to be found from large randomized trials that tell us how to choose the appropriate antithrombotic therapy based on anticipated pathophysiology of future events. If one reviews the entities diagnosed by blood tests (ie, systemic disease and hypercoagulable states), examination of the heart for arrhythmia or cardiogenic source of embolism and the vasculature for changes suggestive of impending thromboocclusion, the current paradigm of red clot vs. white clot (anticoagulant vs. antiplatelet) for choosing therapy seems to apply. The SPAF I trial concluded that aspirin therapy is more effective than placebo for prevention of primary stroke in patients with nonvalvular atrial fibrillation. The second phase of the same trial attempted to compare aspirin with warfarin therapy in the same cohort but did not find any difference between the two therapies in patients younger than 75 years. For those who were older, the hemorrhagic side effects of warfarin outweighed its benefit over aspirin (41). The European Atrial Fibrillation Trial (EAFT) study showed that for recurrent stroke prevention in those with known atrial fibrillation, warfarin is better than aspirin therapy, although both were effective (42). Combination warfarin–aspirin therapy may be useful in this setting, especially for patients too old to take warfarin at doses sufficient to significantly prolong the prothrombin time (PT)—or international normalized ratio (INR)—because of bleeding risk. For other cardiac sources of embolism, the benefit of antiplatelet therapy used alone is less clear. There is evidence that for those patients with mechanical heart valves, combined warfarin–aspirin or warfarin–dipyridamole therapy is more effective than warfarin therapy alone for the prevention of thromboembolism. The incidence of bleeding complications may be slightly higher with the aspirin–warfarin combination when compared with warfarin use alone. Nonetheless, the benefit of combined aspirin–warfarin therapy was not outweighed by bleeding complications. Antiplatelet therapy may have a role in the instance of bacterial endocarditis or other cardiac disease in which the endothelium may be damaged (43–45).

For known arterial disease, there is little information regarding the use of antiplatelet therapy, except for that derived retrospectively from the North American Symptomatic Carotid Endarterectomy Trial (NASCET) study (46). The information derived from that study showed that those patients who underwent carotid endarterectomy followed by best medical therapy (in most patients aspirin therapy) fared better in terms of recurrent ischemic stroke prevention than those who were assigned to best medical therapy alone, which always included aspirin therapy. This trial appears to indicate that in patients with tight carotid stenosis (≥70%) who have had ischemic symptoms, the efficacy of aspirin therapy alone in preventing recurrent stroke was less than that achieved when aspirin was used in conjunction with a specific therapy, carotid endarterectomy, aimed at removing the arterial site of predicted thrombosis or embolism. It should be pointed out that in NASCET the dose of aspirin was not controlled and varied widely. No attempt to individualize or measure a patient's response to aspirin in terms of its antithrombotic effect was made. Examination of the data seems to indicate that of the patients on aspirin alone, those on higher doses of aspirin had a lower incidence of recurrent stroke. In addition, the perioperative morbidity was less in those patients who took higher doses of aspirin than others undergoing this surgical procedure in the trial.

Currently, the ability of antiplatelet therapy to prevent stroke in those patients who harbor hypercoagulable states is unclear. Aspirin would seem to be indicated, at least as adjunct therapy, based on theoretical considerations, but there is no clear evidence that antiplatelet therapy is efficacious in those with hypercoagulable states or other systemic disease states associated with stroke.

CONCLUSION

Important recent findings may bring into question the appropriateness of the white clot–red clot paradigm for choosing antithrombotic therapy to use in an individual patient. Many stroke subtypes are associated with the presence of hyperactive platelets, and this is particularly true in the chronic phase of stroke. In addition, acute stroke itself has been associated with platelet hyperactivity. Finally, the results of all the large randomized trials performed to predict the utility of antiplatelet therapy in those patients who have experienced a recent transient ischemic attack or stroke are significant. These trials have shown that aspirin therapy is effective in reducing stroke recurrence for these patients by at least 22%. Interestingly, ticlopidine has been shown to be more effective than aspirin, especially in the first year after the ictal event (47). The efficacy of aspirin in prevention of stroke recurrence also decreases with time. Thus, regardless of subtyping stroke by etiology, aspirin or ticlopidine may be effective for the prevention of recurrence. Whether the results can be extrapolated to primary stroke prevention is currently not known.

Aspirin is the most commonly prescribed agent for the prevention of thrombotic/thromboembolic stroke. The most common circumstance under which it is prescribed is for prevention of recurrence. However, it is important to point out that no clinical trial has monitored a measurable effect of aspirin thought to be associated with the ability to prevent thrombosis or has correlated this effect with clinical outcome. This is especially important since it has been shown that the efficacy of aspirin is not absolute and there are recurrences of stroke and other vascular events in patients taking aspirin for recurrent stroke prevention. Recent literature concerning normal individuals and patients who have had a cerebral ischemic episode manifested by transient or permanent symptoms indicates that when the antiplatelet effect of aspirin is monitored, different individuals express different degrees of antiplatelet effect when all are given a fixed dose of aspirin. In addition, for patients with previous stroke, the antiplatelet effect of aspirin therapy may vary over time. It is not known whether the same phenomenon will ultimately be described for ticlopidine. We have already observed that the antiplatelet effect of a given dose of ticlopidine is not uniform among individuals. We have not yet done sequential testing of platelet aggregation in these patients to determine if the antiplatelet response to a constant dose of this agent will vary over time.

These recent findings thus suggest that in the prescription of antiplatelet therapy for stroke, in particular recurrent stroke prevention, the dose of aspirin needs to be individualized with regard to some measure of antithrombotic response, and that response should be monitored over time in order to assure maximal and sustained efficacy. The high dose–low dose paradigm for choosing an aspirin dose is no longer sufficient with regard to achieving antiplatelet effect. Nonetheless, it must be shown that attaining the antiplatelet effect is the important parameter to measure when clinical efficacy—stroke prevention—is the goal.

Aspirin has other newly discovered effects that may ultimately be important in the larger framework of stroke prevention. It has been shown in atherosclerotic vessels that transforming growth factor β (TGF-β) levels are depressed and the presence of aspirin may increase these levels (48). This effect of aspirin may inhibit smooth muscle cell proliferation by the arterial wall or inhibit macrophage cytokine release. The end result may be a diminished rate of atherosclerotic plaque formation. Likewise, one effect of cyclooxygenase pathway inhibition may be to enhance the lipoxygenase pathway, a second pathway of arachidonic acid metabolism. The vasoactive and platelet-related activities of metabolites of this pathway are at present unappreciated but may have beneficial effects. Preconditioning with brief periods of ischemia has been shown in laboratory animals to decrease ultimate infarct size in hearts. This protective effect has been shown to be due to lipoxygenase metabolites that increase K^+ channel and decrease Ca^{++} channel activity. This same effect may apply to transient ischemic attack. In addition, aspirin may have some effect on nitric oxide–dependent inhibition of platelet aggregation. Neutrophils have a platelet antiaggregant effect through a nitric oxide–mediated, cyclic guanosine monophosphate (cGMP)–dependent pathway. When blood samples from patients taking aspirin were tested, aspirin facilitated the inhibitory effect of neutrophils on platelet activation by thrombin, ADP, and epinephrine (49,50). In these studies, it was also shown that this effect occurred in the presence of aspirin via a nitric oxide–mediated mechanism. In a recent study, our group has shown that aspirin inhibits the expression of P-selectin when platelets are stimulated by collagen. Others have shown in similar experiments that when epinephrine and ADP are used as activating agents, aspirin is ineffective for the same result (51,52).

Finally, one should address the issue of aspirin resistance and failure in the clinical setting of stroke. Grotemeyer and colleagues (30) measured aspirin effect by a platelet reactivity test in patients who had suffered a stroke. In this study, aspirin nonresponders, as defined by the results of their platelet reactivity test, had a higher likelihood of recurrent stroke. Our group has measured aspirin effect ex vivo by inhibition of platelet aggregation when platelets are stimulated by ADP, AA, collagen, and epinephrine. At repeated measurement over time, one third of patients who once responded to a particular dose of aspirin ultimately lost the effect of the drug at that dosage. We anxiously await the chance to learn that our results have been confirmed.

Most medications are prescribed with the individual's response and disease diagnosis in mind. The efficacy of most medications is monitored over time to insure that the proper dosage adjustments are made. Given the evidence presented in this paper, we believe that it is highly likely that this well known prescribing paradigm also applies to antiplatelet agents. It must also be emphasized that the diagnosis of risk factor, etiology, and mechanism of stroke must be meticulously pursued in the deductive manner in order that a comprehensive therapeutic approach to stroke treatment be achieved (8,53).

REFERENCES

1. Iwamoto T, Kubo H, Takasaki M. Platelet activation in the cerebral circulation in different subtypes of ischemic stroke and Binswanger's disease. *Stroke* 1995;26:52–57.
2. Helgason CM, Brace LD. Issues and problems with existing antithrombotic therapy with warfarin and aspirin in patients with stroke. *Curr Neurol* 1995;15:101–115.
3. Pappas JM. Population variability in the effect of aspirin on platelet function. *Arch Pathol Lab Med* 1994;118:801–804.
4. Hormes JT, Austin JH, James G, et al. Toward an optimal antiplatelet dose of aspirin: Preliminary observations. *J Stroke Cerebrovasc Dis* 1991;1:27–35.
5. Helgason CM, Bolin K, Hoff JA, et al. The development of aspirin resistance in persons with previous ischemic stroke. *Stroke* 1994;25:2331–2336.
6. Hass WK, Easton JD, eds. *Ticlopidine, Platelets and Vascular Disease.* New York: Springer-Verlag, 1993.
7. Steering Committee of the Physician's Health Study Research Group. Final report on the aspirin component of the ongoing physician's health study. *N Engl J Med* 1989;321:129–135.
8. Popper KR, Miller D. A proof of the impossibility of inductive probability. *Nature* 1983;302:687–688.
9. Fitzgerald GA, Jennings LK, Patrono C, eds. *Platelet-Dependent Vascular Occlusion.* New York: New York Academy of Sciences, 1994.

10. Marcus AJ, Safier LB. Thromboregulation: Multicellular modulation of platelet reactivity in hemostasis and thrombosis. *FASEB J* 1993;7:516–522.

11. Ware JA, Heistad DD. Platelet endothelium interactions. *N Engl J Med* 1993;328:628–635.

12. Green K, Vesterqvist O. Activation of thromboxane and prostacyclin biosynthesis in humans. *Adv Prostaglandin Thromboxane Leukot Res* 1990;21:607–610.

13. Ross R. The arterial wall and atherosclerosis. *Annu Rev Med* 1979;30:1–15.

14. Ross R, Glomset J. The pathogenesis of atherosclerosis. *N Engl J Med* 1976;295:420–425.

15. Conrad J, Samama MM. Inhibitors of coagulation atherosclerosis and arterial thrombosis. *Semin Thromb Hemost* 1986;12:87–90.

16. Eldrup-Jorgensen J, Flanigan DP, Brace LD, et al. Hypercoagulable state and lower limb ischemia in young adults. *J Vasc Surg* 1989;9:334–341.

17. Olcott C, Wylie EJ. Platelet aggregation in patients with severe atherosclerosis. *J Surg Res* 1978;83:144–150.

18. Ranke C, Hecker H, Creutzig A, Alexander K. Dose dependent effect of aspirin on carotid atherosclerosis. *Circulation* 1993;87:1873–1879.

19. Schafer AI, Kroll MH. Nonatheromatous arterial thrombosis. *Annu Rev Med* 1993;44:155–170.

20. Khamashta MA, Cuadrado MJ, Mujic F, Taub NA, Hunt BJ, Hughs GRV. The management of thrombosis in the antiphospholipid-antibody syndrome. *N Engl J Med* 1995;332:993–997.

21. Davies J. Defective platelet disaggregation associated with occlusive arterial diseases. *Angiology* 1973;24:391–397.

22. Fitzgerald GA, Smith B, Pedersen AK, Brash AR. Increased prostacyclin biosynthesis in patients with severe atherosclerosis and platelet activation. *N Engl J Med* 1984;310:1065–1068.

23. Patrono C, Davi G. Antiplatelet agents in the prevention of diabetic vascular complications. *Diabetes Metab Rev* 1993;9:177–188.

24. Gomez C. Personal communication.

25. Turpie AGG, Gent M, Laupacis A, et al. A comparison of aspirin with placebo in patients treated with warfarin after heart-valve replacement. *N Engl J Med* 1993:524–529.

26. Fagan SC, Kertland HR, Tietjen GE. Safety of combination aspirin and anticoagulation in acute ischemic stroke. *Ann Pharmacother* 1994;28:441–443.

27. Albers GW. Transoesophageal echocardiographic findings in stroke subtypes. *Stroke* 1994;25:23–28.

28. Helgason CM, Hoff JA, Kondos GT, et al. Platelet aggregation in patients with atrial fibrillation taking aspirin or warfarin. *Stroke* 1993;24:1758–1761.

29. Helgason CM, Tortorice KL, Winkler SR, et al. Aspirin response and failure in cerebral infarction. *Stroke* 1993;24:345–350.

30. Grotemeyer K-H, Scharafinski H-W, Husstedt I-W. Two year follow up of aspirin responder and aspirin non-responder. A pilot study including 180 post-stroke patients. *Thromb Res* 1993;71:397–403.

31. Hardisty RM, Powling MJ, Nokes TJC. The action of ticlopidine on human platelets. Studies on aggregation, secretion, calcium mobilization and membrane glycoproteins. *Thromb Haemost* 1990;64:150–155.

32. Cattaneo M, Lombardi R, Bettega D, Lecchi A, Mannucci PM. Shear-induced platelet aggregation is potentiated by desmopressin and inhibited by ticlopidine. *Arterioscler Thromb* 1993;13:393–397.

33. Ronald HE, Orvim U, Bakken IJ, Barstad RM, Kierulf P, Sakariassen KS. Modulation of thrombotic responses in moderately stenosed arter-ies by cigarette smoking and aspirin ingestion. *Arterioscler Thromb* 1994;14:617–621.

34. Ratnatunga CP, Edmondson SF, Rees GM, Kovacs IB. High dose aspirin inhibits shear-induced platelet reaction involving thrombin generation. *Circulation* 1992;85:1077–1082.

35. Shwu-Luan L, Levitsky S, Feinberg H. Effects of exogenous vasoconstrictors on coronary vascular resistance and prostacyclin production of the quiescent heart: The inhibitory effect of aspirin. *J Pharmacol Exp Ther* 1989;248:44–49.

36. Clarke RJ, Mayo G, Price P, Fitzgerald GA. Suppression of thromboxane A2 but not of systemic prostacyclin by controlled release aspirin. *N Engl J Med* 1991;325:1137–1141.

37. Seccombe JF, Schaff HV, eds. *Vasoactive Factors Produced by the Endothelium. Physiology and Surgical Implications.* Austin, TX: R.G. Landes, 1994.

38. Mohri H, Ohkubo T. Single dose effect of enteric coated aspirin on platelet function and thromboxane generation in middle aged men. *Ann Pharmacother* 1993;27:405–410.

39. Amiral J, Bridey F, Dreyfus M, et al. Platelet factor 4 complexed to heparin is the target for antibodies generated in heparin-induced thrombocytopenia. *Thromb Haemost* 1992;68:95–96.

40. Brace LD, Fared J, Tomeo J, et al. Biochemical and pharmacological studies on the interaction of PK 10169 and its subfractions with human platelets. *Haemostasis* 1986;16:93–105.

41. Stroke Prevention in Atrial Fibrillation Investigators. Warfarin versus aspirin for prevention of thromboembolism in atrial fibrillation. Stroke prevention in atrial fibrillation II study. *Lancet* 1994;343:687–691.

42. European Atrial Fibrillation Trial (EAFT) Study Group. Secondary prevention in non-rheumatic atrial fibrillation after transient ischemic attack or minor stroke. *Lancet* 1993;342:1255–1262.

43. Fatkin D, Herbert E, Feneley MP. Hematologic correlates of spontaneous echo contrast in patients with atrial fibrillation and implications for thromboembolic risk. *Am J Cardiol* 1994;73:672–676.

44. Asherson RA, Cervera R. Antiphospholipid antibodies and the heart. *Circulation* 1991;84:920–923.

45. Tannenbaum SH, Finko R, Cines DB. Antibody and immune complexes induce tissue factor production by human endothelial cells. *J Immunol* 1986;137:1532–1538.

46. Dyken ML, Barnett HJM, Easton JD, Fields WS, et al. Low-dose aspirin and stroke: "It ain't necessarily so." *Stroke* 1992;23:1395–1399.

47. Antiplatelet Trialist's Collaboration. Secondary prevention of vascular disease by prolonged antiplatelet therapy. *BMJ* 1988;296:320–332.

48. Grainger DJ, Kemp PR, Metcalf JC, et al. The serum concentration of active transforming growth factor beta is severely depressed in advanced atherosclerosis. *Nature Med* 1995;1:74–80.

49. Ferri A, Calza R, Pelligrini A, Cattani L. Two distinct mechanisms of inhibition of platelets aggregation by acetylsalicylic acid. *Biochem Mol Biol Int* 1994;32:1101–1107.

50. Lopez-Farre A, Caramelo C, Estaban A, et al. Effects of aspirin on platelet-neutrophil interactions: Role of nitric oxide and endothelin-1. *Circulation* 1995;91:2080–2089.

51. Larsson PT, Wallen NH, Hjemdahl P. Norepinephrine-induced human platelet activation in vivo is only partly counteracted by aspirin. *Circulation* 1994;89:1951–1957.

52. Rinder CS, Student LA, Bonan JL, Rinder HM, Smith BR. Aspirin does not inhibit adenosine diphosphate induced platelet alpha-granule release. *Blood* 1993;82:505–512.

53. Michel PL. Pathologie coronaire: Les benefices de l'aspirin. Quelles doses pour quelles pathologies? *Ann Cardiol Angeiol (Paris)* 1994;43:204–210.

Cerebrovascular Disease, edited by H. Hunt Batjer.
Lippincott-Raven Publishers, Philadelphia © 1997.

CHAPTER 47

Intracranial Embolectomy and Bypass Procedures for Occlusive Disease: Current Indications

Stephen L. Skirboll, David W. Newell, and M. Sean Grady

Surgical intervention for cerebral ischemia due to intracranial occlusive vascular disease has been the subject of great controversy over the past decade. C. Miller Fisher, MD, predicted that "anastomosis of the external carotid artery or one of its branches with the internal carotid artery above the area of narrowing should be feasible" and that "someday vascular surgery will find a way to bypass the portion of the artery during the period of ominous fleeting symptoms" (1). With the development of microsurgical techniques in the 1960s, the first superficial temporal artery–middle cerebral artery (STA-MCA) bypass procedure was performed for cerebrovascular disease by Yasargil and associates (2). In subsequent years, this procedure gained increasing acceptance among neurosurgeons for a variety of indications associated with brain ischemia. In 1985, the EC/IC Bypass Study Group reported a 5-year prospective study of 1377 patients randomly assigned to surgical or medical management for symptoms of transient ischemic attack (TIA) or stroke (3). This study concluded that extracranial-to-intracranial (EC-IC) bypass was no more effective than aspirin therapy in reducing stroke or stroke-related deaths in all categories examined. Subsequently, controversy has surrounded the indications and efficacy of intracranial bypass procedures.

In this chapter, we will review the assessment of brain ischemia, indications for bypass procedures or embolectomy, and surgical techniques for bypass in the anterior or posterior circulations. We will conclude with an overview of the future of these procedures.

RATIONALE FOR SURGICAL BYPASS PROCEDURES

Brain ischemia occurs when cerebral blood flow (CBF) is not sufficient to meet metabolic demands. Reduction of CBF may be caused by narrowing or occlusion of arteries leading to or situated within the intracranial cavity or by a reduction of cardiac output. Occlusion or narrowing of these major arteries may result from cardiac or artery-to-artery embolism, arterial dissection, atherosclerosis, or arterial thrombosis. This chapter will concentrate on the correction of flow-limiting lesions of arteries within the intracranial compartment caused by embolus or atherosclerotic narrowing.

The EC-IC bypass study has been criticized by a number of investigators and clinicians in the field of cerebrovascular disease. (4–6). However, it is clear that indiscriminate use of bypass procedures for brain ischemia is not justified. Over the past 5 years, a more comprehensive understanding of the pathophysiology of cerebral ischemia has been acquired, in no small part due to the EC-IC bypass study and the multicenter clinical trials comparing medical to surgical treatment of carotid artery disease. As a result, the selection of patients who may benefit from bypass procedures has become better defined.

Thromboembolism, the major cause of stroke or TIA, typically does not occur in intracranial vessels of sufficient caliber to permit open surgical embolectomy. For the most part, embolic material originates from the carotid bifurcation in the neck or from the heart. In cases of progressive intracranial arterial narrowing or occlusion, the brain accommodates to the reduction in CBF by developing collateral arterial supply. Patients whose symptoms of cerebral ischemia result

All authors: Department of Neurological Surgery, Harborview Medical Center, Seattle, Washington 98104.

from flow-limiting lesions of intracranial arteries (hemodynamic—rather than thromboembolic-related stroke or TIA) make up a small but important subset. It is the identification of this subset that is the key to determining the population that may benefit from bypass procedures.

PATIENT SELECTION

Clinical Characteristics

Patients should have a history of recurrent symptoms of focal cerebral or retinal ischemia, manifested by TIAs, reversible ischemic neurologic deficits, or mild completed strokes with subsequent fluctuations in neurologic function. Bypass surgery is not indicated in patients with acute or chronic major neurologic deficits. Similarly, an intracranial bypass procedure is not indicated in the asymptomatic patient or in patients with relief of symptoms by anticoagulation or antiplatelet drugs (7). Evaluation should include history and physical examination, chest radiograph, electrocardiography (ECG), and laboratory studies. Identification of stroke risk factors such as cardiac and vascular disease should be fully assessed by the appropriate consultants and tests. Finally, patients must demonstrate evidence of a flow-restricting lesion with insufficient collateral supply and impaired cerebrovascular reserve capacity by a combination of diagnostic anatomic and physiologic imaging techniques as described below.

Diagnostic Imaging

The pattern of damage detected by computed tomography (CT) and magnetic resonance imaging (MRI) can be correlated with the cause of a stroke. Hemodynamic cerebral ischemia or infarction may be distinguished from that caused by thromboembolism by a location limited to transition zones between the vascular territories of the anterior cerebral, middle cerebral, and posterior cerebral arteries. Tissue damage in these regions is often termed a ''border-zone infarction.'' MRI provides greater sensitivity than CT in detecting previous ischemic parenchymal damage, although it may not offer any increase in clinical usefulness. Instead, the degree of parenchymal abnormalities on MRI may better represent an overall description of chronic cerebrovascular disease that may be related to the risk of subsequent stroke (8).

Complete four-vessel cerebral angiography, including images of the external carotid arteries, is mandatory to fully appreciate the pathologic vascular anatomy underlying symptoms of stroke or TIA. Improved catheter design and techniques have reduced the morbidity and mortality associated with angiography, currently at approximately less than 3% in institutions experienced in studying patients for cerebrovascular disease. Only angiography can clearly discern the degree and nature of occlusive lesions, possible embolic

sources, and patterns of cerebral collateral supply. MR angiography has recently become available as a noninvasive technique to visualize the cerebral circulation. At present, this modality may serve as a potentially effective technique for screening or follow-up but does not yet provide optimal dynamic flow information and spatial resolution from which to best determine specific therapeutic interventions.

Advances in physiologic imaging have made the most impact in identifying the patient population that may benefit from an intracranial bypass procedure. Angiography does not provide sufficient insight into the physiologic response of the cerebral vasculature to identify those patients at the greatest risk for hemodynamic ischemia. Dilation of cerebral vessels is an important compensatory mechanism when cerebral perfusion pressure is decreased as a consequence of progressive vascular occlusive disease with poorly developed collateral supply (9,10). In these cases, it is important to evaluate the patient's ability to increase CBF above a resting state by determining the intrinsic vascular capacity to respond to physiologic challenges such as CO_2 or acetazolamide (11–13). This capacity has been termed the cerebrovascular reserve capacity (CRC), or vasomotor reactivity (VMR). Several techniques have been reported, including xenon Xe 133 CT (14) and transcranial Doppler ultrasonography (TCD) with acetazolamide or CO_2 challenge (11,13,15).

Such techniques were not widely available at the time of the EC-IC bypass study. Preliminary reports at that time showed that these tests might be quite important for identifying patients being considered for EC-IC bypass. However, the bypass study was not limited to patients with proven hemodynamic insufficiency and included patients with ischemia associated with a wide range of pathophysiologic conditions. Using techniques to measure cerebrovascular reactivity, investigators have better described and defined hemodynamic ischemia, as well as demonstrating that patients with this type of compromise may be at an increased risk of stroke. A prospective trial of patients with internal carotid artery (ICA) occlusion using TCD with CO_2 challenge found that individuals with diminished or exhausted reactivity had a significantly greater risk (30% vs. 8%) of stroke over a 3-year period compared with individuals with normal reactivity (16). Similar results were established in patients with ICA stenosis or occlusion, using ^{133}Xe-CT with acetazolamide challenge; patients with impaired blood-flow reactivity showed a 36% incidence of stroke over 2 years vs. 4.4% in the normal vasoreactivity group (17).

Significant improvement in CRC was demonstrated following EC-IC arterial bypass surgery in 28 patients with internal carotid artert occlusion and symptomatic hemodynamic cerebral ischemia (18). Before surgery, all patients had recurring episodes of neurologic deficits with angiographically defined ICA occlusion correlating to the side of ischemia, brain CT scans that were either normal or showed border-zone infarction, and severely impaired CRC using ^{133}Xe single-photon emission CT (SPECT) and acetazolamide challenge. The immediate and long-lasting postoperative improvement in CRC was ascribed to the bypass-vessel contribution to CBF. In contrast, Piepgras et al (19) demonstrated no significant improvement after bypass in patients with cerebral occlusive disease and decreased CRC. Resting CBF was essentially unchanged following bypass surgery in this study, suggesting that appropriate candidates for bypass surgery may be those individuals with specific deficits due to ongoing hemodynamic cerebral ischemia and severely impaired CRC that affects the resting CBF.

Cerebrovascular Reactivity Testing

The stages of cerebrovascular compensation for reduced cerebral perfusion pressure caused by proximal arterial obstruction has been well defined using position emission tomography (PET) scan data (10). PET technology has not become widely available to clinicians with an interest in brain ischemia. Other technologies, however, have been able

to provide similar information, albeit not as extensive as PET scan data on reduced CRC in response to proximal arterial lesions. Direct studies of CBF can be performed using radioactive xenon with external detectors, as well as using cold xenon with CT-derived information on the regional distribution, the cold xenon being an index of CBF (17). SPECT can provide regional information on relative blood flow to various brain regions. TCD measurements can monitor the middle cerebral artery (MCA) velocity and thereby detect relative changes in blood flow in response to various stimuli.

To detect changes in cerebrovascular reactivity from proximal arterial obstruction, each of these techniques can be used before and after a vasodilatory or vasoconstrictive stimulus, and the vascular reactivity can be calculated. The commonly used vasodilatory stimuli include inhalation of CO_2 and administration of acetazolamide. In general, as proximal arterial occlusions cause a progressive decrease in perfusion pressure, the first thing to be lost is the vasodilatory response to either acetazolamide or CO_2. Subsequently, the vasocon-

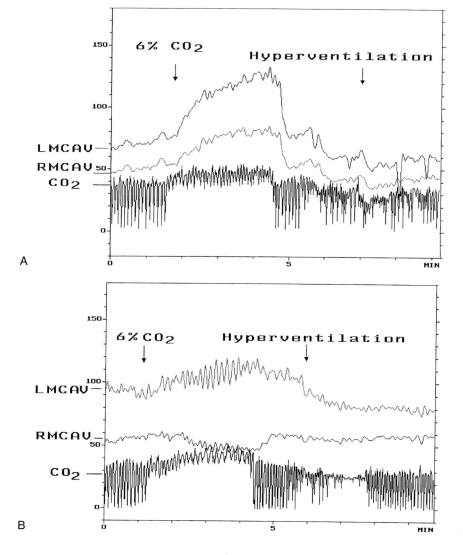

FIG. 1. Example of continuous TCD recordings of both middle cerebral arteries (MCAs) and end-tidal CO_2 in response to changes in CO_2. **(A)** Normal response to inhalation of 6% CO_2 and hyperventilation indicates an increase in blood flow velocity with CO_2 inhalation and a decrease with hyperventilation. **(B)** Abnormal response to changes in CO_2 concentration in the right MCA with more normal response in the left. With inhalation of 6% CO_2, there is an increase in the left MCA velocity and the subsequent paradoxical response in the right MCA velocity with a decrease in flow velocity. With hyperventilation, there is a decrease in flow velocity in the left MCA and no change in the right MCA velocity. This study indicates exhausted vasomotor reserve (VMR) on the right with a paradoxical or "steal" response (LMCAV, left MCA velocity; RMCAV, right MCA velocity; y axis, velocity in cm/sec; x axis, time in minutes).

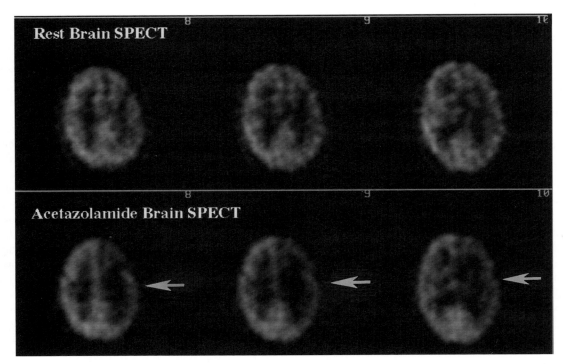

FIG. 2. (A) Normal resting brain SPECT in a patient with limb-shaking TIAs that were brought on by decreases in blood pressure. **(B)** The same patient after administration of acetazolamide exhibits a decrease in perfusion in the MCA territory *(arrows)*.

strictive response to hyperventilation is also affected, and then finally with a vasodilatory stimulus of either acetazolamide or CO_2, there is a paradoxical response of blood flow. In this situation, the blow flow decreases in the affected area with a vasodilatory stimulus. Various scales have been developed to grade responsiveness with each technique. It has now been demonstrated by both TCD with CO_2 and VMR testing, as well as by cold xenon and acetazolamide testing that absent cerebrovascular reactivity in patients with carotid occlusion leads to an increased risk of stroke versus patients with carotid occlusion and intact or only moderately impaired VMR (16,17). Figure 1A shows a normal response in both middle cerebral vessels to hyperventilation and CO_2 inhalation, and Fig. 1B shows an exhausted response with a slight "steal" phenomenon with inhalation of CO_2 in a patient with an intracranial carotid occlusion. Figure 2 shows an example of SPECT imaging before and after acetazolamide administration, indicating a focal area of hypoperfusion during acetazolamide challenge.

Advantages of the TCD imaging include its low cost, ease of test performance, and no requirement of radioisotopes. Disadvantages include the fact that the regional resolution is poorer than tomographic techniques such as SPECT or cold-xenon CT. The direct measurement of autoregulation using TCD has also been performed in patients and is being investigated in those with occlusive disease. Preliminary results indicate that this technique correlates very well with CO_2 reactivity (20). It appears that each of these techniques

is now becoming more readily available and can reliably identify patients with true hemodynamic insufficiency.

Table 1 lists the indications for bypass procedures.

SPECTRUM OF PROCEDURES

Anterior Circulation

Anterior circulation cerebral bypass surgery for occlusive disease is not restricted to a single standard procedure. De-

TABLE 1. *Indications for bypass procedures in atherosclerotic occlusive disease*

TIAs, RINDs, or mild completed strokes with fluctuating neurologic symptoms

Cerebral ischemia or infarction in the border zone or terminal supply territories on imaging studies

Angiographic demonstration of arterial stenosis or occlusion in region that correlates with neurologic symptoms

Failure of medical therapy including modification of risk factors (eg, hypotension) and use of antiplatelet and anticoagulant therapy

Insufficient physiologic collateral blood supply (eg, inadequate ophthalmic, anterior or posterior circle of Willis collaterals, leptomeningeal, or transdural collaterals) associated with impaired cerebrovascular reserve capacity as determined by functional testing (eg, TCD with CO_2/acetazolamide, SPECT-acetazolamide)

TABLE 2. *Bypass procedures for anterior circulation ischemia*

Proximal vessel	Interposition vessel	Recipient vessel
Superficial temporal artery (STA)		Cortical middle cerebral artery (MCA)
STA		M2/M3 of MCA
STA	Vein	M2/M3 of MCA
STA	Vein	Cortical MCA branch
Cervical carotid artery (CCA)	Vein	Cortical MCA branch
CCA	Vein	Supraclinoid internal carotid artery (ICA)
CCA	Vein	Petrous ICA
Petrous ICA	Vein	Intradural ICA
External carotid artery (ECA)	Vein	Cortical MCA branch
Subclavian artery	Vein	Cortical MCA branch
Occipital artery (OA)		Cortical MCA branch
OA	Vein	Cortical MCA branch
Middle meningeal artery		Cortical MCA branch
Retroauricular artery		Cortical MCA branch
STA placed directly on cortex		

pending on the clinical setting, the basic revascularization procedure varies with regard to location of donor vessel, need for an interposition graft, and location of recipient vessel. Donor vessels usually consist of the superficial temporal artery (STA) or its branches, the petrous ICA, or the internal or external cervical carotid artery (CCA). As a general rule, scalp vessels with angiographic lumen diameter <1 mm cannot be used. The patency rates are lower, technical difficulty with anastomosis is greater, and the potential blood-flow augmentation provided by such vessels is reduced. The larger of the two STA branches (anterior or posterior) is usually chosen, although the anterior branch is better situated to facilitate anastomosis to proximal MCA branches. Donor vessels may be directly anastomosed to recipient vessels, as in the STA-MCA bypass or in a petrous ICA–supraclinoid ICA bypass; or they may rely on an interposed vein graft, as in a CCA–petrous ICA or CCA-MCA bypass. Interposition bypass procedures offer the advantage of a larger blood flow channel and can be used when the distal STA is occluded or diseased. Table 2 lists various types of bypass procedures for the anterior circulation.

The advantages of the STA-MCA bypass include its shorter operative time, its less technically challenging nature, and its demonstrated high patency rate of 96% at 1 month after surgery (3). In addition, Schmiedek et al (18) demonstrated a substantial benefit of revascularization for hemodynamic ischemia using the STA-MCA bypass. The

advantages of a saphenous vein bypass graft procedure include a more proximal site of anastomosis, avoidance of abnormal ''watershed'' areas, and greater blood flow. It is particularly advantageous when suitable STA branches are lacking.

Posterior Circulation

While vertebrobasilar insufficiency (VBI) from posterior circulation disease is not as common as anterior circulation ischemia, recurrent TIAs are associated with a similar 25–35% risk of subsequent infarction over the next 4–5 years (21,22). Moreover, posterior circulation infarcts may be associated with an increased morbidity and mortality (23,24). Caplan (25) and others have noted that lesions specific to the vertebrobasilar system compared with other areas are more prone to result in recurrent ischemic symptoms and infarction.

As with the anterior circulation, the most common pathologic process affecting the vertebrobasilar system is atherosclerosis, which can occur at any portion. Natural history studies of atherosclerotic disease in the posterior vs. anterior circulation suggest several possible distinctions (26,27). VBI develops more often secondary to intracranial as compared with extracranial disease (28,29). VBI symptoms usually result from arterial stenosis rather than emboli of the vertebrobasilar system, and ulceration of plaques in general is unusual in the posterior circulation (27–29). Thus, hemodynamic insufficiency, and not emboli, may be more common as a cause of posterior circulation stroke or TIA. In their review of cerebral revascularization, Onesti et al (30) noted that the vertebrobasilar system has fewer naturally occurring collaterals and bypass procedures in this region must perfuse less tissue compared with the anterior circulation. It is these differences that suggest that bypass procedures in the vertebrobasilar system may play a larger role than in the anterior circulation.

As with anterior circulation procedures, numerous surgical options are available for bypass of occlusive disease. Table 3 summarizes the majority of published surgical approaches.

Patient Selection

According to Whisnant et al (31), VBI symptoms include two of the following: (a) motor and/or sensory symptoms occurring bilaterally or simultaneously, (b) dysmetria or gait ataxia, (c) dysarthria, (d) bilateral homonymous hemianopia, (e) diplopia. Other symptoms associated with VBI include tinnitus, vertigo, and multiple cranial nerve deficits, which usually are contralateral to the major sensory deficit. If other symptoms such as dizziness, syncope, drop attacks, or global amnesia occur singly, etiologies other than VBI should be investigated. The diagnosis of VBI should exclude cardiac pathology (dysrhythmias, cardiac insufficiency, emboli), blood disorders (thrombocytosis, sickle cell disease, hyper-

TABLE 3. *Revascularization procedures for the posterior circulation*

Proximal vessel	Interposition vessel	Recipient vessel
Occipital artery (OA)		Posteroinferior cerebellar artery (PICA)
OA		Anteroinferior cerebellar artery (AICA)
Superficial temporal artery (STA)		Superior cerebellar artery (SCA)
STA		Posterior cerebral artery (PCA)
External carotid artery	Saphenous vein	PCA
Cervical carotid artery	Saphenous vein	Vertebral artery
Vertebral artery	Radial artery	PICA

coagulable states), basilar migraine headaches, demyelinating disease, intracranial neoplasms, and in some cases Meniere's disease. A detailed work-up should include complete differential blood count with smear, coagulation profile panel, metabolic screen, a 12-lead ECG, and Holter monitoring for 24–36 hours.

Diagnostic Imaging

A CT scan is useful in delineating strokes and excluding the presence of nonvascular structural lesions. MRI allows a more sensitive description of ischemic areas in the posterior fossa and may afford the possibility of using MR spectroscopy to study these areas. Metabolic function can also be studied with PET, which may provide important physiologic background on the hemodynamic effects in patients with VBI. As with the anterior circulation, complete cerebral angiography remains the gold standard to delineate pathologic vascular disease and collateral supply. TCD has only more recently been used to evaluate vertebrobasilar disease, which is inherently more problematic because of vessel identification and the unusual hemodynamic characteristics of this vascular territory.

COMPLICATIONS OF BYPASS PROCEDURES

Bypass procedures may result in the conversion of an intracranial stenosis to occlusion, leading to an acute neurologic deficit (32). The incidence of this can be reduced by treating with anticoagulants (eg, warfarin or heparin) for 3–6 months prior to surgical consideration (7). Many high-grade lesions will resolve during this treatment, obviating the need for surgical intervention. One theoretical advantage of a proximal placement of anastomosis is the improved perfusion to a greater number of vessels with a lessened chance

of stagnation in the vessel segment just distal to a stenotic site. If a deficit does occur as a result of a proximal intracranial occlusion with a patent graft, the patient can be managed by hydration and increases in the blood pressure. Symptoms persisting or beginning after several days may be treated with anticoagulants to reduce the risk of thrombosis.

Early postoperative deficits following EC-IC bypass have been well described (33). Most are transient and may be caused by cerebral edema, seizures, or dysautoregulation. These pathologic events are considered to be a direct consequence of the redistribution of flow surrounding the anastomotic site. Electroencephalography and close monitoring of anticonvulsant levels should be performed if seizures are suspected, and some groups maintain high steroid doses until the deficit has mostly resolved (34).

Late complications are usually due to ischemia. Delayed stroke may be caused by graft compromise or thrombosis, progression of atherosclerotic disease in the donor vessel, embolization from the graft, or the late conversion of an intracranial stenosis to an occlusion (32). Patients are maintained on daily aspirin to minimize some of these possibilities and control systemic risk factors (eg, hypertension, elevated cholesterol, diabetes, etc). Avoidance of smoking is mandatory. Anticoagulants may be necessary if embolization is suspected. TCD with emboli monitoring may help guide decisions regarding the administration of anticoagulants. If emboli observed by TCD are frequent and persistent, treatment with anticoagulants may be indicated. However, the value of emboli monitoring in this situation has not been established.

As with ischemia, bleeding complications may be seen in both the early and late postoperative periods. Early postoperative hemorrhage can be prevented with tight control of blood pressure (35). The incidence of hemorrhage may be further minimized by delaying the procedure after a recent stroke, if possible, and avoiding the placement of the anastomosis in an area of encephalomalacia. Bleeding from perfusion pressure breakthrough is a theoretical concern when higher flows are reestablished to an ischemic or poorly regulated vascular region. This phenomenon has been more frequently described with higher-flow vein grafts (36).

Early bleeding may occur at the anastomotic site despite strict blood pressure control and is obviously best controlled by preventative measures intraoperatively. Surgical evacuation should be performed when a hematoma causes a substantial degree of mass effect. Repeat bleeding or a new onset of bleeding may suggest the development of a pseudoaneurysm at the anastomotic site, which should be evaluated by angiography and treated with surgical revision.

Other potential complications include fluid collections in the subdural or subgaleal spaces in the early postoperative period; these usually resolve with time. In addition, scalp necrosis, wound infection, and meningitis are all potential issues complicating wound healing. Careful surgical exposure and technique help reduce the incidence of scalp necrosis and wound breakdown.

INTRACRANIAL EMBOLECTOMY

The lodging of an embolus in a major artery in the circle of Willis generally has catastrophic consequences, particularly if there is no well established collateral vascular supply distal to the embolus. Rather than the slow occlusion of focal atherosclerotic disease, which allows time for collaterals to develop, a large embolus causes an immediate reduction in cerebral blood flow. The subsequent stroke is usually large with devastating neurologic consequences. Surgical intervention is limited to arteries with a lumen diameter >1 mm, typically the supraclinoid internal carotid artery (ICA) and middle cerebral artery (MCA). Several critical factors limit the usefulness of intracranial embolectomy, including length of time required to establish diagnosis and operative time required to expose the appropriate vessel and perform the embolectomy. Advances in endovascular neuroradiology and development of thrombolytic drugs such as tissue plasminogen activator (t-PA) and urokinase have relegated intracranial embolectomy to very rare occasions. Circumstances in which embolectomy may be reasonable are limited to identification of a thromboembolism in a major vessel during craniotomy. With the development of intraoperative TCD, major embolic events during carotid endarterectomy have been identified. While embolectomy may have been contemplated for such cases in the past, direct infusion of urokinase through a catheter placed directly into the carotid artery is much faster and consequently likely to be more efficacious (37).

Description of intracranial embolectomy includes case reports and very small series (38–40). All are in agreement that reperfusion must occur within 6–8 hours of onset of symptoms. Mortality and functional results vary considerably in these reports. Ipsilateral ICA occlusion is associated with a poor outcome, and collateral flow on angiography is the best predictor of outcome.

CONCLUSIONS

Subsequent to the EC/IC Bypass Study (3), vascular bypass procedures have most frequently been employed to revacularize the brain when the parent artery must be sacrificed because of tumors or aneurysms. The development of imaging techniques to determine the physiologic response of the cerebral vasculature to stimuli such as CO_2 challenge have enabled physicians interested in cerebrovascular disease to identify patients whose cerebrovascular reserve capacity (CRC) is exhausted. It is this population of patients with "isolated hemispheres," ie, a cerebral hemisphere with poor or absent collateral supply and clinical evidence of ischemia, that will benefit from intracranial bypass procedures. This group is a small subset of the population with cerebral ischemia; careful and thoughtful evaluation of a patient with symptoms of stroke or TIA must occur before the diagnosis of ischemia can be reached on a hemodynamic basis. However, when identified—and after failure of medical treatment—this group of patients can experience relief of their symptoms by intracranial bypass. Intracranial embolectomy, on the other hand, will likely be indicated only rarely but may be needed in certain situations in which acute embolism occurs and there is easy surgical access to the affected vessel.

ACKNOWLEDGMENTS

We would like to thank Colleen Douville, Registered Vascular Technologist, for assistance with TCD studies and Rosetta Marx for preparation of the manuscript.

REFERENCES

1. Fisher CM. Occlusion of the internal carotid artery. *Arch Neurol Psychiatry* 1951;65:346–377.
2. Yasargil MG. Diagnosis and indications for operations in cerebrovascular occlusive diseases. In: Yasargil MG, ed. *Microsurgery Applied to Neurosurgery*. Stuttgart: Georg-Thieme-Verlag, 1969:95–105.
3. The EC/IC Bypass Study Group. Failure of extracranial-intracranial bypass to reduce the risk of ischemic stroke: Results of an international randomized trial. *N Engl J Med* 1985;313:1191–1200.
4. Ausman JI, Diaz FG. Critique of the extracranial-intracranial bypass study. *Surg Neurol* 1986;26:218–221.
5. Awad IA, Spetzler RF. Extracranial-intracranial bypass surgery: A critical analysis in light of the international cooperative study. *Neurosurgery* 1986;19:655–664.
6. Sundt TM JR. Was the international randomized trial of extracranial-intracranial arterial bypass representative of the population at risk? *N Engl J Med* 1987;316:814–816.
7. Day AL. Indications for surgical intervention in middle cerebral artery obstruction. *J Neurosurg* 1984;60:296–304.
8. Awad IA. Extracranial-intracranial bypass surgery: Current indications in techniques. In: Awad IA, ed. *AANS Topics in Cerebrovascular Occlusive Disease and Brain Ischemia*. American Association of Neurological Surgeons; Park Ridge, Illinois 1992:215–230.
9. Gibbs JM, Leenders KL, Wise RJS, et al. Evaluation of cerebral perfusion reserve in patients with carotid-artery occlusion. *Lancet* 1984;1:310–314.
10. Powers WJ, Press GA, Grubb RL Jr, et al. The effect of hemodynamically significant carotid artery disease on the hemodynamic status of the cerebral circulation. *Ann Intern Med* 1987;106:27–35.
11. Ringelstein EB, Sievers C, Ecker S, et al. Noninvasive assessment of CO_2-induced cerebral vasomotor response in normal individuals and patients with internal carotid artery occlusions. *Stroke* 1988;19:963–969.
12. Vorstrup S, Paulson OB, Lassen NA. How to identify hemodynamic cases. In: Spetzler RF, Carter LP, Selman WR, et al, eds. *Cerebral Revascularization for Stroke*. New York: Thieme-Stratton, 1985:120–126.
13. Widder B. The Doppler CO_2 test to exclude patients not in need of extracranial/intracranial bypass surgery. *J Neurol Neurosurg Psychiatry* 1989;52:38–42.
14. Herold S, Brown MM, Frackowiak RS, et al. Assessment of cerebral haemodynamic reserve: Correlation between PET parameters and CO_2 reactivity measured by the intravenous 133 xenon injection technique. *J Neurol Neurosurg Psychiatry* 1988;51:1045–1050.
15. Piepgras A, Schmiedek P, Leinsinger G, et al. A simple test to assess cerebrovascular reserve capacity using transcranial Doppler sonography and acetazolamide. *Stroke* 1990;21:1306–1311.
16. Kleiser B, Widder B. Course of carotid artery occlusions with impaired cerebrovascular reactivity. *Stroke* 1992;23:171–174.
17. Yonas H, Smith HA, Durham SR, et al. Increased stroke risk predicted by compromised cerebral blood flow reactivity. *J Neurosurg* 1993;79:483–489.
18. Schmiedek P, Piepgras A, Leinsinger G, Kirsch C-M, Einhaupl K. Improvement of cerebrovascular reserve capacity by EC-IC arterial

bypass surgery in patients with ICA occlusion and hemodynamic cerebral ischemia. *J Neurosurg* 1994;81:236–244.

19. Piepgras A, Schmiedek P, Leinsinger G, et al. Follow-up studies of cerebrovascular reserve capacity in patients with cerebrovascular disease. In: Schmiedek P, Einhaupl K, Kirsch CM, eds. *Simulated Cerebral Blood Flow*. Berlin: Springer-Verlag, 1992:263–267.

20. Newell DW, Aaslid R, Lam A, et al. Comparison of flow and velocity during dynamic autoregulation testing in humans. *Stroke* 1994;25:793–797.

21. Cartlidge NEF, Whisnant JP, Elveback LR. Carotid and vertebral-basilar transient cerebral ischemia attacks. A community study, Rochester, Minnesota. *Mayo Clin Proc* 1977;52:117–120.

22. Heyman A, Wilkinson WE, Hurwitz BJ, et al. Clinical and epidemiologic aspects of vertebrobasilar and nonfocal cerebral ischemia. In: Berguer R, Bauer RB, eds. *Vertebrobasilar Arterial Occlusive Disease: Medical and Surgical Management*. New York: Raven Press, 1984:27–36.

23. McDowell FH, Potes J, Broch S. The natural history of internal carotid and vertebral-basilar artery occlusion. *Neurology* 1961;11:153–157.

24. Jones HR Jr, Millikan CH, Sandok BA. Temporal profile (clinical course) of acute vertebrobasilar system cerebral infarction. *Stroke* 1980;11:173–177.

25. Caplan LR. Vertebrobasilar disease. Time for a new strategy. *Stroke* 1981;12:111–114.

26. Spetzler RF, Hadley MN, Martin NA, et al. Vertebrobasilar insufficiency. Part 1: Microsurgical treatment of extracranial vertebrobasilar disease. *J Neurosurg* 1987;66:648–661.

27. Hopkins LN, Martin NA, Hadley MN, et al. Vertebrobasilar insufficiency. Part 2: Microsurgical treatment of intracranial vertebrobasilar disease. *J Neurosurg* 1987;66:662–674.

28. Fisher CM, Gore I, Okabe N, et al. Atherosclerosis of the carotid and vertebral arteries—extracranial and intracranial. *J Neuropathol Exp Neurol* 1965;24:455–476.

29. Castaigne P, Lhermitte F, Gautier JC, et al. Arterial occlusions in the vertebrobasilar system. A study of 44 patients with post-mortem data. *Brain* 1973;96:133–154.

30. Onesti ST, Solomon RA, Quest DO. Cerebral revascularization: A review. *Neurosurgery* 1989;25:618–629.

31. Whisnant JP, Cartlidge NEF, Elveback LR. Carotid and vertebral-basilar transient ischemic attacks: Effect of anticoagulants, hypertension, and cardiac disorders on survival and stroke occurrence—A population study. *Ann Neurol* 1978;3:107–115.

32. Gumerlock MK, Ono H, Neuwelt EA. Can a patent extracranial-intracranial bypass provoke the conversion of an intracranial arterial stenosis to a symptomatic occlusion? *Neurosurgery* 1983;12:391–400.

33. Heros RC, Scott RM, Kistler JP, et al. Temporary neurologic deterioration after extracranial-intracranial bypass. Neurosurgery 1984;15:178–185.

34. Day AL, Chandler HN. Cerebral revascularization. In: Apuzzo M, ed. Brain Surgery. New York: Churchill Livingstone, 1993:908–924.

35. Heros RC, Nelson PB. Intracerebral hemorrhage after microsurgical cerebral revascularization. *Neurosurgery* 1980;6:371–375.

36. Sundt TM, Piepgras DG, Marsh WR, et al. Saphenous vein bypass grafts for giant aneurysms and intracranial occlusive disease. *J Neurosurg* 1986;65:439–450.

37. Barr JD, Horowitz MB, Mathis JM, et al. Intraoperative urokinase infusion for embolic stroke during carotid endarterectomy. *Neurosurgery* 1995;36:606–611.

38. Meyer FB, Piepgras DG, Sundt TM, et al. Emergency embolectomy for acute occlusion of the middle cerebral artery. *J Neurosurg* 1985;62:639–647.

39. Gagliardi R, Benvenuti L, Guizzardi G. Acute operation in cases of MCA occlusion. *Neurosurgery* 1983;12:636–639.

40. Galibert P, Delcour J, Grunewald P, et al. Les obliterations de l'arterer Sylvienne. *Neurochirurgie* 1971;17:165–176.

Cerebrovascular Disease, edited by H. Hunt Batjer.
Lippincott-Raven Publishers, Philadelphia © 1997.

CHAPTER 48

Modern Stroke Prevention

Philip A. Teal and John W. Norris

Stroke is an eminently preventable disease. Despite declining stroke mortality documented over several decades, cerebrovascular events remain the third leading cause of death, accounting for 10–12% of deaths in industrialized countries. In the United States alone, there are 500,000 new stroke victims annually, resulting in 150,000 deaths. The economic burden of caring for new cases and the 3 million stroke survivors costs the United States $20 billion a year (1). The human costs in terms of suffering and disability far exceed the dollars and cents of stroke care. Prevention is the most effective strategy to reduce the human and economic burden of cerebrovascular disease.

Several lines of evidence support the concept that stroke is avoidable. First, epidemiologic data, although flawed, suggest that the decline in stroke mortality may, in part, be due to declining stroke incidence (2). Second, prospective studies have identified manageable stroke risk factors such as hypertension and smoking. It is proposed that the control of these risk factors over time may be responsible for the decline in stroke mortality. Third, controlled, randomized trials and metaanalysis of available data have proven the benefits of antiplatelet therapy for the prevention of atherothrombotic stroke, anticoagulation for the prevention of cardioembolic stroke, and carotid endarterectomy for the prevention of stroke associated with high-grade carotid stenosis.

The limited efficacy of currently available interventional therapies for acute stroke underscores the need to optimize stroke prevention strategies. It is commonplace to evaluate a patient with an acute stroke due to inadequately treated hypertension, atrial fibrillation, or symptomatic carotid stenosis, even though it has been estimated that more than 50%

of stroke deaths could be avoided by the appropriate application of currently available knowledge (3).

RISK FACTORS

Epidemiologic studies have identified risk factors for stroke. Risk factors may be classified as nonmodifiable biologic traits, modifiable physiologic factors, and lifestyle or behavioral patterns that have an impact on stroke risk (Table 1). A cornerstone of all stroke prevention strategies is the recognition and manipulation of risk factors through lifestyle changes or active treatment.

Nonmodifiable Biologic Traits

Age, Sex, and Race

Age, sex, and race are inherent biologic risk factors for stroke that are not amenable to treatment. Age is the most powerful predictor of stroke, and stroke incidence rises exponentially with advancing years. After age 55 years, the stroke risk more than doubles with each passing decade (Fig. 1).

Men are more prone to stroke than women in all age groups (approximate risk, 1.3 : 1), except the most elderly. A 45-year-old man has a one-in-four risk of stroke if he lives to reach the age 85; the risk is one in five in women (2). Women, however, are twice as likely as men to suffer a fatal stroke. Among stroke survivors, women are less likely to be discharged home than men. Stroke subtypes also differ based on sex: Women are more likely to suffer subarachnoid hemorrhage, while men are more prone to ischemic infarction (4).

Racial differences exist for stroke incidence and for the site of cerebrovascular pathology. African-Americans have a higher age-standardized incidence of stroke, a higher stroke prevalence, and an almost twofold increase in stroke mortality compared with their white counterparts. The Japanese and Chinese have the highest stroke rates in the world. Cerebrovascular disease was the leading cause of death in Japan

P. A. Teal: Stroke Service, Vancouver Hospital and Health Sciences Center, University of British Columbia, Vancouver, British Columbia, Canada V5Z 4E1.

J. W. Norris: Department of Neurology, University of Toronto, Sunnybrook Health Sciences Centre, Toronto, Ontario, Canada M4N 3M5.

TABLE 1. *Stroke risk factors*

Nonmodifiable biological traits
Age
Sex
Heredity
Race

Potentially modifiable physiologic factors
Hypertension
Diabetes
Lipids
Cardiac disease
Carotid stenosis
Transient ischemic attacks
Homocystinuria
Aortic atheroma

Lifestyle and behavioral factors
Smoking
Obesity
Exercise
Diet
Alcohol use
Oral contraceptives

until only recently, when it was overtaken by cardiovascular causes (5). Intracranial cerebrovascular disease is more prevalent in the Japanese and African-Americans in contrast to the pattern of extracranial occlusive disease found in whites.

Genetic Factors

While family history of stroke is felt to contribute to the risk profile, the strength of genetic determinants for stroke

remain uncertain. Conflicting data suggest that either a maternal or paternal history of stroke may confer an increased stroke risk to offspring. A recent study of over 1200 monozygotic twins and over 1100 dizygotic twins reported a concordance rate for stroke of 17.7% and 3.6%, respectively (6). Familial dyslipidemias, hereditary coagulopathies, and hereditary forms of cerebral amyloidosis are associated with increased stroke incidence. A rare familial form of stroke, cerebral autosomal-dominant arteriopathy with subcortical infarcts and leukoencephalopathy (CADASIL), has been localized to chromosome 19q12 (7).

Potentially Modifiable Risk Factors

Hypertension

Hypertension is the most important risk factor for ischemic and hemorrhagic stroke. Systolic, diastolic, and combined systolic/diastolic hypertension are all powerful independent risk factors. In the Framingham Study, blood pressures >160/95 mm Hg increased the age-adjusted relative risk for stroke by 3.1 for men and 2.9 for women, even in the elderly (4). The risk of stroke increases in proportion to increasing blood pressure. An overview analysis of nine trials involving almost 420,00 patients showed that a prolonged increase of 7.5 mm Hg in the diastolic pressure was associated with a doubling of stroke risk (8). There was no evidence of a lower threshold below which the attributable risk disappeared. The relationship between systolic hypertension and stroke is at least as powerful. Even borderline isolated systolic hypertension between 140 and 160 mm Hg significantly increases the risk of stroke, and stroke incidence rises directly with the level of systolic pressure. It is

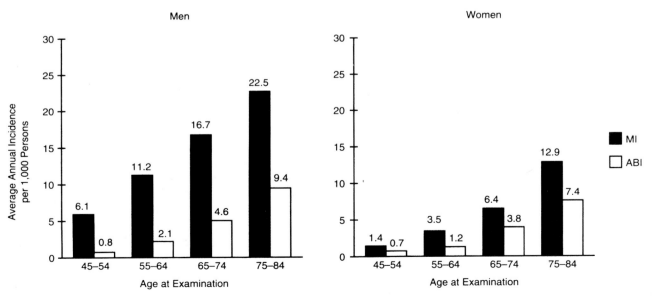

FIG. 1. Incidence of myocardial and brain infarction in men and women according to age categories. (From ref. 4, with permission.)

estimated that about 40% of strokes are due to systolic blood pressure >140 mm Hg. The old clinical maxim that the normal "age-adjusted" systolic blood pressure is 100 mm Hg plus the age in years is invalid.

Lipids

The severity and progression of carotid artery and cerebrovascular atherosclerosis are directly and independently related to cholesterol and low-density lipoprotein (LDL) levels. The connection between serum lipids and stroke, however, remains unclear, reflecting perhaps the heterogeneous nature of cerebrovascular disease and the complex, opposing effects of cholesterol on the risk of ischemic vs. hemorrhagic stroke. Evidence that cholesterol is an independent risk factor for ischemic stroke is beginning to mount. The Multiple Risk Factor Intervention Trial (MRFIT), which screened and followed 350,977 men, reported a positive dose-dependent increased risk for fatal ischemic stroke for cholesterol levels >4.14 mmol/l (>160 mg/dl) (9). An inverse relationship was detected between elevated cholesterol and fatal intracerebral hemorrhage. This apparent paradox may be explained by experimental evidence in hypertensive rats that suggests that low levels of cholesterol weakens the endothelium of cerebral arteries, thus predisposing to intracranial hemorrhage. The number of stroke outcome events in the MRFIT study were too few to permit firm conclusions to be drawn regarding the strength of cholesterol as a risk factor for ischemic stroke. An overview analysis of ten prospective studies found that a total cholesterol level >5.72 mmol/l (>220 mg/dl) was associated with a pooled relative risk for stroke between 1.31 and 2.90 (10).

Conflicting data exist regarding the role of lipoprotein (a) [Lp(a)] as an independent risk factor for stroke. The Physicians Health Study found no association between Lp(a) and stroke in a prospective study of 15,000 middle-aged men, while others have reported that elevated Lp(a) levels may be a major risk factor for ischemic stroke (11,12).

Further studies are required to clarify the relationship between serum lipids and stroke.

Diabetes

Diabetes accelerates atherosclerosis and is associated with both extra- and intracranial arterial disease, thereby predisposing to ischemic stroke. The risk of stroke in diabetics is increased by 1.5–3.5, depending on the type, duration, and severity of disease. Experimental evidence and some human data correlate elevated glucose levels and diabetes with poor stroke outcome. Although biologically plausible, optimal diabetic control has not yet been proven to reduce the risk of initial or recurrent stroke.

Atrial Fibrillation

Atrial fibrillation (AF), chronic or paroxysmal, is the most important cardiac stroke risk factor. Nonvalvular AF

(NVAF) is associated with a fivefold increase in stroke risk, and AF poses a nearly 20-fold increased risk in patients with rheumatic mitral valve disease (13). Based on a pooled data analysis from five contemporary randomized treatment trials, the risk of stroke in untreated patients with NVAF averages 4.5% annually (14). Factors believed to exacerbate the risk of stroke include age 65 years and older, a history of hypertension or diabetes, and a history of previous transient ischemic attacks (TIAs) or strokes. The annual risk of stroke in untreated (control) patients varied from 1.0% in patients younger than 65 years with no other risk factors and no cardiac disease (lone AF) to ≥8.1% in patients older than 75 years with one or more of the risk factors noted above. The risk of recurrent stroke in untreated patients with NVAF was 12% per year in a recent European trial of secondary stroke prevention. Poor left ventricular function, enlarged left atrial size, atrial thrombus, and spontaneous left atrial contrast ("smoke") have been identified as echocardiographic predictors of increased stroke risk in patients with NVAF (15).

Cardiac Disease

Cardiac sources of embolism account for 15–20% of all strokes, with AF accounting for almost half of these events (16). Other high-risk cardiac sources of embolus include prosthetic valves, mitral stenosis, infective endocarditis, marantic endocarditis, atrial myxoma, acute myocardial infarction (especially transmural and anterior wall), left ventricular thrombus, and dilative cardiomyopathy. Lower risks are associated with mitral valve prolapse, mitral annulus calcification, and calcific aortic stenosis. Patent foramen ovale and atrial septal aneurysm may be important cardiac factors, particularly in young stroke patients (17).

Carotid Stenosis

Asymptomatic carotid artery stenosis is associated with only a modest increase in stroke risk. Several observational studies have shown an overall annual risk of stroke ranging from <1% to 2.5% depending on the severity of stenosis. In the Toronto study (18), there was a 1.3% incidence of stroke in patients with <75% stenosis and a 2.5% annual risk of ipsilateral stroke in those with >75% stenosis (Fig. 2). The European Carotid Surgery Trial (ECST) reported an overall annual stroke risk of 0.7% in 2295 patients with asymptomatic carotid stenosis of any degree and a 1.9% annual stroke risk in 127 patients with asymptomatic stenosis >70% (19). Two recently completed randomized surgical trials in asymptomatic patients with >50% and >60% stenosis reported an annual stroke incidence of 2.45% and 2.2%, respectively, in the medically treated control groups (20,21). Curiously, in contrast to the Toronto data (18) and other serial ultrasound studies of asymptomatic patients (22), neither of these trials reported a risk stratification based on severity of stenosis.

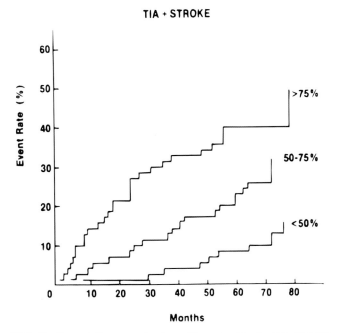

TIA + STROKE

FIG. 2. Cumulative event rates of transient ischemic attacks (TIAs) and strokes in patients with mild (<50%), moderate (50–75%), and severe (>75%) carotid stenosis measured by carotid ultrasound. (From ref. 18, with permission.)

Symptomatic severe carotid artery stenosis has a high risk of stroke. The North American Symptomatic Carotid Endarterectomy Trial (NASCET) (23) reported a 2-year risk of stroke of 26% for patients >70% stenosis on best medical management, and the ECST (24) reported a 3-year stroke incidence of 22%. Further analysis of NASCET data shows that stroke risk increases with the severity of stenosis, the presence of plaque ulceration, intraluminal thrombus, and the occurrence of hemispheric as opposed to retinal ischemic events. The risks become extreme for symptomatic patients with ulcerative plaques of 95% stenosis, as shown by the 2-year stroke incidence of 73.2% in a subgroup analysis of NASCET data (25). The risk of stroke for symptomatic patients with <70% carotid stenosis is uncertain and remains the subject of ongoing investigation by these trials.

Transient Ischemic Attacks

TIAs are a powerful stroke predictor, the 5-year risk being 24–29% (26). The greatest threat occurs early, with a 4–8% risk in the first month and a 12–13% incidence of stroke during the first year after the TIA. Hemispheric TIAs, severity of carotid stenosis >70%, high-risk cardiac sources, increasing frequency of TIAs, crescendo TIA patterns, TIAs upon awakening, advanced age, peripheral vascular disease, and left ventricular hypertrophy are predictors of high stroke risk after a TIA (27).

Aortic Atheroma

Aortic arch atheroma represents an important independent risk factor for stroke, as demonstrated by transesophageal echocardiography and autopsy studies (28). Atherosclerotic plaques >4 mm in thickness and complex atheroma may be particularly high risk, with odds ratios reported at 4.0 and 4.5, respectively. During coronary artery bypass surgery, the greatest frequency of transient embolic signals detected by transcranial Doppler ultrasound occur during declamping of the aorta, supporting the belief that aortic sources are responsible for a portion of the perioperative strokes (29).

Hyperhomocystinemia

Elevated homocysteine levels in homozygotes with cystathionine synthase deficiency are associated with premature atherosclerosis and thromboembolic events including stroke and sinus venous occlusion. Recent reports suggest that heterozygous homocystinemia may also be a stroke risk factor. In one study, high plasma levels of homocystine in the elderly were found to be associated with an increased risk of carotid artery stenosis after adjustment for other risk factors (30). Similar findings have been reported in patients with a history of stroke and from other studies that have linked elevated homocystine levels to ultrasound evidence of carotid atherosclerosis. A recent analysis of data from the Physicians Health Study found a small, nonsignificant association between elevated homocystine levels and the risk of stroke (31). Ongoing prospective studies of stroke risks in heterozygotes will better define the attributable stroke risks.

Lifestyle Factors

Smoking

Cigarette smoking is one of the most powerful independent risk factors for stroke. Stroke risk increases in a dose–response relationship with the number of cigarettes smoked. The Physicians Health Study, a prospective cohort study of 22,071 men, reported a relative risk for stroke of 2.02 for smokers of <20 cigarettes daily and 2.52 for those smoking >20 cigarettes daily, compared with those who never smoked. Women smokers are at similar or even greater risk for stroke due to smoking. A prospective cohort study of 118,539 female nurses 30–55 years old found that, compared with never-smokers, smokers of <15 cigarettes per day had a relative risk for stroke of 2.2, which increased to 3.7 for those who smoked ≥25 cigarettes per day (32). In a metaanalysis of 32 studies, the overall risk of stroke among smokers was increased by 50% compared with nonsmokers (33). The relative risk attributed to smoking was 1.9 for cerebral infarction, 2.9 for subarachnoid hemorrhage, and 0.7 for intracerebral hemorrhage.

The relationship between passive smoking (environmental smoke) and stroke risk has not been adequately addressed. One case–control study reported that the presence of a smoking spouse increased the risk of stroke by 1.7 (34). The Atherosclerosis Risk in Communities Study found that nonsmokers exposed to environmental smoke had increased carotid wall thickness compared with nonexposed nonsmokers (35).

Atherogenic, hematologic, and rheologic effects have been proposed as potential causative factors increasing the risk of stroke in smokers (36). Cigarette smoking, past and present, is significantly related to carotid stenosis. The amount of smoking and particularly the duration of smoking are strong independent predictors of the severity of carotid artery atherosclerosis. Smoking may also act as a precipitating factor for stroke by increasing the hematocrit and fibrinogen and serum viscosity, as well as causing vasoconstriction and altered arterial blood flow patterns.

Obesity

The direct relationship between obesity and stroke is not well established. Obesity promotes atherogenesis and is associated with hypertension, hyperlipidemia, and diabetes. Despite these confounding variables, current evidence suggests that obesity may be an independent risk factor for stroke. The Whitehall Study demonstrated that men aged 40–54 years who had a body mass in the upper quintile had a stroke mortality twice that of men in the thinnest quintile (37). The risk was most pronounced in nonsmokers. A doubling of stroke risk was also found in the Honolulu Heart Program for older men with body mass in the top tertile compared with men in the bottom tertile, even after adjustments for age, hypertension, and diabetes (38). Multivariate analysis of Framingham data revealed that weight >30% above normal was a significant independent stroke risk in men aged 35–64 years and women aged 65–94 years (4). Abdominal adiposity and central fat distribution have been associated with increased stroke risk in both older men and women.

Physical Activity

The impact of a sedentary lifestyle or exercise on stroke risk is uncertain due to conflicting data. Vigorous physical activity is associated with a lower incidence of death due to coronary artery disease, presumably due to salutary effects on the promoters of atherosclerosis. Exercise lowers blood pressure and blood sugar, raises high-density lipoprotein (HDL) cholesterol and lowers LDL cholesterol, promotes weight loss, and encourages smoking cessation. Several studies have failed to establish a significant association between sedentary work and stroke risk or, conversely, a protective effect from physically active trades (eg, longshoremen, carpenters, or baggage handlers). A prospective study of 7735 British men aged 40–59 years found that moderate physical activity significantly reduced stroke risk (39). Another British study suggests that vigorous exercise in early adulthood confers substantial stroke protection in later life and the benefits increase if exercise is continued lifelong (40). Further studies are necessary to better define stroke risk related to inactivity.

Diet

Dietary habits may influence stroke risk by virtue of changes effected in blood pressure, serum cholesterol, blood sugar, and body weight, as well as other precursors of atherosclerosis. Reductions in sodium intake and increases in dietary potassium have been shown in some studies to reduce stroke incidence. The intake of meat and fish may play a role; for instance, the Zutphen Study found that men who consumed >20 g/d of fish had a lower risk of stroke than those who consumed less (41). A recent Australian study found that eating fish more than two times per month also appeared to protect against first-ever stroke and intracerebral hemorrhage, whereas consumption of red meat more than four times weekly was associated with an increased stroke risk (42). A 20-year follow-up of middle-aged men in the Framingham Study found an inverse association between fruit and vegetable intake and the development of stroke (43). Vitamin C levels, whether measured by dietary intake or by plasma concentration, have been correlated with the incidence of fatal stroke in the elderly. Those with vitamin C levels in the upper third of distribution had a relative risk of 0.5 for fatal stroke compared with those in the lowest third (44).

Alcohol

The effects of alcohol consumption on the risk of stroke has been the subject of considerable controversy. Recent epidemiologic evidence indicates that a J- or U-shaped association may exist for alcohol and ischemic stroke, as is the case for coronary artery disease (45). Light to moderate alcohol consumption appears to exert a protective effect for nonhemorrhagic stroke, whereas excessive alcohol consumption, either habitual daily use or binge drinking, increases the risk for both ischemic and hemorrhagic stroke. Racial influences may be interactive, as the protective effect of moderate alcohol consumption demonstrated in predominantly white population studies has not been defined in black populations. Recent reports demonstrate a U-effect in the Japanese, contradicting earlier data. In contrast to ischemic stroke, a positive linear relationship exists between alcohol consumption and intracranial hemorrhage, particularly subarachnoid hemorrhage. In a large prospective study of 87,526 women aged 34–59 years, moderate alcohol consumption carried a relative risk of 3.7 for subarachnoid hemorrhage (46).

Oral Contraceptive and Postmenopausal Hormone Use

Older epidemiologic evidence associated high-estrogen oral contraceptives with an approximately fivefold increased risk for stroke. The risk was greatest in women older than 35 years, especially in smokers and individuals with other vascular risk factors. These reports, based on small patient numbers largely from the era before computed tomography (CT), are methodologically inadequate by today's standards. Evidence linking the current low-estrogen oral contraceptives to stroke is inconclusive. Two recent case–control studies have reported an increased risk of thromboembolic stroke in women with a history of low-dose oral contraceptives use, but the results failed to reach statistical significance (47,48). In one study, the odds ratio for stroke increased with increasing estrogen doses, supporting the concept of a dose–response relationship (49). A large prospective study has shown that the risks associated with oral contraceptives dissipates after discontinuance, and past use does not affect long term-mortality (50). The absolute risk of low-dose oral contraceptives in young nonsmokers with no other vascular risks is extremely low.

Postmenopausal hormone therapy may protect against stroke, although further studies are necessary to resolve conflicting data (49). Cohort studies of more than 23,000 women in Sweden and almost 2000 women in England have reported reduced risks of stroke with postmenopausal hormone use (51,52). The Women's Estrogen for Stroke Trial is in progress to assess the effects of estrogen on the risk of death and stroke in postmenopausal women with a recent TIA or stroke. Based on available data, current American Heart Association guidelines for the management of TIAs do not recommend the discontinuation of postmenopausal estrogen after a TIA.

Multiple Risk Factors

Individuals with multiple stroke risk factors are at particularly high risk for stroke. Epidemiologic evidence indicates that major risk factors such as hypertension, smoking, diabetes, and hypercholesterolemia act in synergy with each other to multiply stroke risk. The combination of smoking and hypertension has been found to increase stroke risk by 12–20-fold compared with the risk for those who neither smoke nor have hypertension. Women smokers older than 35 years who have other vascular risk factors such as hypertension and oral contraceptive use may be at higher stroke risk than women without this risk factor load. Patients with nonvalvular atrial fibrillation are at higher risk of stroke if they are hypertensive, have diabetes, and have suffered a prior embolic event. It has been estimated that the 10% of the population whose composite stroke risk profile includes hypertension, hypercholesterolemia, smoking, and an abnormal electrocardiogram (ECG) account for at least a third of

Table 2. *Stroke prevention strategies*

Primary prevention: Asymptomatic stage
Risk factor management
Aspirin (?)
Warfarin for atrial fibrillation
Carotid endarterectomy

Secondary prevention: Symptomatic stage
Management and investigation of transient ischemic attack and stroke
Risk factor management
Aspirin or ticlopidine
Warfarin for cardioembolic source
Carotid endarterectomy

all strokes. A risk profile to estimate the probability of stroke has been developed based on Framingham data (53).

STRATEGIES FOR STROKE PREVENTION

Therapeutic interventions for the prevention of stroke in individuals at risk are classified based on symptom status (Table 2).

Primary prevention strategies, designed for asymptomatic individuals with no prior history of TIA or stroke, involves risk factor management and the selective use of aspirin, antithrombotic agents, and surgical measures. As the absolute risk of stroke may be relatively low in individuals with only minor stroke risk factors, the selection of active therapy must be based on scientific evidence of benefit over risk. Risk factor modification, often involving lifestyle changes and the low-risk treatment of major stroke contributors such as hypertension or smoking, is the cornerstone of primary prevention.

Secondary stroke prevention—the reduction of stroke risk after a TIA or stroke—employs similar approaches in risk factor management, although the rationale for this must often be extrapolated from epidemiologic studies involving primary prevention. On the other hand, active interventions such as antiplatelet and antithrombotic agents and surgery may be specifically focused on active disease processes. As symptomatic patients generally carry a higher risk of stroke, such treatments are therefore likely to produce greater absolute risk reductions than those seen in asymptomatic individuals.

Risk Factor Modification

Hypertension

Hypertension is the most important stroke risk factor. This distinction is due to its strong association with stroke, the high prevalence of hypertension in the population, and proof that treatment of hypertension is both safe and efficacious. In a metaanalysis of 17 controlled trials, a reduction of 5–6 mm Hg in diastolic blood pressure (DBP) and a 10–12 mm Hg reduction in systolic blood pressure (SBP) produced a 38% reduction in stroke and a 40% reduction in fatal stroke (54). The benefits were similar in patients with severe (DBP >110) or moderate (DBP <110) hypertension. Randomized trials and observational studies suggest that a reduction of even 2 mm Hg in DBP would reduce the incidence of stroke by 15% (55). Stroke prevention by treatment of hypertension in the elderly is effective, as demonstrated by several trials with relative risk reductions for stroke ranging from 25% to 47%. Treatment of isolated systolic hypertension produces comparable results. In the Systolic Hypertension in the Elderly Program, control of isolated systolic hypertension (often only with just low-dose diuretics) resulted in a 36% stroke reduction, a 27% reduction in coronary heart disease, and a 32% reduction in all cardiovascular events. Vigilant treatment of hypertension is a key component of stroke prevention in the young and the old.

Smoking

Cessation of smoking substantially reduces the attributable stroke risk. In a prospective study of nearly 120,000 middle-aged women, the age-adjusted risk of stroke was 2.58 in current smokers, compared with never-smokers, and fell to 1.34 in former smokers (56). The excess risks among former smokers largely disappeared within 2–4 years after cessation. Similar results in men were reported in the Physicians Health Study, current heavy smokers having a relative stroke risk of 2.52, light smokers 2.02, and former smokers 1.20, compared with never-smokers (relative risk, 1.00) (57). The rapid benefits of smoking cessation have been confirmed in other reports. In the Framingham Study, a decline in stroke risk was apparent within 2 years of cessation, and by 5 years the risk had returned to baseline. In the British Regional Heart Study, the reduction in stroke risk was maximal at 5 years. Light smokers reverted to the risks of those who never smoked, while the risk in heavy smokers was considerably reduced by quitting but remained more than twofold the risk of never-smokers (58).

Lipids

Cerebrovascular disease, like coronary artery disease, is related to atherosclerotic processes, and the reduction of cholesterol levels is therefore a biologically plausible but unproven approach to stroke prevention. Statistical overviews of trials of cholesterol lowering have found no significant reduction in stroke risk (59,60). Many of these trials were designed to evaluate the effects of cholesterol reduction on coronary heart disease, and often they were limited to middle-aged men, thus making uncertain the extrapolation of these results to women, older individuals, and patients with previous strokes. The reduction in LDL cholesterol has been demonstrated by prospective serial ultrasound examinations

to produce a regression or stabilization of carotid plaques (61,62). The Scandinavian Simvastatin Survival Study evaluated the effects of cholesterol reduction with simvastatin vs. placebo in 4444 patients with coronary artery disease. A post-hoc analysis found that 98 patients suffered fatal or nonfatal strokes in the placebo arm, compared with only 70 patients in the simvastatin group (relative risk, 0.70). The benefits of newer cholesterol-lowering agents in stroke-prone populations require additional large-scale clinical trials.

Primary Stroke Prevention

Aspirin

Despite widespread use, aspirin has not proven beneficial for the primary prevention of stroke in individuals at low risk. Two studies have evaluated aspirin therapy for the primary prevention of cardiovascular disease and stroke in male physicians (63,64). In the American trial, 22,071 physicians received aspirin 325 mg on alternate days vs. placebo. The relative risk of myocardial infarction was reduced by 44% (63). However, there was a slight increase in the risk of stroke ($p = .06$), primarily due to hemorrhagic stroke. An open-design British trial involving 5139 physicians allocated either aspirin 500 mg/d or aspirin avoidance detected no significant difference in stroke risk, although the aspirin group had a higher incidence of disabling stroke (64). Similarly, aspirin did not reduce the risk of stroke in a prospective study of 87,678 asymptomatic middle-aged women (65). Furthermore, the benefits of aspirin in asymptomatic individuals with atherosclerotic disease or risk factors for stroke remain uncertain. A Canadian study found no significant difference in long term stroke risk in 372 patients with asymptomatic carotid stenosis >50% randomly allocated to either aspirin 325 mg/d or placebo (66).

Warfarin in Atrial Fibrillation

Five randomized or controlled clinical trials comparing warfarin with aspirin or placebo demonstrated that warfarin is effective for the primary prevention of stroke in patients with nonvalvular atrial fibrillation (AF). In a metaanalysis of pooled data from these trials, the annual rate of stroke was 4.5% for the control group and 1.4% for the warfarin group, yielding a risk reduction of 68% (14). Stroke risk was reduced by 84% in women compared with 60% in men. Age greater than 65 years, hypertension, diabetes, previous TIAs or stroke, recent congestive heart failure, and echocardiographic evidence for poor left ventricular function or enlarged left atrial size were associated with an increased risk of stroke in AF. The risk–benefit ratio for warfarin in patients older than 75 years remains uncertain due to the higher risk of hemorrhagic complications of anticoagulation. Risk stratification may aid therapeutic decisions in the elderly.

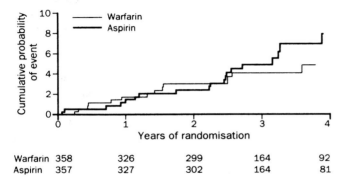

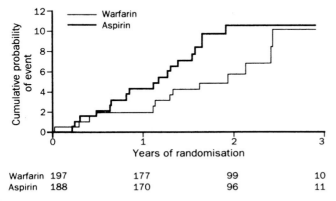

| Warfarin | 197 | 177 | 99 | 10 |
| Aspirin | 188 | 170 | 96 | 11 |

FIG. 3. Cumulative probability of ischemic stroke or systemic embolism in patients with nonvalvular atrial fibrillation (NVAF) based on age and treatment. Patients ≤75 years of age at entry **(top)** and >75 years of age at entry **(bottom)**. (From ref. 67, with permission.)

The benefit of aspirin in the primary prevention of stroke in AF is more uncertain. At present, aspirin is an acceptable alternative to warfarin in young patients with a low stroke-risk profile and in older patients with contraindications to warfarin therapy. In one study, aspirin 75 mg/d did not produce a significant reduction compared with placebo, while in the Stroke Prevention in Atrial Fibrillation (SPAF I) study 325 mg/d produced a risk reduction midway between placebo and warfarin. In the SPAF II trial, warfarin was associated with only a 1.2% absolute stroke reduction over aspirin therapy in the subgroup of patients older than 75 years (67) (Fig. 3). Further studies evaluating the efficacy of aspirin and warfarin alone or in combination are underway.

Primary Surgical Prevention: Carotid Endarterectomy

Carotid endarterectomy for asymptomatic carotid stenosis remains controversial despite three completed randomized trials. The Carotid Artery Stenosis with Asymptomatic Narrowing: Operation versus Aspirin (CASANOVA) trial found no benefit for carotid endarterectomy (68). Unfortunately, patients with >90% stenosis were excluded, and other methodologic shortcomings have largely discounted the results

of this study. The Veterans Administration Trial involving 444 patients found no significant difference in the rate of stroke and death between surgical or medical treatment when the 30-day rate of postoperative stroke or death of 4.4% was included (20). The Asymptomatic Carotid Atherosclerosis Study (ACAS) randomized 1662 patients with asymptomatic stenosis >60% to either medical care or carotid endarterectomy (21). The projected 5-year stroke risk was 11% for patients treated medically and 5.1% for surgical patients, yielding a modest absolute risk reduction of 5.9% over 5 years. With a 2.3% perioperative risk of stroke or death, including a 1.2% complication rate from angiography, the annual risk reduction of 1.2% as a result of surgery in the ACAS study confers only marginal benefit. More data are needed from this and future studies before any definite conclusions can be drawn.

Secondary Stroke Prevention

Aspirin

Aspirin is widely used for the secondary prevention of stroke in patients with TIAs or previous stroke. Analysis of individual studies of aspirin vs. placebo for the prevention of stroke or death using the rules of evidence, however, shows a barely statistically significant benefit. However, when the results were pooled, in the Antiplatelet Trialists' Collaboration (69) metaanalysis, antiplatelet agents, predominantly aspirin, reduced the risk of nonfatal stroke by 23% and reduced the constellation of nonfatal stroke, myocardial infarction, or vascular death by 22%. Aspirin will prevent approximately six strokes for every 1000 patient years of treatment. Optimal aspirin dosage remains controversial, and the evidence that either a high dose (650–1300 mg/d), intermediate dose (325 mg/d), or a low dose (30–80 mg/d) is more effective than the others is inconclusive (70). The benefit of aspirin in patients who have had a previous major stroke remains uncertain, but studies have failed to show any significant effect. Currently, aspirin is indicated for initial therapy of symptomatic patients—those with TIAs or minor strokes—due to noncardiac causes. Aspirin is also recommended for use in patients at risk for cardioembolic events who are unable or unwilling to take warfarin.

Ticlopidine

Ticlopidine is the only other antiplatelet agent proved to reduce the risk of stroke in symptomatic patients. In the Canadian American Ticlopidine Study, ticlopidine reduced the risk of recurrent stroke, myocardial infarction, or vascular death by 23.3% compared with placebo (71) (Fig. 4). In the efficacy analysis, the composite event rate was 15.3% in the placebo group and 10.8% in the ticlopidine group, representing a relative risk reduction of 30.2%. Ticlopidine was beneficial in both men and women. In a randomized

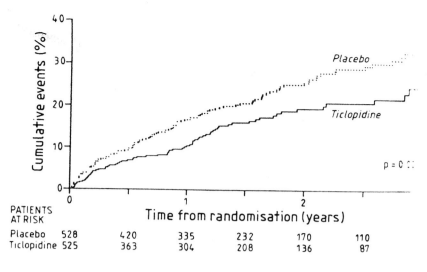

FIG. 4. Occurrence of stroke, myocardial infarction, or vascular death in the placebo and ticlopidine groups from the Canadian American Ticlopidine Study. (From ref. 71, with permission.)

trial comparing ticlopidine and aspirin side by side in over 3000 patients with a recent TIA or minor stroke, the overall risk reduction in favor of ticlopidine over aspirin for fatal and nonfatal stroke was 21% at 3 years based on an intent-to-treat analysis (72). In the first year after the qualifying event, when stroke risk is highest, on-treatment secondary analysis showed a stroke rate of 3.4% for ticlopidine and 6.4% for aspirin, yielding a 48% risk reduction for ticlopidine.

The most distressing factor inhibiting widespread use of ticlopidine was the 2.4% incidence of serious bone marrow depression. The neutropenia is potentially fatal if missed and totally reversible if detected by monitoring the blood count twice for the initial 3 months and discontinuance of the drug. The patient's survival is thus dependent on compliance and the degree of care exercised by his physician.

Ticlopidine is indicated for symptomatic patients at high risk for stroke or recurrent stroke, particularly for those who are intolerant of aspirin or have had cerebrovascular events while on aspirin. Ticlopidine has not been adequately evaluated for use in patients at risk for cardioembolic stroke.

Warfarin

Warfarin is highly beneficial for the secondary prevention of stroke in patients with nonvalvular atrial fibrillation (NVAF) who have had a recent TIA or stroke. In the European Atrial Fibrillation Trial, the incidence of outcome events (vascular death, recurrent stroke, myocardial infarction, systemic embolism) was 17% in the placebo-treated group vs. 8% in warfarin-treated patients. Reduction in the risk of stroke recurrence was even more impressive with annual rates of 12% on placebo vs. 4% per year in the warfarin arm (relative risk, 69%). Anticoagulation was significantly more effective than aspirin, with a risk reduction 62%. Warfarin is recommended for symptomatic patients with NVAF who are candidates for anticoagulation. Currently, there is no evidence to support the routine use of warfarin for the prevention of noncardiac causes of stroke, except for patients with coagulopathies such as the anticardiolipin antibody syndrome.

Warfarin plus aspirin may be beneficial for patients at particularly high risk for cardioembolic strokes. A double-blind, placebo-controlled study of patients with prosthetic valves and AF or a history of embolism found that low-dose aspirin (100 mg) combined with warfarin reduced mortality, particularly from vascular causes, and major systemic emboli (73).

Secondary Prevention by Carotid Surgery

Carotid endarterectomy, skillfully performed, has been demonstrated by two large-scale studies to be highly beneficial for the prevention of stroke in symptomatic patients with >70% carotid stenosis (23,24). In the North American Symptomatic Carotid Endarterectomy Trial (NASCET), the risk of ipsilateral stroke at 2 years was 26% for medically treated patients vs. 9 % for those treated surgically, representing an absolute difference of 17% at 2 years (23). Carotid endarterectomy in the European Carotid Surgery Trial (ECST) resulted in an absolute reduction in stroke of 14% at 3 years (24). The discrepancy between the two studies has been explained by the different methods used to measure the degree of carotid stenosis. Stroke risk and the resulting benefit from surgery are dependent on the severity of carotid stenosis. In NASCET, carotid endarterectomy reduced the annual incidence of ipsilateral stroke from about 18% to 4% in patients with >90% stenosis and from 10% to 3.5% in patients with 70–80% stenosis. The ECST reported similar trends in stroke risk based on the severity of carotid stenosis >70%. In appropriate patients with severe symptomatic carotid stenosis, surgery represents the most effective available strategy for secondary stroke prevention and is strongly recommended.

One of the most interesting findings of this study was a reevaluation of the annual incidence of stroke in patients with TIAs. The NASCET study showed an annual stroke rate of 18% in patients with >90% stenosis, and these patients were already treated with aspirin and risk factor management. The benefits of surgery for symptomatic carotid stenosis <70% remain uncertain and are the subject of ongoing investigation by both NASCET and ECST.

TRENDS AND FUTURE PROSPECTS

Stroke mortality rates have been declining in industrialized countries since the turn of the century. The rate of decline accelerated in the mid-1970s, reaching 5% annually in the United States (2). It has been proposed that the modification of risk factor levels over time is responsible for the changing trends in stroke mortality. Not all of the reduction can be attributed to the treatment of risk factors. For example, it has been estimated that the treatment of hypertension accounts for only 25% of the decline (74). Changing incidence rates for stroke and an improvement in stroke survival reflecting declines in stroke severity and better medical care are possible contributors to the favorable trends in stroke mortality (75,76).

Epidemiologic evidence suggests that we are approaching an end in the decline of stroke incidence and mortality (77). In some populations, increases in stroke incidence have been reported (77,78). It seems paradoxical that such a leveling off would occur now, given the recent explosion in our knowledge of stroke prevention generated by scientifically conducted therapeutic trials and modern epidemiologic studies. The progressive aging of the population is of concern, as it threatens to increase the incidence and prevalence of stroke.

The challenge for the remainder of the "Decade of the Brain" and for the years beyond will be to translate our ever expanding knowledge into effective practice. Both high-risk approaches aimed at individuals threatened by stroke and population-based "mass" approaches designed to reduce stroke precursors in the general population are necessary to limit the human costs and economic burden of stroke to society (79). In a Canadian study, the direct costs of stroke were estimated at $30,000 for first stroke and, assuming equal indirect costs, an overall expense of at least $60,000 (80). Stroke prevention strategies aimed at high-risk individuals must optimize the benefits of risk factor management and the rational use of antithrombotic therapy and surgery. New antiplatelet or antithrombotic agents currently undergoing evaluation and agents yet to be developed will have to be incorporated into treatment regimens. Further refinements in the indications for carotid endarterectomy are anticipated from ongoing trials. The potentials for extra- and intracranial angioplasty are now being explored in multicenter studies. Mass-approach initiatives emphasizing public education on the warning signs and symptoms of stroke, risk factor reduction, and the promotion of healthy lifestyles have the potential to substantially reduce stroke rates. Stroke is preventable.

REFERENCES

1. *Heart and Stroke Facts: 1994 Statistical Supplement.* Dallas, TX: American Heart Association, 1993:1–22.
2. Bonita R. Epidemiology of stroke. *Lancet* 1992;339:342–344.
3. *Stroke Prevention Screening Guidebook.* Englewood, CO: National Stroke Association, 1993.
4. Wolf PA, Cobb JL, D'Agostino RB. Epidemiology of stroke. In: Barnett HJM, Mohr JP, Stein BM, Yatsu FM, eds. *Stroke—Pathophysiology, Diagnosis, and Management.* New York: Churchill Livingstone, 1992:3–27.
5. Norris JW, Bogousslavsky J, Asplund K, et al. Stroke management around the world. *Cerebrovasc Dis* 1994;4:430–440.
6. Brass LM, Isaacsohn JL, Merikangas KR, Robinette CD. A study of twins and stroke. *Stroke* 1992;23:221–223.
7. Bowler JV, Hachinski V. Progress in the genetics of cerebrovascular disease: Inherited subcortical arteriopathies. *Stroke* 1994;25:1969–1975.
8. MacMahon SW, Peto R, Cutler J, et al. Blood pressure, stroke, coronary heart disease: Part 1. Prolonged differences in blood pressure: Prospective observational studies corrected for the regression dilution bias. *Lancet* 1990;335:765–774.
9. Iso H, Jacobs DR, Wentworth D, Neaton JD, Cohen JD. Serum cholesterol levels and six-year mortality from stroke in 350,977 men screened for the multiple risk factor intervention trial. *N Engl J Med* 1989;320:904–910.
10. Qizilbash N, Duffy SW, Warlow C, Mann J. Lipids are risk factors for ischaemic stroke: Overview and review. *Cerebrovasc Dis* 1992;2:127–136.
11. Pedro-Botst J, Senti M, Nogués X, Rubiés-Prat, Roquer J, D'Olhaberriague L, Olivé. Lipoprotein and apolipoprotein profile in men with ischemic stroke. *Stroke* 1992;23:1556–1562.
12. Jurgens G, Taddei-Peters WC, Koltringer P, et al. Lipoprotein (a) serum concentration and apolipoprotein (a) phenotype correlate with severity and presence of ischemic cerebrovascular disease. *Stroke* 1995;26:1841–1848.
13. Wolf PA, Dawber TR, Thomas HE, Kannel WB. Epidemiologic assessment of chronic atrial fibrillation and risk of stroke: The Framingham Study. *Neurology* 1978;28:937–977.
14. Atrial Fibrillation Investigators. Risk factors for stroke and efficacy of antithrombotic therapy in atrial fibrillation: Analysis of pooled data from five randomized controlled trials. *Arch Intern Med* 1994;154:1449–1457.
15. Di Pasquale G, Ubinati G, Pinelli G. New echocardiographic markers of embolic risk in atrial fibrillation. *Cerebrovasc Dis* 1995;5:315–322.
16. Cerebral Embolism Task Force. Cardiogenic brain embolism: The second report of the Cerebral Embolism Task Force. *Arch Neurol* 1989;46:727–743.
17. Van Camp G, Schulze D, Cosyns B, et al. Relation between patent foramen ovale and unexplained stroke. *Am J Cardiol* 1993;71:596–598.
18. Norris JW, Zhu CZ, Bornstein NM, Chambers BR. Vascular risks of asymptomatic carotid stenosis. *Stroke* 1991;22:1485–1490.
19. European Carotid Surgery Trialists' Collaborative Group. Risk of stroke in the distribution of an asymptomatic carotid artery. *Lancet* 1995;345:209–212.
20. Hobson RW, Weiss DG, Fields WS, et al. Efficacy of carotid endarterectomy for asymptomatic carotid stenosis. *N Engl J Med* 1993;328:221–227.
21. Executive Committee for the Symptomatic Carotid Atherosclerosis Study. Endarterectomy for asymptomatic carotid artery stenosis. *JAMA* 1995;273:1421–1428.
22. Roeder GO, Langlois YE, Jager KA, et al. The natural history of carotid arterial disease in asymptomatic patients with cervical bruits. *Stroke* 1984;15:605–613.
23. North American Symptomatic Carotid Endarterectomy Trial Collaborators. Beneficial effect of carotid endarterectomy in symptomatic patients with high-grade carotid stenosis. *N Eng J Med* 1991;325:445–453.
24. European Carotid Surgery Trialists' Collaborative Group. MRC European Carotid Surgery Trial: Interim results for symptomatic patients with severe (70–99%) or with mild (0–29%) carotid stenosis. *Lancet* 1991;337:1235–1243.
25. Eliasziw M, Streifler JY, Fox AJ, Hachinski VC, Ferguson GG, Barnett HJM for the North American Symptomatic Carotid Endarterectomy Trial. Significance of plaque ulceration in symptomatic patients with high-grade carotid stenosis. *Stroke* 1994;25:304–308.

26. Feinberg WM, Albers GW, Barnett HJM, et al. Guidelines for the management of transient ischemic attacks. *Stroke* 1994;25:1320–1335.
27. Hankey GJ, Warlow CP. Incidence, prevalence and risk factors. In: *Transient Ischaemic Attacks of the Brain and Eye.* London: W.B. Saunders, 1994;197–250.
28. Donnan GA, Jones EF. Aortic arch atheroma and stroke. *Cerebrovasc Dis* 1995;5:10–13.
29. Barbut D, Hinton RB, Szatrowski TP, et al. Cerebral emboli detected during bypass surgery are associated with clamp removal. *Stroke* 1994; 25:2398–2402.
30. Selhub J, Jacques PF, Bostom AG, et al. Association between plasma homocysteine concentrations and extracranial carotid-artery stenosis. *N Engl J Med* 1995;332:286–291.
31. Verfhoef P, Hennekens CH, Malinow R, et al. A prospective study of plasma homocyst(e)ine and risk of ischemic stroke. *Stroke* 1994;25:1924–1930.
32. Colditz GA, Bonita R, Stampfer MJ, Willett WC, Rosner B, Speizer FE, Hennekens CH. Cigarette smoking and risk of stroke in middle-aged women. *N Engl J Med* 1988;318:937–941.
33. Shinton R, Beevers G. Meta-analysis of the relation between cigarette smoking and stroke. *BMJ* 1989;298:789–794.
34. Donnan GA, McNeill JJ, Adena MA, Doyle AE, O'Malley JM, Neill GC. Smoking as a risk factor for cerebral ischemia. *Lancet* 1989;2:643–647.
35. Howard G, Burke GL, Szklo M, Tell GS, Eckfeldt J, Evans G, Heiss G. Active and passive smoking are associated with increased carotid wall thickness. *Arch Intern Med* 1994;154:1277–1282.
36. Donnan GA, You R, Thrift A, McNeil JJ. Smoking as a risk factor for stroke. *Cerebrovasc Dis* 1993;3:129–238.
37. Shinton R, Shipley M, Rose G. Overweight and stroke in the Whitehall Study. *J Epidemiol Community Health* 1991;45:138–142.
38. Abbott RD, Behrens GR, Sharp DS, et al. Body mass index and thromboembolic stroke in nonsmoking men in older middle age. *Stroke* 1994; 25:2370–2376.
39. Wannamethee G, Shaper AG. Physical activity and stroke in British middle aged men. *BMJ* 1992;304;597–601.
40. Shinton R, Sagar G. Lifelong exercise and stroke. *BMJ* 1993;307:231–234.
41. Keli SO, Feskens EJM, Kromhout D. Fish consumption and risk of stroke—The Zutphen Study. *Stroke* 1994;25:328–332.
42. Jamrozik K, Broadhurst RJ, Anderson CS, Stewrt-Wynne EG. The role of lifestyle factors in the etiology of stroke: A population-based case-control study in Perth, Western Australia. *Stroke* 1994;25:51–59.
43. Gillman MW, Cupples LA, Gagnon D, Posner BM, Ellison RC, Castelli WP, Wolf PA. Protective effect of fruits and vegetables on development of stroke in men. *JAMA* 1995;273:1113–1117.
44. Gale CR, Martyn CN, Winter PD, Cooper C. Vitamin C and risk of death from stroke and coronary heart disease in cohort of elderly people. *BMJ* 1995;310:1563–1566.
45. Camargo CA. Moderate alcohol consumption and stroke. The epidemiologic evidence. *Stroke* 1989;20:1611–1626.
46. Stampfer MJ, Colditz GA, Willett WC, Speizer FE, Hennekens CH. A prospective study of moderate alcohol consumption and the risk of coronary disease and stroke in women. *N Engl J Med* 1988;319:267–273.
47. Thorogood M, Mann J, Murphy M, Vessey M. Fatal stroke and use of oral contraceptives: Findings from a case-control study. *Am J Epidemiol* 1992;136:35–45.
48. Lidegarrd O. Oral contraception and risk of cerebral thromboembolic attack: Results of a case-control study. *BMJ* 1993; 306:956–963.
49. Belchetz PE. Hormonal treatment of postmenopausal women. *N Eng J Med* 1994;330:1062–1071.
50. Colditz GA for the Nurses' Health Study Research Group. Oral contraceptive use and mortality during 12 years of follow-up: The Nurses' Health Study. *Ann Intern Med* 1994;120:821–826.
51. Falkeborn M, Persson I, Terént A, Adami H, Lithell H, Bergstrom R. Hormone replacement therapy and the risk of stroke. *Arch Intern Med* 1993;153:1201–1209.
52. Finucane FF, Madans, JH, Bush TL, Wolf PH, Kleinman JC. Decreased risk of stroke among postmenopausal hormone users. *Arch Intern Med* 1993;153:73–79.
53. Wolf PA, D'Agostino RB, Belanger AJ, Kannel WB. Probability of stroke: A risk profile from the Framingham study. *Stroke* 1991;22:312–318.
54. Cutler JA, MacMahon S, Furberg CD. Controlled clinical trials of drug therapy treatment for hypertension. *Hypertension* 1989;13(suppl I):I-36–I-44.
55. Cook NR, Cohen J, Hebert PR, Taylor JO, Hennekens CH. Implication of small reductions in diastolic blood pressure for primary prevention. *Arch Inten Med* 1995;155:179–709.
56. Kawaachi I, Coldizt GA, Stampfer MJ, et al. Smoking cessation and decreased risk of stroke in women. *JAMA* 1993;269:232–236.
57. Robbins AS, Manson JE, Lee IM, Satterfield S, Hennekens CH. Cigarette smoking and stroke in a cohort of U.S. male physicians. *Ann Intern Med* 1994;120:458–462.
58. Wannamethee SG, Shaper AG, Whincup PH, Walker M. Smoking cessation and the risk of stroke in middle-aged men. *JAMA* 1995;274:155–160.
59. Atkins D, Psaty BM, Koepsell TD, Longstreth WT, Larson EB. Cholesterol reduction and the risk for stroke in men: A meta-analysis of randomized, controlled trials. *Ann Intern Med* 1993;119:136–145.
60. Hebert PR, Gaziano JM, Henneckens CH. An overview of trials of cholesterol lowering and risk of stroke. *Arch Intern Med* 1995;155:50–55.
61. Hennerici M, Kleophas W, Gries FA. Regression of carotid plaques during low density lipoprotein cholesterol elimination. *Stroke* 1991; 22:989–992.
62. Adams HP, Byington RP, Hoen H, Dempsey R, Furberg CD. Effect of cholesterol-lowering medications on progression of mild atherosclerotic lesions of the carotid arteries and on the risk of stroke. *Cerebrovasc Dis* 1995;5:171–177.
63. Steering Committee of the Physicians' Health Study Research Group. Final report on the aspirin component of the ongoing Physicians' Health Study. *N Engl J Med* 1989;321:129–135.
64. Peto R, Gray R, Collins R, et al. Randomised trial of prophylactic daily aspirin in British male doctors. *BMJ* 1988;296:313–316.
65. Manson JE, Stampfer MJ, Colditz GA, et al. A prospective study of aspirin use and primary prevention of cardiovascular disease in women. *JAMA* 1991;266:521–527.
66. Côte R, Renaldo N, Abrahamowicz M, Langlois Y, Bourque F, Mackey A. Lack of effect of aspirin in asymptomatic patients with carotid bruits and substantial carotid narrowing. *Ann Intern Med* 1995;123:640–655.
67. Stroke Prevention in Atrial Fibrillation Investigators. Warfarin versus aspirin for prevention of thromboembolism in atrial fibrillation: Stroke Prevention in Atrial Fibrillation II Study. *Lancet* 1994;343:687–691.
68. The CASANOVA Study Group. Carotid surgery versus medical therapy in asymptomatic carotid stenosis. *Stroke* 1991;22:1229–1235.
69. Antiplatelet Trialists' Collaboration. Collaborative overview of randomised trials of antiplatelet therapy, I: Prevention of death, myocardial infarction, and stroke by prolonged antiplatelet therapy in various categories of patients. *BMJ* 1994;308:81–106.
70. Dyken ML, Barnett HJM, Easton D, et al. Low-dose aspirin and stroke. *Stroke* 1992;23:1395–1399.
71. Gent M, Blakely JA, Easton JD, et al. The Canadian American Ticlopidine Study (CATS) in thromboembolic stroke. *Lancet* 1989;1:1215–1220.
72. Hass WK, Easton JD, Adams HP, et al. A randomized trial comparing ticlopidine hydrochloride with aspirin for the prevention of stroke in high-risk patients. *N Eng J Med* 1989;321:501–507.
73. Turpie AGG, Gent M, Laupacis A, et al. A comparison of aspirin with placebo in patients treated with warfarin after heart-valve replacement. *N Engl J Med* 1993;329:524–529.
74. Bonita R, Beaglehole R. Increased treatment of hypertension does not explain the decline in stroke mortality in the United States, 1970–1980. *Hypertension* 1989;13(suppl I):I-69–I-73.
75. Broderick JP, Phillip SJ, Whisnant JP, et al. Incidence rates of stroke in the eighties: The end of the decline in stroke? *Stroke* 1989;20:577–582.
76. Wolf PA, D'Agostino RB, O'Neal A, Sytkowski P, Kase CS, Belanger AJ, Kannel WB. Secular trends in stroke incidence and mortality—The Framingham Study. *Stroke* 1992;23:1551–1555.
77. Cooper R, Sempos C, Hsieh SC, Kovar MG. Slowdown in the decline of stroke mortality in the United States, 1978–1986. *Stroke* 1990;21:1274–1279.
78. Trenet A. Increasing incidence of stroke among Swedish women. *Stroke* 1988;19:598–603.
79. Gorelick PB. Stroke prevention. *Arch Neurology* 1995;52:347–355.
80. Smurawaska LT, Alexandrov AV, Bladin CF, et al. Cost of acute stroke care in Toronto, Canada. *Stroke* 1994;25:1628–1631.

SECTION IV
Hemorrhagic Stroke

There have been great strides in our knowledge about vascular malformations, but little progress in other types of hemorrhagic disease, such as hypertensive intracerebral hemorrhage. With the refinements in selective cerebral angiography, magnetic resonance imaging, neuroanesthesia, and microsurgical techniques, the diagnosis and treatment of some hemorrhagic cerebrovascular lesions has been revolutionized. In many instances, theoretical, natural history and outcome data, based on less precise anatomic information and outdated modes of therapy, have become obsolete.

The timing of surgery, optimal surgical approaches, aggressive critical care management of subarachnoid hemorrhage (SAH), and the disposition of poor-grade patients have undergone careful investigation. The treatment of SAH now involves rapid diagnosis and optimization of the patient's medical status, followed by acute microsurgical aneurysm repair. Post-operative care is directed toward detection and treatment of cerebral vasospasm by both physiologic manipulation of the cardiovascular system and endovascular techniques. This multi-modal treatment continues to optimize outcomes.

Cerebral arteriovenous malformations (AVMs) are the most complex of the vascular malformations which have undergone intense study over the past decade; and the advances in treating these complex lesions revolve around precise anatomic localization and a multispecialty management team consisting of the stroke neurologist, neurosurgeon, neuroanesthesiologist, diagnostic and interventional neuroradiologist, radiosurgeon and, in some centers, the neurophysiologist and neuropsychologist. Small, deep, ganglionic AVMs can now be obliterated with radiosurgical techniques. The difficulty of surgically resecting large, superficial AVMs has been vastly reduced by the routine use of preoperative embolization techniques. Further reduction in the risk of intervention (or non-intervention) with AVMs is likely to result from improved understanding of the complex hemodynamics involved with these lesions. With new information, it will become easier to balance the risk of intervention versus the expected patient benefits of prophylaxis against spontaneous AVM rupture.

A paradox in the study of hemorrhagic cerebrovascular diseases is the apparent lack of advancement in the treatment of those diseases not resulting from aneurysm or vascular malformation. In contrast to the declining incidence of ischemic stroke, the incidence of spontaneous intracerebral or hypertensive intracerebral hemorrhage (ICH) has remained unchanged over the past decade, as has the outcome from treatment. Intracerebral hemorrhage is equal in prevalence, slightly more deadly in severity, and more poorly studied than all other causes of intracranial hemorrhage. Presently, no consensus exists regarding treatment, and no national cooperative studies have been successfully performed or are ongoing. Hopefully, future treatment will lie in the identification of structural, biochemical or genetic lesions prior to hemorrhage, thereby minimizing the morbidity and mortality associated with intracranial hemorrhage. Identification and treatment of systemic hypertension and innovative new techniques for clot removal presently appear to offer the best hope for improving outcome and decreasing the cost of caring for patients with spontaneous hemorrhagic cerebrovascular disease. This section is clinically oriented, nonetheless, pathophysiology is discussed. Although many mechanisms, both physiologic and pathologic, are presented as "firm ground," there are still fundamental questions to be answered (Why does "vasospasm" after subarachnoid hemorrhage develop? Why does intravascular volume expansion appear to improve outcome?).

A healthy skepticism for underlying mechanistic assumptions in any medical text is always in order. For example, there are references to "cerebral autoregulation" and its disruption, as if it were a clearly understood phenomenon. On the contrary, the mechanisms involved are poorly understood and "autoregulation" is notoriously difficult to assess dynamically because of a lack of bedside methods to quantitate regional cerebral perfusion. Despite advances in human brain imaging, not every therapeutic decision can hinge on transferring a patient to the radiology suite for an MRI or PET scan. Until we have routine access to imaging of the cerebral circulation, concepts like "cerebral steal" will remain unproven, yet difficult to disprove. Similarly, cerebral protection from ischemic injury by anesthetic agents or mild-hypothermia is a topic that lacks support from rigorous clinical studies, but appears not to cause an increase in morbidity or mortality when used judiciously.

This section reflects an enormous breadth of experience, expertise, and recommendations. The reader should not be misled by the array of views and the large areas of apparent overlap. Different authors present different perspectives of similar case series. Although we strive to order our clinical observations and bundle particulars into classes in order to rationally treat patients, there is no unequivocal correct de-scription of a ''disease,'' as nicely summarized by the dictum attributed to Rousseau, ''There are no diseases, only sick people.'' If any message comes through unmistakably loud and clear it should be that continued improvement in the care of complex cerebrovascular disease will be realized only in a multidisciplinary forum.

Thomas Kopitnik, M.D. and William L. Young, M.D.

Cerebrovascular Disease, edited by H. Hunt Batjer.
Lippincott-Raven Publishers, Philadelphia © 1997.

CHAPTER 49

Hypertensive Intracranial Hemorrhage: Epidemiology and Pathophysiology

Gordon H. Baltuch, Julien Bogousslavsky, and Nicolas de Tribolet

Intracerebral hemorrhage (ICH), or classic apoplexy, has been recognized as a cause of stroke since antiquity and studied in the Western world since the 16th century. The obvious finding of a large intracerebral hematoma with ventricular or subarachnoid extension made the autopsy diagnosis easy and accurate. The concept that ICH was caused by hypertension emerged in the 19th century, although this was not confirmed until formal measurements of blood pressure were made at the turn of this century. Large population studies and the development of stroke registries have resulted in a better comprehension of the risk factors underlying ICH. Furthermore, the advent of computed tomography (CT) in the 1970s and magnetic resonance imaging (MRI) in the 1980s has allowed a more accurate detection and follow up of ICH. This chapter will review the present epidemiology, as well as recent concepts in the pathophysiology of hypertensive ICH.

EPIDEMIOLOGY

Incidence

The true incidence of hypertensive ICH is difficult to determine because the cause, whether it be amyloid, cryptic vascular malformations, arteritis, or hypertension, is not easily determined. The Framingham Study followed 5070 men and women aged 30–62 years over a 36-year period; ICH accounted for a small fraction of total stroke—7.5% in men and 5.6% in women (1). The Lausanne Stroke Registry in Switzerland found that of 1000 patients presenting with a first stroke between 1982 and 1986, 11% occurred secondary to ICH (2). The calculated age-adjusted incidence in the Rochester, Minnesota, study was determined to be 6/100,000

in men, and 7/100,000 in women (total incidence, 13/100,000) for the period 1975–1979 (3) and 15/100,000 for the period of 1980–1984 (4). An evaluation of all ICHs in the Cincinnati area in 1988 revealed the incidence of primary events to be 15/100,000 (5).

The incidence of ICH in Western Europe was similar to the American series. The Oxfordshire Community Stroke Project (England) found the incidence in 1981–1986 to be 14/100,000 (6), and the Dijon Stroke Registry (France) found the incidence in 1985–1989 to be 12/100,000 (7). In contrast to the low relative incidence of ICH compared with total stroke in North America and Western Europe, hemorrhage accounts for approximately 25% of all strokes in Japan, with intraparenchymal hemorrhage accounting for two thirds of the total. The incidence of ICH in the Japanese community of Hisayama was 310/100,000 among men 40 years or older during the period 1961–1970 (8). With time, the incidence fell dramatically to 120/100,000 during the period 1974–1983. However, this incidence was still eight times higher than that in the Cincinnati series.

Interestingly, a recent study from Ecuador demonstrated that the incidence of intraparenchymal hemorrhage per total stroke in their Hispanic population was as high as the incidence in Japan (9). In addition, a recent report has observed a markedly elevated incidence of stroke in the lesser developed European countries (10).

Within the same geographic area, there appears to be a significant difference in the incidence of ICH between racial groups. The Cincinnati group found the sex- and age-adjusted incidence of ICH in African-Americans to be 1.4-fold greater than in Caucasians. If one considers patients younger than 75 years, the incidence is 2.3 times higher in African-Americans (5). The mechanisms underlying these wide variations in hemorrhage rates in different countries, as well as in different racial groups, are still largely unknown. Although racial origin might be a risk factor, control of blood pressure, diet, and socioeconomic conditions are all likely

All authors: Department of Neurology, Neurosurgery, University Hospital (CHUV), Lausanne, Switzerland.

highly important. This is illustrated in studies of Japanese men living in Hawaii and California who had a threefold decrease in incidence of ICH when compared with their cohorts living in Japan (11).

Relationship of Age to Intracerebral Hemorrhage

In the Cincinnati series, the incidence of ICH doubled with each decade after age 35 years (12). In the Rochester series, the incidence went from 0.3/100,000 in the patient population younger than 35 years to an incidence of 57/100,000 in a population older than 75 years. This figure was based on a study conducted between 1955 and 1979 (3). However, it is now thought that in the pre-CT era up to 25% of strokes that were labeled infarcts were in fact ICHs, and therefore the incidence may actually be much higher. This increased incidence appears to parallel the increased incidence of chronic hypertension in older age groups. However, since the incidence of ICH increases with advancing age, and amyloid or congophilic angiopathy generally occurs after age 70 years, distinguishing ''hypertensive'' (or ''primary'') hemorrhage from bleeding as a consequence of amyloid angiopathy is not easily accomplished. Cases considered hypertensive may in fact have been amyloid, and vice versa.

Although these studies indicate a general increase in the incidence of ICH with age, the marked increase in the use of sympathomimetic drugs (especially cocaine), particularly in urban centers, has recently resulted in a significant increase in ICH in young adults (13).

RISK FACTORS

Hypertension

The importance of elevated blood pressure as a risk factor for nonaneurysmal spontaneous ICH is underscored by the name most commonly applied to the condition: *hypertensive* ICH. Interestingly, the degree of hypertension present in patients with ICH varies depending on age. Only 17% of patients 35–55 years of age who present with ICH were not hypertensive, whereas 37% of patients 75 years or older with ICH were normotensive—hypertension being defined as blood pressure >169/90 mm Hg or heart weight >400 g, or both. Younger patients had higher pressures: 28% of those aged 35–55 years had mean pressures >150 mm Hg, whereas no patient older than age 75 had a mean blood pressure at this level (3).

Intracerebral Hemorrhage Secondary to Acutely Raised Blood Pressure Without Chronic Hypertensive Changes

Drugs

Many commonly used decongestants, diet pills, and stimulants known to contain amphetamine-like substances, such as phenylpropanolamine (PPA), have been associated with ICH, especially in women (14). The illicit use of drugs, including cocaine (especially the alkaloid form known as ''crack'') and amphetamines, by oral, nasal, and intravenous routes, causes a dramatic increase in blood pressure and now accounts for a significant and growing proportion of all ICH cases, especially in individuals younger than 35 years (13).

Dental Chair

A common clinical setting that can potentially increase blood pressure markedly is trigeminal nerve stimulation for dental procedures or, less commonly, for trigeminal neuralgia, which can cause ICH (15).

Activity

Onset of ICH has commonly been associated with certain activities such as straining at stool, vomiting, coughing, and coition, as well as strenuous physical activity such as running and weightlifting. Stressful or emotional situations have also been associated with ICH. This likely results from an increase in blood pressure. Interestingly, a recent report from Israel observed an increase in the percentage of hemorrhagic strokes vs. total strokes during the Persian Gulf War (24% of total vs. 12% in peacetime), when the population was highly stressed (16).

Cold

Caplan et al (17) reported a series of patients who developed ICH after exposure to extremely cold temperatures. It is known that immersion of the hands in ice water for one minute is known to cause an elevation of the blood pressure (cold-pressor response), which is more marked in previously hypertensive patients. It is likely that ICH in these cases was secondary to an acute cold-induced elevation in blood pressure.

Associated Factors

Although the disease has often been referred to as *hypertensive* ICH and there is little doubt that elevated blood pressure promotes it, other factors that influence and modify the impact of increased blood pressure are still being identified. It is difficult to assess whether these factors, such as smoking, alcohol consumption, and diet, act independently to affect ICH or through an effect on blood pressure.

Cigarette Smoking

In the Honolulu study of male cigarette smokers, the incidence of ''hemorrhagic'' stroke was 2.5 times greater than in nonsmokers, independent of age, diastolic blood pressure, serum cholesterol, alcohol consumption, hematocrit, and body mass index (18). However, verification of hemorrhage type by imaging, autopsy, or angiography was often not available in this study, so some of the hemorrhages may have been secondary to other etiologies (eg, subarachnoid hemorrhage). In addition, as the study included only men of Japanese origin living in Hawaii, it represents a biased selection group.

Alcohol

The relationship between alcohol and stroke is complex and may be related to many factors, including the population studied, the amount and type of alcohol consumed, and the consumption pattern. Alcohol intake has been shown to be closely associated with hypertension, and acute alcohol intoxication may produce a marked increase in blood pressure resulting in ICH. The Hisayama registry has recently reported an increased incidence of ICH in a nonhypertensive Japanese population who heavily consumed alcohol (>34 g/d ethyl alcohol) (19). Chronic alcohol consumption is associated with platelet and clotting disorders that may result in a tendency to bleed, possibly explaining this increased incidence.

Cholesterol

Iso et al (20) studied the incidence of hemorrhagic stroke as a function of serum cholesterol levels in relation to diastolic blood pressure (DBP) measurements. When deaths from intracranial hemorrhage were examined by entry blood pressure, the age-adjusted rates were significant only in those with low cholesterol whose DBP was >90 mm Hg. The interaction of high DBP and low serum cholesterol in promoting ICH suggested to some investigators "that very low serum cholesterol levels weaken the endothelium of intracerebral arteries, resulting in hemorrhagic stroke in the presence of hypertension" (20). It has been suggested that other factors were also operating to increase hemorrhage risk, including heavy alcohol consumption, protein deficiency, and a higher intake of polyunsaturated fatty acids, both linoleic acid derived from vegetable oils and eicosapentaenoic acid from fish oil, which acts to reduce platelet aggregability.

Seasonal Variations

There appears to be a seasonal variation in ICH, the general incidence of hemorrhage being highest in the winter and lowest in the summer. This has been thought to be secondary to the inverse relationship between blood pressure and temperature (17), but the seasonal variation may be related to other factors such as ambient humidity and hours of sunshine (21).

Declining Mortality and Incidence

Death rates from ICH have fallen dramatically during the past 20 years, paralleling the overall decrease in stroke deaths. A decline in the incidence of ICH has been documented in several populations. In the United States, the reduction has been related to better detection and more effective treatment of hypertension. Although there has been a drop in ICH that corresponds to the treatment of systemic hypertension, it is conceivable that as the population ages, there might be an increase in ICH in the elderly. In addition, the marked increase in ICH secondary to illicit drug use may result in an increased case fatality.

It is as yet unclear whether efforts to reduce cholesterol in Western populations by means of dietary and pharmacologic measures increases the incidence of ICH. The increased use of aspirin for cardiovascular disease may also increase the incidence of ICH, although this remains unproven.

In Japan, including rural areas, substantial changes in diet have occurred in the past 20 years. These include an increase in the percentages of animal fat and animal protein in the diet and a reduction in the amount of sodium chloride. In addition, the prevalence of hypertension in Japan fell and, coincident with it, the incidence of brain hemorrhage (8). There remains a number of unresolved issues and unexplained phenomena in the epidemiology of ICH. An understanding of other yet unidentified risk factors promoting hemorrhage will hopefully lead to a further decrease in stroke incidence.

PATHOPHYSIOLOGY

There appear to be two rather different important mechanisms that result in hypertensive ICH: (a) rupture of small penetrating arteries damaged by chronic hypertension and aging and (b) acute perturbations in blood pressure and blood flow leading to rupture of normal arterioles and capillaries unaccustomed to and unprotected from these circulatory changes.

There is overwhelming evidence that both high blood pressure and aging cause degenerative changes in arteries that make them susceptible to both occlusion and rupture. These pathologic changes include fibrinoid necrosis, medial degeneration, lipohyalinosis, and microaneurysm formation, all of which are found in the penetrating arteries of the brains of hypertensive patients, especially those with ICH. The rupture usually occurs in the middle or distal portions of penetrating arteries at or very near bifurcations. The ruptured arteries show changes in the elastic lamina and degeneration in the vascular media, especially affecting smooth muscle elements.

The issue of whether the hemorrhage is a result of the

rupture of a microaneurysm (Charcot–Bouchard type) has been debated for over a century (22). Current evidence weighs against the theory that rupture is due to breakage of these microaneurysms (14). For example, Charcot–Bouchard type microaneurysms have never been clearly identified as the definitive cause of even a single hematoma, despite very extensive study. In addition, when rupture sites have been identified, they do not usually show a microaneurysm. It is likely that microaneurysms may well represent, at least in some instances, the effects of small vascular rupture rather than the cause.

There is accumulating evidence against the theory that hypertensive ICH is always caused by chronic vascular degenerative changes. In many patients who bled, no pathologic evidence of chronic systemic hypertension (eg, left ventricular hypertrophy or other cardiac, renal, or retinal changes) was found. A possible explanation is that ICH in these patients represents an initial presenting symptom of clinical hypertensive disease (15). In these patients, acute perturbations in blood pressure and blood flow lead to rupture of normal arterioles and capillaries unaccustomed to and unprotected from these circulatory changes. Of course, the more sudden and the more severe the change is, the more likely is the risk of rupture. The combination of a marked increase in cerebral blood flow, as well as a marked increase in blood pressure secondary to manipulation of the carotid bulb, can occasionally be observed following carotid endarterectomy and can lead to ICH (23). It is possible that in some of these patients damage to blood vessels, for example, incurred during protracted but slight hypertension, made the blood vessels more susceptible to breakage when circulatory changes occurred. The pathogenesis of drug-related ICH is widely believed to be the sudden, dramatic increase in blood pressure precipitated by the sympathomimetic effects of the agents used, yet it remains unresolved whether cerebrovascular changes caused by chronic drug use make ICH more likely in the setting of an acute increase in blood pressure.

Location of Hemorrhage

Hypertensive ICH typically occurs in one of five sites: (a) putamen and adjacent internal capsule, (b) lobar, (c) thalamus, (d) pons, and (e) cerebellum. A penetrating artery arising from the middle cerebral artery stem, basilar artery, or circle of Willis is generally the source of hemorrhage; these same vessels are known to be damaged by hypertension.

Controversy exists about the importance of hypertension in the etiology of lobar hemorrhages. Despite various explanations for the predominance of nonhypertensive mechanisms in lobar ICH, Broderick et al (24) have recently provided evidence for the substantial contribution of hypertension to its pathogenesis. They found hypertension as the mechanism in 67% of 66 patients with lobar ICH, a figure that was not significantly different from that of 77

patients with deep hemispheric (73%), 11 with cerebellar (73%), and nine with pontine (78%) hemorrhage. Furthermore, the frequency of hypertension as the mechanism of ICH remained unchanged with advancing age; that is, it did not decrease as the effect of cerebral amyloid angiopathy increased. These observations led the authors to conclude that hypertension is at least as important as cerebral amyloid angiopathy in the pathogenesis of lobar ICH.

Timing of Bleed

In the pre-CT era, it was a popular belief that hypertensive ICH was a monophasic event and that elevated blood pressure did not promote further bleeding. This was based on a study by Herbstein and Schaumberg (25) that indicated that intracerebral bleeding in spontaneous ICH rarely continued beyond 2–3 hours. These investigators injected chromium Cr 51–labeled erythrocytes into 11 patients 2–5 hours after the estimated onset of ICH and measured Cr 51 activity within the hematoma during autopsy. None of the nine patients with ''hypertensive hemorrhage'' showed postmortem evidence of Cr 51 activity within the hematoma, but activity was found within the Duret hemorrhages in the brainstem. The study was limited, however, in that the earliest injection of Cr 51 was 2 hours after the onset of symptoms, the clinical criterion for identification of ICH were not stated, the study was performed before the CT era, and only 11 patients were investigated.

Angiographically, secondary bleeding sites have been demonstrated at the periphery of intracerebral hematomas as late as 20 days after clinical onset (26). Fisher's (27) classic studies of the pathology of ICH provide important insights into the possible mechanism of this continued bleeding. Along the periphery of hemorrhages, Fisher found many small fibrin globes, masses of agglutinated platelets encircled by thin layers of fibrin. He postulated that the initial hemorrhage exerted pressure on adjacent capillaries and arterioles, causing them to break. As they ruptured, blood was added at the circumference of the lesion, gradually expanding the hematoma. As the hematoma grew, local and, later, general intracranial pressure rose, and the surrounding pressure acted to stop the bleeding.

Although edema in the compressed tissue surrounding the hemorrhage often leads to increased mass effect and in some cases worsening of the clinical state, a recent series of reports suggests that the bleeding can continue and clinical deterioration is not due to edema or compression but is secondary to continued bleeding or rebleeding at the initial sight of hemorrhage (Fig. 1). Kelley et al (28), in a study of four patients with hypertensive ICH, demonstrated that there was CT evidence of active bleeding up to 6 hours from the initial bleed. Fehr and Anderson (29) reviewed 56 cases of hypertensive ICH in the basal ganglia and thalamus and documented enlargement of the hematoma by CT in four patients. Poorly controlled hypertension was a factor in two patients

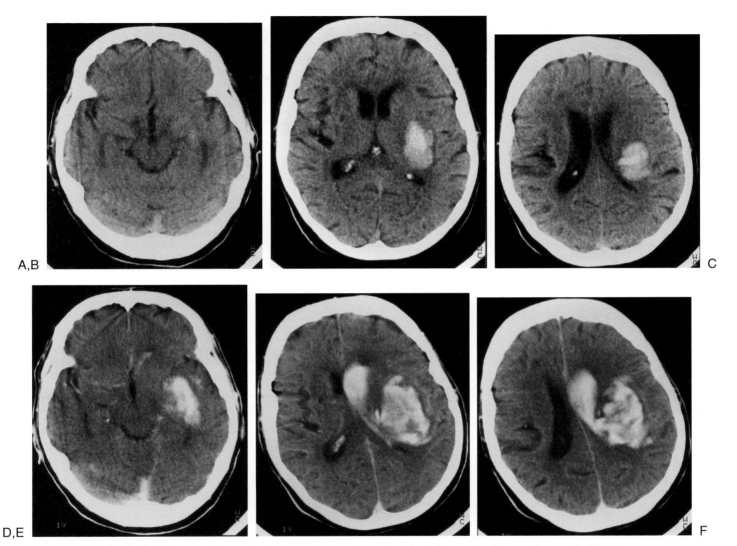

FIG. 1. Serial CT scans demonstrate progression of hypertensive intracerebral hemorrhage: **(A–C)** 180 minutes after the onset of symptoms; **(D–F)** 210 minutes after the onset of symptoms. The patient had deteriorated neurologically in the period between the two CT scans.

who deteriorated within 24 hours. Chen et al (30) noted continued bleeding and clinical deterioration within the first 12 hours in eight patients with ICH. Persistent elevation of blood pressure was noted in six of the eight patients in this series. They concluded that persistent severe hypertension may have been a contributing factor in prolongation of active bleeding or precipitation of rebleeding in their patients. Broderick et al (31) described eight patients who had CT evaluation of ICH within 2 hours of presentation, with a follow-up scan several hours later. They observed that bleeding could continue for up to 5 hours from the initial time of ictus. Deterioration in five of the eight patients was associated with a systolic blood pressure >195 mm Hg. They also observed that the largest increases in the volume of hemorrhage occurred in young hypertensive patients with deep hemorrhages. They stated, "a prospective study of the ultra early time course of ICH is needed in humans to deter-

mine how age, location of bleeding, underlying vascular pathology, blood pressure, and coagulation status affect the duration of bleeding and subsequent clinical outcome" (31). These reports might be clinically important in determining management of patients who deteriorate clinically after initial presentation.

CONCLUSION AND PERSPECTIVES

Although the incidence of intraparenchymal hemorrhage is a relatively small percentage of total stoke, especially in North America and Western Europe (2), it is still, it must be emphasized, twice that of subarachnoid hemorrhage (32). There appear to be two different subgroups of patients with hypertensive ICH: (1) those with a history of hypertension and possibly end-organ changes in the heart, retina, and kidneys, indicative of chronic pressure changes, and (b) those with no history or evidence of prior sustained hypertension who bleed because of relatively recent changes in blood pressure and flow. An unanswered question remains whether the location, size, or outcome of ICH is different between these two groups. One might speculate that chronic hypertension, by causing hypertrophy and increased peripheral resistance in large and medium-sized brain arteries, protects the smaller, more distal arteries from the centrally measured increased blood pressure. This might lead to comparably smaller bleeds (14). Further research into the epidemiology and pathophysiology of ICH is necessary and will hopefully result in the identification of new strategies for the prevention and treatment of this disabling and frequently fatal disease.

REFERENCES

1. Sacco RL, Wolf PA, Bharucha NE, et al. Subarachnoid and intracerebral hemorrhage: Natural history, prognosis, and precursive factors in the Framingham Study. *Neurology* 1984;34:847–854.
2. Bogousslavsky J, Van Melle G, Regli F. The Lausanne Stroke Registry: Analysis of 1000 consecutive patients with first stroke. *Stroke* 1988; 19:1083–1092.
3. Drury I, Whisnant JP, Garraway WM. Primary intracerebral hemorrhage: Impact of CT on incidence. *Neurology* 1984;34:653–657.
4. Broderick JP, Phillips SJ, Whisnant JP, et al. Incidence rates of stroke in the eighties: The end of the decline in stroke? *Stroke* 1989;20:577–582.
5. Broderick JP, Brott T, Tomsick T, Huster G, Miller R. The risk of subarachnoid and intracerebral hemorrhage in blacks as compared with whites. *N Engl J Med* 1992;326:733–736.
6. Bamford J, Sandercock P, Dennis M, et al: A prospective study of acute cerebrovascular disease in the community: The Oxfordshire Community Stroke Project 1981–1986. 2. Incidence, case fatality rates and overall outcome at one year of cerebral infarction primary intracerebral and subarachnoid haemorrhage. *J Neurol Neurosurg Psychiatry* 1990; 53:16–22.
7. Giroud M, Gras P, Chadan N, Beuriat P, Milan C, Arveux P, Dumas R. Cerebral haemorrhage in a French propective population study. *J Neurol Neurosurg Psychiatry* 1991;54:595–598.
8. Ueda K, Hasuo Y, Kiyohara Y, et al. Intracerebral hemorrhage in a Japanese community, Hisayama: Incidence, changing pattern during long-term follow-up, and related factors. *Stroke* 1988;19:48–52.
9. Del Brutto OH, Mosquera A, Sanchez X, Santos J, Noboa CA. Stroke subtypes among Hispanics living in Guayaquil, Ecuador. *Stroke* 1993; 24:1833–1836.
10. Thorvaldsen P, Asplund K, Kuulasmaa K, Rajakangas A-M, Schroll M. Stroke incidence, case fatality, and mortality in the WHO MONICA project. *Stroke* 1995;26:361–367.
11. Takeya Y, Popper JS, Shimizu Y, Kato H, Rhoads GG, Kagan A. Epidemiologic studies of coronary heart disease and stroke in Japanese men living in Japan, Hawaii and California: Incidence of stroke in Japn and Hawaii. *Stroke* 1984;15:15–23.
12. Brott T, Thalinger K, Hertzberg V. Hypertension as a risk factor for spontaneous intracerebral hemorrhage. *Stroke* 1986;17:1078–1083.
13. Kaku DA, Lowenstein DH. Emergence of recreational drug abuse as a major risk factor for stroke in young adults. *Ann Intern Med* 1990; 113:821–827.
14. Kase CS, Caplan LR, eds. *Intracerebral Hemorrhage.* Boston: Butterworth-Heinemann, 1994.
15. Caplan L. Intracerebral hemorrhage revisited. *Neurology* 1988;38: 624–627.
16. Kleinman Y, Korn-Lubetzki I, Eliashiv S, Abramsky O, Eliakim M. High frequency of hemorrhagic strokes in Jerusalem during the Persian Gulf War. *Neurology* 1992;42:2225–2226.
17. Caplan LR, Neely S, Gorelick P. Cold-related intracerebral hemorrhage. *Arch Neurol* 1984;41:227.
18. Abbott RD, Yin Y, Reed DM, et al. Risk of stroke in male cigarette smokers. *N Eng J Med* 1986;315:717–720.
19. Kiyohara Y, Kato I, Iwamoto H, Nakayama K, Fujishima M. The impact of alcohol and hypertension on stroke incidence in a general Japanese population: The Hisayama study. *Stroke* 1995;26:368–372.
20. Iso H, Jacobs DR, Wentworth D, et al. Serum cholesterol levels and six-year mortality from stroke in 350,977 men screened for the multiple risk factor intervention trial. *N Eng J Med* 1989;320:904–910.
21. Bergstrom K, Lodin H. An angiographic observation in intracerebral haematoma. *Br J Radiol* 1967;40:228–229.
21. Capon A, Demeurisse G, Zheng L. Seasonal variation in cerebral hemorrhage in 236 consecutive cases in Brussels. *Stroke* 1992;23:24–27.
22. Charcot JM, Bouchard C. Nouvelles recherches sur la pathogénie de l'hémorrhagie cérébrale. *Arch Physiol Norm Path* 1868;1:110–127, 643–665, 725–734.
23. Caplan LR, Skillman J, Ojemann R, et al. Intracerebral hemorrhage following carotid endarterectomy: A hypertensive complication? *Stroke* 1978;9:457–460.
24. Broderick J, Brott T, Tomsick T, et al. Lobar hemorrhage in the elderly: The undiminished importance of hypertension. *Stroke* 1993;24:49–51.
25. Herbstein DJ, Schaumberg HH. Hypertensive intracerebral hematoma: An investigation of the initial hemorrhage and rebleeding using Cr 51-labeled erythrocytes. *Arch Neurol* 1974;30:412–414.
27. Fisher CM. Pathological observations in hypertensive cerebral hemorrhage. *J Neuropath Exp Neurol* 1971;30:536–550.
28. Kelley RE, Berger JR, Sceinberg P, et al. Active bleeding in hypertensive intracerebral hemorrhage: Computed tomography. *Neurology* 1982;32:852–856.
29. Fehr MA, Anderson DC. Incidence of progression or rebleeding in hypertensive intracerebral hemorrhage. *J Stroke Cerebrovasc Dis* 1991; 1:111–117.
30. Chen ST, Chen SD, Hsu CY, Hogan EL. Progression of hypertensive intracerebral hemorrhage. *Neurology* 1989;39:1509–1514.
31. Broderick JP, Brott TG, Tomsick T, Barsan W, Spilker J. Ultra-early evaluation of intracerebral hemorrhage. *J Neurosurg* 1990;72: 195–199.
32. Broderick JP, Brott T, Tomsick T, Miller R, Huster G. Intracerebral hemorrhage more than twice as common as subarachnoid hemorrhage. *J Neurosurg* 1993;78:188–191.

Cerebrovascular Disease, edited by H. Hunt Batjer.
Lippincott-Raven Publishers, Philadelphia © 1997.

CHAPTER 50

Management of Intracerebral Hemorrhage

Joseph P. Broderick, Thomas Brott, and Mario Zuccarello

Intracerebral hemorrhage is more than twice as common as subarachnoid hemorrhage and much more likely to result in death or major disability than cerebral infarction or subarachnoid hemorrhage. Yet while more than 315 randomized clinical therapeutic trials for acute ischemic stroke and 78 for subarachnoid hemorrhage have been completed or are ongoing (personal communication, Cochran Stroke Review Group, 5/16/95), only four small randomized surgical trials (353 total patients) (1–4) and four small medical trials (513 total patients) (5–8) have been reported. Neither surgery nor medical treatment has been shown to conclusively benefit patients with intracerebral hemorrhage in these small randomized studies.

Despite a lack of proven benefit for surgery, an estimated 7000 operations to remove intracerebral hemorrhages are performed every year in the United States alone (9). Guidelines for operation and medical treatment have been suggested, but the management of intracerebral hemorrhage by neurologists and neurosurgeons throughout the world varies greatly (9,10). The poor outcome for most patients with current management emphasizes that state-of-the-art treatment of intracerebral hemorrhage is inadequate and that new approaches are needed.

EPIDEMIOLOGY

Intracerebral hemorrhage as documented by computed tomography (CT) imaging occurs in approximately 12–29 persons per 100,000 population per year (11). The incidence rate in Greater Cincinnati during 1988 was 15 persons per 100,000 population, which would correspond to 37,000 new cases of intracerebral hemorrhage in the United States every year (12). Intracerebral hemorrhage occurs slightly more frequently among men than women and is significantly more

common among young and middle-aged blacks than whites of similar age (12,13). Although the incidence rate of intracerebral hemorrhage increases exponentially with age (Fig. 1) (11), it still affects nearly as many patients under the age of 65 as does subarachnoid hemorrhage (12). In population studies that have used CT scanning to identify the majority of hemorrhages, ganglionic or periventricular hemorrhages accounted for 30–48% of all intracerebral hemorrhages compared to 34–52% for lobar hemorrhage, 6–11% for cerebellar hemorrhages, and 3–7% for pontine hemorrhages (11,14). The variation in proportions for lobar and deep hemorrhages likely reflects, in part, differences in definitions.

The 30-day mortality for intracerebral hemorrhage ranges from 35% to 52% in population studies during the CT era (11,14). Half of the 30-day mortality occurs within the first 2 days and only a tenth of patients are totally independent by 30 days (11). Only 20% of patients are independent at 6 months (15). Volume of hemorrhage on the baseline CT scan is the most powerful baseline predictor of mortality and morbidity in various population studies and case series (11,16,17). This is true regardless of hemorrhage location (Figs. 2–6) (16). The average volume of intracerebral hemorrhage in the Greater Cincinnati population during 1988, as measured by CT, was 36 cm^3. This is approximately halfway between the volume of a ping-pong ball (28 cm^3) and golf ball (42 cm^3) (Fig. 7).

Other important baseline variables that are significant predictors of mortality include the baseline Glasgow Coma Scale score and the volume of ventricular hemorrhage (11,15,16). In the Greater Cincinnati study, a predictive model incorporating only the volume of parenchymal hemorrhage on the baseline CT and the baseline Glasgow Coma Scale score predicted 30-day mortality with a sensitivity and specificity of 97% (Table 1). In contrast, arterial blood pressure, location of hemorrhage, and age were not independent predictors of mortality (16).

The volume of parenchymal hemorrhage can easily be measured from the CT film by a simple method that correlates well with a sophisticated computerized image analysis

J. P. Broderick and T. Brott: Department of Neurology, University of Cincinnati Medical Center, Cincinnati, Ohio 45267.

M. Zuccarello: Department of Neurosurgery, Mayfield Clinic Medical Center, Cincinnati, Ohio 45219.

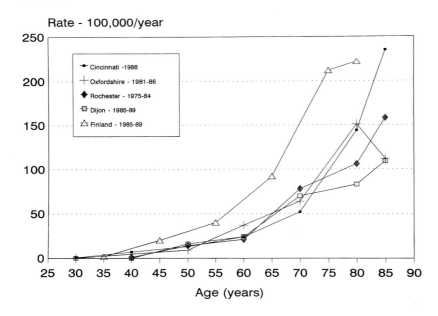

FIG. 1. Age-specific incidence rates of intracerebral hemorrhage. Each data point represents the midpoint of a 10-year age group. The oldest data points represent those persons equal to or older than a given age. (From ref. 11.)

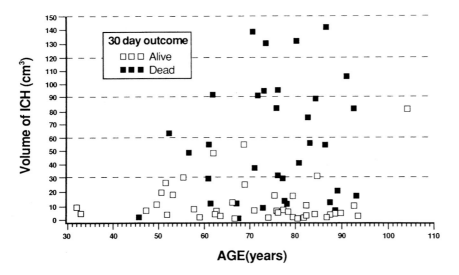

FIG. 2. Plot shows 30-day outcome for the 76 patients with deep hemorrhages according to patient age and volume of parenchymal hemorrhage. ICH indicates intracerebral hemorrhage. (From ref. 16.)

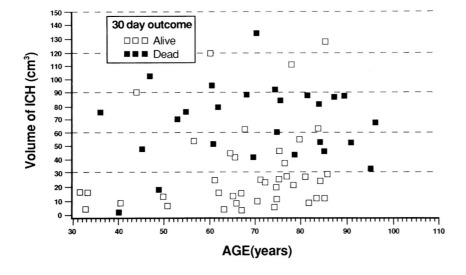

FIG. 3. Plot shows 30-day outcome for the 66 patients with lobar hemorrhages according to patient age and volume of parenchymal hemorrhage. (From ref. 16.)

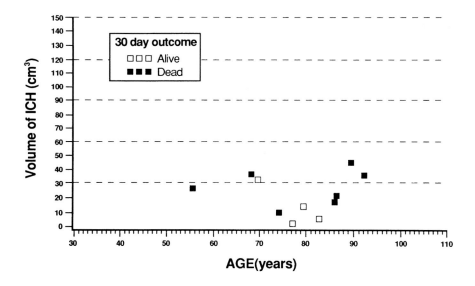

FIG. 4. Plot shows 30-day outcome for the 11 patients with cerebellar hemorrhages according to patient age and volume of parenchymal hemorrhage. (From ref. 16.)

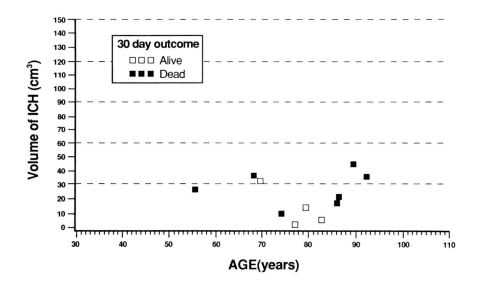

FIG. 5. Plot shows 30-day outcome for the nine patients with pontine hemorrhages according to patient age and volume of parenchymal hemorrhage. (From ref. 16.)

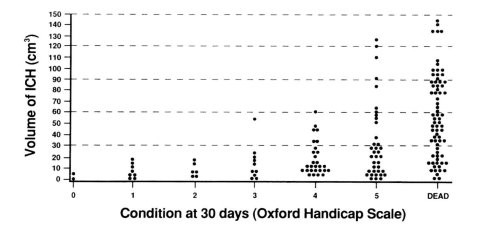

FIG. 6. Plot shows 30-day outcomes for 162 patients with intracerebral hemorrhages as measured by modified Oxford Handicap Scale according to volume of parenchymal hemorrhage. According to the modified Oxford Handicap Scale (113), 0 = no symptoms; 1 = minor symptoms that do not interfere with lifestyle; 2 = minor handicap; 3 = moderate handicap; 4 = moderately severe handicap; 5 = severe handicap; 6 = dead. Grade 3: stupor; grade 4a: semicoma without signs of herniation; grade 4b: semicoma with signs of herniation; grade 5: deep coma. (From ref. 16.)

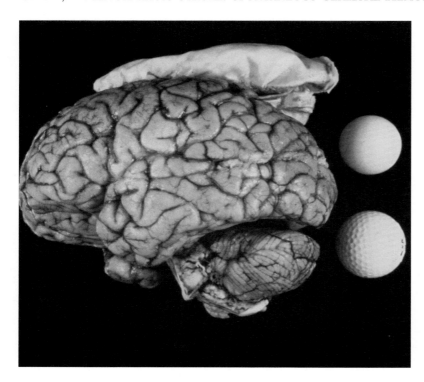

FIG. 7. Normal brain juxtaposed with ping-pong ball and golf ball for size comparison. The average volume of all intracerebral hemorrhages in Greater Cincinnati during 1988 was 36 cm³; approximately halfway between the volume of a ping-pong ball (28 cm³) and golf ball (42 cm³).

measurement of hemorrhage volume (Fig. 8) (16,18). This method can be performed reproducibly by physicians and nurses in a mean time of 38 seconds (18). Thus, a physician using a copy of Table 1, the measurement of hemorrhage volume from the CT film, and the Glasgow Coma Scale score can accurately predict 30-day mortality at the bedside within minutes.

CAUSES OF INTRACEREBRAL HEMORRHAGE

Clinicians have linked the likely cause of a hemorrhage to its location in the brain, the presence of structural abnormalities on brain imaging, associated medical conditions such as hypertension, and age of the patient. Thus, hemorrhages that occur in the basal ganglia, deep periventricular white matter, pons, and cerebellum, particularly if they occur in a patient with known hypertension, are often attributed to hypertensive small vessel disease. In contrast, lobar hemorrhages in the very elderly are often considered to be due

to amyloid angiopathy. These clinical assumptions may be incorrect. However, whatever the cause, the pathogenesis of intracerebral hemorrhage almost always involves abnormal vessels at the site of the hemorrhage. Specific causes of intracerebral hemorrhage are discussed in order of importance.

Hypertensive Vasculopathy

Hemorrhage originating in the thalamus, basal ganglia, deep periventricular white matter, pons, or cerebellum has been linked to prior hypertension and vasculopathy of the small penetrating arteries and arterioles that supply blood to these brain regions (11,19–22). The vasculopathy primarily involves arteries that are 100–600 μm in diameter (19–22) and is characterized by severe degeneration of medial smooth muscle cells, miliary aneurysms associated with thrombus and microhemorrhages, accumulation of nonfatty debris, and hyalinization of the intima (19–22). The reported

TABLE 1. *Model of 30-day mortality using volume of parenchymal hemorrhage and Glasgow Coma Scale*

Glasgow Coma Scale score	ICH volume	No. in risk group	Dead	Expected dead	Probability of being dead at 30 days
≥9	<30	77	13	15	0.19
≥9	31–60	19	11	9	0.46
≥9	>60	17	12	13	0.75
≤8	<30	15	7	7	0.44
≤8	31–60	15	11	11	0.74
≤8	>60	19	17	17	0.91

From ref. 16.

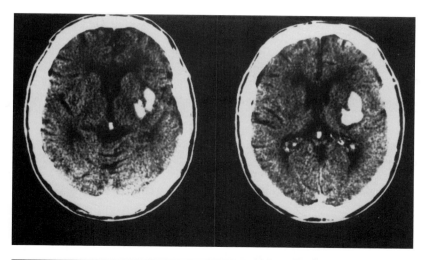

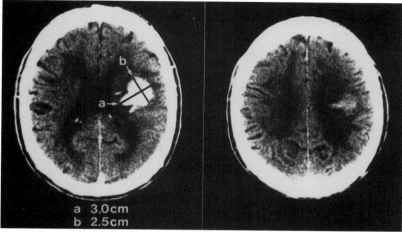

a 3.0cm
b 2.5cm

FIG. 8. CT images illustrate calculation of modified ellipsoid volume = $(A \times B \times C)/2$. A is the largest diameter on the slice with the largest area of hemorrhage. B is the diameter that is 90° to diameter A and is measured at the midpoint of diameter A. Diameter C (vertical diameter) is the number of 1-cm slices on which the hemorrhage is seen. Thus, the estimated volume is $(3 \times 2.5 \times 3.5)/2 = 13$ cm³. (From ref. 16.)

sites of arterial rupture in these cases include both miliary aneurysms and arterial bifurcations where the media was severely degenerated (19–22). Recent pathologic observations indicate that miliary or microaneurysms described by earlier techniques may represent excessive vascular coiling or loops (23).

Similar vascular changes in the long penetrating medullary arteries, which extend from the cortex to the underlying white matter, are seen in patients with lobar hemorrhages without any evidence of amyloid angiopathy. Of 29 lobar hemorrhages removed surgically in the series reported by Wakai and colleagues, 9 were secondary to arteriovenous malformations, 6 had associated amyloid angiopathy, and 11 had associated microaneurysms (24). Of the 11, 6 had a history of hypertension. In a detailed autopsy series by Cole and Yates of 100 hypertensive and 100 normotensive subjects, 30% of all microaneurysms involved the long penetrating medullary arteries (19). The occurrence of microaneurysms was markedly related to the presence of hypertension and advancing age. These data indicate that vascular changes associated with hypertension and advancing age are important causes of lobar hemorrhage. This conclusion is supported by the observation that the proportion of patients with

lobar hemorrhage in the Greater Cincinnati population who had a history of hypertension (67%) was not significantly different from that for locations classically associated with hypertension (73%) (25).

Increased blood pressure not only induces pathologic vascular changes but is also the likely precipitant of vascular rupture in many cases. Blood pressure in hypertensive patients is more variable than in patients without hypertension (26). Sudden changes in blood pressure could result in breakage of a weakened vessel wall, whether the vascular damage was due to hypertension, amyloid angiopathy, or aneurysm. In summary, increased blood pressure plays a major role in the pathogenesis of intracerebral hemorrhage, regardless of location, and the vasculopathy associated with hypertension becomes more evident with advancing age.

Cerebral Amyloid Angiopathy

Cerebral amyloid angiopathy has been increasingly recognized as a cause of lobar intracerebral hemorrhage in the elderly (27–36). Its principal pathologic feature is the deposition of amyloid protein in the media and adventitia of leptomeningeal and cortical small arteries, arterioles, capillaries, and, less often, veins (27–30). The hypothesized pathogenesis of intracerebral hemorrhage due to cerebral amyloid angiopathy involves destruction of normal vascular structure by deposition of amyloid in the media and adventitia and subsequent miliary aneurysmal formation of double barreling and fibrinoid necrosis (27–29). The brittle blood vessels and microaneurysms are then prone to rupture in response to minor trauma or sudden changes in blood pressure.

The presence of amyloid protein in cortical blood vessels in consecutive autopsy series increases markedly with age at death, affecting only 5–8% of those aged 60–69 years and 57–58% of those age 90 years or older (32,33). The vascular deposition of amyloid is most marked in the parietooccipital subcortical regions and is rarely found in the basal ganglia, brainstem, or cerebellum. In a population-based autopsy study of intracerebral hemorrhage, Okazaki and Whisnant reported that amyloid angiopathy was the cause of bleeding in 5 of 17 persons age 65 years or older with a fatal intracerebral hemorrhage during 1970–1979 (27). All hemorrhages originated in the cortex and underlying white matter. Thus, a lobar hemorrhage in a very elderly person without another evident cause is likely due to vascular changes related to age, hypertension, or amyloid.

Vascular Abnormalities: Malformations and Aneurysms

Vascular malformations account for approximately 4–5% of intracerebral hemorrhages if aneurysmal-associated intracerebral hemorrhages are excluded (11). Types of malformations include arteriovenous malformations, cavernous malformations, or venous angiomas. Hemorrhages due to vascular malformations tend to be at the level of the cerebral convexity (subcortical white matter) more often than in the deep portion of the hemisphere, mirroring their typically more superficial location. Vascular malformations accounted for five of nine spontaneous brain hemorrhages in children in Greater Cincinnati during 1988 (37).

Ruptured aneurysms account for 4–11% of intracerebral hemorrhage in population-based studies (11). The intracerebral hemorrhage is almost always associated with subarachnoid bleeding because aneurysms arise from major intracranial arteries within the subarachnoid space.

Brain imaging can provide excellent clues to a structural vascular cause of intracerebral hemorrhage. Abnormal vascular structures such as large flow voids on magnetic resonance imaging (MRI) or serpiginous structures on a CT contrast study can point to a vascular malformation. Location of the intracerebral hemorrhage near the Sylvian fissure or temporal lobe should raise the possibility of a middle cerebral artery aneurysm or arteriovenous malformation. Any lobar hemorrhage, particularly in a young, nonhypertensive patient, should raise the possibility of a structural vascular abnormality.

Disorders of Coagulation and Thrombolysis

In Greater Cincinnati during 1988, 9 (5%) of 188 patients with an intracerebral hemorrhage were receiving anticoagulant therapy at the time of their stroke (11). This proportion is less than the 30% of primary intracerebral hemorrhages reported for Rochester, Minnesota, during 1955–1979 (38). Oral anticoagulants have been associated with a 6- to 11-fold increased risk of intracerebral hemorrhage (38,39). The risk increases with age and the degree of anticoagulation, particularly an International Normalized Ratio of 4 or more (40). The recent increase in warfarin use for patients with atrial fibrillation will likely once again increase the relative frequency of warfarin-associated intracerebral hemorrhage.

Hemorrhage associated with thrombolytic therapy is another increasingly important cause of intracranial bleeding. Two of the 188 hemorrhages in Greater Cincinnati during 1988 were associated with thrombolytic therapy (11). This frequency is likely an underestimate of its importance as a cause of hemorrhage today because the use of thrombolytics for myocardial infarction and other indications has increased substantially over the past 7 years. Other less frequent causes of intracerebral hemorrhage associated with coagulation abnormalities include inherited or acquired disorders of coagulation proteins or platelet abnormalities (11).

Hemorrhage into a Cerebral Infarct

The reported frequency of hemorrhagic transformation depends on the CT criteria for hemorrhage as well as on when and how frequently patients with acute cerebral infarcts are studied by CT. In a prospective study of 65 patients with cerebral infarcts who had standard imaging studies on the 3rd, 7th, 14th, and 21st day after stroke onset, 43% had some evidence of hemorrhage transformation (41). Extensive hematoma within an infarct was much less common. However, intrainfarct hematoma may be difficult to differentiate from primary intracerebral hemorrhage by CT features alone. Bogousslavsky and colleagues recently reported 15 patients with a presumed cerebral infarct "in whom the CT showed no bleeding within 6 hours of stroke onset but showed ganglionic or lobar hemorrhage less than 18 hours later, without visible underlying infarct" (42). In earlier pathologic studies of intracerebral hemorrhage, thrombotic occlusions of small arterioles and microaneurysms coexisted with microhemorrhages and microaneurysms (11). Rupture of an ischemic artery or arteriole may be a more common cause of intracerebral hemorrhage than is presently appreciated.

Other Causes

Bleeding into brain tumors accounts for 2–7% of intracerebral hemorrhages in population studies (11). In adults, the brain tumors most likely to present as an intracerebral hemorrhage are glioblastomas or metastases. Three of the nine intracerebral hemorrhages in children in Greater Cincinnati during 1988–1989 resulted from hemorrhage into longstanding hypothalamic gliomas (37). Heavy alcohol use is a risk factor for intracerebral hemorrhage in several case-control studies (43–45). In addition, intracerebral hemorrhage associated with cocaine, amphetamines, or over-the-counter sympathomimetic agents are no longer considered rare occurrences (46). A large, multicenter, case-control study of the role of these illicit drugs and over-the-counter preparations in the occurrence of intracerebral hemorrhage is currently ongoing.

EVALUATION

Evaluation of the patient with an intracerebral hemorrhage should always include a thorough history and physical examination for possible causes such as prior hypertension, illicit drug use, use of anticoagulants, and a family history of brain hemorrhage or aneurysmal rupture. Baseline laboratory studies should include a complete blood count, prothrombin time, partial thromboplastin time, renal panel, liver functions, serum glucose, electrocardiogram, and chest X ray.

However, the CT scan is the key part of the initial evaluation. The brain CT demonstrates the size and location of the hemorrhage but also may reveal structural abnormalities such as aneurysms, arteriovenous malformations, and brain tumors. If the CT scan is obtained during regular hours, administration of contrast agent by the radiologist can often highlight suspected vascular abnormalities. If the patient is in extremis or requires an immediate operation, further imaging is usually not done.

Halpin and colleagues recently performed a prospective study to examine the role of angiography in patients with intracerebral hemorrhage (47). The mean age of the 102 prospectively evaluated patients was 49 years (range 10–70 years). The very young age of this patient group indicates that this group was composed of referral patients rather than all hemorrhages in the community. However, of the 102 patients, 44 were thought to have an underlying structural lesion as the cause of their hemorrhage. All of these patients were assigned to have cerebral angiography as soon as their respective conditions allowed. CT findings that prompted the impression of a structural lesion were the presence of subarachnoid or intraventricular hemorrhage, abnormal intracranial calcification, prominent vascular structures, and the site of hemorrhage (eg, peri-Sylvian hemorrhage). Of these 44 patients, angiography showed arteriovenous malformations in 23 and aneurysms in 9. Angiography was not performed for clinical reasons in six patients and no abnormality was seen in six patients. Four of the six patients without a cause were under age 35 and had lobar hemorrhages.

Fifty-eight patients were thought not to have an underlying structural lesion on the basis of the CT scan and were assigned to delayed cerebral angiography 3 months after their hemorrhage. Of these, 42 underwent delayed angiography. Angiography showed an arteriovenous malformation in 8 and an aneurysm in 2 patients. No abnormality was found at delayed angiography in 32. Only 11% of elderly hypertensive patients had a structural abnormality, whereas 83% of young normotensive patients had a documented structural abnormality. Of those patients with a basal ganglia hemorrhage, 31% had eventual documentation of a structural vascular abnormality by angiography.

Standard MRI and MR angiography have emerged as useful tools for the detection of structural abnormalities such as malformations and aneurysms (48). Although MRI can miss small aneurysms and vascular malformations, it is superior to CT and angiography in the detection of cavernous malformations as well as in the identification of remote hemorrhage. MRI can provide detailed information concerning the time course of brain hemorrhage (Fig. 9).

Revowden and colleagues recently reported a series of 11 patients with a parenchymal hemorrhage who had a normal cerebral angiogram (49). Four of the patients had an abnormality that was demonstrated only by MRI: a cavernous angioma in the right hippocampus, multiple cavernous angiomas, and a posterior frontal and temporal lobe hemorrhage, as well as a small cystic tumor in association with a posterior fossa midline hematoma and a small thalamic arteriovenous malformation.

Based on the above studies, we recommend that angiography be considered in patients without a clear cause of hemorrhage who are operative candidates; particularly young, normotensive patients who are clinically stable. MR imaging and MR angiography are helpful tests and may obviate the need for cerebral angiography in selected patients. They should also be considered in normotensive patients who are surgical candidates and have lobar hemorrhages and normal angiography. Older hypertensive patients who have hemorrhages in the basal ganglia, cerebellum, or brainstem and without findings on CT that suggest a structural lesion do not require angiography. However, most of these older patients with deep hemorrhages die or have severe morbidity related to their hemorrhage and are not angiographic candidates.

Timing of cerebral angiography depends on the clinical state of the patient and the judgment of the neurosurgeon as to the urgency of surgery, if needed. For example, a young patient with a large lobar hematoma who is herniating acutely is not a candidate for preoperative angiography. In contrast, a stable older patient who has a smaller temporal lobe hematoma, mild focal deficits, and a CT scan suggestive of an arteriovenous malformation should undergo angiography prior to removal of the hemorrhage.

NEW INSIGHTS INTO PATHOPHYSIOLOGY

Bleeding in patients with intracerebral hemorrhage had been thought to be completed within minutes of onset. How-

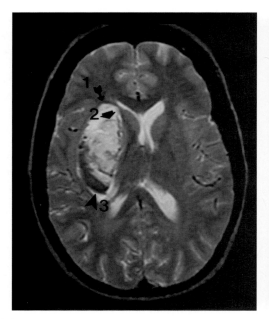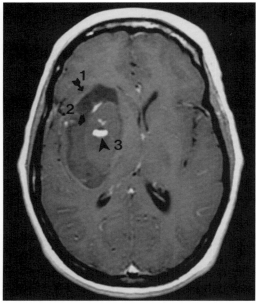

FIG. 9. Magnetic resonance image obtained 6 hours after onset of symptoms in a 24-year-old woman with acute intracerebral hemorrhage. The left (T2-weighted image) and right (T1-weighted, gadolinium contrast) images demonstrates the heterogeneity of the hemorrhage acutely. Area 1 on both images corresponds to the low-density region surrounding the hemorrhage that is often seen on CT images within the first several hours (53). We think that this region represents serum proteins and fluids from blood clot retraction rather than edema due to breakdown in the blood–brain barrier (54,55). Area 2 on both images corresponds to oxyhemoglobin in hyperacute hemorrhage (isodense on T1-weighted images and hyperintense on T2-weighted images). Area 3 on the left image corresponds to a rim where oxyhemoglobin is changing to deoxyhemoglobin (isointense on T1-weighted images and hypointense on T2-weighted images). Area 3 on the right image corresponds to leakage of gadolinium contrast secondary to ongoing bleeding during the time the scan was performed.

ever, several groups have now demonstrated that ongoing bleeding commonly occurs within the first several hours (Fig. 10) (50–52). A prospective study of 103 patients with intracerebral hemorrhage in Greater Cincinnati recently reported that 26% of patients had growth in the volume of hemorrhage of more than a third between the baseline and 1-hour CT. An additional 10% had growth between a 1-hour and 20-hour CT (53). This growth in the volume of hemorrhage was associated with neurologic deterioration. Hemorrhages in the thalamus and basal ganglia were slightly more likely to grow than lobar hemorrhages, although the difference was not significant.

This prospective Greater Cincinnati study also demonstrated that the low-density region surrounding the parenchymal hemorrhage evolves significantly during the first several hours. In fact, 41% of all hemorrhages had a low-density region surrounding the hemorrhage on the baseline CT scan (mean time from onset of less than 2 hours) (54). This low-density region grew by more than a third in 41% of patients between the baseline and 1-hour CT scan, but this growth was not associated with neurologic deterioration.

In a pig model of intracerebral hemorrhage, Wagner and colleagues have demonstrated an abnormal region in the white matter surrounding the brain hemorrhage that corresponds to the low-density region on CT imaging performed

within 1–2 hours after onset (55). This region is due to extravasation of serum from the hemorrhage itself as the blood clot forms and retracts. It is not due to leakage of edema fluid from blood vessels surrounding the hemorrhage. Leakage of edema fluid from surrounding vessels, which has been reported by several experimental investigators, probably does not begin until several hours after onset of hemorrhage (56–58).

PREVENTION

Treatment of mild to moderate hypertension significantly decreases the risk of stroke in both middle-aged and elderly individuals by 36–48% (59–61). Unfortunately, few data concerning the stroke subtype of intracerebral hemorrhage have been reported for these intervention trials. Only the Systolic Hypertension in the Elderly Program Study (SHEP) has reported that treatment of isolated systolic hypertension in the elderly decreases the risk of intracerebral hemorrhage by 50% (62). Despite the lack of conclusive evidence, these intervention studies indicate that treatment of hypertension is probably the most effective means of preventing intracerebral hemorrhage.

A recent report from the Framingham Study indicates that

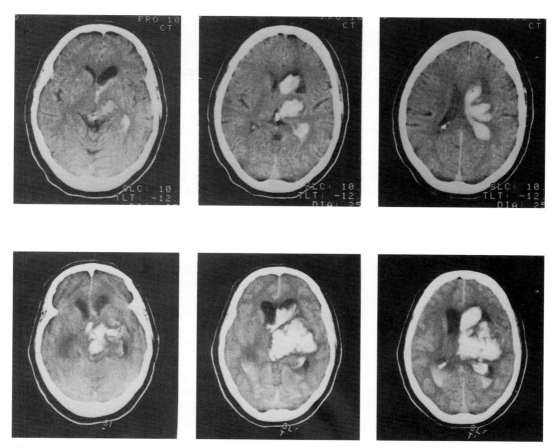

FIG. 10. Serial CT scans in 56-year-old hypertensive black women. An increase in volume of hemorrhage from 8 to 35 cm³ was recorded between the first CT scans *(upper)*, obtained 50 minutes after onset of symptoms, and the second CT scans *(lower)* obtained 210 minutes after onset. (From ref. 50.)

increased daily consumption of fruit and vegetables may decrease the risk of stroke, including hemorrhagic stroke (63). Smoking cessation, while important in the prevention of many diseases, including ischemic stroke and subarachnoid hemorrhage, has not been shown to lower the risk of intracerebral hemorrhage in an interventional or observational cohort study. Because heavy alcohol use is a possible risk factor for intracerebral hemorrhage, control of alcohol intake is a reasonable but unproven recommendation. Finally, one means of preventing iatrogenic intracerebral hemorrhage is the close monitoring of prothrombin times in patients who are treated with warfarin.

Treatment of Acute Intracerebral Hemorrhage

A balanced treatment approach to intracerebral hemorrhage requires an examination of published treatment studies. Randomized studies, if properly performed, provide the best data on which to base clinical decisions. Unfortunately, only eight small studies have been reported. Most of the published reports, many of which are in the Japanese literature, deal with large and small nonrandomized case series

of surgically and medically treated patients. Technical innovations to remove blood clots are evolving but have not been tested in the setting of a randomized trial.

One of the key surgical issues is timing of the operation. Freshly clotted blood is very difficult to remove via standard aspiration techniques during the first hours after onset. Craniotomy removes blood more effectively but is associated with more brain injury from the surgery itself. However, regardless of the type of surgery chosen, most of the damage to the brain and patient due to intracerebral hemorrhage occurs during the first several hours following onset. Ultra-early surgical evacuation of intracerebral hemorrhage has yet to be tested in a randomized trial.

Randomized Medical Studies

There have been four randomized trials of medical therapy for intracerebral hemorrhage (5–8). The first study by Tellez and Bauer compared dexamethasone with placebo in 40 patients in the pre-CT era (6). Because of the lack of CT scanning, the location and clear identification of intracerebral hemorrhage was questionable except for those patients who died. Eleven of the 40 patients were shown to have a hemorrhagic infarction. No benefit was demonstrated for dexamethasone although the difficulties with case identification and the extremely small numbers make this a problematic study.

The second study by Poungvarin and colleagues compared a 9-day course of daily dexamethasone to placebo in a randomized double-blind study (5). Intracerebral hemorrhage was documented by CT. Mortality in the dexamethasone group at 21 days (22 of 46 patients, or 48%) was not significantly different from mortality in the placebo group (21 of 47 patients, or 45%). However, there were 20 complications in the dexamethasone group (13 infections, 2 upper gastrointestinal bleeds, and 5 difficult-to-control hyperglycemia episodes) compared to only 6 complications in the placebo group ($p < 0.001$).

Yu and colleagues compared a 6-day course of glycerol therapy to placebo in a randomized, double-blind trial (8). Treatment consisted of 500 ml of 10% glycerol over 4 hours for 6 days vs. 500 cm^3 of physiologic saline administered in identical fashion (placebo group). Six-month mortality in the glycerol group (37 of 107 patients, or 35%) was not significantly different from the mortality in the placebo group (33 of 109, or 30%). Neurologic outcome as measured by the Scandinavian Stroke Scale and Barthel Index were similar for the two treatment groups. Hemolysis (generally subclinical) was the only adverse effect of glycerol.

Finally, the Italian Acute Stroke Study Group compared hemodilution therapy to best standard medical therapy in a randomized, nonblinded study of patients with acute hemispheric stroke, including 164 patients with intracerebral hemorrhage (7). The hemodilution procedure consisted of blood removal by venesection (350 cm^3) and subsequent dextran (350 cm^3) administration. This procedure was repeated to lower the hematocrit below 35. No patient received more than three hemodilutions. All patients were treated within 12 hours of symptom onset. The proportion of hemodilution patients who were dead or dependent at 6 months (57 of 83, or 69%) was not significantly different from the proportion of placebo patients (52 of 81, or 64%).

Randomized Surgical Studies

McKissock reported the first randomized, nonblinded study of surgical removal of hemorrhage for 180 patients with intracerebral hemorrhage in the pre-CT era (1) (Table 2). Cases were included if the clinical history, physical signs, and angiography supported the diagnosis of intracerebral hemorrhage. Hemorrhages thought to be located in the posterior fossa were excluded. Of 303 potentially eligible cases, 123 were excluded because of death, rapid recovery, structural cause of the hemorrhage, or refusal on the part of the primary physician. Of the 180 randomized cases, 9 patients did not have a hemorrhage or had a posterior fossa hematoma. Most patients underwent operation within 48 hours. The proportion of surgical patients who were dead or totally disabled (71 of 89 cases, or 80%) was higher than the proportion of patients treated medically (60 of 91 cases, or 66%).

Juvela and colleagues reported the second randomized study of surgery vs. best medical therapy for 52 patients with spontaneous supratentorial intracerebral hemorrhage (2). Removal of hemorrhage was accomplished by craniotomy within a mean time of 14.5 hours after onset of the bleed (range 6–48 hours). The proportion of operated patients who were dead or dependent at 6 months (25 of 26, or 96%) was not significantly different from the proportion of patients treated medically (21 of 26, or 81%). Surgically treated patients were significantly more likely to have a worse admission Glasgow Coma Scale score, a larger deep hemorrhage, and intraventricular hemorrhage than medically treated patients.

Batjer and colleagues conducted a randomized trial of three treatment strategies: best medical management, best medical management plus intracranial pressure monitoring, and surgical evacuation (3). Only patients with a significant deficit secondary to a putaminal hematoma at least 3 cm in diameter were eligible. All patients were randomized to treatment group within 24 hours of onset. The proportion of surgical patients who were dead or vegetative at 6 months (4 of 8, or 50%) was not significantly different from the proportion of patients in the monitoring group (4 of 4, or

TABLE 2. *Randomized surgical trials of supratentorial hemorrhage*

Trial	Treatment groups	No. of patients per treatment group	Dead or disabled at 6 months (%)	Distinguishing features of study
McKissock	Craniotomy	89	88	Pre-CT
	Best medical Rx	91	89	
Juvela	Craniotomy	26	96	Mean time to treatment = 14.5 hours, earliest at 6 hours
	Best medical Rx	26	81	
Batjer	Craniotomy	8	75	Randomized only putaminal hemorrhages ≥3 cm in diameter
	Intra. Press. Mon.[a]	4	100	
	Best medical Rx	9	78	
Auer	Endoscopic removal	50	74[b]	Positive benefits limited to patients with lobar hemorrhages
	Best medical Rx	50	90[b]	

[a] Intra. Press. Mon = intracranial pressure monitor
[b] Significant difference at $p < 0.05$ level, percentages estimated from figure 2 in referenced manuscript.

100%) or medical group (7 of 9, or 78%). None of the 21 patients in the study were capable of returning to prestroke activity at 6 months and only 4 were independent at home. The study was prematurely stopped because of poor recruitment and poor outcome in all three patient groups.

Auer and colleagues conducted the only randomized trial of endoscopic aspiration of hemorrhage as compared to best medical treatment (4). Patients had to be between ages 30 and 80, have a hemorrhage greater than 10 cm^3 in volume, receive angiography and treatment within 48 hours of onset, and have no identifiable vascular cause of the hemorrhage. One hundred patients met criteria for study entry, and the 50 patients randomized to surgery had evacuation of the hemorrhage through a burr hole by means of a neuroendoscope. At 6 months, the mortality rate in the surgical group (42%) was significantly lower than that in the medical group (70%, $p < 0.01$). In patients with large hematomas (over 50 cm^3), the quality of survival was not influenced by surgery, whereas the mortality rate was significantly lower. By contrast, in patients with smaller hematomas (<50 cm^3), the quality of survival was improved in the surgical group, whereas the mortality rate was equal between the two groups.

Nonrandomized Surgical Studies: Conventional

Numerous nonrandomized series comparing craniotomy and best medical treatment of intracerebral hemorrhage have been reported (9,64–78). The most consistent finding of these series is the variability in treatment (Table 3) (9). However, a recent population-based study in Greater Cincinnati during 1988 illustrates themes common to many treatment studies. Of the 188 cases of intracerebral hemorrhage in the Greater Cincinnati population during 1988, 26 had a craniotomy to removal an intracerebral hemorrhage and 8 had re-

moval of an arteriovenous malformation in addition to removal of the intracerebral hemorrhage. In 15 patients the operation was performed within 12 hours of onset (9). In comparison to medically treated patients, operated patients were more likely to have a lobar hemorrhage (64% vs. 43%) or a cerebellar hemorrhage (29% vs. 7%). Admission Glasgow Coma Scale scores were similar for operated and medically treated patients but operated patients were significantly younger and had larger parenchymal hemorrhages (Table 4). Operated patients had a borderline lower 30-day mortality (25%) than nonoperated patients (46%) but the overall morbidity and mortality was essentially the same for the two groups. This community experience reflects the opinion of many neurosurgeons that larger cerebellar and lobar hemorrhages should be removed, particularly in younger and otherwise medically healthy patients who are deteriorating clinically. However, it should be noted that this neurosurgical practice is not supported by data from randomized controlled studies.

Even consensus regarding management of younger patients with lobar hemorrhages is lacking (10,76). Masdeu and Rubino surveyed 88 board-certified neurologists and 114 board-certified neurosurgeons about whether they would operate on a 61-year-old man and a 51-year-old man, each with a parietal hemorrhage and no contraindications to surgery (10). Among the neurologists, 24% would have referred both patients for operation, 24% would have referred one of the two, and 52% would have referred neither. Among the neurosurgeons, 47% would have operated on both patients, 25% on one of them, and 28% on neither. Surgical removal of cerebellar hemorrhages has been advocated for patients with cerebellar hemorrhages that are larger than 3 cm in diameter, particularly those that obliterate the brainstem cisterns, cause fourth ventricular compression and obstruction, or are accompanied by neurologic deterioration

TABLE 3. *Operative management of intracerebral hemorrhage during the computed tomographic era*

Location	Time of study	Type of study	Study population	Operative removal (%)
Italy	1982–1983	One center	104 intracerebral hemorrhages	9
Sweden	1982–1986	One center	80 lobar hemorrhages	24
			70 putaminal hemorrhages	9
			32 thalamic hemorrhages	0
			14 cerebellar hemorrhages	0
Germany	1984–1988	One center	146 intracerebral hemorrhages	25
Japan	1981–1989	339 neurosurgical institutes	7010 putaminal hemorrhages	48
Finland	1985–1989	One center	68 basal ganglia or thalamic hemorrhages	0
			53 lobar hemorrhages	15
			17 cerebellar hemorrhages	6
Greater Cincinnati	1988	Population-based 20 hospitals	83 deep hemorrhages	13
			74 lobar hemorrhages	24
			14 cerebellar hemorrhages	29

From ref. 9.
[a] One patient had a ventricular drain.
[b] Three patients had a ventricular drain.

TABLE 4. *Comparisons of patients undergoing surgery with deep or lobar hemorrhage (n = 29) and those patients not undergoing operation (n = 128)*

	Operation	No operation	p value
Mean time from onset to first medical evaluation	5 ± 14 hours	3 ± 5 hours	0.54
Age	58 ± 17 years	72 ± 15 years	0.0001
Initial Glasgow Coma Scale score	11 ± 3	11 ± 3	0.43
Volume of ICH*	50 ± 31 cm³	37 ± 38 cm³	0.10
Volume of IVH**	10 ± 17 cm³	14 ± 26 cm³	0.32
Lobar location	64%	43%	0.05
30-day mortality	25%	46%	0.06
Modified Oxford Handicap Scale score	4.7 ± 1.2	4.6 ± 1.7	0.77

From ref. 9.
[a] Intracerebral hemorrhage.
[b] Intraventricular hemorrhage.

(73–81). A smaller cerebellar hemorrhage in an alert patient without ventricular or brainstem compression will generally have a good outcome with medical management alone.

Treatment of putaminal hemorrhages is particularly controversial (64–72). The largest reported series is a nonrandomized multicenter study from Kanaya and colleagues in Japan that evaluated conservative and surgical treatment of putaminal hemorrhages during the 1980s (69). Of the 7010 patients studied, 3635 received medical treatment alone and 3375 underwent surgery. The majority of patients who were alert or confused were treated medically and included 56% of all medically treated patients. However, 25% of all surgically treated patients also fell into this category. Mortality in alert and confused patients was significantly lower in medically treated patients as compared to those patients treated surgically. However, the mortality in patients who were stuporous or worse was significantly lower in the surgically treated patients. Mortality in patients with hemorrhages less than 10 cm³ was significantly lower in medically treated patients whereas mortality in patients with hemorrhages greater than 30 cm³ was lower in surgically treated patients. Good neurologic outcome in survivors was more common in medically treated patients with good neurologic grades and smaller hemorrhages whereas no difference in morbidity was seen in poorer grade patients with larger hemorrhages.

Based on the results, Kanaya and colleagues recommend surgery for patients with putaminal hemorrhages larger than 30 cm³, particularly if the patient is somnolent or worse. Patients with smaller hemorrhages who are alert are treated medically as are those who are in deep coma (eg, Glasgow of 3 or 4). Their recommendations are similar to those for their earlier multicenter study of 410 patients with putaminal hemorrhage in the 1970s (80).

Craniotomy for surgical removal of brainstem and thalamic hemorrhages has been abandoned by most physicians because of extremely poor outcomes. However, newer approaches have rekindled a surgical approach to some of these patients (see below). In short, the indications for removal of parenchymal hemorrhage due to structural vascular lesions are similar to those for spontaneous parenchymal hemorrhages. However, the decision to remove the hemorrhage and the timing of the operation is tempered by the risks associated with the size and location of the arteriovenous malformation or aneurysm as well as the clinical state of the patient.

In summary, even though some of the reported treatment series are large, the medical and surgical groups in all of these nonrandomized studies contain significant selection biases. The conclusions and recommendations of the authors may or may not be correct.

Nonrandomized Studies: Medical Treatments

Medical treatment for intracerebral hemorrhage centers around blood pressure control, management of increased intracranial pressure, and airway management. Of the 188 patients with intracerebral hemorrhage in Greater Cincinnati during 1988, 38% of patients were treated with mannitol for increased intracranial pressure, 33% underwent intubation during their hospitalization, 78% received treatment for elevated blood pressure, and 13% had placement of an intraventricular catheter for management of intracranial pressure and drainage of cerebrospinal fluid (9). Thus, aggressive medical management is common. However, no randomized studies of blood pressure control or intracranial pressure monitoring have been reported.

The decision of when to monitor intracranial pressure is difficult and controversial. Often patients with an intracerebral hemorrhage who are deteriorating or who have undergone operative removal of the hemorrhage are the best candidates for monitoring since they often receive treatment to reduce intracranial pressure including hyperventilation, mannitol, diuretics, and other more aggressive measures. Monitoring of intracranial pressure enables more rational use of these therapies. Some authors, based on a small series of patients, have recommended the monitoring of intracranial pressure as a guide to whether and when to remove the hemorrhage surgically (64,82)c1.

Nonrandomized Studies: Newer Surgical Approaches

Newer approaches have consisted of two basic principles: earlier removal of hemorrhage and innovative techniques to remove the hemorrhage while limiting brain trauma from the surgical procedure itself. Kaneko and colleagues reported the operative removal of 100 putaminal hemorrhages within 7 hours of symptom onset and 60 hemorrhages within 3 hours of onset (83,84). Patients had a baseline Glasgow of 6–13 with obvious hemiplegia. Of the 100 patients, 68 had a Glasgow score of 10–12 and 10 had a Glasgow score of 13. Most of the patients "had a hematoma volume of more than 20 to 30 cc, with a midline shift of more than 5 mm." The operative technique was craniotomy via a trans-Sylvian or transtemporal approach, depending on the size and location of the hemorrhage. Patients with mild symptoms or with Glasgow Coma Scale scores of 5 or below were treated conservatively. At 6 months, 7 (7%) of the patients had died, 15 (15%) had full recovery, and 35 (35%) were independent at home.

Craniotomy has been the standard approach for removal of intracerebral hemorrhage. Its major advantage is adequate exposure to remove the hemorrhage. More complete clot removal may decrease elevated intracranial pressure and local pressure effects of the blood clot on the surrounding brain. The major disadvantage of a more extensive surgical approach is that it may lead to further brain damage, particularly in patients with deep-seated hemorrhages. In addition, the effectiveness of clot removal using craniotomy is far from ideal. In a prospective serial CT study of intracerebral hemorrhage in Greater Cincinnati, 13 patients were evaluated within 3 hours of onset and underwent craniotomy for surgical removal of the hemorrhage soon thereafter. The

postoperative CT scan at 24 hours from symptom onset showed that the volume of hemorrhage had decreased from a mean of 73 cm^3 to a mean of 38 cm^3 (unpublished data). It is not clear as to whether this residual blood, almost equal to the volume of a golf ball, is due to incomplete removal of hemorrhage, rebleeding, or both.

Technical advances in hemorrhage removal have included improved localization of the hemorrhage by stereotactic devices or intraoperative ultrasound and improved techniques to remove the hemorrhage.

Simple aspiration of intracerebral hemorrhage through a burr hole is relatively noninvasive and associated with lower morbidity than craniotomy. However, early studies reported poor localization of the hematoma and inadequate removal of the hematoma (70).

In 1978, Backlund and Holst reported a new surgical method for aspiration of hematoma using a CT-guided stereotactic technique as well as a specially developed cannula (85). Many kinds of CT-guided stereotactic equipment have been reported subsequently. Innovations in devices to break up and remove the blood clot include modifications of an Archimedes screw inside a cannula (85), a specially designed ultrasonic aspirator (70), a specially designed endoscope (4), a modified nucleotome (86,87), a double-track aspiration (88), intraoperative CT monitoring (89), and repeated instillation of thrombolytics into the bed of a partially aspirated hematoma (Fig. 11). Intraoperative ultrasound has also been used to identify the hemorrhage and monitor removal of the hemorrhage in real time (69). These innovative stereotactic aspiration techniques have been applied to hemorrhages in all brain locations.

Kanno reported that the rebleeding after surgery was seen in 10% of patients who underwent craniotomy, 5% who un-

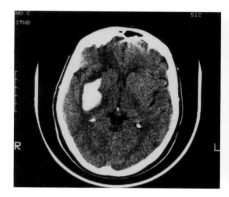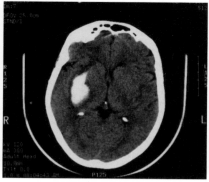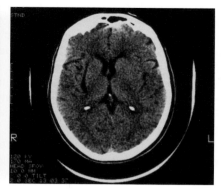

FIG. 11. This 66-year-old woman is a participant in an ongoing pilot randomized study of surgery for intracerebral hemorrhage. The baseline CT *(left)* shows a 19-cm^3 putaminal hemorrhage. She underwent stereotactic aspirations at 7 hours from symptoms onset. Urokinase (6000 units) was instilled after initial aspiration and contents were then aspirated again. The catheter was left in place and the procedure was repeated every 12 hours until the hematoma was removed. The catheter was removed on day 3. The patient's 24-hour CT scan *(middle)* shows a slight decrease in hemorrhage volume (16 cm^3) but her NIH stroke scale score (114) improved from 19 at baseline to 8 at 24 hours (on this scale, 0 is normal and increasing scores indicate neurologic deterioration). Her NIH stroke scale at 3 months was 1 and her Barthel Index score was 100 (normal). A small slit remains at the site of her hemorrhage on the 3-month CT.

derwent CT aspiration, and 6% after ultrasound-guided aspiration (69). On average, CT-guided aspiration removed 71% of the original hematoma whereas ultrasound-guided aspiration removed 81%. The percentage of hemorrhage removed did not vary significantly with the timing of the operation.

Other investigators using various CT-guided aspiration techniques, including thrombolytic instillation, have reported aspiration rates ranging on average from 30% to 90% over the first several days (4,69,70,78,79,85–108). The rebleeding rate in aspiration studies without thrombolytics ranged from 0% to 16% with a mean of 5% among 896 cases (4,69,86,87,91–92,94–95). The rebleeding rate in aspiration studies with installation of thrombolytics ranged from 0% to 10% with a mean of 4% among 392 cases (78,79,87,93,97–108). The most commonly used thrombolytic protocol has been urokinase administered daily or twice daily in a dose of 6000 units via a catheter into the bed of the hematoma with subsequent drainage and aspiration. This procedure is often repeated for several days until the majority of the hematoma has been aspirated. Tissue plasminogen activator has also been used. This agent was instilled via catheter at a dose of 1 mg per cm of maximum hemorrhage diameter on the baseline CT scan (107). The total dose ranged from 5 to 16 mg.

Some investigators have reported that aspiration with thrombolytic agents is less successful in removing clotted blood during the first hours after hemorrhage onset as compared with removal of hemorrhage that has been present for several days (87). Installation of thrombolytics has also been used successfully for hemorrhage within the ventricular system (109–110).

MANAGEMENT GUIDELINES

The lack of a proven medical or surgical treatment for intracerebral hemorrhage has led to great variability among physicians concerning both surgical and medical treatment. Proposed guidelines without definitive studies are uncertain at best and, at worst, can be dead wrong. However, guidelines can provide a rational present treatment plan while outlining questions that require future study. Well-designed and well-executed randomized treatment studies of intracerebral hemorrhage are urgently needed.

Management of blood pressure and intracranial pressure serves two goals: prevention of ongoing bleeding or rebleeding, and maintenance of adequate cerebral perfusion pressure. Control of elevated blood pressure has never been shown to decrease the risk of ongoing or recurrent bleeding. Nevertheless, we recommend treatment of moderate and severe elevations of blood pressure (systolic blood pressure greater than 180 mm Hg or mean arterial blood pressure of >130 mm Hg). The goal of treatment should be to lower blood pressure to a mean pressure of 100–130 mm Hg or in the low hypertensive range (eg, systolic of 140–160 mg Hg). Lower blood pressures may be poorly tolerated because

the cerebral perfusion pressure (CPP) is dependent on the intracranial pressure (ICP) as well as the arterial blood pressure (ABP) (CPP = ABP − ICP). High levels of intracranial pressure require higher blood pressures to maintain a stable cerebral perfusion pressure. If an intracranial pressure monitor is in place, the goal of treatment should be to maintain the cerebral perfusion pressure at 70–100 mm Hg.

The antihypertensive medication should be an agent that is quick in onset and whose effect is easily titratable. Intravenous labetolol is an excellent choice for moderate levels of elevated blood pressure because it is quick, titratable, and has no known adverse effect on either intracranial pressure or autoregulation of local cerebral blood flow (111). Intravenous enalapril is also an excellent choice because it has no known effect on intracranial pressure or autoregulation (112). For more severe elevations (eg, diastolic pressures >130 mm Hg) we use nitroprusside. Theoretically, nitroprusside can increase intracranial pressure because it is a cerebral arterial vasodilator. However, this potential negative has not been demonstrated in clinical use. Nitroprusside has the advantage of being the easiest medication to titrate. Calcium channel blockers, such as sublingual nifedipine, are less predictable and slower in onset and can vasodilate cerebral arteries. They should be used only as second-line medication when the other medications cannot be used. Doses of medication are given in Table 5.

Treatment of suspected increased intracranial pressure should be initiated in patients who have neurologic deterioration even prior to placement of intracranial monitor. Hyperventilation is the fastest available treatment and should be performed until the Pco_2 is between 25 and 30 mm Hg. Mannitol can be administered at a dosage of 12.5 g IV every 5 minutes up to four doses per hour. Its effect should be monitored by serum osmolality every 6 hours. Use of steroids is discouraged. If a patient deteriorates neurologically and is considered potentially salvageable or requires treatment for increased intracranial pressure, an ICP monitor should be used. Preferred monitoring devices include a fiberoptic device inserted into the ipsilateral parenchyma or an intraventricular monitor. Other medical management in-

TABLE 5. *Protocol for antihypertensive agents*

Labetolol	Begin with 10 or 20 mg IVP. If no response, may double dose every 10 minutes up to a maximum total dose of 300 mg.
Enalapril	1.25 mg IVP over 5 minutes. May repeat at q 6 hours. May consider starting with 0.625 mg over 5 minutes in the elderly or hypovolemic patients.
Nitroprusside	Begin with 0.2–0.5 μg/kg min IV. Titrate up or down every 5–10 minutes in similar increments.
Nifedipine	10 mg sublingually. Wait at least 45 minutes to determine whether first dose is effective.

TABLE 6. *Recommendations for surgical treatment of intracerebral hemorrhage*

Not Surgical Candidates
1. Patients with small hemorrhages (<10 cm³) or with minimal neurologic deficits (evidence from randomized clinical trials and natural history studies).
2. Patients with a Glasgow Coma Scale score of 4 or less (evidence from randomized clinical trials and natural history studies).

Surgical Candidates
1. Patients with cerebellar hemorrhage that are greater than 3 cm in diameter, who are neurologically deteriorating, or who have brainstem compression and hydrocephalus from ventricular obstruction, should have their hemorrhages removed surgically as soon as possible (no evidence from randomized trials).
2. Intracerebral hemorrhages that are associated with a structural lesion such as an aneurysm or arteriovenous malformation may be removed if the patient has a chance for a good outcome and the structural vascular lesion is surgically accessible (no evidence from randomized treatment studies).
3. Young patient with moderate- or large-sized lobar hemorrhage who is deteriorating clinically (some evidence from one randomized trial of endoscopic evacuation).

cludes supportive care and prevention and treatment of other medical complications such as deep venous thrombosis, aspiration pneumonia, and infection.

The decision regarding if and when to operate remains controversial. Table 6 lists our recommendations based on the available literature. Patients with small hemorrhages (<10 cm³) or with minimal neurologic deficits should be managed medically since they generally do well with medical treatment alone. Patients with a Glasgow Coma Scale score of 4 or less should also be managed medically because they uniformly die or have extremely poor functional outcome. Patients with cerebellar hemorrhage >3 cm who are neurologically deteriorating or have brainstem compression and hydrocephalus from ventricular obstruction should have their hemorrhages removed surgically as soon as possible. Stereotactic aspiration may be associated with better outcomes than standard craniotomy for moderate-sized cerebellar hemorrhages, but this hypothesis has yet to be tested in a randomized study. Young patients with large lobar hemorrhages who deteriorate during observation often undergo surgical removal of their hemorrhage. However, the efficacy of this approach is supported only by the small endoscopic study of Auer and colleagues (4). Intracerebral hemorrhages that are associated with a structural lesion such as an aneurysm or arteriovenous malformation may be removed if the patient has a chance for a good outcome and the structural vascular lesion is surgically accessible.

The efficacy of surgery is unproven for almost all patients with intracerebral hemorrhage. We think that ultra-early treatment will be critical for both patients with intracerebral hemorrhage just as with patients who have ischemic strokes. Innovative techniques to remove the hemorrhage quickly

and with minimal associated brain injury or rebleeding need to be pursued. Pilot randomized studies of early surgery for intracerebral hemorrhage began in 1994 both at our own institution and at the University of Houston (personal communication, Dr. James Grotta). We are hopeful that future large multicenter randomized studies will demonstrate that very early operative removal of intracerebral hemorrhage may be effective for some patients with intracerebral hemorrhage.

REFERENCES

1. McKissock W, Richardson A, Taylor J. Primary intracerebral haemorrhage. A controlled trial of surgical and conservative treatment in 180 unselected cases. *Lancet* 1961;2:221–226.
2. Juvela S, Heiskanen O, Poranen A, Valtonen S, Kuurne T, Kaste M, Troupp H. The treatment of spontaneous intracerebral hemorrhage. A prospective randomized trial of surgical and conservative treatment. *J Neurosurg* 1989;70:755–758.
3. Batjer HH, Reisch JS, Allen BC, Plaizier LJ, Su CJ. Failure of surgery to improve outcome in hypertensive putaminal hemorrhage. A prospective randomized trial. *Arch Neurol* 1990;47:1103–1106.
4. Auer LM, Deinsberger W, Niederkorn K, et al. Endoscopic surgery versus medical treatment for spontaneous intracerebral hematoma: a randomized study. *J Neurosurg* 1989;70:530–535.
5. Poungvarin N, Bhoopat W, Viriyavejakul A, Rodprasert P, et al. Effects of dexamethasone in primary supratentorial intracerebral hemorrhage. *N Engl J Med* 1987;316:1229–1233.
6. Tellez H, Bauer RB. Dexamethasone as treatment in cerebrovascular disease. 1. A controlled study in intracerebral hemorrhage. *Stroke* 1973;4:541–546.
7. Italian Acute Stroke Study Group. Haemodilution in acute stroke: results of the Italian haemodilution trial. *Lancet* 1988;1:318–320.
8. Yu YL, Kumana CR, Lauder IJ, et al. Treatment of acute cerebral hemorrhage with intravenous glycerol. A double-blind, placebo-controlled, randomized trial. *Stroke* 1992;23:967–971.
9. Broderick J, Brott T, Tomsick T, Tew J, Duldner J, Huster G. Management of intracerebral hemorrhage in a large metropolitan population. *Neurosurgery* 1994;34:882–887.
10. Masdeu JC, Rubino FA. Management of lobar intracerebral hemorrhage: medical or surgical. *Neurology* 1984;34:381–383.
11. Broderick J. Intracerebral hemorrhage. In: Gorelick PB, Alter M, eds. *Handbook of Neuroepidemiology.* New York: Marcel Dekker, 1994; 141–167.
12. Broderick J, Brott T, Tomsick T, Miller R, Huster G. Intracerebral hemorrhage more than twice as common as subarachnoid hemorrhage. *J Neurosurg* 1993;78:188–191.
13. Broderick J, Brott T, Tomsick T, Huster G, Miller R. The risk of subarachnoid and intracerebral hemorrhages in blacks as compared to whites. *N Engl J Med* 1992;326:733–736.
14. Anderson CS, Chakera TMH, Stewart-Wynne EG, Jamrozik KD. Spectrum of primary intracerebral haemorrhage in Perth, Western Australia, 1989–90: incidence and outcome. *J Neurol Neurosurg Psychiatry* 1994;57:936–940.
15. Counsell C, Boonyakarnkul S, Dennis M, et al. Primary intracerebral haemorrhage in the Oxfordshire community stroke project. 2. Prognosis. *Cerebrovasc Dis* 1995;5:26–34.
16. Broderick JP, Brott TG, Duldner JE, Tomsick T, Huster G. Volume of intracerebral hemorrhage. A powerful and easy-to-use predictor of 30-day mortality. *Stroke* 1993;24:987–993.
17. Franke CL, van Swieten JC, Algra A, van Gijn J. Prognostic factors in patients with intracerebral haematoma. *J Neurol Neurosurg Psychiatry* 1992;55:653–657.
18. Kothari RU, Brott TG, Broderick JP, Barsan WG. The abc's of measuring intracerebral hemorrhage volumes. Presented at the 1994 Annual Meeting of SAEM, Washington, DC, 1994.
19. Cole FM, Tates PO. The occurrence and significance of intracerebral microaneurysms. *J Pathol Bacteriol* 1967;93:393–411.
20. Fisher CM. Pathological observations in hypertensive cerebral hemorrhage. *J Neuropathol Exp Neurol* 1971;30:536–550.

21. Ross Russell RW. Observations on intracerebral aneurysms. *Brain* 1963;86:425–442.

22. Takebayashi S. Ultrastructural morphometry of hypertensive medial damage in lenticulostriate and other arteries. *Stroke* 1985;16:449–452.

23. Challa VR, Moody DM, Bell MA. The Charcot–Bouchard aneurysm controversy: impact of a new histologic technique. *J Neuropathol Exp Neurol* 1992;51:264–271.

24. Wakai S, Kumakura N, Nagai M. Lobar intracerebral hemorrhage: a clinical, radiographic, and pathological study of 29 consecutive operated cases with negative angiography. *J Neurosurg* 1992:76:231–238.

25. Broderick J, Brott T, Tomsick T, Leach A. Lobar hemorrhage in the elderly. The undiminishing importance of hypertension. *Stroke* 1993; 24:49–51.

26. Rowe JW, Lipsitz LA. Altered blood pressure. In: Rowe JW, Besdine RW, eds. *Geriatric Medicine*, 2nd ed. Boston: Little, Brown, 1988; 193–207.

27. Okazaki H, Whisnant JP. Clinical pathology of hypertensive intracerebral hemorrhage. In: Mizukami M, Kogure K, Kanaya H, Yamori Y, eds. *Hypertensive Intercerebral Hemorrhage*. New York: Raven Press, 1983:177–180.

28. Vinters HV. Cerebral amyloid angiopathy: a critical review. *Stroke* 1987;18:311–324.

29. Vonsattel JPG, Myers RH, Hedley-Whyte ET, Ropper AH, Bird ED, Richardson EP. Cerebral amyloid angiopathy without and with cerebral hemorrhages: a comparative historical study. *Ann Neurol* 1991; 30:637–649.

30. Mandybur TI, Bates SRD. Fatal massive intracerebral hemorrhage complicating cerebral amyloid angiopathy. *Arch Neurol* 1978;35: 246–248.

31. Maruyama K, Ikeda S, Ishihara T, Allsop D, Yanagisawa N. Immunohistochemical characterization of cerebrovascular amyloid in 46 autopsied cases using antibodies to protein and cystatin C. *Stroke* 1990; 21:397–403.

32. Vinters HV, Gilbert JJ. Cerebral amyloid angiopathy: incidence and complications in the aging brain. II. The distribution of amyloid vascular changes. *Stroke* 1983;14:924–928.

33. Tomonaga M. Cerebral amyloid angiopathy in the elderly. *J Am Geriat Soc* 1981;29:151–157.

34. Masuda J, Tanaka K, Ueda K, Omae T. Autopsy study of incidence and distribution of cerebral amyloid angiopathy in Hisayama, Japan. *Stroke* 1988;19:205–210.

35. Itoh Y, Yamada M, Hayakawa M, Otomo E, Miyatake T. Cerebral amyloid angiopathy: a significant cause of cerebellar as well as lobar cerebral hemorrhage in the elderly. *J Neurol Sci* 1993;116:135–141.

36. Ishihara T, Takahashi M, Yokota T, et al. The significance of cerebrovascular amyloid in the aetiology of superficial (lobar) cerebral haemorrhage and its incidence in the elderly population. *J Pathol* 1991; 165:229–234.

37. Broderick J, Talbot T, Prenger E, Leach A, Brott T. Stroke in children within a major metropolitan area: the surprising importance of intracerebral hemorrhage. *J Child Neurol* 1993;8:250–255.

38. Furlan AJ, Whisnant JP, Elveback LR. The decreasing incidence of primary intracerebral hemorrhage: a population study. *Ann Neurol* 1979;5:367–373.

39. Wintzen AR, de Jonge H, Loeliger EA, Bots GTAM. The risk of intracerebral hemorrhage during oral anticoagulant treatment: a population study. *Ann Neurol* 1984;16:553–558.

40. Hylek EM, Singer DE. Risk factors for intracranial hemorrhage in outpatients taking warfarin. *Ann Intern Med* 1994;120:987–902.

41. Hornig CR, Dorndorf W, Agnoli AL. Hemorrhagic cerebral infarction a prospective study. *Stroke* 1986;17:179–185.

42. Bogousslavsky J, Regli F, Uské A, Maeder P. Early spontaneous hematoma in cerebral infarct: is primary cerebral hemorrhage overdiagnosed? *Neurology* 1991;41:837–840.

43. Donahue RP, Abbott RD, Reed DM, Yano K. Alcohol and hemorrhagic stroke: the Honolulu Heart Program. *JAMA* 1986;255: 2311–2314.

44. Klatsky AL, Friedman GD, Siegelaub AB, Gérard MJ. Alcohol consumption and blood pressure: Kaiser-Permanente multiphasic health examination data. *N Engl J Med* 1977;296:1194–1200.

45. Haut MJ, Cowan DH. The effect of ethanol on hemostatic properties of human blood platelets. *Am J Med* 1974;56:22–23.

46. Feldmann E. Intracerebral hemorrhage. In: Fischer M, ed. *Clinical Atlas of Cerebrovascular Disorders*. London: Wolfe, 1994; 11.1–11.17.

47. Halpin SFS, Britton JA, Byrne JV, Clifton A, Hart G, Moore A. Prospective evaluation of cerebral angiography and computed tomography in cerebral haematoma. *J Neurol Neursurg Psychiatry* 1994; 57:1180–1186.

48. Dul K, Drayer BP. CT and MR imaging of intracerebral hemorrhage. In: Kase CS, Caplan LR, eds. *Intracerebral Hemorrhage*, vol 5. Boston: Butterworth-Heinemann, 1994;73–93.

49. Renowden SA, Molyneux AJ, Anslow P, Byrne JV. The value of MRI in angiogram-negative intracranial haemorrhage. *Neuroradiology* 1994;36:422–425.

50. Broderick JP, Brott TG, Tomsick T, Barsan W, Spilker J. Ultra-early evaluation of intracerebral hemorrhage. *J Neurosurg* 1990;72: 195–199.

51. Fujii Y, Tanaka R, Takeuchi S, Koike T, Minakawa T, Sasaki O. Hematoma enlargement in spontaneous intracerebral hemorrhage. *J Neurosurg* 1994;80:51–57.

52. Kelley RE, Berger JR, Scheinberg P, et al. Active bleeding in hypertensive intracerebral hemorrhage: computed tomography. *Neurology* 1982;32:852–856.

53. Brott T, Broderick J, Barsan W, Kothari R, Tomsick T, Spilker J, Khoury J. Continued bleeding during the first hours of intracerebral hemorrhage. Presented at 1994 Annual Meeting of the American Neurological Association, San Francisco, 1994.

54. Broderick J, Brott T, Kothari R. Very early edema growth with intracerebral hemorrhage. *Stroke* 1995;26(1):184.

55. Wagner K, Xi G, Hua Y, et al. White matter in experimental lobar intracerebral hemorrhage. *Stroke* 1995;26(1):178.

56. Yang G, Betz L, Chenevert T, Brunberg J, Hoff J. Experimental intracerebral hemorrhage: relationship between brain edema, blood flow, and blood brain barrier permeability in rats. *J Neurosurg* 1994;81: 93–101.

57. Mendelow A. Mechanisms of ischemic brain damage with intracerebral hemorrhage. *Stroke* 1993;24(12):I115–I117.

58. Nehls G, Major M, Mendelow D, et al. Experimental intracerebral hemorrhage: progression of hemodynamic changes after production of spontaneous mass lesion. *Neurosurgery* 1988;23:439–444.

59. Phillips SJ, Whisnant JP. Hypertension and stroke. In: Laragh JH, Brenner BM, eds. *Hypertension: pathophysiology, diagnosis, and management*, vol 1. New York: Raven Press, 1990;417–431.

60. SHEP Cooperative Research Group. Prevention of stroke by antihypertensive drug treatment in older persons with isolated systolic hypertension: final results of the Systolic Hypertension in the Elder Program (SHEP). *JAMA* 1991;265:3255–3264.

61. Dahlöf B, Lindholm LH, Hansson L, Scherstén, Ekbom T, Wester P-O. Morbidity and mortality in the Swedish trial in old patients with hypertension (stop-hypertension). *Lancet* 1991;338:1281–1285.

62. SHEP Cooperative Research Group. Prevention of various stroke types by treatment of isolated systolic hypertension. Presented at the International Stroke Society's Second World Congress of Stroke. Washington, DC, 1992.

63. Gillman MW, Cupples LA, Gagnon D, et al. Protective effect of fruits and vegetables on development of stroke in men. *JAMA* 1995;273: 1113–1117.

64. Kase CS, Crowell RM. Prognosis and treatment of patients with intracerebral hemorrhage. In: Kase CS, Caplan LR, eds. *Intracerebral Hemorrhage*. Boston: Butterworth-Heinemann, 1994;467–489.

65. Fujitsu K, Muramoto M, Ikeda Y, Inada Y, Kim I, Kuwabara T. Indications for surgical treatment of putaminal hemorrhage. *J Neurosurg* 1990;73:518–525.

66. Volpin L, Cervellini P, Colombo F, Zanusso M, Benedetti A. Spontaneous Intracerebral hematomas: a new proposal about the usefulness and limits of surgical treatment. *Neurosurgery* 1984;15:663–666.

67. Sawada T, Yamaguchi T, Kikuchi H. Comparison of medical and surgical treatments of hypertensive intracerebral hemorrhage. In: Mizukami M, Kogure K, Kanaya H, Yamori Y, eds. *Hypertensive Intracerebral Hemorrhage*. New York: Raven Press, 1983;233–238.

68. Kalff R, Feldges A, Mehdorn M, Grote W. Spontaneous intracerebral hemorrhage. *Neurosurg Rev* 1992;15:177–186.

69. Kanaya H, Kuroda K. Development in neurosurgical approaches to hypertensive intracerebral hemorrhage in Japan. In: Kaufman HH, ed. *Intracerebral Hematomas*. New York: Raven Press, 1992:197–210.

70. Donauer E, Faubert C. Management of spontaneous intracerebral and

cerebellar hemorrhage. In: Kaufman HH, ed. *Intracerebral Hematomas.* New York: Raven Press, 1992:211–227.

71. Helweg-Larsen S, Sommer W, Strange P, Lester J, Boysen G. Prognosis for patients treated conservatively for spontaneous intracerebral hematomas. *Stroke* 1984;15(6):1045–1048.

72. Zumkeller M, Höllerhage H-G, Pröschl, Dietz H. The results of surgery for intracerebral hematomas. *Neurosurg Rev* 1992;15:33–36.

73. van Loon J, Van Calenbergh F, Goffin J, Plets C. Controversies in the management of spontaneous cerebellar haemorrhage. A consecutive series of 49 cases and review of the literature. *Acta Neurochir (Wien)* 1993;122:187–193.

74. Firsching R, Huber M, Frowein RA. Cerebellar haemorrhage: management and prognosis. *Neurosurg Rev* 1991;14:191–194.

75. Da Pian R, Bazzan A, Pasqualin A. Surgical versus medical treatment of spontaneous posterior fossa haematomas: a cooperative study on 205 cases. *Neurol Res* 1984;6:145–151.

76. Luessenhop AJ. Hypertensive intracerebral hemorrhage in the United States: update on surgical treatment. In: Mizukami M, Kogure K, Kanaya H, Yamori Y, eds. *Hypertensive Intracerebral Hemorrhage.* New York: Raven Press, 1983:123–132.

77. Kase C. Cerebellar hemorrhage. In: Kase CS, Caplan LR, eds. *Intracerebral Hemorrhage.* Boston: Butterworth-Heinemann, 1994: 425–443.

78. Sypert GW, Arpin-Sypert EJ. Spontaneous posterior fossa hematomas. In: Kaufman HH, ed. *Intracerebral Hematomas.* New York: Raven Press, 1992:187–196.

79. Niizuma H, Suzuki J. Computed tomography-guided stereotactic aspiration of posterior fossa hematomas: a supine lateral retromastoid approach. *Neurosurgery* 1987;21:422–427.

80. Kanaya H, Saiki I, Ohuchi T, et al. Hypertensive intracerebral hemorrhage in Japan: update on surgical treatment. In: Mizukami M, Kanaya K, Yamori Y, eds. *Hypertensive Intracerebral Hemorrhage.* New York: Raven Press, 1983:147–163.

81. Kobayashi S, Sato A, Kageyama Y, Nakamura H, Watanabe Y, Yamaura A. Treatment of hypertensive cerebellar hemorrhage surgical or conservative management. *Neurosurgery* 1994;32:246–251.

82. Ropper AH, King RB. Intracranial pressure monitoring in comatose patients with cerebral hemorrhage. *Arch Neurol* 1984;41:725–728.

83. Kaneko M, Tanaka K, Shimada T, Sato K, Uemura K. Long-term evaluation of ultra-early operation for hypertensive intracerebral hemorrhage in 100 cases. *J Neurosurg* 1983;58:838–842.

84. Kaneko M, Koba T, Yokoyama T. Early surgical treatment for hypertensive intracerebral hemorrhage. *J Neurosurg* 1977;46:579–583.

85. Backlund EO, Holst H. Controlled subtotal evacuation of intracerebral haematomas by stereotactic technique. *Surg Neurol* 1978;9:99–101.

86. Nguyen J-P, Decq P, Brugieres P, et al. A technique for stereotactic aspiration of deep intracerebral hematomas under computed tomographic control using a new device. *Neurosurgery* 1992;31:330–335.

87. Kaufman HH. Stereotactic aspiration with fibrinolytic and mechanical assistance. In: Kaufman HH, ed. *Intracerebral Hematomas.* New York: Raven Press, 1992:181–185.

88. Niizuma H, Suzuki J. Stereotactic aspiration of putaminal hemorrhage using a double track aspiration technique. *Neurosurgery* 1988;22: 432–436.

89. Iseki H, Amano K, Kawamura H, et al. A new apparatus for CT-guided stereotactic surgery. *Appl Neurophysiol* 1985;48:50–60.

90. Tanikawa T, Amano K, Kawamura H, et al. CT-guided stereotactic surgery for evacuation of hypertensive intracerebral hematoma. *Appl Neurophysiol* 1985;48:431–439.

91. Zonghui L, Guiquan K, Xiaohan C, Zengmin T, Houzheng C, Yi Z, Shiyu L. Evacuation of hypertensive intracerebral hematoma by a stereotactic technique. *Stereotact Funct Neurosurg* 1990;54-55: 451–452.

92. Kandel EI, Peresedov VV. Stereotaxic evacuation of spontaneous intracerebral hematomas. *J Neurosurg* 1985;62:206–213.

93. Yokote H, Komai N, Nakai E, Ueno M, Hayashi S, Terashita T.

94. Tanizaki Y, Sugita K, Toriyama, Hokama M. New CT-guided stereotactic apparatus and clinical experience with intracerebral hematomas. *Appl Neurophysiol* 1985;48:11–17.

95. Hokama M, Tanizaki Y, Mastuo K, Hongo K, Kobayashi S. Indications and limitations for CT-guided stereotaxic surgery of hypertensive intracerebral haemorrhage, based on the analysis of postoperative complications and poor ability of daily living in 158 cases. *Acta Neurochir (Wien)* 1993;125:27–33.

96. Hondo H, Uno M, Sasaki K, et al. Computed tomography controlled aspiration surgery for hypertensive intracerebral hemorrhage. Experience of more than 400 cases. *Sterotact Funct Neurosurg* 1990;54: 432–437.

97. Zonghui L, Guiquan K, Xiaohan C, et al. Evacuation of hypertensive intracerebral hematoma by a stereotactic technique. *Stereotact Funct Neurosurg* 1990;54–55:451–452.

98. Shitamichi M, Nakamura J, Sasaki T, Suematsu K, Tokuda S. Computed tomography guided stereotactic aspiration of pontine hemorrhages. *Stereotact Funct Neurosurg* 1990;54–55:453–456.

99. Ito H, Muka H, Kitamura A. Stereotactic aqua stream and aspirator for removal of intracerebral hematoma. *Stereotact Funct Neurosurg* 1990;54–55:457–460.

100. Zong-hui L, Zeng-min T, Xiao-han C, et al. CT-guided stereotactic evacuation of hypertensive intracerebral hematoma. *Chinese Med J* 1991;104(5):387–391.

101. Niizuma H, Otsuki T, Johkura H, Nakazato N, Suzuki J. CT-guided stereotactic aspiration of intracerebral hematoma: result of a hematoma-lysis method using urokinase. *Appl Neurophysiol* 1985;48: 427–430.

102. Horimot C, Yamaga S, Toba T, Tsujimura M. Stereotactic evacuation of massive hypertensive intracerebral hemorrhage. *Neurol Surg* 1992; 21(6):512.

103. Matsumoto K, Hondo H. CT-guided stereotaxic evacuation of hypertensive intracerebral hematomas. *J Neurosurg* 1984;61:440–448.

104. Etou A, Mohadjer M, Braus D, Mundinger F. Stereotactic evacuation and fibrinolysis of cerebellar hematomas. *Stereotact Funct Neurosurg* 1990;54-55:445–450.

105. Niizuma H, Yonemitsu T, Jokura H, Nakasato N, Suzuki J, Yoshimoto T. Stereotactic aspiration of thalamic hematoma. Overall results of 75 aspirated and 70 nonaspirated cases. *Stereotact Funct Neurosurg* 1990;54-55:438–444.

106. Ito H, Mukai H, Higashi S, Yamashita J, Kitamura A. Removal of hypertensive intracerebral haematoma with stereotactic aqua-stream and aspirator (SAS &A). *Neurol Surg* 1989;17(10):943.

107. Schaller C, Rohde V, Meyer B, Hassler W. Stereotactic puncture and lysis of spontaneous intracerebral hemorrhage using recombinant tissue-plasminogen activator. *Neurosurgery* 1995;36:328–335.

108. Lippitz BE, Mayfrank L, Spetzger U, Warnke JP, Bertalanffy H, Gilsbach JM. Lysis of basal ganglia haematoma with recombinant tissue plasminogen activator (rtPA) after stereotactic aspiration: initial results. *Acta Neurochir (Wien)* 1994;127:157–160.

109. Findlay JM, Grace MGA, Weir KAB. Treatment of intraventricular hemorrhage with tissue plasminogen activator. *Neurosurgery* 1993; 32:941–947.

110. Mayfrank L, Lippitz B, Groth M, Bertalanffy H, Gilsbach JM. Effect of recombinant tissue plasminogen activator on clot lysis and ventricular dilatation in the treatment of severe intraventricular haemorrhage. *Acta Neurorchir (Wien)* 1993;122:32–38.

111. Brott T, Broderick JP. Intracerebral hemorrhage. *Heart Dis Stroke* 1993;2:59–63.

112. Passmore J, Loomis JH. The role of IV enalapril in lowering blood pressure. *Hosp Formul* 1993;28:173–179.

113. Branford J, Sandercock P, Warlow C, Slattery J. Interobserver agreement for the assessment of handicap in stroke patients. *Stroke* 1989; 20:828.

114. Brott T, Adams HP, Olinger CP. Measurements of acute cerebral infarction: a clinical examination scale. *Stroke* 1989;20:864–870.

Cerebrovascular Disease, edited by H. Hunt Batjer.
Lippincott-Raven Publishers, Philadelphia © 1997.

CHAPTER 51

Cerebral Hemorrhage from Amyloid Angiopathy and Moyamoya Disease

Richard Leblanc

CEREBRAL AMYLOID ANGIOPATHY

Cerebral amyloid angiopathy is the preferred term for a condition that has previously been referred to as *congophylic angiopathy,* reflecting the affinity of the angiopathic vessels for the Congo red stain, and *primary cerebrovascular amyloidosis,* to distinguish amyloid angiopathy, which exclusively affects the nervous system, from other systemic amyloidoses (1). It is considered the most common cause of spontaneous intracranial hemorrhage after arterial hypertension and cerebral aneurysms and may be the commonest cause of intraparenchymal hemorrhage in people beyond their seventh decade (2). Two familial forms, hereditary cerebral hemorrhage of the Icelandic type and of the Dutch type, and a more common sporadic form are recognized. Other diseases of deposition of cerebral amyloid, termed *cerebral amyloidoses,* include Alzheimer's disease and Down's syndrome, and cerebral amyloid is also seen in the transmissible spongiform encephalopathies such as Jakob–Creutzfeldt disease, the Gerstmann–Sträusser–Scheinker syndrome, and kuru (Table 1). Two types of amyloid are recognized in cerebral amyloid angiopathy. Cystatin C (γ trace protein) is implicated in the Icelandic form of hereditary cerebral hemorrhage and β amyloid is primarily involved in the Dutch form of hereditary cerebral hemorrhage and in sporadic cerebral amyloid angiopathy (3,4). Prion protein is the type of amyloid present in the transmissible encephalopathies but these conditions are not associated with cerebral hemorrhage (5).

FAMILIAL CEREBRAL AMYLOID ANGIOPATHY

Hereditary Cerebral Hemorrhage–Icelandic Type

Hereditary cerebral hemorrhage with angiopathy of the Icelandic type (HCHWA-I) was the first familial form of cerebral amyloid angiopathy to be described. The initial description by Gudmundsson et al. in 1972 traced 116 members of one family over three generations and identified 18 nonhypertensive individuals with fatal cerebral hemorrhage (3). It is transmitted as an autosomal dominant trait and is characterized by accumulation of cystatin C (γ trace protein) within cerebral blood vessels. It frequently produces death in the third or fourth decade from repeated intraparenchymal hemorrhages. The amyloid is derived from a precursor protein encoded on chromosome 20, and it has a substitution of leucine for glutamine at position 68 of the γ trace protein, resulting in a variant of cystatin C that is prone to deposition and accumulation within cerebral arteries (6). The concentration of cystatin C in the cerebrospinal fluid in patients with HCHWA-I is diminished as the protein is deposited within arteries and arterioles (7).

Hereditary Cerebral Hemorrhage–Dutch Type

Hereditary cerebral hemorrhage with angiopathy of the Dutch type (HCHWA-D) is also inherited in an autosomal dominant fashion. Thus, a recent study identified 24 normotensive members of the same family with recurrent intracerebral hemorrhages (4). The main amyloid deposited in this condition is the β amyloid protein, which is derived from the amyloid precursor protein encoded on chromosome 21 (8). The β amyloid protein accumulates within cerebral arteries and arterioles as a result of the substitution of the single amino acid glutamine for glutamic acid at position 22 of the protein (9). As in the Icelandic form, patients with HCHWA-D die from repeated cerebral hemorrhages, but at a slightly older age, in their fifth decade on average, than patients with the Icelandic form. They are younger, however, than patients with sporadic cerebral amyloid angiopathy. In the severest cases of HCHWA-D weak immunoreactivity to cystatin C can also be present (10–12).

R. Leblanc: Montreal Neurological Institute and McGill University, Montreal, Quebec H3A 2B4, Canada.

TABLE 1. *Cerebral amyloidoses*

Type of amyloid	Chromosome	Condition
Amyloid β protein	21	• Alzheimer's disease • Down's syndrome • Hereditary cerebral hemorrhage, Dutch type • Sporadic cerebral amyloid angiopathy • Normal aging
Cystatin C (γ trace protein)	20	• Hereditary cerebral hemorrhage, Icelandic type • Sporadic cerebral amyloid angiopathy (severe)
Prion protein		• Hereditary cerebral hemorrhage, Dutch type (severe) • Transmissible spongiform encephalopathies (Creutzfeld–Jakob disease, Gerstmann–Stäussler–Sheinker syndrome, kuru, scrapie)

Sporadic Cerebral Amyloid Angiopathy

The hereditary forms of cerebral hemorrhage with amyloid angiopathy are important for the insight that they have provided and will continue to provide into the etiology and the pathophysiology of cerebral amyloid angiopathy. However, much more common is the sporadic form of cerebral amyloid angiopathy.

Prevalence

The prevalence of cerebral amyloid angiopathy is a function of the age of the population. It may be present in over 40% of patients 60 years or older (2). There is a stepwise increase in the incidence of cerebral amyloid angiopathy with increasing age, from 5% to 8% in the seventh decade to 23–43% in the eighth decade to 37–46% in the ninth decade and to approximately 60% of patients older than 90 years (2,13). Most patients with the severest form of amyloid angiopathy have coexisting Alzheimer's disease (14). Indeed the amyloids in blood vessels and in senile plaques share antigenicity and have a similar amino acid sequence (14–16). The occurrence of cerebral hemorrhage from amyloid angiopathy is also age-related (15). Cerebral hemorrhage from amyloid angiopathy accounts for 4–10% of cases of spontaneous cerebral hemorrhage and cerebral hemorrhage can be seen in 40–70% patients with amyloid angiopathy (14,18–20). With the advancing age of our population, neurosurgeons will encounter patients with cerebral hemorrhage from amyloid angiopathy with increasing frequency in the coming decades.

Etiology and Pathophysiology

By analogy with the Dutch form of hereditary cerebral hemorrhage with angiopathy (HCHWA-D), sporadic cerebral amyloid angiopathy is felt to result from the substitution of glutamine for glutamic acid at position 22 of the amyloid β protein (15,16). The amyloid β protein is an approximately 40-amino-acid-long peptide that is partly intramembranous and partly extracellular. It is produced by a larger amyloid precursor protein encoded on the long arm of chromosome 21 (9). When normally metabolized the amyloid precursor protein residues may be cytoprotective. However, the substitution of glutamine for glutamic acid at codon 693 in the amyloid precursor protein results in the massive deposition of the amyloid β protein as an insoluble, extracellular deposit within the media and adventitia of leptomeningeal and cortical arteries and arterioles (9). Cystatin C can colocalize with the amyloid β protein (10–12) and its presence seems to correlate with more extensive amyloid β protein deposition leading to clinically more severe spontaneous, sporadic cerebral hemorrhages (10). Others have suggested, especially for the amyloid deposition associated with the transmissible spongiform encephalopathies, that a spontaneous, random, posttranslational alteration of the precursor protein might cause a collapse of the amyloid β protein into β-pleated sheets. These would then serve as a template for ongoing alterations, as seen in protein polymerization induced by similar but altered protein templates, and promote deposition and accumulation of amyloid (5).

The amyloid protein is deposited within the media and adventitia of the leptomeningeal and cortical arteries, replacing the contractile elements, and within the elastic lamina, which it fragments, splits, or destroys. The structural integrity of the amyloid-laden vessels can be further compromised by fibrinoid degeneration and microaneurysm formation, especially if there is associated arterial hypertension. Thus weakened, the brittle and fragile cortical arteries are prone to spontaneous, often massive, cerebral hemorrhage or to cerebral hemorrhage after cerebral trauma or cortical surgery. Replacement of the contractile elements by noncontractile amyloid interferes with vasoconstriction, the first response to vascular trauma and the initial phase of hemostasis, promoting the development of large, sometimes multicompartmental and multilobar, hematomas (14) (Fig. 1). It has been suggested that the endothelium of amyloid-laden vessels may be functionally deficient (21). A deficient endothelium might promote thrombolysis, the replacement of collagen by amyloid in the subendothelial layer might interfere with platelet adhesion and aggregation, and the accumulated amyloid might bind factors XII and IX and prothrombin, interfering with their role in the hemostatic cascade. However, although the internal elastic lamina is frequently fragmented and split in patients with cerebral amyloid angiopa-

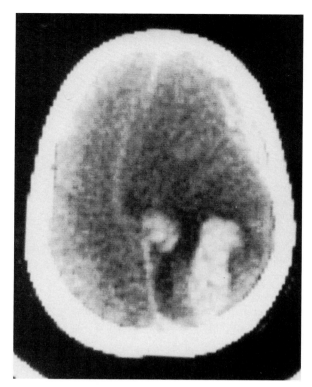

FIG. 1. Noninfused CT scan of a 72-year-old woman with a history of transient visual disturbances 3 weeks prior to a sudden collapse. The CT scan demonstrates two hematomas in the occipital region proven histologically to be of different ages, the smaller, medial one being the older of the two. A prominent subdural hematoma is noted as is subarachnoid hemorrhage. Histologic examination confirmed the presence of severe amyloid angiopathy. (From ref. 17.)

thy, the endothelium itself is usually spared except in the severest cases. Another possible mechanism promoting spontaneous hemorrhage in cerebral amyloid angiopathy is suggested by the inhibitory effect of the amyloid precursor protein on serine proteases, including coagulation factors XIa and IXa (23,24). Such functional factors combined with the structural deficiencies of the amyloid-laden vessels might act in consort to promote cerebral hemorrhage (Table 2).

TABLE 2. *Factors contributing to hemorrhage in cerebral amyloid angiopathy*

Amyloid deposition in tunica media	• Disruption of vascular integrity • Interference with contractile response to hemorrhage
Endothelial dysfunction	• Promotion of thrombolysis • Interference with platelet adhesion and aggregation • Binding of coagulation factors XII, IX, and prothrombin by amyloid
β-Amyloid precursor protein	• Inhibition of coagulation factors XIa and IXa

Data from refs. 14, 17, 21, 23, 24, 27.

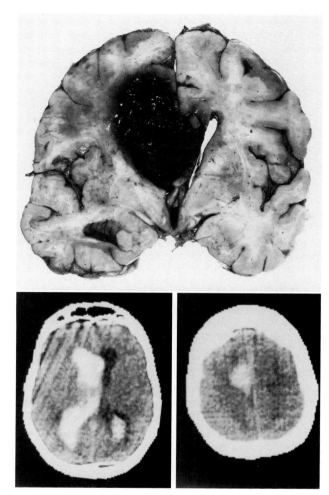

FIG. 2. Postmortem specimen *(top)* and noninfused CT scans *(bottom)* of a 75-year-old woman who died 10 days after an initial collapse. Histologic examination confirmed the presence of cerebral amyloid angiopathy as the source of the large cingulate hematoma that ruptured through the ependyma to produce intraventricular hemorrhage and through the cortex to produce subarachnoid hemorrhage. (From ref. 58.)

Cerebral hemorrhage from amyloid angiopathy is lobar and involves the cortex. The hematoma frequently ruptures through the cortex into the subarachnoid space and through the arachnoid membrane into the subdural space (Fig. 1). More severe hemorrhages breech the ependyma and rupture into the ventricle (Fig. 2). Multiple hematomas can be seen and recurrent hemorrhage is common.

Pathology

Amyloid is strongly eosinophilic and the presence of amyloid within cerebral arteries can be readily demonstrated by its affinity for Congo red and by the characteristic apple green birefringence that it produces under polarized light (Figs. 3 and 4). Staining after immunoprocessing with amyloid directed antibodies also can demonstrate the presence

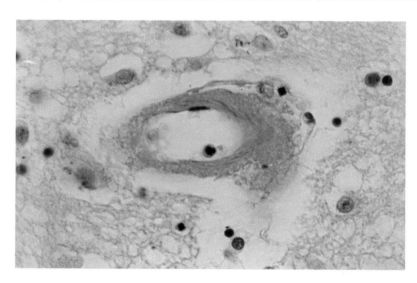

FIG. 3. Hematoxylin-and-eosin stain of a cortical artery from the case illustrated in Fig. 1 demonstrating extensive, strongly eosinophilic amyloid deposition. (From ref. 17.)

of amyloid within cerebral blood vessels (Fig. 4). Electron microscopy reveals characteristically elongated fibrils that accumulate as β-pleated sheets. These replace smooth muscle cells and may produce separation of the internal elastic lamina and of the external basement membrane (19). Fibrinoid degeneration and fibrinoid necrosis as well as microaneurysm formations are also sometimes seen (22). These may be related to arterial hypertension, which is present in up to 30% of patients with amyloid angiopathy (14). "Double barreling" of the lumen occurs subsequent to proliferation of connective tissue and splitting of the internal elastic lamina into two layers (22). The accumulating amyloid can encroach on the lumina and occlude cortical arteries, producing small, coalescing cortical infarcts (14,18). Small cortical petechial hemorrhages and perivascular gliosis can also be seen (25,26). Larger, frequently multiple lobar hemorrhages occur in 40–70% of patients with cerebral amyloid angiopathy. Older hematomas are generally smaller than more recent ones (Fig. 1). As the arteries and arterioles affected are cortical or subcortical, the hematomas are based on the cortex (Figs. 4–6). The hematoma usually ruptures through the cortex to produce subarachnoid hemorrhage (Fig. 4). If the hemorrhage is especially severe, blood having ruptured through the arachnoid membrane can accumulate in the subdural space producing a subdural hematoma. Similarly, the ependyma can be breached producing intraventricular hemorrhage. Amyloid β protein is also implicated in Alzheimer's disease and this frequently coexists with cerebral amyloid angiopathy (14). Thus senile plaques and neurofibrillary tangles may be present in enough quantity to reach the histologic diagnosis of Alzheimer's disease (14).

Clinical Presentation

Sporadic cerebral amyloid angiopathy can remain clinically silent and be seen only incidentally at autopsy. Cerebral hemorrhage can also be clinically silent and may produce mild focal neurologic deficits or extensive cerebral damage and death.

Small, numerous cortical hemorrhages without mass effect can be demonstrated by magnetic resonance imaging (MRI) in some patients with dementia of acute onset and with generalized seizures (25,26). Larger but still clinically silent hemorrhages have been well documented in patients with the familial Dutch form who underwent follow-up computed topography (CT) scanning weeks after an initial hemorrhage (4). During the follow-up period the initial hemorrhages had resolved but new, clinically silent hemorrhages had appeared. More extensive, unilobar cerebral hemorrhages, producing focal neurologic signs that can be quantitated as Hunt and Hess grades II–III, are common (17). These hemorrhages are not associated with significant mass effect or intracranial hypertension. Because of their location, atypical for other common etiologies of cerebral hemorrhage such as arterial hypertension or cerebral aneurysms, they are often believed to represent hemorrhages within a tumor, especially if the patients are investigated some days after the initial hemorrhage when, because of the breakdown of the blood–brain barrier, infused CT scanning demonstrates enhancement. Still more extensive cerebral hemorrhages, quantitated as Hunt and Hess grades IV–V, occur frequently (17). The severity of these hemorrhages is related to the extent and severity of the amyloid deposition within the cortical arteries. These larger, often multilobar, life-threatening hemorrhages frequently are associated with cortical rupture and extension into the subarachnoid and subdural spaces. An arterialized subdural hematoma then adds to the mass effect of the initial hemorrhage. The hematoma also can rupture through the ependyma to produce intraventricular hemorrhage, with poor prognosis.

An individual patient can pass through successive grades of severity over a relatively short time as the cerebral hematoma enlarges as a result of interference with hemostasis

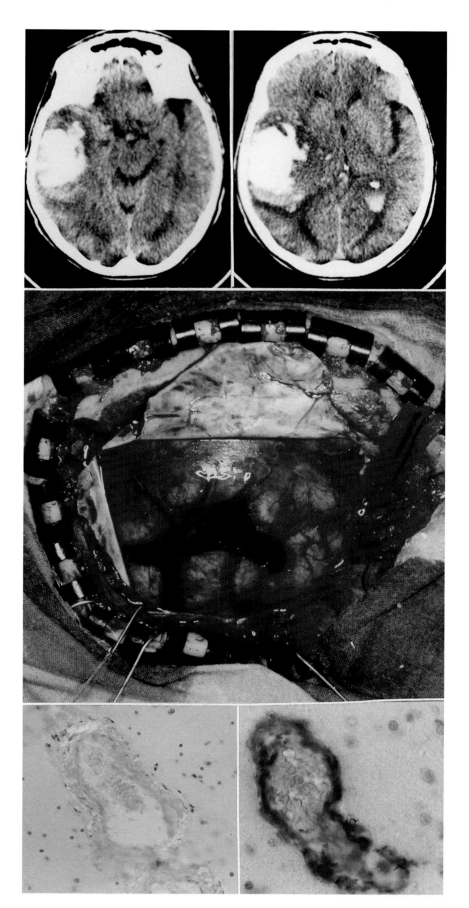

FIG. 4. Noninfused CT scans *(top)* of a 73-year-old woman with the acute onset of stupor and hemiplegia. A large temporal hematoma with extension to the cortex and subarachnoid space is demonstrated. These findings were confirmed at craniotomy *(middle)*, showing the exposed temporal lobe with focal disruption of the temporal cortex and associated subarachnoid hemorrhage. Histologic examination of the resected temporal lobe *(bottom)* showed the presence of birefringence under polarized light after staining with Congo red *(left)* and positive immunostaining directed at amyloid *(right)*.

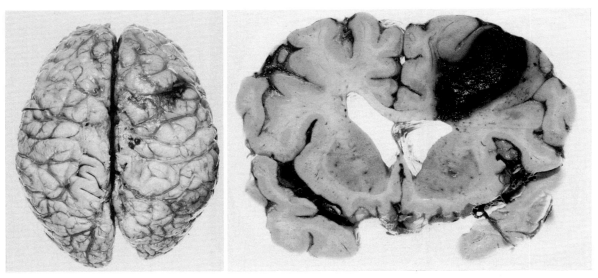

FIG. 5. Postmortem specimen demonstrating a unilobar hematoma extending through the cortex and subarachnoid space but without breaching the ependyma. The patient died of cardiorespiratory complications. Autopsy confirmed the presence of cerebral amyloid angiopathy.

from deficient vasoconstriction and, possibly, from interference with the thrombotic cascade (14,17,21,23,24,27) (Table 2, Fig. 7).

Posttraumatic Cerebral Hemorrhage

The occurrence of cerebral hemorrhage from amyloid angiopathy after head injury has been well documented (14,28–30). This is frequently associated with a subdural hematoma, and cerebral amyloid angiopathy may be responsible for the so-called arterial subdural hematoma sometimes seen in older individuals. Posttraumatic cerebral hemorrhage associated with amyloid angiopathy is frequently fatal.

Iatrogenic Cerebral Hemorrhage

Cortical Surgery

Cerebral hemorrhage from amyloid angiopathy can be iatrogenic, occurring in the immediate postoperative phase after cortical biopsy and ventriculostomy for the diagnosis and treatment of presumed normal pressure hydrocephalus (29,30). Following ventriculostomy the hematoma extends from the biopsy site along the pathway of the catheter into the lateral ventricles. Rebleeding in the resection cavity of an evacuated hematoma is common and may be responsible for clinical deterioration in the early postoperative phase (14,32–37).

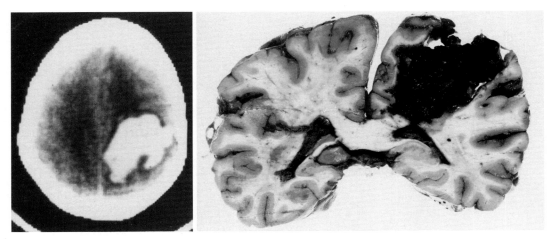

FIG. 6. A noninfused CT scan *(left)* showing a large parietooccipital intracerebral hematoma with characteristic finger-like projections, confirmed at autopsy *(right)* to have arisen from cerebral amyloid angiopathy. (From ref. 44.)

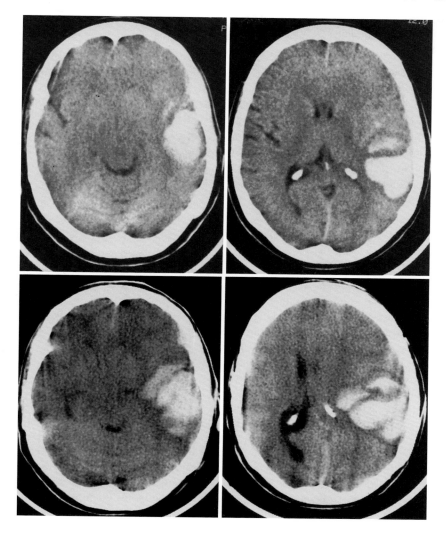

FIG. 7. Noninfused CT scan *(top)* demonstrating a large temporal hematoma with finger-like projections associated with subarachnoid hemorrhage, surrounding edema, and mass effect in a 74-year-old woman with progressive dysphasia and hemiparesis. Repeat CT scan 16 hours later *(bottom)* demonstrates enlargement of the hematoma, extension of the associated subarachnoid hemorrhage, and worsening of the cerebral edema and mass effect. Autopsy confirmed the presence of amyloid angiopathy. (From ref. 27.)

Anticoagulation

Cerebral hemorrhage from amyloid angiopathy has been associated with the use of antiplatelet agents and anticoagulants (4,14,17,22). It is unlikely that these medications directly caused the hemorrhages because hemorrhages have recurred despite the withdrawal of these medications in individual patients (4).

Thrombolysis

Amyloid angiopathy–related cerebral hemorrhages have been reported with the use of streptokinase, urokinase, and tissue plasminogen activators for coronary thrombolysis (21,38–40) (Fig. 8). The hemorrhages become symptomatic 6–8 hours after treatment and are associated with subarachnoid, intraventricular, and subdural extension. Treatment of cerebral hemorrhage associated with thrombolysis for myocardial ischemia is especially difficult because of the high mortality associated with major intracranial surgery in patients with acute coronary ischemia and infarction. Treatment is directed first at correcting the hypocoagulation (38). Since thrombolytic agents have a short half-life and cerebral hemorrhage may become manifest some hours after their use, treatment directed at reversing their effect is usually unnecessary. As treatment protocols for myocardial thrombolysis call for the concomitant use of heparin, the effects of this medication must be counteracted, if the PT and PTT are abnormally elevated, by the use of appropriate agents such as protamine, fresh-frozen plasma, cryoprecipitate, and aminocaproic acid. Surgery is directed at evacuation of the intracerebral hematoma (38). Intracranial surgery is further complicated in the presence of cerebral amyloid angiopathy because hemostasis can be difficult to achieve.

Investigation and Differential Diagnosis

In the absence of cerebral hemorrhage, CT scans and MRIs of patients with amyloid angiopathy may reveal only nonspecific cortical atrophy and ex vacuo ventriculomegaly

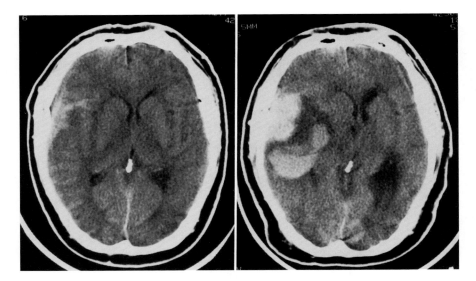

FIG. 8. Noninfused CT scans of a 66-year-old man who underwent coronary thrombolysis for myocardial infarction. The scan at left was obtained 18 hours after treatment when the patient began to complain of headache and demonstrates a small temporal lobe hematoma associated with subarachnoid extension. The scan at right was taken 18 hours later when the patient had developed stupor and left hemiplegia. It demonstrates marked enlargement of the hematoma and increased mass effect. Despite evacuation of the hematoma the patient died of recurrent cardiac ischemia in the early postoperative phase. Histologic examination of the resected specimen confirmed cerebral amyloid angiopathy. (From ref. 38.)

(41,42). There may be no specific radiologic finding, therefore, to suggest the presence of cerebral amyloid angiopathy in patients who may be considered for a cortical biopsy and/or ventricular shunting for presumed normal pressure hydrocephalus. Neurosurgeons should be aware of the possibility of cerebral amyloid angiopathy in these patients and should advise them and their families of the possible occurrence of postoperative cerebral hemorrhage after these procedures.

In some cases MRI can demonstrate multiple punctate cortical hemorrhages as well as ferritin and hemosiderin deposits from prior petechial cortical hemorrhages (25,26). It has been suggested that the demonstration by MRI of recent or remote multiple petechial cortical hemorrhages associated with periventricular leukoencephalopathy may be predictive of cerebral amyloid angiopathy.

CT scanning in patients with a cerebral hematoma can often suggest the diagnosis of amyloid angiopathy because the hematomas occur at sites uncommon for other conditions that produce cerebral hemorrhage (14,17,42,43). In amyloid angiopathy, the hematomas originate from the cortex and produce a lobar or multilobar hemorrhage. The hematoma can be single or multiple and may have characteristic finger-like extension on CT scanning. The hemorrhage can be of such severity as to rupture through the cortex into the subarachnoid space and even through the subarachnoid membrane into the subdural space. The hematoma can also disrupt the white matter and rupture through the ependyma into the ventricles. In arterial hypertension the hematomas frequently involve the basal ganglia, the pons, and the cerebellum. Sporadic cerebral amyloid angiopathy almost never involves these structures. Hypertensive lobar hematomas are usually confined to the white matter, sparing the cortex, whereas the hematomas originate and extend from the cortex in amyloid angiopathy. Hematomas from cerebral aneurysms have a predilection for the anterior temporal and mesial frontal lobes as a result of rupture of middle cerebral and anterior communicating artery aneurysms, respectively,

and are almost invariably associated with extensive subarachnoid hemorrhage involving the basal cisterns and the Sylvian and interhemispheric fissures. Although amyloid angiopathy is frequently associated with subarachnoid hemorrhage, this is less extensive and is maximal over the area of cortical disruption. A cerebral hemorrhage from an arteriovenous malformation or from a cavernous angioma can also occur at unusual sites in the brain and be associated with subarachnoid hemorrhage. These underlying lesions can almost always be demonstrated by MRI or infused CT scanning. The latter, however, especially if performed some days after the hemorrhage, can be associated with luxury perfusion and enhancement suggesting the misdiagnosis of hemorrhage within a tumor. Angiography excludes an aneurysm or cerebrovascular anomaly as the cause of the cerebral hemorrhage, although coexistent atherosclerosis can be demonstrated. The differential diagnosis of blood dyscrasia, iatrogenic hemorrhage from anticoagulation, leukemia, vasculitis, and multiple hemorrhages associated with the smoking of cocaine can be elucidated by history taking, physical examination, and ancillary laboratory tests (44). In patients who survive an initial hemorrhage the occurrence of repeated hemorrhages, either at the same or at other sites, strongly supports the diagnosis of amyloid angiopathy.

Treatment

Spontaneous Hemorrhage

The role of surgery in the treatment of patients with cerebral hemorrhage from amyloid angiopathy is still to be defined, although most have observed a high mortality and morbidity of surgery for this condition (14,17,45,46). Over a third of patients will die post-operatively from the initial hemorrhage or from the complications of debilitation in these old and sometimes demented individuals with a major intracranial hemorrhage. Up to half of the survivors will have severe neurologic deficits and many of these will suffer subsequent, ultimately fatal rehemorrhages within months or years after the initial event. Many of the patients who are reported to have survived surgery were in good clinical condition at the time of operation (17,45,46). In many cases they underwent surgery some days or weeks after the hemorrhage because of the misdiagnosis of hemorrhage within a tumor and surgery was undertaken not to relieve mass effect and intracranial hypertension but to obtain tissue diagnosis. In our own clinical material a third of the patients died postoperatively from the initial hemorrhage or from its complications, and a quarter were neurologically disabled (17). The patients who are well at the time of discharge from hospital may go on to have repeated hemorrhages that produce neurologic and cognitive deficits that are progressively more severe and ultimately fatal (16,34,36,37,47,48) (Fig. 9). All of our patients who survived to leave the hospital in good condition were grades II and III at the time of surgery and most had undergone surgery more than 10 days after the hemorrhage for the misdiagnosis of hemorrhage within a tumor. All patients who were in poor condition (grades IV and V) and who were operated on acutely died or were severely disabled.

Our experience and the experience gleaned from the literature suggest that surgery has a limited role to play in the treatment of cerebral hemorrhage from amyloid angiopathy. In patients who are in good neurologic condition, surgical evacuation is most often unnecessary to relieve intracranial hypertension. In patients with malignant intracranial hypertension from the mass effect of the hematoma, surgery is associated with a high mortality and morbidity from difficult hemostasis, recurrent hemorrhage in the immediate or late postoperative phase, and the cardiorespiratory complications of debilitation in elderly, sometimes demented, patients who have sustained a catastrophic cerebral event. Operative mortality and morbidity are a function of the severity of the amyloid angiopathy and the extent of the cerebral hemor-

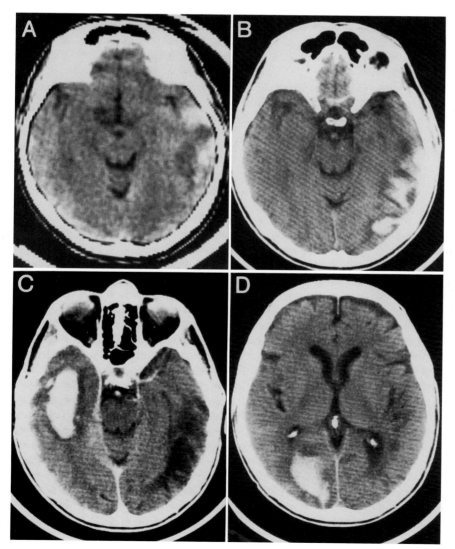

FIG. 9. Noninfused CT scan **(A)** of a 71-year-old man who presented to hospital 3 weeks after the onset of dysphasia. A mixed-density left temporal intracerebral hematoma is seen. Because of enhancement after infusion of intravenous contrast material a diagnosis of hemorrhage within a tumor was formulated and craniotomy was performed. No tumor cells were present but there was extensive amyloid angiopathy. The patient returned to hospital 28 months later with headache and recurrent dysphasia. CT scanning at that time **(B)** revealed a new, more extensive left temporal intracerebral hematoma. His condition improved but he returned to hospital 22 months later because of the acute onset of confusion. CT scanning **(C)** revealed a right temporal hematoma from which he recovered. Readmission was precipitated 6 months later by a new right occipital hemorrhage **(D)**. The patient suddenly died a month later of unexplained causes. (From ref.17.)

rhage that it produces, especially as it extends into the ventricular or subdural spaces, and the age and medical condition of the patient, especially as these affect the cardiorespiratory system (17).

If surgery is necessary to relieve mass effect, then it should be undertaken with the expectation of difficult hemostasis. Amyloid-laden vessels are refractory to bipolar diathermy. Nonetheless it has been our experience that hemostasis can be achieved with the extensive use of polyanhydrous glucuronic acid (Oxygel, Beckton-Dickinson, Sandy, UT) covered with absorbable gelatin sponges (Gelfoam, Upjohn, Don Mills, Ontario, Canada) and wet, fluffy cottonoid sponges for gentle tamponing.

Hemorrhage After Thrombolysis

As amyloid angiopathy may be present in elderly or demented patients undergoing coronary thrombolysis, surgeons should be aware that patients with a cerebral hemorrhage associated with thrombolysis may have underlying amyloid angiopathy and anticipate difficult hemostasis if surgery is undertaken (21,38–40). These hematomas can progressively enlarge (36) and exhibit layering and a fluid level on CT scan (36,38). Despite evacuation of the hematoma patients remain at risk of recurrent coronary events or of recurrent cerebral hemorrhage.

Prognosis

As cerebral hemorrhage from amyloid angiopathy is a function of advancing age, and with the increased longevity of our populations, neurosurgeons will encounter cerebral hemorrhage from amyloid angiopathy with increasing frequency. The clinical presentation is related to the extent and severity of the amyloid angiopathy: the more severe and extensive the angiopathy the poorer the clinical condition and the graver the prognosis (17). Patients in better clinical condition have unilobar hematomas without ventricular involvement. Patients in poorer condition have hemorrhages that are more extensive and often multilobar, with frequent rupture into the ventricles and into the subdural space. Surgical evacuation of the hematoma in the latter group is associated with a high incidence of death and severe neurologic disability. If surgery is undertaken as a life-saving procedure the surgeon should expect difficult hemostasis with the likelihood that there will be repeated hemorrhage, either at the operative site or elsewhere, in the early or late postoperative phase.

The demonstration that familial cerebral amyloid angiopathies are associated with specific genetic lesions suggests that there will be continued interest in this condition at a molecular level. Herein lies the best hope of preventing the putative age-related mutation that leads to the deposition of amyloid within the brain and cerebral blood vessels and its two major associations, dementia and cerebral hemorrhage.

MOYAMOYA DISEASE

Moyamoya disease is a frequent cause of cerebral ischemia and stroke. Cerebral hemorrhage is part of the natural history of moyamoya disease and is usually fatal. Indeed, cerebral hemorrhage frequently results from the rupture of the puff-of-smoke collaterals that give this condition its evocative name.

Moyamoya disease is characterized by multiple, progressive, ultimately symmetric stenoses and occlusions of the anterior part of the circle of Willis with sparing of the vertebrobasilar system. The progressive stenosis and occlusion of the internal carotid, middle cerebral, and anterior cerebral arteries promote the development of basal, transcortical, transethmoidal, and transdural anastomoses responsible for the characteristic puff-of-smoke appearance of the anastomotic webs on cerebral angiography (49). The two related phenomena of progressive occlusion and secondary collateralization account for the two cardinal features of moyamoya disease: repeated, multifocal cerebral infarction and cerebral hemorrhage.

Epidemiology

Moyamoya disease has been described in both black and white races and has been seen on all continents. Nonetheless the highest yearly incidence at 1 per million most likely occurs in the Japanese (50). The age distribution is bimodal, the first peak occurring in the first decade and the second in the third and fourth decades (49,50). The first peak reflects the onset of the disease with progressive arterial stenoses and occlusions and is characterized by transient cerebral ischemia, strokes, cerebrovascular dementia, and epilepsy. The second peak reflects rupture of the collateral web and is associated with intracerebral, intraventricular, and subarachnoid hemorrhage. Moyamoya disease is more common in women than in men. A familial occurrence is recognized in approximately 10% of cases, affecting mostly a parent and child with a lesser occurrence in siblings, and moyamoya disease has been reported in twins (50). This familial occurrence suggests a possible genetic etiology for moyamoya disease, a possibility strengthened by its association with von Recklinghausen's disease and with specific human leukocyte antigens. An inflammatory etiology has been suggested by the occurrence of tonsillitis and other infections of the oropharynx prior to the onset of moyamoya disease, and an auto-immune etiology has been suggested by the presence of histologic changes similar to those of periarteritis nodosa in the affected blood vessels. Others have suggested that overactivity of the sympathetic nervous system is responsible for prolonged vasoconstriction leading to stenosis and occlusion of the arteries of the anterior circle of Willis.

Cerebral Hemorrhage and Moyamoya Disease

Cerebral hemorrhage occurs in 40–60% of adults with moyamoya disease. It is more common in females, in a pro-

TABLE 3. *Cerebral hemorrhage in moya-moya disease*

- Fibrinoid necrosis of anastomotic vessels
- Rupture of microaneurysms on anastomotic arteries
- Rupture of pseudoaneurysms of the anterior and posterior choroidal arteries
- Rupture of a saccular aneurysm of the basilar artery or of the proximal internal carotid artery

portion of 7:3, and it is usually fatal (50). Up to one third of survivors will suffer repeat hemorrhages days to years after the initial event.

Cerebral hemorrhage results from rupture of the anastomotic web, micro- and pseudoaneurysms, and true saccular aneurysms as increasing hemodynamic stresses are applied to the anastomotic vessels, the internal carotid artery proximal to the occlusion, and the vertebrobasilar system as blood flow is redirected from the anterior to the posterior circle of Willis (49–52) (Table 3). Small-diameter collateral vessels of the basal ganglia are weakened by fibrinoid deposits, fragmentation of the elastic lamina, and attenuation of the media. Microaneurysms also occur on these vessels and are associated with focal fibrinoid deposition and thinning of the arterial wall and of the elastic lamina (50,53). Rupture within the anastomotic web produces ganglionic hemorrhage. Slightly larger pseudoaneurysms occur on the distal anterior and posterior choroidal arteries as these are submitted to increased hemodynamic stresses (50,53). The micropseudoaneurysms are composed of concentric layers of fibrin and red blood cells and can disappear on follow-up angiography (54). True saccular aneurysms account for 50% of the aneurysms seen in moyamoya disease (49,55–57). They occur on the internal carotid artery proximal to the occlusion, frequently within the cavernous sinus, where they can be multiple, and most commonly on the distal basilar artery as a response to the hemodynamic stresses placed on the vertebrobasilar system as the intracranial circulation is redirected away from the occluded carotid circulation. Anterior and middle cerebral artery aneurysms are distinctly unusual in moyamoya disease.

The cerebral parenchyma and ventricular system are the commonest sites of hemorrhage in moyamoya disease (49,50,51). Parenchymal hemorrhages affecting the basal ganglia and thalamus and the subcortical white matter account for approximately 60% of hemorrhages in this condition, whereas subependymal and intraventricular hemorrhages account for approximately 35%. Isolated, arterial subdural hematomas resulting from the rupture of transdural anastomoses and isolated subarachnoid hemorrhage from the rupture of a saccular aneurysm occur in the remainder of cases.

Investigation and Treatment

As cerebral hemorrhage in moyamoya disease occurs principally in the adult form, the underlying diagnosis will usually be known. Routine hematologic tests are normal with the exception of an over-representation of HLA-B40 in the juvenile form and of HLA-B54 in the adult form of moyamoya disease. Intracerebral, intraventricular, subdural, or subarachnoid hematomas are identified by CT scanning. If not previously known, the diagnosis of moyamoya disease is established by cerebral angiography. This demonstrates bilateral, symmetric stenoses or occlusions of the large vessels forming the anterior two thirds of the circle of Willis, in association with an extensive collateral web involving characteristically the basal ganglia, the small orbital vessels via the ophthalmic, posterior, and anterior ethmoidal and external carotid arteries, and the middle meningeal and superficial temporal arteries in the region of the cranial sutures (49,50). Cortical-intraparenchymal anastomoses are also frequent. Pseudoaneurysms and true saccular aneurysms may also be identified.

The treatment of intracranial hemorrhage from moyamoya disease is directed at the site of involvement, either intraparenchymal, intraventricular, subdural, or subarachnoid. Subdural and cerebral hemorrhages are treated by surgical evacuation and intraventricular hemorrhage by ventricular drainage. Subarachnoid hemorrhage from a ruptured saccular aneurysm is treated by clipping of the aneurysm or by interventional neuroradiologic procedures, if warranted. A thorough understanding of the anastomotic network and great care in their preservation are essential in the surgical treatment of cerebral hemorrhage in moyamoya disease as the surgical approach may damage collateral channels, most notably the superficial temporal and middle meningeal arteries and transcortical anastomoses.

REFERENCES

1. Griffiths RA, Mortimer TF, Oppenheimer DR, Spalding JMK. Congophilic angiopathy of the brain: a clinical and pathological report of two siblings. *J Neurol Neurosurg Psychiatry* 1982-:396–408.
2. Vinters HV, Gilbert JJ. Amyloid angiopathy: its incidence and complications in the aging brain. *Stroke* 1983;14:915–923.
3. Gudmundsson G, Hallgrimsson J, Jonasson TA, et al. Hereditary cerebral hemorrhage with amyloidosis. *Brain* 1972;95:387–404.
4. Haan J, Algra PR, Roos RAC. Hereditary cerebral hemorrhage with amyloidosis–Dutch type. Clinical and computed tomographic analysis of 24 cases. *Arch Neurol* 1990;47:649–653.
5. Gajdusek DC, Beyreuther K, Brown P, et al. Regulation and genetic control of brain amyloid. *Brain Res Rev* 1991;16:83–114.
6. Barrett AJ, Davies ME, Grubb A. The place of human γ-trace (cystatin C) amongst the cysteine proteinase inhibitors. *Biochem Biophys Res Commun* 1984;120:631–636.
7. Löfberg H, Grubb AO, Nilsson EK, et al. Immunohistochemical characterization of the amyloid deposits and quantitation of pertinent cerebrospinal fluid proteins in hereditary cerebral hemorrhage with amyloidosis. *Stroke* 1987;18:431–440.
8. Van Broeckhoven C, Haan J, Bakker E, et al. Amyloid beta protein precursor gene and hereditary cerebral hemorrhage with amyloidosis (Dutch). *Science* 1990;248:1120–1122.
9. Levey E, Carman M, Fernandez-Madrid IJ, et al. Mutation of the Alzheimer's amyloid gene in hereditary cerebral hemorrhage, Dutch type. *Science* 1990;248:1124–1126.
10. Maruyama K, Ikelda S, Ishihara T. Allsop D, Yanagisawa N. Immunohistochemical characterization of cerebrovascular amyloid in 46 autopsied cases using antibodies to protein and cystatin C. *Stroke* 1990;21: 397–403.

11. Shimode K, Fujihara S, Nakamura M, Kobayashi S, Tsunematsu T. Diagnosis of cerebral amyloid angiopathy by enzyme-linked immunosorbent assay of cystatin C in cerebrospinal fluid. *Stroke* 1991;22:860–866.

12. Vinters HV, Secor DL, Pardridge WM, Gray F. Immunohistochemical study of cerebral amyloid angiopathy. III. Widespread Alzheimer A4 peptide in cerebral microvessel walls colocalizes with gamma trace in patients with leukoencephalopathy. *Ann Neurol* 1990;28:34–42.

13. Tomonga M. Cerebral amyloid angiopathy in the elderly. *J Am Geriatr Soc* 1981;29:151–157.

14. Cosgrove GR, Leblanc R, Meagher-Villemure K, Ethier R. Cerebral amyloid angiopathy. *Neurology* 1985;35:625–631.

15. Coria F, Castaño EM, Frangione B. Brain amyloid in normal aging and cerebral amyloid angiopathy is antigenically related to Alzheimer's disease beta protein. *Am J Pathol* 1987;129:422–428.

16. Coria F, Prelli F, Castano EM, et al. Beta protein deposition: a pathogenetic link between Alzheimer's disease and cerebral amyloid angiopathies. *Brain Res* 1988;463:187–191.

17. Leblanc R, Preul M, Robitaille Y, Villemure J-G, Pokrupa R. Surgical considerations in cerebral amyloid angiopathy. *Neurosurgery* 1991;29:712–718.

18. Okazaki H, Reagan TH, Campbell RJ. Clinicopathologic studies of primary cerebral amyloid angiopathy. *Mayo Clin Proc* 1979;54:22–31.

19. Lee SS, Stemmerman GN. Congophilic angiopathy and cerebral hemorrhage. *Arch Pathol Lab Med* 1978;102:317–321.

20. Jellinger K. Cerebrovascular amyloidosis with cerebral hemorrhage. *J Neurol* 1977;214:195–206.

21. Ramsay DA, Penswick JL, Robertson DM. Fatal streptokinase-induced intracerebral hemorrhage in cerebral amyloid angiopathy. *Can J Neurol Sci* 1990;17:336–341.

22. Mandybur TI. Cerebral amyloid angiopathy: the vascular pathology and complications. *J Neuropathol Exp Neurol* 1986;45:79–90.

23. Smith PP, Higuchi DA, Brooze GJ Jr. Platelet coagulation factor XIa inhibitor, a form of Alzheimer amyloid precursor protein. *Science* 1990;248:1126–1128.

24. Schmaier AH, Dahl LD, Rozemuller AJM et al. Protease nexin-2/amyloid beta protein precursor: a tight-binding inhibitor of coagulation factor IXa. *J Clin Invest* 1993;92:2540–2545.

25. Case records of the Massachusetts General Hospital: case 27-1991. *N Engl J Med* 1991;325:42–54.

26. Hendricks HT, Franke CL, Theunissen PHMH. Cerebral amyloid angiopathy: diagnosis by MRI and brain biopsy. *Neurology* 1990;40:1308–1310.

27. Leblanc R, Carpenter S, Steart J, Pokrupa R. Subacute enlarging cerebral hematoma from amyloid angiopathy: case report. *Neurosurgery* 1995;36:403–406.

28. Kalyran-Raman UP, Kalyan-Raman K. Cerebral amyloid angiopathy causing intracranial hemorrage. *Ann Neurol* 1984;16:321–329.

29. Regli F, Von Satel JP, Perentes E, Assal G. L'angiopathie amyloid cérébrale. *Rev Neurol* 1981;137:181–184.

30. Ulrich G, Taghavy A, Schmidt H. The nosology and etiology of congophilic angiopathy (shape of vessels of the cerebral amyloidosis). *J Neurol* 1973;206:39–59.

31. Torack RM. Congophilic angiopathy complicated by surgery and massive hemorrhage. *Am J Pathol* 1975;81:349–366.

32. Rengachary SS, Racela LS, Watanabe I, Abdou N. Neurosurgical and immunological implications of primary cerebral amyloid (congophilic) angiopathy. *Neurosurgery* 1980;7:1–9.

33. Filloux FM, Townsend JJ. Congophilic angiopathy with intracerebral hemorrhage. *West J Med* 1985;143:498–502.

34. Gilbert JJ, Vinters HV. Cerebral amyloid angiopathy: incidence and complications in the aging brain. I. Cerebral hemorrhage. *Stroke* 1983;14:915–923.

35. Gilles C, Brucher JM, Khoubesserian P, Vanderhaeghen JJ. Cerebral amyloid angiopathy as a cause of multiple intracerebral hemorrhages. *Neurology* 1984;34:730–735.

36. Tucker WS, Bilbao JM, Klodawsky H. Cerebral amyloid angiopathy and multiple intracerebral hematomas. *Neurosurgery* 1980;611–614.

37. Tyler KL, Poletti CE, Heros RC. Cerebral amyloid angiopathy with multiple intracerebral hemorrhages. *J Neurosurg* 1982;57:286–289.

38. Leblanc R, Haddad G, Robitaille Y. Cerebral hemorrhage from amyloid angiopathy and coronary thrombolysis. *Neurosurgery* 1992;31:586–590.

39. Pendlebury WW. Iole ED, Tracey RP, et al. Intracerebral hemorrhage related to cerebral amyloid angiopathy and t-PA treatment. *Ann Neurol* 1991;29:210–213.

40. Wijdicks EFM, Jack Jr CR. Intracerebral hemorrhage after fibrinolytic therapy for acute myocardial infarction. *Stroke* 1993;24:554–557.

41. Gauthier S, Robitaille Y, Quirion R, et al. Antemortem labortory diagnosis of Alzheimer's disease. *Prog Neuro-Psychopharmacol Biol Psychiatry* 1986;10:391–403.

42. Brown RT, Coates R, Gilbert JJ. Radiographic-pathologic correlation in cerebral amyloid angiopathy: a review of 12 patients. *J Can Assoc Radiol* 1985;36:308–311.

43. Leblanc R, Cosgrove RG, Meagher-Villemure K, et al. Cerebral amyloid angiopathy: the role of CT scanning in diagnosis and management. Presented at the Annual Meeting of the American Association of Neurological Surgeons, San Francisco, April 1984.

44. Leblanc R. Intracranial hemorrhage from vasculitides, vasculopathies and coagulopathies. In: Tindall GJ, Cooper P, Barrow DL, eds. *The Practice of Neurosurgery,* Williams and Wilkins, 1996;2:2313–2343.

45. Greene GM, Godersky JC, Biller J, et al. Surgical experience with cerebral amyloid angiopathy. *Stroke* 1990;21:1545–1549.

46. Matkovic Z, Davis S, Gonzales M, et al. Surgical risk of hemorrhage in cerebral amyloid angiopathy. *Stroke* 1991;22:456–461.

47. Finelli PF, Kessimian N, Bernstein PW. Cerebral amyloid angiopathy manifesting as a recurrent intracerebral hemorrhage. *Arch Neurol* 1984;41:330–333.

48. Seitelberger F. Dementia following nonarteriosclerotic vascular processes of the CNS. In: Meyer JS, Lechner H, Reivich M, et al., eds. *Cerebral Vascular Disease.* St. Louis: CV Mosby, 1972:200–206.

49. Suzuki J, Kodama N. Moyamoya disease: a review. *Stroke* 1983;14:104–109.

50. Yonekawa Y, Handa J, Okuno T. Moyamoya disease: Diagnosis, treatment, and recent achievement. In: Barnette HJM, Stein BM, Mohr JP, et al., eds. *Stroke: Pathophysiology, Diagnosis and Management,* 2nd ed. New York: Churchill Livingstone, 1992:721–747.

51. Okamoto J, Mukai K, Kashihara M, et al. A case of atypical moyamoya disease with a ruptured aneurysm on moyamoya vessel. *Surg Neurol* 1982;10:897–903.

52. Yamashita M, Oka K, Tanaka K. Histopathology of the brain vascular network in moyamoya disease. *Stroke* 1983;14:50–58.

53. Aoki N, Mizutani H. Does moyamoya disease cause subarachnoid hemorrhage? Review of 54 cases with intracranial hemorrhage confirmed by computerized tomography. *J Neurosurg* 1984;60:348–353.

54. Yuasa H, Tokito S, Izumi K, et al. Cerebrovascular moyamoya disease associated with an intracranial pseudoaneurysm. Case Report. *J Neurosurg* 1982;56:131.

55. Debrun G, Lacour P. A new case of moyamoya disease associated with several intracavernous aneurysms. *Neuroradiology* 1974;7:277–282.

56. Nagamine Y, Takahashi S. Sonobe M. Multiple intracranial aneurysms associated with moyamoya disease. Case report. *J Neurosurg* 1981;54:673–676.

57. Waga S, Tochio H. Intracranial aneurysms associated with moyamoya disease in childhood. *Surg Neurol* 1985;23:237–243.

58. Leblanc R. Cerebral amyloid angiopathy and moyamoya disease. In: Batjer HH, ed. Spontaneous intracerebral hemorrhage. *Neurosurg Clin North Am* 1992;3:625–636.

Cerebrovascular Disease, edited by H. Hunt Batjer.
Lippincott-Raven Publishers, Philadelphia © 1997.

CHAPTER 52

Spontaneous Cerebral Hemorrhage: Innovative New Techniques for Decompression

Thomas A. Kopitnik, Jr.

Stroke is the third leading cause of death in the United States and accounts for an annual health care expenditure of approximately 30 billion dollars (1). Spontaneous intracerebral hematoma (SICH) (Fig. 1) as a cause of stroke occurs at a rate of between 6% and 13% of all strokes in the United States and accounts for approximately one fourth to one half of all stroke-related deaths in the United States (2–5). A 1988 population-based survey of SICH in Cincinnati found an annual incidence of 15 per 100,000 population (7). Despite the passage of over 125 years since Charcot and Bouchard described SICH associated with miliary aneurysms, very little progress has been made in the overall outcome of this disease process (8). The morbidity and mortality of SICH remains high, with more than 50% mortality and at least 75% moderate to severe morbidity (9–11). The expected outcome of both medical and surgical management is poor, with outcome primarily dependent on both the location and magnitude of the hemorrhage. The 30-day mortality is approximately 40%, whereas only 12% who survive will merely have a minor residual neurologic deficit (12). SICH related specifically to hypertension may decrease in the future as diagnosis and treatment of hypertension improves. Because SICH is more common in older patient populations, as life expectancy in the United States increases and the population ages, SICH will likely remain a major health issue in the future. This chapter will address some of the future prospects and possibilities for innovative treatment of this complex condition.

The issue of whether spontaneous SICH should be evacuated remains a controversial issue and is presently the subject of study on a national level. Some studies have suggested that surgical outcome is related to the patient's preoperative condition. Kanaya reported a retrospective study that found patients who were alert, confused, or somnolent had out-

comes that were independent of the treatment modality used. Similarly, those patients who were stuporous or semicomatose had surgical results significantly improved over those of medical management (13). A similar study in 1977 reported 38 patients who presented with SICH and underwent surgery within 7 hours of presentation (14). Of the 38 patients, 35 were stuporous or comatose prior to surgery. Twelve of the 38 patients reportedly made a complete recovery whereas 12 patients suffered mild residual neurologic impairment. The remaining 14 patients (37%) were either severely disabled or died secondary to the hemorrhage. The authors later published a similar report in 1983 in which 100 patients underwent a similar treatment protocol of surgical evacuation of the hematoma within 7 hours of onset. They reported similar outcomes and theorized that improved results compared with historical controls resulted from rapid removal of the hematoma (15). The principal of immediate operative removal in properly selected patients may afford improved outcome and lessen the morbidity and mortality, although non-randomized studies retrospectively compared to historical controls have not been widely accepted as definitively determining the best treatment for SICH.

The standard operative treatment for SICH has typically consisted of a large craniotomy under general anesthesia and clot evacuation under direct vision. Because clot location and associated medical conditions are strongly related to patient outcome, advances in operative instrumentation, microsurgery, and anesthesia related to a standard open procedure have had little impact on patient outcome. Operative mortality can be extremely high, ranging from 20% to 90% in deeply comatose patients with ganglionic and thalamic hemorrhages (16–19). These suboptimal results have stimulated an interest in both a search for less traumatic and safer methods of clot removal, as well as a renewed interest in definitive, well-designed studies that could reveal which techniques potentially benefit specific patient populations with SICH.

T. A. Kopitnik, Jr.: Department of Neurological Surgery, University of Texas Southwestern Medical Center, Dallas, TX 75235.

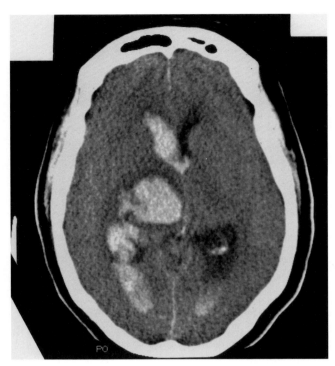

FIG. 1. CT scan of typical thalamic spontaneous intracerebral hematoma with intraventricular extension.

Methods to evacuate clot from SICH that are less invasive and potentially less traumatic than open craniotomy have typically focused on simple aspiration, mechanically assisted aspiration, stereotactic methods, installation of fibrinolytic agents, and, more recently, endoscopic and laser-assisted methods. To date, no randomized controlled study has demonstrated superiority of any treatment regimen compared to either best medical treatment or conventional open craniotomy. As new and innovative treatments are introduced, it is best to remember that decreased procedural morbidity will likely be unaffected unless the necessity of general anesthesia and a prolonged operative procedure can be eliminated.

SIMPLE ASPIRATION

Conceptually, the optimal approach to remove SICH would be a simple procedure that is rapid, has a low cost, and has a high success rate. Simple aspiration through either a twist drill or a burr hole is economical and rapidly carried out but has a limited success rate due to a variety of factors. Attempts at aspiration as the primary treatment regimen are unpredictable due to difficulty aspirating solid portions of the hematoma and problems with rebleeding following the procedure. Within hours of experimental clot genesis, at least 80% of the hematoma is in the form of a dense, fibrinous clot, whereas only 20% remains liquid (20). Aspiration as a form of treatment of intracranial hematomas has been most successful when used to aspirate chronic or subacute hematomas that were composed mostly of liquid clot (21,22).

McKissock attempted to treat SICH with simple aspiration, finding that only a small portion of the clot could be aspirated and that open craniotomy was superior with regard to the amount of hematoma that could be removed (17,23). Most reports of successful aspiration of SICH as the sole treatment have related to aspiration of deep ganglionic or brainstem hemorrhages in which the aspiration was performed no more than 24 hours after onset (24–26). In 1989, Niizuma reported a study of 175 patients with putaminal hemorrhages treated with aspiration. One hundred thirty-four (75%) of these patients had >50% of the clot removed whereas 13 (7.4%) of the patients suffered rebleeding after the procedure (27). It appears as though simple aspiration may be a viable but limited option in treating those patients at highest risk for surgical intervention or present with SICH primarily involving the brainstem. Simple freehand aspiration may be of optimal value in an emergency salvage procedure, where possible functional survival may occur, but open craniotomy cannot be performed despite catastrophic neurologic deterioration. The major limitation of aspiration is the unpredictable amount of hematoma that may be aspirated and the high incidence of immediate rebleeding. With brainstem hematomas, aspiration would mandate incorporating stereotactic techniques to ensure a safe and reliable trajectory to the hematoma cavity.

STEREOTACTIC ASPIRATION

The limitation of freehand clot aspiration of SICH is the unpredictable trajectory to approach the hematoma and the inability to position the aspiration cannula precisely in a specific portion of the clot. Clot aspiration using stereotactic techniques and intraoperative imaging has been shown to be useful in some instances. This was reported by Benes in 1965 to have met with some limited success in aspirating nontraumatic hematomas (28). Several characteristics of hematomas render them suitable for stereotactic aspiration. The size, shape, and location can be easily determined on computed tomography (CT) and magnetic resonance imaging (MRI), the hematoma can be readily targeted using CT- and MR-compatible stereotactic frames, and the procedure could be performed under local anesthesia.

There has been an increasing interest in treatment of SICH through stereotactic aspiration, particularly in the Japanese literature. Niizuma has published three consecutive reports regarding stereotactic clot aspiration between 1985 and 1989 (27,29,30). He reported that over this time period, volumes of hematoma that could be aspirated increased from 50% in 1985 to 77% in 1989. In these reports, rebleeding occurred in approximately 7.4% of patients and the procedure was performed no earlier than 6 hours following the ictus to allow local hemostasis to theoretically occur. In managing patients in this manner, Niizuma reported that the percentage of patients with fair or better outcomes who were able to return to useful lives was 80.9% (27). The results of this study are difficult to interpret with regard to the efficacy of stereotactic aspiration as the sole treatment. One hundred twenty-two (70%) of the patients also had instillation of urokinase into the hematoma cavity after initial attempt at aspiration was unsuccessful. Matsumoto has also found similar results with the use of CT-guided stereotactic aspiration in the treatment of SICH (31). He found the procedure to be well tolerated under local anesthesia, safe, and successful at removing the majority of the hematoma, but, similar to the reports of Niizuma, Matsumoto added instillation of thrombolytic medication to facilitate hematoma dissolution. He went on to report that his results, although not statistically significant due to the low number of patients, compared favorably with historical reports of conventional craniotomy from the previous decade.

Despite the potential advantages of stereotactic aspiration under local anesthesia, this procedure remains a blind technique in which the presence of active rebleeding or change in the configuration of the hematoma cannot be appreciated as the aspiration is being performed. Stereotactic aspiration is less traumatic and less stressful to a critically ill patient who may not tolerate a general anesthetic and potential blood loss involved with open craniotomy for SICH. Despite the inherent limitations, stereotactic aspiration probably has some limited role in the treatment of deep-seated hematomas, including those involving the diencephalon and brainstem.

FIBRINOLYTIC THERAPY

An adjunct to stereotactic aspiration of SICH has been the use of fibrinolytic medications instilled directly into the hematoma cavity. Both first- and second-generation fibrinolytic medications in the forms of urokinase (UK) and recombinant tissue plasminogen activator substance (r-TPA), respectively, have been evaluated both experimentally and in humans (32–39). Both thrombolytic drugs function to facilitate the dissolution of clot by biochemical activation of intrinsic fibrinolytic activity. This occurs with both thrombolytic agents through the activation of plasminogen, which is an inactive proenzyme. Plasminogen is activated and converted to plasmin, which then dissolves fibrin into fibrin degradation products (40). Urokinase activity is not specific to fibrinolysis activity but is also fibrinogenolytic, therefore inhibiting formation of new fibrin clot by dissolving fibrinogen, a precursor molecule of fibrin (41). The most important intrinsic tissue plasminogen activator is tissue plasminogen activator (TPA) or its synthetic analog r-TPA, which is fibrin-specific but does not interfere with fibrinogenic activity and thereby does not theoretically inhibit new clot formation. TPA is synthesized and secreted by endothelial cells and has very low concentrations in the cerebrospinal fluid, subarachnoid space, and ventricular system (42,43).

In experimental animal studies of subarachnoid, intracerebral, and intraventricular injections of UK mixed with blood,

UK appeared to promote clot reabsorption and appeared safe (32–37). Pang studied the effects of intraventricular UK on an experimentally produced intraventricular hemorrhage in a placebo-controlled canine model. He instilled 20,000 IU of UK into the ventricles of his canine model twice a day until a CT scan demonstrated complete clot lysis. Clot lysis was usually seen in 3–6 days in the UK group of animals but rarely seen prior to 7 days in the control group. Only mild systemic fibrinolysis was seen in the doses employed (35–37). Several Japanese groups have reported extensive experience with the use of UK in the treatment of SICH in humans, although no randomized, placebo-controlled study has been reported (39). Although the UK treatment regimens vary among published reports, most investigators report administration of 6000 IU of UK two to four times a day through a stereotactically placed catheter within the hematoma cavity. Aspiration of the liquified hematoma and repeat instillation of UK is continued for several days until clot lysis is complete as visualized on CT scanning. In 1985, Niizuma reported 97 cases of SICH treated with UK injection and aspiration within 24 hours of hematoma genesis and showed improved outcomes compared to patients managed either medically or with conventional craniotomy (29). He reported a rebleeding rate of 4% with the use of UK. A more recent report by the same author reviewed 122 patients with putaminal hemorrhages who underwent stereotactic aspiration and instillation of 6000 IU UK into the hematoma cavity (27). Over 80% of the hematoma was removed in 82% of the patients. Although removal of the hematomas was achieved over a period of days in this study, no statistical difference in outcome was found compared to craniotomy. In fact, functional outcome was improved in the patients who underwent open craniotomy in the larger hematomas, possibly due to rapid decompression of the surrounding viable brain tissue. The strategy of aspiration and use of fibrinolytic medication has been reviewed in large Japanese studies involving thousands of patients and is now used extensively in that country due to promising results with this type of treatment (44).

Several studies have investigated the utility of r-TPA, which is fibrin-specific, to facilitate aspiration of SICH (45). TPA appears to be safe when injected into the subarachnoid space for subarachnoid hemorrhage and into the ventricular system to dissolve intraventricular hematomas (33,46–49). TPA is a naturally occurring substance and is generally regarded as not producing an immunogenic response (50). The initial half-life of r-TPA is 3–5 minutes, whereas its terminal half-life ranges from 39 to 57 minutes (42). The disadvantages of r-TPA are the high cost due to manufacture through recombinant DNA techniques and the relatively short half-life. TPA cannot distinguish between hematoma and protective fibrin cap on a bleeding site and therefore has a similar potential risk of rebleeding as other thrombolytic medications. Investigations into other thrombolytic medications are ongoing and it is likely that new drugs with optimal half-lives, increased specificity, and more desirable chemical properties will be developed in the future that will greatly improve the treatment of SICH through stereotactic aspiration methodology (40,42,51–54).

MECHANICALLY ASSISTED ASPIRATION

The mechanical properties of clot formation have determined to a large extent the efficacy of aspiration to decompress a SICH. Because portions of the clot may solidify shortly after clot genesis, techniques have been used to either dissolve chemically or fragment the clots by physical means. Various devices have been used to mechanically morcellate the hematoma and facilitate aspiration through stereotactic methods. One of the earliest devices developed for such a use was a long-twist drill bit passed through a cannula through which regulated suction was applied. As clot was suctioned into the cannula, the rotating drill bit would theoretically cut portions of the clot and facilitate aspiration. This technique was patterned after the water screw principle of Archimedes, and introduced by Backlund and Holst in 1978 (55). The procedure was performed with the use of a 20-cm-long drill through a 4-mm cannula that was referred to as the Archimedes water screw device .

In 1982 Broseta described the use of the water screw method to evacuate SICH in 16 patients, but with a postoperative mortality of 81% (56). To improve the safety and increase the efficacy of clot removal, modifications have been made to this device by various surgeons. Modifications have included adding a thin-walled tube within the cannula to prevent clogging, addition of a motor, and use of a very thin screw (57–59). Kandel used this technique to evacuate hematomas in 32 patients presenting in ''grave condition'' and reported complete removal in 28 patients (88%) with a rebleeding rate of 16% and a mortality rate of 22% (58). The use of the water screw device has continued to the present but the procedure is time consuming, has variable and unpredictable yield with regard to clot decompression, has not been shown to be superior to either medical management or craniotomy, and remains a blind procedure during which active rebleeding cannot be easily detected.

Other devices have been investigated to aid in mechanical clot fragmentation but have not been widely accepted as safe, efficacious, or practical. Among the devices tested are water irrigation systems, ultrasonic aspirators, and oscillating cutters introduced through a cannula (60–62). A high-pressure water irrigation and suction system, referred to as the stereotactic aquastream and aspirator (SAS&A), has been shown to aspirate clot more efficiently than the Archimedes screw in an in vitro model but has not been widely used in the treatment of SICH (60). An ultrasonic device similar to the cavitron was developed in Japan to be used as an ultrasonic hematoma aspiration system (61). The ultrasonic device consisted of a 2-mm probe introduced stereotactically into the clot and has the capability of both ultrasonically dissolving a hematoma and efficiently aspirating the liquified clot. The devise was used in 375 patients with SICH of widely variable locations and sizes. Although the study was not randomized or controlled, the authors claimed improved outcome compared to either medical management or conventional craniotomy and open evacuation of the hematoma (61).

One of the more recent developments to facilitate stereotactic hematoma aspiration has been a modification of existing percutaneous diskectomy equipment that was initially designed to remove lumbar disks percutaneously under local anesthesia. The device is a modification of the nucleotome system (Surgical Dynamics, San Leandro, CA) and has been used to treat SICH primarily in France and rarely by a few investigators in the United States (62,63). The device consisted of an oscillating guillotine cutting blade in an enclosed cannula with the combined ability to apply suction and irrigation. The original nucleotome was modified by reducing the size and precisely regulating the suction applied to the tip of the probe. The resultant modified instrument, the hematome, could adjust the irrigation rate (0.3–1.0 cm^3/min), vacuum (0–593 mm Hg), and cutting speed (0–180 cpm), as needed to optimally remove the hematoma. The cannula has a closed tip and an open side port through which clot is theoretically aspirated, amputated, suspended in saline irrigation, and subsequently aspirated through an inner cannula into a collection reservoir. When used with vacuums of 150 mm Hg or less, it did not aspirate significant amounts of brain in a rat model, although the cutting rate was limited because cutting rates over 120 cpm experimentally decreased aspiration (64). In studies using an in vitro clot model with a vacuum of 150 mm Hg, the device could aspirate 75% of a 4-hour-old clot in approximately 15 minutes (64). A national U.S. trial of the device was attempted although investigator interest rapidly declined when the device was found to be time consuming, cumbersome, and impractical to apply. Despite improvement in technology, the hematome system remained a blind technique in which real-time anatomic monitoring to assess if active rebleeding was occurring was impractical, even if the procedure was performed in the CT suite.

NEUROENDOSCOPIC TECHNIQUES

There has been very little interest in use of endoscopic techniques in the treatment of SICH. A single randomized study of 100 patients treated with either best medical management or endoscopic decompression of SICH has been reported (65). The patient subgroups were well distributed in terms of size, location, age, and neurologic status. The hematomas were located in the putamen, thalamus, or the subcortical region. Outcome was assessed 6 months following the hemorrhage. The patients in this study with subcortical hematomas fared the best, with significant differences in outcome compared to the medically treated patients with hematomas in similar locations. Forty percent of the patients with subcortical hematomas who were treated with endoscopic hematoma decompression had good outcomes compared to 25% good results in the medical group. Unfortunately, patients with SICH within the putamen or thalamus had no difference in outcome with endoscopic surgery than those treated medically without decompression of the hematoma. This study seems to support that hematoma evacuation may be of some benefit in selected patients with lobar hematomas. This study did not address whether these patients

underwent a general anesthetic, had stereotactic methods employed, or the duration of the procedure required to achieve significant decompression of the hematoma. Endoscopic decompression of SICH may afford a simple, safe, reliable method of rapidly evacuating intracerebral hematomas without the risks of conventional craniotomy, but clearly further evaluation of this promising technology needs to be performed.

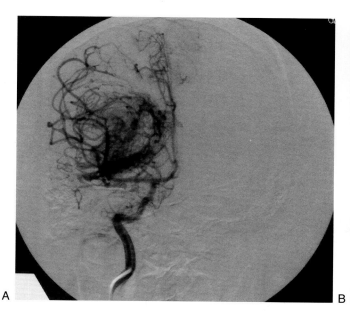

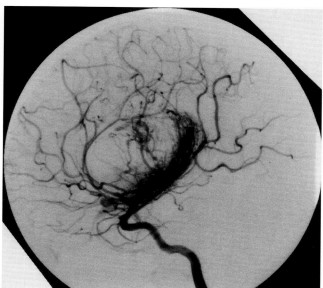

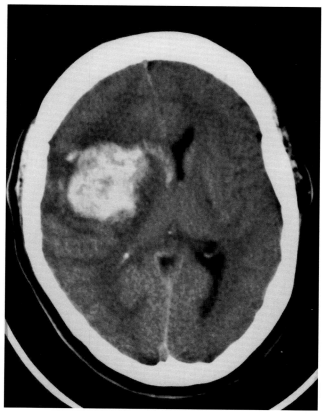

FIG. 2. (A) AP and **(B)** lateral cerebral arteriogram demonstrating ganglionic arteriovenous malformation as the etiology of apparent spontaneous intracerebral hematoma visualized with **(C)** CT scanning.

CONCLUSIONS

Despite significant advances in the technological and physiologic aspects of microvascular surgery, neuroanesthesia, and computer-assisted imaging techniques, very little progress has been made over the past 20 years in the treatment of SICH. Many questions remain unanswered as to the best form of treatment, which is surprising given that SICH is more common than subarachnoid hemorrhage and carries significantly higher morbidity and mortality. One of the difficulties in assessing new technological advances to potentially treat this condition is the lack of well-designed, controlled, randomized studies to determine which patients potentially benefit from a particular treatment. The diagnostic tests required to confirm the diagnosis remains controversial. It is not clear as to which patients should undergo MRI scanning and/or cerebral arteriography. Most of the innovative new techniques are blind techniques in which active rebleeding during hematoma evacuation cannot be immediately recognized, which is not the case with open craniotomy. If a previously unrecognized arteriovenous malformation (Fig. 2) or cavernous malformation (Fig. 3) is the etiology of the intracerebral hemorrhage in a patient with a history of longstanding hypertension, disastrous rebleeding could occur if any of the above-mentioned innovations are attempted for obvious reasons.

In a similar manner, the timing of optimal hematoma decompression, if elected, remains undetermined despite many attempts to answer this question experimentally and clinically. In order for future prospects of treatment to be rationally evaluated and ultimately accepted by physicians treating SICH, large cooperative studies will be needed to determine if surgical clot decompression has any significant impact on a particular group of patients and when decompression should be performed. Only then can the individual innovations for SICH decompression be scientifically evaluated as practical and generally applicable techniques to assist in the treatment of this common and severely disabling disease process.

REFERENCES

1. Matchar D, Duncan P. Cost of stroke. *Stroke Clin Updates* 1994;5: 9–12.
2. Bozzola FG, Gorelick PB, Jensen JM. Epidemiology of intracranial hemorrhage. *Neuroimag Clin North Am* 1992;2:1.
3. Drury ID, Whisnant JP, Garraway WM. Primary intracerebral hemorrhage: impact of CT on incidence. *Neurology* 1984;34:653.
4. Furlan AJ, Whisnant JP, Elveback LR. The decreasing incidence of primary intracerebral hemorrhage: a population study. *Ann Neurol* 1979;5:367.
5. Broderick JP, Brott T, Tomsick T, et al. Intracerebral hemorrhage more than twice as common as subarachnoid hemorrhage. *J Neurosurg* 1993;78:188–191.
6. Frankowski RF. Epidemiology of stroke and intracerebral hemorrhage. In: Kaufman HH, ed. *Intracerebral Hematomas.* New York: Raven Press, 1992;1–11.
7. Broderick JP, Brott T, Tomsick T, Huster G, Miller R. The risk of subarachnoid and intracerebral hemorrhages in blacks as compared with whites. *N Engl J Med* 1992;326:733–736.
8. Charcot JM, Bouchard C. Nouvelles recherches sur la pathogenia de l'hemorrhage cerebrale. *Arch in Physiol* 1868;1:110–127.
9. Ducker TB. Spontaneous intracerebral hemorrhage. In: Wilkins RH, Rengachary SS, eds. *Neurosurgery,* vol 2. New York: McGraw-Hill, 1985; 1510–1517.
10. Lisk D, Pasteur W, Rhoades H, Putnam R, Grotta J. Early presentation of hemispheric intracerebral hemorrhage: prediction of outcome and guidelines for treatment allocation. *Neurology* 1994;44:133–139.
11. Tuhrim S, Dambrosia JM, Price TR, et al. Prediction of intracerebral hemorrhage survival. *Ann Neurol* 1988;24:258–263.
12. Broderick J, Brott T, Tomsick T, Tew J, Kuldner J, Huster G. Management of intracerebral hemorrhage in a large metropolitan population. *Neurosurgery* 1994;34:882–887.
13. Kanaya H, Uijawa H, Itoh Z, et al. Grading and indications for treatment in ICH of the basal ganglia (cooperative study in Japan). In: Pia HW, Langmaid C, Zierski J, eds. *Spontaneous Intracerebral Hematomas: Advances in Diagnosis and Therapy.* Berlin: Springer-Verlag, 1980; 268–274.
14. Kaneko M, Koba T, Yokayama T. Early surgical treatment for hypertensive intracerebral hemorrhage. *J Neurosurg* 1977;46:579–583.
15. Kaneko J, Tanaka K, Shimada T, et al. Long-term evaluation of ultra-early operation for hypertensive intracerebral hemorrhage in 100 cases. *J Neurosurg* 1983;58:838–842.
16. Paillas JE, Alliez B. Surgical treatment of spontaneous intracerebral hemorrhage. Intermediate and long-term results in 250 cases. *J Neurosurg* 1973;39:145–151.
17. McKissock W, Richardson A, Taylor J. Primary intracerebral hemorrhage. A controlled trial of surgical and conservative treatment in 180 unselected cases. *Lancet* 1961;2:221–226.
18. Luessenhop AJ, Shevlin WA, Ferrero AA, et al. Surgical management of primary intracerebral hemorrhage. *J Neurosurg* 1967;27:419–427.
19. Batjer H, Reisch H, Allen B, Plaizier LJ, Su CJ. Failure of surgery to improve outcome in hypertensive putaminal hemorrhage. *Arch Neurol* 1990;47:1103–1106.
20. Kaufman HH, Schochet SS. Pathology, pathophysiology, modeling. In: Kaufman HH, ed. *Intracerebral Hematomas: Etiolooy. Pathophysiology, Clinical Presentation, and Treatment.* Raven Press: New York, 1992;13–22.
21. Acampora S, Profeta G, Troisi F. Stereotaxic evacuation of hematomas (Letter to the Editor). *J Neurosurg* 1985;62:460.
22. Shirakata S, Ohi Y, Fujita K, et al. Surgical treatment of hypertensive intracerebral hematoma in subacute stage. Aspiration method by needle

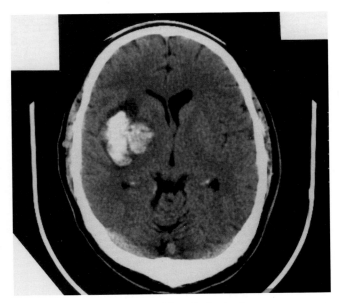

FIG. 3. CT scan of patient with pathologically proven cavernous malformation as the etiology of spontaneous intracerebral hematoma.

puncture into hematoma cavity. In: *Proceedings of the Fifth Conference of Surgical Treatment of Stroke.* Tokyo: Neuron, 1976;137–139 (Japan).

23. McKissock W, Richardson A, Walsh L. Primary intracerebral hemorrhage. Results of surgical treatment in 244 consecutive cases. *Lancet* 1959;2:683–686.

24. Beatty RM, Zervas NT. Stereotactic aspiration of a brain stem hematoma. *Neurosurg* 1973;13:207–207.

25. Nakai E, Komai N, Itakura T, et al. Stereotactic aspiration surgery for hypertensive pontine hemorrhage (poster). American Association of Neurological Surgeons, Dallas, May 3–7, 1987.

26. Bosch D, Beute GN. Successful stereotaxic evacuation of an acute pontomedullary hematoma. *J Neurosurg* 1985;62:153–156.

27. Niizuma H, Shimizu Y, Yonemitsu T, Nakasoto N, Suzuki J. Results of stereotactic aspiration in its cases of putaminal hemorrhage. *Neurosurgery* 1989;24:814–819.

28. Benes B, Vladyka V, Zverina E. Stereotaxic evacuation of a typical brain hemorrhage. *Acta Neurochir* 1965;13:419–426.

29. Niizuma H, Otsuki T, Jokura H, Nakazato N, Suzuki J. Ct guided stereotactic aspiration of intracerebral hematoma; result of a hematomalysis method using urokinase. *Appl Neurophysiol* 1985;48:427–430.

30. Niizuma H, Suzuki J. Stereotactic aspiration of putaminal hemorrhage using a double track aspiration technique. *Neurosurgery* 1988;22:432–436.

31. Matsumoto K, Hondo H. CT-guided stereotaxic evacuation of hypertensive intracerebral hematomas. *J Neurosurg* 1984;61:440–448.

32. Dujovny M, Yokoh A, Cuevas P, et al. Experimental intracerebral hematoma: urokinase treatment. *Stroke* 1987;18:280. (abstr)

33. Findlay JM, Weir BKA, Gordon P, Grace M, Baughman R. Safety and efficacy of intrathecal thrombolytic therapy in a primate model of cerebral vasospasm. *J Neurosurg* 1989;24:491–498.

34. Narayan RK, Narayan TM, Katz DA, Kornblith P, Murano G. Lysis of intracranial hematomas with urokinase in a rabbit model. *J Neurosurg* 1985;62:580–586.

35. Pang D, Sclabassi RJ, Horton JA. Lysis of intraventricular blood clot with urokinase in a canine model: 1. *Neurosurgery* 1986;19:540–546.

36. Pang D, Sclabassi RJ, Horton JA. Lysis of intraventricular blood clot with urokinase in a canine model: 2. *Neurosurgery* 1986;19:547–552.

37. Pang D, Sclabassi RJ, Horton JA. Lysis of intraventricular blood clot with urokinase in a canine model: 3. *Neurosurgery* 1986;19:553–572.

38. Segal R, Dujovny M, Nelson D, Meyer J. Local urokinase treatment for spontaneous intracerebral hematoma. *Clin Res* 1982;30:412A (abstr).

39. Kaufman HH. Stereotactic aspiration with fibrinolytic and mechanical assistance. In: Kaufman HH, ed. *Intracerebral Hematomas: Etiolocy, Pathophysiology, Clinical Presentation, and Treatment.* Raven Press: New York, 1992;181–186.

40. Collen D, Lijnen HR. Basic and clinical aspects of fibrinolysis and thrombolysis. *Blood* 1991;78:3114–3124.

41. Duckert F. Urokinase. In: Markwarot F, ed. *Fibrinolysis and Antifibrinolytics.* New York: Springer-Verlag, 1978;209–238.

42. Loscalo J, Braunwald E. Tissue plasminogen activator. *N Engl J Med* 1988;319:925–931.

43. Collen D, Lijnen HR. The fibrinolytic enzyme system. In: Sawaya R, ed. *Fibrinolysis and the Central Nervous System.* Philadelphia: Hanley and Belfus, 1990;14–25.

44. Kanaya H, Kuroda K. Development in neurosurgical approaches to hypertensive intracerebral hemorrhage in Japan. In: Kaufman HH, ed. *Intracerebral Hematomas.* New York: Raven Press, 1992;197–209.

45. Lippitz BE, Mayfrank L, Spetzger U, Warnke JP, Bertalanffy H, Gilsbach JM. Lysis of basal ganglia haematoma with recombinant tissue plasminogen activator (rtPA) after stereotactic aspiration: initial results. *Acta Neurochir* 1994;127:157–160.

46. Brinker T, Seifert V, Stolke D. Effect of intrathecal fibrinolysis on cerebrospinal fluid absorption after experimental subarachnoid hemorrhage. *J Neurosurg* 1991;74:789–793.

47. Brinker T, Seifert V, Dietz H. Subacute hydrocephalus after experimental subarachnoid hemorrhage: its prevention by intrathecal fibrinolysis with recombinant tissue plasminogen activator. *Neurosurgery* 1992;31:306–312.

48. Findlay JM, Weir BKA, Stollery DE. Lysis of intraventricular hematoma with tissue plasminogen activator. *J Neurosurg* 1991;74:803–807.

49. Findlay JM, Weir BKA, Kassell NF, Disney LB, Grace MGA. Intracisternal recombinant tissue plasminogen activator after aneurysmal subarachnoid hemorrhage. *J Neurosurg* 1991;75:181–188.

50. Jang IK, Vanhaechke J, DeGeest H, et al. Coronary thrombolysis with recombinant tissue-type plasminogen activator: patency rate and regional wall motion after 3 months. *J Am Coll Cardiol* 1986;8:1455–1460.

51. Collen D. Towards improved thrombolytic therapy. *Lancet* 1993;342:34–36.

52. DelZoppo GJ. Thrombolytic therapy in cerebrovascular disease. *Stroke* 1988;19:1174–1179.

53. Haber E, Quertermous T, Matsueda GR, Runge MS. Innovative approaches to plasminogen activator theory. *Science* 1989;243:51–56.

54. Marder VJ, Sherry S. Thrombolytic therapy: current status. *N Eng J Med* 1988;318:1512–1520, 1585–1595.

55. Backlund EO, Von Holst H. Controlled subtotal evacuation of intracerebral haematomas by stereotactic technique. *Surg Neurol* 1978;9:99–101.

56. Broseta J, Gonzalez-Darder J, Garcia-Salorio J. Stereotactic evacuation of intracerebral hematoma. *Appl Neurophysiol* 1982;45:443–448.

57. Higgins AC, Nashold BS. Stereotactic evacuation of intracerebral hematoma. *Appl Neurophysiol* 1980;43:96–103.

58. Kandel EI, Peresedov V. Stereotaxic evacuation of spontaneous intracerebral hematomas. *J Neurosurg* 1985;62:206–213.

59. Pan DH-C, Lee L-S, Chen M-S, et al. Modified screw and suction technique for stereotactic evacuation of deep intracerebral hematomas. *Surg Neurol* 1986;25:540–544.

60. Itoh H, Muka H, Kitamura A. Removal of hypertensive intracerebral hematoma with stereotactic aquastream and aspirator (SAS&A) for removal of intracerebral hematoma. *Neurol Surg* 17:939–943, 1989

61. Matsumoto K, Hondo H, Tomida K. Aspiration surgery for hypertensive brain hemorrhage in the acute stage. In: Suzuki J, ed. *Advances in Surgery for Cerebral Stroke. Proceedings of the International Symposium on Surgery for Cerebral Stroke*, Sendai, 1987. Tokyo: Springer-Verlag, 1988.

62. Nguyen JP, Decq P, Brugieres P, Yepes C, Melon E, Gaston A, Keravel Y. A technique for stereotactic aspiration of deep intracerebral hematomas under computed tomographic control using a new device. *Neurosurgery* 1992;31:330–334.

63. Onik G, Helms CA, Ginsburg L, et al. Percutaneous lumbar diskectomy using a new aspiration probe. *AJNR* 1985;6:290–293.

64. Kaufman HH, Herschberger J, Maroon J, Wilberger JE, Onik GM. Mechanical aspiration of hematomas in an in vitro model. *Neurosurgery* 1989;25:347–350.

65. Auer L, Deinsberger W, Niederkorn K, et al. Endoscopic surgery vs. medical treatment for spontaneous intracerebral hematoma: a randomized study. *J Neurosurg* 1989;70:530–535.

Cerebrovascular Disease, edited by H. Hunt Batjer.
Lippincott-Raven Publishers, Philadelphia © 1997.

CHAPTER 53

Hemorrhagic Infarction

Mark B. Rorick and Robert J. Adams

The term "hemorrhagic infarction" (HI) refers to a brain lesion in which evidence for hemorrhage is found either as multiple petechial areas or confluent zones within an area of necrosis caused by arterial occlusion (1,2). This process is fundamentally different from intracerebral hematoma (ICH), which is initiated by arterial rupture and is characterized by dense hematoma formation with mass effect. The two can be distinguished by radiologic and pathologic criteria and this distinction is important because of differences in etiology, prognosis, and management.

The typical computed tomography (CT) appearance of HI is a mottled mixture of hypodense and hyperdense areas in the cortical or deep gray matter (3) (Fig. 1). HI tends to be heterogeneous centrally and peripherally, irregular in contour, surrounded by a wide zone of low attenuation, and usually shows little evidence of mass effect. ICH is usually associated with a dense, homogeneous area with mass effect and often extension into the ventricular system (4). Location may help in differentiating HI from ICH. For example, hypertensive ICH usually involves the putamen, thalamus, cerebellum, or pons, and HI is most common in cortical areas. However, there is considerable variability in the appearance of HI on CT, ranging from a limited area of faint hyperdensity to a nearly confluent high-signal area that can be difficult to differentiate from an ICH. Subacute contrast enhancement may be present in both types of lesions but is usually "gyral" in pattern with HI and more of a "ring" enhancement with ICH (4). In some lesions there may be both hematoma and HI in the same affected area. Serial CT scans beginning in the early hours after a stroke are optimal for the accurate detection of HI.

On magnetic resonance imaging (MRI) hemorrhagic infarction has a high-signal appearance on T1-weighted images and a patchy signal void within a high-signal region on T2-weighted images. A cortical HI may consist of a serpiginous signal void in the cortical zone of affected gyri. MRI is more sensitive than CT in revealing small amounts of blood, and the characteristic MRI properties of blood breakdown products are visible for months after a hemorrhage (5).

PATHOLOGY, PATHOPHYSIOLOGY, AND ASSOCIATION WITH CEREBRAL EMBOLISM

The pathologic appearance is similar to that of cerebral infarction without hemorrhage and only the unique features will be mentioned here. Pathologists have long distinguished pale (anemic) and red (hemorrhagic) infarcts, the only difference being that the latter have numerous petechiae (6). The landmark studies of Fisher and Adams (1) provided a detailed pathologic picture of HI and established a causal link with reperfusion, which accompanied many cases of infarct due to cerebral embolism. They reported that 18% of 373 cases with cerebral vascular occlusion showed evidence of HI and that the vast majority of these were seen in cases of cerebral embolism (2). The hemorrhagic portion of HI was noted to be composed of multiple, small (0.2–2.0 mm in diameter), irregular petechial hemorrhages found typically in the gray matter of the basal ganglia or cerebral cortex (Fig. 2A). On microscopic section the hemorrhages surrounded or were found in relation to small blood vessels thought to be capillaries, venules, or small arterioles. The earliest observation of HI was in a patient who survived only 6 hours after cerebral infarction. They also documented the appearance at various stages from early neutrophil infiltration to ingestion of red cells by macrophages and astrocytic and fibroblastic reactive processes that were similar to infarctions without hemorrhagic change except for the presence of pigment-laden macrophages (Fig. 2B).

Based on their 57 cases in which the infarct was caused by embolism, they developed the theory of "migratory embolism." They reported that hemorrhagic areas were most often observed proximal to pale areas and that emboli were

M. B. Rorick: Department of Neurology, MetroHealth Medical Center, affiliated with Case Western Reserve University, Cleveland, Ohio 44109-1998.

R. J. Adams: Department of Neurology, Medical College of Georgia, Augusta, Georgia 30912.

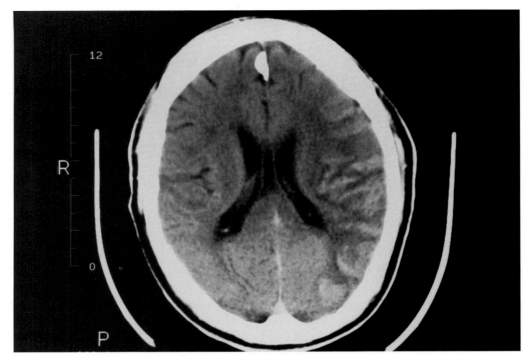

FIG. 1. Repeat CT 9 days later shows hemorrhagic infarction in the cortical gray matter.

usually found distally in the arterial tree to the point where occlusion, and subsequent infarction, was thought to first have occurred. The embolus first occludes the artery proximally, then fragments or otherwise moves distally leaving a (distal) part of the arterial distribution deprived of blood but allowing reperfusion of a more proximal part. The HI occurs in the reperfused part due to exposure of vessels damaged by ischemia to restored blood flow or sometimes at the periphery of the pale area due presumably to collateral flow to the rim of the infarct. In general, with HI the architecture of the infarcted tissue is preserved, which is in contrast to a primary cerebral hemorrhage where tissue is replaced or displaced by homogeneous clot (7).

Other autopsy studies supported the findings of Fisher and Adams and strengthened the association with embolism. In an autopsy series of Jorgansen and Torvik (8), 58 (or 42%) of 138 cases with recent cerebral infarcts were hemorrhagic and of these 42 (or 72%) were attributed to an embolic mechanism. Some of the hemorrhagic lesions were contained within the territories of branches proximal to the site of arterial occlusion, but others had embolic occlusions proximal to the entire infarcted area. They observed blood in various stages of resolution and suggested that bleeding may occur in stages. In an autopsy study of 48 patients dying within 15 days of supratentorial cerebral infarct, Lodder et al. reported a prevalence of HI of 33% of which 10, or 63%, were reported due to cardiac embolism (9). Hemorrhagic infarction was especially common in large infarcts associated with brain herniation.

Hemorrhagic infarction has been reported with persistent occlusion of the parent artery proximally indicating that hemorrhagic transformation is not always associated with migration of embolic material. Of 21 cases of HI with verified emboli on autopsy, the entire infarcted area was distal to the embolus in 7 cases (8). Yamaguchi (1987) recorded a few cases of "massive hemorrhagic infarction" in which repeat angiography and CT showed complete arterial occlusions that were confirmed by autopsy (10). Ogata et al. studied the brains of 14 patients who died of brain herniation after cardioembolic stroke and identified HI in 7 brains, pale infarct in 7 brains, and correlated these findings with the sites of occlusion of either or both the internal carotid and middle cerebral artery proximal to the lesion (11). Five of the 7 HI cases had occlusions of various sites in the middle cerebral artery whereas in 6 of 7 pale infarcts the arterial occlusions were in the internal carotid artery extending into the middle cerebral artery thus obstructing the proximal anterior cerebral artery and presumably a major pathway for collateral circulation. These findings were interpreted to suggest that HI in middle cerebral artery infarctions occurs when collateral circulation via leptomeningeal collaterals (12) reaches the periphery of an otherwise pale infarction. The location of the obstruction either allowed or blocked access via the proximal anterior cerebral artery and resulted in the presence or absence of hemorrhage. They also noted blood pressure elevations in 5 of 7 HI cases leading to speculation that poststroke hypertension may contribute to the incidence or severity of HI.

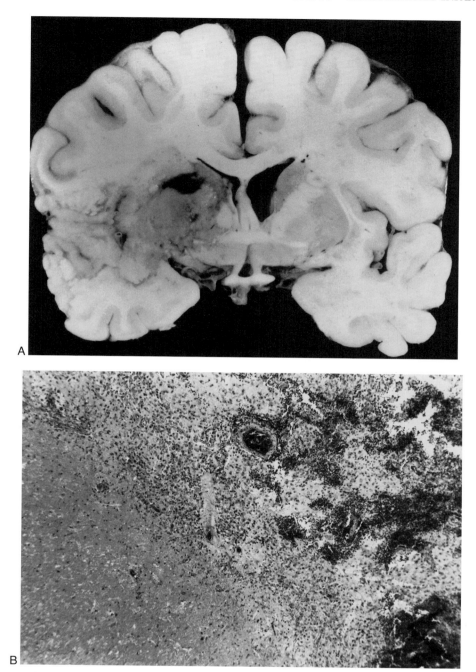

FIG. 2. Hemorrhagic infarct in a patient with atrial fibrillation and hypertrophic cardiomyopathy. **A:** Coronal brain slice shows hemorrhagic portions in the basal ganglia area within a large left middle cerebral artery infarct. **B:** Coagulation necrosis in tissue adjacent to an area with perivascular hemorrhage and foamy macrophages. Hematoxylin and eosin, ×4.

In summary, autopsy series have defined the location of hemorrhage and documented a common but not universal association with proximal patency of the involved arterial circulation. The majority of cases studied at autopsy have been attributed to embolism. Examples of HI on the periphery of infarcts in the presence of persistent arterial occlusion have been accounted for by reperfusion from leptomeningeal collaterals (7,11).

Angiographic studies have provided ample evidence that migratory embolism after stroke is a common occurrence that is often accompanied by HI. In an early (pre-CT) angiographic-autopsy series of patients with cerebral embolism the cerebral infarction was primarily hemorrhagic in one case where angiography was normal and in two cases where fragmentation of an embolus had been demonstrated on repeated angiography (13). In a series of 15 stroke patients with initially occluded internal carotid or middle cerebral arteries, bloody cerebrospinal fluid indicating development of HI occurred in 6 of 7 patients with recanalization and only in 1 of 8 without recanalization (14). Of 36 patients studied with CT and angiography within 6 hours of stroke onset, 18 developed HI on follow-up CT at 1 week (15). All cases of HI had initial angiographic occlusion of the middle cerebral artery (15 cases) or internal carotid artery (3 cases) acutely. There was follow-up angiography in only 3 of the 36 patients, but the authors used the presence of middle cerebral artery hyperdensity as a surrogate marker for middle cerebral artery occlusion. Based on this evidence, 15 of 18 patients had at least proximal recanalization. This study also supported the notion that the location of the hemorrhage may be related to the mechanism of reperfusion. Hemorrhage in the basal ganglia, not well supplied by collateral circulation, was always associated with apparent recanalization of the middle cerebral artery. Cortical hemorrhage could be seen either with recanalization or persistence of occlusion presumably because reperfusion in the latter cases came from leptomeningeal collaterals (15). Because recanalization, especially in cases of embolism, is not uncommon and leptomeningeal collaterals are potentially present in all patients, it is unclear as to why HI is not the rule rather than the exception in clinical practice.

NATURAL HISTORY

The range in prevalence of HI in autopsy series is 33–67%. Autopsy series are biased toward patients with large cerebral infarcts, particularly those developing herniation, and these series indicate a higher prevalence of HI than estimates based on CT or MRI studies of stroke survivors (2). The accuracy of estimates based on neuroimaging cannot be separated from the issue of timing of CT because most studies reporting HI in cerebral infarction using CT did not employ sequential or delayed imaging. The autopsy data suggest that HI is rare in the first few days after stroke and the CT data support this concept. Most series using early scanning (24–48 hours) report that about 4–8% of early scans in ischemic stroke patients show evidence of HI (16,17). How many ''convert'' to showing evidence of hemorrhage on delayed scanning is hard to determine. The study of Hornig et al. (18) remains the only study with multiple, sequential scans performed at regular intervals. While 6% of their 65 cases were positive for HI before day 3, a total of 28 were positive by the end of 4 weeks. Sequential scanning picked up 7 between the 3rd and 7th days, 15 between the 7th and 14th days, and 2 more between days 14 and 21. No cases were added after 21 days. This study suggests that CT scanning would have to be delayed until at least day 14 to include the majority of those cases likely to undergo hemorrhagic conversion. A study of 50 consecutive patients with acute ischemic strokes included initial CT scans performed within 5 hours of ictus. Scanning was repeated at 5–7 days.

Hemorrhagic infarctions were not diagnosed from any acute (<6 hours) scans but were present in 26% of second CT scans (19). A recent study compared CT and MRI in a prospective study of 50 consecutive patients scanned within 72 hours of stroke (20). None of the patients were treated with anticoagulation or thrombolytic treatment. Eighteen of 50 (36%) patients had HI on the basis of MRI criteria but only 8 had clear evidence from CT, supporting the notion that MRI estimates of HI may significantly exceed those based on CT due to increased sensitivity.

Studies with larger numbers of stroke patients may underestimate the occurrence of HI in stroke due to timing of CT scanning and incomplete rates of repeat study. In the NINDS stroke data bank CT scans from 1267 patients with ischemic stroke were stratified on the basis of each patient's risk for cardiogenic embolism. The presence of HI increased from 3.8% for low- and medium-risk groups to 8.9% for high-risk groups (N.S.) (16). The median times from stroke onset to the last CT were 72 hours, 75 hours, and 66 hours for the low-, medium-, and high-risk groups, respectively.

In summary, about 5% of ischemic stroke patients have HI on their initial CT scans but with delayed scanning this figure increases to the range of 26–43%, a figure closer to the estimates of prevalence from autopsy studies. Estimates from MRI are likely to be higher due to increased sensitivity. Hemorrhagic conversion, at least by CT, takes place largely between the 1st and 21st day after onset. Most of these are clinically asymptomatic (2).

RISK FACTORS FOR HI

Embolism

The pathophysiologic link between HI and cerebral embolism and reperfusion due to clot migration has been discussed. While cardioembolic strokes are thought to have a propensity for hemorrhagic transformation on this basis (2), it has been more difficult to firmly link CT evidence of HI with presumed cardiogenic embolism in large clinical series. Both the Lausanne (17) and the NINDS stroke data banks (16) have looked at the issue of whether HI on CT can predict the presence of cardiogenic stroke risk factors. In the larger (n = 1267) NINDS experience there was no significant difference in the rate of hemorrhagic infarcts on CT scanning (from 1 to about 3 days from onset) between low- and high-risk groups defined by clinical, electrocardiographic, and echocardiographic criteria. In the Lausanne registry (n = 305 for this analysis), patients with a presumed cardiac source of embolus had about twice the rate of hemorrhage on CT (7.9 vs. 4%, $p < 0.05$).

Infarct Features

There is considerable evidence linking HI with infarct size (2,19,23,24). Features of acute CT associated with higher risk of HI include volume of infarction, edema, and mass effect (19,22) and the appearance of hypodensity within 4 hours of symptom onset (15).

Hypertension

Although it seems reasonable that hypertension would predispose to HI, a history of hypertension or elevated blood pressure after stroke does not emerge as a risk factor for HI in clinical series (21,22,24,25).

Hyperglycemia

Hyperglycemia has been suggested as a possible risk factor for development of HI (19,25,26) but support for this association is unconvincing. While diabetes was more common among patients with HI compared to a case-control group with cerebral infarction (odds ratio 1.85) in the study of Beghi et al., the difference was not significant (25). Horowitz et al. found a higher glucose in their acute stroke patients with CT evidence of HI but glucose was also positively related to infarct size and clinical severity (27) confounding the issue. Overall, hyperglycemia has not stood out when other factors were considered.

Age

Increased age was found to be a risk factor for HI in one study, a finding that may have been confounded by infarct size (24). Other reports, however, do not suggest that age is an independent risk factor for HI (21,22,28)

In summary, most studies have shown a greater risk for HI in patients with presumed embolic infarcts and in those with early and large lesions, especially with mass effect. Other clinical features, such as age and hypertension, are possible but as yet not convincingly related to HI risk.

Anticoagulation

There has been much concern about the role of anticoagulation in either causing HI or promoting conversion of a hemorrhagic area into a dense hematoma that could cause clinical deterioration. Because there are many potential confounding factors the issue remains in question. The evidence ideally would come from randomized, controlled trials of anticoagulation in acute stroke using early and delayed CT observations. The one randomized trial comparing anticoagulation with no anticoagulation in early cardioembolic stroke reported two delayed hemorrhagic conversions in the control group and none among 24 anticoagulated patients (28). A randomized controlled trial of acute (< 48 hours) ischemic stroke not restricted to cardioembolic stroke compared the outcome in 112 patients given heparin with 113 patients treated with placebo. CT was done at entry but was repeated only in those in which neurologic progression occurred. They reported that no patients in either group had progression because of hematoma or hemorrhagic conversion of an infarct. A retrospective, nonrandomized series comparing 49 patients with acute cardioembolic stroke who received early anticoagulation with 41 similar patients who were not anticoagulated showed an equally low incidence of total hemorrhage (6 vs. 5) and the same number of hemorrhages associated with worsening (2 each group) (29). The case-control study of HI reported by Beghi et al. (25) did not identify anticoagulation as a significant risk despite the fact that more HI patients were on anticoagulation. The retrospective review of 41 cases presented by Hornig et al. (18) and 160 cases by Okada et al. (24) also failed to link anticoagulation with HI. However, there are many anecdotal and small series reporting hemorrhagic transformation in anticoagulated acute stroke patients, most of which are detected because of clinical worsening (21,30–32). This has led some authors to conclude that while the incidence of HI is not increased by anticoagulation, the consequences when it occurs may be more significant (2,21,33). In most of these reports the cases associated with worsening are of hematoma formation, not of HI, but the distinction may be irrelevant in this setting. Selected case series have been used to argue hazards of early anticoagulation counseling a waiting period of 24–48 hours or more and avoidance of anticoagulation in cases with large infarcts for 7 days or longer in cases with early CT evidence of hemorrhage (21). Others report good outcome (22) even with continued anticoagulation in the face of HI on CT scan (33). The issue remains unresolved.

Thrombolysis

Use of thrombolytics for myocardial infarction (Fig. 3) is associated with intracranial hemorrhage, and intracranial bleeding has posed a major concern in the use of thrombolytics for cerebral infarction. However, overall hemorrhage rates in patients with cerebral infarction given thrombolytics have been relatively low. This is in keeping with experimental data that has not generally shown an increase in conversion of ischemic to hemorrhagic infarcts in animals (34). Data from stroke treatment trials using thrombolytics in humans indicates a range of HI from 2% to 28% and of ICH from 0 to 11% (35–41). Some of these studies may underestimate the occurrence of HI because follow-up CT timing ranged from 24 hours to 4 weeks and the indication was clinical deterioration rather than scheduled surveillance. Analysis of all randomized and nonrandomized studies published for thrombolytic drugs given for acute ischemic stroke showed a mean incidence of petechial hemorrhage of only 10% (42). This estimate was based on widely variable rates with some studies possibly showing a lower occurrence of HI due to less sensitive CT screening methods and lower dosing of thrombolytic drugs. Despite a low overall incidence most studies contain cases with early deterioration

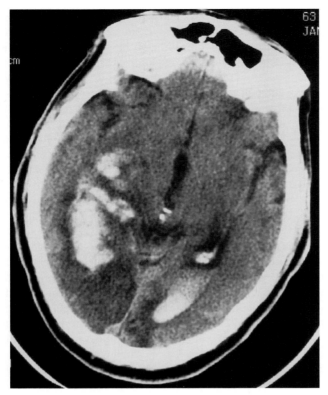

FIG. 3. Cranial CT showing a hematoma in the territory of a posterior cerebral infarction with intraventricular extension. This CT was performed 24 hours after the hospital admission and 18 hours after administration of tissue plasminogen activator (tPA) followed by heparin. The patient was a 70-year-old man who was brought to the emergency room by family members because of acute behavior change and confusion a day earlier. He was noted to have ECG changes consistent with myocardial infarction and treated with tPA. No CT scan was performed on admission or before thrombolytic therapy. The appearance of the scan indicates that the initial problem of this patient was a top of the basilar infarct producing confusion and visual symptoms. The hematoma was discovered on a CT performed because of persistent confusion. The patient's neurologic condition had not deteriorated and he remained alert for the next 3 weeks in the hospital and was eventually discharged.

including death from hematoma formation, which is likely related to treatment dose (40), and probably the time elapsed from the start of symptoms to treatment (38). The angiographic data acquired during the use of thrombolytic agents after stroke have given conflicting information on the importance of recanalization and presumed reperfusion in triggering HI. In a group of 77 patients treated within 6 hours of symptom onset with intraarterial urokinase, tissue plasminogen activator, or intravenous tissue plasminogen activator, HI more often developed in patients with recanalization by angiography at <8 hours or between 8 and 24 hours compared to patients without recanalization at those time periods (43). However, this study did not indicate that delayed recanalization, ie, between 8 and 24 hours after stroke onset, had

a greater likelihood of leading to HI than early recanalization. The duteplase study also used angiography and demonstrated no relationship between recanalization and the development of hemorrhagic transformation or discrete hematoma (38). The other thrombolytic trial with angiographic data (37) reported that three of four brain hemorrhages occurred in patients with no evidence of recanalization with treatment.

SUMMARY

Most studies indicate that HI is a frequent occurrence in stroke, especially with large infarcts of cardioembolic etiology but most of these are not associated with clinical deterioration. Neurologic deterioration occurring after stroke that is associated with cerebral hematoma while rare is probably more common with anticoagulation and thrombolytic treatment than when these agents are not used. The optimal strategy for the use of anticoagulation for the prevention of early recurrence of embolic stroke is not clear. Recommendations suggesting a delay of anticoagulation in cases with large infarcts until repeat CT scanning can be performed and further deferral of anticoagulation if HI is present are reasonable guidelines for most patients (44). Exceptions can be made for patients with particularly high recurrence risks and anticoagulation has been continued despite CT evidence of bleeding in some cases with clinical determination. Although excessive anticoagulation, hypertension, and hyperglycemia have not been consistently associated with HI, cautious control of these aspects of the stroke patient's care is certainly prudent. Although HI is often associated with embolism and reperfusion, CT evidence of HI alone is insufficient evidence to conclude the mechanism of a patient's cerebral infarction or the patency of the arteries supplying the area of infarction.

REFERENCES

1. Fisher CM, Adams RD. Observations on brain embolism with special reference to the mechanism of hemorrhagic infarction. *J Neuropathol Exp Neurol* 1951;10:92–94.
2. Hart RG, Easton JD. Hemorrhagic infarcts. *Stroke* 1986;17:586–589.
3. Savoiardo M, Grisoli M. Computed tomography scanning. In: Barnett HJM, Mohr JP, Stein BM, Yatsu FM, eds. *Stroke: Pathophysiology, Diagnosis, and Management*, 2nd ed. New York: Churchill Livingstone, 1992;155–187.
4. Kase CS, Mohr JP, Caplan LR. Intracranial hemorrhage. In: Barnett HJM, Mohr JP, Stein BM, Yatsu FM, eds. *Stroke: Pathophysiology, Diagnosis, and Management*, 2nd ed. New York: Churchill Livingstone, 1992;561–616.
5. Hesselink JR, Healy ME, Dunn WM, Rothrock JF, McCreight PHB, Brahme F. Magnetic resonance imaging of hemorrhagic cerebral infarction. *Acta Radiol Suppl* 1986;369:46–48.
6. Garcia JH. Circulatory disorders and their effects on the brain. In: Davis RL, Roberson DM, eds. *Textbook of Neuropathology*. Baltimore: Williams and Wilkins, 1985;548–631.
7. Fisher CM, Adams RD. Observations on brain embolism with special reference to hemorrhagic infarction. In: Furlan AJ, ed. *The Heart and Stroke*. New York: Springer-Verlag, 1987;17–36.
8. Jorgensen L, Torvik A. Ischemic cerebrovascular diseases in an autopsy series, Part 2. Prevalence, location, pathogenesis, and clinical course of cerebral infarcts. *J Neurol Sci* 1969;9:285–320.
9. Lodder J, Krijne-Kubat B, Broekman J. Cerebral hemorrhagic infarc-

tion at autopsy: cardiac embolic cause and the relationship to the cause of death. *Stroke* 1986;17:626–629.

10. Yamaguchi T, Minematsu K, Choki J. Arterial embolism. In: Wood JH, ed. *Cerebral Blood Flow: Physiological and Clinical Aspects.* New York: McGraw-Hill, 1987;503–517.

11. Ogata J, Yutani C, Imakita M, et al. Hemorrhagic infarct of the brain without reopening of the occluded arteries in cardioembolic stroke. *Stroke* 1989;20:876–883.

12. Vander Eecken HM, Adams RD. The anatomy and functional significance of the meningeal arterial anastomoses of the human brain. *J Neuropathol Exp Neurol* 1953;12:132–157.

13. Dalal PM, Shah PM, Sheth SC, Deshpande CK. Cerebral embolism: angiographic observations on spontaneous clot lysis. *Lancet* 1965;1: 61–64.

14. Irino T, Taneda M, Minami T. Sanguineous cerebrospinal fluid in recanalized cerebral infarction. *Stroke* 1977;8:22–24.

15. Bozzao L, Angeloni U, Bastianello S, Fantozzi LM, Pierallini A, Fieschi C. Early angiographic and CT findings in patients with hemorrhagic infarction in the distribution of the middle cerebral artery. *AJNR* 1991;12:1115–1121.

16. Kittner SJ, Sharkness CM, Sloan MA, et al. Features on initial computed tomography scan of infarcts with a cardiac source of embolism in the NINDS Stroke Data Bank. *Stroke* 1992;23:1748–1751.

17. Bogousslavsky J, Cachin C, Regli F, Despland PA, Van Melle G, Kappenberger L. Cardiac sources of embolism and cerebral infarction-clinical consequences and vascular concomitants: the Lausanne Stroke Registry. *Neurology* 1991;41:855–859.

18. Hornig CR, Dorndorf W, Agnoli AL. Hemorrhagic cerebral infarction—a prospective study. *Stroke* 1986;17:179–185.

19. Horowitz SH, Zito JL, Donnarumma R, Patel M, Alvir J. Computed tomographic-angiographic findings within the first five hours of cerebral infarction. *Stroke* 1991;22:1245–1253.

20. Weingarten K, Filippi C, Zimmerman RD, Deck MDF. Detection of hemorrhage in acute cerebral infarction. Evaluation with spin-echo and gradient-echo MRI. *Clin Imag* 1994;18:43–55.

21. Cerebral Embolism Study Group: Immediate anticoagulation of embolic stroke: brain hemorrhage and management opinions. *Stroke* 1984; 15:779–789.

22. Hornig CR, Bauer T, Simon C, Trittmacher S, Dorndorf W. Hemorrhagic transformation in cardioembolic cerebral infarction. *Stroke* 1993;24:465–468.

23. Lodder J, Van Der Lugt. Evaluation of the risk of immediate anticoagulant treatment in patients with embolic stroke of cardiac origin. *Stroke* 1983;14:42–46.

24. Okada Y, Yamaguchi T, Minematsu K, et al. Hemorrhagic transformation in cerebral embolism. *Stroke* 1989;20:598–603.

25. Beghi E, Boglium G, Cavaleti G, et al. Hemorrhagic infarction: risk factors,clinical and tomographic features, and outcome: a case-control study. *Acta Neurol Scand* 1989;80:226–231.

26. Broderick JP, Hagen T, Brott T, Tomsick T. Hyperglycemia and hemorrhagic transformation of cerebral infarcts. *Stroke* 1995;26:484–487.

27. Horowitz SH, Zito JL, Donnarumma R, Patel M, Alvir J. Clinical-radiographic correlations within the first five hours of cerebral infarction. *Acta Neurol Scand* 1992;86:207–214.

28. Cerebral Embolism Study Group. Immediate anticoagulation of embolic stroke: a randomized trial. *Stroke* 1983;14:668–676.

29. Rothrock JF, Dittrich HC, McAllen S, Taft BJ, Lyden PD. Acute anticoagulation following cardioembolic stroke. *Stroke* 1989;20:730–734.

30. Shields RW, Laureno R, Lachman R, Victor M. Anticoagulant-related hemorrhage in acute cerebral embolism. *Stroke* 1984;15:426–437.

31. Babikian VL, Kase CS, Pessin MS, Norrving B, Gorelick PB. Intracerebral hemorrhage in stroke patients anticoagulated with heparin. *Stroke* 1989;20:1500–1503.

32. Calandre L, Ortega JF, Bermejo F. Anticoagulation and hemorrhagic infarction in cerebral embolism secondary to rheumatic heart disease. *Arch Neurol* 1984;41:1152–1154.

33. Pessin MS, Estol CJ, LaFranchise F, Caplan LR. Safety of anticoagulation after hemorrhagic infarction. *Neurology* 1993;43:1298–1303.

34. del Zoppo GJ, Copeland BR, Anderchek K, Hacke W, Koziol JA. Hemorrhagic transformation following tissue plasminogen activator in experimental cerebral infarction. *Stroke* 1990;21:596–601.

35. del Zoppo GJ, Ferbert A, Otis S, et al. Local intra-arterial fibrinolytic therapy in acute carotid territory stroke. A pilot study. *Stroke* 1988; 19:307–313.

36. Hacke W, Zeumer H, Ferbert A, Bruckmann H, del Zoppo GJ. Intra-arterial thrombolytic therapy improves outcome in patients with acute vertebrobasilar occlusive disease. *Stroke* 1988;19:1216–1222.

37. Mori E, Tabuchi M, Yoshida T, Yamadori A. Intracarotid urokinase with thromboembolic occlusion of the middle cerebral artery. *Stroke* 1988;19:802–812.

38. del Zoppo GJ, Poeck K, Pessin MS, et al. Recombinant tissue plasminogen activator in acute thrombotic and embolic stroke. *Ann Neurol* 1992; 32:78–86.

39. von Kummer R, Hacke W. Safety and efficacy of intravenous tissue plasminogen activator and heparin in acute middle cerebral artery stroke. *Stroke* 1992;23:646–652.

40. Brott TG, Haley EC, Levy DE, et al. Urgent therapy for stroke. Part I. Pilot study of tissue plasminogen activator administered within 90 minutes. *Stroke* 1992;23:632–640.

41. Haley EC, Levy DE, Brott TG, et al. Urgent therapy for stroke. Part II. Pilot study of tissue plasminogen activator administered 91–180 minutes from onset. *Stroke* 1992;23:641–645.

42. Wardlaw JM, Warlow CP. Thrombolysis in acute ischemic stroke: does it work? *Stroke* 1992;23:1826–1839.

43. von Kummer R, Holle R, Rosin L, Forsting M, Hacke W. Does arterial recanalization improve outcome in carotid territory stroke? *Stroke* 1995;26:581–587.

44. Yatsu FM, Hart RG, Mohr JP, Grotta JC. Anticoagulation of embolic strokes of cardiac origin: an update. *Neurology* 1988;38:314–316.

Cerebrovascular Disease, edited by H. Hunt Batjer.
Lippincott-Raven Publishers, Philadelphia © 1997.

CHAPTER 54

Intracranial Vascular Malformations: Clinical Presentations

Winfield S. Fisher III

Arteriovenous malformations (AVMs) are about one seventh to one tenth as common as aneurysms; approximately 2500 new cases occur per year and 280,000 people in the United States harbor one of these lesions (1,2). There seems to be a male predominance varying from an incidence of just over 1:1 (male-to-female) to 2:1 (3). The embryonic formation of AVMs appears to be related to either retained fistulous communications between primordial vessels or development of abnormal channels during a very early stage suggesting a genetic role in the development of this disease (4). Additional evidence for a genetic contribution is the finding that AVMs may occur in conjunction with other AVMs (Fig. 1), venous and cavernous angiomas, and known familial relationships (although few in number) have been reported (5).

Hemorrhage, seizures, and increasing neurologic deficits are the clinical triad of important presentations for AVMs. Since clinical decision making for therapy of these lesions is dictated by knowing the natural history of these lesions, a full knowledge of their clinical presentations and their long-term risks is required. This chapter will deal solely with the clinical presentations of true AVMs and not deal with other "cerebral vascular malformations" such as telangiectasias, venous varices, venous angiomas, or cavernous angiomas (cavernomas).

CHRONOLOGICAL PRESENTATION OF ARTERIOVENOUS MALFORMATIONS

Luessenhop has developed an eloquent temporal presentation of symptoms according to age of presentation (6). For young children (less than 1 year of age) the major presentation is that of congestive failure. Later in childhood hydrocephalus due to venous compression becomes an important

presentation. As shown in a schematic format in Fig. 2, headache, hemorrhage, and seizures become more prominent presentations at later ages. In addition, neurologic manifestations presumed secondary to steal (ischemia) become more prominent with age as well.

Headache

Many AVM patients and their families report a longstanding history of headaches. Headaches are frequently reported

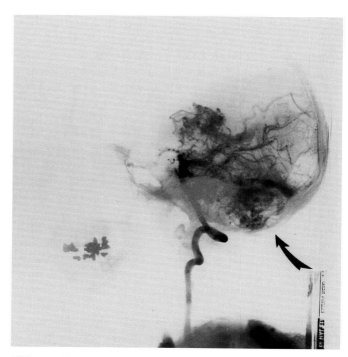

FIG. 1. Patient with two arteriovenous malformations (AVMs). One AVM is present in the thalamus and the other in the posterior fossa *(arrow)*. Such findings in the same patient suggest a genetic predisposition to AVM formation.

W. S. Fisher III: Division of Neurosurgery, University of Alabama at Birmingham, Birmingham, Alabama 35294.

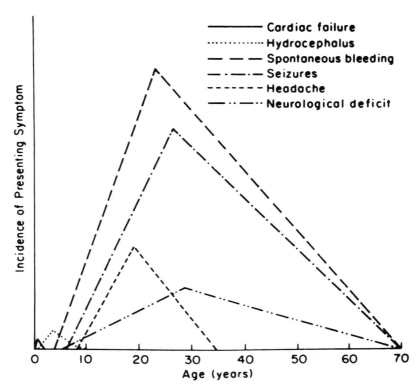

FIG. 2. Estimated rate of first appearance of symptoms correlated with the age at which they appear. (From ref. 6, p. 19.)

to be hemicranial, or occipital, leading to the description of the headaches as "migraines" (3). Troost and Newton reported headaches as a common initial presentation, with many of the features of migraine headache (scintillating scotomata, etc.) (7). Many of these patients did not have other more classical symptoms of migraine: the headaches did not affect the alternate side, the visual symptoms persisted during the headache, and the headaches persisted for a longer time than is common for migraine (7). On the other hand, common migraines occur in 10% of the population and classical migraines in 2% (3,7). The incidence of migraines among patients with AVMs does not seem to exceed that of the normal population, making it difficult to associate an elevated incidence of migraine headaches in AVM patients (3,7).

The pathologic etiology of these headaches is thought to be related to longstanding meningeal arterial involvement and recruitment of blood supply by the AVM. Drake reported the successful treatment of intractable headaches by embolization, supporting the theory of this meningeal contribution (8). Others have commented on the AVM location as a determinant in headache causation (other than due to obvious hemorrhage) (3). In Drake's series the majority of his patients' headaches were located in the occipital region. AVM location in the occipital area has been reported to be associated with increased frequency of headaches, presumably because of its regional association with the posterior

cerebral arteries, although the relationship between location and incidence of headaches remains controversial (3,8).

Hemorrhage

The primary reason to consider surgical intervention in any patient with an AVM is to prevent recurrent or future crippling hemorrhage. The annual risk of hemorrhage from an unruptured AVM is low, on the order of 2–4%, making it comparable to any other chronic disease with a long time horizon (2,9–16). However, the cumulative effects of this low rate over many years has been examined at length, and it has been determined that patients harboring AVMs do not enjoy as long a life expectancy compared to their non-AVM counterparts (2,9–16).

The frequency of hemorrhage from AVMs has been well studied. Pool reported the incidence of hemorrhage as 42% and epilepsy 33% (17). Svien and McRae in their study of 95 patients reported hemorrhage in 53%, epilepsy in 46%, and progressive neurologic deficit in 21% (16). The Cooperative Study of Intracranial Aneurysms and Subarachnoid Hemorrhage included a large number of patients in the collective grouping of all "cerebral vascular malformations." Of these, hemorrhage was a frequent presentation in 68% of cases, although this group included other etiologies such as cavernous malformations, etc. (15). Hemorrhage peaked between the ages of 15 and 20; by age 40, 72% of the hemorrhages had occurred (15).

A long time horizon of follow-up was established in Helsinki where patients were followed on average for 24 years by Ondra et al. (13). In this study a large series of 163 unoperated AVM patients, representing over 90% of the entire Finnish population presenting with symptoms from an AVM, were enrolled. Of this group of patients, 71% presented with hemorrhage and 24% presented with seizures. Interestingly, patients presenting with seizures had the same long-term incidence of hemorrhage as patients presenting with hemorrhage. Of further note, the average time between initial presentation and secondary hemorrhagic event was 7.7 years. A constant rate of hemorrhage (4% per year) was maintained for the first 20 years of the study followed by a 50% decline thereafter (2% per year) (13).

The consequences of hemorrhage in Ondra's series were underscored at follow-up. Approximately 43% of the original 160 patients had died, with 23% dying from a cause directly related to their AVM (13). The mean age of death in the study population for those patients dying from their AVM hemorrhage was 44 years of age compared to the mean age of death for the Finnish population of 73 years. Twenty-three percent of all patients in the Ondra study suffered either death or major morbidity with their first hemorrhage. The overall combined morbidity and mortality rates for their patients were 2.7% and 1% per year, respectively (13).

The clinical presentation of hemorrhage in a patient with an AVM may vary anywhere from simple mild headache to coma. Symptoms are related to the location of the hemorrhage; some of symptoms may be quite variable, depending on AVM location. Most patients will initially describe the acute onset of headache, which may rapidly worsen into weakness, neurologic deficit, or coma (as a reflection of an expanding hematoma). Subarachnoid blood may cause meningismus with signs of increased intracranial pressure. However, at times no intraparenchymal blood nor subarachnoid blood can be identified on scanning procedures. In this group of patients the headaches may be due to minor hemorrhage ("leakage") reflected in the degree of hemosiderin surrounding the AVM seen frequently at the time of surgical resection (18). Rare reports of subdural hematomas have also occurred (19).

The type of hemorrhage, be it subarachnoid, intracerebral, or subdural, really lends no clear clues that the etiology of the hemorrhage is an AVM. However, certainly if the symptoms of photophobia, meningismus, or focal neurologic deficit occur with sudden onset headache, an AVM needs to be included as part of the differential diagnosis. Location of the AVM dictates the type of presentation as well; hemorrhage is by far the most common presentation regardless of location, although with superficial supratentorial lesions seizures occur frequently (2,9–16).

Often the anatomic location of the hemorrhage is first detected by computed tomography (CT) scanning since such scanning is expedient and can accommodate patients who

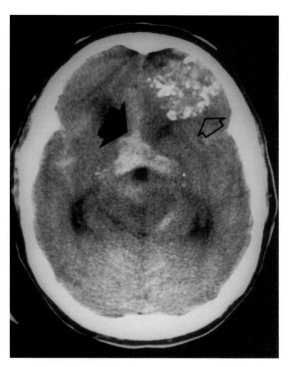

FIG. 3. Typical appearance of arteriovenous malformation (AVM) on noncontrast CT. This patient had a concomitant aneurysm with subarachnoid hemorrhage (SAH). Note calcification of AVM *(open arrow)* and SAH *(closed arrow)*.

are critically ill. The location and configuration of the hemorrhage on initial CT scanning can be helpful in guiding the physician into performing further diagnostic testing. Anatomically, AVMs have an inverted conical shape; the enlarged vascular loops, which may be calcified, can often be identified on simple CT scanning (see Fig. 3). Hemorrhage around the AVM may enhance this configuration and lend visual clues to the diagnosis (Fig. 4). Ventricular extension of hemorrhage with "casting" of the ventricles indicates that indeed the AVM is large enough to extend to the ventricular system (most cases) (Fig. 5). Unfortunately, most AVM patients usually present with a lobar hemorrhage, and a diagnostic arteriogram is required to differentiate these lesions from a hypertensive or other pathologic cause.

Morphologic and angiographic determinants of hemorrhage have been investigated. Concomitant aneurysms, AVM size, AVM location, angiographic findings (of intranidal aneurysm, venous stenosis, periventricular location, central venous drainage, and angiomatous change), and pregnancy have all been investigated for risk of AVM hemorrhage. Approximately 8–9% of all patients with an AVM also harbor an aneurysm. The majority of these aneurysms are located on feeding vessels, lending some credence to the developmental theory of aneurysm formation (20,21). It is impossible to determine from the literature which of these concomitant lesions (the aneurysm or the AVM) causes hemorrhage most frequently. Three hypothetical scenarios

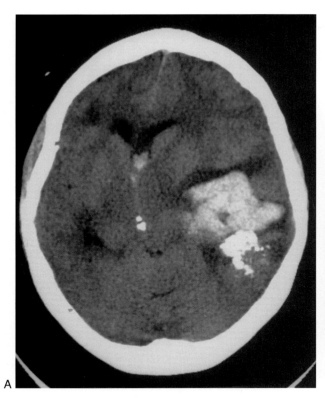
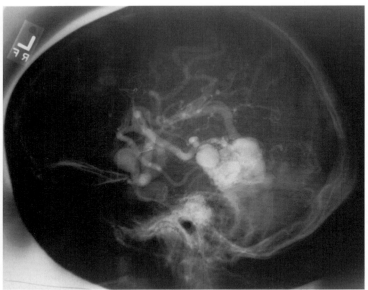

FIG. 4. A: CT (noncontrast) of patient with concomitant AVM and aneurysm. Note parenchymal hemorrhage contiguous with the AVM. **B:** Arteriogram of the same patient. Middle cerebral artery broad-based aneurysm is present. In addition, an intranidal aneurysm is present as well.

can occur with concomitant AVMs and aneurysms. First, the AVM is the source of hemorrhage (Fig. 4). In this group of patients clot is frequently contiguous with the AVM itself or intraparenchymal as seen on diagnostic studies. In the second scenario, the aneurysm has hemorrhaged with evidence of subarachnoid (or parenchymal) blood remote or distant to the site of the AVM (Fig. 6). The third scenario includes patients in whom it is impossible to tell which lesion bled (AVM or aneurysm). Therapy is usually directed to the symptomatic lesion because the risk of rehemorrhage for AVMs in the short term is quite low, whereas the risk of rebleed in the concomitant aneurysm is much higher and may actually be greater than that of a solitary aneurysm due to increased blood flow through the AVM.

Multiple authors have reported on the increased risk of hemorrhagic presentation in patients who have concomitant aneurysms. Brown et al. found that for patients with both lesions the risk of hemorrhage was statistically different than for patients without aneurysms who harbored an AVM (7% and 1.7% over 5 years, respectively) (21). Marks et al. found that intranidal aneurysms (aneurysms detected early in the angiogram and that fell into the confines of the nidus of the AVM) played a significant role in predicting risk of hemorrhage (22) (Fig. 7). Intranidal aneurysms were detected in 14% of their patients compared to 8% of their patients who had arterial aneurysms on feeding vessels (22).

The size of AVMs and their likelihood of hemorrhage was evaluated by Waltimo and others and remains a controversial issue. Waltimo's analysis of 45 patients revealed that lesions greater than 7 cm^3 were prone to seizures, whereas smaller lesions were prone to hemorrhage (23). Other larger series of small AVMs show no increased incidence of hemorrhage (21). Whether patients with small AVMs have not achieved a size sufficient to cause other symptoms (such as seizures or loss of neurologic function) remains the issue. Spetzler reported significance in his series of small AVMs (3 cm) vs. those greater than 6 cm for hemorrhage. In his patients they found higher intraarterial pressures in the smaller AVMs, suggesting a role in the more frequent incidence of hemorrhage (24). However, neither Brown nor Marks et al. found any association between size and risk of rupture (9,22).

Central AVMs may be more prone to hemorrhage than their superficial counterparts. This may be directly related again to selection bias in that most central AVMs are smaller and therefore may not have achieved a size adequate to cause other symptoms. Marks et al. described central venous drainage and periventricular location as statistically proven markers for predicting risk of hemorrhage; however, anatomic location was found to be a poor predictor (22). Most central AVMs have periventricular locations and central venous drainage.

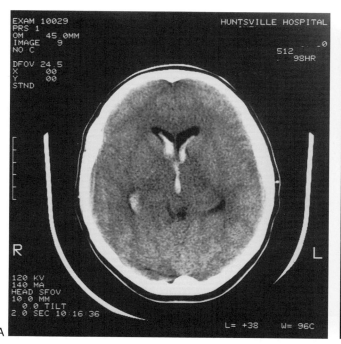

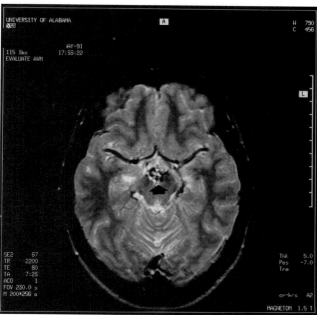

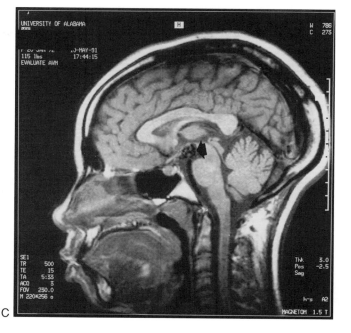

FIG. 5. **A:** Ventricular extension ("casting of ventricle") of hemorrhage from an AVM. **B, C:** Axial and sagittal MRI images of same AVM as in A, revealing its interpeduncular location.

Cerebellar AVMs have been identified to bleed more frequently than their counterparts located in the supratentorial spaces. Drake described a high percentage (92%) of hemorrhage in patients who presented with cerebellar AVMs (25). This high number is verified by other authors as well (26). In addition, posterior fossa AVMs seem to have a higher number of concomitant aneurysms as well (12 of 66 in Drake's series), possibly lending to the high incidence of hemorrhage (25). As with smaller cortical AVMs, the cerebellar AVMs may be recognized more frequently for hemorrhage than their supratentorial counterparts simply because

of the anatomic constraints of the posterior fossa (a small hemorrhagic lesion is less well tolerated) and the neurologic function of the tissue involved. Posterior fossa AVMs of the brainstem, however, frequently present with a more indolent course of increasing neurologic dysfunction as is seen in demyelinating diseases or neoplasms (25).

As previously mentioned, strong angiographic correlation for risk of hemorrhage has been found for central venous drainage, intranidal aneurysm, and periventricular location (22). In addition, strong negative correlation has been found for "angiomatous change," a term applied by Marks et al.

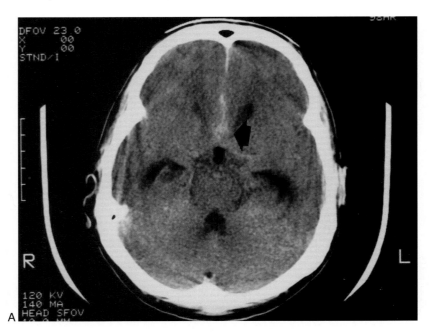

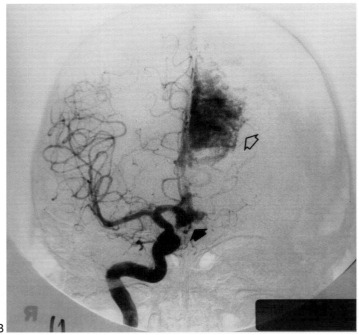

FIG. 6. A: CT (noncontrast) of patient with SAH from an anterior communicating artery aneurysm who also had a concomitant AVM. Solid arrow identifies the blood in the interhemispheric fissure. **B:** Arteriogram of same patient (*closed arrow*, aneurysm of the anterior communicating artery; *open arrow*, AVM).

to describe recruitment of cortical vessels other than direct feeding vessels to the AVM (22). It has been hypothesized that these patients may actually have lower pressures within their AVMs, making them less prone to hemorrhage, ie, the "angiomatous change" was a marker of low perfusion pressures and high degree of shunt.

A frequently declared but less strongly proven angiographic predictor of hemorrhage is that of venous stenosis (particularly of deep AVMs) (22,27). Vinuela described a high degree of venous stenosis of deep AVMs, particularly involving the vein of Galen (27). No mention of increased

bleeding frequency was reported, however. Marks et al. found a trend toward hemorrhage with venous stenosis (but no significance [$p = 0.09$]) in the presence of venous stenosis (22).

The question of increased risk of hemorrhage of AVMs during pregnancy remains controversial (28–30). Frequently categorized with aneurysms as a source of intracranial hemorrhage in the pregnant female, it is difficult to discern the most common time period during pregnancy for AVM presentation. It appears that the incidence of hemorrhage is approximately equal for both lesions (AVMs and aneurysms)

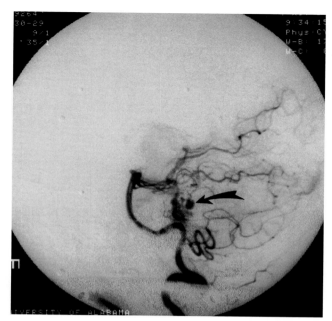

FIG. 7. Lateral arteriogram of AVM. Note intranidal aneurysm (arrow).

and that pregnancy has an adverse effect on incidence. Despite the implication that increased blood volume may play a role, no good data exist to suggest that the third trimester in particular is a time prone to AVM hemorrhage. Soft data seem to suggest that pregnant females are susceptible to rehemorrhage on the order of 25% during the same pregnancy (28–30).

Children present as an interesting subgroup of patients with AVMs. The leading cause of intracranial (nontraumatic) hemorrhage in children are AVMs, especially in young children where aneurysm rupture is rare. Patients less than 1 year of age frequently present with congestive high-output heart failure rather than hemorrhage simply because of the fistulous shunt through the AVM. Hydrocephalus can also play a prominent role due to compression of cerebrospinal fluid paths due to enlarging venous outflow channels (6,31–37) (Fig. 8). After the first year, pediatric AVMs mimic those of adults in that the sex ratio and location are not particularly different than they are for adults (32). Ostergaard reported two cases of his series of 16 pediatric patients who harbored concomitant aneurysm and AVM (36). Celli et al. reported that in their series of patients outcome was worse than in a comparable adult population. Mortality rates in the pediatric group was approximately doubled that of the adults (23% vs. 14.5%). In addition, the pediatric patients were more prone to coma (31%) compared to their adult counterparts (11–17%) after hemorrhagic presentation (32).

Seizures

Seizures are clearly the second most common presentation of AVMs, occurring in approximately 70% of AVM patients.

The percentage of patients presenting with seizures is remarkably constant across most series: Drake (18%), Heros (24%), Stein (26%), Yasargil (33.1%), and Ondra and Troupp (24%) (1,8,13,38,39). The seizure itself may represent dynamic processes occurring within the AVM (a small hemorrhage, "leakage," or thrombosis [Fig. 9]), and more often than not present focally (45–59% of the time).

The factors influencing the development of seizures were described by Crawford et al. (40). Of 343 patients, the AVMs of 61 patients with seizures were significantly larger (>6 cm) and more superficial than patients with hemorrhage. The majority of the patients with seizures had supratentorial AVMs (90%). Of a small number of patients followed prospectively who were not operated on, there was a trend to develop seizures in the superficial lesions vs. the deep lesions. Younger patients had a higher risk of developing seizures, and statistical significance was found with decreasing susceptibility to development of epilepsy with age (40).

Progression in Neurologic Dysfunction

Progression of neurologic dysfunction has often been ascribed to long-term effects of recurrent small hemorrhages, mass effect of the AVM, hydrocephalus, ischemic complications, and "steal." Steal is a term used to describe blood flow away from a region of the brain in order to flow toward the shunt (area of reduced intraarterial pressure) of the AVM. This flow may cause symptoms in an area remote from the AVM and typically causes hypoperfusion, ischemia, and symptoms in the region where the blood was "stolen."

Vascular ischemia caused by steal does seem to have a patho-physiologic basis (41–44). Constantino and Vinters reported a case of a patient with an occipital lobe AVM who died from a pulmonary embolus. This patient's AVM was discovered because of temporal lobe seizures. On autopsy the patient was found to have neuronal changes in the temporal lobe presumed to be due to the ischemia caused by steal from the occipital lobe AVM (41).

Other supporting evidence for progression of neurologic dysfunction is supported by the evidence that AVMs enlarge as patients get older (6). With this enlargement there is an associated decline in neurologic function that may also be related to steal. Feeding vessels to the AVM also elongate and enlarge as they approach the AVM and resume a more normal size after resection of the AVM (42). These radiographic findings suggest that the AVM shunt enhances progressive enlargement of feeding vessels due to low intraluminal pressure and high flow. Elegant studies using intraoperative Doppler techniques have identified high flow velocities of feeding vessels to AVMs (42). Nornes has demonstrated by means of direct intraarterial puncture, low intraarterial feeding pressures (42). Cerebral perfusion pressure (CPP: inflow pressure − outflow pressure) is reduced in patients with AVMs not only because of a reduced arterial feeding vessel pressure but because of elevated venous out-

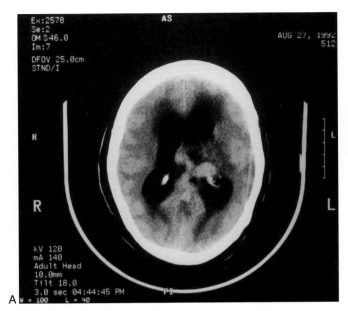

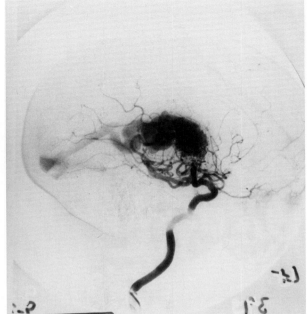

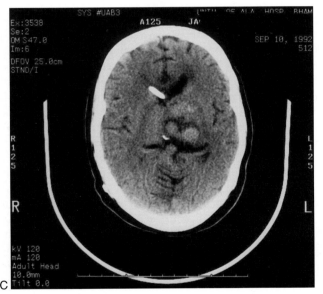

FIG. 8. A: CT (noncontrast) of a developmentally delayed adult, with slowly progressive decline in level of consciousness. Note large venous outflow channels. **B:** Arteriogram of the same patient. **C:** CT after treatment of hydrocephalus.

flow pressure as well (42). Adjacent arteries to the AVM are maximally dilated because of the low CPP. Therefore, surrounding cerebral tissue near the AVM remains in a state of constant chronic ischemia with the potential of causing associated progressive and stepwise neurologic deficits (42). Physiologic demonstration of the steal phenomenon with its associated hypoperfusion exists (42,43) and will be discussed at length in other chapters in this text. However with treatment, patients with steal have been reported to improve in their neurologic function. Luessenhop reported such a case of a patient who had an embolization of her lesion with dramatic improvement of a left spastic paraparesis (3,44).

The incidence of steal and increasing neurologic dysfunction varies from series to series, probably because the precise

definition of the entity is unclear, and the only way to clearly define the presence of induced ischemia by steal is to document reversal of its effects after resection. Yasargil reported an even distribution between those individuals who had neurologic dysfunction and those who did not in his patients who did not present with hemorrhage (10.6% versus 9.9%) (45). Brown described 12 patients of a series of 146 whose primary reason for investigation was ischemia caused by AVM (8%) (9). Fults and Kelley reported a much lower incidence of symptoms related to nonhemorrhagic and nonepileptic causes; hemiparesis not associated with hemorrhage occurred in 2.3% of their patients (12). Crawford et al. reported an incidence of 7% of all patients who presented with neurologic (nonhemorrhagic, nonepileptic) symptoms

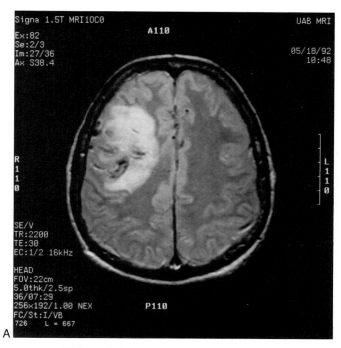
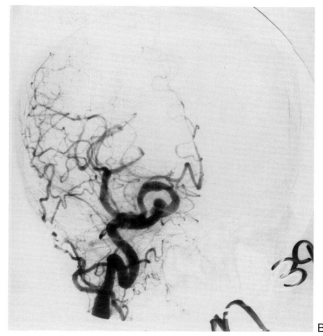

FIG. 9. A: MRI of elderly patient presenting with seizures and the acute onset of confusion that persisted over several weeks. Note the degree of edema surrounding the lesion and the hint of multiple vascular loops. **B:** Arteriogram of the same patient. Note the vessel tortuosity. This was considered to be a case of a truly angiographically occult AVM.

at diagnosis (10). Drake reported 5 patients of 166 who presented with steal (3%) (8). Although identifiable with sophisticated cerebral blood flow exams (43), the clinical diagnosis becomes difficult in light of the alternative diagnosis of small subclinical but incremental hemorrhages experienced by the patient. Although frequently described, the true incidence of steal is not known.

SPECIAL TYPES OF AVMS

Vein of Galen

Two types of AVMs that fall under the domain of intracranial vascular malformations are vein of Galen aneurysms and dural AVMs. Vein of Galen aneurysms can be considered a misnomer because the venous aneurysm per se is a direct result of the venous outflow for a high arteriovenous shunt system (31,33,34,37). Vein of Galen aneurysms are thought to occur between vessels of choroidal origin. Since the high-flow shunt occurs in the midst of a developing and pliable brain, the vein of Galen can reach sizes of tremendous proportions. Categorization of the vein of Galen aneurysms has been divided into two types: primary, those true fistulas that drain directly into the vein of Galen; and secondary, where a nidus is usually in close proximity to the vein of Galen, which is the dilated venous outflow for the AVM shunt (31).

The presentation of patients with vein of Galen aneurysms depends very much on the age of the patient. Young neonatal patients present with congestive failure, hydrocephalus, or both (31,33,34,37). Therapy is directed to converting the high-output failure to that which is more controllable. Johnston et al. reviewed the world's literature of vein of Galen aneurysms and found, as others have, that circulatory symptoms are the most prominent presentation of neonates, that young children (less than age five) present with symptoms of hydrocephalus, and thereafter the presentation can become one of recurrent subarachnoid or intracranial hemorrhage (34).

Dural AVMs

Dural AVMs are a developmental entity whereby the nidus of the AVM is restricted entirely to the leaves of the dura. At times, the clinical presentation may be difficult to detect, and the natural history of these lesions is not well established. Spontaneous remissions are possible (46,47). Nevertheless, the consensus is that these lesions are acquired, ie, they either occur spontaneously or are associated with other events such as trauma, surgery, or viral prodromes. Similar to intradural AVMs, the symptoms of presentation of DAVMs are directly related to the location of the lesion. Clinically the presentation of these patients involves one of three major presentations: subjective murmur or bruit, ophthalmologic symptoms (either painful and/or with paralysis), or symptoms secondary to increased intracranial pressure and focal neurologic symptoms. Hemorrhage, although rare, is one of the feared complications of the more aggressive types of DAVMs (46,47).

By far the most common symptom reported by patients is that of a subjective bruit, usually heard over the transverse sinus where venous stenosis or occlusion has occurred. These patients commonly present with the complaint of insomnia and anxiety associated with this murmur. Whether because of postural changes or lack of nocturnal noises, patients report that the bruit disrupts sleep and causes elevation of anxiety. Occasionally, the patient will report an antecedent episode of a viral prodrome or illness but the relationship of these symptoms is unclear.

Patients with ocular symptoms may also complain of bruit, which can be difficult to auscultate on exam. Although at times painless, frequently ophthalmologic symptoms are associated with pain. Intraocular pressure can be elevated because of venous congestion; more commonly patients present with ophthalmoplegic symptoms requiring intervention because of the degree of diplopia. Scleral injection and proptosis may also occur if the degree of venous hypertension is significant. Papilledema may be present as an indirect effect of increased intracranial hypertension from venous pressure elevation, hydrocephalus, or pseudotumor.

Venous congestion with local ischemic changes have been the hypothesized etiology for patients with focal neurologic deficits. Certainly hemorrhage of the lesion into adjacent regions can cause focal deficits, headaches, and neurologic dysfunction, but documented cases of steal as seen in intradural AVMs have not been reported.

Face pain may be a presentation of symptoms related to DAVMs involving the leaves of dura in close proximity of the fifth cranial nerve. In addition to face pain, patients periodically present with signs and symptoms of SAH, which at times may be severe with extension of blood into the ventricular cavities. Predicting which of these patients will go to become more aggressive has been reviewed by Awad and co-workers. In their report (a meta-analysis of over 360 DAVMs) the features of 100 aggressive DAVMs were assessed. Leptomeningeal retrograde venous drainage, variceal or aneurysmal venous structures, and Galenic venous drainage were all found to have significance in predicting aggressive lesions (47). Further discussion regarding the analysis and care of these lesions will occur in later chapters.

REFERENCES

1. Stein BM, Kader A. (Honored Guest Lecture) Intracranial arteriovenous malformations. *Clin Neurosurg* 1992;39:76–113.
2. Wilkins RH. Natural history of intracranial vascular malformations; a review. *Neurosurgery* 1985;16:421–430.
3. Mohr JP. Neurological manifestations and factors related to therapeutic decisions. In: Wilson CB, Stein BM, eds. *Intracranial Arteriovenous Malformations.* Baltimore: Williams and Wilkins, 1984;1–11.
4. Yasargil MG. Pathological considerations. In: Yasargil MG, ed. *Microneurosurgery. vol IIIA. AVM of the Brain, History, Embryology, Pathological Considerations, Hemodynamics, Diagnostic Studies, Microsurgical Anatomy.* New York: Georg Thieme Verlag, 1987;49–56.
5. Yokoyama K, Asano Y, Murakawa T, Takada M, Ando T, Sakai N, Yamada H, Iwata. Familial occurrence of arteriovenous malformation of the brain. *J Neurosurg* 1991;74:585–589.
6. Luessenhop AJ. Natural history of cerebral arteriovenous malformations. In: Wilson CB, Stein BM, eds. *Intracranial Arteriovenous Malformations.* Baltimore: Williams and Wilkins, 1984;12–23.
7. Troost BT, Newton TH. Occipital lobe arteriovenous malformations: clinical and radiologic features in 26 cases with comments on differentiation from migraine. *Arch Ophthalmol* 1956;93:250–256.
8. Drake CG. Cerebral ateriovenous malformations: considerations for and experience with surgical treatment in 166 cases. *Clin Neurosurg* 1979;26:145–208.
9. Brown RD, Wiebers DO, Forbes G, O'Fallon WM, Piepgras DG, Marsh WR, Maciunas RJ. The natural history of unruptured intracranial arteriovenous malformations. *J Neurosurg* 1988;68:352–357.
10. Crawford PM, West CR, Chadwick DW, Shaw MDM. Arteriovenous malformations of the brain: natural history in unoperated patients. *J Neurol Neurosurg Psychiatry* 1986;49:1–10.
11. Forster DMC, Steiner L, Hakanson S. Arteriovenous malformations of the brain. A long-term clinical study. *J Neurosurg* 1972;37:562–570.
12. Fults D, Kelly DL. Natural history of arteriovenous malformations of the brain: a clinical study. *Neurosurgery* 1984;15:658–662.
13. Ondra SL, Troupp H, George ED, Schwab K. The natural history of symptomatic arteriovenous malformations of the brain: a 24-year follow-up assessment. *J Neurosurg* 1990;73:387–391.
14. Graf CJ, Perret GE, Torner JC. Bleeding from cerebral arteriovenous malformations as part of their natural history. *J Neurosurg* 1983;58:331–337.
15. Perret G, Nishioka H. Arteriovenous malformations: an analysis of 545 cases of cranio-cerebral arteriovenous malformations and fistulae reported to the cooperative study. *J Neurosurg* 1966;25:467–490.
16. Svien HJ, McRae JA. Arteriovenous anomalies of the brain: fate of patients not having definitive surgery. *J Neurosurg* 1965;23:23–28.
17. Pool JL. Treatment of arteriovenous malformations of the cerebral hemispheres. *J Neurosurg* 1962;19:136–141.
18. McCormick WF. The pathology of vascular (''arteriovenous'') malformations. *J Neurosurg* 1966;24:807–816.
19. Martin NA, Wilson CB. Preoperative and post-operative care. In: Wilson CB, Stein BM, eds. *Intracranial Arteriovenous Malformations.* Baltimore: Williams and Wilkins, 1984;234–245.
20. Stehbens WE. Etiology of intracranial berry aneurysms. *J Neurosurg* 1989;70:823–831.
21. Brown RD, Wiebers DO, Forbes GS. Unruptured intracranial aneurysms and arteriovenous malformations: frequency of intracranial hemorrhage and relationship of lesions. *J Neurosurg* 1990;73:859–863.
22. Marks MP, Lane B, Steinberg GK, Chang PJ. Hemorrhage in intracerebral arteriovenous malformations: angiographic determinants. *Radiology* 1990;176:807–813.
23. Waltimo O. The relationship of size, density and location of intracranial arteriovenous malformations to the type of initial symptom. *J Neurol Sci* 1973;19:13–19.
24. Spetzler RF, Hargraves RW, McCormick PW, Zabramski JM, Flom RA, Zimmerman RS. Relationship of perfusion pressure and size to risk of hemorrhage from arteriovenous malformations. *J Neurosurg* 1992;76:918–923.
25. Drake CG, Friedman AH, Peerless SJ. Posterior fossa arteriovenous malformations. *J Neurosurg* 1986;64:1–10.
26. Batjer H, Samson Duke. Arteriovenous malformations of the posterior fossa. Clinical presentation, diagnostic evaluation, and surgical treatment. *J Neurosurg* 1986;64:849–856.
27. Vineula F, Nombela L, Roach MR, Fox AJ, Pelz, DM. Stenotic and occlusive disease of the venous drainage system of deep brain AVM's. *J Neurosurg* 1985;63:180–184.
28. Dias MS, Sekhar LN. Intracranial hemorrhage from aneurysms and arteriovenous malformations during pregnancy and the puerperium. *Neurosurgery* 1990;27:855–866.
29. Horton JC, Chambers WA, Lyons SL, Adams RD, Kjellberg RN. Pregnancy and the risk of hemorrhage from cerebral arteriovenous malformations. *Neurosurgery* 1990;27:867–872.
30. Robinson JL, Hall CS, Sedzimir CB. Arteriovenous malformations, aneurysms, and pregnancy. *J Neurosurg* 1974;41:63–70.
31. Amacher AL. Vein of Galen aneurysms. In: Wilkins RH, Rengachary SS, eds. *Neurosurgery.* New York: McGraw-Hill, 1985;1459–1465.
32. Celli P, Ferrante L, Palma L, Cavedon G. Cerebral arteriovenous mal-

formations in children. Clinical features and outcome of treatment in children and in adults. *Surg Neurol* 1984;22:43–49.

33. Hoffman HJ, Chuang S, Hendrick EB, Humphreys RP. Aneurysms of the vein of Galen. Experience at the Hospital for Sick Children, Toronto. *J Neurosurg* 1982;57:316–322.

34. Johnston IH, Whittle IR, Besser M, Morgan MK. Vein of Galen malformation: diagnosis and management. *Neurosurgery* 1987;20:747–758.

35. Kelly JJ, Mellinger JF, Sundt TM. Intracranial arteriovenous malformations in childhood. *Ann Neurol* 1978;3:338–343.

36. Ostergaard JR. Association of intracranial aneurysm and arteriovenous malformation in childhood. *Neurosurgery* 1984;14:358–362.

37. Yasargil MG, Antic J, Laciga R, Jain KK, Boone SC. Arteriovenous malformations of vein of Galen: microsurgical treatment. *Surg Neurol* 1976;6:195–200.

38. Heros RC, Korosue K, Diebold PM. Surgical excision of cerebral arteriovenous malformations: late results. *Neurosurgery* 1990;26:570–578.

39. Yasargil MG. Clinical considerations. In: Yasargil MG, ed. *Microneurosurgery. vol IIIB. AVM of the Brain, Clinical Considerations, General and Special Cooperative Techniques, Surgical Results, Nonoperated Cases, Cavernous and Venous Angiomas, Neuroanesthesia.* New York: Georg Thieme Verlag, 1988;19–20.

40. Crawford PM, West CR, Shaw MDM, Chadwick DW. Cerebral arteriovenous malformations and epilepsy: factors in the development of epilepsy. *Epilepsia* 1986;27:270–275.

41. Constantino A, Vinters HV. A pathologic correlate of the 'steal' phenomenon in a patient with cerebral arteriovenous malformation. *Stroke* 1986;17:103–106.

42. Nornes H. Quantitation of altered hemodynamics. In: Wilson CB, Stein BM, eds. *Intracranial Arteriovenous Malformations.* Baltimore: Williams and Wilkins, 1984;32–43.

43. Batjer HH, Devous MD, Seibert GB, Purdy PD, Ajmani AK, Delarosa M, Bonte FJ. Intracranial arteriovenous malformation: relationships between clinical and radiographic factors and ipsilateral steal severity. *Neurosurgery* 1988;23.322–328.

44. Luessenhop AJ, Mujica P. Embolization of segments of the circle of Willis and adjacent arteries for management of certain inoperable cerebral arteriovenous malformations. *J Neurosurg* 1981;54:573–582.

45. Yasargil MG. Clinical considerations. In: Yasargil MG, ed. *Microneurosurgery. vol IIIB, AVM of the Brain, Clinical Considerations, General and Special Operative Techniques, Surgical Results, Nonoperated Cases, Cavernous and Venous Angiomas, Neuroanesthesia.* New York: Georg Thieme Verlag, 1988;21–22.

46. Lasjaunias P, Chiu M, Brugge KT, Tolia A, Hurth M, Bernstein M. Neurologic manifestations of intracranial dural arteriovenous malformations. *J Neurosurg* 1986;64:724–730.

47. Awad IA, Little JR, Akrawi WP, Ahl J. Intracranial dural arteriovenous malformations: factors predisposing to an aggressive neurologic course. *J Neurosurg* 1990;72:839–850.

Cerebrovascular Disease, edited by H. Hunt Batjer.
Lippincott-Raven Publishers, Philadelphia © 1997.

CHAPTER 55

Cavernous Malformations: Natural History and Indications for Treatment

J. Nozipo Maraire and Issam A. Awad

The existence of intracranial vascular malformations has been known for over 100 years. The first reported case of an intracranial arteriovenous malformation (AVM) dates to the works of Steinheil in 1895 (1), whereas the classic study of "angiomatous angiomas" by Virchow constitutes the first comprehensive work on cerebral vascular malformations (2). Over the past century the understanding of these anomalies has challenged the most illustrious minds in neurosurgery and neuropathology. In 1928 Cushing and Bailey made the critical distinction between true vascular tumors and congenital malformation of blood vessels (2). Olivecrona subsequently devised a classification system for the latter based on etiology and pathology. He distinguished racemose lesions, which included arteriovenous, venous, and capillary malformations (1). In their landmark studies, Russel and Rubenstein and McCormick proposed more stringent classification systems for cerebral vascular malformations that form the basis of modern nomenclature. They recognized four discrete entities: (a) capillary telangiectasias, (b) venous malformations, (c) AVMs, and (d) cavernous malformations (CMs) (3,4). Only AVMs and CMs are typically manifested clinically, predisposing to epilepsy, neurologic deficit, and hemorrhagic stroke.

The current accepted definition of a CM is a low-flow vascular anomaly consisting of sinusoidal vascular channels lined by a single layer of endothelium (Fig. 1). Characteristically, these lesions lack intervening brain parenchyma within the collagenous stroma that separates individual channels. Grossly they are discrete, well-circumscribed lesions with a reddish purple, multilobulated appearance that has often been likened to a cluster of mulberries. The surrounding neural parenchyma often has evidence of prior microhemorrhage, hemosiderin discoloration, and hemosiderin-filled macrophages. Within the lesion, hyalinization, thrombosis with varying degrees of organization, calcification, cysts, and cholesterol crystals are common. A gliotic reaction of the surrounding parenchyma is characteristic and may form a pseudocapsule around the lesion.

EPIDEMIOLOGY

There is variability in the estimates of lesion prevalence of CMs. Such estimates have been determined through lesion prevalence at autopsy or on serial imaging studies including computed tomography (CT) and magnetic resonance imaging (MRI). In some cases the prevalence has been projected from relative frequency ratio between AVMs, aneurysms, and CMs with questionable validity. The major autopsy data document a calculated prevalence of 0.02–0.53% (5,6), whereas more recent serial MR studies that examine lesions with imaging characteristics typical of CMs calculate a prevalence rate 0.39–0.9% (5,7–9).

The existence of a familial form characterized by multiple lesions and an autosomal dominant inheritance pattern is well documented (10–14). The prevalence of familiality and lesion multiplicity is notably higher than suggested in earlier scattered clinical reports. Multiplicity in familial lesions is as high as 73%, compared to less than 33% for apparently sporadic lesions (10,12,13). It has been suggested that Hispanic patients may have a higher predilection for familial CMs (11,12).

Intracranial CMs affect both sexes with equal frequency, except in the middle cranial fossa where there is a female preponderance. Lesions have been described at all ages, with a majority of patients presenting in the second to fourth decades of life. It has been suggested that there is a male predominance among patients presenting at less than 30 years of age, a female preponderance among patients aged 30–60, and a more equal ratio thereafter (9). Data from virtually all clinical series demonstrate that symptomatic lesions are rare

I. Awad: Section of Neurosurgery, Yale University School of Medicine, New Haven, Connecticut 06511.

J. N. Maraire: Department of Neurology, Yale University Hospital, New Haven, Connecticut 06571.

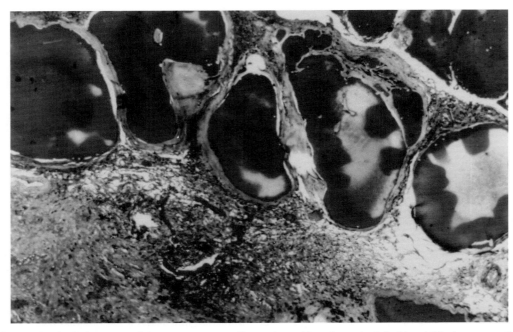

FIG. 1. Histologic features of the cavernous malformations. The characteristic blood-filled caverns, lined by a single endothelial layer, are separated by a fibrous stroma devoid of mature vessel wall elements.

in the elderly. It is not known as to why CMs manifest so rarely later in life. It is possible that lesions invariably become symptomatic early in life or not at all, or that senescence may be associated with lesion regression or quiescent behavior.

CMs have been reported to range in size from <0.1 cm to >9 cm (3,5,7,15,16). The majority of intracranial CMs are supratentorial with a distribution frequency reflecting the volume of the brain region. The pons and the cerebellum are the most common infratentorial sites (5,9,15,17). Other, less common intracranial locations include the cerebellopontine angle, the pineal gland, the middle fossa, the cavernous sinus, the optic nerve and chiasm, and dural-based lesions. Most CMs appear as solitary lesions, however, multiple lesions occur in up to 33% of sporadic cases and up to 73% in familial clusterings (3,5,9,13,15). CMs have been reported in association with other vascular lesions such as capillary telangiectasias, arteriovenous and venous malformations, with a frequency of 8–44% (3,9,12,15,18–22). Initial studies suggest that CMs are more likely to be part of a mixed lesion than other vascular malformations, the most common association being between CMs and venous malformations. The associated venous anomaly is usually clinically silent (18,20). Intracranial CMs may rarely be found in conjunction with intraspinal, extracerebral soft tissue and visceral hamartomas (3,5) and other central nervous system tumors such as meningiomas and astrocytomas (5).

NATURAL HISTORY

Our understanding of the mechanisms governing the natural history of CMs is rudimentary. Current knowledge is based largely on case reports, selected series and retrospective studies with relatively small sample sizes. Few studies have followed large patient cohorts in a prospective fashion. CMs are known to be dynamic lesions that display growth and involution through a variety of morphologic changes, thereby manifesting a wide clinical spectrum. Lesions may remain quiescent for years or they may bleed repeatedly, leading to severe cumulative neurologic disability. At present it is not possible to fully predict which lesions will become symptomatic or which subgroup of patients will have poor outcomes. A review of the literature does, however, demonstrate the broad clinical features of CMs and identifies factors that affect their natural history.

It is well known that CMs are dynamic lesions. Multiple clinical series have demonstrated neuroimaging changes in lesion size and signal characteristics as well as the appearance of new lesions over time (3,8,11,13,15). These changes are thought to be attributable to intralesional hemorrhage, thrombosis, organization, calcification, cyst formation, and involution of the caverns (13,17,21,23). Our current understanding of the factors governing the biologic behavior of CMs is rudimentary. A review of the literature demonstrates several features, some intrinsic to the lesion itself and others to the host, that influence the natural history and biological behavior of CMs.

DIAGNOSIS

There is at present no pathognomonic clinical syndrome or diagnostic test for the establishment of a diagnosis of CM. However, a synthesis of clinical history, presentation, and neuroimaging can suggest the presence of this lesion, which ultimately can only be proven by pathological specimen. Traditional neuroimaging may easily miss a CM. CT scanning has a high sensitivity but a low specificity. It may reveal calcifications, cystic components, or acute hemorrhage, but it does not accurately reveal the underlying lesion or lesion type. Along with thrombosed AVMs, CMs are angiographically occult. The few non specific angiographic findings are an avascular mass or, less commonly, a capillary blush, evidence of neovascularity, or an associated venous anomaly without arteriovenous shunting (10,15,23,24).

MRI is the most sensitive diagnostic tool for the evaluation of CMs. The appearance is sufficiently characteristic to allow confident preoperative evaluation of symptomatic lesions; identification, screening, and follow-up of incidental lesions; and depiction of lesion behavior including expansion, hemorrhage, and thrombosis (8,9,12,25). Cavernous malformations typically appear as well-defined, lobulated lesions on MR with a classic T2-weighted image of a central core of reticulated mixed density surrounded by a rim of signal hypointensity (8,9,25) (Fig. 2). Pathologically confirmed lesions have an 80–100% radiographic correlation.

The mixed signal intensities reflect chronic lesion behavior and the hemodynamics of CMs. The spectrum of behavior of CMs ranges from quiescence to gross hemorrhage. Repeated subclinical intralesional hemorrhages lead to the deposition of heme products secondary to erythrocyte breakdown. The reticulated low T2 signal also reflects speckled intralesional calcification. There is infiltration of macrophages laden with ferritin. The paramagnetic effects of iron

appear to account for the characteristic rim of low signal intensity seen on T2 images (8,9,19,20,25). Areas of hyperintensity correspond to focal hemorrhages and different stages of thrombus organization. Associated cysts most likely represent residua of previously expanded hemorrhagic caverns that have since involuted with thrombus organization and resolution (15).

The classic T2-weighted MR image while characteristic is not pathognomonic. Other lesions may manifest an indistinguishable appearance. Differential diagnosis should include AVMs, mixed vascular lesions, thrombosed AVMs, primary hemorrhagic and metastatic tumors, infectious and granulomatous diseases, and inflammatory lesions (25). Hemorrhagic primary or metastatic tumors and nonhemorrhagic tumors with melanin and fat may also confound the diagnosis. Absence of signs of systemic neoplasm and surrounding edema with the presence of multiple lesions, calcifications, and ossification offer clues distinguishing neoplasms from CMs and substantially increase diagnostic accuracy. Most AVMs, with the notable exception of small thrombosed AVMs, are readily distinguished from CMs by the presence of serpiginous signal void abnormalities, dilated arteries, and draining veins.

Clinically Silent Lesions

Solitary and multiple CMs of all sizes and locations may be clinically silent. These include cases with incidentally discovered lesions. Patients presenting with mild headaches and nonspecific symptoms are considered asymptomatic. The range of asymptomatic patients ranges from up to 44% in MR series to 95% in autopsy series. In one study, 40% of patients with initially clinically silent lesions became symptomatic within an interval of 6 months to two years (9). There are insufficient data at present to identify which patients progress to develop symptoms, provoking local or systemic factors and risk factors associated with symptomatic transformation. Headache alone, while difficult to attribute specifically to CMs, may be the sole clinical manifestation of lesion hemorrhage, especially in non-eloquent brain regions (13,21).

Seizures

The most common manifest clinical association of CMs is seizures, found in 38–100% of cases in clinical series. All seizure types have been observed. In order of frequency, generalized seizures predominate followed by complex partial seizures and simple seizures. CMs account for a disproportionately high fraction of intractable seizures associated with cerebrovascular malformations (26). CMs have almost double the frequency of seizures compared with other lesions, such as AVMs and tumors with similar volume densities and virtually identical locations. CMs located in the temporal lobes are more commonly associated with medically

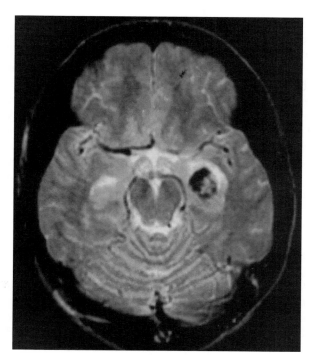

FIG. 2. T2-weighted axial MR displaying characteristic reticulated core surrounded by a low-density hemosiderin ring.

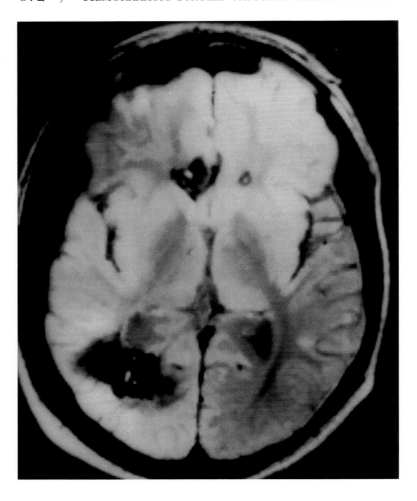

FIG. 3. T1-weighted MR displays multiple lesions.

refractory epilepsy. In one series of vascular malformations excised for intractable epilepsy, 74.7% were CMs and only 14.8% were AVMs (26). Given that the prevalence of the latter is at least 50% greater, this is particularly suggestive of a greater epileptogenic potential of CMs (26). Overall the data suggest that the majority of patients with seizure disorder are controlled on medication (26,27).

The pathophysiology of seizures in CMs is postulated to be related to irritation and compression secondary to mass effect, multiple local hemorrhages with exposure of surrounding brain to blood breakdown products, particularly iron and the subsequent local gliotic reaction (12,26). In experimental models, the deposition of heavy metals, including iron, has been shown to be epileptogenic (28). The pathway may include calcium influx and cytotoxicity, free radical formation, or an alteration of excitatory and inhibitory neurotransmitter balance. Furthermore, the ensuing reactive gliosis, a common feature of mesial temporal lobe sclerosis, is associated with intractable seizures (28). In CMs, calcification, temporal lobe location, and extensive hemosiderin deposition are frequently associated with a clinical presentation of epilepsy rather than gross hemorrhage (15,29).

It is important to adequately localize the epileptogenic zone before ascribing CM as the cause of seizures. In multi-

ple lesions it is especially important to be able to identify the lesion causing clinically significant epilepsy. Unfortunately, in nearly half of the cases it is not possible to localize or even lateralize the seizure focus by scalp electroencephalography (EEG) as the study may be normal or of indeterminate localizing value (26). Prolonged EEG monitoring with video correlation of seizures and interictal and ictal positron emission tomography (PET) or single photon emission computed tomography (SPECT) may be synthesized to yield convergent data and thus enhance the accuracy and validity of localization (26). In some cases, invasive electrode monitoring may be required for optimal mapping of epileptogenicity (26).

Hemorrhage

Hemorrhagic stroke is potentially the most debilitating consequence of CMs. A distinction must be made between apoplectic or gross hemorrhage and ongoing microhemorrhages and intralesional hemorrhagic expansion in CMs. The characteristics of a hemorrhagic lesion are depicted in Fig. 4.

Repeated subclinical intralesional hemorrhages are a uni-

TABLE 1. *Clinical outcomes of CM excision in selected large series*

Author Year (Number of patients in series)	Clinical Outcome (percent of cases in reported series)		
	Excellent	Good/Fair	Poor/Dismal
Voigt and Yasargil* 1976 (21)	—	100	—
Giombini 1978 (14)	64	29	7
Simard 1986 (23)	52	39	9
(Detailed follow up data for epilepsy patients only)			
Vaquero 1987 (25)	76	8	16
Weber 1989 (11)	20	79	1
Robinson 1991 (21)	57	33	10
Zimmerman 1991 (16)	6	75	19
Brainstem only			
Wascher 1993 (22)	77	23	—
Infratentorial			
Maraire & Awad 1995 (45)	73	25	2

* all had "successful surgical outcomes"

versal feature of CMs and are part of their dynamic behavior (10,12,15–17,19,20,30,31). The frequency of gross hemorrhage, however, is a less common but clinically more significant event. It has been reported in 8–37% of lesions in clinical series (7,10–12,19–21,30,32). A higher association has been reported in children with a range of 36–60% (22,3). Annual clinically significant hemorrhagic risk has been estimated at 0.1–2.7% per lesion per year (7,9,13,16,17).

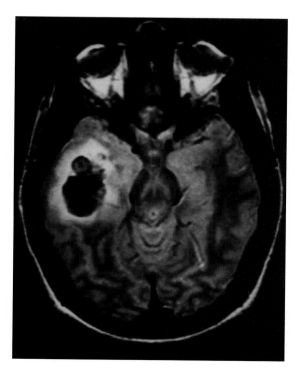

FIG. 4. MR of a cavernous malformation with gross hemorrhage and mass effect.

The majority of hemorrhages are intraparenchymal within the region of the CM. They are rarely subarachnoid (frequently seen with optic nerve or chiasmal CMs) or intraventricular (21). In mixed lesions composed of a CM and a venous malformation, the hemorrhage is invariably secondary to the former (21). In contrast to AVMs, a bleeding episode from a CM is rarely life threatening. However, there are documented cases of patient demise from an acute apoplectic episode and few cases of rapid neurologic deterioration (15,17). More recent large series have also reported rare mortality attributable to a first hemorrhage from a CM (9,15,21). The precise clinical presenting syndrome depends on the location of the lesion. Typically, there is acute onset of headache, which may be accompanied by a neurologic deficit and occasionally a change in the level of consciousness (21). In the posterior fossa, hemorrhages cause neurologic sequelae with greater frequency due to the concentration and clustering of vital tracts and nuclei and the possibility of obstruction of cerebrospinal fluid pathways. In the cerebellum patients present with headache, emesis, ataxia, vertigo, and nystagmus whereas in the brainstem typical signs include diploplia, hemiparesis, sensory deficits, and a change in mental status (9,17,34). In general, however, initial bleeds are self-limited and patients have a good to fair neurologic outcome (9,17,21). In contrast, recurrent clinically overt hemorrhages are associated with progressive neurologic decline and severe residual deficits. In the brainstem there may be periods of exacerbation followed by remission, mimicking demyelinating disease. Regardless of the presentation, data from several studies suggest that there is an increased risk of recurrent hemorrhage after an initial bleed (8–10,15–17,21,23,34). Preliminary reports also suggest that women may have a higher risk of hemorrhage, particularly during pregnancy (3,9,20,21).

Neurologic Deficit

The third common clinical presentation of CMs is acute or progressive neurologic deficit. This is usually associated with intralesional or perilesional hemorrhage documentable by MR imaging. The frequency in clinical series ranges from 15% to 47% (3,7–10,12,13,15,19,20,23,34). The precise syndrome depends on the size and location of the lesion. The deficit may be transient, progressive, recurrent, or fixed. Aggressive and recurrent hemorrhagic episodes leave heightened degrees of disability often resulting in severe fixed impairments (3,7–10,12,19–21,23,32,34).

Morphologic Features

Several large series have failed to find any correlation between lesion size and neurologic disability or propensity for hemorrhage (9,20). One series suggests that patients with multiple lesions have an earlier onset and higher frequency of seizures (7). It has been suggested that the presence of dense calcifications, ossifications, a thick glial capsule and a greater degree of intralesional organization are associated with a less aggressive clinical course (15,27,29). Calcifications are associated with greater epileptogenicity (15). In an attempt to find prognostic features on neuroimaging, one study found that only 69% of MR lesions in a mean follow-up of 18 months matched the clinical course of the patient, whereas 31% were discordant (35). The only correlation between MR characteristics and the biological behavior of CMs was the observation that as long as gross hemorrhage occurred within the hypodense hemosiderin landmark the patient would remain asymptomatic. However, if the bleed ruptured through this margin or the glial capsule, then the patient presented with acute symptoms (35).

Location

Although the majority of lesions occur in the supratentorial compartment, substantially greater neurologic sequelae occur with CMs in the infratentorial compartment (9,17,20,21,23,24). This correlation remains significant even after lesion size is controlled for. Brainstem lesions have a high rate of recurrent symptomatic hemorrhage, up to 69%, and a significant cumulative morbidity (9,20,21,23,36). They present as a characteristic pattern of exacerbations and remission of symptoms (17,21,23,24). In one study, 21% of cases with initially mild episodes in this region had subsequent devastating hemorrhages (36). Seizures occur almost exclusively in the supratentorial compartment. However, some authors have suggested that temporal lobe lesions are more likely to be epileptogenic. A rigorous analysis of 86 patients found no clinically significant variance in seizure frequency between the supratentorial locations (9).

Associated Pathology

Mixed cerebrovascular malformations have been described from histopathologic and neuroimaging data (3,9,12,18–24,27,30,31). The most common association between CM and venous malformations is reported in 8–36% of lesions (9,12,19,30,34). The natural history of CMs with an existing AVM, a venous malformation, or capillary telangiectasia has not been adequately studied, although preliminary data suggest that the clinical course mirrors that of CMs alone (9,12,18,27,30,36). Thus, although such heterogeneous histology may affect the complexity of clinical decisions, there is little evidence to suggest that it alters biological lesion behavior.

Previous Hemorrhage

There is an increased risk of recurrent hemorrhage and progressive neurologic decline after an initial bleed from a CM (16,19,20,23,24). Series of both infratentorial and supratentorial lesions report a 20–80% frequency of rebleed in the same lesion with intervals between episodes ranging from weeks to years (8,10,16,23,33,36). This is significantly greater than the risk of 0.39–2.7% risk of initial hemorrhage in reported series. It has been demonstrated in one study that among infratentorial cases three quarters of patients presenting with sudden onset of acute hemorrhage rebled within 26 months (37). A recent study also demonstrated that young women were at a statistically significant higher risk of recurrent bleed than other cohort groups, including older women (16). The histopathologic evidence of prior gross hemorrhage has also been associated with increased recurrent hemorrhagic risk. Lesion growth and hemorrhage correlated with a poor outcome. A series examining certain pathological features at surgery and autopsy with a retrospective analysis of the clinical and biological behavior of the lesion found that lesions with calcifications, evidence of chronic intralesional hemorrhage with thrombus organization, and a thicker glial pseudocapsule were more likely to present with seizures than gross hemorrhage (29). These findings are supported by numerous case reports and histopathologic observations. It is possible that the slow ooze of blood, thrombus organization, and the consequent glial reaction may be protective from gross hemorrhage while predisposing to seizures.

Lesion Growth

The dynamic nature of CMs is well documented (11,13,15,17,21,27,35,37). Growth of lesions and CT or MR changes over time are reported in up to 38% of patients (9,11,13,17,35). In a recent familial study of CMs, with an average follow-up of 2.2 years, 29% of patients developed new lesions with an average rate of 0.4 new lesion per patient per year (13). In the brainstem, lesion expansion has been associated with progressive and severe neurologic sequelae including death (17). Interestingly, in multiple lesions, the removal of one previously active lesion does not appear to deter the growth, dynamics, or development of symptoms from novel or previously quiescent lesions. Recurrent hemorrhages may even occur from different lesions sequentially (11). The pathophysiology of lesion expansion and evolution may be passive, secondary to hemorrhage and the dynamics of clot and thrombus organization, or attributable to active proliferation. It may be that a causal relationship exists between the two mechanisms such that repeated microhemorrhages may promote hemorrhagic angiogenic proliferation.

Age

Age appears to play a significant role in the natural history of CMs. In contrast to adult series, there is a greater preponderance of hemorrhage and acute neurologic deficits as presenting symptoms in children, accounting for 43–78% of symptomatic patients (33). The pediatric population displays two age peaks of symptoms, at 3 and 11 years. Reportedly, younger children display more active lesion growth compared to the older age group. It has been suggested that pediatric patients have a greater propensity for overt hemorrhage (22,33). In familial clusterings of CMs, successive generations appear to manifest symptoms at an earlier age. Only rarely are CMs symptomatic in the elderly.

Gender

There is a marked sex difference in the clinical presentation and neurologic disability of CMs. Women are more likely to manifest with gross hemorrhage and neurologic deficits whereas men are more likely to present with epilepsy (3,8,15,16,38). A review of the literature demonstrates that women comprise 50–100% of those patients presenting with acute neurologic symptoms compared to 11–50% of those with seizures (3,8,15,16,27,37). There is evidence that young women are at significantly greater risk of recurrent hemorrhage from a symptomatic lesion (16). In one study of brainstem CMs, 80% presented with gross hemorrhage and all of these were women (37). Two larger mixed series have corroborated these findings, suggesting that even in supratentorial lesions, women are more likely to present with clinically significant overt hemorrhage (16,39). This trend is also demonstrable in pediatric cases. Furthermore, women with CMs display a significantly greater degree of neurologic disability compared to men (9,19). There is also a notable female preponderance among mixed vascular malformations. Women have also been reported to have a greater propensity to form multiple lesions. This association between aggressive lesion behavior and female gender in CMs is further supported by the overwhelming female preponderance in middle fossa extradural lesions, which are extremely vascular and tend to bleed profusely at surgery, unlike other intracranial CMs. It is unclear as to whether this is attributable to the local lesion milieu or circulating host factors such as hormones.

Female Reproductive Cycle

Several preliminary studies have suggested that women's reproductive cycle may have an impact on the rate of growth and the hemorrhagic risk of CMs. One recent large retrospective analysis found a significant difference in hemorrhage rates between women less than and those greater than 40 years of age (16). Case reports of intracranial and systemic CMs document an aggressive clinical course during pregnancy (8,9,36). In one series where women composed 86% of the cohort presenting with hemorrhage, one third were in their first trimester of pregnancy (9). This is corroborated by a second study of 2000 consecutive MRIs that found that 75% of patients with acute onset of neurologic deficits were women, and two thirds were pregnant (8).

The dynamic risk of pregnancy and CM with regard to the cardiovascular changes, fluctuating hormone levels, dif-

ferent trimesters of pregnancy, and risk of recurrent hemorrhages in single or multiple pregnancies has not been carefully characterized.

Familial Inheritance

Most of the epidemiologic data regarding familial CMs are concordant with sporadic cases. The most notable exception is the markedly higher prevalence of multiple lesions, reported to be as high as 73% in familial CMs, compared to less than 33% among sporadic cases (3,9,12,13,15,20,27). Several studies suggest that successive generations may manifest symptoms at an earlier age (11,38). Earlier studies reported a high incidence of sudden death among familial cases. Several studies report an increased prevalence of familial CMs among populations of Hispanic origin (11,12)

As in sporadic cases, a single "dominant" lesion is usually responsible for epileptic and hemorrhagic symptoms in multiple cases. There is no statistically demonstrable propensity for greater or less neurologic disability with multiple lesions (11,20).

THERAPEUTIC OPTIONS

Patients with CMs may be divided into distinct clinical categories that correlate with their risk of hemorrhage and neurologic disability. Each clinical scenario proposes a distinct management approach aimed at weighing treatment risk against the best estimate of the cumulative natural risk.

Expectant Follow-Up

Asymptomatic patients with single or multiple lesions and only vague complaints such as headache or dizziness in the absence of neurologic deficits present a low annualized risk of a first debilitating hemorrhage. There are no current data to support an aggressive approach in this group, or in purely incidental lesions, in either sporadic or familial cases. Yet surgical intervention for solitary lesions carries a very small risk and virtually eliminates all subsequent serious risk from the lesions (40). It appears reasonable to follow these patients clinically and with sequential MR imaging. Alternatively, elective excision of readily accessible lesions may be considered in younger patients whose cumulative risk over time may not be negligible. Young patients with mild or non-disabling symptoms and solitary, accessible (usually supratentorial or cerebellar) lesions should be followed closely, with consideration of lesion excision at the first manifestation of lesion growth or an exacerbation of symptoms. Cases involving less accessible lesions dictate a correspondingly higher threshold for lesion excision.

The major role of medical management in CMs is in the control of epilepsy. Often the epileptogenicity may be localized to a single lesion. The clinical spectrum ranges from patients who respond well to anticonvulsant medication to those with medically intractable and functionally debilitating seizures. Several studies have shown that patients with severe epilepsy who were given anticonvulsant treatment only had their symptoms persist unabated with significant clinical and social disability from seizures (9,26).

Surgical Treatment

It is currently agreed that accessible symptomatic CMs should be resected. The current firmly established indications for surgical management are overt hemorrhage, focal neurologic symptoms, and/ or uncontrolled epilepsy. The overall results in both adult and pediatric patients are generally favorable Table 1.

Patients presenting with an initial bleed are at greater risk for recurrent hemorrhage. Resection of symptomatic supratentorial accessible lesions has been accompanied by a very low rate of morbidity (9,15,16,18–22,40). Favorable results have also been reported in resection of brainstem lesions that present to a pial or ventricular surface (7,16,34,37,40). There is no consensus as to whether these lesions should be excised after a first bleed or should await symptom recurrence or progression. Lesion accessibility clearly affects surgical risk (7,10,16,17,40). Mortality risk with surgery for brainstem CMs has ranged from 0% to 20%, with transient neurologic worsening in 20–40% and permanent worsening in <20% of cases (7,15,17,34,40). In one series of brainstem lesions presenting with neurologic deficits that were misdiagnosed, mistreated, and not operated on, 70% of patients had an unremitting or fatal outcome (15). A recent study corroborated the poor outcome with recurrent hemorrhages of the posterior fossa (17). In patients with multiple lesions only the offending lesion should be resected whereas those not readily accessible through the same exposure should be followed expectantly as with asymptomatic lesions. Recurrences have been reported with subtotal removal and are found more commonly in less accessible and infratentorial locations. There is evidence to suggest de novo lesion genesis in certain cases (13,40).

Patients with uncontrolled epilepsy are candidates for surgical excision of the lesion. Overall analysis of the data demonstrates improvement of symptoms in the majority of patients (7,9,10,26,27). Of groups treated with surgical resection of the offending lesion 50–91% were reportedly seizure-free with or without anticonvulsant therapy (7,9,10). Persistent seizures are reported with incomplete lesion resection. Excision of CMs should be accompanied by resection of grossly abnormal surrounding brain parenchyma whenever possible, to enhance seizure outcome (7,18,26). Excision of additional epileptogenic brain is only recommended for severe intractable cases or in those where prior lesion surgery was unsuccessful (8,21,26,40).

Radiosurgery has been established as an alternative, effective treatment option for small AVMs in eloquent and inaccessible areas. With the standard dosages as used for AVMs, CMs exhibit a poor clinical response and a high complication rate (10,15). In one series of 16 patients (13 with a CM alone and 3 with a CM associated with a venous malformation), there was no radiographic change in 80%, but 37.4% eventually developed radiation induced changes, one patient rebled, and 12.5% had persistent neurologic deficits (41). When lower margin doses are utilized, the results may be more promising (42–44). One such report used doses of 12–16 Gy for 39 deep-seated CMs with an average follow-up of 23 months. The authors reported temporary neurologic sequelae with MR changes secondary to radiation in ten patients (25.4%). There were four deaths, two reportedly unrelated to radiosurgery and two after delayed microneurosurgery. After 15 months there were no cases of delayed hemorrhage (42–44). Clearly, the use of radiosurgery needs further investigation. In particular, issues of patient selection, follow-up, long-term risks, and safe dose levels must be addressed. Endpoints of therapeutic success or failure have been difficult to establish in view of the variability of natural behavior of the lesions.

LESION BEHAVIOR AND FUTURE OPTIONS

The interface of basic and clinical sciences has led to synergy of research. In CMs the study of the familial form has led to the localization of the genetic abnormality for familial CMs on chromosome 7q (14,45). Much remains to be done to find the precise localization of the gene, its sequence and gene product. In addition, preliminary studies using probes for vascular maturity and cellular adhesion have supported the hypothesis that CMs are immature vessels that undergo continuing dysangiogenesis (31). Further research may lead to improved screening, perhaps through a blood test in patients at risk (ie, family members) and innovative therapeutic modalities aimed at preventing lesion genesis, inhibiting aggressive behavior, or inducing lesion regression.

REFERENCES

1. Olivecrona H, Ladenheim J. *Congenital Arteriovenous Aneurysms of the Carotid and Vertebral Artery Systems.* Berlin: Springer-Verlag, 1957.
2. Cushing H, Bailey P. *Tumors Arising from the Blood Vessels of the Brain.* Springfield, IL: Charles C Thomas: 1928.
3. Russel D, Rubenstein L. *The Pathology of Tumours of the Nervous System.* 4th ed. London: Edward Arnold, 1977;126–145.
4. McCormick WF. The pathology of vascular (''arteriovenous'') malformations. *J Neurosurg* 1966;24(4):807–816.
5. Hsu F, Rigamonti D, Huhn SL. Epidemiology of cavernous malformations. In: Awad I, Barrows D, eds. *Cavernous Malformations.* Park Ridge: AANS, 1993:13–23.
6. Otten P, Pizzolato GP, Rilliet B, Berney J. 131 cases of cavernous angioma (cavernomas) of the CNS, discovered by retrospective analysis of 24,535 autopsies [Review] [French]. *Neurochirurgie* 1989;35(2):82–83.
7. Del Curling O, Kelly DL, Elster AD, Craven TE. An analysis of the

natural history of cavernous angiomas. *J Neurosurg* 1991;75(5): 702–708.

8. Sage MR, Brophy BP, Sweeney C, Phipps S, Perrerr LV, Sandhu A, Albertyn LE. Cavernous haemangiomas (angiomas) of the brain: clinically significant lesions. *Australasian Radiol* 1993;37(2):147–155.

9. Robinson JR, Awad IA, Little JR. Natural history of the cavernous angioma. *J Neurosurg* 1991;75(5):709–714.

10. Giombini S, Morello G. Cavernous angiomas of the brain. *Acta Neurochirurgica* 1978;40(1–2):61–82.

11. Hayman LA, Evans RA, Ferrell RE, Fahr LM, Ostrow P, Riccardi VM. Familial cavernous angiomas: natural history and genetic study over a 5-year period. *Am J Medi Genet* 1982;11(2):147–160.

12. Rigamonti D, Hadley M, Drayer B, Johnson PC, Hoenig-Rigamonti K, Knight JT, Spetzler RF. Cerebral cavernous malformations. *N Engl J Med* 1988;319(6):343–347.

13. Zabramski JM, Wascher TM, Spetzler RF, Johnson B, Golfinos J, Drayer BP, Brown B, Rigamonti D, Brown GB. The natural history of familial cavernous malformations: results of an ongoing study. *J Neurosurg* 1994;80(3):422–432.

14. Gunel M, Awad I, Anson J, Lifton RP. Mapping a gene causing cerebral cavernous malformations to 7q11.2-q21. *Proc Natl Acad Sci USA* 1995; 92:6620–6624.

15. Simard MJ, Garcia-Bengochea F, Ballinger WE Jr, Mickle JP, Quisling RG. Cavernous angioma: a review of 126 collected and 12 new clinical cases. *Neurosurgery* 1986;18(2):162–172

16. Aiba T, Tanaka R, Koike T, Kameyama S, Takeda N, Komata T. Natural history of intracranial cavernous malformations. *J Neurosurg* 1995; 83:56–59.

17. Fritschi JA, Reulen HJ, Spetzler RF, Zabramski JM. Cavernous malformations of the brain stem. A review of 139 cases (review). *Acta Neurochirurgica* 1994. 130:35–46.

18. Awad IA, Robinson JJ, Mohanty S, Estes ML. Mixed vascular malformations of the brain: clinical and pathogenetic considerations. *Neurosurgery* 1993;33(2):179–188.

19. Robinson J, Awad I. Clinical spectrum and natural course. In: Awad I, Barrow D, eds. *Cavernous Malformations*. Park Ridge, IL: AANS, 1993:25–36.

20. Robinson JJ, Awad IA, Magdinec M, Paranandi L. Factors predisposing to clinical disability in patients with cavernous malformations of the brain. *Neurosurgery* 1993;32(5):730–735.

21. Barrow D, Krisht A. Cavernous malformations and hemorrhage. In: Awad I, Barrow D, eds. *Cavernous Malformations*. Park Ridge, IL: AANS, 1993:65–80.

22. Voigt K, Yasargil MG. Cerebral cavernous haemangiomas or cavernomas. Incidence, pathology, localization, diagnosis, clinical features and treatment. Review of the literature and report of an unusual case. *Neurochirurgia* 1976;19(2):59–68.

23. Lobato RD, Perez C, Rivas J, Cordobes F. Clinical, radiological, and pathological spectrum of angiographically occult intracranial vascular malformations. *J Neurosurg* 1988;68:518–531.

24. Lobato RD, Rivas JJ, Gomez PA, Cabrera A, Sarabia R, Lamas E. Comparison of the clinical presentation of symptomatic arteriovenous malformations (angiographically visualized) and occult vascular malformations. *Neurosurgery* 1992;31(3):391–396.

25. Perl J, Ross J. Diagnostic imaging of cavernous malformations. In: Awad I, Barrow D, eds. *Cavernous Malformations*. Park Ridge, IL: AANS, 1993:37–48.

26. Awad I, Robinson J. Cavernous malformation and epilepsy. In: Awad IA, Barrow DL editors. *Cavernous Malformations*. Park Ridge, IL: AANS, 1993:49–63.

27. Weber M, Vespignani H, Bracard S, et al. Les angiomes caverneux intracerebraux. *Revue Neurologique* 1989;145(6–7):429–36.

28. Kraemer DL, Awad IA. Vascular malformations and epilepsy: clinical considerations and basic mechanisms. *Epilepsia* 1994;35(suppl 6): S30–43.

29. Steiger HJ, Markwalder RV, Reulen HJ. Is there a relationship between the clinical manifestations and the pathologic image of cerebral cavernomas? *Neurochirurgie* 1989;35(2):84–88.

30. Robinson JJ, Awad IA, Masaryk TJ, Estes ML. Pathological heterogeneity of angiographically occult vascular malformations of the brain. *Neurosurgery* 1993;33(4):547–554.

31. Robinson JR, Awad IA, Zhou P, Barna BP, Estes ML. Expression of basement membrane and endothelial cell adhesion molecules in vascular malformations of the brain: preliminary observations and working hypothesis. *Neurological Research* 1995;17(1):49–58.

32. Vaquero J, Salazar J, Martinez R, Martinez P, Bravo G. Cavernous malformations of the central nervous system: clinical syndromes, CT scan diagnosis, and prognosis after surgical treatment in 25 cases. *Acta Neurochirurgica* 1987;85(1–2):29–33.

33. Mazza C, Scienza R, Dalla BB, Beltramo A, Bontempini L, Dapian R. Cerebral cavernpous malformations (cavernomas) in children. *Neurochirurgie* 1989;35(2):106–108.

34. Zimmerman RS, Spetzler RF, Lee KS, Zabramski JM, Hargraves RW. Cavernous malformations of the brain stem. *J Neurosurg* 1991;75(1): 32–39.

35. Sigal R, Krief O, HouttevilleJP, Halimi P, Doyon D, Pariento D. Occult cerebrovascular malformations: follow up with MR imaging. *Radiology* 1990;!76(3):815–819.

36. Abe M. Clinical presentations of vascular malformations of the brain stem: comparison of angiographically positive and negative types. *J Neurol Neurosurg Psychiatry* 1989;52:167–175.

37. Sakai N, Yamada H, Tanigawara T, et al. Surgical treatment of cavernous angiomas involving the brainstem and review of the literature. *Acta Neurochir* 1991;113(3– 4):138–143.

38. Maraire JN, Awad IA. Intracranial cavernous malformations: Lesion behaviour and management strategies. *Neurosurgery* 1995;(in press).

39. Farmer JP, Cosgrove GR, Villemure JG, Meagher VK, Tampieri D, Melanson D. intracerebral cavernous angiomas. *Neurology* 1988; 38(11):1699–1704.

40. Barrow D, Awad I. Conceptual overview and management strategies. In: Awad I, Barrow D, eds. *Cavernous Malformations*. Park Ridge, IL: AANS, 1993:205–213.

41. Steiner L, Lindquist L, Steiner M. In: Symon L, Calliauw L, Cohadon F, Antunes JL, Loew F, Nornes H, Pasztor E, Pickard JD, Strong AJ, Yasargil MG, eds. *Advances and Technical Standards in Neurosurgery*. Wien: Springer-Verlag, 1992:57–59.

42. Coffey R, Lunsford L. Radiosurgery of cavernous malformations and other angiographically occult vascular malformations. In: Awad I, Barrow D, eds. *Cavernous Malformations*. Park Ridge, IL: AANS, 1993: 187–200.

43. Lunsford LD, Kondziolka D, Bissonette DJ, Maitz AH, Flickinger JC. Stereotactic radiosurgery of brain vascular malformations. *Neurosurg Clin North Am* 1992;3(1):79–98.

44. Lunsford LD, Kondziolka D, Flickinger JC. Stereotactic radiosurgery: current spectrum and results [review]. *Clin Neurosurg* 1992;38(405): 405–444.

45. Dubovsky J, Zabramski JM, Kurth J, Spetzler RF, Rich SS, Orr HT, Weber JL. *Hum Mol Genet* 1995;4:453–458.

46. Wascher TM, Spetzler RF. Microsurgical treatment of infratentorial cavernous malformations. In: Awad I, Barrow D, eds. *Cavernous Malformations*. Park Ridge, IL: AANS, 1993:117–132.

Cerebrovascular Disease, edited by H. Hunt Batjer.
Lippincott-Raven Publishers, Philadelphia © 1997.

CHAPTER 56

Intracranial Arteriovenous Malformations: Patient Evaluation and Considerations for Treatment

Warren R. Selman, Robert W. Tarr, and Robert A. Ratcheson

The identification of patients suspected of harboring an arteriovenous malformation (AVM) has been simplified by the use of diagnostic studies such as computed tomography (CT) and magnetic resonance imaging (MRI) and angiography (MRA). These modalities have also contributed to an improved understanding of the natural history of these lesions. Nonetheless, the determination of whether a particular treatment is likely to provide a better outcome than expected without such treatment remains complex.

Contemporary noninvasive imaging techniques have allowed more precise determination of the location of the malformation with respect to functionally important structures. Invasive cerebral angiography remains necessary to provide architectural details of the malformation and its nidus, which can help to determine the therapeutic alternatives and optimal treatment of individual patients with an AVM. Physiologic assessment of the impact of the AVM on the surrounding brain may also provide important information affecting the management of selected patients. Thus, a knowledge of the anatomic detail of the AVM, the physiologic impact on the surrounding brain, and the natural history with and without different therapeutic regimens are required when advising patients of the optimal management of a specific AVM.

NATURAL HISTORY

In general, patients with AVMs may seek medical attention for one or a combination of the following reasons: intracranial hemorrhage, seizure, focal neurologic deficit, impairment of higher cortical function, headache, and bruit. With the widespread use of noninvasive imaging techniques, it is apparent that some AVMs remain relatively asymptomatic and are discovered only incidentally.

Recommendations for treatment must be evaluated in light of the natural history of AVMs. Samson and Batjer have divided the natural history of AVMs into four critical components: (a) risk of death; (b) risk of hemorrhage; (c) risk of significant neurologic morbidity; and, finally, (d) those characteristics unique to the patient, the mode of presentation, and the malformation, which influence the previous three risks (1).

Risk of Death, Hemorrhage, and Neurologic Morbidity

Prior to 1980, studies on the natural history of AVMs suffered from a lack of standardized entry criteria, insufficient numbers of patients, and a lack of long-term follow-up. Wilkins reviewed these studies and synthesized a report on 1500 patients (2). From this amalgamation of patients it appeared that AVMs were associated with a significant morbidity due to an annualized risk of hemorrhage of 2–3% and mortality of 1%. Recent reports have further refined our understanding of the natural history of these lesions (3,4). The results of these and earlier studies, which have been summarized in several excellent reviews (1,5), demonstrate that AVMs are associated with an even higher risk of hemorrhage (approximately 4% per year) and significant long-term morbidity and mortality. These studies also provide increased evidence that specific, identifiable characteristics of the patient and the lesion affect the natural history and ultimately the decision of when and how to treat the patient.

The important report by Ondra and co-workers updated the population-based study first reported by Troupp and col-

W. R. Selman, R. W. Tarr, and R. A. Ratcheson: Department of Neurological Surgery, and Division of Neuroradiology, Case Western Reserve University and University Hospital of Cleveland, Cleveland, Ohio 44106

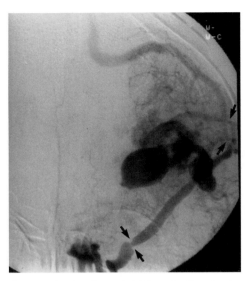

FIG. 1. Superselective lateral right pericallosal artery angiogram demonstrates two small intranidal aneurysms *(arrows)*.

leagues in the 1970s (4,6,7). Ondra and colleagues analyzed 160 patients with AVMs; the mean follow-up was 24.7 years, the average age of presentation was 33 years, and the majority of patients presented with a hemorrhage. There was a 4% per year risk of rebleeding after entry into the study. The mean interval between the presenting event and a subsequent hemorrhage was 7.7 years (range 6 weeks–22 years). The interval to new hemorrhage did not vary between patients who presented with bleeding, seizures, or headaches. The yearly risk of significant morbidity was 1.7% and the yearly mortality was 1%. It is important to emphasize that the risk

of hemorrhage and death were the same regardless of the initial mode of presentation.

Patient Characteristics

Particular characteristics of the patient and the malformation may be of help in determining the natural history of a given lesion in a specific patient. For example, AVMs are slightly more common in women than men, although the figure is not statistically significant, and women have a slightly increased incidence of hemorrhage compared to men (63.9% vs. 56.4%) (8). Most AVMs become symptomatic between the second and fourth decades of life, at which time there is the greatest risk of initial hemorrhage. The risk of recurrent hemorrhage is greatest between the fourth and sixth decades of life (5,9). There has been considerable controversy regarding the management of AVMs in pregnant women. However, Horton reported that of 451 women with AVMs undergoing 540 pregnancies, all of whom were referred for stereotactic radiation, the risks of hemorrhage from the AVM was 3.5% and that labor and delivery had no adverse effect on the rate of hemorrhage (10).

AVM Characteristics

Specific characteristics of the AVM that have been suggested to influence the natural history include size, intranidal anatomy, and configuration of the venous drainage. Recent engineering advances in microcatheter systems have enabled superselective angiographic analysis of AVM anatomy. Superselective analysis is useful to differentiate intranidal

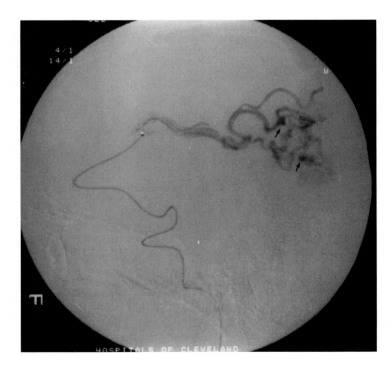

FIG. 2. Posterior-anterior venous phase from a left internal carotid artery angiogram shows several points of arteriovenous malformation (AVM) venous outflow stricture *(arrows)*.

aneurysms from ectasia, estimate intranidal arteriovenous fistula, and determine the extent of nidal compartmentalization. Superselective angiography is critical for providing detail of the angioarchitecture of microarteriovenous malformations (less than 1 cm) for which conventional angiography does not provide adequate resolution (11).

Smaller AVMs have generally been considered more likely to present with hemorrhage. Whether this represents a selection bias influenced by larger AVMs presenting with other clinical manifestations is not entirely clear. Hemodynamic assessment of small AVMs has revealed evidence of distinct differences in flow patterns and pressure within the nidus that may render small lesions more likely to hemorrhage than large ones (12,13). Intraoperative measurements have demonstrated that in small AVMs that have hemorrhaged the feeding artery pressure was significantly higher than in large AVMs that had not hemorrhaged.

The association of aneurysms on feeding vessels has been identified as a risk factor for hemorrhage (14). It has been determined that intranidal aneurysms and segments of venous occlusion contribute to an increased risk of hemorrhage from the malformation itself (Figs. 1–3) (15–17). Intraoperative pressure measurements have demonstrated evidence on increased pressure at prestenotic sites of venous drainage

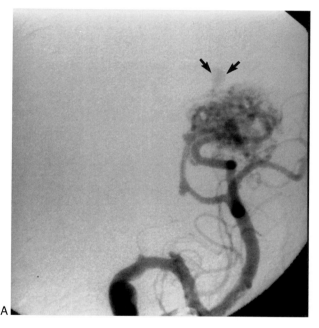

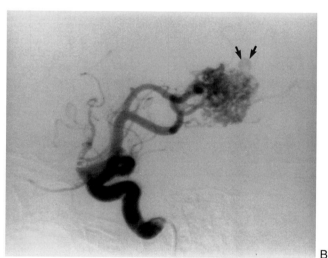

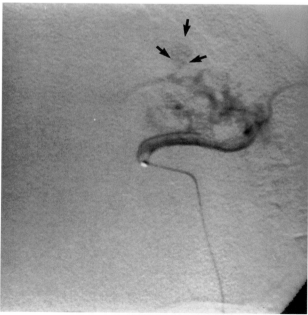

FIG. 3. (A) Posterior-anterior and **(B)** lateral left internal carotid artery angiogram is suspicious for a large intranidal aneurysm *(arrows)*. **(C)** Superselective left middle cerebral artery angiogram demonstrates this dysplastic segment to be a proximal venous varice rather than an intranidal aneurysm *(arrows)*.

(18). Marks and co-workers retrospectively analyzed angiograms of 65 patients with AVMs. Forty-five of these patients had a history of hemorrhage. Angiographic findings significantly correlated with hemorrhage included central venous drainage, periventricular or intraventricular nidus location, and the presence of intranidal aneurysms. Angiomatous change, which is defined as dilated cortical and leptomeningeal collateral supply to the AVM nidus, was inversely correlated with a history of hemorrhage (16).

THERAPEUTIC ASSESSMENT

Anatomy

When evaluating an AVM size and location are the most important factors to consider with respect to therapeutic options. Newer CT imaging algorithms and standard sequence MRIs can provide anatomic detail of the lesion (Figs. 4 and 5). These three-dimensional studies not only delineate the internal architecture of the malformation but also reveal the relationship of the lesion to surrounding anatomic landmarks (19).

While the value of determining the relation of the lesion to identifiable anatomic structures is not to be underestimated, modern MR techniques can provide information on the relation of the lesion to functionally important regions. Functional MRI is a relatively new technique that can localize sensorimotor and visual cortex (Fig. 6). MR sequences that are sensitive to changes in blood flow or deoxyhemoglobin concentration may be used to image increases in regional blood flow or changes in venous deoxyhemoglobin concentration secondary to increased metabolism of activated neurons (20,21). The sensorimotor cortex can be localized using tactile stimulation and motor tasks. The visual cortex can be localized using light or pattern stimulation. Functional MR has been shown to correlate well with invasive cortical mapping techniques for determination of motor and sensory cortex location (22). Functional MR localization has some advantage over positron emission tomography in providing better spatial and temporal resolution. It must be stressed, however, that both techniques require superimposition of anatomic and physiologic images and thereby have some potential for inaccuracy.

Precise localization of functionally important cortex may be needed for determination of therapeutic alternatives of some AVMs. In these situations, direct cortical mapping should be used. The Rolandic cortex may be identified by recording short latency evoked potentials from the cortical surface following the stimulation of large peripheral sensory nerves (23). From identification of phase reversal across the central sulcus, the location of the motor cortex may be inferred. The use of a more complex electrode array or more complete stimulation mapping with a bipolar electrode may be used for more detailed identification of the Rolandic cortex, adjacent motor pathways, and localization of language function (24–26).

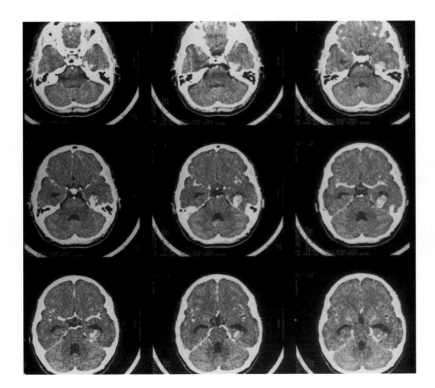

FIG. 4. High-resolution (2.0 mm slice thickness) dynamic CT during bolus contrast injection allows good fidelity nidus measurement determinations to be made.

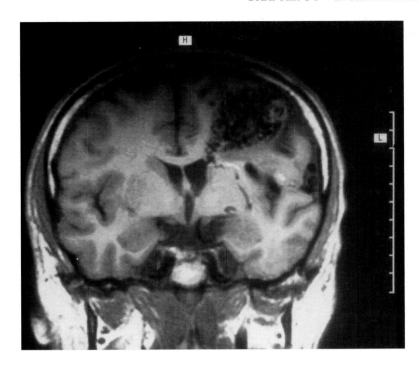

FIG. 5. Coronal T1-weighted MRI shows the deep periventricular extent of this left frontoparietal AVM.

PHYSIOLOGY

A variety of studies can be used alone or in combination to assess the physiologic impact of the AVM and therapeutic intervention on the surrounding brain. These studies include cerebral angiography, MR angiographic flow determinations, transcranial Doppler (TCD), positron emission tomography (PET), single photon emission tomography (SPECT), and endovascular diagnostic studies.

Angiographic Determination of Cerebral Blood Flow Patterns

In addition to standard anatomic features, the angiogram is also routinely used to assess the physiologic impact of the lesion on the surrounding brain. Historically, one of the most important characteristics of the arterial phase of the angiogram was cerebral steal. This term was introduced by Murphy in 1954 (27). Feindel and Perot were the first to apply the term to AMVs when they reported the occurrence of bright red veins at the time of surgery to describe the reduction in nutrient flow through the surrounding brain caused by low-resistance shunt flow through the AVM (28). Feindel and co-workers (29) quantitated the reduction in flow in the brain surrounding an AVM. Nornes later described the pressure changes that occur along a feeding vessel, which may result in a diminution of perfusion pressure in nutrient branches that supply the surrounding normal brain (30). The effect of such changes is to place the surrounding brain at risk for ischemic damage. The clinical application of cerebral steal syndrome to symptoms related to ischemia remains in use, although the incidence of the clinical steal syndrome in AVMs appears to be rare.

It has been suggested that such alterations in perfusion pressure to the surrounding brain are associated with an increased risk of post-treatment hemorrhage from normal perfusion pressure breakthrough (31). The role of this putative phenomenon in the etiology of hemodynamic complications following treatment of AVMs must be reevaluated in light of the theory of occlusive hyperemia, whereby obstruction of the venous outflow system is believed to be a primary cause of postoperative hemorrhage and edema (32,33).

MRI/MRA

As noted previously, standard sequence MRI provides information on the size and location of the AVM. The relationship of feeding arteries and draining veins to the nidus can be demonstrated non-invasively using MRA. Three-dimensional time-of-flight techniques are best suited for depicting arterial inflow, whereas two-dimensional time-of-flight techniques are best suited for demonstrating the relatively slower flow of the venous drainage (34,35). Delineation of venous drainage may be optimized by the administration of contrast agents. Dephasing artifacts due to turbulent flow often causes signal dropout in portions of the AVM that prevents MRA from replacing detailed standard angiography for accurate delineation of AVM angioarchitecture (Fig. 7). MR angiogram sequences can, however, provide some estimate of not only the vessel anatomy but also the flow in particular vessels (Fig. 8) (36). The role of MRA flow determinations in helping to

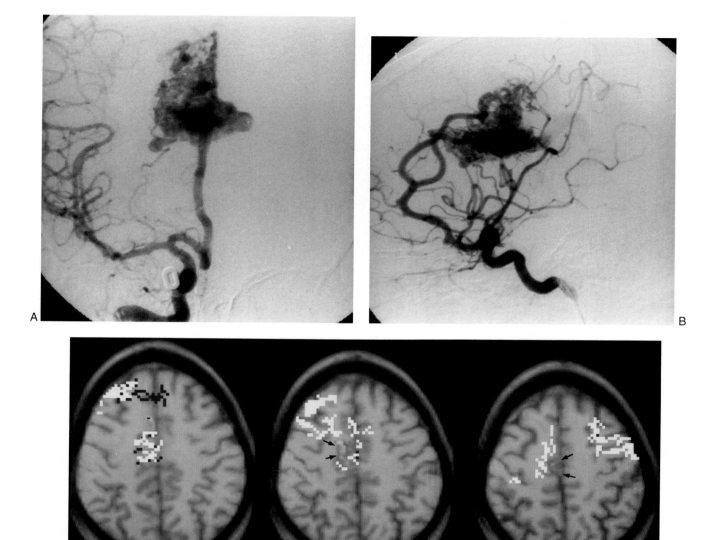

FIG. 6. (A, B) Posterior-anterior and lateral right internal carotid artery angiogram demonstrates a posterior right frontal AVM. **(C)** Functional MRI during bilateral lower extremity motor tasks. Note the proximity of the AVM nidus *(arrows)* to the left lower extremity motor cortex.

predict the response to treatment based on alterations of either feeding artery or draining vein flow rates, however, needs to be clarified by further studies.

TCD

Transcranial Doppler assessment of patients with AVMs suggests that some of the observed hemodynamic patterns may have therapeutic implications (37). TCD studies have also been used in conjunction with physiological challenges. Impaired CO_2 reactivity in some feeding arteries, as compared to contralateral vessels, was demonstrated after hyperventilation (38). Further experience with this technique is

needed to determine if such information can predict the possible development of hemodynamic complications and lead to modifications in treatment strategies.

PET/SPECT/CT XENON CBF

Batjer and Devous used xenon cerebral blood flow (CBF) determinations before and after an acetazolamide challenge in 35 patients with AVMs. Patients with hyperemic complications were noted to have vasodilatation to acetazolamide in territories surrounding the AVM, perforating vessel feeding, and evidence of angiographic steal (39). Tarr and colleagues (40) used acetazolamide challenge xenon CT CBF analysis

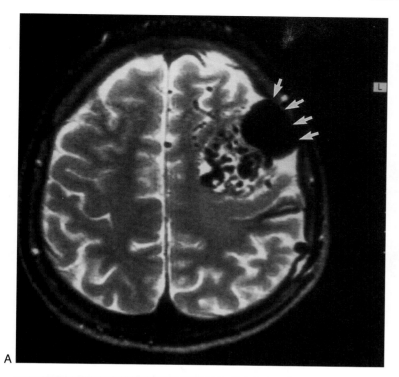

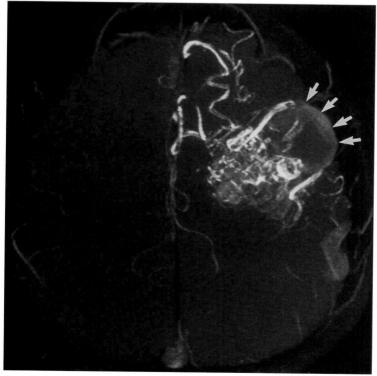

FIG. 7. A: Axial T2-weighted MRI demonstrates a left frontal AVM associated with a large venous varix *(arrows).* **B:** Three-dimensional time-of-flight magnetic resonance angiography demonstrates the feeding arterial pedicles as well as the nidus. However, note the signal dropout in the venous varix due to turbulent flows *(arrows).*

in the evaluation of patients with AVMs. They noted abnormal vasoreactivity in parenchymal areas in proximity and at a distance from the AVM nidus, suggesting that AVMs may affect the hemodynamic milieu of both proximal and distal vascular territories (Fig. 9). These authors also documented impaired vasoreactivity following partial AVM emboliza-

tion, which returned to normal in a time-dependent fashion (41).

PET scans have also been utilized in an attempt to determine whether a particular AVM was associated with alterations in either the blood flow or regulatory capacity of the surrounding brain (Fig. 10) (42). Further studies are needed

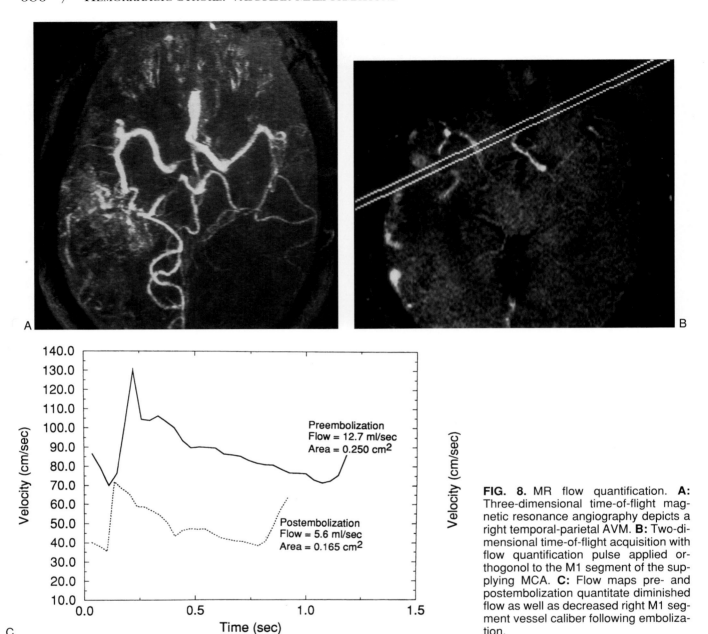

FIG. 8. MR flow quantification. **A:** Three-dimensional time-of-flight magnetic resonance angiography depicts a right temporal-parietal AVM. **B:** Two-dimensional time-of-flight acquisition with flow quantification pulse applied orthogonol to the M1 segment of the supplying MCA. **C:** Flow maps pre- and postembolization quantitate diminished flow as well as decreased right M1 segment vessel caliber following embolization.

to determine if imaging of blood flow changes with TCD, xenon CT, SPECT, or PET in response to physiologic challenges can serve as a guide to determine the safety of a particular treatment or the optimal time between staged embolizations.

Endovascular Diagnostics

Functional Importance

The use of amytal testing to determine dominance of language function is well recognized (43). With refinement of microcatheter techniques, the supraselective amytal test has

been used to determine the safety of therapeutic intervention with respect to specific vessels (44). There are, however, no objective studies of the accuracy or reliability of this method for determining the functional importance of specific vessels, especially in the presence of high-flow AVMs where flow may be partially diverted from functionally important cortex; reliance on this method alone may not be warranted.

Pedicle pressures

Endovascular determination of feeding artery pressures reported by Norbash and colleagues helped to provide a physiological basis for the relationship between angio-

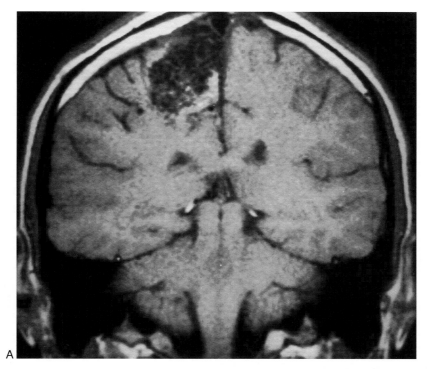

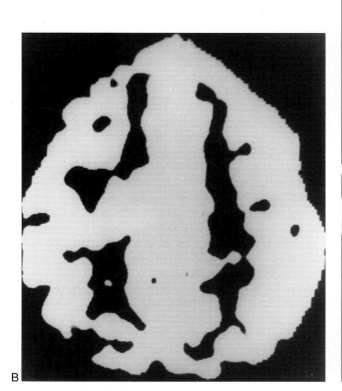

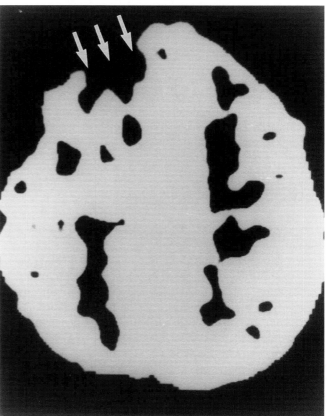

FIG. 9. A: T1-weighted coronal MRI depicts a medial right parietal AVM nidus. **B:** Baseline stable xenon CT cerebral blood flow (CBF) map. **C:** Post-acetazolamide (Diamox) stable xenon CT CBF map. Following acetazolamide administration, there is evidence of steal in the right ACA–MCA watershed distribution *(arrows)*. (White = CBF ≥ 30 cm³/100 g/min; black = CBF < 30 cm³/100 g/min.)

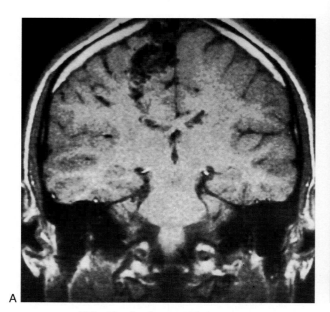

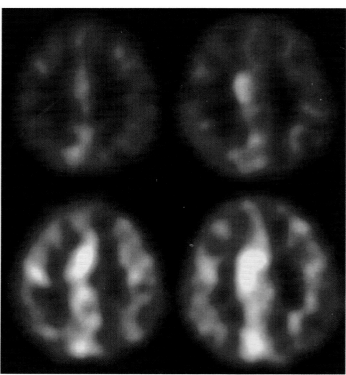

FIG. 10. A: Coronal T1-weighted MRI demonstrates medial right frontal AVM. **B:** Functional positron emission tomography scan during left leg motor tasks maps the left leg motor cortex. (Top row = baseline; bottom row = left arm motor task.)

graphic characteristics and the risk of hemorrhage and steal symptoms (12). Several investigators have also used measurements of pedicle pressures in an attempt to determine the risk of rupture of an AVM during or immediately following therapeutic embolization (45).

CONSIDERATIONS FOR TREATMENT

The natural history of AVMs underscores the need for therapeutic intervention. While no treatment is without risk, deferring therapy until the AVM becomes symptomatic from hemorrhage carries significant risks in that the morbidity and mortality rates from an initial hemorrhage are approximately 40% and 17%, respectively (5). Prevention of hemorrhage, while certainly a prime consideration in the management of patients with AVM, is not the only therapeutic goal. Seizures can be a devastating problem, and approximately 38% of patients present with seizures (46,47). Previous reports had suggested that there was no substantial improvement in seizure control after AVM resection (27). Recent studies suggest that successful surgical AVM extirpation can reduce seizure frequency (48,49).

As will be detailed in subsequent chapters, microsurgical, radiosurgical, and endovascular techniques have been used successfully in the treatment of AVMs. The appropriate role of each of these therapies, either alone or in combination,

is emerging. Because of better understanding of the natural history of AVMs and refinements in therapeutic options, treatment should be considered for almost all patients who harbor an AVM.

Several classifications, based predominantly on size and location, have been proposed to correlate the type of AVM with the risk of neurologic deficit or mortality following treatment (39,50–53). The system proposed by Spetzler and Martin in 1986 seems to have received the widest acceptance (53). This grading assigns a numeric value to the AVM size, the functional importance (described by the authors as eloquence) of the adjacent brain, and the pattern of venous drainage. The classification of inoperable (grade VI) may not be accurately reflected in the strict application of this system. Thus, as Heros has pointed out, a small brainstem AVM with no surface presentation is usually considered inoperable, although receiving only a grade III (54). While most would agree that an experienced surgeon could remove lesions in grades I, II, or III with a high degree of safety, the decision to operate on patients with grade IV or V lesions is considerably more complex. The treatment of patients with larger, more deeply situated AVMs (grades IV and V) is associated with an increase in neurologic deficit in at least 20% of patients (55,56). The management of patients in this subgroup mandates that a more precise analysis of the AVM that takes into account the nature and extent of the arterial input, the specific patterns and characteristics of the venous drainage, the degree of cortical representation, and the configuration of the nidus needs to be developed to determine which patients have a greater risk of neurologic damage from operative intervention. Whether the physiologic studies detailed in the previous section are capable of providing this information is currently being evaluated.

With respect to which mode of therapy is optimal, Steiner and colleagues have suggested that microsurgery, radiosurgery, and endovascular surgery are compatible and complementary (57). This may be especially true in deep, centrally located AVMs, which are often difficult to treat by any single mode of therapy. Hurst and colleagues reviewed the role of endovascular treatment in these lesions (58). The role of microsurgery was documented by Sisti and colleagues, who reviewed their experience with 67 AVMs <3 cm in diameter and reported angiographic obliteration in 94% with a surgical morbidity of 1.5% and no operative mortality. Forty-five percent of these lesions were in regions that some would consider surgically inaccessible, such as the thalamus, brainstem, medial hemisphere, and paraventricular regions. The immediate protection against hemorrhage provided by microsurgical removal is a real advantage, and the avoidance of the theoretical risk of development of delayed radiation-related brain injury is an advantage over stereotactic radiosurgery (59,60). The results of this series emphasize that size alone should not dictate which form of treatment is offered to a patient. Similarly, some large lesions previously classified as unresectable may also be safely managed surgically. By using a regimen of staged preoperative embolizations it may be possible to avoid hemodynamic consequences of acute resection and render very large lesions manageable.

The importance of a comprehensive team approach, which includes specialists in microvascular neurosurgery, endovascular neuroradiology, and stereotactic radiosurgery, cannot be overemphasized in ensuring that patients receive appropriate therapy. Large lesions previously classified as unresectable may be successfully managed with a combination of endovascular techniques followed by surgical excision or radiosurgery, and many small lesions can be immediately and effectively eliminated with microsurgery.

ACKNOWLEDGMENTS

The authors gratefully acknowledge the editorial assistance of Larimee Cortnik and Kathleen Hammer.

REFERENCES

1. Samson DS, Batjer HH. Preoperative evaluation of the risk/benefit ratio for arteriovenous malformations of the brain. In: Williams RH, Rengachary SS, eds. *Neurosurgery Update II. Vascular, Spinal, Pediatric, and Functional Neurosurgery.* New York: McGraw-Hill, 1991; 129–133.
2. Wilkins RH. Natural history of intracranial vascular malformation: a review. *Neurosurgery* 1985;16:421–430.
3. Brown RD, Wiebers DO, Forbes G, et al. The natural history of unruptured intracranial arteriovenous malformations. *J Neurosurg* 1988;68: 352–357.
4. Ondra SL, Troupp H, George ED, Schwab K. The natural history of symptomatic arteriovenous malformations of the brain: 24 year follow-up assessment. *J Neurosurg* 1990; 73:387–391.
5. Barrow DL. Intracranial aneurysms and vascular malformations. *Clin Neurosurg* 1992;40:3–39.
6. Troupp H. Arteriovenous malformations of the brain: What are the indications for operation? In: Morley TP, ed. *Current Controversies in Neurosurgery.* Philadelphia: W.B. Saunders, 1976;210–216.
7. Troupp H, Marttila I, Halonen V. Arteriovenous malformations of the brain. Prognosis without operation. *Acta Neurochir* (Wein) 1970;22: 125–128.
8. Graf CJ, Perret GE, Torner JC: Bleeding from cerebral arteriovenous malformations as part of their natural history. *J Neurosurg* 58:331–337, 1983.
9. Leussenhop AJ: Natural history of cerebral arteriovenous malformations. In: Wilson CB, Stein BM, eds. *Intracranial Arteriovenous Malformations.* Baltimore: Williams and Wilkins, 1984;24–31.
10. Horton JC, Chambers WA, Lyons SL, Adam RD, Kjellberg RN. Pregnancy and the risk of hemorrhage from cerebral arteriovenous malformations. *Neurosurgery* 1990;27:867–872.
11. Willinsky R, TerBrugge K, Montanera W, Wallace C, Aggarwal S. Micro-arteriovenous malformations of the brain: superselective angiography in diagnosis and treatment. *Am J Neuroradiol* 1992;13:325–330.
12. Norbash AM, Marks MP, Lane B. Correlation of pressure measurements with angiographic characteristics predisposing to hemorrhage and steal in cerebral arteriovenous malformations. *Am J Neuroradiol* 1994;15:809–813.
13. Spetzler RF, Hargraves RW, McCormick PW, Zambramski JM, Flom RA, Zimmerman RS. Relationship of perfusion pressure and size to risk of hemorrhage from arteriovenous malformations. *J Neurosurg* 1992;76:918–923.
14. Batjer H, Suss RA, Samson D. Intracranial arteriovenous malformations associated with aneurysms. *Neurosurgery* 1986;18:29–35.
15. Garcia-Monaco R, Rodesch G, Alvarez H, Iizuka Y, Hui F, Lasjaunias P. Pseudoaneurysms within ruptured intracranial arteriovenous malformations: diagnosis and early endovascular management. *Am J Neuroradiol* 1993;14:315–321.
16. Marks MP, Lane B, Steinberg GK, Chang PJ. Hemorrhage in intracerebral arteriovenous malformations: angiographic determinants. *Radiology* 1990;176:807–813.
17. Vinuela F, Nombela L, Roach MR, Fox A, Pelz DM. Stenotic and occlusive disease of the venous drainage system of deep brain AVMs. *J Neurosurg* 1985;63:180–184.
18. Miyasaka Y, Kurata A, Tokiwa K, Tanaka R, Yada K, Ohwada T. Draining vein pressure increases and hemorrhage in patients with arteriovenous malformation. *Stroke* 1994;25:504–507.
19. Berger MS, Cohen W, Ojemann GA. Correlation of motor cortex using intraoperative brain mapping data with preoperative magnetic resonance imaging anatomy. *J Neurosurg* 1990;72:383–387.
20. Connelly A, Jackson GD, Frackowiak RS, Belliveau JW, Vargha-Khadem F, Gadian DG. Functional mapping of activated human primary cortex with a clinical MR imaging system. *Radiology* 1993;188: 125–130.
21. Yetkin FZ, Mueller WM, Hammeke TA, Morris GE, Haughton VM. Functional magnetic resonance image mapping of the sensorimotor cortex with tactile stimulation. *Neurosurgery* 1995;36:921–925.
22. Jack CR, Thompson RM, Butts RK, et al. Sensory motor cortex: Correlation of presurgical mapping with functional MR imaging and invasive cortical mapping. *Radiology* 1994;190:85–92.
23. Kelly DL, Goldring S, O Leary JL. Averaged evoked somatosensory responses from the exposed cortex of man. *Arch Neurol* 1965;73:1–9.
24. Gregori EM, Goldring S. Localization of function in the excision of lesions from the sensorimortor region. *J Neurosurg* 1984;61: 1047–1054.
25. King RB, Schell GR. Cortical localization and monitoring during cerebral operations. *J Neurosurg* 1987;67:210–214.
26. Ojemann GA, Ojemann J, Lettich E, Berger M. Cortical language localization in left, dominant hemisphere. An electrical stimulation mapping investigation in 117 patients. *J Neurosurg* 1989;71:316–326.
27. Murphy JP. *Cerebrovascular Disease.* Chicago: Year Book; 1954.
28. Feindel W, Perot P. Red cerebral veins: A report on arteriovenous shunts in tumors and cerebral scars. *J Neurosurg* 1986;22:315–325.

29. Feindel W, Yamamoto YL, Hodge CP. Red cerebral veins and the cerebral steal syndrome. *J Neurosurg* 1971;35:167–179.

30. Nornes H, Grip A. Hemodynamic aspects of cerebral arteriovenous malformations. *J Neurosurg* 1980;53:456–464.

31. Spetzler RF, Wilson CB, Weinstein P, Mehdorn M, Townsend J, Tellis. Normal perfusion pressure breakthrough theory. *Clin Neurosurg* 1978; 25:651–672,

32. Al-Rodhan NRF, Sundt TM Jr, Piepgras DG, Nichols DA, Rufenacht D, Stevens LN. Occlusive hyperemia: a theory for the hemodynamic complication following resection of intracerebral arteriovenous malformations. *J Neurosurg* 1993;78:167–175.

33. Wilson CB, Hieshima G. Occlusive hyperemia: a new way to think about an old problem. *J Neurosurg* 1993;78:165–166.

34. Edelman RR, Wentz KU, Mattle HP, et al. Intracerebral arteriovenous malformations: Evaluation with selective MR angiography and venography. *Radiology* 1989;173:831–837.

35. Marchal G, Bosmans H, Van-Fraeyenhoven L, et al. Intracranial vascular lesions: optimization and clinical evaluation of three dimensional time-of-flight MR angiography. *Radiology* 1990;179:443–448.

36. Wasserman BA, Lin W, Tarr RW, Haacke EM, Müller E. Cerebral arteriovenous flow quantification by means of two-dimensional cardiac gated phase-contrast MR imaging. *Radiology* 1995;194:681–686.

37. Manchola IF, DeSalles AAF, Foo TK, Ackerman RH, Candia GT, Kjellberg RN. Arteriovenous malformation hemodynamics: a transcranial Doppler study. *Neurosurgery* 1993;33:556–562.

38. DeSalles AAF, Manchola I. CO_2 reactivity in arteriovenous malformations of the brain: a transcranial Doppler ultrasound study. *J Neurosurg* 1994;80:624–630.

39. Batjer HH, Devous MD, Seibert GB, et al. Intracranial arteriovenous malformation: relationship between clinical factors and surgical complications. *Neurosurgery* 1989;24:75–79.47.

40. Tarr RW, Johnson DW, Rutigliano M, et al. Use of acetazolamide-challenge xenon CT in the assessment of cerebral blood flow dynamics in patients with arteriovenous malformations. *Am J Neuroradiol* 1990; 11:441–448.

41. Tarr RW, Johnson DW, Horton JA, et al. Impaired cerebral vasoreactivity after embolization of arteriovenous malformations: assessment with serial acetazolamide challenge from Xenon CT. *Am J Neuroradiol* 1991;13:417–423.

42. Tyler JL, Leblanc R, Meyer E, et al. Hemodynamic and metabolic effects of cerebral arteriovenous malformations studied by positron emission tomography. *Stroke* 1989;20:890–898.

43. Wada J, Rasmussen T. Intracarotid injections of sodium amytal for the lateralization of cerebral speech dominance. *J Neurosurg* 1960;17: 266–282.

44. Rauch RA, Vinuela F, Dion J, et al. Preembolization functional evaluation in brain arteriovenous malformations: the superselective amytal test. *AJNR* 1992;13:303–308.

45. Jungreis CA, Horton JA, Hecht ST. Blood pressure changes in feeders to cerebral arteriovenous malformations during therapeutic embolization. *Am J Neuroradiol* 1989;10:575–577.

46. Martin NA, Vinters HV. Arteriovenous Malformations. In: Carter LP, Spetzler RF, Hamilton MG, eds. *Neurovascular Surgery*. New York: McGraw-Hill, 1994;875–904.

47. Weiland ME: Arteriovenous malformations and epilepsy. In: Carter LP, Spetzler RF, Hamilton MG, eds. *Neurovascular Surgery*. New York: McGraw-Hill, 1994;875–904.

48. Hwa-Shain Y, Tew JM Jr, Gartner M. Seizure control after surgery on cerebral arteriovenous malformations. *J Neurosurg* 1993;78:12–18.

49. Piepgras DG, Sundt TM Jr, Ragoowansi AT, Stevens L. Seizure outcome in patients with surgically treated cerebral arteriovenous malformations. *J Neurosurg* 1993;78:5–11.

50. Garretson HD. Intracranial arteriovenous malformations. In: Wilkins RH, Rengachary SS, eds. *Neurosurgery*. New York: McGraw-Hill, 1985;1448–1458.

51. Luessenhop AJ, Gennarelli TA. Anatomical grading of supratentorial arteriovenous malformations for determining operability. *Neurosurgery* 1:30–35, 1977.

52. Shi Y, Chen X. A proposed scheme for grading intracranial arteriovenous malformations. *J Neurosurg* 1986;65:484–489.

53. Spetzler RF, Martin NA. A proposed grading system for arteriovenous malformations. *J Neurosurg* 1986;65:476–483.

54. Heros RC. Commentary. *Neurosurgery* 1994;34:7.

55. Hamilton MG, Spetzler RF. The prospective application of a grading system for arteriovenous malformations. *Neurosurgery* 1994;34:2–7.

56. Heros RC, Kosrosue K, Diebold PM. Surgical excision of cerebral arteriovenous malformations: late results. *Neurosurgery* 1990;26: 570–578.

57. Steiner L, Lindquist C, Cail W, Karlsson B, Steiner M. Microsurgery and radiosurgery in brain arteriovenous malformations. *J Neurosurg* 1993;79:647–652.

58. Hurst RW, Berenstein A, Kupersmith MJ, Madrid M, Flamm ES. Deep central arteriovenous malformations of the brain; the role of endovascular treatment. *J Neurosurg* 1995;82:190–195,.

59. Sisti MB, Kader A, Stein BM. Microsurgery for 67 intracranial arteriovenous malformations less than 3 cm in diameter. *J Neurosurg* 1993; 79:653–660.

60. Yasargil MG. Microneurosurgery, vol III B: AVM of the brain, clinical considerations, general and specific operative techniques, surgical results, nonoperated cases, cavernous and venous angiomas. *Neuroanesthesia*. New York: Georg Thieme Verlag, 1988.

Cerebrovascular Disease, edited by H. Hunt Batjer.
Lippincott-Raven Publishers, Philadelphia © 1997.

CHAPTER 57

Principles of Interventional Neuroradiology

Fernando Viñuela, Gary Duckwiler, and Guido Guglielmi

Explosive technical developments in the manufacturing of microcatheters have been associated with marked improvements in intracranial navigation and superselective catheterization of cerebral arteries and veins beyond the circle of Willis. These techniques require appropriate technical and clinical training to keep iatrogenia at a minimum. Intracranial manipulation of microcatheters and microguidewires by inexperienced hands can result in catastrophic complications such as arterial perforation, arterial dissection, and cerebral thromboemboli. The properly trained interventional neuroradiologist is an important member of an interdisciplinary neurovascular team composed of vascular neurosurgeon, stroke neurologist, neuroanesthesiologist, and neurophysiologist.

The interventional neuroradiologist also works in close association with the diagnostic neuroradiologist. Neuroimaging tools such as brain computed tomography (CT), magnetic resonance imaging (MRI), magnetic resonance angiography (MRA), functional MR, positron emission tomography (PET), as well as standard and superselective digital angiography allow the gathering of important anatomic, functional, and dynamic information about the vascular pathology as well as the underlying normal brain or spinal cord. This information allows the neurotherapeutic team to elaborate a plan of action with less iatrogenia when dealing with complex intracranial vascular abnormalities such as arteriovenous malformations, arteriovenous fistulae, aneurysms, and vascular tumors.

The ability to perform safe intracranial vascular navigation opens a world of research and therapeutic alternatives. The interventional neuroradiologist may block abnormal arteriovenous communications as seen in arteriovenous malformations and fistulae, occlude arterial aneurysms, lyse a clot producing an acute ischemic stroke, or dilate an arterial

stenosis related to posthemorrhagic vasospasm or atheromatous plaque. This technology may be applied alone or in association with other therapeutic modalities such as microvascular or stereotactic neurosurgery.

The interventional neuroradiologist also profits from the explosive development of dedicated sophisticated neuroangiography suites with modern electronic technology such as biplane fluoroscopy, rapid-sequence digital angiography, electronic magnification, and road mapping capabilities. This technology permits an appropriate and permanent identification of intracranial vascular geometry, microcatheter position, and localization of the therapeutic target.

ARTERIOVENOUS MALFORMATIONS OF THE BRAIN

Cerebral arteriovenous malformations (AVMs) are the most common vascular malformations of the central nervous system (1). They are located in the brain (pial AVMs), the dura mater (dural AVMs), or both (mixed AVMs).

AVMs may be supra- or infratentorial and they frequently recruit blood supply from more than one arterial territory (anterior, middle, and posterior cerebral arteries) and from perforators (lenticulostriate, thalamoperforators, anterior and posterior choroidal, etc.) (2). AVMs may be associated with aneurysms in the circle of Willis in 6–9% of cases (3).

The utilization of superselective angiography of arterial pedicles of AVMs has shown intranidal aneurysms in more than 12% of cases. Not infrequently, a plexiform AVM may also be associated with arteriovenous fistulae in the same arterial territory (4).

Patients harboring a brain AVM may present with an intracranial hemorrhage (parenchymal, subarachnoid, intraventricular, or mixed), seizures, progressive neurologic deficit, headaches, and progressive mental deterioration (5).

The natural history of the disease is unclear. Forster et al. reported that 10–17% of patients may die from a hemorrhage whereas 40–50% may have a neurologic deterioration and become invalids over 20–40 years (6).

F. Viñuela, G. Duckwiler, and G. Guglielmi: Department of Radiology, University of California at Los Angeles, Los Angeles, CA 90024.

The choice of therapy for AVMs of the brain depends on the patient's clinical presentation and the size and topography of the lesion. Modern neuroimaging modalities permit the collection on important pretherapeutic anatomic, functional, and dynamic information, which influences the type of therapy selected.

CT and MRI-MRA demonstrate anatomic information such as size and location of the AVM nidus and status of the surrounding brain parenchyma. MRA shows promise for evaluating the number and size of feeders and drainers as well as the angioarchitecture of the AVM nidus.

Digital, rapid sequence, standard cerebral angiography remains the gold standard for the anatomic evaluation of brain AVMs.

Modern imaging technology also allows the collection of functional information with particular attention to the detection of cortical eloquent/essential areas such as motor-sensory, language, and visual cortexes. Such technology includes two- and three-dimensional MRI (detection of central sulcus), somatosensory evoked potentials, high-resolution electroencephalography, superselective amobarbital (Amytal) testing, and PET. Functional MRI and magnetoencephalography have now been incorporated as important functional tests and they may help to map brain activity in higher cognitive functions (7).

Hemodynamic changes associated with brain AVMs such as arterial steal, venous hypertension, and the breakthrough phenomenon may be the source of neurologic symptoms or iatrogenia. Dynamic neuroimaging tools such as PET, single photon emission tomography, xenon CT transcranial Doppler ultrasonography, and intravascular pressure monitoring have been utilized to observe blood flow dynamics before, during, and after endovascular or surgical therapy of brain AVMs.

Technical Considerations

Most endovascular embolizations of brain AVMs are performed in the neuroangiography suite with the patient under neuroleptic analgesia, systemic heparinization, and utilization of a transfemoral arterial approach. In exceptional cases (the pediatric population and very uncooperative patients) general anesthesia is utilized.

The intraoperative catheterization and embolization of AVM arterial feeders is now an exceptional procedure due to the development of new generations of microcatheters that can be positioned very close to the AVM nidus (8). In most cases, flow-guided catheters are utilized. They do not need microguidewires and the morbidity related to its intravascular manipulation is low.

The embolic occlusion of an arterial pedicle and corresponding AVM nidus may be preceded by superselective amobarbital testing. This functional testing is useful for detecting brain cortical eloquent areas (motor-sensory cortex, language cortex, etc.) or the functional role of perforators such as lenticulostriate perforators, thalamoperforators, or anterior and posterior choroidal arteries (9,10).

Materials used to embolize brain AVMs include particles (polyvinyl alcohol foam), liquid agents (acrylics, alcohol), and detachable balloons or coils (11–13). It is essential to deposit the embolic material in the AVM nidus to minimize the possibility of AVM recanalization. The occlusion of AVM arterial feeders without nidus occlusion may complicate final surgical removal of the lesion due to the development of collateral circulation from leptomeningeal, transmedullary, and transdural arteries (14).

After the embolization procedure is finished, systemic heparinization is reversed with protamine (10 mg protamine/1000 U heparin) and the patient is admitted to an intermediate care unit for 12 hours. Discharge is performed 3 days later, if clinically warranted.

A staged, preoperative embolization may be performed in large or giant AVMs. The time between embolizations varies from patient to patient but is approximately 3–5 days. The lapse between embolization and final surgical removal of the residual AVM is approximately 7–10 days. Emergency surgical removal of the residual AVM is recommended if there is postembolization angiographic evidences of untoward embolic occlusion of a dominant draining vein. This hemodynamic situation may precipitate an acute or delayed hemorrhagic complication.

Goals of Embolization

Endovascular embolization of brain AVMs may be performed alone or in combination with surgery or stereotactic neurosurgery (15). Six specific goals may be identified:

1. Presurgical embolization of large and giant cortical AVMs (Fig. 1).
2. Prestereotactic embolization in nonsurgical cortical or deep AVMs (Fig. 2).
3. Palliative embolization in large AVMs presenting with progressive neurologic deficit.
4. Palliative embolization in large cortical AVMs presenting with seizures resistant to medical therapy.
5. Palliative embolization in deep AVMs presenting with hemorrhage or progressive neurologic deficit.
6. Intravascular embolization of small AVMs as the single therapeutic modality (Fig. 3).

In our experience with 456 patients, 55% of them had postembolization complete surgical resection of the residual AVM. This therapeutic strategy is particularly useful in large AVMs receiving blood supply from multiple arterial territories. The endovascular occlusion of deep feeders such as anterior or posterior perforators, anterior or posterior choroidal and posterior cerebral feeders facilitates the intraoperative control of hemorrhage and complete resection of the AVM nidus.

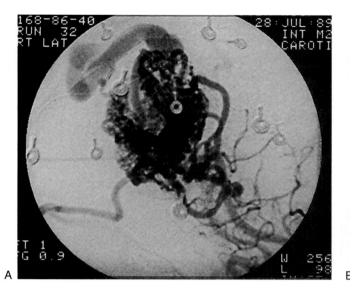

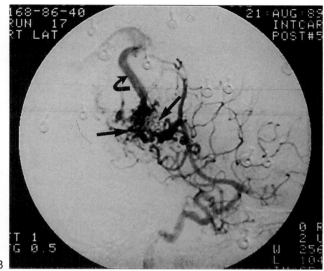

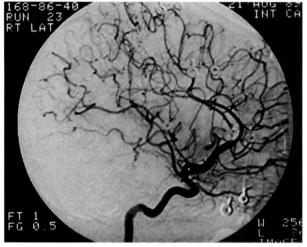

FIG. 1. Presurgical embolization of brain AVM. A) Lateral right internal carotid angiogram shows a large cortical parietal AVM. B) Immediate post-embolization angiogram shows small residual AVM (straight arrow) and slow flow into dominant draining vein (curved arrow). C) Post-surgical internal carotid angiogram shows complete surgical removal of residual AVM. The patient remained neurologically intact.

Morbidity and Mortality

The morbidity related to endovascular embolization of brain AVMs may be related to ischemic or hemorrhagic complications occurring during or immediately after the procedure. Ischemic complications have been reduced dramatically with the new generation of microcatheters and improved superselective catheterization, and with the utilization of preembolization superselective amobarbital testing. We have identified hemorrhagic complications in 19 of 456 patients (4%) who had endovascular embolization of brain AVMs. The cause of these hemorrhagic complications were arterial perforation in 8 patients (1.75%), intranidal aneurysm rupture in 3 (0.65%), untoward venous occlusion in partially embolized AVMs in 4 (0.877%), and undetermined in 4 (0.877%).

The mortality in our series of 456 patients may be separated into two distinct groups. In our first 128 patients in whom we used calibrated-leak balloons and intraoperative embolization, the mortality rate was 3.9%. The following

328 patients were embolized with the new generation of microcatheters and a more intensive use of superselective amobarbital testing. The mortality rate related to embolization alone in this group of patients was 0.9% and the surgical mortality was 1.52%. All cases were large or giant AVMs with pre-surgical embolic occlusion of 50% or less of the AVM nidus.

DURAL ARTERIOVENOUS FISTULAE

Dural arteriovenous fistulae (DAVFs) are abnormal arteriovenous communications located within the dura mater. These may drain into dural sinuses, dural veins, or adjacent cortical veins.

They are most often acquired and seen in the adult population. However, they can also be found in neonates, sometimes mimicking the clinical presentation of a high-flow Galenic arteriovenous fistula.

DAVFs may be located anywhere in the dura mater, al-

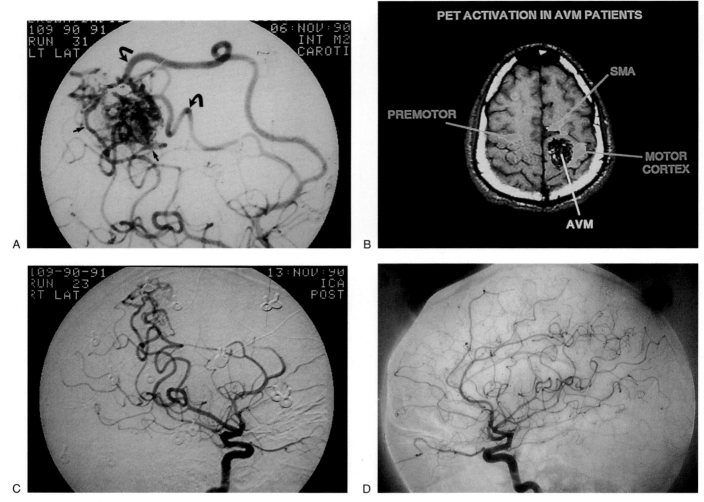

FIG. 2. AVM embolization followed by stereotaDFIGic radiosurgery. A) Lateral left internal carotid angiogram shows a posterior fronto-parietal AVM fed by anterior (curved arrows) and middle (straight arrows) cerebral artery feeders. B) MRI/PET imaging combination shows the AVM nidus intimately related to the left motor cortex. C) Immediate postembolization angiogram shows obliteration of anterior cerebral artery feeders and a small residual AVM supplied by middle cerebral artery feeders. D) One year follow-up angios after stereotatactic radiosurgery of residual AVM shows complete occlusion of avm nidus and preservation of normal cerebral circulation.

though they most often involve the transverse/sigmoid sinuses, cavernous sinus, superior sagittal sinus, the dura of anterior fossa (ethmoidal dural AVF), the superior petrosal sinus and tentorium. They are less frequently observed involving the inferior petrosal sinus and marginal sinus (16–18)

Selective and superselective digital angiography remain the gold standard for the topographic and anatomic diagnosis of DAVFs. They show the anatomic localization and arterial supply of the DAVFs, critical anastomosis between extra- and intracranial circulations, partial or complete thrombosis of dural sinuses, and recruitment of brain cortical veins with venous hypertension.

The blood supply of the dura mater is complex. It is important to emphasize important extra- and intracranial contribu-

tions (19,20). The intracranial blood supply arises from the meningeal branches of the intracavernous internal carotid artery (meningohypophyseal and infero-lateral trunks), the ophthalmic artery (ethmoidal and anterior falcine branches), and the vertebral artery (anterior and posterior meningeal arteries). The extracranial blood supply originates from the meningeal branches of the external carotid artery (dural branches from occipital, ascending pharyngeal, middle meningeal, and internal maxillary arteries) and the transosseous branches of superficial temporal and posterior auricular arteries.

The clinical presentation of DAVFs depends on their location, low- or high-speed arteriovenous shunting, the presence of dural sinus thrombosis, and recruitment of cortical veins. The recruitment of cortical veins and development of

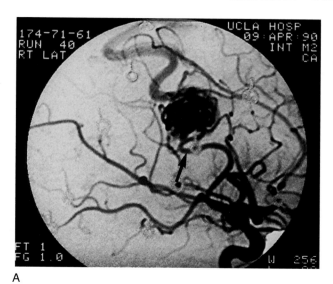

FIG. 3. Complete AVM occlusion by embolization alone. A) Right lateral internal carotid angiogram shows a small posterior frontal AVM supplied by a single arterial feeder (straight arrow) and draining through a single vein. B) Immediate post-embolization angiogram shows complete AVM occlusion. The patient remained neurologically intact after the procedure.

varices may produce mass effect or intracranial hemorrhage (21,22).

DAVFs of transverse/sigmoid sinuses may present with intracranial, pulse-synchronous bruit; moderate or severe headaches; or symptoms related to venous hypertension such as seizures, progressive neurologic deficit, or intracranial hemorrhage.

Cavernous sinus DAVFs classically present with progressive exophthalmos, chemosis and conjunctival edema, increased intraocular pressure, diplopia, headaches, and intracranial bruit. Decreased visual acuity may be related to

chronic venous hypertension and ischemia of the optic nerve. An intracranial hemorrhage may occur if there is flow diversion into cortical veins such as the superficial Sylvian or perimesencephalic veins (23).

DAVFs of superior petrosal sinus and tentorium commonly present with mass effect from perimesencephalic varices compressing the brainstem or intracranial hemorrhage. DAVFs of anterior fossa classically present with subarachnoid hemorrhage or intraparenchymal hemorrhage due to rupture of an enlarged or varicose cortical vein.

The therapeutic options in DAVFs include conservative therapy, compressive maneuvers in the neck, transarterial embolization, transvenous embolization, surgical sinus exposure and intraoperative embolization, direct surgical resection of the lesion, and a combination of the above.

The conservative therapy or compressive maneuvers in the neck are adopted when a DAVF presents with minor symptoms that are well tolerated by the patient (intracranial bruit or headaches) and digital angiography shows a slow-flow dural fistula without recruitment of cortical veins and venous hypertension. DAVFs may thrombose spontaneously and an aggressive therapeutic option with potential iatrogenia is not appropriate in these cases.

The transarterial embolization of DAVFs was the primary endovascular approach until the development of the now more popular transvenous embolization (24–26). This therapeutic modality was more successful in achieving 100% anatomic cure in intracavernous DAVFs and less successful in those in another locations such as transverse/sigmoid sinuses, tentorium, and superior sagittal sinus.

A complete digital cerebral angiography is followed by superselective angiography of dural arterial feeders such as middle meningeal, ascending pharyngeal, internal maxillary, or occipital arteries. The superselective embolization of the intracavernous branches of the internal carotid artery may also be performed in special situations, although they may be related to more severe clinical complications (27). A provocative test with the injection of amobarbital or xylocaine can precede the embolization in order to decrease the possibility of postembolization cranial nerve palsies (28).

Embolic materials utilized in DAVF transarterial embolization includes particles such as polyvinyl alcohol or gel foam, liquid agents such as pure ethanol or acrylics, and coils and balloons for large DAVFs mostly observed in congenital cases.

The aim of transarterial embolization is to decrease the sinus arteriovenous shunting, promote further thrombosis, and either cure the patient or prepare him or her for a transvenous or surgical procedure. Transarterial embolization has a limited anatomic success due to the difficulty of delivering the embolic material right at the arteriovenous fistula site. The proximal occlusion of arterial feeders elicits a very rapid and generous development of ipsilateral and contralateral dural collaterals that reestablishes the abnormal shunt with a more complex angioarchitecture.

The technical and clinical morbidity of this therapeutic

modality is low when performed by well-trained endovascular therapists. Risks include endovascular damage of arteries in the neck, brain ischemia or infarction due to embolization through critical (dangerous) arterial anastomosis, and cranial nerve palsies.

The critical or dangerous arterial anastomosis between extra- and intracranial circulations is very well described in the literature and may be the source of such catastrophic complications as monocular blindness, brain stroke, or death (29).

Postembolization cranial nerve palsy is related to nerve ischemia. It is produced by the untoward occlusion of critical neuromeningeal arteries that supply the cranial nerves when they pierce the dura at the skull base foramina (29). Examples are IXth, Xth, and XIth cranial nerve palsy, due to untoward embolization of neuromeningeal branch of ascending pharyngeal artery, and VIIth nerve palsy, due to emboliza-

tion of superior tympanic branches of middle meningeal artery or stylomastoid branch of occipital artery.

The transvenous embolization of DAVF was popularized by Halbach et al (30). The intracranial navigation into dural sinuses using a transfemoral, transjugular, or surgical approach is safe and allows positioning of a catheter, microcatheter, and embolic material at the dural fistula site without the need of a more dangerous transarterial navigation. For example, it is possible to embolize a transverse sinus DAVF by utilizing an ipsilateral venous approach if the sinus is partially thrombosed (Fig. 4). The contralateral transjugular-transtorcular navigation can be used in a completely thrombosed transverse-sigmoid sinus.

A cavernous sinus DAVF may be embolized through inferior petrosal or superior ophthalmic vein navigations or direct surgical puncture of the wall of the sinus (31–34).

The complete transvenous occlusion of the DAVF and

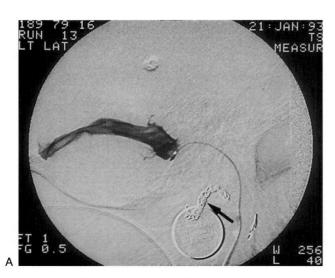

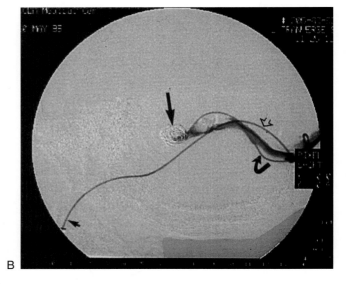

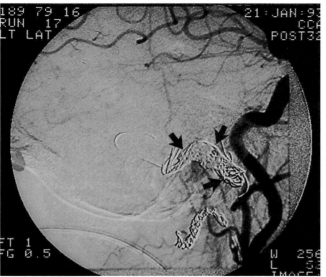

FIG. 4. Transvenous embolization of dural arteriovenous fistula. A) Ipsilateral retrograde catheterization of left dural sinus in a transverse/sigmoid DAVF. Platinum microcoils fill a large occipital feeder (arrows). B) Controlateral catheterization of distal part of left tranverse sinus through right jugular vein (small straight arrow), right transverse sinus (open arrow) and left transverse sinus (curve arrow). Metallic coils have been deposited at the fistula site (large straight arrow). C) Left common carotid angiogram shows complete obliteration of the left transverse/sigmoid DAVF. A cast of coils is seen filling the transverse/sigmoid junction (arrows).

diseased sinus may be achieved using stainless steel coils, platinum single or fibered microcoils, balloons, or acrylics. The diseased sinus may be completely occluded if it is not utilized by the normal brain in an anterograde fashion. The untoward endovascular occlusion of a dural sinus utilized by normal cortical veins may have catastrophic clinical complications such as severe cortical vein infarction or hemorrhage due to acute, irreversible venous hypertension.

The surgical treatment of DAVFs is now utilized as the last resort when the endovascular techniques have failed to completely occlude a fistula with cortical venous drainage and signs of venous hypertension. Surgery is very useful in DAVFs involving the superior petrosal sinus and tentorium and it is the primary therapeutic modality in ethmoidal (anterior fossa) DAVFs (35–37).

Presurgical embolization of DAVFs has dramatically reduced the surgical morbidity of these lesions, which was mainly related to uncontrollable blood loss (36).

INTRACRANIAL HIGH-FLOW ARTERIOVENOUS FISTULAE

In 1928, Walter Dandy was the first to diagnose and treat a cerebral arteriovenous fistula (38). Intracranial high-flow arteriovenous fistulae (IAVFs) may be defined as congenital or acquired single-hole arteriovenous communications producing important hemodynamic changes with neurologic and/or cardiovascular implications. The best known congenital IAVF is the Galenic malformation. The posttraumatic carotid cavernous arteriovenous fistula is the acquired arteriovenous fistula most commonly described in the adult population.

IAVF produces local hemodynamic changes common to all congenital or acquired types. Large, single, or multiple dilated arterial feeders drain directly into dural sinuses (congenital/acquired DAVFs), cortical pial veins (congenital non-Galenic pial arteriovenous fistulae), or vein of Galen (Galenic arteriovenous fistulae), producing massive arteriovenous shunting, turbulent flow, and increased intravenous pressure. These hemodynamic changes at the fistula site produce anatomic changes such as dilatation of arteries, involvment of dural sinuses or cortical veins, and recruitment of surrounding venous pathways (39–41). The clinical presentation of IAVF varies with age, localization (supra- or infratentorial, intra- or extradural, etc.), anatomic characteristics, severity of arteriovenous shunting, and dilatation of its venous outlet with frequent development of giant varices. The spectrum of clinical presentation includes congestive heart failure, mass effect, seizures, and, less commonly, intracranial hemorrhage (41–44).

Congestive heart failure is more commonly seen in neonatal Galenic, non-Galenic, and dural arteriovenous fistulae. It is related to the presence of a high-flow intracranial arteriovenous shunting with concomitant right heart overload. Seizure is more often seen in infants and children and is often related to brain compression by a large or giant varix and/or development of chronic venous hypertension. Mental retardation is more often observed in Galenic and congenital DAVFs than in congenital non-Galenic pial arteriovenous fistulae. It appears to be related to the development of uncontrollable seizures secondary to chronic venous hypertension, subcortical venous infarction, and dystrophic calcifications. Severe headache prevails in children and adults and may be explained on the basis of mass effect and/or chronic venous hypertension. Intracranial hemorrhage is rarely observed in this type of intracranial vascular abnormality and it may be related to a significant anatomic obstruction to the IAVF venous outlet (36,45).

Mass effect and severe venous hypertension are two factors that explain most clinical manifestations observed in acquired carotid cavernous fistulae (pulsating exophthalmos, double vision due to cranial nerve palsy, increased intraocular pressure, and decreased vision) (46,47).

Digital, standard, and superselective cerebral angiography remain the gold standard to achieve accurate information on localization of the arteriovenous shunting, size and number of arterial feeders, and identification of varices and collateral venous pathways. It is mandatory to perform a complete cerebral angiography with inclusion of anterior and posterior circulations as well as dural and pial arterial and venous circulations.

Yasargil classifies Galenic malformations according to their arterial supply (48). Type I includes Galenic malformations supplied by choroidal and pericallosal feeders. Type II is defined by the presence of transdiencephalic feeders. Type III is a combination of types I and II and type IV Galenic malformations are mesencephalic, diencephalic, and cerebellar arteriovenous malformations that drain preferentially into an enlarged vein of Galen.

In the non-Galenic arteriovenous fistulae, the arterial feeders may arise from middle, anterior, or posterior cerebral circulations or from participation of the three vascular territories (41). Varices are extraparenchymal and they may be located in the subarachnoid space of the interhemispheric fissure, cerebral convexity, basal cisterns, or in the posterior fossa extending through the tentorium or in the Galenic system (41).

The angiographic findings in congenital DAVFs include large dural arterial feeders arising from external and internal carotid and vertebral arteries draining into widely dilated dural sinuses, persistent embryonic venous sinuses, dural sinus stenosis or occlusions, and recruitment of cerebral veins with severe diffuse supra- and/or infratentorial venous hypertension.

The therapeutic modalities used to treat IAVF includes craniotomy and clipping of the feeding arteries. The surgical excision of the varix is no longer performed because proximal occlusion of arterial feeders has resulted in dramatic shrinkage of even giant varices (41).

The single or multiple arterial feeders may also be occluded by endovascular route (41,49). Using high-speed digital substraction angiography and road mapping, it is possible to identify the exact location of the arteriovenous fistulae in relation to the wall of the varix and occlude it with nondetachable or detachable balloons, standard or detachable microcoils, or acrylics (41,49,50) (Fig. 5). This procedure may be done in one therapeutic session or in stages. An abrupt occlusion of this type of vascular pathology may have deleterious effect in the brain (intracerebral hemorrhage or severe edema due to breakthrough phenomenon) or in the heart (intractable biventricular heart failure).

The surgical or endovascular occlusion of IAVFs must be performed as close as possible to the varix (Fig. 6). The proximal arterial occlusion is rapidly followed by distal re-

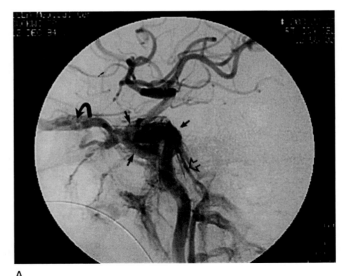

A

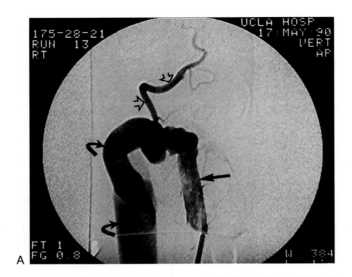

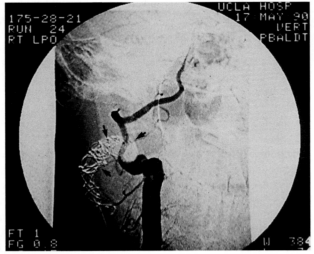

FIG. 5. Embolization of congenital, high flow skull base arteriovenous fistula. A) Frontal view of right vertebral angiogram shows a giant arteriovenous fistula between right vertebral artery (straight arrow) and right jugular vein (curved arrows). Notice the change in caliber of the vertebral artery distal to the fistula site (open arrow). B) Postembolization right vertebral angiogram shows complete coil obliteration of the AV fistula (arrows) with preservation of the normal vascular anatomy.

B

FIG. 6. Endovascular balloon occlusion of traumatic carotid cavernous fistula. A) Right internal carotid angiogram shows typical traumatic C-C fistula with abnormal filling of cavernous sinus (straight arrows), superior ophthalmic vein (curved arrow) and inferior petrosal sinus (open arrow). B) Postembolization carotid angiogram shows complete balloon obliteration of the CC fistula (arrows) with preservation of the lumen of the internal carotid artery.

constitution of the arteriovenous shunting by cortical, transmedullary, and transdural collaterals.

The most important technical/clinical complication associated with the endovascular treatment of IAVF is the untoward migration of the embolic material with acute occlusion of the varix or collateral venous circulation (intracerebral venous hemorrhage or infarction) or the pulmonary circulation (pulmonary thromboembolism).

The clinical and therapeutic aspects of traumatic skull base IAVF and, in particular, carotid cavernous fistulae are very well described in the literature (51,52). Endovascular occlusion of this vascular pathology has become the gold standard and the surgical option is utilized when endovascular techniques have failed to occlude completely the arteriovenous fistula.

Endovascular techniques includes transarterial, transvenous, and combined embolizations with deposit of embolic material in the venous side of the fistula, preserving the lumen of the injured artery.

In traumatic carotid cavernous fistulae, the classical technique of transarterial navigation and utilization of detachable balloons described by Serbinenko and Debrun remains a very effective endovascular modality with a high anatomic cure and low morbidity and mortality (53,54) (Fig. 6). Similar anatomic results are obtained with the transarterial or transvenous delivery in the injured cavernous sinus of standards or detachable coils and in limited occasions of acrylics.

The combination of all these endovascular techniques accomplish a complete anatomic cure of skull base, congenital or traumatic high-flow arteriovenous fistulae in more than 95% of cases with a very low morbidity and mortality.

ANEURYSMS

There is a relatively long history of endovascular techniques in the treatment of cerebral aneurysms. In the 1970s and 1980s the endovascular approach using detachable balloons emerged as a therapeutic alternative in selected cases of nonclippable intracranial aneurysms. The balloon was inserted into the aneurysm, excluding it from the circulation. Although this technique was effective in some cases, the risk of subarachnoid hemorrhage was significant and this balloon aneurysmal occlusion is no longer utilized (55,56). However, parent artery occlusion with detachable balloons in patients harboring skull base or intracranial giant or fusiform aneurysms remains a very valuable endovascular technique (57–59). Proximal artery occlusion or arterial balloon trapping may only be therapy for very complex aneurysms. Before permanently occluding the parent artery, it is mandatory to assure that the brain will have sufficient collateral arterial supply using anatomic visualization of the circle of Willis, functional evocative testing (temporary balloon occlusion without or with hypotensive testing), or quantitation of cerebral blood flow with test occlusion (HMPAO, SPECT, xenon CT), or simple neurologic monitoring during temporary balloon occlusion (60–62).

Currently, a new embolic material, the Guglielmi detachable coils (GDCs) (Target Therapeutic, Fremont, CA) is available for endosaccular occlusion of intracranial aneurysms. These are soft platinum coils that may be inserted into the aneurysm lumen, and after position is assured they are detached using a small direct current of 1 mA (63,64) (Fig. 7). This technique includes several steps. A Tracker microcatheter is introduced into the aneurysm using road mapping capabilities. The largest GDC coil is selected for that particular aneurysm in order to cross the neck of the aneurysm and influence the aneurysm inflow zone from the beginning of the procedure. The platinum coil is very soft and adapts to the shape of the aneurysm with a minimal increase in intraluminal pressure. The interstices of the first coil are then filled with smaller GDC coils until a compact packing of the aneurysm is obtained (Fig. 8).

Currently there are more than 30 types of GDC coils in small (Tracker 10 type) and large (Tracker 18 type) versions. The latest generation of GDC coils (soft coils type) allows a denser packing of the aneurysm and it appears to decrease

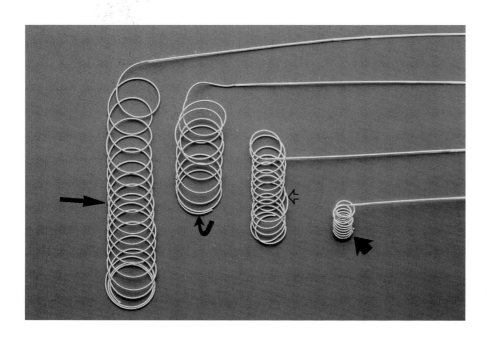

FIG. 7. GDC coils. Examples of 8x40 cm (straight arrow), 8x20 cm (curved arrow), 5x15 cm (open arrow) and 2x8 cm (fat arrow).

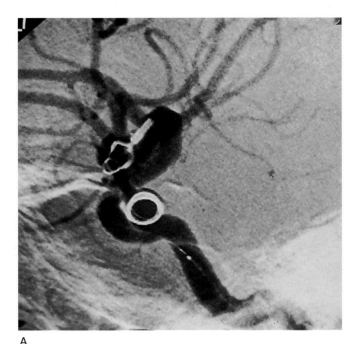

A

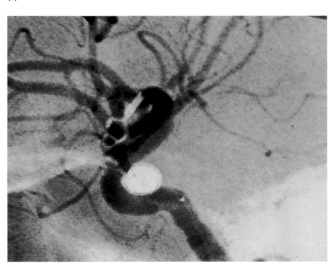

B

FIG. 8. Dense GDC packing of superior hypophyseal aneurysm. A) Example of deposit of first coil in superior hypophyseal aneurysm crossing across the neck of the aneurysm. B) Complete, dense GDC packing of the aneurysm with preservation of the lumen of the internal carotid artery.

the chance of perforating acutely ruptured aneurysms. The GDC endovascular material is now FDA-approved for use in surgically difficult intracranial aneurysms (Fig. 9).

The technique appears to be mostly effective in small aneurysms with a small neck (90% complete aneurysm occlusion and 7% re-canalization rate at 6 months) and in acutely ruptured aneurysms in neurologically deteriorated patients (Fig. 10). In wide-neck and in large aneurysms complete aneurysm occlusion falls to 50% and a 6-month follow-up

angiogram shows aneurysm recanalization in approximately 30% of cases.

We reviewed immediate anatomic and clinical results in GDC embolization of 403 acutely ruptured aneurysms (Tables 1–3). In this large multicenter phase III investigation the short-term reduction in rehemorrhage rate in the aneurysm population was very favorable when compared with the natural history of the disease, and there was a low complication rate.

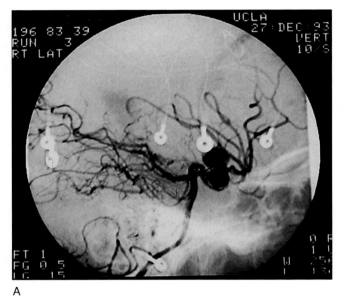

A

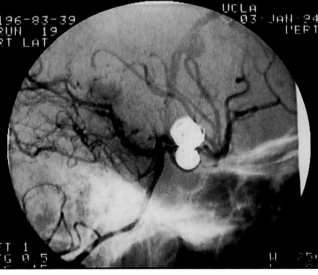

B

FIG. 9. GDC embolization of unclippable aneurysm. A) Lateral view of right vertebral angiogram shows a posterior communicating/P1 junctional, bilobulated aneurysm and retrograde filling of anterior circulation due to spontaneous occlusion of right internal carotid artery. B) Immediate post-embolization angiogram shows complete and dense GDC packing of the aneurysm with preservation of the lumen of the posterior communicating artery.

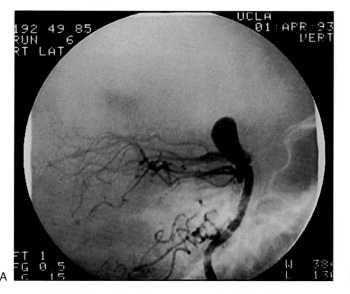

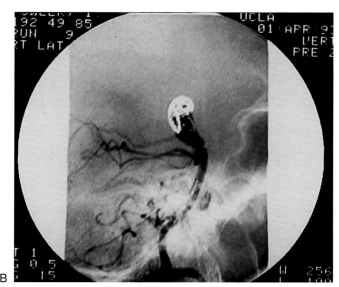

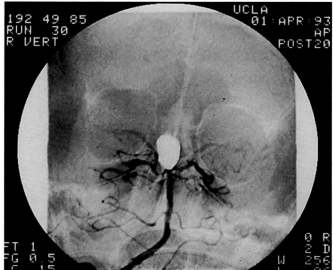

FIG. 10. GDC occlusion of acute ruptured aneurysm. A) Lateral view of right vertebral angiogram shows a large basilar tip aneurysm. B) GDC occlusion of dome of the aneurysm with GDC coils. C) Complete GDC occlusion of basilar tip aneurysm with preservation of lumen of basilar and posterior cerebral arteries. Patient remained neurologically unchanged at the end of procedure.

CEREBROVASCULAR ISCHEMIC DISEASE

The major neurointerventional methods for treatment of cerebrovascular ischemia include percutaneous angioplasty and intra-arterial thrombolysis. Percutaneous angioplasty may then be subdivided in angioplasty for atherosclerotic stenosis and angioplasty for symptomatic vasospasm following subarachnoid hemorrhage (SAH).

Vasospasm occurs after SAH with a relatively high frequency but it becomes symptomatic in 15–30% of cases. It peaks at approximately 7–10 days post-SAH but it can occur anywhere from 3 to 21 days after aneurysm rupture. Most

TABLE 1. *GDC Embolization in acutely ruptured aneurysms experience with 403 patients*

	Anatomical Results			
Size	Complete	Neck Remnant	Body Filling	Attempt
Small/small neck	70.8%	21.4%	4.3%	3.5%
Small/wide neck	31.4%	41.5%	10.3%	6.8%
Large aneurysm	35%	57.2%	5%	2.8%
Giant aneurysm	50%	50%	0%	0%

TABLE 2. *GDC embolization of acutely ruptured aneurysms; experience with 403 patients*

Technical Complications	
Type	Percentage
Aneurysm perforation	2.72%
Cerebral embolization	2.62%
Parent artery occlusion	2.9%
Coil migration	0.49%
Increased mass effect	0.49%
Total	9.22%

patients respond well to hypertension, hemodilution, and hypervolemia (HHH) medical therapy but in those patients who remain symptomatic after intensive immediate medical therapy endovascular therapy has a significant role to play. At our institution the patient's status post-SAH is monitored from the onset of symptomatic vasospasm by clinical examination, transcranial Doppler examination, and bedside hot xenon cerebral blood flow monitoring. If after a short while the clinical deficit is not reversed the patient is brought for cerebral angiography and endovascular treatment for vasospasm. In some cases, embolization of the ruptured aneurysm is performed immediately before endovascular treatment of vasospasm.

There are two primary endovascular methods for treatment of cerebral vasospasm: chemical and mechanical angioplasty. Chemical angioplasty is usually performed with papaverine. Papaverine infusion is most effective when given early in the course of vasospasm and when delivered superselectively at the site of vasospasm. The effect of papaverine is temporary and multiple infusions may be needed during the period of most severe vasospasm. Papaverine is incompatible with heparinized blood and needs to be mixed in normal saline. The typical dilution is 300 mg papaverine in 100 cm^3 normal saline and a typical dose per arterial territory would be 300 mg. The infusion rate of papaverine depends on systemic blood pressure. However, the total dose is typically infused over a 60-minute period (65,66). When infused below the ophthalmic artery, pupillary dilatation may occur and it must be distinguished from acute tentorial herniation. There have been reports of respiratory depression in the posterior fossa.

TABLE 3. *GDC embolization of acutely ruptured aneurysms; experience with 403 patients*

H&H grading/immediate morbi−mortality			
Grade	Unchanged	Deterioration	Death
I	92.8%	6%	1.2%
II	91.41%	8.6%	0%
III	83.6%	10.7%	5.7%
IV	53.8%	8.6%	11.6%
V	53.8%	11.6%	34.6%
Total	84.8%	8.9%	6.2%

Chemical angioplasty may be performed in conjunction with mechanical angioplasty. Although a variety of endovascular systems are available, the most commonly used in the United States would be the nondetachable silicone occlusion balloon with 0.2-cm^3 volume manufactured by Interventional Therapeutics Corporation (South San Francisco, CA). This nondetachable silicone balloon is typically mounted on a Tracker microcatheter. This nondetachable silicone balloon has a convenient low lateral wall. Angioplasty of cerebral vasospasm does not require high-pressure inflation and, in fact, should be avoided to prevent rupture of intracranial arteries. Mechanical angioplasty is usually limited to the carotid, basilar, M1, A1, and P1 segments. Angioplasty distal to these sites increases the risk of arterial rupture. Typically, a single inflation is all that is necessary. The balloon may be supported by an internal guidewire to advance, retrieve, and stabilize its position. When there is an insecure aneurysm, care must be taken to avoid the aneurysm neck and lumen. Mechanical angioplasty is typically more effective and its effects persist better than chemical angioplasty (67–70).

Angioplasty for atherosclerotic disease is entirely different from angioplasty for cerebral vasospasm. Atherosclerotic disease requires high-pressure balloon systems that are available in large sizes from a number of manufacturers. Target Therapeutics and Microinterventional Systems (Sunnyvale, CA) provides small vessel angioplasty systems that are flexible enough to enter the intracranial circulation. Coronary artery balloons are also available but tend to be less flexible for traversing the C1–2 region of the vertebral artery and the carotid siphon.

Brachiocephalic angioplasty at the origins of the great vessels can typically be carried out with a high degree of success (90% range) and a low rate of complications (1–2% range) (71,72). Vertebral origin angioplasty has some unique anatomic characteristics that are not observed in the remainder of the brachiocephalic arteries. Proximal vertebral artery angioplasty may require a very high inflation pressure and may have a higher rate of dissection than the remaining brachiocephalic arteries.

As expected, smaller arteries angioplasty does have inherently more risk than large arteries angioplasty and as angioplasty is performed more peripherally in the intracranial circulation, the risks of arterial damage go up considerably. Much recent work has been performed in the common carotid and internal carotid territories in the cervical region. Complication rates appear to be low with a high rate of anatomic success. Occasionally, stenting has been utilized in association with angioplasty. The initial results are promising, although long-term follow-ups will be necessary to determine the patency rate using this technique (73). Distal in the vascular system, intracranial internal carotid or vertebrobasilar territories angioplasty is feasible using the more flexible microangioplasty systems as mentioned above. However, it should be noted that the rate of anatomic failure and complications is much higher. Rates of complications

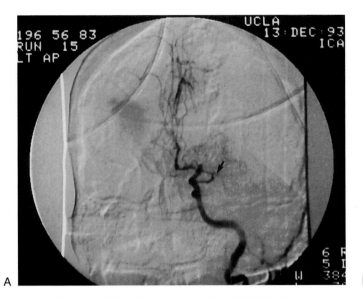

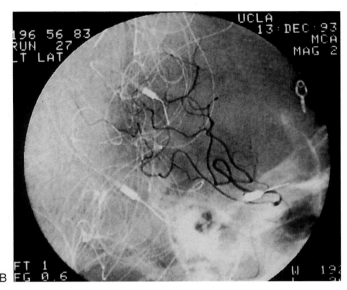

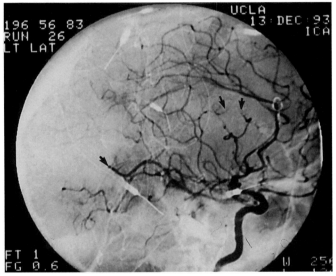

FIG. 11. Intra-arterial thrombolysis in embolic stroke. A) Left internal carotid angiogram shows embolic occlusion of M1 portion of left middle cerebral artery (arrow). B) Superselective left middle cerebral artery angiogram after M1 recanalization with intraarterial infusion with urokinase. C) Left internal carotid angiogram inmediately after thrombolytic therapy shows recanalization of most of left hemisphere circulation and presence of isolated, distal branch occlusions (arrows).

may go up to as high as 25% in the basilar territory. However, given the high degree of morbidity and mortality associated with intracerebral vascular occlusive disease and the lack of alternative treatment modalities, in selected patients, this may be an acceptable risk (74).

Stroke is the third most common cause of death and the most common cause of long-term nursing home care in the United States. In general, analysis of the small reported series of patients would indicate that intraarterial therapy is more effective than intravenous therapy, although a combination of both therapies may eventually prove to be most beneficial. In fact, multiple trials are ongoing, using intraarterial therapy alone, intraarterial therapy combined with intravenous therapy, and intravenous therapy alone. The technicalities of the intraarterial therapy does vary from protocol to protocol and from institutions to institutions. However,

the general intraarterial approach involves microcatheterization of the occluded intracranial artery and subsequent infusion of tissue plasminogen activator (Genentech, South San Francisco, CA) or urokinase (Abbott, North Chicago, IL). or similar thrombolytic agents (75–78). Intraarterial thrombolysis is typically instituted within 6 hours after onset of stroke symptoms (79) (Fig. 11). The potential complications of such therapy includes reperfusion hemorrhage and arterial perforation (80). An analysis of this series at our institution shows a rate of improvement in neurologic deficits of approximately 50% with a 10% complication rate. However, these are based on small numbers and large-scale protocols are necessary to fully identify the risks and benefits.

Intraarterial thrombolysis may be combined with angioplasty in cases of thrombotic occlusion of arteries with superimposed atherosclerotic disease.

REFERENCES

1. McCormick WF. The pathology of vascular (arteriovenous) malformations. *J Neurosurg* 1966;24(4):807–816.
2. Kaplan HA, Aronson SM, Browder EJ. Vascular malformations (angiomas) of the brain: an anatomical study. *J Neurosurg* 1961;8:630–635.
3. Stehbens WE. Ultrastructure of aneurysms. *Arch Neurol* 1975;32: 798–807.
4. Viñuela F, Fox AJ, Debrun GM, et al. Preembolization superselective angiography: role in the treatment of brain arteriovenous malformations with isobutyl-2-cyanacrylate. *AJNR* 1984;5:765–769.
5. Wilkins RH. Natural history of anrteriovenous malformations: a review. *Neurosurgery* 1985;16:421–430.
6. Forster DM, Steiner L, Hakanson S. Arteriovenous malformations of the brain. A longterm clinical study. *J Neurosurg* 1972;37(5):562–70.
7. Martin N, Grafton S, Viñuela F, et al. Imaging techniques for cortical functional localization. *Clin Neurosurg* 1992;38:132–165.
8. Girvin JP, Fox AJ, Viñuela F, et al. Intraoperative embolization of cerebral arteriovenous malformations in the awake patient. *Clin Neurosurg* 1983;31:188–247.
9. Rauch RA, Viñuela F, Dion J, et al. Preembolization functional evaluation in brain arteriovenous malformations: the superselective Amytal test. *AJNR* 1992;13(1):303–308.
10. Rauch RA, Viñuela F, Dion J, et al. Preembolization functional evaluation in brain arteriovenous malformations: the ability of superselective Amytal test to predict neurologic dysfunction before embolization. *AJNR* 1992;13(1):309–314.
11. Debrun G, Viñuela F, Fox AJ, et al. Embolization of cerebral arteriovenous malformations with bucrylate. Experience in 46 cases. *J Neurosurg* 1982;56:615–627.
12. Purdy PD, Samson D, Batjer HH, et al. Preoperative embolization of cerebral arteriovenous malformations with polyvinyl alcohol particles: experience in 51 adults. *AJNR* 1990;11:501–510.
13. Halbach VV, Higashida RT, Yang P, et al. Preoperative balloon occlusion of arteriovenous malformations. *Neurosurgery* 1988;22:301–308.
14. Viñuela F, Fox AJ, Pelz D, et al. Angiographic follow-up of large cerebral AVMs incompletely embolized with isobutyl-2-cyanoacrylate. *AJNR* 1986;7(5):919–925.
15. Dion JE, Mathis JM. Cranial arteriovenous malformations: the role of embolization and stereotactic surgery. *Neurosurg Clin N Am* 1994;5: 459–474.
16. Houser OW. Intracranial dural arteriovenous malformations. *Radiology* 1972;105(1):55–64.
17. Garcia MR. Multifocal dural arteriovenous shunts in children. *Childs Nerv Syst* 1991;7(8):425–431.
18. Picard L, Bracard S, Moret J. Spontaneous dural arteriovenous fistulas. *Semin Interv Radiol* 1987;4:219–236.
19. Doyon D, Metzger J. Malformations vasculaires duremeriennes sustentorielles. *Acta Radiol* 1973;13:792–800.
20. Castaigne P, Bories J, Brunet P, et al. Fistules arterio-veineuses de la dure-mere. *Ann Med Interne* 1975;126:813–817.
21. Obrador S, Soto M, Silvela J. Clinical syndromes of arteriovenous malformations of the transverse-sigmoid sinus. *J Neurol Neurosurg Psychiatry* 1975;38(5):436–451.
22. Viñuela F, Fox AJ, Pelz D, et al. Unusual clinical manifestations of dural arteriovenous malformations. *J Neurosurg* 1986;64:554–558.
23. Halbach VV, Higashida RT, Hieshima GB. Dural fistulas involving the cavernous sinus: results of treatment in 30 patients. *Radiology* 1987; 163:437–442.
24. Lasjuanias P, Halimi P, Lopez-Ibor L, et al. Traitement endovasculaire des malformations vasculararies durales (MVD) pures spontannees. *Neurochirurgie* 1983;30:207–223.
25. Halbach VV, Higashida RT, Hieshima GB, et al. Dural fistulas involving the cavernous sinus: results of treatment in 30 patients. *Radiology* 1987;163:437–442.
26. Halbach VV, Higashida RT, Hieshima GB, et al. Treatment of dural arteriovenous malformations involving the superior sagittal sinus. *AJNR* 1988;9:337–343.
27. Halbach VV, Higashida RT, Hieshima GB et al. Embolization of branches arising from the cavernous portion of the internal carotid artery. *AJNR* 1989;10:143–150.
28. Horton JA, Kerber CW. Lidocaine injection into the external carotid branches: provocative test to preserve cranial nerve function in therapeutic embolization. *AJNR* 1986;7:105–108

29. Lasjuanias P, Berenstein A. *Surgical Neuroangiography. Functional Anatomy of Craniofacial arteries.* Berlin: Springler-Verlag, 1987.
30. Halbach VV, Higashida RT, Hieshima GB, et al. Transvenous embolization of dural arteriovenous fistulas involving the transverse and sigmoid sinuses. *AJNR* 1989;10:377–384.
31. Mullan S. Treatment of carotid cavernous fistulas by cavernous sinus thrombosis. *J Neurosurg* 1979; 50:131–144.
32. Hosobuchi Y. Electrothrombosis of carotid-cavernous fistula. *J Neurosurg* 1975; 42–76–85.
33. Teng MM, Guo WY, Huang CI, et al. Occlusion of arteriovenous malformations of the cavernous sinus via the superior ophthalmic vein. *AJNR* 1988;9(3):539–546.
34. Halbach VV, Higashida RT, Hieshima GB, et al. Transvenous embolization of dural fistulas involving the cavernous sinus. *AJNR* 1989;10: 377–384.
35. Sundt TM, Piepgras DG. The surgical approach to arteriovenous malformations of the lateral and sigmoid dural sinuses. *J Neurosurg* 1983; 59:32–39.
36. Barnwell SL, Halbach VV, Higashida RT, el al. Complex dural arteriovenous fistulas: results of a new combined neurosurgical and interventional neuroradiology treatment in 16 patients. *J Neurosurg* 1989;7(13): 352–258.
37. Kobayashi H, Hayashi M, Noguchi Y, et al. Dural arteriovenous malformations in the anterior cranial fossa. *Surg Neurol* 1988;30(5):396–401.
38. Dandy WE. Arteriovenous aneurysms of the brain. *Arch Surg* 1928; 17:190-243.
39. Litvak J, Yahr MD, Ransohoff J. Aneurysms of the great vein of Galen and midline cerebral arteriovenous anomalies. *J Neurosurg* 1960;17: 945–954.
40. Barnwell SL, Cirillo SF, Halbach VV, et al. Intracerebral arteriovenous fistulas associated with intraparenchymal varix in childhood: case report. *Neurosurgery* 1990;26(1):122–125.
41. Lownie SP, Ducwiler GR, Fox AJ, et al. Endovascular therapy of non-Galenic cerebral arteriovenous fistulas. In: Viñuela F, ed. *Interventional Neuroradiology: Endovascular Therapy of the Central Nervous System.* New York: Raven Press, 1992;87–106.
42. Silverman BK, Breck T, Craig J, et al. Congestive failure in the newborn caused by cerebral arteriovenous fistulas. *Am J Dis Child* 1955; 89:539–543.
43. Long DM, Seljeskog EL, Chou SN, et al. Giant arteriovenous malformations of infancy and childhood. *J Neurosurg* 1974;40:304–312.
44. Godersky JC, Menezes AH. Intracranial arteriovenous anomalies of infancy: modern concepts. *Pediatr Neurosci* 1987;13:242–250.
45. Lasjuanias P, Berenstein A. *Surgical Neuroangiography*, vol 1. Berlin: Springer–Verlagσ87:266–267.
46. Jorgensen JS, Guthoff R. Ophthalmoscopic findings in spontaneous carotid cavernous fistula: an analysis of 20 patients. *Graefes Arch Clin Exp Ophthalmol* 1988;226(1):34–36.
47. Sanders MD, Hoyt WF. Hypoxic occular sequelae of carotid cavernous fistulae. *Br J Ophthalmol* 1969;53:82–97.
48. Yasargil MG. *Microneurosurgery*, vol IIIB. Stuttgart: Thieme, 1988.
49. Halbach VV, Higashida RT, Hieshima GB, et al. Transarterial occlusion of solitary intracerebral arteriovenous fistulas. *AJNR* 1989;10: 747–752.
50. Lasjuanias P, Terbrugge K, Piske R, et al. Dilatation de la veine de Galien. Formes anatomo-cliniques et traitements endovasculaires. A pròpos de 14 cas explores et/ou traites entre 1983–86. *Neurochirurgie* 1987;133:315–333.
51. Debrun GM, Viñuela F, Fox AJ, et al. Indications for treatment and classification of 132 CCFs. *Neurosurgery* 1988;22:285–289.
52. Higashida RT, Halbach VV, Tsai FX, et al. Interventional neurovascular treatment of traumatic carotid and vertebral artery lesions. Results in 234 cases. *AJR* 1989;153:577–582.
53. Serbinenko FA. Balloon catheterization and occlusion of major cerebral vessels. *J Neurosurg* 1974;41:125–145.
54. Debrun G, Lacour P, Caron J, et al. Detachable balloon and calibrated-leak balloon techniques in the treatment of cerebral vascular lesions. *J Neurosurg* 1978;49:635–649.
55. Higashida RT. Treatment of intracranial aneurysms with preservation of the parent vessel: results in 84 patients. *AJNR* 1990;11(4):633–640.
56. Higashida RT. Endovascular detachable balloon embolization therapy of cavernous carotid artery aneurysms: results in 87 cases. *J Neurosurg* 1990;72(6):857–863.

57. Debrun G, Fox AJ, Drake CC, et al. Giant unclippable aneurysms: treatment with detachable balloons. *AJNR* 1981;2:167–173.

58. Berenstein A, Ransohoff A, Kuppersmith M, et al. Transvascular treatment of giant aneurysms of the cavernous carotid and vertebral arteries: functional investigation and embolization. *Surg Neurol* 1984;21:3–21.

59. Fox AJ, Viñuela F, Pelz D, et al. Use of detachable balloons for proximal artery occlusion in the treatment of unclippable cerebral aneurysms. *J Neurosurg* 1987;66:40–46.

60. Barker DW, et al. Balloon test occlusion of the internal carotid artery: change in stump pressure over 15 minutes and its correlation with xenon CT cerebral blood flow. *AJNR* 1993;14(3):587–590.

61. Cloughesy TF, et al. Monitoring carotid test occlusions with continuous EEG and clinical examination. *J Clin Neurophysiol* 1993;10(3):363–369.

62. Mathis JM, et al. Temporary balloon test occlusion on the internal carotid artery: experience in 500 cases. *AJNR* 1995;16(4):749–754.

63. Guglielmi G, Viñuela F, Duckwiler G, et al. Electrothrombosis of saccular aneurysms via endovscular approach. 2: Preliminary clinical experience. *J Neurosurg* 1991;75(1):8–14.

64. Guglielmi G, Viñuela F, Duckwiler G, et al. Endovascular treatment of posterior circulation aneurysms by electrothrombosis using electrically detachable coils. *J Neurosurg* 1992;77(4):515–24.

65. Kaku Y, et al. Superselective intra-arterial infusion of papaverine for the treatment of vasospasm after subarachnoid hemorrhage. *J Neurosurg* 1992;77(6):842–847.

66. Kassell NF, et al. Treatment of cerebral vasospasm with intraarterial papaverine. *J Neurosurg* 1992;77(6):848–852.

67. Brothers MF, Holgate RC. Intracranial angioplasty for treatment of vasospasm after subarachnoid hemorrhage: technique and modifications to improve branch access. *AJNR* 1990;11(2):239–247.

68. Dion JE, et al. Pre-operative microangioplasty of refractory vasospasm secondary to subarachnoid hemorrhage. *Neuroradiology* 1990;32(3):232–236.

69. Eskridge JM, Newell DW, Pendlenton GA. Transluminal angioplasty for treatment of vasospasm. *Neurosurg Clin North Am* 1990;1(2):387–399.

70. Eskridge JM, Newell DW, Winn HR. Endovascular treatment of vasospasm. *Neurosurg Clin N Am* 1994;5(3):437–447.

71. Motarjeme A, Gordon GI. Percutaneous transluminal angioplasty of the brachiocephalic vessels: guidelines for therapy. *Int Angiol* 1993;12(3):260–269.

72. Theron J, et al. Intravascular techis of cerebral revascularization. *J Mal Vasc* 1990;15(3):245–256.

73. Becker GJ. Should metallic vascular stents be used to treat cerebrovascular occlusive diseases. *Radiology* 1994;191(2):309–312.

74. Clark WM, et al. Safety and efficacy of percutaneous transluminal angioplasty for intracranial atherosclerotic stenosis. *Stroke* 1995;26(7):1200–1204.

75. Barr JD, et al. Acute stroke intervention with intraarterial urokinase infusion. *J Vasc Interv Radiol* 1994;5(5):705–713.

76. Zeumer H. Local thrombolysis in the management of acute cerebral ischemia. *Arzneimittelforschung* 1991;41(3A):352–354.

77. Del Zopppo G, Pessin MS, Mori E. Thrombolytic intervention in acute thrombotic and embolic stroke. *Z Kardiol* 1993;2(89):89–104.

78. Frey JL, et al. Intrathrombus administration of tissue plasminogen activator in acute cerebrovascular occlusion. *Angiology* 1995;46(8):649–656.

79. Barnwell SL, et al. Safety and efficacy of delayed intraarterial urokinase therapy with mechanical clot disruption for thromboembolic stroke. *AJNRd* 1994;15(10):1817–1822.

80. Ueda T, et al. Evaluation of risk of hemorrhagic transformation in local intra-arterial thrombolysis in acute ischemic stroke by initial SPECT. *Stroke* 1994;25(2):298–303.

Cerebrovascular Disease, edited by H. Hunt Batjer.
Lippincott-Raven Publishers, Philadelphia © 1997.

CHAPTER 58

Intracranial Arteriovenous Malformations: Endovascular Strategies and Methods

Richard E. Latchaw, Michael T. Madison, Donald W. Larsen, and Patricia Silva

The evolution of endovascular techniques to embolize a cerebral arteriovenous malformation (AVM) is a paradigm for the somewhat recent development of the subspecialty of interventional neuroradiology. Cerebral AVMs have always represented a formidable challenge to the cerebrovascular surgeon because of the surgical morbidity and mortality related to the surgical resection of these lesions. Long ago it had been theorized that presurgical embolization might decrease the blood flow in an AVM, facilitating surgical removal. In 1960, Luessenhop (1) embolized AVMs using silastic beads, but that embolization had to be performed from the extracranial vasculature because technically there was no way to navigate the intracranial arteries. This nonselective approach meant that the beads usually would go to only those portions of the AVM having the fastest blood flows and largest feeding arteries. A more selective approach occurred in 1974 when Serbinenko (2) used detachable balloons to occlude large arteries feeding intracranial malformations. In 1976 Kerber (3) and in 1977 Pevsner (4) developed calibrated leak balloons attached to silastic microcatheters. Blood flow propelled these microcatheters to the areas of highest flows and a liquid tissue adhesive was embolized into the AVM. However, there was no control of these microcatheters beyond that provided by blood flow, and their small lumina required the use of a liquid agent.

The significant breakthrough came in 1986 with the development of the wire-directed microcatheter for intracranial arterial navigation. Large or small intracranial vessels could now be catheterized selectively, the angioarchitecture of a malformation could be studied, and a variety of materials could be injected to occlude the AVM. In the last 10 years, there has been progressive development of the microcatheter/microguidewire systems, along with marked improvement in the angiographic equipment, allowing the endovascular surgeon to perform the embolization procedure more safely and more efficaciously.

During the same time interval, the operating microscope was developed and microsurgical techniques were perfected. Focused radiosurgical techniques were also developed and found to be particularly effective for small, deep malformations not easily resected. The rapidly developing embolization techniques have aided the evolution of microsurgery. Although it is still too early to obtain definitive results, embolization also may be a significant supplement to radiosurgery by decreasing the lesion size, thereby increasing the efficacy of the radiation therapy with fewer complications.

This chapter will discuss the indications for endovascular treatment, and the endovascular materials and techniques that allow the embolization procedure to be conducted safely and efficaciously. The strategies and techniques of embolization differ, depending on whether endovascular therapy is to be followed by microsurgery, radiosurgery, or, in unusual cases, to be the sole therapy. Inherent in a discussion of these strategies and techniques is the need to understand the angioarchitecture of the AVM. The efficacy of the embolization procedure and the potential complications will be presented, along with some concepts regarding future developments of the essential tools for these procedures.

R. E. Latchaw and D. W. Larsen: Departments of Radiology and Neurosurgery, University of Miami School of Medicine, Miami, FL 33101.

M. T. Madison: Departments of Radiology and Neurosurgery, University of Minnesota Hospital and Clinics, Minneapolis, Minnesota 55455.

P. Silva: Neuroradiologist, Departamento de Neuroimagen y Terapía Endovascular, Instituto Nacional de Neurología y Neurocirugia, Mexico City, Mexico 14269.

INDICATIONS FOR ENDOVASCULAR TREATMENT

The natural history of untreated AVMs is dismal. There is a 3% per year chance of hemorrhage, a 10–29% chance of death from rupture, and up to a 50% incidence of morbidity for those who survive. The yearly mortality rate is estimated at 2%, morbidity at 3.5%, and combined morbidity and mortality at 5% (5–12). Hemorrhage, seizures, neurologic deficit, and headache are the most frequent presenting symptoms, which are most common in the third decade of life. By age 70, 95% of AVMs will have become symptomatic (12).

Based on this natural history, the most common indications for treatment of an AVM are hemorrhage, intractable seizure disorder, and progressive neurologic deficit. The size and location of an AVM greatly influence the indications for and the type of definitive therapy. Spetzler and Martin developed a grading system combining the variables of AVM size, contiguity to eloquent tissue, and direction of its draining veins (13). They also used this grading system to evaluate surgical outcomes (13), but the influence of presurgical embolization was not incorporated.

There are eight treatment potentials for a given AVM: microsurgery alone, radiosurgery alone, embolization alone, embolization and surgery, embolization and radiosurgery, surgery and radiosurgery, all three techniques, and no treatment (14–26). Today there is no definitive study that scientifically proves the efficacy of embolization alone to improve the natural history of an AVM, nor the efficacy of embolization as either a preoperative or preradiosurgical technique. It is extremely difficult to devise a study that can separate the role of the embolization from the microsurgical or radiosurgical treatment that follows, particularly given the many different sizes, locations, and structural components of AVMs. Cerebrovascular surgeons prefer to have a decreased flow rate in an AVM, particularly when it is medium to large in size, less distension of veins, obliteration of arterial feeders that would be difficult to control with a given surgical approach, and possibly a better defined margin between the AVM and normal tissues. The radiosurgeon has a very high chance of totally obliterating an AVM when its volume is 10 cm^3 or less. An AVM of larger size might be made smaller by the embolization of a permanent material in order to improve the efficacy of the radiosurgery, if there were no recurrence in the embolized portion. However, a controlled study proving the efficacy of this combination of therapies had yet to be performed. Embolization alone rarely produces total obliteration of an AVM, and there are no data to indicate that partial obliteration of an AVM by endovascular therapy decreases the risk of intracranial hemorrhage. Hence, obliteration of the lesion by either microsurgery or radiosurgery following embolization is usually necessary. Embolization alone is usually reserved for very large lesions producing symptoms of progressive neurologic deficit in which neither conventional surgery nor radiosurgery is considered feasible with an acceptable degree of morbidity and mortality. In such a case, embolization may decrease the flow rate sufficiently to decrease symptoms, at least temporarily (27).

In summary, the indications for and the type of therapy for a given cerebral AVM are determined by the cerebrovascular team, consisting of individuals with expertise in microsurgery, radiosurgery, and endovascular surgery. Once a particular course of therapy is agreed on, specific strategies of endovascular therapy can be employed using a variety of materials, depending on the experience of the endovascular therapist and the needs of the microsurgeon or radiosurgeon.

ENDOVASCULAR MATERIALS AND PROCEDURES

Navigation of the endovascular pathways is accomplished using a wire-directed or flow-directed microcatheter system. Once the catheter has reached the AVM, a variety of embolic agents can be used, depending on the malformation angioarchitecture, the rapidity of flow within the lesion, the size and type of microcatheter used, and the position of the catheter tip relative to the nidus of the AVM. A variety of medications, including patient sedation and anesthesia, are of value, as are various endovascular techniques such as intravascular pressure measurements. Excellent angiographic equipment is essential for the performance of these intricate procedures.

Microcatheter Systems

The wire-directed microcatheter systems utilize a microcatheter between 2.0 and 2.7 French (Fr) in external diameter and a variety of flexible microguidewires with diameters ranging from 0.010 to 0.018 in. The propulsion of the microcatheter is along the microguidewire, which is manipulated into the intracranial vessel of choice under fluoroscopic control. The technology of microcatheter production has advanced dramatically since its introduction in 1986. Microcatheters are generally made of lengths of extruded polymer of varying stiffness that are bonded together to give an extremely soft and flexible distal portion to navigate tortuous vessels, and more stiffness in the middle and lower portions for torque control and pushability. The microguidewires vary in their degree of radiopacity and their flexibility, and the tip of most can be manually curved to provide directionality. The microcatheter system is usually passed through a guiding catheter, most commonly 6 Fr, with the nontapered tip of the guiding catheter placed near the skull base. The relatively large size of the guiding catheter permits the injection of contrast material around the microcatheter for angiography during the procedure, particularly for the purpose of obtaining a road map, which is a single negative image of the cerebral vasculature on which fluoroscopy is superimposed to visualize the superselective catheterization process.

The wire-directed microcatheter system has certain advantages over a flow-guided system. In particular, the microcatheter has a size that allows the injection of a variety of embolic agents, and it can be directed into small vessels without depending upon the fast flow in larger arteries feeding the AVM. The major disadvantage of this system is the force necessary to propel the microcatheter, leading to pressure on the intracranial vessels that can produce headache, possible vascular dissection, potential perforation of a feeding artery aneurysm or a fragile artery feeding the AVM, and back pressure on the guiding catheter, which may dissect the catheterized extracranial vessel.

The flow-guided microcatheter must be propelled by cerebral blood flow, and its destination is usually dictated by the rapid flow to the AVM, although various curves can be placed on the tip of the catheter to influence its direction. It is difficult to manipulate and direct when the flow rate diminishes. It is made of extremely soft polymer and hence is less traumatic to the intracranial vasculature than the wire-directed systems. There is also significantly lower back pressure on the guiding catheter during its propagation so that there is less chance of injury to the extracranial catheterized artery. However, its relatively smaller lumen relative to a wire-directed microcatheter means that liquid agents or very small particles must be used for embolization.

Frequently, the two microcatheter systems are used in complementary fashion in a given case. If there are very fast flows to an AVM, particularly if an arteriovenous fistula is present, or if the feeding arteries are extremely tortuous, a flow-directed system can be used first to inject a tissue adhesive to eliminate the fistulous component. If there is an aneurysm on a feeding pedicle, it is safer to use a flow-directed microcatheter than a wire-directed one, which could produce aneurysm rupture. A wire-directed system can then be used for embolizing the rest of the malformation, particularly via slower flowing vessels and small deep feeders into which a catheter must be directed.

Embolic Materials

Tissue Adhesives

The most commonly used tissue adhesives are isobutyl (IBCA) and n-butyl cyanoacrylate (NBCA). Cyanoacrylates polymerize rapidly, from a fraction of a second to a few seconds, once they come in contact with ionic fluids such as blood. The polymerization time can be altered with the addition of glacial acetic acid or with Pantopaque, Ethiodol, or Lipiodol (28,29) (which are also contrast agents for opacification of the adhesive mixture and which may be supplemented by tantalum or tungsten powder). Control of the glue is a major issue because it takes significant experience to gauge the rapidity of the flow in the feeding pedicle, to adjust the polymerization time accordingly, and to place the tissue adhesive in a precise location, all within a second or two, but without having the material flow through the nidus to produce significant venous occlusion distal to the nidus and without gluing the microcatheter in place (30).

Two techniques of injection are used: the sandwich technique and the full-column technique (31). In both, the lumen of the microcatheter is initially bathed with nonionic dextrose in water (D$_5$W) to prevent polymerization in the catheter. In the sandwich technique, an amount of tissue adhesive less than the dead space of the microcatheter is placed into

the catheter and pushed with the D$_5$W. In the full-column technique, a larger volume of tissue adhesive has to be prepared to accommodate the dead space of the microcatheter and is injected under fluoroscopy until the desired degree of embolization has been achieved.

The permanency of an embolic agent is a significant issue, especially if the AVM is going to be irradiated after embolization rather than operatively removed. Complete filling of a vessel with the embolic agent is necessary to ensure permanency, rather than a mixture of the embolic material and clotted blood, the latter being metabolized within a few weeks to months, which allows recanalization of the vessel. A full cast of NBCA is the most permanent embolic agent currently available, although there have been reports of recanalization even with this agent (32–35). Another cause for apparent recanalization is the recruitment of collateral circulation to the still patent nidus, especially if only proximal vascular occlusion of a feeding artery has been achieved rather than an intranidal deposition of the adhesive.

Particulate Materials

The most commonly used particulate material, and probably the most commonly used embolic agent overall, is polyvinyl alcohol (PVA or Ivalon). This is a biologically inert plastic polymer, originally used as a baffle for cardiac surgery, which can be made into particles of variable size, ranging from 150 to 1150 μm (36). The size of the particles to be used depends on the relative sizes of the intranidal vessels, the intranidal arteriovenous (AV) shunts, and the microcatheter used. A size large enough to block the AV shunts and not simply pass through to the lungs must be used (37), yet not so large that only proximal feeder occlusion is achieved, allowing collateral vessels to increase in size. Choosing a size larger than small (and often unseen) normal branches of the arterial pedicle will decrease the potential for ischemic injury of normal tissues. Because the particles are not opacified, they must be placed in a solution of a nonionic contrast agent and saline, usually mixed 1:1.

The great advantage of particulate material embolization is the control of the procedure. The interventionalist injects small amounts of PVA in contrast/saline and continually watches the progress of the vascular occlusion. The rate of injection can be slowed or stopped at any time, particularly if the flow through the nidus appears to be decreasing, there is visualization of reflux of contrast material and particles indicating too forceful injection for the existing flow rate, or there is opacification of vessels feeding normal parenchyma. One disadvantage is that particulate materials may not block fast-flowing fistulae, so that other methods of blocking the fistula may be necessary, followed by PVA embolization of the slower flowing components. Another disadvantage is the lack of permanency relative to a tissue adhesive. PVA particles have a stellate contour (36), so that their projections stick to the endothelium and to other PVA particles, but red blood cells accumulate between them, producing a clot. Over a time of weeks to months, the red cells and the clot are lysed, and the blood vessel recanalizes unless significant intravascular sclerosis has occurred.

There are other particulate materials, such as microspheres of a plastic polymer, that can be made as small as a few micrometers in size. Lyophilized dura has been used in Europe but not in North America. Particles of Gelfoam are generally not used because of their dissolution within a few days.

Microcoils

When it is not possible to reach the nidus of an AVM because of vascular tortuosity, platinum coils ranging in size from a few millimeters to a centimeter or more in diameter (with variable lengths and configurations) can be injected through the microcatheter proximal to the nidus, allowing the flow to take them to the fistulous component of the malformation. Although it may not be possible to occlude completely a fistulous component even using many microcoils, the flow rate may be diminished sufficiently to allow PVA embolization to be successful. This technique also can be used when there is such rapid flow through a fistula that there is fear that even rapidly polymerizing glue will pass through to the veins. In this situation, the coils can be injected with the catheter near the nidus to slow the flow, followed by a more controlled deposition of the tissue adhesive.

Microcoils also can be used to occlude the feeding artery after embolizing tissue adhesives or particles into the nidus to decrease the likelihood of recanalization preoperatively. Simply occluding the feeding artery with coils, even if near the nidus, usually predisposes to the formation of collaterals in the surrounding brain, making surgery even more difficult. However, this technique can be used selectively if surgery is imminent and there is fear of embolizing surrounding normal brain with more deeply penetrating tissue adhesives or particles.

Silk Sutures

This is another material for slowing down the rapidity of blood flow, producing a result similar to that of microcoils, preceding the injection of a tissue adhesive or particles. Silk suture of 2-0 size and 1 cm or more in length can be injected, producing stagnation of flow as the threads form intravascular masses. Unfortunately, the silk sutures are not opacified and their location cannot be defined radiographically. They may pass through a fistulous component to produce venous occlusion more distally, leading to increased intranidal pressure and subsequent hemorrhage.

Alcohol

Absolute alcohol produces severe damage to the endothelium. When there is relatively slow flow, such as with venous malformations (38) or arterial flow slowed by the inflation of a balloon proximal to the catheter tip or the placement of microcoils or silk suture proximal to the AVM nidus, the alcohol produces significant vascular damage and occlusion of the AVM. It is not opacified, however, and its location cannot be defined radiographically. If an opacifying agent such as a liquid contrast material is added, it dilutes the effectiveness of the alcohol. Metrizamide powder (which still can be obtained even though it has been replaced by other myelographic contrast agents) can be dissolved in the alcohol, without diluting its effectiveness.

Alcohol may perfuse small branches to normal brain, producing demyelination; these branches are too small to be seen angiographically and may not fill with even the liquid amobarbital (Amytal) during provocative testing because of the preferential flow to the AVM. Therefore, when using alcohol, it is essential that provocative testing be performed frequently during the embolization procedure as the flow rate to the AVM diminishes. We do not use alcohol in areas of known rich anastamoses, or near eloquent tissues or vital structures, for fear of producing complications.

Balloons

Releasable balloons may be used in vessels large enough to accommodate them in order to block the direct AV communication of a fistula. There are other materials that are cheaper and easier to use, such as microcoils, if there is a need to block only a feeding artery.

A nonreleasable balloon may be used to provide flow control during the embolization of a very fast-flowing fistula. The microcatheter for embolization is placed as near the AVM nidus as possible, and a second catheter with the nondetachable balloon is inflated more proximally. A tiny balloon on a very flexible catheter, and a rapidly deflating balloon on the distal shaft of a microcatheter, would be very useful for flow control of AVM embolization and are under development.

Angiographic Equipment

Although many embolization procedures can be performed with a single-plane angiographic system, we find that embolization of a cerebral AVM is greatly facilitated by the use of a biplane system. Biplane fluoroscopy facilitates superselective catheterization by viewing the course of the microcatheter system in two directions in rapid succession. A C-arm allows visualization from any direction, and hence a biplane C-arm fluoroscopic unit greatly facilitates the safety and efficacy of the embolization procedure.

Rapid filming sequences of high resolution are essential, with a minimum of 4, and preferably 8–10, frames per second necessary to locate fistulous components and intranidal microaneurysms, which may be obscured by the rest of the AVM nidus unless detected early in the sequence. Digital subtraction angiography (DSA) is a requisite for rapid decision making.

Low-noise road mapping, preferably in both projections with a biplane system, is essential for guiding the microcatheter. Blanking the road map allows the superimposition of real-time fluoroscopy on a totally subtracted background, so that injections of contrast agents and embolic materials can be monitored more accurately.

The more the interventionalist can see, the safer and more efficacious will be the procedure.

Adjuvant Medications and Techniques

Provocative Testing

Once superselective catheterization of a pedicle feeding the AVM has been achieved, with the catheter tip as close to the nidus as possible, a drug such as sodium amobarbital (39) or other short-acting barbiturate such as sodium methohexital (Brevital) (40) can be injected through the microcatheter to test if the catheterized artery also feeds normal brain and whether a neurologic deficit might occur during the embolization. Although an angiographic sequence performed via microcatheter injection may not show vessels feeding normal brain, such blood flow may be present but not visible because of the sump effect of the AVM. Subsequent occlusion of a portion of the malformation may lead to redirection of blood flow and embolic material to these normal structures. The test is performed by injecting the amobarbital into the pedicle and testing the patient for a neurologic deficit appropriate to the neuroanatomy being evaluated. EEG may be added to detect more subtle changes. The location of eloquent brain tissue can also be mapped preoperatively using this technique (39).

Both false-positive and false-negative amobarbital tests can be obtained. The amobarbital may have an effect on noneloquent tissues, producing EEG abnormalities that are not apparent clinically. In addition, the liquid amobarbital may penetrate tiny vessels that would remain patent by collateral flow if particulate material were used for embolization. Most importantly, a false-negative sense of security may be provided in that an artery may be feeding both the AVM and normal tissue, but not be predicted by the amobarbital test because of the AVM sump effect. Therefore, it is essential that the test be repeated during the course of embolization as the flow rate diminishes. A combination of intravascular pressures and amobarbital testing might be used to predict that an artery feeds both the AVM and normal tissue. A higher intravascular pressure than the very low pressures normally present within a pedicle purely feeding an AVM suggests that the pedicle might be perfusing normal tissues in addition to the AVM. The presence of a negative amobarbital test but with higher than expected preembolization pressures suggests the possibility of late ischemic effects in eloquent tissues, especially if a single-shot embolization

technique is used such as the administration of a tissue adhesive rather than particles, the latter allowing repeat testing during progressive embolization.

New imaging techniques can also be used to map the location of eloquent tissues contiguous to an AVM. Functional magnetic resonance imaging (MRI) depends on the activation of eloquent areas during a prescribed physical or mental paradigm, with the increased blood flow to the activated neural tissue detected with specific MR sequences. The location of eloquent tissues relative to the AVM can then be predicted before the embolization procedure (41). Magnetoencephalography can provide similar localization of eloquent tissues; it is based on the magnetic effects of neural transmission during activation rather than increased blood flow (42).

General Anesthesia Versus Conscious Sedation

General anesthesia has the advantage of eliminating patient pain and motion during superselective catheterization, particularly with a wire-directed microcatheter system. This is particularly important because fluoroscopic road mapping is sensitive to misregistration from patient motion. Road mapping is extremely important for visualizing the vascular structures feeding the AVM, particularly the smaller cerebral arteries, during superselective catheterization. General anesthesia also provides motionless angiographic sequences for better identification of tiny vessels feeding normal brain. However, general anesthesia does not permit testing a patient during amobarbital injection or for continuous neurologic evaluation during the embolization procedure. Therefore, although general anesthesia may produce a more rapid procedure because of less patient discomfort and the intermittent treatment of that discomfort, there is a decreased safety margin. Hence, we perform the majority of the procedures with intravenous conscious sedation, which can be rapidly augmented or decreased according to the needs of the procedure.

Heparin

Systemic heparinization is used when there is prolonged intravascular catheterization, such as an embolization procedure, to prevent clot formation around the catheter and guidewires and subsequent thromboembolic complications. We perform a baseline activated clotting time (ACT), administer 5000 units of heparin intravenously (IV), and augment that dose with 2500 units every hour. After termination of the procedure, the amount of heparinization remaining is determined by calculating the time since the last dose, knowing that the half-life of heparin is 1 hour. Ten milligrams of protamine sulfate per 100 remaining units of heparin is given slowly IV and the ACT is repeated, which must achieve baseline levels before the catheter sheath is removed.

The argument against using systemic heparinization is the risk of converting a minor subarachnoid or intracerebral hemorrhage from vascular perforation or rupture to a significant hematoma. Using proper techniques and the newer microcatheter systems, vascular trauma is uncommon. Thromboembolic complications pose a greater risk, in our opinion, necessitating the use of heparin.

Steroids

Steroids are used for decreasing the inflammatory reaction of the embolic material and the potential swelling of the periangiomatous tissues after embolization. However, it is known that steroids are not helpful, and can be detrimental, for cerebral ischemia. They may also produce hyperglycemia in the diabetic patient, and avascular necrosis of bone has been reported with even small doses. If steroids are to be used, they should be started in advance of the procedure, usually the day before, with augmentation immediately before and continuation for a few days after the procedure. We use dexamethasone (Decadron), 4 mg every 6 hours before and immediately after the procedure, gradually tapering the dose before cessation.

Antispasmodic Agents

Vascular spasm can decrease blood flow to vital structures and can limit the ability to manipulate or propel a microcatheter. It is usually secondary to vascular irritation by the microcatheter or guiding catheter.

Nitropaste is given by skin patch for extracranial vasospasm, with the length of the strip determining the amount of administered drug. It is not particularly effective for intracranial vasospasm, for which 10 mg of sublingual nifedipine can be administered. Oral nimodipine (the parenteral form is not available in the United States) is effective at reducing vascular spasm following subarachnoid hemorrhage, which may be produced by inadvertent vascular perforation. Hypotension may occur, however, requiring close monitoring of the patient's vital signs.

Intravascular Pressure Measurements

Pressure measurements through the microcatheter can be used to monitor the progress of embolization during the injection of embolic materials and help determine the point at which to terminate embolization in a given arterial feeder (43–45). The intravascular pressure of a pedicle feeding an AVM is substantially lower than systemic pressure but rises to that pressure as intranidal occlusion is achieved. In addition, with particulate material embolization, the effectiveness of a given particle size can be monitored with this technique, although the injection of many aliquots of embolic material may be necessary to change the pressure within a feeding pedicle to a large malformation. These measurements may help to detect the presence of a fistulous compo-

nent producing very low pressures, so that a tissue adhesive mixture can be adjusted for very rapid polymerization. Finally, intravascular pressure measurements can also help to predict whether a pedicle feeds both the malformation and surrounding normal brain or just the AVM, as previously discussed.

Intravascular Velocity Measurements

Transcranial Doppler (TCD) has gained acceptance as an ideal noninvasive way to detect vasospasm following subarachnoid hemorrhage, surgery, or other vascular insults.

TCD can also be used to evaluate intravascular velocities within arteries at the skull base, potentially helping to detect the slowing of intravascular flows during progressive embolization of a malformation (46). A Doppler probe the size of a 0.018-in. microguidewire has recently been developed, which can be placed through a microcatheter to monitor the intravascular velocities within a pedicle feeding a malformation (47). Its ability to monitor the effectiveness of an embolization procedure is under evaluation.

STRATEGIES AND TECHNIQUES OF EMBOLIZATION

The first goal of the cerebrovascular team is to decide whether a given AVM should receive therapy, and if so, the type of definitive therapy, whether microsurgery or radiosurgery. This will in large part dictate the need for and type of embolization procedure. Some AVMs are relatively small and located on the surface in noneloquent areas, making them excellent candidates for microsurgery. Embolization may not be needed because all of the essential feeders can be clipped under direct visualization at the time of surgery. Patients with larger AVMs may also be candidates for microsurgery but may benefit from preoperative embolization, which can decrease the flow rate and the venous distension, occlude pial feeders not easily visualized with the surgical approach, and access small delicate perforating arteries that may be difficult to control at the time of surgery. Some AVMs are relatively small but are deeply situated or contiguous to vital structures, making them excellent candidates for radiosurgery. Some AVMs may be too large for radiosurgery to be statistically successful at total obliteration, but might be made smaller by embolization of a permanent material, thereby increasing the efficacy of the radiosurgery. Some AVMs are so large (Spetzler–Martin grade 4 or 5) that a high morbidity and mortality from microsurgery might be expected. However, some of these AVMs (especially those that receive a high grade in part because of deep venous drainage or a location near eloquent cortex) can be successfully embolized so that they become more amenable to microsurgery with an acceptate degree of morbidity. Finally, some may be so large and complex that neither microsurgery nor radiosurgery can be considered potentially efficacious with an acceptable degree of morbidity. If the patient with such a large malformation has symptoms of progressive neurologic deficit, suggesting a vascular steal, there may be benefit from partial embolization to decrease that steal.

The techniques of embolization differ for each of these AVM categories and for the definitive therapy to follow. The techniques of embolization and the materials to be used are highly dependent on the vascular components of a malformation, including vascular feeders, fistulae, aneurysms, and venous outflow. Therefore, it is essential that the *angioarchitecture* of the AVM be thoroughly evaluated, so that the strategies and techniques for embolization can be determined.

Evaluation of the Angioarchitecture

It is difficult, or impossible, to evaluate adequately the angioarchitecture of an AVM by selective internal carotid or vertebral artery catheterization, even using rapid filming sequences. The rapidly filling nidus masks the presence of intranidal aneurysms and arteriovenous fistulae, and it may be impossible to determine if a vessel gives feeders en passage before supplying normal parenchyma. Superselective catheterization and mapping of the AVM is usually required. Doing this before the formal embolization procedure adds morbidity and expense. Instead, we usually attempt to determine from the rapidity of venous filling on the extracranial injection if a fistula is probably present or if there are prenidal or intranidal microaneurysms. When superselective catheterization is performed for embolization, many observations and therapeutic decisions usually have to be made during the procedure. Hence, there is the need for excellent angiographic equipment and technical capabilities, as previously discussed.

AVMs differ in terms of being relatively compact or diffuse. A tightly compact lesion is easier to obliterate with both microsurgery and radiosurgery, and is easier to embolize, than the more diffuse variety. It is essential that the multiple compartments and multiple feeders be thoroughly understood. An AVM may have direct arterial feeders only to the AVM, and these may come from one or more major cerebrovascular territories. En passage or transitional feeders supply both the AVM and normal surrounding parenchyma. Embolization of these feeders may result in ischemic damage of normal tissue. If this is eloquent tissue, the patient may suffer a significant neurologic deficit. The third category of feeders is collateral circulation. Such collateral is frequently seen in AVMs located close to the boundary zones between major cerebrovascular territories. Enlarged arteries may be acting simply as collateral to the primary feeders of an AVM or an arteriovenous fistula. If the malformation were obliterated, the arteries would decrease to a normal size feeding normal tissues. It is frequently difficult to differentiate collateral vessels from direct AVM feeders, but the presence of enlarged vessels at the border zone should arouse suspicion.

These collateral vessels should not be embolized for fear of harming normal parenchyma.

The detection of an arteriovenous fistula within the AVM, or as the primary lesion, is essential. This large connection between a feeding artery and a draining vein means that some types of embolic material, such as particles, will pass preferentially through the fistula to the lungs without successfully occluding the malformation. Such a fistula needs to be eliminated early in the embolization process in order to facilitate further embolization of the smaller vessels and shunts of the AVM (Fig. 1). If the lesion is essentially an arteriovenous fistula, therapy is achieved by simply closing the fistula with balloons, coils, or a tissue adhesive.

Intranidal or prenidal aneurysms related to AVMs occur in 23–50% of cases (48–51) and are important etiologic factors in the incidence of hemorrhage in patients with AVMs (48,49). Intranidal aneurysms can be embolized and/or surgically removed with the rest of the AVM. Prenidal aneurysms are either saccular or fusiform in nature and are related to either the increased flow in the feeding arteries or to dysplasia of the vascular pedicles feeding the malformation. These aneurysms are fragile, and care must be taken if a microcatheter is to pass through or beside them. It is our feeling that all such aneurysms should be secured during the embolization procedure, for fear of producing increased pressure in the feeding pedicle with embolic occlusion of the low-pressure AVM, resulting in aneurysmal rupture. If the aneurysm is saccular, it can be occluded before AVM embolization with detachable coils. If fusiform, the parent artery can be occluded after AVM embolization, allowing collateral circulation to perfuse any normal tissues fed by that artery. The incidence of aneurysms on vessels not feeding the AVM appears to be the same as the general population (48), and these aneurysms can be occluded either surgically or with detachable coils.

It is extremely important to evaluate the venous drainage of an AVM. Stenosis of a draining vein may lead to the presence of more proximal venous dilatations and varices. Venous stenosis is thought to be a significant risk factor for AVM hemorrhage, due to increased intranidal pressure (51, 52). The presence of venous stenosis and intra- or prenidal aneurysms may make the chances of hemorrhage higher than for AVMs without such components, and may suggest the need for embolization and definitive therapy even if there has never been a clinically documented hemorrhage.

Preoperative Embolization Techniques

The goal of preoperative embolization is not necessarily complete angiographic occlusion of the AVM nidus. Rather, a major goal is to eliminate vessels that will be difficult to visualize and to control at the time of surgery (Figs. 1 and 2). For example, an AVM in the parieto-occipital region may have both middle and posterior cerebral feeders. Whereas the middle cerebral vessels may be relatively easy to clip at

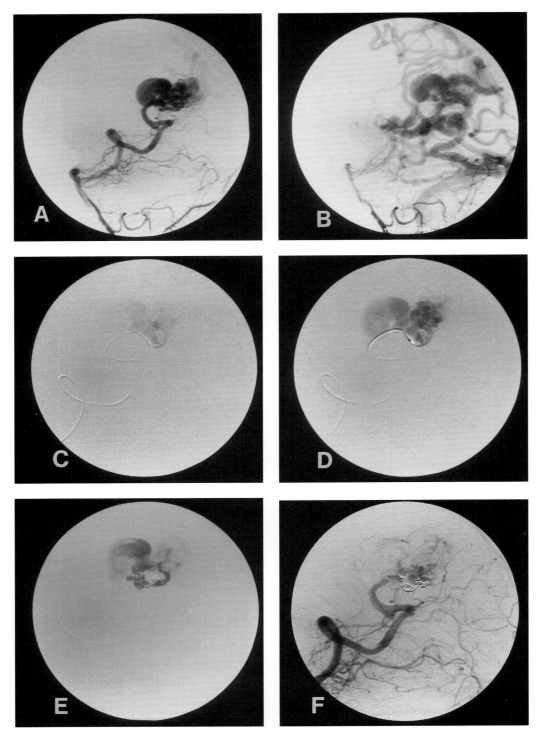

FIG. 1. Embolization of right parietal arteriovenous malformation (AVM) with multiple materials. This right parietal AVM was fed primarily from the right posterior cerebral artery **(A)**, with very fast flow into a large venous varix and subsequent outflow into multiple dilated venous channels **(B)**. It was difficult to demonstrate probable venous stenosis near the superior sagittal sinus as a cause for so many dilated veins over the hemisphere. Selective catheterization of the feeding pedicle **(C)**, and subsequent superselective angiography demonstrated filling of the venous varix in 0.25 second **(D)**, indicating the presence of a large fistulous component. Platinum microcoils were embolized to decrease the flow rate **(E)**, which facilitated the deposition of a tissue adhesive into the fistula without movement more distally into draining veins. Lateral **(F)** and anteroposterior (AP) (*continued*)

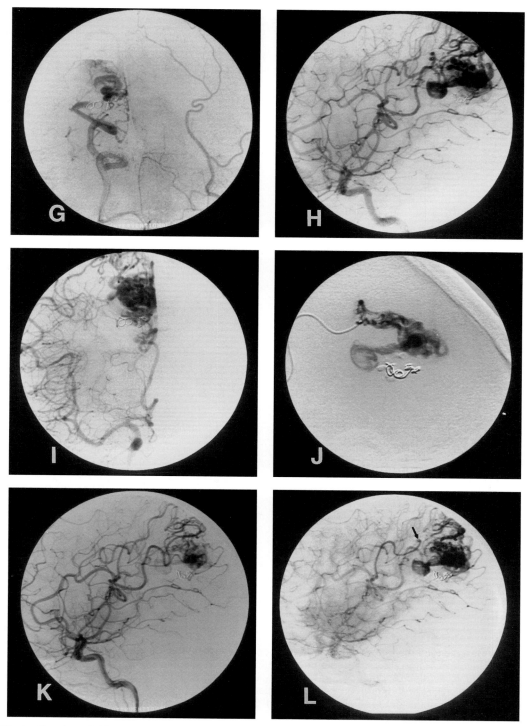

FIG. 1. *Continued.* **(G)** views demonstrated the very slow filling of the AVM from small branches of the parieto-occipital artery and slow filling of the venous varix, but the preservation of the calcarine artery. Two days later, repeat angiography demonstrated no change in the embolized portion of the AVM on left vertebral angiography, but filling from the right anterior and middle cerebral arteries on the lateral **(H)** and AP **(I)** views during right internal carotid angiography, which was unchanged from the preembolization study. Selective catheterization of the distal portion of the right callosomarginal artery demonstrated slow filling of AVM vessels **(J)**, which were subsequently embolized with PVA. The postembolization right carotid study demonstrated slow filling of a portion of the AVM by right middle cerebral collateral branches **(K)** and slow filling of the preserved distal right callosomarginal artery **(L,** *arrow).* The middle cerebral artery feeders were easily clipped at surgery, which totally devascularized the lesion, greatly facilitating resection.

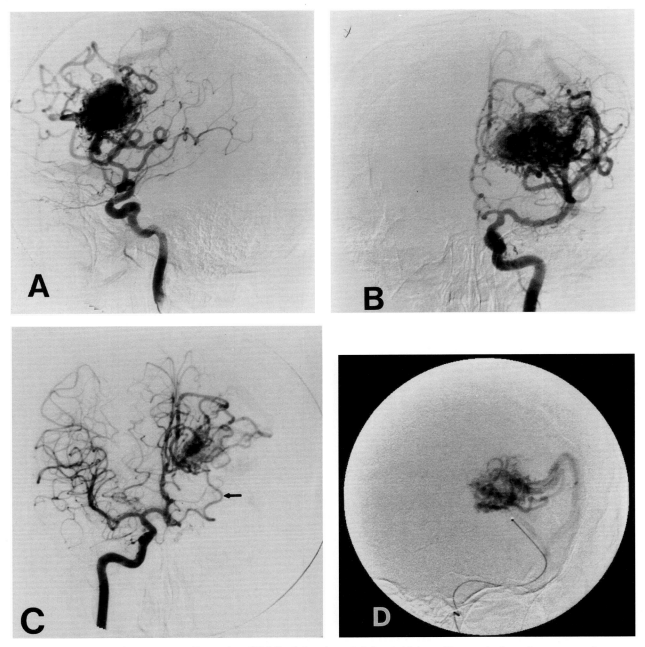

FIG. 2. Arteriovenous malformation (AVM) of the deep left frontal lobe with supply from the recurrent artery of Huebner. This AVM in the region of the left caudate nucleus and contiguous white matter has supply from left middle and anterior cerebral artery branches, as demonstrated on the lateral **(A)** and anteroposterior **(B)** views during left carotid injection. The right carotid injection also showed supply from the left recurrent artery of Huebner **(C, arrow).** Selective catheterization of a right middle cerebral artery branch was performed **(D)**, with embolization of PVA particles. Multiple other middle cerebral arteries branches were subsequently embolized. Three separate anterior cerebral branches were selectively catheterized and embolized with PVA.

the time of surgery, the posterior cerebral feeders may be difficult to visualize due to the operative approach. Hence, it may be sufficient to embolize the posterior cerebral branches preoperatively, allowing the surgeon to clip the middle cerebral feeders.

A second goal is to decrease the flow rate so that there is less intraoperative hemorrhage from feeding vessels as they are coagulated, and less venous distension, which may block visualization and access to the arterial components (Figs. 1 and 3). A third goal is the elimination of arteriovenous fistulae, and intra- and prenidal aneurysms. The fistulae produce very high flow rates and venous distention, and

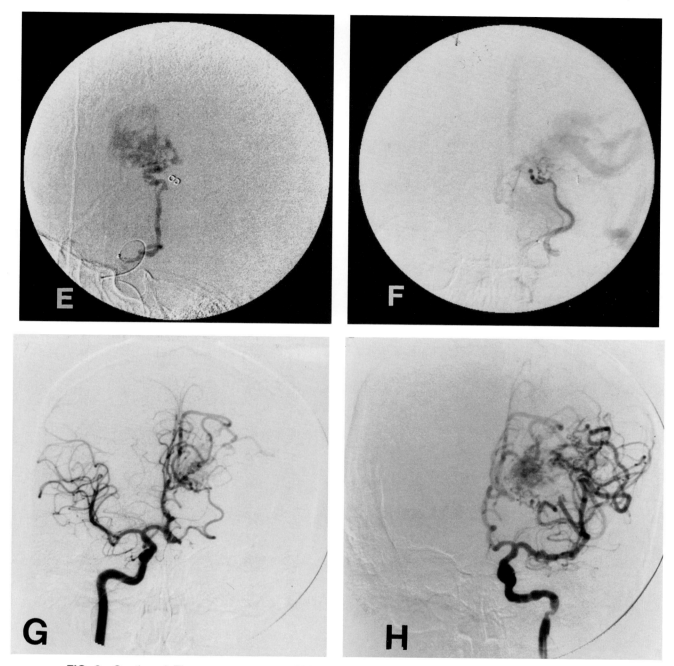

FIG. 2. *Continued.* The recurrent artery of Huebner was catheterized **(E)** and embolized with PVA, which markedly diminished flow to the AVM but preserved the parent vessel **(F)**. Postembolization right **(G)** and left **(H)** carotid angiograms showed marked diminution in the flow through the AVM, but some spasm of the distal left cervical internal carotid artery **(H)**, which did not result in complications. Total surgical resection was subsequently performed, and the patient was neurologically intact upon discharge.

the aneurysms represent a potential source of catastrophic hemorrhage. If the AVM is near eloquent tissue, a fourth goal is the mapping of the feeding arteries to the AVM relative to those to the eloquent tissue, using the amobarbital test as previously described (39). Embolization of vessels feeding the AVM directly, sparing vessels that feed eloquent tissue, may give the surgeon a critically important plane for dissection.

In general, we prefer to perform preoperative AVM embolization with particles (see Figs. 1 and 2) because they are easy to use, are given slowly over a period of time, and their administration can be stopped if there is visualization of normal arteries or early neurologic deficit. Because the surgeon will resect the AVM by staying on the periphery of the lesion, there is usually no need to fill the nidus totally with a tissue adhesive, which is more difficult to use. How-

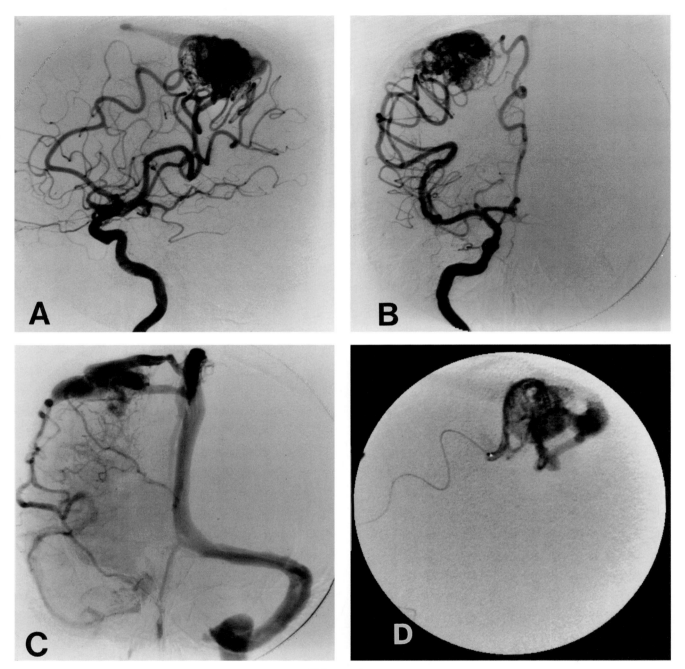

FIG. 3A–D.

ever, the angioarchitecture of the AVM may dictate the use of other embolic materials. An arteriovenous fistula must be closed first so that particles to occlude the rest of the AVM are not simply passed through to the venous circulation. This closure may require the use of a rapidly polymerizing tissue adhesive. This is best delivered with the microcatheter close to the fistula and the use of a very short polymerizing time to decrease the amount of tissue adhesive that might flow into draining veins. The flow can be slowed with the initial use of microcoils (see Fig. 1) or silk suture, or with a more

proximal nondetachable balloon for flow control while injecting the tissue adhesive to prevent too much glue from passing into draining veins and producing increased intranidal pressure. If the microcatheter cannot be brought close enough to the fistula to use a tissue adhesive without simply occluding the parent artery, thereby allowing collateral circulation to keep the fistula open, it is possible to eliminate the fistula using microcoils or silk suture, possibly followed by PVA, although this technique may not be successful. Intranidal aneurysms are most confidently eliminated with a

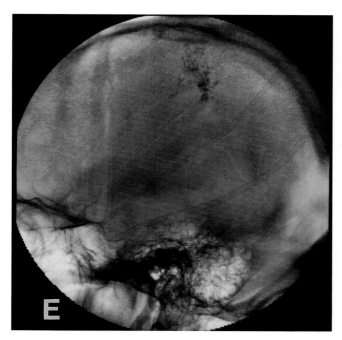
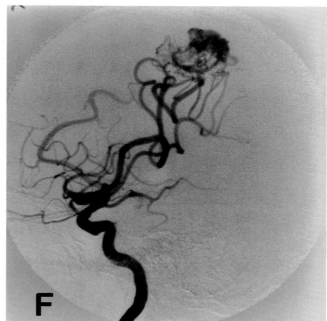

FIG. 3. Right parietal arteriovenous malformation (AVM) initially considered for microsurgery but subsequently treated with radiosurgery. This patient presented with seizures due to an AVM in the region of the right high-convexity motor strip on the lateral **(A)** and anteroposterior **(B)** views of the right carotid angiogram. The venous phase **(C)** demonstrated large veins overlying the AVM. The location of the AVM near eloquent tissue and the prominent overlying veins were thought to make microsurgery difficult, but the lesion was borderline in size for the use of radiosurgery. If embolization could safely but significantly decrease the flow rate and venous distension, surgery could be performed. Catheterization of a callosomarginal feeder to the AVM was performed **(D)**, with subsequent intranidal deposition of a tissue adhesive, as seen on the plain skull film **(E)**. The postembolization angiogram demonstrated persisting feeders from tortuous right middle cerebral branches **(F)**. Reconsideration was made at this point to perform radiosurgery on this lesion, which was significantly smaller and slower in flow rate (F) than before embolization. The use of a permanent tissue adhesive facilitated using a radiotherapeutic isocenter of smaller size than would have been necessary before embolization.

tissue adhesive, but particles can also be used. Particulate material can then be used for the rest of the AVM, especially after the flow rate has been decreased. Prenidal saccular aneurysms can be eliminated before AVM embolization with detachable coils. Fusiform prenidal aneurysms can be eliminated by occluding the parent artery after AVM embolization. A large artery directly feeding an AVM can be totally occluded with detachable microcoils following particulate material embolization if there is concern about recanalization of that vessel preoperatively.

If there are obvious en passage vessels angiographically (Fig. 4), embolization of these feeders may be impossible for fear of producing neurologic deficit. The cerebrovascular surgeon using the operating microscope can frequently separate the small branches that directly supply the AVM from such an en passage parent vessel, sparing the blood supply to normal parenchyma. Pedicles that are not initially characteristic of en passage vessels because of the sumping effect of the AVM, but in the vicinity of eloquent tissue, should be tested with amobarbital as the embolization procedure progresses. Excellent visualization during embolization as provided by high-resolution DSA and road mapping, along

with multiple amobarbital tests, will protect against unwanted ischemic damage of normal structures.

It may be appealing to start the embolization process with the largest vessel feeding the highest flow component to the AVM. However, this may make it more difficult to embolize the periphery of the AVM fed by smaller arteries, which may, in reality, be en passage vessels. Embolization might be performed from the outside in utilizing the sumping effect of the fast flow component internally to facilitate embolization of the periphery of the AVM in order to decrease the chance of ischemic injury to normal tissues. Once the periphery has been successfully embolized, the fast-flow internal components fed only by direct AVM feeders can be occluded. Such a technique also facilitates demarcating the AVM and its feeders from the surrounding normal parenchyma.

Some neurointerventionalists find the use of intravascular pressure measurements to be helpful during embolization in order to determine the efficacy of the selected particle size and to aid in the decision making as to when to stop embolizing a given arterial feeder (43–45). We have tried such techniques but have found that excellent visualization during

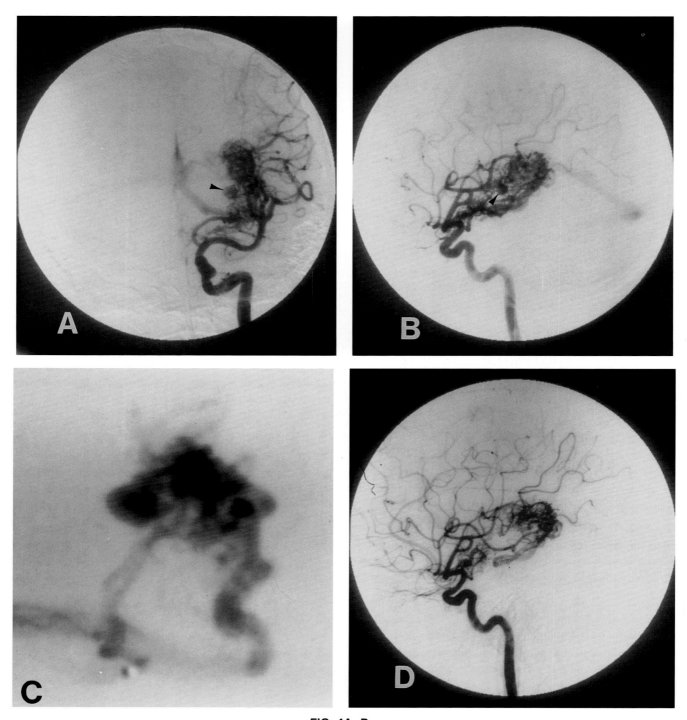

FIG. 4A–D.

slow, careful particle embolization makes pressure measurement unnecessary in most cases.

Some large AVMs are best embolized in multiple stages (22,24,53,54). Total or near-total embolization of a large AVM may divert the chronically increased AVM blood flow into the vessels feeding the normal contiguous brain, vessels that may have lost their ability to autoregulate due to chronic

relative ischemia (55), producing the so-called normal perfusion pressure breakthrough (NPPB) phenomenon (56,57). This may lead to edema and hemorrhage, and severe neurologic deficit or death. However, the existence of NPPB is conjectural; such a complication is probably more often the result of occlusion of draining veins and secondary increased back pressure to both the AVM and normal surrounding

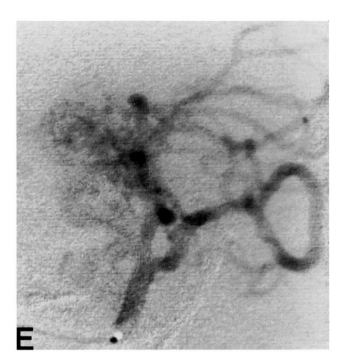
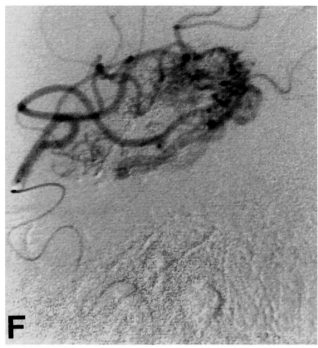

FIG. 4. Arteriovenous malformation(AVM) with a microaneurysm, treated with embolization and radiosurgery. The anteroposterior **(A)** and lateral **(B)** views on left carotid angiography demonstrated a diffuse left Sylvian AVM containing a microaneurysm *(arrowheads)*, most likely responsible for the recent hemorrhage. The angioarchitecture of the AVM on this left carotid injection suggested that en passage vessels were probably present. The anterior choroidal artery was catheterized, the microaneurysm was angiographically demonstrated **(C)**, and a tissue adhesive was embolized to permanently eliminate that microaneurysm. Subsequent postembolization angiography demonstrated a reduction in filling of much of the AVM and angiographic ablation of the microaneurysm. Superselective angiography of multiple middle cerebral artery branches **(E, F)** demonstrated en passage filling of the AVM from branches to normal tissues, making further embolization, or microsurgery, impossible without producing significant neurologic deficit. It was elected to perform radiosurgery on the residual AVM. Most importantly, the microaneurysm had been eliminated, probably reducing the chance of recurrent hemorrhage while awaiting the sclerosis from radiosurgery.

tissues (58,59), although we believe that NPPB occurs with some large AVMs. The appropriate time interval between the stages of embolization and the interval between embolization and surgery is unknown (23,24,53,54). We would prefer to wait 3–5 days between embolization stages but are frequently forced by logistical considerations to embolize every second or third day. There is usually a 2-day interval between the last embolization procedure and surgery.

Embolization of a very large AVM may produce stasis of blood in large draining veins, with progressive thrombosis of smaller venous tributaries, leading to venous infarction, edema, and hemorrhage (58,59). If the feeding artery is large as a result of very fast flow, significant decrease in that flow by embolization can result in flow stagnation, back thrombosis, and occlusion of normal branches. The use of anticoagulants following embolization of AVMs with these large feeding arteries or draining veins may be warranted, realizing that there is an increased risk for postembolization hemorrhage. The presence of venous stasis may also indicate the need for immediate surgery after embolization to remove

the chance of hemorrhage due to high back pressures in the AVM.

Embolization Before Radiosurgery

There are three goals for embolization before radiosurgery. The first is to make the AVM nidus smaller to increase the efficacy of radiosurgery, particularly for AVMs that are >10 cm^3 (see Fig. 3). The second goal is to eliminate intranidal or prenidal aneurysms, which are thought to increase the risk of hemorrhage (Fig. 4). The risk of hemorrhage does not decrease during the 2 or 3 years following radiosurgery, until the AVM has become totally sclerotic (60). There is no evidence that partial embolization decreases that risk. However, it appears reasonable to attempt to eliminate high-risk aneurysms if this can be done with low morbidity. The third goal is the elimination of large arteries, particularly those feeding a fistula, theoretically because these vessels are less likely to respond to radiosurgery than the smaller vessels of the AVM nidus.

While it might appear desirable to make the AVM as small as possible by embolization, this is sometimes impossible and even unnecessary, if it can be made 10 cm^3 or less, which translates into a radiosurgical cure rate of 85% (16). It is necessary either to decrease the overall size of the AVM or to split it into a few components that can be treated with multiple radiosurgical isocenters. It is absolutely essential that the angioarchitecture be thoroughly understood to facilitate either occluding a significant portion of the AVM without leaving a patent rim or to split it into isocenters of manageable size. To embolize the center of the AVM without eliminating a significant portion of the margin makes radiosurgical planning extremely difficult or impossible. The outside-in technique would be of value to prevent leaving such a rim.

It is essential that a permanent embolic material be used for preradiosurgical embolization, if the embolized component is not to be included in the radiation field. A tissue adhesive is the best material to utilize for permanence (61). While there have been rare reports of recanalization using tissue adhesives (32–35), there has been more experience of recanalization with particulate materials. How long should the radiosurgeon wait to see that there is no recanalization in the embolized portion before undertaking radiotherapy planning? That is a difficult question to answer and is frequently obviated by the logistics of the case. It would be desirable to wait a number of weeks to months before repeating angiography to ensure that recanalization has not occurred in the embolized portion. However, the patient frequently comes from far away, and it is necessary to perform radiosurgery soon after embolization. It might be assumed that the embolized portion will not recanalize, so that only the angiographically patent portion is irradiated, with follow-up angiography in a number of months to years. All patients undergoing radiosurgery are followed with MRI until there is no apparent flow in the AVM. The patients then undergo repeat angiography to ensure that the AVM has been obliterated. If it appears on the MRI or subsequent angiogram that the embolized portion has recanalized, that portion can then undergo irradiation. Obviously, the risk for hemorrhage has not been eliminated during this entire time. Some radiosurgeons prophylactically irradiate both the embolized and nonembolized portions of these large AVMs, for fear of recanalization of the embolized portion, or decline the use of embolization altogether, fearing that even a tissue adhesive is not permanent enough and hence embolization adds nothing but risk to the treatment. The overall efficacy of irradiating AVM volumes >10 cm^3, and the incidence of necrosis of normal surrounding tissues, is undergoing further evaluation.

Intranidal aneurysms in an AVM to be irradiated should be embolized with a tissue adhesive because the AVM is not going to be resected and recanalization might occur with particulate material embolization. Saccular prenidal aneurysms can be eliminated with detachable coils, but fusiform aneurysms will require parent artery occlusion.

Embolization as the Sole Treatment

There are four conditions in which embolization is used as the sole treatment. The first is the presence of an arteriovenous fistula without an AVM component. In such a case, a microcatheter is placed at the point of the fistula and detachable balloons, microcoils, or a tissue adhesive, singly or in combination, are used to occlude the fistula. If these materials can block the arteriovenous shunt, no further therapy is required.

The second condition is the presence of a single feeding artery to, and draining vein from an AVM, similar to an arteriovenous fistula. Injection of a tissue adhesive may successfully occlude the entire AVM nidus including the proximal portion of the draining vein, again producing a total cure. Cure of an AVM by embolization alone occurs in 10% or less of cases (22).

The third condition is severe headache, where embolization of the middle meningeal artery and other feeders to the dura may decrease the pain. Usually these dural collaterals accompany large pial malformations, which may be too large for microsurgery or radiosurgery. If temporary relief is given by PVA embolization, the procedure can be repeated with a more permanent agent if symptoms recur.

The fourth reason for embolization without other therapy is for palliation because a very large AVM is producing progressive neurologic deficit, dementia, or other neurologic symptoms. Here the goal is to decrease the flow rate and relative steal from the normal tissues (27,62). Decreasing the high flow rate in a large AVM is most permanent with a tissue adhesive. A variety of other materials including particles and microcoils also may be used, although recanalization and collateral formation may occur and relief of neurologic signs and symptoms may be only temporary.

COMPLICATIONS

The major complications are intracerebral hemorrhage, ischemic stroke, vascular dissection leading to thromboembolism, and perforation producing subarachnoid hemorrhage and vasospasm. Hemorrhage and swelling may occur from normal perfusion pressure breakthrough (56,57), but this, as previously stated, is a rare occurrence related to embolizing large AVMs. Postembolization hemorrhage and swelling probably occur more commonly because large portions of the venous outflow are occluded (58,59). Hemorrhage more commonly occurs from increased intranidal pressure with secondary rupture of intranidal aneurysms or small fragile vessels. Finally, hemorrhage may occur from perforation of the fragile feeding arteries or prenidal aneurysms, particularly when using a wire-directed microcatheter system. The complications of hemorrhage can be decreased by recognizing and avoiding or treating prenidal aneurysms, by avoiding the venous occlusions, by staging the embolization procedure, and by using both flow-directed catheters and the newer, more flexible wire-directed microcatheter systems.

Ischemic stroke is usually secondary to occluding arteries feeding normal brain tissue with embolic material. Assuming that embolization is not made into vessels that obviously supply normal parenchyma, this usually occurs because embolic material refluxes into the normal vessels or because the embolized artery is really an en passage vessel. This complication can be decreased by excellent visualization throughout the procedure, particularly with high-resolution fluoroscopy, road mapping techniques, and frequent short DSA sequences, in order to evaluate the continuous changes in vascular filling and perfusion. The frequent use of provocative techniques such as the amobarbital test also helps to avoid embolizing normal brain. Ischemia rarely occurs as a technical complication such as a fracture of the embolizing catheter or gluing the microcatheter in place with secondary compromise of a vessel lumen. There is also the 1% or less incidence of ischemic complications attendant to any cerebral angiographic diagnostic procedure.

A major problem during an endovascular procedure is the trauma to either the intracranial or the extracranial vasculature, leading to vasospasm, dissection, embolization, occlusion, and cerebral ischemia. Trauma to the intracranial vasculature can be decreased by using flow-directed microcatheters or relatively soft and flexible wire-directed microcatheter systems. Experience in the embolization of AVMs leads to the knowledge of how much force can be exerted on the delicate arterial structures. Extreme force with wire-directed microcatheter systems, particularly when attempting to navigate the pronounced tortuosity of arteries feeding the AVM, produces back pressure on the guiding catheter, which is forced in a cephalocaudad direction, with subsequent trauma to the extracranial vascular endothelium and possible dissection and thromboembolism. The more supple flow-directed and newer wire-directed catheters produce less, or no, back pressure. Newer guiding catheters with softer tips and more flexible distal segments that are less traumatic are now being produced.

The overall complication rate for the embolization of AVMs varies in the literature (22,63–66) but is probably from 5–10%. The mortality is approximately 1%. Such complication rates must be added to the surgical morbidity and mortality, and compared to the potential risk of hemorrhage and other causes of morbidity and mortality in the natural history of the AVM, so that the combination of embolization and definitive therapy becomes warranted in the risk–benefit ratio.

EFFICACY OF EMBOLIZATION

The efficacy of embolization before microsurgery or radiosurgery has not been accurately determined. It is extremely difficult to evaluate the efficacy of preoperative embolization; measuring the amount of operative hemorrhage with or without embolization is misleading because the amount of blood loss also depends on the type and location of the lesion, the experience of the cerebrovascular surgeon, and other factors. Most cerebrovascular surgeons, however, feel that embolization frequently makes surgery easier by making the lesion more controllable, and may even make a high morbidity and potentially nonsurgical case into a surgical one (24,53). Embolization also may decrease the size of a lesion, increasing the efficacy of radiosurgery, although no reliable statistical data are available, and there are the problems of recanalization and bleeding during the interval between treatment and sclerosis.

The relative efficacy of the various embolic materials has not been adequately determined. This is primarily because there are different roles for each of the embolic agents. For example, a tissue adhesive may be necessary to close a fistulous component but the rest of the AVM may be successfully occluded with either the tissue adhesive or a particulate material. It would be extremely difficult to devise a randomized evaluation of two embolic materials for a given series of AVMs because each AVM will have different components requiring different embolic materials and strategies.

It has been found that the frequency of seizures and the degree of progressive neurologic deficit may decrease with palliative embolization (27). This occurs either because of a relative decrease in the amount of arterial steal or because of a decrease in the degree of venous hypertension in the surrounding normal parenchyma. Unfortunately, these benefits may be temporary.

DEVELOPMENT OF NEW EMBOLIZATION MATERIALS AND TECHNIQUES

There is a continuing need for even more supple microcatheters to negotiate the tortuous intracranial vasculature. As large a lumen as possible within such a microcatheter facilitates the embolization of large particles without occluding the microcatheter. Braided microcatheters maintain their luminal dimensions despite multiple sharp bends, but the braiding must not decrease catheter flexibility Even more flexible guidewires are necessary to negotiate the vascular tortuosity and to decrease the vascular trauma. Most wire-directed microcatheters now have hydrophilic coating to decrease the friction between the microcatheter and the microguidewire. While significant advances in microcatheter system technology have been made in the last few years, there is still a need for even better systems.

The perfect embolic material has yet to be devised. The current tissue adhesives are difficult to control. The polymerization time is difficult to predict. The use of a radiopaque colloidal suspension of variable density may permit more control of the intravascular flow rate of the embolic material and the size of the vessels that are occluded.

There is a need for better, more supple guiding catheters that produce less trauma to the extracranial vasculature.

Highly flexible or formable distal segments may permit them to lock in place to decrease their movement and subsequent dissection of a vessel. The use of a double-lumen microcatheter with a rapidly deflatable balloon may facilitate relative flow control within the feeders to the AVM, allowing a tissue adhesive to permeate more of the AVM with less chance of polymerization due to contact with blood. However, the interventionalist must be cognizant that such a technique may produce increased intravascular pressure, disseminating the embolic material into arteries feeding normal brain.

New imaging techniques to monitor the effects of embolization procedures, and of subsequent therapy, will be forthcoming. Perfusion and diffusion MRI will provide the earliest evidence of ischemic changes, and it is conceivable that embolization procedures might be performed on a hybrid MR-fluoroscopy system. MR angiography will continue to improve, helping to evaluate the status of the AVM after radiosurgery.

In summary, technology must continue to evolve in order for the morbidity from these high-risk procedures to continue to decrease. There has been such a rapid evolution of the technology, however, that there is every reason to believe it will continue.

REFERENCES

1. Leussenhop AJ, Spence WT. Artificial embolization of cerebral arteries. Report of use in a case of arteriovenous malformation. *JAMA* 1960; 172:1153–1155.
2. Serbinenko FA. Balloon catheterization and occlusion of major cerebral vessels. *J Neurosurg* 1974;41:125–145.
3. Kerber C. Balloon catheter with a calibrated leak. A new system for superselective angiography and occlusive catheter therapy. *Radiology* 1976;120:547–550.
4. Pevsner PH. Micro-balloon catheter for superselective angiography and therapeutic occlusion. *AJR* 1977;128:225–230.
5. Wilkins RH. Natural history of intracranial vascular malformations: a review. *Neurosurgery* 1985;16:421–430.
6. Wilkins RH. Natural history of arteriovenous malformations. In: Barrow DL, ed. *Neurosurgical Topics: Intracranial Vascular Malformations.* AANS, 1990;31–43.
7. Crawford PM, West CR, Chadwick DW, et al. Arteriovenous malformations of the brain: natural history in unoperated patients. *J Neurol Neurosurg Psychiatry* 1986;49:1–10.
8. Ondra SL, Troupp H, George ED, et al. The natural history of symptomatic arteriovenous malformations of the brain: a 24-year follow-up assessment. *J Neurosurg* 1990;73:387–91.
9. Troupp H. Arteriovenous malformations of the brain. What are the indications for operation? In: Morley TP, ed. *Current Controversies in Neurosurgery.* Philadelphia: WB Saunders, 1976:210–216.
10. Troupp H, Marttila I, Halonen V. Arteriovenous malformations of the brain. Prognosis without operation. *Acta Neurochir (Wien)* 1970; 22:125.
11. Brown RD, Wiebers DO, Forbes G, et al. The natural history of unruptured intracranial arteriovenous malformations. *J Neurosurg* 1988;68:352–357.
12. Luessenhop AJ. Natural history of cerebral arteriovenous malformations. In Wilson CB, Stein BM, eds. *Current Neurosurgical Practice, Vol 1. Intracranial Arteriovenous Malformations.* Baltimore: Williams and Wilkins, 1984;12–21.
13. Spetzler RF, Martin NA. A proposed grading system for arteriovenous malformations. *J Neurosurg* 1986;65:476–483.
14. Deruty R, Pelissou-Guyotat I, Mottolese C, Amat D, Bascoulergue Y. Prognostic value of the Spetzler's grading system in a series of cerebral AVMs treated by a combined management. *Acta Neurochirurgica* 1994;131(3–4):169–175.
15. Hurst RW, Berenstein A, Kupersmith MJ, Madrid M, Flamm ES. Deep central arteriovenous malformations of the brain: the role of endovascular treatment. *J Neurosurg* 1995;82(2):190–195.
16. Friedman WA, Bova FJ, Mendenhall WM. Linear accelerator radiosurgery for arteriovenous malformations: the relationship of size to outcome. *J Neurosurg* 1995; 82:180–189.
17. Cromwell LD, Harris AB. Treatment of cerebral arteriovenous malformation: combined neurosurgical and neuroradiological approach. *AJNR* 1983;4:366–368.
18. Dawson RC III, Tarr RW, Hecht ST, et al. Treatment of arteriovenous malformations of the brain with combined embolization and stereotactic radiosurgery: results after 1 and 2 years. *AJNR* 1990; 11:857–864.
19. Deruty R, Pelissou-Guyotat I, Mottolese C, et al. The combined management of cerebral arteriovenous malformations experience with 100 cases and review of the literature. *Acta Neurochir* 1993;123:101–112.
20. Lasjaunias P, Manelfe C, Terbrugge K, et al. Endovascular treatment of cerebral arteriovenous malformations. *Neurosurg Rev* 1986;9:265–275.
21. Marks MB, Lane B, Steinberg GK, et al. Endovascular treatment of cerebral arteriovenous malformations following radiosurgery. *AJNR* 1993;14:297–303.
22. Viñuela F, Dion JE, Duckwiler G, et al. Combined endovascular embolization and surgery in the management of cerebral arteriovenous malformation: experience in 101 cases. *J Neurosurg* 1991; 75:856–864.
23. Westphal M, Cristante L, Grzyska U, Freckmann N, Zanella F, Zeumer H, Herrmann HD. Treatment of cerebral arteriovenous malformations by neuroradiological intervention and surgical resection. *Acta Neurochirurgica* 1994;130(1–4):20–27.
24. Spetzler RF, Martin NA, Carter LP, et al. Surgical management of large AVMs by staged embolization and operative excision. *J Neurosurg* 1987;67:17–28.
25. Grzyska U, Westphal M, Zanella F, Freckmann N, Herrmann H-D, Zeumer H. A joint protocol for the neurosurgical and neuroradiologic treatment of cerebral arteriovenous malformations: indications, technique, and results in 76 cases. *Surg Neurol* 1993;40:476–484.
26. Nakstad PH, Nornes H. Superselective angiography, embolization and surgery in treatment of arteriovenous malformations of the brain. *Neuroradiology* 1994;36(5):410–413.
27. Wolpert SM, Barnett FJ, Prager RJ. Benefits of embolization without surgery for cerebral arteriovenous malformations. *AJR* 1982;138:99–102.
28. Brothers MF, Kaufmann JC, Fox AJ, et al. n-Butyl 2-cyanoacrylate substitute for IBCA in interventional neuroradiology: histopathologic and polymerization time studies. *AJNR* 1989;10:777–786.
29. Spiegel SM, Viñuela F, Goldwasser JM, et al. Adjusting the polymerization time of isobutyl-2 cyanoacrylate. *AJNR* 1986;7:109–112.
30. Takasugi JE, Shaw C. Inadvertent bucrylate pulmonary embolization: a case report. *J Thorac Imaging* 1989;4:71–73.
31. Viñuela F, Fox AJ, Pelz D, et al. Angiographic follow-up of large cerebral AVMs incompletely embolized with isobutyl-2-cyanoacrylate. *AJNR* 1986;7:919–925.
32. Vinters HV, Lundie MJ, Kaufmann JC. Long-term pathological follow-up of cerebral arteriovenous malformations treated by embolization with bucrylate. *N Engl J Med* 1986;314:477–483.
33. Rao VRK, Mandalam KR, Gupta AK, et al. Dissolution of isobutyl 2-cyanoacrylate on long-term follow-up. *AJNR* 1989;10:135–141.
34. Henderson AM, Stephenson M. 3-Methoxybutyl-cyanoacrylate: evaluation of biocompatibility and bioresorption. *Biomaterials* 1992;13:1077-1084.
35. Fournier D, Terbrugge K, Rodesch G, et al. Revascularization of brain arteriovenous malformations after embolization with bucrylate. *Neuroradiology* 1990;21:497–501.
36. Latchaw RE, Gold LHA. Polyvinyl foam embolization for vascular and neoplastic lesions of the head, neck and spine. *Radiology* 1979; 131:669–679.
37. duCret RP, Adkins MC, Hunter DW, et al. Therapeutic embolization: enhanced radiolabeled monitoring. *Radiology* 1990;177:571–575.
38. Yakes WF, Haas DK, Parker SH, et al. Symptomatic vascular malformations: ethanol embolotherapy. *Radiology* 1989;170:1059–1066.
39. Rauch RA, Viñuela F, Dion J, et al. Preembolization functional evaluation in brain arteriovenous malformations: the superselective Amytal test. *AJNR* 1992;12:303–308.

40. Peters KR, Quisling RG, Gilmore R, et al. Intraarterial use of sodium methohexital for provocative testing during brain embolotherapy. *AJNR* 1993;14:171–174.
41. Latchaw RE, Hu X, Ugurbil K, Hall WA, Madison MT, Heros RC. Functional magnetic resonance imaging as a management tool for cerebral arteriovenous malformations. *Neurosurgery* 1995;37(4):619–626.
42. Orrison WW Jr, Rose DF, Hart BL, Maclin EL, Sanders JA, Willis BK, Marchand EP, Wood CC, Davis LE. Noninvasive preoperative cortical localization by magnetic source imaging. *AJNR* 1992;13:1124–1128.
43. Duckwiler GR, Dion JE, Viñuela F, et al. Intravascular microcatheter pressure monitoring: experimental results and early clinical evaluation. *AJNR* 1990;11:169–175.
44. Jungreis CA, Horton JA. Pressure changes in the arterial feeder to a cerebral AVM as a guide to monitoring therapeutic embolization. *AJNR* 1989;10:1057–1060.
45. Norbash A, Marks M, Lane B. Correlation of pressure measurements with angiographic characteristics predisposing to hemorrhage and steal in cerebral arteriovenous malformations. *AJNR* 1994;15:809–813.
46. Fleischer LH, Young WL, Pile-Spellman J, et al. Relationship of transcranial Doppler flow velocities and arteriovenous malformation feeding artery pressures. *Stroke* 1993;24:189–1902.
47. Chaloupka JC, Viñuela F, Malanum RP, Ji Ch, Goller DE, Robert J, Duckwiler G. Technical feasibility and performance studies of a Doppler guide wire for potential neuroendovascular applications. *AJNR* 1994;15:503–507.
48. Turjman F, Massoud TF, Viñuela F, Sayre JW, Guglielmi G, Duckwiler G. Aneurysms related to cerebral arteriovenous malformations: superselective angiographic assessment in 58 patients. *AJNR* 1994;15:1601–1605.
49. Marks MP, Lane B, Steinberg GK, et al. Intranidal aneurysms in cerebral arteriovenous malformations: evaluation and endovascular treatment. *Radiology* 1992;183:355–360.
50. Batjer H, Suss RA, Samson D. Intracranial arteriovenous malformations associated with aneurysms. *Neurosurgery* 1986;18:29–35.
51. Marks MP, Lane B, Steinberg GK, et al. Hemorrhage in intracerebral arteriovenous malformations: angiographic determinants. *Radiology* 1990;176:807–813.
52. Viñuela F, Nombela L, Roach MR, et al. Stenotic and occlusive disease of the venous drainage system of deep brain AVMs. *J Neurosurg* 1985;63:180–184.
53. Stein BM, Kader A. Intracranial arteriovenous malformations. *Clin Neurosurg* 1992;39:76–113.
54. Livingston KL, Hopkins LN. Endovascular treatment of intracerebral arteriovenous malformations. *Clin Neurosurg* 1992;39:331–347.
55. Tarr RW, Johnson DW, Horton JA, et al. Impaired cerebral vasoreactivity after embolization of arteriovenous malformations: assessment with serial acetazolamide challenge xenon CT. *AJNR* 1991;12:417–423.
56. Spetzler RF, Hargraves RW, McCormick PW, et al. Relationship of perfusion pressure and size to risk of hemorrhage from arteriovenous malformations. *J Neurosurg* 1992;76:918–923.
57. Spetzler RF, Wilson CB, Weinstein P, et al. Normal perfusion pressure breakthrough theory. *Clin Neurosurg* 1978;25:651–672.
58. Duckwiler GR, Dion JE, Viñuela F, et al. Delayed venous occlusion following embolotherapy of vascular malformations in the brain. *AJNR* 1992;13:1571–1579.
59. Tomlinson FH, Rüfenacht DA, Sundt TS, Nichols DA, Fode NC. Arteriovenous fistulas of the brain and the spinal cord. *J Neurosurg* 1993;79:16–27.
60. Lunsford LD, Kondziolka D, Flickinger JC, Bissonette DJ, Jungreis CA, et al. Stereotactic radiosurgery for arteriovenous malformations of the brain. *J Neurosurg* 1991;75:512–524.
61. Dion JE, Mathis JM. Cranial arteriovenous malformations. *Neurosurg Clin N Am* 1994;5:459–474.
62. Fox AJ, Girvin JP, Viñuela F, et al. Rolandic arteriovenous malformations: improvement in limb function by IBC embolization. *AJNR* 1985;6:575–582.
63. Berenstein A, Choi JS, Kupersmith M, et al. Complications of endovascular embolization in 182 patients with cerebral AVMs. *AJNR* 1989;10:876.
64. Pelz DM, Fox AJ, Viñuela F, et al. Preoperative embolization of brain AVMs with isobutyl-2-cyanoacrylate. *AJNR* 1988;9(4):757–765.
65. Lasjaunias P, Hui F, Zerah M, Garcia-Monaco R, Malherbe V, Rodesch G, Tanaka A, Alvarez H. Cerebral arteriovenous malformation in children. Management of 179 consecutive cases and review of the literature (review). *Child Nerv Syst* 1995;11(2):66–79.
66. Schweitzer JS, Chang BS, Madsen P, Viñuela F, Martin NA, Marroquin CE, Vinters HV. The pathology of arteriovenous malformations of the brain treated by embolotherapy. II. Results of embolization with multiple agents. *Neuroradiology* 1933;35(6):468–474.

Cerebrovascular Disease, edited by H. Hunt Batjer.
Lippincott-Raven Publishers, Philadelphia © 1997.

CHAPTER 59

Intracranial Arteriovenous Malformation: Therapeutic Options

Gary K. Steinberg and Michael P. Marks

The last decade has witnessed a marked evolution in new therapeutic options for treating intracranial arteriovenous malformations (AVMs), and the appropriate application of these advanced techniques has significantly improved the clinical outcome for patients harboring these vascular lesions. While conventional microsurgical resection has been successfully utilized for more than 25 years in cases of small AVMs in noncritical cerebral locations, innovations in surgical and anesthetic techniques have extended the surgical limits to complex AVMs in critical, functional ("eloquent") regions with good results. These innovations include improved irrigating bipolar coagulation, delicate micro-AVM clips, stereotactic microsurgical approaches, intraoperative cortical mapping and electrophysiologic monitoring, and better control of intraoperative blood pressure and brain relaxation. Stereotactic radiosurgery (Bragg peak charged particle, gamma knife, or LINAC) and endovascular embolization have recently proven to be highly successful treatment modalities. They are used as the primary treatment modality in some cases, and in others as adjuncts, allowing safe cure of difficult intracranial AVMs compared to a higher risk if microsurgery alone were employed.

The benefits of endovascular embolization include immediate reduction in AVM volume and decrease in AVM flow. Embolization is usually performed with the patient awake during the procedure, obviating the need for general anesthesia, open craniotomy, or prolonged hospital stay, and improving clinical assessment at the time of embolization. Occasionally, in the case of some smaller AVMs, embolization alone is curative but more commonly, it is used as an adjunct to open microsurgery, stereotactic radiosurgery, or both. In some cases, we have employed embolization following microsurgery and/or stereotactic radiosurgery, but generally it

is used as a prelude to further microsurgery or radiosurgery. Disadvantages of embolization are the small risks of causing hemorrhage from residual AVM, dissections of cervical or intracranial arteries, infarcts from errant embolic material or excessive thrombosis in normal cerebral vessels, gluing of a catheter in cerebral vessels, and local minor complications at the femoral arterial cannulation site. In our experience, the risks of embolization can be minimized by meticulous attention to technical details; staging of embolization procedures (not obliterating too large a volume of AVM at any one session); close neurologic, clinical monitoring during the procedure; and the use of Amytal provocative testing prior to permanent embolization. Monitoring of somatosensory evoked potentials (SEPs) or brainstem auditory evoked potentials (BAERs) has sometimes proved useful in assessing patients undergoing embolization of AVMs in highly eloquent territories. We prefer glue embolization using *N*-butylcyanoacrylate (NBCA) because of its versatility and permanence as well as its easy delivery through flow directed microcatheters. We have seen several cases of AVM recanalization after polyvinyl alcohol (PVA) embolization.

Microsurgical resection is the preferred mode of therapy for small AVMs in nonfunctional brain areas. For AVMs in functional cerebral regions, microsurgical resection still holds certain advantages: immediate and permanent cure of the lesion with elimination of future hemorrhage risk, and often improvement in other neurologic symptoms and signs (1–9). However, the risks of causing new neurologic deficit with microsurgery can be significant when the AVM is situated in a critical brain area, especially if the AVM is larger than 3 cm diameter or has deep venous drainage (1–5,8,9). Furthermore, open microsurgery requires general anesthesia and more prolonged hospitalization than either embolization or radiosurgery.

We have found a stereotactic approach, using the Cosman–Roberts–Wells (CRW) system and, more recently, the frameless robotic arm (Radionics), to be extremely useful

G. K. Steinberg and M. P. Marks: Department of Neurosurgery and Radiology and Stanford Stroke Center, Stanford University Medical Center, Stanford, California 94305.

for microsurgical resection of deep-seated or small-surface AVMs. These techniques provide precise localization of the AVM (within a few millimeters) and allow for small craniotomy, limited dural opening, and minimal brain manipulation or unnecessary exposure. In our experience, it results in lower morbidity and shorter hospitalization compared with more conventional, larger craniotomies. Intraoperative cortical mapping of functional areas (motor, sensory, language), with the patient asleep but nonparalyzed or the patient awake, is also extremely valuable at the time of craniotomy. This procedure requires close collaboration with an intraoperative neurophysiology team and helps to determine if an AVM is situated within, rather than adjacent to, a critical functional region. Often an AVM will displace normal brain function to an atypical location. Our preliminary experience with preoperative functional MR imaging in AVM patients suggests that this technique may also be useful in localizing functional areas.

Stereotactic, Bragg peak (helium ion, proton beam) or photon (gamma knife, LINAC) radiosurgery has distinct advantages for the treatment of AVMs in functional brain areas, in patients who are poor surgical candidates and in patients who refuse surgery. There is a high obliteration rate for small and moderate-sized AVMs (<3.5 cm diameter), a low morbidity rate and radiosurgery does not require general anesthesia or hospitalization. Stereotactic radiosurgery demonstrates a high rate of improvement in symptoms of headaches, seizures, and stabilization or improvement of progressive neurologic deficit (5,7,10–16). The radiosurgery procedure has some disadvantages: there is a latency period of 1–3 years before complete obliteration of the AVM occurs, during which time the AVM can bleed; and there exists a small risk (1–3%) of temporary or permanent delayed radiation complications with small and moderate-sized AVMs. These complications are due to radiation-induced white matter changes or vasculopathy (17). Larger AVMs (>3.5 cm diameter) are more difficult to cure safely with stereotactic radiosurgery alone because their complete obliteration rate is lower (42% at 2 years), and the risk of complications is higher than for smaller AVMs, even using the Bragg peak helium ion technique (5,7,10–12).

Since each procedure (embolization, microsurgery, and stereotactic radiosurgery) has its own risks of complications and use of combined therapy subjects the patient to cumulative risks, it is important to judicially apply these various therapies to each patient. In the past 13 years we have treated over 750 intracranial AVMs, with 80% of the AVMs located in critical, functional (eloquent) regions, including brainstem, corpus callosum, thalamus, basal ganglia, or motor, sensory, language, and visual cortical areas (8). Approximately one half of the AVMs have been >3.5 cm in diameter. As we gained more experience utilizing these various therapeutic techniques in different combinations, we evolved an individualized approach to each patient with an intracranial AVM. The choice of modality and order of treatment is determined by an assessment of the relative risks of each

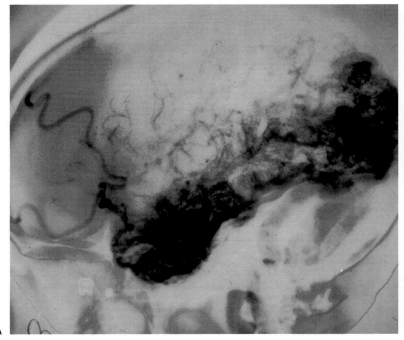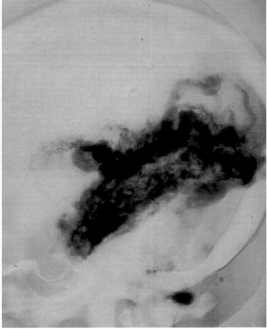

A   B

FIG. 1. A 20-year-old woman presenting with occasional migraine headaches. **A:** Lateral projection from right internal carotid artery angiogram. **B:** Lateral projection from right vertebral artery angiogram. These views demonstrate a very large AVM (approx. 7 cm longest diameter) occupying the right temporal and occipital lobes. Venous drainage was deep. This patient was advised to receive symptomatic treatment of her migraines and clinical follow-up.

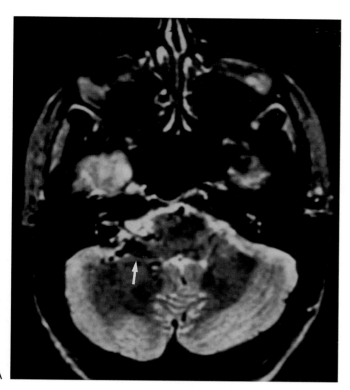

A

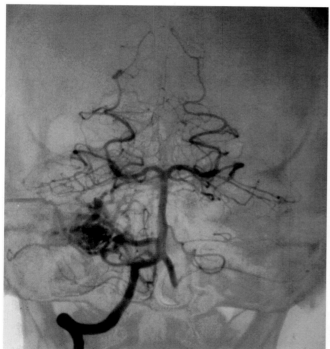

B

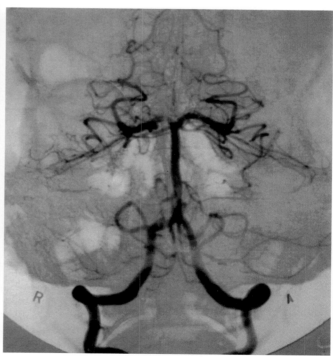

C

FIG. 2. A 50-year-old woman with a right cerebellar peduncle arteriovenous malformation (AVM) extending into the cerebellopontine angle. She presented with intermittent left hemiparesis and right visual field scintillations. **A:** Axial T1-weighted MRI demonstrates AVM flow voids in the cerebellar peduncle and CP angle *(arrow)*. **B:** Anteroposterior (AP) view from a right vertebral artery injection demonstrates filling of a 2-cm nidus from the anterior inferior and posterior inferior cerebellar arteries. **C:** Angiogram perform 2 months following a single embolization session with *N*-butylcyanoacrylate (NBCA) demonstrates complete obliteration of the AVM nidus. The patient developed a partial right visual field defect that resolved over several months.

treatment and each combination of therapies, in conjunction with our analysis of the natural history of the individual patient's AVM and the patient's preference. After reviewing the radiologic studies (angiogram, MR, and CT), clinical presentation, medical condition, and age of each patient, our multidisciplinary AVM team assesses the natural history of the AVM in the particular patient under consideration.

The angiogram is analyzed carefully to identify certain angiographic characteristics of AVMs that have been shown to correlate with increased risk of hemorrhage: intranidus aneurysms, central venous drainage, small size, and the absence of angiomatous change (anomalous transcortical arterial supply to the AVM) (18–20). The presence of angiomatous change is also taken into consideration for treatment

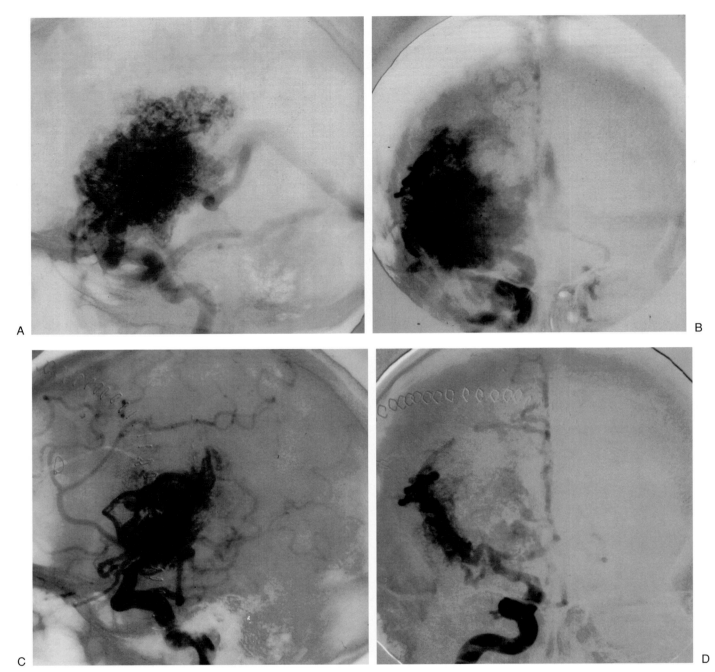

FIG. 3. A 15-year-old boy presenting with mild left-sided weakness from a large right basal ganglia AVM. He underwent helium ion radiosurgery (15 GyE to 70,000 mm³) 3 years previously that did not alter the size of the AVM. Percutaneous endovascular embolization was unsuccessful due to the myriad small perforating arteries. **A:** Lateral projection from a right internal carotid artery angiogram. **B:** Anterior projection from a right internal carotid artery angiogram. The A and B views demonstrate the unchanged AVM nidus following radiotherapy and attempted endovascular embolization. The patient was taken to the operating room where the right anterior and middle cerebral arteries were exposed. Temporary clips were placed on the proximal right middle cerebral artery M2 segments, just distal to the bifurcation, and distal right A1 anterior cerebral artery adjacent to the anterior communicating artery, and the right posterior communicating artery using somatosensory evoked potential monitoring. Small-particle polyvinyl alcohol (50–150 μm) was then embolized through a microcatheter that had been endovascularly guided into the supraclinoid carotid artery at its bifurcation. **C:** Lateral projection from a right internal carotid artery angiogram postoperatively. **D:** Anterior projection from a right internal carotid artery angiogram postoperatively. The C and D views demonstrate significant reduction in the AVM nidus using this intraoperative embolization technique. The patient remained neurologically unchanged. Following this study the patient was reradiated using Bragg peak proton beam radiosurgery. Postradiosurgery follow-up is pending.

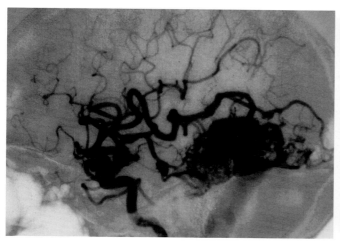

A

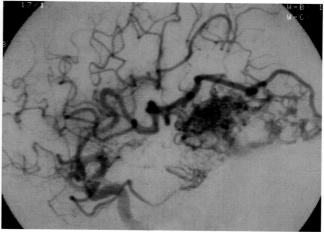

B

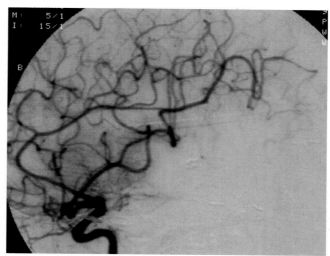

C

FIG. 4. A 58-year-old woman with a large right temporal AVM. She presented with a left superior quandrantanopsia and migraine headaches. **A:** Lateral projection from a right internal carotid artery angiogram demonstrates filling of the AVM nidus measuring approximately 4 cm in diameter. **B:** Lateral projection from the right internal carotid artery angiogram following a single session of embolization with *N*-butylcyanoacrylate (NBCA) demonstrates a greater than 50% reduction in the size of the AVM nidus. Embolization achieved a significant flow reduction and reduced the number of feeding pedicles. **C:** Lateral projection from a right internal carotid artery angiogram following surgical resection showing complete excision of the AVM. The patient developed an additional left inferior quandrantanopsia post-operatively, but this resolved over 4 months.

TABLE 1. *Therapeutic options for AVM treatment*

AVM size	Noncritical location	Critical location[a]
Small AVMs (≤3.0 cm diam.)	1. Microsurgical resection 2. Stereotactic radiosurgery if poor surgical risk 3. Occasionally, embolization aimed at complete thrombosis	1. Stereotactic radiosurgery 2. Occasionally, microsurgical resection or embolization if multiple hemorrhages
Large AVMs (>3.0 cm diam.)	1. Embolization followed by microsurgical resection 2. Embolization followed by stereotactic radiosurgery if poor surgical risk	1. Embolization followed by stereotactic radiosurgery 2. Stereotactic radiosurgery alone if poor embolization candidate (proton beam XRT for AVMs >3.5 cm)

AVM, arteriovenous malformation; XRT, radiosurgery.
[a] Motor/sensory cortex, corona radiata, thalamus, internal capsule, brainstem.

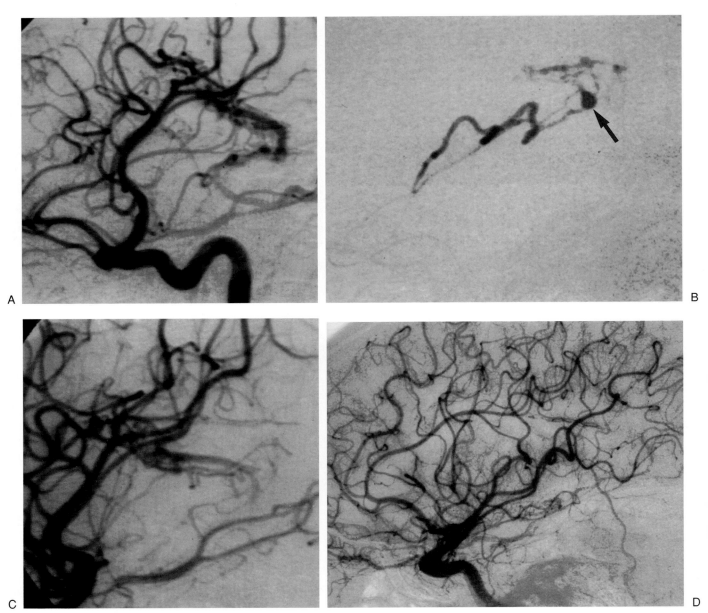

FIG. 5. A 27-year-old man with a left temporal AVM. He had previously hemorrhaged and developed an aphasia that partially cleared. **A:** Lateral projection from a left internal carotid artery angiogram. This demonstrates supply to a small AVM from temporal opercular vessels and the anterior choroidal artery. A small intranidal aneurysm was noted. **B:** Lateral projection from a superselective anterior choroidal artery angiogram at the time of embolization. This view better demonstrates filling of the inferior portion of the nidus and a small intranidal aneurysm *(arrow)*. **C:** Lateral projection from a left internal carotid artery angiogram postembolization. This demonstrates continued partial filling of the AVM, but the inferior portion of the nidus containing the intranidal aneurysm is thrombosed. Patient then underwent radiotherapy using LINAC radiosurgery (15 GyE). **D:** Lateral projection from a left internal carotid artery angiogram 12 months following embolization and radiosurgery shows complete thrombosis of the AVM. The patient remained unchanged neurologically, with only mind anomia. (Reprint with permission from ref. 19.)

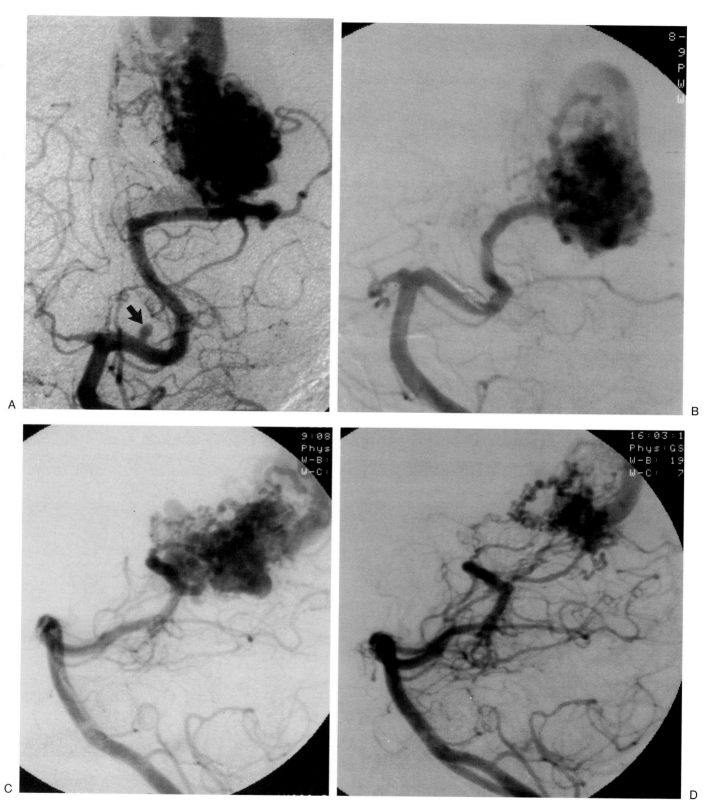

FIG. 6. A 26-year-old women with a left occipital AVM. She presented with a right inferior quandrantanopsia and migraine headaches. **A:** Towne projection from a left vertebral artery angiogram demonstrates filling of the AVM nidus from a dilated posterior cerebral artery. An aneurysm was noted on the left P1 segment *(arrow)*. The aneurysm was clipped through a pterional approach prior to initiating embolotherapy. **(B)** Anterior and **(C)** lateral projection from a left vertebral artery angiogram. These views show filling of the nidus following aneurysm clipping prior to embolization. **D:** Lateral projection from a left vertebral artery angiogram following a single session of embolization with *N*-butylcyanoacrylate (NBCA) demonstrates approximately a 75% reduction in the AVM nidus size prior to further therapy.

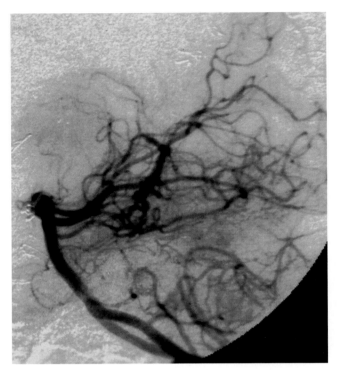

FIG. 6. *Continued.* **E:** Lateral projection from a left vertebral artery angiogram following surgical excision of the remainder of the AVM, demonstrating complete excision of the lesion. The patient was neurologically unchanged after treatment.

modality selection because it has a high correlation with the development of clinical steal neurologic symptoms and signs, including progressive neurologic deficit (21). Other AVM characteristics, including size, location, and pattern of venous drainage, as well as the patient's age, presenting symptoms, neurologic status, and medical condition, are factored into treatment planning because these parameters are

predictors for risks of microsurgery or radiosurgery (3,5,8). The relative risks of embolization, microsurgery, and stereotactic radiosurgery are estimated and discussed with the patient and family, along with our assessment of the AVM's expected natural history. The patient's preference for a particular treatment modality or combination of modalities is carefully considered at the time of treatment recommendation.

A decision regarding no treatment (except anticonvulsants or analgesics for symptomatic therapy) vs. definitive treatment for the AVM is made by the members of the AVM team and the patient. In cases where the risks of treatment obviously outweigh the probable natural history of the AVM, a choice of no treatment is appropriate. For instance, a woman whom we evaluated, who was 20 years old with a 7-cm left temporo-occipital AVM fed by anterior and posterior circulation and draining centrally, who suffered occasional migraine headaches, was advised to receive symptomatic treatment for her migraines and clinical follow-up but no other treatment for her AVM (Fig. 1). Likewise, a 1.5-cm diameter perimesencephalic cistern AVM that was discovered incidentally in a 77-year-old man was not treated. Once a decision to treat a particular patient is made, our multidisciplinary team discusses the relative goals, benefits, and risks of each treatment modality separately and the additive benefits and risks of combined therapies. The overall aim of all treatments is to achieve complete angiographic obliteration of the AVM, eliminating the potential for future hemorrhage, progressive neurologic deficit, intractable seizures, or incapacitating headaches, with minimal risk of neurologic complications.

Smaller AVMs (≤3.0 cm diameter) may be treated using various modalities. We will consider treatment with endovascular embolization aimed at complete AVM thrombosis and cure for some smaller AVMs (Fig. 2). Seven patients with AVMs in functional areas were treated in this manner

TABLE 2. *AVM therapeutic options: benefits and risks*

Treatment modality	Advantages	Disadvantages
Microsurgery	1. Immediate and permanent cure 2. Immediate elimination of hemorrhage risk	1. Risk of neurologic deficits, especially with large or critically located AVMs 2. Invasive (general anesthesia and craniotomy) 3. Longer hospitalization (3–5 days)
Embolization	1. Immediate reduction in AVM volume and obliteration of intranidus aneurysms 2. Less invasive (local anesthesia) 3. Shorter hospitalization (1 day)	1. Rarely cures AVM 2. Risk of neurologic deficits from hemorrhage or infarct
Stereotactic radiosurgery	1. Virtually no immediate risk 2. No hospitalization 3. Noninvasive (no anesthesia or craniotomy)	1. Latency of 1–3 years before complete AVM obliteration 2. Risk of hemorrhage during latency period 3. Risk of delayed neurologic deficits from radiation complications

AVM, arteriovenous malformation.

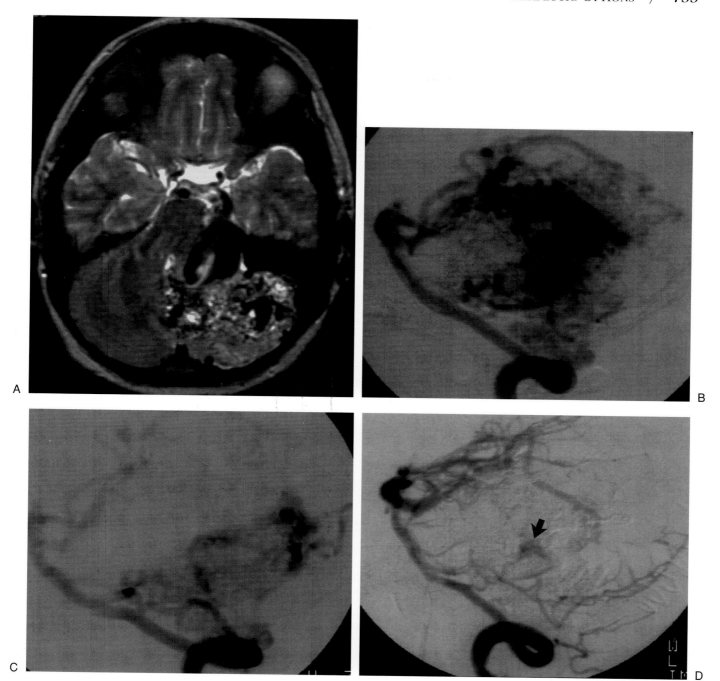

FIG. 7. A 15-year-old girl with a large left cerebellar AVM. She presented with headaches and diplopia. **A:** A T2-weighted axial MR demonstrates the flow voids from a left cerebellar AVM occupying the entire left cerebellar hemisphere. **B:** Lateral projection from a left vertebral artery angiogram (pretreatment), showing the large ACM supplied by the superior cerebellar, anterior inferior cerebellar, and posterior inferior cerebrellar arteries. **C:** Lateral projection from a left vertebral artery angiogram following two-staged embolizations using N-butylcyanoacrylate (NBCA) demonstrates a greater than 50% reduction of the AVM nidus size. **D:** Lateral projection from a left vertebral artery angiogram following surgery demonstrates a small residual portion of the AVM nidus which was deep and adjacent to the brainstem (arrow). The patient's headaches and diplopia resolved completely. She underwent radiosurgery using LINAC to this small residual. Postradiosurgery follow-up studies are pending.

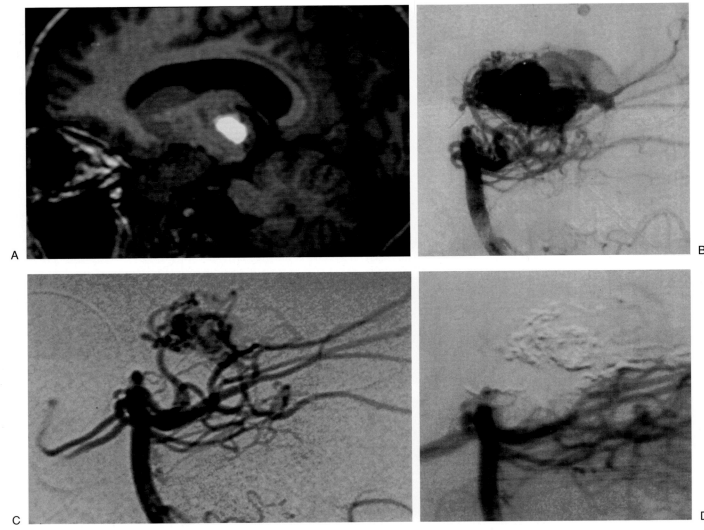

FIG. 8. A 17-year-old woman with a thalamic AVM presenting with hemorrhage, dense right hemiparesis, and coma prior to treatment. She made an excellent clinical recovery. **A:** Sagittal T1-weighted MRI demonstrates high signal in the medial aspect of the thalamus from methemoglobin deposited at the time of AVM hemorrhage. **B:** Lateral projection from a left vertebral artery angiogram shows a left thalamic AVM fed by thalamoperforators. The patient underwent Bragg peak helium ion radiosurgery (20 GyE to 4400 mm³). **C:** Lateral projection from a left vertebral artery angiogram performed approximately 36 months following radiosurgery demonstrates some reduction in the AVM nidus flow, but continued filling of the deep central lesion. The patient also suffered additional hemorrhages 17 and 30 months following radiosurgery with temporary right hemiparesis. Embolization was therefore used to treat the AVM. **D:** Lateral projection from a left vertebral artery angiogram performed 3 months following two-staged embolization procedures with *N*-butylcyanoacrylate (NBCA) demonstrates complete obliteration of the AVM nidus. The patient remained neurologically unchanged with slight right-sided spasticity.

using NBCA; this resulted in complete angiographic AVM obliteration. None of these patients have angiographically recanalized their AVM or suffered a hemorrhage in follow-up 1–5 years after embolization. One patient suffered a new aphasia and hemiparesis at the time of embolization but made a good recovery over 6 months. If we conclude that endovascular embolization does not have a high potential for complete obliteration of these small AVMs, it generally is not used. We favor microsurgical resection if the small

AVM is in a non-eloquent area, presents to a pial or ependymal surface, or can be approached safely through noneloquent brain. Approximately 175 patients had complete resection of their small AVM (1–3 cm diameter) with microsurgery alone. Intraoperative angiography was often used to assess complete AVM resection and a postoperative angiogram performed 5–14 days postoperatively confirmed complete AVM resection in all of these patients. In our series, microsurgical resection of most small AVMs, even in func-

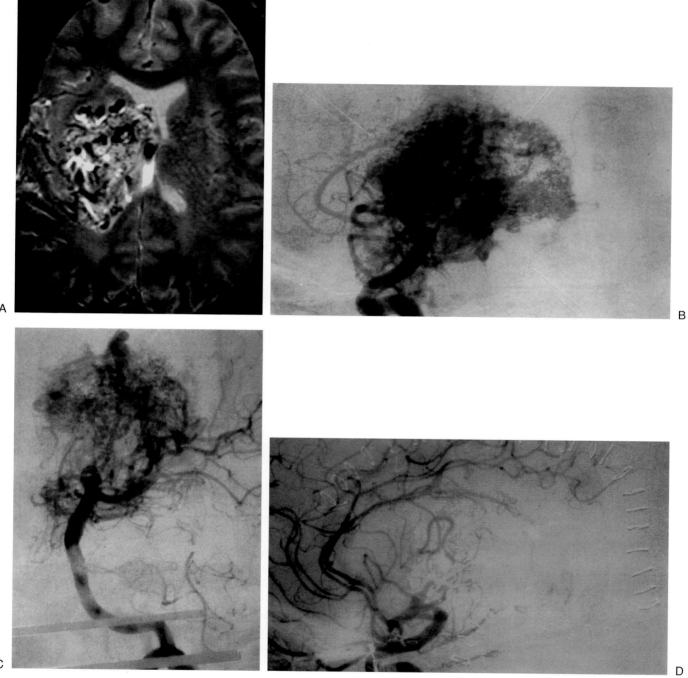

FIG. 9. A 32-year-old man with a large right basal ganglia, thalamic AVM. He had presented 16 years previously with hemorrhage causing left hemiparesis and intractable seizures. He underwent treatment with helium ion Bragg peak radiosurgery (17.5 GyE to 80,000 mm³) 3 years previously and had no change in the AVM size. **A:** Axial T2-weighted image through the basal ganglia and thalamus demonstrates the flow voids of the AVM which measured approximately 5 cm in diameter. **B:** Lateral projection from a right internal carotid artery angiogram. **C:** Lateral projection from a left vertebral artery angiogram. These views demonstrate filling of the AVM nidus from the anterior and posterior circulation. The patient underwent two-staged embolization procedures using N-butylcyanoacrylate (NBCA), followed by surgical resection of the AVM. **D:** Lateral projection from a right internal carotid artery angiogram following embolization and surgery.

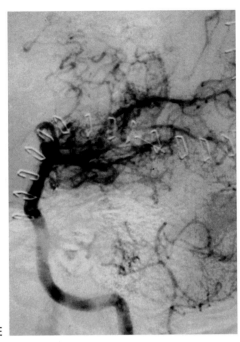

FIG. 9. *Continued.* **E:** Lateral projection from a left vertebral artery angiogram following embolization and surgery. These views demonstrate complete thrombosis and excision of the AVM without residual arterial venous shunting. The patient's seizurs were well controlled and he was otherwise neurologically unchanged (mild hemiparesis) following his multimodality treatment.

tional regions like corpus callosum, language cortex, and visual cortex, has been very successful in achieving complete AVM cure with low risk of permanent neurologic deficits (8). This confirms the results of other reports (1,6,9). About 85% of these patients remained neurologically normal or unchanged following surgery. While approximately 15% of the patients were worsened immediately postoperatively, most of them made excellent recoveries over several weeks to months. We have never observed rebleeding after complete AVM resection. We have found the use of a stereotactic technique (CRW or frameless Radionics system) to be extremely helpful in localizing and resecting some of these small AVMs.

Small AVMs (≤3.0 cm diameter) in the motor-sensory cortex, corona radiata, thalamic areas, internal capsule, or brainstem are usually treated with radiosurgery (20–25 GyE), unless there is more urgency to obliterate the AVM sooner than 1–3 years (eg, multiple recent bleeds) or the patient is unwilling to accept a 1- to 3-year latency period before AVM obliteration occurs. In our experience, open microsurgery for AVMs in these particular functional areas carries higher risk of neurologic deficit than does radiosurgery (8). Radiosurgery is also often recommended for small AVMs in other functional or noneloquent areas, if the patient is considered a poor surgical risk (eg, elderly or in poor medical condition) or the patient declines open surgery. Ap-

proximately 350 AVM patients were treated solely with radiosurgery. Our previous publications document good results after helium ion radiosurgery for small AVMs with a 3-year complete obliteration of 90–95%, significant improvement in clinical symptoms and signs and low risk of complications (5,7,10–12). With our current dose of 20–25 GyE about 1–3% of patients develop new delayed neurologic deficits from radiation-induced edema or necrosis; half of these complications were transient or minor. However, there is still a latency period of 1–3 years for achieving complete obliteration, during which time bleeding can occur and neurologic symptoms persist. A few of our patients suffered a hemorrhage from their AVMs during this latency period. Once complete angiographic obliteration of the AVM had been demonstrated, no patients suffered either subsequent recanalization of the AVM or subsequent hemorrhage. Although much of our radiosurgery experience has been with the Bragg peak helium ion method, gamma knife or LINAC radiosurgery appears to be comparable in terms of their success for treating smaller AVMs (≤3.0 cm diameter) (13–16).

AVMs that are >3.0 cm diameter are usually treated with endovascular embolization prior to microsurgical resection or prior to stereotactic radiosurgery. The rationale underlying this approach is that larger volume AVMs carry higher risks of complications with either microsurgery or radiosurgery and have lower obliteration rates with radiosurgery than smaller AVMs. In our patients, AVMs greater than 3.7 cm diameter had 3-year complete obliteration of only 50–60% with a higher complication rate than radiosurgically treated small AVMs (5,7). The goal of embolization is tailored to each case. If embolization is being used as a presurgical adjunct, our aims are to decrease AVM volume and flow as well as close deep AVM feeders that may be difficult to reach during the initial phase of surgery. We obliterate as much volume of AVM with embolization as is considered safely possible, but we will often use two or three different embolization sessions separated by at least 1 week to achieve this goal. We prefer to wait at least a week between embolization sessions and between the last embolization and surgery to allow hemodynamic stabilization of the AVM and surrounding vasculature. In our experience this has substantially decreased the incidence of ischemic and hemorrhagic complications associated with both embolization and surgery. Typically, large AVM volumes are reduced 50–85% by embolization. In selected cases of deep hemisphere or basal ganglia AVMs, we use intraoperative embolization (sometimes with temporary occlusion of normal arteries) to gain access to particular feeding vessels and inject NBCA or PVA into an otherwise inaccessible nidus (Fig. 3).

The combination of embolization followed by microsurgery resulted in complete AVM obliteration in more than 40 patients harboring AVMs in functional regions (Fig. 4). These AVMs measured up to 6 cm diameter. In most cases, the entire AVM (embolized plus nonembolized portions)

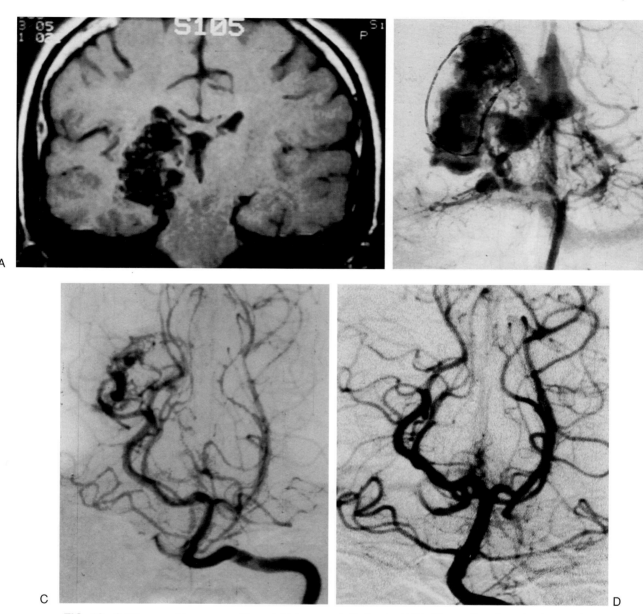

FIG. 10. A 23-year-old woman with a right temporal–thalamic AVM. She suffered a prior hemorrhage resulting in a homonymous hemianopsia. **A:** Coronal T1-weighted MRI demonstrates the AVM occupying the mesial right temporal lobe and extending into the thalamus. **B:** Anterior projection from a left vertebral artery angiogram demonstrates filling of the AVM with marks delineating the nidus for radiosurgery treatment planning. The patient underwent helium ion radiosurgery (25 GyE to 7000 mm³). **C:** Anterior projection from a left vertebral artery angiogram performed 36 months following radiosurgery demonstrates significant reduction in the AVM nidus, but without complete thrombosis. The patient underwent surgical excision of the residual AVM seen in the pulvinar of the thalamus. **D:** Anterior projection from a left vertebral artery angiogram done postoperatively demonstrates complete excision of the AVM without residual shunting. The patient developed a mild left sensory deficit that resolved after 2 months.

was resected. However, in a few cases, portions of AVM thrombosed by embolization alone were not resected. Postoperative angiography at 5–14 days following surgery confirmed complete angiographic AVM obliteration in all patients. No AVMs rebled or showed recanalization following embolization plus microsurgical resection. A few of these patients had new neurologic deficits following embolization

and surgery; however, most deficits were temporary with recovery over weeks to months.

Preradiosurgery embolization is designed to decrease the volume of AVM that will need to be treated with radiosurgery. We try to achieve residual volumes of <3.5 cm diameter if possible, since our radiosurgery results are better for these small to moderate-sized AVMs (5,7,10–12). In certain

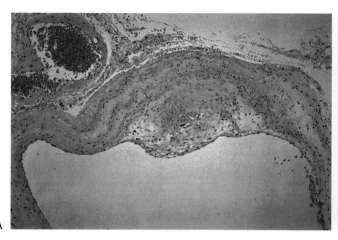
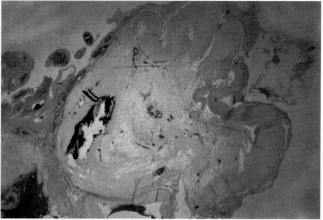

A

B

FIG. 11. Photomicrograph (hematoxylin and eosin) of AVM vessels in two patients 37 months **(A)** or 40 months **(B)** following helium ion radiosurgery treatment (A: 18 GyE to 35,000 mm^3; B: 20 GyE to 14,200 mm^3). No angiographic change in the appearance of the AVM was seen in either case. **A:** Extensive endothelial proliferation, thickening of vessel wall, and luminal narrowing. **B:** Thickening of vessel wall with hyaline and calcium deposition; complete thrombosis of vessel. These changes likely accounted for the ease of AVM resection in these cases compared to our experience with nonradiosurgery treated AVMs.

cases, we use preradiosurgery embolization to obliterate portions of the AVM predisposed to hemorrhage, such as intranidus aneurysms (Fig. 5). Similarly, microsurgery may be used to clip aneurysms on feeding vessels prior to radiosurgery or embolization (Fig. 6). Reduction of flow only without AVM volume reduction might theoretically increase the rate and extent of obliteration following radiosurgery. However, this approach is not of proven benefit, and treating the larger AVM volume would still carry some increased risk of complications unless a lower treatment dose were used. When AVM volume cannot be reduced below 25 cm^3 (3.7 cm diameter) we will still often treat with stereotactic Bragg peak radiosurgery (proton beam), using a lower therapeutic dose (20 GyE).

Embolization followed by helium or proton beam radiosurgery was used in over 50 patients. Although complete long-term follow-up is not available on these patients, total angiographic obliteration has been achieved in several patients at 2–3 years following radiosurgery. In all cases, only the nonembolized portion of the AVM received radiosurgery. We have observed recanalization following embolization with PVA which was used early in our experience. No AVMs embolized with NBCA and subsequently radiated have recanalized in follow-up angiograms. The AVMs in the embolization/radiosurgery group measured up to 6 cm diameter. None of the patients with complete angiographic AVM obliteration rebled or recanalized in long-term follow-up. We have observed a few rebleeds after embolization and radiosurgery but before complete AVM thrombosis has been achieved.

In some cases we plan one or several stages of microsurgery or both endovascular embolization and microsurgery before employing stereotactic radiosurgery for a particular AVM. This combined approach is used for especially large and complex AVMs in functional regions. Twenty-five patients underwent staged treatment using initial embolization followed by partial microsurgical resection and, finally, helium ion radiosurgery for the residual AVM (Fig. 7). These AVMs measured up to 7 cm in diameter. In these cases only angiographically demonstrable residual AVM was irradiated. Partial microsurgical AVM resection followed by radiosurgery was utilized in 30 patients. The surgical procedure was performed to reduce AVM volume in noncritical areas, leaving a small AVM in a functional area for treatment with radiosurgery. Some of the AVMs have been completely obliterated with this combination of modalities, but many of these patients have not yet had their 2-year follow-up angiogram. One potential problem in leaving some residual AVM after deliberate partial AVM resection is bleeding. We take special precautions postoperatively, including induced hypotension and hypovolemia, for several days to avoid this complication. Since instituting this policy, we have experienced only two perioperative hemorrhages from residual AVM left deliberately. One patient bled fatally after the combined treatment with embolization, microsurgery, and radiosurgery but before AVM obliteration was complete. Another patient had a minor bleed after surgery, before undergoing radiosurgery.

Approximately 15% of the AVMs we treated with radiosurgery alone did not obliterate completely after 3 years. These were mostly large AVMs and, in a few cases, AVMs treated with low doses (11–18 GyE) or incomplete nidus coverage. We have never observed an AVM unobliterated 3 years after radiosurgery that went on to complete obliteration in subsequent years. Also, there were no AVMs unchanged angiographically at 2 years following radiosurgery

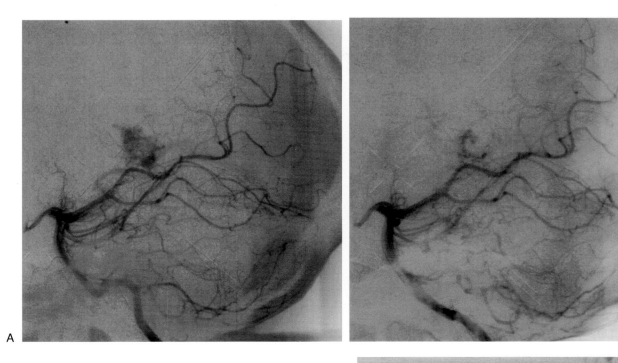

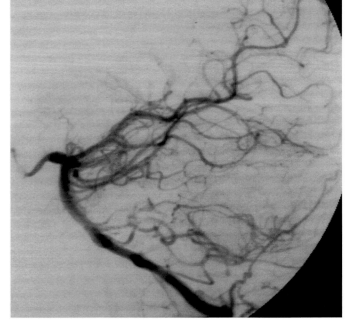

FIG. 12. A 27-year-old woman with a right choroid plexus AVM. She suffered two intraventricular hemorrhages prior to treatments. **A:** Lateral projection from a left vertebral artery angiogram demonstrates filling of the 1.5-cm AVM nidus. The patient underwent therapy with helium ion radiosurgery (15 GyE to 700 mm³). **B:** Lateral projection from a left vertebral artery angiogram performed 44 months following radiosurgery demonstrates decreased filling of the nidus but a residual is present. The patient underwent a second treatment with helium ion radiosurgery (20 GyE to 200 mm³). **C:** Lateral projection from a left vertebral artery angiogram 12 months following the second treatment with radiosurgery demonstrates complete thrombosis of the AVM without residual shunt. The patient remained neurologically normal following both radiosurgery treatments.

that obliterated completely in subsequent years. For these AVMs we usually recommend further treatment with embolization, microsurgery, or both modalities. We have successfully cured 26 of these previously radiated but unobliterated AVMs with microsurgery alone (16 patients), embolization alone (2 patients), or combined embolization and microsurgery (8 patients) (22,23) (Figs. 8–9). Embolization of these lesions has suggested that these AVMs previously radiated had large shunts (22). Some of these patients showed partial angiographic obliteration reducing the volume of AVM to

be resected or embolized and resected (Fig. 10). Surgical observations and histopathology findings in many of the patients suggested that although radiosurgery did not always alter the angiographic appearance of these large AVMs, many of the smaller vessels within the AVM were completely or partially thrombosed (Fig. 11). At surgery the previously irradiated AVM was found to be markedly less vascular and easier to resect, compared with similar AVMs that had not been radiated. In some cases, the radiosurgery appeared to obliterate the fine vessel AVM components, leaving larger AV fistulous elements. In many cases the radiosurgery transformed a high-risk, difficult resection into a straightforward, safe procedure with minimal blood loss and low morbidity (23).

There are also some large AVMs that have failed to obliterate after radiosurgery, where we still consider embolization or microsurgery too risky. We usually recommend a second course of stereotactic radiosurgery for these patients, recognizing that they may have a slightly higher risk of radiation-induced complications. This retreatment with radiosurgery is usually reserved for symptomatic patients with complex, large AVMs in the corona radiata, basal ganglia, internal capsule, thalamus, or brainstem. Thus far, 22 patients whose AVMs were not obliterated 2–3 years after initial helium ion radiosurgery received a second helium ion or proton beam radiosurgical treatment. Follow-up is short on these patients, but three have gone on to complete angiographic obliteration within 2–3 years after the second radiosurgery treatment (Fig. 12). One patient has developed radiation-induced white matter edema and transient hemiparesis after the second radiosurgery. However, it does not appear that these reirradiated patients have an excessively high complication rate due to repeat radiosurgery. Other groups have also utilized a second radiosurgery procedure for incompletely obliterated AVMs (24).

Untreated intracranial AVMs, particularly when located in critical functional brain regions, continue to cause significant morbidity and mortality. Their successful treatment remains a challenge. The use of individualized, multimodality therapy with different combinations of embolization, microsurgery, and radiosurgery has increased the chances for safe, complete obliteration and improved clinical outcome in many of these patients. It is important to constantly review our patient selection criteria, radiologic results, and clinical outcomes, and continually redesign our treatment strategies, in an effort to successfully treat patients with the largest and most complex intracranial AVMs.

ACKNOWLEDGMENTS

This work was supported in part by funding from the William Randolph Hearst Foundation (G.K.S). We thank Mary Marcellus for assistance with the clinical data, Phil Verzola for technical help with the figures, and Liz Aysm for preparation of the manuscript.

REFERENCES

1. Drake CG. Cerebral arteriovenous malformations: considerations for and experience with surgical treatment in 166 cases. *Clin Neurosurg* 1979;26:145-208.
2. Drake CG, Friedman AH, Peerless SJ. Posterior fossa arteriovenous malformations. *J Neurosurg* 1986;64:1-10.
3. Spetzler RM, Martin NA. A proposed grading system for arteriovenous malformations. *J Neurosurg* 1986;65:476-483.
4. Batjer H, Samson D. Arteriovenous malformations of the posterior fossa: clinical presentation, diagnostic evaluation, and surgical treatment. *J Neurosurg* 1986;64:849–856.
5. Steinberg GK, Fabrikant JI, Marks MP, et al. Stereotactic heavy-charged-particle Bragg-peak radiation for intracranial arteriovenous malformations. *N Engl J Med* 1990;323:96–101.
6. Stein BM. Surgical decisions in vascular malformations of the brain. In: Barnett HJM, Mohr JP, Stein BM, et al., eds. *Stroke: Pathophysiology, Diagnosis, and Management*. New York: Churchill-Livingstone, 1992; 1093–1133.
7. Steinberg GK, Levy RP, Marks MP, Fabrikant JI. Vascular malformations: charged-particle radiosurgery. In: Alexander E, Loeffler JS, Lunsford LD, eds. *Stereotactic Radiosurgery*. New York: McGraw-Hill, 1993;122–135.
8. Steinberg GK, Marks MP, Levy RP, Fabrikant JI. Multimodality treatment of vascular malformations in functional brain areas using stereotactic radiosurgery, embolization and microsurgery. In: Yamada S, ed. *Arteriovenous Malformations in Functional Brain Areas*. Mt. Kisco: Futura Publishing, 1996. In press.
9. Heros RC, Korosue K, Diebold PM. Surgical excision of cerebral arteriovenous malformations: late results. *Neurosurgery* 1990;26:570–578.
10. Fabrikant JI, Levy RP, Steinberg GK, et al. Charged-particle radiosurgery for intracranial vascular malformations. *Neurosurg Cinic North Am* 1992;3:99–103.
11. Levy RP, Fabrikant JI, Frankel KA, Phillips MH, Lyman JT. Stereotactic heavy-charged particle Bragg peak radiosurgery for the treatment of intracranial arteriovenous malformations in childhood and adolescence. *Neurosurgery* 1989;24:841–852.
12. Levy RP, Fabrikant JI, Frankel KA, et al. Charged-particle radiosurgery of the brain. *Neurosurg Clin North Am* 1990;1:955–990.
13. Steiner L. Radiosurgery in cerebral arteriovenous malformations. In: Fein JM, Flamm ES, eds. *Cerebrovascular Surgery*. vol 4. New York: Springer-Verlag, 1985;1161–1215.
14. Kondziolka D, Lunsford LD, Flickinger JC. Gamma knife stereotactic radiosurgery for cerebral vascular malformations. In: Alexander E, Loeffler JS, Lunsford LE, eds. *Stereotactic Radiosurgery*. New York: McGraw-Hill, 1993;136–146.
15. Betti OO, Munari C, Rosler R. Stereotactic radiosurgery with the linear accelerator: treatment of arteriovenous malformations. *Neurosurgery* 1989;24:311–321.
16. Friedman WA, Bova FJ. LINAC radiosurgery for arteriovenous malformations. In: Alexander E, Loeffler JS, Lunsford LD, eds. *Stereotactic Radiosurgery*. New York: McGraw-Hill, 1993;147–155.
17. Marks MP, Delapaz RL, Fabrikant JI, et al. Intracranial vascular malformations: imaging of charged-particle radiosurgery, Part II complications. *Radiology* 1988;168:457–462.
18. Marks MP, Lane B, Steinberg GK, Chang P. Hemorrhage in intracerebral arteriovenous malformations: angiographic determinants. *Radiology* 1990;176:807–813.
19. Marks MP, Lane B, Steinberg GK, Snipes GJ. Intranidal aneurysms in cerebral arteriovenous malformations: evaluation and endovascular treatment. *Radiology* 1992;183:355–360.
20. Marks MP, Bracci PM, Steinberg GK. The correlation of risk factors of hemorrhage with the natural history of brain arteriovenous malformations. Annual Meeting of Congress of Neurological Surgeons Program 1993;43:95.
21. Marks MP, Lane B, Steinberg GK, Chang P. Vascular characteristics of intracerebral arteriovenous malformations in patients with clinical steal. *AJNR* 1991;12:489–496.
22. Marks MP, Lane B, Steinberg GK, Fabrikant JI, Levy RP, Frankel KA, Phillips MH. Endovascular treatment of cerebral arteriovenous malformations following radiosurgery. *AJNR* 1993;14: 297–303.
23. Steinberg GK, Chang SD, Levy RP, Marks MP, Frankel K, Marcellus M. Surgical resection of intracranial arteriovenous malformations following stereotactic radiosurgery. *J Neurosurg*. 1996;84:920–928.
24. Pollock BE, Kondziolka D, Lunsford LD, Bissonette D, Flickinger JC. Repeat stereotactic radiosurgery of arteriovenous malformations: factors associated with incomplete obliteration. *Neurosurgery* 1996; 38:318–324.

Cerebrovascular Disease, edited by H. Hunt Batjer.
Lippincott-Raven Publishers, Philadelphia © 1997.

CHAPTER **60**

Special Problem: AVM Associated with Aneurysm

R. A. de los Reyes and Matthew E. Fink

INTRODUCTION

The patient with an arteriovenous malformation (AVM) associated with aneurysm(s) presents a special clinical problem. Although the surgeon is commonly thinking about each of these lesions individually, their simultaneous occurrence raises clinically relevant questions regarding, among other things, their effect on the natural history and the order and type of treatment for each lesion. We shall attempt to review the literature regarding the incidence, pathophysiology, natural history, and treatment of these vascular anomalies and make recommendations based on the above.

INCIDENCE

The reported incidence of AVMs associated with aneurysms varies from a low of 2.7 (1) to 23% (2) of cases, with the majority of series being in the 5–15% range. It is likely that the true incidence is somewhere towards the upper range because later series, presumably employing pan- and selective angiography, tend to report higher percentages. In particular, intranidal aneurysms may be missed without sophisticated angiographic techniques. There does not appear to be any overall sex predominance.

Age, on the other hand, shows a definite, positive correlation. Berenstein and Lasjaunias (3) noted a distinct increase in the association of AVM and arterial aneurysm with increasing age: the combination was present in 8% of patients under 25 years of age, 24% of patients 25–49 years of age, and 37% of patients over the age of 50. This represents a fourfold increase in the association between aneurysm and AVM in patients between the ages of 10 and 50, which they

R. A. del los Reyes: Department of Neurosurgery, Beth Israel Medical Center North Division, New York, NY 10128

M. E. Fink: Department of Neurology, Beth Israel Medical Center North Division, New York, New York 10128

attributed to "the role played by chronic high flow and the aging of the vascular system." It is interesting that in the same series the incidence of multiple aneurysm was 44%.

Although we could find no studies specifically evaluating the role of size (and, by implication, the flow) on the incidence of the aneurysm/AVM association, the majority of reported cases were in larger, higher flow AVMs (4,5). More importantly, aneurysms associated with smaller or lower flow AVMs tended to occur with greater frequency in non flow-related vessels. The role of flow will be covered in the section on pathophysiology.

It appears, then, that aneurysms are associated with AVMs in around 10–15% of patients, and that this association increases with increasing age of the patient and size of the lesion.

PATHOPHYSIOLOGY (CLASSIFICATION)

Numerous hypotheses have been presented in the past regarding the association, or lack thereof, between aneurysms and AVMs. These may be summarized as follows:

1. The lesions occur together by pure chance and are independent of each other.
2. The association is due to parallel expression of multiple disorders of vascular development.
3. The aneurysm is the result of hemodynamic stress on the arterial wall resulting from increased blood flow due to the presence of the AVM.

Although the first hypothesis can, and probably does, explain the presence of non-flow-related aneurysms (approximately 25% of cases) (3), the numerous studies showing the disproportionately increased incidence of aneurysms associated with AVMs (3,6–8) would seem to indicate that chance alone is an insufficient explanation.

The second hypothesis is intriguing, particularly in regard

to the possible association of medial defects in the arteries, which ultimately lead to the formation of arterial aneurysm, but this remains to be proven.

The third hypothesis is most attractive, particularly with respect to aneurysms on the feeding vessels to an AVM. Somach and Shenkin (9) reviewed six patients who had undergone carotid artery ligation for the treatment of intracranial aneurysms. Repeat angiography 3–10 years later revealed that two of the patients had developed an aneurysm on the contralateral internal carotid artery. Conversely, Hayashi et al (10) and Shenkin et al (11) described significant decreases in the size of previously imaged aneurysms on feeding vessels to AVMs after surgical excision of the AVM. Whether the arteriographic changes were due to intraluminal thrombosis or intimal thickening is unclear, as is the long-term fate of the aneurysm. Other conditions that increase flow, such as the hemodynamic stress on the posterior circulation associated with moya-moya disease, are also associated with an increased incidence of aneurysm formation (7).

Nornes et al (12) examined 16 patients who underwent total excision of cerebral AVMs. Pressure recordings were made from feeding arteries at the entrance to the AVM. The pressure was well below the systemic arterial pressure in all cases, ranging from 40 to 77 torr (average 56 torr). On temporary occlusion, this stump pressure rose instantly from 55 to 95 torr (average 76 torr). Drainage vein pressure before occlusion ranged from 8 to 23 torr (average 15 torr) and fell to zero in all patients when the AVM was excised. These data and other clinical observation support the hypothesis that hemodynamic stresses associated with increased flow play an important role in the genesis of aneurysms in patients with AVMs.

Regardless of their origin, it seems clear that there are differences in the types and locations of aneurysms associated with AVMs. Because these differences may affect the natural history (eg, propensity to hemorrhage) as well as the treatment strategies, numerous attempts at classification (2, 8,13) have been made. The classification system of Perata et al (13) seems reasonable, and it is depicted in Fig. 1. According to their scheme, aneurysms associated with AVMs should be classified as follows:

1. *Dysplastic* or remote, unrelated to inflow vessels
2. *Proximal*, arising at the circle of Willis origin of a vessel supplying the AVM
3. *Pedicular*, arising from the midcourse of a feeding pedicle
4. *Intranidal,* within the AVM nidus itself

Whether intranidal aneurysms represent true aneurysms, pseudo-aneurysms, or both is debatable, but we shall adopt the above classification in our discussion of natural history and treatment (Figs. 2 and 3).

NATURAL HISTORY

The most serious and frequent complication of AVM associated with aneurysm is hemorrhage. The incidence of hemorrhage has important implications in the therapeutic algorithm: lesions that might be considered "unapproachable" might be considered for palliative or alternative therapies if characteristics could be identified that would place them in a "high-risk" hemorrhage category. Alternatively, surgery might be deferred for low-risk lesions.

Marks et al (8) analyzed the vascular characteristics of AVMs that correlated with hemorrhage in 65 cases. The following lesion characteristics were evaluated at angiography: size, location, peri- or intraventricular location, arterial aneurysm, arterial stenosis, angiomatous change, intranidal aneurysm, arteriovenous fistula, central venous drainage,

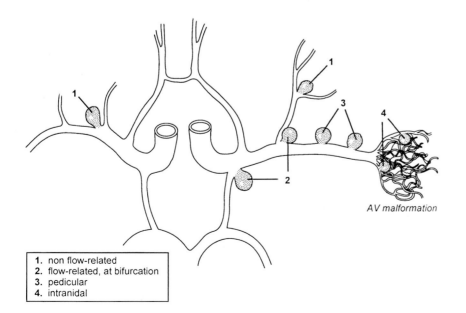

1. non flow-related
2. flow-related, at bifurcation
3. pedicular
4. intranidal

AV malformation

FIG. 1. Examples of locations of dysplastic (1), proximal flow related (2), pedicular (3), and intranidal (4) aneurysms in association with a middle cerebral artery arteriovenous malformation.

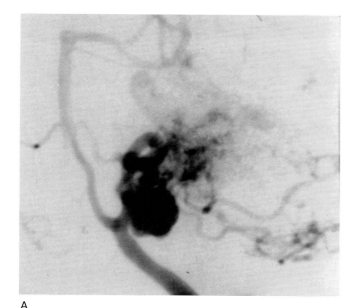

A

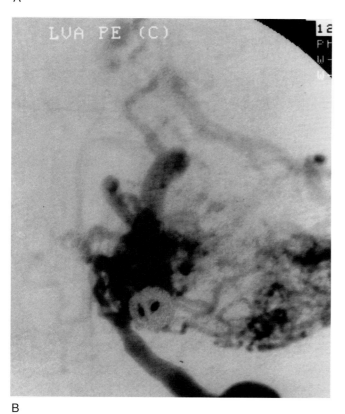

B

FIG. 2. A: Lateral left vertebral angiogram showing large left posterior inferior cerebellar artery aneurysm in association with a cerebellar arteriovenous malformation. **B:** Same patient after coiling of the aneurysm in preparation for embolization and subsequent excision of the malformation. (Courtesy of Alex Berenstein, M.D.)

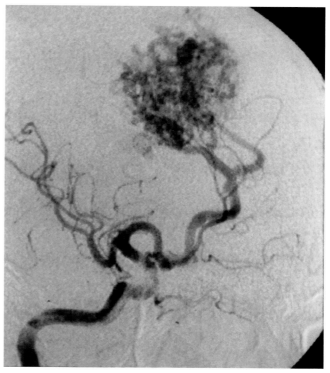

FIG. 3. Right internal carotid angiogram revealing pedicular *(open arrow)* and intranidal *(closed arrow)* aneurysms in a patient with an anterior cerebral distribution arteriovenous malformation. (Courtesy of Alex Berenstein, M.D.)

cortical venous drainage, cortical mixed venous drainage, delayed drainage, venous stasis, venous ectasia or aneurysm, and venous variation. Of the lesion characteristics evaluated, four were found to be the most predictive: central venous drainage, intranidal aneurysm, and periventricular or intraventricular location strongly correlated with history of hemorrhage, and the angiomatous change had a strong *negative* correlation. Similarly, Turjman et al (14) evaluated 100 consecutive patients with cerebral AVMs and found that deep venous drainage, feeding by perforators, intranidal aneurysm(s), multiple aneurysm, feeding by the vertebrobasilar system, and location in the basal ganglia all correlated positively with a clinical presentation of hemorrhage. Thus, it would appear that the presence of an intranidal aneurysm should prompt a more aggressive posture with respect to resection or palliation. Perata et al (13) and Cunha et al (15) suggest the same for pedicular aneurysms, as do Brown et al (16) who reported a fourfold (7% vs. 1.7%) increase in the incidence of intracranial hemorrhage in AVM patients with associated aneurysms.

The above data have obvious implications with respect to the workup of patients with CT or MRI evidence of arteriovenous malformation. To date, MRI/MRA do not have the capability of demonstrating aneurysms that are small or intranidal. Refinements in MRA, 3D CT angiography, or rise of new technology may one day render conventional angiography unnecessary. However, for now conventional angiography should be performed on most patients for a complete evaluation regarding their risk of hemorrhage.

A number of series have attempted to quantify the actual incidence and source of subarachnoid hemorrhage (SAH) in combined cases. Subarachnoid hemorrhage occurred in 29 of 37 patients (78%) with coexisting aneurysms and AVMs in the series of Perret and Nishioka (17). The presumed source of bleeding was the AVM in 9 patients, the aneurysm in 7 patients, and uncertain in the remaining 13 patients. Suzuki and Onuma (18) reported that SAH was the initial symptom in 7 of 9 patients: three hemorrhages from the AVM, three from the aneurysm, and one from both.

Thus, it would appear that aneurysms in association with an AVM increase the risk of hemorrhage and that this may be particularly so for intranidal aneurysms. This should be taken into account when assessing the potential risks in the AVM patient, whether or not the AVM is symptomatic or asymptomatic.

TREATMENT

The therapeutic approach to the patient with combined aneurysm/AVM depends to a great extent on whether or not there has been a hemorrhage. In the setting of a hemorrhage, it has been our policy to treat the lesion responsible for the hemorrhage first. While this is frequently more easily said than done, certain features can help: Is the hemorrhage subarachnoid, intraparenchymal, or both? If intraparenchymal, is it adjacent to the aneurysm or closer to a vein? Is there vasospasm on the angiogram? If the offending lesion is still indeterminate, we assume that the aneurysm, with its higher incidence of rehemorrhage and greater mortality, has bled and treat accordingly, either by open surgery or endovascularly.

For unruptured aneurysm/AVM combinations (and for some ruptured ones as well), the overall approach varies in the literature. These can be summarized as follows:

1. Treat both lesions at the same time.
2. Treat the aneurysm first.
3. Treat the AVM first.
4. Vary the treatment according to set criteria.

In Suzuki and Onuma's (18) series of 1979, 8 of 9 patients underwent a one-stage resection of both lesions and all returned to "a useful life." They advocate simultaneous treatment whenever possible. Most authors, however, prefer a staged approach, citing higher morbidity with simultaneous treatment.

Batjer et al (6) evaluated 22 patients with combined aneurysm and AVM. They suggested that a sudden increase in vascular resistance associated with abrupt elimination of an AVM shunt places a proximal aneurysm on a feeding artery at immediate risk of distention and rupture, and they cite instances of such occurrences. They advocate treatment of proximal aneurysm prior to resection of AVM.

Shenkin et al (11), Hayashi et al (10), and Lasjaunias et al (2) take the opposite view, describing instances of shrinkage or disappearance of aneurysms following resection of associated AVMs.

While, as previously discussed, increased flow associated with an AVM appears to promote aneurysmal formation, aneurysms outside of the angioarchitecture of the AVM (ie, dysplastic aneurysms) would not seem to be flow-related and should not be considered in the same category. Given the redistribution of flow following AVM resection, it may be reasonable to treat dysplastic (non-flow-related) aneurysms first.

Although much remains to be elucidated regarding these interesting and challenging combination lesions, our present treatment algorithm is as follows:

1. If there is a hemorrhage, the lesion believed responsible should be treated first.
2. In the absence of hemorrhage:
   a. Non-flow-related (dysplastic) aneurysms are treated first
   b. Pedicular and intranidal aneurysms are treated by embolization of the aneurysms when possible, followed by embolization of the AVM. If the AVM has multiple feeders, those associated with aneurysms are treated first (3).
   c. Proximal, flow-related aneurysms may be treated before *or*, if necessary, after the AVM depending on such factors as size and angioarchitecture of the AVM, location and configuration of the aneurysm(s), and other adjunctive factors such as the effect on the feasibility of interventional procedures such as AVM embolization.

REFERENCES

1. Paterson JH, McKossoch W. A clinical survey of intracranial angiomas with special reference to their mode of progression and surgical treatment: a report of 110 cases. *Brain* 1956;79:233–266.
2. Lasjaunias P, Piske R, Terbrugge K, et al. Cerebral arteriovenous malformations (C.AVM) and associated arterial aneurysms (AA). *Acta Neurochir* 1988;91:29–36.
3. Berenstein A, Lasjaunias P. *Surgical Neuroangiography*. New York: Springer-Verlag, 1992:1–88.
4. Kondziolka D, Nixon BJ, Lasjaunias P, et al. Cerebral arteriovenous malformations with associated arterial aneurysms: hemodynamic and therapeutic considerations. *Can J Neuro Sci* 1988;15: 130–134.
5. Miyasaka K, Wolpert SM, Prager RJ. The association of cerebral aneurysms, infundibula, and intracranial arteriovenous malformations. *Stroke* 1982;13:196–203.
6. Batjer H, Suss RA, Samson D. Intracranial arteriovenous malformations associated with aneurysms. *Neurosurgery* 1986;18:29–35.
7. Konishi Y, Kadowaki C, Hara M, et al. Aneurysms associated with moyamoya disease. *Neurosurgery* 1985;16:484–490.
8. Marks MP, Lane B, Steinberg GK, et al. Hemorrhage in intracerebral arteriovenous malformations: angiographic determinants. *Radiology* 1990;176:807–813.
9. Somach FM, Shenkin HA. Angiographic end-results of carotid ligation in the treatment of carotid aneurysm. *J Neurosurg* 1966;24: 966–974.
10. Hayashi S, Arimoto T, Itakura T, et al. The association of intracranial aneurysms and arteriovenous malformations of the brain. Case report. *J Neurosurg* 1981;55:971–975.

11. Shenkin HA, Jenkins F, Kim K. Arteriovenous anomaly of the brain associated with cerebral aneurysms. Case report. *J Neurosurg* 1971; 34:225–228.

12. Nornes H, Grip A. Hemodynamic aspects of cerebral arteriovenous malformations. *J Neurosurg* 1980;53:456–464.

13. Perata HJ, Tomsick TA, Tew JM. Feeding artery pedicle aneurysms: association with parenchymal hemorrhage and arteriovenous malformation in the brain. *J Neurosurg* 1994;8:631–634.

14. Turjman F, Massoud TF, Vinuela F, Sayre JW, Guglielmi G, Duckwiler G. Correlation of the angioarchitectural features of cerebral arteriovenous malformations with clinical presentation of hemorrhage. *Neurosurgery* 1995;37:856–862.

15. Cunha e Sa MJ, Stein BM, Solomon RA. McCormick PC. The treatment of associated intracranial aneurysms and arteriovenous malformations. *J Neurosurg* 1992;77:853–859.

16. Brown RD, Wiebers DO, Forbes GS. Unruptured intracranial aneurysms and arteriovenous malformations: frequency of intracranial hemorrhage and relationship of lesions. *J Neurosurg* 1990;73:859–863.

17. Perret G, Nishioka H. Report on the Cooperative Study of Intracranial Aneurysms and Subarachnoid Hemorrhage: Section VI. Arteriovenous malformation. An analysis of 545 cases of craniocerebral arteriovenous malformations and fistulae reported to the Cooperative Study. *J Neurosurg* 1966;25:467–490.

18. Suzuki J, Onuma T. Intracranial aneurysms associated with arteriovenous malformations. *J Neurosurg* 1979;50: 742–746.

Cerebrovascular Disease, edited by H. Hunt Batjer.
Lippincott-Raven Publishers, Philadelphia © 1997.

CHAPTER 61

Radiosurgery for Arteriovenous Malformations

William A. Friedman

The concept of radiosurgery was first espoused more than 40 years ago by Lars Leksel (2,3). Recent developments in computer technology for dose planning, as well as refinements in radiation delivery systems, have led to a veritable explosion of interest in this treatment method. Perhaps of equal importance is the fact that increasing amounts of scientific evidence have persuaded the majority of the international neurosurgical community that radiosurgery is a viable treatment option for selected patients suffering from a variety of challenging neurosurgical disorders, including arteriovenous malformations (AVMs) of the brain.

THE HISTORY OF RADIOSURGERY

Gamma Knife Systems

In 1951, Lars Leksell, a Swedish neurosurgeon already known for the development of his enduring stereotactic frame and his previous discoveries in the field of neurophysiology, described the concept of focusing many beams of external radiation on a stereotactically defined intracranial target (2). He coined the term "radiosurgery" to describe this process. He and his colleagues (physicists, engineers, and radiation oncologists) experimented with a variety of radiation sources, including orthovoltage X-ray machines, particle beams (3), and early linear accelerators, before designing a completely new device, called the "gamma knife."

The first gamma knife was installed in Stockholm in 1968. It contained 179 ^{60}Co sources, all collimated and focused on one point (Fig. 1). The unit was designed to produce an elliptically shaped lesion, similar to that produced by a radiofrequency lesion electrode, primarily as a functional neurosurgery tool (pain, movement disorders, psychiatric disease). It subsequently became clear that the inability to stimulate or record before lesion making, as well as the long

latency until the lesion developed, limited the use of radiosurgery in functional neurosurgery.

The second gamma knife was installed in 1974 at the Karolinska Institute in Stockholm. It contained 201 ^{60}Co sources and utilized two "primary" collimators for each beam. Secondary circular collimators of 4 mm, 8 mm, and

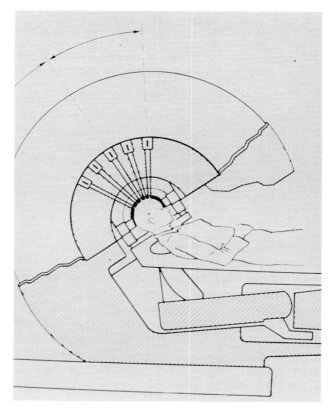

FIG. 1. The gamma knife is a hemispheric device that contains 201 cobalt sources, all collimated and focused on one point. The patient is stereotactically positioned within one of four collimator helmets (producing 4-, 8-, 14-, or 18-mm radiation beams) such that the intracranial target coincides with the focal point of the machine. This results in a high target dose with relatively little radiation to surrounding structures.

W. A. Friedman: Department of Neurosurgery, University of Florida, Gainesville, FL 32610

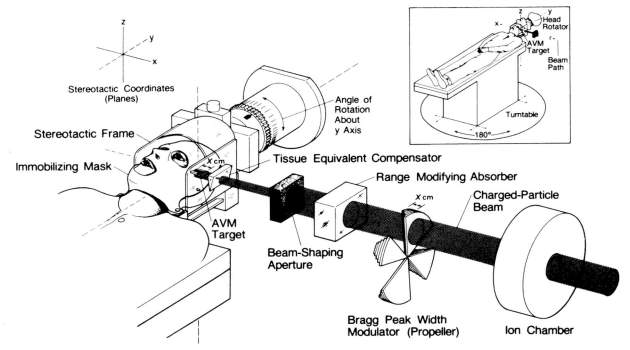

FIG. 2. Charged particle beam delivery system at the University of California at Berkeley–Lawrence Laboratory 184-in. synchrocyclotron. The stereotactic positioning system allows translation along three orthogonal axes and rotation around the *y* and *z* axes. The width of the Bragg ionization peak can be spread to the prescribed size by interposing a modulating filter (here a propeller with variable-thickness blades) in the beam path. The depth in tissue is determined by a range-modifying absorber. Individually designed apertures shape the beam cross-section to conform to the shape of the lesion. Multiple beams at different angles are used to produce the lowest possible dose to sensitive adjacent brain structures.

14 mm were used, producing spherical lesions more suitable for the treatment of anatomic brain lesions (arteriovenous malformations and tumors). More recent versions of the gamma knife have included an 18-mm collimator. These units have been installed at multiple institutions worldwide. The first U.S. gamma knife was installed at the University of Pittsburgh in 1987 (4,5).

Particle Accelerator Systems

Wilson, a physicist, has been credited with first suggesting the medical usage of particle beams (1940s) (27). As mentioned above, early radiosurgical groups used the proton beam produced by synchrocyclotrons. Workers in Sweden (Uppsala) employed high-energy intersecting proton beams in a fashion analogous to the intersecting cobalt beams of the gamma knife. Groups in Boston and Berkeley, however, used the Bragg peak effect (see below) to maximize the radiosurgical effectiveness of the proton beam. Single-dose and fractionated treatments have been devised (Fig. 2).

A 160-MeV proton beam with a 10-mm-wide Bragg peak is used in Boston (7). Generally, the radiation is delivered via 12 portals in one fraction. Since 1980, 130-MeV helium ion beams have been used at the Berkeley installation (8). The limiting factor on the use of particle beam radiosurgery appears to be the requirement for a synchrocyclotron to generate the radiation source. These facilities are currently available only at a small number of high-energy physics research institutes.

Linear Accelerator Systems

Linear accelerators (LINACs) were simultaneously developed in the United States and Great Britain in the 1950s. They are devices that accelerate electrons to nearly the speed of light. The electron beam is aimed at a heavy-metal alloy target. The resulting interactions produce X rays, which can be collimated and focused on a patient. LINACs have over the ensuing decades become the favored treatment device for conventional radiation therapy.

In 1984 Betti and his colleagues described a radiosurgical system using the LINAC as the source of radiation (9). Colombo et al described their system in 1985 (10). Multiple investigators have subsequently modified LINACs in a variety of ways to achieve the aforementioned requirements of radiosurgical systems (11–13). In 1988, the University of Florida radiosurgery system was built based on the work of Winston and Lutz, who first developed methods for quantifying the accuracy of linear accelerator radiosurgery systems (14,15), eliminating the inherent inaccuracy of the linear

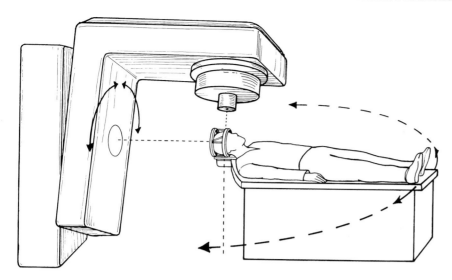

FIG. 3. A linear accelerator (LINAC) is a device that accelerates electrons nearly to the speed of light. The electrons collide with a heavy metal alloy, producing a beam of photon energy, called X rays. The target is stereotactically positioned to coincide with the isocentric rotation point of the LINAC gantry. After one arc of radiation is delivered, the patient is horizontally repositioned at a new "table angle" and another arc performed. Typically, five to nine arcs of radiation are used per isocenter.

accelerator bearings and incorporating ultra-high-speed computer dose planning (16).

All LINAC radiosurgical systems rely on the following basic paradigm (Fig. 3): A collimated X-ray beam is focused on a stereotactically identified intracranial target. The gantry of the LINAC rotates over the patient, producing an arc of radiation focused on the target. The patient couch is then rotated in the horizontal plane and another arc performed. In this manner, multiple, non-coplanar intersecting arcs of radiation are produced. In a fashion exactly analogous to the multiple intersecting cobalt beams in the gamma knife, the intersecting arcs produce a high target dose, with minimal radiation to the surrounding brain.

PHYSICS OF RADIOSURGERY

Radiosurgery delivers high doses (large amounts of energy) to treatment volumes while delivering smaller, consequently less effective, doses to nontarget tissues. One basic radiosurgery technique used by all teletherapy units, such as isotope units (the gamma knife) and electronically produced photon units (linear accelerators, LINACs), relies on averaging the effects of multiple photon beams focused at a single point. Both X rays and gamma rays are photons. The only difference between these two types of radiation is the source: gamma rays, such as those produced by cobalt-60, originate in the nuclei of that isotope. Each time a cobalt-60 atom decays, it produces two photons that have an average energy of 1.25 MeV.

Linear accelerators do not use stored isotopes but produce their photons through the slowing down of high-energy electrons. Through the use of microwave power, LINACs accelerate electrons to high energies. For stereotactic radiosurgery, energies between 4 MeV and 15 MeV have been used. These electrons are focused onto a target, usually a high-atomic-number alloy (a heavy metal). As electrons interact

with the target, they are slowed down. In this slowing down process they give off their energy through two mechanisms: collisional losses and radiative losses. The collisional losses result in heat and produce no therapeutic radiation. The radiation losses, however, produce photons. These photons, which are produced outside the nucleus, are called X rays. While these X rays are produced over a spectrum of energies up to the maximum energy of the LINAC, their effective energy is equal to approximately one third of the maximum energy. Hence, a 6-MeV LINAC produces an X-ray beam with an average energy of approximately 2 MeV.

Since the energies of both the gamma knife and the LINAC are similar, their photon absorption characteristics in tissue are also similar. In tissue of unit density, the cobalt-60 beam will lose approximately 5% of its intensity per centimeter whereas the 6-MeV LINAC will lose approximately 4% of its intensity per centimeter. Since this loss is constant, after a small initial buildup depth, the photon beam possesses no special properties that allow any significant concentration of its energy over a target volume. The technique used for concentration of the energy at the target site is a simple averaging process (Fig. 4). For example, if six beams are aimed at a target at the center of a 15-cm sphere, each beam will be attenuated by tissue absorption of energy to approximately 70% of its surface value. The intersection of the six beams, however, will have a value of 6 × 70%, or 420% of the surface dose. This averaging process is accomplished in the gamma knife by using 201 separate cobalt-60 sources, all focused at the same point. For LINACS, multiple non-coplanar arcs of radiation are used to achieve the same effect.

The second physics approach to radiosurgery involves the use of heavy charged particle beams. Particle beams lose energy uniformly until the particle nears the end of its range. At this point the particle sharply increases its energy loss, depositing a well-defined maximum dose. This region of increased dose is termed the "Bragg peak." The depth at which the Bragg peak occurs can be varied by changing

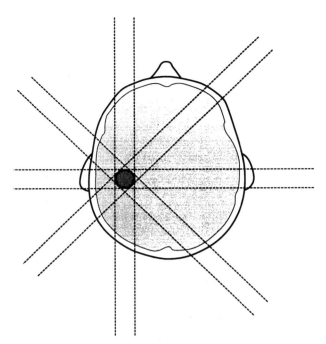

FIG. 4. In this example, four stationary beams of radiation are cross-fired at the same target point. Along each beam path, the dose decreases in an exponential fashion with depth through tissue. The doses are additive only at the target, where the beams intersect. As a simplified example, imagine 100 beams of radiation, all taking a different pathway through the brain but coming together at the target point. Each beam pathway will receive approximately 1% of the maximum dose, whereas the target receives 100%.

the entrance energy of the particle beam. In practice, this is achieved through the use of absorbers. Absorbers are also used to spread the width of the Bragg peak to match the target width. While the Bragg peak effect has an advantage over the exponentially decreasing dose profile of photon beams, it alone does not produce a satisfactorily steep dose gradient at the target site. As with photon beams, an averaging technique is employed. Because of the Bragg peak, fewer cross-bred beams are necessary to produce a steep gradient.

RADIOSURGICAL TREATMENT PARADIGM

Although the details of radiosurgical treatment techniques differ somewhat from system to system, the basic paradigm is quite similar everywhere. Below is a detailed description of a typical radiosurgical treatment at the University of Florida.

Almost all radiosurgical procedures in adults are performed on an outpatient basis. The patient reports to the neurosurgical clinic at 8:15 a.m. There a stereotactic head ring is applied under local anesthesia. No skin shaving or preparation is required. If the treatment is for an arteriovenous malformation, the patient may be transported to the angiography suite for stereotactic angiography. Subse-

quently, stereotactic computed tomography (CT) and/or stereotactic magnetic resonance imaging (MRI) is performed. A bolus of intravenous contrast material is given through the lesion just before imaging to maximize resolution. Because the stereotactic angiogram is a relatively poor three-dimensional database (17–19), we also rely on the appearance of the nidus on contrast-enhanced CT scans for treatment planning. Others have recommended stereotactic magnetic resonance angiography (MRA) techniques for the same purpose (20). After CT scanning, the patient is transported to the outpatient radiology area for postangiographic observation.

The stereotactic angiogram, stereotactic CT, scan and/or stereotactic MRI (transferred via ethernet) are taken to the radiation physics suite for dosimetry. The nidus of the AVM is outlined on the angiogram, which is then mounted on a digitizer board. A mouse-like device is used to identify the stereotactic fiducial markers and trace the nidus; they simultaneously appear on the computer screen. The computer then generates anteroposterior, lateral, and vertical coordinates of the center of the lesion as well as its demagnified diameter. Next, the computer quickly determines the position of all of the CT and/or MR images within the stereotactic coordinate system. The angiographic target center point is displayed on the CT/MR image. Dosimetry then begins and continues until the neurosurgeon, radiation therapist, and radiation physicist are satisfied that an optimal dose plan has been developed (Fig. 5). A final computer printout shows all of the treatment parameters in a checklist format.

After dose planning is completed, the radiosurgical device is attached to the LINAC. The patient then is attached to the device and treated. The actual radiation treatment time averages approximately 20 minutes. Afterward the head ring is removed, and after a short observation period the patient is discharged. The radiosurgical device is disconnected from the LINAC, which is then ready again for conventional usage.

RADIOSURGERY FOR ARTERIOVENOUS MALFORMATIONS

Multiple studies have demonstrated a substantial (3–4% per year) risk of hemorrhage, often associated with morbidity or mortality, in patients harboring AVMs (21). Refinements in microsurgical technique as well as the development of increasingly effective endovascular treatments render many of the lesions amenable to successful, safe, surgical cure (22–25). Those AVMs that are not suitable for surgical removal are often considered for radiosurgical management.

Angiographic Thrombosis Rates

Radiosurgery appears to produce AVM thrombosis by inducing a pathologic process in the AVM nidus, leading to gradual thickening of the vessels until thrombosis occurs

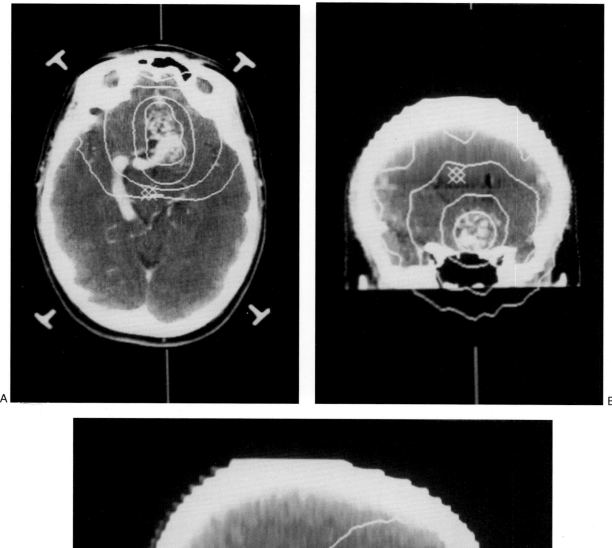

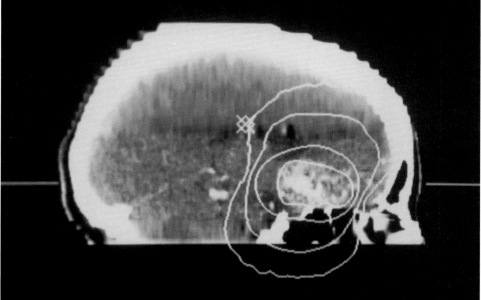

FIG. 5. This patient presented with seizures secondary to a left frontal arteriovenous malformation (AVM). The irregular contour of her lesion nidus, seen here on contrast-enhanced CT scan, was treated conformally by using a combination of four isocenters (28 mm, 28 mm, and 28 mm, and 16 mm in diameter). The total treatment volume was 21.7 cm^3. The isodose lines displayed are the 70%, 35%, 14%, and 7% doses, as seen on axial **(A)**, coronal **(B)**, and sagittal **(C)** views. CT scans are routinely used for AVM dosimetry planning because they represent an anatomic-radiographic database easily understood by neurosurgeons and because of inherent limitations of stereotactic angiography (see text).

(26,27). Several radiosurgical series have systematically evaluated this process by obtaining 1- and 2-year follow-up angiograms. Steiner has published multiple reports on gamma knife radiosurgery for AVMs (28–31). He has reported 1-year occlusion rates ranging from 33.7% to 39.5% and 2-year occlusion rates ranging from 79% to 86.5%. However, these results were "optimized" by retrospectively selecting patients who received a minimum treatment dose. For example (32), in a recent report he stated that "a large majority of patients received at least 20–25 Gy of radiation . . . . Of the 248 patients treated before 1984, the treatment specification placed 188 in this group." The reported thrombosis rates in this paper only applied to these 188 patients (76% of his total series). Interestingly, Yamamoto and colleagues recently reported on 25 Japanese patients treated on the gamma unit in Stockholm but followed in Japan (58). The 2-year thrombosis rate in those AVMs that were completely covered by the radiosurgical field was 64%. One additional patient had complete thrombosis at 3-year angiography and one additional at 5-year angiography, for a total cure rate of 73%. In another paper (33), these authors reported angiographic cures in six of nine (67%) children treated in Stockholm or Buenos Aires and followed in Japan.

Kemeny reported on 52 AVM patients treated with gamma knife radiosurgery (34). They all received 2500 cGy to the 50% isodose line. At 1 year, 16 patients (31%) had complete thrombosis and 10 patients (19%) had "almost complete" thrombosis. He found that the results were better in younger patients and in patients with relatively lateral location of AVMs. There was no difference in outcome between small (<2 cm³), medium (2–3 cm³), and large (>3 cm³) AVMs.

Lunsford and colleagues reported on 227 AVM patients treated with gamma knife radiosurgery (35). The mean dose delivered to the AVM margin was 21.2 Gy. Multiple isocenters were used in 48% of the patients. Seventeen patients underwent 1-year angiography, which confirmed complete thrombosis in 76.5%. As indicated in the paper, "this rate may be spurious since many of these patients were selected for angiography because their MR image had suggested obliteration." Among 75 patients who were followed for at least 2 years, 2-year angiography was performed in only 46 (61%). Complete obliteration was confirmed in 37 of 46 patients (80%). This thrombosis rate strongly correlated with AVM size, as follows: <1 cm³, 100%; 1–4 cm³, 85%; 4–10 cm³, 58%. This group more recently reported on a group of 65 "operable" AVMs, treated with radiosurgery (36). Of 32 patients who subsequently underwent follow-up angiography, 84% showed complete thrombosis.

In a recent analysis on 86 AVMs treated with a particle beam radiosurgical system, Steinberg reported a 29% 1-year thrombosis, 70% 2-year thrombosis, and 92% 3-year thrombosis rate (37). The best results were obtained with smaller lesions and higher doses. Initially a treatment dose of 34.6 Gy was used but a higher than expected neurologic complication rate (20% for the entire series) led to the currently

used dose range of 7.7–19.2 Gy. No patients treated with the lower dose range had complications.

Betti reported on the results of 66 AVMs treated with a linear accelerator radiosurgical system (7,38). Doses of "no more than 40 Gy" were used in 80% of patients. He found a 66% 2-year thrombosis rate. The percentage of cured patients was highest when the entire malformation was included in the 75% isodose line (96%) or the maximum diameter of the lesion was less than 12 mm (81%).

Colombo reported on 97 AVM patients treated with a linear accelerator system (12,39). Doses from 18.7 to 40 Gy were delivered in one or two sessions. Of 56 patients who were followed longer than 1 year, 50 underwent 12-month follow-up angiography. In 26 patients (52%) complete thrombosis was demonstrated. Fifteen of 20 patients (75%) undergoing 2-year angiography had complete thrombosis. He reported a definite relationship between AVM size and thrombosis rate, as follows: lesions <15 mm in diameter had a 1-year obliteration rate of 76% and a 2-year rate of 90%. Lesions 15–25 mm in diameter had a 1-year thrombosis rate of 37.5% and a 2-year rate of 80%. Lesions greater than 25 mm in diameter had a 1-year thrombosis rate of 11% and a 2-year rate of 40%. In a more recent report (40), Colombo and colleagues reported follow-up on 180 radiosurgically treated AVMs. The 1-year thrombosis rate was 46% and the 2-year rate was 80%.

Souhami (41) reported on 33 AVMs treated with a linear accelerator system. The prescribed dose at isocenter varied from 50 to 55 Gy. A complete obliteration rate of 38% was seen on 1-year angiography. For patients whose arteriovenous malformation nidus was covered by a minimum dose of 25 Gy, the total obliteration rate was 61.5% whereas none of the patients who had received less than 25 Gy at the edge of the nidus obtained a total obliteration.

Loeffler (42) reported on 16 AVMs treated with a linear accelerator system. The prescribed dose was 15–25 Gy, typically to the 80–90% line. The total obliteration rate was 5 of 11 (45%) at 1 year and 8 of 11 (73%) at 2 years after treatment.

Between May 18, 1988 and February 7, 1995, 216 AVMs were treated on the University of Florida radiosurgery system (43). There were 105 men and 111 women in the series. The mean age was 39 (range 7–70). Presenting symptoms included hemorrhage (44), seizure (45), headache/incidental (19), and progressive neurologic deficit (17). Twenty-three patients had undergone prior surgical attempts at AVM excision. Nineteen patients had undergone at least one embolization procedure. All patients were screened by a vascular neurosurgeon prior to consideration of radiosurgery.

The mean radiation dose to the periphery of the lesion was 1500 cGy (range 1000–2500 cGy). This treatment dose was almost always delivered to the 80% isodose line (range 70–90%). One hundred seventy-five patients were treated with one isocenter, 26 patients with two isocenters, 12 patients with three isocenters, 2 patients with four isocenters, and 1 patient with five isocenters. The mean lesion volume

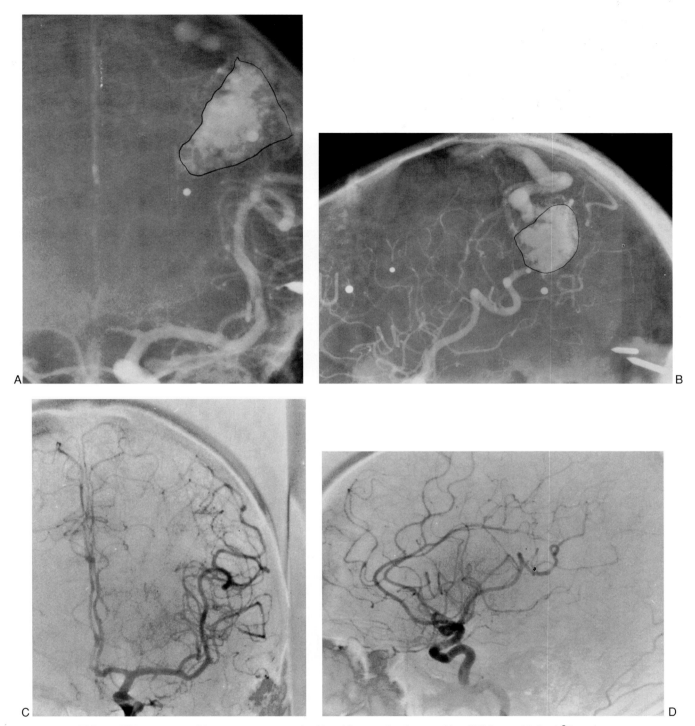

FIG. 6. This 27-year-old woman presented with a history of seizures. Her AVM was 11.3 cm^3 in volume and located in the left parietal region (**A,** anteroposterior angiogram; **B,** lateral angiogram, nidus outlined). Since it was 28-mm in diameter and had no deep venous drainage, it was only a Spetzler–Martin grade 2 lesion. Yet it was felt because of location that surgery had a not insignificant risk of at least temporary neurologic deficits. Angiography 24 months posttreatment revealed complete thrombosis (**C,** anteroposterior angiogram; **D,** lateral angiogram).

was 9.6 cm³ (0.5–45.3 cm³). Median lesion volume was 7.2 cm³. In an effort to provide data comparable to other publications in the radiosurgical literature, the following size categories were used in this report: A (<1 cm³), B (1–4 cm³), C (4–10 cm³), D (>10 cm³). The treatment volume was determined in all cases by performance of a computerized dose volume histogram of the treatment isodose shell (which was constructed to be conformal to the AVM nidus).

Mean follow-up duration for the entire AVM group is 36 months (3–82 months). Follow-up consisted of clinical examination and MRI scanning 6–12 months after treatment (46). If possible, follow-up was performed in Gainesville; otherwise scan and exam results were forwarded by the patient's local physician. Clinical information is available on 210 of 216 patients.

Initially, all patients were asked to undergo angiography

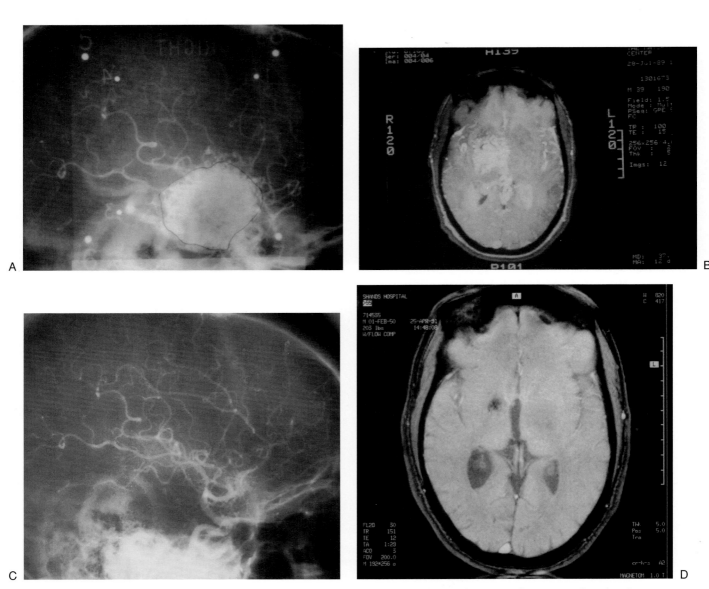

FIG. 7. This 39-year-old man presented with a history of headaches, seizures, and a progressive visual field cut. He was referred for radiosurgery. He received 1000 cGy to the 70% isodose line, through a 35-mm collimator (**A,** lateral view, pretreatment angiogram; **B,** pretreatment MRI scan). One-year angiography revealed substantial but incomplete thrombosis of the lesion. Two-year angiography revealed complete nidus thrombosis (**C,** lateral view, post-treatment angiogram; **D,** posttreatment MRI scan). The posttreatment MRI scan reveals complete resolution of the AVM nidus, with only a small hemosiderin signal near the genu of the internal capsule, with no apparent effect on normal brain structures.

at yearly intervals, regardless of the MRI findings. After the first 50 patients were treated, it was decided to defer angiography until MRI/MRA strongly suggested complete thrombosis. Furthermore, if complete thrombosis was not identified 3 years after radiosurgery, repeat radiosurgery was undertaken in an effort to obliterate any remaining nidus.

An angiographic cure required that no nidus or shunting remain on the study, as interpreted by a neuroradiologist and the treating neurosurgeon (Figs. 6 and 7). A total of 61 patients had angiographic cures out of 80 angiograms performed (76%). These patients are considered to have achieved a definitive successful endpoint for radiosurgery. The following angiographic cure rates were seen in the various size categories: A, 100%; B, 84%; C, 90%; D, 57%.

Of interest is the observation that three patients with 2-year angiograms showing small amounts of remaining nidus had complete occlusion on 3-year follow-up angiograms.

COMPLICATIONS

Hemorrhage

Multiple series report that the hemorrhage rate for AVMs treated but not yet obliterated with radiosurgery is the same as if they had not been treated (26). Most recently, Steiner et al analyzed clinical outcomes in 247 consecutive cases of AVM treated with the gamma knife (47). No patient with angiographically proven thrombosis had a hemorrhage. The protective effect of radiosurgery against hemorrhage in incompletely obliterated lesions was evaluated, using both the person-year and Kaplan–Meier life table methods of analysis. The person-year method showed a rebleed rate of 2–3% per year, very similar to the known natural history of the disease. The Kaplan–Meier analysis showed a risk of 3.7% per year until 5 years after radiosurgery. At that point the risk seemed to ''plateau.'' As discussed by the authors, this plateau, which has long been the source of controversy in the radiosurgery literature, may be an artifact of this statistical method when applied to a relatively small group of patients.

Colombo (40) recently studied the risk of hemorrhage after radiosurgery of 180 patients. In totally irradiated AVMs ($n = 163$) the bleeding rate decreased from 4.8% in the first 6 months to 0% from 12 months on. In subtotally irradiated AVMs, the bleeding risk increased from 4% in first 6 months to 10% from 12 to 18 months and then decreased to 5.5% from 18 to 24 months. There were no hemorrhages observed in this group after 24 months had elapsed.

In their report on 65 patients with ''operable'' AVMs treated with radiosurgery, the Pittsburgh group noted a 7.7% incidence of hemorrhage, all within the first 8 months of treatment (36). In the University of Florida experience, 12 patients have had a hemorrhage after radiosurgical treatment (Fig. 8). All hemorrhages have occurred in the first 19 months after radiosurgery. The incidence of hemorrhage in the first year after treatment is 6% higher than predicted

from natural history studies. Despite the fact that many AVMs take 2–3 years to thrombose after this treatment, no hemorrhage thus far has occurred later than 19 months after treatment.

Does radiosurgery increase the risk of hemorrhage during the first year after treatment? Does radiosurgery provide a protective effect against hemorrhage in subtotally obliterated lesions after that one year interval has passed? These questions remain the subject of debate and investigation. Regardless, it remains clear that hemorrhage is the major drawback of radiosurgery when compared to microsurgical treatment.

Radiation-Induced Complications

Several authors have previously reported that radiosurgery can acutely exacerbate seizure activity. Others have reported nausea, vomiting, and headache occasionally occurring after radiosurgical treatment (48).

Delayed radiation-induced complications have been reported by all groups performing radiosurgery. Steiner found symptomatic radiation necrosis in approximately 3% of his patients (29). Statham described one patient who developed radiation necrosis 13 months after gamma knife radiosurgery of a 5.3-cm^3 AVM with 25 Gy to the margin (49). Lunsford reported that 10 patients in his series (4.4%) developed new neurologic deficits thought to be secondary to radiation injury (35). Symptoms were location-dependent and developed 4–18 months after treatment. All patients were treated with steroids and all improved. Only two patients were reported to have residual deficits that appeared permanent. The radiation dose and isodose line treated did not correlate with this complication. As he noted, the failure of correlation of dose and complications may very well relate to the fact that the dose was selected to fall below Flickinger's computed 3% risk line. This is a mathematically derived line that prescribes lower doses for larger lesions (50,51).

Steinberg reported a definite correlation between lesion dose and complications (37). As indicated above, the initial treatment dose of 34.6 Gy led to a relatively high complication rate. No patients treated with the subsequently used lower dose range had complications. In an earlier report on 75 AVM patients treated with helium particles, at a dose of 45 Gy, 7 of 75 patients (11%) experienced radiation-induced complications (52). Kjellberg (7,53) constructed a series of log-log lines, relating prescribed dose and lesion diameter using a compilation of animal and clinical data. His 1% isorisk line is similar to Flickinger's mathematically derived 3% risk line.

In Colombo's series 9 of 180 (5%) patients experienced symptomatic radiation-induced complications (40). Four (2.2%) were permanent. Loeffler reported that 1 of 21 AVM patients developed a similar problem, which responded well to steroids (42). Souhami reported ''severe side-effects'' in 2 of 33 (6%) patients (41). Marks recently reviewed six radiosurgical series and found a 9% incidence of clinically

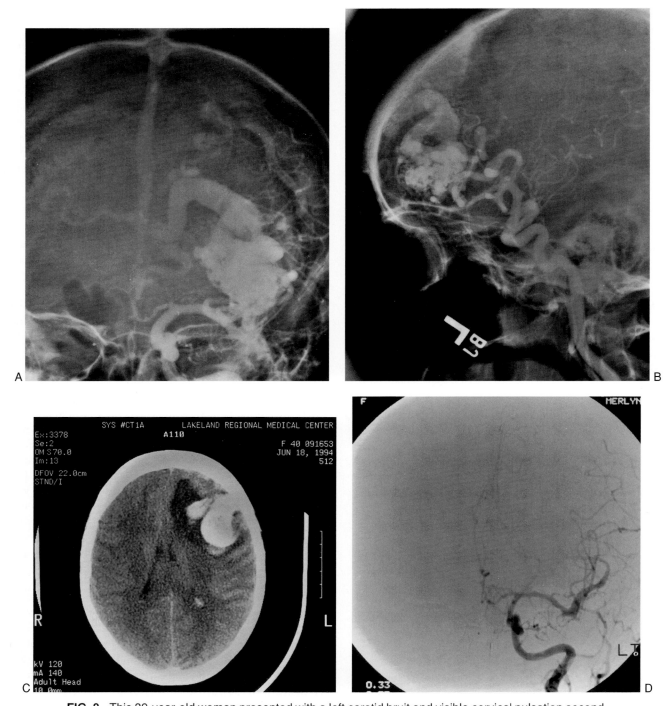

FIG. 8. This 39-year-old woman presented with a left carotid bruit and visible cervical pulsation secondary to a high-flow left frontal arteriovenous malformation (AVM) (**A,** pretreatment anteroposterior arteriogram; **B,** pretreatment lateral arteriogram). She underwent radiosurgical treatment (1500 cGy, 80% isodose line, 26-mm collimator). She remained well until 19 months posttreatment, when she experienced an intracerebral hemorrhage (**C,** CT scan). Fortunately, she made a good neurologic recovery, without surgical intervention. An arteriogram performed 2 months after the hemorrhage revealed complete occlusion of the AVM (**D,** anteroposterior arteriogram).

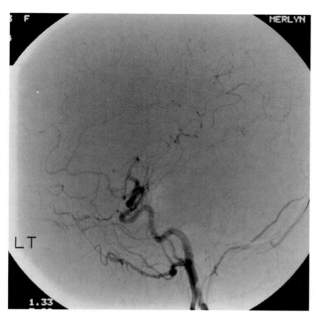

FIG. 8. *Continued.* (**E,** lateral arteriogram).

significant radiation reactions (54). Seven of 23 cases received doses below Kjellberg's 1% risk line.

In the University of Florida series, six patients (3%) experienced transient delayed complications directly attributable to radiosurgery. One of these patients experienced headache, three dysphasia, one hemiparesis, and 1 monoparesis. The onset of symptoms was at 10–14 months postradiosurgery. All had documented areas of edema around their AVMs, which resolved after short courses (several months) of steroid therapy. Five have fully recovered; one is still under treatment. Four of these patients have subsequently been documented to have angiographic cures. Three patients (1%) have experienced permanent radiation-induced complications. One patient has a mild lower extremity weakness, one has a Parinaud's syndrome and hemibody analgesia, and one has a fourth-nerve palsy. The onset of symptoms was 10, 11, and 14 months after radiosurgery, respectively. Two patients have subsequently been documented to have angiographic cures; one has refused angiography but has an MRI cure. Figure 9 shows the treatment dose and lesion size of all patients treated. Two patients with permanent complications received doses higher than were subsequently used in other AVMs of similar volume. Conversely, the three patients with transient complications received doses that have been safely used in other patients with similar sized AVMs.

Others have reported that asymptomatic radiation-induced changes appear frequently (24% in Lunsford's series) on MR images (55). We have also observed this phenomenon. These changes tend to be asymptomatic if the lesion is located in a relatively "silent" brain area and symptomatic if the lesion is located in an "eloquent" brain area. Thus, lesion location may be another important consideration in radiosurgical treatment planning and dose selection.

Most radiosurgical series report their radiation-induced complications as a percentage of the total patient population

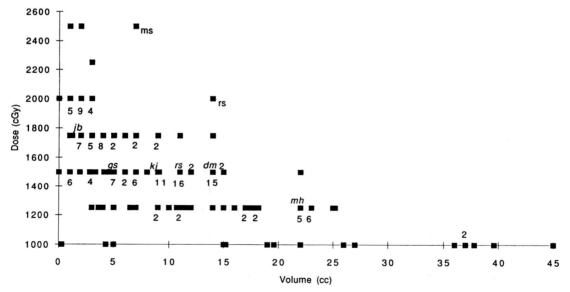

FIG. 9. This figure displays the dose prescribed to the periphery of every arteriovenous malformation (AVM) vs. that AVM's volume. Numbers displayed adjacent to data points indicate the number of patients treated at that particular volume and dose. In general, the larger the volume, the lower the dose that can be safely prescribed. The three patients with minor, permanent neurologic complications are indicated with bold initials (ms, rs, gs). Two of the three were treated early in the series and received doses that are higher than those we now employ for lesions of similar volume. The six patients with transient radiation-induced complications are indicated with non-bold initials. They received doses that have been safely employed in other patients.

treated. Since most radiation-induced complications do not appear for 12–18 months after treatment, this results in a systematic underestimate of the true complication rate.

Multimodality AVM treatment

Radiosurgery may be used alone in the treatment of AVMs <3.5 cm in diameter. Occasionally, larger AVMs are treated with a combination of endovascular therapy, surgery, and radiosurgery (56). Embolization and radiosurgery have been applied with increasing frequency (Fig. 10). Many questions remain to be answered regarding this combination of thera-

pies. For example, what type of embolic material is best? Currently, we treat the nidus that remains after embolization. Since radiosurgery frequently takes 2 years to produce nidus thrombosis, the possibility exists that the embolic material will "wash out" during this latent period.

Guo et al reported 46 patients treated with embolization and gamma knife radiosurgery (57). In 16 cases, collateral vessels developed that made subsequent delineation of the nidus for radiosurgery difficult. In addition, nine patients had neurologic complications for embolization. Only 19 of 35 large AVMs were reduced in size enough to be subsequently treatable with radiosurgery.

It does seem reasonably clear at this point that radiosur-

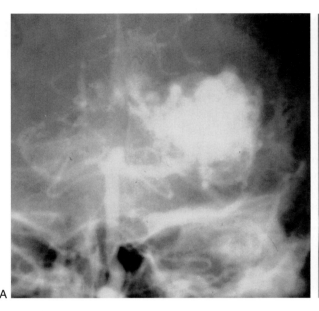

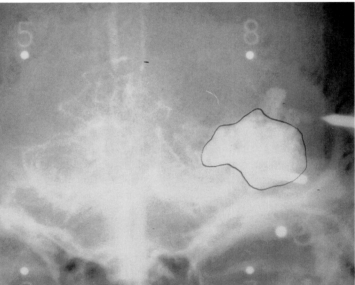

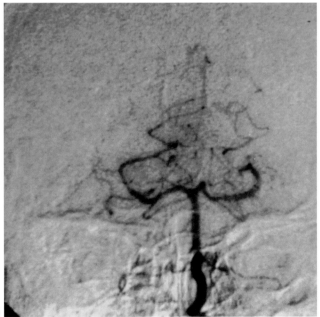

FIG. 10. This 40-year-old man presented with a history of headaches and seizures. He underwent multiple endovascular treatments for a large left occipital parietal arteriovenous malformation (**A,** preembolization anteroposterior angiography). The residual nidus (**B,** postembolization anteroposterior angiography, with nidus outlined) was treated with radiosurgery (1500 cGy, 80% isodose line, 28-mm collimator). One year posttreatment angiography (anteroposterior digital angiogram) showed complete thrombosis.

gery combined with embolization exposes the patient to the risk of both procedures. Since embolization alone rarely produces a cure, it should be used in combination with radiosurgery, only when the AVM is too large to be safely treated with radiosurgery alone. It should be noted that radiosurgery can also be used in combination with surgery to produce complete AVM obliteration. Conversely, surgery may be used to remove an AVM remnant when radiosurgery does not result in complete occlusion. Of course, embolization, surgery, and radiosurgery may occasionally all be employed in a single patient.

Francel and colleagues reported repeat radiosurgical treatment of 60 patients who experienced incomplete obliteration after one radiosurgical treatment (58). Of those patients who underwent follow-up angiography, 72% were cured. At the University of Florida, all patients who have incomplete obliteration 3 years after radiosurgical treatment are asked to undergo retreatment. Thus far, 11 patients have been retreated. The first two patients have been followed long enough to undergo 2-year follow-up angiography; both now show complete occlusion (Fig. 11).

Cavernous Malformations

The advent of MRI scanning as a neurologic screening test has resulted in the identification of substantial numbers of cavernous malformations. This vascular malformation differs pathologically from true AVMs. The role of radiosurgery in the treatment of angiographically occult vascular malformations (AOVMs) is not well defined. Kondziolka reported on 24 patients treated on the gamma knife at the University of Pittsburgh (59). Radiosurgery was used conservatively; each patient had sustained two or more hemorrhages and had a MRI-defined AOVM located in a region of the brain where microsurgical removal was judged to pose an excessive risk. Fifteen malformations were in the medulla, pons, and/or mesencephalon, and 5 were located in the thalamus or basal ganglia. Follow-up ranged from 4 to 24 months. Nineteen patients either improved or remained clinically stable and did not hemorrhage again during the follow-up interval. One patient suffered another hemorrhage 7 months after radiosurgery. Five patients experienced temporary worsening of preexisting neurologic deficits that sug-

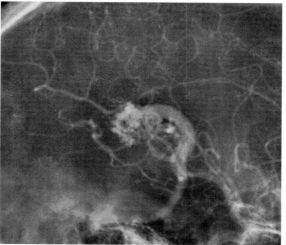

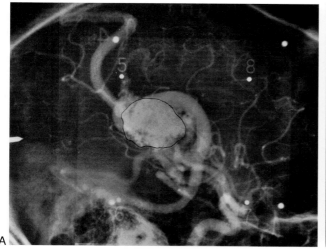

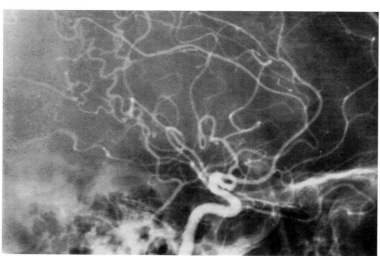

FIG. 11. This 37-year-old man presented with a long history of grand mal seizures. He underwent radiosurgical treatment of his arteriovenous malformation (**A,** treatment arteriogram, nidus outlined). The 11.4-cm³ nidus received 1500 cGy through a 28-mm collimator. Three years later, an arteriogram (**B,** lateral view) revealed a reduced but persistent nidus, which was retreated. This 3.4-cm³ nidus received 1500 cGy through a combination of two 14-mm collimators. Arteriography 2 years later (**C,** lateral view) revealed complete occlusion.

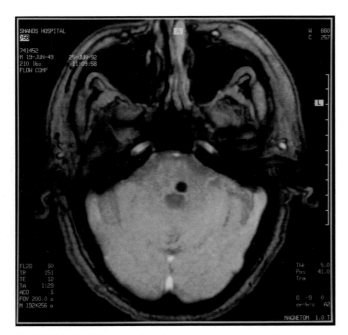

FIG. 12. This 41-year-old white man experienced three hemorrhages from this pontine cavernous malformation. He was surgically explored, but at the time of surgery no evidence of malformation could be seen on the fourth ventricular floor. The surgeon elected to refer the patient for radiosurgery, whereupon he received 1500 cGy to the 80% line of a 1-cm collimator. Nine months after radiosurgery the patient developed a facial nerve palsy. At 2-year follow-up this deficit remained but the patient was otherwise well and had not experienced further hemorrhage.

gested delayed radiation injury. MRI demonstrated signal changes and edema surrounding the radiosurgical target.

Steinberg (60) reported 35 patients treated for "angiographically occult vascular malformations." The clinical outcome was excellent or good in 80% and poor in 14%. Six percent of the patients died. Six patients experienced recurrent hemorrhage. Four patients worsened from probable radiation injury.

These reports clearly indicate a significantly higher complication rate for radiosurgical treatment of cavernous malformations than for true AVMs. In addition, the fact that they are angiographically occult means that no objective criteria for "successful" treatment exist. Only by following patients with a proven propensity for hemorrhage and demonstrating a significant decrease in hemorrhage rate can benefit be shown. Proof of such benefit does not currently exist. At the University of Florida, aggressive surgical therapy is used on the majority of symptomatic cavernous malformation (Fig. 12). Radiosurgery is regarded as a last resort.

CONCLUSIONS

In summary, many reports indicate that approximately 80% of AVMs in the radiosurgery size range will be angio-

graphically obliterated 2 years after radiosurgical treatment. Permanent neurologic complications are rare (2–3%). The major drawback of this treatment method is that patients are unprotected against hemorrhage during the 2- to 3-year latent period. Although radiosurgery has been used primarily as a single modality of treatment in previous studies, it has more recently been increasingly employed as part of a multimodality treatment approach incorporating surgical and endovascular methods. Radiosurgery is currently of unproven value in the treatment of cavernous malformations.

REFERENCES

1. Backlund EO, Johansson L, Sarby B. Studies on craniopharyngiomas. 11. Treatment by stereotaxis and radiosurgery. *Acta Chir Scand* 1972; 138:749–759.
2. Leksell L. The stereotaxic method and radiosurgery of the brain. *Acta Chir Scand* 1951;102:316–319.
3. Leksell L, Larsson B, Andersson B, Rexed B, Sourander P, Mair W. Lesions in the depth of the brain produced by a beam of high energy protons. *Acta Radiol* 1960;54:251–264.
4. Lunsford LD, Flickinger JC, Lindner G, Maitz A. Stereotactic radiosurgery of the brain using the first United States 201 cobalt-60 source gamma knife. *Neurosurgery* 1989;24:151–159.
5. Maitz AH, Lunsford LD, Wu A, Lindner G, Flickinger JC. Shielding requirements on-site loading and acceptance testing on the Leksell gamma knife. *Int J Radiat Oncol Biol Phys* 1990;18:469–476.
6. Levy RP, Fabrikant JI, Frankel KA, Phillips MH, Lyman JT. Charged-particle radiosurgery of the brain. *Neurosurg Clin North Am Stereotact Surg*. Philadelphia: WB Saunders, 1990;955–990.
7. Kjellberg RN, Abbe M. Stereotactic Bragg peak proton beam therapy. In Lunsford LD, ed. *Modern Stereotactic Neurosurgery*. Boston: Martinus Nijhoff, 1988;463–470.
8. Lyman JT, Phillips MH, Frankel KA, Fabrikant JI. Stereotactic frame for neuroradiology and charged particle Bragg peak radiosurgery of intracranial disorders. *Int J Radiat Oncol Biol Phys* 1989;16: 1615–1621.
9. Betti OO, Derechinsky VE. Hyperselective encephalic irradiation with a linear accelerator. *Acta Neurochir Suppl* 1984;33:385–390.
10. Colombo F, Benedetti A, Pozza F, Avanzo RC, Marchetti C, Chierego G, Zanardo A. External stereotactic irradiation by linear accelerator. *Neurosurgery* 1985;16:154–160.
11. Hartmann GH, Schlegel W, Sturm V, et al. Cerebral radiation surgery using moving field irradiation at a linear accelerator facility. *Int J Radiat Oncol Biol Phys* 1985;11:1185–1192.
12. McGinley PH, Butker EK, Crocker IR, Landry JC. A patient rotator for stereotactic radiosurgery. *Phys Med Biol* 1990;35:649–657.
13. Podgorsak EB, Olivier A, Pla M, Lefebvre PY, Hazel J. Dynamic stereotactic radiosurgery. *Int J Radiat Oncol Biol Phys* 1988;14: 115–126.
14. Lutz W, Winston KR, Maleki N. A system for stereotactic radiosurgery with a linear accelerator. *Int J Radiat Oncol Biol Phys* 1988;14: 373–381.
15. Winston KR, Lutz W. Linear accelerator as a neurosurgical tool for stereotactic radiosurgery. *Neurosurgery* 1988;22:454–464.
16. Friedman WA, Bova FJ. The University of Florida radiosurgery system. *Surg Neurol* 1989;32:334–342.
17. Blatt DL, Friedman WA, Bova FJ. Modifications in radiosurgical treatment planning of arteriovenous malformations based on CT imaging. *Neurosurgery* 1993;33:588–596.
18. Bova FJ, Friedman WA. Stereotactic angiography: an inadequate database for radiosurgery? *Int J Radiat Oncol Biol Phys* 1991;20:891–895.
19. Spiegelmann R, Friedman WA, Bova FJ. Limitations of angiographic target localization in radiosurgical treatment planning. *Neurosurgery* 1992;30:619–624.
20. Kondziolka D, Lunsford LD, Kanal E, Talagala L. Stereotactic magnetic resonance angiography for targeting in arteriovenous malformation radiosurgery. *Neurosurgery* 1994;35:585–591.
21. Ondra SL, Troupp H, George ED, Schwab K. The natural history of

symptomatic arteriovenous malformations-nations of the brain: a 24-year follow-up assessment. *J Neurosurg* 1991;73:387–391.

22. Hamilton MG, Spetzler RF. The prospective application of a grading system for arteriovenous malformations. *Neurosurgery* 1994;34:2–7.

23. Heros RC, Korosue K, Diebold PM. Surgical excision of cerebral arteriovenous malformations: late results. *Neurosurgery* 1990;26:570–578.

24. Sisti MB, Kader A, Stein BM. Microsurgery for 67 intracranial arteriovenous malformations less than 3 cm in diameter. *J Neurosurg* 1993; 79:653–660.

25. Spetzler RF, Martin NA. A proposed grading system of arteriovenous malformations. *J Neurosurg* 1985;65:476–483.

26. Ogilvy CS. Radiation therapy for arteriovenous malformations: a review. *Neurosurgery* 1990;26:725–735.

27. Yamamoto M, Jimbo M, Kobayashi M, Toyoda C, Ide M, Tanaka N, Lindquist C, Steiner L. Long-term results of radiosurgery for arteriovenous malformation: neurodiagnostic imaging and histological studies of angiographically confirmed nidus obliteration. *Surg Neurol* 1992; 37:219–230.

28. Nedzi LA, Kooy H, Alexander E, Gelman RS, Loeffler JS. Variables associated with the development of complications from radiosurgery of intracranial tumors. *Int J Radiat Oncol Biol Phys* 1991;21:591–599.

29. Steiner L. Treatment of arteriovenous malformations by radiosurgery. In Wilson CB, Stein BM, eds. *Intracranial Arteriovenous Malformations.* Baltimore: Williams and Wilkins, 1984;295–313.

30. Steiner L. Radiosurgery in cerebral arteriovenous malformations. In: Fein JM, Flamm ES, eds. *Cerebrovascular Surgery.* vol 4. Wien: Springer-Verlag, 1985;1161–1215.

31. Steiner L, Leksell L, Greitz T, Forster DM, Backlund EO. Stereotaxic radiosurgery for cerebral arteriovenous malformations. Report of a case. *Acta Chir Scand* 1972;138:459–464.

32. Lindquist C, Steiner L. Stereotactic radiosurgical treatment of malformations of the brain. In Lunsford LD, ed. *Modern Stereotactic Neurosurgery.* Boston: Martinus Nijhoff, 1988;491–506.

33. Yamamoto M, Jimbo M, Ide M, Tanaka N, Lindquist C, Steiner L. Long-term follow-up of radiosurgically treated arteriovenous malformations in children: report of nine cases. *Surg Neurol* 1992;38:95–100.

34. Kemeny AA, Dias PS, Forster DM. Results of stereotactic radiosurgery of arteriovenous malformations: an analysis of 52 cases. *J Neurol Neurosurg Psychiatry* 1989;52:554–558.

35. Lunsford LD, Kondziolka D, Flickinger JC, Bisonette DJ, Jungreis CA, Maitz AH, Horton JA, Coffey RJ. Stereotactic radiosurgery for arteriovenous malformations of the brain. *J Neurosurg* 1991;75: 512–524.

36. Pollock BE, Lunsford LD, Kondziolka D, Maitz A Flickinger JC. Patient outcomes after stereotactic radiosurgery for ''operable'' arteriovenous malformations. *Neurosurgery* 1994;35:1–8.

37. Steinberg GK, Fabrikant JI, Marks MP, Levy RP, Frankel KA, Phillips MH, Shuer LM, Silverberg GD. Stereotactic heavy-charged particle Bragg peak radiation for intracranial arteriovenous malformations. *N Engl J Med* 1990;323:96–101.

38. Betti 00, Munari C, Rosler R. Stereotactic radiosurgery with the linear accelerator: treatment of arteriovenous malformations. *Neurosurgery* 1989;24:311–321.

39. Linskey ME, Lunsford LD, Flickinger JC. Radiosurgery for acoustic neurinomas: early experience. *Neurosurgery* 1990;26:736–744.

40. Colombo F, Pozza F, Chierego G, Casentini L, De Luca G, Francescon P. Linear accelerator radiosurgery of cerebral arteriovenous malformations: an update. *Neurosurgery* 1994l,:14–21.

41. Souhami L, Olivier A, Podgorsak EB, Pla M, Pike GB. Radiosurgery of cerebral arteriovenous malformations with the dynamic stereotactic irradiation. *Int J Radiat Oncol Biol Phys* 1990;19:775–782.

42. Loeffler JS, Alexander E III, Siddon RL, Saunders WM, Coleman CN, Winston KR. Stereotactic radiosurgery for intracranial arteriovenous malformations using a standard linear accelerator. *Int J Radiat Oncol Biol Phys* 1989;17:673–677.

43. Friedman WA, Bova FJ. LINAC radiosurgery for arteriovenous malformations. *J Neurosurg* 1992;77:832–841.

46. Quisling RG, Peters KR, Friedman WA Tart RP. Persistent nidus blood flow in cerebral arteriovenous malformation after stereotactic radiosurgery: MR imaging assessment. *Radiology* 1991;180:785–791.

47. Steiner L, Lindquist C, Adler JR, Torner JC, Alves W, Steiner M. Clinical outcome of radiosurgery for cerebral arteriovenous malformations. *J Neurosurg* 1992;77:1–8.

48. Alexander E III, Siddon RL, Loeffler JS. The acute onset of nausea and vomiting following stereotactic radiosurgery: correlation with total dose to area postrema. *Surg Neurol* 1989;32:40–44.

49. Statham P, Macpherson P, Johnston R, Forster DM, Adams JH, Todd NV. Cerebral radiation necrosis complicating stereotactic radiosurgery for arteriovenous malformation. *J Neurol Neurosurg Psychiatry* 1990; 53:476–479.

50. Flickinger JC. An integrated logistic formula for prediction of complications from radiosurgery. *Int J Radiat Oncol Biol Phys* 1989;17: 879–885.

51. Flickinger JC, Schell MC, Larson DA. Estimation of complications for linear accelerator radiosurgery with the integrated logistic formula. *Int J Radiat Oncol Biol Phys* 1990;19:143–148.

52. Hosobuchi Y, Fabrikant JI, Lyman JT. Stereotactic heavy-particle irradiation of intracranial arteriovenous malformations. *Appl Neurophysiol* 1987;50:248–252.

53. Kjellberg RN, Hanamura T, Davis KR, Lyons SL, Adams RD. Bragg-peak protonbeam therapy for arteriovenous malformations of the brain. *N Engl J Med* 1983;309:269–274.

54. Marks LB, Spencer DP. The influence of volume on the tolerance of the brain to radiosurgery. *J Neurosurg* 1991;75:177–180.

55. Marks MP, Delapaz RL, Fabrikant JI, Frankel KA, Phillips MH, Levy RP, Enzmann DR. Intracranial vascular malformations: imaging of charged-particle radiosurgery. Part 11. Complications. *Radiology* 1988; 168:457–462.

56. Dawson RC, III, Tarr RW, Hecht ST, Jungreis CA, Lunsford LD, Coffey R, Horton JA. Treatment of arteriovenous malformations of the brain with combined embolization and stereotactic radiosurgery: results after I and 2 years. *Am J Neuroradiol* 1990;11:857–864.

57. Guo WY, Wikholm G, Karlsson B, Lindquist C, Svendsen P, Ericson K. Combined embolization and gamma knife radiosurgery for cerebral arteriovenous malformations. *Acta Radiol* 1993;34:600–606.

58. Francel PC, Steiner L, Steiner M, Lindquist C. Repeat radiosurgical treatment in arteriovenous malformations following unsatisfactory results of initial single high-dose radiation. *J Neurosurg* 1991;74: 352A(abstr).

59. Kondziolka D, Lunsford LD, Coffey RJ, Bissonette DJ, Flickinger JC. Stereotactic radiosurgery of angiographically occult vascular malformations: indications and preliminary experience. *Neurosurgery* 1990; 27:892–900.

60. Steinberg GK, Levy RP, Fabrikant JI, Frankel KA, Phillips MH, Marks MP. Stereotactic helium ion bragg peak radiosurgery for angiographically occult intracranial vascular malformations-nations. *J Stereo Func Neurosurg* 1991;57:64–71.

Cerebrovascular Disease, edited by H. Hunt Batjer.
Lippincott-Raven Publishers, Philadelphia © 1997.

CHAPTER 62

Surgical Techniques for Lobar Arteriovenous Malformations: Frontal, Temporal, Parietal, Occipital

Daniel L. Barrow and Michael Cawley

GENERAL BACKGROUND

Early attempts to operate on arteriovenous malformations (AVMs) of the brain were associated with discouraging results (1,2). In 1943, Olivecrona and Riives reported the first large series in which AVMs of the brain were successfully managed by surgery (3). Initial successes in the surgical management of AVMs were restricted to convexity malformations sparing critical areas of the brain. The introduction of microsurgical techniques in the 1960s and further refinement of surgical methods has greatly expanded the role of surgery in the treatment of AVMs (4). Pioneering work in the embolization of AVMs (5) led to the development of modern endovascular techniques that now provide an important adjunct to the surgical management of selected lesions. Likewise, investigators building on the early work of Leksell have established stereotactic radiosurgery as a promising alternative to surgery for some AVMs (6).

Lobar AVMs typically appear on or near the surface of the frontal, temporal, parietal, or occipital lobes. These lesions almost always extend in an inverted cone-shaped fashion to the surface of the ventricular system and have a predictable arterial supply. Although a number of variables influence the degree of surgical difficulty in the treatment of lobar AVMs, these lesions represent the group of malformations most readily amenable to surgical resection.

CLINICAL DECISION MAKING

Clinical decision making involves careful comparison between the risks of the natural history of a given disorder and the risks of the various treatment options. Overall the risk of bleeding from an AVM is about 3–4% per year with a 1% annual risk of death from the AVM (7,8). The risk of rebleeding rises to 6–18% in the year following AVM hemorrhage (7,9–11). This risk is evenly distributed throughout the first year and declines to 3–4% after the first year.

As our knowledge of the natural history of intracranial AVMs has evolved, it has become apparent that patients harboring these lesions live with a significant cumulative morbidity. Despite the significant risks associated with the natural history, some of these lesions cannot be treated without unacceptable risk and should remain. Thus, the initial challenge in the management of patients with intracranial AVMs is the decision of whether or not the patient should be offered any treatment.

In considering the decision to treat an AVM, the clinician must choose from a variety of therapeutic modalities, including surgical excision, embolization, radiosurgery, and various combinations of these treatments. Of paramount importance in selecting an optimal, individualized treatment plan is the realization that each modality carries its own inherent risk, which is cumulative when combined with other modalities. Furthermore, the optimal management involves a multidisciplinary approach. The ultimate challenge centers on an honest assessment of the available technology vis-à-vis the risk factors for each treatment option from each of the involved disciplines. When contemplating the surgical treatment of a lobar AVM, the surgeon must consider a number of characteristics of both the patient and the lesion.

Characteristics of the Patient

As with any other decision to recommend surgery, the counseling of a patient harboring an AVM must take into

D. L. Barrow and M. Cawley: Department of Neurosurgery, Emory University School of Medicine, Atlanta, Georgia 30322.

account the patient's age, overall physical and mental health, occupation, and expectations. Age is of paramount importance. Although there is some evidence that the annual risk of recurrent hemorrhage from an AVM increases with advancing years (12), if a patient has reached the seventh decade without a hemorrhage, the risk of hemorrhage during the remainder of his or her life may not justify the risks of surgery (13,14). On the other hand, a young patient diagnosed with an AVM faces a considerable cumulative lifetime risk of morbidity and mortality. The patient's physical health is also of utmost importance in considering surgical treatment of an AVM. There are very few more risky and stressful procedures undergone by our patients and their families. This stress necessitates a healthy mental outlook as well. The patient and his family must be fully aware of the reasons for aggressive surgical treatment of these lesions and must have a realistic appreciation of the length of convalescence and the severe consequences of certain complications. Likewise, consideration of the patient's occupation and leisure activities must be part of a decision weighing the risks and benefits of treatment. A day laborer might tolerate a postoperative visual field cut that an air traffic controller could not.

Characteristics of the AVM

It has been suggested that the mode of presentation of an AVM has some effect on its risk of rupture; lesions that have bled in the past are said to be more likely to rupture in the future (15). Other studies have shown that the natural history is unaffected by the mode of presentation (7). However, several features of the malformation itself can assist in predicting the chances of operative morbidity and mortality; size, configuration, location, arterial supply, and venous drainage pattern of a particular AVM are all critical variables that determine the hazards of surgical resection. In general, the larger the lesion is the more difficult the resection will be. More diffuse AVMs are less easily removed than those with a compact nidus (Fig. 1). Deep arterial and venous supply to the malformation should also alert the surgeon to the difficulty inherent in surgical treatment. Location also plays an enormous role in the decision to recommend for or against surgery. A lobar AVM that is situated near the central sulcus, the dominant posterior frontotemporal areas, or the occipital white matter tracts and pole requires that the surgeon recognize the possible serious consequences of even the most technically sublime procedure.

Spetzler and Martin (16) have devised a grading scale for AVMs in order to more clearly stratify the risks involved in the surgical excision of any one particular lesion. Their scale is based on the malformation's size, venous drainage pattern, and location, and is to date the most useful system in predicting surgical difficulties and comparing the results of different modes of treatment.

GOALS OF TREATMENT

The most commonly cited goal in the treatment of cerebral AVMs is the prevention of a first or recurrent hemorrhage. Regardless of which therapeutic modality is employed, only complete obliteration of the lesion achieves this goal. It has

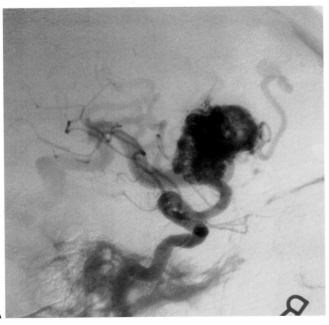
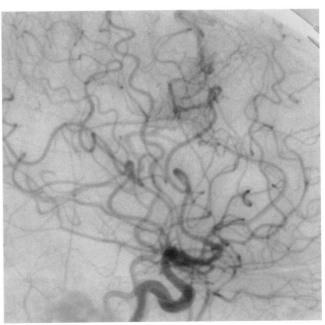

FIG. 1. A: Lateral right carotid angiogram demonstrates a frontal AVM with a well-circumscribed, compact nidus. **B:** Lateral right carotid angiogram of a poorly circumscribed, "loose" arteriovenous malformation (AVM).

become clear that if even the smallest residual fragment of malformation remains, the risk of hemorrhage is unchanged (17). Surgical excision provides the most immediate and complete protection from hemorrhage whereas the less invasive endovascular embolization as a single therapy has proved useful for small lesions only (18–21). Even these small lesions have been shown to have an unacceptably high rate of recanalization after variable periods of time (22,23). It is our opinion that embolization should play a role primarily as a preoperative surgical adjunct if the goal of treatment is elimination of the risk of hemorrhage.

Radiosurgical techniques have also been employed in the treatment of certain AVMs. Several studies have shown an obliteration rate of 80–85% for small AVMs; however, at least 2 years is usually required to reach the goal of complete obliteration, and no protection from a first or recurrent hemorrhage is conferred during this time (24–27). Radiosurgery may be an excellent option for small, deep-seated lesions that cannot be approached surgically without prohibitive risk but is not as commonly recommended for the treatment of lobar AVMs.

Another goal in the treatment of an AVM may be the amelioration of intolerable headache. Quite often embolization of external carotid system feeding arteries will accomplish this for a variable period. Progressive neurologic deficits may also be a feature of some larger AVMs. This decline in function is presumably due to chronic ischemia in the normal brain adjacent to the lesion. An AVM is a direct arterial to venous shunt without any resistance vessels and thus acts as a sump siphoning blood from nearby areas of higher resistance. These areas suffer the so-called intracerebral vascular steal phenomenon. Removal of an AVM should halt the progression of deficits and in some cases may reverse it. In those patients with lesions not amenable to surgical cure, partial embolization or even partial surgical resection may alter the amount of steal enough to stabilize or improve an ischemic neurologic deficit. Of course, neither partial embolization nor partial resection has any effect on the risk of future hemorrhage.

DIAGNOSTIC AND PREOPERATIVE EVALUATION

AVMs have a characteristic appearance on neuroimaging studies. Computed tomography (CT), magnetic resonance imaging (MRI), and angiography all play an important role in the diagnosis of these lesions and the formulation of a therapeutic plan.

Computed Tomography

On non-contrast-enhanced CT, acute and subacute hemorrhage is most readily apparent. This hemorrhage is usually intraparenchymal or intraventricular and lies adjacent to the malformation; AVM rupture rarely results in subarachnoid hemorrhage alone (28,29). Hydrocephalus, mass effects, and encephalomalacia resulting from recent or distant AVM rupture are imaged well on CT (30). Up to 25% of larger AVMs will also show some degree of calcification (31). Contrast-enhanced CT will often demonstrate the AVM nidus, feeding arteries and draining veins as a serpentine intraparenchymal enhancing lesion. The addition of contrast may also evidence a small malformation not previously seen on plain CT images.

Magnetic Resonance Imaging

MRI has largely replaced CT in delineating the precise anatomic relationships of an individual lesion. Its sensitivity to flowing blood makes MRI ideal for detailed demonstration of the malformation's nidus, arterial feeders, and draining veins (32–34). The ability to construct multiplanar images is of enormous benefit in gaining an anatomic understanding of the AVM vis-à-vis other intracranial structures and/or any intraparenchymal hemorrhage. This in-depth anatomic understanding is essential when deciding if a particular lesion should be operated on and, if so, in constructing an operative plan. T1-weighted images are especially helpful in delineating the malformation's relationship to the deep temporal lobe, claustrum, basal ganglia, thalamus, hypothalamus, internal capsule, ventricles, corpus callosum, and interhemispheric fissure. Cohen et al. (35) have described a deep sulcus sign on MRI that acts as a reliable landmark for the Rolandic fissure and the sensorimotor cortices (Fig. 2).

Angiography

Angiography remains the gold standard in the imaging of AVMs. Whereas MRI may be more valuable in deciding if surgery is appropriate, angiography may be more helpful in planning the surgical attack. With the use of superselective catheterization and digital subtraction techniques, an exquisite understanding of the anatomy of the feeding arteries, draining veins, and nidus of even the largest lesions may be gained (30,36). A subjective judgment may be reached regarding the compactness of the nidus, an important factor in determining operative risk. Angiography also allows a qualitative assessment of flow: rapid passage of contrast through the malformation indicates the presence of high-flow shunting and may be circumstantial evidence of intracerebral steal. Angiography may also demonstrate aneurysms associated with enlarged arterial feeders. It is estimated that aneurysms will be encountered in approximately 6–30% of AVMs (28,29,37,38). Venous anomalies such as stenoses, thromboses, and varices are also associated with as many as 30% of AVMs (38,39). The presence and location of such associated lesions has great impact on both the endovascular and surgical approaches to the parent AVM.

A complete study must include images of both internal carotid arteries, as well as adequate images of the vertebrobasilar system. The external carotid artery systems must also

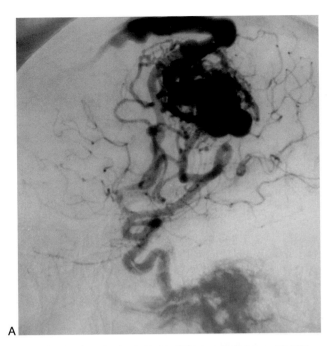

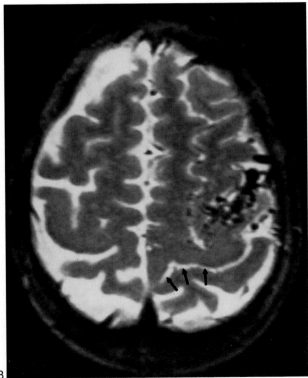

FIG. 2. A: Lateral left carotid angiogram of a posterior frontal AVM. From the angiogram, the relationship to the motor strip is uncertain. **B:** Axial T2-weighted MRI shows the central sulcus *(arrows)* and the AVM a full gyrus anterior to the central sulcus and thus anterior to the motor strip.

be visualized as they may contribute blood supply to some AVMs and provide collateral flow to normal brain surrounding the lesion (40,41). When studying the preoperative angiogram, the surgeon must become intimately familiar with the AVM's location and size, arterial input, venous drainage, and associated vascular abnormalities. However, as noted above, in some high-flow malformations details of the angioarchitecture may be obscured. In this situation, super-selective catheterization of specific feeding arteries may be helpful in delineating the precise anatomy of these lesions (Fig. 3).

With these superselective studies, one may reveal arteries en passage that provide small branches to the lesion itself but then continue on to supply blood to adjacent normal brain. In such cases it may also be useful to introduce small doses of short-acting barbiturates into specific feeding arteries. This mini–Wada test often provides physiologic information regarding the malformation's relationship to functionally important adjacent brain tissue that may prove useful in determining the likelihood of complications arising during embolization or surgical resection (42).

Any angiograms performed more than 2–3 weeks prior to a proposed surgical excision should be repeated because AVM architecture can evolve markedly after hemorrhage or attempts at endovascular obliteration. Indeed, thrombosis and complete obliteration of AVMs without any treatment has been documented (43). Up-to-date angiographic studies also allow the surgeon to identify any newly arisen aneurysms that may have an impact on the operative plan.

Functional Imaging

More sensitive quantitative determination of regional cerebral blood flow may be obtained using single-photon emission computed tomography (SPECT), xenon-enhanced CT, or positron emission tomography (PET). Specific cerebral blood flow tests may include acetazolamide or CO_2 challenges to evaluate the risk of postoperative vasomotor paralysis. PET will also localize the functional areas of brain tissue activated by specific behavioral tasks. As with the more crude mini–Wada test, these studies help delineate the relationship of an AVM to functionally important areas of the brain and are thus useful in predicting the risks of treatment.

OPERATIVE MANAGEMENT

Timing of Surgery

Unlike aneurysmal subarachnoid hemorrhage, hemorrhage after AVM rupture is usually intraparenchymal or intraventricular. Therefore, the risk of delayed ischemic deficits from cerebral vasospasm is small. Likewise, the risk of rebleeding after AVM rupture differs from that of aneurysmal rupture. There is no immediate acute increase in the rate of hemorrhage after an AVM has bled. Therefore, unless an

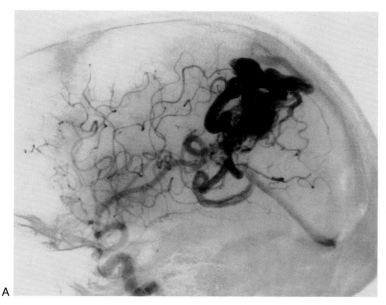
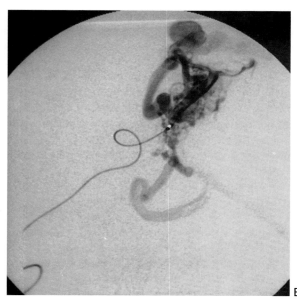

A   B

FIG. 3. **A:** Lateral left carotid angiogram of a parietal AVM fed by the middle cerebral artery with superficial and deep venous drainage. **B:** Superselective angiography of the dominant middle cerebral feeding artery more clearly demonstrates the anatomy of the AVM prior to surgery.

intracerebral or subdural hemorrhage creates a mass lesion requiring urgent removal, we delay surgical intervention for 2–4 weeks to allow the patient to recover from the initial ictal event. In most cases, if the clot does require urgent evacuation, the AVM is left intact and removed at a later date. Only small, obvious surface malformations are resected at the time of clot evacuation.

The timing of surgery following adjunctive endovascular embolization is more controversial. After embolic occlusion of a significant portion of a malformation, there occurs a redistribution of blood flow to surrounding normal brain tissue. This may lead to acute or subacute brain swelling due to the reintroduction of blood flow to chronically hypoperfused, dysautoregulated normal brain. Subclinical ischemia from dislodged fragments of embolic material may also contribute to adjacent brain edema. These factors have led us to delay surgical resection after adjunctive embolization for 2–4 days to allow the brain to accommodate the new local cerebral hemodynamics. Only in the case of acute venous side occlusion during the embolization procedure do we advocate urgent surgical excision. Barring this eventuality, delays should, in any case, not extend more than 1–2 weeks because the malformation may recruit additional blood supply and/or its arterial feeders and nidus may recanalize.

Anesthesia

We routinely employ general anesthesia as it allows for better brain relaxation and control of blood pressure. Some surgeons have advocated awake surgical excision of those AVMs residing in eloquent areas. We believe that the length and delicacy of the procedure makes this strategy undesir-

able. As an alternative, on occasion we have performed awake surgical mapping of the cortex surrounding an AVM and resected the lesion at a later date under general anesthesia or placed subdural electrodes for more chronic mapping prior to resection.

Prior to induction, central venous and arterial lines are placed to allow close monitoring and control of central venous filling and systemic arterial pressures. We prefer that the arterial blood pressure be kept at normal levels as the dysautoregulated adjacent brain is already chronically ischemic and may be predisposed to further compromise from necessary retraction during the resection. If the surgical approach necessitates that the head be placed above the heart, a precordial or esophageal Doppler monitor is placed to detect and treat any venous air emboli. A Foley catheter and lower extremity pneumatic compression devices are also utilized.

An osmotic diuretic is used judiciously and the patient is ventilated to maintain normocarbia. Lumbar drainage is used infrequently as, in most cases, access to the ventricular or cisternal systems may be achieved early in the course of the operation. Perioperative antibiotics are routinely administered due to the increased risks of infection in a lengthy procedure. Dexamethasone and anticonvulsants are also used, and the latter must be present in therapeutic levels as an early postoperative seizure may have catastrophic consequences.

Positioning

For lobar convexity AVMs, we position the patient so that the malformation is uppermost in the field and parallel to the floor. This allows the surgeon to take a perpendicular line of attack. Whenever possible, the head is positioned to allow gravity to assist in brain retraction. For instance, in approaching an interhemispheric lobar AVM, we place the patient's head in a lateral position with the ipsilateral side down, allowing the surrounding cortex to fall away from the malformation; for a sub- or transtemporal exposure, we tilt the vertex slightly down to again allow gravity to assist in temporal lobe retraction. Of course, no position should be allowed to compromise venous return because this will result in both congested brain tissue and an engorged malformation. Radiolucent pins and head holder are used to facilitate the routine use of intraoperative angiography.

Equipment and Instruments

Due to the length of the procedure and its delicate, often frustrating nature, the surgeon should assume a sitting position with the arms well supported. A femoral arterial sheath is placed prior to draping in anticipation of later intraoperative angiographic studies. Intraoperative electroencephalography and somatosensory evoked potential equipment are only occasionally required. A cell saver device may be useful as there exists the potential for significant blood loss in these operations.

The initial cranial and dural opening as well as some of the initial gross dissection of the AVM itself may be done under loupe magnification. However, the majority of the resection is carried out under the operating microscope, which affords far superior magnification and illumination. A self-retaining retractor system with numerous malleable tapered and nontapered blades should be available, as should a full set of microsurgical instruments.

Of utmost importance is the availability of multiple sets of non-sticking bipolar electrocoagulators. On the surface of the brain, small-tipped coagulators should be used to minimize the spread of current. Deeper into the brain and malformation, broader tipped bipolars are superior as the greater dispersion of current allows for more effective coagulation of the abnormal, thin-walled vessels of the malformation. A selection of small aneurysm clips should be on hand to help secure larger arterial feeding vessels. AVM microclips with jaw lengths of 1–4 mm should also be available to secure the small diaphanous vessels encountered at the apex of the malformation in the deep white matter or near the ependymal surface of the ventricular system. Several suction tips of varying sizes should be available with both tapered tips and ball tips. We find suction tips with graduated thumb control of suction strength to be most helpful in minimizing trauma. Hemostasis is also greatly assisted by the judicious use of several sizes and shapes of cottonoid patties and pledgets.

Bone and Dural Flaps

In general, a wide field of exposure should be pursued. To do this, a generous bone flap to allow easier identification of important anatomic landmarks should be made. If the approach requires midline or interhemispheric exposure, we advocate placing the medial burr holes directly over the superior sagittal sinus. In most cases the dura here is thicker and more easily stripped than in the paramedian regions. Additionally, one may avoid the enlarged and adherent paramedian draining veins and venous lakes frequently engendered by the altered venous outflow of AVMs.

Unlike the bone flap, the dura is opened only around the periphery of the malformation. This allows the surrounding brain to be kept moist and protected from intraoperative trauma. Care must be taken to avoid injury to enlarged surface draining veins as they may be adherent to the undersurface of the dura. If dissection of such vessels cannot proceed without undue trauma, the dura may be cut away around the vein in question and left attached to the malformation. Care must also be taken to adequately secure any external carotid system arterial feeders reaching the AVM via the dura.

Resection of the AVM: General Considerations

After a thorough review of the preoperative angiogram, the surgeon should be able to anticipate the architecture of an individual AVM as the dura is opened. Most of these lobar lesions describe an inverted cone shape extending from the cortical surface, or just below it, to the wall of the ventricular system. If the malformation is not readily apparent on the surface of the brain, any apparent arterialized veins should be followed into a sulcus to find the AVM itself. Once the surgeon is oriented as to the location of the malformation, resection may follow in a relatively simple, stepwise fashion.

First, accessible superficial feeding arteries are secured using bipolar coagulation along a 3- to 5-mm segment of vessel prior to division. If the feeding vessel is greater than 2 mm in diameter, a small aneurysm clip may be applied, followed by careful coagulation and division. It is important that these feeding arteries be followed to the point where they enter the malformation itself; only then should they be divided. Care must also be taken to assure that no arteries en passage are divided (Fig. 4). Such arteries are more commonly encountered in resection of corpus callosal and Sylvian fissure AVMs and should be meticulously spared.

During the identification and sacrifice of the superficial feeding arteries the surgeon must be sure to leave all significant draining veins intact to allow continued decompression of the nidus of the malformation. If a question arises as to whether a reddish-appearing vessel is an arterial feeder or an arterialized draining vein, light compression may be applied with a forceps or temporary clip. If back-pressure pulsations appear away from the nidus, the vessel is most likely an arterial feeder. If back-pressure pulsations appear between the point of compression and the nidus, or if the malformation becomes enlarged and tense, the vessel may be assumed to be a draining vein.

Once all accessible superficial arterial feeders have been

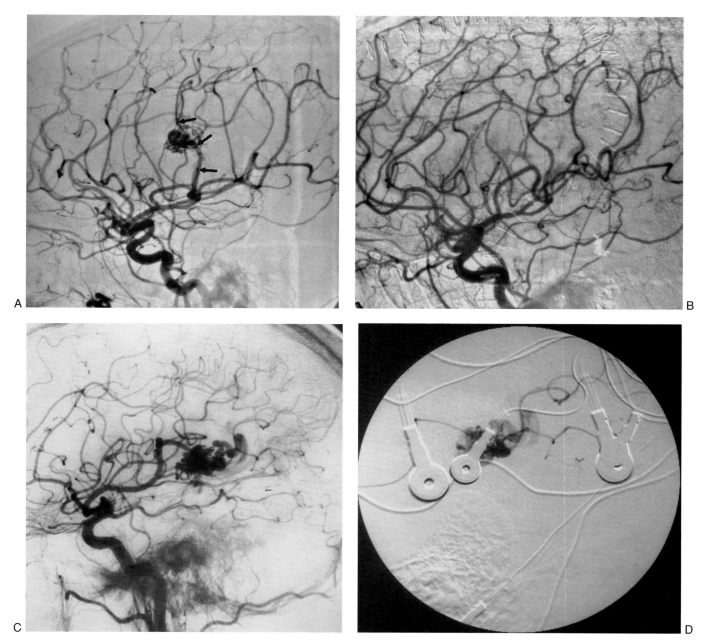

FIG. 4.   A: Lateral left carotid angiogram of a small cortical AVM fed by an artery "en passage" *(arrows).* **B:** Postoperative angiogram documents patency of the same artery and complete obliteration of the AVM. **C:** Left lateral angiogram shows an AVM fed by the middle cerebral artery. **D:** Superselective angiography of a feeding artery demonstrates an artery en passage that feeds the AVM and proceeds on to supply eloquent cortex.

secured, a circumscribing cortical incision is made around the AVM. Often the surgeon will encounter a plane of gliotic tissue immediately adjacent to the malformation itself. Circumferential dissection should be carried out in this area using a bipolar cautery in the dominant hand and a fine-tipped sucker in the nondominant hand. Dissection should be carried to a depth of 2–3 cm, never too deep in one area. This will allow most of the small feeders to be coagulated and divided. Larger vessels should be secured with small

straight aneurysm clips. The surgeon who wanders into a completely avascular plane has most likely strayed into normal white matter and should reestablish a plane of dissection closer to the malformation. Likewise, straying into the malformation will result in vigorous bleeding. In this situation, one should back-track and reestablish the aforementioned gliotic plane. Any hemorrhage from the rent made in the malformation may be tamponaded using a cottonoid patty and compression with the self-retaining retractor blade.

As the dissection is carried deeper toward the apex of the lesion, self-retaining retraction blades may be placed deeper into the field. Such retractors should rest only on the malformation itself—which can take a surprising amount of distortion—rather than the brain tissue. This maneuver, along with adequate brain relaxation, should provide optimal exposure of most lobar AVMs. At the apex of the AVM, the surgeon is likely to encounter the most difficulty in terms of dissection and hemostasis. Many deep, friable, diaphanous vessels feeding the apex of the malformation arise from the ependymal surface of the ventricular system. The surgeon should carefully and patiently coagulate such vessels using continuous light irrigation and broad-tipped, nonsticking bipolar coagulators. If these vessels are prematurely torn or divided, they will instantly retract into the surrounding white matter. The temptation to chase such bleeders should be resisted as this often results in significant trauma to normal brain. In some cases, gentle suction may be used to lift up these vessels, exposing 2–3 mm of vessel that can then be secured with AVM microclips. Coagulation is then applied as an additional hemostatic measure. Hemostatic agents such as gel foam or Avitene should never be employed at this stage of the operation as they may merely hide a source of bleeding.

Once the arterial feeders to the malformation are interrupted, the AVM should soften noticeably and shrink away from the surrounding brain. At this point the draining veins may be taken. In some cases, it is wise to temporarily occlude the final draining vein for several minutes and observe the reaction of the AVM. As with the sacrifice of arterial feeders, the draining veins should be occluded at a point close to the nidus so as not to compromise the venous drainage of nearby

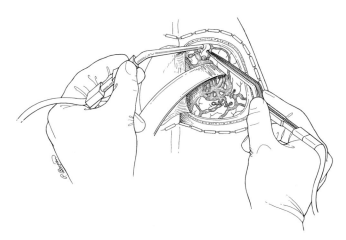

FIG. 6. Initial stages of AVM resection. A self-retaining retractor is used to retract the AVM rather than the adjacent brain. Using a bipolar in the dominant hand and a graduated suction in the nondominant hand, circumferential dissection is carried out around the periphery of the malformation, maintaining the plane of dissection immediately adjacent to the AVM. Superficial feeding arteries are coagulated and divided only as they enter the AVM. Larger feeding arteries are occluded with clips.

brain tissue. Occasionally, with the interruption of the draining veins, the malformation may be seen to swell or continue bleeding from multiple points. In this case, a persistent arterial feeder adherent to the undersurface of a draining vein is often found. Once this rogue artery is divided, order is restored.

Having thus secured both the arterial supply and the venous drainage of the AVM, it may be pronounced dead. Every effort should be made to remove the malformation en bloc. This avoids unnecessary bleeding and obscuration of the anatomy, both of which increase the risk of leaving residual AVM behind.

At the authors' institution, we routinely perform intraoperative angiography to document complete obliteration of the AVM prior to closure. In experienced hands, we have found that this adds only 15–25 minutes to the operative time. If any residual malformation is seen, reexploration is carried out immediately. Intraoperative angiography may also prove useful in differentiating a true feeding artery from an artery en passage or to help localize a small AVM not apparent on the cortical surface. Alternatively, intraoperative ultrasound or frameless stereotactic techniques may be helpful in this last scenario.

Resection of the AVM: Specific Considerations

Frontal Lobe AVMs

AVMs of the frontal lobe may be based on any or all of the lobe's three cortical surfaces. Frontal lobe malformations of the inferior or orbital cortical surface are most often fed

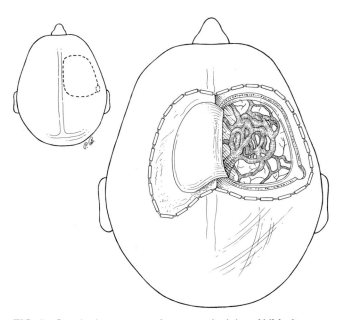

FIG. 5. Surgical exposure of a convexity lobar AVM after craniotomy and dural opening. Inset shows position of burr hole and craniotomy.

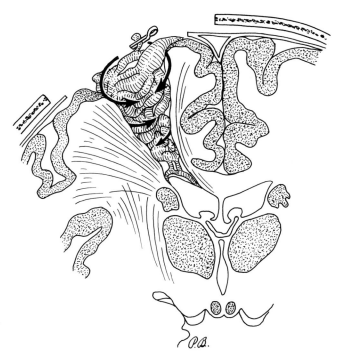

FIG. 7. Once the superficial feeders are controlled, the surgeon continues a circumferential dissection around the AVM, following the gliotic plane along the edge of the lesion. Near the ependymal surface of the ventricle, one commonly encounters small, diaphanous vessels that are very difficult to coagulate and tend to retract into the adjacent white matter.

by arterial branches of the first and second segments of both the middle and anterior cerebral arteries (MCAs and ACAs). If these lesions are situated near the frontal pole, significant arterial contributions may arise from the internal carotid system via the ethmoidal arteries and from the external carotid system via dural feeders and the anterior falcine artery. Venous drainage is usually anterior into the superior sagittal sinus or posterior into the basal vein of Rosenthal and the galenic system.

In addition to the general concepts discussed above, several recommendations can be made regarding orbital frontal lobe AVMs in particular. After performing a standard pterional craniotomy, the sphenoid ridge should be carefully drilled off. This facilitates wide opening of the proximal Sylvian fissure and early access to the first two segments of the MCA. After gentle subfrontal retraction, with or without orbital corticotomy or corticectomy, the AVM may be identified as the surgeon follows the enlarged arterial feeding branches from the MCA to the malformation. Care must be taken to positively identify any feeding vessels and secure these only at their entrance to the malformation. Failure to do so may result in the inadvertent sacrifice of crucial lenticulostriate vessels (Fig. 8).

AVMs of the lateral frontal lobe are usually fed by Sylvian branches of the MCA. If the lesion is situated more postero-laterally, it may also receive arterial supply from deep perfo-

rators of the MCA and ACA. Venous drainage is superior into the superior sagittal sinus or inferior into the Sylvian veins. After completion of a large pterional-frontal bone and dural flap, the Sylvian fissure is widely opened to expose feeding arteries and normal vessels alike. The sphenoid ridge does not need to be drilled off as exposure of the proximal MCA is not usually required in these cases (Fig. 9). Occasionally, more medial exposure of the parasagittal area may be required if there are any arterial feeding arteries from the second part of the ACA.

Malformations of the mesial frontal lobe are usually supplied by branches of the ACA; their venous drainage is into the superior and inferior sagittal sinuses. Most often these lesions require a parasagittal craniotomy crossing the midline. It may be difficult to secure the deep mesial feeding arteries arising from the ACA. These vessels are often obscured by large critical draining veins bridging from the malformation to the sagittal sinuses. Unless these deep-feeding arteries have been secured by preoperative embolization, a generous anteroposterior parasagittal exposure must be made to provide several alternative avenues for approaching these vessels (Fig. 10). Alternatively, a parasagittal corticotomy may allow earlier access to the malformation itself. At this point some deeper arterial feeders may be secured and some ACA branches may be temporarily occluded. The surgeon may then return to the interhemispheric fissure and carefully sacrifice a few draining veins to provide direct visualization of arterial feeders, which are then taken as they enter the malformation.

Temporal Lobe AVMs

The arterial supply of most temporal lobe AVMs is derived from branches of the MCA. However, if these lesions extend to the periventricular or posterior temporal regions, significant feeding vessels may arise from the anterior choroidal or posterior cerebral arteries, respectively. The venous drainage of AVMs of the temporal lobe may be as complex as its arterial supply. These lesions may drain into the Sylvian fissure system, the sphenoparietal sinus, the vein of Labbé, and often into the galenic system via the basal vein of Rosenthal. The key to successful exposure and resection of temporal lobe malformations is an initial wide opening of the Sylvian fissure. If the lesion involves the temporal tip, proximal dissection of the sphenoidal segment of the fissure allows early identification of the anterior temporal artery. If the malformation is located more laterally, the insular portion of fissure is opened to afford exposure of the second segment of the MCA. Once this is accomplished, isolation of feeding arteries from the MCA may proceed.

If preoperative angiography indicates that significant arterial supply arises from either the posterior cerebral artery (PCA) or the anterior choroidal artery, early definition of the nidus's cortical and subcortical margins precedes identification of deep-feeding vessels. Proximal to distal dissec-

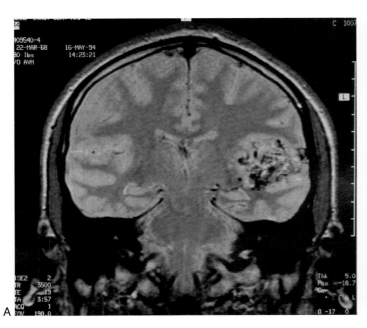

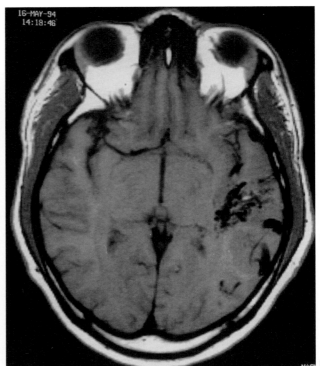

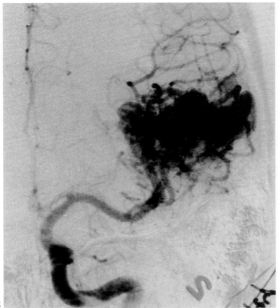

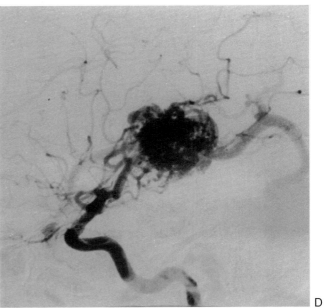

FIG. 8. **(A)** Coronal and **(B)** axial MRI of an AVM on the frontal side of the Sylvian fissure. **(C)** Anteroposterior (AP) and **(D)** lateral angiogram demonstrates the arterial supply to the AVM from branches of the middle cerebral artery. This AVM was approached through the Sylvian fissure via a pterional craniotomy and drilling of the lesser wing of the sphenoid. This allowed for the wide opening of the Sylvian fissure to place the feeding arteries to the malformation on stretch so they could be differentiated from normal vessels.

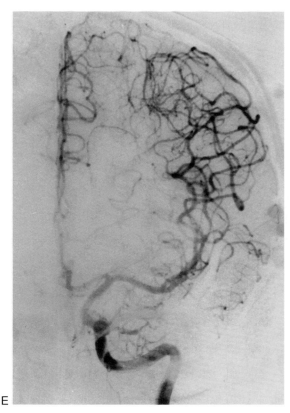

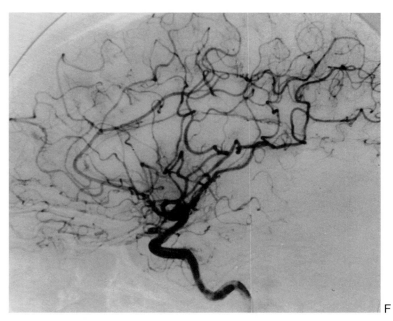

E

F

FIG. 8. *Continued.* **(E, F)** Postoperative AP and lateral right carotid angiograms, respectively.

tion of the anterior choroidal artery is not wise as the artery courses deep in the ventricles and gives off many critical perforators. Likewise, proximal dissection of the PCA may require significant elevation of the temporal lobe and runs the risk of injuring the vein of Labbé. The usual circumferential dissection of the malformation itself will usually allow a transcortical approach to these deep feeders (Fig. 11).

Parietal Lobe AVMs

These malformations are approached in a manner similar to posterior frontal lobe AVMs. They are usually supplied by branches of the distal MCA or ACA. Occasionally, large lesions may derive arterial input from both the MCA and ACA, as well as the vertebrobasilar system via the posterior pericallosal artery and penetrators from the second and third segments of the PCA. Venous drainage is usually into the superior sagittal sinus and the Sylvian venous system. As with most lobar AVMs, exposure should be wide; in most parietal malformations the posterior Sylvian fissure and paramedian regions should be exposed. For parietal AVMs supplied by both ACA and MCA feeders, preoperative embolization of the ACA contribution allows the surgeon to address the more superficial and accessible MCA feeders by placing the head in a lateral position to provide for a perpendicular approach to the lesion. Circumferential dissec-

tion proceeds from the surface toward the falx (Fig. 12). In this functionally important area of the brain, the utmost care must be taken in positively identifying arterial feeding vessels and minimizing retraction. Even in the most experienced hands, the risks of devastating neurologic deficits inherent in the resection of malformations of the parietal lobe may preclude surgical excision as a viable option.

Occipital Lobe AVMs

Like parietal lobe malformations, the excision of these lesions poses a challenge to the surgeon because of the functional importance of the surrounding brain tissue. The visual cortex and the optic radiations are at significant risk in any dissection of the occipital lobe. The arterial supply of these AVMs is derived from distal PCA and MCA branches. If the malformation involves the splenial region, significant contributions may also arise from terminal ACA branches. In addition, occipital AVMs will often recruit external carotid system feeding arteries either through the meningeal system or as direct calvarial perforators.

Occipital lobe malformations are associated with a high incidence of venous anomalies. These may include sinus occlusion or stenosis and bizarre superficial and galenic venous architecture (39,44). Most often, the venous drainage of lateral lesions will be into the superior sagittal and transverse

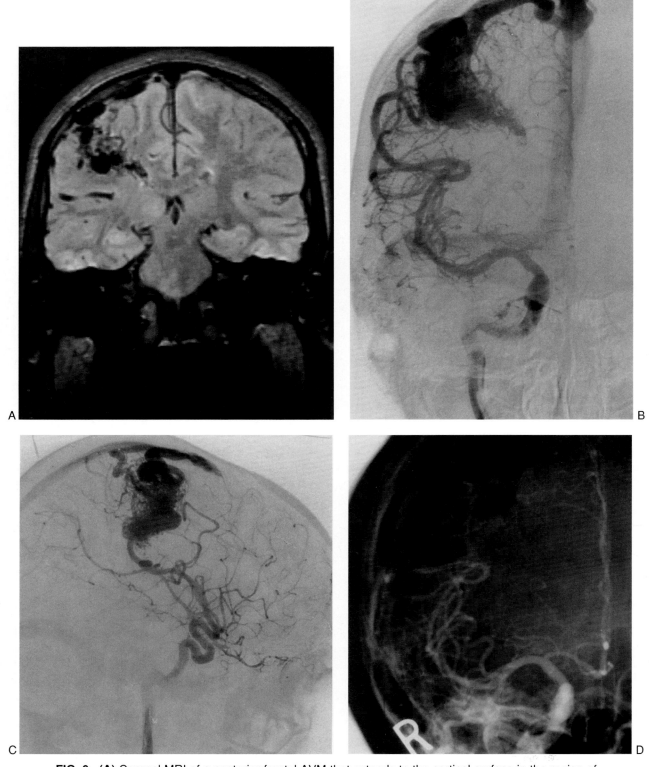

FIG. 9. (A) Coronal MRI of a posterior frontal AVM that extends to the cortical surface in the region of the motor strip. **(B)** Anteroposterior (AP) and **(C)** lateral right carotid angiogram shows the AVM fed by branches of the middle cerebral artery with superficial venous drainage. The compact nature of this AVM contributed to the safety of surgical resection despite its location within functionally important brain. The AVM was removed with the patient in the supine position and the head parallel to the floor for a perpendicular approach to the lesion. **(D)** Postoperative AP right carotid angiogram documents complete resection of the AVM. The patient had transient infacility of the left hand that resolved completely.

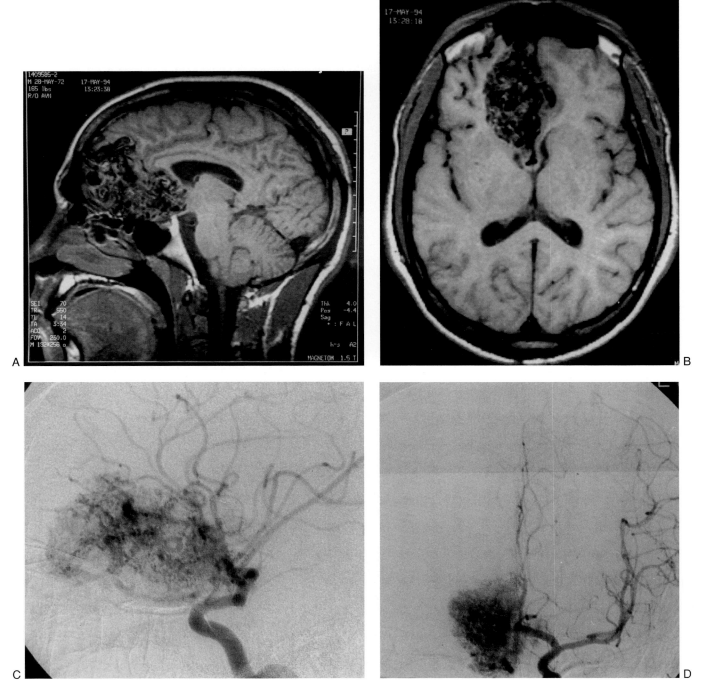

FIG. 10. Mesial frontal AVM. **(A)** Sagittal and **(B)** axial MRI demonstrates a large AVM located in the mesial portion of the frontal lobe extending into the subfrontal region and hypothalamus. **(C)** lateral and **(D)** anteroposterior carotid angiograms reveal the extensive blood supply to the malformation from the anterior cerebral arteries. The extensive arterial supply to this malformation requires a large parasagittal craniotomy to allow for a variety of approaches to secure the arterial supply.

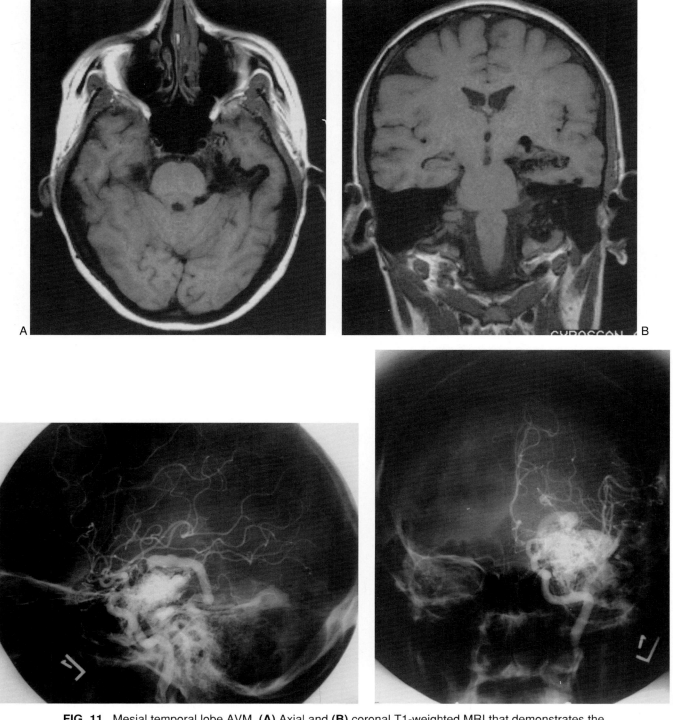

FIG. 11. Mesial temporal lobe AVM. **(A)** Axial and **(B)** coronal T1-weighted MRI that demonstrates the precise location of the AVM. **(C)** Lateral and **(D)** anteroposterior (AP) left carotid angiogram of the AVM fed by branches of the middle cerebral, anterior choroidal, and posterior communicating arteries with both superficial and deep venous drainage.

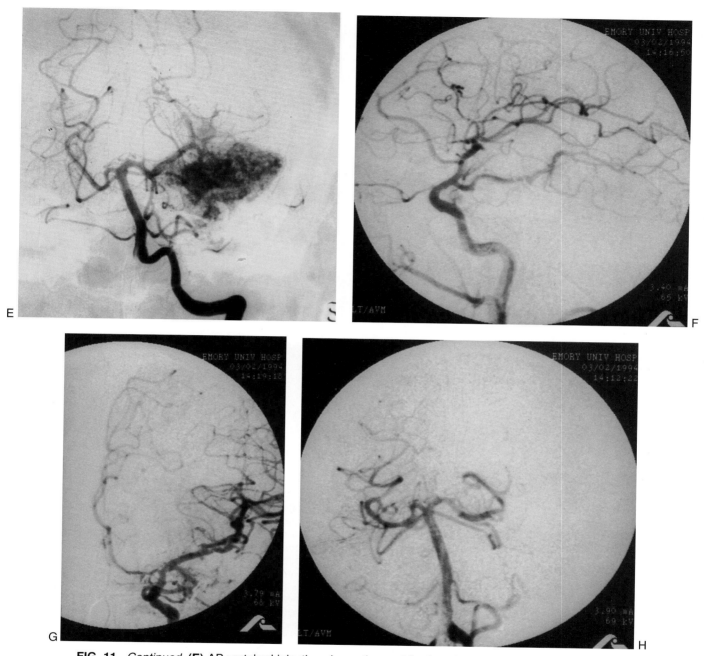

FIG. 11. *Continued.* **(E)** AP vertebral injection shows the contribution of the posterior temporal branch to the AVM. **(F–H)** Intraoperative angiograms documenting complete resection of the AVM.

sinuses; mesial lesions will drain into the galenic system and—often far anteriorly—into the superior sagittal sinus; polar lesions drain into the transverse sinus.

We prefer the lateral park bench position for lateral occipital lesions and the prone position for more mesial lesions requiring an interhemispheric approach. During turning of the scalp, bone, and dural flaps, care should be taken to adequately secure any external carotid system arterial feeders. Preoperative embolization may prove a helpful adjunct

in eliminating these bothersome feeding arteries. Resection of laterally placed malformations then continues much as for frontal convexity lesions. More mesially located AVMs require an interhemispheric approach after any obvious MCA feeding arteries have been taken. Once in the interhemispheric fissure, the surgeon should identify the PCA proximally as it emerges beneath the splenium and dissect proximally to distally, elevating the medial occipital lobe out to the pole. Feeding arteries from the PCA may be

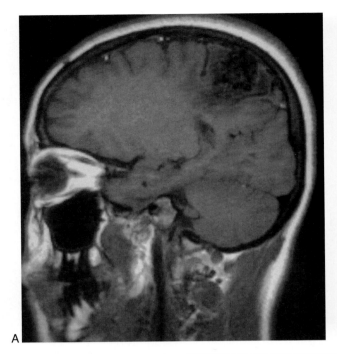

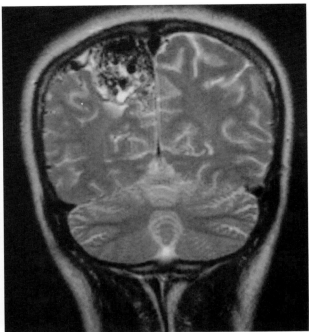

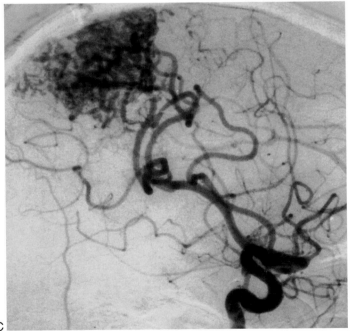

FIG. 12. Parietal AVM. **(A)** Sagittal and **(B)** coronal MRI of a right parietal AVM that presented with a progressive left hemiparesis. **(C)** Lateral and **(D)** antero-posterior (AP) right carotid angiograms demonstrate both middle and anterior cerebral feeding arteries. The patient underwent preoperative embolization of the anterior cerebral feeders with cyanoacrylate. Following embolization, the AVM was resected with the patient's head in the lateral position so that the remaining middle cerebral feeding arteries could be circumferentially dissected and secured. The plane of dissection was carried to the falx where the few remaining anterior cerebral feeding arteries were obliterated. **(E)** Postoperative AP right carotid angiogram documents complete resection with normal filling of the surrounding vasculature.

taken as they are identified entering the malformation (Fig. 13).

Circumferential dissection of these mesial lesions often proves difficult as any retraction on the surrounding brain must be limited to avoid severe postoperative visual field defects. In this situation, it is wise to retract the medial dura over the sagittal sinus to increase the angle of attack without further retraction on the occipital lobe. Light coagulation of the malformation may shrink it somewhat and allow quick delivery of the AVM into the interhemispheric fissure.

Intraoperative Angiography

Once the malformation has been removed, intraoperative angiography is performed to be certain that complete obliteration of the AVM with normal filling of the surrounding vasculature has been accomplished. If any portion of the malformation remains, the residual AVM can be removed to avoid the need for another operative procedure. Assurance of complete removal eliminates the risk of early postoperative rebleeding due to an unknown residual AVM. The reso-

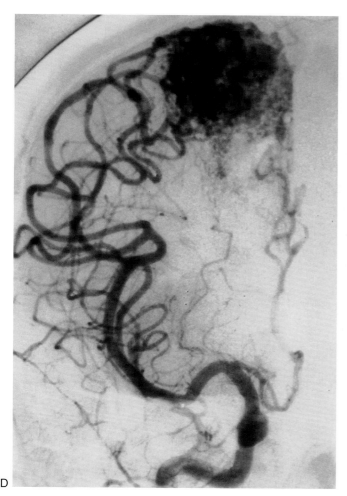

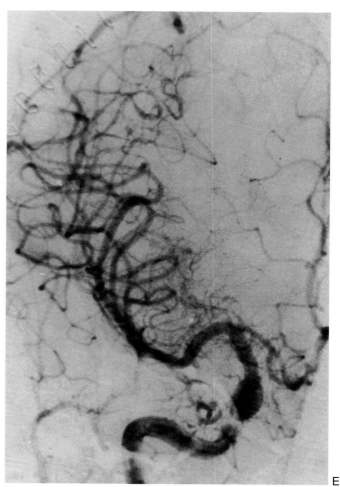

D

E

FIG. 12. *Continued.*

lution of modern, portable, digital, subtraction, intraoperative angiography is adequate to make this intraoperative determination without adding significant length to the operation (Fig. 13E). Occasionally, intraoperative angiography is used to assist in intraoperative localization of small AVMs and to identify arteries en passage intraoperatively.

Hemostasis and Closure

It is impossible to overemphasize the importance of achieving a meticulously dry operative field. Even the slightest ooze from the smallest unsecured vessel may result in a catastrophic postoperative hemorrhage in the recently traumatized and dysautoregulated resection bed. After intraoperative angiography, the operating microscope is reintroduced and a close inspection of the resection cavity is performed. Vigorous irrigation, followed by suction with a small cotton ball affixed to the suction tip allows extensive examination of the field. At this stage of the operation, we prefer the systemic blood pressure to be normal or slightly elevated.

Once all bleeding points have been addressed, the resec-

tion bed may be lined with a single layer of Surgicel. Any red staining apparent as the Surgicel is applied indicates an uncontrolled bleeding point. A Valsalva maneuver is then performed to confirm the absence of any venous bleeding points, the resection cavity is filled with saline, and a watertight dural closure is achieved. The bone flap is reapproximated using 2-0 Nurulon sutures and the wound is closed in layers.

Postoperative Care

The patient is awakened in the operating room immediately after the procedure and examined for any new neurologic deficits. During emergence from anesthesia, emphasis is placed on a smooth awakening and strict control of blood pressure. Transfer to the recovery room is followed in 1–2 hours by transfer to the intensive care unit. During the first 48 hours normotension is maintained; in the case of some larger AVMs slight hypotension is preferred. Therapeutic levels of anticonvulsants are continued for a variable period depending on the patient's preoperative seizure history. Ste-

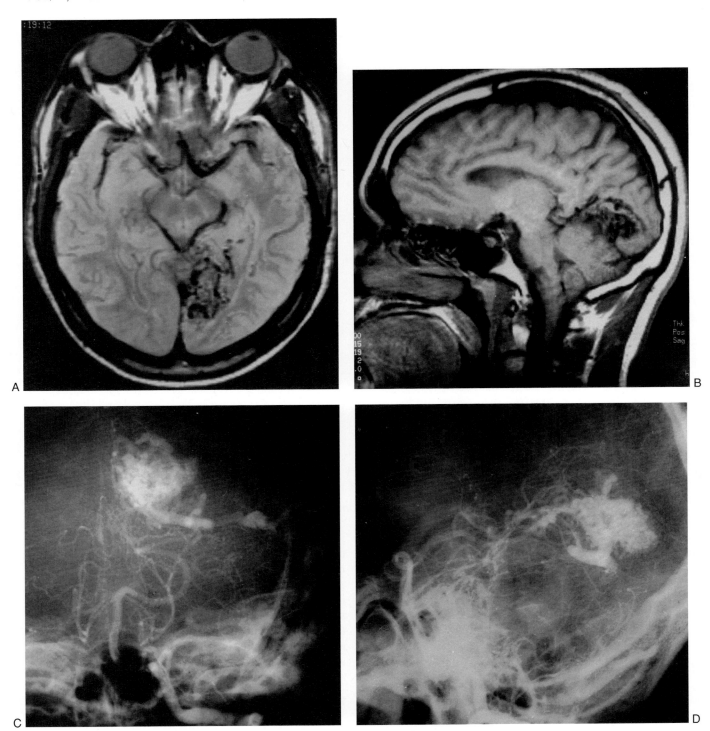

FIG. 13. Mesial occipital AVM. **(A)** Axial and **(B)** sagittal MRI of an AVM on the mesial surface of the occipital lobe, medial to the trigone of the lateral ventricle. **(C)** Anteroposterior (AP) and **(D)** lateral vertebral angiogram shows the supply to the malformation from the posterior cerebral artery. This AVM was approached through an interhemispheric operation with the patient's head in the lateral position and side-of-the-AVM-dependent to allow gravity to assist with retraction. The AVM was exposed by opening the calcarine fissure and circumferentially dissecting the nidus from medial to lateral.

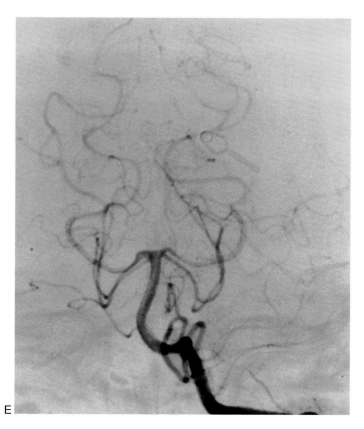

E

FIG. 13. *Continued.* **(E)** Postoperative angiogram demonstrating the normal filling of the distal branches of the posterior cerebral artery and absence of the AVM.

roids are not routinely continued postoperatively, but perioperative antibiotics are continued for 24 hours after surgery. Barring any complications, the patient may be discharged within a week of the procedure. Just prior to discharge, a repeat cerebral angiogram is performed to formally document complete obliteration of the malformation if there remains any doubt as to the completeness of resection from the intraoperative angiogram.

COMPLICATION MANAGEMENT AND AVOIDANCE

Surgical management of intracranial AVMs presents some of the most complex decision making and technical challenges in neurosurgery. A number of potential intraoperative and postoperative complications may result in an adverse outcome in the management of these potentially curable lesions. As with most surgical complications, avoidance is of paramount importance. Unfortunately, avoidance is not always possible. In such cases, the appropriate management of complications that do arise becomes mandatory.

Intraoperative Complications

Direct Parenchymal Injury

As mentioned above, the brain surrounding most AVMs suffers from chronic hypoperfusion due to preferential flow through the malformation, resulting in a local intracerebral steal. This steal may decrease the perfusion of the adjacent brain to 25–35 ml/100 g/min (38,45) and severely derange normal autoregulatory mechanisms. These factors combine to make direct parenchymal injury a real danger in the resection of AVMs.

As some malformations will not come to the cortical surface, occasionally one must access the lesion via corticotomy. While this is not always avoidable, close preoperative examination of the MRI usually allows the surgeon to plan an avenue of attack through adjacent sulci or in a tangential manner so as to avoid critical brain regions. However, a tangential approach requiring undue retraction may be a Pyrrhic victory as the dysautoregulated brain tolerates any retraction poorly. Once the malformation has been located, the surgeon may stray out of the gliotic plane during circumferential dissection around the AVM. If dissection suddenly becomes avascular, the surgeon may have wandered into normal white matter. In this case every effort should be made to back-track and dissect closer to the loops of the malformation.

Sacrifice of arterial feeding vessels at a point too remote from the malformation may likewise lead to catastrophe. In these situations, many small arteries nourishing adjacent brain may be inadvertently occluded, leading to further ischemia in already compromised brain. To avoid this complication, diligent efforts must be made toward meticulous dissection of each suspected feeding artery. If necessary, temporary clips may be used to facilitate identification of the feeder's point of entry into the nidus. The feeding vessel should be definitively taken only at this point.

Venous infarction is equally damaging to the surrounding brain. This complication is often the result of the sacrifice of a normal draining vein misidentified as a part of the malformation. This is most catastrophic in the interhemispheric region and around the vein of Labbé. Once again, meticulous dissection is the key to avoidance.

Hemorrhage

Bleeding during operation of an AVM may have many sources. During placement of the head frame, skull pins may pierce enlarged external carotid system feeding arteries causing copious scalp hemorrhage. Subdural hematomas may rapidly accumulate during dural opening if an enlarged dural draining vein is torn. In both cases, the bleeding point should be isolated and repaired; especially in the case of a ruptured draining vein, every effort should be made to maintain its patency early on in the operation.

During resection of the AVM, bleeding may arise from the malformation or from the adjacent brain parenchyma. Entrance into the nidus is usually the result of dissection into an outpouching tuft of vessels encountered in the gliotic plane. With careful bipolar cautery and irrigation, the bleeding can usually be controlled long enough to reestablish the proper plane of dissection. A small cottonoid patty may then be placed over the rent and held secure with a retractor blade while attention is turned to another area. Bleeding from the cortical side of the resection bed is most likely due to inadequately secured feeding vessels. One should attempt to draw such vessels up into the suction tip and place an appropriate microclip; the surgeon must not be tempted to chase these vessels deep into the surrounding brain. Likewise, one should not elect to pack off these bleeders as this may result in unrecognized intraparenchymal or intraventricular hematoma formation. In the rare case of uncontrollable bleeding, rapid suction decompression of the malformation and any associated hematoma may be followed by the judicious use of temporary clips or a limited lobectomy.

Brain Swelling

During the course of even the most straightforward dissection, the surgeon may note an abrupt diffuse swelling of the brain in the field. Left unchecked, this may markedly increase the difficulty of dissection and result in potentially life-threatening pressure effects on brainstem regulatory centers. As a first response to such swelling, the surgeon should direct the anesthesiology staff to check for ventilatory insufficiency or venous drainage compromise in the neck. Having ruled out these etiologies, the surgeon is faced with the likelihood that the swelling is due to occult bleeding, acute hydrocephalus, or edema secondary to dysautoregulation (38).

Occult bleeding is most often due to an unsecured feeding artery or to an isolated residual AVM fragment that has ruptured. The management of the former has already been discussed; the management of the latter entails establishment of the proper plane of dissection and rapid removal. Acute hydrocephalus is most often due to unrecognized intraventricular bleeding. This usually results from overanxious dissection into the periventricular area around the malformation's apex or from rupture of a retained AVM fragment into the ventricle. In this situation, the ventricle should be opened widely, the clot removed, and the bleeding point addressed. All attempts should be made to clear blood from the ventricle to decrease the risk of postoperative obstructive hydrocephalus.

Edema secondary to cerebral dysautoregulation is often termed *normal perfusion pressure breakthrough* (NPPB). While this phenomenon is more often seen in the postoperative period, occasionally it may occur intraoperatively. NPPB, first outlined by Spetzler et al. (45), results from the abrupt obliteration of a high-flow, low-resistance arteriovenous shunt, which leads to increased blood flow to adjacent brain that has been chronically hypoperfused. This chronic state of hypoperfusion theoretically results in impaired autoregulatory mechanisms that may not be able to accommodate the abruptly increased blood flow. Grossly, the surgeon may observe a distended brain herniating beneath the pial margins, punctate and confluent hemorrhages, or evidence of new arteriovenous shunting in pial vessels remote from the AVM (38).

The treatment of NPPB in the acute intraoperative setting revolves around lowering cerebral blood flow. Systolic blood pressure may be lowered with an agent such as sodium nitroprusside to 80–90 mm Hg. If necessary, further decreases in cerebral blood flow may be achieved with the induction of barbiturate coma to the point of electroencephalographic burst suppression. Having taken these measures, the surgeon should debride any devitalized tissue, achieve meticulous hemostasis, complete any further resection required, and place an intracranial pressure monitoring device prior to transfer from the operating room.

Premature Occlusion of Venous Drainage

It is axiomatic in the performance of AVM resection that adequate venous drainage be maintained until all arterial feeding vessels have been interrupted. If this basic tenet is violated, one will be faced with a tense, engorged malformation hemorrhaging from multiple sites and obscuring important surgical anatomy. In this situation, if the AVM cannot be delivered quickly, one may cannulate one of the larger draining veins inadvertently sacrificed and decompress the malformation by diverting effluent blood to a cell saver device. However, avoidance of this particular complication is far easier than its remedy.

Occlusion of an Artery En Passage

Many AVMs, especially those of the corpus callosum and Sylvian fissure, are supplied by arterial branches from parent arteries that continue on to nourish normal brain. Though these parent vessels may often be closely adherent to the malformation itself, meticulous dissection allows differentiation between the two. Should doubt continue as to whether a particular artery is a feeder or is en passage, radiopaque orientation markers may be left in place and an intraoperative angiogram performed to better delineate the precise arterial anatomy. In any case, a vessel should only be taken after positively identifying it as a feeding artery and then only at its point of entry into the malformation. Care should also be exercised in cauterizing adjacent to arteries en passage as the proximate heat may result in their thrombosis.

Postoperative Complications

Hemorrhage

Postoperative hemorrhage is usually heralded by an abrupt decline in the patient's neurologic status and is most often due to rupture of residual AVM. The most effective way to avoid postoperative hemorrhage is to meticulously examine the resection bed prior to closure for any residual AVM fragments. Intraoperative angiography is also of invaluable assistance in confirming complete obliteration of the malformation. Bleeding from the resection bed may also be the result of poor hemostatic efforts during the closing phase of the operation. But even with the most meticulous hemostasis, acutely elevated systemic blood pressure may result in the reopening of small coagulated vessels. Thus, having assured complete removal of the AVM and having achieved a dry resection bed, the most important maneuver in avoiding postoperative hemorrhage is to strictly control systemic blood pressure, maintaining it at normal or slightly hypotensive levels. To this end, anticonvulsant levels must be kept in the therapeutic range as postoperative seizures may cause acute elevations in blood pressure and lead to hemorrhage. If hemorrhage is suspected, immediate CT scanning is appropriate, as is emergency evacuation, if warranted.

Normal Perfusion Pressure Breakthrough

In the postoperative period, NPPB manifests itself with acute or subacute neurologic decline or seizures due to severe brain swelling or hemorrhage. As discussed above, this phenomenon results from the acutely increased blood flow directed into the dysautoregulated, chronically hypoperfused brain surrounding a recently resected AVM. While the existence of this phenomenon remains controversial (4,46) and its etiology and precise hemodynamics are still unclear, there are factors that can be used to predict which patients may suffer more severely from NPPB. Though most patients probably suffer some degree of NPPB after AVM resection, those who may suffer more fulminant episodes include those patients whose malformations have a large nidus, contralateral arterial supply, long and tortuous large-bore arterial feeders, and high-flow, low-resistance hemodynamics. Radiographic or clinical evidence of intracerebral steal also may indicate that a particular patient may be at increased risk for postoperative NPPB. Once NPPB is suspected, efforts should be aimed at carefully decreasing cerebral blood flow and decreasing intracranial pressure with a head-up position, osmotic diuretics, and hyperventilation as necessary.

Several strategies have been devised to avoid NPPB and its sequelae. Pertuiset has advocated partial occlusion of the carotid artery at the time of resection to decrease the blood flow seen by the dysautoregulated vessels (47). More recently, several studies have examined the efficacy of preoperative embolization and staged resection with or without intraoperative embolization (13,15,19–21,43,48–51). We have relied primarily on the use of preoperative embolization either in single or multiple stages to gradually throttle the malformation and more slowly redistribute blood to the surrounding normal brain prior to excision. In highly selective cases, we have used the strategy of staged intraoperative embolization and resection. With the advent of new microcatheters and better embolization materials, the need for such staged procedures with intraoperative embolization has declined.

Retrograde Thrombosis of a Feeding Artery

The abrupt interruption of a large-caliber, high-flow feeding artery to an AVM may result in proximal sludging of flow if there is no adequate outflow conduit. This sludging may lead to thrombosis in the postoperative period with consequent ischemia or infarction. As no effective treatment exists for such an eventuality, emphasis is placed on prevention. The judicious use of preoperative embolization may help to more slowly close down some of the larger feeders and allow collateral outflow channels to develop.

Cerebral Vasospasm

This is rarely noted to be a significant complication in the management of cerebral AVMs as their rupture deposits little blood in the subarachnoid space, unless the malformation presents secondary to an associated aneurysmal rupture. If encountered, care should be taken in the institution of hypervolemic hypertensive therapy until it is reasonably certain that those divided vessels in the resection bed have sufficiently scarred closed.

Seizure

In a patient without any preoperative history of epilepsy, the risk of postoperative seizures has been variably estimated to be 6.5–50% (52). Given the unenlightening range of these figures, suffice it to say that most patients with preoperative seizures will improve at least somewhat and that a small number of patients will develop new seizures. Most of these new seizures will diminish with time. What is of utmost importance is the prevention of early postoperative seizures, as these ictal events may increase the risk of postoperative hemorrhage.

Hydrocephalus

Postoperative hydrocephalus is most often caused by the presence of blood products in the ventricular system. This may occur during initial hemorrhage or surgical resection. Preventive measures include the avoidance of intraoperative intraventricular hemorrhage as outlined above and the thorough evacuation of any intraventricular clot encountered. Early postoperative hydrocephalus may be treated with ventricular drainage until the blood products have resorbed. Weaning off ventricular drainage should be followed by close neurologic examination and serial CT scans. However, a significant percentage of these patients, as well as most patients developing late hydrocephalus, will require indwelling cerebrospinal fluid shunts.

Infection

The risk of developing a wound infection, meningitis, or ventriculitis during operation for resection of an AVM may be slightly higher than for more routine intracranial procedures due to the length of the procedure. Care must also be taken to maintain sterility of the numerous ancillary devices the surgeon may require, and traffic through the operating suite should be kept to a minimum. In an attempt to further ensure a clean operative field, we routinely use perioperative antibiotics.

CONCLUSION

The appropriate management of patients with AVMs requires a knowledge of the natural history of the lesion, considerable skill in clinical decision making, excellent judgment, and estimable surgical aptitude. Optimal consultation and treatment is provided if a multidisciplinary approach is utilized, where individuals with expertise in the various treatment options are involved in the evaluation, arbitration, and application of therapeutic options. If the decision is made to offer surgical resection as the treatment of an AVM, it is imperative that the surgeon utilize appropriate preoperative imaging studies to assist in operative planning and employ meticulous surgical techniques in order to provide an outcome that is significantly improved over the natural history of the disorder.

REFERENCES

1. Cushing H, Bailey P. *Tumors Arising from the Blood Vessels of the Brain. Angiomatous Malformations and Hemangioblastomas.* vol 3. Springfield, IL: Charles C Thomas, 1928;219.
2. Dandy WE. Arteriovenous aneurysm of the brain. *Arch Surg* 1928;17: 190–243.
3. Olivecrona H, Riives J. Arteriovenous aneurysms of the brain: Their diagnosis and treatment. *Arch Neurol Psychiatry* 1948;59:567–602.
4. Yasargil MG. *Microneurosurgery. vol IIIB. AVM of the Brain: Clinical Considerations, General and Special Operative Techniques, Surgical Results, Non-operative Cases, Cavernous and Venous Angiomas, Neuroanesthesia.* Stuttgart: George Thieme Verlag, 1988.
5. Luessenhop AJ, Spence WT. Artificial embolization of cerebral arteries. Report of case in care of arteriovenous malformation. *JAMA* 1960; 172:1153–1155.
6. Leksell L. The stereotaxic method and radiosurgery of the brain. *Acta Chir Scan* 1951;102:316–319.
7. Ondra SL, Troupp H, George ED. The natural history of symptomatic arteriovenous malformations of the brain: A 24-year follow-up assessment. *J Neurosurg* 1990;73:387–391
8. Samson D, Batjer HH. Preoperative evolution of the risk/benefit ratio for arteriovenous malformations of the brain. In: Wilkins RH, Rengechary SS, eds. *Neurosurgery Update II.* New York: McGraw-Hill, 1991; 129–133.
9. Anderson EB, Petersen J, Mortensen EL, et al. Conservatively treated patients with cerebral arteriovenous malformation: mental and physical outcome. *J Neurol Neurosurg Psychiatry* 1988;51:1208–1212.
10. Brown RD, Jr, Wiebers DO, Forbes G, et al. The natural history of unruptured intracranial arteriovenous malformations. *J Neurosurg* 1988;68:352–357.
11. Fults D, Kelley DL Jr. Natural history of arteriovenous malformations of the brain: a clinical study. *Neurosurgery* 1984;15:658–662.
12. Graf GH, Perret GE, Torner JC. Bleeding from cerebral arteriovenous malformations as part of their natural history. *J Neurosurg* 1983;58: 331–337.
13. Luessenhop AJ, Rosa L. Cerebral arteriovenous malformations: indications for and results of surgery, and the role of intravascular techniques. *J Neurosurg* 1984;60:14–22.
14. Perret G, Nishioka H. Report on cooperative study on intracranial aneurysms and subarachnoid hemorrhage. Section VI: arteriovenous malformations. Analysis of 545 cases of cranio–cerebral arteriovenous malformations and fistulae reported to cooperative study. *J Neurosurg* 1966;25:467–490.
15. Crawford PM, West CR, Chadwick DW, et al.: Arteriovenous malformations of the brain: natural history in unoperated patients. *J Neurol Neurosurg Psychiatry* 1986;49:1–10.
16. Spetzler RF, Martin NA. A proposed grading system for arteriovenous malformations. *J Neurosurg* 1986;65:476–483.
17. Drake CG. Cerebral arteriovenous malformations: considerations for and experience with surgical treatment in 166 cases. *Clin Neurosurg* 26:145–208, 1979.
18. Abad JM, Alvarez F, Manrique M, et al. Cerebral arteriovenous malformations: comparative results of surgical vs. conservative treatment in 12 cases. *J Neurosurg Sci* 1993;27:203–210.
19. Debrun G, Vinuela F, Fox A, et al. Embolization of cerebral arteriovenous malformations with bucrylate: experience in 46 cases. *J Neurosurg* 1982;56:615–627.
20. Samson D, Ditmore QM, Beyer CW, Jr. Intravascular use of isobutyl-2-cyanoacrylate. I. Treatment of intracranial arteriovenous malformations. *Neurosurgery* 1981;8:43–51.
21. Stein BM, Wolpert SM. Surgical and embolic treatment of cerebral arteriovenous malformations. *Surg Neurol* 1977;7:359–369.
22. Germano IM, Davies RL, Wilson CB, et al. Histopathological follow-up study of 66 cerebral arteriovenous malformations after therapeutic embolization with polyvinyl alcohol. *J Neurosurg* 1992;76:607–614.
23. Viners HV, Lundie MJ, Kaufmann JCE. Long-term pathological follw-up of cerebral arteriovenous malformations treated by embolization with bucrylate. *N Engl J Med* 1986;314:477–483.
24. Heros RC, Korosue K. Radiation treatment of cerebral arteriovenous malformations. *N Engl J Med* 1990;323:127–129.
25. Kemeney AA, Dias PS, Forster DMC. Results of stereotactic radiosurgery of arteriovenous malformations: an analysis of 52 cases. *J Neurol Neurosurg Psychiatry* 1989;52:554–558.

26. Ogilvy CS. Radiation therapy for arteriovenous malformations: a review. *Neurosurgery* 1990;26:725–735.
27. Pellettieri L, Carlsson CA, Grensten S, et al. Surgical versus conservative treatment of intracranial arteriovenous malformations. A study in surgical decision making. *Acta Neurochir [Suppl]* 1980;29:1–86.
28. Batjer HH, Suss R, Samson D. Intracranial arteriovenous malformations associated with aneurysms. *Neurosurgery* 1986;18:29–35.
29. Kondziolka D, Nixon BJ, Lasjaunias P, et al. Cerebral arteriovenous malformations with associated arterial aneurysms: hemodynamic and therapeutic considerations. *Can J Neurol Sci* 1988;15:130–134.
30. Terbrugge K, Scotti G, Ethier R, et al. Computed tomography in intracranial arteriovenous malformations. *Radiology* 1977;122 [2 Suppl]: 703–705.
31. Kumar AJ, Fox AJ, Vinuela F, et al. Revisited old and new findings in unruptured larger arteriovenous malformations of the barin. *J Comput Assist Tomogr* 1984;3:648–655.
32. Kucharczyk W, Lemme-Pleghos L, Uske A, et al. Intracranial vascular malformations: MR and CT imaging. *Radiology* 1985;56:383–389.
33. Noorbehesht B, Fabrikant JI, Enzmann DR. Size determination of supratentorial arteriovenous malformations by MR, CT, and angiography. *Neuroradiology* 1987;29:512–518.
34. Smith HJ, Strother CM, Kikuchi Y, et al. MR imaging in the management of supratentorial intracranial AVMs. *AJNR* 1988;150:1143–1153.
35. Cohen WA, Berger MS, Ojemann GA. Preoperative localization of sensory-motor cortex [abstract]. *AJNR* 1988;9:1025.
36. Vinuela F. Endovascular therapy of brain arteriovenous malformations. *Semin Interv Radiol* 1987;4:269–280.
37. Martin NA, Wilson CB. Medial occipital arteriovenous malformations. Surgical treatment. *J Neurosurg* 1982; 56:798.
38. Samson D, Batjer HH. Surface lesions: lobar arteriovenous malformations. In: Apuzzo MLJ, ed. *Brain Surgery.* New York: Churchill Livingstone, 1993;1142–1175.
39. Yasargil MG. *Microneurosurgery. vol IIIA. AVM of the Brain: History, Embryology, Pathological Considerations, Hemodynamics, Diagnostic Studies, Microsurgical Anatomy.* Stuttgart: George Thieme Verlag, 1988.
40. Lasjaunias P, Berenstein A, Moret J. The significance of dural supply of central nervous system lesions. *Neurosurgery* 1983;10:31–42.
41. Newton TH, Cronqvist S. Involvement of dural arteries in intracranial arteriovenous malformations. *Radiology* 1969;93:1071–1078.
42. Vinuela F, Fox AJ, Debrun G. Pre-embolization superselective angiography in the treatment of brain arteriovenous malformations. *AJNR* 1984;5:765–769.
43. Nornes H, Grip A. Hemodynamic aspects of cerebral arteriovenous malformations. *J Neurosurg* 1980;53:456–464.
44. Megison P, Batjer H, Purdy P, Samson D. Spontaneous resolution of arteriovenous malformation without hemorrhage: a case report. *AJNR* 1989;10:204.
45. Spetzler RF, Wilson CB, Weinstein P, et al. Normal perfusion pressure breakthrough theory. *Clin Neurosurg* 1978;25:651–672.
46. Morgan MK, Sundt TM Jr. The case against staged operative resection of cerebral arteriovenous malformations. *Neurosurgery* 1989;25:429–436.
47. Pertuiset B, Ancri D, Arthuis F, et al.: Shunt induced hemodynamic disturbances in supratentorial arteriovenous malformations. *J Neuroradiol* 1985;12:165–178.
48. Andrews BT, Wilson CR. Staged treatment of arteriovenous malformations of the brain. *Neurosurgery* 1987;21:314–323.
49. Pasqualin D, Scienza R, Cioffi F, et al. Treatment of cerebral arteriovenous malformations with a combination of preoperative embolization and surgery. *Neurosurgery* 1991;29:358–368.
50. Spetzler RF, Martin NA, Carter, LP. Surgical management of AVMs by staged embolization and operative excision. *J Neurosurg* 1987;67: 17–28.
51. Vinuela F, Dion JE, Duckwiler G, et al. Combined endovascular embolization and surgery in the management of cerebral arteriovenous malformations: experience with 101 cases. *J Neurosurg* 1991;75:856–864.
52. Korosue K, Heros RC. Complications of complete surgical resection of AVMs of the brain. In: Barrow DL, ed. *Intracranial Vascular Malformations.* Parkridge, IL: American Association of Neurological Surgeons, 1990:157–168.

Cerebrovascular Disease, edited by H. Hunt Batjer.
Lippincott-Raven Publishers, Philadelphia © 1997.

CHAPTER 63

Surgical Techniques for Deep Arteriovenous Malformations: Ganglionic, Callosal, Paraventricular

Michael B. Sisti and Bennett M. Stein

GENERAL BACKGROUND

The surgical management of deep-seated supratentorial arteriovenous malformations (AVMs) is a formidable therapeutic challenge. As with all AVMs, the goals of treatment are twofold: first, the complete removal of the malformation and, second, the preservation of neurologic function. Because of the deep and frequently critical anatomic location of AVMs situated within the paraventricular region, corpus callosum, and basal ganglia, deep operative exposures are required to expose and resect these malformations. As a result, achieving the goals of treatment for these AVMs is particularly hazardous.

Multidisciplinary cooperation and multimodality treatment are required to manage these AVMs. Occasionally, despite the devastating natural history of these lesions, no treatment can be offered. The management of deep AVMs thus requires considerable clinical experience, judgment, and the combined skill of neurologists, neuroradiologists, neurosurgeons, and radiation oncologists who are thoroughly familiar with the management of AVMs.

Reported series of the management of deep supratentorial AVMs reveal that the optimal therapeutic outcome can best be achieved by individuals and institutions possessing the requisite experience. Recent reports on the surgical management of large series of deep AVMs reflect not only on the uncommon occurrence of this condition but the skills of physicians involved in treating them. Stein reported in 1984 on 25 AVMs located in the medial aspect of the cerebral hemispheres and limbic system (13). He accomplished complete surgical removal of the 25 AVMs in this location with

no mortality and a morbidity of 4%. In 1987, Solomon and Stein reported a series of 22 AVMs of the thalamocaudate region; total removal was accomplished in 18 patients, with none suffering permanent neurologic injury (11). Barrow et al in 1994 reported a series of 26 AVMs of the ventricular trigone completely removed by surgery. In this group, 21 patients resumed premorbid activities, 2 had a fair result, 2 had a poor result, and 1 patient died (2). Tew et al in 1995 reported on a series of 65 vascular lesions affecting the thalamus and basal ganglia. Forty-five patients underwent surgery, 10 patients were observed, and 10 patients received radiosurgery (14). Among the 39 patients undergoing surgery for their AVMs, 5 patients worsened and 1 died. Long and his colleagues at the Barrow Neurological Institute in 1995 reported on the multimodality treatment of 32 AVMs in the thalamus, basal ganglia, and brainstem (5). For patients treated prior to the use of stereotactic radiosurgery, the complete removal rate was 43% as opposed to 72% after the introduction of radiosurgery at this institution. Overall treatment morbidity was 9% and there was no mortality. These recent surgical series indicate that acceptable morbidity and mortality can be achieved for these treacherous lesions when a multimodality and individualized approach is employed by physicians experienced in the management of AVMs.

PERTINENT NEUROLOGIC AND VASCULAR ANATOMY AND VARIATIONS

The defining feature of this group of AVMs is their deep anatomic location. The anatomic position of this AVM determines the clinical presentation of the patient, the severity of risk of the natural history of the disease to the patient, and risks of therapeutic interventions on the patient. Thus, to understand the clinical risks and properly evaluate treatment

M. B. Sisti and B. M. Stein: Department of Neurological Surgery, Columbia University College of Physicians & Surgeons, New York, New York 10032-2603.

options, complete understanding of neuroanatomic relationships of involved brain regions is essential. Obviously, a complete review of the pertinent anatomic and clinical features of these regions is beyond the scope of this chapter. However, several pertinent anatomic features should be noted. The most important of these is the AVM's relationship to ventricular anatomy. Paraventricular AVMs, including those in the corpus callosum, reside in the brain parenchyma immediately outside this ventricular system and thus involve the temporal lobe, trigone, medial parietal and frontal lobes, basal ganglia, and the limbic system. The clinical presentation and vascular anatomy of these AVMs is directly related to where along the ventricular system the AVM is located. The most pertinent arterial relationship to AVMs abutting the ventricular system is to the choroidal vascular system. In the temporal lobe, the anterior choroidal branches are the most significant whereas in the trigone branches of the posterior lateral choroidal artery predominate. For AVMs located in the deep thalamocaudate region, branches of posterior medial choroidal artery and deep penetrating branches of the thalamoperforate system provide major arterial supply and are integral to the AVM's treatment. Venous drainage is likewise intimately related to ventricular anatomy with subependymal veins and choroidal veins draining to the internal cerebral veins, thalamostriate veins, and the Galenic system. Because of the numerous vascular variations and anastomoses of the choroidal arterial system in each AVM, complete preoperative angiographic study of this system is essential to understanding the blood supply to and venous drainage from any AVM in juxtaposition to the ventricles. This has great operative significance as the choroidal blood supply to paraventricular AVMs is deep to the AVM and thus surgically difficult to access in the preliminary dissection of the AVM.

Clinical disorders of movement, sensation, and memory are frequent sequelae of AVMs in these areas, and bleeding into the ventricular system that results in hydrocephalus is common. AVMs of the basal ganglia reside below the lateral ventricular system and project deep within the caudate nucleus, internal capsule, and thalamus. In addition to the clinical presentation within a ventricular hemorrhage, disorders of consciousness and memory are more common among these malformations than AVMs in paraventricular or parenchymal locations. Complete neurologic recovery is less frequently encountered due to the greater sensitivity of the brain tissue to injury in these deeper locations.

This group of AVMs is notable for an increased risk of presentation with hemorrhage. This may be due in part to the hemodynamic features of these AVMs that predispose them to bleeding (12). The smaller size of these AVMs may be associated with higher perfusion pressures and thus increased rate of bleeding. Venous drainage into the deep venous system may also increase the risk of both venous hypertension and venous stenosis that is associated with increased rate of bleeding from AVMs. Additionally, these AVMs have a higher incidence of both venous and arterial aneurysms that predisposes them to bleeding. Also, seizures are less common in deep AVMs and thus these lesions may not be detected prior to bleeding as with cortical AVMs, where seizures are more frequently encountered.

Radiographic Evaluation

The cornerstone of evaluation of the patient with a deep AVM is the radiographic analysis of the AVM's anatomy and its relationship to surrounding brain structures. A combination of MRI scanning and cerebral angiography, occasionally with stereoscopic views, provides the necessary anatomic details to analyze the vascular anatomy of the AVM and associated vascular anomalies and to define regional anatomic relationships of the AVM to the brain parenchyma (8). The MRI has been an invaluable aid in determining the operative approach to the AVMs as the relationship with the nidus of the AVM to the ventricular system is well visualized on these studies. Of course, the diagnostic angiogram defines the arterial supply, venous drainage, and associated vascular lesions and suggests whether superselective studies or embolization may be necessary for further treatment. Knowledge of the location of the nidus of the AVM and its relationship to the arterial feeders and venous drainage is critical in designing the optimal operative approach to the AVM as frequently early isolation and cauterization of the arterial feeders where possible and preservation of the venous drainage from the AVM is required to safely resect the malformation. If radiosurgery is to be performed, these angiographic and anatomic features are no less important for the proper delivery of radiation dosimetry to the anatomic boundaries of the AVM nidus and to avoid incorporating normal surrounding brain parenchyma.

Due to the multiplanar views obtainable, the preoperative MRI scan frequently suggests the most efficacious surgical route to the AVM that will ensure adequate exposure of the malformation while simultaneously minimizing injury to the surrounding brain tissue. The relationship of the AVM and the surgical exposure to known functional brain regions, sulci, cerebral fissures, and the presence of associated hematomas can be exploited to select the optimal operative exposure for each AVM. Frequently, this information can be used in conjunction with stereotactic guidance to further ensure the identification of deep or obscure malformations (9).

GENERAL SURGICAL PRINCIPLES AND STRATEGIES

Arteriovenous malformations that occupy the deep paraventricular regions of the brain and basal ganglia require detailed analysis of the risks and benefits of treatment prior to surgical intervention. The possible therapeutic options that may be offered include observation, microsurgical excision, embolization, stereotactic radiosurgery, staged treatments, and multimodality management. The selection process for these modalities requires a thorough understanding of each patient's individual clinical, anatomic, and surgical risk considerations. Complete AVM removal with preservation of neurologic function necessitates a complete understanding of the AVM's operative anatomy and surgical technique and a need to individualize treatment strategy to the specific and individual circumstances of each patient. This requires considerable judgment and experience, given the remarkable variability of this particular class of AVMs.

Perhaps the most critical factor in recommending surgery to these patients is the surgical accessibility of the AVM. Surgical accessibility is predominantly a function of the location of the AVM and the risk of the operative approach to remove it at that location. Adjuncts to enhance the operability of the AVM are preoperative embolization, intraoperative stereotactic or ultrasonic localization, and intraoperative angiography (1,9). Alternatives to surgery may be considered if it is likely that the operative approach will result in incomplete resection of the malformation, injure normal brain structures, or if the patient has already sustained major neurologic damage from the hemorrhage of the AVM. For those circumstances where surgery possesses too grave an operative or clinical risk, radiosurgery can be considered for small AVMs. Those that possess a reasonably regular nidus or geometry and are <3 cm in diameter can help to predict the successful outcome of radiation several years after treatment (4,6). The disadvantage of radiosurgery, such as the inability to protect against rebleeding from the AVM until thrombosis has occurred, and the appreciable failure rate of this technique may be outweighed when the short-term operative risks are prohibitively high.

Some large, bilateral, or diffuse AVMs in these regions will defy all therapeutic options. In these circumstances, the natural history of the disease may be preferable to offering a futile and potentially risk-laden treatment to the patient having such an AVM. Occasionally embolization may be used in inoperable AVMs if associated aneurysms are responsible for bleeding or if occluding deep feeders to the AVM will significantly reduce blood flow to the malformation.

Arteriovenous malformations that are surgically accessible require the selection of an optimal operative approach. The optimal operative approach to this class of AVMs should ensure the following: first, complete exposure of the AVM; second, the shortest distance to the AVM; third, avoidance of functional brain territories; fourth, utilization of hematoma cavities to enhance the operative exposure of the AVM; fifth, attempted single-stage removal of the AVM wherever possible; and finally, utilization of intraoperative localization techniques for AVMs that may be difficult to locate based upon small size deep within the operative exposure. Exposing these AVMs shares much in common with the general principles of AVM surgery (10). Avoidance of venous outflow obstruction reduces pressure in the brain and AVMs. Thus positioning the head above the level of the heart and minimizing rotation of the neck is essential. Positioning the head to view the AVM perpendicular to the operative field

will also facilitate the operative microsurgical dissection. The brain should be as relaxed as possible, and the spinal drainage of 60–100 cm³ of cerebrospinal fluid is routinely employed during the procedure to avoid injury to the brain from retraction to expose the AVM. The use of a beam splitter on the operating microscope allows two surgeons a 3D view of the operative field, and this significantly enhances operative teamwork by allowing one surgeon to work with a cautery and a suction while the second surgeon simultaneously assists with microscissors and retraction. This cosurgeon approach reduces operative fatigue and time and is thus invaluable in most AVM procedures.

In general, AVMs of the frontal, temporal, and parietal regions are approached in the supine or lateral position whereas AVMs in the corpus callosum and thalamocaudate regions are approached in a semi-sitting slouch position. Skin incisions and bone flaps should be extensive so as not to minimize the exposure and retraction required to identify and resect deeply situated AVMs. Of particular importance in intrahemispheric approaches to medial AVMs is that the superior sagittal sinus be fully exposed. This requires the bone flap to cross the midline to the side opposite the AVM to achieve the necessary medial exposure of the sinus and falx. Intraoperative hypotension is used when dealing with small, deep, thin-walled arterial feeding vessels in the white matter at the base of the malformation, and post-resection hypertension may be used to check operative hemostasis in the operating room prior to closure of the wound.

MICROSURGICAL DISSECTION AND PRINCIPLES

Paraventricular AVMs

Arteriovenous malformations involving the anterior aspect of the paraventricular region of the temporal lobe involve the hippocampus and uncus and are supplied predominantly by the anterior choroidal, posterior communicating, and thalamoperforating arteries. Occasionally, there may be minor contributions from the middle cerebral artery as well. These lesions are best approached by a pterional craniotomy in which the Sylvian fissure is opened to identify feeding arteries medial to the AVM and particularly to interrupt branches of the anterior choroidal artery that feed the AVM. Once identification and isolation of the appropriate accessible arterial feeders has been accomplished, the anterior aspect of the temporal lobe, which contains the malformation, can be excised as one would in an anterior temporal lobectomy. The venous drainage is either into sphenoparietal sinus or the veins medial to the temporal lobe, particularly the basal vein of Rosenthal. After circumscribing the interior aspect of the temporal lobe and isolation of all arterial feeders, the draining veins may be interrupted as the final operative step.

Arteriovenous malformations located in the midportion of

the temporal lobe, particularly involving the parahippocampal gyrus and hippocampus, require a posterior temporal craniotomy with exposure of the midtemporal lobe back to the vein of Labbé. The opening should allow access to the floor of the temporal lobe. These AVMs frequently require resection of the inferior temporal gyrus to gain access to the midportion of the hippocampus or parahippocampal gyrus. In the dominant hemisphere, great care must be taken not to resect portions of the inferior or middle temporal gyrus more than 4.5 cm posterior to the anterior temporal tip to avoid postoperative disturbances of language and naming functions. The cortical resection required to expose these AVMs will interrupt the major arterial feeders being received from the inferior branches of the middle cerebral artery and, most importantly, feeders from the inferior temporal branch of the posterior cerebral artery. When the ventricle is entered, the choroid plexus should be heavily cauterized and divided both rostrally and caudally to the AVM. Any branches coming through the choroidal tissue from more distal branches of the anterior choroidal artery can be cauterized at this time. When the nidus of the malformation has been separated from the arterial feeders the deep venous drainage may be interrupted. Venous drainage into the basilar vein of Rosenthal and subependymal veins within the wall of the ventricle is frequently encountered, and they are divided at the conclusion of the operative procedure.

Moving posteriorly in the ventricular system the region of the ventricular trigone is encountered where the temporal and frontal portions of the ventricular system join. Trigonal AVMs are the most deeply situated of ventricular AVMs and three basic operative approaches can be used to access AVMs in this region (2,3,15,16). These routes are the direct transtemporal, parasagittal-interhemispheric, and transcortical parietal occipital approaches. The direction of operative approach to the malformation is dependent on the location of the nidus of the malformation with respect to the trigone and the location of associated arterial feeders, venous drainage, and associated hematoma cavities. In the majority of these malformations are laterally situated and may be approached from the posterior aspect of the temporal lobe through the middle temporal gyrus and occasionally in the nondominant hemisphere through the superior temporal gyrus (Fig. 1). This exposure may be facilitated and directed by lateral cystic hematoma cavities that are frequently associated with these malformations. The arterial supply first encountered is usually from the choroidal fissure of the temporal horn and usually can be interrupted initially. Unlike the case with most parenchymal AVMs, malformations of the trigone are exposed at the more central region of the malformation rather than at the margins of the lesion where the arterial supply enters into it. These malformations drain almost exclusively into the internal cerebral vein system to multiple subependymal veins, some of which may be interrupted early in the operative approach. This can increase risk of intraoperative bleeding due to the interruption of the venous drainage to some sections of the AVM early in the

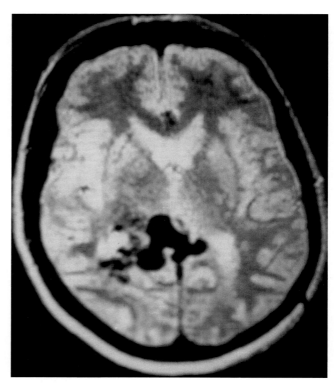

FIG. 1. T2 MRI scan demonstrating an arteriovenous malformation (AVM) lateral to the ventricular trigone with a large medial hematoma cavity.

operative exposure. Occasionally, if the malformation is sufficiently large, the procedure may need to be staged with an operative approach from another direction depending on the projection of the AVM on the brain. As the medial border of the AVM is deep to the operative exposure from the transtemporal route, staging is sometimes necessary for larger malformations. As much of the AVM should be secured as possible, followed at a later stage by an interhemispheric approach to the more medial projection of the malformation. For lesions located on the more posterior aspect of the trigone, a parietal-occipital approach through the superior parietal lobule may be utilized. As the distance is somewhat greater than from the temporal lobe to the trigone, intraoperative ultrasound for identification of the nidus or hematoma cavity or stereotactic localization may be employed. Resection along this route ensures proper identification of the nidus of the malformation without deviation into uninvolved brain regions. Malformations located medial to the trigone of the lateral ventricle present the most difficult operative challenge in these types of AVM. They require a parasagittal-interhemispheric approach in the sitting slouch or prone position. A large horseshoe-shaped skin incision crossing the midline is made to facilitate intrahemispheric exposure. The bone flap must cross the sagittal sinus to allow for retraction of the falx medial to the trigone and medial cerebral hemisphere. Mannitol and spinal drainage are necessary to provide sufficient brain relaxation to expose the interhemispheric fissure. Great care must be taken with superficial cortical parietal veins on the side of the operative approach to prevent postoperative superficial cortical venous infarction. This requires adjusting the operative approach at the time of surgery to take into account the individual variations in the venous drainage from cortex to the sagittal sinus. The lateral retraction of the cerebral hemisphere can be optimized by dissecting sharply along the arachnoid surrounding these veins to improve their mobilization as the brain is retracted. This approach is particularly hazardous because the arterial feeder to these malformations is from the posterior choroidal and posterior cerebral arteries where these vessels come around the cerebral peduncle. At this point the feeding arteries are deep to the nidus of the malformation itself and thus deep to the operative exposure. In addition, venous drainage is to the internal cerebral veins and Galenic system, which is medial to the malformation and is exposed early in the operative approach. Frequently, this approach may be used as part of a staged procedure to a large malformation projecting into this region, which has previously been approached by the transtemporal route.

Arteriovenous malformations located in the paraventricular and splenial region of the corpus callosum are approached in analogous fashion to the parasagittal interhemispheric approach for medial trigonal AVMs (Fig. 2). Patients are placed in the semi-sitting-slouch position and large U-shaped skull incisions are made crossing on the midline to provide adequate exposure of the sagittal sinus. Again, great care must be taken with superficial cortical draining veins to prevent postoperative venous infarction from retraction injury to these veins during the surgery. Normally one self-retaining retractor holding the falx medially and two self-retaining retractors holding the cortex laterally are necessary to achieve adequate deep exposure. Both mannitol and spinal drainage are used to facilitate the safe retraction of the medial cerebral hemisphere. Care must be taken not to put excessive tension on the medial retractor as this may obstruct venous drainage in the sagittal sinus and increase the pressure throughout the cerebral hemisphere. The vessels supplying these malformations come predominantly from the medial and lateral choroidal arteries and distal branches of both the posterior cerebral artery and the anterior cerebral artery. Frequently, these malformations will not only involve splenium and cingulate gyrus but will also extend laterally in the direction of the trigone. The limited retraction that can be placed on the medial parietal lobe impedes access to the lateral aspect of these malformations. Occasionally, a small resection of the cingulate gyrus is necessary to improve operative exposure in this area. The venous drainage is generally deep to the malformation itself into the internal cerebral brain, vein of Galen, or straight sinus and the veins should be ligated after the nidus of the malformation has been resected from the corpus callosum and posterior cingulate gyrus.

Malformations presenting more rostrally in the body of the corpus callosum and the cingulate gyrus are approached

in an analogous fashion to splenial AVMs, except that the skin incision and bone flaps are more rostrally placed. For malformations involving the posterior aspect and body of the corpus callosum, cingulate gyrus, and medial aspect to the parietal lobe, arterial supply is predominantly from the distal branches of the pericallosal and callosal marginal arteries and occasionally from distal branches of the posterior cerebral artery. Venous drainage of these malformations is predominantly along the medial aspect of the hemisphere to the superior sagittal sinus and occasionally to the deep internal cerebral system and the vein of Galen. Care must be taken when retracting the falx and the parietal lobe laterally so that medial venous drainage to the superior sagittal sinus is not compromised in the operative exposure. Involvement with the motor and sensory cortex for AVMs in this location is, of course, of great significance. All brain tissue in this area not directly associated with the malformation should be left undisturbed by the operative resection to prevent postoperative dysfunction of movement or sensation.

Lesions located in the anterior aspect of the corpus callosum and the anterior aspect of the cingulate gyrus on the medial portions of the frontal lobe are approached in an analogous fashion to AVMs on the posterior corpus callosum. The operative approach is an interhemispheric parasagittal one centered at the coronal suture. AVMs in this region are predominantly fed by branches of the anterior cerebral artery with occasional contributions from distal branches in the middle cerebral artery from leptomeningeal collaterals. Venous drainage of these malformations is principally to the superior sagittal sinus and occasionally into the draining ependymal veins going into the deep venous system. As the arterial input to these malformations is predominantly from the anterior aspect of the AVM and the venous drainage is predominantly posterior, these lesions can be circumscribed from a rostral-caudal direction. This will allow sequential isolation of the arterial supply anteriorly and interruption of the draining veins posteriorly as the final stage of the step of the operative procedure. As in AVMs in the body of the corpus callosum, motor and sensory deficits can occur through the lateral retraction of the medial aspects of the frontal and anterior parietal lobes as well as the interruption of the venous drainage in this area. In general, these deficits are transient and resolve several weeks after the operative procedure. Intraoperative functional localization has not significantly affected the surgical technique in managing these malformations as the general principle is to focus on the resection of the malformation with maximum preservation of any uninvolved surrounding cortical or white matter regions in this area not associated with the AVM. For AVMs located beneath the genu of corpus callosum or in the septal and medial frontal regions, an approach by a low bifrontal craniotomy is required. Frequently, a bilateral interhemispheric approach is necessary to adequately expose these malformations as they receive frequent anastomotic arterial supply from both anterior cerebral artery trunks. These lesions frequently drain both to the sagittal sinus superficially

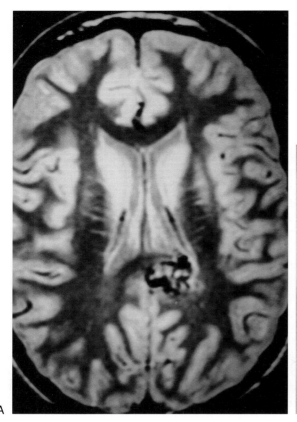
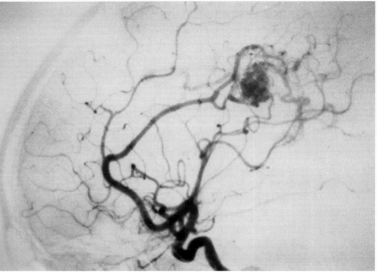

A   B

FIG. 2. A: T2 MRI scan of brain demonstrating the AVM nidus in the splenium of the corpus callosum medial to the ventricular trigone. The interhemispheric approach would provide surgical access to the AVM. **B:** Lateral carotid angiogram revealing distal anterior cerebral pericallosal supply to the AVM with early venous drainage toward the vein of Galen.

and deep into the internal cerebral vein system in the anterior aspect of the third ventricle. Frequent involvement with the hypothalamic and septal area in this region may lead to disturbances of autonomic and electrolyte balance in these patients and requires a careful monitoring during and after the operative procedure.

Thalamocaudate AVMs

AVMs of the thalamocaudate region predominantly occupy the floor of the ventricular system where the caudate nucleus, internal capsule, and thalamus project dorsally. The principal arterial feeders to these malformations are from several sources; however, the majority are fed by branches of the posterior lateral and posterior medial choroidal arteries. More anteriorly situated malformations may receive supply from the anterior choroidal artery, whereas the posteriorly situated malformations may receive branches from the pericallosum as well as penetrating branches from the posterior cerebral artery in the region of the fusiform gyrus. Thalamoperforate arteries entering into the malformations ventrally from the posterior cerebral arteries and basilar apex also feed these malformations. Venous drainage is almost

exclusively into the intraventricular system to the internal cerebral veins, thalamostriate vein, vein of Galen, or straight sinus. The surgical excision of these lesions is predominantly a function of the projection of the malformation to the ependyma of the interior of the ventricular system (5,7,14). Malformations that are deeply situated within the substance of the caudate nucleus, internal capsule, or thalamus are generally treated with stereotactic radiosurgery as normal, critical intervening brain structures would need to be transgressed to achieve visualization of malformations for microsurgical excision. For those malformations presenting to the ventricular surface, their anatomy can be readily visualized with an interhemispheric parasagittal approach as has been previously described. Unlike paraventricular or callosal AVMs, the operative exposure is deeper and requires a larger opening into the corpus callosum to expose the AVM's intraventricular anatomy. The rostral one third of the corpus callosum is generally the preferred route into the ventricle as this is the safest portion of the corpus callosum to section without causing disabling neurologic dysfunction. The incision in the corpus callosum is made not only in a rostral caudal direction but also in a medial to lateral direction so that an elliptical opening is created running a length of 1.5–3 cm on the corpus callosum. This provides adequate exposure in the intraventricular space allowing correct identification of the intraventricular anatomy and the AVM. Great care must be taken when resecting ventral portions of the septum pellucidum as the body of the fornix is located at the base of this structure and injuring the fornix bilaterally will create postoperative short-term memory deficits. When the corpus callosum has been opened, cottonoids may be placed along the opening in the corpus callosum with retractors placed into the ventricle from both the lateral and medial directions. This will give adequate intraventricular exposure, which is necessary to work on the malformation deep within the floor of the ventricular system. Care must be taken not to compress distal branches of the anterior cerebral artery over the corpus callosum during this retraction. AVMs in this location can generally be grouped into an anterior caudothalamic location and posterior caudothalamic or thalamostriate location.

For AVMs located in the anterior caudothalamic location, the relationships to the foramen of Monro, thalamostriate vein, caudate veins, and caudate nucleus are all critical (Fig. 3). Fortunately, AVMs in this location can generally be visualized circumferentially. The AVM must first be mobilized from the caudate nucleus laterally and the region of the foramen of Monro and thalamostriate vein medially along the floor of the ventricle. In this area great care must be taken not to injure the fornix along the anterior border of the foramen of Monro or the genu of the internal capsule laterally at the junction of the caudate nucleus and the rostral aspect of the medial thalamus. Mobilization of the AVM is accomplished by cauterizing and sectioning the thalamostriate and the associated choroid plexus posterior to it. Access may then be gained into the choroidal fissure where the posterior medial choroidal arteries feeding the AVM may be isolated. The lateral aspect of the AVMs may receive arterial inputs through the caudate nucleus from deep penetrating lenticulostriate arteries of the anterior or middle cerebral arteries, and these are separated from more surrounding normal tissue after cauterization of the nidus of the malformation to facilitate exposure of the margins of the malformation deep in the white matter. Ultimately, the AVM may be isolated on its venous drainage into the internal cerebral vein, which will be at the posterior medial border of the malformation.

Posterior caudothalamic AVMs or thalamostriate AVMs are positioned more posterior on the floor of the lateral ventricular system behind the caudate nucleus and may be approached by either the anterior transcallosal approach or by a posterior transcallosal exposure, depending on the location of the nidus of the AVM. When exposure of the nidus of the malformation has been achieved, initial cauterization of the choroidal vessels supplying the malformation is accomplished. Frequently the inferior aspect of the septum pellucidum and fornix ipsilateral on the side of the AVM may be resected in obtaining operative exposure of the malformation if they are involved with the malformation medially. Dissection along the margins of the malformation exposes the posterior aspect of the hippocampus, the posterior limb of the internal capsule, and the dorsal thalamus. Once the

nidus of the malformation has been isolated from the surrounding brain tissue, the deep venous drainage, which is frequently medial the internal cerebral vein, may be exposed and coagulated.

AVMs involving the lateral striate area, such as the globus pallidus, and external capsule require an operative approach through a frontal temporal craniotomy for a trans-Sylvian approach to the insular cortex (14). Malformations that are considered operable in this region project toward the deep recesses of the insular cortex within the Sylvian fissure. It is therefore necessary to open the Sylvian fissure widely to achieve exposure of the insular cortex for malformations that project laterally sufficiently to enable their identification and separation from uninvolved surrounding brain tissue. These malformations are fed predominantly from branches of the middle cerebral artery in the Sylvian fissure, the lateral lenticulostriate vessels of the middle cerebral artery, and occasionally anterior or posterior choroidal feeders along its deep medial borders. Preoperative embolization of the deep medial feeders of the lenticulostriate and choroidal system is a useful adjunct in securing these deep, small arterial feeders because identifying them during the operation is quite difficult. Great care must be taken during the exposure of these malformations not only to identify the exact portion of the insular cortex where the malformation projects superficially but to preserve normal, uninvolved middle cerebral branches that are passing by the nidus of the malformation. Frequently, these lesions drain into the region of the Sylvian fissure; therefore early exposure of their venous drainage must be preserved to prevent occlusion of the drainage if adequate venous collaterals are not present.

POSTOPERATIVE MANAGEMENT AND COMPLICATIONS

The commonly encountered complications in the postoperative period include hemorrhage, stroke, cerebral edema, and hydrocephalus. The most common cause of postoperative bleeding is incomplete resection of the malformation, which may be detected through intraoperative angiography or early postoperative angiography before hemorrhage occurs (1). Any small residual AVM presents a potentially significant risk to the patient and may be managed by repeat operation or radiosurgery, depending on the condition of the patient and the degree of difficulty anticipated in completely removing the remaining AVM if surgery is selected. Other causes of postoperative bleeding include perfusion pressure breakthrough and inadequately secured vessels encountered at the time of surgery. The use of microclips on larger feeding vessels may help to reduce the chance of postoperative bleeding from these sources. If the potential for perfusion pressure breakthrough is anticipated or if significantly elevated postoperative blood pressures are encountered, a period of postoperative blood pressure control with β blockers may be indicated. Postoperative edema from brain retraction

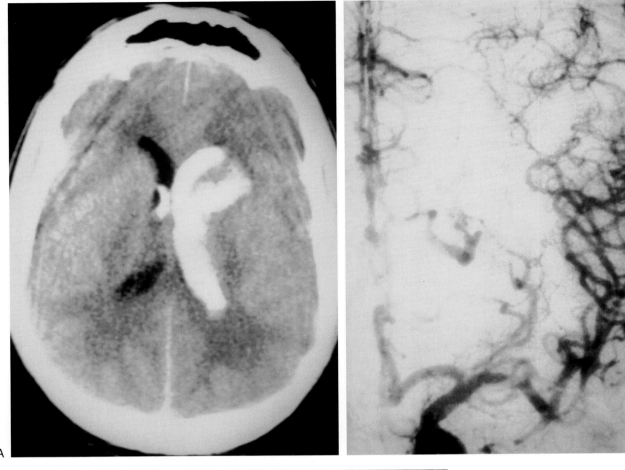

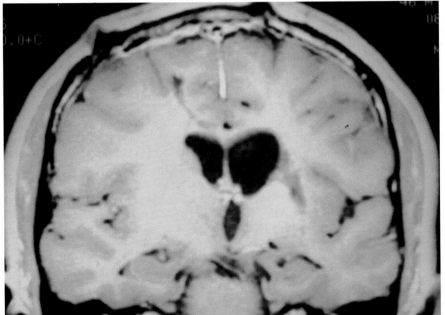

FIG. 3. A: CT scan demonstrating intraventricular hemorrhage with blood in the left caudate nucleus. **B:** Left AP carotid angiogram demonstrating deep lenticulostriate blood supply from the middle cerebral AVM to the small AVM nidus. Note the early venous drainage to the thalamostriate vein indicating the dorsal position of the AVM in the caudate nucleus. **C:** Postoperative coronal T1 MRI revealing resection of the malformation on the floor of the dilated left ventricle. Note the operative approach from the right with a bone flap crossing the midline.

is generally transient and may be treated with corticosteroids. Stroke from interruption of normal vessels is generally recognized from postoperative deficits and CT scans. The prognosis is not as good as for cerebral edema and early institution of rehabilitation may help to potentiate the patient's maximum potential neurologic recovery. Postoperative hydrocephalus may result in bleeding into the ventricles or the obstruction of the flow of cerebrospinal fluid from operative and hemostatic materials placed near the ventricle. This complication can be minimized by placing minimum hemostatic agents within the ventricular system, thereby facilitating the free flow of CSF within the ventricles. Keeping the ventricles free of operative debris and blood may help to reduce not only the short-term risk of hydrocephalus and ventriculitis in the perioperative period, but also the possibility of delayed communicating hydrocephalus months after the operative procedure. Ventricular drainage is particularly useful in the transcallosal approaches to interventricular AVMs for 1–3 days after the operative procedure to prevent acute hydrocephalus. Occasionally intraventricular air will cause alteration in mental status or seizures and this may be prevented by irrigating the air out of the ventricle prior to the dural closure.

All patients should undergo postoperative angiography to document the complete removal of the AVM as small and unexpected residual pieces of the malformation require additional treatment.

OVERVIEW

Arteriovenous malformations of the paraventricular region, corpus callosum, and basal ganglia represent a formidable clinical challenge. The complete removal of such malformations requires an intimate knowledge of the AVM's anatomy and its relationship to cerebral structures that is gleaned from preoperative MRI scans and angiograms. Given each patient's unique set of clinical variables, anatomic relationships, and treatment risk factors, the clinician must select the appropriate therapeutic option or combination of options consisting of observation, microsurgery, embolization, or radiation. To reduce the morbidity of the disease, the treatment regimen and recommended therapy must be individualized for each patient. If surgery is selected, it is anticipated that the malformation can be completely removed with minimal risk to the normal surrounding brain structures. The proper operative approach encompasses the most direct route for the complete exposure of the AVM, minimizes injury to uninvolved areas of the brain, and takes advantage of the AVM's hemorrhage to expose and separate the AVM from surrounding brain tissue. Prior to or during operative intervention the use of embolization and stereotactic localization and the identification of associated vascular anomalies is critical. For small, surgically inaccessible AVMs, radiosurgery should be considered. For certain large, bilateral, or diffuse lesions, particularly in patients who have been neurologically devastated by hemorrhage from the AVMs, only observation and supportive treatment can be offered.

REFERENCES

1. Barrow DL, Boyer KL, Joseph GJ. Intraoperative angiography in the management of neurovascular discorders. *Neurosurgery* 1992;30: 153–159.
2. Barrow DL, Dawson R. Surgical management of arteriovenous malformations in the region of the ventricular trigone. *Neurosurgery* 1994; 35:1046–1054.
3. Batjer JJ, Samson D. Surgical approaches to trigonal arteriovenous malformations. *J Neurosurg* 1987;67:511–517.
4. Friedman WA, Bova, FJ. Linear accelerator radiosurgery for arteriovenous malformations. *J Neurosurg* 1992;77:832–841.
5. Lawton MT, Hamilton MG, Spetzler RF. Multimodality treatment of deep arteriovenous malformations: thalamus, basal ganglia, and brain stem. *Neurosurgery* 1995;37:29–36.
6. Lunsford LD, Kondziolka D, Flickinger JC, Bissonette DJ, Jungreis CA, Maitz AH, Horton JA, Coffey RJ. Stereotactic radiosurgery for arteriovenous malformations of the brain. *J Neurosurg* 1991;75: 512–524.
7. Malik GM, Umansky F, Patel S, Ausman JI. Microsurgical removal of arteriovenous malformations of the basal ganglia. *Neurosurgery* 1988;23:209–217.
8. Sisti MB, Kader A. Stein BM. Microsurgery for 67 intracranial arteriovenous malformations less than 3 cm in diameter. *J Neurosurg* 1993; 79:653–660.
9. Sisti MB, Solomon RA, Stein BM. Stereotactic craniotomy in the resection of small arteriovenous malformations. *J Neurosurg* 1991;75: 40–44.
10. Solomon RA, Stein BM. Surgical management of arteriovenous malformations that follow the tentorial ring. *Neurosurgery* 1986;18:708–714.
11. Solomon RA, Stein BM. Interhemispheric approach for the surgical removal of thalamocaudate arteriovenous malformations. *J Neurosurg* 1987;66:345–351.
12. Spetzler RF, Hargraves RW, McCormick PW, Zabramski JM, Flom RA, Zimmerman RS. Relationship of perfusion pressure and size to risk of hemorrhage from arteriovenous malformations. *J Neurosurg* 1992;76:918–923.
13. Stein BM. Arteriovenous malformations of the medial cerebral hemisphere and the limbic system. *J Neurosurg* 1984;60:23–31.
14. Tew JM, Lewis AI, Reichert KW. Management strategies and surgical techniques for deep seated supratentorial arteriovenous malformations. *Neurosurgery* 1995;36:1065–1072.
15. U HS. Microsurgical excision of paraventricular arteriovenous malformations. *Neurosurgery* 1985;16:293–303.
16. U HS, Kerber CW, Todd MM. Multimodality treatment of deep periventricular cerebral arteriovenous malformations. *Surg Neurol* 1992; 38:192–203.

Cerebrovascular Disease, edited by H. Hunt Batjer.
Lippincott-Raven Publishers, Philadelphia © 1997.

CHAPTER **64**

Intracranial Dural Arteriovenous Fistula

Nicholas S. Little and David G. Piepgras

Dural arteriovenous fistulas (DAVFs) or dural arteriovenous fistulous malformations (DAVFMs) describe a lesion that consists of one or more fistulous connections within the dura mater. Those who propose the term DAVFM do so because the lesions often comprise more than one fistula (1–4), whereas those who prefer DAVF believe that the term malformation implies that the lesions are congenital when in fact the majority are almost certainly acquired (5–7). This chapter will deal with lesions thought to be acquired, not known congenital lesions such as vein of Galen malformations.

DAVFs are commonly described with respect to the venous sinus to which they are related or the anatomic location of the fistula. Several further classification and grading systems have been described and will be discussed. Treatment options have included carotid/jugular compression therapy, feeder ligation, surgical excision, angiographic embolization, and, more recently, radiosurgery. The type of therapy recommended for each lesion depends on location and characteristics of the fistulae themselves.

Between 1931 and 1994 over 400 patients with DAVF were reported and are thought to represent 10–15% of cranial AVMs (8). Both anterior fossa and tentorial DAVF are twice as common in men than in women, in contrast to dural carotid-cavernous and transverse/sigmoid fistulae, which have a female predominance (3). Of reported cases, >50% are related to the transverse/sigmoid whereas the next most common site is the cavernous sinus. Anterior fossa/falx, tentorial incisura, and sagittal sinus/convexity are among less common regions and comprise <10% of cases each. Multiple fistulae may occur either concurrently or at different times in the same patient (9). Direct carotid-cavernous fistulae with flow from the internal carotid artery (ICA) into the surrounding cavernous sinus is a well-known complication of skull base fracture and penetrating injury and, less commonly, rupture of a cavernous carotid

aneurysm. These are not included in this discussion of dural-based AVF.

ETIOLOGY

Most DAVFs are believed to be acquired and idiopathic (1,2,5). The minority of cases appear to be related to a specific factor such as trauma, surgery, infection, or dural sinus thrombosis. The site and characteristics of the fistula may provide a clue to the particular etiology.

Trauma with associated skull fracture has been reported to lead to DAVF. These are usually linear fractures of the vault that cross the superior sagittal, transverse, or sigmoid sinus (10,11). Cranial surgery, like trauma, has been reported to predispose to DAVF (12,13). There have been several reports in the literature of DAVF in association with meningiomas. These were either noted prior to tumor removal or seen postoperatively. Their colocation close to venous sinuses may have been coincidental but more likely causally related. It is likely that these fistulae developed as a result of meningioma-induced sinus thrombosis (at least partial) or possibly as a result of a tumor angiogenic factor (14–17).

Infection of the cranial air sinuses, notably mastoid and sphenoid, have been reported to precede sinus thrombosis and subsequent fistula development. In cases of idiopathic DAVF, especially that associated with sinus thrombosis, a condition of preexisting procoagulant state, such as exists with antiphospholipid antibody syndrome, should be suspected.

Some pathologic studies of DAVF demonstrate the presence of thrombosis in association with DAVF (18). Whether thrombosis is a cause or an effect of coexistent flow abnormalities is still controversial. The prevailing view holds that fistulae develop as a secondary phenomenon to sinus thrombosis, due to the opening up of small physiologic AV pathways in the wall of the sinus or abnormal connections forming during recanalization (19,20). Others believe that

N. S. Little and D. G. Piepgras: Department of Neurological Surgery, Mayo Clinic, Rochester, MN 55905

thrombosis might be an epiphenomenon that can occur at any stage of the fistula progression and might be due to stenosis and thickening of sinus walls leading to turbulence and subsequent thrombosis (21). This theory is supported by the fact that neither thrombosis, stenosis, or occlusion is present in all patients with fistula. The observation that spontaneous cures may occur secondary to thrombosis also implies that thrombosis is, at least in some cases, a later phenomenon.

Experimental studies in rats with a carotid-jugular fistula venous hypertension model have shown the development of DAVF in several of these animals (22). This again suggests that thrombosis is not a necessary intermediary. The heterogeneity of fistulas in location, complexity, and relative involvement of a venous sinus (or in many cases only the wall of the sinus) suggests that multiple etiologies are likely responsible for fistula formation. The possibility that local angiogenic factors may be involved in the fistula evolution is intriguing but until now has not been demonstrated.

Syndromes associated with vascular fragility such as fibromuscular dysplasia, neurofibromatosis type 1, and Ehlers–Danlos syndrome have all been associated with dural AV fistulae of the spine or cranium (5,23,24).

CLASSIFICATION

A universal scheme to classify DAVFs has not been accepted yet. All proposed systems rely largely on the angiographic features, most notably the venous system characteristics.

Factors considered in most grading systems include the following:

Presence/absence venous stenosis or occlusion
Direction of flow, either anterograde or retrograde
Presence of cortical leptomeningeal venous drainage
Aneurysm (especially on the venous side)
Single/multiple fistulae
Fistula involving sinus/wall of sinus

A recent and relatively straightforward grading system has been proposed by Borden et al (25) in which there are three main types with two subtypes each.

Type 1 DAVFs drain directly into dural sinuses or meningeal veins.
Type 2 are similar to type 1 but also have retrograde drainage into subarachnoid veins.
Type 3 drain exclusively in a retrograde fashion through subarachnoid veins.

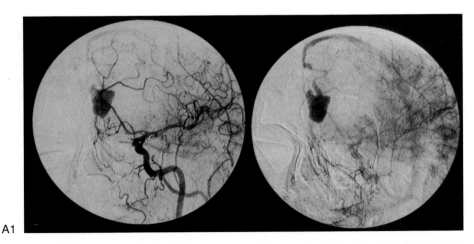

A1

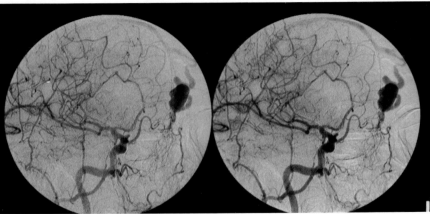

A2

FIG. 1. A: Common carotid angiograms (left and right oblique views) from a 55-year-old patient with headache. These demonstrate a subfrontal cribriform region dural arteriovenous fistula (DAVF) fed predominantly by ethmoidal branches of the ophthalmic arteries. There is a large intradural varix as part of the pial venous drainage to the superior sagittal sinus.

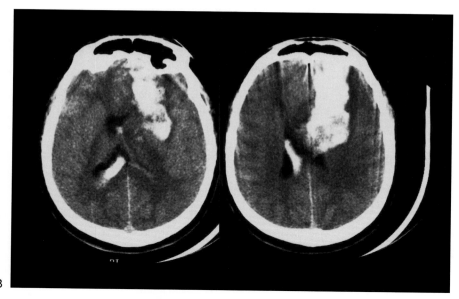

B

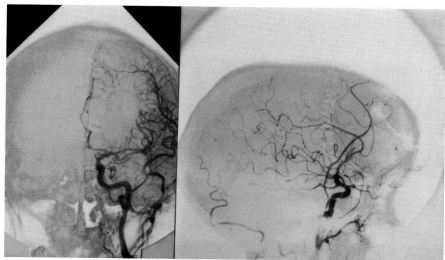

C

FIG. 1. B: A CT scan of the same patient 1 year later showing a large left frontal intracerebral hemorrhage that resulted from rupture of the untreated DAVF. The patient recovered from the hemorrhage and after delayed referral underwent craniotomy and intradural disconnection of the draining vein. **C:** Postoperative anteroposterior and lateral common carotid angiogram confirming complete obliteration of the fistula.

The presence of single or multiple fistulae further indicates subtype A or B, respectively. In the intracranial lesion the presence of subarachnoid venous drainage appears to be the single determinant of the risk for hemorrhage. Essentially if there is no cortical venous drainage, the risk of hemorrhage is negligible. If subarachnoid drainage exists, then the risk of hemorrhage becomes significant and likely increases with the presence of other factors such as venous stenosis/occlusion and venous aneurysms. It is interesting to note that although leptomeningeal venous drainage is an established risk factor for hemorrhage of cranial DAVF, this is not the case with spinal DAVF. Intradural hemorrhage from a spinal DAVF with medullary draining veins is extremely rare.

It is the angiographically determined venous characteristics of the fistula that determine risk for hemorrhage, not simply location per se. It has been recognized that fistulae involving the anterior fossa and tentorial incisura are at greater risk for hemorrhage owing to their propensity for drainage through leptomeningeal veins (1,18,25,26) (Fig. 1). In general, fistulae involving the cavernous sinus and transverse/sigmoid sinus tend to have a more benign course as their venous drainage is usually contained within the sinus. However, no lesion or location is immune from hemorrhage or other serious complications, if there is progression to cortical venous drainage or major intracranial venous hypertension. Awad in a review of the literature claimed that all fistulae with an aggressive neurologic course had at least one of three features (1):

Leptomeningeal retrograde venous drainage
Variceal or aneurysmal venous structures
Galenic venous drainage

These features are present in the majority of cases at the tentorium or anterior falx, rarely in dural cavernous AVF, and variably in fistula at other sites (27–30). Other grading schemes have been proposed by Djindjian (31), Lasjaunias

(29), Piton (32), and Lalwani et al (33). All are angiographically based grading systems similar to the aforementioned.

The Barrow system of classification of carotid-cavernous fistulae is well accepted (34) and will not be discussed further except to mention that origin of arterial supply is emphasized and has implications for therapy. Dural cavernous AVF usually present with eye symptoms and signs including pain, diplopia, and scleral venous dilatation. In chronic cases they may jeopardize vision due to increased intraocular tension. Natural history is usually favorable and these lesions in particular have a high rate of spontaneous cure presumably through thrombosis (which may be associated with transient paradoxical worsening of eye signs).

PATHOPHYSIOLOGY

In several histologic series the site of the fistula was demonstrated to be in the wall of the involved sinus. This appeared to be a common finding in the presence of direct sinus luminal involvement as well as fistulae that drained via other pathways. Associated sinus thrombosis was an inconsistent finding (4,18,35). Fistulae may have a high or low flow and unilateral or bilateral supply, neither of which correlate with the risk for hemorrhage (1). Fistulae not involving the lumen of the associated sinus may have an increased likelihood of leptomeningeal venous drainage attributed to venous outflow recruitment (36).

Demyelination in the vicinity of distended leptomeningeal veins has been demonstrated in pathologic studies, presumably secondary to venous hypertension (37). The histologic characteristics of the draining vein are similar to those seen in AVM vessels with thickening and sometimes mineralization of the vessel wall.

Reversal of flow and venous hypertension in leptomeningeal draining veins account for the majority of neurologic manifestations (29). Nonhemorrhagic manifestations may include global and/or focal deficit, which may be transient or progressive, seizures, papilledema, and headache. Cervical myelopathy may occur due to venous hypertension affecting the spinal cord through medullary veins distant from the cranial DAVF (38) (Fig. 2).

As already stated, hemorrhage from a DAVF occurs almost exclusively from those lesions with leptomeningeal draining veins. Bleeding is thought to arise from the venous side of the malformation, there being an increased risk if there is aneurysmal dilatation of the vein or accompanying venous outflow stenosis and/or thrombosis.

CLINICAL FEATURES

DAVF may present in a number of ways primarily related to the site of the fistula, the magnitude of flow, and the mode of venous drainage. The angiographic and radiographic features usually correlate with presentation. Occasionally they are asymptomatic and found incidentally (39). Due to the heterogeneity of presentation, a high index of suspicion must be maintained to guide investigation in those patients with subtle clinical signs and radiologic findings.

Hemorrhage is the most devastating and feared complication. As already discussed, its risk is predicted by the venous anatomy of the fistula. Intracranial hemorrhage is typically manifested by sudden, severe headache, possible loss of consciousness with or without neurologic deficit. It may mimic other causes of intracranial hemorrhage such as aneurysm and potentially be overlooked on conventional carotid and vertebral angiography, which does not include the external carotid system. The site of the hemorrhage may be intraventricular, intraparenchymal, subarachnoid, or subdural and may be distant from the DAVF nidus (25). Several authors suggest that the risk of early recurrent bleeding from DAVF is high (1,26,29).

Pulse synchronous tinnitus or bruit is the most common presenting symptom. It is frequently associated with transverse/sigmoid location and as such is more likely to be associated with a benign course. However, other symptoms and signs related to venous hypertension may be present. Large, high-flow fistulae with minimal venous obstruction characteristically have loud bruits that may interfere with patients sleep. On auscultation they may be heard over the entirety of the cranium. Small, low-flow fistulae may have soft bruit only heard with direct auscultation in the ipsilateral mastoid/retromastoid area. It is necessary to exclude transmitted bruit from the heart and cervical vessels; therefore the whole cranium along with neck and chest must be examined.

Various compressive maneuvers of the extracranial vessels may change the character of the bruit. It has been advocated as first-line therapy for some fistulae, but this would seem contraindicated in those lesions with risk factors for hemorrhage, especially cortical venous drainage. Direct compression of the carotid and/or jugular vein on the ipsilateral side may act to decrease the bruit intensity. In some cases of transverse/sigmoid region fistulae, compression of the occipital artery (often hypertrophied) will produce a diminution of the bruit.

A sustained change in the character or intensity of the bruit may herald a change in the nature of the fistula. This may occur spontaneously following angiography or compressive maneuvers. Change or disappearance of the bruit does not necessarily mean obliteration of the fistula and may in some cases signal development of alternate venous pathways such as via leptomeningeal veins. Therefore any changes in the bruit of a benign DAVF warrants reevaluation of the lesion and probably is an indication for repeat angiography.

Headache is a common complaint of patients with DAVF. They may localize to the side of the fistula or be generalized and may be multifactorial in their origin. Possible mechanisms for headache with DAVF include dural distension at the fistula site, brain edema secondary to venous hypertension, hydrocephalus, fifth nerve compression/ischemia, and

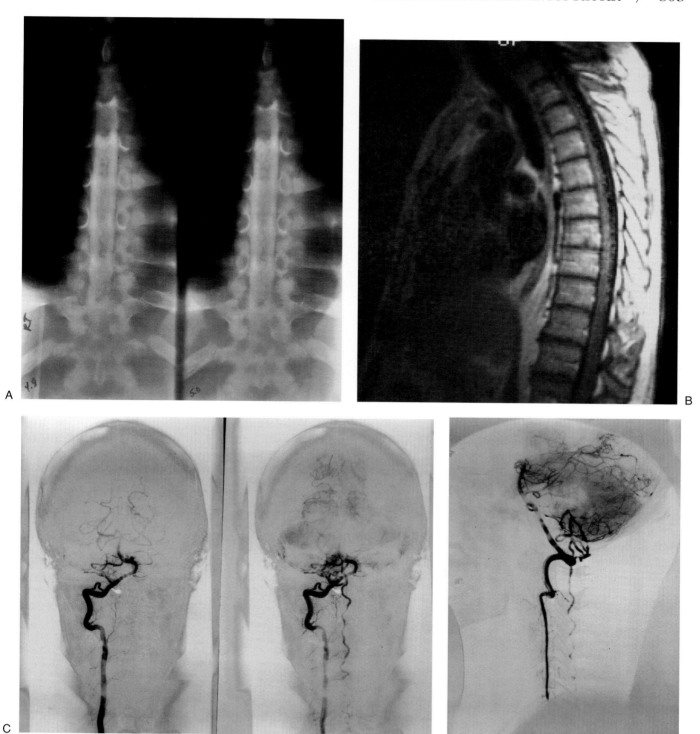

FIG. 2. **(A)** Tomographic myelogram (anteroposterior view) and **(B)** sagittal MRI in a patient with progressive cervical-thoracic myelopathy. **(C)** Anteroposterior and lateral vertebral angiograms showing early venous drainage from the posterior fossa and descending along the posterior aspect of the cervical cord. The responsible lesion was a dural-based arteriovenous fistula (AVF) located on the right side of the foramen magnum with venous drainage exclusively onto the spinal cord at the cervicomedullary junction. Disconnection of the draining vein from the site of the AVF resulted in angiographically confirmed obliteration of the AVF and reversal of the myelopathy.

inflammation secondary to ongoing thrombosis and hemorrhage.

Hydrocephalus is an uncommon finding of DAVF and is usually due to venous sinus hypertension leading to a disturbance of cerebrospinal fluid absorption. Rarely it may result from aqueductal obstruction by a dilated galenic venous system or venous aneurysm. Repeated small episodes of subarachnoid hemorrhage may also lead to arachnoid fibrosis and resulting decrease in cerebrospinal fluid absorption (15,40,41).

Dementia, presumably secondary to the effects of venous hypertension, has been reported to improve following obliteration of the DAVF, an observation shared in our case material. In these cases, diffuse white matter changes on MRI have been demonstrated preoperatively (42).

A pseudotumor-like syndrome with normal brain CT, papilledema, and symptoms of increased intracranial pressure occurs rarely. This also likely due to the result of impaired intracranial venous outflow (21,43).

Cranial nerve palsies may also result due to various mechanisms. In dural cavernous AVF, mechanical factors may limit globe motility and mimic extraocular nerve palsy; however, true nerve palsies may occur at this and other sites. An arterial steal phenomenon has been suggested and palsies have been shown to improve with reduction of the shunt (34). Improved function may also result from a decrease in venous hypertension postembolization. Actual compression by the pathologically dilated draining veins may also be a rare cause of nerve dysfunction. Lasjaunias et al reported a visual field deficit secondary to direct compression of the optic apparatus by engorged olfactory veins draining a frontal dural AVF (29).

DIAGNOSIS

The mainstay in the diagnosis of cranial DAVF is cerebral angiography with selective internal carotid, external carotid, and vertebral injection. The condition is especially important to consider in cases of "idiopathic" subarachnoid hemorrhage investigated by internal carotid and vertebral injections only. Such a scenario is illustrated in the case portrayed in Fig. 3. In DAVF the angiogram is crucial in determining diagnosis, prognosis, and treatment. The angiographic features constitute the basis for the various proposed grading schemes that have already been discussed.

Other standard neuroradiographic investigations in descending order of utility are MRI/MRA, CT scan, and plain skull X ray.

MRI is of great value in showing the extent, if any, of brain parenchymal abnormality. It is most sensitive in evaluating hemorrhage, ischemia, and edema of the brain (Figs. 4 and 5). MRI will show characteristic dilated and tortuous draining veins that may exist in both the subarachnoid cisterns and over the hemispheres as well as venous aneurysms (Fig. 6). Dilated veins within the parenchyma are strongly suggestive of DAVF with venous hypertension. MRI is less useful in the diagnosis of subarachnoid hemorrhage. At present magnetic resonance angiography (MRA) is not of sufficient resolution to fully characterize the lesion but will often indicate the location and extent of the fistula (44). MRI/MRA may be normal in a significant number of cases but in general is a useful adjunct to angiography in diagnosis and guiding treatment (45).

CT scanning may reveal the same abnormalities as seen on MRI but, except for detection of subarachnoid hemorrhage, has decreased sensitivity for demonstrating other pathologic changes.

Skull X ray may show enlarged vascular grooves in the calvarium but adds little to the evaluation for this condition.

TREATMENT

The decision to treat a DAVF depends on both the clinical profile and the angiographic characteristics. A lesion that is "benign" both clinically and angiographically may warrant no treatment and just observation. Fistulae with troubling but not medically serious symptoms such as pulsatile tinnitus, and an angiogram showing no cortical venous drainage may not demand treatment. Alternatively, a trial of noninvasive and potentially less definitive therapy such as compression or partial embolization may be appropriate. A significant number of benign DAVF will spontaneously thrombose, occasionally following angiography (7,46). Patients with hemorrhage and/or neurologic deficit, as well as those with angiographically determined risk factors, require definitive therapy.

Therapeutic options are arterial vascular compression, endovascular therapy, direct surgery, radiosurgery, or a combination of these. In general, the angiographic features guide the selection of the most appropriate techniques.

The most amenable site for treatment with compression therapy are the cavernous sinus and lateral/sigmoid sinuses. Manual carotid/jugular compression in the neck by the patient is appropriate as first-line therapy in cases of carotid-cavernous fistula where there is no contraindication and the natural history is considered to be favorable. Although benefit is unpredictable, compression therapy has been associated with obliteration of these lesions, which also tend to have the highest incidence of spontaneous remission (11). Transverse/sigmoid fistulae will often have a large supply via the occipital artery and other external carotid branches. Manual compression of this vessel in the retromastoid region by the patient for periods of up to 30 minutes has led to obliteration of the fistula in a surprising number of patients reported by Halbach et al (7). Concomitant ipsilateral jugular compression may be an important factor in promoting fistula thrombosis. Compressive maneuvers are contraindicated in patients whose lesions show risk factors of hemorrhage.

Embolization has contributed greatly to the overall management of DAVF. It may be employed as a single therapy to achieve permanent thrombosis, to reduce flow for symptom

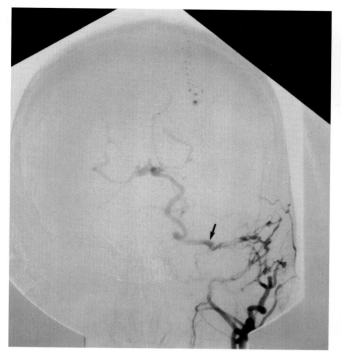

A1

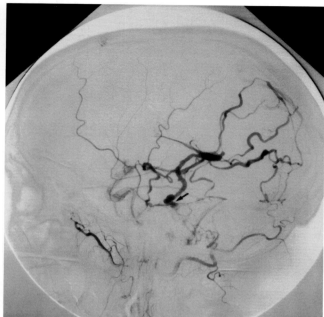

A2

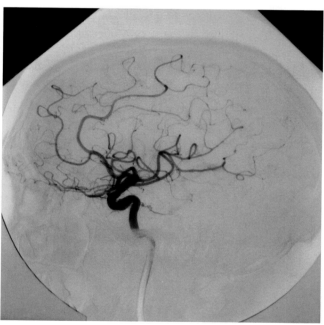

B

FIG. 3. A: Anteroposterior and lateral views, selective left external carotid angiograms in a patient suffering two subarachnoid hemorrhages. There is external carotid artery supply to a petrous arteriovenous fistula that drains into the deep venous system through a single subarachnoid draining vein. **B:** The single lateral view of the left internal carotid artery study shows an enlarged tentorial branch of the meningohypophyseal trunk that also contributed to the fistula. Complete obliteration of the fistula and cure of the patient was achieved by operative subtemporal intradural approach to the petrous apex and division of the draining vein. Postoperative angiogram confirmed complete obliteration of the fistula.

palliation, or as an adjunct therapy preoperatively. Both transvenous and transarterial approaches may be utilized and a variety of agents including glue, particulate matter, and endovascular coils may be appropriate. If complete thrombosis and cure of the fistula is to be achieved, it is necessary that the thrombosis occur immediately at the fistula site and necessarily the proximal venous egress. In general, for transarterial embolization, the closer the site of occlusion to the actual fistula site, the greater the chance of success in obliterating the fistula. Proximal arterial occlusion or ligation is

highly unlikely to provide cure or lasting palliation due to the likelihood of collateral development and is mentioned only to be condemned.

With arterial embolization, consideration and care must be given to avoiding ischemic injury to the cranial nerves and brain parenchyma. Pre-embolization testing with lidocaine has been advocated to assess risks for damage to neural structures. Characteristics of the embolic agents such as particle size and glue set rate are factors affecting both safety and efficacy of embolization therapy. Potential complica-

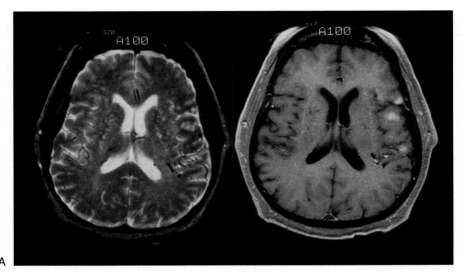

A

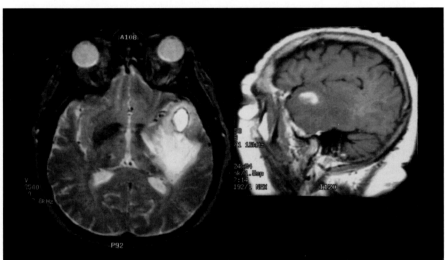

B

FIG. 4. A: T1- and T2-weighted axial MRI scans of a 60-year-old man presenting with seizures and dysphasia. The erroneous diagnosis at this time was lacunar infarction. Intracerebral dilated veins in the posterior temporal region are readily apparent. **B:** T2-weighted axial and parasagittal MRI scans of the same patient 2 months later after continuing seizures, progressive dysphasia, and right hemiparesis. There is now marked left temporal edema with focal hemorrhage.

tions include inadvertent arterial embolization of the brain arteries; however, a greater concern is thrombosis of venous drainage without occlusion of the fistula resulting in cerebral hemorrhage. Hydrocephalus has been reported as a complication of several cases involving embolization of the galenic venous system (47).

Transvenous embolization is most likely to be successful in those cases in which the normally existing venous flow has been either obliterated or reversed (48). If there is normal directional flow from the parenchymal veins into an involved sinus, this route should not be used for fear of complications related to acutely sacrificing normal venous drainage. Routes for transvenous embolization may be via femoral vein catheterization or by direct surgical exposure of the involved sinus or tributary. An example of the latter is the operative exposure of the superior ophthalmic vein to pass coils into a dural cavernous fistula as described by Mullan (49). Similarly, a burr hole over the transverse sinus or torcula may allow direct access for packing of the involved sinus. Patients with

low-flow, low-risk, uncomplicated fistulae are generally not candidates for transvenous therapy. In all cases there must be concern that venous or sinus thrombosis at a site other than the fistula itself may aggravate venous hypertension and increase risk for cerebral hemorrhage.

Direct operative treatment of DAVF has included local packing, complete excision of the fistula, isolation of the fistula, or disconnection of arterialized leptomeningeal venous drainage from the site of the AVF. Currently surgery is often facilitated by preoperative embolization. Prior to the use of adjuvant embolization, particularly for large transverse/sigmoid sinus fistulae, surgery carried increased morbidity and risks of mortality due to major blood loss (50).

Especially in cases of complex fistulae of the transverse/sigmoid DAVF with multiple arterial feeders and extensive retrograde venous drainage, excision of the fistulous segment constitutes the most definitive treatment option. However, anatomic and pathologic/angiographic features of fistulae may preclude such therapy. Fistulae located in the

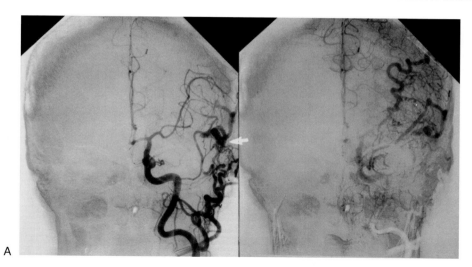

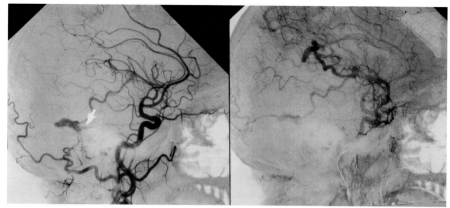

FIG. 5. Anteroposterior and lateral views, left common carotid angiogram of the patient shown in Fig. 4. There are changes consistent with major left temporal mass secondary to a small transverse sinus–based DAVF draining into the vein of Labbé (site of the fistula indicated by arrows). Surgical disconnection of the draining vein from the fistulous site was easily accomplished with gradual resolution of the patient's signs and symptoms.

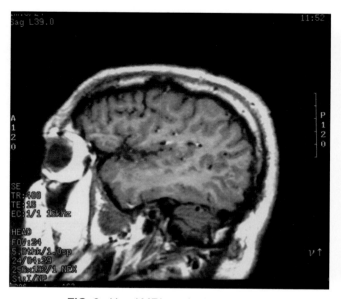

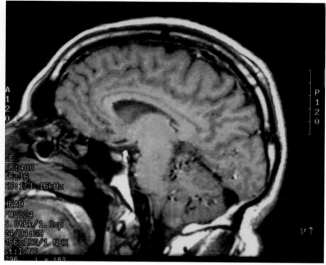

FIG. 6. Head MRI, sagittal views of lateral and midline regions demonstrating dilated intracerebral veins secondary to venous hypertension. Common carotid angiogram showed a transverse dural arteriovenous fistula with sinus occlusion and retrograde sinus drainage that was felt to be the etiology for venous hypertension.

cavernous sinus or in the wall of a patent sagittal sinus or torcula would be inappropriate for complete excision. Adequate collateral venous pathways must be present if complete excision of the fistulous segment is to be accomplished with safety.

For simple AV fistulae, particularly those with a single draining vein, simple disconnection of the draining vein from the site of the fistula constitutes safe and effective therapy. Such treatment not only is effective in relieving the venous hypertension and preventing serious neurologic consequences but usually will induce complete thrombosis of the fistula itself (27,51). Such treatment is appropriate for those fistulae with arterialized leptomeningeal veins with retrograde flow. Example cases are demonstrated in Figs. 1–5.

Early experience with radiosurgery as definitive treatment for DAVF has been encouraging. This treatment modality has special appeal for those fistulae that because of location (eg, cavernous sinus or jugular bulb) are difficult to treat via embolization or surgery alone (52). In selected cases radiosurgery has produced obliteration of most DAVF after 12–24 months (6,20,53). For patients with troubling symptoms related to flow or venous hypertension, arterial embolization *after* radiosurgery can reduce inflow and thereby possibly reduce risks for hemorrhage until obliteration occurs. Decrease of inflow will also diminish symptoms and signs such as pulsatile tinnitus or those related to orbital and ophthalmic venous congestion.

CONCLUSION

Dural-based AV fistulae are rare and often complex lesions. They may have a favorable or highly dangerous natural history depending on their specific characteristics, particularly their venous dynamics. Most of the lesions with hazards for hemorrhage and neurologic impairment can be successfully treated but may require multidisciplinary modalities. In the less straightforward cases or if uncertainty exists regarding their nature or best treatments, referral to an experienced cerebrovascular surgery team is highly appropriate.

REFERENCES

1. Awad IA, Little JR, Akrawi WP, et al. Intracranial dural arteriovenous malformations: factors predisposing to an aggressive neurological course. *J Neurosurg* 1990;72:839–850.
2. Barnwell SL, Halbach VV, Dowd CF, et al. Complex dural arteriovenous fistulas: results of combined endovascular and neurosurgical treatment in 16 patients. *J Neurosurg* 1989;71:352–358.
3. Cognard C, Gobin YP, Pierot L, et al. Cerebral dural arteriovenous fistulas: clinical and angiographic correlation with a revised classification of venous drainage. *Radiology* 1995;194: 671–680.
4. Findlay JM, Mielke BW. Fatal rebleeding from a dural arteriovenous malformation of the posterior fossa: case report with pathological examination. *Can J Sci* 1994;21:67–71.
5. Bahar S, Chiras J, Carpena JP, et al. Spontaneous vertebro-vertebral arteriovenous fistula associated with fibromuscular dysplasia. *Neuroradiology* 1984;26:45–49.
6. Chandler HC, Friedman WA. Successful radiosurgical treatment of a dural arteriovenous malformation: case report. *Neurosurgery* 1993; 33(1).
7. Halbach VV, Higashida RT, Hieshima GB, et al. Dural fistulas involving the transverse and sigmoid sinuses: results of treatment in 28 patients. *Radiology* 1987;163:443–447.
8. Luessenhop AJ. Dural arteriovenous malformations. In: Wilkins RH, Rengachary SS, eds. *Neurosurgery*. New York: McGraw-Hill, 1986: 1473–1477.
9. Kuwayama N, Takaku A, Nishijima M, et al. Multiple dural arteriovenous malformations. Report of two cases. *J Neurosurg* 1989;71: 932–934.
10. Dennery JM, Ignacio BS. Post-traumatic arteriovenous fistula between the external carotid arteries and the superior longitudinal sinus: report of a case. *Can J Surg* 1967;10:333–336.
11. Halbach VV, Higashida RT, Hieshima GB, et al. Dural fistulas involving the cavernous sinus: results of treatment in 30 patients. *Radiology* 1987;163:437–442.
12. Nabors MW, Azzam CJ, Albanna FJ, et al. Delayed postoperative dural arteriovenous malformations. Report of two cases. *J Neurosurg* 1987; 66:768–772.
13. Pappas CT, Zabramski JM. Iatrogenic arteriovenous fistula presenting as a recurrent subdural hematoma. Case report. *J Neurosurg* 1992; 76(1):134–136.
14. Davie JC, Hodges F. Arteriovenous fistula after removal of meningioma. Case report. *J Neurosurg* 1967;27:364–369.
15. Sawamura Y, Janzer RC, Fankhauser H, et al. Arteriovenous malformation in meningothelial meningioma: case report. *Neurosurgery* 1991; 29(1).
16. Ugrinovski J, Vrcakovski M, Lozance K. Dural arteriovenous malformation secondary to meningioma removal. *Br J Neurosurg* 1989;3: 603–608.
17. Yokota M, Tani E, Maeda Y, et al Meningioma in sigmoid sinus groove associated with dural arteriovenous malformation: case report. *Neurosurgery* 1993;33(2).
18. Nishijima M, Takaku A, Endo S. Etiological evaluation of dural arteriovenous malformations of the lateral and sigmoid sinuses based on histopathological examinations. *J Neurosurg* 1992;76:600–606.
19. Houser OW, Campbell JK, Campbell RJ, et al. Arteriovenous malformation affecting the transverse dural venous sinus-an acquired lesion. *Mayo Clin Proc* 1979;54:651–661.
20. Mironov A. Pathogenetical considerations of spontaneous dural arteriovenous fistulas. *Acta Neurochir* 1994;131(1–2):45–58.
21. Lamas E, Lobato RD, Espaerza J, et al. Dural posterior fossa AVM producing raised sagittal sinus pressure. Case report. *J Neurosurg* 1977; 46.
22. Terada T, Higashida R, Halbach V, et al. Development of acquired arteriovenous fistulas in rats due to venous hypertension. *J Neurosurg* 1994;80:884–889.
23. Deans WR, Bloch S, Leibrock L, et al. Arteriovenous fistula in patients with neurofibromatosis. *Radiology* 1982;144:103–107.
24. Schievink WI, Piepgras DG. Cervical vertebral artery aneurysms and arteriovenous fistulae in neurofibromatosis type 1: Case reports. *Neurosurgery* 1991;29:760–765.
25. Borden JA, Wu JK, Shucart WA. A proposed classification for spinal and cranial dural arteriovenous fistulous malformations and implications for treatment. *J Neurosurg* 1995;82:166–179.
26. Martin NA, King WA, Wilson CB, et al. Management of dural arteriovenous malformations of the anterior cranial fossa. *J Neurosurg* 1990; 72:692–697.
27. Grisoli F, Vincentelli F, Fuchs S, et al. Surgical treatment of tentorial arteriovenous malformations draining into the subarachnoid space. *J Neurosurg* 1984;60:1059–1066.
28. Ito J, Imamura H, Kobayashi K, et al. Dural arteriovenous malformations of the base of the anterior cranial fossa. *Neuroradiology* 1983; 24:149–154.
29. Lasjaunias P, Chiu M, Ter Brugge K, et al. Neurological manifestations of intracranial dural arteriovenous malformations. *J Neurosurg* 1986; 64:724–730.
30. Terada T, Kikuchi H, Karasawa J, et al. Intra cerebral arteriovenous malformation fed by the anterior ethmoidal artery: case report. *Neurosurgery* 1984;14:578–582.

31. Djindjian R, Cophignon J, Theron J. Embolization by superselective angiography from the femoral route; review of 60 cases: technique, indications, complications. *Neuroradiology* 1973;6:20–26.

32. Piton J, Guile MH, Guibert-Traniel F, et al. Fistules du sinus lateral. *J Neuroradiol* 1984;11:143–159.

33. Lalwani AK, Dowd CF, Halbach VV, et al. Grading venous restrictive disease to predict the clinical presentation and guide therapy in patients with dural arteriovenous fistulas of the transverse/sigmoid sinus. *J Neurosurg* 1993;79:11–15.

34. Barrow DL, Spector RH, Braun IF, et al. Classification and treatment of carotid-cavernous sinus fistulas. *J Neurosurg* 1985;62:248–256.

35. Hinokuma K, Ohama E, Ikuta F, et al. Dural arteriovenous malformations with abnormal parenchymal vessels: an autopsy study. *Acta Neuropathologica* 1990;80(6):656–659.

36. Barnwell SL, Halbach VV, Higashida RT, et al. A variant of arteriovenous fistulas within the wall of dural sinuses. Results of combined surgical and endovascular therapy. *J Neurosurg* 1991;74:199–204.

37. Friede RL, Shubiger O. Direct drainage of extracranial arteries into the superior sagittal sinus associated with dementia. *J Neurol* 1981;225:1–8.

38. Wrobel CJ, Oldfield EH, Di Chiro G, et al. Myelopathy due to intracranial dural arteriovenous fistulas draining intrathecally into spinal medullary veins. Report of three cases. *J Neurosurg* 1988;69:934–939.

39. Aminoff MJ, Kendall BE. Asymptomatic dural vascular anomalies. *Br J Radiol* 1973;46:662–667.

40. Hirono N, Yamadori A, Komiyama M, et al. Dural arteriovenous fistula: a cause of hypoperfusion-induced intellectual impairment. *Eur Neurol* 1993;33(1):5–8.

41. Kuhner A, Krastel A, Stoll W. Arteriovenous malformations of the transverse venous sinus. *J Neurosurg* 1976;45:12–19.

42. Zeidman S M, Monsein L H, Aroserena O, et al. Reversibility of white matter changes and dementia after treatment of dural fistulas. *AJNR* 1995;16(5):1080–1083.

43. Gelwan MJ, Choi IS, Berenstein A, et al. Dural arteriovenous malformations and papilledema. *Neurosurgery* 1988;22(6)Part 1.

44. Chen JC, Tsuruda JS, Halbach VV, et al. Suspected dural arteriovenous fistula: results with screening MR angiography in seven patients. *Radiology* 1992;183(1):265–271.

45. De Marco JK, Dillon W, Halbach VV, et al. Dural arteriovenous fistulas: evaluation with MR imaging. *Radiology* 1990;175:193–190.

46. Newton TH, Hoyt WF. Dural arteriovenous shunts in the region of the cavernous sinus. *Neuroradiology* 1979;1:71–81.

47. Halbach VV, Higashida RT, Hieshima GB, et al. Treatment of dural fistulas involving the deep cerebral venous system. *AJNR* 1989;10:393–399.

48. Halbach VV, Higashida RT, Hieshima GB, et al. Transvenous embolization of dural fistulas involving the transverse and sigmoid sinuses. *AJNR* 1989;10:385–392.

49. Mullan S. Treatment of carotid cavernous fistulas by cavernous sinus thrombosis. *J Neurosurg* 1979;50:131–144.

50. Sundt TM, Piepgras DG. The surgical approach to arteriovenous malformations of the lateral and sigmoid dural sinuses. *J Neurosurg* 1983;59:32–39.

51. Thompson GB, Doppman JL, Oldfield EH. Treatment of dural arteriovenous fistula by interruption of leptomeningeal venous drainage. *J Neurosurg* 1994;80:617–623.

52. Hidaka H, Terashima H, Tsukamoto Y, et al. Radiotherapy of dural arteriovenous malformation in the cavernous sinus. *Radiat Med* 1989;7(3):160–164.

53. Coffey RJ, Link MJ, Nicholls DA, et al. The role of radiosurgery and particulate embolization in the treatment of dural arteriovenous fistulas. *J Neurosurg* 1996;84:804–809.

Cerebrovascular Disease, edited by H. Hunt Batjer.
Lippincott-Raven Publishers, Philadelphia © 1997.

CHAPTER **65**

Technical Features of the Management of Arteriovenous Malformations of the Brainstem and Cerebellum

Duke S. Samson, Thomas A. Kopitnik, Jr., H. Hunt Batjer, and Phillip D. Purdy

GENERAL BACKGROUND

Arteriovenous malformations (AVMs) of the vertebral basilar system located in the cerebellum or brainstem are relatively uncommonly vascular anomalies and represent approximately 15–20% of all intracranial parenchymal arteriovenous malformations (1–5). Malformations of the brainstem and cerebellum have been generally considered as similar lesions because of their common subtentorial location and close proximity, although they have relatively distinct natural histories and vary in their clinical presentations. There are significant differences with regard to vascular anatomy and parenchymal representation between cerebellar and brainstem AVMs, and for this reason they should be considered as separate and distinct pathologic entities. Cerebellar malformations are four to five times as common as those of the brainstem, and although large cerebellar AVMs may encroach on the middle cerebellar peduncle, experience suggests that in most instances AVMs of the vertebral basilar system are sharply circumscribed in either the cerebellar or the brainstem parenchyma. Thus, the preoperative performance and evaluation of high-quality imaging studies, including magnetic resonance imaging (MRI) and selective cerebral angiography, are critical in the planning and execution of operative procedures directed at AVMs located in the posterior fossa. It is essential that the surgeon develop a three-dimensional conceptual awareness of the location of the AVM and its relationship to surrounding and overlying neural structures prior to surgery. Precise determination of the location, number, and size of feeding arterial branches and draining vascular channels is of paramount importance. This requirement may necessitate the repetition of preliminary angiographic studies, especially when performed in the presence of significant cerebellar hematomas that compress, obscure, or distort the angiographic nidus of the vascular malformation. The use of superselective angiography has been especially useful in determining the precise vascular contribution of each feeding arterial pedicle leading to the AVM. This has generally been accomplished with superselective catheterization of each major feeding vessel to the AVM during preoperative embolization (Fig. 1).

AVMs of the posterior fossa, including both brainstem and cerebellar locations, frequently present with spontaneous hemorrhage (1,2,4,6). There is some controversy as to whether AVM size can be used as a factor in determining the propensity for the lesion to hemorrhage. Several reports have noted that small AVMs present with hemorrhage more frequently than large AVMs (7,8), although small AVMs may often remain asymptomatic except for hemorrhage, especially with lesions in the cerebellum. Others have found no relationship between size and risk of subsequent hemorrhage (9,10). When spontaneous hemorrhage is the presentation of a posterior fossa AVM, the initial goal of acute management should be treatment of significant mass effect or hydrocephalus. Definitive surgical therapy of the malformation should be deferred if possible for a period of 6–8 weeks from the time of the last hemorrhage to allow parenchymal swelling to decrease and some liquification of the hematoma to occur. There is a small subpopulation of patients who present with life-threatening intraparenchymal hematomas and require immediate surgical attention and clot de-

D. S. Samson and T. A. Kopitnik Jr.: Department of Neurological Surgery, The University of Texas, Southwestern Medical Center, Dallas, Texas 75235.

P. D. Purdy: Department of Radiology, The University of Texas, Southwestern Medical Center, Dallas, Texas 75235.

H. H. Batjer: Division of Neurosurgery, Northwestern Medical School, Chicago, IL 60611.

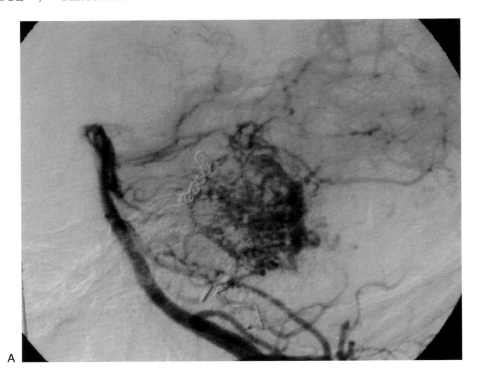

A

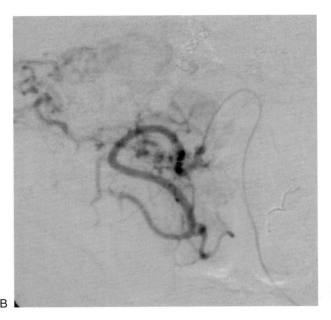

B

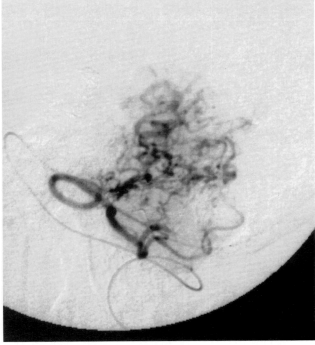

C

FIG. 1. Vertebral angiogram of cerebellar arteriovenous malformation with **(A)** partial embolization of superior cerebellar artery (SCA) and posterior inferior cerebellar artery (PICA) feeding, **(B)** anteroposterior, and **(C)** lateral superselective catheterization of large anterior inferior cerebellar artery (AICA) feeder prior to AICA embolization.

compression. The surgical goal during acute emergency surgery for posterior fossa mass effect from an AVM hematoma should be subtotal removal of clot and relief of associated mass effect without an attempt being made to disturb or remove the AVM (Fig. 2). Patients treated with hematoma evacuation can be subsequently managed medically until there is both clinical and radiographic evidence of resolution

of the initial hemorrhage and any associated mass effect. Definitive radiographic studies can then be performed as required as the patient becomes clinically stable.

Preliminary endovascular embolization of cerebellar and, to a lesser extent, brainstem AVMs represents an important adjunct to surgical treatment that has made atraumatic resection of almost all posterior fossa malformations simpler and

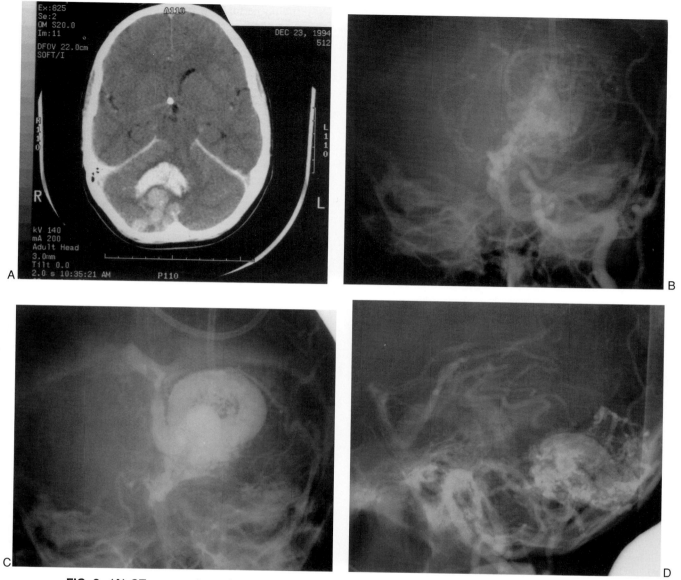

FIG. 2. (A) CT scan and vertebral angiogram **(B)** anteroposterior (arterial phase), **(C)** anteroposterior (venous phase), **(D)** lateral (arterial phase), of patient presenting with life-threatening posterior fossa hematoma from cerebellar hemispheric arteriovenous malformation.

more straightforward (11,12). The overwhelming majority of infratentorial malformations are amenable to at least partial devascularization by embolization, which in our unit is routinely performed several days prior to definitive operation. Unfortunately, malformations located in the brainstem are problematic because of their unique arterial supply and are not optimal candidates for preliminary embolization due to the high risk of resultant hemorrhage or brainstem infarction in our experience. Currently, we restrict embolization of brainstem AVMs to lesions with a large angiographically demonstrable arterial supply that are not deemed amenable to complete surgical resection due to location.

SURGICAL PRINCIPLES AND STRATEGIES

The basic tenets of AVM surgery in the posterior fossa are no different from those applied to the more common malformations located in the supratentorial space. A balanced anesthetic technique with attention to normotension and reduction of intracranial pressure is employed and preliminary provision made for the infusion of large volumes of colloid, crystalloid, and blood, if necessary. In general, patients are operated on in the lateral, park bench, prone, or Concorde position, as will be discussed in regard to individual AVMs. The sitting position, which previously was favored for malformations in the posterior fossa, is generally avoided because of hemodynamic risk and surgeon fatigue during protracted operative procedures. We prefer to use a relatively large bony exposure to aid in early identification of the vascular anatomy and facilitate exposure of the feeding and draining vessels at some distance from the nidus of the AVM. Surgically, attention is focused early in the procedure to the isolation of the afferent arterial supply and a rigorous attempt is made to preserve all draining veins until the malformation dissection has been completed. Microsurgical spiral or circumferential dissection of the periphery of the malformation, regardless of its location, is a basic tenet of surgical removal of these lesions. Careful attention to hemostasis in the periependymal area is required where

very friable perforating vasculature is easily ruptured and difficult at times to control. The use of small aneurysm clips is invaluable in obtaining hemostasis in the periependymal region for most AVMs.

Immediate postoperative angiography is recommended in all cases of AVM resection to document complete resection of the AVM and prepare for appropriate diagnosis and early treatment of any postoperative complication, including hemorrhage. We perform postoperative angiography prior to termination of general anesthesia and re-explore the resection site immediately in the event residual AVM is angiographically apparent.

Malformations of the cerebellum are anatomically divisible into lesions of the cerebellar hemisphere, the vermis, and

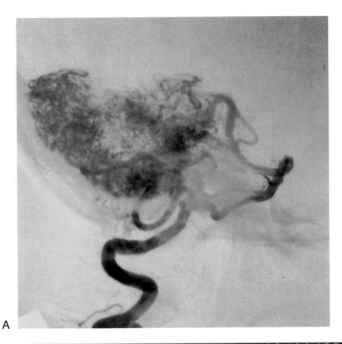

A

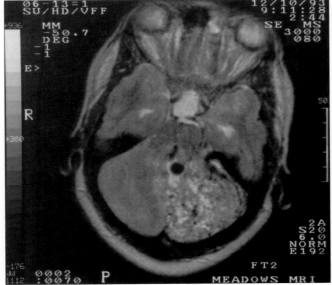

B

FIG. 3. (A) Lateral vertebral angiogram, **(B)** axial MRI, and **(C)** sagittal MRI of patient with large holohemispheric cerebellar arteriovenous malformation.

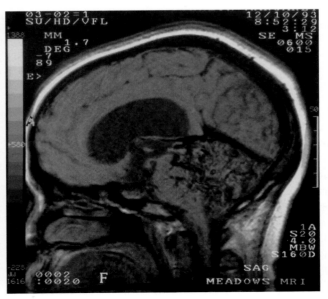

C

the tonsils, with vermian and hemispheral lesions being by far the most common (13). Malformations of the cerebellar hemisphere may vary in size from quite small to very large lesions with dramatic blood flow (Fig. 3). The arterial supply of these malformations is almost always unilateral in nature and frequently includes contributions from both the superior cerebellar (SCA) and posterior inferior cerebellar arteries (PICA), both of which may be the site of associated and sometime symptomatic arterial aneurysms. If on the preoperative arteriogram the anterior inferior cerebellar artery (AICA) can be demonstrated to supply the malformation, MRI studies will most commonly demonstrate involvement of not only the cerebellar hemisphere but the lateral aspect of the roof of the fourth ventricle and the adjacent middle cerebral peduncle. Venous drainage of large cerebellar AVMs is often via both the lateral hemispheric veins and the midline vermian venous plexus (Fig. 4).

Surgical Management of Malformations of the Cerebellar Hemisphere

When surgically treating AVMs of the cerebellar hemisphere superior to the major horizontal fissure, positioning the patient in the Concorde position coupled with a large superiorly located bony exposure will provide a wide operative approach that does not usually necessitate the use of normal brain tissue retraction (14). In more laterally or inferiorly placed lesions we have employed the lateral position with a large laterally situated bone flap that exposes the transverse and sigmoid sinuses. The initial approach to cerebellar hemispheric AVMs should be to identify and divide the arterial supply as early as possible in the operative procedure. When the AICA is a major source of arterial supply, the artery can be most reliably identified at or near the foramen of Luschka. The AICA should be followed into the brain parenchyma to the margin of the malformation prior to sacrifice to avoid possible ischemia to the lateral pons or middle cerebellar peduncle. After the primary feeding vessels to the AVM have been identified and divided, the dissection is optimally started on the medial margin of the malformation with subsequent circumferential dissection. Retraction of the AVM nidus in a lateral direction will lift the malformation out of the hemisphere and avoid retraction of the normal cerebellar tissue. Dissection in this manner essentially hinges the AVM on the lateral venous pedicle and permits access to the anterior pial margins through the brain by elevation and dissection of the deepest portion of the malformation. Because AVMs of the cerebellar hemisphere, regardless of their size, infrequently have ventricular representation, it is unnecessary to routinely expose the ependyma and open the fourth ventricle unless preoperative radiographs suggest periependymal involvement.

Surgical Management of Malformations of the Vermis

Vermian malformations, on the other hand, very commonly involve the roof of the fourth ventricle and in some cases extend into the ventricular chamber. AVMs of the cerebellar vermis receive arterial supply from the SCA and PICA and often, if not always, have bilateral arterial supply. Venous drainage is usually primarily via the vermian venous plexus with secondary lateral venous drainage across the cerebellar hemisphere into the petrosal vein or directly superior into the Galenic system (Fig. 5).

The Concorde position coupled with an extensive midline bony exposure provides an excellent view of these malformations and their attendant vasculature. Opening of the arachnoid over the cisterna magnae early in the surgical exposure permits the cerebellum to be gently displaced into the inferior aspect of the posterior fossa and facilitates exposure of the superior vermis without the use of cerebellar retraction. When surgically resecting AVMs of the cerebellar vermis, we initially expose the SCA feeders on the superior surface of the cerebellar hemisphere. These vessels should be followed into the vermis and the nidus of the malformation prior to sacrifice to prevent infarction of the cerebellar nuclei. Branches of the PICA supplying vermian AVMs can typically be accessed at the medial margins of the cerebellar tonsils near the midline. The very high frequency of bilateral PICA feeding should be kept in mind, especially if the AVM remains turgid after occlusion of all other recognized arterial input.

Once the major feeding vessels have been accessed, the cerebellar vermis can be opened in the sagittal plane and circumferential dissection of the malformation begun. With a long vermian incision, potentially harmful cerebellar retraction can often be avoided and the malformation can be gently displaced away from the site of dissection. If the malformation remains turgid following seemingly complete circumferential dissection, inspection of the vermian venous pedicle will often demonstrate branches of the SCA entering the malformation within the arachnoid sheath of the superior venous drainage. Sequential identification and sacrifice of these vessels will permit further collapse and atraumatic resection of the nidus of the AVM. Because of the frequency that the fourth ventricular wall is involved with vermian malformations it is necessary to open the roof of the fourth ventricle in almost each case. After the fourth ventricle has been entered, the floor of the ventricle should be carefully marked with cottonoid strip and following resection of the AVM the ventricular wall carefully inspected to ensure that residual malformation is not present.

Surgical Management of Malformations of the Tonsils

Malformations located in the cerebellar tonsil are the third variety of cerebellar AVMs. In our experience these are relatively limited in size and most commonly present with subarachnoid and intraventricular hemorrhage (Fig. 6). Tonsillar malformations produce problems in exposure only if the surgeon fails to appreciate their very caudal location and the necessity for a wide opening of the foramen magnum and

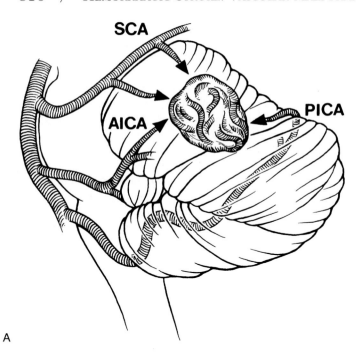

A

FIG. 4. Blood supply to arteriovenous malformations (AVMs) of the cerebellar hemisphere. **(A)** Artist schematic of potential sources of supply. **(B)** Lateral vertebral angiogram demonstrating SCA, AICA, and PICA supply. **(C)** AP vertebral angiogram. **(D)** Axial MRI. **(E)** Sagittal MRI. All demonstrate involvement of middle cerebellar peduncle with AVM nidus.

occasional resection of the ring of the atlas. Our general approach to lesions within the cerebellar tonsil has been with positioning the patient in the lateral position with a low paramedian incision and an extensive, inferiorly located, suboccipital craniectomy. After opening the cisterna magna, the obex and floor of the fourth ventricle are identified and protected with a surgical cotton strip and the involved cerebellar tonsil is elevated to identify the lateral and posterior medullary segments of the feeding PICA. The artery is then followed to its entry into the tonsil with sequential sacrifice of the enlarged perforating vessels entering the nidus and ultimate clipping of the PICA vessel itself is performed as it terminates in the AVM. If necessary, a limited incision in the caudal aspect of the inferior vermis will provide additional exposure of the rostral aspect of the cerebellar tonsil. With sacrifice of the feeding artery, it is most expeditious to simply resect the involved tonsil along with the AVM nidus. This is accomplished by displacing the tonsil laterally and sequentially cauterizing the inferior vermian veins, which generally represent the malformation's sole venous outflow.

Surgical Management of Malformations of the Brainstem

Arteriovenous malformations of the brainstem, to include the mesencephalon, pons, medulla, floor of the fourth ventricle, and cerebellopontine (CP) angle, are rare lesions that can present with subarachnoid or intraparenchymal hemorrhage or a variety of fluctuating neurologic signs and symptoms mimicking a demyelination process (2,15,16). Even those malformations that initially come to clinical attention because of episodic neurologic deficits are prone to hemor-

rhage if their diagnosis and treatment is delayed, and in general, the natural history of these malformations as a group appears to be relatively ominous (17). Anatomically, malformations of the brainstem are best divided into two separate and relatively distinct groups: (a) brainstem AVMs with a superficial or pial representation, and (b) brainstem AVMs located within the parenchymal or deep-brain substance. Although no significant difference in the clinical presentation of these two types has yet to be identified, from a conceptual and therapeutic point of view they are quite distinct.

Superficial AVMs of the brainstem are typified by brainstem AVMs that occur in the CP angle. These are located on the lateral aspect of the pons and can be entirely epipial in location or have a variable degree of parenchymal involvement, including extension into the foramen of Luschka. As a rule, these malformations are supplied from arterial branches derived from enlarged AICA that enter the malformation directly in the subarachnoid space. Superficial brainstem AVMs within the CP angle usually have no deep penetrating arterial supply to the depths of the AVM. The venous drainage of these lesions is via lateral pontine veins, which also occupy the subarachnoid space of the CP angle and ultimately drain to the Galenic or petrosal systems. The presence of the enlarged afferent and efferent vasculature, the pial presentation of the malformation itself, and the surrounding and associated cranial nerves make for a potentially confusing and crowded CP angle during attempts at microsurgical exposure. Malformations such as these are routinely approached with the patient in the true lateral position with the head positioned lateral with respect to the floor. The bony exposure is carried lateral to the sigmoid sinus to permit slight elevation of the posterior aspect of the sinus and ensure maximal access to the CP angle cistern. The cistern

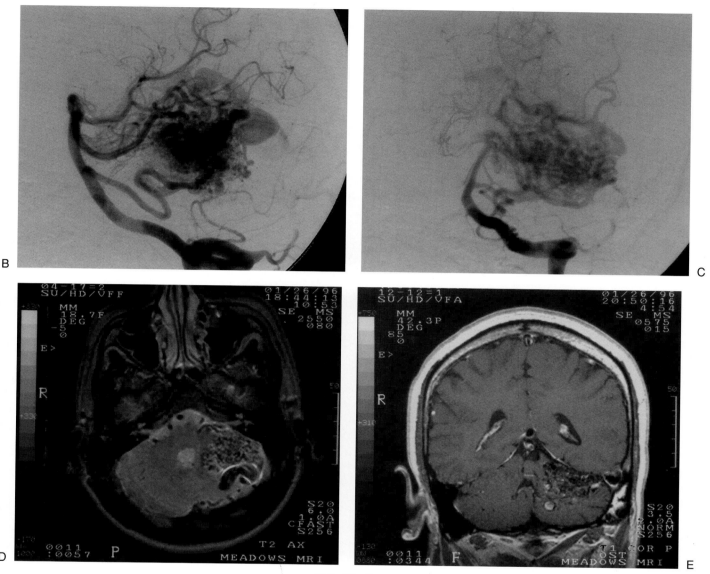

FIG. 4B–E.

of the angle is widely opened from the level of the vertebral artery to the petrosal vein, with evacuation of spinal fluid from the cisterna magna providing additional nontraumatic exposure. Although sequential sacrifice of the feeding branches of the malformation is the ideal initial step during resection, the nature of the anatomic puzzle in the CP angle often precludes preliminary circumnavigation of the lesion. In this situation, the posterior aspect of the malformation, at the junction of the brainstem and cerebellum, can be identified and the malformation can be gently dissected from its bed in the subpial space with sequential occlusion of the marginal entering arteries. This approach is possible because of the superficial location of almost all such brainstem AVMs and requires sequential elevation and lateral retraction of the nidus as it is undercut by the microsurgical exposure. Such an approach permits sequential cauterization of

the entering arteries and will preserve the venous drainage until the malformation has been completely elevated. Often displacement of the associated cranial nerves is necessary for visualization of the entire circumference of the malformation and postoperative transient cranial nerve palsies are quite common, although almost never permanent.

A similar conceptual approach used for brainstem AVMs of the CP angle can be applied to superficial malformations located in the region of the tectal plate, the anterior or lateral aspect of the cerebral peduncles, or to the rare AVM found on the lateral aspect of the medulla. Preoperative confirmation of the superficial nature of these malformations by high-quality MRI scans is a mandatory prerequisite for treating this type of lesion. Superficially located AVMs of the brainstem have an entirely different operative risk than AVMs within the parenchyma of the brainstem.

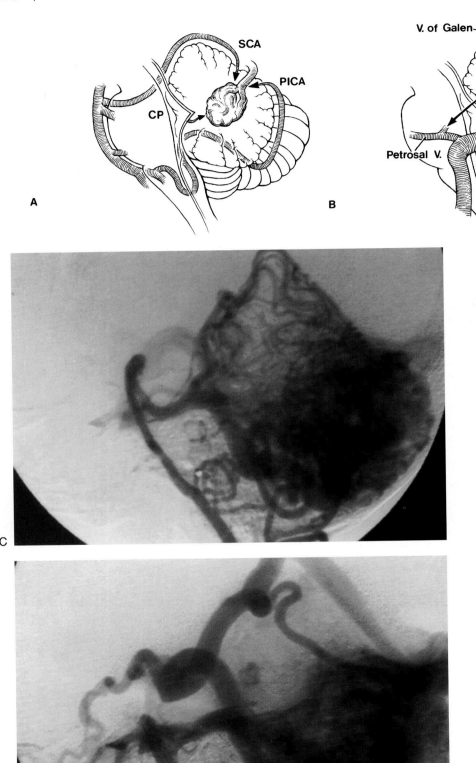

FIG. 5. Blood supply to vermian arteriovenous malformations (AVMs). **(A)** Artist's schematic of potential arterial supply and **(B)** venous drainage. Lateral vertebral angiogram **(C)** arterial, **(D)** venous, of large vermian AVM.

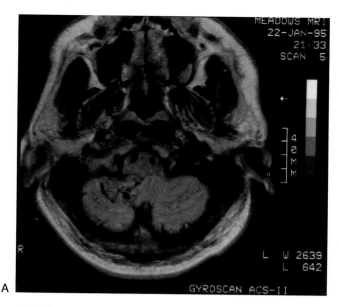

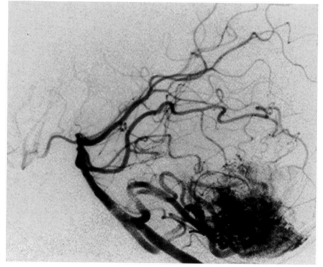

FIG. 6. Arteriovenous malformation of cerebellar tonsil. **A:** Axial MRI. **B:** Lateral vertebral angiogram. **C:** Anteroposterior vertebral angiogram.

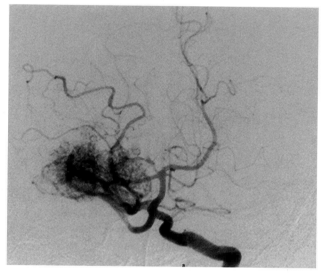

Deeply located or parenchymal lesions of the anterior basis pontis, medullary and pontine floors of the fourth ventricle, and the deeper aspect of the cerebellar peduncles and midbrain represent a second and distinct type of brainstem malformation. These lesions uncommonly present with subarachnoid hemorrhage and more frequently come to clinical attention because of progressive neurologic syndromes more commonly seen with demyelinating disorders or intrinsic gliomas of the brainstem. These lesions receive their arterial input directly from perforating vessels of the parent vertebral and basilar systems and are uncommonly fed by distal branches of the superior cerebellar, anterior inferior cerebellar, or posterior inferior cerebellar arteries. The afferent supply to these malformations enters the lesion on the ventral or parenchymal aspect and most commonly passes through the normal brainstem en route to the malformation (Fig. 7). The venous drainage of deep parenchymal brainstem AVMs

is principally by intraventricular ependymal veins draining into the Galenic system. These malformations are unique because of their intimate association with brainstem parenchyma and because of their deep arterial supply, which cannot be accessed beyond the border of the arteriovenous malformation itself. The small size and coexisting normal brainstem distribution of these vessels makes preoperative embolization difficult and dangerous. In a similar manner, surgical resection of these malformations is fraught with risk to essential midbrain, pontine, and medullary structures. Occasionally, when a small lesion of this type is associated with a prior intraparenchymal hemorrhage, the lesion may be amenable to complete surgical resection with no significant neurologic sequela because the associated hematoma cavity may provide access to the malformation without significant resection of normal brainstem tissue. Unfortunately, the usual degree of surgical trauma and iatrogenic ischemia ne-

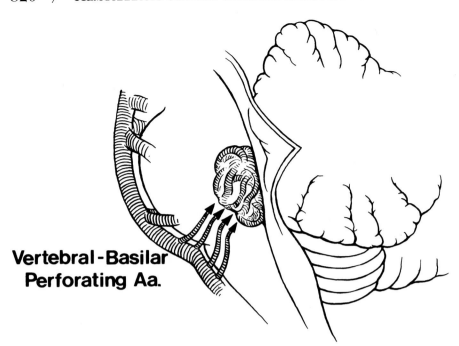

Vertebral-Basilar Perforating Aa.

FIG. 7. Artist's schematic of potential arterial supply to brainstem arteriovenous malformations.

cessitated by the resection of a parenchymal brainstem malformation produces significant, if not disabling, neurologic morbidity.

When surgical treatment is deemed necessary, these lesions can be approached via the previously mentioned hematoma cavity or via the margins of the malformation itself without an attempt being made to address the feeding vessels initially. Under high-power magnification the lateral borders of the lesion must be carefully identified and the lesion sequentially cauterized and circumferentially dissected until the deep penetrating arterial supply can be identified and divided. Such an approach is most frequently attended by considerable and persistent arterial bleeding that can only be managed by cautery, tamponade, and persistent dissection. The deeper structures of the brainstem must not be transgressed in an attempt to transect the arterial feeding beyond the margins of the malformation. In general, patients with parenchymal brainstem AVMs are poor candidates for microsurgical resection and should be considered candidates for stereotactic focused radiation.

SUMMARY

At the University of Texas Southwestern Medical Center from 1977 through 1995, we have surgically managed 103 malformations of the posterior fossa, 23 of which were located in the brainstem. Selective preoperative embolization has been performed in 60% of the cases and routinely employed over the past 8 years. Of these 103 patients, 100 have had complete resection of their AVM and management mortality has been 6% with management morbidity of 8%. This surgical experience suggests that AVMs of the cerebel-

lum (hemispheres, vermis, tonsils) and AVMs of the superficial or pial aspect of the brainstem, most especially those presenting in the cerebellopontine angle, are good candidates for surgical resection with relatively low morbidity and mortality. On the other hand, microsurgical resection of deep or parenchymal AVMs of the mesencephalon, pons, and medulla is attended by prohibitively high morbidity and mortality. These intrinsic brainstem malformations, which receive their exclusive arterial input from perforating branches of the parent vertebral and basilar arteries, cannot be reliably accessed or dissected without attendant injury and ischemia to surrounding brainstem structures and should only be considered as surgical candidates in the presence of a demonstrable adjacent hematoma cavity. Routine preoperative embolization facilitates the management of almost all AVMs of both cerebellum and brainstem and should be considered an intrinsic part of the treatment protocol.

REFERENCES

1. Batjer H, Samson D. Arteriovenous malformations of the posterior fossa: clinical presentation, diagnostic evaluation, and surgical treatments. *J Neurosurg* 1986;64:849–856.
2. Drake CG, Friedman AH, Peerless SJ. Posterior fossa malformations. *J Neurosurg* 1986;64:1–10.
3. Garcia MR, Alvarez H, Eoulou A, et al. Posterior fossa arteriovenous malformations: angioarchitecture in relation to their hemorrhagic episodes. *Neuroradiology* 1990;31:471–475.
4. Yasargil MG. *Microneurosurgery,* vol IIIB. New York: Thieme Verlag, 1988;168–169.
5. Kellinger K. Vascular malformations of the central nervous system: a morphological overview. *Neurosurg Rev* 1986;9:177–216.
6. Martin NA, Stein BM, Wilson CB. Arteriovenous malformations of the posterior fossa. In: Wilson CB, Stein BM, eds. *Intracranial Arteriovenous Malformations.* Baltimore: Williams and Wilkins, 1984; 209–221.

7. Fults D, Kelly DL Jr. Natural history of arteriovenous malformations of the brain: a clinical study. *Neurosurgery* 1984;15:658–662.

8. Gentilli F, Schwartz M, TerBrugge K, et al. A multidisciplinary approach to the treatment of brain vascular malformations. *Adv Tech Stand Neurosurg* 1992;19:179–188.

9. Brown RD Jr, Wiebers D, Forbes G. The natural history of unruptured intracranial arteriovenous malformations. *J Neurosurg* 1988;68: 352–357.

10. Crawford P, West C, Chadwick D, Shaw M. Arteriovenous malformations of the brain: natural history in unoperated patients. *J Neurol Neurosurg Psychiatry* 1986;49:1–10.

11. Purdy PD, Batjer HH, Kopitnik TA, Risser R, Samson DS. Use of ethanol in preoperative AVM embolization. In: Da Pian R, ed. New Trends in Management of Cerebrovascular Malformations. New York: Springer-Verlag, 1994;446–451.

12. Purdy PD, Batjer HH, Kopitnik TA, Samson DS. The team approach to combined embolization and resection of arteriovenous malformation. In: Da Pian R, ed. *New Trends in Management of Cerebrovascular Malformation.* New York: Springer-Verlag, 1994;503–506.

13. Yasargil MG. *Microneurosurgery,* vol IIIB. New York: Thieme Verlag, 1988;201–203.

14. Samson DS, Batjer HH. Posterior fossa arteriovenous malformations. In: Carter LP, Spetzler RF, Hamilton MG, eds. *Neurovascular Surgery.* New York: McGraw-Hill, 1995;1006–1007.

15. Drake CG. Cerebral arteriovenous malformations: considerations for and experience with surgical treatment in 166 cases. *Clin Neurosurg* 1979;26:145–208.

16. Stahl SM, Johnson KP, Malamed N. The clinical and pathological spectrum of brain stem vascular malformations. Long-term course simulates multiple sclerosis. *Arch Neurol* 1980;36:25–29.

17. Samson DS, Batjer HH, Kopitnik TA. Arteriovenous malformations of the brainstem: surgical management and classification. *J Neurosurg* 1996;84:365A.

Cerebrovascular Disease, edited by H. Hunt Batjer.
Lippincott-Raven Publishers, Philadelphia © 1997.

CHAPTER 66

Vein of Galen Aneurysms

Michael B. Horowitz, Charles A. Jungreis, and Ronald G. Quisling

The term *vein of Galen aneurysm* (VGA) encompasses a diverse group of vascular anomalies sharing a common feature, ie, dilatation of the vein of Galen. The name is therefore a misnomer. Although some investigators speculate that VGAs compose up to 33% of giant arteriovenous malformations (AVMs) of infancy and childhood (1), the true incidence of this anomaly remains uncertain. A review of the literature reveals fewer than 300 reported cases since Jaeger, Forbes, and Dandy's clinical description in 1937 (2). As will be outlined below, our understanding of the embryology, anatomy, clinical presentation, and management of these difficult vascular malformations has progressed significantly over the past 50 years.

EMBRYOLOGY AND VASCULAR ANATOMY OF THE VEIN OF GALEN

The development of the human cerebrovascular system is complex and a thorough analysis has been conducted by Padget (3). Cerebral vascularization begins during gestational week 4, at the time of neural tube closure. By the end of week 5, the main afferens to the VG, the choroidal and quadrigeminal arteries, are well developed (4). During week 6 the circle of Willis is completed. The anterior cerebral artery (ACA) supplies the choroid plexus of the lateral ventricles and the middle cerebral artery (MCA) supplies the striatum (4). Meanwhile, at the roof of the diencephalon, the median prosencephalic vein (MPV), or primitive internal cerebral vein, develops as the main draining structure for the telencephalic choroid plexus. By week 10, the MPV is largely replaced by the paired internal cerebral veins (ICV),

which then become the predominant means of choroidal drainage (4). Although the MPV regresses, its most caudal portion joins the ICV to form the VG (4).

Differentiation of the venous sinuses occurs concurrently with development of arterial and venous drainage systems. By week 4, a primitive capillary network is drained by anterior, middle, and posterior meningeal plexi (3,4). Each plexus has a stem that drains into one of the paired longitudinal head sinuses which in turn drain into the jugular veins (3,4). Atresia of the longitudinal sinuses leads to the development of the transverse and sigmoid sinuses by week 7 (3,4). At birth, only the superior and inferior sagittal, straight, transverse, occipital, and sigmoid sinuses remain, along with a still plexiform torcula (3,4). On occasion, a transient falcine sinus extending from the VG to the superior sagittal sinus is seen (4). Such sinuses represent persistent intradural channels located within the falx cerebri.

Under normal circumstances, the mature VG persists as a bridge between the deep parenchymal venous system and the venous sinuses. As such, it serves as a conduit between the internal cerebral veins, basal veins of Rosenthal, precentral cerebellar vein, vermian veins, and straight sinus (5). Lying within the subarachnoid space in an area known as the great transverse cleft, the VG is bordered superiorly by the free margin of the falx, posteriorly by the tentorium cerebelli, anteriorly and inferiorly by the roof of the third ventricle, and laterally by the choroidal fissures of the lateral ventricles (4) (Fig. 1).

Arterial Supply

In a series of 23 patients with VGAs, Raybaud et al. found the posterior choroidal arteries to be the primary feeders (4). The anterior cerebral arteries were the second most commonly involved vessels, generally providing bilateral blood supply. The anterior thalamoperforators were common secondary tributaries, joining primary afferens at the level of the choroidal fissure. Perimesencephalic vessels were constantly involved in neonates and frequently involved in older chil-

M. B. Horowitz: Departments of Neurosurgery and Radiology, Division of Neuroradiology, University of Texas Southwestern Medical Center, Dallas, Texas 75235.
C. A. Jungreis: Departments of Radiology and Neurosurgery, University of Pittsburgh Medical Center, Pittsburgh, Pennsylvania 15213.
R. G. Quisling: Department of Radiology, University of Florida, Gainesville, Florida 32610.

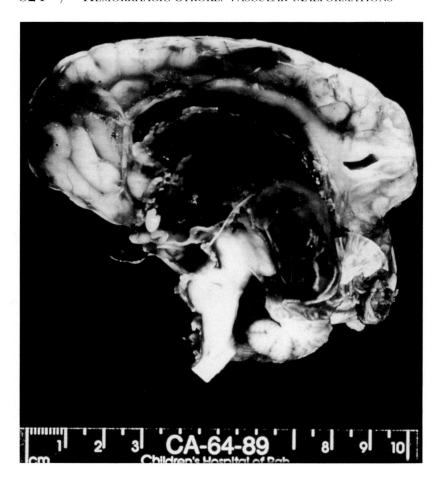

FIG. 1. Midsagittal section of the brain illustrating the large thrombosed vein of Galen (VGA) *(open arrows)* overlying the cerebellum and the collicular plate. The ventricles are distended with recent hemorrhage. Multifocal subarachnoid hemorrhage is also seen. Yellow streaks represent a postmortem attempt at perfusing the arteries with yellow silicone. Note the small size of the brain and cerebellum. White fibrotic meninges cover the medial occipital lobe adjacent to the malformation *(curved arrow)*. (Courtesy of Dr. M. A. Barmada, Children's Hospital of Pittsburgh.)

dren. Distal branches of the posterior cerebral arteries and posterior thalamoperforators supplied the malformation in a moderate number of neonates. In approximately 50% of patients, the meningeal arteries were significant.

Venous Drainage

In normal individuals the VG drains the internal cerebral veins, basal vein of Rosenthal, posterior mesencephalic vein, superior vermian vein, precentral cerebellar vein, and superior cerebellar veins (5). Sixty-eight percent of Raybaud's patients had major venous anomalies including an absent or interrupted straight sinus, a straight sinus divided into two segments, and a straight sinus judged too small in relationship to the sac (4). A small number of patients demonstrated both a falcine and a patent straight sinus. An equally small number of individuals presented with a falcine loop. This arrangement consisted of a falcine sinus draining the sac into the superior sagittal sinus. From the superior sagittal sinus, blood flowed posteriorly into the torcula and then into one transverse sinus. Some blood, however, flowed anteriorly within the superior sagittal sinus, entered a second falcine sinus that angiographically appeared to cross the first (in a separate dural sheet), and finally discharged into the

torcular or other transverse sinus. In these situations blood may drain via petrosal and tentorial venous channels into the cavernous sinus. Falcine sinuses were generally associated with high-flow shunts. Five of Raybaud's cases revealed an angiographic absence of straight, falcine, transverse, and sigmoid sinuses with stasis of contrast within the sac and lack of jugular vein opacification. In terms of nonsinus venous drainage, the authors at no time demonstrated dilatation of the internal cerebral veins although they did see retrograde flow in these structures. Large choroidal veins and an engorged subependymal system drained into the basal veins, uncal veins, and cavernous sinuses. Lateral mesencephalic venous drainage entered the transverse sinus.

CATEGORIZATION

Yasargil divides VGAs into four categories (6). Type 1 represents pure fistulas between arteries and the VG with the nidus of the lesion being the ampulla of the VG. This entire lesion is extrinsic to the brain parenchyma. Type 2 are composed of thalamoperforators that travel through normal parenchyma and both supply brain tissue and give branches to the VG. These lesions are both intrinsic and extrinsic to the central nervous system. Type 3 malformations are mixed lesions with characteristics of both type 1 and type 2 lesions. Type 4 lesions have malformations proximal to the VGA that drain into veins that then empty into the VG.

A further modification of these classifications has been provided by Quisling and Mickle who categorized galenic vascular malformations on the basis of several factors: nidus complexity, afferent supply, and efferent drainage patterns (7). Type 1 represents "true" galenic fistulas with direct arteriovenous communication via a unilateral, choroidal arterial trunk. As it approaches the VGA this trunk can be divided into as many as five smaller distal branches. When an angiomatous matrix is present, it is usually less than 1 cm at its greatest diameter and is typically in direct continuity with the galenic aneurysm. Type 2 galenic fistulas are actually "ordinary" deep AVMs located within the thalamus and/or hypothalamus. They are supplied by the thalamoperforating arteries and drain via the superior thalamic veins and galenic system. AVM matrix size in such cases ranges from 1 to 2 cm at the greatest diameter. Type 3 galenic vascular malformations are similar to type 1 fistulas but have significantly more afferent vascular complexity. Instead of a single feeding artery, type 3 malformations are supplied by both anterior and posterior choroidal arteries and the persistent embryonic remnants of the distal anterior cerebral arteries. The authors observed that their angiographic distinctions correlated with the clinical presentation of the lesion. For example, no patients in categories 1 or 2 had overt cardiac decompensation (7), whereas the type 3 galenic fistulas, which as a group exhibited the most shunting, were more likely to present with high-output cardiac failure in the newborn period.

In addition to categorizing the arterial supply to the VGA, these authors also favored using a grading system for the venous aspect of the malformation. In grade 1 venous morphology, the degree of ectasia of the straight sinus is proportional to that of the VG, with both being only minimally enlarged. Grade 2 morphology occurs when the VG is more dilated than the straight sinus, with both structures moderately increased in size. Grade 3 lesions demonstrate marked dilatation of both structures, and grade 4 have a significant enlargement of the VG with a normal, stenotic, or absent straight sinus (7). These angiographic findings correlated well with measurements of venous pressure within the malformation. Whereas the mean venous pressure within galenic aneurysms in individuals with venous restrictions was 40 cm of water, the pressure in patients without venous restrictions averaged 25 cm of water (7). These angiographic findings and pressure measurements were related in a logical way to a number of clinical features. For example, no patient with obstructed drainage was in cardiac failure at the time of presentation, thus confirming that some measure of cardiac protection is provided by restriction of venous outflow from the malformation. Conversely, no case in which the efferent venous pressure was less than 20 cm of water had brain calcifications, implicating elevated venous pressure in the development of the finding. Finally, grade 4 patients with severe outflow restriction were more likely to undergo spontaneous thrombosis of their malformation, suggesting that a lower flow rate is present in those fistulas that have a high-grade efferent stenosis. Taken together, these observations provided the rationale for initial attempts to treat galenic malformations via the venous route particularly in patients with high-output cardiac failure.

DEVELOPMENTAL THEORY

Raybaud proposes that VGAs are not a result of dilatation of the VG but rather a consequence of dilatation of a persistent median prosencephalic vein. The evidence he cites supporting this statement includes the following: (a) The VG develops late and lacks connections to the choroidal branch of the anterior cerebral artery which is a primary feeder in most VGA. (b) The typical VGA directly drains both the prosencephalic and mesencephalic arteries in a pattern typical for the MPV while the normal mature VG does not. Anomalous venous drainage as described in previous sections probably represents persistent fetal drainage that remains intact because it effectively deals with the high flow system. Such persistent fetal drainage may prevent the development of the normal sinus system. Alternatively, persistent falcine sinuses may be a consequence of straight sinus occlusion early in the developmental period (4).

Lasjuanias et al have proposed additional theories concerning the development of VGA (8). They agree that VGA may develop secondary to proximal angiomatous malformations. However, they also bring to light the frequency of sinus obstruction (especially the straight sinus) associated with VG malformations, thus speculating that increased resistance to outflow at an early stage may lead to proximal venous ectasia. These authors felt that venous agenesis was a more likely mechanism of outflow obstruction than was sinus thrombosis since acquired thrombosis usually fails to produce subsequent VGA. Mayberg, however, has reported a case of a 64-year-old man with a dural AVM, VGA, and straight sinus thrombosis (9). It is his contention that the straight sinus thrombosis was the primary event leading to the development of both vascular abnormalities.

CLINICAL PRESENTATION

The association in neonates of intractable congestive heart failure (CHF) and a cranial bruit provides the most striking manifestation of VGA; however less fulminant modes of presentation are the norm in older infants, children, and adults. Although attempts have been made to subdivide clinical presentation on a strictly age related basis, it is readily apparent that, between age groups, signs and symptoms overlap (10,11). For example, in Amacher's classification schema, group 1 consists of neonates with a cranial bruit and severe congestive heart failure (CHF). Group 2 consists of neonates and infants with mild heart failure who develop craniomegaly and cranial bruits within 1–6 months. Group 3 comprises children 1–12 months old with craniomegaly and cranial bruit, but no heart failure. Group 4 consists of individuals age 3.5–27 years who present with headache, exercise syncope, and subarachnoid hemorrhage (10). In addition, certain presenting signs such as visual deterioration, proptosis, seizures, hemiparesis, seizures, developmental retardation, facial vein enlargement, epistaxis and vertigo do not necessarily coincide with age-related groupings. Nonetheless, the above classification schema provides a useful basis for categorizing patients with VGA.

Congestive Heart Failure

Congestive heart failure is the major cause of mortality and morbidity in neonates and infants harboring a VGA. In severe cases, as much as 80% of left ventricular output may be delivered to the head as a consequence of the low vascular resistance within the malformation (12). Because this output returns directly to the right ventricle, right heart failure from volume and work overload may ensue. Myocardial ischemia is further promoted by decreased afterload induced by the AVM. Consequent reduction in diastolic pressures jeopardizes myocardial perfusion (8). Other cardiac anomalies reported in association with VGAs include transposition of the great vessels and aortic stenosis (13,14).

Heart failure generally presents not prior to but shortly after birth. The explanation for this may reside in the fact that in utero, the placenta's low vascular resistance reduces the amount of blood that is "stolen" by the abnormal, low-resistance cerebral shunt (12). On examination, the neonate or infant with cardiac decompensation from VGA may manifest cyanosis, decreased peripheral pulses, and, in some cases, audible cranial bruits (12). In the absence of an obvious bruit, the correct diagnosis may initially be missed unless a high index of suspicion is maintained.

Hydrocephalus

The etiology of hydrocephalus is multifactorial and includes Sylvian aqueduct obstruction, resorptive blocks, hydrocephalus ex vacuo (a consequence of encephalomalacia and cerebral atrophy) (15), and abnormal transependymal cerebrospinal fluid resorption. Resorptive blocks may be attributable to increased pressure within the sagittal sinus (7,8).

Developmental Retardation

Developmental retardation is common with VGA and is often used as an argument against offering treatment to severely affected infants. Mechanisms implicated for such damage are arterial steal, ischemia due to compression from engorged draining veins and an enlarged VG, and increased venous pressure with subsequent venous infarction following spontaneous, partial or complete VGA thrombosis (7,8,16). Grossman recognized the role of arterial steal after

noting resolution of optic disc pallor in two patients undergoing VGA excision (17). He concluded that early surgery might abort ischemic brain damage in those individuals who were fortunate enough to be born with normal parenchyma.

Failure To Thrive

Many neonates and infants with VGA fail to thrive. Cardiac decompensation undoubtedly plays a tremendous role in such failure. However, hypothalamic and hypophyseal dysfunction secondary to venous congestion within these structures must also be considered a potential mechanism (8).

VGA Thrombosis

Spontaneous thrombosis of VGA may be heralded by the development of obstructive hydrocephalus or by the onset of intraventricular hemorrhage (18–24). Heinz, the first to describe thrombosis of VGA, felt it occurred in utero or during birth (20). However, later reports clearly indicated that thrombosis could take place throughout infancy and, in some cases, in adulthood (18,25). There is no typical presentation of thrombosed VGA except for the nearly ubiquitous presence of hydrocephalus and its attendant signs and symptoms.

Associated Illnesses

Both Turner's syndrome and blue rubber bleb nevus syndrome have been reported to occur in conjunction with VGA (26,27). The former involves the absence of a single X chromosome in females and has been associated with other vascular anomalies including coarctation of the aorta and pulmonic stenosis. The latter presents with blue, nipple-like, compressible skin lesions composed of blood-filled venous and cavernous angiomas. Whether or not the association of these diseases with VGA is a chance occurrence is not known at this time. Other malformations reported in association with VGA include supernumerary digits, hypospadias, transposition of the great vessels (28), and aortic stenosis (13,14).

EVALUATION AND DIAGNOSTIC STUDIES

Ultrasound

Ultrasound represents an excellent method of screening for and evaluating VGA, both in utero and during the neonatal period (29—31). Ultrasonic demonstration of vascular pulsations helps differentiate VGA from other possible midline structures (30) (Figs. 2 and 3). Color Doppler ultrasound permits the characterization of blood flow within the malformation and, while useful in delineating feeding and draining

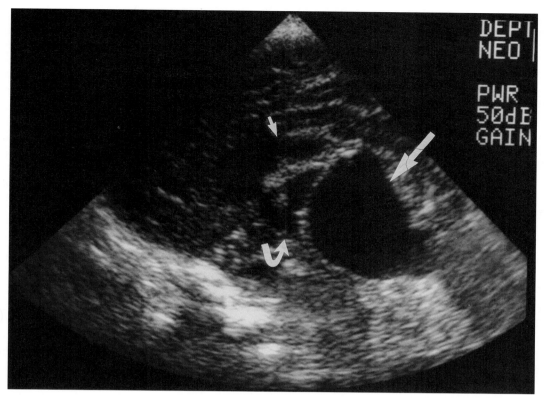

FIG. 2. Sagittal view head ultrasound revealing dilated lateral ventricle *(small arrow)*, dilated and anteriorly displaced third ventricle *(curved arrow)*, and VGA *(large arrow)*.

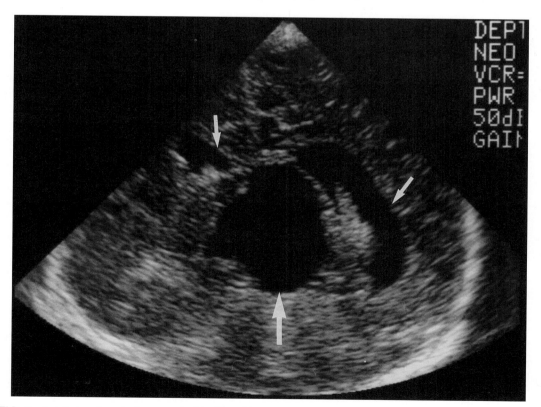

FIG. 3. Axial view head ultrasound with dilated lateral ventricles *(small arrows)* and midline VGA *(large arrow)*.

vessels, is especially valuable in evaluating the effectiveness of therapy (32,33).

Chest Radiographs

Chest radiographs may reveal cardiomegaly with right-sided chamber enlargement, widening of the superior mediastinum retrosternal fullness, posterior displacement of the upper trachea, and retropharyngeal soft tissue prominence due to encroachment on this space by dilated carotid arteries and jugular veins (34).

Skull Radiographs

Radiographs of the skull are of minimal utility in the diagnosis and evaluation of suspected VGA. Occasionally they demonstrate a rim of calcium corresponding to a calcified VGA sac (35).

Computed Tomography (CT)

CT images of VGA generally reveal a round mass lying in the quadrigeminal cistern behind the posterior border of an anteriorly displaced third ventricle (Fig. 4A). High density within the lesion may suggest VGA thrombosis (5,22,36). Following administration of contrast, dense, homogeneous opacification of both the VGA and the adjacent tentorial vessels and draining sinuses is seen (5,36) (Fig. 4B, C). When the malformation is thrombosed contrast tends to enhance the aneurysm wall and opacify small zones within the aneurysmal pouch (5,36). A "target sign" has been described in this circumstance. Calcification of the malformation wall, seen in approximately 14% of patients, is rarely seen in individuals younger than 15 years (18). Cerebral parenchymal calcifications are generally attributed to ischemia especially when located in watershed regions and as such, may be an index of cerebral damage.

Magnetic Resonance Imaging (MRI) and Angiography (MRA)

The ability of MR to image noninvasively in sagittal, coronal, and axial planes makes it an invaluable tool in the characterization of arterial afferens, venous drainage, malformation position and size, and appearance of surrounding brain. MR allows for the early identification of sinus abnormalities

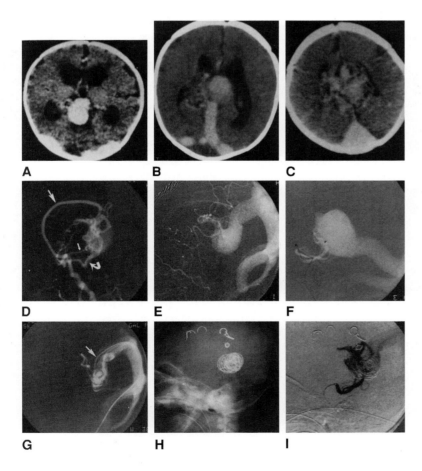

FIG. 4. Newborn with VGA. **A:** Contrast-enhanced axial head CT scan revealing 2.5-cm midline VGA anteriorly displacing the third ventricle with accompanying hydrocephalus. **B:** Contrast-enhanced axial head CT in the same patient demonstrating an enlarged straight sinus. **C:** Contrast-enhanced axial head CT more superiorly demonstrating the extensive surrounding vascular plexus. **D:** Lateral internal cerebral artery angiogram revealing the anterior cerebral artery *(large arrow)*, anterior choroidal artery *(small arrow)*, and posterior choroidal artery *(curved arrow)* supply to the VGA. **E:** Lateral angiographic view showing VGA drainage via enlarged falcine, transverse, and sigmoid dural sinuses. Note that the junction of the falcine sinus with the superior sagittal sinus is not at the torcula. **F:** Lateral angiogram via superselective catheterization of posterior circulation. Posterior choroidal artery supply is opacified. Prominent venous drainage via the straight sinus is apparent. **G:** Lateral angiogram displaying transvenous approach with the catheter *(arrow)* in the sinus system and the catheter tip in the VGA. Some coils have been deposited in the VGA. **H:** Lateral skull radiograph demonstrating minicoils within both VGA and right pericallosal artery. A transvenous approach had been utilized for coil deposition in the VGA, and a transarterial approach had been utilized for coil deposition in the pericallosal artery. **I:** Lateral view of a right posterior cerebral artery angiogram demonstrating residual posterior choroidal artery supply to the VGA. Endovascular coils have been deposited in the VGA and anterior pericallosal artery. The flow through the malformation has been decreased sufficiently by the coils to resolve the congestive heart failure in this infant.

and venous drainage patterns, which not only facilitates therapeutic planning of transvenous or transtorcular endovascular approaches but also helps guide the angiographer to the most important vessels for study (37). This is particularly critical in neonates where venous access is difficult and total acceptable contrast loads are low. However, MRI has not obviated the need for catheter angiography, especially when intervention is planned (38,39). MRA, on the other hand, has begun to provide substantial insight into the anatomy of many vascular diseases and as it improves it will become the primary tool for the evaluation of VGAs.

Angiography

Angiography remains the gold standard for the evaluation of VGAs (Fig. 4D, E).

MANAGEMENT

The primary indication for treating neonates with a VGA is CHF refractory to medical management. In many cases, surgery or endovascular treatment can be postponed by medical management until the child is older, at which point intervention is safer and easier. In those patients requiring invasive treatment, the goal of therapy is not necessarily the complete obliteration or extirpation of the VGA but rather the arrest of CHF. Relative contraindications to treatment include medically controlled CHF or uncontrollable systemic failure. Finally, imaging evidence of brain damage has been considered a contraindication by some (40).

Surgery

Jaeger, Forbes, and Dandy performed carotid ligation in an attempt to control the degree of blood flow through a galenic malformation (2). This procedure provided no clear protection against further cardiovascular compromise and eventual death. Subsequent to that initial case report, numerous other reports have described surgical approaches to galenic malformations (6,11,15,41,42). Certain issues must be considered before undertaking any planned ablative procedure. The retraction necessary to adequately visualize and deal with the VGA and its arterial supply is potentially more dangerous in the poorly myelinated and delicate neonatal brain than in older children. Moreover, the risks of life-threatening blood loss is accentuated in such patients because of their limited blood volumes. Accordingly, where feasible, every attempt should be made to deal with such lesions nonsurgically in this age group with the thought that surgery, if required, can be undertaken more safely in an older patient.

Theoretical risks of normal perfusion pressure breakthrough (NPPB) must be considered when planning any treatment of vascular malformation. Following obliteration

of some vascular malformations, previously hypoperfused peripheral brain tissue experiences increased blood flow. Sudden increases in blood flow to these regions has been reported to result in brain swelling, hemorrhage, and seizures (43,44). Normal perfusion pressure breakthrough has been associated with malformations >4 cm in largest dimension, with angiograms showing steal, and with individuals who manifest possible steal-related neurologic deficits (45). Many surgeons and interventionalists therefore feel that staged treatment of complicated galenic malformations should be considered, especially when the above-mentioned risk factors are present.

The need for and timing of ventricular drainage in conjunction with primary treatment of VGA remains controversial. Schneider et al. have described a number of complications associated with ventriculoperitoneal shunts in children with hydrocephalus and a VGA. These included status epilepticus, intraventricular hemorrhage, subdural collections, and new neurologic deficits (46). In Yasargil's series two postoperative deaths were heralded by intraventricular hematomas in hydrocephalic patients shunted at the time of surgery. The author felt that all individuals requiring shunts should have catheter placement performed prior to malformation ablation because following ablation the subependymal veins may become distended and thus possibly prone to rupture if a catheter is passed through the ventricular wall (42). Distended ependymal veins, however, may be present prior to malformation ablation and the risks of shunt placement may be high at this time as well.

In many patients, particularly those with obstructive hydrocephalus secondary to thrombosed VGAs, cerebrospinal fluid shunting is the only therapy required (21). In such patients, attempts to resect the thrombosed aneurysm sac have been associated with unacceptable morbidity (20–23,25,42).

Endovascular Approaches

Advances in catheter design and embolization materials have brought neuroradiologic endovascular approaches to the forefront of therapeutic options in VGA management. Berenstein's indications for embolization include (a) preoperative obliteration of less surgically accessible feeding vessels in the hope of reducing surgical morbidity; (b) postoperative obliteration of smaller feeding vessels after surgical ligation of major arterial suppliers; (c) definite therapy of VGA using a staged technique (47). Lasjaunias has made an important distinction in his discussions of endovascular treatment of VGA. In those patients with VGA secondary to a parenchymal or choroidal AVM, he emphasizes the necessity of avoiding venous embolization. Approaches to such malformations should be from the arterial side to avoid venous hypertension/congestion and its associated morbidity and mortality (40).

Various techniques have been described for VGA obliteration including transarterial, transvenous, and transtorcular embolization (8,40,47–52) (Fig. 4F–I). The specific endovascular approach has depended on the specific anatomy of the given case. Arteriovenous fistulas can be occluded on the arterial side from either a transarterial or transvenous approach using embolic agents such as coils, acrylics (cyanoacrylates), and endovascular balloons. Fistulas pose the technical challenge of depositing emboli at the site of the shunt in such a way as to maintain their position. High-flow fistulas are notorious for transmitting even large emboli to the venous side and to the pulmonary circulation with fatal results. As a consequence of such "pass-through" phenomena, venous occlusion therapy has gained popularity. In cases of multiple fistulas converging on the vein of Galen, the transvenous and transtorcular approaches have even more appeal. The goal in these approaches is to occlude the outflow in the VG thus inducing retrograde thrombosis and obliteration of the fistulas. Many embolic agents have been used although coils are currently the primary agent utilized in this approach. Complete cure is not usually required and partial occlusion of the dilated vein frequently reverses the cardiovascular compromise (Ron Quisling, personal communication).

When approaching these lesions from a transarterial route with primary arterial embolizations the interventionalist must be aware of the risks of NPPB. Mickle tried to avoid NPPB by reducing blood flow 50% in stage 1 and then returning 3–21 days later, if necessary, to completely eliminate all residual flow (51). If total obliteration could not be achieved, embolization was aimed at stabilizing the patient's cardiovascular status in the hope of converting a neonate or infant into an older age group member in whom surgery or embolization has a better outcome (47).

An unusual but potentially fatal complication of endovascular therapy is a consumptive coagulopathy manifested by a precipitous postembolization thrombocytopenia that is followed by intracranial hemorrhage. The etiology of such coagulation abnormalities may rest in the rapid deposition of large amounts of thrombus within the recently treated vascular anomaly. As in the related Kasabach–Merritt syndrome (53) treatment consists of clotting factors and platelet replacement.

OUTCOME

Johnston reviewed 232 cases of VGA reported in the literature prior to 1987 and recorded cases involving 80 neonates, 82 infants (1–12 months), 39 children (1–5 years), 22 children and young adults (6–20 years), and 22 adults (>20 years). Of these patients, 110 presented with CHF, 94 with increased ICP, 57 with cranial bruit, 37 with focal neurologic deficit, 26 with seizures, and 25 with hemorrhage (41). Ninety-one individuals underwent direct surgical treatment, 29 received a shunt and remote vessel ligation, 46 had medical management alone, and 79 had no therapy or no details of therapy in their reports. Overall mortality was 55.6% with 37.4% mortality for surgical cases and a 46.3% incidence of significant morbidity in postoperative survivors. Neonates had a 91.4% surgical mortality, which approximated the nonsurgical outcome. The 1- to 12-month age group suffered a 31.7% operative mortality and the >1 year age group had a 25.6% surgical mortality and a 42.3% major morbidity. Yasargil's series consisting of 70 patients showed a 67% neonatal (<1 month old) postoperative mortality, a 40% infant (1–24 months old) postoperative mortality, and a 27% child/adult postoperative mortality (6). Total survival in this series of operated and nonoperated patients included 10% for neonates, 47% for infants, and 56% for child/adult. An inescapable conclusion from these studies, which include cases spanning many eras of neurosurgical, medical, and radiologic advances, is that neonates have a profoundly worse outcome than other age groups, most likely as a consequence of cardiac decompensation with resultant multisystem failure. Fortunately, in the current era of endovascular therapy, morbidity and mortality rates have improved. Lasjaunias has reported 36 cases treated by endovascular approaches (78% pediatric; 22% adult) with a mortality of 13% (40). Casasco et al. reported 100% survival in seven infants treated via transvenous embolization (54). Dowd et al. reported transvenous approaches to the venous and/or arterial side of VGA in three neonates who survived and were stable at 9–12 months follow-up (52). Mickle's experience with transtorcular embolization in 15 infants and older children and 9 neonates was favorable. Forty-four percent of the latter and 93% of the former survived (55). Lylyk et al. utilized endovascular therapy in 28 children. Forty-five percent of those <1 year of age had good outcomes, 61.5% of those age 1–2 had good outcomes, and 100% of those older than 2 had good outcomes (56).

SUMMARY AND CONCLUSIONS

Our philosophy in managing a patient with a VGA is, of course, greatly influenced by the age of the patient, the clinical symptomatology, and the angioarchitecture of the malformation. Therapeutic options are primarily based on whether or not a true AVM is present or if the malformation represents an arteriovenous fistula involving the vein of Galen. Arterial endovascular approaches, microneurosurgery, and/or radiosurgery are preferred for management of the former, whereas the transvenous endovascular approach has become the cornerstone of treatment in the latter. The most critical group, however, is the neonate in extreme cardiovascular distress. In this type of case our therapeutic intervention is initially endovascular from the venous side, either transfemoral or transtorcular. The immediate goal is to increase resistance to right ventricular output. Advantages of this approach over a transarterial approach include a shorter anesthesia time, minimal fluid and/or contrast administration, and creation of a wire "basket" or "bird's nest" on the venous side that helps to prevent emboli that may be deposited on the arterial side in subsequent embolizations from passing through the malformation. The transvenous approach can be easily repeated multiple times and may be supplemented by transarterial embolizations. Endovascular coils have been the mainstay for such venous embolizations. The endpoint of treatment is not complete occlusion of the fistula but improvement in cardiac function. Often more than one stage is required to reach our goal.

The results in recent years have been encouraging and are to a large degree attributable to the advances in endovascular approaches. With future improved tools for diagnosis and treatment perhaps the prognosis for this difficult malady will also continue to improve.

ACKNOWLEDGMENTS

Thanks to Leslie Mihal for help in the preparation of this manuscript, Alison Russell for photographic assistance, and Ian Pollack, M.D. for editorial expertise.

REFERENCES

1. Long DM, Seljeskoge El, Chous SN, French LA. Giant arteriovenous malformations and childhood. *J Neurosurg* 1974;40:304.
2. Jaegar JR, Forbes RP, Dandy WE. Bilateral congenital cerebral arteriovenous communication aneurysm. *Trans Am Neurol Assoc* 1937;63:173–176.
3. Padget DH. Cranial venous system in man in reference to development, adult configuration and relation to arteries. *Am J Anat* 1956;98:307–355.
4. Raybaud CA, Strother CM, Hald JK. Aneurysms of the vein of Galen: embryonic considerations and anatomical features relating to the pathogenesis of the malformation. *Neuroradiology* 1989;31:109–128.
5. Skirkhoda A, Whaley RA, Boone SC, Scatliff JH, Schnapf D. Varied CT appearance of aneurysms of the vein of Galen in infancy. *Neuroradiology* 1981;21:265–270.
6. Yasargil MG. *Microsurgery.* vol IIIB. New York: Thieme Verlag, 1988:323–357.
7. Quisling RG, Mickle JP. Venous pressure measurements in vein of Galen aneurysms. *AJNR* 1989;10:411–417.
8. Lasjaunias P, Ter Brugge K, Lopez Ibor L, et al. The role of dural anomalies in vein of Galen aneurysms: report of six cases and review of the literature. *AJNR* 1987;8:185–192.
9. Mayberg MR, Zimmerman C. Vein of Galen aneurysm associated with dural AVM and straight sinus thrombosis. Case Report. *J Neurosurg* 1988;68:288–291.
10. Amacher AL, Shillito J Jr. The syndromes and surgical treatment of aneurysms of the great vein of Galen. *J Neurosurg* 1973;39:89–98.
11. Hoffman HJ, Chuang S, Hendrick EB, Humphreys RP. Aneurysms of the vein of Galen. Experience at the Hospital for Sick Children. Toronto. *J Neurosurg* 1982;57:316–322.
12. Pellegrino PA, Milanesi O, Saia OS, Carollo C. Congestive heart failure secondary to cerebral arterio-venous fistula. *Childs Nerv Syst* 1987;3:141–144.
13. Gomez JR, Whitten CF, Nolke A. Bernstein J, Meyer JS. Aneurysmal malformation of the great vein of Galen causing heart failure in early infancy. *Pediatrics* 1983;31:400.
14. Hirano A, Solomon S. Arteriovenous aneurysm of the vein of Galen. *Arch Neurol* 1960;3:589.
15. Rosenfeld JV, Fabinyi GC. Acute hydrocephalus in an elderly woman with an aneurysm of the vein of Galen. *Neurosurgery* 1984;15:852–854.
16. Norman MG, Becker LE. Cerebral damage in neonates resulting from arteriovenous malformation of the vein of Galen. *J Neurol Neurosurg Psychiatry* 1974;37:252–258.
17. Grossman RI, Bruce DA, Zimmerman RA, Goldberg HI, Bilaniuk LT. Vascular steal associated with vein of Galen anerysm. *Neuroradiology* 1984;26:381–386.
18. Chapman S, Hockley AD. Calcification of an aneurysm of the vein of Galen. *Pediatr Radiol* 1989;19:541–542.
19. Dean DF. Management of clotted aneurysm of the vein of Galen. *Neurosurgery* 1981;8:589–592.
20. Heinz RE, Schwartz FJ, Sears RA. Thrombus in the vein of Galen malformation. *Br J Radiol* 1968;41:424–428.
21. Mancuso P, Chiaramonte I, Pero G, Tropea R, Guarnera F. A case of thrombosed aneurysm of the vein of Galen associated with superior sagittal sinus thrombosis. *J Neurosurg Sci* 1989;33:305–309.
22. Six EG, Cowley AR, Kelly DL Jr, Laster DW. Thrombosed aneurysm of the vein of Galen. *Neurosurgery* 1980;7:274–278.
23. Weir BK, Allen PB, Miller JD. Excision of thrombosed vein of Galen aneurysm in an infant. Case report. *J Neurosurg* 1968;29:619–622.
24. Whitaker JB, Latack JT, Venes JL. Spontaneous thrombosis of a vein of Galen aneurysm. *AJNR* 1987;8:1134–1136.
25. Lazar ML. Vein of Galen aneurysm: successful excision of a completely thrombosed aneurysm in an infant. *Surg Neurol* 1974;2:22–24.
26. Jarrell HR, Schochet SS Jr, Krous H, Barnes P. Turner's syndrome and vein of Galen aneurysm—a previously unreported association. *Acta Neuropathol* 1981;55:189–191.
27. Rosenblum WI, Nakoneczna I, Konderding HS, Nochlin D, Ghatak NR. Multiple vascular malformation in the "blue rubber bleb naevus" syndrome: a case with aneurysm of vein of Galen and vascular lesions suggesting a link to the Weber–Osler–Rendu syndrome. *Histopathology* 1978;2:301–311.
28. Eide J, Folling M. Malformation of the great vein of Galen with neonatal heart failure. Report of two cases. *Acta Paediatr Scand* 1978;67:529–532.
29. Jeanty P, Kepple D, Roussis P, Shah D. In utero detection of cardiac failure from an aneurysm of the vein of Galen. *Am J Obstet Gynecol* 1990;163:50–51.
30. Mendelsohn DB, Hertzanu Y, Butterworth A. In utero diagnosis of a vein of Galen aneurysm by ultrasound. *Neuroradiology* 1984;26:417–418.
31. Rodemyer CR, Smith WL. Diagnosis of a vein of Galen aneurysm by ultrasound. *JCU* 1982;10:297–298.
32. Deeg KH, Scarf J. Colour Doppler imaging of arteriovenous malformation of the vein of Galen in a newborn. *Neuroradiology* 1990;32:60–63.
33. Tessler FN, Dion J, Vinuela F, et al. Cranial arteriovenous malformations in neonates: color Doppler imaging with angiographic correlation. *AJR* 1989;153:1027–1039.
34. Swischuk LE, Crowe JE, Mewborns EJ Jr. Large vein of Galen aneurysms in the neonate. A constellation of diagnostic chest and neck radiologic findings. *Pediatr Radiol* 1977;6:4–9.
35. Agee OF, Musella R, Tweed CG. Aneurysm of the great vein of Galen. Report of two cases. *J Neurosurg* 1969;31:346–351.
36. Martelli A, Scotti G, Harwood-Nash DC, Fitz CR, Chuang SH. Aneurysms of the vein of Galen in children: CT and angiographic correlations. *Neuroradiology* 1980;20:123–133.
37. Seidenwurm D, Berenstein A, Hyman A, Howalski H. Vein of Galen malformation: correlation of clinical presentation, arteriography and MR imaging. *AJNR* 1991;12:347–354.
38. Leff SL, Kronfeld G, Leonidas JC. Aneurysm of the vein of Galen. Ultrasound, MRI and angiographic correlations. *Pediatr Radiol* 1989;20:98–100.
39. Roosen N, Schirmer M, Lins E, Bock WJ Stork W, Gahlen D. MRI of an aneurysm of the vein of Galen. *AJNR* 1986;7:733–735.
40. Lasjaunias P, Rodesch G, Terbrugge K, et al. Vein of Galen aneurysmal malformations. Report of 36 cases managed between 1982 and 1988. *Acta Neurochir* 1989;99:26–37.
41. Johnston IH, Whittle IR, Besser M, Morgan MK. Vein of Galen malformation: diagnosis and management. *Neurosurgery* 1987;20:747–758.
42. Yasargil MG, Antil J, Laciera R, Jain KK, Boone SC. Arteriovenous malformations of vein of Galen: microsurgical treatment. *Surg Neurol* 1970;6:195–200.
43. Barrow DL (ed). Intracranial vascular malformations. Neurosurgical Topics AANS 1990:91.
44. Spezler RF, Wilson CB, Weinstein P, Mehdorn J, Townsend J, Telles D. Normal perfusion pressure breakthrough theory. *Clin Neurosurg* 1978;25:651–672.

45. Barrow DL (ed). Intracranial vascular malformations. Neurosurgical Topics AANS 1990:160.
46. Schneider SJ, Wisoff JS, Epstein FJ. Complications of ventriculoperitoneal shunt procedures or hydrocephalus associated with vein of Galen malformations in childhood. *Neurosurgery* 1992;30(5):706–708.
47. Berenstein A, Epstein F. Vein of Galen malformations: combined neurosurgical and neuroradiologic intervention in American Association of Neurological Surgeons (eds). *Pediatric Neurosurgery: Surgery of the Developing Nervous System*. New York: Grune and Stratton, 1982; 638–647.
48. Hawkins J, Quisling RG, Mickle JP, Hawkins IF. Retrievable Gianturco-coil introducer. *Radiology* 1986;158:262–264.
49. King WA, Wackym PA, Jinuela F, Peacock WJ. Management of vein of Galen aneurysms: combined surgical and endovascular approach. *Child's Nerv Syst* 1989;5:208–211.
50. McCord FB, Shields MD, McNeil A, Halliday HL, McClure G, Reid MM. Cerebral arteriovenous malformation in a neonate: treatment by embolization. *Arch Dis Child* 1987;62:1273–1275.
51. Mickle JP, Quisling RG. The transtorcular embolization of vein of Galen aneurysms. *J Neurosurg* 1986;64:731–735.
52. Dowd CF, Halbach W, Barnwell SL, Higashida RT, Edwards MSB, Hieshema EM. Transfemoral venous embolization of vein of Galen malformations. *AJNR* 1990;11:643–648.
53. Kasabach HH, Merritt KK. Capillary hemangioma with extensive purpura: report of a case. *Am J Dis Child* 1940;59:1063–1080.
54. Casasco A, Lylyk P, Hodes JE, Kohan G, Aymard A, Merland JJ. Percutaneous transvenous catheterization and embolization of vein of Galen aneurysms. *Neurosurgery* 1991;28:260–265.
55. Mickle AP. The transtocular embolization of vein of Galen aneurysms and update on the use of this technique in twenty-four patients. In: Marlin AE, ed. *Concepts in Pediatric Neurosurgery*. Basel: Karger, 1991;11:69–78.
56. Lylyk P, Vinuela F, Dion JE, Duckwiler G, Guslielmi G, Peacock W, Maretin N. Therapeutic alternatives for vein of Galen vascular malformations. *J Neurosurg* 1993;78:438–445.

Cerebrovascular Disease, edited by H. Hunt Batjer.
Lippincott-Raven Publishers, Philadelphia © 1997.

CHAPTER **67**

Intracranial Arteriovenous Malformations: Cerebrovascular Hemodynamics

Adam P. Brown and Robert F. Spetzler

GENERAL CHARACTERISTICS

Arteriovenous malformations (AVMs) are congenital in origin and probably occur due to an aberrancy in development during the initial 2–3 months of embryogenesis (1). The underlying lesion appears to represent a perpetuation of primitive arteriovenous communications, which normally should be replaced by an intervening capillary network. The feeding arteries and draining veins are, however, normal vessels of the region. Due to the abnormal hemodynamic conditions, the arteriovenous shunts result in an enlargement of the involved arterial and venous channels. Generally, as the mass of the malformation matures, it takes on a wedge-shaped form with its apex directed toward the ventricular surface (Fig. 1). Studies of embryogenesis may reveal the basis for this appearance (2). Transcerebral veins course throughout the white matter of the hemispheres in the direction of myelinated fibers from the cerebral cortex to the subependymal venous system. These vessels are extremely fine and may actually function as capillaries. Hence, in a malformation with defective capillary development, these vessels may play a central role in lesion formation and shape.

Histologically, an AVM has three morphologic components: the dysplastic vascular nidus, the feeding arteries, and the draining veins. The dysplastic nidus is a coiled tangle of abnormal vessels acting as a low-resistance shunt. The vessels of the nidus contain markedly attenuated walls with focal areas of dilatation. This nidus serves as the recipient of the feeding arterial flow and is thus exposed to high intravascular pressures due to the lack of a high-resistance arteriolar bed. Hence the AVM nidus is presumably the source of hemorrhage in most of these lesions. Conversely, the feeding arteries and draining veins are not congenitally abnormal

but become pathologic secondary to the hemodynamic properties of the nidus. Both vessel types dilate due to abnormally high blood flow, whereas the abnormally high pressures encountered by the venous system cause arterialization of these vessels. As a whole, the coiled AVM mass is partially separated by thin islands of sclerotic neural tissue in a bed formed by displacement rather than invasion of the brain (3).

AVMs are the most commonly recognized of the cerebral vascular malformations. This is in part due to their clinical appearance and in part to the therapeutic options available. Their autopsy incidence, however, makes them about half as common as venous malformations and slightly more common than capillary telangiectases and cavernous malformations. In the Cooperative Study of Subarachnoid Hemorrhage (SAH), symptomatic AVMs were found in 549 of almost 6400 cases, representing an 8.6% incidence of SAH. With SAH accounting for up to 10% of all strokes, AVMs make up less than 1% of these symptomatic occurrences. With respect to autopsy studies, however, AVMs may have a higher prevalence than suggested above. McCormick and Rosenfield (3) performed 4530 consecutive neural autopsies and uncovered 196 AVMs, for an incidence of 4.3%. Though not strictly a population-based study, these data suggested a higher prevalence of AVMs than previously believed. In reviewing the patient data in McCormick's series, it was found that only 12% of patients had symptoms attributed to their AVM. Therefore, for the autopsy group as a whole, this symptomatic stroke incidence of 0.53% approached that of the clinically based Cooperative Study.

PHYSIOLOGY

Kaplan and colleagues (1) proposed that an AVM consists of two physiologic components. The first is the nidus itself, or the shunt proper. Poorly developed vessels at the precapillary and capillary level make up this component. The other

A. P. Brown and R. F. Spetzler: Division of Neurological Surgery, Barrow Neurological Institute, St. Joseph's Hospital and Medical Center, Phoenix, Arizona 85013.

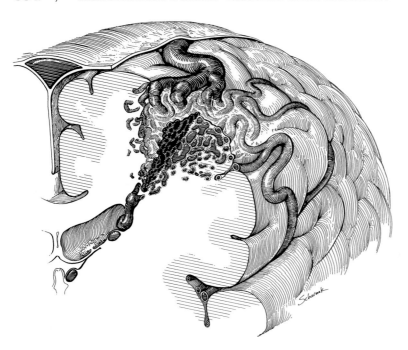

FIG. 1. Diagrammatic representation of classic hemispheric arteriovenous malformation. The lesion consists of feeding arterial branches, draining veins, and a nidal mass. The conical-shaped lesion extends from the cortical surface to the ventricular region with intervening sclerotic neural tissue. (Reprinted with permission from Barrow Neurological Institute.)

portion of the AVM consists of the blood vessels conducting flow to (feeding arteries) and from (draining veins) the high-flow, low-resistance shunt. These authors suggested that the AVM component structures are individually normal and are therefore able to respond to the altered local hemodynamics incident on the shunt. The exact physiologic significance of this statement is difficult to ascertain because no data were presented in their manuscript from which to draw conclusions. Therefore, whether these authors felt that AVMs were passive pressure conduits or systems capable of regulating pressure and blood flow is unknown.

In 1971, Feindel et al (4) reported their results utilizing intraoperative xenon blood flow measurements, during the resection of an AVM. Using four gamma detector probes distributed ipsilaterally both near and far from the angioma, they demonstrated shunt or nonnutritional flow for a wide region of the involved hemisphere. The greatest peaks were noted over the lesion and its draining veins. With closure of the arterial feeders, the shunt peaks disappeared and were replaced by perfusion flow in all four regions. Significant flow increases were seen both in the region of the occluded AVM (increase of 88%) and far from the AVM (mean increase of 69%). These phenomena were validated both quantitatively and qualitatively using several methods, including the observation of improved watershed filling on angiographic studies following AVM resection. Subsequently, other authors have confirmed these findings of poor ipsilateral and contralateral hemispheric blood flow preoperatively, except in the AVM region, with significant bilateral increases following AVM elimination (5–8).

Nornes and Grip (9) used pulsed echo Doppler flow meters to measure feeding artery velocities in 16 AVM patients. Using specially designed 3-mm probe tips, they found a clear

tendency to higher flow velocities in larger arteries. Additionally, in the 11 patients with more than one AVM feeding artery, 8 showed higher flow velocities in the larger vessels. They were also able to calculate bulk flow through the AVM in 9 patients and determined a range of 150–900 ml/min, with a mean flow of 490 ml/min. With respect to AVM feeding artery pressures, the authors measured a mean pressure of 56 mm Hg in the 8 patients studied with a corresponding mean systemic arterial pressure of about 105 mm Hg. This difference in arterial pressure is in contrast to normal cerebral arteries which sustain about 90% of systemic pressure (10–12). Studying the venous outflow of the AVM, the authors noted mean velocities and waveforms indicative of arterial flow. This suggested, as other studies had, that arterial pulses were mediated through the AVM shunt to the venous side (13,14). Upon sequential occlusion of all inflow to the AVM, the pulsatile venous flow disappeared along with a marked fall in outflow venous pressure (toward zero). After occlusion of all arterial feeders, Nornes and Grip noted an extreme rise in the surrounding nutrient vessel blood flow. The mean increase in perfusion pressure to these vessels was greater than 50 mm Hg, or almost a 100% increase over baseline pressure. Interestingly, the three patients in their series who developed moderate to marked cerebral swelling following feeder occlusion also demonstrated the largest increases in perfusion pressure with the occlusion.

Barnett and colleagues (15) measured local cerebral blood flow (CBF) intraoperatively in 18 patients using thermistor/Peltier (Flotronics, Phoenix, AZ) stack arrays applied to the cortex both near (<2 cm) and far (>2 cm) from the AVM margin. Comparing pre- and postresection CBF values revealed 18 of 21 measurement increases in CBF at far sites, from a preoperative mean of 43 ml/100 g/min to a postexcision value of 57 ml/100 g/min ($p < 0.05$). In contrast, blood flow changes at near sites showed the same number of flow increases and decreases between the two measurements. However, difficulty with such near-area blood flow measurements may have been due to intraoperative retraction and surgical trauma. Overall, mean flows in the pre-excision AVM cortex were approximately two thirds of those of control patients undergoing asymptomatic aneurysm clipping.

These authors also compared CO_2 reactivity and vascular pressure measurements in AVM patients vs. control subjects. No significant differences in CO_2 reactivity were obtained when comparing pre- and postoperative values (6). In the six patients, a complete set of arterial pressure measurements were available. Three demonstrated low feeding artery pressures of 38–63% of mean systemic arterial pressure. Following feeding artery occlusion and AVM excision, measurement of these stump pressures approximated systemic mean arterial pressure (MAP). At the same time, draining vein pressures fell from a preocclusion mean of 8 mm Hg greater than central venous pressure (CVP) to just 1–2 mm Hg greater than CVP following resection.

Postoperatively, two patients in this study developed severe generalized swelling in the ipsilateral hemisphere surrounding the resection bed. One patient had a large AVM (>4 cm) and the other a small AVM (<2 cm). Interestingly, both patients demonstrated >30 ml/100 g/min increase in CBF (the largest increases in the population studied) at far sites as well as impaired CO_2 reactivity at both near and far sites. One of the two had progressive neurologic deficits preoperatively. No direct vessel pressure measurements were available in these two patients.

Cerebral hemodynamics in AVM patients were also studied by Hassler and Steinmetz (16) using intraoperative intravascular pressure recordings (6 operations) and microvascular Doppler sonography (33 operations). Mean feeding artery pressures ranged between 45% and 62% of MAP preoperatively. Following arterial occlusion and AVM resection, feeding artery pressures increased by 52–69% whereas the pCO$_2$ was held stable. No correlation in feeding artery pressures with AVM size or length or diameter of feeding vessels was shown. In evaluating flow velocities before AVM resections, feeding arteries exhibited very high flow velocities with elevated systolic and markedly elevated diastolic components indicating low peripheral resistance (Fig. 2). Draining veins displayed arterialized spectra. Brain-supplying arteries off feeding arteries but distal to the AVM also demonstrated elevated diastolic velocities, suggesting that surrounding parenchymal arterioles were dilated secondary to abnormally low intravascular pressures. Remote arteries (not supplying the angioma) showed normal Doppler spectra. The authors also examined CO_2 reactivity in each of these vessels. Preoperatively, they found that responses in angioma suppliers were almost abolished with only a small velocity increase with hypercapnia and with no change after hypocapnia. The brain supplying arteries off the feeders demonstrated approximately normal flow acceleration with

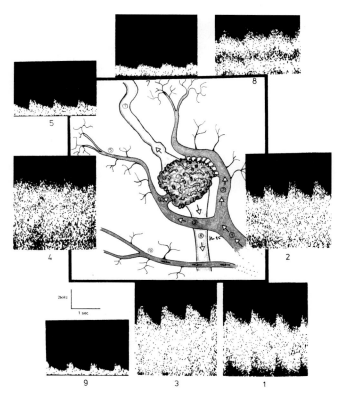

FIG. 2. Preresection intraoperative Doppler tracings of blood flow velocities surrounding an arteriovenous malformation. Feeding arteries 1–4 depict typical Doppler waveforms with high systolic and diastolic velocities and low pulsatility. An en passage vessel (5) demonstrates an elevated velocity throughout diastole due to decreased peripheral vascular resistance. An unassociated artery (9) shows normal Doppler patterns. Draining veins (7 and 8) have arterialized spectra. (From ref. 16.)

hypercapnia but impaired reduction with hypocapnia perhaps due to lack of vasoconstriction in the peripheral brain distribution. Remote arteries had normal reactivities. Following AVM resection, the feeding artery velocities markedly diminished, as expected, the remote arteries were unaffected, and the distal brain supplying arteries showed evidence of slightly elevated peripheral resistance. No flow accelerations were ever observed in these vessels. For CO_2 reactivity following AVM resection, some element of normal vasomotor responses was seen in all arteries measured (Fig. 3). In the brain supplying arteries off the angioma feeders, normal spectra following excision were apparent, whereas feeding arteries demonstrated some, albeit blunted, responses. These changes in CO_2 reactivities in the distal brain supplying vessels demonstrated the stronger autoregulative effect of hypotension (or low intravascular pressures) caused by the downstream AVM over CO_2 autoregulation in surrounding cerebral tissues.

In 1990, Muraszko et al (17) performed several important laboratory experiments on isolated segments of feeding arteries in 24 AVM patients. These data were correlated to the

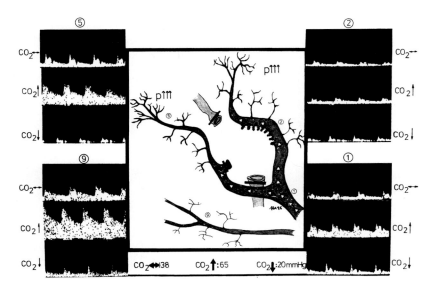

FIG. 3. Intraoperative postresection Doppler sonograms of CO_2 reactivity in the surrounding resection bed. The feeding arteries have been eliminated. The en passage vessel (5) has a normal vasomotor response. Arterial dilatation and flow acceleration occur with hypercapnia; constriction and flow deceleration occur with hypocapnia. These responses were not seen before arteriovenous malformation resection. (From ref. 16.)

patients' postoperative clinical course. The authors selected feeding artery segments just proximal to the AVM nidus. Each was at least 1 cm in length and 0.8 mm in internal diameter. These segments were taken at the time of the operation and immediately placed in a perfusion chamber. Studies were then performed to assess spontaneous muscular activity as well as isometric contraction of the rings to various vasoactive substances. As control vessels, the authors used canine basilar artery segments along with eight fresh, normal human cadaver vessels. Feeding artery segments from 4 of the 24 patients were clearly abnormal. None of these four patients developed any spontaneous contractile activity in the perfusion bath, while all other vessels demonstrated contractile abilities. Furthermore, in testing these vessels against numerous vasoactive substances, the same four vessels failed to show a contractile response. All other specimens demonstrated isometric contractions to at least three of the compounds tested. Clinically, each of the four patients with poor feeding artery muscular activity had Spetzler–Martin grade IV or V AVMs (18). All had continued ectasia of their feeding arteries on postoperative angiography, vs. 7 of the 19 normal contractile group. Also, three of the four patients in the nonreactive group had complicated postoperative courses characterized by hemispheric swelling, edema, and/or hemorrhage. When those patients with normally reactive vessels were examined postoperatively, only one of nine with grade IV and V AVMs was noted to have postoperative difficulties. Thus, this in vitro feeding artery analysis was able to detect clear abnormalities in several AVM-feeding arteries and successfully correlate these deficiencies to clinical outcome, though clearly not in a rigorous scientific manner. An important question left unanswered by this study, however, was the relationship of these findings to the surrounding brain nutrient arteries. Most likely, it is these latter vessels that are responsible for the postoperative sequelae.

Further examination of feeding artery pressures was performed by Spetzler and associates (19). They studied arterial pressures and CBF in large AVMs (≥ 6 cm) subjected to staged embolization and operative excision. As with the study by Nornes and Grip (9), these authors found that low feeding artery pressures existed in large, high-flow AVMs. These pressures ranged from 26% to 38% of mean systemic pressure. After clipping the feeding arteries, intraoperative measurements proximal to the occlusion demonstrated an immediate increase in arterial pressure that approximated systemic pressure (Fig. 4). Given the decrease in shunt flow to the nidus following occlusion, a concomitant reduction in draining venous pressure was expected. Each of these pressure changes should increase cerebral perfusion pressure and hence increase CBF to the ipsilateral hemisphere. The authors confirmed this finding by utilizing the thermal diffusion technique or by xenon CT (these flow increases have also been noted to occur in the contralateral hemisphere) (6,20,21). In the portion of the feeding artery distal to the occlusion, pressures were noted to fall considerably (Fig. 4). These same pressures increased markedly following the embolization procedure. This pressure increase was most likely due to a decrease in venous runoff or an increased peripheral resistance caused by the embolic material. Furthermore, if the occluding clip was then removed from the embolized feeding artery, a higher feeding artery pressure in combination with an increased peripheral (nidal) resistance was encountered. This created a system with a potentially increased risk of hemorrhage (see below).

Data from several of the above studies suggest that large, high-flow AVMs are fed by low-pressure arteries. Coupled to this is the observation that larger AVMs more often present with neurologic deficits or seizures whereas hemorrhage is the more common presentation of small AVMs (22,23). This latter relationship seems counterintuitive when one considers that nidus volume increases geometrically with respect to AVM radius and that the nidus is presumably the source of hemorrhage for most lesions. Spetzler and colleagues (23) examined this apparent paradox prospectively

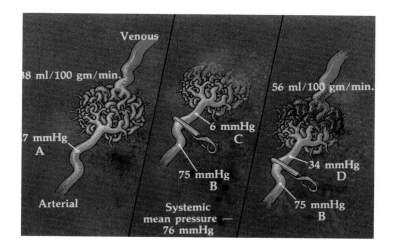

FIG. 4. Schematic presentation with actual measurements from a single patient. The change in cortical cerebral blood flow from 38 to 56 ml/100 g/min was recorded with the thermal diffusion flow probe. The other measurements were those recorded directly from the feeding artery. The perfusion pressure in the artery feeding the arteriovenous malformation (AVM) was 27 mm Hg **(A)**. Following placement of a clip on the feeding vessel the perfusion pressure rose proximally to 75 mm Hg **(B)**, approaching systemic arterial pressure, while the pressure distal to the clip dropped to 6 mm Hg **(C)**. After embolization of the AVM through the feeding vessel the distal perfusion pressure actually rose to 34 mm Hg **(D)** as the venous runoff was largely obliterated. The increased risk of hemorrhage if the proximal clip had been removed can be appreciated, as the AVM would have been changed from a relatively low-pressure system of 27 mm Hg (A) to a higher pressure system of 75 mm Hg (B). The importance of proximal vessel occlusion following embolization is thus emphasized. (From ref. 19.)

in a group of 92 AVM patients looking at lesion size, clinical presentation, and arterial perfusion pressure. Figure 5 (23) summarizes a portion of their data and reveals that small AVMs (0–3 cm in greatest dimension) presented with hemorrhage significantly more often than medium-sized (3–6 cm) or large AVMs (>6 cm). Moreover, hematoma size, as measured by the greatest diameter on the presenting CT scan, was inversely proportional to the AVM size (Fig. 6) (23). Twenty-four patients in this study were then available for intraoperative feeding artery pressure measurements by the strain gauge technique. Ten of these patients presented with hemorrhage whereas 14 developed other neurologic symptoms. In patients with hemorrhage, mean feeding artery pressure was 90% of mean systemic pressure vs. 47% in those

without hemorrhage. In addition, the mean feeding artery pressure was significantly higher, 64 ± 12 mm Hg, in AVMs that bled as opposed to pressures of 36 ± 17 mm Hg in those with other presentations. Furthermore, mean feeding artery pressure was significantly higher in patients with small AVMs (66 ± 12 mm Hg) compared to medium-sized AVMs (47 ± 17 mm Hg) and large AVMs (35 ± 17 mm Hg), regardless of the mode of presentation. In none of the above groups did systemic arterial pressures differ significantly. Hence, because smaller AVMs had higher feeding artery pressures that closely approximated mean systemic pressure, Spetzler and colleagues (23) suggested this as the pathophysiologic reason for their presenting more commonly with hemorrhage. In contrast, larger AVMs, with

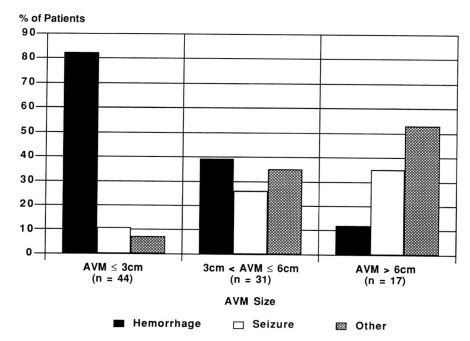

% of Patients

FIG. 5. Relationship between the size and type of clinical presentation of arteriovenous malformations (AVMs). Small AVMs ruptured significantly more often ($p < 0.001$, χ^2 test) than medium-sized and large AVMs. There was no significant difference in the type of clinical presentation of medium-sized and large lesions. Similar data have been corroborated by other AVM studies, including that of Kader et al. (21) in this manuscript. (From ref. 23.)

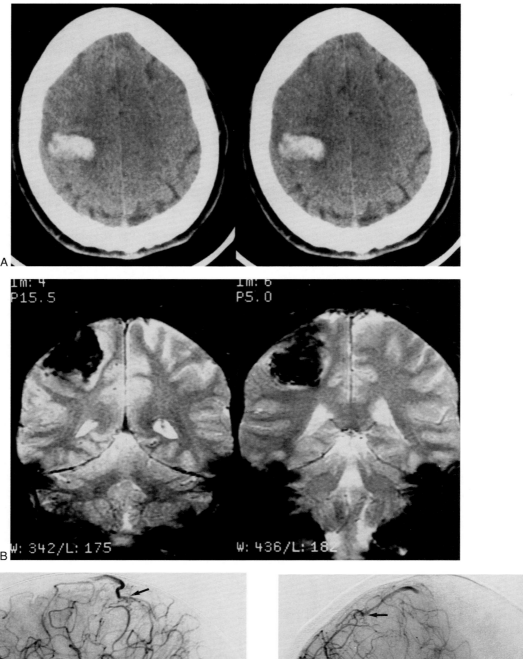

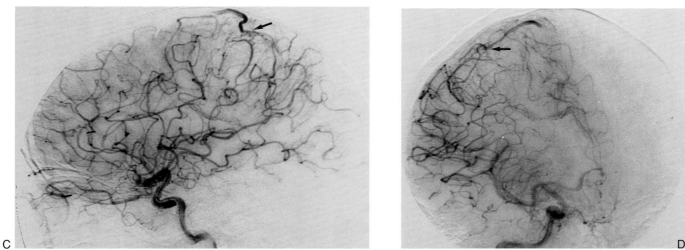

FIG. 6. A 29-year-old man presented with left hemiparesis and dysphasia. **(A)** A noncontrasted CT scan shows an intracerebral hemorrhage. **(B)** The coronal MR image depicts the extent of the acute bleed. **(C)** Lateral and **(D)** oblique subtracted angiograms demonstrate a very small AVM *(arrows)* with its associated early draining vein. This case shows the inverse relationship between AVM size and hematoma volume.

the lower resistance shunts, more often present with neurologic symptoms secondary to decreased nutritive (surrounding) blood flow.

The study of AVM venous physiology is scant in the recent literature. Young and colleagues (24) reported their studies of draining vein physiology in 1994. Their purpose was to assess pressure transmission across the AVM nidus as well as to identify the variables influencing the draining vein(s). All pressure measurements were made intraoperatively using the strain gauge technique. Two thirds of the patients had undergone preoperative embolization. In general, they found no influence of size, clinical presentation, presence of deep venous drainage, angiographic venous stenosis, or location of the AVM on their analyses. Following AVM resection, the authors found a significant decrease in the draining vein pressure (DVP). However, this result was more pronounced and consistent when the central venous pressure (CVP) was factored into the comparison. The authors then examined the relationship between feeding artery pressure and DVP in 21 of their patients. As in previous studies (9,15), a positive correlation between the two was confirmed. This association was even more significant when pressures were referenced to the head as opposed to the right atrium. Although this relationship suggested some element of a passive pressure conduit across the nidus, the correlation was much less than identity. Therefore, an inherent buffering capacity of the nidus was suggested. This buffer may be no more than the existence of significant venous capacitance within the fistula. When systemic arterial pressure and CVP were each experimentally increased, the draining vein behaved more as a venous rather than an arterial structure with little effect transmitted across the nidus. Hence, in this instance, the AVM did not appear to behave as a simple conduit for pressure transmission. Finally, the authors also demonstrated that the net perfusion pressure, or transnidal pressure, across the AVM (feeding artery pressure − draining vein pressure) was inversely correlated to AVM size (ie, higher in small AVMs). The authors suggested that this higher transnidal pressure across smaller sized AVMs may be another explanation as to why smaller AVMs present more often with hemorrhage.

CEREBRAL STEAL, AUTOREGULATION, AND THE NORMAL PERFUSION PRESSURE BREAKTHROUGH SYNDROME

One conclusion that can be drawn from the hemodynamics of AVMs is that these lesions induce feeding artery hypotension coupled with draining vein hypertension amounting to a net reduction in surrounding brain perfusion pressure. The total effect these pressure changes induce in the cerebral circulation, and hence function, however, is unknown. From a clinical standpoint, AVMs may present with symptoms due to intracranial hemorrhage. They may also cause neurologic deficits due to pulsatile compression of surrounding tissue,

hydrocephalus, seizures, headaches, or cerebral steal. This latter term was first coined by J. P. Murphy (4) when he noted that feeding artery diameters decreased following AVM resection, whereas the remaining arterial tree filled more completely. The steal syndrome thus refers to the shunting of blood from branching nutrient vessels to the AVM secondary to lowered intravascular resistance and pressures engendered by the high-flow malformation. Furthermore, although they are congenital lesions, AVMs have been shown to progress via recruitment of collateral blood supply from adjacent circulations (ie, from the posterior circulation in an anterior circulation-based lesion) and/or from the contralateral circulation (25). Thus, steal and ischemia occur when collateral blood flow and autoregulation fail to compensate for the diminishing perfusion of the brain adjacent to an AVM. Clinically, this phenomenon may be illustrated by motor, sensory, visual, or language deficits, or, alternatively, as a slowly progressive dementia. Seizure activity is another potential clinical manifestation. Once interruption of the steal occurs, as with AVM resection or sometimes with selective embolization, dramatic clinical improvement is possible, suggesting an increase in local blood flow as the principle factor.

In 1978, Spetzler et al (26) suggested that certain large AVMs exhibiting chronic steal symptoms from surrounding tissue may impair the autoregulatory capacity of the brain. They reasoned that with large lesions the nutrient vessels of normal brain adjacent to the AVM must chronically dilate their arterial trees in order to usurp blood from the AVM. Following AVM resection, however, this chronically ischemic arterial tree, now exposed to a much greater perfusion pressure, may not retain its ability to regulate this increased blood flow. The increased hydrostatic pressure seen by the capillaries could therefore result in significant edema, and perhaps hemorrhage, due to capillary breakthrough. This clinical picture was termed the normal perfusion pressure breakthrough (NPPB) syndrome. This mechanism may be similar to the infrequent hyperperfusion syndrome found after carotid endarterectomy (27).

NPPB is a rare complication in most series. It occurred in only 2 of 166 cases of Drake (28), in 2 of 65 cases reported by Wilson et al (29), and in 3 of 90 cases reported by Luessenhop and Rosa (30). In this latter report, however, NPPB occurred in 3 of the 16 patients with AVMs greater than 4 cm. Other authors continue to report the occurrence, complications, and treatment of NPPB (6,15,17,31,32). A compilation of this data suggest an increased risk of NPPB in AVMs with (a) large size, (b) rapid shunt flow (high-flow AVMs), (c) large caliber of feeding arteries, (d) poor CBF to areas adjacent to the AVM (paucity of filling of normal vasculature on angiography), (e) reduced feeding pressure relative to mean systemic pressure on preoperative studies, especially if this pressure is less than 50% of MAP, (f) substantially increased feeding artery pressure following excision, (g) angiographic steal from ipsilateral and contralateral circulations including the external circulation, (h) feeding arteries with impaired CO_2 reactivity, (i) feeding arteries greater than 8 cm in length, and (j) a history of progressive or fluctuating neurologic deficits. In patients with these AVM characteristics, consideration should be given to staged obliteration and resection (see below, "Practical Considerations").

Although Spetzler first questioned the status of cerebral autoregulation in patients with large AVMs, much recent work on this subject has been performed by Young and associates at Columbia University (6,21,33). These authors found preserved pressure autoregulation in a group of 25 patients undergoing 28 procedures for moderate to large AVMs (21). Using the xenon-133 method, CBF was measured intraoperatively in both hemispheres following AVM exposure, after gross total resection, and following an increase in MAP of 20 mm Hg using phenylephrine. Their results demonstrated the well-described increase in CBF between the first two measurements but failed to show further increases in perfusion given the phenylephrine challenge. They concluded that, given the lack of augmentation of flow with phenylephrine, the increase in CBF seen between pre- and postoperative measurements was not due to paralyzed resistance arterioles passively accepting an increased perfusion pressure. However, several caveats to this study should be noted. First, 11 of the 25 patients underwent preoperative embolization. It is possible that this staging of procedures was successful in restoring cerebral autoregulation prior to the intraoperative monitoring. Second, 23 of the 25 patients had uncomplicated postoperative courses. Hence these patients may never have been at risk of developing NPPB because of (previously) intact autoregulation. Third, two patients developed postoperative swelling and hemorrhage. These same two patients demonstrated the largest absolute increases in CBF from pre- to postoperative measurements, though without a significant pressure-passive CBF response. Nonetheless, this finding, in accordance with that of others (9,15), is predictive of those patients at risk for NPPB. The authors did caution that the intraoperative findings, under general anesthesia and with modest hypocapnia in the presence of a craniotomy, may not be applicable to the awake state at normocapnia. Finally, the resolution of the CBF technique, as well as the areas of measurement, must be questioned. The detector probes were placed bilaterally 5–6 cm from the nidus margin in the same major arterial territory. Most likely, however, the arterioles at greatest risk for vasomotor paralysis are those immediately adjacent to the AVM nidus. Hence, changes attributable to those vessels were almost certainly missed by this technique. Therefore, whether autoregulation is truly preserved in these regions may still be unanswered.

The same authors took this information one step further and hypothesized that the cerebral autoregulatory curve is displaced to the left in these hypotensive cortical territories adjacent to AVMs (24). This shift is analogous to the upward displacement of the autoregulatory curve noted in chronic hypertension. The methodology employed allowed feeding artery pressure measurements and xenon-133 CBF calculations during feeding artery pedicle embolization. Baseline pressure and CBF measurements were taken and compared with those same measurements following a phenylephrine challenge that increased feeding artery pressures by more than 33%. Only 1 of 14 patients in 15 procedures demonstrated a significant increase in CBF and this individual had a 4 mm Hg increase in pCO_2 between the two measurements. When individuals were stratified into those with severe feeding artery hypotension relative to systemic pressure (feeding artery pressure less than 54% of systemic pressure) and those with moderate hypotension, no significant change in CBF was again demonstrated. These findings allowed the authors to conclude that insofar as the limits of their technique, autoregulation was maintained in areas adjacent to an AVM (30). Further, they postulated that, given the significant feeding artery hypotension measured in this study (and in their previous studies), a shift of the lower limit of MAP to the left in the autoregulatory curve may account for the lack of signs of ischemia in these patients despite the significant hypotension. Similar difficulties existed in this study as with the previous one, however, including a lack of patients who demonstrated clinical NPPB (and hence their pressure and CBF measurements). Additionally, their severe hypotensive group displayed feeding artery pressures that were not nearly as hypotensive as previous studies (19). Nonetheless, these two studies demonstrated that given the limits of current techniques, the majority of patients undergoing AVM treatment do not experience CBF changes that are pressure passive. Hence, some degree of autoregulation must be preserved in these instances. For those few patients whose postoperative course is complicated by breakthrough, however, little information is available.

PRACTICAL CONSIDERATIONS

Little doubt remains regarding the need for treatment in patients found to harbor an AVM. Although once thought to be somewhat benign in nature, many series have reported and concluded that these lesions possess a yearly rebleeding rate of 2–4% (34–36) as well as annual morbidity and mortality rates both in the range of 1–2.5% (34–36). Furthermore, based on a literature review, each hemorrhagic episode from an AVM carries a 10–15% mortality rate and a 20–30% permanent morbidity rate (37).

The current recommendations for treatment in AVM patients is based on our results in two recent series comprising 220 patients (18,38) in association with other major AVM series in the recent literature (39,40). For patients in suitable neurologic condition with Spetzler–Martin grade I and II lesions, complete microsurgical resection is recommended regardless of whether the lesion is or has been symptomatic (18). Based on the prospective application of this grading system for 120 total patients, grade I and II patients suffered no treatment-associated morbidity or mortality given a mean follow-up of 1 year (38). Spetzler–Martin grade III AVMs are evaluated individually with regard to neurologic and medical condition, presenting features, and AVM components. Nonetheless, based on the fact that no new major neurologic morbidity occurred for this AVM grade in the prospective report, asymptomatic patients are frequently suggested for surgery, whereas symptomatic individuals are routinely recommended for resection. For these three patient grades, the risks of the natural history of the AVM are greater than the associated treatment, and cure, of the lesion. Given the current risks of embolization therapy of 5–10% (41–43), this treatment is not recommended in grade I or II lesions, and only exceptionally for grade III AVMs.

More difficult recommendations arise for patients harboring grade IV and V AVMs. Multiple factors must be taken into account for these patients to determine whether surgical or nonsurgical care is warranted. These include patient's age and medical condition, neurologic presentation and current neurologic status, occurrence of repetitive intracerebral hemorrhages, the patient's desires, and the surgeon's operative experience. Since the majority of these lesions will require preoperative and perhaps intraoperative transarterial embolization, the risks of this treatment must be included as well (41–43). Surgery is currently recommended for such patients only if they present with progressive neurologic disability, repetitive AVM hemorrhage, or have a fixed neurologic deficit in the distribution of the AVM. Given these stringent criteria, approximately 25% of patients with these AVMs are selected for surgery.

Once surgery is indicated, a multidisciplinary approach is required. This includes the microneurosurgical and endovascular teams initially, perhaps the radiosurgeons if a residual nidus remains, and the important support staff for the patient. It has been the experience of the senior author that most of these lesions require staged surgical management. Staging these procedures is critical because of their large size, high flow, propensity to have multiple feeders, and other characteristics that put these patients at high risk for developing NPPB (see above). Obliterating these lesions in stages allows a stepwise adaptation in cerebral hemodynamics that potentially avoids the disastrous consequences of abrupt resection.

Most often this staged approach begins with one or more episodes of transfemoral embolization followed by intraoperative embolotherapy. Aggressive transfemoral embolization should be avoided in favor of intraoperative transarterial therapy because the latter approach provides better control, permits extensive embolization of the selected portion of the nidus, and allows ligation of the feeding artery. This ligation prevents the elevated proximal pressure, due to embolization, from being transmitted to nonoccluded portions of the AVM in the distribution of the feeding artery (Fig. 4). This remains a key factor in avoiding postembolization hemorrhage (44). Most often, one major group of feeding vessels is embolized during each stage. Once extensive embolization has been accomplished, the final stage(s) is (are) reserved for microsurgical resection. All intraoperative procedures are performed under barbiturate anesthesia (thiopental) and mild

hypothermia for cerebral protection during periods of temporary ischemia. Despite embolization, all of these lesions remain viable and pose technically challenging surgery. The small, deep penetrating vessels are the most difficult to control. They require patience and persistence. Occasionally, mild hypotension is necessary to control bleeding. Once excision is complete, a thorough inspection of the resection bed is mandatory. Postoperative hemorrhage is more commonly due to residual AVM or precarious hemostasis in fragile vessels than from NPPB. Postoperatively, four-vessel angiography should be performed in all cases. Additional treatment is based on this information.

In our recent prospective AVM series, 44 patients with grade IV and V lesions required surgical therapy. Grade IV patients underwent a mean of 2.9 procedures each (embolization plus surgery), compared to 4.4 in the grade V patients. In late follow-up (mean 1 year), 78% and 86% of patients in grades IV and V, respectively, were improved or unchanged neurologically. For grade IV lesions, the remaining 22% deteriorated by one grade based on the Glasgow Outcome Scale (GOS). In the 17% (2 patients) who developed a new deficit with grade V lesions, one patient deteriorated by one grade and the other by two grades on the GOS. No deaths occurred in either group.

REFERENCES

1. Kaplan HA, Aronson SM, Browder EJ. Vascular malformations of the brain. An anatomical study. *J Neurosurg* 1961;18:630–635.
2. Kaplan HA. The transcerebral venous system. An anatomical study. *Arch Neurol* 1959;1:148–152.
3. McCormick WF, Rosenfield DB. Massive brain hemorrhage: A review of 144 cases and an examination of their causes. *Stroke* 1973;4: 946–954.
4. Feindel W, Yamamoto YL, Hodge CP. Red cerebral veins and the cerebral steal syndrome. Evidence from fluorescein angiography and microregional blood flow by radioisotopes during excision of an angioma. *J Neurosurg* 1971;35:167–179.
5. Takeuchi S, Kikuchi H, Karasawa J, Naruo Y, Hashimoto K, Nishimura T, Kozuka T, et al. Cerebral hemodynamics in arteriovenous malformations: evaluation by single-photon emission CT. *AJNR* 1987;8: 193–197.
6. Young WL, Prohovnik I, Ornstein E, Ostapkovich N, Sisti MB, Solomon RA, Stein BM. The effect of arteriovenous malformation resection on cerebrovascular reactivity to carbon dioxide. *Neurosurgery* 1990; 27:257–267.
7. Homan RW, Devous MD, Sr., Stokely EM, Bonte FJ. Quantification of intracerebral steal in patients with arteriovenous malformation. *Arch Neurol* 1986;43:779–785.
8. Tyler JL, Leblanc R, Meyer E, Dagher A, Yamamoto YL, Diksic M, Hakim A. Hemodynamic and metabolic effects of cerebral arteriovenous malformations studied by positron emission tomography. *Stroke* 1989;20:890–898.
9. Nornes H, Grip A. Hemodynamic aspects of cerebral arteriovenous malformations. *J Neurosurg* 1980;53:456–464.
10. Little JR, Tomsak RL, Ebrahim ZY, Furlan AJ. Retinal artery pressure and cerebral artery perfusion pressure in cerebrovascular occlusive disease. *Neurosurgery* 1986;18:716–720.
11. Spetzler RF, Roski RA, Zabramski J. Middle cerebral artery perfusion pressure in cerebrovascular occlusive disease. *Stroke* 1983;14: 552–555.
12. Bakay L, Sweet WH. Cervical and intracranial intra-arterial pressures with and without vascular occlusion. *Surg Gynecol Obstet* 1952;95: 67–75.

13. Nornes H, Grip A, Wikeby P. Intraoperative evaluation of cerebral hemodynamics using directional Doppler technique. *J Neurosurg* 1979; 50:145–151.

14. Dandy WE. Venous abnormalities and angiomas of the brain. *Arch Surg* 1928;17:715–793.

15. Barnett GH, Little JR, Ebrahim ZY, Jones SC, Friel HT. Cerebral circulation during arteriovenous malformation operation. *Neurosurgery* 1987;20:836–842.

16. Hassler W, Steinmetz H. Cerebral hemodynamics in angioma patients: An intraoperative study. *J Neurosurg* 1987;67:822–831.

17. Muraszko K, Wang HH, Pelton G, Stein BM. A study of the reactivity of feeding vessels to arteriovenous malformations: correlation with clinical outcome. *Neurosurgery* 1990;26:190–200.

18. Spetzler RF, Martin NA. A proposed grading system for arteriovenous malformations. *J Neurosurg* 1986;65:476–483.

19. Spetzler RF, Martin NA, Carter LP, Flom RA, Raudzens PA, Wilkinson E. Surgical management of large AVMs by staged embolization and operative excision. *J Neurosurg* 1987;67:17–28.

20. Okabe T, Meyer JS, Okayasu H, Harper R, Rose J, Grossman RG, Centeno R, et al. Xenon-enhanced CT CBF measurements in cerebral AVMs before and after excision. *J Neurosurg* 1983;59:21–31.

21. Young WL, Kader A, Prohovnik I, Ornstein E, Fleischer LH, Ostapkovich N, Jackson LD, et al. Pressure autoregulation is intact after arteriovenous malformation resection. *Neurosurgery* 1993;32:491–497.

22. Kader A, Young WL, Pile-Spellman J, Mast H, Sciacca RR, Mohr JP, Stein BM, et al. The influence of hemodynamic and anatomic factors on hemorrhage from cerebral arteriovenous malformations. *Neurosurgery* 1994;34:801–808.

23. Spetzler RF, Hargraves RW, McCormick PW, Zabramski JM, Flom RA, Zimmerman RS. Relationship of perfusion pressure and size to risk of hemorrhage from arteriovenous malformations. *J Neurosurg* 1992;76:918–923.

24. Young WL, Kader A, Pile-Spellman J, Ornstein E, Stein BM, the Columbia University AVM Study Project. Arteriovenous malformation draining vein physiology and determinants of transnidal pressure gradients. *Neurosurgery* 1994;35:389–396.

25. Luessenhop AJ. Natural history of cerebral arteriovenous malformations. In: Wilson CB, Stein BM, eds. *Intracranial Arteriovenous Malformations.* Baltimore: Williams and Wilkins, 1984;12–23.

26. Spetzler RF, Wilson CB, Weinstein P, Mehdorn M, Townsend J, Telles D. Normal perfusion pressure breakthrough theory. *Clin Neurosurg* 1978;25:651–672.

27. Bernstein M, Fleming JFR, Deck JHN. Cerebral hyperperfusion after carotid endarterectomy: a cause of cerebral hemorrhage. *Neurosurgery* 1984;15:50–56.

28. Drake CG. Cerebral arteriovenous malformations: considerations for and experience with surgical treatment in 166 cases. *Clin Neurosurg* 1979;145–208.

29. Wilson CB, Sang H, Domingue J. Microsurgical treatment of intracranial vascular malformations. *J Neurosurg* 1979;51:446–454.

30. Luessenhop AJ, Rosa L. Cerebral arteriovenous malformations: indications for and results of surgery, and the role of intravascular techniques. *J Neurosurg* 1984;60:14–22.

31. Day AL, Friedman WA, Sypert GW, Mickle JP. Successful treatment of the normal perfusion pressure breakthrough syndrome. *Neurosurgery* 1982;11:625–630.

32. Batjer HH, Devous MD, Sr., Meyer YJ, Purdy PD, Samson DS. Cerebrovascular hemodynamics in arteriovenous malformation complicated by normal perfusion pressure breakthrough. *Neurosurgery* 1988;22:503–509.

33. Young WL, Pile-Spellman J, Prohovnik I, Kader A, Stein BM, the Columbia University AVM Study Project. Evidence for adaptive autoregulatory displacement in hypotensive cortical territories adjacent to arteriovenous malformations. *Neurosurgery* 1994;34:601–611.

34. Brown RD Jr, Wiebers DO, Forbes G, O'Fallon WM, Piepgras DG, Marsh WR, Maciunas RJ. The natural history of unruptured intracranial arteriovenous malformations. *J Neurosurg* 1988;68:352–357.

35. Crawford PM, West CR, Chadwick DW, Shaw MDM. Arteriovenous malformations of the brain: natural history in unoperated patients. *J Neurol Neurosurg Psychiatry* 1986;49:1–10.

36. Ondra SL, Troupp H, George ED, Schwab K. The natural history of symptomatic arteriovenous malformations of the brain: a 24-year follow-up assessment. *J Neurosurg* 1990;73:387–391.

37. Samson DS, Batjer HH. Preoperative evaluation of the risk/benefit ratio for arteriovenous malformations of the brain. In: Wilkins RH, Rengachary SS, eds. *Neurosurgery Update II. Vascular, Spinal, Pediatric, and Functional Neurosurgery.* New York: McGraw-Hill, 1991; 129–133.

38. Hamilton MG, Spetzler RF. The prospective application of a grading system for arteriovenous malformations. *Neurosurgery* 1994;34:2–7.

39. Heros RC, Korosue K, Diebold PM. Surgical excision of cerebral arteriovenous malformations: late results. *Neurosurgery* 1990;26:570–578.

40. Stein BM, Kader A. Intracranial arteriovenous malformations. *Clin Neurosurg* 1991;76–113.

41. Purdy PD, Batjer H, Samson D. Management of hemorrhagic complications from preoperative embolization of arteriovenous malformations. *J Neurosurg* 1991;74:205–211.

42. Benati A. Interventional neuroradiology for the treatment of inaccessible arterio-venous malformations. *Acta Neurochir (Wien)* 1992;118:76–79.

43. Viñuela F, Dion JE, Duckwiler G, Martin NA, Lylyk P, Fox A, Pelz D, et al. Combined endovascular embolizatioin and surgery management of cerebral arteriovenous malformations: experience with 101 cases. *J Neurosurg* 1991;75:856–864.

44. Mullan S, Kawanaga H, Patronas NJ. Microvascular embolization of cerebral arteriovenous malformations. A technical variation. *J Neurosurg* 1979;51:621–627.

Cerebrovascular Disease, edited by H. Hunt Batjer.
Lippincott-Raven Publishers, Philadelphia © 1997.

CHAPTER 68

Neuroanesthetic Considerations for Surgical and Endovascular Therapy of Arteriovenous Malformations

William L. Young, Eugene Ornstein, Kristy Z. Baker, and John Pile-Spellman

GENERAL CONSIDERATIONS

Arteriovenous malformations (AVMs) are a treatable cause of neurological morbidity usually found in young adults (1). The primary goal of treatment is to decrease the risk of spontaneous bleeding and this is best accomplished by total surgical obliteration. The risk of spontaneous hemorrhage from an AVM is in the range of 3% per year. Although the numbers vary with the particular series, approximately one third of these patients will die from the bleed, one third will have a significant stroke, and one third will escape unscathed. Risk for bleeding is probably higher in smaller, higher pressure AVMs that include aneurysms in the nidus or have periventricular venous drainage, especially if venous occlusive disease is present (2).

There are several important differences between aneurysms and AVMs that the anesthesiologist should note. Approximately 10% of patients with AVMs also harbor intracranial aneurysms. However, the converse is not true; the incidence of AVMs in aneurysm patients is probably much closer to the incidence of AVMs in the general population. Intracerebral hemorrhage from aneurysms is usually associated with subarachnoid hemorrhage, whereas AVMs more commonly bleed into the ventricle or into parenchyma. This explains why the occurrence of vasospasm is distinctly uncommon in AVM cases. Spontaneous hemorrhage during the perioperative period as a result of variations in systemic blood pressure are probably less likely as well (3), due to a buffering capacity of the fistula on changes in systemic pressure (4).

There are three modes for treatment of AVMs: endovascular embolization, radiosurgery, and surgical excision. Treatment strategies, especially for complex lesions, frequently involve more than one modality. In general, endovascular therapy is performed as a preparatory adjunct to surgery. Using various glues or other embolic materials, the blood supply to the fistula can be pared down, most commonly in several stages. This has the advantage of allowing surrounding brain regions to adapt to the circulatory changes (discussed below). As a preoperative adjunct, embolization is thought to facilitate operative removal, with less bleeding (5). Embolization also can eliminate deep vascular pedicles that might be difficult to control surgically. The application of radiosurgery is controversial at present; it is probably ideally reserved for smaller lesions that are surgically inaccessible (6).

Obliteration of high-flow feeders is beneficial in patients with progressive neurologic deficits or intractable seizures, probably due to the expanding mass effect of abnormal vascular structures.

CEREBRAL CIRCULATORY CHANGES IN AVM PATIENTS

AVMs may exert a deleterious effect on brain function by several mechanisms, including mass effects (eg, hematoma, edema, or gradually expanding abnormal vascular structures such as venous aneurysms), metabolic depression (diaschisis), and seizure activity. However, a largely unproven but conceptually attractive paradigm is often discussed to ex-

W. L. Young: Departments of Anesthesiology, Neurological Surgery, and Radiology, Columbia University College of Physicians and Surgeons, New York, New York 10032.

E. Ornstein and K. Z. Baker: Department of Anesthesiology, Columbia University College of Physicians and Surgeons, New York, New York 10032.

J. Pile-Spellman: Departments of Radiology and Neurological Surgery, Columbia University College of Physicians and Surgeons, New York, New York 10032.

plain many instances of pretreatment defects—ascribed to cerebral ''steal''—and certain catastrophic posttreatment complications of brain swelling and intracerebral hemorrhage (ICH). This has been termed ''normal perfusion pressure breakthrough'' (NPPB) (7) or ''circulatory breakthrough.'' These models propose that (a) perfusion pressure is reduced to the lower limit of autoregulation by both arterial hypotension and venous hypertension in neighboring vascular territories; (b) arteriolar resistance in these adjacent territories is at or near a state of maximal vasodilatation (if perfusion pressure decreases, steal ensues); (c) chronic hypotension results in ''vasomotor paralysis'' and deranged autoregulatory capability; and (d) reversal of arterial hypotension after treatment is not matched by a corresponding increase in cerebrovascular resistance and results in hyperemia and, in its worst case, swelling or ICH.

Such a model implies that it is not the AVM itself but rather decreased perfusion pressure in adjacent, functional tissue, which is responsible for both pretreatment ischemic and posttreatment hyperemic symptoms. In principle, this model assumes mechanisms encountered in other conditions of reduced perfusion pressure, eg, occlusive atherosclerotic disease (8).

The intraoperative appearance of diffuse bleeding from the operative site or brain swelling and the postoperative occurrence of hemorrhage or swelling have been attributed to NPPB or ''hyperemic'' complications. A difficulty in studying the problem arises due to the very heterogenous set of criteria used by different authors in defining exactly what a hyperemic complication is. Although the incidence of postoperative hyperemic complications has been estimated to be as high as 25–50%, it is probably lower than 5% (9).

However, not only is autoregulation of increases in perfusion generally maintained in cerebral tissue adjacent to AVMs preoperatively and postsurgically, but the lower limit of autoregulation appears to be shifted to the left (10). This adaptive shift to the left places the lower limit at a level considerably lower than the lower limit postulated for normal brain (50 or 60 mm Hg) (7,11). Therefore, the presence of chronic hypotension does not necessarily result in vasoparalysis in the arteriolar resistance bed. Although CO_2 reactivity may be impaired in brain regions surrounding AVMs, there is generally a preserved responsiveness to CO_2 pre- and postsurgical resection, which lends further support to the notion of intact autoregulatory capacity (10).

Cerebral steal is felt by many authors to explain focal neurologic deficits in AVM patients; steal is attributed to local hypotension. As we have recently described (12), focal deficits are a rare presentation (<10%) and not necessarily associated with localized cerebral hypotension. It is highly likely that local mass effects from the abnormal vessels of the AVM are more important than local hemodynamic failure to account for symptomatic focal neurologic deficit unrelated to ICH.

Therefore the diagnoses of steal and NPPB are, if they exist, the exception rather than the rule. As regards intraoperative management, the diagnosis of NPPB should be a diagnosis of exclusion after all other correctable causes for malignant brain swelling or bleeding have been excluded. Our empirical bias is that autonomic or adrenergic blockade may be of use, in addition to other supportive and resuscitative measures, in preventing and treating this syndrome. This has indirect support from reports of both sympathetic activation after AVM resection (13) and the potential activation of perivascular autonomic innervation to the cerebral vasculature after treatment (14).

ANESTHETIC MANAGEMENT DURING SURGERY

Preoperative Management

Since AVM resection is almost never emergent, a careful review of the patient's perioperative status and assessment of potential intraoperative difficulties is possible. Preexisting medical conditions should be optimized and neurologic dysfunction, either as a result of presenting hemorrhage, presumed effect of the AVM, or preoperative embolization (infarction or edema), should be factored into the intraoperative management plan regarding choice of monitoring, vascular access, anesthetic agents, vasoactive drugs, and muscle relaxants. A critical consideration throughout the operative period is the potential for massive and rapid blood loss. Choice of intraoperative monitoring is tempered by this eventuality and adequate blood, along with access for its administration, must be at hand.

Intraoperative Management

Monitoring

In addition to routine monitors, such as electrocardiogram (ECG), pulse oximeter, end-tidal CO_2, temperature probe, and direct arterial pressure transduction, central access should be considered for resection of larger lesions. Although not necessary for uncomplicated cases, it is not always possible to predict pre-operatively which patient is going to become a complicated case during resection, subsequently requiring extraordinary levels of induced hypotension or aggressive volume therapy. Such cases are a minority, but central venous or pulmonary artery catheters are useful for management of complicated patients. Central access is easily obtained by using the antecubital fossa for both central venous pressure (using a commercially available kit) and pulmonary artery lines (we use a short, rapid infusion catheter instead of the longer neck introducer).

Monitoring cerebral hemodynamics during AVM resection is desirable for several reasons. The ideal goals for cere-

TABLE 1. *Ideal goals for cerebral hemodynamic monitoring*

Ability to titrate drug effects for cerebral protection (barbiturate) or brain relaxation (hypocapnia)
To monitor for the occurrence of regional cerebral ischemia during vascular manipulation
To monitor for the occurrence of global cerebral ischemia during induced hypotension
To monitor for the occurrence of cerebral hyperperfusion
To assist the surgeon in differentiating arterial and venous structures
To identify patients at high risk for postoperative complications (no good guidelines exist at present)

bral hemodynamic monitoring are shown in Table 1. (This is discussed in more detail in the following chapter.) Unfortunately, our ability to monitor the central nervous system lags far behind our ability to monitor other systems and the development of suitable technologies is still in its infancy. There is no consensus about optimum monitoring techniques, primarily because there is a dearth of commercially available technologies.

Transduction of vascular pressures in the operative field may aid the surgeon in differentiating arterial and venous structures. In certain cases, it may assist in the decision as to whether a draining vein that interferes with surgical access to the nidus can be sacrificed. Proximal arterial pressure is measured during a temporary occlusion of the vein; if the pressure does not change it implies that alternate venous pathways are sufficient to prevent distention of the nidus and rupture. Technically, direct puncture of feeding arteries and draining veins in the operative field using 26-gauge needles is a simple procedure with little if any risk. Vascular pressure measurements have been reported by several groups (see ref. 15).

Anesthetic Technique

Intracranial pressure control, often discussed regarding anesthetic care of neurosurgical patients, is rarely a problem with the AVM patient coming for elective resection. Notwithstanding, these patients may have decreased intracranial compliance, so the usual caveats about avoiding cerebral vasodilators are reasonable.

Excepting cerebral vasodilators, the specific choice of anesthesia may be guided primarily by other cardio- and cerebrovascular considerations. We generally employ an isoflurane/N₂O technique because it offers superior systemic blood pressure control over most techniques. Total intravenous anesthetic techniques, or combinations of inhalational and intravenous methods, can be effectively used as well (16). Some centers use additional barbiturate loading during the resection to afford additional protection against cerebral ischemia, resulting in perhaps a greater degree of brain relaxation and protection against acute hyperemia (17). Barbiturates can be titrated to an electroencephalographic endpoint

of burst suppression. The main price to be paid for barbiturate use is delayed emergence and the forgoing of early postoperative neurologic exams. There is no compelling evidence that outcome is effected. If metabolic suppression is desired (and we by no means endorse this as a unique, effective method of intraoperative protection; see ref. 18), propofol or etomidate may be considered. The use of metabolic suppression may be useful in the event of an intraoperative catastrophe, as described under in the section on induced hypotension.

A detailed description of the induction sequence is given in chapter 91 by Ornstein et al; the same general considerations apply to AVMs, although the risk of rupture during induction is much lower. However, it should be borne in mind that approximately 10% of AVM patients harbor intracranial aneurysms.

The goals of a modern neuroanesthetic should not revolve around provision of pharmacologic brain protective therapy per se. There are a number of basic considerations that will maximize nonpharmacologic cerebral protection and provide protection from injury (summarized in Table 2). There are two general types of damage that protective efforts are guided toward: neurosurgical (anatomic) and anesthetic (physiologic) trespass. Possible mechanisms of injury from the neurosurgeon include brain retraction, direct vascular injury (ischemia, thrombosis, venous occlusion), and mechanical disruption of neuronal tissue or white matter tracts. Anesthetic injury may result from systemic hypo- or hypertension, decreased O₂ content, hypoosmolarity, or hyperglycemia. It must be stressed that mechanisms of damage are interactive. For example, trivial amounts of brain retraction coupled with modest reduction of systemic blood pressure may have pronounced synergistic effects on emergence or neurologic outcome.

Management goals should include a relaxed brain, controlled systemic and cerebral hemodynamics, maintenance

TABLE 2. *Nonpharmacologic brain protection*

Relaxed brain:
    Good head position
    CSF drainage
    Diuretics/osmotherapy
    Avoid excessive cerebral vasodilators
    Modest hypocapnia
Controlled systemic and cerebral hemodynamics:
    Euvolemia
    Optimal cerebral perfusion pressure
Fluid and electrolyte management:
    Isotonicity
    Euglycemia
Temperature management:
    Toleration of modest hypothermia intraoperatively
    Prevention of hyperthermia postoperatively
Controlled emergence:
    Tailored awakening
    Autonomic control

of isotonicity and euglycemia, mild hypothermia, and a controlled emergence.

Brain Relaxation

Adequate brain relaxation begins with good head position to promote intracranial venous drainage. The least amount of flexion and rotation necessary for the operative approach should be planned with the surgeon. Careful positioning of the head may also prevent postoperative tongue swelling, a rare but morbid occurrence. A rule of thumb might be given as "two fingerbreadths per 70 kg" between the mandible and clavicle (not the sternum) after the head is positioned in rigid pin fixation. The head of the table should be positioned to prevent venous engorgement.

Cerebral spinal fluid removal is an effective means of brain relaxation, obtained by direct lumbar puncture or ventricular drainage. Diuretic therapy with mannitol and/or furosemide is widely applied. The most important consideration for anesthetic choice intraoperatively is the avoidance of cerebral vasodilators. Modest hypocapnia should be used sparingly as an adjunct to brain relaxation, but levels below 30 mm Hg should have a specific indication.

Controlled Systemic and Cerebral Hemodynamics

Fluid restriction was a time-honored means of guarding against brain swelling in the neurosurgical patient. Adequate volume status to maintain stable systemic hemodynamics, especially with the application of induced hypotension, may require liberal fluid administration. Recent evidence reconciles these two apparently divergent goals (the influence of serum tonicity on fluid movement into the brain is discussed below).

Control of cerebral hemodynamics begins with control of systemic arterial pressure, which in turn is predicated on adequate cardiac preload (euvolemia). Iatrogenic dehydration, as practiced in years past, has no place in modern neurosurgical practice. Indeed in the setting of aneurysmal subarachnoid hemorrhage, it is clearly deleterious. During manipulation of the intracranial contents or their vascular supply, the anesthesiologist should strive to maintain the "optimal cerebral perfusion pressure (CPP)," ie, the highest clinically acceptable blood pressure for the particular clinical circumstance. Brain relaxation is probably also served by maintenance of a normal arterial pressure. Cerebral blood volume is kept to a minimum by appropriate autoregulatory vasoconstriction (19).

In contrast to the current trend to strictly maintain normotension during aneurysm clipping, induced hypotension is frequently useful during AVM resection. This is especially pertinent to large AVMs that have a deep arterial supply. Bleeding from these small, deep-feeding vessels may be difficult to control and decreasing arterial pressure facilitates surgical hemostasis. The subject of induced hypotension is discussed extensively in the neuroanesthesia literature. There is little to add here regarding the choice of agents except our bias that cerebral vasodilators are best avoided in the AVM patient. In the setting of the AVM patient posttreatment, vasodilators have the theoretical disadvantage of exacerbating cerebral hyperemia. The prevalence, extent, and clinical significance of such effects are far from clear at present. But in the already murky waters that surround the cerebral hemodynamic changes in the perioperative period, one less unknown is preferable. For perioperative induced hypotension, we prefer to use α- and β-adrenergic antagonists such as labetolol and esmolol, often in conjunction with modestly increasing the inspired concentration of isoflurane.

The interaction of induced hypotension and hypocapnia remains an ill-defined area. The lower limit of pressure autoregulation is not adversely affected by hypocapnia (20). Although we routinely maintain modest hypocapnia (approximately ≈30 mm Hg) during hypotension, some authors recommend normocapnia (21).

An important interface between anesthesia and blood pressure control is likely to develop with the advent of newer α_2-adrenergic agonists. Clonidine is the prototype of this class of agents. Not only does it appear to smooth out the course of intraoperative blood pressure changes but it has additional anesthetic properties. Dexmedetomidine, a more specific α_2 agonist, is under investigation for human use.

During uncontrolled bleeding, the surgeons may be forced to place clips blindly in an attempt to stem hemorrhage. In this event, barbiturate therapy may be indicated and could be used as a means of or as an adjunct to the induction of mild or moderate temporary arterial blood pressure reduction until bleeding is brought under control. Induction of systemic hypotension with a pure vasodilator has theoretical disadvantages. In the setting of emergent intracranial vascular occlusion to control hemorrhage, the distal perfusion field of the occluded artery will have little or no opportunity to recruit collateral flow from neighboring (relatively vasodilated) normal arterial supply regions. However, the clinician should use whatever means with which he or she is comfortable and adept to expeditiously reduce blood pressure as demanded by the clinical situation.

Fluid and Electrolyte Management

There is a convincing body of evidence that it is tonicity of replacement therapy, not oncotic pressure, that determines water movement into both normal and damaged brain (22). Even mildly hypotonic fluids such as lactated Ringer's solution, if given in sufficient quantity, may aggravate brain swelling more than do isotonic crystalloids or colloids. Isotonic fluid replacement with either blood, saline, or hetastarch after forebrain ischemia in the rat appears to yield similar results in terms of cerebral edema formation (23). The most important point is that fluid should never be withheld at the expense of a stable cardiovascular status. Serum osmolarity can be easily monitored if large volumes of crystalloid are needed.

The choice of colloids is not a clear one. Although hetastarch has been implicated as a cause of coagulation disorders, this is probably not important for volumes under 1 L used intraoperatively. Cost is the primary concern when choosing between hetastarch and human serum albumin. Postoperatively, hetastarch use is more controversial (24).

There is considerable evidence that glucose aggravates cerebral injury (25). Routine perioperative steroid may cause some degree of hyperglycemia. In the absence of clear guidelines, the most rational approach is to avoid glucose-containing fluids, unless there is a specific indication. One such indication would be a diabetic patient receiving insulin therapy. In this case, ''tight'' rather than ''loose'' control of serum glucose seems reasonable; it is probably not worth risking hypoglycemia in an anesthetized patient for any presumptive protective effect of lowering a mildly elevated glucose level.

Toleration of Modest Hypothermia

Mild hypothermia (with core temperature decreases as little as 1.5–3°C) confers dramatic cerebral protection against ischemic insult in animal models (26). This protective effect is greater than would be expected from metabolic suppression alone and may be related to a decrease in excitatory neurotransmitter release from ischemic cells (27). Hypothermia appears to play a more significant role in determining outcome from ischemic insult than choice of anesthetic agents (28). Recent investigations reveal that anesthetized patients can be easily cooled to the cerebroprotective range (33–34°C), although complete intraoperative rewarming may be difficult to achieve (29).

Even mild degrees of hypothermia are not without potential risk. Passive rewarming is associated with peripheral vasoconstriction, shivering, and subsequent increases in oxygen consumption and myocardial work. Drug metabolism is decreased, prolonging the effect of even short-acting anesthetic drugs. Postoperative hypothermia (<35°C) is complicated by increased rates of myocardial ischemia, angina, and arterial hypoxemia in populations at risk for coronary artery disease (30). Moderate hypothermia (<33°C) has other well-documented potential effects, including increased susceptibility to infection, cardiac arrhythmias, hypocoagulability, thrombocytopenia, impaired platelet aggregation, and activation of fibrinolysis, all of which reverse with rewarming (see refs. 29 and 30).

Most of these adverse effects have been observed in patients leaving the operating room while still hypothermic. It is unclear as to whether the potential benefits of cerebral protection gained from mild hypothermia and partial rewarming are offset by the systemic physiologic stress induced, particularly if shivering occurs upon emergence. Intraoperative safety and efficacy studies are currently

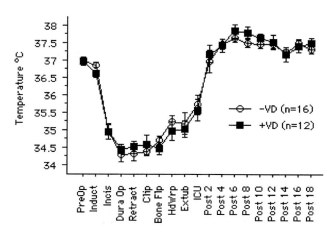

FIG. 1. Tympanic membrane temperature vs. operative stage. Patients were actively cooled during neurosurgical procedures and rewarmed with convective devices and circulating water blankets. Twelve patients (+VD group) received sodium nitroprusside (1.5 ± 1.4 μg/kg/min) during intraoperative rewarming. Although vasoconstriction impairs heat transfer, intraoperative vasodilatation with nitroprusside did not speed rewarming after deliberate mild hypothermia for craniotomy. −VD, without vasodilator; +VD, with vasodilator; PreOp, preoperative; Induc, induction; Incis, incision; Dura Op, dura opening; Retract, retraction; Clip, aneurysm clipping; Bone Flp, bone flap; HdWrp, completion of the head wrap; Extub, extubation; ICU, arrival in the ICU; Post 2, eg, postoperative 2 hours. (Data from ref. 42.)

underway, but preliminary trials of mild hypothermia for head trauma victims appear promising (31).

The induction of general anesthesia results in an obligatory core temperature decrease as peripheral vasodilatation redistributes heat to the periphery. Rather than struggling to maintain normothermia, we currently believe that this temperature reduction (34–35°C) should be encouraged until closure is imminent and only then should active rewarming with water blankets and convective devices begin. Better strategies will be needed to more effectively cool and especially rewarm patients. An example of a preliminary study that attempted to use nitroprusside to facilitate rewarming is shown in Fig. 1. Careful temperature monitoring should continue throughout the perioperative period. Hyperthermia must be avoided as it potentiates ischemic damage (32).

Emergence and Initial Recovery: Blood Pressure Control

A particularly challenging aspect of perioperative care is emergence and initial recovery. It is our impression that the AVM patient tends to be systemically (and in the worst case, cerebrally) hyperdynamic (13). We typically use a moderate phenylephrine-induced blood pressure augmentation (20–30% above normal mean arterial pressure) during drying of the operative bed to inspect for hemostasis. After hemostasis is achieved and the volatile agent is discontinued, we routinely use large doses of labetolol (approximately 300) and, after a 0.5–1 mg/kg loading dose, a variable esmolol infusion to maintain the patient's blood pressure within 10% below the usual ward values.

We would emphasize that, without firm outcome data, in order to insist on one drug regimen or another, choice of agent to manipulate blood pressure must be placed in the context of the clinical situation (eg, avoiding β-adrenergic blockers with bronchospastic airway disease or use of nitroglycerin with coronary artery disease) and the experience of the practitioner.

The most sensitive monitor of cerebral function remains the neurologic examination. A prompt emergence will ensure that drug residua are not confused with and do not obscure focal neurologic damage. Control of systemic hemodynamics is of critical importance during the emergence phase as the patient makes the transition from the anesthetized to the conscious state.

Postoperative Management

The points related to intraoperative blood pressure management apply here. We find esmolol to be an effective agent to smoothly cap blood pressure swings common in the initial intensive care period. However, there are seemingly refractory cases of postoperative hypertension, and the clinician must be prepared to draw on all of the agents in the available armamentarium. A possible advantage of barbiturate loading may be a smoother emergence from anesthesia, although more protracted and without the benefit of neurologic exams.

The sword of aggressive blood pressure control can cut both ways. There are rare cases of ischemic deficits due to intraoperative sacrifice of, for example, an en passage feeding vessel (a vessel feeding the AVM and also sending distal branches to normal brain), which may result in a deficit ascribed to brain retraction or the resection itself. Marginally perfused areas may be critically dependent on collateral perfusion pressure. Maintenance of low or even normal blood pressure may be inadequate and result in infarction if unrecognized. Unfortunately, the only reliable means of verifying borderline perfusion states at the present time in most centers is immediate postoperative angiography or, more rarely, intraoperative angiography.

Postoperative hyperthermia may be detrimental (32) and even exacerbated by intraoperative mild induced hypothermia (29). Therefore, careful attention should be paid to control of patient temperature in the ICU.

ANESTHETIC MANAGEMENT DURING INTERVENTIONAL NEURORADIOLOGIC PROCEDURES

The three primary functions of the anesthesiologist in the interventional suite are (a) provision of a physiologically stable and immobile patient, (b) manipulation of the systemic blood pressure as dictated by the needs of the procedure, and (c) disaster management. In adults, this may be accomplished by traditional methods of general anesthesia with endotracheal intubation or intravenous sedation to render the patient unaware of his or her surroundings yet allow for rapid return to consciousness for intermittent assessment of neurologic function during manipulation of the vasculature. Deep intravenous sedation implies that the patient breathes spontaneously with an unprotected airway. There is no good nomenclature for such an anesthetic state so we will, for the sake of simplicity, refer to it as intravenous sedation in the following discussion. "Conscious sedation" can be a misleading term that does not adequately communicate the concerns of the anesthesiologist to the rest of the operative team regarding airway management. Small children and uncooperative adult patients will require general anesthesia with endotracheal intubation.

Intravenous Sedation vs. General Anesthesia

Choice of anesthetic technique is a controversial area; there are generally two schools of thought on how to manage the patient undergoing embolization of an AVM. One is to rely on the knowledge of neuroanatomy and vascular architecture to ascertain the likelihood of neurologic damage after deposition of glue. The "anatomy" school therefore will prefer to embolize under general anesthesia. Arguments for this approach include improved visualization of structures with the absence of patient movement, especially under temporary apnea. Further, it is argued that if the glue is placed intranidally, then by definition no normal brain is threatened.

The other school, which we might call the "physiologic" school, trades off the potential for patient movement for the increased knowledge of the true functional anatomy of a given patient. Localization of cerebral function may not always follow textbook descriptions. Furthermore, the AVM nidus or a previous hemorrhage may result in a shift or relocalization of function. The physiologic approach demands, at the present, deep intravenous sedation in order to wake the patient for selective Wada testing before injection of embolic material (discussed below). Because reversible intravenous sedation and functional evaluation is our preferred approach, our discussion is presented with this bias in mind.

Preprocedure Considerations

In addition to the usual preanesthetic evaluation of the neurosurgical patient, previous experience with angiography and contrast reactions (including general atopy and iodine/shellfish allergies) should be noted. Neck, back, or joint problems may influence the ability to secure the airway or patient tolerance to lying supine for several hours. Because of significant radiation exposure, the possibility of pregnancy in female patients should be explored.

An anxiolytic may be given, if appropriate to the patient's sensorium. Prophylaxis for cerebral ischemia is in a state of development. We have routinely placed patients on oral nimodipine in those cases that entail an appreciable risk of cerebral ischemia. Nimodipine is also felt to lessen the incidence of traumatic vessel spasm during catheter passage. The above notwithstanding, the efficacy of nimodipine for such prophylactic purposes has not been documented to be effective by randomized, controlled studies.

Additional considerations for premedication include corticosteroids, anticonvulsants, aspirin, and antibiotics.

Conduct of Anesthesia

Patient Positioning

Because the procedures may take many hours, having the patient as comfortable as possible before beginning sedation is essential. No amount of intravenous sedation can substitute for careful patient positioning. A comfortable air or foam mattress and some type of device for good head and neck positioning are needed. After the femoral introducer sheath has been placed (Fig. 2), a pillow is placed under the knees to obtain a modest amount of flexion, which may improve patient tolerance to prolonged periods of lying supine. Because patients may return for multiple treatments, continued patient acceptance is important. Since head position needs to be maintained constant, a headrest that discourages movement or paper tape across the patient's forehead is used as a reminder. Use of rigid fixation should be avoided as it might increase the likelihood of aspiration if emesis occurs.

Vascular Access and Arterial Pressure Monitoring

Secure intravenous access should be available with adequate extension tubing to allow drug and fluid administration at maximal distance from the image intensifier during fluoroscopy. When the patient is draped with arms restrained and advanced toward the image intensifier, access to intravenous sites is difficult.

Direct transduction of arterial pressure is indicated for intracranial embolization procedures, especially with manipulation of systemic pressure with vasoactive agents. Three arterial pressures may easily be monitored from the typical triaxial catheter system used to access the distal cerebral circulation (Fig. 2). Pressure transducers and access stopcocks for blood withdrawal and zeroing are mounted, depending on local preferences, either on the sterile field or toward the anesthesia team.

Although some institutions also perform radial artery catheterizations, the femoral artery introducer sheath is easily used to monitor arterial pressure. This spares the patient from radial artery cannulation. A disadvantage is that it frequently underestimates the systolic and overestimates the

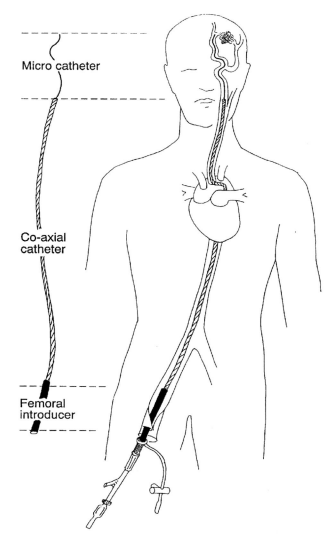

FIG. 2. Representation of a typical arrangement of the transfemoral coaxial catheter system showing the femoral introducer, the coaxial catheter, and the microcatheter (superselective catheter). (Adapted from W. L. Young, Clinical Neuroscience Lectures, Cathenart Publishing, Munster, IN, 1995, used with permission.)

diastolic pressure, due to the coaxial catheter passing through it. However, the mean pressures are reliable and may be used to safely monitor the induction of either hyper- or hypotension. The femoral catheter is continually flushed with an intraflow device at 3 ml/hr of heparinized saline, which does not appreciably influence the mean pressure recording.

Arterial pressure may also be monitored from the coaxial catheter in the carotid or the vertebral artery and may provide early warning of thrombus formation, vascular spasm at the catheter tip, or catheter migration and may be suggested by damping of the waveform. The coaxial catheter is flushed with heparinized saline at a high flow rate, which may artifactually increase the measured pressure. In addition, the pressure at the tip of the superselective catheter may be monitored to gain information about AVM feeding artery pressure. The use of microcatheters for mean pressure measurements has been validated by Duckwiler et al. (33).

Other Systemic Monitoring and Patient Preparation

Other monitors should include five-lead ECG (ideally with automated ST segment trending) and automatic blood pressure cuff. In patients at risk for myocardial ischemia, a baseline recording of the ECG may be helpful for later comparisons during hemodynamic manipulation. A pulse oximeter probe is placed on the great toe of the leg that will receive the femoral catheters. This can give an early warning of femoral artery obstruction or distal thromboembolism. It is also useful when the femoral sheath must be removed and the site compressed for hemostasis, particularly in smaller children where overvigorous compression can lead to permanent occlusion of the vessel.

Oxygen (O_2 2–4 L/min) is given by nasal cannula with a system to sample and monitor partial pressure of end-tidal CO_2 ($PetCO_2$). Humidification of the O_2 may improve patient tolerance. For the spontaneously breathing patient, an indicator of respiratory rate is recommended if $PetCO_2$ is not available and may be useful for detecting abnormal respiratory patterns during procedures involving the posterior fossa. Temperature may be monitored in a number of ways, such as an axillary probe or bladder catheter thermistor. Shivering is a troublesome problem because it results in patient motion and image degradation, and every effort should be made to keep the patient's temperature near normal (except in the case of a neurologic catastrophe).

Bladder catheters assist in fluid management as well as patient comfort. A significant volume of heparinized flush solution may be necessary over the course of the procedure and radiographic contrast is an osmotic diuretic. Administration of other diuretics such as mannitol or furosemide may also be required for fluid management or in the event of a catastrophe.

When the patient's condition warrants placement of a central venous or pulmonary artery catheter, central catheters may be positioned with the use of fluoroscopy. Similarly, the endotracheal tube position for general anesthesia cases is easily verified by the fluoroscopy of the chest during passage of the coaxial catheters.

Anesthetic Management

Primary goals of anesthetic choice for intravenous sedation include alleviation of pain or discomfort, anxiolysis, and patient immobility, along with a rapid decrease in the level of sedation when neurologic testing is required.

The procedures, in general, are not painful. There may be an element of pain (burning) associated with injection of contrast into the cerebral arteries and by distention or traction on them (headache). However, discomfort from long periods of lying still is the rule. Insertion of the bladder catheter and, to a lesser extent, the initial groin puncture for the femoral cannulation are two notable points of discomfort. The procedure is also psychologically stressful. There is a risk of serious stroke or death. This may be particularly important in a patient who has already suffered a preoperative hemorrhage or stroke.

Movement by the patient will decrease the usefulness of the digital image subtraction (road mapping) techniques. For example, a wire or catheter could penetrate a vessel wall and still appear to reside within the lumen (Fig. 3).

Anesthetic agents are selected to meet the goals listed above. Our primary approach to intravenous sedation is to establish a base of neurolept anesthesia by titration (per 70 kg) of 100–150 $\mu g/kg$ of fentanyl, 2–4 mg of droperidol, and 3–5 mg of midazolam after intravenous access and O_2 administration has been started. The goal of this initial drug titration is to render the patient immobile and generally unaware of the surroundings, but still arousable with adequate spontaneous ventilation.

Droperidol may be useful in a neurolept technique because of its antiemetic effect, α-adrenergic blockade, and our impression that it renders a calmer, more motionless patient than do benzodiazepines alone. Postprocedure dysphoria is a theoretical concern and dopadrenergic blockade can result in extrapyramidal symptoms in normal patients as well as in those with Parkinson's disease. For antiemesis, some practitioners expectantly give odansatron in procedures that involve induced hypotension in sedated patients.

When the patient is in final position and draping begins, a propofol infusion is started at very low levels (10–20 $\mu g/kg/min$) and then titrated slowly to result in an unconscious patient with a patent airway. The use of propofol gives the anesthesiologist some degree of control when a rapid return to consciousness is needed for neurologic assessment.

A variety of other sedation regimens and variations are certainly possible and must be based on the experience of the practitioner and the aforementioned goals of anesthetic management. Common to all intravenous sedation techniques is the potential for upper airway obstruction. Placement of nasopharyngeal airways may cause troublesome bleeding in anticoagulated patients and is generally avoided. If the need for a nasopharyngeal airway is expected, it is prudent to place it before anticoagulation and observe meticulous hemostasis.

Laryngeal mask airways may have a place in the management of deep intravenous sedation in these cases (Irene Osborn, MD and David Stone, MD, personal communication). If they are used, care must be taken to ensure that there is not excessive motion during the period when the depth of anesthesia is decreased to remove the airway. Coughing or bucking with the large, stiff introducer catheters in the neck vessels may result in vascular injury.

An additional anesthetic technique that we have used in certain difficult cases is a variation of the traditional "wake-up test" used for spinal surgery; the method is a combination

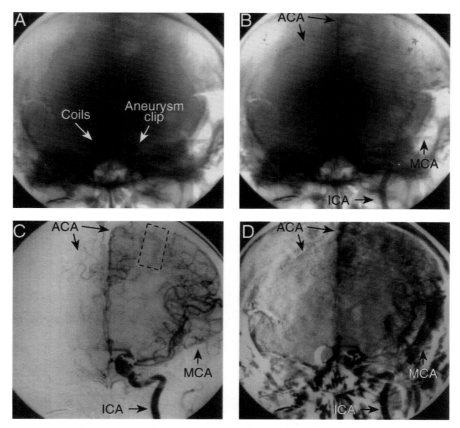

FIG. 3. Digital subtraction angiography: movement artifact. **A:** Scout anteroposterior skull film. **B:** Same view with contrast injected through the internal carotid artery. **C:** Contrast injection with bone subtraction. This image may be used as a backdrop during live fluoroscopy to serve as a "road map" for the passage of microcatheters into the distal circulation. **D:** An example of how patient motion profoundly degrades the image.

of traditional general anesthesia and intravenous sedation. The patient is nasotracheally intubated and maintained using a nitrous-narcotic technique. Before neurologic testing is needed, 4% lidocaine is instilled around the cuff of the endotracheal tube, the N$_2$O discontinued, and the narcotic infusion titrated down. The patient will be able to follow commands but tolerate the presence of the endotracheal tube.

Careful management of coagulation is required to prevent thromboembolic complications during and after the procedures, although algorithms for anticoagulation remain controversial (34–36). Whether heparinization should be used for every case of intracranial catheterization is not clear. Some would argue that anticoagulation increases the risk of intracranial hemorrhage. We feel strongly that heparinization should be routinely performed during any superselective catheterization. In addition to thrombus formation from foreign bodies in the circulation, a considerable amount of thrombogenic endothelial damage may be done by the passage of the superselective catheter.

After placement of the femoral introducer catheter, a baseline activated clotting time (ACT) is obtained. Heparin, 5000 units/70 kg, is given and another ACT is checked to verify

a target prolongation of at least 2–3 times baseline. ACT is monitored at least every hour. If an ACT is not drawn on schedule due to some extenuating circumstance, heparin, 2000 units, is given empirically every hour. The risk of overdosing the patient on heparin in this fashion is minimal compared to the risk of inadvertent thrombus formation. Heparin dose and ACT may be entered in a graphic manner on the anesthesia record so that it is easier to follow trends at a glance.

In our practice, heparin is continued through the first postprocedure night. The rationale for postprocedure anticoagulation is to protect against both the thrombogenic effects of endothelial trauma and the inherently thrombogenic nature of the materials instilled, such as glue or coils, which can cause retrograde thrombosis in embolized vessels. A period of 24 hours is felt to be sufficient for a "pseudoendothelial" layer to form and prevent either retrograde or anterograde thrombus formation that may propagate along arterial and venous pathways with potentially disastrous results. The heparin effect is then allowed to wane on the first postprocedure day. Because the patient is heparinized, the large introducer sheath in the groin is left in place for the first postprocedure night and removed before discharge to the floor on the following morning.

An occasional patient may be refractory to attempts to obtain adequate anticoagulation. Switching from bovine to porcine heparin or vice versa may be of use. If antithrombin III deficiency is suspected, administration of fresh frozen plasma may be necessary.

Depending on the tortuosity of the vascular pathway and other technical considerations, it may either be very difficult or extremely easy for the radiology team to place the catheter tip exactly where they want it. The ease of passing the superselective catheter will determine, in part, how many pedicles can be embolized on a given day. The patients, despite best efforts, usually will not tolerate more than 4–5 hours of intravenous sedation and remain still enough to allow satisfactory performance of the neuroimaging procedures.

As the superselective catheter is passed distally, pressure measurements may be made at the tip of the catheter. The pressure will typically decrease in a stepwise fashion as it is advanced distally (33,37).

When the catheter has been placed in position for potential glue injection, the level of sedation is decreased and a baseline neurologic exam is performed. A superselective anesthesia functional examination (SAFE) is then performed as described below. If this test is positive, ie, a focal neurologic deficit is encountered, then the catheter is repositioned or embolization of that pedicle may be aborted. If negative, the glue or embolic material can be injected.

SAFE is carried out to determine, if prior to therapeutic embolization, the tip of the catheter has been inadvertently placed proximal to the origin of nutritive vessels to eloquent regions (38). Such testing is an extension of the Wada and Rasmussen test, in which amobarbital is injected into the internal carotid artery to determine hemispheric dominance and language function.

Before testing, the level of sedation should be decreased, eg, by stopping the propofol infusion. In rare instances, it may be necessary to use naloxone or flumazenil to antagonize other intravenous agents, but this should be avoided by not oversedating the patient with fixed agents. A baseline, focused neurologic exam under residual light sedation is performed by the interventional neuroradiology (INR) team. Sodium amobarbital (30 mg) or lidocaine (30 mg), mixed with contrast, is then given via the superselective catheter and an angiogram of the distribution of the drug/contrast mixture is obtained. Sodium amobarbital is used for investigating gray matter areas. Lidocaine may be used for evaluating the integrity of white matter tracts. Injection of lidocaine may result in seizures when used in the brain, particularly in areas such as motor strip. Besides being disquieting to the patient and increasing the risk of aspiration, seizure activity can result in a transient focal neurologic deficit. A postictal paralysis, for example, can confuse interpretation of the test. For this reason, the barbiturate is usually given first, followed by lidocaine. If the amobarbital is negative, it may protect against cortical seizure but not significantly interfere with assessment of lidocaine's effect on white matter tracts.

Not all authors agree on the use of lidocaine for intracerebral testing (38).

After drug injection, the neurologic examination is repeated. Attention is directed to areas at risk as well as "quiet areas" where a deficit might be missed if only a motor or sensory exam is performed, such as dominant parietal lobe.

SAFE is generally reliable, but false-positive tests can occur with overinjection and reflux into normal vessels. Underinjection, or a "sump" effect from an AVM, may lead to false-negative results. Systemic recirculation of the anesthetic may result in generalized sedation. Rauch et al described the use of EEG monitoring, coupled with a clinical exam, to enhance the sensitivity of SAFE (38).

Once the superselective catheter is in optimal position, profound but tolerable systemic hypotension is induced while the radiologist prepares the glue for injection. Hypotension slows the flow through the fistula and provides for a more controlled deposition of embolic material, the glues in particular. Deliberate hypotension is used to achieve flow arrest. Ideally, there would be zero flow through the AVM, so that the distribution of glue would be totally controlled by the radiologist injecting the glue. (Complications of glue injection are described at the end of this section.)

Adequate flow arrest appears to occur at a different systemic pressure for each patient. In fact, it seems that flow through the fistula remains relatively constant until a certain pressure is reached, when it drops off sharply. As the pressure is lowered, the radiologist will perform several contrast injections with fluoroscopy and visually determine the optimal systemic pressure to slow the flow through the fistula. Typically, we will reduce systemic MAP to approximately 50 mm Hg, but greater or lesser degrees depend on the speed of the contrast transit through the fistula.

This subject has not been rigorously studied. Consequently, it is not clear as to whether systemic hypotension decreases shunt flow solely on the basis of a reduction in pressure or by limiting total (and, in the case of an AVM, increased) flow to the brain or some combination of both factors. In any event, in the presence of a cerebral fistula, reducing systemic pressure does not affect downstream feeding artery pressure to the same degree, and different patients may require different degrees of hypotension to adequately slow flow through the fistula for glue deposition (4,5).

In awake patients, nausea and vomiting can be a major problem. It is for this reason that droperidol is an attractive choice as part of the sedative regime. An additional dose of droperidol (1.25 mg) may be given for antiemesis just before starting hypotension (which usually begins at least 2 hours after the initial dose). If nausea is known to be a problem from prior experience, odansatron may be considered. Before beginning hypotension, one should confirm that the patient is fully oxygenated and the airway unobstructed.

Most of the AVM patients treated are relatively young and fit. Most importantly, they are not under general anesthesia and the adjunctive hypotensive effect of general anesthesia is absent during intravenous sedation. Therefore, it may be considerably more challenging to induce hypotension in this setting. Sometimes surprisingly large doses of hypotensive agents may be necessary.

Our first-line agent is usually esmolol, given as a 1 mg/kg bolus and titrated to target systemic blood pressure at an infusion rate beginning at 0.5 mg/kg/min. High levels of infusion are often needed and boluses of labetolol (approximately 50–100 mg) are useful as an adjunct. Adrenergic blockers have the advantage of not directly affecting cerebral blood flow and have the theoretical advantage of shifting the autoregulatory curve to the left, ie, flow is maintained normal until a lower pressure is reached. Trimethaphan probably also shares such an effect. Disadvantages of trimethaphan include tachyphylaxis and the large doses needed for awake patients. Use of large doses may result in pupillary dilatation (this may confound the neurologic exam) and inhibition of plasma pseudocholinesterase.

Sodium nitroprusside (SNP) and nitroglycerin may be used in interventional neuroradiology, but we tend to avoid these cerebral vasodilators, including dihydralazine, unless there is some specific indication (eg, coronary artery disease for nitroglycerin). As discussed above, there is a theoretical potential for interfering with collateral perfusion to an ischemic region. A relative disadvantage of nitroglycerin and SNP is that it is easy to overshoot and render the patient momentarily severely hypotensive. Although this can be treated without incident in the patient under general anesthesia with endotracheal intubation, the onset of hypotension-induced emesis and nausea in an awake patient can be disastrous in the INR setting from several standpoints. It can decrease the total amount of time available to the team for the procedure because of continued discomfort and interfere with angiographic visualization because of motion artifact (see Fig. 3). The nausea may be confused with acute intracranial hypertension from vascular perforation. Retching can cause movement or migration of the coaxial or intracranial catheters from the desired location, cause further endothelial damage, or produce vessel perforation.

Another technique used to achieve flow arrest is to place a balloon catheter via the other femoral artery. The balloon is positioned proximal to the superselective catheter to be used for gluing. Prior to glue injection, the balloon may be inflated to either slow or completely arrest distal flow. But this necessitates passage of another intracranial catheter from the contralateral femoral artery and the attendant risks of vessel rupture from balloon overinflation.

Although any injected embolic material can occlude normal vessels, injection of the glue is fraught with particular hazards. The injection of glue is a critical moment (not unlike the moment when a surgeon closes the clip on the neck of an aneurysm). The catheter may become glued to the vessel. If the catheter cannot be removed by intermittent firm, gentle traction, it may be necessary to leave the catheter intravascularly, where it will eventually endothelialize.

Similarly, the catheter, as it is withdrawn, may drag a piece of glue into the proximal part of the artery and occlude it. In this event, territories fed by nutrient vessels distal to the occlusion may become ischemic. Glue that is carried into the draining vein can cause venous outflow obstruction and result in ICH.

Glue may also pass into the pulmonary circulation. Small amounts (<0.5 ml) may not be clinically significant. Larger amounts, however, may result in a syndrome akin to acute pulmonary thromboembolism. Because the glue is extremely thrombogenic, it may pick up thrombus en route and form more clot once lodged in the pulmonary vasculature. This is of particular concern in small children with large AVMs. At the time of gluing, the anesthesiologist must be ready to intervene immediately in the event of catastrophe.

Measurement of immediate postembolization pressures has been suggested as a means of following the course of hemodynamic changes (33) and predicting postprocedure complications because large increases in feeding artery pressure appear to be associated with ICH. Additional studies are needed to further define the clinical utility of such measurements. At the present time immediate postembolization pressure measurements are only practical with thread, coils, or polyvinyl alcohol particles. When glues such as N-butyl cyanoacrylate (NBCA) are used, currently available superselective catheters must be withdrawn immediately after glue injection (so that they are not cemented into place). It is possible to "chase" glue from the microcatheter with non-ionic solutions, but this reduces the operator control over glue deposition.

Typically, the pressures in the proximal feeding artery are quite low, ie, 40–60% of MAP. The proximal portion of the artery usually feeds large areas of functional eloquent brain. The mean pressure in feeding arteries near the entry to a high-flow AVM nidus is usually 15–25% of MAP. Pressure may be transmitted to the cerebral venous system and may pressurize normal venous drainage areas. There is not a direct relationship between AVM feeding artery and draining vein pressures. Outflow pressure from the nidus is probably primarily determined by the architecture of the venous drainage (4).

Since AVM feeding arteries supply variable degrees of normal brain, abrupt restoration of normal systemic pressure to a chronically hypotensive vascular bed may overwhelm autoregulatory capacity and result in hemorrhage or swelling (NPPB). It is for this reason, in part, that the target range for posttreatment blood pressure is strict maintenance of ≈10% below the patient's normal ward blood pressure. An alternative approach to explain hemorrhage and swelling after AVM treatment has been termed "venous overload" or "occlusive hyperemia" (39), emphasizing that venous outflow obstruction can also result in complications. The exact pathophysiology of hemodynamic complications after treatment of AVMs remains controversial (40).

Postprocedure nausea and vomiting can be due to anesthetic agents or the large volumes of contrast agent. This general topic is reviewed elsewhere (41). For procedures in the posterior fossa, small degrees of ischemia and swelling from contrast not infrequently result in symptomatic local brain swelling in the postprocedure period. In the more capacious supratentorial compartment, such minor swelling is rarely symptomatic. In the posterior fossa, this may present as delayed deficits or decreased sensorium during the course of the first evening after the procedure, particularly if cerebrospinal fluid pathways become obstructed. This eventuality should be factored into decisions regarding airway management.

Complications and Special Considerations

Management of Neurologic Catastrophes

Complications during instrumentation of the cerebral vasculature can be rapid and dramatic and require a multidisciplinary collaboration. Having a well-thought-out plan for dealing with intracranial catastrophe may make the difference between an uneventful outcome and death.

If a neurologic catastrophe occurs, rapid and effective communication between the anesthesia and radiology teams is critical. The primary responsibility of the anesthesia team is to preserve gas exchange and, if indicated, secure the airway. If endotracheal intubation is necessary, a thiopental and relaxant induction should not be avoided because of the possibility of a transient decrease in perfusion pressure.

Simultaneous with airway maintenance, the first branch in the decision-making algorithm is for the anesthesiologist to communicate with the INR team and determine whether the problem is hemorrhagic or occlusive.

In the setting of vascular occlusion, a method to increase distal perfusion is by blood pressure augmentation with or without direct thrombolysis. If the problem is hemorrhagic, immediate reversal of heparin is indicated. Protamine is given as rapidly as possible to reverse heparin without undue regard for the systemic blood pressure.

As an emergency reversal dose, 1 mg protamine can be given for each 100 units of apparent heparin activity at the time. The ACT can then be used to fine-tune the final protamine dose.

Bleeding catastrophes are usually heralded by headache, nausea, vomiting, and vascular pain related to the area of perforation. Sudden loss of consciousness is not always due to ICH. Seizures, as a result of contrast or temporary ischemia, and the resulting postictal state can also result in an obtunded patient.

Blood Pressure Augmentation (Deliberate Hypertension)

Not infrequently a situation will arise where the patient will experience cerebral ischemia from either a planned or inadvertent vascular occlusion. The systemic blood pressure may be increased to drive adequate flow via collaterals to the area of ischemia as a temporizing measure (5). The primary routes of collateral circulation are the large vessels that make up the circle of Willis (anterior communicating artery and

posterior communicating artery and the ophthalmic via the external carotid artery) and the surface connections between pial arteries that bridge major arterial territories (anterior cerebral artery–posterior cerebral artery/anterior cerebral artery–middle cerebral artery/middle cerebral artery–posterior cerebral artery).

Our first-line agent is phenylephrine (approximately 1 μg/kg) bolus followed by titrated infusion to increase the pressure up to levels that reverse the neurologic deficit, empirically, 30–40% above baseline. The ECG and ST segment monitor should be carefully inspected for signs of myocardial ischemia. Blood pressure goals must be tempered by the patient's preexisting medical status. Based on the best available evidence, deliberate hypertension in the face of symptomatic cerebral ischemia from vascular occlusion during AVM embolization should not be avoided because of fear of rupturing the malformation (3).

If the heart rate is very low to start, eg, due to preoperative β blockade or sinus node disease, an alternate choice would be ephedrine or dopamine, with or without phenylephrine.

ACKNOWLEDGMENTS

The authors thank Lotfi Hacein-Bey, M.D. for comments and suggestions and the Neuroanesthesia Section of the Department of Anesthesiology and the technologist and nursing staff of the Neuroradiology Division for their part in patient care and development of protocols. We also thank Joyce Ouchi for expert assistance in preparation of the manuscript and Bennett M. Stein, M.D., J. P. Mohr, M.D., and the other members of the Columbia University AVM Project for their continued support. Portions of this work were supported by PHS RO1 NS27713 and NS34949.

REFERENCES

1. Stein BM, Wolpert SM. Arteriovenous malformations of the brain: I. Current concepts and treatment. *Arch Neurol* 1980;37:1–5.
2. Kader A, Young WL, Pile-Spellman J, et al. The influence of hemodynamic and anatomic factors on hemorrhage from cerebral arteriovenous malformations. *Neurosurgery* 1994;34:801–808.
3. Szabo MD, Crosby G, Sundaram P, Dodson BA, Kjellberg RN. Hypertension does not cause spontaneous hemorrhage of intracranial arteriovenous malformations. *Anesthesiology* 1989;70:761–763.
4. Young WL, Kader A, Pile-Spellman J, Ornstein E, Stein BM, Columbia University AVM Study Project. Arteriovenous malformation draining vein physiology and determinants of transnidal pressure gradients. *Neurosurgery* 1994;35:389–396.
5. Young WL, Pile-Spellman J. Anesthetic considerations for interventional neuroradiology (review). *Anesthesiology* 1994;80:427–456.
6. Sisti MB, Kader A, Stein BM. Microsurgery for 67 intracranial arteriovenous malformations less than 3 cm in diameter. *J Neurosurg* 1993;79:653–660.
7. Spetzler RF, Wilson CB, Weinstein P, Mehdorn M, Townsend J, Telles D. Normal perfusion pressure breakthrough theory. *Clin Neurosurg* 1978;25:651–672.
8. Powers WJ. Cerebral hemodynamics in ischemic cerebrovascular disease. *Ann Neurol* 1991;29:231–240.
9. Young WL, Ornstein E, Baker KZ, Kader A, Stein BM, The Columbia

University AVM Project. Cerebral hyperemia after AVM resection is related to ''break-through'' complications but not to feeding artery pressure (abstract). *Anesth Analg* 1995;80:S573.

10. Young WL, Pile-Spellman J, Prohovnik I, Kader A, Stein BM, Columbia University AVM Study Project. Evidence for adaptive autoregulatory displacement in hypotensive cortical territories adjacent to arteriovenous malformations. *Neurosurgery* 1994;34:601–611.

11. Nornes H, Grip A. Hemodynamic aspects of cerebral arteriovenous malformations. *J Neurosurg* 1980;53:456–464.

12. Mast H, Mohr JP, Osipov A, et al. ''Steal'' is an unestablished mechanism for the clinical presentation of cerebral arteriovenous malformations. *Stroke* 1995;26:1215–1220.

13. Porembka D, Ebrahim Z, Bloomfield E, Stuebing R. The postoperative hyperdynamic cardiovascular response following intracranial excision of arterial venous malformation (AVM) (abstract). *Anesthesiology* 1991;75:A215.

14. Macfarlane R, Moskowitz MA, Sakas DE, Tasdemiroglu E, Wei EP, Kontos HA. The role of neuroeffector mechanisms in cerebral hyperperfusion syndromes (review article). *J Neurosurg* 1991;75:845–855.

15. Fleischer LH, Young WL, Pile-Spellman J, et al. Relationship of transcranial Doppler flow velocities and arteriovenous malformation feeding artery pressures. *Stroke* 1993;24:1897–1902.

16. Ravussin P, Tempelhoff R, Modica PA, Bayer-Berger M-M. Propofol vs. thiopental-isoflurane for neurosurgical anesthesia: Comparison of hemodynamics, CSF pressure, and recovery. *J Neurosurg Anesth* 1991; 3:85–95.

17. Spetzler RF, Martin NA, Carter LP, Flom RA, Raudzens PA, Wilkinson E. Surgical management of large AVMs by staged embolization and operative excision. *J Neurosurg* 1987;67:17–28.

18. Todd MM, Warner DS. A comfortable hypothesis reevaluated: cerebral metabolic depression and brain protection during ischemia (editorial). *Anesthesiology* 1992;76:161–164.

19. Rosner MJ. Cerebral perfusion pressure: link between intracranial pressure and systemic circulation. In: Wood JH, ed. *Cerebral Blood Flow: Physiologic and Clinical Aspects*. New York: McGraw-Hill, 1987; 425–448.

20. Paulson OB, Strandgaard S, Edvinsson L. Cerebral autoregulation. *Cerebrovasc Brain Metab Rev* 1990;2:161–192.

21. Drummond JC, Shapiro HM. Cerebral physiology (Chapter 19). In: Miller RD, ed. *Anesthesia*. vol 1. New York: Churchill Livingstone, 1990;621–649.

22. Zornow MH, Todd MM, Moore SS. The acute cerebral effects of changes in plasma osmolality and oncotic pressure. *Anesthesiology* 1987;67:936–941.

23. Warner DS, Boehland LA. The effects of iso-osmolal hemodilution on post-ischemic brain water content in the rat. *Anesthesiology* 1988;68: 86–91.

24. Trumble ER, Muizelaar JP, Myseros JS, Choi SC, Warren BB. Coagulopathy with the use of hetastarch in the treatment of vasospasm. *J Neurosurg* 1995;82:44–47.

25. Lanier WL. Glucose management during cardiopulmonary bypass: Cardiovascular and neurologic implications (editorial). *Anesth Analg* 1991; 72:423–427.

26. Busto R, Dietrich WD, Globus MY-T, Valdes I, Scheinberg P, Ginsberg MD. Small differences in intraischemic brain temperature critically determine the extent of ischemic neuronal injury. *J Cereb Blood Flow Metab* 1987;7:729–738.

27. Busto R, Dietrich WD, Globus MY-T, Ginsberg MD. The importance of brain temperature in cerebral ischemic injury. *Stroke* 1989;20: 1113–1114.

28. Sano T, Drummond JC, Patel PM, Grafe MR, Watson JC, Cole DJ. A comparison of the cerebral protective effects of isoflurane and mild hypothermia in a model of incomplete forebrain ischemia in the rat. *Anesthesiology* 1992;76:221–228.

29. Baker KZ, Young WL, Stone JG, Kader A, Baker CJ, Solomon RA. Deliberate mild intraoperative hypothermia for craniotomy. *Anesthesiology* 1994;81:361–367.

30. Frank SM, Beattie C, Christopherson R, et al. Unintentional hypothermia is associated with postoperative myocardial ischemia. *Anesthesiology* 1993;78:468–476.

31. Marion DW, Obrist WD, Carlier PM, Penrod LE, Darby JM. The use of moderate therapeutic hypothermia for patients with severe head injuries: a preliminary report. *J Neurosurg* 1993;79:354–362.

32. Chen H, Chopp M. Effect of mild hyperthermia on the ischemic infarct volume after middle cerebral artery occlusion in the rat. *Neurology* 1991;41:1133–1135.

33. Duckwiler G, Dion J, Vinuela F, Jabour B, Martin N, Bentson J. Intravascular microcatheter pressure monitoring: experimental results and early clinical evaluation. *AJNR* 1990;11:169–175.

34. Eskridge JM. Interventional neuroradiology. *Radiology* 1989;172: 991–1006.

35. Purdy PD, Batjer HH, Samson D. Management of hemorrhagic complications from preoperative embolization of arteriovenous malformations. *J Neurosurg* 1991;74:205–211.

36. Vinuela F, Halbach VV, Dion JE. *Interventional Neuroradiology: Endovascular Therapy of the Central Nervous System*. New York: Raven Press, 1992.

37. Fogarty-Mack P, Pile-Spellman J, Hacein-Bey L, et al. The effect of arteriovenous malformations on the distribution of intracerebral arterial pressures. *AJNR: Am J Neuroradiol*. 1996;17: in press.

38. Rauch RA, Vinuela F, Dion J, et al. Preembolization functional evaluation in brain arteriovenous malformations: the ability of superselective amytal test to predict neurologic dysfunction before embolization. *AJNR* 1992;13:309–314.

39. Al-Rodhan NRF, Sundt TM Jr, Piepgras DG, Nichols DA, Rufenacht D, Stevens LN. Occlusive hyperemia: a theory for the hemodynamic complications following resection of intracerebral arteriovenous malformations. *J Neurosurg* 1993;78:167–175.

40. Young WL, Kader A, Prohovnik I, et al. Pressure autoregulation is intact after arteriovenous malformation resection. *Neurosurgery* 1993; 32:491–497.

41. Watcha MF, White PF. Postoperative nausea and vomiting: its etiology, treatment, and prevention. *Anesthesiology* 1992;77:162–184.

42. Baker KZ, Stone JG, Jackson L, et al. Intraoperative nitroprusside does not speed rewarming from mild hypothermia (abstract). *Anesthesiology* 1995;83:A177.

Cerebrovascular Disease, edited by H. Hunt Batjer.
Lippincott-Raven Publishers, Philadelphia © 1997.

CHAPTER 69

Arteriovenous Malformations: Considerations for Perioperative Critical Care Monitoring

Abraham Kader and William L. Young

The surgical treatment of cerebral arteriovenous malformations (AVMs) carries a significant risk of morbidity and mortality, especially for larger lesions and those in eloquent areas of the brain (1,2). A potential source of morbidity from treatment has been attributed to hemodynamic derangements from interruption of high shunt flow through the malformation; these hemodynamic changes may be related to certain cases of postoperative hyperemia and hemorrhage (3). Therefore, an understanding of the cerebral hemodynamic consequences of shunt flow through cerebral AVMs and the changes that occur after resection is important for a rational approach to the perioperative care of these patients. This chapter will review aspects of cerebral and systemic hemodynamics pertinent to intra- and postoperative monitoring.

CEREBRAL HEMODYNAMIC CONSIDERATIONS

Pathophysiology of Perioperative Cerebral Hyperemia and Intraoperative Cerebral Blood Flow Monitoring

The hemodynamic effects of shunt flow through an AVM are incompletely understood and controversial. One of the major challenges to studying the relationship between hemodynamic derangements and postoperative complications is the very low incidence of catastrophic outcomes. Therefore, statistical power is difficult to achieve. Nevertheless, many attempts have been made and much has been written on the subject (4–8). A conceptually attractive but unproven paradigm prevails to explain many instances of pretreatment deficits—cerebral steal (9,10)—and certain catastrophic posttreatment complications of brain swelling and intracere-

A. Kader: Department of Neurosurgery, Albert Einstein College of Medicine; Montefiore Medical Center, Bronx, New York 10467.

W. L. Young: Departments of Anesthesiology, Neurological Surgery, and Radiology, College of Physicians and Surgeons of Columbia University, New York, New York 10032.

bral hemorrhage (5). This paradigm assumes that in some patients high feeding-artery flow reduces perfusion pressure in neighboring vascular territories. Further, this reduction in perfusion pressure places these vascular territories at or near the lower limit of autoregulation by a combination of arterial hypotension and venous hypertension. A compensatory and chronic arteriolar vasodilation will result in "vasomotor paralysis," both at sites near and distant from the AVM. In other words, maximally dilated arteriolar resistance vessels will have lost their ability to vasoconstrict to an acute increase in net perfusion pressure. Therefore, after AVM removal, increased perfusion pressure can cause hyperemia and, in the worst case, swelling or hemorrhage (11–17). Such a mechanism has also been proposed in the setting of carotid endarterectomy (18) and carotid–jugular fistula ablation (19). Evidence for the pathophysiologic link between hyperemia and subsequent swelling and hemorrhage is lacking. Presumably, hyperemia results in acute vascular engorgement with breakdown of the blood–brain barrier, leading to vasogenic edema and vessel rupture.

This phenomenon has been termed *circulatory breakthrough* (6,20) and *normal perfusion pressure breakthrough* (NPPB) (5). Briefly stated, breakthrough occurs when a chronically hypotensive bed is acutely repressurized after treatment. The model further implies that it is not the mass of the AVM itself but rather decreased perfusion pressure in adjacent functional tissue that is responsible for both preoperative ischemic symptoms and postoperative hyperemic complications. This perception greatly influences both the interpretation of clinical phenomena and treatment choices. For example, one of the primary reasons for the current approach to staged treatment of AVMs—either by embolization or staged surgery—is to prevent complications resulting from too rapid a redistribution of blood flow after shunt obliteration (15). There is considerable empiric evidence that high-flow AVMs induce arterial hypotension and venous hypertension in the input and outflow conduits to the fistula

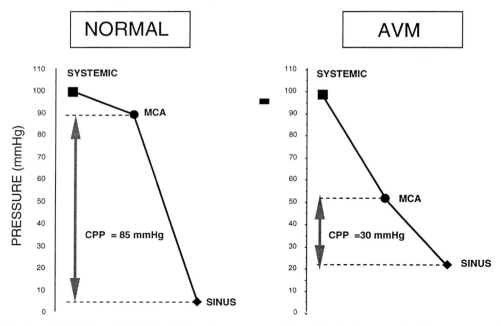

FIG. 1. Hypothetical worst-case depiction of pressure relationships between arterial and venous sides of the circulation in the middle cerebral artery (MCA) territory from a normal **(A)** and an arteriovenous malformation (AVM) **(B)** hemisphere. The low arterial and high venous pressures, eg, sagittal sinus, that may be observed at the inflow and outflow of the AVM may be transmitted to functional brain regions, reducing the available cerebral perfusion pressure (CPP) to the adjacent normal vascular territories. The values represent an extreme case, based on previously reported data (6,15,22,24,35). (Adapted from ref. 85, with permission.)

(15,21–32). A "worst-case" is depicted in Fig. 1. It should be emphasized that there is not an inverse relationship between arterial and venous pressure; that is, low arterial pressure is not necessarily accompanied by venous hypertension. On the contrary, we found a positive correlation between feeding-arterial and superficial draining venous pressure (Fig. 2) (31). Our studies suggest that arterial pressure appears to decrease gradually as one proceeds distally out along the arterial tree, although the pressure changes are exaggerated at major branch points (33,34) (Fig. 3). It is notable that relatively large arterial distributions are subjected to relative hypotension, as shown in Figs. 3 and 4. Holohemispheric hypotension is rarely if ever present. In a study of 41 patients undergoing surgery or embolization, 56% of patients had a distal feeding-artery pressure ≤40 mm Hg (35). Therefore, the incidence of severe reductions in distal-field cerebral arterial pressure is relatively high. It would therefore be expected that normalization of these arterial pressures after AVM resection would place a large number of patients at risk of breakthrough complications. With some exceptions (3,36,37), however, most surgical series show that the incidence of NPPB is very low, in the range of 0–3% (2,38–41). One of the problems is that there is no universally acceptable way to independently verify the existence of "hyperemic" complications or NPPB, since brain swelling and hemorrhage may be due to other causes.

To study the incidence and etiology of perioperative hy-

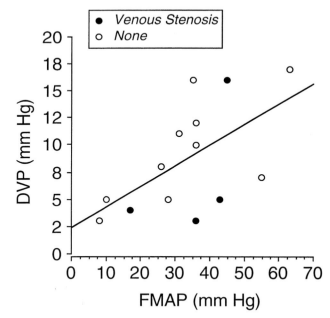

FIG. 2. Superficial draining vein pressure (DVP) as a function of feeding mean arterial pressure (FMAP). Pressures referenced to the site of measurement at head level were recorded from cortical surface vessels intraoperatively before AVM resection. There is a positive correlation between FMAP and DVP (y = .2x + 2.4, r = .59, n = 14, $p < .05$). Patients who had venous stenosis are indicated as shown in the key. (From ref. 31, with permission.)

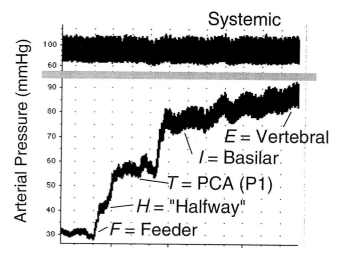

FIG. 3. Recording made of vascular pressures in a patient with an occipital AVM fed by the posterior cerebral artery (PCA). Pressure was measured using a 1.5-French superselective catheter prior to transfemoral liquid polymer embolization. The zones were defined as follows: E, extracranial; I, intracranial; T, transcranial Doppler (TCD) insonation site (eg, M1, A1, or P1); H, pressure measured at half the distance from zone T to zone F, supplying functional tissue and shunt; and F, feeder. The catheter was positioned in the feeding artery (zone F) and slowly pulled back through zone H, the P1 segment (zone T), the basilar artery (zone I) and finally into the extracranial vertebral artery (zone E). As the catheter was withdrawn slowly from the distal feeding artery adjacent to the fistula, the pressure can be seen to increase, with step increases at branch points. The simultaneously recorded systemic arterial pressure is also shown. Note that the pressure in the proximal portion of the posterior cerebral artery (PCA), which irrigates a large area of normal, eloquent tissue, is moderately hypotensive in this asymptomatic patient. Data are taken from ref. 35. (Adapted from ref. 85, with permission.)

peremic complications, our group prospectively evaluated 235 patients undergoing AVM surgery, of whom 143 had intraoperative cerebral blood flow (CBF) measurements (42). There were very few cases (n = 6) of possible NPPB: two immediate (<24 hours) postoperative cases of intracerebral hemorrhage (one fatal, one devastating), two cases of severe brain swelling resulting in coma, and two cases of mild brain swelling, one of which was intraoperative but necessitated staging the surgery. The maximal incidence was therefore no higher than 2.3%. In the above subset of patients with presumptive "hyperperfusion" complications, ^{133}Xe hemispheric CBF increased to a greater degree from before to after resection than it did in patients without such complications. Both AVM groups had a greater increase in CBF than did a control group undergoing craniotomy for tumor (Fig. 5). However, intraoperative CBF monitoring did not appear to have great sensitivity in discriminating potential cases of NPPB. For the breakthrough group, 60% (3 of 5 patients) had a >2-standard-deviation increase of CBF from pre- to postresection vs. 4% of the rest of patients.

Importantly, if repressurization of previously hypotensive territories explained perfusion increases after treatment, then these increases should be limited to the areas of preoperative regional cerebral hypotension. In our studies, the increases in CBF were bilateral, even though arterial hypotension was limited to the vascular territories supplying the AVM. Furthermore, CBF changes were not related to the degree of hypotension caused by the shunt (Fig. 6). In another study of 25 patients undergoing AVM resection, even though CBF increased from pre- to postresection, increasing systemic arterial pressure with phenylephrine after resection did not increase CBF further (43) (Fig. 7). Therefore, it is unlikely that the hyperemia after resection was due to the presence of a paralyzed arteriolar bed presented with an acute increase

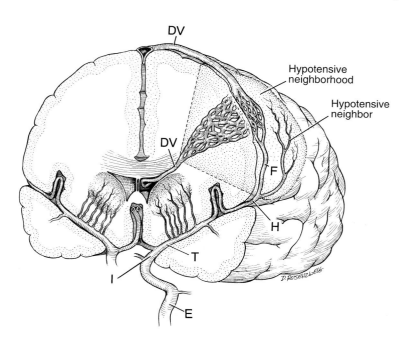

FIG. 4. Schematic depiction of the distribution of arterial hypotension in the parent arteries of AVM-feeding vessels. Coronal oblique view of intracranial circulation to AVM demonstrates anatomic vascular zones (see Fig. 3) and surrounding functional area subject to chronic hypotension ("hypotensive neighborhood"). One vessel perfusing the hypotensive neighborhood, labeled the "hypotensive neighbor," is illustrated. The zones (E, I, T, H, F), explained in Fig. 3, are illustrated here. Draining veins (DV) are also shown. Note that there is also a hypotensive neighborhood, perfused by hypotensive neighbors, in the volume of brain that has been cut away for illustrative purposes. (Adapted from ref. 85, with permission.)

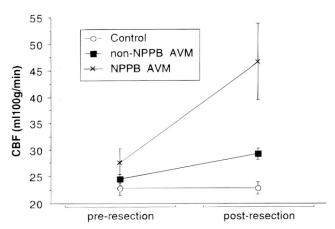

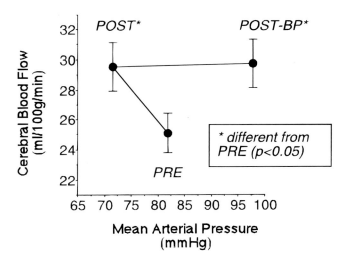

FIG. 5. Mean changes ± SEM in uncorrected cerebral blood flow (CBF) from pre- to postresection in 95 patients undergoing AVM resection under relative hypocapnia. Patients with normal perfusion pressure breakthrough (NPPB) (n = 5) had a greater increase in CBF from pre- to postresection than AVM patients without NPPB (n = 90) ($p <. 0001$). Both NPPB ($p <.001$) and non-NPPB ($p < .05$) patients had a greater increase in CBF postresection than control patients (n = 22).

FIG. 7. Studies were performed during resection of moderate to large AVMs in 25 patients undergoing 28 procedures under isoflurane anesthesia. Cerebral blood flow (CBF) was measured (^{133}Xe method) in the hemisphere adjacent to the nidus before resection after dural exposure *(PRE)*, after AVM removal before dural closure at spontaneous systemic blood pressure *(POST)*, and finally with mean arterial pressure increased by 20 mm Hg using intravenous phenylephrine *(POST-BP)*. CBF is shown as a function of mean arterial pressure (MAP) before and after resection. Values are expressed as mean ± SE. Despite a significantly lower MAP, CBF increased from PRE to POST. In contrast, increasing MAP with phenylephrine did not further increase CBF. Both POST and POST-BP CBF values are greater than PRE ($p < .05$). (From ref. 43, with permission.)

in perfusion pressure. If the increase from pre- to postresection was due to a paralyzed vascular bed, then pressure-passive flow increases should have been observed with phenylephrine-induced augmentation of systemic arterial pressure.

We have also investigated the response of cerebral autoregulatory function to acute phenylephrine-induced increases in systemic arterial pressure in superselectively catheterized middle cerebral artery pedicles adjacent to AVMs using the ^{133}Xe-CBF method (32). Our studies suggest that chronic hypotension does not invariably result in "vasomotor paralysis" with loss of the ability to vasoconstrict to acute increases in perfusion pressure. Instead, chronic hypotension appears to adaptively displace the lower limit of autoregulation in affected vascular territories by a shift of the

autoregulatory curve to the left (Fig. 8). Such a shift in autoregulatory function is conceptually analogous but opposite to the adaptive displacement seen with chronic systemic hypertension (44,45). In other words, the pressure at which the resistance vessels of the brain become maximally dilated is reset to a lower pressure; autoregulatory vasoconstriction is intact. Therefore, chronic arterial hypotension may be a

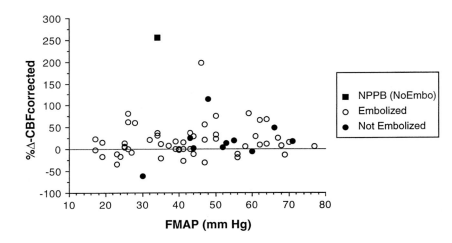

FIG. 6. Individual values for percentage change in corrected CBF from pre- to postresection in 64 patients who had feeding mean arterial pressure (FMAP) measured during craniotomy or during the last embolization session before surgery. There was no relationship ($y = .2x + 13$, $r = .07$, $p = .57$). The findings were similar when patients were restricted to only those who had pressure measured during craniotomy.

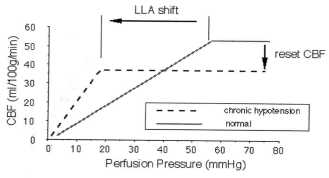

FIG. 8. Schematic depiction of adaptive autoregulatory displacement. Cerebral blood flow (CBF) is shown as a function of cerebral perfusion pressure. It appears that the lower limit of autoregulation is reset to a lower point in chronically hypotensive vascular territories adjacent to AVMs and that there is a minimal, nonischemic reduction in CBF in such territories (see reference 32). (Adapted from ref. 85, with permission.) LLA, lower limit of autoregulation.

necessary, but not a sufficient, condition for the occurrence of postoperative hyperemic brain swelling. In addition to casting doubt on repressurization injury, these observations also call into question the existence of pretreatment cerebral steal (46).

If hyperemic complications are not due to repressurization of hypotensive vascular territories, what then may be the etiology? Besides the NPPB theory, probably the most important cause of complications confused with breakthrough are technical in nature and include retraction injury, inadvertent nutrient-artery sacrifice and hemorrhage resulting from inadequate hemostasis or residual AVM (47–49). Venous insufficiency and hypertension may also play a role. The terms *occlusive hyperemia* (41) and *venous overload* (50) have been proposed to describe this phenomenon. The relationship between venous insufficiency and cerebral hyperemia is unclear, however. CBF should decrease in the setting of edema from venous congestion.

Acute reversal of decreased pulsatility has also been proposed as a possible mechanism for hemodynamic changes in the postoperative period (23,25,51). Another speculative mechanism might be related to autonomic perivascular innervation, which can profoundly influence CBF in various pathophysiologic states (52,53). A derangement in autonomic perivascular innervation to normal circulatory beds in AVM patients is compatible with certain paradoxical CBF responses to pharmacologic challenges in AVM patients (43,54,55). Batjer et al. (56) argues that posttreatment hyperemia is due to a deranged vascular bed that actively participates in swelling, and not simply to passive behavior of a paralyzed vascular bed. Although feeding vessels themselves appear to be devoid of all autonomic or peptidergic innervation (57,58), local changes in peptidergic activity in adjacent circulatory regions may somehow affect distant beds by collateral innervation. Such a mechanism might explain why in many cases of AVM resection there appear to

be global increases in CBF that cannot be explained by local changes in perfusion pressure. Schroeder et al. (59,60) reported global CBF increases after carotid endarterectomy, another instance in which repressurization of a previously hypotensive vascular territory should, intuitively, lead to regional rather than global changes in perfusion. However, the regionality of CBF increases after carotid endarterectomy remains unclear. In a subsequent study, Jorgensen and Schroeder (61) reported only ipsilateral hyperemia by transcranial Doppler ultrasonography.

Management of Perioperative Cerebral Edema and Hemorrhage

Since the syndrome of NPPB is rare, other causes of brain hemorrhage or swelling should be excluded first. In the event of intraoperative brain swelling, respiratory insufficiency or impairment of cerebral venous drainage should be ruled out. During AVM dissection, occult intracerebral or intraventricular hemorrhage must also be investigated, as well as acute hydrocephalus. Significant intraoperative cerebral swelling that could be ascribed to "breakthrough hyperemia" is a rare event. In such cases, intraoperative CBF monitoring could support the diagnosis of hyperemia. Faced with acute intraoperative brain swelling that cannot be medically managed by standard maneuvers to decrease brain volume, we favor staging the surgery and instituting cerebroprotective measures in the intensive care unit (ICU), as discussed below.

The cause of an acute neurologic deterioration in the postoperative AVM patient must first be investigated with computed tomography (CT). Although the most common cause of hemorrhage is residual AVM, hemorrhage may also occur as a result of rupture of previously coagulated stumps of feeding arteries to the AVM. Patients with neurologic deterioration as a result of postoperative bleeding must immediately return to the operating room for clot evacuation. After this is accomplished, an intracranial pressure monitor is helpful in management, as cerebral edema may develop in these patients as a result of the hematoma.

A CT scan obtained within the first 24 hours after surgery may be useful in the management of patients felt to be at high risk for complications. Examples might be an exceedingly difficult and prolonged dissection, intraoperative brain swelling, or difficulty with surgical hemostasis. If CT demonstrates a hematoma in the operative bed and the patient is stable neurologically, an angiogram should be performed to determine the presence of residual AVM. Any residual AVM should be surgically removed as soon as possible. If no AVM is found and the hematoma is not causing significant mass effect or neurologic deficit, the patient may be managed conservatively with frequent CT scans and close neurologic observation in the ICU.

Hypodense areas on the postoperative CT scan may be the result of intraoperative retraction, venous congestion, or ischemia. When they are restricted to the immediate area around the operative bed, they are most likely due to brain retraction and improve with conservative management. Moderate cerebral edema may be treated with mannitol or furosemide. Diuretic therapy should be undertaken with care not to render patients hypovolemic (see below), as hypovolemia may predispose to cerebral venous thrombosis. Edema from venous congestion may occur as a result of delayed thrombosis of draining veins or dural sinuses after AVM resection.

When other causes of cerebral edema and/or bleeding have been excluded, NPPB may be considered. The diagnosis of cerebral hyperemia can be confirmed by bedside ^{133}Xe-CBF measurements (62) or single-photon emission computed tomography (SPECT). Although there is no proven way to best treat this syndrome, the main goal of treatment is, intuitively, to decrease cerebral blood volume. Hyperventilation can be of benefit in patients with NPPB because there is evidence that CO_2 reactivity remains intact in patients after AVM resection (55). Specifically, even in a case of a patient with presumed NPPB who had a large increase in CBF after resection, CO_2 reactivity was not altered (55).

Case reports suggest that barbiturates such as pentobarbital or thiopental are effective in treating swelling attributed to NPPB (4,11,36). Burst suppression on electroencephalogram (EEG) is a convenient clinical endpoint for drug infusion that can be monitored at the bedside. CBF reduction should be maximal when the EEG achieves burst suppression. The cerebral vasoconstrictive effects of barbiturates are an indirect effect of cerebral metabolic depression; cerebral metabolic oxygen consumption ($CMRO_2$) cannot be reduced further, once EEG silence is achieved. (It should be borne in mind, however, that there is no experimental evidence that burst suppression on the EEG corresponds to maximal cerebral protection.) Barbiturate coma is not without untoward effects. Careful monitoring of systemic arterial pressure is important since barbiturates induce hypotension in about 50% of patients; barbiturates are potent arterial and venous vasodilators and may depress myocardial contractility. Adequate cerebral perfusion pressure must be maintained. Monitoring central volume status and cardiac output with a pulmonary artery catheter and an arterial line for continuous systemic blood pressure monitoring are needed to optimally manage systemic hemodynamics. In cases of prolonged coma, intravenous hyperalimentation should be instituted and a nasogastric tube should be placed, as many patients develop a paralytic ileus. Deep venous thrombosis (DVT) surveillance with frequent lower-extremity ultrasound tests is recommended. Patients with documented DVTs should be treated with inferior vena cava interruption, since anticoagulation may be contraindicated in the immediate perioperative period. Finally, patients in burst-suppression coma require intracranial pressure monitoring and frequent CT scans because the neurologic examination cannot be followed. The induction of barbiturate coma, as in all general anesthetic states, has the additional side effect of

inhibiting peripheral thermoregulatory vasoconstriction, thereby lowering core body temperature. This may mask fevers from pneumonia, urinary tract infections, and meningitis; therefore, close monitoring and early treatment of these infections should be undertaken. Temperature control and monitoring may have general application to the postoperative patient. There is increasing laboratory evidence that mild hypothermia (33–35°C) may decrease neuronal injury in the setting of cerebral ischemia (63–65). Intraoperatively, studies evaluating the safety and efficacy of mild hypothermia have recently been published (66), and preliminary data from patient trials in the ICU suggest that mild hypothermia may positively affect outcome in patients with traumatic brain injury (67). Intuitively, mild hypothermia may therefore be beneficial in patients with postoperative hemorrhage, marked cerebral edema, and/or NPPB.

Cerebral Hemodynamic Monitoring Options

^{133}Xe-CBF Monitoring

We have described our experience above. Unfortunately, ^{133}Xe monitoring is not generally available except as a research procedure. However, CBF measurements are well suited for bedside monitoring and have been used extensively in the setting of head trauma (62,68,69).

Tomographic CBF Methods

Both SPECT (54) and ^{133}Xe-enhanced CT (70) have been used to assess cerebral hemodynamics in the care of AVM patients. The main drawback to their use is the transport of either anesthetized or ICU patients to the imaging suite.

Transcranial Doppler Ultrasonography

Transcranial Doppler (TCD) is a noninvasive technique that measures blood velocity in the major cerebral arteries at the level of the circle of Willis. As a result of the increased flow into the low-resistance fistula, parent vessels of feeding arteries to the AVM have higher velocities and low pulsatility indices (a measure of downstream resistance) (71). These values return toward normal after AVM removal (51,72).

One might suspect hyperemia if the high velocities seen before surgery remain elevated postoperatively or initially normalize after resection and then increase in the postoperative period. Such an increase in TCD velocities in the setting of hyperemia has been reported with the hyperperfusion syndrome after carotid endarterectomy (73). Although the use of TCD has not been reported to monitor for cerebral hyperemia after AVM resection, it has been used as a guide to endovascular treatment of arteriovenous fistulae. Giller et al (74) reported a case in which absence of TCD evidence of hyperemia during test occlusion of the fistula emboldened them to obliterate the lesion in one stage.

TCD imaging has been useful in the management of vasospasm after subarachnoid hemorrhage, in which an increase in velocity signifies arterial narrowing (as opposed to increased flow). However, vasospasm seldom occurs during the acute period after AVM hemorrhage. Since most AVM patients are operated on weeks after hemorrhage, vasospasm is almost never seen after elective AVM resection.

Jugular Bulb Arterial Oxygen Saturation (SaO₂) Measurement: AVDO₂ Monitoring

The arteriovenous difference in oxygen content ($AVDO_2$) is the ratio of metabolism to flow or:

$$AVDO_2 = CMRO_2/CBF \qquad [1]$$

If $CMRO_2$ remains constant, then relative changes in $AVDO_2$ reflect global CBF, and a "CBF equivalent" can be calculated:

$$CBF = 1/(Ca - Cv) \qquad [2]$$

where Ca and Cv are the arterial and venous oxygen contents, respectively. The blood content of arterial or venous blood can be estimated by considering the quantity of oxygen bound by hemoglobin and the smaller portion that is dissolved in blood by the formula in equation 3:

$$(\% \text{ saturation} \times 1.39 \times \text{hemoglobin concentration}) + (.003 \times Po_2) \qquad [3]$$

Assuming unchanged $CMRO_2$ is a great leap of faith in most circumstances and should always be interpreted cautiously. It is, however, a very practical way of assessing global CBF changes. Both intermittent jugular bulb SaO_2 sampling and continuous oximetric catheters have been described. $AVDO_2$ monitoring can be useful as an "early warning system" for disturbances in flow–metabolism coupling (71); the method has been extensively employed in patients with traumatic brain injury (75).

It should be noted that the term *hyperemia* is imprecise because it does not distinguish "luxury perfusion" and coupled increases in CBF and $CMRO_2$. To date, there are no studies that have examined cerebral metabolism after AVM resection and, more specifically, in patients who have had "hyperemic" complications.

Laser Doppler and Thermal Diffusion Flow Probes

Laser Doppler flowmetry has been used extensively in animal studies of cerebral pathophysiology. It provides a good estimate of relative changes in CBF but not an absolute value. The probe's laser energy is reflected from moving red cells, and the Doppler shift is used to estimate cortical blood flow. There is, however, a paucity of clinical studies

with this method (76). Its main disadvantage is that it measures flow in only a very small area of cortex and minor movements in relation to the brain surface result in significant artifact and changes in flow. With currently available instruments, we have been unable to obtain in AVM patients consistently reliable results in the operating room with concomitant measurements using ^{133}Xe. Further improvements in probe design that will allow adaptation to the operating-room environment should allow this method to be developed into a clinically useful modality.

Thermal diffusion monitoring estimates CBF by measuring the temperature gradient between two plates in the probe that are in contact with the cortical surface. The heat generated in one of the plates is washed out by cortical blood flow. Although this technique has been more widely used in the operating room (22,77), it shares some of the disadvantages of laser Doppler flowmetry; these include its measuring only a small area of cortex with resulting artifacts from slight movements of the probe, as well as error introduced if the probe migrates to an area over an artery or vein. Although both of these techniques hold promise in the future for continuous monitoring of CBF in the ICU setting, further study is needed to assess their reliability.

Intracranial Pressure Monitoring

In a study of 32 patients in whom intracranial pressure (ICP) was monitored routinely after AVM resection, most patients had elevations of ICP >25 mm Hg. These ICP elevations responded to sedative or diuretic therapy (36). Interestingly, nine of the 32 had sustained elevations of ICP >30 mm Hg associated with neurologic deterioration. These nine patients were treated with barbiturates, with titration of the dose to achieve ICP control, from 2 to 5 days. This treatment was successful in decreasing ICP in all patients and resulted in good outcome in eight of nine patients. The incidence of neurologic deterioration as a result of marked cerebral edema and/or hemorrhage in this study was significantly higher than in most surgical series in the literature (2,38,39,41), although no other series has routinely monitored ICP.

As mentioned earlier, in our prospective study of 235 patients, only six had significant neurologic deterioration that could be attributed to "hyperemic" complications (42). In addition, there were four other patients who had postoperative hemorrhage: One had residual AVM, one an epidural hematoma, and two had blood collections in the bed of the AVM without mass effect on CT scan or neurologic deterioration. Since these complications are rare, we feel that routine ICP monitoring is not necessary in the vast majority of AVM patients. ICP monitoring may be of use in the management of patients who have had postoperative hematomas, significant cerebral edema, or breakthrough complications, especially if burst-suppression coma has been induced. In the routine postoperative AVM patient, the neurologic examination in the awake state remains a sufficiently sensitive measure of cerebral function.

Seizure Prophylaxis

Patients undergoing surgery for supratentorial AVMs must have perioperative therapeutic levels of anticonvulsants. Serum levels should be monitored at the time of surgery, as well as daily postoperatively. Postoperative seizures usually represent the presence of other complications such as hematoma, venous infarction, or postoperative edema, and therefore patients should be stabilized and taken immediately for CT scan to rule out any structural lesions that may require further intervention. Because of the detrimental increases in cerebral metabolic rate and CBF, it is most important to control the epileptic activity rapidly with a short-acting barbiturate (eg, thiopental) or benzodiazepine (eg, midazolam), followed by administration of an additional dose of the patient's anticonvulsant, especially if the serum levels are not therapeutic. Barbiturate coma is reserved for the patient with refractory status epilepticus.

SYSTEMIC HEMODYNAMIC CONSIDERATIONS

Perioperative Monitoring of Systemic Blood Pressure

Precise and accurate beat-to-beat monitoring of arterial blood pressure is a prerequisite for optimal care of the AVM patient, both intraoperatively and in the immediate postoperative period. At present, an indwelling arterial catheter is the only reliable way to achieve this goal. In the vast majority of cases, the radial artery offers the easiest and safest access to the circulation. Alternate choices include the dorsalis pedis, axillary, and femoral arteries. The morbidity from modern small-gauge indwelling arterial catheters is exceedingly low. Arterial catheterization also allows intermittent sampling of blood for arterial blood gas analysis and other laboratory studies.

Intraoperative Deliberate Hypotension

During the deep dissection of large, complex AVMs, difficulty with coagulation of thin-walled feeding arteries is commonly encountered. Inducing moderate systemic hypotension can be quite helpful in this endeavor. Hypotension appears to decrease the flow through these small, abnormal feeding vessels and facilitates cauterization (78). Our preferred agent is esmolol, given as a 1 mg/kg bolus followed by a constant infusion beginning at 0.5 mg/kg/min and titrated to achieve the desired level of blood pressure. Esmolol is a rapid-acting β-adrenergic blocker that has a short plasma half-life (approximately 8 minutes) due to metabolism by plasma cholinesterase. Its hypotensive effect lasts somewhat longer due to inhibition of the renin–angiotensin cascade.

Boluses of the mixed α- and β-adrenergic blocker, labetalol (5–100 mg), are frequently useful as an adjunct. On theoretical grounds, we tend to avoid cerebral vasodilators such as hydralazine, nitroglycerin, or sodium nitroprusside, as they could exacerbate cerebral edema from brain retraction or worsen the postoperative hyperemia seen in some AVM patients. The clinician, however, should use whichever agent he or she is most adept at using to achieve the blood goals necessary for safe and expeditious control of blood pressure.

Mean systemic arterial pressures in the neighborhood of 50 mm Hg are well tolerated by patients. Occasionally, to secure hemostasis, brief periods of a mean arterial pressure in the neighborhood of 40 mm Hg may be necessary. In our experience, deliberate hypotension does not pose a risk of cerebral ischemia in the AVM patient. This may be because their autoregulation curve has been shifted to the left, allowing the brain to maintain blood flow in the nonischemic range in spite of low systemic pressures (32). Furthermore, intravascular pressure measurements suggest that there is a "buffering effect" caused by the fistula of the AVM, so that changes in systemic arterial pressures are not completely transmitted to the cerebral arteries (31) (Figs. 9 and 10). Our frequent use of intraoperative arterial hypotension has not resulted in an increased incidence of hyperemic complications as postulated by others (79) or postoperative evidence

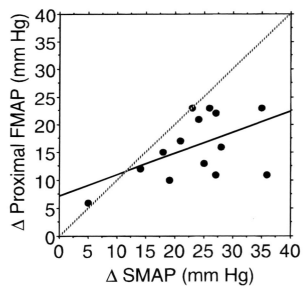

FIG. 9. Change in proximal feeding-artery pressure (ΔProximal FMAP) as a function of changes in simultaneously recorded internal carotid pressure (ΔSMAP) with phenylephrine-induced hypertension ($y = .4x + 7.2$, $r = .54$, $p < .05$, $n = 14$). Both the regression line *(solid)* and the line of identity *(dotted)* are shown. Although the relative percentage change in feeding and systemic arterial pressure may be similar, there is no direct transmission of systemic pressure changes to the circulation nearer to the AVM fistula, effectively acting as a "pressure buffer" to the distal circulation. Data are taken from ref. 32. (From ref. 31, with permission.)

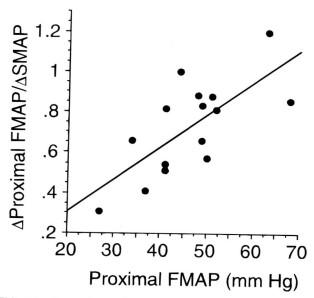

FIG. 10. The ratio of the change in feeding artery to the change in systemic pressure (ΔProximal FMAP/ΔSMAP) is positively correlated with the fistula-induced hypotension at the baseline measurement in the feeding artery (y = .02x − .02, r = .71, p < .003, n = 14); that is, the lower the feeding-artery pressure is, the less absolute will be the change with systemic hypertension and the more apparent (or effective) the "pressure buffer." Data are taken from ref. 32. (From ref. 31, with permission.)

of cerebral ischemia due to decreased flow to previously ischemic territories (80).

Deliberate Augmentation of Blood Pressure to Verify Hemostasis

After removal of the AVM, the operative bed is inspected for hemostasis after elevating mean arterial pressure 20–30% above normal for 10–15 minutes. This may be accomplished with 1–2 μg/kg of the relatively pure α-adrenergic agonist, phenylephrine, given as divided doses and titrated to the desired blood pressure. A modest reflex bradycardia is seen in most patients, which subsides as the increase in pressure abates. This maneuver may identify poorly coagulated stumps or possibly a nest of residual AVM. In our experience, increasing arterial pressure in this range has no effect on CBF as measured by the ^{133}Xe technique (43).

Postoperative Systemic Blood Pressure Monitoring

After hemostasis, during emergence from anesthesia and the first 24 hours after surgery, blood pressure should be maintained within 10% below the patient's baseline blood pressure. The purpose of maintaining the blood pressure in the slightly subnormal range is not to reduce perfusion pres-

sure per se, but rather to scrupulously prevent episodes of uncontrolled hypertension. Maintaining systemic blood pressure at a very modest reduction gives some degree of leeway, should an unforeseen stimulus cause an episode of increased systemic pressure. Control of hypertension is most probably important in preventing postoperative hematomas caused by rupture of cauterized stumps of dysplastic feeding vessels to the AVM or an unidentified residual nidus.

Our preferred regimen is similar to that used for intraoperative deliberate hypotension; a somewhat larger loading dose of labetalol (300–1000 mg) is used, and a continuous infusion with esmolol is given during the patient's stay in the ICU. These adrenergic blockers are very effective in preventing the peaks in blood pressure commonly seen during extubation and in the ICU. Intraoperative barbiturate administration may help in blood pressure control; however, it slows emergence from anesthesia, thereby obscuring the neurologic examination. Adequate cardiac preload is essential for any application of vasoactive drugs to maintain a constant systemic blood pressure.

Aggressive hypotensive therapy after surgery has not been documented to prevent hemorrhagic complications and may cause complications itself. In rare cases where en-passage vessels have been sacrificed at surgery, induction of even mild arterial hypotension may critically reduce collateral perfusion pressure to ischemic areas (Fig. 11). Although deliberate modest blood pressure augmentation may be necessary to treat such cases of "collateral failure," at least as a temporizing measure, great care should be exercised when augmenting arterial blood pressure in the perioperative period. As mentioned, there is the risk of disrupting coagulated vessels stumps or residual AVM. Additionally, it is also possible that hypertension could overwhelm autoregulatory vasoconstriction. The upper limit of autoregulation has never been tested in humans in this setting, but it should probably be assumed to be shifted to a lower systemic pressure (analogous to the leftward shift of the lower limit of pressure autoregulation) (32).

Angiograms performed in the operating room or immediately after surgery while the patient is still under general anesthesia can rationally guide treatment in circumstances where inadvertent nutrient-artery sacrifice or residual AVM is suspected. There are, however, many disadvantages of early angiography. The logistics of intraoperative angiography are complicated, as is transport of the postoperative patient who is intubated and still under general anesthesia. Interpretation of acute angiograms is difficult in some cases. They may show suspicious dysplastic vasculature and abnormal shunting, which may disappear days after surgery, but a repeat angiogram would be required to rule out residual AVM. Additionally, early angiography may miss a small residual nidus as a result of spasm or swelling.

Fluid Management

Postoperative AVM patents should be kept euvolemic. Hypovolemia may increase the risk of cerebral venous

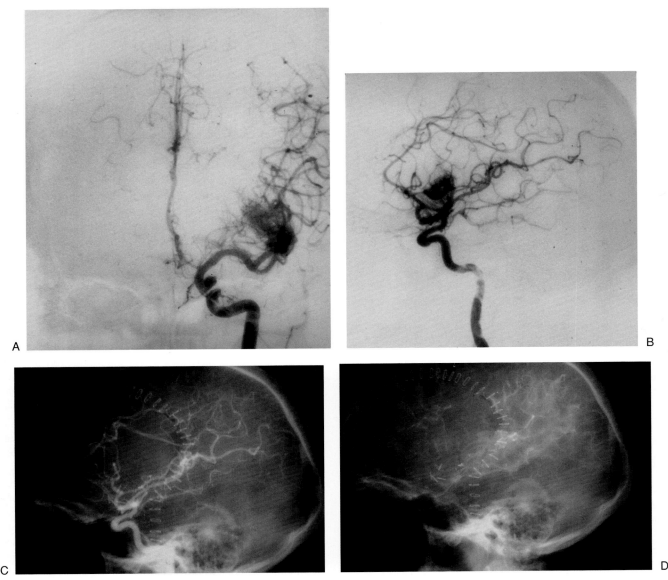

FIG. 11. Preoperative anteroposterior **(A)** and lateral **(B)** views of a left internal carotid angiogram demonstrate an AVM in the sylvian fissure fed by middle cerebral artery (MCA) branches. During the first 48 hours after surgery, the patient was globally dysphasic. The deficit was attributed to brain retraction at the operative site. His systemic blood pressure during this period was controlled in the low-normal range using an infusion of esmolol. On the third postoperative day, an angiogram was obtained. It was noted that an MCA en-passage branch was sacrificed at surgery **(C)**. There is late arterial-phase filling of the ischemic regions by collateral pathways **(D)**. The patient's deficit improved immediately after his systemic blood pressure was increased and resolved completely within 4 days. (Courtesy of Dr. B. Stein.)

thrombosis. Dilated draining veins that have tributaries from surrounding brain may thrombose as a result of the sluggish flow after AVM resection. Severe hypervolemia, conversely, may exacerbate cerebral edema. If loop diuretics or mannitol is used to treat brain swelling, central volume status must be carefully monitored.

Most AVM patients are young and otherwise healthy and can be maintained euvolemic with careful monitoring of fluid balance and serum electrolytes. Complicated cases may benefit from central venous pressure monitoring and, if left

ventricular dysfunction is suspected, pulmonary artery catheter monitoring. Preliminary evidence suggests that postoperative AVM patients are systemically hyperdynamic (81); therefore, in some cases, systemic monitoring may be beneficial in managing cardiac output and blood pressure. If colloid is indicated to maintain cardiac preload, human serum albumin is preferred in spite of its modestly higher cost. Recent evidence suggests that hetastarch may result in coagulation disorders that might predispose to hemorrhage (82).

Hypotonic fluid therapy will result in water movement

across the blood–brain barrier in structurally intact brain (83). Isotonic fluid replacement is mandatory. Even large volumes of mildly hypotonic fluids such as lactated Ringer's solution may exacerbate cerebral edema. We avoid glucose-containing fluids because of evidence that they aggravate cerebral injury (84), especially since routine perioperative steroid use may cause some degree of hyperglycemia. Aggressive lowering of mildly elevated plasma glucose, however, is not recommended for fear of inducing hypoglycemia, and evidence is lacking that it is efficacious in improving outcome after brain injury.

SUMMARY

In both the intraoperative and the immediate postoperative periods after AVM resection, it is essential to have beat-to-beat assessment of systemic arterial pressure. Further, clinically appropriate assessment of central volume status is also necessary. Optimal cerebral perfusion pressure and, necessarily, adequate cardiac preload must be provided. "Optimal" will be defined according to the specific clinical circumstances, ie, whether surgical manipulation requires deliberate hypotension or the intraoperative bed needs to be assessed for evidence of adequate hemostasis by increasing systemic pressure.

The occurrence of perioperative idiopathic brain swelling or hemorrhage (NPPB) as a result of AVM surgery is uncommon. The mechanism for the observed postoperative hyperemia is unclear, but it appears that increases in CBF are usually global and not necessarily related to the degree of preresection feeding-artery hypotension. It also appears that, instead of "vasomotor paralysis," the lower limit of autoregulation of chronically hypotensive vascular beds is shifted toward the left. This shift of the autoregulation curve allows the brain to maintain blood flow in the nonischemic range in spite of low systemic pressures and prevents massive hyperemic responses with normalization of pressures after AVM resection in most patients. The status of the upper limit of autoregulation is unclear.

The above notwithstanding, a significant source of serious morbidity from AVM surgery results from postoperative complications such as cerebral edema and hemorrhage; the precise mechanisms are unclear. Hemorrhage is most commonly due to residual AVM or rupture of coagulated vessel stumps. For this reason, a critical consideration in the early postoperative period is continual assessment of the patient's neurologic examination for signs of acute deterioration and tight control of the systemic blood pressure. Cerebral edema may result from brain retraction, venous thrombosis, and ischemia, as well as hyperemia from NPPB. Therefore, an understanding of the pathophysiology of these complications is important for a rational approach to the perioperative management of these patients. Future progress in techniques to monitor CBF and cerebral metabolism in both the operating room and ICU will provide further improvements in the management of these patients.

ACKNOWLEDGMENTS

Supported in part by PHS grants RO1 NS27713 and NS34949. The authors wish to thank Joyce Ouchi for expert assistance in preparation of the manuscript; and the members of the Columbia University AVM project for their continued support.

REFERENCES

1. Hamilton MG, Spetzler RF. The prospective application of a grading system for arteriovenous malformations. *Neurosurgery* 1994;34:2–7.
2. Heros RC, Korosue K, Diebold PM. Surgical excision of cerebral arteriovenous malformations: Late results. *Neurosurgery* 1990;26: 570–578.
3. Pasqualin A, Barone G, Cioffi F, Rosta L, Scienza R, Pian RD. The relevance of anatomic and hemodynamic factors to a classification of cerebral arteriovenous malformations. *Neurosurgery* 1991;28: 370–379.
4. Batjer HH, Devous MD Sr, Meyer YJ, Purdy PD, Samson DS. Cerebrovascular hemodynamics in arteriovenous malformation complicated by normal perfusion pressure breakthrough. *Neurosurgery* 1988;22: 503–509.
5. Spetzler RF, Wilson CB, Weinstein P, Mehdorn M, Townsend J, Telles D. Normal perfusion pressure breakthrough theory. *Clin Neurosurg* 1978;25:651–672.
6. Nornes H, Grip A. Hemodynamic aspects of cerebral arteriovenous malformations. *J Neurosurg* 1980;53:456–464.
7. Brown AP, and Spetzler RF. Intracranial arteriovenous malformations: cerebrovascular hemodynamics. In: Batjer HH et al. *Cerebrovascular Disease.* New York: Lippincott-Raven Publishers, 1997;833–842.
8. DeMeritt JS, Pile-Spellman J, Mast H, Moohan N, Lu DC, Young WL, Hacein-Bey L, Mohr JP, Stein BM. Outcome analysis of preoperative embolization with N-butyl cyanoacrylate in cerebral arteriovenous malformations. *Am J Neuroradiol* 1995;16:1801–1807.
9. Mast H, Mohr JP, Soussis IA, et al. Hemodynamic "steal" remains an unestablished mechanism for clinical presentation of arteriovenous malformations (abstract #P177). *Ann Neurol* 1994;36:303–304.
10. Wade JPH, Hachinski VC. Cerebral steal: Robbery or maldistribution? In: Wood JH, ed. *Cerebral Blood Flow: Physiologic and Clinical Aspects.* New York: McGraw-Hill, 1987:467–480.
11. Day AL, Friedman WA, Sypert GW, Mickle JP. Successful treatment of the normal perfusion pressure breakthrough syndrome. *Neurosurgery* 1982;11:625–630.
12. Feindel W, Yamamoto YL, Hodge CP. Red cerebral veins and the cerebral steal syndrome: Evidence from fluorescein angiography and microregional blood flow by radioisotopes during excision of an angioma. *J Neurosurg* 1971;35:167–179.
13. Nagao S, Ueta K, Mino S, et al. Monitoring of cortical blood flow during excision of arteriovenous malformations by thermal diffusion method. *Surg Neurol* 1989;32:137–143.
14. Okabe T, Meyer JS, Okayasu H, et al. Xenon-enhanced CT CBF measurements in cerebral AVM's before and after excision: Contribution to pathogenesis and treatment. *J Neurosurg* 1983;59:21–31.
15. Spetzler RF, Martin NA, Carter LP, Flom RA, Raudzens PA, Wilkinson E. Surgical management of large AVM's by staged embolization and operative excision. *J Neurosurg* 1987;67:17–28.
16. Tamaki N, Lin T, Asada M, et al. Modulation of blood flow following excision of a high flow cerebral arteriovenous malformation: Case report. *J Neurosurg* 1990;72:509–512.
17. Yamada S, Cojocaru T. Arteriovenous malformations. In: Wood JH, ed. *Cerebral Blood Flow: Physiologic and Clinical Aspects.* New York: McGraw-Hill, 1987:580–590.
18. Piepgras DG, Morgan MK, Sundt TM Jr, Yanagihara T, Mussman LM.

Intracerebral hemorrhage after carotid endarterectomy. *J Neurosurg* 1988;68:532–536.

19. Halbach V, Higashida RT, Hieshima G, Norman D. Normal perfusion pressure breakthrough occurring during treatment of carotid and vertebral fistulas. *Am J Neuroradiol* 1987;8:751–756.

20. Nornes H, Grip A, Wikeby P. Intraoperative evaluation of cerebral hemodynamics using directional Doppler technique: Part I. Arteriovenous malformations. *J Neurosurg* 1979;50:145–151.

21. Ahuja A, Gibbons KJ, Guterman LR, Hopkins LN. Pedicle pressure changes in cerebral arteriovenous malformations during therapeutic embolization: Relationship to delayed hemorrhage (abstract). *Stroke* 1993;24:185.

22. Barnett GH, Little JR, Ebrahim ZY, Jones SC, Friel HT. Cerebral circulation during arteriovenous malformation operation. *Neurosurgery* 1987;20:836–842.

23. Duckwiler G, Dion J, Vinuela F, Jabour B, Martin N, Bentson J. Intravascular microcatheter pressure monitoring: Experimental results and early clinical evaluation. *Am J Neuroradiol* 1990;11:169–175.

24. Hassler W, Steinmetz H. Cerebral hemodynamics in angioma patients: An intraoperative study. *J Neurosurg* 1987;67:822–831.

25. Jungreis CA, Horton JA, Hecht ST. Blood pressure changes in feeders to cerebral arteriovenous malformations during therapeutic embolization. *Am J Neuroradiol* 1989;10:575–578.

26. Kader A, Young WL, Pile-Spellman J, et al. The influence of hemodynamic and anatomic factors on hemorrhage from cerebral arteriovenous malformations. *Neurosurgery* 1994;34:801–808.

27. Marks MP, Steinberg GK, Norbash A, Lane B. Vascular characteristics predictive of hemorrhage in cerebral AVM's (abstract). *J Neurosurg* 1993;78:346A.

28. Miyasaka Y, Kurata A, Tokiwa K, Tanaka R, Yada K, Ohwada T. Draining vein pressure increases and hemorrhage in patients with arteriovenous malformation (case report). *Stroke* 1994;25:504–507.

29. Miyasaka Y, Yada K, Kurata A, et al. Correlation between intravascular pressure and risk of hemorrhage due to arteriovenous malformations. *Surg Neurol* 1993;39:370–373.

30. Spetzler RF, Hargraves RW, McCormick PW, Zabramski JM, Flom RA, Zimmerman RS. Relationship of perfusion pressure and size to risk of hemorrhage from arteriovenous malformations. *J Neurosurg* 1992;76:918–923.

31. Young WL, Kader A, Pile-Spellman J, Ornstein E, Stein BM, Columbia University AVM Study Project. Arteriovenous malformation draining vein physiology and determinants of transnidal pressure gradients. *Neurosurgery* 1994;35:389–396.

32. Young WL, Pile-Spellman J, Prohovnik I, Kader A, Stein BM, Columbia University AVM Study Project. Evidence for adaptive autoregulatory displacement in hypotensive cortical territories adjacent to arteriovenous malformations. *Neurosurgery* 1994;34:601–611.

33. Young WL, Pile-Spellman J. Anesthetic considerations for interventional neuroradiology (Review). *Anesthesiology* 1994;80:427–456.

34. Fogarty-Mack P, Pile-Spellman J, Hacein-Bey L, Osipov A, DeMeritt J, Jackson EC, Young WL, Columbia University AVM Study Project. The effect of arteriovenous malformations on the distribution of intracerebral arterial pressures. *Am J Neuroradiol* 1996;17: in press.

35. Fleischer LH, Young WL, Pile-Spellman J, et al. Relationship of transcranial Doppler flow velocities and arteriovenous malformation feeding artery pressures. *Stroke* 1993;24:1897–1902.

36. Awad IA, Magdinec M, Schubert A. Intracranial hypertension after resection of cerebral arteriovenous malformations: Predisposing factors and management strategy. *Stroke* 1994;25:611–620.

37. Batjer HH, Devous MD Sr, Seibert GB, Purdy PD, Bonte FJ. Intracranial arteriovenous malformation: Relationship between clinical factors and surgical complications. *Neurosurgery* 1989;24:75–79.

38. Drake CG. Cerebral arteriovenous malformations: Considerations for and experience with surgical treatment in 166 cases. *Clin Neurosurg* 1979;26:145–208.

39. Yasargil MG. *Microneurosurgery*. Vol IIIA. AVM of the brain, history, embryology, pathological considerations, hemodynamics, diagnostic studies, microsurgical anatomy. New York: Thieme Medical, 1988; 221–226.

40. Morgan MK, Johnston IH, Hallinan JM, Weber NC. Complications of surgery for arteriovenous malformation of the brain. *J Neurosurg* 1993; 78:176–182.

41. Al-Rodhan NRF, Sundt TM Jr, Piepgras DG, Nichols DA, Rufenacht D, Stevens LN. Occlusive hyperemia: A theory for the hemodynamic

42. Young WL, Kader A, Ornstein E, Baker KZ, Ostapkovich N, Pile-Spellman J, Fogarty-Mack P, Stein BM, The Columbia University AVM Project. Cerebral hyperemia after arteriovenous malformation resection is related to "breakthrough" complications but not to feeding artery pressure. *Neurosurgery* 1996;38:1085–1095.

43. Young WL, Kader A, Prohovnik I, et al. Pressure autoregulation is intact after arteriovenous malformation resection. *Neurosurgery* 1993; 32:491–497.

44. Paulson OB, Strandgaard S, Edvinsson L. Cerebral autoregulation. *Cerebrovasc Brain Metab Rev* 1990;2:161–192.

45. Strandgaard S. Autoregulation of cerebral circulation in hypertension. *Acta Neurol Scand Suppl* 1978;66:1–82.

46. Mast H, Mohr JP, Osipov A, et al. "Steal" is an unestablished mechanism for the clinical presentation of cerebral arteriovenous malformations. *Stroke* 1995;26:1215–1220.

47. Stein BM, Wolpert SM. Arteriovenous malformations of the brain: I. Current concepts and treatment. *Arch Neurol* 1980;37:1–5.

48. Hassler W. *Hemodynamic Aspects of Cerebral Angiomas*. Vienna: Springer-Verlag, 1986 (*Acta Neurochir [Wien]* [suppl 37]).

49. Peerless SJ. Comment on Day AL, Friedman WA, Sypert GW, Mickle JP: Successful treatment of the normal perfusion pressure breakthrough syndrome. *Neurosurgery* 1982;11:629–630.

50. Wilson CB, Hieshima G. Occlusive hyperemia: A new way to think about an old problem (editorial). *J Neurosurg* 1993;78:165–166.

51. Lindegaard K-F, Grolimund P, Aaslid R, Nornes H. Evaluation of cerebral AVM's using transcranial Doppler ultrasound. *J Neurosurg* 1986; 65:335–344.

52. Macfarlane R, Moskowitz MA, Sakas DE, Tasdemiroglu E, Wei EP, Kontos HA. The role of neuroeffector mechanisms in cerebral hyperperfusion syndromes (review article). *J Neurosurg* 1991;75:845–855.

53. Macfarlane R, Tasdemiroglu E, Moskowitz MA, Uemura Y, Wei EP, Kontos HA. Chronic trigeminal ganglionectomy or topical capsaicin application to pial vessels attenuates postocclusive cortical hyperemia but does not influence postischemic hypoperfusion. *J Cereb Blood Flow Metab* 1991;11:261–271.

54. Batjer HH, Devous MD Sr. The use of acetazolamide-enhanced regional cerebral blood flow measurement to predict risk to arteriovenous malformation patients. *Neurosurgery* 1992;31:213–218.

55. Young WL, Prohovnik I, Ornstein E, et al. The effect of arteriovenous malformation resection on cerebrovascular reactivity to carbon dioxide. *Neurosurgery* 1990;27:257–267.

56. Batjer HH. Comment on Young WL, Pile-Spellman J, Prohovnic I, Kader A, Stein B, the Columbia University AVM Study Project. Evidence for adaptive autoregulatory displacement in hypotensive cortical territories adjacent to arteriovenous malformations. *Neurosurgery* 1994;34:610.

57. Maynard KI, Ogilvy CS. Patterns of peptide-containing perivascular nerves in the circle of Willis: Their absence in intracranial arteriovenous malformations. *J Neurosurg* 1995;82:829–833.

58. Muraszko K, Wang HH, Pelton G, Stein BM. A study of the reactivity of feeding vessels to arteriovenous malformations: Correlation with clinical outcome. *Neurosurgery* 1990;26:190–200.

59. Schroeder T, Holstein PE, Engell HC. Hyperperfusion following endarterectomy (letter to the editor). *Stroke* 1984;15:758.

60. Schroeder T, Sillesen H, Sorensen O, Engell HC. Cerebral hyperperfusion following carotid endarterectomy. *J Neurosurg* 1987;66:824–829.

61. Jorgensen LG, Schroeder TV. Defective cerebrovascular autoregulation after carotid endarterectomy. *Eur J Vasc Surg* 1993;7:370–379.

62. Martin NA, Doberstein C. Cerebral blood flow measurement in neurosurgical intensive care. *Neurosurg Clin N Am* 1994;5:607–618.

63. Ginsberg MD, Sternau LL, Globus MY-T, Dietrich WD, Busto R. Therapeutic modulation of brain temperature: Relevance to ischemic brain injury. *Cerebrovasc Brain Metab Rev* 1992;4:189–225.

64. Kader A, Brisman MH, Maraire N, Huh J-T, Solomon RA. The effect of mild hypothermia on permanent focal ischemia in the rat. *Neurosurgery* 1992;31:1056–1061.

65. Sano T, Drummond JC, Patel PM, Grafe MR, Watson JC, Cole DJ. A comparison of the cerebral protective effects of isoflurane and mild hypothermia in a model of incomplete forebrain ischemia in the rat. *Anesthesiology* 1992;76:221–228.

66. Baker KZ, Young WL, Stone JG, Kader A, Baker CJ, Solomon RA.

Deliberate mild intraoperative hypothermia for craniotomy. *Anesthesiology* 1994;81:361–367.

67. Marion DW, Obrist WD, Carlier PM, Penrod LE, Darby JM. The use of moderate therapeutic hypothermia for patients with severe head injuries: A preliminary report. *J Neurosurg* 1993;79:354–362.

68. Obrist WD, Langfitt TW, Jaggi JL, Cruz J, Gennarelli TA. Cerebral blood flow and metabolism in comatose patients with acute head injury: Relationship to intracranial hypertension. *J Neurosurg* 1984;61:241–253.

69. Bouma GJ, Muizelaar P, Bandoh K, Marmarou A. Blood pressure and intracranial pressure-volume dynamics in severe head injury: Relationship with cerebral blood flow. *J Neurosurg* 1992;77:15–19.

70. Tarr RW, Johnson DW, Rutigliano M, et al. Use of acetazolamide-challenge xenon CT in the assessment of cerebral blood flow dynamics in patients with arteriovenous malformations. *Am J Neuroradiol* 1990; 11:441–448.

71. Young WL, Ornstein E. Cerebral and spinal cord blood flow (review). In: Cottrell JE, Smith DS, ed. *Anesthesia and Neurosurgery,* 3rd ed. St. Louis, MO: Mosby-Year Book, 1994:17–57.

72. Petty GW, Massaro AR, Tatemichi TK, et al. Transcranial Doppler ultrasonographic changes after treatment for arteriovenous malformations. *Stroke* 1990;21:260–266.

73. Powers AD, Smith RR. Hyperperfusion syndrome after carotid endarterectomy: A transcranial Doppler evaluation. *Neurosurgery* 1990;26:56–60.

74. Giller CA, Batjer HH, Purdy PD, Walker B, Mathews D. Interdisciplinary evaluation of cerebral hemodynamics in the treatment of arteriovenous fistulae associated with giant varices. *Neurosurgery* 1994;35:778–784.

75. Ritter AM, Robertson C. Cerebral metabolism. *Neurosurg Clin N Am* 1994;5:633–665.

76. Rosenblum BR, Bonner RF, Oldfield EH. Intraoperative measurement of cortical blood flow adjacent to cerebral AVM using laser Doppler velocimetry. *J Neurosurg* 1987;66:396–399.

77. Carter LP. Surface monitoring of cerebral cortical blood flow. *Cerebrovasc Brain Metab Rev* 1991;3:246–261.

78. Stein BM, Kader A. Intracranial arteriovenous malformations. *Clin Neurosurg* 1992;39:76–113.

79. Morgan MK, Sundt TM Jr. The case against staged operative resection of cerebral arteriovenous malformations. *Neurosurgery* 1989;25:429–436.

80. Samson DS, Batjer HH. Surface lesions: Lobar arteriovenous malformations. In: Apuzzo MLJ, ed. *Brain Surgery.* New York: Churchill Livingstone, 1993:1142–1174.

81. Porembka D, Ebrahim Z, Bloomfield E, Stuebing R. The postoperative hyperdynamic cardiovascular response following intracranial excision of arterial venous malformation (AVM) (abstract). *Anesthesiology* 1991;75:A215.

82. Trumble ER, Muizelaar JP, Myseros JS, Choi SC, Warren BB. Coagulopathy with the use of hetastarch in the treatment of vasospasm. *J Neurosurg* 1995;82:44–47.

83. Zornow MH, Scheller MS, Todd MM, Moore SS. Acute cerebral effects of isotonic crystalloid and colloid solutions following cryogenic brain injury in the rabbit. *Anesthesiology* 1988;69:180–184.

84. Lanier WL. Glucose management during cardiopulmonary bypass: Cardiovascular and neurologic implications (editorial). *Anesth Analg* 1991; 72:423–427.

85. Young WL. Clinical Neuroscience Lectures. Munster, IN: Cathenart Publishing, 1996 in press.

Cerebrovascular Disease, edited by H. Hunt Batjer.
Lippincott-Raven Publishers, Philadelphia © 1997.

CHAPTER 70

Intracranial Arteriovenous Malformations: Causes and Management of Perioperative Hemorrhage

Lee R. Guterman, Kevin J. Gibbons, Gregory J. Castiglia, and L. Nelson Hopkins

Cerebral arteriovenous malformations (AVMs) are tenacious entities presumed to begin formation during human embryonic development (1). These vascular lesions can continue to enlarge after birth and into adult life. The mechanisms responsible for formation and growth remain unknown (2).

The natural history of these lesions was defined by Ondra et al (3). They observed 166 patients with asymptomatic AVMs over a period of 23.7 years. They reported a combined morbidity and mortality of 2.7% per year, a major bleed rate of 4% per year, and mortality of 1% per year. Over 80% of the patients who hemorrhaged after enrollment in the study sustained new neurologic deficits. Over half of the deaths were attributed directly to hemorrhage.

For years, the mainstay of treatment for AVMs has been surgical resection. Over the past decade microcatheter-based delivery of thrombogenic material into the malformation has gained popularity (4). More recently, stereotactic radiosurgery has been used for primary treatment of these lesions or as an adjunct to embolization. The perioperative period is associated with risk of intracranial hemorrhage regardless of the modality or combination of modalities chosen.

Management of perioperative hemorrhage is problematic and fraught with obstacles. Perioperative embolization is associated with a 5–15% rate of hemorrhage per session (5). The majority of malformations require multiple endovascular procedures preoperatively. Stereotactic radiosurgery requires 12–24 months for radiation-induced vessel sclerosis to completely occlude the malformation. During this period the AVM is unprotected from hemorrhage. Complete surgical resection is the only method that protects the patient from

rebleeding in the postoperative period. Yet AVMs resected in patients under 13 years of age have been reported to recur even after postoperative angiography demonstrated no malformation (6).

In this chapter we will examine the anatomic features of AVMs that contribute to perioperative bleeding. Each treatment modality will be examined and potential hemorrhagic complications will be identified. Methods for managing perioperative hemorrhage as a means of minimizing secondary damage will be outlined.

ANGIOGRAPHIC/ANATOMIC FEATURES OF AVM AS A SOURCE OF HEMORRHAGE

Specific features of a cerebral AVM's angioarchitecture help define the propensity of a malformation to hemorrhage. These features can exist pretreatment or be induced by the intervention. Vinuela et al examined the angioarchitecture of 53 patients with deep-seated AVMs. Over 70% of the patients presented with intracranial hemorrhage (ICH) (7). Forty-one patients in their series presented with ICH, and 14 of these had stenosis in the region of the vein of Galen. Seven patients had complete occlusion of the deep venous system. These AVMs showed numerous collateral venous pathways through enlarged medullary and cortical venous pathways. There was dominant drainage via the basal vein of Rosenthal. Marks et al examined the angioarchitecture in 65 patients, 45 of whom presented with ICH (8). They found that positive predictors of ICH at presentation included central venous drainage, periventricular or intraventricular location, or the presence of intranidal aneurysms. The later had a high correlation with ICH. More central anatomic position ie, basal ganglia, thalamus, and corpus callosum, correlated with an increased risk of ICH at presentation. Approximately

L. R. Guterman, K. J. Gibbons, G. Castiglia, and L. N. Hopkins: Department of Neurosurgery, State University of New York at Buffalo, School of Medicine and Biomedical Sciences, Buffalo, NY 14209.

36% of patients presenting with ICH had venous stenosis, with the region of the vein of Galen being the most common site. They found that angiomatous change and cortical venous drainage were negative predictors of ICH.

Review of the literature and our personal series indicates that the following angiographic factors are associated with an increase risk of perioperative ICH:

Aneurysms on arterial feeding pedicles
Venous aneurysms and ectasias
Venous outflow obstruction
Venous drainage pattern
Anatomy of the nidus

Alteration of the angioarchitecture of cerebral AVMs with embolization, radiosurgery, or surgical excision can result in development of a physical property that increases the likelihood of postprocedural hemorrhage. In treating cerebral AVMs, especially in a staged fashion, it is essential that changes in the angioarchitecture be monitored. In this way therapeutic intervention can be adjusted to prevent perioperative hemorrhagic complications.

The presence of saccular aneurysms on the feeding pedicles of AVMs have been implicated as a source of intracranial hemorrhage (9). Okamoto et al reported on 78 patients with aneurysms on feeding pedicles to cerebral AVMs. They concluded that abnormal hemodynamic stresses on the arteries that feed malformations play a significant role in the formation of AVM-associated aneurysms (10). Garcia-Manaco reported on 189 patients who presented with ICH from cerebral AVMs. Fifteen of these were found to have aneurysms. Nine aneurysms were located on the feeding pedicle proximal to the nidus whereas six aneurysms were located on the draining vein distal to the nidus. They advocated endovascular treatment of these lesions. Embolization of AVMs with particles was considered hazardous. Therefore a nonwedge technique for delivery of liquid polymer adhesives is used. In each case the AVM and the aneurysm were treated simultaneously (11). Lasjaunias et al reported a twofold increase in ICH in cerebral AVM with associated aneurysms (12). Kondziolka et al differentiated between aneurysms associated with feeding pedicles of AVM and those on distant branches coexistent with the AVM, called "dysplastic aneurysms." They concluded that dysplastic aneurysms will not regress with treatment of the AVM and can even enlarge. They suggest that these aneurysms be treated separately (13).

It has become our routine to treat aneurysms associated with AVM aggressively. Distant or dysplastic aneurysms not associated with AVM-feeding pedicles are treated by open surgical ligation. They are unlikely to regress or thrombose after the AVM has been occluded. Although these aneurysms may be flow-related, they still carry a risk of SAH. Aneurysms deemed inoperable secondary to surgical inaccessibility, poor neurologic grade, or difficult aneurysm anatomy can be treated by endovascular coil occlusion (Fig. 1).

Aneurysms on feeding pedicles of malformations are treated by endovascular coil occlusion prior to embolization of the AVM (Fig. 2). Introduction of particles into the nidus of a malformation results in increased feeding pedicle pressures (14). As a result, flow and pressure in the aneurysm proximal to the nidus will change. In some cases the pedicle and aneurysms may thrombose. If this does not occur the aneurysms would be at increased risk of hemorrhage secondary to hemodynamic changes. A similar situation would occur if liquid polymer adhesives were being used. Therefore we have chosen to perform endovascular occlusion of aneurysms on feeding pedicles to AVMs.

Venous ectasias and outflow obstruction can be implicated as a potential source of perioperative hemorrhage after embolization although no quantitative studies have been performed to define the relationship (Fig. 3). The goal of embolization varies significantly among practitioners. In our institution we attempt to occlude the portion of the nidus supplied by the pedicle being embolized. We strive to leave the venous drainage undisturbed so that the pressure and flow in remaining pedicles does not change. Outflow obstruction of the venous drainage for the remaining nidus can result in devastating hemorrhage. After embolization, inspection of the venous drainage pattern of the remaining malformation is performed. If significant change has occurred we leave patients anticoagulated with intravenous heparin until collateral venous drainage can be established. This practice can potentiate bleeding should it occur. Therefore anticoagulation and neurologic status are monitored in an intensive care unit. Alternatively, aggressive embolization of the remaining pedicles can be performed. In smaller AVMs or in larger lesions in the later phase of staged treatments this practice can prevent perioperatve hemorrhage. In large AVMs in the early phase of staged treatments this practice can be disastrous. It has been our experience that large changes in flow induced by embolizing multiple feeding pedicles in one session cannot be tolerated. Either residual AVM or surrounding cerebral vessels with incompetent autoregulation can hemorrhage under the stress of the flow alteration induced by excessive embolization.

Angiomatous change in the nidus can be associated with hemorrhage. This fine feathery appearance of the nidus is associated with increased fragility of its vasculature. Alterations in flow are not well tolerated by these thin abnormal vessels. As a result, hemorrhage after embolization can be seen (Fig. 4).

VASCULAR PERFORATIONS DURING ENDOVASCULAR INTERVENTIONS

Perforation of AVM vessels during embolization procedures occurs regardless of technique employed. Attempts have been made to compare over-the-wire catheter tech-

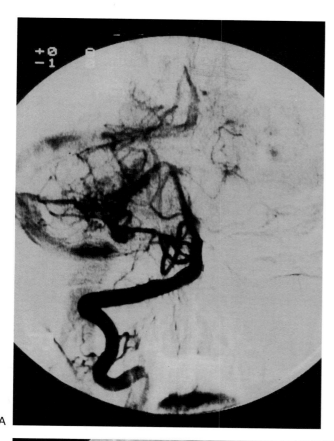

A

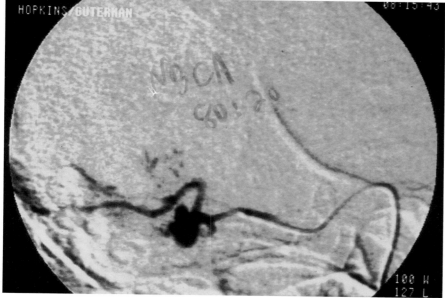

B

FIG. 1. A 62-year-old white man who presented with a posterior fossa intracranial hemorrhage, ataxia, and right-sided past pointing. The left vertebral artery injection is pictured in **(A)**. Note an aneurysm on the left anterior inferior cerebellar artery (AICA) feeding pedicle to the cerebellar malformation. A microcatheter was flow-directed into the left AICA and the artery embolized with NBCA **(B)**. The patient returned in 3 weeks for embolization of the remaining superior cerebellar artery feeders to the malformation. The initial hemorrhage was felt to be from the aneurysm on the AICA feeding pedicle.

niques to flow-directed catheter systems. No conclusive differences could be obtained (15). Halbach et al reviewed their series of AVM embolizations in 400 patients (16). They reported seven perforations resulting in one death. The remaining patient had no neurologic sequelae surrounding the event. They report that the anterior choroidal artery has a high frequency of perforation. This may be due to its acute takeoff from the middle cerebral artery and its small diameter. Purdy et al reported seven cases of life-threatening hemorrhages occurring during staged embolization of AVM (17). Five patients were taken to the operating room for emergent craniotomy. There were two deaths and one significant neurologic deficit. Four patients were unaffected by the hemorrhage.

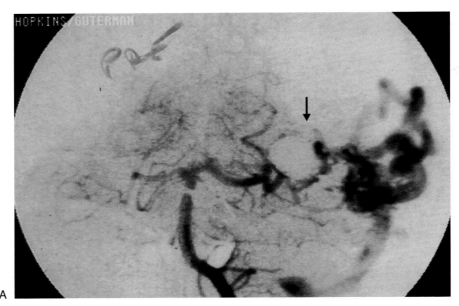

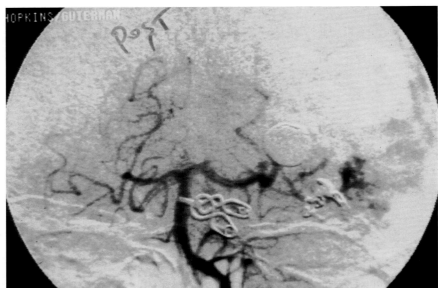

FIG. 2. This 52-year-old white woman presented with acute subarachnoid hemorrhage and was found to have three anterior circulation aneurysms in addition to a cerebellar arteriovenous malformation fed by the right posterior cerebral artery (PCA). A large aneurysm was noted on the proximal segment of the PCA feeding the malformation. This was occluded using electrically detachable coils (*arrow*) **(A)**. The feeding pedicle was then embolized with NBCA **(B)**. A small amount of nidus remained to be embolized at a latter date. The aneurysm was coiled prior to embolization of the PCA feeding pedicle with NBCA.

In our experience vessel perforations can be the result of:

Transvascular wire and/or catheter placement
High-pressure injections into catheters that are wedged completely or partially
Rupture of a aneurysm or dysplastic vessel during embolization
Venous outflow obstruction

In our practice AVM embolization is performed under systemic anticoagulation with intravenous heparin. We routinely monitor anticoagulation with activated clotting time (ACT). This technique provides a quantitative measure of clotting within 5 minutes of sampling and can be performed in the angio suite. We maintain the ACT as close to 300 seconds as possible (normal <130 seconds).

Perforation is recognized by signs and symptoms in awake patients and extravasation of contrast into the subarachnoid space during digital subtraction angiography. If a vessel perforation occurs with a guide wire and/or microcatheter the device is not removed immediately. Protamine is administered intravenously until the ACT is normalized. This usually requires 50–75 mg in an adult. Repeat angiography is performed through the guide catheter. If extravasation has not ceased, measures are taken to occlude the feeding pedicle using coils or liquid polymer adhesives (ie, glue).

Immediately after perforation, pharmacologic control of blood pressure is crucial to prevent secondary damage and limit extension of the hemorrhage. Intravenous beta blockade is preferred to nitrates unless bradycardia is present. Hypotension is induced. Efforts are made not to compromise

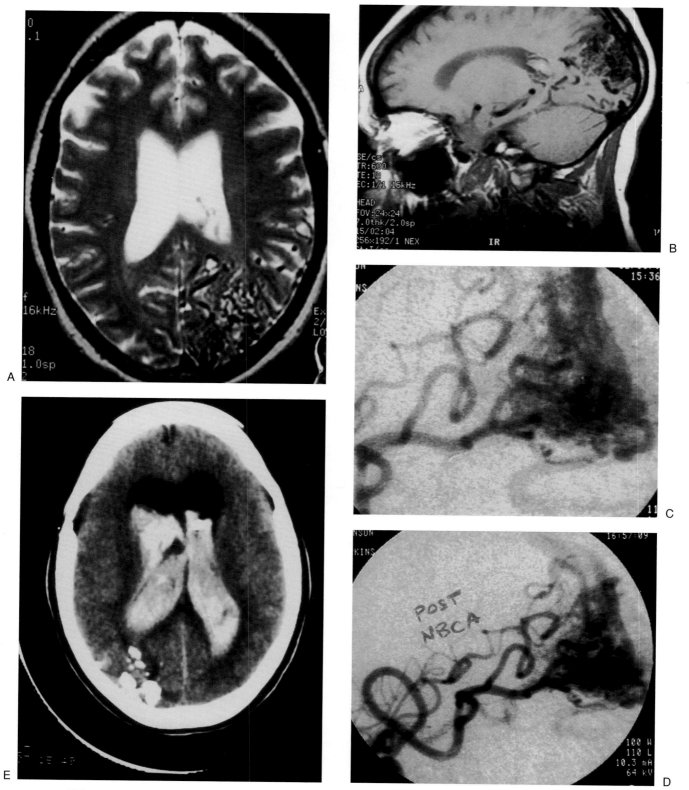

FIG. 3. This 37-year-old black woman presented after two intraventricular hemorrhages. She was found to have a large posterior parietal/occipital arteriovenous malformation fed by branches of the middle cerebral artery and posterior cerebral artery. The axial **(A)** and sagittal **(B)** MRIs are pictured. A pretreatment anterior posterior internal carotid artery angiogram is depicted in **(C)**. After embolization of two feeding pedicles, repeat carotid angiogram is presented showing a decrease in the size of the nidus **(D)**. Within 12 hours of endovascular treatment she suffered a massive intraventricular hemorrhage **(E)** and herniated shortly thereafter. Venous outflow obstruction was felt to be the cause of the hemorrhage.

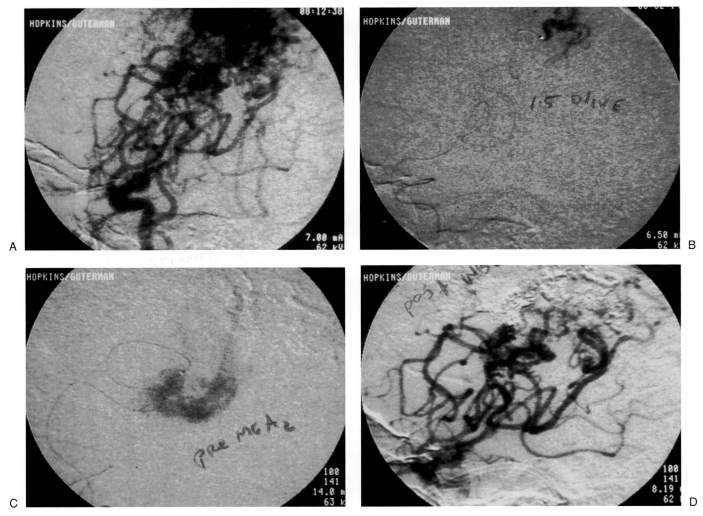

FIG. 4. A 42-year-old white man with a long history of left frontoparietal arteriovenous malformation (AVM). Patient presented with a mixed aphasia and right-sided weakness. A left internal carotid angiogram **(A)** reveals large fine nidus with multiple middle cerebral artery (MCA) feeders. The nidus demonstrates angiomatous change. In **(B)** a selective lateral MCA angiogram is performed through a flow-directed microcatheter. This pedicle was embolized with hitoacryl (NBCA). In **(C)** a selective lateral MCA angiogram is performed through another flow-directed microcatheter. This pedicle was also embolized with NBCA. In **(D)** a lateral internal carotid artery angiogram is pictured after embolization of these two pedicles. The patient suffered an intracranial hemorrhage shortly after the embolization despite rigorous blood pressure control and ICU monitoring. He tolerated the hemorrhage well and demonstrated no change in neurologic status. The angiomatous change in the AVM nidus did not tolerate flow alterations induced by embolization.

perfusion pressure. If neurologic deterioration requires intubation and sedation then intracranial pressure monitoring is mandatory. If not previously established, seizure prophylaxis should be instituted. Mean arterial pressure should be balanced with intracranial pressure measurements to maintain cerebral perfusion above 70 mm Hg.

Perforation in AVM vessels can be more problematic than perforation of a normal cerebral vessel. Absence of the muscular or elastic layers can prevent spontaneous closure. In these cases transvascular deployment of a coil can help close the defect. The coil can be deployed partially in the subarach-

noid space with the remainder in the vessel lumen. It may not always be necessary to occlude the vessel lumen completely, although subtotal occlusion may potentiate embolic phenomena in a delayed fashion. If the perforation occurs downstream of the catheter position, it may be necessary to completely occlude the feeding pedicle. Either Dacron-coated coils or liquid polymer adhesives can be used. In the latter case great care must be taken to avoid proximal reflux during injection.

Typically during glue injection distal flow carries the polymer away from the injection site. After a perforation flow is dramatically reduced in the pedicle. Forceful injection of glue can easily result in reflux and occlusion of eloquent vascular supply.

SURGICAL RESECTION OF AVM

Hemorrhage during or after surgical treatment of intracranial AVM remains the major cause of operative morbidity and mortality. Careful analysis of the many potential causes of hemorrhage in this setting is required in the effort of each surgeon to provide the best possible outcome. This section reviews the incidence of operative and postoperative hemorrhage, the causes and contributing factors, and the means of avoiding this complication.

Incidence

Overall, hemorrhage as a perioperative complication may occur in 3–22% of cases in reported series (18). A cautionary note is required in interpreting these reports. These series reflect the accumulated experience from centers with specialized interest and expertise in AVM. As a result, they experience a higher volume of cases. In addition, these centers also are exposed to AVMs that require greater technical and clinical skills to maintain low operative morbidity and mortality.

Intraoperative Hemorrhage

Intraoperative hemorrhage, interpreted as uncontrolled or excessive hemorrhage, is difficult to define and is therefore rarely reported in great detail. The resection of most AVMs of moderate to large size will at some point involve significant bleeding, which if not readily controlled greatly increases the difficulty of resection. Morgan's series of 112 patients reports intraoperative hemorrhage in 3 of 4 patients who died and in 1 of 24 patients described as having complicated cases, producing an overall incidence of 3.6% (19). Pasqualin's series report severe intraoperative hemorrhage in 21 of 248 patients (8%) (18).

Causes of intraoperative hemorrhage are usually not mysterious. Most often significant, readily apparent vessel injury has occurred. Injury usually involves the nidus or the venous side of the lesion and can occur during craniotomy and dural opening, initial dissection, removal of nidus, final hemostasis, or closure. The events that may lead to hemorrhage during each of the above stages of the procedure are reviewed below. An important early step to avoid and control potentially devastating hemorrhage at any stage is careful planning and placement of a bone flap that provides adequate exposure of the entire lesion. This should permit adequate control and visualization of arterial feeders, visualization of the nidus from as many angles as feasible, and exposure of the venous drainage. Although vessels are not routinely sacrificed at a distance from the nidus, inspection of vessels away from the nidus permits more accurate identification and assessment.

Injury During Exposure

Early hemorrhage, occurring during opening, usually involves the venous system. Simple maneuvers that usually obtain hemostasis, such as Surgicel tamponade of a small sinus rent or venous lake injury, often fail when arterialized blood under high pressure is encountered. Careful placement of burr holes and flaps to avoid parasagittal arterialized venous lakes, meticulous attention to dural dissection from the inner table of the skull prior to craniotomy, and careful placement of dural flaps, with sharp dissection of arachnoidal adhesions between dura and cortical vessels, particularly draining veins, all help to avoid early trouble. If encountered, early venous hemorrhage must be carefully assessed and controlled, without sacrifice or complete occlusion of the vessel.

Dissection

Beyond inadvertent vessel injury during exposure, the causes of intraoperative hemorrhage during resection of the lesion usually involve basic errors in judgment. These include sacrifice of a major draining vein prior to gaining control of all inflow to the lesion. An arterialized vein can be mistaken for a feeding artery. A loss of perspective often related to reliance on excessive magnification can result in dissection into the nidus. Retraction or compression of the nidus before adequate reduction in arterial inflow can result in perforation. In addition, inadequate hemostasis, particularly of fine deep vessels, can result in continued bleeding during resection. The technical aspects of surgical resection used when treating a large AVM are beyond the scope of this chapter. The surgeon must adhere to a controlled, methodical approach that includes adequate exposure, arterial isolation, circumferential nidus dissection, and, finally, venous dissection.

Hemostasis

In addition to the arterial feeders seen on preoperative angiography, AVMs may receive additional supply from fine networks of vessels contributing to the nidus. This is particularly true in the deeper portions of the lesion, usually extending from the ependymal surface. Difficulty in obtaining satisfactory results with bipolar cautery, fear of injury to normal deep vessels, and inadequate recognition of their contribution to the AVM may contribute to a tendency to pack and hide arterial inflow and/or hemorrhage from these small vessels. Additionally, a moderate-sized arterial feeder may piggy-back in along the deep draining vein and can be overlooked on preoperative angiography of a large AVM. Failure to adequately secure this vessel prior to division results in a deep source of hemorrhage that is potentially difficult to visualize.

Residual AVM

Hemorrhage from retained AVM is less frequent now that intraoperative angiography is readily available. No postoperative hemorrhages due to retained AVM have occurred in our recent consecutive series of 43 patients undergoing surgery for AVM since the routine utilization of intraoperative angiography. A single case of residual AVM occurred, in which intraoperative angiography could not be obtained for technical reasons, and the patient was returned to surgery within 24 hours for successful completion of surgery.

Late Hemorrhage

After apparent resection of the lesion, hemorrhage intraoperatively or postoperatively is usually related to one of three causes: residual AVM, inadequate hemostasis in the surgical bed, and ''remote'' hemorrhage into adjacent or distant brain parenchyma. The latter may be due in part to hemodynamic effects of rapid elimination of a large shunt. This latter condition has been termed normal perfusion pressure breakthrough (20) or, alternatively, relative hyperemia (21). Less common causes to consider include coagulopathy, inadequate blood pressure control, and venous infarction.

Remote Hemorrhage, Perfusion Pressure Breakthrough, and Reactive Hemorrhage

Uncontrolled hemorrhage and edema formation may occur after successful complete excision, without evidence of coagulopathy or other apparent reason. Observation of this complication, particularly after successful sudden obliteration of a large high-flow AVM, prompted Spetzler et al (20) to theorize that the sudden restoration of normal blood flow or perfusion pressure to vessels and parenchyma long hypoperfused was the cause of hemorrhage (normal perfusion pressure breakthrough, NPPB). This breakthrough theory is supported by several observations in our surgical and endovascular experience. The problem is usually seen only after obliteration of high-flow lesions. Embolization to reduce flow decreases the risk after surgical resection but embolization is accompanied by a risk of hemorrhage if flow is changed dramatically in one session. The largest lesions have the lowest feeding pedicle pressures prior to treatment. After particle embolization the pressure rises abruptly. Perfusion-related complications, termed hyperemic complications, may be seen in up to 21% of patients (22).

Some controversy exists concerning the exact pathophysiologic basis for reactive hyperemia or NPPB. Loss of effective autoregulation implies passive elevation in blood flow in response to pressure elevation. Work by Young et al clearly demonstrated a 20% increase in global cerebral blood flow after AVM resection but without any further increase with a pharmacologic pressure challenge (23). This implies that autoregulation remains intact in the vessels adjacent to the resected malformation. However, the sensitivity of the measurements do not completely exclude the possibility of pressure passive flow in some areas. Of note, in that series the two patients with complications (hemorrhage and uncontrolled edema) had the highest increases in blood flow noted. An alternative theory, attempting to move away from controversies about autoregulation, was proposed by Al-Rodhan et al (21). They define this problem as occlusive hyperemia, ie, as hemorrhage and/or edema resulting from a combination of arterial and venous stagnation or obstruction. There is agreement that blood flow is abnormal after resection, involves both arterial and venous circulations, is time-dependent, and that the abnormality is proportional to the preocclusive shunt through the lesion.

RADIOSURGERY FOR AVM

Radiation treatment has long been considered a treatment for AVM, although patients remain at risk for ICH from the AVM until the malformation is completely obliterated. Approximately 80% of the patients have complete angiographic obliteration within a latency interval of 2–3 years, at which point the risk of AVM hemorrhage is eliminated. Obliteration is not an instantaneous effect of radiosurgery, and patients have been known to have patent malformations for years following radiation treatment (24). The bleeding risk after irradiation and before obliteration have been reported to equal or slightly exceed that of the natural history of an untreated AVM (25). Unfortunately, some studies rely on magnetic resonance imaging (MRI) for their generating flow arrest endpoint (26). Radiation appears to have its greatest effect on vascular endothelium. At the cellular level, radiosurgery results in AVM obliteration via endothelial cell proliferation, progressive vessel wall thickening, and eventual lumen closure. Small blood vessel endothelia are more sensitive to radiation than those found in larger vessels. The vasovasorum in large vessels becomes occluded resulting in endarteritis obliterans. Subsequent hyaline thickening of the vessel wall leads to occlusion (27).

Until complete obliteration occurs, the risk of hemorrhage is not significantly reduced by radiation therapy. In considering the results of large series reporting radiation therapy for cerebral AVMs, the morbidity and mortality that results from hemorrhage during the latency period prior to AVM obliteration must be considered. Lundsford et al report ICH in 4% of their series (28). Two of these hemorrhages were fatal. Colombo et al (25) report five fatal hemorrhages in addition to two patients suffering permanent neurologic deficit from bleeding. The mortality rate was 2.7% with an overall complication rate of 3.3%. Steiner et al (24) reported 85 cases where the AVM was noted to be angiographically patent more than 2 years following treatment. Nine hemorrhages occurred yielding a calculated bleed rate of 6.5% per year. In Friedman's series 12 of 225 patients sustained a posttreatment hemorrhage after radiosurgery. There was no evidence to support a statistically significant departure from the natural hemorrhage rate at any time after radiosurgical treatment (26).

These results indicate that after radiosurgery of AVM the risk of bleeding remains unchanged over a period of approximately 2 years. At that time, if the malformation is completely obliterated angiographically, the risk of hemorrhage is zero. Prior to angiographic obliteration patients remain at risk of hemorrhage.

CONCLUSION

Treatment of cerebral AVMs is fraught with potential hemorrhagic complications. Periprocedural complications associated with embolization can be minimized with careful delivery of embolic agents and careful postoperative management. Surgical resection can result in perioperative hemorrhage unless meticulous microsurgical technique is utilized. Radiosurgery imparts protection from hemorrhage only after angiographic confirmation of obliteration of the lesion.

REFERENCES

1. Mullan S, Mojtahedi S, Johnson D, MacDonald RL. Embryological basis of some aspects of cerebral vascular fistulas and malformations. *J Neurosurg* 1996;85:1–8.
2. Mullan S, Mojtahedi S, Johnson D, MacDonald RL. Cerebral venous malformation–arteriovenous malformation transition forms. *J Neurosurg* 1996;86:9–13.
3. Ondra SL, Troupp H, George ED, Schwab K. The natural history of symptomatic arteriovenous malformations of the brain: a 24-year follow-up assessment. *J Neurosurg* 1990;73:387–391.
4. Gobin YP, Laurent A, Merienne L, et al. Treatment of brain arteriovenous malformations by embolization and radiosurgery. *J Neurosurg* 1996;85:19–28.
5. Personal communication, Complications Conference, July 1995, Jackson Hole, Wyoming.
6. Kader A, Goodrich JT, Sonstein WJ, Stein BM, Carmel PW, Michelsen WJ. Recurrent cerebral arteriovenous malformations after negative postoperative angiograms. *J Neurosurg* 1996;85:14–18.
7. Vinuela F, Nombela L, Roach M, Roach MR, Fox AJ, Pelz DM. Stenotic and occlusive disease of the venous drainage system of deep brain AVMs. *J Neurosurg* 1985;63:180–184.
8. Marks MP, Lane B, Steinberg GK, Chang Pj. Hemorrhage in intracerebral arteriovenous malformations: angiographic determinants. *Radiology* 1990;176:807–813.
9. Miyasaka, K, Wolpert SM, Prager RJ. The association of cerebral aneurysms, infundibula, and intracranial arteriovenous malformations. *Stroke* 1982;13(2):196–203.
10. Okamoto S, Handa H, Hashimoto N. Location of intracranial aneurysms associated with cerebral arteriovenous malformations: statistical analysis. *Surg Neurol* 1984;22:335–40.
11. Garcia-Monaco R, Rodesch G, Alvarez H Lizuka Y, Hui F, Lasjaunias P. Pseudoaneurysms within ruptured intracranial arteriovenous malformations: diagnosis and early endovascular management. *AJNR* 1993;14:315–321.
12. Lasjaunias P, Piske R, Terbrugge K, Willinsky R. Cerebral arteriovenous malformations (C.AVM) and associated arterial aneurysms (AA). *Acta Neurochir* 1988;91:29–36.
13. Kondziolka D, Nixon BJ, Lasjaunias P, Tucker W, TerBrugge, K, Spiegel SM. Cerebral arteriovenous malformations with associated arterial aneurysms: hemodynamic and therapeutic considerations. *Can J Neurol Sci* 1988;15:130–134.
14. Ahuja A Gibbons KJ, Guterman LR, Hopkins LN. Pedicle pressure changes in cerebral arteriovenous malformations during therapeutic embolization: relationship to delayed hemorrhage. *Stroke* 1993;24;1:185.
15. Wallace RC, Flom RA, Khayata MH, et al. The safety and effectiveness of brain arteriovenous malformation embolization using acrylic and particles: the experiences of a single institution. *Neurosurgery* 1995;37(4):606–618.
16. Halbach VV, Higashida RT, Dowd CF, Barnwell SL, Hieshima GB. Management of vascular perforations that occur during neurointerventional procedures. *AJNR* 1991;12:319–327.
17. Purdy PD, Batjer HH, Samson D. Management of hemorrhagic complications from preoperative embolization of arteriovenous malformations. *J Neurosurg* 1991;74:205–211.
18. Pasqualin A, Barone G, Cioffi F, Rosta Luisa, Scienze R, Da Pian R. The relevance of anatomic and hemodynamic factors to a classification of cerebral arteriovenous malformations. *Neurosurgery* 1991;28(3):370–379.
19. Morgan MK, Johnston IH, Hallinan JM, Weber NC. Complications of surgery for arteriovenous malformations of the brain. *J Neurosurg* 1993;78:176–182.
20. Spetzler RF, Wilson CB, Weinstein P, et al. Normal perfusion pressure breakthrough theory. *Clin Neurosurg* 1978;25:651–672.
21. Nayef R, Al-Rodhan F, Sundt TM, et al. Occlusive hyperemia: a theory for the hemodynamic complications following resection of intracerebral arteriovenous malformations. *J Neurosurg* 1993;78:167–175.
22. Batjer HH, Devous MD, Seibert GB, Purdy PD, Bonte FJ. Intracranial arteriovenous malformation: relationship between clinical factors and surgical complications. *Neurosurgery* 1989;24(1):75–79.
23. Young WL, Kader A, Prohovnik I, et al. Pressure autoregulation is intact after arteriovenous malformation resection. *Neurosurgery* 1993;32(4):491–497.
24. Steiner L, Lindquist C, Adler JR, Torner JC, Alves W, Steiner M. Clinical outcome of radiosurgery for cerebral arteriovenous malformations. *J Neurosurg* 1992;77:1–8.
25. Colombo F, Pozza F, Chierego G, Casentini L, De Luca G, Francescon P. Linear accelerator radiosurgery of cerebral arteriovenous malformations: an update. *Neurosurgery* 1994;34(1):14–21.
26. Friedman WA, Blatt DL, Bova FJ, Buatti JM, Mendenhall WM, Kubilis PS. The risk of hemorrhage after radiosurgery for arteriovenous malformations. *J Neurosurg* 1996;84:912–919.
27. Redekop JG, Elisevich KV, Gaspar LE, Wiese KP, Drake CG. Conventional radiation therapy of intracranial arteriovenous malformations: long-term results. *J Neurosurg* 1993;78:413–422.
28. Lunsford LD, Kondziolka D, Flickinger JC, et al. Stereotactic radiosurgery for arteriovenous malformations of the brain. *J Neurosurg* 1991;75:512–524.

Cerebrovascular Disease, edited by H. Hunt Batjer.
Lippincott-Raven Publishers, Philadelphia © 1997.

CHAPTER 71

Intracranial Aneurysm: Clinical Manifestations

Hector W. Ho, James P. Chander, and H. Hunt Batjer

EPIDEMIOLOGY

The prevalence of intracranial aneurysms is not entirely clear. Radiographic and autopsy studies suggest a figure of about 5% in the general population or about 10–15 million people in the United States (1–4). The incidence of aneurysmal subarachnoid hemorrhage is 6–16 per 100,000 population per year with an annual prevalence estimated to be 30,000 persons per year (5). Patients who sustain an aneurysmal subarachnoid hemorrhage have a poor prognosis with a mortality rate of 25% and a significant morbidity rate of 50% (5). Current statistics reveal that aneurysmal rupture accounts for approximately 0.4–0.6% of all deaths (6). In a review article examining the impact of unruptured intracranial aneurysms on the public health in the United States, Wiebers et al found that despite an overall decrease in stroke rate, the incidence of aneurysmal subarachnoid hemorrhage remains the same (7). This report estimated that $522,500,000 and $1,755,600,000 are spent each year in the United States for care of patients with unruptured and ruptured aneurysms, respectively.

Most reviews indicate a clear female preponderance for ruptured intracranial aneurysms ranging from 54% to 61% (8). They rarely occur in more than one family member; however, an inheritance factor has been suggested (9). When aneurysms are presented in more than one family member, a known hereditary syndrome is often present. In particular, patients with autosomal dominant polycystic kidney disease, Ehlers–Danlos syndrome, pseudoxanthoma elasticum, and coarctation of the aorta are at significantly increased risk of aneurysm formation (10).

Approximately 20–30% of patients will have multiple aneurysms (11–14). They tend to occur more often in females. In Suzuki's series of 1080 cases, multiple aneurysms were present in 15% of the cases (15). He reviewed 6 autopsy

studies totaling 1404 cases in which multiple aneurysms were present in 23.5% cases (range 18.9–50%). In his review of 7 clinical series involving 10,795 patients, the incidence of multiple aneurysms was 14.1% with a range of 7.7–29.8%. In the Cooperative Study (Sahs et al), the autopsy rate was 22.1% whereas that determined angiographically was 18.6% (16). In Suzuki's study, two aneurysms were present in 77% of cases, 3 aneurysms in 15% of cases, and 4 or more aneurysms in 8% of cases. This same study determined that 47% of multiple aneurysms are on opposite sides, 21% are on the same side, 29% have one in the midline and one on the side, and 3% have both in the midline (15). There is a 3–5% chance in finding a posterior circulation aneurysm in association with an anterior circulation aneurysm. When multiple internal carotid or middle cerebral artery aneurysms exist, there is a greater tendency for the aneurysms to occur symmetrically as opposed to on the same vessel.

NATURAL HISTORY

For the asymptomatic unruptured aneurysm, the risk of rupture is estimated to be 1.0–1.4% per year (17,18). The cumulative rate of rupture is 10% at 10 years, 26% at 20 years, and 32% at 30 years (18). The size of the aneurysm has been implicated as a risk factor for rupture. Wieber's review of saccular aneurysms revealed that aneurysms >10 mm in diameter had a higher risk of rupture at 5.9% per year (19). Juvela et al reported the risk of rupture to be inversely associated with age (18). Intracranial aneurysmal rupture is extremely uncommon in the first decade of life. The incidence increases with each passing decade, reaching its peak in the sixth decade. According to Pakarinen's review of the literature (15 series, 5679 patients), the incidence in the first decade is <10%, second 2%, third 6%, fourth 15%, sixth 28%, seventh 16%, and eighth 6% (6). Death from subarachnoid hemorrhage not uncommonly occurs between 40 and 60 years of age.

Numerous reports have documented aneurysmal growth,

H. W. Ho, J. P. Chander and H. H. Batjer: Division of Neurological Surgery, Northwestern University Medical School, Chicago, IL 60611

but growth rates have been found to vary considerably during follow-up periods (18,20,21). Aneurysmal thrombosis has been related to both the geometry of the neck and fundus as well as to turbulent flow resulting from distortion of the vessel intimal surface (22,23). The incidence of spontaneous aneurysmal thrombosis varies considerably. Schunk has reported a greater tendency toward partial thrombosis in larger aneurysms (24). Thrombosed aneurysms may be a source of emboli and subsequent transient ischemic attacks (25–27). The risk factors for subarachnoid hemorrhage and the natural history of ruptured intracranial aneurysms are discussed in the next chapter.

PATHOLOGY

Pathogenesis

Aneurysms most likely arise from a complex multifactorial set of circumstances involving both a congenital predisposition as well as local environmental factors that weaken the arterial wall and ultimately lead to aneurysm formation (28). Evidence supporting genetic factors in the pathogenesis of aneurysms includes reports of familial cases of intracranial aneurysms and the high incidence of aneurysms in pathologic disorders such as polycystic kidney disease and type III collagen deficiency (29–31). Supporting an acquired component of aneurysm formation are the observations that the incidence of intracranial aneurysm is age-dependent (32), de novo development and growth of aneurysms occur particularly after unilateral carotid occlusion (33,34), and the typical location is at points of bifurcation where hemodynamic stress is the greatest. Crawford and later Sekhar made key observations on the pathogenesis of intracranial aneurysms (35,36). Histologic and pathologic features of the aneurysms described by these authors include degenerative changes, thinning of the media (muscular layer), inflammatory changes, atherosclerosis, location at points of hypertensive and hemodynamic stress, and presence of medial and elastic defects of the aneurysmal wall.

Associated Conditions

Although the pathogenic basis of the association between some medical conditions and intracranial aneurysms is not well established, the features described above provide a plausible explanation for many of these conditions. Table 1 outlines medical conditions associated with various types of aneurysms. It is estimated that about 10% of patients with polycystic kidney disease will have an aneurysmal subarachnoid hemorrhage whereas the overall prevalence of ruptured and unruptured aneurysms occurring in these patients may be as high as 40% (29). Polycystic kidney disease is an autosomal dominant disease characterized by abnormalities in arterial walls as well as hypertension. Fibromuscular dysplasia is a vasculopathic condition with presumed associated congenital defects in the media and internal elastic mem-

TABLE 1. *Configuration and etiologies of intracranial aneurysms*

I. Saccular
  A. Hemodynamic
    1. Variable pulsatile pressure at bifurcation points
    2. Increased flow (AVMs, absent or hypoplastic contralateral vessel)
    3. Coarctation of the aorta
      Polycystic kidney disease (autosomal dominant)
      Fibromuscular dysplasia
  B. Structural: media and elastic defects
  C. Genetic
    1. Familial inheritance
    2. Syndromes: Ehlers'–Danlos syndrome, Marfan's syndrome, Type III collagen deficiency, pseudoxanthoma elasticum, Rendu–Osler–Weber syndrome, Klippel–Trenauny–Weber syndrome
  D. Infections: bacterial, fungal
  E. Traumatic
  F. Neoplastic
  G. Miscellaneous conditions: moyamoya disease, systemic lupus erythematous, sickle cell disease, radiation
II. Fusiform
  A. Atherosclerosis
  B. Trauma
  C. Infection
  D. Neoplasia
  E. Hemodynamic
  F. Fibromuscular dysplasia
  G. Radiation
III. Dissecting-Trauma
IV. False-Trauma

brane. The reported incidence of intracranial aneurysm associated with fibromuscular dysplasia is approximately 21% (37). Conditions that result in hemodynamic stress of intracranial arteries may lead to aneurysm formation. Some of these conditions include arteriovenous malformations (AVMs) (38), moyamoya disease (39), coarctation of the aorta (40), and unilateral carotid agenesis or occlusion (41). Connective tissue disorders such as Ehlers–Danlos syndrome, Marfan's syndrome, and pseudoxanthoma elasticum are also associated with a higher incidence of developing intracranial aneurysms (42).

Injury to the wall of cerebral vessels by any mechanism can potentially lead to development of intracranial aneurysms. Conditions included in this category are trauma, infection, and neoplastic growth (43). Aneurysms caused by these factors generally occur at a more distal site of the vessel rather than the basal vessels near the circle of Willis. Exceptions to this generalization are internal carotid artery aneurysms resulting form trauma to the skull base.

Classification

In a recent review by Meyer et al, a reasonable classification scheme for intracranial aneurysms is presented (44). All aneurysms have four classifying characteristics that may ultimately determine management strategy. These characteristics include (a) etiology, (b) size, (c) location, and (d) configuration.

Etiology

The causes of intracranial aneurysms have been reviewed under the heading of pathogenesis. They can be classified as idiopathic, associated with a specific medical condition, or secondary to vessel injury (Table 1).

Size

An aneurysm's size is determined by measuring the largest diameter of the dome. Sundt (45) categorizes them as follows: saccular is <15 mm; globular is 15–25 mm; giant is >25 mm (Table 2). Others have categorized them as small (<10 mm), large (10–24 mm), and giant (>25 mm). Although unruptured intracranial aneurysms tend to be smaller than ruptured aneurysms, and asymptomatic aneurysms smaller than those that are symptomatic, no pathologic studies have yet been able to correlate these findings. This may be due to the inherent methodologic flaws related to the change in size after rupture and fixation artifact (46).

Location

As mentioned previously, aneurysms are usually located at bifurcation points of large arteries where hemodynamic stress is the greatest. Various clinical and autopsy studies have provided us with information on intracranial aneurysm location by artery (32,47,48). The frequency distribution of aneurysms is illustrated in Table 2. In general, approximately 90–95% of all aneurysms arise from the carotid system whereas the other 5–10% arise from the vertebrobasilar system. In a report of the Cooperative Aneurysm Study (49), 41% of the patients had aneurysms in the internal carotid artery, 34% in the anterior communicating or anterior cerebral artery, 20% in the middle cerebral artery, 4% in the vertebrobasilar circulation, and 1% in other sites. In a review of 2873 cerebral aneurysms, Fox found that 36% were located at the midline, 33% on the right side, and 32% on the left side (50).

Configuration

Intracranial aneurysms can be categorized according to shape as saccular, fusiform, dissecting, or false (Table 1). Saccular aneurysms are the most common and are described as having a defined neck and dome. They are probably acquired by hemodynamically induced degeneration of the arterial wall. Fusiform aneurysms are diffuse dilatations of the cerebral vessels with no definable neck. These are often associated with atherosclerotic disease and occasionally with trauma, infection (mycotic), and neoplasia. Dissecting aneurysms are fusiform dilatations of a parent artery usually due to trauma. These occur more often in the extracranial segments of the internal carotid and vertebral arteries and more often in the posterior circulation than the anterior circulation. Patients with dissecting aneurysms frequently present with evidence of cerebral ischemia; however, occasionally they will experience a hemorrhagic event. False aneurysms or pseudoaneurysms are characterized by the absence of vessel wall components in their dome. The new wall typically consists of surrounding blood clot, reactive connective tissue, or other cerebral structures. As one can imagine, these aneurysms are very tenuous and difficult to reconstruct. False aneurysms are often a result of trauma.

CLINICAL FEATURES OF ANEURYSMS IN A SPECIFIC LOCATION

Clinical manifestations associated with intracranial aneurysms are mainly attributed to the subarachnoid hemorrhage that occurs after rupture. In general, these signs and symptoms can be categorized into five groups based on its mechanism of development. The possible mechanisms are (a) meningeal irritation; (b) compression by aneurysm; (c) increased intracranial pressure secondary to edema or hydrocephalus; (d) focal cerebral injury; and (e) other causes (51). The clinical signs and symptoms produced by meningeal irritation may present as mild and early warning leak headaches to severe excruciating headaches. In addition, meningeal irritation may produce nuchal rigidity, nausea, and vomiting. With the exception of third nerve palsy, most other compressive syndromes such as visual field defects, brainstem compression signs, and other cranial nerve deficits are due to giant aneurysms. Cerebral edema and hydrocephalus lead to signs of increased intracranial pressure. Headache,

TABLE 2. *Classification of intracranial aneurysms*

I. Sizes
  A. Sundt
    1. Saccular—<15 mm
    2. Globular—15–25 mm
    3. Giant—>25 mm
  B. Others
    1. Small—<10 mm
    2. Large—10–24 mm
    3. Giant—≥25 mm
II. Location

	Series (percentages)			
Vessel	Sahs (32)	Stehbens (10) (autopsy)	Stehbens (10) (clinical)	Kassell (47)
Internal carotid	41	24	38	30
Anterior cerebral	34	30	31	39
Middle cerebral	20	33	20	22
Vertebrobasilar	4	12	5	8

nausea and vomiting, papilledema, third and sixth nerve palsies, and depressed or altered mental status are key features of increased pressure. Focal signs such as weakness, aphasia, visual field deficits may result from vasospasm, localized hematoma, or thrombosis and embolism. Other less specific signs and symptoms that may be associated with intracranial aneurysms include seizures; syndrome of inappropriate antidiuretic hormone secretion; pituitary insufficiency; increased body temperature, heart rate, blood pressure, white blood count, sedimentation rate, and blood glucose; and electrocardiogram changes. This section will briefly describe the common clinical features of aneurysms at specific locations. Clinical features related to subarachnoid hemorrhage will be discussed in the next chapter.

Internal Carotid Artery Aneurysms

Aneurysms arising from the petrous portion of the carotid artery are very rare. These aneurysms are usually caused by trauma or infection, although they may develop spontaneously or through an atherosclerotic process. Often, petrous aneurysms are large by the time they are detected and come to the attention of the otorhinolaryngologist due to earache, hearing loss, and subjective bruit. In addition, patients with aneurysms in this location may also have vertigo and dizziness, facial weakness, and pulsatile tinnitus due to the close proximity to cranial nerves, especially VII and VIII (52). On examination through an otoscope, a retrotympanic mass may be seen and the examiner must be astute and not attempt to biopsy these lesions. Rupture of these aneurysms may lead to massive bleeding from the ear and/or nose in these patients.

Intracavernous carotid artery aneurysms account for approximately 3–5% of all cerebral aneurysms (53). In Yasargil's series of 13 patients with cavernous internal carotid artery aneurysms, 9 patients complained of ipsilateral retroorbital pain and 11 had cranial nerve deficits (54). Slow enlargement of unruptured intracavernous aneurysms may result in compression of the oculomotor, trochlear, and abducens nerves leading to extraocular palsies and diplopia. In addition, the ophthalmic and maxillary divisions of the trigeminal nerve may be compressed producing ocular and upper facial pain. Although rare, further upward extension of an unruptured aneurysm may lead to compression of the optic nerve and chiasm giving the patient a visual field deficit or blindness. Lateral extension of the mass to involve the superior orbital fissure can cause proptosis or exophthalmos. The rupture of an intracavernous carotid aneurysm classically produces ophthalmoplegia and sudden onset of retroorbital pain. A carotid-cavernous fistula usually develops after rupture leading to scleral injection, pulsatile exophthalmos, periorbital bruit, and blindness. Less frequently, subarachnoid hemorrhage, stroke, or massive epistaxis may occur after rupture of these lesions.

Paraclinoidal aneurysms represent approximately 2–8%

of all intracranial aneurysmal cases (54–56). Aneurysms located in this region have a higher association with multiplicity and are commonly large or giant in size. These aneurysms tend to occur in younger patients and more frequently in females. In Yasargil's series, the mean age for these patients was 44 and 91% were female (54). Like other intracranial aneurysms, these paraclinoidal aneurysms most frequently present with subarachnoid hemorrhage. Either through direct compression by aneurysmal enlargement or by rupture of the aneurysm, patients with these aneurysms often present with visual complaints such as central scotomas, hemianopsias, or distortion of color (57,58). On examination, optic atrophy, papilledema, decrease in visual acuity, and an afferent pupillary defect may be seen.

Aneurysms arising near or just distal to the origin of the posterior communicating artery make up approximately 50% of all internal carotid artery aneurysms and 25% of all intracranial aneurysms (54,59–61). Beside the signs and symptoms arising from subarachnoid hemorrhage, the most common presentation for these patients is a third cranial nerve palsy with ptosis, dilated pupil or mydriasis, and down- and out-deviation of the ipsilateral eye. These manifestations usually present themselves early in the course of the aneurysmal expansion, thus explaining the low incidence of giant aneurysms in this region. Hypothalamic dysfunction, ipsilateral orbital pain, hemiparesis, and seizures have also been reported but these features have minimal localizing value.

Anterior choroidal artery aneurysms account for approximately 5–10% of all internal carotid artery aneurysms and 2% of all intracranial aneurysms (54,61). Most of these patients have sustained a subarachnoid hemorrhage on presentation. Manifestations reported for these aneurysms include signs and symptoms similar to those of posterior communicating aneurysms (62), hemiparesis (54), Abbie's syndrome consisting of contralateral sensory and motor deficits with homonymous hemianopsia (63), and retroorbital pain (64).

Aneurysms arising from the internal carotid artery bifurcation make up approximately 10–15% of internal carotid artery aneurysms and 3–7% of all intracranial aneurysms (54). In one series >80% of patients with aneurysms at this location were <30 years of age (54). In addition to the signs of subarachnoid hemorrhage, some of these patients present with a syndrome suggestive of a basal ganglia hemorrhage. This is due to the proximity of aneurysmal dome to the orbital basal portion of the frontal lobe. Rupture in this region can produce hematomas deep into the brain parenchyma leading to hemiparesis and seizures.

Middle Cerebral Artery Aneurysms

Middle cerebral artery aneurysms represent approximately 15–20% of all cerebral aneurysms (60,65). These aneurysms most commonly arise in the Sylvian fissure at the bifurcation of the M1 segment of the middle cerebral artery. The most common presentation for patients with aneurysms at this location is subarachnoid hemorrhage with its associated headache (66).

Unruptured middle cerebral artery aneurysms may result in symptoms due to mass effect or emboli. As the aneurysms enlarge, compression of the frontal and temporal lobe may lead to contralateral hemiparesis and seizures, respectively. Transient ischemic attacks or infarction, although uncommon, may occur as emboli are dislodged from a more proximal intraluminal thrombus in these unruptured aneurysms (56).

Upon rupture of a middle cerebral artery aneurysm, approximately 60% of the patients experience a loss of consciousness (67). Other clinical features of ruptured middle cerebral artery aneurysms include contralateral hemiparesis and sensory deficits, aphasia when the dominant hemisphere is affected, contralateral visual field defect, and seizures. When hemiparesis is involved, the arm is usually affected more than the leg. Of all aneurysms at various sites, middle cerebral artery aneurysms are most commonly associated with development of seizures, especially when associated with an intracerebral hematoma (68). Intracerebral hematomas in the frontal, temporal, or parietal lobes have been reported to be as high as 50% of middle cerebral artery aneurysm ruptures (52). Most often, these hematomas are located in the temporal lobe. On the computed tomographic (CT) scan, unilateral sylvian fissure hemorrhage associated with extension of hematoma into the frontal and temporal lobes is almost pathognomonic for a middle cerebral artery aneurysm rupture.

Anterior Communicating Artery Aneurysms

Aneurysms located in the anterior communicating artery represent approximately 30–37% of all intracranial aneurysms making this location the most common site for aneurysmal subarachnoid hemorrhage (55,69). In Yasargil's series, aneurysms at this location were found more frequently in men (62%) than women (38%) (69). Patients with these lesions most commonly present with subarachnoid hemorrhage with accompanying headache. Although the headaches are usually non-localizing, sometimes they can present as headaches that are bifrontal or retroorbital.

As with aneurysms at other locations, many of the clinical features related to anterior communicating artery aneurysms may be explained by their relationship to surrounding anatomic structures. Unruptured large anterior communicating artery aneurysms may compress the frontal lobe leading to abulia, personality changes, and dementia. Compression of the optic nerve and chiasm may lead to visual symptoms. Slow progressive visual loss with or without field cuts may be an indicator of an unruptured expanding aneurysm at this location.

Hypothalamic-pituitary-adrenal dysfunction may occur as a result of rupture of these aneurysms upward into the third ventricle and hypothalamus (70). Pituitary insufficiency, especially diabetes insipidus, is commonly seen when endocrinologic disturbances occur. Amnesic syndromes have also been described and Yasargil postulated that perforators originating from the anterior communicating artery may have been disrupted leading to infarctions in structures such as fornix and anterior commissure (71). Medial hemispheric involvement through injury to the pericallosal and callosomarginal arteries may lead to hemiparesis with the leg affected more than the arm. In addition, disturbances of micturition and defecation have been associated with anterior communicating artery aneurysms (72).

Rupture of anterior communicating artery aneurysms is frequently associated with frontal lobe hematomas and 53–79% of these bleeds are associated with intraventricular hemorrhage (70). Mechanisms of intraventricular hemorrhage include dissection of blood through the medial frontal lobe, corpus callosum, and lamina terminalis. Approximately 25% of the patients with intraventricular hemorrhage will develop hydrocephalus. In severe rupture, blurred vision and even blindness may result from retinal, subhyaloid, and vitreous hemorrhages (73).

Distal Anterior Cerebral Artery Aneurysms

Aneurysms located in the distal anterior cerebral artery compose 2–4% of all intracranial aneurysms (74). Most of these aneurysms arise near the genus of the corpus callosum at the bifurcation between the pericallosal and callosomarginal arteries. Less commonly, the aneurysm may originate near or at the frontopolar artery origin. Unruptured anterior cerebral artery aneurysms when thrombosed can present with embolic transient ischemic attacks. Frontal lobe and optic nerve compression by an enlarging aneurysm in the distal anterior cerebral artery may lead to mental deterioration or visual loss, respectively (75). Ruptured aneurysms located at or near the frontoorbital artery origin may have similar clinical findings to those patients who have anterior communicating artery aneurysms. Frequently, more distal anterior cerebral artery aneurysm rupture produces pyramidal tract signs with lower extremity monoparesis as well as transient incontinence or diarrhea due to medial superior frontal lobe and paracentral lobule dysfunction (76). Although the lower extremity weakness is usually contralateral to the vessel involved, bilateral or even ipsilateral weakness may result due to vasospasm or clot formation more proximally. Intracerebral hemorrhage in the interhemispheric fissure may be seen on CT scans and is helpful in raising the suspicion for a distal anterior cerebral artery aneurysmal rupture. These aneurysms are often associated with other cerebrovascular lesions.

Basilar Artery Aneurysms

Aneurysms of the posterior circulation make up approximately 5–10% of all intracranial aneurysms (70,77,78). This includes both the basilar and vertebral arteries and their branches. Upper basilar aneurysms at the bifurcation lie in the interpeduncular fossa of the midbrain near all perforating vessels in this region. Because of this anatomic relationship, symptoms are related to injuries to the midbrain, pons, lower thalamus, and hypothalamus. Compression of corticobulbar and corticospinal tracts by an enlarging aneurysm of the basilar artery can lead to dysphagia, hoarseness, and hemi- or quadriparesis (70). Ocular signs secondary to basilar aneurysm compression include ptosis, diplopia, mydriasis, internuclear ophthalmoplegia, and gaze palsies. Commonly seen after basilar artery aneurysmal rupture are occipital headaches, impaired level of consciousness, hemiparesis, and cranial nerve palsies (79). Profound alteration of consciousness in about 50% of the cases has been reported by Duvoisin and Yahr (80). In addition, oculomotor and abducens nerve palsies with ocular bobbing may be a presentation with basilar bifurcation aneurysm rupture. This reflects the involvement of the midbrain and pons. In 25–40% of basilar artery bifurcation aneurysm ruptures, intraventricular hemorrhage into the third ventricle has been reported (79).

Aneurysms at the lower basilar trunk may lead to the anterior inferior cerebellar artery syndrome, which will be described in the section below. Other pontine syndromes that have been reported to occur after lower basilar artery trunk aneurysm rupture include Millard–Gubler syndrome, Foville's syndrome, Grenet's syndrome, and syndrome of Marie–Foix (81).

Posterior Cerebral Artery Aneurysms

Aneurysms of the posterior cerebral artery accounts for 0.8–1.3% of all intracranial aneurysms (82,83). Compression of the parietal, temporal, or occipital lobes from an unruptured expanding aneurysm in this region can lead to a presentation of memory loss, seizures, hemianopsia, and hemiplegia. Rupture of these aneurysms can result in a spectrum from a Weber's syndrome to a severely debilitating brainstem syndrome with deep coma. Severe ischemia to the territory of the distal posterior cerebral artery may lead to occipital lobe and thalamic infarctions. Homonymous hemianopsia and the syndrome of Dejerine–Roussy may result from these infarctions. The thalamic syndrome named above may include contralateral hemiparesis, impairment or loss of superficial and deep sensation, spontaneous burning pain and dysesthesias, choreoathetoid movements, ataxia, and tremor (66). Approximately 25% of posterior cerebral artery aneurysms are either giant or fusiform (83).

Superior Cerebellar Artery Aneurysms

Aneurysms of the superior cerebellar artery are uncommon. When they occur, they frequently arise at the junction between the basilar artery and the superior cerebellar artery projecting laterally and posteriorly. Superior cerebellar ar-

tery aneurysms often nestle into the cerebral peduncles and in close contact with the oculomotor nerve. Compression by enlargement of the aneurysm may lead to Weber's syndrome consisting of ipsilateral oculomotor nerve palsy coupled with contralateral hemiparesis. Ipsilateral cerebellar signs and Horner's syndrome with contralateral loss of sensation may also be present in these patients. Rupture of the aneurysm at this site can lead to a comatose state with decorticate or decerebrate posturing (56).

Anterior Inferior Cerebellar Artery Aneurysms

Aneurysms located in the anterior inferior cerebellar artery are uncommon and in older literature may have been termed ''internal auditory artery aneurysms.'' Branches off this artery help supply the pons and pontomedullary junction. Aneurysms of the anterior inferior cerebellar artery are often in the cerebellopontine angle and thus symptoms arising from this aneurysm often affect the facial and vestibulocochlear nerve. Ipsilateral facial weakness, tinnitus, vertigo, and hearing loss are hallmarks of anterior inferior cerebellar artery aneurysms (84–86). Other clinical signs include loss of taste in the anterior two thirds of the tongue, nausea and vomiting, horizontal nystagmus, and a weak corneal reflex. Many of these signs may be secondary to compression by the aneurysm before they rupture.

Vertebral and Posterior Inferior Cerebellar Artery Aneurysms

Vertebral artery aneurysms are relatively uncommon. They arise at points of bifurcation such as the vertebral/posterior inferior cerebellar artery (PICA) or vertebral/basilar artery junction. These points of bifurcation are in proximity to the lower medulla oblongata and pontomedullary junction, respectively. Vertebral/basilar junction aneurysms produce symptoms similar to those of anterior inferior cerebellar artery aneurysms. They include VIth, VIIth, and VIIIth cranial nerve palsies with horizontal nystagmus, facial weakness, vertigo, and sometimes ipsilateral hemiataxia and contralateral hemiparesis (56).

Vertebral/PICA aneurysms represent about 1% of all intracranial aneurysms (87). Because of the variability in which the PICA may arise, any of the lower cranial nerves may be affected. Often these aneurysms have an intimate relationship with the vagal and hypoglossal nerves. Occipital headaches that are exacerbated by recumbency are frequent complaints in patients with large PICA aneurysms (67). Medullary compression by the PICA aneurysm may cause hoarseness, dysphagia, ataxia, and hemiparesis. Infarction of the territory supplied by the distal PICA can lead to lateral medullary syndrome (Wallenberg's syndrome). The characteristics of this syndrome include ipsilateral hemiataxia, facial pain and dysesthesia, Horner's syndrome, dysphagia and hoarseness, contralateral hemisensory loss of pain and temperature, and vertigo.

Radiographically, the CT scan alone may suggest a PICA aneurysm rupture when the hemorrhage is concentrated in the cisterna magna around the lower brainstem and in the fourth ventricle. In addition, blood is often minimal or absent in the cisterns of the circle of Willis.

CONCLUSION

These malignant lesions may result in the complete spectrum of neurologic states from the completely awake and normal patient to the deeply comatose. Although certain syndromes are reasonably common with aneurysms in specific sites, a high index of suspicion must be exercised by the clinician. It is known that many aneurysm patients present initially with mild heralding symptoms. Modern neuroimaging techniques must be used aggressively to screen these individuals to rule out this life-threatening condition.

REFERENCES

1. Atkinson JLD, Sundt TM, Houser OW, Whisnant JP. Angiographic frequency of anterior circulation intracranial aneurysms. *J Neurosurg* 1989;70:551–555.
2. Inagawa T, Hirano A. Autopsy study of unruptured incidental intracranial aneurysms. *Surg Neurol* 1990;34:361–365.
3. McCormick WF, Acosta-Rua GJ. The size of intracranial saccular aneurysms: an autopsy study. *J Neurosurg* 1970;33:422–427.
4. Nakagawa T, Hashi K. The incidence and treatment of asymptomatic, unruptured cerebral aneurysms. *J Neurosurg* 1994;80:217–223.
5. Mayberg MR, Batjer HH, Dacey R, Diringer M, Haley EC, Heros RC, Sternau LL, Torner J, Adams HP Jr, Feinberg W, Thies W. Guidelines for the management of aneurysmal subarachnoid hemorrhage. *Circulation* 1994;90:2592–2605.
6. Pakarinen S. Incidence, etiology, and prognosis of primary subarachnoid hemorrhage: a study based on 589 cases diagnosed in a defined population during a defined urban period. *Acta Neurol Scand* 1967; 43(Suppl 29):1–28.
7. Wiebers DO, Torner JC, Messner I. Impact of unruptured intracranial aneurysms on the public health in the United States. *Stroke* 1992;23: 1416–1419.
8. Weir BK: Intracranial aneurysms and subarachnoid hemorrhage: an overview, In: Wilkins RH, Rengarchy SS, eds. *Neurosurgery*. New York: McGraw-Hill, 1985:1308–1329.
9. Sakai N, Sakata K, Yamanda H, Aiba T, Takeda F. Familial occurrence of intracranial aneurysms. *Surg Neurol* 1974;2:25.
10. Stebhens WE. Etiology of intracranial berry aneurysms. *J Neurosurg* 1989;70:823–831.
11. Inagawa T. Multiple intracranial aneurysms in elderly patients. *Acta Neurochir* 1990;106:119–126.
12. McCormick WF, Schmalstieg EJ. The relationship of arterial hypertension to intracranial aneurysms. *Arch Neurol* 1977;34:285–287.
13. Nehls DG, Flom RA, Carter LP, Spetzler RF. Multiple intracranial aneurysms: determining the site of rupture. *J Neurosurg* 1985;63: 342–348.
14. Ostergaard JR, Hog E. Incidence of multiple intracranial aneurysms: influence of arterial hypertension and gender. *J Neurosurg* 1985;63: 49–55.
15. Suzuki J. Multiple aneurysms: treatment. In: Pia HW, Langmaid C, Zierski J, eds. *Cerebral Aneurysms: Advances in Diagnosis and Therapy*. Berlin: Springer-Verlag, 1979;352–363.
16. Sahs AL, Perret GE, Locksley HB, Nishioka H, eds. Intracranial aneurysms and subarachnoid hemorrhage: a cooperative study. Philadelphia: JB Lippincott, 1969.
17. Jane JA, Kassell NF, Torner JC, Winn HR. The natural history of aneurysms and arteriovenous malformations. *J Neurosurg* 1985;62: 321–323.
18. Juvela S, Porras M, Heiskanen O. Natural history of unruptured intracranial aneurysms: a long-term follow-up study. *J Neurosurg* 1993;79: 174–182.
19. Wiebers DO, Whisnant JP, Sundt TM Jr, O'Fallon WM. The significance of unruptured intracranial saccular aneurysms. *J Neurosurg* 1987; 66:23–29.
20. Allcock JM, Canham PB. Angiographic study of the growth of intracranial aneurysms. *J Neurosurg* 1976;45:617-621.
21. Sarwar M, Batnitzky S, Schechter MM, Liebeskind A, Zimmer AE. Growing intracranial aneurysms. *Radiology* 1976;120:603–607.
22. Black SPW, German WJ. Observation of the relationship between the volume and the size of the orifices of experimental aneurysms. *J Neurosurg* 1960;17:984–990.
23. Roach MR. Blood flow and thrombosis, particularly in aneurysms. In: Deutsch E, Brinkhous KM, Lechner K, Hinnom S, eds. *Thrombosis: Pathogenesis and Clinical Trials*. New York: Thieme and Springer Verlag 1974:123–138.
24. Schunk H. Spontaneous thrombosis of intracranial aneurysms. *AJR* 1964;91:1327–1338.
25. Antunes JL, Correll JW. Cerebral emboli from intracranial aneurysms. *Surg Neurol* 1976;6:7–10.
26. Fukuoka S, Suematsu K, Nakamura J, Matsuzaki T, Satoh S, Hashimoto I. Transient ischemic attacks caused by unruptured intracranial aneurysms. *Surg Neurol* 1982;17:464–467.
27. Stewart RM, Samson D, Diehl J, Hinton R, Ditmore QM. Unruptured cerebral aneurysms presenting as recurrent transient neurologic deficits. *Neurology* 1980;30:47–51.
28. Batjer HH. Intracranial aneurysm. In: Rengachary SS, Wilkins RH, eds. *Principles of Neurosurgery*. St. Louis: Mosby–Wolfe, 1994; chapter 11.
29. Fehlings MG, Gentili F. The association between polycystic kidney disease and cerebral aneurysms. *Can J Neurol Sci* 1991;18:505–509.
30. Lozano AM, Leblanc R. Familial intracranial aneurysms. *J Neurosurg* 1987;66:522–528.
31. Neil-Dwyer G, Bartlett JR, Nicholls AC, Narcisi P, Pope FM. Collagen deficiency and ruptured cerebral aneurysms: a clinical and biochemical study. *J Neurosurg* 1983;59:16–20.
32. Sahs AL. Observation on the pathology of saccular aneurysms. In: Sahs AL, ed. *Intracranial Aneurysms and Subarachnoid Hemorrhage: A Cooperative Study*. Philadelphia: JB Lippincott, 1969;22–36.
33. Rinne JK, Hernesniemi JA. De novo aneurysms: special multiple intracranial aneurysms. *Neurosurgery* 1993;33:981–985.
34. Somach FM, Shenkin HA. Angiographic end results of carotid ligation in the treatment of carotid aneurysm. *J Neurosurg* 1966;24:966–974.
35. Crawford T. Some observations on the pathogenesis and natural history of intracranial aneurysms. *J Neurol Neurosurg Psychiatry* 1959;22: 259–266.
36. Sekhar LN, Heros RC. Origin, growth, and rupture of saccular aneurysms: a review. *Neurosurgery* 1981;8:248–260.
37. Mettinger KL. Fibromuscular dysplasia and the brain. II. Current concept of the disease. *Stroke* 1982;13:53–58.
38. Crawford PM, West CR, Chadwick DW, Shaw MD. AVM of the brain: natural history in unoperated patients. *J Neurol Neurosurg Psychiatry* 1986;49:1–10.
39. Kodama N, Suzuki J. Moyamoya disease associated with aneurysm. *J Neurosurg* 1978;48:565–569.
40. Bigelow NH. The association of polycystic kidney disease with intracranial aneurysms and other related disorders. *Am J Med Sci* 1953;225: 485–494.
41. Kunishio K, Yamamoto Y, Sunami N, Asari S. Agenesis of the left internal carotid artery, common carotid artery, and main trunk of the external carotid artery associated with multiple cerebral aneurysms. *Surg Neurol* 1987;27:177–181.
42. Weir B. Medical, neurologic, and ophthalmologic aspects of aneurysms. In: Weir B, ed. *Aneurysms Affecting the Nervous System*. Baltimore: Williams and Wilkins, 1987;54–133.
43. Weir B. Special aneurysms (nonsaccular and saccular). In: Weir B, ed. *Aneurysms Affecting the Nervous System*. Baltimore: Williams and Wilkins, 1987;134–208.
44. Meyer FB, Morita A, Puumala MR, Nichols DA. Medical and surgical

management of intracranial aneurysms. *Mayo Clin Proc* 1995;70: 153–172.

45. Sundt TM Jr, ed. *Surgical Techniques for Saccular and Giant Intracranial Aneurysms.* Baltimore: Williams and Wilkins, 1990.

46. Barrow DL, Reisner A. Natural history of intracranial aneurysms and vascular malformations. *Clin Neurosurg* 1993;40:3–39.

47. Kassell NF, Torner JC, Haley EC Jr, Jane JA, Adams HP, Kongable GL. The International Cooperative Study on the Timing of Aneurysm Surgery. I. Overall management results. *J Neurosurg* 1990;73:18–36.

48. Stehbens WE. *Pathology of Cerebral Blood Vessels.* St. Louis: CV Mosby, 1972;351–470.

49. Sahs AL, Nibbelink DW, Torner JC, eds. Aneurysmal subarachnoid hemorrhage: report of the cooperative study. Baltimore: Urban and Schwarzenberg, 1981.

50. Fox JL. *Intracranial Aneurysms.* vol 1. New York: Springer-Verlag, 1983;76-77.

51. Fox JL, Albin MS, Bader DCH, Davis DO, Korczynski SL, Malis LI, Reichman OH, Rhoton AL, Wilson CB. Microsurgical treatment of neurovascular disease. *Neurosurgery* 1978;3:285–337.

52. Morantz RA, Kirchner FR, Kishore P. Aneurysms of the petrous portion of the internal carotid artery. *Surg Neurol* 1976;6:313–318.

53. Berenstein A, Ransohoff J, Kupersmith M, Flamm E, Graeb D. Transvascular treatment of giant aneurysms of the cavernous carotid and vertebral arteries. *Surg Neurol* 1984;21:3–12.

54. Yasargil MG. Internal carotid aneurysms. In: Yasargil MG, ed. *Microneurosurgery.* vol 2. Stuttgart: Georg Thieme Verlag, 1984;33–123.

55. Locksley HB. Report on cooperative study of intracranial aneurysms and subarachnoid hemorrhage. Section V, I: Natural history of subarachnoid hemorrhage, intracranial aneurysms and arteriovenous malformations. *J Neurosurg* 1966;25:219–239.

56. Rodman KD, Awad IA. Clinical presentation. In: Awad IA, ed. *Current Management of Cerebral Aneurysms.* American Association of Neurological Surgeons 1993;21–41.

57. Almeida GM, Shibata MK, Bianco E. Carotid-ophthalmic aneurysms. *Surg Neurol* 1976;5:41-45.

58. Yasargil MG, Gasser JC, Hodosh RM, Rankin TV. Carotid-ophthalmic aneurysms: direct microsurgical approach. *Surg Neurol* 1977;8: 155–165.

59. Kudo T. An operative complication in a patient with a true posterior communicating artery aneurysm. *Neurosurgery* 1990;27:650–653.

60. Kassell NF, Torner JC. Size of intracranial aneurysms. *Neurosurgery* 1983;12:291–297.

61. Ojemann RG, Heros RC, Crowell RM. *Surgical Management of Cerebrovascular Disease.* 2nd ed. Baltimore: Williams and Wilkins, 1988; 147–449.

62. Drake CG, Vanderlinden RG, Amacher AL. Carotid-choroidal aneurysms. *J Neurosurg* 1968;29:32–26.

63. Okawara S. Aneurysm of the anterior choroidal artery. *Brain Nerve* 1967;19:1185–1192.

64. Perria L, Viale GL, Rivano C. Further remarks on the surgical treatment of carotid-choroidal aneurysms. *Acta Neurochir* 1971;24:253–262.

65. Yasargil MG, Smith RD. Middle cerebral artery aneurysms. In: Youmans JR, ed. *Neurological Surgery.* vol 3. 2nd ed. Philadelphia: WB Saunders, 1982;1663–1696.

66. Fox JL. *Intracranial Aneurysms.* vol 1. New York: Springer-Verlag, 1983;133–162.

67. Hudgins RJ, Day AL, Quisling RG, Rhoton AL Jr, Sypert GW, Garcia-Bangochea F. Aneurysms of the posterior inferior cerebellar artery. *J Neurosurg* 1983;58:381–387.

68. Sengupta RP, Saunders M, Clarke PRR. Unruptured intracranial aneurysms: an unusual source of epilepsy. *Acta Neurochir* 1978;40:45–53.

69. Yasargil MG. Anterior cerebral and anterior communicating artery aneurysms. In: Yasargil MG, ed. *Microneurosurgery.* vol 2. Stuttgart: Georg Thieme Verlag, 1984;165–231.

70. Ojemann RG, Crowell RM. *Surgical Management of Cerebrovascular Disease.* Baltimore: Williams and Wilkins, 1983;127–265.

71. Yasargil MG, Fox JL. Operative approach to aneurysm of the anterior communicating artery. In: Krayenbuhl HLH, ed. *Advanced and Technical Standards in Neurosurgery.* vol 2. New York: Springer–Verlag, 1975;115–128.

72. Andrew J, Nathan PW, Spanos NC. Disturbances of micturition and defecation due to aneurysms of the anterior communicating or anterior cerebral artery. *J Neurosurg* 1966;24:1-10.

73. Norlen G, Barnum AS. surgical treatment of aneurysms of the anterior communicating artery. *J Neurosurg* 1953;10:634–650.

74. Yasargil MG, Carter LP. Saccular aneurysms of the distal anterior cerebral artery. *J Neurosurg* 1974;40:218–223.

75. Norwood EG, Kline LB, Chandra-Sekhar B, Harsh GR III. Aneurysmal compression of the anterior visual pathway. *Neurology* 1986;36: 1035–1041.

76. Becker DH, Newton TH. Distal anterior cerebral artery aneurysm. *Neurosurgery* 1979;495–503.

77. Drake CG. Further experience with surgical treatment of aneurysms of the basilar artery. *J Neurosurg* 1968;29:372–392.

78. Nijensohn DE, Saez RJ, Reagan TJ. Clinical significance of basilar artery aneurysms. *Neurology* 1974;24:301–305.

79. Fisher CM. Clinical syndromes in cerebral thrombosis, hypertensive hemorrhage, and ruptured saccular aneurysm. *Clin Neurosurg* 1975; 22:117–147.

80. Duvoisin RC, Yahr MD. Posterior fossa aneurysms. *Neurology* 1965; 15:231–241.

81. Loeb C, Meyer JS. Strokes due to vertebro-basilar disease. Springfield, IL: Charles C Thomas, 1965.

82. Locksley HB. Report on cooperative study of intracranial aneurysms and subarachnoid hemorrhage, section V, II: Natural history of subarachnoid hemorrhage, intracranial aneurysms and arteriovenous malformations based on 6838 cases in the cooperative study. *J Neurosurg* 1966;25:321–368.

83. Pia HW, Fontana H. Aneurysm of the posterior cerebral artery. *Acta Neurochir (Wien)* 1977;38:13–35.

84. Mori K, Miyazaki H, Ono H. Aneurysm of the anterior inferior cerebellar artery at the internal auditory meatus. *Surg Neurol* 1978;10: 297–304.

85. Nishimoto A, Fujimoto S, Tsuchimoto S, Matsumoto Y, Tabuchi K, Higashi T. Anterior inferior cerebellar artery aneurysm: report of three cases. *J Neurosurg* 1983;59:697–702.

86. Zlotnik EI, Sklyut JA, Smejanovick AF, Stasenko EN. Saccular aneurysm of the anterior inferior cerebellar-internal auditory artery. *J Neurosurg* 1982;57:829–832.

87. Drake CG. The treatment of aneurysms of the posterior circulation. *Clin Neurosurg* 1979;26:96–144.

Cerebrovascular Disease, edited by H. Hunt Batjer.
Lippincott-Raven Publishers, Philadelphia © 1997.

CHAPTER 72

Aneurysmal Subarachnoid Hemorrhage: Pathophysiology and Sequelae

Hector W. Ho and H. Hunt Batjer

EPIDEMIOLOGY

Subarachnoid hemorrhage (SAH) secondary to rupture of an intracranial aneurysm is a common problem that accounts for approximately 80% of nontraumatic SAHs, 6–8% of all strokes, and 22–25% of cerebrovascular deaths (1). Recent data from the National Hospital Discharge Survey (2) and published reports on the epidemiology of SAH (3–5) estimate the annual prevalence of aneurysmal SAH in the United States to be in excess of 30,000 persons. The population-based incidence rate is reported to range from 6 to 16 per 100,000 with the highest rates in Japan (6) and Finland (7). The incidence of aneurysmal SAH, unlike that of other types of stroke, has not declined over time. However, some studies support that population-based mortality rates have declined since 1970 (5,8). The outcome from aneurysmal SAH remains poor despite considerable advances in diagnostic, surgical, and anesthetic techniques. The overall mortality rate is estimated to be 25%. For the patients who survive the initial hemorrhage, approximately 50% will have significant morbidity.

RISK FACTORS

It is estimated from autopsy studies that up to 5% of the general population harbor unruptured intracranial aneurysms. In 15–20% of these cases, multiple aneurysms were found (9–11). This combined with the fact that rupture of these aneurysms carries a high mortality rate has inspired many to study and define the population at risk for aneurysmal SAH. Many risk factors have been implicated in the pathogenesis of aneurysmal SAH. They include age, gender, race, smoking, alcohol use, arterial hypertension, atherosclerosis, oral contraceptive use, drug abuse, body mass index, vascular asymmetry in the circle of Willis, analgesic use,

collagen vascular disease, size of unruptured aneurysm, and other genetic factors (10,12–21).

The incidence of aneurysmal SAH increases with age reaching a peak in the sixth decade of life. The mean age for this population is approximately 50 years. In adults, woman are affected more than men by a ratio of 3:2. Aneurysmal SAH is rare in children and boys are affected more than girls by a ratio of 3:1. This conversion of gender predominance with age prompted some to suggest that pediatric and adult aneurysms are governed by different pathogenic mechanisms (22). Recent data suggest that African-Americans are at a higher risk than white Americans. One study found that young and middle-aged African-Americans had 2.1 times the risk of spontaneous SAH when compared to age-matched white Americans (13). Smoking and heavy alcohol consumption were found to be independent risk factors for aneurysmal SAH (15). Although some cohort studies suggest that hypertension may be a risk factor for aneurysmal SAH, other case-control studies did not confirm these findings. At the present time, the relationship between hypertension and aneurysmal SAH remain uncertain (23,24). In prospective and retrospective studies, the size of an aneurysm appears to be a risk factor for rupture leading to SAH (9, 21,25,26). The critical size of aneurysms determining the risk of rupture was reported to be between 5 and 7 mm. Aneurysms <3 mm have a low chance of rupture whereas ones that are >10 mm have the greatest risk of rupture (24, 26). Evidence that genetic factors play a role in aneurysmal SAH exists. In a large autopsy series, de la Monte and his colleagues reported that 11% of patients with either a ruptured or unruptured aneurysm had a family history of cerebrovascular disease compared with 4% of matched controls (14). In a Swedish study, approximately 500 patients treated for intracranial aneurysms were reported to have a higher incidence of blood relatives with aneurysmal SAH than expected in the general population (27). Human leukocyte antigen (HLA) factors (28,29), certain complement genes (30),

H. W. Ho and H. H. Batjer: Division of Neurological Surgery, Northwestern University Medical School, Chicago, IL 60611

and secretion of proteolytic enzymes (31) have all been implicated as genetic factors that play a role in aneurysmal SAH. Conditions associated with intracranial aneurysms have been presented in the previous chapter and will not be revisited here.

A task force, formed by the Stroke Council of the American Heart Association, reviewed these and other data (24). Their findings and recommendations for modification of risk factors for SAH have been summarized in the following four statements:

1. The relationship between hypertension and SAH is uncertain. The treatment of high blood pressure with antihypertensive medication is strongly recommended to prevent stroke of varying etiology.
2. Cessation of smoking may reduce the risk of SAH, although evidence for this association is indirect.
3. In patients with acceptable surgical risk, clipping of unruptured aneurysms larger than 5–7 mm is recommended. Further studies are recommended to address these issues.
4. Screening of certain high-risk populations for unruptured aneurysms is of uncertain value; advances in magnetic resonance angiography (MRA) may facilitate screening in the future.

NATURAL HISTORY

Understanding the natural history and common sequelae of aneurysmal SAH will allow the physician to formulate rational treatment strategies. One of the most feared complications of an initial hemorrhage is recurrent bleeding. The mortality rate for rebleeding is estimated to be approximately 70%. The greatest risk for rebleeding is in the first 24 hours after the initial hemorrhage. This is estimated based on a report from a prospective Cooperative Aneurysm Study to be 4.1% (32). The rate then decreases steadily until the third day when it remains constant at 1–2% per day. Several studies have shown that untreated ruptured aneurysms have a 20–30% risk of rebleeding in the first month and 50% of the patients rehemorrhage 6 months following their initial hemorrhage (32–34). Thereafter, the rate of rebleeding stabilizes at 3% per year (35).

CLINICAL FEATURES

Signs and Symptoms

Although intracranial aneurysms can manifest in various ways, the clinical presentation of a major aneurysmal SAH is one of the most distinctive in medicine. Despite the characteristic history for a major hemorrhage, misdiagnosis of SAH is common (36,37). This may be due to the fact that between 40% and 50% of patients give a history of distressingly mild symptoms of the warning or sentinel leak prior to a major SAH (38,39). Reports have demonstrated that when these warning signs are missed, patients suffer a higher mortality rate (40–50%) (40). Because of the devastating sequelae that may follow an SAH, it should be treated as a medical emergency. Thus, it is imperative that emergency medical personnel, nurses, and physicians recognize the clinical manifestations and institute immediate diagnostic and therapeutic measures.

The history given by a patient with a warning leak is often erroneously attributed to migraine, sinusitis, meningitis, seizures, or hypertension (41,42). Okawara reported the highest incidence of warning sign presentation to have occurred in young adults, especially women in the third to fourth decade of life (43). A warning headache can be described as being moderate to severe, often unremitting, and lasts for 1–2 days. These headaches may have localizing value with associations of bifrontal headaches accompanying anterior communicating artery aneurysms, hemicranial headaches with middle cerebral artery aneurysms, and severe occipital headaches with posterior circulation aneurysms (38,44). Other symptoms that may accompany the warning headache include dizziness, nausea, vomiting, neck pain, transitory sensory and/or motor deficits, change in the level of consciousness, and oculomotor or visual disturbances (45).

The classic clinical presentation for SAH is sudden severe headache frequently described by the patients as explosive and the worst headache of their life. This may be accompanied by other common signs such as nuchal rigidity, neck pain, nausea and vomiting, and lethargy. Loss of consciousness may reflect the acute rise of intracranial pressure equaling or exceeding mean arterial pressure at the time of aneurysmal rupture. This occurs in approximately 45% of patients with SAH (46). In addition, IIIrd and VIth nerve palsies, subhyaloid retinal hemorrhages, and papilledema may result from increased intracranial pressure. The occurrence of seizures after an SAH (26%) usually does not reflect the location of hemorrhage or the patient's prognosis (47). Less common presentations of SAH include fever, chest pain, back pain, coma, photophobia, hyperacusis, focal neurologic deficits, vertigo and ataxia, and visual hallucinations (48,49). Electrocardiogram (ECG) changes after an SAH have been reported with the hypothesis of a resultant adrenergic storm leading to arrhythmias and accelerated pacing (50,51). Abnormal ECG patterns recorded in patients following hemorrhage include inverted T waves, prolonged Q-T interval, ST depression, and occasional Q waves.

It must be kept in mind that the outcome for patients with an aneurysmal SAH is disappointing. It is estimated that 8–60% of the patients die before they reach the hospital (6, 52,53).

Grading and Prognosis

The history and initial physical and neurologic examination are critical in determining the patient's suitability for early neurosurgical intervention as well as the patient's prognosis. A variety of grading systems have been devised to

TABLE 1. *Hunt–Hess clinical grading scale for subarachnoid hemorrhage (48)*

Grade	Patient's condition
1	Asymptomatic or mild headache and mild nuchal rigidity
2	Cranial nerve palsy, nuchal rigidity, and moderate to severe headache
3	Drowsy, confused, or mild focal deficit
4	Stupor, moderate to severe hemiparesis, and early decerebrate posturing
5	Comatose and decerebrate posturing

TABLE 3. *Computed tomographic scan classification of subarachnoid hemorrhage (34)*

Group	Description
1	No blood detected
2	Diffuse deposition or thin layer of blood, with all vertical layers of blood (interhemispheric fissure, insular cistern, and ambient cistern) <1 mm thick
3	Localized clots or vertical layers of blood 1 mm or more in thickness (or both)
4	Diffuse or no subarachnoid blood but with intracerebral or intraventricular clots

predict outcome after SAH. The two most commonly used grading systems are the Hunt and Hess Clinical Grading Scale (54) (Table 1) and the World Federation of Neurological Surgeons Clinical Grading Scale (55) (Table 2). In both grading systems, the morbidity and mortality of patients increases as their clinical grade ascends. A study from the Mayo Clinic revealed that approximately 48% of the patients presented with Hunt–Hess grades 1 and 2, 20% presented with grade 3, and 30% presented with grades 4 and 5 (56). The breakdown in the percentage of patients for each grade will vary depending on the hospital and its referral pattern. In addition to these clinical grading scales based on the history and examination, a computed tomographic (CT) scan classification for SAH has also been devised to predict the incidence of cerebral vasospasm (57) (Table 3).

Besides the initial clinical grade, other factors influence the outcome of patients who suffer from aneurysmal SAH. They include medical and neurologic complications that result from the hemorrhage. This will be discussed in the later sections below.

Diagnosis

The initial diagnostic evaluation of a patient suspected of having an SAH should include a non-contrast-enhanced CT scan. Although initial CT scans have been reported to be negative in up to 35% of patients with a sentinel hemorrhage (38), a high-density clot in the subarachnoid space can be detected in 92% of cases if the CT scan is performed within 24 hours of the initial hemorrhage (58). Due to the changes in the density of blood on CT over time, the sensitivity for diagnostic purposes decreases and the scan may be negative

TABLE 2. *World Federation of Neurological Surgeons clinical grading scale for subarachnoid hemorrhage (29)*

Grade	Glasgow coma scale	Motor deficit
0	15	Absent
1	15	Absent
2	13–14	Absent
3	13–14	Present
4	7–12	Present or absent
5	3–6	Present or absent

for the SAH. CT scans have the inherent advantage of disclosing intracerebral hemorrhages and early hydrocephalus when present. It may also add important information such as calcification of the aneurysm neck and the presence of thrombus within the aneurysm, which has surgical implications. The pattern and distribution of blood on the CT scan may have predictive value to the location of the aneurysm (59–61). The location of the hemorrhage generally corresponds to the area of which the aneurysm has bled. Whereas intraparenchymal hemorrhages are more commonly seen with middle cerebral artery aneurysms, interhemispheric hemorrhages may indicate an anterior communicating artery aneurysm. Intraventricular hemorrhages are more prevalent in basilar apex, posterior inferior cerebellar artery, and anterior communicating artery aneurysmal rupture. Hemorrhage within the Sylvian fissure suggests an aneurysmal rupture in the distal internal carotid artery, middle cerebral artery, or posterior communicating artery. Perimesencephalic SAHs with extension only to the ambient cistern or basal portion of the Sylvian fissure are often nonaneurysmal in nature (62, 63). SAH of unknown etiology will be presented in depth in a section to follow. Conventional CT scan performed with contrast enhancement is of limited value at this time, although high-resolution CT with three-dimensional reconstruction may play a significant role in the near future.

A lumbar puncture for examination of the cerebral spinal fluid (CSF) is indicated if the history is suggestive and the CT scan nondiagnostic or unavailable. Barrows in 1955 was the first to document changes in red blood cells, protein, and pigment in the CSF of patients following SAH (64). CSF findings in normal, traumatic, and subarachnoid hemorrhage have been presented in recent literature (65,66) (Table 4). The characteristics of CSF for the patient with SAH include increased red blood cell count with xanthochromic supernatant when centrifuged, elevated protein level, and normal or mildly depressed glucose level. The opening pressure of the lumbar puncture after SAH is often elevated especially during the first 2 weeks of the initial hemorrhage. Xanthochromia of the CSF occurs approximately 2 hours after the initial hemorrhage and may persist for several weeks.

Currently, the standard for diagnosing cerebral aneurysms as a cause of SAH is cerebral angiography. A four-vessel

TABLE 4. *Cerebrospinal fluid findings in traumatic tap and subarachnoid hemorrhage (103)*

Condition	Opening pressure	Appearance	Cells	Protein (mg/dl)	Glucose (mg/dl)
Normal	7–18	Clear	None	15–45	50
Traumatic tap	Normal	Bloody with supernatant clear	RBC/WBC ratio equal to peripheral blood count	Mildly elevated	Normal
SAH	Increased	Bloody with supernatant xanthochromic	Early increase of RBCs, late increase of WBCs	Moderate to severe elevation	Normal to mild decrease

SAH, subarachnoid hemorrhage; RBC, red blood cells; WBC, white blood cells.

cerebral angiogram is the most accurate method to characterize an aneurysm's location, size, direction of dome and neck, and relationship with the parent vessel. In addition, the presence of multiple aneurysms, associated vascular malformations, and extent of vasospasm can be determined through the angiogram. The sensitivity of detecting an aneurysm when present exceeds 90%. False-negative rates are estimated to range from 12% to 16% (67,68). Possible mechanisms for false-negative angiograms include vasospasm, inaccurate interpretation, aneurysmal obliteration by a thrombus, and inadequate studies. A negative angiogram with strong evidence of an SAH through CT scan and/or CSF studies places the surgeon in a predicament. This problem will be further explored in the section "SAH of Unknown Etiology." Intraoperative angiography is a useful tool in facilitating proper clip placement especially in difficult cases (69). With advances in technology and contrast media, the complication rate for a patient undergoing an intraarterial digital subtraction angiography procedure was estimated by a recent study to be approximately 0.01% for persistent neurologic deficits and 0.5% for transient deficits (70).

Currently, the use of magnetic resonance imaging (MRI) in the diagnosis of acute SAH diagnosis is controversial (71). However, it may be useful in detecting aneurysms >5 mm as well as demonstrating intraluminal thrombosis in giant aneurysms (72,73). With the combination of rapid advancement in MRI and MRA technology, the low morbidity associated with MRI/MRA, decreasing cost for its use, and higher sensitivity, it is possible that MR modalities will be used at a higher frequency for the diagnosis of intracranial aneurysms in the near future.

Transcranial Doppler ultrasonography (TCD) is currently recommended for diagnosis and monitoring of cerebral vasospasm. Good correlation with cerebral angiography has been documented, especially to the proximal segments of the anterior cerebral, middle cerebral, posterior cerebral arteries (74, 75). Evaluation of the distal branches are more limited and as many as 10% of the patients do not have an adequate ultrasonic window for an adequate study. Experience with insonation depths and angulation for identification of particular vessels will allow for reliability and consistency in sequential studies. The critical velocity for severe clinical vasospasm and a high risk of infarction is reported to be at 200 cm/sec (76,77). The clinical significance of cerebral vasospasm will be discussed in a later chapter. Although TCD is an effective noninvasive technique for evaluating cerebral vasospasm, cerebral angiography may still be necessary for definitive diagnosis. The effect of TCD use in the overall outcome of patients who suffer from SAH remains to be determined.

The use of positron emission tomography, single-photon emission tomography, and xenon computed tomography for the measurement of regional cerebral blood flow requires further studies to determine their role in the management of patients with SAH. Electroencephalograms and evoked potentials do not have the specificity and sensitivity for SAHs and currently are not routinely used in the management of this disorder (24).

COMPLICATIONS AND INITIAL MANAGEMENT

A myriad of medical and neurologic complications may occur hours to days after a patient suffers from an SAH. These complications are more common in patients with poorer clinical grade and can lead to devastating or even fatal outcomes. A good understanding of the management principles of the most common entities can help to substantially reduce the morbidity and mortality for these patients. Weir emphasized the importance of neurologic preservation through prevention of systemic complications (39). He noted from a series of 100 patients who had aneurysmal SAH that 54% suffered from pulmonary complications, 23% from cardiovascular complications, 26% from genito-urinary complications, and 3% from gastrointestinal complications. Other systemic complications may include electrolyte disturbances, infections, and venous thromboembolism (Table 5). The major neurologic complications after an aneurysmal

TABLE 5. *Common secondary complications of subarachnoid hemorrhage*

Medical complications	Neurological complications
Pulmonary complications	Rehemorrhage
Cardiovascular complications	Cerebral vasospasm
Electrolyte abnormalities	Hydrocephalus
Gastrointestinal complications	Seizures
Infections	
Venous thromboembolism	
Genitourinary complications	

SAH are rehemorrhage, cerebral vasospasm, hydrocephalus, and seizures (Table 5). The management goals for SAH can be categorized into four areas. First, the patient must be accurately evaluated to determine his or her initial condition. Second, stabilization and monitoring of the patient's general neurologic and systemic complications from the initial hemorrhage must be accomplished. Third, efforts must be made to prevent rehemorrhage because this is a major cause of morbidity and mortality. Fourth, a plan should be devised for the monitoring and treatment of vasospasm.

General medical monitoring and support should be provided after the initial evaluation. The patient should be kept in an intensive care setting with staff familiar with neurologic assessment of patients. Frequent vital sign and neurologic evaluations are important for early detection of possible complications. Patients should be restrained from oral intake and provided intravenous fluids such as normal saline with supplemental potassium chloride or dextrose. The type and amount of fluid used should take into consideration the patient's condition such as presence of hypertension or hypotension, hyperglycemia, or hyponatremia. If the patient is lethargic, nasogastric tube placement may be helpful in avoidance of gastric reflux leading to aspiration. Quiet bedrest with the head of the bed at 30° to facilitate intracranial venous drainage should be provided. Monitoring through the use of continuous ECG, pulse oximetry, arterial line for blood pressure, and record of intake and output is important. The use of a Foley catheter may be helpful for the accurate measurement of urinary output as well as sampling of urine for electrolyte disturbances and infections. Periodic blood sampling for electrolytes and osmolarity, complete blood count with platelets, prothrombin time and partial thromboplastin time, and arterial blood gas should be instituted. Good pulmonary toilet and periodic chest X ray are important for avoidance of pulmonary complications. For prophylaxis against thrombophlebitis, knee-high TED hose and pneumatic compression boots are beneficial.

Use of antiemetics, stool softeners, H2 blockers, and analgesics will also reduce the risk of complications and provide comfort to patients. The phenothiazine-derived antiemetics should be avoided due to their potential role in lowering the seizure threshold of these patients. H2 blockers may help reduce the risk of stress ulcer development. If sedation is necessary, phenobarbital is commonly used because it has additional properties to reduce hypertension and serve as an anticonvulsant. For SAH patients with cerebral infarction, previous seizure, hypertension, or intraparenchymal hematoma, the risk for development of seizures is heightened (78–81). For patients without seizures, infarctions, or hematomas, the efficacy of prophylactic anticonvulsant drug use has not been established (47,82). Because of the increased risk for rebleeding with a generalized seizure and the associated devastation that may result, many authorities recommend the use of prophylactic anticonvulsant drugs in the management of aneurysmal SAH (24,83). Dexamethasone use may relieve patients from their headaches and neck pain secondary to meningeal inflammation, but its effect on cerebral edema under this circumstance is controversial. Currently, the daily use of calcium channel blockers such as nimodipine for vasospasm management is recommended (24).

Medical Complications

Pulmonary Complications

Pulmonary complications following SAH are not uncommon. Infection, aspiration, atelectasis, edema, and emboli of the pulmonary system are all potential complications in these patients. In the elderly population, many have preexisting pulmonary and cardiac compromise in function. Sputum culture, aggressive pulmonary toilet, and initiation of antimicrobial therapy may be necessary to optimize the patient's oxygenation. Approximately 17% of cases treated with hypertensive hypervolemic hemodilution therapy have been reported to be complicated by pulmonary edema (84). The mechanism is fluid overload which can be avoided with careful monitoring of pulmonary artery wedge pressure. Neurogenic pulmonary edema is thought to be due to increased cardiac filling pressures and/or leaky capillary bed secondary to an elevated catecholamine release (85). As with other causes, severe neurogenic pulmonary edema should include the use a Swan–Gantz catheter to help monitor pulmonary wedge pressures as well as ventilatory support with continuous positive airway pressure or positive end-expiratory pressure. Occasionally, these complications can lead to full-blown adult respiratory distress syndrome and cause severe morbidity and mortality. Early and aggressive treatments of pulmonary complications can minimize further hypoxic injury to the brain. Patients with poor clinical grade require endotracheal intubation and ventilatory support early on in the course of treatment. Pulmonary embolus is estimated to occur in approximately 1% of patients after aneurysmal SAH. Prevention of deep venous thrombosis with passive exercise, elastic stockings, pneumatic compression boots, and early mobilization is beneficial. A vena cava filter placement may be necessary for patients in the preoperative or early postoperative period with a deep venous thrombosis.

Cardiac Complications

Cardiac complications might also be a result of the massive rise in circulating catecholamine levels occurring at the time of the hemorrhage. Any ECG changes following an aneurysmal SAH must by viewed as evidence of cardiac dysfunction and treated accordingly. Cardiac arrhythmias, occurring in 20–40% of patients following SAH, have been reported to result in cardiac infarction and sudden death (86, 87). Cardiac isoenzymes should be obtained when ECG changes show evidence of cardiac ischemia or infarction. The use of β-adrenergic blocking agents have been shown to reduce these catecholamine-mediated complications (88). These agents should not be used if the patient has asthma or a hypersensitivity to β blockers. In addition, development of heart blocks with bradycardia and hypotension may result from the use of these agents. A cardiologist is commonly consulted by the neurosurgeon for perioperative care when ECG changes are noted in a patient suffering from a SAH.

Electrolyte Disturbances

Electrolyte disturbances are not an uncommon complication after SAH affecting 10–30% of patients (89,90). As with many other complications following aneurysmal SAH, hyponatremia occurs more frequently in patients with poor clinical grade. Hyponatremia usually develops several days after the initial hemorrhage. This drop in sodium depresses a patient's level of consciousness and lowers their seizure threshold. Hyponatremia following SAH has mainly been attributed to the syndrome of inappropriate secretion of antidiuretic hormone (SIADH), but recent uncontrolled prospective studies suggest a relationship of hyponatremia to excessive natriuresis and volume contraction (91,92). The syndrome of cerebral salt wasting was recently reviewed and the treatment is opposite from that of SIADH (93). Others have associated fluid restriction to an increased incidence of delayed ischemic deficits and volume contraction to symptomatic vasospasm (94,95). Guidelines from the American Heart Association strongly advise against the use of volume contraction and hypotonic solution in the treatment of hyponatremia after SAH (24). Management should include intravascular administration of isotonic solution and close monitoring of the patient's volume status aiming for normal or slight hypervolemia. Progressive hypernatremia with diabetes insipidus may be seen in patients who have massive hemorrhage and elevated intracranial pressure after SAH. On occasion, patients with giant anterior communicating artery aneurysms or had surgery in that area may develop hypernatremia. The diagnosis of diabetes insipidus should be considered when urine output is excessive (>250 ml/hr for 2 hr) and the urine osmolarity is <1.005. Administration of antidiuretic hormone may be indicated in these patients.

Gastrointestinal Complications

Following aneurysmal SAH, approximately 3–4% of patients develop gastrointestinal bleeding secondary to stress ulceration. The mechanism proposed to account for this includes an increase in acid and gastrin secretion combined with a breakdown of protective lining of the gastrointestinal tract. Prophylaxis and treatment consist of nasogastric tube placement with low intermittent suction, antacids, and H2-blocking agents. Monitoring of the hematocrit and fluid status is also important.

Infections and Deep Venous Thrombosis

Infections are common in these patients, many of whom have indwelling catheters in their veins, arteries, urinary bladder, stomach, and trachea. In addition, these patients are immobile and carry a higher risk for development of deep venous thrombosis as mentioned above. Both of these complications need to be treated in an expeditious manner because they can lead to more serious conditions such as sepsis and pulmonary embolism.

Neurologic Complications

Rebleeding

Rebleeding is one of the most dreaded complications of aneurysmal SAH. As described in the section on natural history of aneurysmal SAH, aneurysmal rerupture risk is the highest within the first 24 hours after the initial hemorrhage (4.1%) and remains at approximately 1–2% per day for the next 4 weeks. The cumulative risk of rebleeding at 2 weeks is 19% and at 6 months is 40–50%. The mortality rate associated with a rehemorrhage is estimated to be as high as 78% (96). A Cooperative Aneurysm Study reported a higher risk of rehemorrhage in women compared to men with a ratio of 2.2:1, in poorer clinical grade patients, and in patients with a systolic blood pressure of >169 mm Hg at presentation (97). Clinical signs of rebleeding include depression of level of consciousness, increased headaches, nausea and vomiting, seizures, and new neurologic deficits. Reducing the incidence of rebleeding will clearly have a major impact on the outcome of these patients. Securing the aneurysm surgically as early as possible is the most effective strategy to minimize the risk of a rerupture. The timing and techniques of operation for ruptured aneurysm will be discussed in a later chapter. In addition to aneurysm clipping, other strategies to reduce the risk of rebleeding have been studied.

Although bedrest and a quiet environment should remain as part of the current treatment protocol, bedrest alone was found in the Cooperative Aneurysm Study to be inferior to drug-induced hypotension, intracranial surgery, and carotid ligation in prevention of rebleeding (98). Antihypertensive use for prevention of rebleeding remains controversial with some reports of increased (99), no change (98), and decreased (100) rebleeding rates. Both regulated bedrest or antihypertensive therapy alone are not recommended to prevent rebleeding after SAH, but they may be included as part of an overall treatment (24).

Although carotid ligation was commonly used before 1970 for the treatment of intracranial aneurysms, more recent studies examining its usefulness in rebleeding prevention were not able to clearly determine its value (98,101, 102). The risk of complications from carotid ligation must also be taken into consideration when planning to treat patients by this method.

Antifibrinolytic therapy has been available for >25 years. The most commonly used agents are ϵ-aminocaproic acid and tranexamic acid. The Cooperative Aneurysm Study showed a rebleeding rate of 11.7% in the antifibrinolytic-treated group compared to 19.4% in the non-treated group (103). However, focal ischemic deficits were increased in the antifibrinolytic-treated group with a rebleeding rate of 32.4% compared to the non-treated group with a rebleeding rate of 22.7%. The use of these agents consistently showed an increase in cerebral ischemic deficits from numerous studies especially in patients with significant vasospasm (104–106). Recent guidelines given by the American Heart Association state that use of antifibrinolytic therapy for prevention of rebleeding is recommended in certain situations. These circumstances include patients with low risk for vasospasm and/or patients who may benefit from delaying surgery. However, the guidelines warn that the risk for cerebral ischemia is higher, thus resulting in no benefit of overall outcome (24).

Endovascular therapy with the use of intraluminal coils for prevention of rebleeding have been investigated and short-term occlusion of the aneurysm ranges from 48% to 96% (107–109). These preliminary results suggest that coils can promote thrombosis of the aneurysm in many cases, but the long-term follow-up results are not yet available. Intraluminal coils were approved by the Food and Drug Administration in the fall of 1995 for use in the treatment of inoperable intracranial aneurysms or in patients who are unfit for surgery. This topic will be further considered in a later chapter.

Vasospasm

Vasospasm is a major cause of morbidity and mortality in patients following aneurysmal SAH. Biller noted that as many as 70% of these patients show angiographic signs of cerebral vasospasm, but only about 36% of them are symptomatic (83). Despite maximal therapy, 15–20% of patients suffer from stroke or die from cerebral vasospasm after an SAH (110,111). Intensive investigative efforts have been made to determine the pathophysiologic characteristics of cerebral vasospasm and the mechanism underlying this phenomenon is becoming clearer (112–114). Vasospasm follows a typical temporal pattern with the onset at day 3–5 after the initial hemorrhage. A period of maximal luminal narrowing occurs between days 5 and 14 and resolution of the spasm by 2–4 weeks (115). Symptoms and signs of delayed ischemic neurologic deficit corresponds to the course of angiographic vasospasm. The diagnosis and monitoring of cerebral vasospasm are accomplished with the aid of cerebral angiograms and transcranial Doppler ultrasonography. Currently, the treatments for cerebral vasospasm include the use of hypertension/hypervolemia/hemodilution (H/H/H) therapy, calcium channel antagonists, surgical clot removal from the subarachnoid space, application of cisternal plasminogen

activators, transluminal angioplasty, antioxidant and anti-inflammatory agents (24). Detailed discussion of this topic will appear in a later chapter.

Hydrocephalus

Hydrocephalus may occur shortly after SAH due to the a blockage of the ventricles or cisterns by a blood clot. This acute hydrocephalus was found to be present in 20–27% of the patients who survived the initial hemorrhage (116,117). As with other complications that follow an SAH, the incidence of acute hydrocephalus increases with the poorer clinical grade patients. Ventriculostomy is recommended when a patient presents with a depressed level of consciousness and ventriculomegaly. With an unsecured aneurysm, attention must be given to the rate of CSF drainage. Rapid change of intracranial pressure through CSF drainage may precipitate aneurysmal rerupture. A gradual lowering of intracranial pressure to 15–20 cm water is recommended. Long-term or chronic hydrocephalus was found to occur in about 20% of patients 30 days after the initial hemorrhage (118), although some have reported this finding in up to 60% of patients (119). This is likely due to the scarring of arachnoid granulation tissue and disturbance of CSF absorption. In symptomatic patients, chronic hydrocephalus secondary to an SAH can be treated by placement of a ventricular shunt for CSF diversion. As with all shunting procedures, a 5–10% risk of infection applies.

Seizures

Seizures may occur after an aneurysmal SAH especially if it involves a middle cerebral artery aneurysmal rupture with an associated intracerebral hematoma. Other risk factors for seizures after SAH include infarction and a history of hypertension (78,80). The overall incidence is estimated to be approximately 25% (47,120). Most seizures occur within 18 months after the initial hemorrhage and may present as focal, generalized, or partial complex. Although the need for and efficacy of routine use of an anticonvulsant have not been firmly established, most would agree to its use because of the potential risk of rebleeding after the initial hemorrhage (24,121). Patients who have not had a prior seizure could be tapered off a few months after starting. Otherwise, extended therapy and EEG monitoring are employed. The anticonvulsants phenytoin and phenobarbital are commonly used for this condition.

SAH OF UNKNOWN ETIOLOGY

Overview

Although the etiology of SAH can be determined in the majority of cases, there remains a substantial group of patients who fail to reveal any structural abnormalities on angiographic studies. It is estimated that in 20–25% of these cases cerebral angiograms performed to identify source of bleeding after SAH will be negative (122). Many possible causes may present with this situation, including inadequate angiogram, obliteration of the lesion by the hemorrhage, thrombosis of the aneurysm, aneurysm that is too small to be detected on angiogram, and cervical or upper thoracic arteriovenous malformation. Although trauma is the most common cause of nonaneurysmal SAH, there are times when it is difficult to discern whether the patient's SAH was the result or cause of his or her injury. A thorough history will greatly help identify other possible causes. Other causes to consider in the differential diagnosis should include angiographically occult vascular malformations, intracranial tumors, hemorrhagic infarctions, venous thrombosis, hypertensive hemorrhages, drug use (especially amphetamines), and medical conditions such as coagulopathies, sickle cell anemia, and collagen vascular diseases.

A cooperative study examining patients who had no identifiable etiology for their SAH found that the long-term prognosis is significantly better than for patients with an aneurysmal SAH (123). Controversy exists as to whether to perform a second cerebral angiogram after an initial negative study (24,124). Forster and colleagues reported that only one patient of the 56 (1.8%) in his study was found to have an aneurysm on the second study (125). However, the patients in that study were not examined by CT scan for the initial diagnosis of SAH and 3 of the 94 patients did have a second hemorrhage as a result of an aneurysm but were not studied by a second angiogram. A review by Friedman of 15 studies showed that 3.6–22% of these patients were found to have an aneurysm on the second angiogram (126). At this institution, when a pattern other than a classic perimesencephalic SAH is identified on CT scan, a repeat cerebral angiogram is per-

formed 1 week, 2 weeks, and 1 month after the initial hemorrhage.

The goals for treatment of patients with SAH of unknown etiology are prevention of secondary injury and administration of symptomatic relief. Bedrest, monitoring, blood pressure control, and analgesics are provided to the patients whereas the administration of anticonvulsants, corticosteroids, and calcium channel blockers is decided on an individual basis. CT scans should be performed daily for the first few days after SAH to determine whether rebleeding or hydrocephalus has developed. If hydrocephalus develops, a rational approach is to initially place an external ventricular drain followed by an attempt to wean the patient off the drainage. If the patient fails to tolerate the challenge, permanent diversion with the use of a ventriculoperitoneal shunt is performed. Cerebral vasospasm occurs much less frequently in these patients than in those with an aneurysmal SAH (68). Even when vasospasm was angiographically observed, many of the patients in this specific group were not symptomatic (127). Treatment of cerebral vasospasm for this group is the same as for patients with an aneurysmal SAH.

Perimesencephalic SAH

A separate and distinct condition considered to be benign and associated with a very low rebleeding risk and good outcome is perimesencephalic SAH (128,129). These patients are usually not critically ill, have a normal level of consciousness, and have a low risk for major complications or death. In a study by Rinkel, of the 37 patients followed for at least 18 months (mean of 45 months), none had rebleeding or persistent neurologic deficits (128). Although the exact anatomic source of bleeding is still unknown, it has been suggested that perimesencephalic SAH is due to a venous or capillary rupture at the level of the tentorial hiatus

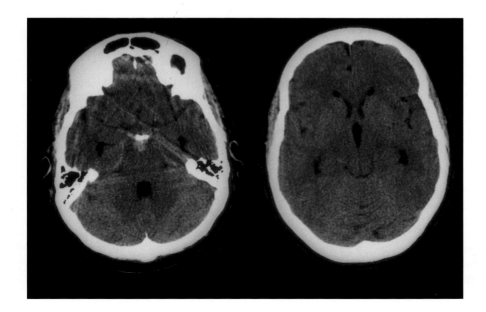

FIG. 1. Computed tomographic scan of a perimesencephalic subarachnoid hemorrhage. Note the characteristic pattern of blood distribution in the interpeduncular cistern. (Courtesy of Dr. Jordan M. Prager, Division of Neuroradiology, Evanston Hospital, Evanston, Illinois.)

(63). A characteristic blood distribution pattern on CT and MRI for this condition has been described. In one study, 100% of these patients had the epicenter of bleeding located immediately anterior to the midbrain and pons or in the interpeduncular cisterns extending to the anterior part of the ambient cisterns (62) (Fig. 1). Although debate continues regarding whether a repeat angiogram should be performed in this subset of patients with a classic perimesencephalic SAH, many advocate that a second angiogram is unnecessary especially in the absence of cerebral vasospasm (130,131). The optimal treatment for these patients is not known but aggressive therapies are not indicated because the risk of rehemorrhage or ischemic stroke is extremely low. Symptomatic relief, bedrest, and blood pressure control on admission and follow-up monitoring for signs of hydrocephalus by examination and CT scan might be warranted.

REFERENCES

1. Mohr JP, Caplan LR, Melski JW, et al. The Harvard Cooperative Stroke Registry: a prospective registry. *Neurology* 1978;28:754–762.
2. *Detailed Diagnosis and Procedures,* National Hospital Discharge Survey, 1990. Hyattsville, MD: US Dept of Health and Human Services, 1992, PHS 92–1774. Series 13.
3. Broderick JP, Brott T, Tomsick T, Miller R, Huster G. Intracerebral hemorrhage more than twice as common as subarachnoid hemorrhage. *J Neurosurg* 1993;78:188–191.
4. Davis PH, Hachinski V. Epidemiology of cerebrovascular disease. In: Anderson DW, ed. Neuroepidemiology: a tribute to Bruce Schoenberg. Boca Rotan: CRC Press, 1991.
5. Ingall TJ, Wiebers DO. Natural history of subarachnoid hemorrhage. In: Whisnant JP, ed. *Stroke: Populations, Cohorts, and Clinical Trials.* Boston: Butterworth-Heinemann Ltd, 1993.
6. Kiyohara Y, Ueda K, Hasuo Y, Wada J, Kawano H, Kato I, Sinkawa A, Ohmura T, Iwamoto H, Omae T. Incidence and prognosis of subarachnoid hemorrhage in a Japanese rural community. *Stroke* 1989; 20:1150–1155.
7. Sarti C, Tuomilehto J, Salomaa V, Sivenius J, Kaarsalo E, Narva EV, Salmi K, Torppa J. Epidemiology of subarachnoid hemorrhage in Finland from 1983 to 1985. *Stroke* 1991;22:848–853.
8. Ingall TJ, Whisnant JP, Wiebers DO, O Fallon WM. Has there been a decline in subarachnoid hemorrhage mortality? *Stroke* 1989; 20: 718–724.
9. McCormick WF, Acosta-Rua GJ. The size of intracranial saccular aneurysms: an autopsy study. *J Neurosurg* 1970;33:422–427.
10. Sacco RL, Wolf PA, Bharucha NE, Meeks SL, Kannel WB, Charette LJ, McNamara PM, Palmer EP, D Agostino R. Subarachnoid and intracerebral hemorrhage: natural history, prognosis, and precursive factors in the Framingham Study. *Neurology* 1984;34:847–854.
11. Stehbens WE. Aneurysms and anatomic variation of cerebral arteries. *Arch Pathol* 1963;75:45–64.
12. Bonita R. Cigarette smoking, hypertension and the risk of subarachnoid hemorrhage: a population-based case-control study. *Stroke* 1986; 17:831–835.
13. Broderick JP, Brott T, Tomsick T, Huster G, Miller R. The risk of subarachnoid and intracerebral hemorrhages in blacks as compared with whites. *N Engl J Med* 1992;326:733–736.
14. de la Monte SM, Moore GW, Mong MA, Hutchins GM. Risk factors for the development and rupture of intracranial berry aneurysms. *Am J Med* 1985;78:957–964.
15. Juvela S, Hillbom M, Numminen H, Koskinen P. Cigarette smoking and alcohol consumption as risk factors for aneurysmal subarachnoid hemorrhage. *Stroke* 1993;24:639–646.
16. Knekt P, Reunanen A, Aho K, Heliovaara M, Rissanen A, Aromaa A, Impivaara O. Risk factors for subarachnoid hemorrhage in a longitudinal population study. *J Clin Epidemiol* 1991;44:933–939.
17. Longstreth WT Jr, Koepsell TD, Yerby MS, van Belle G. Risk factors for subarachnoid hemorrhage. *Stroke* 1985;16:337–385.
18. Oyesiku NM, Colohan AR, Barrow DL, Reisner A. Cocaine-induced aneurysmal rupture: an emergent factor in the natural history of intracranial aneurysms? *Neurosurgery* 1993;32:518–526.
19. Thorogood M, Mann J, Murphy M, Vessey M. Fatal stroke and use of oral contraceptives: findings from a case-control study. *Am J Epidemiol* 1992;136:35–45.
20. Torner JC. Epidemiology of subarachnoid hemorrhage. *Semin Neurol* 1984;4:354–369.
21. Wiebers DO, Whisnant JP, Sundt TM Jr, O Fallon WM. The significance of unruptured intracranial saccular aneurysms. *J Neurosurg* 1987;66:23–29.
22. Meyer FB, Sundt TM Jr, Fode NC, Morgan MK, Forbes GS, Mellinger JF. Cerebral aneurysms in childhood and adolescence. *J Neurosurg* 1989;70:420–425.
23. Chyatte D. The epidemiology, genetics, and clinical behavior of intracranial aneurysms. In: Awad IA, ed. *Current Management of Cerebral Aneurysms.* American Association of Neurological Surgeons, 1993; 1–20.
24. Mayberg MR, Batjer HH, Dacey R, Diringer M, Haley EC, Heros RC, Sternau LL, Torner J, Adams HP Jr, Feinberg W, Thies W. Guidelines for the management of aneurysmal subarachnoid hemorrhage. *Stroke* 1994; 25:2315–2328.
25. Ferguson GG. Physical factors in the initiation, growth, and rupture of human intracranial saccular aneurysms. *J Neurosurg* 1972; 37: 666–677.
26. Kassell NF, Torner JC. Size of intracranial aneurysms. *Neurosurgery* 1983; 12:291–297.
27. Norrgard O, Angquist KA, Fodstad H, Forsell A, Lindberg M. Intracranial aneurysms and heredity. Neurosurgery 1987;20:236–239.
28. Lye RH, Dyer PA, Sheldon S, Antoun N. Are HLA antigens implicated in the pathogenesis of nonhemorrhagic deterioration following aneurysmal subarachnoid hemorrhage. *J Neurol Neurosurg Psychiatry* 1989;52:1197–1199.
29. Mellergard P, Ljunggren B, Brandt L, Johnson U, Holtas S. HLA-typing in a family with six intracranial aneurysms. *Br J Neurosurg* 1989;3:479–485.
30. Ostergaard JR, Brunn-Petersen G, Kristensen BO. The C3-F gene in patients with intracranial saccular aneurysms. *Acta Neurol Scand* 1986;74:356–359.
31. Chyatte D, Brophy C, Reilly J, et al. Metabolism of the extracellular matrix in cerebral aneurysm disease. In: *Proceedings of the American Association of Neurological Surgeons 58th Annual Meeting* May 2, 1990. Nashville, Tennessee. 1990;321.
32. Kassell NF, Torner JC. Aneurysmal rebleeding: a preliminary report from the Cooperative Aneurysm Study. *Neurosurgery* 1983;13: 479–481.
33. Henderson WG, Torner JC, Nibbelink DW. Intracranial aneurysms and subarachnoid hemorrhage: report on a randomized treatment study, IV-B: regulated bedrest: statistical evaluation. *Stroke* 1977;8: 579–589.
34. Jane JA, Winn HR, Richardson AE. The natural history of intracranial aneurysms: rebleeding rates during the acute and long term period and implication for surgical management. *Clin Neurosurg* 1977;24: 176–184.
35. Jane JA, Kassell NF, Torner JC, Winn HR. The natural history of aneurysms and arteriovenous malformations. *J Neurosurg* 1985;62: 321–323.
36. Kassell NF, Kongable GL, Torner JC, Adams HP Jr, Mazuz H. Delay in referral of patients with ruptured aneurysms to neurosurgical attention. *Stroke* 1985;16:587–590.
37. Mayberg MR. Warning leaks and subarachnoid hemorrhage. *West J Med* 1990;153:549–550.
38. LeBlanc R. The minor leak preceding subarachnoid hemorrhage. *J Neurosurg* 1987;66:35–39.
39. Weir B, ed. *Aneurysms Affecting the Nervous System.* Baltimore: Williams and Wilkins, 1987.
40. Chan BSH, Dorsch NWC. Delayed diagnosis in subarachnoid hemorrhage. *Med J Aust* 1991;154:509–511.
41. Dorsch NW. Cerebral aneurysms and the missed hemorrhage. *Aust NZ J Med* 1986;16:486–490.
42. Ostergaard JR. Headache as a warning symptom of impending aneurysmal subarachnoid hemorrhage. *Cephalgia* 1991;11:53–55.
43. Okawara SH. Warning signs prior to rupture of an intracranial aneurysm. *J Neurosurg* 1973;38:575–580.

44. Waga S, Otsubo K, Handa H. Warning signs in intracranial aneurysms. *Surg Neurol* 1975;3:15–20.

45. Bassi P, Bandera R, Loiero M, Tognoni G, Mangoni A. Warning signs in subarachnoid hemorrhage: a cooperative study. *Acta Neurol Scand* 1991;84:277–281.

46. Weaver JP, Fisher M. Subarachnoid hemorrhage: an update of pathogenesis, diagnosis, and management. *J Neurol Sci* 1994;125:119–131.

47. Hart RG, Byer JA, Slaughter JR, Hewett JE, Easton JD. Occurrence and implications of seizures in subarachnoid hemorrhage due to ruptured intracranial aneurysms. *Neurosurgery* 1981;8:417–421.

48. Adams HP Jr, Jergenson DD, Kassell NF, Sahs AL. Pitfalls in the recognition of subarachnoid hemorrhage. *JAMA* 1980;244:794–796.

49. Fontanarosa PB. Recognition of subarachnoid hemorrhage. *Ann Emerg Med 1989;*18:1199–1205.

50. Barton CW. Subarachnoid hemorrhage presenting as acute chest pain: a variant of le coup de poignard. *Ann Emerg Med* 1988;17:977–978.

51. Marion DW, Segal R, Thompson ME. Subarachnoid hemorrhage and the heart. *Neurosurgery* 1986;18:101–106.

52. Freytag E. Fatal rupture of intracranial aneurysms: survey of 250 medicolegal cases. *Arch Pathol* 1966;81:418–424.

53. Pakarinen S. Incidence, aetiology, and prognosis of primary subarachnoid hemorrhage: a study based on 589 cases diagnosed in a defined urban population during a defined period. *Acta Neurol Scand* Suppl 1967;29:1–28.

54. Hunt WE, Hess RM. Surgical risk as related to time of intervention in the repair of intracranial aneurysms. *J Neurosurg* 1968;28:14–20.

55. Drake CG (Chairman). Report of World Federation of Neurological Surgeons Committee on a Universal Subarachnoid Grading Scale (letter). *J Neurosurg* 1988;68:985–986.

56. Phillips LH 2d, Whisnant JP, O'Fallon WM, Sundt TM Jr. The unchanging pattern of subarachnoid hemorrhage in a community. *Neurology* 1980;30:1034–1040.

57. Fisher CM, Kritler JP, Davis JM. Relation of cerebral vasospasm to subarachnoid hemorrhage visualized by computerized tomographic scanning. *Neurosurgery* 1980;6:1–9.

58. Kassell NF, Torner JC, Haley EC Jr, Jane JA, Adams HP, Kongable GL. The International Cooperative Study on the Timing of Aneurysmal Surgery. I. Overall management results. *J Neurosurg* 1990;73: 18–36.

59. Chou SN. Critical care of patients with spontaneous subarachnoid hemorrhage. In: Thompson RA, Green JR, eds. *Critical Care of Neurologic and Neurosurgical Emergencies*. New York: Raven Press, 1980;15–23.

60. Laissy JP, Normand G, Monroc M, Duchateau C, Alibert F, Tiebot J. Spontaneous intracerebral hematomas from vascular causes: predictive value of CT compared with angiography. *Neuroradiology* 1991; 33:291–295.

61. Silver AJ, Pederson ME Jr, Ganti SR, Hilal SK, Michelson WJ. CT of subarachnoid hemorrhage due to ruptured aneurysm. *AJNR* 1981; 2:13–22.

62. Rinkel GJE, Wijdicks EFM, Vermeulen M, Ramos LMP, Tanghehl HL, Hasan D, Meiners LC, van Gijn J. Nonaneurysmal perimesencephalic subarachnoid hemorrhage: CT and MR patterns that differ from aneurysmal rupture. *AJNR* 1991;12:829–834.

63. van Gijn J, van Dongen KJ, Vermeulen M, Hijdra A. Perimesencephalic hemorrhage: a nonaneurysmal and benign form of subarachnoid hemorrhage. *Neurology* 1985;35:493–497.

64. Barrows LJ, Hunter FT, Banker BQ. The nature and clinical significance of pigments in the cerebral spinal fluid. *Brain* 1955;78:59–80.

65. Rodman KD, Awad IA. Clinical presentation. In: Awad IA, ed. *Current Management of Cerebral Aneurysms*. American Association of Neurological Surgeons, 1993;21–41.

66. Wood JH. *Subarachnoid Hemorrhage: Neurobiology of Cerebral Spinal Fluid.* vol 1. New York: Plenum Press, 1980;279–286.

67. Iwanaga H, Wakai S, Ochiai C, Narita J, Inoh S, Nagai M. Ruptured cerebral aneurysms missed by initial angiographic study. *Neurosurgery* 1990;27:45–51.

68. Juul R, Fredricksen TA, Ringkjob R. Prognosis in subarachnoid hemorrhage of unknown etiology. *J Neurosurg* 1986;64:359–362.

69. Barrow DL, Boyer KL, Joseph GJ. Intraoperative angiography in the management of neurovascular disorders. *Neurosurgery* 1992;30: 153–159.

70. Grzyska U, Freitag J, Zeumer H. Selective cerebral intraarterial DSA:

71. Atlas SW. MR imaging is highly sensitive for acute subarachnoid hemorrhage . . . not! *Radiology* 1993;186:319–322.

72. Meyer FB, Morita A, Puumala MR, Nichols DA. Medical and surgical management of intracranial aneurysms. *Mayo Clin Proc* 1995;70: 153–172.

73. Olsen WL, Brant-Zawadzki M, Hodes J, Norman D, Newton TH. Giant intracranial aneurysms: MR imaging. *Radiology* 1987;163: 431–435.

74. Aaslid R, Huber P, Nornes H. Evaluation of cerebrovascular spasm with transcranial Doppler ultrasound. *J Neurosurg* 1984;60:37–41.

75. Sloan MA, Haley EC Jr, Kassell NF, Henry ML, Stewart SR, Beskin RR, Sevilla EA, Torner JC. Sensitivity and specificity of transcranial Doppler ultrasonography in the diagnosis of vasospasm following subarachnoid hemorrhage. *Neurology* 1989;39:1514–1518.

76. Hutchison K, Weir B. Transcranial Doppler studies in aneurysm patients. *Can J Neurol Sci* 1989;16:411–416.

77. Seiler RW, Reulen HJ, Huber P, Grolimund P, Ebeling U, Steiger HJ. Outcome of aneurysmal subarachnoid hemorrhage in a hospital population: a prospective study including early operation, intravenous nimodipine, and trancranial Doppler ultrasound. *Neurosurgery* 23; 1988:598–604.

78. Kotila M, Waltimo O. Epilepsy after stroke. *Epilepsia* 1992;33: 495–498.

79. Kvam DA, Loftus CM, Copeland B, Quest DO. Seizure during the immediate postoperative period. *Neurosurgery* 1983;12:14–17.

80. Ohman J. Hypertension as a risk factor for epilepsy after aneurysmal subarachnoid hemorrhage and surgery. *Neurosurgery* 31990;27: 578–581.

81. Rose FC, Sarner M. Epilepsy after ruptured intracranial aneurysm. *Br Med J* 1965;1:18–21.

82. Deutschman CJ, Haines SJ. Anticonvulsant prophylaxis in neurological surgery. *Neurosurgery* 1985;17:510–517.

83. Biller J, Godersky JC, Adams HP Jr. Management of aneurysmal subarachnoid hemorrhage. *Stroke* 1988;19:1300–1305.

84. Origitano TC, Wascher TM, Reichman OH, Anderson DE. Sustained increased cerebral blood flow with prophylactic hypertensive hypervolemic hemodilution (triple-H therapy) after subarachnoid hemorrhage. *Neurosurgery* 1990;27:729–739.

85. Kennedy SK. Airway management and respiratory support. In: Ropper AH, Kennedy SF, eds. *Neurological and Neurosurgical Intensive Care.* 2nd ed. Rockville, MD: Aspen Publishers, 1988;57–84.

86. Andreoli A, de Pasquale G, Pinelli G, Grazi P, Tognetti F, Testa C. Subarachnoid hemorrhage: frequency and severity of cardiac arrhythmias—a survey of 70 cases studied in the acute phase. *Stroke* 1987; 18:558–564.

87. Feibel JH, Campbell RG, Joynt RJ. Myocardial damage and cardiac arrhythmias in cerebral infarction and SAH: correlation with increased systemic catecholamine output. *Trans Am Neurol Assoc* 1976;101: 242–244.

88. Neil-Dwyer G, Walter P, Cruickshank JM. Beta-blockade benefits patients following a subarachnoid hemorrhage. *Eur J Clin Pharmacol* 33 1985;28(suppl 1):25–29.

89. Doczi T, Bende J, Huzka E, Kiss J. Syndrome of inappropriate secretion of antidiuretic hormone after subarachnoid hemorrhage. *Neurosurgery* 1981;9:394–397.

90. Fox JL, Falik JL, Shalhoub RJ. Neurosurgical hyponatremia: the role of inappropriate antidiuresis. *J Neurosurg* 1971;34:506–514.

91. Nelson PB, Seif SM, Maroon JC, Robinson AG. Hyponatremia in intracranial disease: perhaps not the syndrome of inappropriate secretion of antidiuretic hormone (SIADH). *J Neurosurg* 1981;55: 938–941.

92. Wijdicks EF, Vermeulen M, ten Haaf JA, Hijdra A, Bakker WH, van Gijn J. Volume depletion and natriuresis with a ruptured intracranial aneurysm. *Ann Neurol* 1985;18:211–216.

93. Harringan MR. Cerebral salt wasting syndrome: a review. *Neurosurgery* 1996;38:152–160.

94. Solomon RA, Post KD, McMurtry JG III. Depression of circulating blood volume in patients after subarachnoid hemorrhage: implications for the management of symptomatic vasospasm. *Neurosurgery* 1984; 15:354–361.

95. Wijdicks EF, Vermeulen M, Hijdra A, van Gijn J. Hyponatremia and

cerebral infarction in patients with ruptured intracranial aneurysms: is fluid restriction harmful? *Ann Neurol* 1985;17:137–140.

96. Nishioka H, Torner JC, Graf CJ, Kassell NF, Sahs AL, Goettler LC. Cooperative study of intracranial aneurysms and subarachnoid hemorrhage: a long term prognostic study. II. Ruptured intracranial aneurysms managed conservatively. *Arch Neurol* 1984;41:1142–1146.

97. Torner JC, Kasell NF, Wallace RB, Adams HP Jr. Preoperative prognostic factors for rebleeding and survival in aneurysm patients receiving antifibrinolytic therapy: report of the cooperative aneurysm study. *Neurosurgery* 1981;9:506–513.

98. Torner JC, Nibbelink DW, Burmeister LF. Statistical comparisons of end results of a randomized treatment study. In: Sahs AL, Nibbelink DW, Torner JC, eds. *Aneurysmal Subarachnoid Hemorrhage: Report of the Cooperative Study.* Baltimore: Urban and Schwarzenberg, 1981: 249–276.

99. Nibbelink DW. Antihypertensive and antifibrinolytic therapy following subarachnoid hemorrhage from ruptured intracranial aneurysm. In: Sahs AL, Nibbelink DW, Torner JC, eds. *Aneurysmal Subarachnoid Hemorrhage: Report of the Cooperative Study.* Baltimore: Urban and Schwarzenberg, 1981;287–296.

100. Wijdicks EF, Vermeulen M, Murray GD, Hijdra A, van Gijn J. The effects of treating hypertension following aneurysmal subarachnoid hemorrhage. *Clin Neurol Neurosurg* 1990;92:111–117.

101. Perret GE, Nibbelink DW. Randomized treatment study: carotid ligation. In: Sahs AL, Nibbelink DW, Torner JC, eds. *Aneurysmal Subarachnoid Hemorrhage: Report of the Cooperative Study.* Baltimore: Urban and Schwarzenberg, 1981;121–143.

102. Taylor W, Miller JD, Todd NV. Long-term outcome following anterior cerebral artery ligation for ruptured anterior communicating artery aneurysms. *J Neurosurg* 1991;74:51–54.

103. Kassell NF, Torner JC, Adams HP Jr. Antifibrinolytic therapy in the acute period following aneurysmal subarachnoid hemorrhage: preliminary observations from the Cooperative Aneurysm Study. *J Neurosurg* 1984;61:225–230.

104. Pinna G, Pasqualin A, Vivenza C, Da Pian R. Rebleeding, ischemia and hydrocephalus following anti-fibrinolytic treatment of ruptured cerebral aneurysms: a retrospective clinical study. *Acta Neurochir* 1988;93:77–87.

105. Tsementzis SA, Hitchcock ER, Meyer CH. Benefits and risks of antifibrinolytic therapy in the management of ruptured intracranial aneurysms: a double-blind placebo-controlled study. *Acta Neurochir* 1990; 102:1–10.

106. Wijdicks EF, Hansan D, Lindsay KW, Brouwers PJ, Hatfield R, Murray GD, van Gijn, Vermeulen M. Short term tranexamic acid treatment in aneurysmal subarachnoid hemorrhage. *Stroke* 1989;20:1674–1679.

107. Casasco AE, Aymard A, Gobin YP, Houdart E, Rogopoulos A, George B, Hodes JE, Cophignon J, Merland JJ. Selective endovascular treatment of 71 intracranial aneurysms with platinum coils. *J Neurosurg* 1993;79:3–10.

108. Fernandez-Zubillaga A, Guglielmi G, Vinuela F, Duckwiler GR. Endovascular occlusion of intracranial aneurysms with electrically detachable coils: correlation of the aneurysm neck size and treatment results. *AJNR* 1994;15:815–820.

109. Guglielmi G, Vinuela F, Duckwiler GR, Dion J, Lylyk P, Berenstein A, Strother C, Graves V, Halbach V, Nichols D, et al. Endovascular treatment of posterior circulation aneurysms by electrothrombosis using electrically detachable coils. *J Neurosurg* 1992;77:515–524.

110. Haley EC Jr, Kassell NF, Torner JC. The International Cooperative Study on the Timing of Aneurysm Surgery: the North American experience. *Stroke* 1992;23:205–214.

111. Longstreth WT Jr, Nelson LM, Koepsell TD, van Belle G. Clinical course of spontaneous subarachnoid hemorrhage: a population-based study in King County, Washington. *Neurology* 1993;43:712–718.

112. Cook DA. Mechanisms of cerebral vasospasm in subarachnoid hemorrhage. *Pharmacol Therapeut* 1995;66:259–284.

113. Ehrenreich H, Schilling L. New developments in the understanding of cerebral vasoregulation and vasospasm: the endothelin–nitric oxide network. *Clev Clin J Med* 1995;62:105–116.

114. Macdonald RL, Weir BKA. A review of hemoglobin and the pathogenesis of cerebral vasospasm. *Stroke* 1991;22:971–982.

115. Heros RC, Zervas NT, Varsos V. Cerebral vasospasm after subarachnoid hemorrhage: an update. *Ann Neurol* 1983;14:599–608.

116. Rajshekhar V, Harbaugh RE. Results of routine ventriculostomy with external ventricular drainage for acute hydrocephalus following subarachnoid hemorrhage. *Acta Neurochir* 1992;115:8–14.

117. van Gijn J, Hijdra A, Wijdicks EF, Vermeulen M, van Crevel H. Acute hydrocephalus after aneurysmal subarachnoid hemorrhage. *J Neurosurg* 1985;63:355–362.

118. Vassilouthis J, Richardson AE. Ventricular dilatation and communicating hydrocephalus following spontaneous subarachnoid hemorrhage. *J Neurosurg* 1979;51:341–351.

119. Black PM. Hydrocephalus and vasospasm after subarachnoid hemorrhage from ruptured intracranial aneurysms. *Neurosurgery* 1986;18: 12–16.

120. Sundaram MB, Chow F. Seizures associated with spontaneous subarachnoid hemorrhage. *Can J Neurol Sci* 1986;13:229–231.

121. Crowell RM, Gress DR, Ogilvy, Kistler JP. Principles of management of subarachnoid hemorrhage: general management. In: Ratcheson RA, Wirth FP, eds. *Ruptured Cerebral Aneurysms: Perioperative Management.* Baltimore: Williams and Wilkins, 1994;59–76.

122. Cioffi F, Pasqualin A, Cavazzani P, Da Pian R. Subarachnoid haemorrhage of unknown origin: clinical and tomographical aspects. *Acta Neurochir* 1989;97:31–39.

123. Nishioka H, Torner JC, Graf CJ, Kassell NF, Sahs AL, Goettler LC. Cooperative study of intracranial aneurysms and subarachnoid hemorrhage: a long term prognostic study. III. Subarachnoid hemorrhage of undetermined etiology. *Arch Neurol* 1984;41:1147–1151.

124. Gilbert JW, Lee C, Young B. Repeat cerebral pan-angiography in subarachnoid hemorrhage of unknown etiology. *Surg Neurol* 1990; 33:19–21.

125. Forster DMC, Steiner L, Hakanson S, Bergvall U. The value of repeat pan-angiography in cases of unexplained subarachnoid hemorrhage. *J Neurosurg* 1978;48:712–716.

126. Friedman AH. Subarachnoid hemorrhage of unknown etiology. In: Wilkins RH, Rengachary SS, eds. *Neurosurgery. Update II.* New York: McGraw-Hill, 1991;73–77.

127. Kopitnik TA, Samson DS. Management of subarachnoid hemorrhage. *J Neurol Neurosurg Psychiatry* 1993;56:947–959.

128. Rinkel GJE, Wijdicks EFM, Vermeulen M, Hageman LM, Tans JTJ, van Gijn J. Outcome in perimesencephalic (nonaneurysmal) subarachnoid hemorrhage: a follow-up study in 37 patients. *Neurology* 1990; 40:1130–1132.

129. Van Calenbergh F, Plets C, Goffin J, Velghe L. Nonaneurysmal subarachnoid hemorrhage: prevalence of perimesencephalic hemorrhage in a consecutive series. *Surg Neurol* 1993;39:320–323.

130. Adams HP Jr, Gordon DL. Nonaneurysmal subarachnoid hemorrhage (editorial). *Ann Neurol* 1991;29:461–462.

131. Rinkel GJE, Wijdicks EFM, Vermeulen M, Hasan D, Brouwers PJ, van Gijn J. The clinical course of perimesencephalic nonaneurysmal subarachnoid hemorrhage. *Ann Neurol* 1990;29:463–468.

Cerebrovascular Disease, edited by H. Hunt Batjer.
Lippincott-Raven Publishers, Philadelphia © 1997.

CHAPTER **73**

Intracranial Aneurysm: Surgical Principles

Ralph G. Dacey

Care of the aneurysm patient requires an optimal combination of pre-, intra-, and postoperative management. Decisions made prior to surgery affect intraoperative events and different strategies may be chosen during surgery to reduce postoperative complications. Therefore it is somewhat arbitrary to separate surgical care from other aspects of care. Nonetheless, surgical technique is of critical importance in the achievement of good results.

The goal of aneurysm surgery is to obliterate the aneurysm while preserving flow through the parent vessels and the perforators arising from them. This goal can be achieved with little difficulty in a small aneurysm with a simple and pliant neck. It may be much more difficult in a giant lesion where thrombus and calcification make clipping more complicated. Meticulous attention to technique during aneurysm surgery is essential in order to prevent rebleeding and preserve cerebral perfusion.

OPERATIVE EQUIPMENT

The operative microscope makes surgery for intracranial aneurysms safe and effective. It provides magnification, stereoscopic perspective, and ample illumination to the constricted surgical fields developed by dissection of the basal subarachnoidal cisterns (1). A counterbalanced stand allows unimpeded motion of the microscope and stability during microdissection (1). Most surgeons find it useful to project the operative view through a video monitor so that the scrub nurse can follow and anticipate events during microdissection.

The operative field, retractors, microscope, and surgeon's hands must remain stable relative to one another during surgery, necessitating complete head immobilization by a three-point skeletal fixation pin head holder. Microsurgical linked-socket-type retractors are in turn affixed to the table or head holder to provide steady, gentle brain retraction.

R. G. Dacey: Department of Neurosurgery, Washington University School of Medicine, Saint Louis, Missouri 63110.

Many surgeons sit on a hydraulically controlled mobile stool and rest their hands or wrists on the patient's head or the retractor ring for comfort and to remove large, proximal motor units in the surgeon's arms from microsurgical movement. The field and microscope must be in position and configuration such that the surgeon is comfortable during the microdissection.

Microsurgical instruments vary according to the surgeon's preference. The most important instruments are the bipolar forceps, suction tips, and microscissors. Diamond knives, dissecting spatulas, and hooks in various shapes are also available. Most surgeons use a small number of instruments and become very familiar with their use in a variety of situations. Curved suction tips with thumb slots to precisely control suction force are essential to protect perforators and cranial nerves. Fenestrated and blunt tips allow the suction to be used to gently retract tissue, placing appropriate tension on arachnoidal bands so that they can be cut sharply.

In recent years a large variety of aneurysm clips have become available in many sizes and configurations. Yasargil, Sugita, and Sundt clips all have features that may be advantageous in various operative situations, and many surgeons maintain an inventory of different clip combinations for specific situations. Often one type of clip will be needed for a particular type of aneurysm, and if tandem clipping is necessary several identical clips will be required.

ANESTHETIC CONSIDERATIONS

Anesthetic considerations in the management of intracranial aneurysms are discussed in detail in Chapter 26. It is critical that the neurosurgeon communicate effectively with the anesthesiologist to produce optimal conditions for successful aneurysm clipping.

Electrophysiologic monitoring, including compressed spectral array, electroencephalogram (EEG), somatosensory evoked potentials, and brainstem evoked potentials, are used on a selective basis depending on the neurophysiologic systems to be assessed in the vascular territory at risk (2). The use of the compressed spectral assay/EEG is helpful in determining the dosage requirements for the induction of burst suppression should temporary occlusion be necessary in the course of the procedure. Decisions regarding the use of neurophysiologic monitoring should be discussed with the anesthesiologist prior to surgery. In selected patients where ventriculostomy is not indicated, a spinal drain placed in the lumbar theca can be effective in aiding with brain relaxation. Mannitol, 0.5–1 g/kg body weight, is administered with the skin incision with a small dose of Lasix. After the aneurysm has been clipped, fluids are administered to produce a state of euvolemia or mild hypervolemia, extending into the postoperative period. For this reason, placement of a Swan–Ganz catheter is often desirable, especially in older patients or patients with significant cardiopulmonary dysfunction.

During the initial portion of the craniotomy, the anesthesiologist and surgeon must communicate regarding the conditions of the brain during dissection and retraction. Should the surgeon elect to use temporary arterial occlusion in the management of the aneurysm, a modest rise in the mean arterial pressure should be induced by the anesthesiologist, and burst suppression is induced by the administration of propofol or etomidate (3,4). Although no randomized studies have proven that such pharmacologic management of temporary occlusion is helpful, significant experimental and clinical data support this practice.

THE PTERIONAL APPROACH

Most cerebral aneurysms can be approached by the pterional approach or modifications of it. This surgical corridor allows microdissection of aneurysms involving the internal carotid artery, anterior cerebral artery, middle cerebral artery, and basilar apex. Extensions of the approach can expose proximal A2 segment-ACA (anterior cerebral artery) aneurysms and aneurysms extending to the midbasilar artery region. Midline and right-sided lesions are generally accessed via a right pterional approach in patients with left cerebral dominance. Exceptions to this include certain basilar artery aneurysms and aneurysms of the anterior communicating artery region associated with a dominant left A1 segment.

Precise positioning of the patient will facilitate optimal surgical exposure with minimal brain retraction. In general, the head should be rotated approximately 15° to 45° to the contralateral side. For anterior communicating aneurysms, more head rotation is required. Aneurysms of the basilar apex and middle cerebral artery require less rotation. Minimal temporal retraction is required when the degree of rotation is optimal to expose aneurysms at different sites (5). The neck is flexed somewhat to the contralateral side and the head is extended to place the maxillary eminence as the highest point on the properly positioned patient. Three-point skeletal fixation headrest (either the Mayfield Keys or Radiolucent Headholder for intraoperative angiography) is then used to fix the patient's position. The head should be placed just slightly above the heart to enhance venous return.

A skin incision is made behind the patient's hairline extending to the midline. The incision extends from the level of the zygomatic process of the temporal bone, in close proximity to the ear to avoid injury to the frontalis branch of the facial nerve. It is usually necessary to divide the anterior branch of the superficial temporal artery; however, the posterior branch should be preserved for extracranial–intracranial (ECIC) anastomosis in this case. After hemostatic galeal clips are applied in a way that preserves the superficial temporal artery, the scalp flap is rotated somewhat anteriorly, and the temporalis muscle and fascia are divided so the anterior aspect of the muscle can be reflected anteriorly with the skin flap. This protects and preserves the frontalis branch of the facial nerve and usually leads to less postoperative atrophy of the anterior aspect of the temporalis muscle. As the scalp flap is rotated anteriorly, fishhooks are applied over a folded laparotomy sponge.

As the pterion is exposed, the uppermost portion of the fronto-zygomatic process is dissected down to the orbital rim. Three burr holes are usually sufficient to allow adequate bone dissection. One hole is made in the keyhole, one in the temporal fossa above the temporal zygomatic process, and one just above the superior temporal line posteriorly. It is usually not necessary to place a burr hole on the forehead as this may lead to an undesirable cosmetic deformity. It is essential that the anterior-most cut be low at the level of the floor of the frontal fossa. Occasionally, the frontal sinus will be entered during this portion of the bone dissection. If this occurs, the mucosa should be carefully removed from the bone flap. A vascularized flap of pericranium is then reflected down to seal the opening into the sinus. Using the rongeurs, a subtemporal craniectomy and resection of the lateral third of the sphenoid wing is then performed. This dissection can also be done or augmented with the high-speed cutting burr (6).

Once hemostasis has been achieved in the extradural plane, a crescent-shaped incision is made in the dura, extending from the frontal to the temporal regions, across the Sylvian fissure. The dura is then tented up over the modified contour of what is left of the sphenoid wing so as to provide unimpeded observation of the basal cisterns. At this point, it is essential that some brain relaxation be achieved. Often a spinal drain placed in the lumbar theca can be opened to drain cerebrospinal fluid and further augment brain relaxation. This serves the added purpose of obviating continuous aspiration of cerebrospinal fluid with the sucker tip. In patients with significant hydrocephalus or those with a temporal mass lesion, the anterior horn of the lateral ventricle can be drained with a ventriculostomy tube inserted through the middle or superior frontal gyrus at the posterior medial aspect of the craniotomy opening. This is often an effective maneuver to obtain brain relaxation in a patient undergoing early surgery who has a tight, swollen brain.

The microscope is then brought into position and used for

the remainder of the procedure. The exposed brain is covered with surgical sponge and dissection of the Sylvian fissure is initiated. For most anterior circulation and basilar artery aneurysms approached by the pterional route, it is usually most efficient to begin the dissection laterally by incising the superficial arachnoid, just medial to the superficial middle cerebral vein with the diamond knife. The bipolar forceps are then used to spread and coagulate small veins that traverse the Sylvian fissure in this region. There is variability in the ease with which the Sylvian fissure can be opened at this point, but the M2 branches of the middle cerebral are quickly identified and dissection is continued to expose the M1 segment of the middle cerebral artery. For middle cerebral artery aneurysms, care must obviously be taken at this point in the dissection, but it is usually not necessary to conduct the dissection from proximal to medial because proximal control can easily be obtained after the fissure has been widely opened. For large middle cerebral artery aneurysms, the fundus of the aneurysm often impedes the surgeon's view of the proximal middle cerebral artery if the fissure is opened medially, and therefore a wide opening of the Sylvian fissure starting laterally is usually the safest and the most efficient means of initiating the dissection.

At this point, the blade of the microsurgical retractor can be gently placed on the inferior surface of the frontal lobe to visualize the optic nerve and proximal internal carotid artery. The dissection is continued across the proximal portion of the Sylvian cistern and into the cistern of the lamina terminalis. Wide dissection of the basal cisterns in this manner is desirable, somewhat irrespective of the site of the aneurysm, because more effective and less traumatic brain retraction can be achieved in this way. The surgeon should gently advance the frontal retractor and maintain a consciousness of the degree of retraction throughout the entire procedure. Firm, but gentle retraction is usually all that is required. At the medial aspect of the Sylvian cistern there is often a vein that traverses the proximal-most aspect of the Sylvian fissure. This vein can usually be safely coagulated and divided. It is often not necessary to separate the branches of the superficial middle cerebral vein from their attachment to the sphenoparietal sinus. In situations where the temporal lobe needs to be retracted to a greater extent, these veins can usually be divided safely after their thorough coagulation. A certain amount of stress relaxation occurs due to the viscoelastic characteristics of the brain, and it is often possible to decrease the gentle retraction pressure as the dissection continues.

Aneurysms at the apex of the basilar artery can be approached via the pterional trans-Sylvian approach through a number of terminal access intervals. Often the configuration of the carotid artery and its branches will facilitate approach through the carotico-ophthalmic interval. In other cases, the carotico-optic interval provides the most suitable avenue of approach. In a few cases, the basilar apex can be approached above the carotid bifurcation and the proximal portion of the A1 segment. The membrane of Liliequist is divided sharply to reveal the termination of the basilar artery. The choice of the pterional, subtemporal, or other approaches to intracranial aneurysms must be carefully planned as part of the preoperative evaluation of the patient (6).

MICRODISSECTION AND PREPARATION FOR CLIP PLACEMENT

Once the Sylvian, carotid, and lamina terminalis cisterns have been opened widely and adequate brain relaxation is achieved, microsurgical dissection focuses on preparing the aneurysm for clip placement. The subarachnoid cisterns containing the aneurysm, parent vessels, and perforators are opened using sharp dissection. The blunt suction tip held in the nondominant hand can be used to manipulate the arachnoid to allow sharp dissection with the microscissors, diamond knife, or beaver blade. Dissection should generally begin on the parent vessel proximal to the aneurysm. The arachnoid and appropriate branches and perforators should be dissected so as to prepare a position on the parent vessel proximally for the placement of a temporary clip should it be needed.

For many aneurysms of the proximal internal carotid artery (ophthalmic artery aneurysms, superior hypophyseal artery aneurysms, carotid cave aneurysms), it will be desirable to isolate the internal and external carotid arteries in the cervical region. Although it is possible to obtain proximal control by placing a temporary clip proximal to the distal dural ring or in the intrapetrous section of the artery, the most straightforward approach to obtaining proximal control is isolation of the cervical vessels (7). A suction decompression device described by Batjer and Samson is also useful and can be inserted in the cervical internal carotid artery to provide retrograde decompression of a proximal carotid artery aneurysm after temporary carotid occlusion (8).

In aneurysms of the anterior communicating artery, one A1 segment is frequently larger than the other. If the larger A1 segment is on the nondominant hemisphere side, then proximal control can easily be obtained upon opening of the lamina terminalis cistern, with care being taken to avoid damage to or temporary occlusion of the recurrent artery of Heubner or other perforators arising from this segment. If the larger A1 segment is present on the dominant hemisphere side, then proximal control can be established either by making the operative approach to the dominant hemisphere or by carrying the exposure of the lamina terminalis cistern contralaterally to the A1 segment, opposite the side of approach. This may be difficult for aneurysms that project anteriorly in the region of the chiasm and/or limbus sphenoidale.

Proximal control can usually be easily established for aneurysms of the middle cerebral artery bifurcation. Large aneurysms in this region may obscure the proximal artery immediately adjacent to the neck of the aneurysm, but with patient dissection the aneurysm fundus can be manipulated to observe the proximal vessel. Again, care must be taken here not to injure small perforating vessels arising from the distal M1 or M2 segments. A site for temporary occlusion should also be prepared when approaching aneurysms of the basilar apex. When using the pterional approach, aneurysms whose necks are at the level of or below the posterior clinoid process may be difficult to establish a site for temporary vessel occlusion and the establishment of proximal control. In these cases, the subtemporal approach will often afford a visualization of the more proximal segment of the basilar artery just below the origin of the superior cerebellar arteries, or the interventional radiologists may be called on to insert a temporary balloon in the midbasilar artery via the transfemoral route. In cases where the patient has been prepared for intraoperative angiography, this adds relatively little to the complexity of the procedure and can be a useful adjunct. In aneurysms of the vertebral artery, a far lateral cervicomedullary approach (9,10) can be used to establish proximal control. Here dissection involves separating medullary perforators and rootlets of the ninth, tenth, and eleventh nerves from the artery to allow temporary clip placement.

Once the cisterns surrounding the proximal parent vessel have been opened and preparations made for the application of a temporary clip, attention should be turned to the distal parent artery and/or branches arising in close proximity to the aneurysm. Dissection of these vessels should begin at a position some distance away from the fundus and distal neck. Again, a relatively wide opening of the cistern is important to allow appropriate observation of perforators and distal branches arising near the neck and fundus of the aneurysm. Positions for the later placement of a temporary clip should also be considered on the distal branches at this point in the dissection. In some situations, establishing control of the efferent vessels is more difficult than others. The distal supraclinoid internal carotid artery and the posterior communicating artery and anterior choroidal artery or arteries are relatively easily identified. The distal neck of ventrally projecting aneurysms in this region may abut the anterior choroidal artery and require meticulous dissection from the aneurysm fundus. Exposure of the A2 segments distal to anterior communicating artery aneurysms is facilitated by opening the interhemispheric fissure after some resection of the gyrus rectus. The ipsilateral and then contralateral A2 can then usually be identified at a site somewhat distal to the apex of the aneurysmal fundus. It is sometimes difficult to separate efferent branches of the M2 segments from the fundus and neck of the middle cerebral artery aneurysm. Sometimes the distal M1 segment is aneurysmal and the dissection and reconstruction of aneurysms of this type can be challenging. The efferent P1 and P2 segments adjacent to basilar apex aneurysms are often easily visualized and dissected on the side ipsilateral to the operative approach. However, especially with the subtemporal approach, visual-

ization of the contralateral P1 and P2 segments may be difficult. Gentle manipulation of the aneurysm fundus with a blunt suction tip and/or dissectors may aid in the dissection of this vessel. Similarly, it may be somewhat difficult to adequately visualize and therefore dissect the vertebral artery and basilar artery distal to vertebral artery-PICA (posterior inferior cerebellar artery) and vertebral confluence aneurysms.

Aneurysms of the proximal carotid artery often require extensive microsurgical bone removal prior to successful clip application (Fig. 1) (11). This is true of aneurysms arising at the ophthalmic artery and superior hypophyseal artery aneurysms. The dura overlying the lateral portion of the planum sphenoidale and roof of the optic canal should be incised. The incision should then be extended in a semilunar

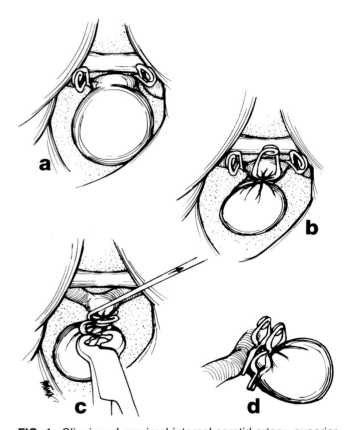

FIG. 1. Clipping of proximal internal carotid artery–superior hypophyseal artery aneurysm. **A:** The anterior clinoid process and medial sphenoid wing have been removed with a high-speed diamond bit drill. Temporary clips are placed proximal and distal to the neck. An initial straight aneurysm clip is placed across the neck of the aneurysm. It was not possible to place a clip parallel to the main axis of the parent vessel. **B:** The aneurysm is noted to still fill after this primary clip application. **C:** A blunt, right angle hook is placed behind the medial-most aspect of the neck of the aneurysm and a secondary straight fenestrated clip is placed across the medial-most aspect of the aneurysm neck, reinforcing it. **D:** Note that the fenestrated clip reinforces the medial-most aspect of the aneurysm neck.

fashion to the tip of the anterior clinoid process lateral to the internal carotid artery and aneurysm fundus. The dura is then stripped form the anterior clinoid process and using the high-speed diamond bit drill, the anterior clinoid process is removed. Care must be taken to initially and carefully unroof the optic canal and then resect the falciform fold of dura over the optic nerve. Attention can then be turned to the anterior clinoid process itself, which is removed with the high-speed diamond bit drill. Usually its last connection is to the optic strut, which separates the superior orbital fissure from the optic canal. The optic strut must be carefully removed down to a position somewhat beneath the optic nerve to allow adequate exposure of the anterior loop of the internal carotid artery. At this point, the dural dissection is continued and the distal dural ring is opened to reveal the clinoidal segment of the internal carotid artery. For most aneurysms in this region, this degree of bone resection will provide adequate exposure. The fundus of the superior hypophyseal artery aneurysm must then be separated for the medial most aspect of the cavernous sinus in the carotid cave. This will allow the development of a plane for the proximal clip jaw application in a position beneath the anterior loop of the internal carotid artery. Clip application prior to adequate dissection of the dura and bone in this region can be fraught with complications.

Once the afferent and efferent vessels have been controlled and provision made for the application of temporary clips, attention is turned to the dissection of the arachnoidal planes around the fundus and neck of the aneurysm. By using either the blunt-tipped suction or a dissector, the parent artery and aneurysmal fundus can be manipulated gently to allow the use of the scissors or arachnoid knife to sharply develop the plane between the aneurysm fundus and the surrounding vessels. Blunt dissection should generally be avoided because it is associated with significant complications when intraoperative rupture of the aneurysm occurs (12). Unless the plane between surrounding vessels and the neck of the aneurysm requires no significant dissection, it is generally advisable to begin the separation of surrounding branches and the wall of the parent vessel from the midportion of the fundus, carefully developing the plane and extending the dissection proximal on the fundus to the neck of the aneurysm, thereby separating it from associated branches. For most nongiant aneurysms, gentle manipulation of the vessels and aneurysm fundus will allow adequate visualization of surrounding branches and perforators and allow the surgeon to develop a plane around the neck of the aneurysm for passage of a smooth dissector to simulate passage of the aneurysm clip blade. Once a free plane has been established to allow placement of the aneurysm clip with little traction or tension on the fundus or surrounding vessels, the neck is ready to accept a clip. Since most aneurysms arise distal to a branch just after a curve in the artery (13), the fundus is usually closely associated with branches and these must be separated from the neck and fundus of the aneurysm prior to satisfactory clipping.

Intraoperative rupture sometimes complicates surgery for intracranial aneurysms. Reports of this complication have ranged from 15% to 50%, with most surgeons reporting rates in the 15–20% range. If the occurrence of this complication prevents satisfactory clip application resulting in injuries to surrounding parent vessels or emerging branches, the neurologic morbidity and mortality for the procedure is significantly elevated (12,14). Aneurysm ruptures that occur prior to dissection, such as with the induction of anesthesia or the opening of the craniotomy, are difficult to manage and have been associated with a high mortality. Batjer and Samson (12) and Giannotta et al. (14) have proceeded with an emergent operative procedure in patients who had rupture of the intracranial aneurysm during the induction of anesthesia. Three of their eight patients made a good recovery after this ''rescue clipping.''

Batjer and Samson (12) reported that most of their intraoperative ruptures occurred during dissection of the aneurysm or clip application. Aneurysmal ruptures were more common and associated with greater morbidity if they were due to blunt dissection. Aneurysmal rents, in these cases, tended to be larger and associated with more profuse hemorrhage. Intraoperative ruptures complicating sharp dissection were usually much easier to handle and were not associated with significantly more neurologic morbidity.

A variety of strategies are available to manage an intraoperative aneurysm rupture. Rapid application of a clip in a suboptimal fashion in this situation should be avoided. Such an application in the absence of adequate dissection and visualization of surrounding branches, the aneurysm neck, and perforators may result in worse morbidity. The surgeon should use two suctions initially to clear the operative field of blood, locate the rent, and place a suction immediately adjacent to the rent to allow adequate visualization during subsequent maneuvers. The surgeon should then place a cottonoid over the aneurysmal rent and tamponade the aneurysmal fundus. If this maneuver is initially effective in controlling the hemorrhage, continued sustained pressure for several minutes will often allow removal of the cottonoid without the recurrence of a hemorrhage. If the aneurysmal rent is large and tamponade does not rapidly control the situation, temporary clips should be placed on the afferent and efferent vessels, with care being taken to prevent injury to surrounding perforators and other structures. The blood pressure should then be elevated approximately 10% by the anesthesiologist during the period of temporary occlusion (see below). The use of hypotension as a means of managing intraoperative hemorrhage should generally be avoided. Giannotta et al. (14) reported that, in their experience, the use of hypotension during the management of an intraoperative rupture was associated with poor neurologic outcomes. Once temporary clips have been applied, the slack aneurysm fundus can be manipulated and the aneurysmal rent visualized. The clip can then be placed proximally on the neck to occlude the aneurysm. Occasionally it is necessary to place one or two microsutures when the aneurysmal rent extends

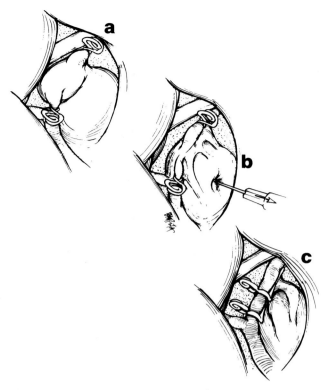

FIG. 2. Tandem clipping for large internal carotid artery aneurysm. **A:** temporary clips are applied to the proximal and distal internal carotid artery. The aneurysm is then aspirated **(B)** with a Flamm scalp vein needle apparatus. **C:** right angle curved fenestrated Fujita clips are then placed in tandem along the length of the broad aneurysm neck.

into the parent vessel. The repair is then completed with the application of an aneurysm clip.

Adequate dissection and clip application with large globular or thick-walled aneurysms often requires decompression of the aneurysm fundus. A variety of techniques have been reported. Batjer and Samson (8) advocated the use of suction applied to a catheter inserted in the cervical internal carotid artery for retrograde decompression of ophthalmic segment aneurysms after temporary cervical carotid artery occlusion. Flamm (15) advocated the use of a butterfly scalp vein needle attached to suction to decompress the aneurysm during the final portions of dissection and clip application (Fig. 2). Temporary balloon occlusion introduced by a transfemoral route has been used in the management of carotid and basilar artery aneurysms where proximal temporary clipping was not feasible (16,17).

MANAGEMENT OF THROMBUS AND CALCIFICATION

Partial thrombosis often occurs in large and giant cerebral aneurysms. The Italian Cooperative Study (4) found that 48% of aneurysms with diameters between 2 and 2.5 cm

had partial, subtotal, or total thrombosis. For aneurysms greater than 22.5 cm in maximal dimension, the incidence of thrombosis was 76% (18). The presence of intraluminal thrombosis often makes manipulation of the aneurysm during dissection more difficult because the aneurysm fundus is less pliant and its mass prevents adequate mobilization during dissection. Similarly, during subsequent clip application, the relatively rigid fundus and neck of the aneurysm may force the clip jaws down on the parent vessel, thereby occluding the lumen. For this reason, it is usually necessary to open the aneurysm fundus and remove the thrombus from such aneurysms prior to definitive clip application (Fig. 3). Significant thrombosis occurs most frequently in large or giant aneurysms of the internal carotid and middle cerebral arteries. Control of the afferent and efferent circulation should be obtained as described above. Often the mass of the aneurysm will make the last portions of the dissection somewhat difficult, and complete dissection may have to wait until the aneurysm has been at least partially decompressed. Very large aneurysms with multiple layers of laminated thrombus may be opened prior to the application of temporary clips thereby decreasing the total duration of local circulatory arrest. The ultrasonic aspirator is frequently a helpful adjunct in rapidly removing the thrombus from the aneurysm fundus. When the filling lumen of the aneurysm is reached during this type of dissection, temporary clips can be applied. For smaller aneurysms where the resection of the thrombus will be extremely quick, temporary clips are applied just prior to incising the fundus of the aneurysm. It is important that a careful and complete removal of the thrombus be performed, especially in the neck of the aneurysm. If residual thrombus were to be present on the intimal surface of the reconstructed lumen of the parent vessel, the risk of distal embolization would exist. Similarly, the surgeon must make sure that a smooth, nonduplicated intimal surface remains after the complete removal of thrombus. This sometimes requires partial resection of intramural atheroma (see below). Once a satisfactory intimal surface has been assured, the parent vessel can be reconstituted using the clip application methods described below.

Atheroma in the neck of a cerebral aneurysm will often cause similar problems with definitive clip application (19). A calcified, irregular, and thick aneurysm neck will usually not readily accept a clip and the clip jaws may be deflected either proximally encroaching on the parent lumen or distally on the aneurysm fundus producing suboptimal aneurysm obliteration. The incidence of calcification was 19% in a series of large and giant aneurysms reported by Rosta et al. (4). If calcification and atheroma are extensive enough to preclude satisfactory clip positioning, the surgeon has two options. One is to apply temporary clips, open the aneurysm, and perform an aneurysmectomy. Sufficient atheroma and calcification are removed, usually from one side of the aneurysm neck, to allow satisfactory positioning of the clip. Alternatively, the surgeon may elect to prepare the site of a clip application by placing a hemostat across the neck of the

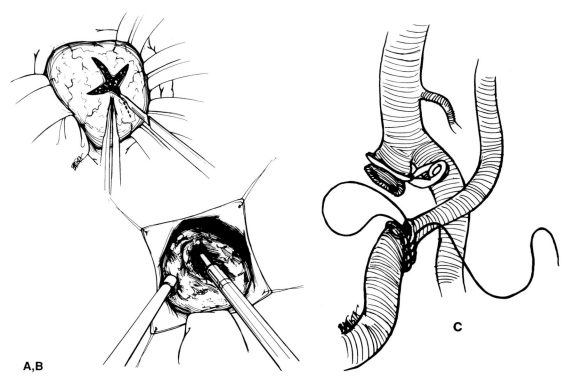

A,B

C

FIG. 3. A: A giant thrombosed middle cerebral artery aneurysm is exposed by dividing the Sylvian fissure. A cruciate incision is made in the wall of the fundus of the aneurysm. **B:** Traction sutures are placed on the wall and the ultrasonic aspirator is used to remove laminated clot from within the fundus of the aneurysm. **C:** The residual origin of the aneurysm (arising from the superior division of the middle cerebral artery) is clipped after the aneurysm fundus has been resected. The superior division, which had been amputated from the base of the aneurysm, is then anastomosed end to end to the anterior temporal branch of the middle cerebral artery.

aneurysm and partially crushing the atheroma in such a way as to make the neck accept eventual permanent clip application. This latter maneuver carries the risk of damaging the neck and parent vessel and the risk of introducing embolic material into the distal territory of the parent artery. Nonetheless, it may be an effective maneuver in selected circumstances.

Occasionally, calcification in the neck of a smaller and otherwise uncomplicated aneurysm will prevent satisfactory opposition of the clip jaws and cause persistent filling of the aneurysm in circumstances where the surgeon has determined that the jaws of the clip completely encompass the neck of the aneurysm. Tandem clips may be helpful in this situation.

TEMPORARY ARTERIAL OCCLUSION

Temporary vessel occlusion is often a helpful adjunct in the management of somewhat large and/or complex aneurysms (3). As mentioned above, it is frequently critical in the management of a large intraoperative aneurysm rupture. Temporary clips have closing pressures of <70 g. In studies of endothelial injury, the extent of clip-related endothelial

damage is somewhat less extensive than that seen with balloon-occluded vessels. Temporary vessel occlusion can be associated with interruption of somatosensory evoked potentials, but if the period of occlusion is relatively short, these abnormalities are not usually manifest as permanent neurologic deficits. A variety of cerebral protective agents have been advocated for use during temporary arterial occlusion and aneurysm surgery. Volpentol and propofol have been administered, in addition to vitamin C, mannitol, and diphenylhydantoin. The most common agent used is etomidate administered to induce burst suppression (6 to 8 bursts per minute) (3,20). Some authors have advocated the use of pressors to elevate systemic arterial pressure during the period of temporary occlusion (20). These pharmacologic maneuvers, although not proven to be effective, appear to be associated with a small incidence of permanent neurologic deficit.

Care should be taken in gently applying the temporary clip to the normal vessel. The perforating vessels, such as the recurrent artery of Huebner, the lenticulostriate branches of the A1 and M1 segments, and perforators related to the basilar artery, should be carefully spared as the temporary clips are applied. Often, curved clips or clips applied with angled pistol-grip appliers may be helpful in assuring that the head of the clip does not obscure the surgeons view or access for definitive permanent clip application. If the aneurysm is to be opened or in cases of intraoperative rupture, both the efferent as well as the afferent arteries should be clipped to prevent impairment of perfusion of the distal territory of the parent vessel. Temporary arterial occlusion using balloon catheters introduced via a transtemporal approach has been described as an adjunct in the treatment of basilar artery aneurysms (16).

Durations of temporary clipping up to 90 minutes have been reported. Batjer and Samson have indicated that a gradient of tolerance to temporary occlusion exists with up to 60 minutes of internal carotid artery occlusion, 35 minutes of middle cerebral artery occlusion, 19 minutes of upper basilar artery occlusion, 4-½ minutes of lower basilar artery occlusion, having been well tolerated by their patients (21). There is some controversy about whether intermittent temporary vessel occlusion should be used. Conflicting data from experimental animals exist on this point at the present time (22). In aneurysms where more than 20 minutes of temporary arterial occlusion can be predicted, circulatory arrest with profound hypothermia may be a useful technique. Large basilar apex lesions are the most frequent lesions treated by this set of techniques (23).

STRATEGIES FOR DEFINITIVE CLIP APPLICATION

When an aneurysm clip is placed across the neck of an aneurysm, the walls of the neck of the lesion are opposed in such a way that flowing blood is excluded from the aneurysmal fundus. Exclusion of flowing blood from the fundus of the aneurysm removes the hemodynamic stresses on the aneurysm fundus, which result in hemorrhage. In addition, the external application of the clip to the dilated neck of the aneurysm serves to reconstitute the normal arc of curvature of the parent vessel so that the hoop stress in the vessel is distributed over an arc with a smaller radius than was present under the circumstances where the aneurysm was growing. In this way, clipping is fundamentally different than an endovascular approach, such as the use of detachable coils since the small residual, unclipped portion of the neck continues to have a configuration that had been associated with growth of the aneurysm prior to its treatment (Fig. 4).

An aneurysm clip must have sufficient force to withstand the hemodynamic sheer stress at the orifice of the aneurysm and the forces that tend to expand the vessel in a radial fashion with each cardiac cycle. Minimal clip occlusive forces are a function of several variables including the length of the neck of the aneurysm, the transmural pressure to which the aneurysm is exposed, and the width of the clip blade (24). Therefore, minimal clip occlusive forces vary depending on the configuration of the aneurysm. A small, thin-walled aneurysm with a narrow neck arising at the origin of the calloso-marginal branch of the anterior cerebral artery might

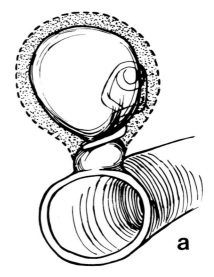

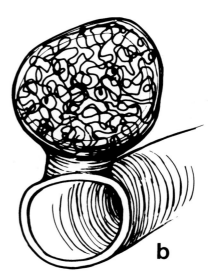

FIG. 4. Residual aneurysm neck. **A:** In this schematic view of the theoretical aneurysm, a clip is placed across the neck of the aneurysm. Some residual neck of the aneurysm persists, proximal to the clip jaws. A similar situation exists in **(B)** where a detachable coil has been placed in the fundus of the aneurysm, again leaving some residual neck. Both of these situations are not optimal but may be necessary in certain situations for technical reasons. In (A) the walls of the neck of the aneurysm are brought together by the aneurysm clip in contrast to the situation in (B). This configuration may be more stable and less likely to result in proximal aneurysm regrowth (see text for discussion).

be satisfactorily occluded with a very small aneurysm clip having a closing force of less than 200 g. In contrast, a large, thick-walled ophthalmic artery aneurysm with a long, broad-based neck might require the application of several strong tandem clips having forces exceeding 400 g and supplemented by booster clips. In general, large proximal carotid artery aneurysms tend to require aneurysms with higher clip-closing forces than smaller, more distally placed aneurysms.

Currently available aneurysm clips are manufactured in a variety of shapes, lengths, and configurations with a corresponding variety of clip-closing forces. Clip-closing forces diminish as one proceeds more distally along the clip blades away from the hinge, or base, of the clip (Fig. 10) (25). Clip application strategies therefore must take this into account. If a high clip-closing pressure is required at a significant distance from the base of the clip, the primary clip application may need to be supplemented with either a tandem clip to augment the closing force or the application of a booster clip (26,27). Several examples of strategies that can be effective are illustrated below.

In general, the surgeon should attempt to place the aneurysm clip blades parallel to the long axis of the neck of the aneurysm along the parent vessel wall. For some aneurysms, such as a posterior communicating artery aneurysm (Fig. 5), satisfactory clipping of the aneurysm can be accomplished by placing the clip blades perpendicular to the long axis of the internal carotid artery. The length of the clip blade to be applied to the aneurysm should be carefully estimated by the surgeon. The length of the clipped neck will be about 20–30% longer than the diameter of the unclipped aneurysm fundus, but care should be taken to avoid excessive clip blade lengths because they may damage perforators or adjacent neural structures. In tight microsurgical quarters, such as the approach to a basilar apex aneurysm, longer clips may

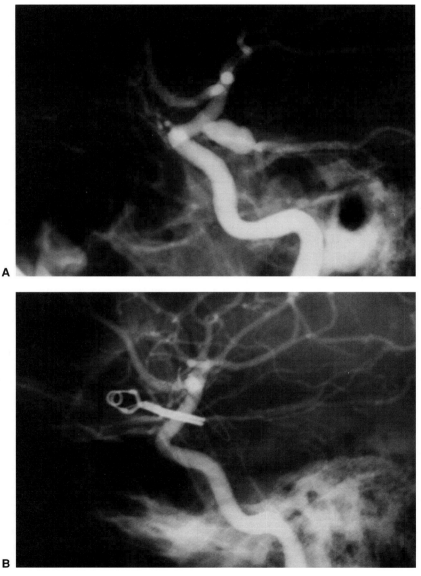

FIG. 5. Internal carotid artery aneurysm at the posterior communicating artery before **(A)** and after **(B)** clip application. Note that the clip in this situation is perpendicular to the long axis of the parent vessel. The configuration and narrow neck of the aneurysm make this clip application satisfactory.

use of a fenestrated clip is for ventrally projecting aneurysm of the internal carotid artery (1,14), such as those occurring at the superior hypophyseal arteries or posterior carotid wall aneurysm, where right angle fenestrated clips are applied so the aperture of the clip encompasses the internal carotid artery (Figs. 2 and 7) (28). The medially convex curvature of the supraclinoid internal carotid artery is matched by the curved clip blades of some right angle fenestrated clips to provide a more anatomic reconstitution of the normal configuration of the parent vessel while producing lower sheering forces (Figs. 2 and 7).

It is often necessary to apply multiple clips to an aneurysm neck or fundus to satisfactorily obliterate the aneurysm. Such tandem clip applications can be used to augment the closing force or the length over which the closing force is exerted in various clip application situations. For example, for a large ventrally projecting internal carotid artery aneurysm, right angle fenestrated clips can be applied in tandem so that sufficiently high clip closing forces can be exerted over the entire length of the neck (Fig. 2). Depending on the locations of the origin of the branches, right angle fenestrated clips can be applied in opposing directions (Figs. 7 and 8). Fenestrated clips with larger apertures can be used to place the blades of the clip below (more distal in the fundus) the primary clip blades to reinforce the clip construct. Straight aneurysm clips can also be placed in tandem fashion. A fenestrated straight clip may be used immediately adjacent to a primarily placed nonfenestrated straight clip to supplement clip closing forces in the distal-most portion of the neck (Fig. 1). This is often a helpful maneuver when the aneurysm fills despite an apparently adequate initial clip placement. Alternatively, as noted by Samson and Batjer (5), the use of a small, short, nonfenestrated straight clip in tandem fashion will obliterate residual small filling of the neck immediately adjacent to the clip spring (Fig.1). Occasionally, the placement of multiple tandem clips will be necessary to satisfactorily obliterate large, thick-walled aneurysms (Fig. 7). When a primary clip is placed very close to the neck of an aneurysm, it is possible for the clip to occlude the parent vessel, if the wall of the aneurysm neck is thick or if atheroma is present in the parent vessel immediately adjacent to the aneurysm. In this situation, a tandem clip can be placed immediately distal to the primary clip to satisfactorily obliterate the aneurysm and the initial clip can then be removed, thereby permitting adequate filling of the parent vessel. A similar problem can occur when a straight clip is used to obliterate an aneurysm with "dog ears," which extend on either side of the neck of an aneurysm arising in a major bifurcation, such as at the anterior communicator or middle cerebral artery site. The use of a long bayonetted clip or shank clip, as advocated by Osawa, Obinata, Kobayashi, and Tanaka (29), can often be a satisfactory solution to this problem. The apex of the shank of the clip accommodates the main channel of the parent vessel while the angled clip blades, proximal and distal to the main angle of the clip,

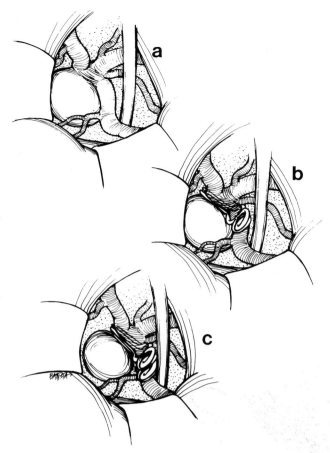

FIG. 6. A: A large, somewhat globular basilar apex aneurysm is exposed via a pterional trans-Sylvian approach. The thalamoperforating trunks arising from the P-1 segments are seen bilaterally. **B:** An initial fenestrated straight clip is placed across the neck of the aneurysm with the fenestration encompassing a portion of the neck of the aneurysm and the P-1 segment. **C:** A second shorter fenestrated clip is then placed across the more proximal portion of the neck of the aneurysm to completely obliterate it.

need to be used and may need to be applied with pistol grip appliers to better visualize the tips of the clip during clip application. The various complex shapes and configurations of today's aneurysm clips are of great advantage to the surgeon, but the simplest straight clip that can be applied to an aneurysm is generally the best one.

When a major parent vessel or branch lies between the surgeon and the neck of the aneurysm, a fenestrated or aperture clip, as originally devised by Drake, is often extremely useful. Care must be taken to assure that the portion of the aneurysm fundus that lies within the aperture is completely clipped. Often straight, smaller clips can be used to supplement the clipping of this portion of an aneurysm. The commonest application of fenestrated clips are with the use of a straight, fenestrated clip for aneurysms of the basilar apex, where the aperture includes the ipsilateral P1 segment of the posterior cerebral artery (Fig. 6). The other most frequent

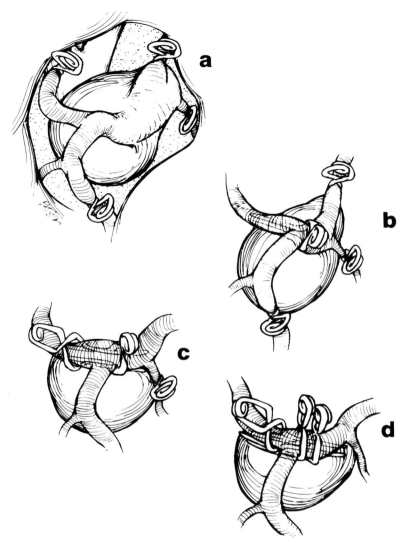

FIG. 7. Sequential tandem clipping of complex distal internal carotid artery aneurysm. **A:** Temporary clips are applied to the proximal internal carotid artery, posterior communicating artery, middle cerebral artery, and A-1 segment of the anterior cerebral artery. **B:** An initial curved right angle fenestrated Fujita clip is placed on the distal neck beneath the A-1 segment of the anterior cerebral artery. **C:** A second curved, right angle fenestrated Fujita clip is placed over the proximal neck with the clip blades beneath the internal carotid artery just distal to the posterior communicating artery. **D:** A third permanent right angle fenestrated clip is placed to reinforce the area where the heels of the two primary clips are in close apposition.

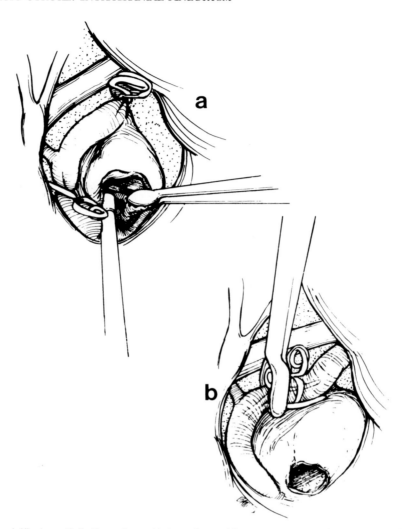

FIG. 8. A: A calcified, partially thrombosed internal carotid artery aneurysm is exposed. After temporary clips are applied on the internal carotid artery proximally and distally, the aneurysm fundus is opened and atherothrombotic plaque removed from the lateral-most wall of the aneurysm neck using blunt dissectors and forceps. **B:** right angle fenestrated Fujita clips are then placed across the neck of the aneurysm.

obliterate the lobes of the aneurysm, extending above and below the bifurcation (Fig. 9).

Intraoperative angiography has proved to be very useful in assessing appropriate clip placement for intracranial aneurysms (30,31). Because residual aneurysm or aneurysm rests are to be avoided (32), intraoperative angiography serves the dual purpose of demonstrating adequate filling of the parent vessels and their branches as well as assuring satisfactory obliteration of the aneurysm. In general, the right femoral artery is prepared with the placement of a sheath after induction of general anesthesia. After clip application, the angiographer then accesses the previously placed sterile draped sheath and performs the arteriogram with digital C-

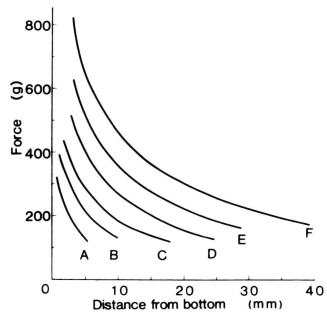

FIG. 10. Relationship between aneurysm clip closing force and distance from the bottom of the clip. As one procedes greater distances from the base of the clip, clip closing force decreases.

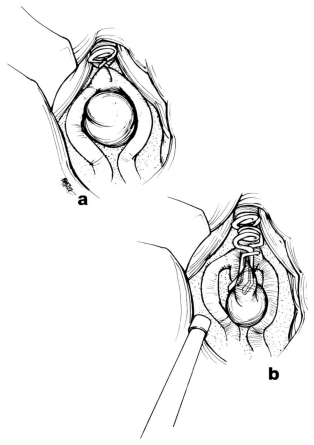

FIG. 9. "Shank clipping" of middle cerebral artery bifurcation aneurysm. **A:** The Sylvian fissure has been opened and a temporary clip has been placed across the M-1 portion of the middle cerebral artery. The "dog ear" of the aneurysm extends toward the surgeon, perpendicular to the plane of the M-2 branches. **B:** In order to clip this portion of the aneurysm as well as the neck of the aneurysm between the two M-2 branches, a superbayonetted Sundt clip is placed across the neck of the aneurysm. The shank of the bayonet clip encompasses that part of the aneurysm that projects toward the surgeon. Note that a small portion of the proximal-most aneurysm neck lies proximal to the clip blades. Attempts to place the clips more proximally on the neck resulted in kinking of the superior division of the middle cerebral artery.

arm fluoroscopic equipment. If clip placement is not optimal, the clip can be repositioned and the angiogram repeated. A number of authors have described the advantages of this approach and have indicated that in a small but significant number of cases, changes were made in the operative management based on the intraoperative angiography. Further refinements of the use of this technique will depend on appropriate preoperative criteria for the selection of patients who might most benefit from the use of this technique (30,31).

REFERENCES

1. Yasargil MG, ed. *Microneurosurgery. vol II. Clinical Considerations, Surgery of the Intracranial Aneurysms and Results.* New York: Thieme Stratton, 1987.
2. Friedman WA, Chadwick GM, Verhoeven FJ, Mahla M, Day AL. Monitoring of somatosensory evoked potentials during surgery for middle cerebral artery aneurysms. *Neurosurgery* 1991;29:83–88.
3. Batjer HH, Frankfurt AL, Purdy PD, Smith SS, Samson DS. Use of etomidate, temporary arterial occlusion, and intraoperative angiography in surgical treatment of large and giant cerebral aneurysms. *J Neurosurg* 1988;68:234–240.
4. Rosta L, Battaglia R, Pasqualin A, Beltramello A. Italian cooperative study on giant intracranial aneurysms: 2. Radiological data. *Acta Neurochir Suppl* 1988;42:53–59.
5. Samson DS, Batjer HH. *Intracranial Aneurysm Surgery: Techniques.* New York: Futura, 1990.
6. Yasargil MG, Fox JL, Ray MW. The operative approach to aneurysms of the anterior communicating artery. In: Krayenbuhl H, et al., eds. *Advances and Technical Standards in Neurosurgery.* vol 2. New York; Springer-Verlag, 1975;113–168.
7. Tanaka Y, Kobayashi S, Kyoshima K, Sugita K. Multiple clipping technique for large and giant internal carotid artery aneurysms and complications: angiographic analysis. *J Neurosurg* 1994;80:635–642.

8. Batjer HH, Samson DS. Retrograde suction decompression of giant paraclinoidal aneurysms. Technical note. *J Neurosurg* 1990;73: 305–306.

9. Baldwin HZ, Miller CG, van Loveren HR, Keller JT, Daspit CP, Spetzler RF. The far lateral/combined supra- and infratentorial approach. A human cadaveric prosection model for routes of access to the petroclival region and ventral brain stem. *J Neurosurg* 1994;81: 60–68.

10. Heros RC. Lateral suboccipital approach for vertebral and vertebrobasilar artery lesions. *J Neurosurg* 1986;64:559–562.

11. Day AL. Aneurysms of the ophthalmic segment. A clinical and anatomical analysis. *J Neurosurg* 1990;72:677–691.

12. Batjer HH, Samson DS. Intraoperative aneurysmal rupture: incidence, outcome, and suggestions for surgical management. *Neurosurgery* 1986;18:701–707.

13. Rhoton AL, Saeki N, Perlmutter D, Zeal A. Microsurgical anatomy of common aneurysm sites. *Clin Neurosurg* 1979;26:248–306.

14. Giannota SL, Oppenheimer JH, Levy ML, Zelman V. Management of intraoperative rupture of aneurysm without hypotension. *Neurosurgery* 1991;28:531–536.

15. Flamm ES. Suction decompression of aneurysms. Technical note. *J Neurosurg* 1981;54:275–276.

16. Mizoi K, Yoshimoto T, Takahashi A, Ogawa A. Direct clipping of basilar trunk aneurysms using temporary balloon occlusion. *J Neurosurg* 1994;80:230–236.

17. Shucart WA, Kwan ES, Heilman CB. Temporary balloon occlusion of a proximal vessel as an aid to clipping aneurysms of the basilar and paraclinoid internal carotid arteries. Technical note. *Neurosurgery* 1990;27:116–119.

18. Atlas SW, Grossman RI, Godberg HI, Hackney DB, Bilaniuk LT, Zimmerman RA. Partially thrombosed giant intracranial aneurysms: correlation of MR and pathologic findings. *Radiology* 1987;162:111–114.

19. Hylton PD, Reichman OH. Endoneurysmal microendarterectomy in the treatment of giant cerebral aneurysms: technical note. *Neurosurgery* 1988;23:674–679.

20. Rosenwasser RH, Jimenez DF, Wending WW, Carlsson C. Routine use of etomidate and temporary vessel occlusion during aneurysm surgery. *Neurol Res* 1991;13:224–228.

21. Samson D, Batjer HH, Bowman G, Mootz L, Krippner WJ Jr, Meyer YJ, Allen BC. A clinical study of the parameters and effects of temporary arterial occlusion in the management of intracranial aneurysms. *Neurosurgery* 1994;34:22–28.

22. Steinberg GK, Panahian N, Sun GH, Maier CM, Kunis D. Cerebral damage caused by interrupted, repeated arterial occlusion versus uninterrupted occlusion in a focal ischemic model. *J Neurosurg* 1994;81: 554–559.

23. Richards PG, Marath A, Edwards JM, Lincoln C. Management of difficult intracranial aneurysms by deep hypothermia and elective cardiac arrest using cardiopulmonary bypass. *Br J Neurosurg* 1987;1:261–269.

24. Rosenbaum TJ, Sundt TM Jr. Interrelationship of aneurysm clips and vascular tissue. *J Neurosurg* 1978;48:929–934.

25. Atkinson Jl, Anderson RE, Piepgras DG. A comparative study in opening and closing pressures of cerebral aneurysm clips. *Neurosurgery* 1990;26:80–85.

26. Sundt TM Jr, Piepgras DG, Marsh WR. Booster clips for giant and thick based aneurysms. *J Neurosurg* 1984;60:751–762.

27. Sundt TM Jr. *Surgical Techniques for Saccular and Giant Intracranial Aneurysms.* Baltimore: Williams and Wilkins, 1990.

28. Fujita, S. Fenestrated clips for internal carotid artery aneurysms. Technical note. *J Neurosurg* 1986;65:122–123.

29. Osawa M, Obinata C, Kobayashi S, Tanaka Y. Newly designed bayonet clips for complicated aneurysms: technical note. *Neurosurgery* 1995; 36:425–426.

30. Martin NA, Bentson J, Vinuela F, Hieshima G, Reicher M, Black K, Dion J, Becker D. Intraoperative digital subtraction angiography and the surgical treatment of intracranial aneurysms and vascular malformations (see comments). *J Neurosurg* 1990;73:526–533.

31. Derdeyn CP, Moran CJ, Cross DT, Grubb RL Jr, Dacey RG Jr. Intraoperative digital subtraction angiography: a review of 112 consecutive examinations. *AJNR* 1995;16:307–318.

32. Lin T, Fox AJ, Drake CG. Regrowth of aneurysm sacs from residual neck following aneurysm clipping. *J Neurosurg* 1989;70:556–560.

Cerebrovascular Disease, edited by H. Hunt Batjer.
Lippincott-Raven Publishers, Philadelphia © 1997.

CHAPTER 74

Endovascular Treatment of Intracranial Aneurysms

Joseph H. Introcaso and Antoine Uské

Endovascular treatment of intracranial aneurysms began in 1973, with the use of detachable latex balloons by Serbenenko (1). These were used primarily for parent artery occlusion, but selective aneurysm occlusion with preservation of the parent artery was also performed in selected cases. Refinements in the design of latex balloons and development of silicone detachable balloons improved the technique of parent artery occlusion and allowed further attempts at selective endovascular occlusion of intracranial aneurysms (2–5).

However, the inability of balloons to conform to the shape of the lumen of the aneurysm and the forces they exert on the aneurysm wall limited the success of this technique for selective occlusion of intracranial aneurysms (5–7). Detachable balloons remain the principle therapeutic device in performing endovascular parent artery occlusion and in the treatment of cavernous-carotid fistulae (8).

Development of a wide variety of shapes and sizes of fibered platinum microcoils made further attempts at selective endovascular occlusion of aneurysms possible (9,10). The relatively unpredictable and uncontrollable nature of deployment of these types of coils made the final outcome of these cases uncertain. Selective occlusion of intracranial aneurysms made a very significant advance with the development of electrolytically detachable coils (Guglielmi detachable coils, GDCs) (11), which may be repositioned or withdrawn prior to final deployment. This technique made coil occlusion of intracranial aneurysms safer and more predictable than could be achieved with standard fibered platinum microcoils. Several types of mechanically detachable coils are now also available; however, they remain investiga-

tional devices in the United States (12). These devices provide a greater degree of control than the standard fibered microcoils, but somewhat less than the GDC system.

Several liquid embolic agents for selective occlusion of intracranial aneurysms are currently in the early stages of laboratory testing and one has been tested in humans in Japan (13–15). Non-resorbable materials, such as cellulose acetate polymer (CAP) dissolved in dimethyl sulfoxide (DMSO), can be injected directly into the aneurysm during flow arrest within the parent artery. These materials rapidly solidify and flow can be restored within the parent artery in several minutes. The possibility of completely occluding an aneurysm with a nonresorbable material which conforms to the lumen of the aneurysm is one of the most promising methods for endovascular treatment of intracranial aneurysms in the future. However, many technical problems must be overcome before this technique can be applied to general clinical practice.

The possibility of aneurysm treatment using stents has also been explored with regard to sidewall aneurysms (16–20); however, this technique is not currently applicable for the treatment of bifurcation aneurysms. Once again, technical limitations involving stent deployment, flexibility, and wall coverage have limited the success of this approach to the treatment of intracranial aneurysms. Rapid progress in the development of newer types of covered stents provides the greatest hope for future progress of this technique.

PARENT ARTERY OCCLUSION

Frequently aneurysms involving the petrous and cavernous segments of the internal carotid arteries are fusiform in nature or have very wide necks, making them unsuitable for selective endovascular occlusion (Fig. 1A, B). Surgical approaches to these lesions are often difficult, even in the hands of the most experienced surgeon. In these cases, the

J. H. Introcaso: Department of Radiology, Northwestern University Medical School, Northwestern Memorial Hospital, Chicago, IL 60611.

A. Uské: Department of Radiology, University of Lausanne, Centre Hopitalier Universitaire Vaudois, Lausanne, Switzerland CH-1011.

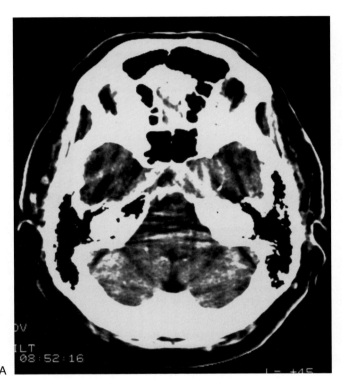
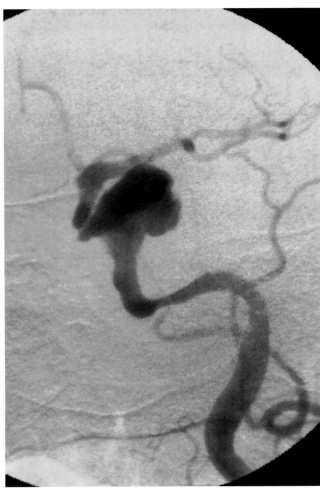

FIG. 1. Fusiform aneurysm involving the petrous and cavernous portion of the internal carotid artery. The patient is a 72-year-old woman who presented to her primary care physician with diplopia and the CT scan **(A)** shown above was obtained. This demonstrates a crescentic ring of calcification bordering a slightly high attenuation mass involving the left cavernous sinus. An angiogram was then performed **(B)**, which revealed a giant fusiform aneurysm of the petrous and cavernous portion of the left internal carotid arteries. After passing a balloon occlusion test, this patient was treated by parent artery sacrifice using latex balloons to occlude the left internal carotid artery.

treatment of choice is endovascular occlusion of the internal carotid artery (parent artery occlusion), following functional testing (balloon occlusion test) to demonstrate the adequacy of collateral circulation. If the balloon occlusion test demonstrates inadequate or marginal cerebral perfusion through collateral pathways, a surgical bypass procedure may be performed prior to sacrifice of the parent vessel (4). This strategy is also applicable to aneurysms involving the posterior circulation (21).

Endovascular occlusion of large arteries, such as the internal carotid artery, is most quickly and easily achieved using detachable balloon devices. Balloons may be made of either latex (Nycomed, Paris, France) or silicone (Interventional Therapeutics Corporation, Freemont, California). These devices are available in a wide variety of shapes and sizes, with valve mechanisms fabricated by either the manufacturer

or the operator. The physical properties of the two types of balloons vary significantly. Latex balloons require relatively high inflation pressures and do not allow diffusion across their wall. Therefore, they may be inflated with a mixture of contrast material and will not change in size following detachment, given proper function of the valve mechanism. However, silicone balloons allow diffusion across their wall and thus must be inflated with either isotonic solution or, preferably, a polymerizing substance (2-hydroxyethyl-methyl methacrylate, HEMA), to avoid a change in size over time following detachment (22). The amount of force required to detach the balloon is variable for both types of devices. This is determined by the manufacturer, the catheter on which the balloon is mounted, or the technique of fabrication utilized by the operator (''hand-tied'' balloons). The regulatory status of these devices in the United States remains unclear at this time, making availability and use difficult in the current health care environment.

Metallic coils may also be used for large vessel occlusion. Coils were first utilized by Gianturco et al and were intended for use in medium-sized vessels, such as renal arteries and the mesenteric circulation (23). These were delivered through a catheter by pushing them with a guide wire. Yang et al refined the design, making coils suitable for delivery through a microcatheter system for occlusion of smaller vessels (24). Today many different types of coils are currently available from several manufacturers in almost every conceivable shape and size. Most commonly, the metallic framework of the coil is made of a platinum alloy to ensure magnetic resonance imaging (MRI) compatibility. Dacron fibers are frequently attached to the metallic framework of the coil to increase thrombogenicity. Several types of coils have been developed, which may be repositioned prior to final deployment. These designs do not incorporate Dacron fibers and are principally intended for selective endovascular occlusion of intracranial aneurysms. However, they may be useful in parent artery occlusion in cases where optimal control of coil size and position is required. The attributes of these detachable coil systems will be discussed further with regard to selective endovascular occlusion of intracranial aneurysms.

Functional Testing

Assessment of adequacy of the collateral circulation is essential when considering parent vessel occlusion (4). This begins with a complete selective diagnostic arteriogram including cross-compression views, providing information about the integrity of the circle of Willis and the presence of congenital anatomic variants. Anatomic information obtained will not only help to plan the endovascular approach but will also allow planning of possible surgical bypass procedures if the patient fails trial balloon occlusion.

The balloon occlusion test is performed under full anticoagulation monitored by activated clotting times (ACTs). A non-detachable balloon catheter is placed under road map guidance into the vessel to be occluded. Often a double-lumen catheter is utilized to allow monitoring of distal stump pressures, as well as infusion of heparinized saline distal to the balloon within the occluded segment. Care must be taken to limit the rate of saline infusion because this may influence the result of the occlusion test by dilution of flow from collateral pathways. The balloon is inflated to occlude flow in the vessel and serial clinical neurologic examinations are performed. The balloon remains inflated for a period of at least 30 minutes or until a neurologic deficit is observed. Several groups have advocated a period of ''hypotensive challenge'' during this period of observation in an effort to increase the sensitivity of the test to marginal levels of perfusion. Many additional methods of monitoring have been advocated as adjuncts to clinical examination (25–27).

These include electroencephalography (EEG), quantitative xenon CT, positron emission tomography (PET), single photon emission computed tomography (SPECT), and, more recently, functional MRI perfusion studies (fMRI). All of these techniques can increase the reliability of balloon occlusion test results, but also may increase risk to the patient through lengthened procedure times and movement of the patient from one examination table to another with a balloon catheter within a critical vessel. The cost and availability of these monitoring modalities may also pose a problem, especially with regard to PET. Currently, protocols for monitoring during balloon occlusion testing vary widely between centers and practitioners.

When the balloon occlusion test results in a clinical neurologic deficit, placement of a high-flow bypass graft (saphenous vein graft) may be considered for flow augmentation prior to parent artery sacrifice. However, the situation of a marginal quantitative monitoring test without clinical deficit or a questionable clinical finding poses a more difficult therapeutic decision. In these cases a relatively low-flow bypass procedure, such as a superficial temporal artery bypass, may be considered prior to proceeding with definitive parent artery occlusion.

SELECTIVE ANEURYSM OCCLUSION

The current standard for selective endovascular occlusion of intracranial aneurysms is the GDC system (28). The concept behind this system includes the principles of both electrothrombosis and electrolysis. Several studies have demonstrated that negatively charged blood elements (red blood cells, white blood cells, platelets, and fibrinogen) will migrate to the positive electrode off an electrical circuit, thus promoting thrombosis (29–31). Platinum proved to be many times more thrombogenic in this electrical circuit than stainless steel (32). Electrolysis comes into play at the detachment zone of the coil, where it is attached to the delivery wire. The process of electrolysis is defined as the migration of ions (ie, Fe^{2+}) through an electrolytic solution (ie, blood) from one electrode to another having opposite charge. This results in decomposition of one of the electrodes. Noble metals, such as platinum, do not participate in this process. The system devised by Guglielmi involved the placement of a positively charged platinum electrode into an aneurysm resulting in electrothrombosis while at the same time detaching itself from the delivery device by electrolytic action (11,28). In vitro experiments confirmed the efficacy of electrothrombosis associated with this system; however, further examination revealed minimal effect of electrothrombosis with electrical currents in the 0.5- to 1.0-mA range utilized in humans. Therefore, the goal in selective endovascular occlusion of aneurysms is to fill the lumen as completely as possible with coils, which will result in thrombosis of the aneurysm due to disruption of the flow pattern within the aneurysm. Organization of the thrombus by fibroblasts will provide long-

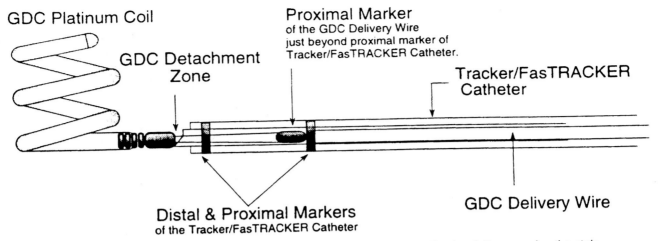

FIG. 2. Guglielmi detachable coil (GDC). Note the small gap in the Teflon insulation covering the stainless steel delivery wire at the detachment zone. (Courtesy of Target Therapeutics Inc., Freemont, California.)

term stability through a dense fibrous network binding the coil mass to the aneurysm, which is functionally excluded from the parent vessel (33). Clearly, this assumes complete packing of the aneurysm with coils.

GDC coils are helical nonfibered platinum alloy coils attached to a stainless steel delivery wire, which is used to control delivery of the coil into the aneurysm. The distal portion of the stainless steel wire is coated with Teflon for electrical insulation, except for a tiny portion of the most distal segment to allow for electrolytic detachment of the platinum coil. Platinum markers are incorporated into the delivery wire and the microcatheter to allow reliable positioning of the detachment zone just beyond the catheter tip (Figs. 2 and 3). These coils are available in diameters varying from 2 mm to 20 mm and lengths from 4 cm to 30 cm. They are also available in four types, which vary in stiffness based on the diameter of the platinum alloy wire utilized in their fabrication. The larger, stiffer coils are used to fabricate a spherical framework. Smaller diameter, softer, pliable coils are then used to pack the central portion of the aneurysm.

GDC Results and Discussion

Over the past 6 years more than 6000 patients with intracranial aneurysms have been treated worldwide using the GDC system. The results have been quite promising. As with any new technology there is a period of learning and refinement of technique (Fig. 4A–G). In addition, as we carefully examine our successes and failures we refine case selection criteria, which will further improve success rates. Although the GDC technique is still in its infancy, we must compare our results with the established clinical standard of surgical clipping, which has proven effectiveness with more than 60 years of experience.

Based on information proveded by Target therapeutics Inc. (Freemont, CA), Tables 1–10 summarize the North American experience with GDCs for the treatment of intracranial aneurysms in the first 735 patients (770 aneurysms). This group was composed of patients who were evaluated by experienced vascular neurosurgeons and felt not to be surgical candidates. Review of these data reveals that "complete" occlusion of the aneurysm is achieved most frequently (87%) in small aneurysms, ≤10 mm (Fig. 5A–D). This is comparable to reported results of surgical clipping by Drake (87% complete occlusion) and Stevens (82.4% complete occlusion) (34,35). However, the GDC technique is less successful with larger aneurysms. Size of the neck of the aneurysm relative to the dome is also a good predictive factor for successful occlusion (36). Aneurysms with narrow necks relative to the aneurysm dome are very suitable for endovascular occlusion with GDC (85% success), whereas wide-necked aneurysms are relatively poor candidates.

Procedure related morbidity of this series is detailed in

TABLE 1. *Number of patients*

Total no.	735
Males	209
Females	526
Mean age	54.5 years
Age range	0.3–90.6 years

TABLE 2. *Number of aneurysms*

Total no.	770
Ruptured aneurysms	370
Hunt & Hess grade I, II, III	296
Hunt & Hess grade IV	52
Hunt & Hess grade V	22
Unruptured aneurysms	400
Symptomatic	352

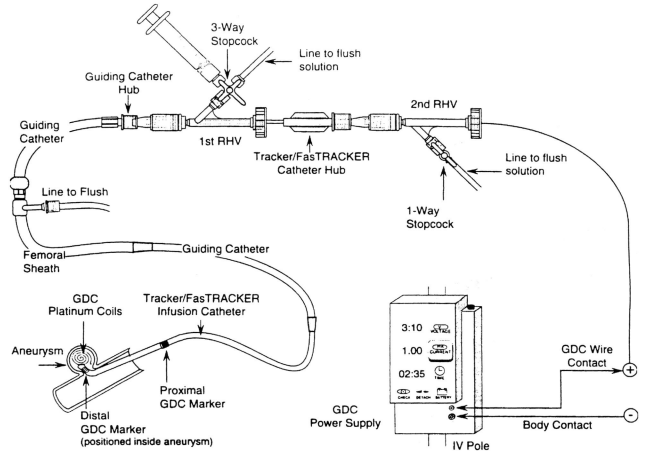

FIG. 3. Diagrammatic representation of the Guglielmi detachable coil delivery system. (Courtesy of Target Therapeutics Inc., Freemont, California.)

Table 8. Morbidity statistics reported represent all patients combined, ie, ruptured aneurysms, symptomatic unruptured aneurysms, and asymptomatic unruptured aneurysms. Total procedure-related morbidity was 8.7%, with 3.8% categorized as severe. Direct comparison to surgical series is difficult due to the mixed patient population. However, these figures are near the range reported for surgical series limited to asymptomatic unruptured aneurysms (3.6–7.3%) (37).

The greatest problem resulting in device-related morbidity was cerebral embolism, experienced in 4.6% of cases. Although thrombolysis may be considered for treatment of distal emboli, even the risk of local catheter-directed thrombolysis is high in the presence of an aneurysm acutely treated with coils. Cerebral emboli have been reduced in part by refinement of the coil detachment zone; however, it appears that case selection is also a significant factor. Higher rates

of distal embolization have been reported in cases of middle cerebral artery aneurysms. Therefore, fewer cases of middle cerebral artery aneurysm will likely be undertaken in the future, without further refinements in the GDC technique.

Intracranial hemorrhage was the second most common problem encountered with GDC treatment, seen in 1.2% of cases. Other problems encountered were parent vessel thrombosis (1.0%), aneurysm perforation (0.5%), and worsening of symptoms related to mass effect (0.5%). Unspecified types of morbidity were encountered in 0.9% of cases. Periprocedural mortality experienced with GDC treatment in unruptured aneurysms (0.9%) is comparable to that reported in surgical series (0.3–2%) (37).

The large majority of patients were treated with a single procedure (80%), whereas some patients (20%) required multiple procedures. Patients required multiple procedures

TABLE 3. *Aneurysm location*

Anterior circulation	60%
Posterior circulation	38%
Other	2%

TABLE 4. *Aneurysm size (dome)*

10 mm or less	51%
11–25 mm	38%
>25 mm	11%

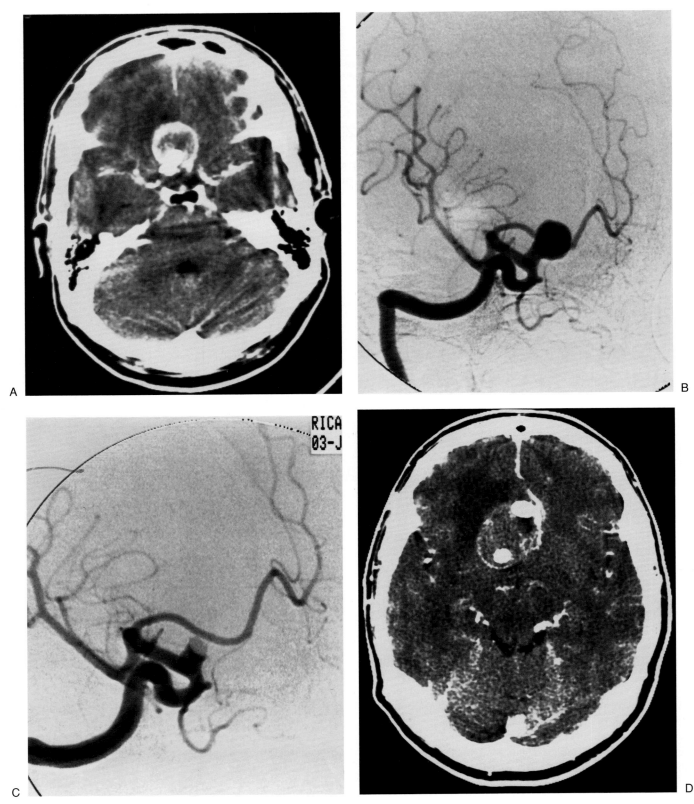

FIG. 4. A–D

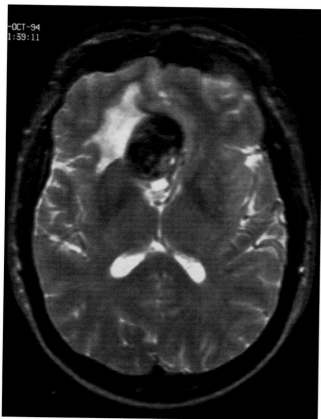

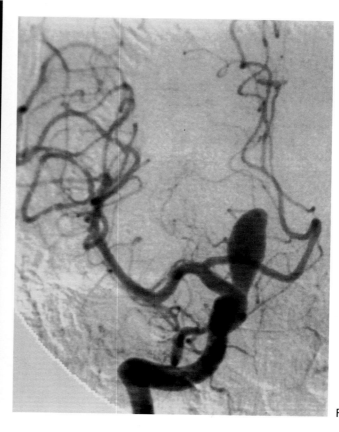

E

F

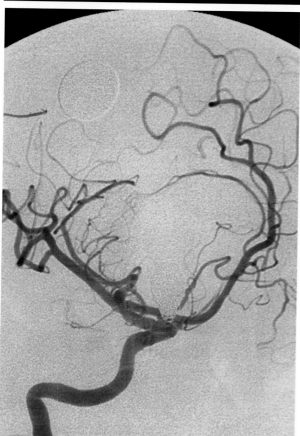

G

FIG. 4. Giant supraclinoid internal carotid artery aneurysm in a young man. **A:** This contrast-enhanced CT scan demonstrated a giant supraclinoid internal carotid artery aneurysm containing considerable mural thrombus. Marked enhancement of the wall of the aneurysm is noted. **B:** Same patient as in 4A. An angiogram was performed, again demonstrating this giant saccular aneurysm. **C:** Same patient. This time the patient declined surgery; instead, endovascular treatment was attempted with placement of a detachable silicone balloon within the lumen of the aneurysm, sparing the parent artery. A significant portion of the neck of the aneurysm remained patent. **D:** Same patient. The patient was lost to follow-up for several years, until he presented again to our Emergency Department following a seizure. He also exhibited signs and symptoms of increasing mass effect. This contrast-enhanced CT scan was obtained. Clearly, the aneurysm has enlarged. The ovoid high attenuation structure adjacent to the anterior cerebral arteries is the silicone balloon, which has migrated to the periphery of the aneurysm. Mild enhancement of the wall of the aneurysm is again noted. The small patent lumen of the aneurysm is posteriorly located. Moderate mass effect is present with displacement of the anterior cerebral arteries to the left and low attenuation within the right frontal white matter. **E:** Same patient. This T2-weighted MRI image demonstrates considerable edema within the white matter of the right frontal lobe surrounding the aneurysm. **F:** Same patient. An angiogram was obtained demonstrating the patent lumen of the aneurysm. **G:** Same patient. The patient again declined surgical treatment and was referred for Guglielmi detachable coil (GDC) therapy. Endovascular occlusion of the aneurysm was performed in two procedures with the final result shown above. At follow-up 3 months after treatment the angiographic appearance was stable. The patient experienced some improvement in symptoms related to mass effect. (Final GDC treatment angiogram courtesy of Dr. Victor A. Aletich, University of Illinois Hospital, Chicago.)

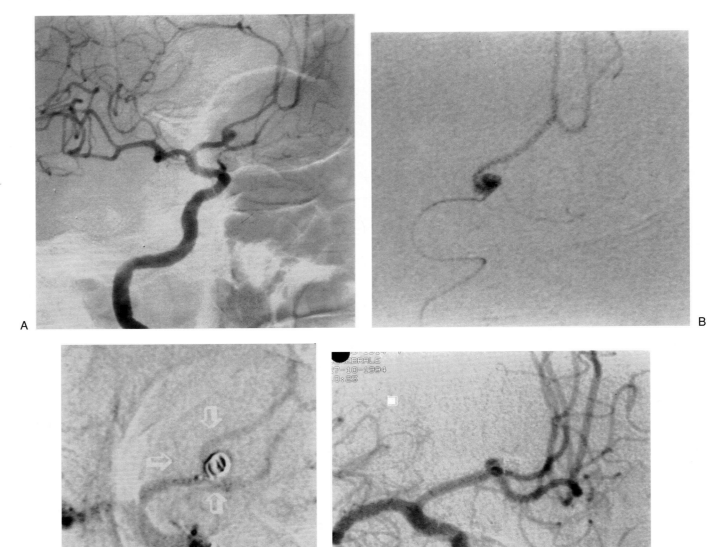

FIG. 5. Anterior communicating artery aneurysm in a 79-year-old woman presenting with subarachnoid hemorrhage (Fisher grade III, Hunt & Hess grade III). **A:** The transorbital oblique projection demonstrated a right anterior communicating artery aneurysm approximately 4 mm in diameter. B: Same patient as in 5A. Due to the patient's history of coronary artery disease she was not considered a surgical candidate. Therefore, endovascular therapy was undertaken using GDC coils 1 day after rupture. A microcatheter was positioned into the aneurysm and the above angiogram performed. **C:** Same patient. This angiogram was performed by injection through the guiding catheter immediately prior to detachment of the first coil. After the procedure she experienced moderate left upper extremity weakness, which fully resolved by postoperative day 4. This was likely due to distal embolization during the procedure. **D:** Same patient. A follow-up angiogram performed 15 months after treatment demonstrated angiographic cure.

TABLE 5. *Aneurysm neck size*

4 mm or less	60%
>4 mm	40%

TABLE 6. *Aneurysm occlusion (90% of dome volume or greater at last follow-up angiogram)*

10 mm or less	87%
11–25 mm	76%
>25 mm	78%

TABLE 7. *Glasgow outcome scale (combination of ruptured and unruptured cohorts at last follow-up)*

Grade I	73%
Grade II	6%
Grade III	3%
Grade IV	1%
Grade V	17%

TABLE 8. *Morbidity: device-related (combination of ruptured and unruptured cohorts)*

	Total	Severe
Cerebral embolism	4.6%	1.5%
Intracranial hemorrhage	1.2%	1.1%
Thrombosis	1.0%	0.14%
Worsening symptoms	0.5%	0.3%
Aneurysm perforation	0.5%	0.3%
Other	0.9%	0.5%
Total	**8.7%**	**3.8%**

TABLE 9. *Mortality*

Patient with *ruptured* aneurysms	
Periprocedural	2.6%
Rehemorrhage after treatment	1.6%
Other cerebrovascular events	6.6%
Total cerebrovascular	**10.8%**
Patient with *unruptured* aneurysms	
Periprocedural	0.9%
Rehemorrhage after treatment	0.9%
Other cerebrovascular events	2.2%
Total cerebrovascular mortality	**4.0%**

TABLE 10. *Hemorrhage*

During treatment	
Ruptured	3.3%
Unruptured	0.94%
After treatment	
Ruptured[a]	3.7%
Unruptured[b]	1.9%

[a] Average length of follow-up 7.3 months.
[b] Average length of follow-up 7.7 months.

due to deliberate staging of treatment, recanalization within the interstices of the coil mass, or continued growth of the aneurysm. Several studies suggest that flow dynamics at the aneurysm neck plays a significant role in recanalization and aneurysm growth, leading to the need for retreatment (38, 39). Specifically, basilar tip and internal carotid bifurcation aneurysms appear to have higher rates of treatment failure due to extreme forces applied at the aneurysm neck by blood flow patterns within the parent vessel. The force of the inflow jet appears to result in either compression of the coils mass or continued growth of the aneurysm adjacent to the coil mass. When aneurysms contain significant amounts of mural thrombus the likelihood of compaction of the coil mass and continued growth of the aneurysm is increased.

The results of the clinical GDC trial demonstrate that selective endovascular coiling of intracranial aneurysms can be performed safely, with acceptable risk of morbidity and mortality. However, we must continue to examine the data to determine if this treatment favorably alters the natural history of the disease over the patient's lifetime. Autopsy studies have demonstrated that the vast majority of aneurysms rupture at the apex of the aneurysm dome (40,41). Therefore, it is postulated that placement of coils within an aneurysm occluding the dome may protect the patient from rupture, despite the possibility of a small portion of the neck remaining patent. Drake et al examined the outcomes of patients with incompletely clipped aneurysms in three reports (42–44). In these series rehemorrhage from incompletely treated aneurysms varied from 21% to 44% with the vast majority of these events being fatal. One series reported in 1987 by Feuerberg et al demonstrated that 17.8% (5 of 28) of incompletely clipped aneurysms demonstrated complete occlusion on follow-up angiograms (45). No change in size of the aneurysm remnant was observed in 46.4% (13 of 28). They estimated the annual risk of rehemorrhage from an incompletely clipped aneurysm to be between 0.38% and 0.79% per year. This suggests less risk than the estimated risk of hemorrhage of an untreated aneurysm (1–5% per year) (37). Although the exact risk of hemorrhage from incompletely treated aneurysms remains controversial, it is clear that the risk is significant. An aneurysm cannot be considered cured unless there is no remnant demonstrated on long-term (1-year) follow-up angiograms. Further study is needed to more closely identify the risk of incompletely treated aneurysms and possible differences in risk with either surgical or endovascular techniques.

One factor often cited as a benefit of surgical aneurysm treatment over endovascular techniques is the ability to remove a blood clot from the subarachnoid space at the time of craniotomy. However, clinical studies have thus far failed to demonstrate a decreased incidence of cerebral vasospasm when blood clots are removed from the cisterns, even when thrombolytic agents are utilized. When symptomatic vasospasm does occur, there may be less risk associated with hypertensive therapy in a patient treated by surgical clipping compared to endovascular coiling, but this remains un-

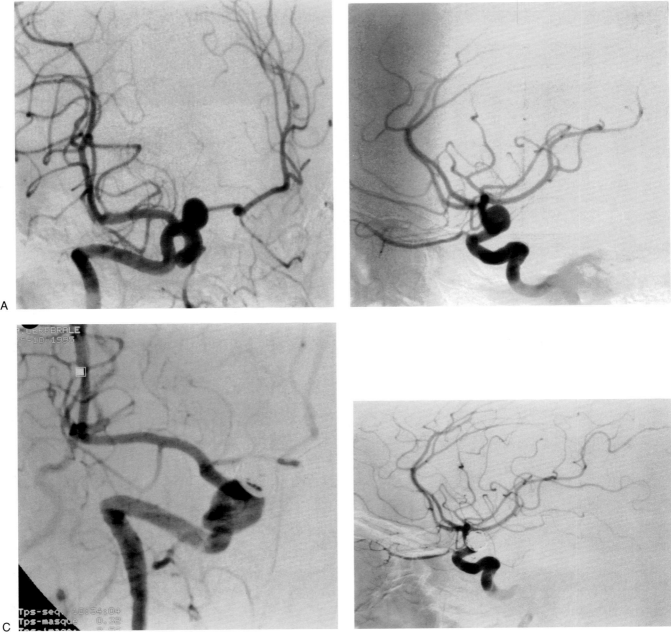

FIG. 6. A, B: Supraclinoid internal carotid aneurysm in a patient with a pituitary macroadenoma. This incidental supraclinoid internal carotid aneurysm was discovered on an MRI examination performed for evaluation of acromegaly and decreased visual acuity in a 51-year-old woman. The presence of a very extensive pituitary macroadenoma influenced the decision to undertake endovascular treatment of this aneurysm (A, frontal projection; B, lateral projection.) **C, D:** Supraclinoid internal carotid aneurysm in a patient with a pituitary macroadenoma; same patient as in 6A and B. Endovascular occlusion of the aneurysm was performed using three Guglielmi detachable coils, without evidence of residual aneurysm. One month later the patient underwent uneventful transsphenoidal resection of the pituitary adenoma. At follow-up examination several months later there was no evidence of recurrent aneurysm. The patient's growth hormone levels and visual acuity had also improved. (C, frontal projection; D, lateral projection.)

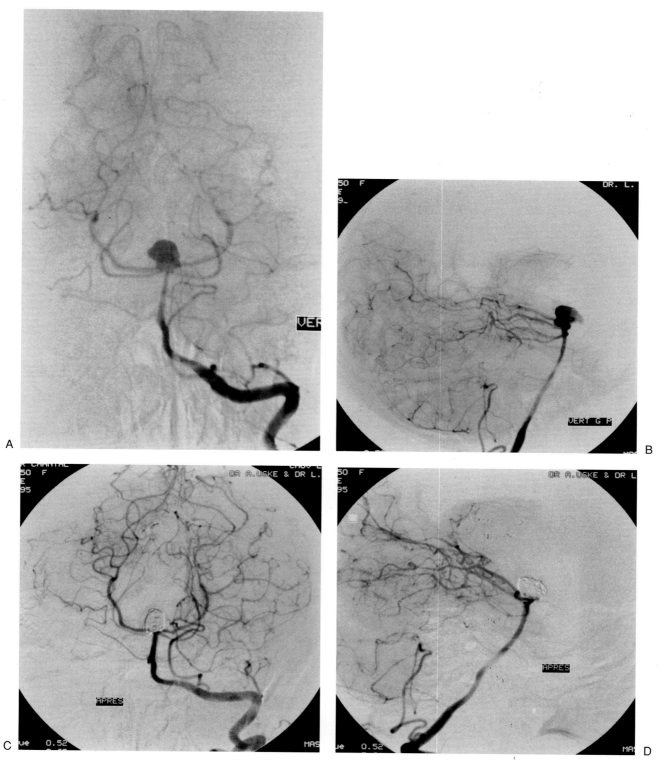

FIG. 7. A, B: Ruptured basilar bifurcation aneurysm in a patient with unruptured right middle cerebral and posterior communicating artery aneurysms. This 46-year-old woman presented with acute subarachnoid hemorrhage (Fisher grade III, Hunt & Hess grade IV). (A, frontal projection; B, lateral projection.) **C, D:** Ruptured basilar bifurcation aneurysm in a patient with unruptured right middle cerebral and posterior communicating artery aneurysms; same patient as in 7A and B. Endovascular occlusion of the basilar bifurcation aneurysm was performed at the time of the diagnostic angiogram. Ventricular drainage was performed and the patient's condition improved, until 6 days following hemorrhage. She developed severe symptomatic vasospasm treated by angioplasty of the internal carotid and middle cerebral arteries bilaterally, as well as the basilar artery. Her condition steadily improved and she was discharged with mild neurologic deficit. She returned 3 months later for surgical clipping of the asymptomatic right middle cerebral and posterior communicating artery aneurysms. (C, frontal projection; D, lateral projection.)

925

proved. Symptomatic vasospasm may be treated with either papaverine infusion or angioplasty following either endovascular coiling or surgical clipping. However, the greatest advantage of surgical clipping is the ability to reconstruct vessels that may be involved in the aneurysm. Surgical bypass procedures may be needed in some cases and can be achieved at the same time as treatment of the aneurysm.

CONCLUSION

Endovascular techniques for the treatment of intracranial aneurysms have rapidly evolved over the past 20 years. When indicated, parent artery occlusion can be achieved by an endovascular approach for the treatment of intracranial aneurysms. Selective endovascular occlusion of intracranial aneurysms is also possible using controlled deployment coils systems, such as the GDC. The clinical role of selective endovascular coil occlusion of intracranial aneurysms is continually being redefined. However, it is clear that endovascular techniques will not replace surgical clipping in the near future. Endovascular techniques currently remain an alternative for those patients who, for many reasons, may not be candidates for surgical treatment (Fig. 6A–D). In some cases, it may be optimal to utilize a combined approach involving both surgical and endovascular techniques (46). A staged approach with stabilization of the patient's condition by endovascular coiling followed by surgical clipping may be beneficial in a number of circumstances (Fig. 7A–D). It is clear that endovascular techniques will play an increasingly important role in the treatment of intracranial aneurysms. Continued close cooperation between surgeons and endovascular neuroradiologists will help to advance this technology and ensure optimal patient care.

REFERENCES

1. Serbenenko FA. Balloon catheterization and occlusion of major cerebral vessels. *J Neurosurg* 1974;41:125–145.
2. Debrun G, Fox A, Drake C, et al. Giant unclippable aneurysms: treatment with balloons. *AJNR* 1981;2:167–173.
3. Hieshima GB, Grinnell VS, Mehringer CM. A detachable balloon for therapeutic transcatheter occlusions. *Radiology* 1981;138:227–228.
4. Fox A, Vinuela F, Pelz DM, et al. Use of detachable balloons for proximal artery occlusion in the treatment of unclippable cerebral aneurysms. *J Neurosurg* 1987;66:40–46.
5. Higashida RT, Halbach VV, Barnwell SL, et al. Treatment of intracranial aneurysms with preservation of the parent vessel: results of percutaneous balloon embolization in 84 patients. *AJNR* 1990; 11:633–640.
6. George B, Aymard A, Gobin P, et al. Traitement endovasculaire des anéurysmes intracrâniens: intérêt et perspective d'après une série de 92 cas. *Neurochirurgie* 1990;36:237–278.
7. Konovalov AN, Serbinenko FA, Filatov JM, et al. Endovascular treatment of arterial aneurysms. *AJNR* 1990;11:225.
8. Hopkins LN, Guterman LR, Livingston K, et al. Endovascular management of intracranial aneurysms. In: Tindall GT, Cooper PR, Barrow DL, eds. *The Practice of Neurosurgery*. vol. 2. Baltimore: Williams and Wilkins, 1996;2143–2154.
9. Graves VB, Partington CR, Rüfenacht DA, et al. Treatment of carotid artery aneurysms with platinum coils: an experimental study in dogs. *AJNR* 1990;11:249–252.
10. Dowd CF, Halbach VV, Higashida RT, et al. Endovascular coil emboli-

11. Guglielmi G, Vinuela F, Sepetka I, et al. Electrothrombosis of saccular aneurysms via endovascular approach. I. Electrochemical basis, technique and experimental results. *J Neurosurg* 1991;75:1–7.
12. Marks MP, Chee H, Lidell RP, et al. A mechanically detachable coil for the treatment of aneurysms and occlusion of blood vessels. *AJNR* 1994;15:821–827.
13. Sugiu K, Kinugasa K, Mandai S, et al. Direct thrombosis of experimental aneurysms with cellulose acetate polymer (CAP): technical aspects, angiographic follow up, and histologic study. *J Neurosurg* 1995;83(3): 531–538.
14. Tereda T, Nakamura Y, Nakai K, et al. Embolization of arteriovenous malformations with peripheral aneurysms using ethylene vinyl alcohol copolymer: report of three cases. *JVIR* 1992;3:149.
15. Park S, Perl J, Gribenko A, et al. New polymers for therapeutic embolization. Proceedings of the 32nd Annual Meeting of the ASNR, May 1994. Published by American Society of Neuroradiology (ASNR) Oakbrook, Illinois.
16. Massoud TF, Turjman F, Vinuela F, et al. Endovascular treatment of fusiform aneurysms with stents and coils: technical feasibility in a swine model. *AJNR* 1995;16(10):1953–1963.
17. Grotenhuis JA, de Vries J, Tacl S. Angioscopy guided placement of balloon expandable stents in the treatment of experimental carotid aneurysms. *Min Invas Surg* 1994;37(2):56–60.
18. Geremia G, Haklin M, Brennecke L. Embolization of experimentally created aneurysms with intravascular stent devices. *AJNR* 1994;15(7): 1223–1231.
19. Szikora I, Gutterman LR, Wells KM, et al. Combined use of stents and coils to treat experimental wide-necked carotid aneurysms: preliminary results. *AJNR* 1994;15(6):1091–1102.
20. Wakhloo AK, Schellhammer F, de Vries J, et al. Self expanding and balloon expandable stents in the treatment of carotid aneurysms: an experimental study in a canine model. *AJNR* 1994;15(3):493–502.
21. Higashida RT, Halbach VV, Cahan LD, et al. Detachable balloon embolization therapy of posterior circulation intracranial aneurysms. *J Neurosurg* 1989;71:512–519.
22. Goto K, Halbach VV, Hardin CW, et al. Permanent inflation of detachable balloons with a low-viscosity hydrophilic polymerizing system. *Radiology* 1988;169:787–790.
23. Gianturco C, Anderson JH, Wallace S. Mechanical devices for arterial occlusion. *AJR* 1975;124(3):428–435.
24. Yang PJ, Halbach VV, Higashida RT, et al. Platinum wire: a new transvascular embolic agent. *AJNR* 1988;9(3):547–550.
25. Monsein LH, Jeffrey PJ, van Heerden BB, et al. Assessing adequacy of collateral circulation during balloon test occlusion of the internal carotid artery with 99m Tc-HMPAO SPECT. *AJNR* 1991; 12:1045–1051.
26. Peterman SB, Taylor A, Hoffman JC. Improved detection of cerebral hypoperfusion with internal carotid balloon test occlusion and 99m Tc-HMPAO cerebral perfusion SPECT imaging. *AJNR* 1991; 12:1035–1041.
27. Erba SM, Horton JA, Latchaw RE, et al. Balloon test occlusion of the internal carotid artery with stable xenon/CT cerebral blood flow imaging. *AJNR* 1988;9:533–537.
28. Guglielmi G. Endovascular treatment of intracranial aneurysms. *Neuroimag Clin North Am* 1992;2(2):269–278.
29. Sawyer PN, Pate JW. Bio-electric phenomena as an etiologic factor in intravascular thrombosis. *Am J Physiol* 1953;175:103–107.
30. Sawyer PN, Pate JW, Weldon CS. Relations of abnormal and injury electric potential differences to intravascular thrombosis. *Am J Physiol* 1953;175:108–112.
31. Sawyer PN, Pate JW. Electric potential differences across the normal aorta and aortic grafts of dogs. *Am J Physiol* 1953;175:113–117.
32. Miller MD, Johnsrude IS, Limberakis AJ, et al. Clinical use of transcatheter electrocoagulation. *Radiology* 1978;129:211–214.
33. Mawad ME, Mawad JK, Cartwright J, et al. Long-term histologic changes in canine aneurysms embolized with Guglielmi detachable coils. *AJNR* 1995;16:7–13.
34. Drake CG, Allcock JH. Postoperative angiography and the "slipped" clip. *J Neurosurg* 1973;39:683.
35. Stevens JL. Postoperative angiography in treatment of intracranial aneurysms. *Acta Radiol* 1966;5:536.
36. Zubillaga A, Guglielmi G, Vinuela F, et al. Endovascular occlusion of

intracranial aneurysms with electrically detachable coils: Correlation of aneurysm neck size and treatment results. *AJNR* 1994;15:815–820.

37. King JT, Flamm ES. Management of asymptomatic, unruptured, intracranial aneurysms. In: Tindall GT, Cooper PR, Barrow DL, eds. *The Practice of Neurosurgery.* vol 2. Baltimore: Williams and Wilkins, 1996;1997–2004.

38. Graves VB, Strother CM, Partington CR, et al. Flow dynamics of lateral carotid aneurysms and their effect on coils and balloons: an experimental study in dogs. *AJNR* 1992;13:189–196.

39. Strother CM, Graves VB, Rappe A. Aneurysm hemodynamics: an experimental study. *AJNR* 1992;13:1089–1095.

40. Crompton MR. Mechanism of growth and rupture in cerebral berry aneurysms. *Br Med J* 1966;1:1138–1142.

41. Suzuki J, Ohara H. Clinicopathological study of cerebral aneurysms. Origin, rupture, repair and growth. *J Neurosurg* 1978;48:505–514.

42. Drake CG, Vanderlinden RG. The late consequences of incomplete surgical treatment of intracranial aneurysms. *J Neurosurg* 1967;27: 226–238.

43. Drake CG, Friedman AH, Peerless SJ. Failed aneurysm surgery. Reoperation in 115 cases. *J Neurosurg* 1984;61:848–856.

44. Allcock JM, Drake CG, Postoperative angiography in cases of ruptured intracranial aneurysm. *J Neurosurg* 1963;20:752–759.

45. Feuerberg I, Lindquist C, Lindqvist M, et al. Natural history of postoperative aneurysm rests. *J Neurosurg* 1987;66:30–34.

46. Marks MP, Steinberg GK, Lane B. Combined use of endovascular coils and surgical clipping for intracranial aneurysms. *AJNR* 1995; 16: 15–18.

Cerebrovascular Disease, edited by H. Hunt Batjer.
Lippincott-Raven Publishers, Philadelphia © 1997.

CHAPTER **75**

Intracranial Aneurysm: Temporary Arterial Occlusion

Robert J. Dempsey

The principles behind temporary arterial clipping for aneurysm surgery are relatively straightforward. During the evolution of surgical techniques for aneurysms, the primary emphasis has always been on the accurate placement of a permanent clip at the base of the aneurysm to exclude the abnormal aneurysm wall from the circulation. Several authors, primarily Drake and Yasargil, have stressed the importance of accurate clip placement, excluding all essential perforators from the clip (1,2). During the dissection of an aneurysm, however, intraoperative rupture and the bulbous nature of larger aneurysms limit visibility and accurate clip placement. In addition, a turgid or calcific aneurysm may cause the clip to slide down the neck obstructing the parent artery.

Historic attempts to improve the safety of dissection included the routine use of controlled hypotension. However, the risk of infarction in an acutely injured brain subjected to hypotension after subarachnoid hemorrhage remained high. Several authors described the use of normal blood pressure with temporary arterial clipping of either the parent vessel or all vessels entering and exiting the aneurysm during surgery. Pool described sequential temporary clips as dissection progressed for an anterior communicating aneurysm (3). Peerless and Drake described springing a permanent clip to decrease its closing pressure and using that as a temporary artery clip to enhance dissection (4). As these techniques proved their utility, surgeons used this protected time to open giant aneurysms and remove clot or calcific debris to form a clippable neck. This method also allows critical final dissection about the dome to proceed protected from intraoperative rupture for aneurysms of any size.

USE OF TEMPORARY ARTERIAL CLIPPING

Temporary arterial clipping enhances the safety of aneurysm surgery in several ways. Pool described the sequential

movement of temporary clips closer and closer to the aneurysm neck until it could be safely manipulated (3). Presently most surgeons use the technique described in Fig. 1: An anterior communicating artery aneurysm is exposed. Considerable manipulation of the aneurysm dome may be needed to identify prominent collateral vessels such as the contralateral A1 segment. In addition, the surgeon must clear small perforators from the aneurysm neck to exclude them from the permanent clip. Temporary clipping is first placed on the primary feeding vessel to allow increased safety of the subsequent dissection. Further clips complete interruption of blood flow from all major vessels leading to and exiting from the region of the neck (Fig. 1A). The neck may then be manipulated and quickly cleared of perforators to allow permanent clip placement (Fig. 1B). In addition to decreasing the risk of inadvertent rupture, such temporary clipping also allows the dome of the aneurysm to become sufficiently soft, which decreases the possibility that the permanent clip will migrate down onto the parent vessel and occlude it near the aneurysm neck. Although the angiogram had shown that the primary supply of this aneurysm was the ipsilateral A1 segment, it is advisable to temporary occlude the opposite A1 and both A2 segments. Without such a maneuver, rupture of the aneurysm with incomplete temporary clipping would allow the aneurysm to back-bleed through other collaterals. This would obscure the operative field as well as steal blood from collateral vascular territories and increase the likelihood of creating an ischemic deficit. Finally, as in the case of a giant partially thrombosed or calcified aneurysm, complete temporary clipping allows the aneurysm dome to be opened and evacuated of thrombus to form an appropriate neck for clipping.

Figure 2 illustrates an endovascular adaptation of temporary clipping in a basilar tip aneurysm. The surgeon's visibility for proximal vascular control is quite limited. In addition, the working space is small and excessive use of temporary clips may obscure the operative field. In this case, an endo-

R. J. Dempsey: Department of Neurological Surgery, University of Wisconsin Hospital, Madison, Wisconsin 53792.

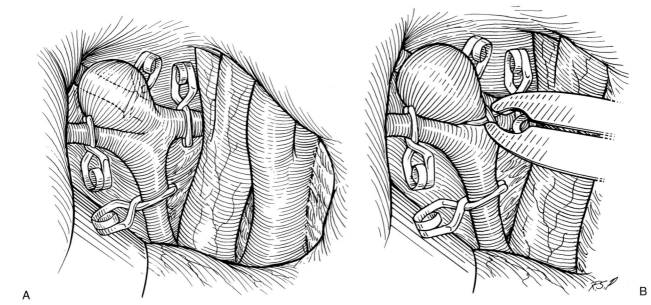

FIG. 1. Schematic diagram of the use of temporary arterial clips in the repair of an anterior communicating artery aneurysm. **A:** Aneurysm location obscures distal blood supply. **B:** Placement of temporary clips allows complete trapping of the aneurysm for safe placement of a single permanent clip. The aneurysm is slack and the neck is easily formed.

vascular balloon is placed within the basilar artery, allowing proximal control. If complete trapping is needed to open the aneurysm dome, temporary clips may be placed on the posterior cerebral arteries exiting the aneurysm. In addition, this technique allows the surgical team to withdraw blood from the region of the temporary clips. In the case of a large or giant aneurysm, temporary clipping with aspiration would then allow the dome to become flaccid and more easily formed into a neck for permanent clip application.

Successful placement of temporary clips greatly facilitates the safety of permanent clip application and reduces the risk of excessive hemorrhage from premature rupture. However, the appropriate vessels on which to place temporary clips may not be easily identifiable. In this case, endovascular

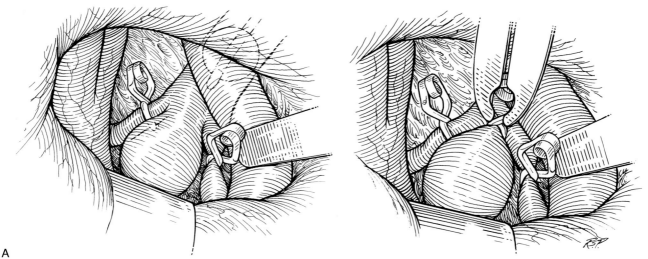

FIG. 2. Endovascular adaptation of temporary arterial clipping. **A:** The approach to the basilar tip aneurysm allows limited surgical room and limited visibility of proximal vascular control. **B:** The use of temporary clips on the posterior cerebral arteries is demonstrated. In addition, temporary control of the proximal basilar segment is maintained with an endovascular balloon. Aspiration of the aneurysm dome may also be accomplished through this technique to deflate a larger giant aneurysm to increase visibility of the neck and the surrounding perforators.

applications can assist with proximal vascular control. The final concern, however, must be the possibility of creating a permanent ischemic lesion during the period of temporary arterial clipping. It is this question that has generated the major research regarding the design of clips, the safe temporal limits of clipping, and the likelihood of ischemic infarction. These are questions that are best answered by examining the pathophysiology of transient cerebral ischemia.

Two lines of investigation have advanced our understanding of temporary arterial clipping. First, clip manufacturers have designed a series of temporary aneurysm clips based on studies of clip closing pressure. Along with investigations of temporary clip biomechanics came a second line of investigation into the appropriate duration of temporary clip pins and the tolerance of the injured brain to this maneuver.

Temporary Aneurysm Clips

Aneurysm clips are now available in a wide variety of sizes, materials, and closing pressures. Clip lengths ranging from 1 to 25 mm are readily available. Materials include nonferromagnetic metals and alloys designed for decreased reactivity to biological tissues and inertness within the magnetic field of a magnetic resonance imaging (MRI) scanner (5).

A considerable concern with permanent aneurysm clips is clip slippage, if arterial pressure results in sufficient turgidity within the aneurysmal dome to force the clips open and allow the aneurysm to refill. Therefore, closing pressures may be considerable in permanent clips. In the case of the reinforcing clips used in large or giant aneurysms, a closing force of 300 g of pressure is useful.

Permanent clip characteristics require sufficient force to maintain closure against arterial pressure. However, several histologic studies, including those of Sugita, have showed fragmentation of elastic and muscular fibers and infiltration of neutrophils into the internal muscular layer of the artery after even brief temporary clipping of an artery if a "permanent" aneurysm clip is used (6). Such histologic injuries to the vessel wall lead to a concern of late thrombosis, vasospasm, or intimal separation if a clip is placed and then removed. As the use of temporary clipping during procedures has become more popular, specialized clips have been devised to interrupt flow with minimal intimal injury. These temporary clips generally include closing pressure from 50 to 90 g. A wide variety are available with sizes and shapes similar to those of the permanent clip systems (Fig. 3). Dr. Sundt has also devised a microclip system primarily for use in arteriovenous malformations (AVMs) with clip blade lengths ranging from 1 to 4 mm and closing pressures ranging from 10 to 50 g (Johnson and Johnson Professional, Inc., Raynham, MA). The surgeon then has the possibility of a wide range of closing pressures and should take them into account when considering temporary vascular occlusion. The minimum force capable of securing interruption in flow is recommended. In the series of Samson and Batjer, an important predictor of poor outcome was the inclusion of perforator-laden segments in the temporary clip (7). Their studies would suggest that clinically important damage may be done to these vessels with excessive pressure or duration of temporary clipping. The surgeon is advised to take advantage of the variety of clips and to tailor their use to the situation at hand.

Avoiding Permanent Deficit During Temporary Arterial Clipping

In order to understand the use of temporary clips and the possibilities for pharmacologic cerebral protective therapies provided by such clips, it is necessary to examine the pathophysiology of transient cerebral ischemia.

The history of neurosurgery represents a continuous strug-

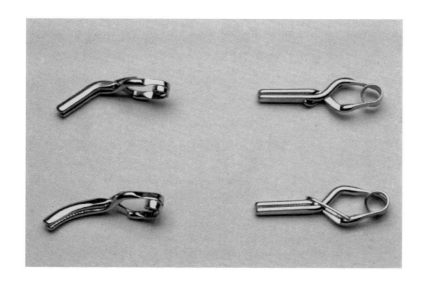

FIG. 3. Curved and straight versions of both temporary and permanent clips. Temporary clips *(top)* are typically plated in gold. Permanent clips are on the bottom row. The clips differ primarily in closing pressure. A variety of blade lengths and closing pressures are available. (Courtesy of Mizuho America, Beverly, MA.)

gle to perfect surgical methods so they result in minimal or no postoperative deficit. There are numerous causes of postoperative deficits, and focal or cerebral ischemia is a common determinant of outcome (8,9). Several noted authorities in the field of intracranial aneurysm surgery have shown the utility of temporary arterial clipping (3,4,10). The permissible duration of temporary arterial clipping is an important issue and requires one to:

1. Understand the pathophysiology of cell death after transient cerebral ischemia.
2. Examine physiologic methods to extend limits of vulnerability.
3. Study anesthetics that increase tolerance to planned ischemia.
4. Study experimental drugs that attempt to extend ischemic tolerance by targeting facets of the pathologic response to ischemia.
5. Study the clinical experience with temporary arterial occlusion and durations tolerated without stroke.

BIOCHEMICAL EVENTS OF TRANSIENT ISCHEMIA

The limits of cerebral tolerance to ischemia have been established in multiple laboratory models. During a no-flow state, the brain rapidly exhausts its reserves of available oxygen within <15 seconds and available glucose and adenosine in <5 minutes (11). In this condition a series of pathologic events are set into motion. The most important of these involve disruption of the normal ionic membrane pumps (Fig. 4). Under normal conditions ionic pumps maintain extracellular concentrations of sodium and calcium that are respectively 10- and 10,000-fold higher than intracellular levels. At the same time, the intracellular concentration of potassium is 40-fold higher than the extracellular level (9).

A loss of the ATP-derived energy necessary to maintain these ionic pumps allows the cell to start to normalize these gradients. The results are catastrophic. Although the neuron depends on the potassium-sodium gradient for its electrical activity, the influx of calcium into the cytosol may have several additional adverse effects. First, the influx of calcium alters calcium-dependent phospholipases, resulting in a change in the biochemical nature and structure of cellular membranes. Intracellular transport mechanisms are also altered. The result is a progressive loss of cellular function coupled with further disruption of membrane integrity and the development of cellular and brain edema. Calcium may enter the cytosol from intracellular sources such as mitochondria and endoplasmic reticulum, and, in addition, enter the cell through voltage-dependent and receptor-gaited calcium channels. Prominent among these receptors are those stimulated by glutamate at the N-methyl-D-aspartate (NMDA) receptor (Fig. 5). Strategies to extend tolerance to ischemia therefore commonly target the maintenance of energy, the stability of cellular membranes, and the limitation of calcium influx.

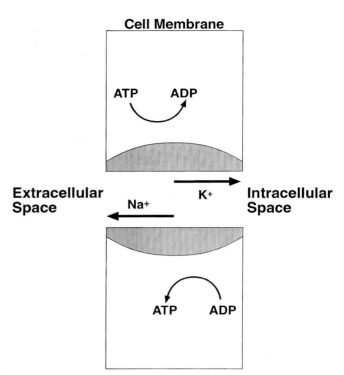

FIG. 4. The normal ionic gradient of the neuron is maintained by sodium-potassium ionic pumps. These along with calcium pumps maintain a 10-fold extracellular sodium gradient, a 10,000-fold extracellular calcium gradient, and a 40-fold intracellular potassium gradient. These gradients are necessary for normal electrical activity of the neuron as well as normal enzymatic and metabolic function.

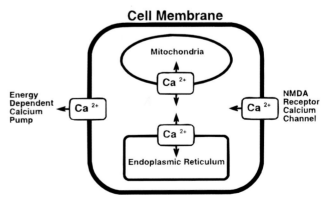

FIG. 5. Calcium fluxes in normal function and ischemia. During ischemia, calcium influx into the cytoplasm may occur at voltage-gaited and agonist-gaited calcium channels as well as by mobilization of calcium from intracellular organelles. Excessive intracellular calcium may disrupt normal neuronal function and lead to rapid cell death.

Ischemic Penumbra

The greatest amount of information pertinent to the clinical question of acceptable limits for temporary clipping during aneurysm surgery has come from the research laboratory in studies of the ischemic penumbra. This concept, expressed by Symon, denotes a region of collaterally perfused tissue surrounding a more dense ischemic core (12). In the penumbra region infarction is not inevitable as long as ATP maintains membrane ion pumps, keeping calcium and sodium extracellularly. Multiple laboratory studies have suggested that functional recovery of cortical neurons is related to both the degree and duration of ischemia. Therefore, both are equally important (13). It is estimated that approximately 55% of the neuronal metabolic needs are utilized to meet activation, ie, synaptic transmission of action potentials. However, 45% of the metabolic needs are used to maintain cellular integrity, such as protein, lipid, and nucleic acid synthesis. Hossmann (14) has shown that after a period of transient ischemia, protein synthesis may be inhibited by minimal decreases in blood flow. Although normal levels are 60 cm^3/100 g/min, the threshold for altered protein synthesis may be as close to normal levels as 55 cm^3/100 g/min.

Neurotransmitters are released at approximately 35 cm^3/100 g/min, beginning a disturbance in energy metabolism and potentially opening calcium channels. Finally, neuron depolarization occurs at 15 cm^3/100 g/min and may be further stimulated by the release of the neurotransmitter glutamate. Therefore, glutamine release in the injured area presents a challenge in the face of inadequate metabolic supply. The result is a gradual expansion of the infarct core into areas in which ATP is depleted. After a few hours, the penumbra has disappeared and become purely infarct (14). In primate models it has been suggested that penumbra may be defined as a region of ischemia with blood flows of 10–23 cm^3/100 g/min, with normal being approximately 60. In these models, irreversible ischemia may be present at flows below 10 cm^3/100 g/min. The penumbra flows may be survived if flow is restored within one-third to three hours, depending on the study. However, permanent flows below 18 cm^3/100 g/min are not tolerated, perhaps due to suppression of normal protein synthesis. These concepts are the scientific basis of therapeutic windows for brain viability. They also explain the limitations on the duration of reversibility in the transient ischemia seen clinically in temporary aneurysm clipping (15).

In looking at the limits of ischemia for temporary aneurysm clipping, the question that must be asked is why an infarct will expand into a region of penumbra or potentially idling brain. A possible explanation is the generation of spreading depression-like depolarization in the injured brain. Glutamate might trigger such depolarization, increasing the metabolic demand on ionic pumps. This process has been shown to increase glucose and oxygen demands to 200% of normal. In addition, when the temporary clip is released, the metabolic processes of reperfusion, including the generation of leukotrienes, result in the presence of free radicals as a byproduct of these reactions (16). These free radicals attack vulnerable membrane lipids. The resulting peroxidation acts as a spreading chain reaction compromising normal membrane function and neuronal viability.

INTRAOPERATIVE MONITORING

Laboratory studies show that vulnerability to infarction is related to local cerebral blood flow. Therefore monitoring cerebral blood flow during temporary clipping is ideal. However, accurate measurement of cerebral blood flow is difficult during aneurysm surgery because of the open cranial vault and the difficulties of applying xenon studies in this setting. Thermal diffusion flow probes have been used to correlate cerebral blood flow to electrical function (17). These laboratory studies have suggested that reductions of blood flow sufficient to cause the loss of neuronal and electrical activity as measured by electroencephalogram (EEG) or evoked potential (approximately 15 cm^3/100 g/min) are sufficient to threaten infarction if these levels are continued indefinitely. For this reason EEG and somatosensory evoked potentials have been used to alert the surgeon to an ischemia-related loss of function (18). A further estimate of cerebral flows is given by transcranial Doppler. With this technology ultrasound Doppler may be used to detect a precipitous drop in flow velocity that may be associated with vessel occlusions. This technique is extremely helpful in carotid endarterectomy but its utility in aneurysm operations appears to be primarily to monitor collateral flow during a therapeutic occlusion of proximal vessels (19,20).

Each of these monitoring technologies has limitations. EEG may remain normal in the face of clinically important deep lesions as with perforator occlusions. Somatosensory evoked potential conduction times may not predict clinical changes and transcranial Doppler velocity changes are not well characterized. Nevertheless, the utility of mechanisms such as EEG allows continuous monitoring and early notification of the onset of ischemia as well as a well-standardized method for measuring the depth of anesthesia and the use of cerebroprotective agents.

Cerebral Protection During Temporary Aneurysm Clipping

With the advent of temporary vessel clipping for aneurysm repair and its resultant planned transient cerebral ischemia, a series of strategies have been proposed for brain protection. These clinical strategies have been derived from the research studies on the brain's tolerance to experimental transient ischemia discussed above.

Anesthetic Protective Agents

The primary strategy for cerebral protection involves the use of general anesthetics. Early experiments with barbiturates suggested that agents that decrease the metabolic demand of the brain during the period of ischemia would extend the tolerance of that brain region to an anticipated period of ischemia. This protection is not generalized to all anesthetics. Inhalational agents such as isoflurane, ifenprodil, and halothane have not shown consistent protection (21,22). When effective during ischemia the neuroprotective effects of barbiturates appear to be associated with anesthesia to depths sufficient to obtain EEG burst suppression. This anesthetic state correlates with a reduction in cerebral metabolic demand to approximately one half. Barbiturates also offer protection from ongoing depolarization and the associated additional metabolic demand. It is felt that these agents also may act by scavenging free radicals and the stabilizing neuronal membranes.

Barbiturates are logical protective interventions given the pathophysiology of transient ischemia illustrated above (23,24). Unfortunately, these agents may cause significant cardiovascular and respiratory depression and prolonged emergence from anesthesia at the conclusion of the operation. In addition, experimental studies and clinical experience have shown little benefit if treatment is delayed.

There has been considerable interest in other possible protective anesthesia agents. Etomidate has shown the greatest clinical experience. It is a nonbarbiturate carboxylated imidazole that is capable of metabolic suppression without significant cardiac side effects (25). Laboratory studies have shown a decrease in cerebral blood flow as well as $CMRO_2$. At increasing doses, metabolic suppression increases until EEG silence is obtained. At this point normal metabolic activity has been decreased by approximately 48% (25,26). Significant cortisol output may be blocked at these levels of etomidate, requiring perioperative steroid replacement (26).

Batjer et al. have published a series of patients with large and giant aneurysms in whom temporary arterial occlusion was used under etomidate protection. In their initial studies they suggested that tolerance to ischemia was variable depending on the region of the brain perfused. Intervals of up to 60 minutes of internal carotid artery occlusion were tolerated. This was contrasted with limits of 35 minutes of middle cerebral artery occlusion and 19 minutes of basilar artery occlusion. A minimal period of 4-½ minutes of lower basilar artery occlusion was considered to be safe (27).

Other anesthetic agents, including propofol and ketamine, a noncompetitive glutamate antagonist, have been studied in the laboratory. Ketamine directly attacks the glutamate-responsive NMDA receptor for calcium channels. It has been shown to be protective in the laboratory but use for aneurysmal surgery has not been developed. Other agents remain in development.

Hypothermia

It is logical next to study the mechanism by which anesthetic agents protect against arterial occlusion. The primary agents showing clinical utility, barbiturates and etomidate, reduce the metabolic demand as part of their proposed protective mechanism (28). While other mechanisms of action, including free radical scavenging and membrane lipid stabilization, are possible, a reduction in $CMRO_2$ to approximately 50% of normal levels is a consistent finding. As seen earlier, approximately 50% of neuronal energy demand is spent maintaining electrical activity. This presumably may be transiently suspended. The other half of metabolic activity, however, is necessary for maintaining vital functions such as membrane stabilizing ionic pumps.

These observations have been instrumental in the renewed interest in the potential role of hypothermia as a protective modality during planned cerebral ischemia (29). Laboratory studies have shown that small decreases in brain temperature confer striking protection during ischemic brain injury. Conversely, small elevations of brain temperature during ischemia markedly extend pathologic changes and promote an earlier disruption of the blood–brain barrier. The mechanism of protection is believed to be the retardation of the rate of ATP depletion as well as the attenuation of the release of excitatory neurotransmitters such as glutamate into the extracellular space. In addition, catabolic enzyme systems may be inhibited by such hypothermia.

In some cases previous studies of protective pharmacologic agents are now interpreted to at least partially exert their beneficial effects through the maintenance of mild hypothermia (16,30). The exact target temperatures during ischemia remain controversial. Minimal decreases in temperature, eg, to 33°C, are believed to be protective (31). Studies in children undergoing thoracic surgery suggest that an increased benefit as measured by tolerance of longer periods of ischemia may be seen with cooling to 18°C. From an experimental standpoint, the reduction of metabolic demand ($CMRO_2$) to 50% of normal (equivalent to that of EEG burst suppression during barbiturate or etomidate) is seen with cooling to 28°C. However, significant cardiopulmonary compromise may be seen with excessive cooling and require support even to the level of cardiopulmonary bypass.

Additional Cerebral Protective Agents

Analysis of the pathophysiology of neuronal death after transient cerebral ischemia suggests several other sites of possible therapeutic intervention. Areas that have attracted the most attention have been the abnormal influx of calcium into the damaged cell, the postischemic mobilization and metabolism of free fatty acids, and the resulting generation of free radicals capable of further damaging membrane and enzymatic function. At present calcium channel blockers enjoy the greatest popularity. Nimodipine has been suggested to be beneficial in multiple animal and human trials (32,33,34). The extent of this protection, however, is limited as postischemic calcium intracellular accumulation may occur from multiple mechanisms including the voltage-sensitive calcium channels that nimodipine targets as well as agonist-operated calcium channels. For this reason, both NMDA and AMPA (α-amino-3-hydroxy-5-methyl-4-isoxazole propionic acid) receptor antagonists to restrict the pathologic influx of calcium at agonist-operated calcium channels are undergoing trials in laboratory models (35). Finally, a series of trials have suggested the potential benefits of inhibitors of free radical damage, specifically iron-catalyzed lipid peroxidation. These agents have shown success in animal models and are now undergoing trials for clinical utility in ischemia and vasospasm (36).

CLINICAL APPLICATION OF PROTECTIVE STRATEGIES

The use of temporary artery clipping to improve the safety of intraoperative dissection and final clip placement during aneurysm surgery has been used sporadically for many years. First applied in a systematic fashion by Pool, Drake, and Symon, these strategies derive primarily from surgical experience and the logical application of the knowledge of ischemic pathophysiology at the time (3,4,10,37,38). Symon suggested that during temporary arterial occlusion the effects were individual to the patient. In his studies some patients showed a loss of electrical activity that suggested that only brief periods of ischemia could be tolerated. In addition, it had been known that animal models showed selective regional vulnerability in certain areas such as the hippocampus. Symon felt that local cerebral flow measurements enhanced the ability to predict tolerance, or the lack of it, to temporary clipping (10). Other investigators have reinforced the experimental observation that both the duration and depth of local ischemia were important predictors of infarction. Ogawa suggested that after the placement of temporary clips, residual cerebral blood flow below 15 cm³/100 g/min resulted in transient postoperative symptoms if temporary clipping continued for more than 10 minutes. In these studies, if decreased local cerebral blood flow continued for more than 20 minutes, irreversible neurologic deficits were observed (39).

A more recent study of 121 patients undergoing elective temporary arterial occlusion during aneurysm dissection demonstrated the development of a standardized protective regime. This included etomidate to induce EEG burst suppression and the maintenance of normal blood pressure and body temperature. Within these parameters patients were found to routinely tolerate temporary clipping up to 14 minutes in duration. All patients occluded for more than 31 minutes suffered at least some evidence of a neurologic deficit. It was suggested that conditions that would increase the likelihood of a postoperative infarct included increased age of the patient, worsening preoperative neurologic condition (Hunt and Hess grades III and IV), and the occlusion of perforator segments of the middle cerebral or basilar arteries (7). The study did not resolve several questions including

the use of hypothermia, alternative protective agents, and the sequence and completion of temporary clip placement.

Among the issues regarding the actual mechanism of clipping is the question of complete trapping of the aneurysm vs. proximal occlusion alone. Samson et al. suggested that incomplete occlusion was statistically associated with the development of postoperative infarction (7). In the event of intraoperative disruption of the dome of the aneurysm a complete occlusion would eliminate bleeding. However, rupture under conditions of proximal occlusion alone would allow the formation of a steal phenomenon with distal branches back-bleeding into the aneurysm and further rendering ischemic the collaterally fed distal vascular bed (7). This study further suggested that temporary clipping of perforator segments may be damaging, which would be consistent with irreversible endothelial damage by temporary clips when small perforators are included. The question of repetitive brief periods of ischemia vs. a single prolonged period is not resolved, although some evidence suggests that intermittent reperfusion during temporary focal ischemia may be better tolerated (40).

OVERALL MANAGEMENT STRATEGIES

The avoidance of infarction during aneurysmal surgery requiring temporary arterial clipping is an evolving process based on our present understanding of the pathophysiologic events leading to infarction during transient ischemia. Management should include control of increased intracranial pressure and brain swelling to avoid the addition of retractor ischemia to the region of interest. Hyper- and hypotension should be avoided and adequate oxygenation maintained. On induction of anesthesia, the goal must be to minimize transmural aneurysmal pressure while maintaining cerebral perfusion pressure. Induction medications therefore may include thiopental, a short-acting barbiturate combined with a narcotic agent such as fentanyl that is added to blunt the blood pressure rise of laryngoscopy. Multiple other combinations are possible (41).

Intraoperative monitoring is essential for determining if metabolic demands are being met. These include standard electrocardiogram, capnography, esophageal stethoscope, and temperature. Arterial blood pressure and, if possible, intracranial pressure (ICP) measurements allow continuous monitoring of cerebral perfusion pressure. EEG or one of its derivatives allows for the early warning of focal ischemia and is useful for determining the presence of EEG burst suppression prior to temporary clipping. Optional monitoring methods include the placement of pulmonary artery catheters to follow myocardial function, jugular bulb oxygen saturation to determine changing cerebral metabolic needs suggesting focal ischemia, and transcranial Doppler to show alterations in blood flow velocity.

Maintenance goals during the operation include the presence of a normal cerebral perfusion pressure with a ''slack'' brain and the reversibility of agents to allow prompt postoperative awakening if clinically possible. Maintenance agents generally include a narcotic and an inhalation agent such as isoflurane at low concentrations. Isoflurane has been shown to have a dose-dependent decrease in $CMRO_2$.

If temporary artery occlusion can be anticipated, anesthetic preparation proceeds with the protective agent thiopental or etomidate and the presence of moderate hypothermia, generally 32°C. During these maneuvers maintenance of mean arterial pressure is important. With thiopental delayed postoperative awakening may be expected. Cardiac depression also needs to be monitored. Some centers use mannitol as a potential protective agent during temporary clipping whereas others use it prior to clipping in an attempt to minimize brain swelling and retractor ischemia. During emergence at the completion of surgery it is important to avoid hypotension and maintain cerebral perfusion and steady oxygenation through the extubation period.

The use of temporary arterial clipping has proven to be a significant advance in the microsurgery of intracranial aneurysms. It allows a softened aneurysm dome. It also allows the surgeon to open and/or excise large aneurysms and facilitates accurate placement of permanent clips. However, the cost of temporary clipping is the development of transient cerebral ischemia. This results in the unique clinical circumstance of planned cerebral ischemia, which allows scientific study, and the application of concepts developed in laboratory models to the operative setting. Principles developed from the laboratory involve the maintenance of normal cerebral perfusion pressure, the limitation of the duration of temporary clipping, hypothermia, and anesthetic methods to decrease metabolic demand during ischemia, and several potential strategies to pharmacologically limit neuronal vulnerability to infarction. By applying available experimental evidence our understanding of these protective mechanisms can evolve and our surgical technique improve.

Acknowledgments

I would like to thank Janet Harney and Michael Liebman, M.S. for their editorial assistance, Mustafa K. Baskaya, M.D. for proofreading, and Richard Penell for the drawings and graphic images in this chapter.

REFERENCES

1. Drake CG, Vanderlinden RG, Amacher AL. Carotid-ophthalmic aneurysms. *J Neurosurg* 1968;29:24–31.
2. Yasargil MG. Clinical Considerations, Surgery of the Intracranial Aneurysms and Results. In: *Microneurosurgery* vol 2. Stuttgart: Thieme Verlag, 1984.
3. Pool JL. Aneurysms of the anterior communicating artery: bifrontal craniotomy and routine use of temporary clips. *J Neurosurg* 1961;18:98–112.
4. Peerless SJ, Drake CG. Surgical techniques of posterior cerebral aneurysms. In: Schmidek HH, Sweet WH, eds. *Operative Neurosurgical Techniques: Indications, Methods, and Results.* vol 2. Philadelphia: WB Saunders, 1988;973–989.
5. Tew JM Jr, Steiger HJ. Aneurysm clips. In: Wilkins RH, Rengachary SS, eds. *Neurosurgery.* vol 1. New York: McGraw-Hill, 1985; 1372–1376.
6. Sugita K, Hirota T, Iguchi I, Mizutani T. Comparative study of the pressure of various aneurysm clips. *J Neurosurg* 1976;44:723–727.
7. Samson D, Batjer HH, Bowman G, Mootz L, Krippner WJ, Meyer YJ, Allen BC. A clinical study of the parameters and effects of temporary arterial occlusion in the management of intracranial aneurysms. *Neurosurgery* 1994;34(1):22–29.
8. O Sullivan K, Cunningham AJ. Intraoperative cerebral ischaemia. *Br J Hosp Med* 1989;42:288–296.
9. Siesjö BK. Pathophysiology and treatment of focal cerebral ischemia. *J Neurosurg* 1992;77:169–184.
10. Symon L. Thresholds of ischaemia applied to aneurysm surgery. *Acta Neurochirurgica* 1985;77:1–7.
11. Aitkenhead AR. Cerebral protection after cardiac arrest. *Resuscitation* 1991;22:197–202.
12. Symon L. Flow thresholds in brain ischaemia and the effects of drugs. *Br J Anaesth* 1985;57:34–43.
13. Heiss W-D, Rosner G. Functional recovery of cortical neurons as related to degree and duration of ischemia. *Ann Neurol* 1983;14(3):294–301.
14. Hossmann K-A. Viability thresholds and the penumbra of focal ischemia. *Ann Neurol* 1994;36(4):557–565.
15. Jones TH, Morawetz RB, Crowell RM, Marcoux FW, FitzGibbon SJ, DeGirolami U, Ojemann RG. Thresholds of focal cerebral ischemia in awake monkeys. *J Neurosurg* 1981;54:773–782.
16. Dempsey RJ, Combs DJ, Maley ME, Cowen DE, Roy MW, Donaldson DL. Moderate hypothermia reduces postischemic edema development and leukotriene production. *Neurosurgery* 1987;21(2):177–181.
17. Mizoi K, Yoshimoto T. Intraoperative monitoring of the somatosensory evoked potentials and cerebral blood flow during aneurysm surgery. *Neurol Med Chir (Tokyo)* 1991;31:318–325.
18. Symon L, Momma F, Murota T. Assessment of reversible cerebral ischaemia in man: intraoperative monitoring of the somatosensory evoked response. *Acta Neurochirurgica* 1988;42 (Suppl):3–7.
19. Spencer MP, Thomas GI, Nicholls SC, Sauvage LR. Detection of middle cerebral artery emboli during carotid endarterectomy using transcranial Doppler ultrasonography. *Stroke* 1990;21(3):415–423.
20. Giller CA, Steig P, Batjer HH, Samson D, Purdy P. Transcranial doppler ultrasound as a guide to graded therapeutic occlusion of the carotid artery. *Neurosurgery* 1990;26(2):307–311.
21. Kurihara J, Tomita H, Ochiai N, Kato H. Protection by halothane of the vagal baroreflex system from transient global cerebral ischemia in dogs. *Jpn J Pharmacol* 1992;60:63–66.
22. Baughman VL, Hoffman WE, Thomas C, Miletich DJ, Albrecht RF. Comparison of methohexital and isoflurane on neurologic outcome and histopathology following incomplete ischemia in rats. *Anesthesiology* 1990;72:85–94.
23. Araki T, Kogure K, Nishioka K. Comparative neuroprotective effects of pentobarbital, vinpocetine, flunarizine and ifenprodil on ischemic neuronal damage in the gerbil hippocampus. *Res Exp Med* 1990;190:19–23.
24. Sano T, Patal PM, Drummond JC, Cole DJ. A comparison of the cerebral protective effects of etomidate, thiopental, and isoflurane in a model of forebrain ischemia in the rat. *Anesth Analg* 1993;76:990–997.
25. Batjer HH. Cerebral protective effects of etomidate: experimental and clinical aspects. *Cerebrovasc Brain Metab Rev* 1993;5(1):17–32.
26. Kenyon CJ, McNeil LM, Fraser R. Comparison of the effects of etomidate, thiopentone and propofol on cortisol synthesis. *Br J Anaesth* 1985; 57:509–511.
27. Batjer HH, Frankfurt AI, Purdy PD, Smith SS, Samson DS. Use of etomidate, temporary arterial occlusion, and intraoperative angiography in surgical treatment of large and giant cerebral aneurysms. *J Neurosurg* 1988;68:234–240.
28. Kuroiwa T, Bonnekoh P, Hossmann K-A. Therapeutic window of CA1 neuronal damage defined by an ultrashort-acting barbiturate after brain ischemia in gerbils. *Stroke* 1990;21(10):1489–1493.
29. Silverberg GD, Reitz BA, Ream AK. Hypothermia and cardiac arrest in the treatment of giant aneurysms of the cerebral circulation and hemangioblastoma of the medulla. *J Neurosurg* 1981;55:337–346.
30. Ginsberg MD, Sternau LL, Globus MY-T, Dietrich WD, Busto R. Therapeutic modulation of brain temperature: relevance to ischemic brain injury. *Cerebrovasc Brain Metab Rev* 1992;4:189–225.

31. Busto R, Globus MY-T, Dietrich WD, Martinez E, Valdés I, Ginsberg MD. Effect of mild hypothermia on ischemia–induced release of neurotransmitters and free fatty acids in rat brain. *Stroke* 1989;20(7)904–910.

32. Hakim AM, Evans AC, Berger L, Kuwabara H, Worsley K, Marchal G, Biel C, Pokrupa R, Diksic M, Meyer E, Gjedde A, Marrett S. The effect of nimodipine on the evolution of human cerebral infarction studied by PET. *J Cereb Blood Flow Metab* 1989;9:523–534.

33. Andrews RJ, Muto RP. Retraction brain ischaemia: mannitol plus nimodipine preserves both cerebral blood flow and evoked potentials during normoventilation and hyperventilation. *Neurol Res* 1992;14:19–25.

34. Hadley MN, Major MC, Zabramski JM, Spetzler RF, Rigamonti D, Fifield MS, Johnson PC. The efficacy of intravenous nimodipine in the treatment of focal cerebral ischemia in a primate model. *Neurosurgery* 1989;25(1):63–70.

35. Nellgård B, Wieloch T. Cerebral protection by AMPA- and NMDA-receptor antagonists administered after severe insulin-induced hypoglycemia. *Exp Brain Res* 1992;92:259–266.

36. Hall ED, Pazara KE, Braughler JM, Linseman KL, Jacobsen EJ. Nonsteroidal lazaroid U78517F in models of focal and global ischemia. *Stroke* 1990;21 (Suppl III):III-83–III-87.

37. Drake CG. Giant intracranial aneurysms: experience with surgical treatment in 174 patients. In: *Clin Neurosurg* 1979;26:12–95.

38. Symon L, Vajda J. Surgical experiences with giant intracranial aneurysms. *J Neurosurg* 1984;61:1009–1028.

39. Ogawa A, Sato H, Sakurai Y, Yoshimoto T. Limitation of temporary vascular occlusion during aneurysm surgery. *Surg Neurol* 1991;36:453–457.

40. Goldman MS, Anderson RE, Meyer FB. Effects of intermittent reperfusion during temporal focal ischemia. *J Neurosurg* 1992;77:911–916.

41. Sundt TM Jr, Piepgras DG. Surgical approach to giant intracranial aneurysms. *J Neurosurg* 1979;51:731–742.

Cerebrovascular Disease, edited by H. Hunt Batjer.
Lippincott-Raven Publishers, Philadelphia © 1997.

CHAPTER 76

Cavernous Carotid Aneurysm: Direct vs. Indirect Approaches

Vinko V. Dolenc and Anton Valavanis

Although numerous anatomic studies of the parasellar region have been carried out during the last 50 years (1–14), aneurysms of the cavernous internal carotid artery (ICA) are still difficult to treat successfully. Neurospecialists such as neurologists, neuroradiologists, and neurosurgeons disagree as to the need for and the method of active management of this demanding and fairly rare pathology.

Neuroradiologists, who favor the active endovascular approach (15–22), and neurosurgeons, who favor the direct approach (4,6,8,9,23–34), are opposed by neurologists who favor the wait-and-see policy. The arguments for and against each policy seem reasonable. Patients with intracavernous ICA aneurysms that are rather large, even giant, and in most cases do not produce a difficult clinical picture are usually referred directly to neurologists. In the vast majority of cases, the symptoms precede the signs. Being aware of the possibility of permanent deficits (hemiparesis or even hemiplegia and/or cranial nerve palsies) or late deficits due to occlusion of the ipsilateral ICA by endovascular treatment, neurologists have reason to support the wait-and-see doctrine. Neuroradiologists, who strongly favor endovascular treatment, also have good reasons for defending their modality of treatment of cavernous ICA aneurysms, which is a modification of the surgical treatment of such lesions. Neurosurgeons who initiated treatment of cavernous ICA aneurysms are in turn under constant attack from neurologists and neuroradiologists. However, it was the neurosurgeons who conducted most of the anatomic studies of the parasellar region in order to understand normal and pathologic anatomy and deal with the pathology of this region (1–14,27). There is no doubt that seeing the anatomic structures and their relationships in a specimen or during live surgery is superior to viewing

images on a screen. It is also true that long-term follow-up studies have proved that so far the surgical approach can best solve the problem in the majority of patients with cavernous ICA aneurysms.

All specialists involved will have to seriously consider the cost–benefit ratio of each modality of approach and bear in mind the increasingly active role played by patients regarding their course of treatment. It goes without saying that such an approach will place considerable responsibility both on the decision made and on the implementation of the chosen modality of treatment. The patient's more active role will bring physicians from different specialties together, thus making their role complementary rather than dividing them and fueling their antagonism. It is also true that in the long run the accumulation of experience, the increasing number of cases, and complementary studies will narrow the place for "personal opinions" as the available objective analytic data will not only dictate the treatment of choice but will shape the cutting edge for the understanding of the development of this pathology and its elimination with the most appropriate modality of treatment. In the future it is likely that the treatment of choice will consist of a combination of the best elements of those currently available.

SURGICAL ANATOMY

Internal Carotid Artery

The ICA enters the petrous canal and courses through the skull base extradurally to entering the intradural space underneath the optic nerve (ON) medial to the anterior clinoid process (ACP) making four loops (Fig. 1): posterior (PL), lateral (LL), medial (ML), and anterior loop (AL). The planes in which the loops are positioned are not parallel; they are inclined toward each other at a sharp angle so that finally the planes of the PL and the AL are almost perpendic-

V. V. Dolenc: Department of Neurological Surgery, University of Ljubljana, 61105 Ljubljana, Slovenia

A. Valavanis: Institute for Neuroradiology, University Hospital Zurich, CH-8091 Zurich, Switzerland

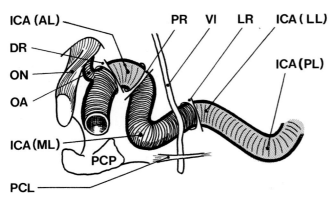

FIG. 1. Schematic drawing of the ICA course on the right side through the skull base. The covered intrapetrous segment (segment A), the cavernous or "free" segment (segment B) and the covered infraclinoid segment (segment C) of the ICA are schematically presented. The dural rings around the ICA: the lateral (LR), proximal (PR), and distal ring (DR)—the important anatomic landmarks between segments A, B, and C—are presented. The loops of the ICA—posterior (PL), lateral (LL), medial (ML), and anterior (AL)—are adjusted to the surrounding bony and dural structures. These four loops are in different planes. The only properly intracavernous cranial nerve is VI, which is fairly intimately related to the free segment of the ICA.

ular to one another. Awareness of the planes of the individual loops of the ICA greatly enhances intraoperative orientation. Of main surgical importance is the so-called "free" segment of the ICA in the parasellar venous network (Fig. 1), which extends between the lateral (LR) and the proximal ring (PR). The segment of the ICA extending from its entry point into the petrous bone to the LR, ie, to its exit point from the carotid canal, is "encased" in the canal, which in 80% of cases is formed by bone around the circumference and in 20% of cases is partially formed by the fibrous membrane from the peripheral leg of the PL to the LR. The other segment of the ICA, which is also encased in the bony canal, is the AL of the ICA (Fig. 1), ie, the ICA underneath the ACP, from the PR to the distal (dural) ring (DR). The topography of the three segments of the ICA, the covered ICA in the petrous bone (segment A), the free segment in the parasellar venous plexus (segment B), and the covered segment between the ACP and the wall of the sphenoid bony sinus extending from the PR to the DR (segment C) (Fig.1), determines the etiology of the artery wall aneurysm disease or trauma along the ICA. The covered segments of the ICA are seldom affected by an aneurysmal change, an exception being the distal covered segment C, where most of the traumatic extradural ICA aneurysms occur after fracture of the surrounding bones, or iatrogenic injury of the ICA (AL) wall on its medial side during transsphenoidal surgery for pituitary adenomas (Figs. 2 and 3). Such false (iatrogenic) aneurysms project medialward into the sphenoid bony sinus or occasionally into the sella but never laterally or superiorly where the ACP is located.

Aneurysms along the free segment of the ICA vary in

type (saccular, fusiform, traumatic), size (small, large, giant), location (from the LR to the PR), and in relation to the circumference of the artery, although they most frequently occur on the horizontal part of the free segment of the ICA and on the lateral side of the artery circumference (Figs. 4–7). It is important first to find out whether the aneurysm is thrombosed and, if so, to what extent, and second to gage the condition of the ICA wall proximal and distal to the origin of the aneurysm in the ICA (arteriosclerotic, compressed by the overlying large or giant aneurysm, or both) (Figs. 8 and 9). Any type of aneurysm, of any size and location, may be without an intraaneurysmal clot or thrombus, and it is very important to diagnose this before any treatment, whether endovascular and/or direct surgical. Nothing less than a thorough knowledge of the condition of the ICA wall proximal and distal to the aneurysm, the extent of the aneurysmal neck, the size of the aneurysm, its location, and possible thrombus in the aneurysm will lead to the institution of the correct mode of treatment, ie, endovascular and/or direct surgical (25–38). Furthermore, a careful study of the angiograms before surgery will enable the surgeon to

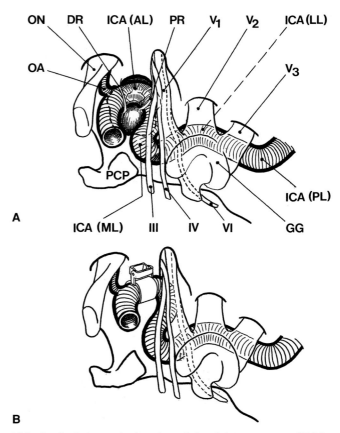

FIG. 2. A: Schematic drawing of the right cavernous ICA in its AL with the aneurysm located on the medial side of its wall and projecting into the sella. **B:** A cuff clip is shown around the ICA at the site of the resected aneurysm. The aneurysm is excluded and the patency of the ICA preserved.

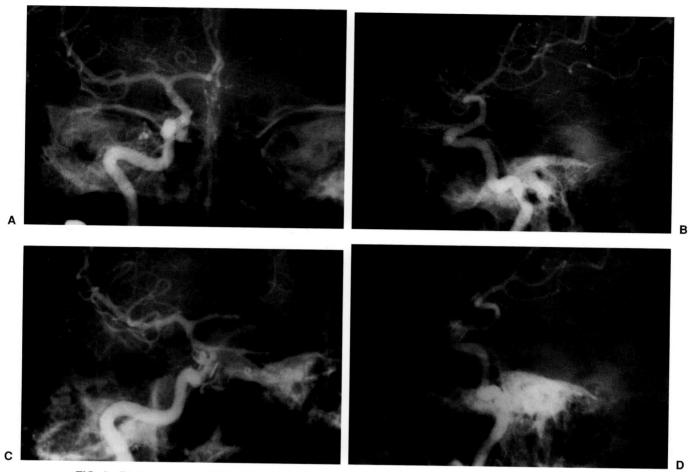

FIG. 3. Right-sided carotid angiography demonstrating a false aneurysm at the AL preoperatively, the AP view **(A)**, and the lateral view **(B)**; and a cuff clip situated on the AL postoperatively, the AP view **(C)**, and the lateral view **(D)**. The ICA is patent.

select the appropriate type of surgical exclusion of the aneurysm and reconstruction of the ICA wall (11): local (Figs. 2–7), direct (Fig.10), or complete (Figs. 8 and 9).

Cranial Nerves III–VI

Oculomotor nerves III, IV, and VI, as well as nerve V with all its segments, Gasserian ganglion (GG), V1, V2, and V3, are described in detail elsewhere (3,6,10–14). The relation of the individual nerves to the dural layers and their relation to the ICA and other important anatomic structures are also described in detail elsewhere (10–13). Of surgical importance is the knowledge of the topography of the areas between the nerves and the dural and/or bony structures, as these represent the ''windows'' through which access to different segments of the ICA is possible (3,4,6,7,27). The anteromedial triangle (3) affords access to the AL in its entirety (Fig. 2); the paramedian triangle (Fig. 6) and Parkinson's triangle (Fig. 4) allow the free segment of the ICA from the LR to the PR to be adequately explored around

its circumference and in its entire length, and any type of aneurysm can be dealt with appropriately (Figs. 4–7). The anterolateral, lateral, and posteromedial triangular windows are not of particular relevance in dealing with cavernous ICA aneurysms (3,4). However, of great importance is the posterolateral (Glasscock's) triangle (3,5), through which the ICA in the petrous canal can be visualized and prepared for temporary and/or permanent occlusion, as well as for complete reconstruction when required (4,37). In all cases of cavernous ICA aneurysms, the removal of the ACP is mandatory (Figs. 3, 5, 7, 9) and so is the opening of the optic canal on its dorsal, lateral, and under aspects—the last mentioned representing the complete removal of the optic strut. Through the anteromedial triangle, the AL of the ICA can be dissected around its circumference without opening either the DR or the PR. In this way the AL of the ICA is prepared for temporary clipping. The exposure of the ICA in the posterolateral (Glasscock's) triangle (5) is mandatory in all cavernous ICA aneurysms in order to provide proximal control by temporary occlusion of the ICA. All of these triangles, formed by individual nerves and representing the

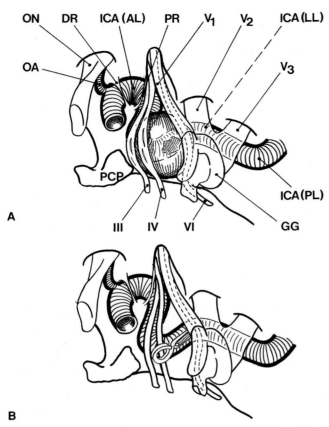

FIG. 4. A: Schematic drawing of the right cavernous ICA with the aneurysm on its free segment. The orifice of the aneurysm neck is on the lateral side of the ICA wall. The aneurysm displaces nerves III and IV medialward and nerves V1 and VI lateralward. **B:** The aneurysm has been clipped and the sac of the aneurysm resected through Parkinson's triangle. The patency of the ICA is preserved and the nerves released from the pressure from the aneurysm.

windows to the extradural parasellar and intrapetrous ICA, can be well visualized without opening the dura. Also, most of the berry aneurysms and/or fusiform aneurysms of the cavernous ICA can be treated without opening the dura (4). The opening of the dura and visualization of the ophthalmic artery (OA) and the intradural ICA is necessary only in large and/or giant aneurysms involving the cavernous ICA wall, which can also be found along the segment of the AL, or in cases where the cavernous ICA proximal and/or distal to the aneurysm is significantly diseased, thus necessitating complete reconstruction of the ICA with a graft from the petrous to the intradural segment of the ICA (Figs. 8 and 9). The dura should also be opened in cases of traumatic aneurysms involving the distal leg of the AL of the ICA. This type of traumatic (false) aneurysm necessitates the placement of a cuff clip (Figs. 2 and 3) or resection of a short segment of the ICA and direct end-to-end reconstruction of the artery (Fig. 10). Taking into consideration the normal relationship between the individual nerves and the ICA, and the dural

layers in the lateral wall of the parasellar space, combined with the location, size, and other characteristics of the cavernous ICA aneurysms, even before treatment of such an aneurysm one can pinpoint the most probable displacement of each individual nerve and/or distension of it over or around the large and/or giant aneurysm. It is well known that in most cases nerve VI is usually stretched and displaced laterally and inferiorly, whereas nerves III and IV are displaced and stretched medially and upward, and V₁ is usually stretched laterally over the aneurysmal sac. During surgery, when the aneurysmal sac is entered, one should be aware of the displacement of the nerves around the aneurysmal sac; the section of the aneurysmal wall at the neck may not be dangerous for the nerves unless one tries to pull the sac of the aneurysm away from the displaced, stretched, and thinned nerves (which, in fact, is not necessary).

Venous Plexus of the Parasellar Space

The venous plexus of the parasellar space will be reduced in its volume around the ICA according to the position and the size of the aneurysm arising from the ICA. In cases of large and even more so in cases of giant aneurysms, the venous compartments in the parasellar space will be completely occluded by the mass of the aneurysm. In cases where part of the venous plexus is still preserved it is important to be aware of the varying possibilities for performing hemostasis during the operation. Otherwise, in cases of large and giant aneurysms, venous hemostasis during surgery will not be a problem, but the surgeon should be aware of the risk of opening the intercavernous sinuses and the superior and inferior petrous sinus while excising the aneurysmal sac; the channels should be plugged to prevent any possible retrograde bleeding after surgery, which may occur due to the patient's strain and accordingly increased intrathoracic and intravenous intracranial pressure. It should also be mentioned that in cases of small aneurysms and persisting venous network in the parasellar space, acute occlusion of all of these veins will cause pronounced nonpulsating exophthalmos though short-lasting on that side after surgery. This in fact will never happen when the venous plexus has been progressively reduced and finally completely occluded due to the "growing" of the aneurysmal mass.

Types of Aneurysms and Clinical Presentation

The aneurysms of the cavernous ICA can manifest themselves only when they become large enough to stretch or compress the nerves (39). For this reason, the first of all nerves to be affected is nerve VI because it is the only one that courses through the cavernous sinus (CS) (Fig. 1) and, in addition, it is "fixed" to the ICA by the sympathetic fibers (3). When the aneurysm grows from the ICA so it is located between the individual sympathetic fibers coursing from the ICA to nerve VI, it may push against nerve VI. The fixed nerve may then

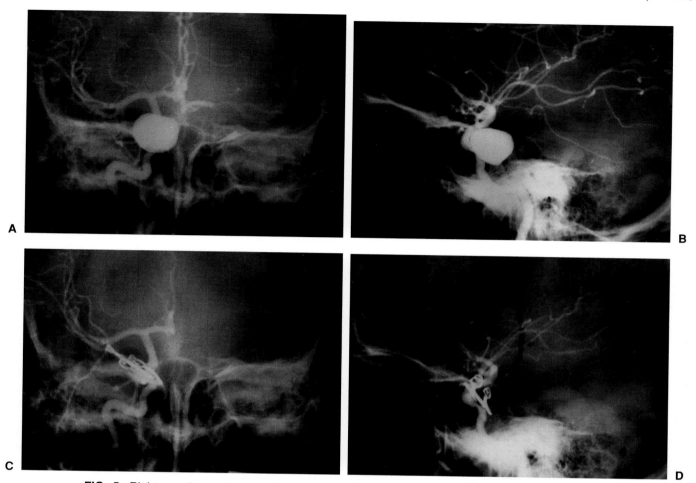

FIG. 5. Right carotid angiogram showing an aneurysm on the free segment of the cavernous ICA preoperatively, the AP view **(A)**, and the lateral view **(B)**. Postoperative angiograms show three clips on the horizontal part of the free segment of the ICA and no aneurysm, the anterior view **(C)**, and the lateral view **(D)**. Stenosis of the diameter of the ICA is present as a result of the broad neck and thick wall of the aneurysm neck, necessitating placement of three clips.

lose its function partially or completely for long enough that tearing of one or more sympathetic fibers occurs due to the increased size of the aneurysm, or the fibers may slide along the wall of the aneurysm and so too will nerve VI. Only in this way can a transitory nerve VI palsy be explained on an anatomopathologic basis. When the aneurysm becomes larger, it will push and stretch nerve VI further laterally and downward and will press it against the bone at the exit point from Dorello's canal. Pareses of nerves III, IV, and V1 are rare, and if they occur they are slight to moderate. In berry aneurysms and fusiform aneurysms, even in large and/or giant ones, the symptoms due to the compression (stretching) of V1, V2, V3, and the GG are occasional. A sudden onset of severe, sometimes agonizing pain in the V1 and V2 distribution, as well as palsy of nerves III, IV, and VI, may only occur when a small aneurysm, usually of the berry type, ruptures and a large or giant false aneurysm results. In such cases, sudden severe pain, complete ophthalmoplegia, and exophthalmos

are characteristic clinical features. In most unruptured large and/or giant aneurysms, the symptoms and signs are very few and of mild intensity. There is a slight difference between large and giant aneurysms that are filled with a thrombus, either partially (Fig. 9) or completely, and those that have no thrombus inside the sac (Figs. 5 and 7). In the latter case, the patients experience discomfort and/or tension that may be associated with physical and/or psychological stress. Traumatic and false aneurysms are in most cases located on the AL of the ICA and occur as a result of a fracture of the wall of the sphenoid sinus, the ACP, and/or the sphenoid wing. In most of these cases, ipsilateral blindness is associated with a massive nose bleed, which may occur days or even weeks after the trauma (40,41). These nose bleeds may frighten the patient and also cause hemorrhagic shock because of the loss of up to 1 L or more of arterial blood. In this kind of traumatic aneurysm other nerves (III, IV, VI, V1) may also be affected. In cases of iatrogenic traumatic aneurysms of the ICA, the aneu-

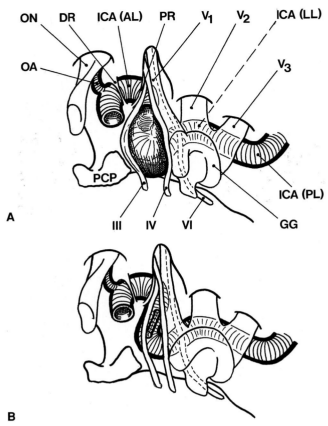

FIG. 6. A: Schematic drawing of the cavernous ICA with the aneurysm on the free segment displacing nerve III medialward and nerves IV, V1, and VI lateralward. **B:** Schematic drawing of the situation after resection of the aneurysm and reconstruction of the artery wall with separate sutures. The patency of the artery is preserved and the pressure exerted by the aneurysm on the nerves has been removed by resection of the neck of the aneurysm.

rysms are confined to the medial side of the distal leg of the AL of the ICA (Figs. 2 and 3) or to the medial side of the horizontal part of the free segment of the ICA in cases when this is positioned "inside" the sella. The iatrogenic traumatic aneurysms usually do not cause neurologic deficits but may cause a nose bleed and/or a caverous carotid fistula (CCF).

Large and/or giant cavernous ICA aneurysms may also rupture into the intradural space; if they do, the hemorrhage is usually large and the outcome might be fatal (42). Partially thrombosed aneurysms, especially when associated with the diseased ICA wall, can be the origin of emboli and the cause of aneurysm-to-artery embolism (Fig. 9). The usual neurologic deficit is transient ischemic attack; however, a major stroke may also be the end result.

The Diagnostic Workup

Computed tomography (CT), magnetic resonance imaging (MRI), and MR angiography are indispensable for the preliminary workup of the patients. These imaging techniques provide information on the size and extension of the aneurysm, the presence of an intraluminal thrombus, and the state of the wall of the aneurysm. MR angiography provides information regarding the flow pattern within the aneurysmal lumen. Four-vessel selective angiography should be performed in every case, not only to delineate the aneurysm and its relationship to the ICA but to exclude further aneurysms, particularly of the contralateral ICA. Following the angiographic examination, functional angiographic investigation with the balloon occlusion test should be performed in order to assess the collateral circulation. For that purpose, a bifemoral approach is used. Through one femoral artery a guiding catheter is inserted into the ipsilateral ICA. This catheter is used as the guiding catheter for the microballoon. A regular angiographic catheter is introduced through the contralateral femoral artery through which angiography of the contralateral ICA, ipsilateral external carotid artery (ECA), and dominant vertebral artery will be performed during the balloon occlusion test. Through the guiding catheter, a microballoon is inserted into the ICA and navigated into the cavernous segment. The ICA is occluded by balloon inflation at the level of the aneurysm. During the balloon occlusion of the ICA, heparinized saline is infused through the guiding catheter into the occluded proximal ICA in order to prevent thrombus formation. The state of the anterior communicating artery (Acom) and the posterior communicating artery (Pcom) is investigated by contralateral internal carotid and dominant vertebral artery angiography. Particular attention is given to the venous phase. Simultaneous appearance of the veins of both hemispheres indicates sufficient collaterals. The circulation through the ophthalmic artery is investigated by ipsilateral external carotid angiography during the balloon occlusion of the ICA. Usually, retrograde flow in the ophthalmic artery from the facial or internal maxillary arteries is observed. During the balloon occlusion test the patient is also examined neurologically. The patient is in the supine, flat position, and the ICA is occluded for 20 minutes. If there is good angiographic patency of either the Acom or Pcom and there is simultaneous appearance of the cortical veins of both hemispheres in the venous phase, no neurologic deficits should be observed during the balloon occlusion test.

NONSURGICAL APPROACH

Endovascular Treatment of Large or Giant Fusiform Cavernous Aneurysms

Several techniques of balloon occlusion of the ICA can be applied, depending on the size and extension of the aneurysm as well as on the local vascular anatomy. The balloon occlusion is performed by inserting a detachable latex balloon into the cavernous segment of the ICA. Usually, occlusion of the ICA at the proximal end of the aneurysm will suffice in producing complete obliteration of the aneurysm

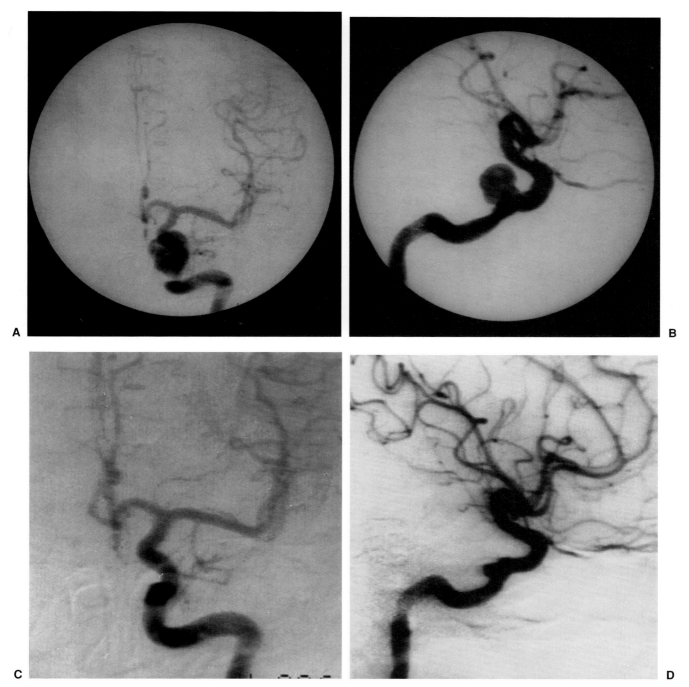

FIG. 7. Left carotid angiogram demonstrating a broad-neck aneurysm on the free segment of the ICA preoperatively, the AP view **(A)**, and the lateral view **(B)**. The postoperative angiogram shows a more intense shadow at the site of the resected aneurysm and reconstructed artery, in the AP view **(C)**, and in the lateral view **(D)**; a small remaining part of the aneurysm is seen.

and the distal ICA up to the origin of the ophthalmic artery. If there is retrograde filling of the aneurysm, as demonstrated by contralateral internal carotid or vertebral artery angiography, two balloons may be used to trap the segment of the ICA from which the aneurysm arises. If it is technically impossible to place a balloon distal to the aneurysm, the

following alternative technique has proved to be most reliable: a microcatheter is inserted into the distal part of the aneurysm while the ICA is occluded proximally at the proximal origin of the aneurysm with the balloon. Through the microcatheter, Guglielmi detachable coils are inserted at the exit area of the fusiform aneurysm in order to prevent retro-

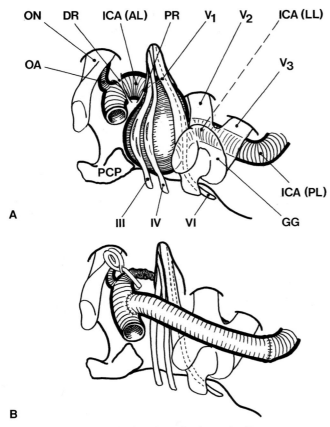

ON DR ICA (AL) PR V₁ V₂ ICA (LL)

OA V₃

PCP ICA (PL)

A III IV VI GG

B

FIG. 8. A: Schematic drawing of a large fusiform aneurysm of the cavernous ICA exerting significant pressure toward nerves III, IV, V1, and VI. **B:** Schematic drawing of the reconstruction of the ICA with a venous graft inserted between the proximal (intrapetrous) segment of the ICA and the intradural ICA. The graft has been placed lateral to nerves III, IV, V, and VI. A permanent clip is on the ICA proximal to the ophthalmic artery (OA).

grade flow into the aneurysm and promote thrombosis. After detachment of a few coils at the exit area of the aneurysm the proximally located balloon is detached. Following balloon detachment at the level of the cavernous segment of the ICA, a second balloon is always inserted into the proximal ICA and detached in order to avoid extensive thrombus formation at the stump of the ICA with the potential risk of thromboembolism through the external carotid artery into the ophthalmic or cerebral circulation. Following balloon occlusion of the ICA the patient is monitored for 24 hours in the intensive care unit. It is imperative that the blood pressure be kept at least at normal levels. Plasma expanders are very useful in this initial postocclusion phase. Early postocclusion CT or MRI performed within a few days after balloon occlusion will demonstrate complete thrombosis of the aneurysm. Follow-up CT or MRI after 6 and 12 months usually reveals complete shrinkage of the aneurysm mass.

Selective Endosaccular Obliteration of Saccular Aneurysms of the Cavernous ICA Aneurysms

For this type of cavernous ICA aneurysms selective obliteration with platinum microcoils (15) provides an alternative technique to the direct surgical approach. The aneurysmal sac is selectively catheterized with an appropriate microcatheter. Following selective catheterization of the aneurysm lumen, Guglielmi detachable coils of appropriate size are introduced into the aneurysm and detached by electrolysis. The number and size of the coils needed depends on the volume of the aneurysm. The initial results of this technique are promising (Fig. 11). However, no data on long-term follow-up are available for this technique.

SURGICAL APPROACH

The patient is in the supine position on the operating table with his or her head fixed in the Mayfield tripoint headrest. The patient's head is rotated by 25–30° to the opposite direction of the lesion (Fig. 12) in order that the frontotemporal region on the side of the lesion in the CS can be exposed. The skin incision is made in a curved line running from the point in front of the tragus of the ear in an upward direction to the midline, behind the hairline. The concavity of the skin incision is directed anteriorly. Care should be taken that the incision of the skin is made close to the tragus of the ear, ie, behind the line of the external temporal artery and the facial nerve. The skin flap with the subcutaneous tissue is then separated from the periosteum and the fascia of the temporalis muscle and reflected anteriorly over the edge of the orbit. The incision of the periosteum curves around the insertion line of the temporalis muscle so that the insertion of the temporalis muscle is not damaged (Fig. 13). At the joining point of the orbital edge and the superior leg of the zygoma the muscle is peeled off from the bone so the bone at the pterion is exposed. At this point, the bone is drilled off with a diamond drill to enable simultaneous opening of the orbit, the anterior cranial fossa, and the middle cranial fossa (Fig. 14). The incision of the temporalis muscle in its posterior part runs along the longitudinal axis of the muscle fibers. The incised section of the temporalis muscle is then peeled off from the squama of the temporal bone where two burr holes are introduced: the first one in the squama of the temporal bone itself, and the second one at the borderline between the squama of the temporal bone and the frontal and the parietal bone (Fig. 14). The bone is then cut from the first burr hole in an anterior and downward direction into the squama for a distance of approximately 2 cm, ie, as much as the temporalis muscle overlying this bone allows without the muscle being damaged (Fig. 14). The bone is then cut from the first burr hole in the direction of the second burr hole toward the border of the squama of the temporal bone, and then from the second burr hole over the frontal bone as far as the pterion. The next step is the placement of

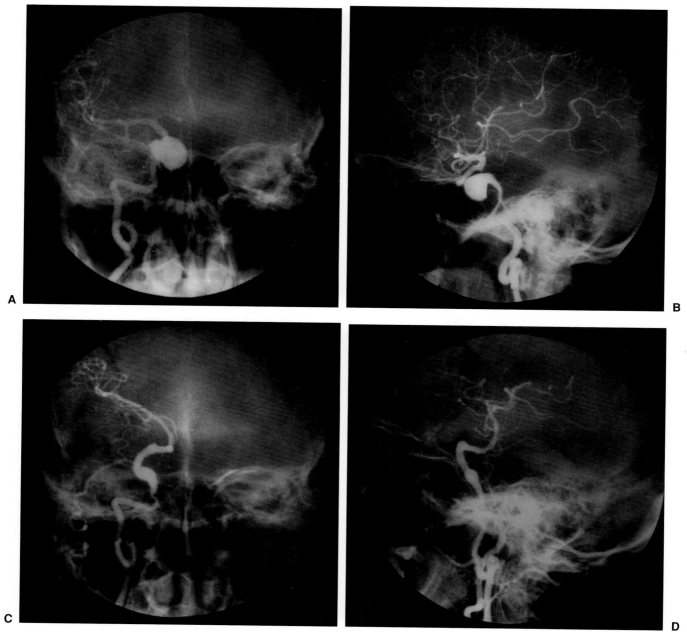

FIG. 9. Preoperative right carotid angiogram demonstrating a large cavernous ICA aneurysm, partially thrombosed and exerting pressure against the ICA proximal to the aneurysm, causing stenosis of this part of the ICA, the AP view **(A)**, and the lateral view **(B)**. Postoperative angiograms show the ICA reconstructed with a venous graft and no aneurysm, the AP view **(C)**, and the lateral view **(D)**. The cavernous ICA proximal to the graft is rather narrow, but patent, after surgery. The venous graft used is very short as it is placed between the proximal intracavernous free segment of the ICA and the supraclinoid intradural ICA, and not from the petrous to the supraclinoid ICA as is the customary procedure.

small holes symmetrically on each side of the bone cut in a diagonal direction so as to enable the surgeon to fix the bone flap correctly at the end of surgery. The second purpose of these small holes is to ensure that the dura is suspended over the borders of the bone before it is incised so as to prevent any epidural hemorrhage (Fig. 15). The next step is lifting

the osteomuscular flap by breaking off the bone at the level of the anterior part of the squama of the temporal bone over the proximal part of the temporal lobe, ie, lateral to the Sylvian fissure. When the bone flap is divided at its base from the squama of the temporal bone, additional peeling of the temporalis muscle from the squama of the temporal bone is

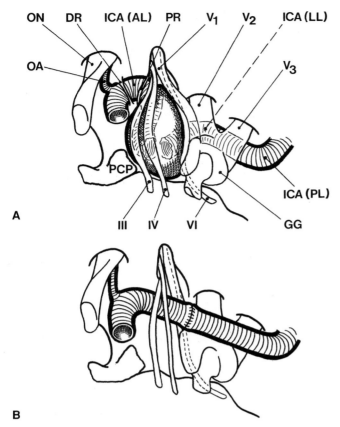

A

B

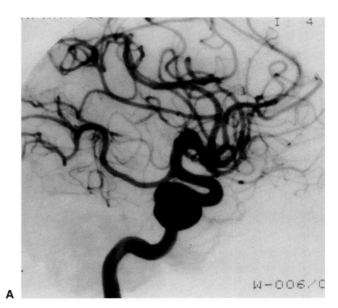

A

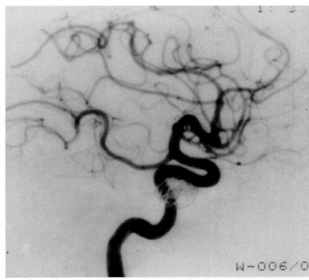

B

FIG. 10. A: Schematic drawing of the cavernous ICA with a large aneurysm, where the entry point of the ICA into the aneurysm is several millimeters away from the exit point from the aneurysm into the distal segment of the ICA. Nerves III and IV are displaced and stretched medialward, whereas on the other side, nerves VI and V1 are displaced and stretched lateralward. **B:** The aneurysm sac is resected, and the distal part of segment A and the proximal part of segment B are dissected free and transposed from the medial aspect of nerves V3, V2, V1, and VI to their lateral aspect. The distal part of the free segment B is mobilized in the peripheral direction, so that the PR is cut around the ICA, and the distal part of the free segment B and segment C are extended in a lateral direction, and the distal stump of the ICA is drawn through Parkinson's triangle and anastomosed directly (end-to-end) with the proximal stump of the ICA.

FIG. 11. Left carotid angiogram, the lateral view, demonstrating a cavernous ICA saccular aneurysm before endovascular obliteration **(A)**; after treatment with Guglielmi detachable coils, a shadow of packed coils is seen, and there is no aneurysm filling. The ICA is patent and of a normal diameter **(B)**.

carried out, and the bone flap and the temporal muscle are reflected over the skin flap in a dorsolateral direction. If necessary, the base of the bone flap is additionally trimmed with a rongeur to ensure that the borders are properly rounded and kept clear of the operative field so they do not disturb the surgeon as he or she works over the temporal lobe toward the base of the middle fossa (Fig. 15). Once the osteomuscular flap has been fixed in a lateral direction, the dura over the temporal lobe is peeled off from the temporal bone toward the base of the middle fossa. Additional trimming of the squama of the temporal bone is performed so that the foramen spinosum (FS), the anterior surface of the

petrous bone, the foramen ovale (FO), and the foramen rotundum (FR) are all well exposed. The dura over the temporal lobe should not be compressed with a spatula: it should be fixed with stitches and pulled away from the bone. The orbital roof is resected on the posterior aspect of the superior orbital fissure (SOF) so that the dural continuation from the temporal lobe and the CS into the periorbita through the SOF is preserved undamaged. While removing the orbital roof, great attention should be paid to ensure that the periorbita is not damaged. If the periorbita is lacerated and the fatty tissue released, this tissue can be "pushed" back into the orbit by bipolar coagulation. The roof of the orbit on the

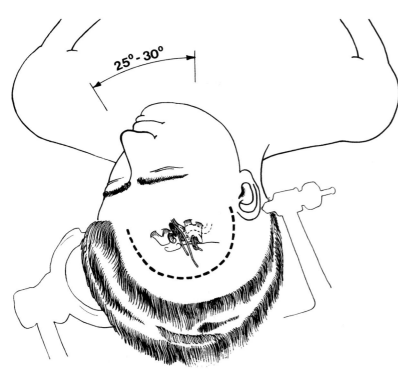

FIG. 12. Schematic drawing of the initial positioning of the patient's head in a tripoint headrest. A schematic drawing of structures on one side of the skull base represents the actual targeting of the surgical approach. The initial positioning of the head is for the skin incision, formation of the skin and osteomuscular flaps, and initial unroofing of the orbit. For the approaches to bony, dural, neural, and vascular structures and to the lesion, the position of the head will be appropriately changed. It is mandatory that the operating table and the headrest rotate easily to the left and right as well as tilt in the Trendelenburg and reverse Trendelenburg direction.

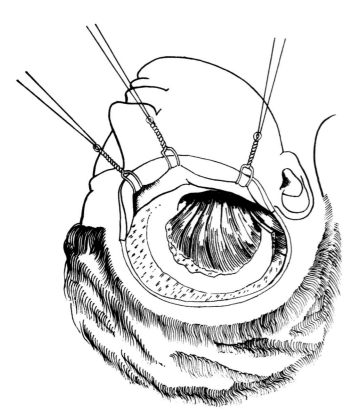

FIG. 13. Schematic drawing of the reflected skin flap on the right side. The periosteum is incised around the insertion area of the temporalis muscle to the bone, and the incision of the temporalis muscle in its posterior portion is made in a radial direction, ie, the muscle fibers are split longitudinally as to their longitudinal axis rather than cut in a perpendicular direction. The temporalis muscle together with the periosteum is peeled off from the bone at the joining point of the ascending leg of the zygomatic bone to the orbital rim, and the pterion is exposed.

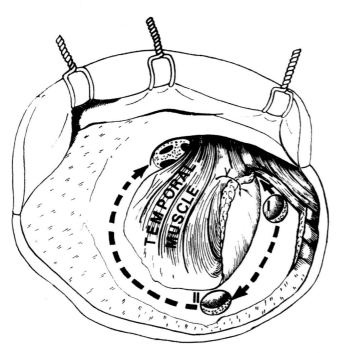

FIG. 14. Schematic drawing of further steps of the formation of the osteomuscular flap. The periosteum is stripped off the bone at the pterion and is further cut around the insertion area of the temporalis muscle, and then the fibers of the temporalis muscle are split in the posterior part so the bone is well visualized. The bone is first drilled off with a cutting drill behind the joining point of the upper leg of the zygoma and the orbital rim so that the middle cranial fossa, the orbit, and the anterior cranial fossa are opened at the same time. A burr hole (I) is then made in the squama of the temporal bone. The second burr hole (II) is made on the borderline of the squama of the temporal bone and the frontal bone. The next step is cutting of the bone in the direction as indicated by the arrows, ie, lateralward, medialward, and around the insertion of the temporalis muscle.

anterior aspect of the sphenoid wing is also removed all the way down to the peripheral end of the optic canal. The sphenoid wing is removed as far as the ACP. The dura should be carefully peeled from the planum sphenoidale so the falciform ligament over the optic nerve (ON) is well exposed and the dorsal wall of the optic canal may be safely drilled away with the diamond drill. It is important that before opening the optic canal and removing the ACP, the duplicature of the dura covering the nerves coursing from the CS into the orbit is cut and the cleavage line is found; also the dura on the under aspect of the temporal lobe is preserved (Fig. 15). While the dura is being peeled from the lateral wall of the CS, the ACP is visualized from its lateral side, and then the drilling of the ACP from its midportion in an outward direction can be started. Once the bulk of the ACP has been drilled off, its wall can be easily fractured with a microdissector and removed from the neural and vascular structures. The optic strut is removed in its entirety by a diamond drill. The lateral and dorsal walls of the optic canal are also drilled

off with the diamond drill under continuous irrigation. In order to avoid damaging the ON by overheating, it is advisable to perform the drilling at short intervals and to check the thickness of the bone with the microdissector. In this way one will avoid not only damage to the ON by overheating but also direct mechanical damage to the ON by the drill. While removing the last piece of the ACP behind the AL of the ICA it is possible that the CS may be entered accidentally. In such cases venous bleeding occurs, but this can be easily stopped by plugging the hole in the CS with Surgicel. Care should be taken not to drill off the lateral wall of the sphenoid sinus above and medial to the AL of the ICA. Peeling the dura away from the lateral wall of the CS and from the lesion in the CS will reveal nerves III, IV, and V1, and by peeling the dura more laterally and in a posterior direction nerves V2 and V3 will be visualized (Fig. 16). The middle meningeal artery (MMA) is coagulated and cut close to the FS, and its proximal stump is pushed into the canal. The canal of the MMA is additionally plugged with Surgicel and sealed with bone wax. By carefully peeling the dura from the lateral wall of the CS, ie, by splitting the outer layer from the inner layer of the lateral wall of the CS, all the nerves (III, IV, V1, V2, V3, and GG) can be well visualized (Fig. 16).

The ICA is exposed in the petrous bone medial to the

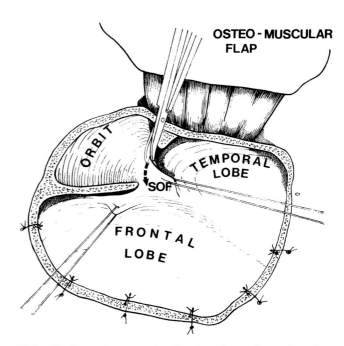

FIG. 15. An osteomuscular flap has been formed and reflected to the lateral side over the zygoma. The dura of the temporal and frontal lobes is exposed. The orbital roof has been partially removed and the dural tent of the superior orbital fissure (SOF) is exposed. The dura has been fixed to the edge of the bone around the craniotomy line. Additional stay sutures of the dura have been placed on the duplicature of the dura of the SOF tent. Curved scissors over the dural duplicature of the SOF point at the direction *(arrow)* in which cutting the duplicature is carried out in order not to damage nerves III, IV, V1, and VI inside the dural duplicature.

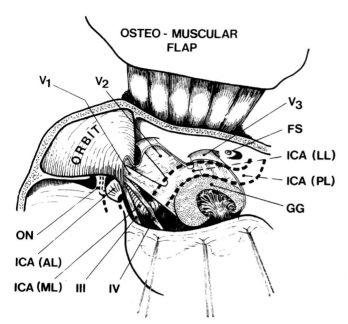

FIG. 16. Schematic drawing of the exposure of the right cavernous sinus (CS) structures after splitting the outer layer of its lateral wall. The dura on the under aspect of the right temporal lobe is fixed with stay sutures. Nerves V1, V2, V3, GG, and even the plexiform segment of the root of nerve V, as well as the optic nerve and nerves III and IV, are visualized. The anterior clinoid process (ACP) together with the sphenoid wing has been removed and the anterior loop (AL) of the ICA is shown. The orbit is unroofed anterior and posterior to the sphenoid wing together with the removal of the sphenoid wing itself. The osteomuscular flap is reflected laterally over the zygoma. The middle meningeal artery (MMA) has been cut and the foramen spinosum (FS) packed with Surgicel and bone wax.

eustachian tube (5). The drilling of the bone over the carotid canal should be started 5–8 mm medial to the FS and dorsal to V3 and GG (4). In most cases, the ICA is covered with bone, although in 20% of cases the bone is very thin or nonexistent. Therefore, while drilling the bone over the ICA, care should be taken not to drill too far laterally, ie, too close to the FS, or the eustachian tube might be entered first. The easiest way to enter the carotid canal is by drilling the petrous bone behind the GG in the anteromedial direction. In this way, the ICA will be found from its medial side. When the ICA is exposed, it should be peeled off from the walls of the carotid canal circumferentially. The periarterial fibrous tissue, consisting of the periosteal outer layer, the softer regular tissue, the sympathetic fibers, and the venous plexus, should not be damaged. The exposed segment of the ICA should be long enough to permit placement of the temporary clips or insertion of the balloon into the carotid canal between the bony wall and the wall of the ICA (21). The periarterial connective tissue (periosteum, venous plexus, sympathetic fibers, and fibrous tissue) should be disrupted and resected only in cases of grafting of the ICA from the petrous

bone to the ICA proximal to the OA or distal to it (Figs. 8 and 9).

In cases of smaller or medium-sized cavernous ICA aneurysms that do not involve the AL of the ICA, distal exposure of the ICA is carried out at the AL, ie, also circumferentially, with the preservation of the periarterial fibrous tissue and the periosteum of the ACP forming the floor of the anteromedial triangle (3). However, in cases of large or giant cavernous ICA aneurysms, also involving the AL of the ICA, exposure of the ICA intradurally, proximal to the PCom, is necessary. In these cases the ACP is usually thin. The exposure of the intradural ICA proximal to the PCom is also necessary in all cases of diseased ICA, either proximal or distal to the aneurysm in the CS, regardless of the size of the aneurysm because in such cases a complete reconstruction (4,35) of the ICA is necessary with a graft (Figs. 8 and 9). The location of the ''neck'' of the cavernous ICA aneurysm as well as the size of the aneurysm and the quality of the artery proximal and distal to the exit of the aneurysm from the ICA dictate the approach into the cavernous space, ie, which window(s) will be used. However, in most cases the most suitable approach will be through Parkinson's triangle (Fig. 4). In cases where it is necessary to completely mobilize the horizontal part of the cavernous ICA, additional mobilization of nerve IV will have to be done, and the entrance through the paramedian triangle (3) will be needed (Fig. 6). Whenever possible, nerve III should be left attached to the PR and not dissected completely out of the dural layers. However, mobilization of nerve III is necessary in most cases in order to permit the placement of clip(s) or sutures. In cases of large and giant cavernous aneurysms, it is preferable to enter the cavity of the aneurysm after placing the proximal and distal temporary clips and visualizing the proximal and distal orifices of the aneurysm. The aneurysm should then be mobilized from all sides and resected close to the artery (providing the artery wall has been preserved). The artery wall should then be reconstructed by direct suturing (Fig. 7). The individual types of reconstruction of the ICA are (a) local (Figs. 2, 4, 6), (b) direct (Fig. 10), and (c) complete (Fig. 8). Local reconstruction of the ICA is performed by clipping the aneurysm or resecting it and that in cases where the aneurysm neck does not occupy more than one half of the circumference of the ICA. The permanent clip(s) must be placed along the longitudinal axis of the ICA on the neck of the aneurysm (Fig. 4). The sac of the aneurysm may be left in place or resected. In cases where the sac is not resected, it should be punctured and the blood evacuated from it, thus providing reduction of compression against the neighboring nerves. In other cases of larger aneurysms with broader necks, the aneurysm may be entered and the neck resected; separate sutures along the longitudinal axis should then be made using the walls of the neck of the aneurysm for reconstruction of the ICA, thus restoring more or less the normal diameter of the ICA at the site of reconstruction and avoiding stenosis of the artery (Figs. 6 and 7).

In cases where the artery wall is diseased or the whole

circumference of the ICA is changed into the aneurysm (fusiform), the diseased or aneurysmatically dilated segment of the ICA is resected and the proximal and distal stumps are pulled together (after mobilization of the proximal and distal adjacent loops); the stumps are then sutured directly, proximal to the distal stump. This type of reconstruction is only possible when the diseased or dilated segment of the ICA is <5 mm (Fig. 10). Complete reconstruction of the ICA is necessary in a sclerotic or diseased wall of the ICA proximal and/or distal to the aneurysm, as well as in large and giant intracavernous fusiform aneurysms (Fig. 8). In these cases, a graft (venous or arterial) is placed between the petrous or proximal cavernous portion of the ICA and distally sutured to the ICA either proximal or distal to the OA, depending on the diseased segment of the ICA (Fig. 9). A possible clot or a thrombus in the aneurysm should be removed from the aneurysmal sac, although there is no need to remove the sac itself. After exclusion of the aneurysm it is necessary to plug the CS with Surgicel toward the intercavernous sinuses around the pituitary gland in the sella, as well as toward the superior and inferior petrous sinus and toward the plexus over the clival region. This packing is done to prevent the occurrence of hemorrhage after surgery when the patient may suffer from some physical strain.

In cases of complete reconstruction of the ICA after the resection of the cavernous ICA aneurysm and the artery itself, a graft is placed over the cranial nerves of the CS (Figs. 8 and 9). The patency of the ICA—after it has been reconstructed locally and/or directly, and particularly in cases of complete reconstruction of the ICA with a graft—should be intraoperatively checked angiographically or at least with intraoperative Doppler.

RESULTS OF NONSURGICAL TREATMENT OF CAVERNOUS ICA ANEURYSMS

A series of 74 aneurysms of the cavernous segment of the ICA have been treated by the endovascular balloon occlusion technique by Valavanis at the Neuroradiological Institute, University Hospital, Zurich, since 1982. In 9 cases, an EC–IC bypass had to be performed prior to balloon occlusion due to insufficient collateral circulation at the level of the circle of Willis. In 69 cases, long-term follow-up CT or MRI was performed and showed complete shrinkage of the aneurysm in 66 cases, partial shrinkage in 2, and no significant shrinkage in 1. The remaining 5 patients were lost to follow-up. Two patients suffered an ocular thromboembolic complication resulting in partial visual loss and 3 patients suffered hemispheric infarctions for a total morbidity of 6.7%. No mortality attributable to the procedure occurred in this series.

RESULTS OF SURGICAL TREATMENT OF CAVERNOUS ICA ANEURYSMS

From 1981 through 1995, 86 patients with cavernous ICA aneurysms were treated by direct surgical approach. Cavernous ICA aneurysms were small in 52 patients, large in 18 patients, and in the remaining 16 patients they measured >2.5 cm in diameter.

In 5 of 9 patients with a traumatic aneurysm, the characteristic nose bleed and ipsilateral blindness occurred immediately after trauma, whereas in the remaining 4 patients the optic nerve was not injured and the visual function was preserved. Out of the latter 4 patients, 2 had nose bleed that occurred several weeks following the trauma. In 1 of the 4 patients, the aneurysm was situated on the free segment of the cavernous ICA (Fig. 7). In this patient, initially complete ophthalmoplegia was present, and 6 months after the trauma all the nerves except nerve VI had regained their function. The cavernous ICA traumatic aneurysm was larger than initially; it was on the dominant left side and endovascular exclusion of the aneurysm with preservation of the patency of the ICA was not successful. Nerve VI palsy persisted, so that surgery was indicated. The lesion was excised by the direct surgical approach and the artery wall reconstructed with separate sutures (Figs. 6 and 7). Six months after resection of the aneurysm, the function of nerve VI was restored and diplopia had ceased. In another case of false aneurysm, the AL of the ICA was injured during transsphenoidal surgery and bleeding was stopped intraoperatively. In this case, no neurologic deficits were found prior to surgery of the aneurysm. Repeated carotid angiography after surgery showed the aneurysm located on the medial side of the AL. The patient underwent reoperation, tolerated the procedure well, and there were no neurologic deficits postoperatively (Figs. 2 and 3). All traumatic aneurysms of the series were small, ie, <15 mm in diameter.

In the series of 43 small saccular aneurysms, the aneurysms were located on the free segment B of the ICA. Twenty of these were excluded from the circulation by clipping, 15 by resection of the aneurysm and reconstruction of the ICA wall with separate sutures, 5 by a combination of suturing and clipping, and in 3 cases—following resection of the aneurysm and part of the diseased artery wall—direct reconstruction (end-to-end) of the ICA was performed by suturing the proximal and distal stumps of the ICA (Fig. 10). In 16 patients of 34 with large or giant aneurysms, a graft was inserted between the proximal and the distal stump of the ICA after the resection of the aneurysm. One of these 16 patients—on whom during the first surgery a resection of the aneurysm and local reconstruction of the ICA with separate sutures had been performed—was reoperated on the next day after the first surgery because the follow-up angiography showed occlusion of the ICA. During the reoperation, the segment of the cavernous ICA harboring the aneurysm, as well as the adjacent proximal and distal segments of the sclerotic ICA, were resected and a saphenous graft was interposed that has remained patent (Fig. 9). In 12 cases of large aneurysms, following the resection of the aneurysm, the artery wall was reconstructed with separate sutures. In 5 cases, large aneurysms were removed by clipping, and in 3 cases, following the resection of the aneurysm and part of the artery wall, direct reconstruction was performed (Fig. 10). Of 86 patients of the whole series of cavernous ICA aneurysms, 3 died following surgery; 2 patients had traumatic aneurysms and severe associated lesions of the brain. The third patient died as a result of pulmonary infection after surgery for a giant cavernous ICA aneurysm. Six patients treated for large or giant aneurysms have remained with permanent hemiparesis on the contralateral side. Three patients have a permanent nerve III palsy and two have nerve VI palsy. Three patients with traumatic ICA aneurysms who were blind before surgery have remained blind. Five patients who noticed visual deterioration prior to surgery due to expansion of the aneurysm had significant improvement of the visual function following resection of the aneurysm. None of the patients operated on for cavernous ICA aneurysms had postoperative impairment of visual function, either temporary or permanent. In all but 5 patients of the series, operated on by direct approach, nerve III palsy was postoperatively present. In 77 cases, this palsy disappeared within 3–4 months postoperatively.

Postoperative carotid angiography was performed in 80 patients. The ICA proved to be nonpatent in 6 cases: 2 of local reconstruction of the ICA, 1 of direct end-to-end anastomosis, and 3 of an interposed graft. In one patient, occlusion of the ICA occurred after local reconstruction; the patient was reoperated and the graft, which was inserted during the second surgery, has remained patent (Fig. 9).

DISCUSSION

Each type of cavernous ICA aneurysm requires a different approach. Traumatic (false) aneurysms necessitate urgent treatment. Surgery is the optimum option as most of the aneurysms are located along the AL of the ICA and reconstruction of the artery wall is necessary. Endovascular treatment for false aneurysms is not advisable unless the patient's medical condition does not permit the direct surgical approach; the patient must also be able to tolerate definite ICA occlusion. Traumatic aneurysms that are situated on the "free" segment of the cavernous ICA (Fig. 7) as well as those that follow rupture of a small aneurysm, causing acute ophthalmoplegia and in most cases very severe trigeminal pain (which may last from several weeks to 2 months), require surgery because of the better possibility for reconstruction of the artery wall, with preservation of the patency of the ICA, as well as pain relief and improvement of neurologic deficits after removal of the clot. In cases where a patient does not tolerate the balloon occlusion test, endovascular occlusion of the ICA preceded by extra-intracranial anastomosis is an alternative to the direct surgical approach and reconstruction of the ICA.

From the neurosurgeon's point of view, small and asymptomatic saccular aneurysms of the cavernous ICA do not necessitate immediate treatment and can be followed for a period of time until they produce local and/or distant symptoms. Local symptoms are usually the result of direct compression of the nerves due to enlargement of the aneurysm, whereas distant symptoms are due to embolisms because the turbulence of blood in the aneurysm may lead to the formation of a clot that may be dislodged, thereby directing the emboli to the periphery. However, certain saccular aneurysms should be excluded from circulation, ie, those in patients in whom repeated angiographies confirm that the small aneurysm is growing and those with a clot in patients who have a history of aneurysm-to-artery embolisms.

In the opinion of neuroradiologists, however, treatment of all small saccular aneurysms of the cavernous ICA, even asymptomatic ones, is indicated because of the risk of rupture causing a large or giant false cavernous aneurysm, a CCF, or even fatal intradural bleeding (42). In such cases, the diagnostic procedures may immediately be followed by an endovascular attempt at exclusion of the aneurysm from the circulation, with preservation of the patency of the ICA (Fig. 11), which is a must in incidentally found cavernous aneurysms. If it is impossible to preserve ICA patency the preferable treatment is direct surgery. In such cases, local reconstruction of the artery wall is performed and the ICA is preserved patent (Fig. 5). If in the above-mentioned cases surgery is not feasible, endovascular treatment with permanent occlusion of the ICA is the treatment of choice provided that the patient can tolerate the balloon occlusion test.

Large and giant fusiform aneurysms without a thrombus do not call for immediate treatment. From the neuroradiologic point of view, in cases where a patient tolerates the balloon occlusion test, endovascular treatment is advocated; the cavernous segment of the ICA together with the aneurysm is excluded by inserting two balloons, the distal one being put into the AL of the ICA proximal to the OA and the proximal one into the ICA proximal to the aneurysm.

There are three possible ways of surgically treating fusiform cavernous ICA aneurysms: modification of local reconstruction can be performed by resecting the sac of the aneurysm and reconstructing the ICA with separate sutures; in those cases where a fusiform dilatation of the ICA is on the short segment of the ICA (<5 mm), resection of the aneurysm can be performed and direct reconstruction of the ICA can be achieved by end-to-end suture of the ICA (Fig. 10); and in cases where a longer segment of the ICA is involved in a fusiform aneurysm, a saphenous vein or arterial graft can be placed between the proximal and the distal stump of the ICA after resection of the aneurysm and the diseased segment of the ICA (Figs. 8,9). A combination of endovascular occlusion of the ICA distal and proximal to the aneurysm, with precedent extra–intra anastomosis, can be adopted in cases where the balloon occlusion test is not tolerated and the direct surgical approach is not feasible, which might well occur in elderly patients and/or in patients with severe medical problems.

In large and giant saccular aneurysms containing a thrombus—which is the origin for emboli—surgical bypass of the cavernous ICA is preferable. Such an approach is even more imperative in cases where the artery wall of the ICA proximal and/or distal to the aneurysm is also diseased (arteriosclerotic) (Fig. 9). In such cases, endovascular placement of a balloon distal to the aneurysm may be difficult and cause partial dislodging of the thrombus, which will cause embolism(s). The occlusion of the ICA proximal to the aneurysm alone is not sufficient because the thrombus will grow in a peripheral direction; and at the origin of the ophthalmic artery it runs the risk of being dislodged in the direction of the periphery due to the reversed bloodstream in the ophthalmic artery. In large and giant aneurysms with an old and firm thrombus the aneurysm mass in the cavernous space exerts compression of the nerves. Surgical removal of the mass will lead to improvement of local neurologic deficits. Bilateral cavernous ICA aneurysms do not double the problem of unilateral ones but rather place the risk on an exponential scale (29,34). It goes without saying that in such cases there is little place for occlusion of the ICA(s). Such patients require a direct surgical approach, which should be in two stages. Where elderly patients and patients with serious medical problems are concerned, monitoring of the aneurysm is probably preferable to surgery.

Mycotic aneurysms located in the cavernous ICA initially require appropriate antibiotic treatment before any endovascular or surgical treatment can be carried out (28). In cases where the balloon occlusion test is tolerated, surgical occlusion of the ICA is preferable. Endovascular occlusion of the ICA with preceding extra–intra anastomosis has been suggested by some authors for patients who are unable to tolerate this test. Where the ICA is extensively diseased, eg, in cases of Marfan's syndrome, a graft from the petrous to the supraclinoid ICA or an even longer one, running from the ECA to the intradural ICA or even to the MCA, is preferable.

In conclusion, it must be stressed that many types of cavernous ICA aneurysms remain difficult to treat, and each one should be discussed as a separate case by all of the members of the team, taking into account all data obtained from the diagnostic workup. Such discussion and decision making should be held by the neuroradiologists, neurosurgeons, and neurologists involved, who should be able to foresee all immediate possible outcomes and potential future neurologic symptoms and signs prior to carrying out any modality of treatment. In order to be able to conduct such a team approach, it is highly advisable that patients with cavernous ICA aneurysms be treated in centers where a great deal of experience has been accumulated through previous treatment of such cases.

REFERENCES

1. Dolenc VV. Direct microsurgical repair of intracavernous vascular lesions. *J Neurosurg* 1983;58:824–831.
2. Dolenc VV. A combined epi- and subdural approach to carotid-ophthalmic artery aneurysms. *J Neurosurg* 1985;62:667.
3. Dolenc VV. *Anatomy and Surgery of the Cavernous Sinus.* New York: Springer-Verlag, 1989.
4. Dolenc VV. Intracavernous carotid artery aneurysms. In: Spetzler RF, Carter LP, eds. *Neurovascular Surgery.* New York: McGraw-Hill, 1994;659–673.
5. Glasscock ME. Exposure of the intra-petrous portion of the carotid artery. In: Hamberger CA, Wersaal J, eds. *Disorders of the Skull Base Region.* Proceedings of the 10th Nobel Symposium. Stockholm: Almqvist and Wiksell, 1969;135–143.
6. Parkinson D. A surgical approach to the cavernous portion of the carotid artery. Anatomical studies and case report. *J Neurosurg* 1965;23:474.
7. Parkinson D. Carotid cavernous fistula. History and anatomy. In: Dolenc VV, ed. *The Cavernous Sinus: A Multidisciplinary Approach to Vascular and Tumorous Lesions.* New York: Springer-Verlag, 1987; 3–29.
8. Parkinson D. Transcavernous repair of carotid cavernous fistula. *J Neurosurg* 1969;26:420.
9. Parkinson D. Carotid cavernous fistula: direct repair with preservation of the carotid artery. *J Neurosurg* 1973;38:99.
10. Taptas JN. La loge du sinus caverneux, sa constitution et les rapports des elements qui la traversent. *Semin Hop Paris* 1949;25:1719.
11. Taptas JN. Loge du sinus caverneux et sinus caverneux. Rapports meninges des nerfs craniens et de l'artere carotide interne dans leur traversee de la fosse cerebrale moyenne. *Semin Hop Paris* 1960;36:1853.
12. Taptas JN. The so-called cavernous sinus: a review of the controversy and its implications for neurosurgeons. *Neurosurgery* 1982;11:712.
13. Taptas JN. Must we still call cavernous sinus the parasellar vascular and nervous crossroads? The necessity of a definite topographical description of the region. In: Dolenc VV, ed. *The Cavernous Sinus: A Multidisciplinary Approach to Vascular and Tumorous Lesions.* New York: Springer-Verlag, 1987;30–40.
14. Umansky F, Nathan H. The lateral wall of the cavernous sinus, with special reference to the nerves related to it. *J Neurosurg* 1982;56:228.
15. Berenstein A, Ransohoff J, Kupersmith M, Flamm E, Graeb D. Transvascular treatment of giant aneurysms of the cavernous carotid and vertebral arteries. Functional investigation and embolization. *Surg Neurol* 1984;21:3–12.
16. Debrun G. Detachable balloon and calibrated leak balloon technique in the treatment of cerebral vascular lesions. *J Neurosurg* 1978;49:635.
17. Debrun GM. Embolization techniques in the treatment of vascular lesions involving the cavernous sinus. In: Dolenc VV, ed. *The Cavernous Sinus: A Multidisciplinary Approach to Vascular and Tumorous Lesions.* New York: Springer-Verlag, 1987;1973–1981.
18. Kupersmith MJ, Berenstein A. Percutaneous transvascular treatment of giant carotid aneurysms. Neuroophthalmic findings. *Neurology* 1984; 34(3):328–335.
19. Lasjaunias P, Berenstein A. Aneurysms of the cavernous segment of the internal carotid artery. In: *Surgical Neuroangiography. vol 2. Endovascular Treatment of Craniofacial Lesions.* Berlin: Springer-Verlag, 1987;248–264.
20. Serbinenko F. Wound catheterization and occlusion of major cerebral vessels. *J Neurosurg* 1974;41:125.
21. Spaziante R. Intracavernous giant fusiform aneurysm of the carotid artery treated with Gianturco coils. *Neurochirurgia* 1986;29:34.
22. Vinuela F, Lylyk P. Endovascular therapy of vascular lesions of the cavernous sinus. Experience with 129 cases. In: Dolenc VV, ed. *The Cavernous Sinus: A Multidisciplinary Approach to Vascular and Tumorous Lesions.* New York: Springer-Verlag, 1987;182–197.
23. Diaz FG, Ohaegbulam MD, Ausman JI. Surgical management of aneurysms in the cavernous sinus. *Acta Neurochir* 1988;91:25.
24. Diaz FG. Surgical alternatives in the treatment of cavernous sinus aneurysms. *J Neurosurg* 1989;71:846.
25. Dolenc VV, Cerk M, Sustersic J. Treatment of intracavernous aneurysms of the ICA and CCFs by direct approach. In: Dolenc VV, ed. *The Cavernous Sinus: A Multidisciplinary Approach to Vascular and Tumorous Lesions.* New York: Springer-Verlag, 1987;297–310.
26. Dolenc VV. Surgery of vascular lesions of the cavernous sinus. *Clin Neurosurg* 1990;36:240.
27. Dolenc VV. Carotid ophthalmic aneurysms. In: Spetzler RF, Carter LP, eds. *Neurovascular Surgery.* New York: McGraw-Hill, 1994;673–686.
28. Eguchi T, Nakagomi T, Teraoka A. Treatment of bilateral mycotic intracavernous carotid aneurysms. Case report. *J Neurosurg* 1982;56: 443.
29. Faria MA, Fleischer AS, Spector RH. Bilateral giant intracavernous carotid aneurysms treated by bilateral carotid ligation. *Surg Neurol* 1980;14:207.

30. Gelber BR, Sundt TM Jr. Treatment of intracavernous and giant carotid aneurysms by combined internal carotid ligation and extra- to intracranial bypass. *J Neurosurg* 1980;52:1.

31. Heros RC, Nelson P, Ojemann RG. Large and giant paraclinoid aneurysms. Surgical techniques, complications and results. *Neurosurgery* 1983;12:153–163.

32. Johnston I. Direct surgical treatment of bilateral intracavernous internal carotid artery aneurysms. Case report. *J Neurosurg* 1979;51:98.

33. Nakao S, Fukumitsu T, Ogata M. Transient total ophthalmoplegia following internal carotid artery ligation for treatment of intracavernous giant aneurysm. Case report. *Surg Neurol* 1981;17:458.

34. Sano H. Bilateral giant intracavernous aneurysms. Technique of unilateral operation. *Surg Neurol* 1988;29:35.

35. Dolenc VV. The necessity for intracavernous ICA reconstruction. In: Sato K, ed. *Neurosurgeons 10.* Proceedings of the Japanese Congress of Neurological Surgeons. Tokyo: SciMed Publications, 1991;299–307.

36. Linskey ME, Sekhar LN, Horton JA. Aneurysms of the intracavernous carotid artery. A multidisciplinary approach to treatment. *J Neurosurg* 1991;75:525.

37. Spetzler RF, Fukushima T, Martin N, Zabramski JM. Petrous carotid-to-intradural carotid saphenous vein graft for intracavernous giant aneurysm, tumor, and occlusive cerebrovascular disease. *J Neurosurg* 1990; 73:496.

38. Sundt TM Jr. *Surgical Techniques for Saccular and Giant Intracranial Aneurysms.* Baltimore: Williams and Wilkins, 1990.

39. Dandy WE, Follis RH Jr. On the pathology of carotid-cavernous aneurysms (pulsating exophthalmos). *Am J Ophthalmol* 1941;24:365.

40. Liu MY, Shih CJ, Wang YC, Tsai SH. Traumatic intracavernous carotid aneurysms with massive epistaxis. *Neurosurgery* 1985;17:569.

41. Maurer JJ, Mills M, German WJ. Triad of unilateral blindness, orbital fracture and massive epistaxis after head injury. *J Neurosurg* 1961;18: 837.

42. Hodes JE, Fletcher WA, Goodman DF, Hoyt WF. Rupture of cavernous carotid artery aneurysms causing subdural hematoma and death. *J Neurosurg* 1988;69:617.

Cerebrovascular Disease, edited by H. Hunt Batjer.
Lippincott-Raven Publishers, Philadelphia © 1997.

CHAPTER 77

Paraclinoid Carotid Aneurysms: Surgical Techniques

Mark B. Renfro and Arthur L. Day

Intracranial internal carotid artery aneurysms have been classically divided into two large categories, depending on their relationship to the anterior clinoid process. Infraclinoid aneurysms are generally considered to be within the cavernous sinus, produce cranial neuropathies, rarely rupture and bleed, and therefore rarely require urgent intervention. Supraclinoid aneurysms, arising or projecting above the anterior clinoid process into the subarachnoid space, have much higher risks of subarachnoid hemorrhage or visual pathway compression. New anatomic viewpoints derived from the growth of skull base surgery and refinements in neurodiagnostic studies now allow a reclassification of internal carotid artery aneurysms into precise clinical categories, a separation that is useful in defining their clinical features, risks of future hemorrhage, and methods and indications of safe and effective treatment.

Internal carotid artery aneurysms arising in the region of the anterior clinoid process are collectively referred to as paraclinoid aneurysms. Using the broadest definition, clinoidal segment, ophthalmic segment, and certain intracavernous and posterior communicating artery aneurysms may be included in this category (1–8) (Table 1). Posterior communicating artery aneurysms may arise near the anterior clinoid process when the ophthalmic segment is foreshortened or when the anterior clinoid process is elongated, and in such circumstances, it may be necessary to remove the clinoid tip to gain proximal internal carotid artery visualization and vascular control prior to surgical clipping. Giant intracavernous aneurysms may expand upward and erode the anterior clinoid process from below, primarily because of their large size. If such lesions are treated with open surgery and trapping, clinoidal removal is generally required to allow distal clip placement proximal to the ophthalmic artery origin.

This chapter defines paraclinoid aneurysms as including only those lesions whose origins, even when small, have a direct relationship to the anterior clinoid process. This discussion, therefore, is limited to aneurysms arising from the ophthalmic and clinoidal segments, whereas the clinical variants of posterior communicating and true intracavernous aneurysms are discussed in other chapters.

ANATOMY AND TERMINOLOGY

The area near the anterior clinoid process (the paraclinoid region) represents a complex anatomic point of confluence, where such vascular structures as the internal carotid artery (ICA), ophthalmic artery (OphArt), superior hypophyseal artery perforators (SupHypArt), veins of the superior orbital fissure, and cavernous sinus meet with traversing nerves (optic, oculomotor, trochlear, abducens, trigeminal, parasympathetic, and sympathetic), and several bony ridges and dural folds (9). Removal or manipulation of the osseous and dural structures greatly facilitates exposure of the various underlying neural and vascular elements, and familiarity with the anatomy is essential in dealing effectively with the various vascular lesions that arise in this region.

Osseous and Dural Anatomy

The anterior clinoid process (ACP) represents the most medial extension of the lesser wing of the sphenoid bone and is the epicenter of the paraclinoid region (Fig. 1). The lesser wing and the ACP together form and protect the roof of the superior orbital fissure (SOF) and anterior cavernous sinus. Medially, the ACP partially encases the lateral and anterior portions of the ICA as the vessel nears the subarachnoid space. The ACP tip is also attached to the optic strut (OS), which projects from the medial and inferior surfaces of the clinoid to the body of the sphenoid, separating the optic canal from the SOF. The ACP and OS collectively

M. B. Renfro and Arthur L. Day: Department of Neurosurgery, University of Florida, Gainesville, FL 32610.

TABLE 1. *Four types of aneurysms arising or expanding near the anterior clinoid process (see also Figs. 3A, 3B, 4A, 4B)*

Dural relationship	Aneurysm type	Anatomic separation point
Extradural (within cavernous sinus)	1. "True" intracavernous	Carotid oculomotor membrane

"Inter dural"	2. Clinoid segment
	   a. Anterolateral
	   b. Medial
		Dural ring

Intradural (subarachnoid)	3. Ophthalmic segment
	   a. Ophthalmic
	   b. Superior hypophyseal
	   c. Dorsal
		Dural ring

	4. Communicating segment	Posterior communicating artery

form a portion of the superomedial wall of the SOF and the inferolateral wall of the optic canal. The ACP is normally solid but may contain air cells that communicate through the OS with the sphenoid sinus.

The middle clinoid process (MCP) is situated lateral to the tuberculum sella and medial to the carotid sulcus, and the posterior clinoid process (PCP) is located at the superolateral margin of the dorsum sellae. Multiple dural folds attach to and extend from these clinoid processes, including the anterior petroclinoid fold (petrous apex to the ACP), the interclinoid fold (PCP to the ACP), and posterior petroclinoid fold (petrous apex to the PCP) (9). These dural folds may become ossified, creating calcified bridges (ie, the caroticoclinoid foramen between the ACP and the MCP) that increase the difficulty of clinoidal removal and the risks of ICA injury or premature aneurysm disruption.

Another dural fold, the falciform ligament, extends from the superomedial base of the ACP medially across the superior surface of the optic nerve to merge with the dura of the tuberculum and dorsum sella. This ligament lengthens the optic nerve ensheathment for several millimeters posterior to the termination of the bony optic canal; aneurysms or tumors may cause visual loss by elevating the optic nerve against its free sharp edge.

Two anatomically distinct dural membranes reflecting off the ACP separate the adjacent ICA into distinct segments (Fig. 2). One is composed of periosteal reflections from the superomedial edge of the ACP, which passes medially to, radially attaches to and encircles the ICA, and fuses medially with the diaphragma sellae and anteriorly with the dural floor of the optic canal (10–14). The site of penetrance of the ICA through this membrane is called the dural ring. Circumferential section of the dural ring allows mobilization of the carotid artery and exposes the medial aspect of the clinoidal segment of the ICA (see below). From a lateral view, the dural ring lies below the level of the ACP superior surface and marks the true point of ICA penetrance into the subarachnoid space. The dural ring is usually thicker laterally, thins medially, and surrounds the ICA in an oblique plane that slopes downward from anterior to posterior and lateral to medial directions (6,13,14). This downward slant of the thinned medial portion of the ring creates a small subarachnoid pocket medial to the ICA called the carotid cave (14).

The second membrane, representing the thin periosteal layer covering the inferomedial surface of the ACP, also attaches to the ICA (9). This layer, termed the carotid-oculomotor membrane, bridges medially from the ICA laterally to the oculomotor nerve and marks the point of ICA exit

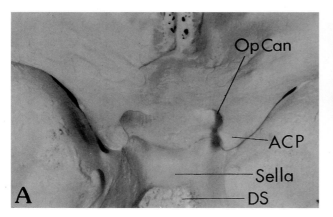
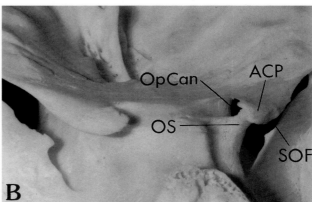

FIG. 1. Osseous anatomy of the "paraclinoid" region, dorsal **(A)** and posterior oblique **(B)** views: The anterior clinoid process (ACP) represents the medial extension of the lesser wing of the sphenoid bone, and abuts the lateral and anterolateral surfaces of the clinoidal segment of the internal carotid artery. Note the optic strut (OS), extending from the inferomedial clinoid base to the sphenoid bone and separating the optic canal (OpCan) from the superior orbital fissure (SOF). DS, dorsum sella.

from its encasing venous surroundings within the cavernous sinus.

Vascular Anatomy

Segments

Several ICA sections are closely related to the paraclinoid region, including the intracavernous, clinoidal, and ophthalmic segments (see Fig. 2).

Cavernous Segment

The intracavernous carotid artery is classically thought to lie, entirely within the venous channels of the cavernous sinus. It can be divided into five parts: (a) the posterior vertical segment, (b) the posterior bend, (c) the horizontal portion, (d) the anterior bend, and (e) the anterior vertical portion (9). True intracavernous ICA (CavSeg) aneurysms arise from the first four parts of the intracavernous vessel proximal to the anterior ascending vertical segment, in close proximity to cranial nerves III, IV, V, VI, and the ocular sympathetics.

Clinoidal Segment

Removal of the ACP exposes an ICA segment that is neither within the cavernous sinus nor the subarachnoid space (Fig. 2C) (9–11). This vessel segment, herein termed the clinoidal segment (ClinSeg), lies between the dural ring and carotid-oculomotor membrane and corresponds to the distal part of the anterior vertical portion of the intracavernous carotid artery. This ICA segment is normally completely obscured by the ACP, which rests on the lateral surface of the vessel. Spanning a distance of approximately 5 mm, the clinoidal segment ICA wall is stippled by thin periosteal attachments off the medial ACP surface and a few small venous channels.

Ophthalmic Segment

The ophthalmic segment (OphSeg) is generally the longest subarachnoid ICA segment, usually spanning a distance of 1–1.5 cm (15). This segment begins as the ICA penetrates the dural ring to enter the subarachnoid space and ends at the origin of the posterior communicating artery.

Bends

Two major ICA bends in the paraclinoid region create hemodynamic stresses that predispose to aneurysm formation (see Fig. 2). The first and most obvious (on lateral view, Fig. 2B) is a superiorly directed hemodynamic vector arising as the ICA ascends and bending sharply posteriorly after penetrating the dural ring. The second, best seen from a dorsal or AP view (Fig. 2A, C), is a gentle medial-to-lateral curve that begins at the anterior intracavernous bend and continues as the artery approaches its terminal bifurcation, causing a medially directed stress vector along the entire paraclinoid ICA region.

Branches

Two major named arterial branches arise from the paraclinoid portions of the ICA, most commonly from the OphSeg. The first, largest, and best known is the ophthalmic artery (OphArt). This branch usually arises from the dorsal or dorsomedial ICA surface just above the dural ring (16,17). The OphArt typically originates beneath the lateral portion of the overlying optic nerve and subsequently travels through the optic canal to reach the orbit.

Several large perforating vessels also arise within the paraclinoid region, the largest of which has been named the superior hypophyseal artery (SupHypArt) (18,19). These perforators supply the dura around the cavernous sinus, the superior aspect of the pituitary gland and stalk, and the optic nerves and chiasm (18–20). They typically arise from the medial or inferomedial surface of the OphSeg, usually along the second (medial-to-lateral) ICA bend, just above the dural ring and proximal to the posterior communicating artery origin. The gentle downward slope of the dural ring posteriorly often places the SupHypArt origin on a horizontal plane below the level of both the ACP and OphArt.

The ophthalmic and superior hypophyseal arteries occasionally arise from the ClinSe in which case the OphArt reaches the orbit either through a foramen in the OS or by piercing the carotid-oculomotor membrane and passing through the superior orbital fissure. When a SupHypArt arises from the ClinSeg, it passes medially to supply the dura and pituitary gland, and may provide some blood supply to the optic nerve within the optic canal.

Terminology

Most ICA aneurysms are saccular and derive their name from an intimate hemodynamic association with a branch of the parent vessel. As outlined by Rhoton, most saccular aneurysms arise from a curve of the parent vessel, in the angle between it and a significant arterial branch, and point in the direction that flow would have continued in the parent vessel if the curve had not been present (21). Paraclinoid aneurysms generally conform to these rules, and they are herein classified according to the site of origin (including the segment, branch, and curve), the direction of projection (which defines the propensity of hemorrhage and cranial nerve compressive effects), and the specific type of treatment for that particular lesion location.

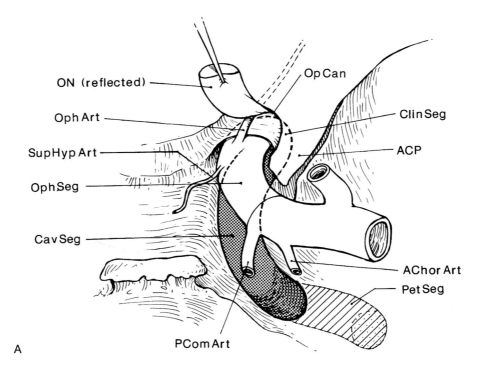

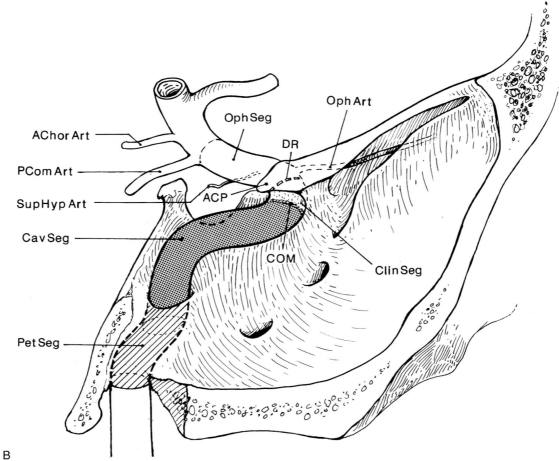

FIG. 2A–B.

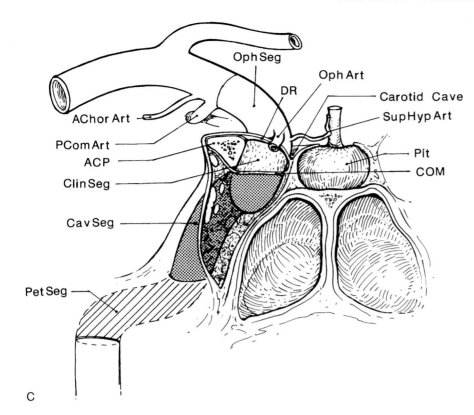

FIG. 2. ICA anatomy: bends, branches, dural attachments, segments (schematic), including dorsal (A), lateral (B), and antero-posterior (AP) views. Note the lateral to medial bend of the internal carotid artery (ICA), seen best on dorsal and AP views, which begins at the distal portion of the cavernous segment (CavSeg) and continues until the terminal bifurcation. The superior hypophyseal arteries (SupHypArt) arise from the medial surface of this bend, usually from the ophthalmic segment (OphSeg) just above the dural ring (DR). Also note the posterior ICA bend as the vessel ascends from the cavernous sinus, seen best on lateral view. The ophthalmic artery (OphArt) arises from this curvature, usually from the OphSeg just above the DR. PComArt, posterior communicating artery; AChorArt, anterior choroidal artery; ACP, anterior clinoid process; OpCan, optic canal; ON, optic nerve; COM, carotid-oculomotor membrane; ClinSeg, clinoidal segment; PetSeg, petrous segment.

Ophthalmic Segment Aneurysms

Three variations of OphSeg aneurysms have been described: (a) ophthalmic, (b) superior hypophyseal, and (c) dorsal types (Fig. 3). Aneurysms arising in clear relation to the OphArt are termed OphArt aneurysms. These lesions typically originate from the dorsal ICA bend above the dural ring just distal to the OphArt origin and initially project dorsally or dorsomedially toward the lateral half of the optic nerve (2,4,7,22,23). The optic nerve is usually displaced superiorly and medially, often elevated firmly against the sharp edge of the falciform ligament.

SupHypArt aneurysms arise from the medial-to-lateral ICA bend, incorporate the perforating branches to the hypophysis in their origins, and have no direct relationship to the ophthalmic artery (23). Small SupHypArt aneurysms usually arise from the inferior or inferior medial ICA surface just distal to the dural ring, lateral to the sella, and medial to the carotid and ACP (parasellar or paraclinoid variant). Some will burrow partially beneath the ACP and diaphragma sella and expand within the carotid cave. Because the space medial to the ICA is limited, however, most larger lesions will eventually expand medially or superomedially above the diaphragma sella into the suprasellar space.

On rare occasions, aneurysms arise more distally from the OphSeg and exhibit no clear association with the ophthalmic or superior hypophyseal arteries. These lesions, termed "dorsal" carotid artery aneurysms, appear to be pure hemo-dynamically induced lesions originating at the dorsal ICA surface several millimeters distal to the OphArt takeoff.

Clinoidal Segment Aneurysms

The same two hemodynamic forces that promote aneurysm development in the OphSeg also act on the ICA as it traverses the ClinSeg. The neck of ClinSeg aneurysms, however, arises in the interval between the carotid-oculomotor membrane and the dural ring, below the plane of the ACP, above the venous compartment of the cavernous sinus, and outside of the subarachnoid space (Fig. 4). As the anterior vertical portion of the intracavernous ICA ascends from the cavernous sinus, a superior vector projects flow upward, away from the cranial nerves of the cavernous sinus and against the overlying dura, ACP, and OS. The lateral-to-medial curve produces a second hemodynamic vector medially. Two variants of ClinSeg aneurysms have been clarified, the anterior-lateral and medial types (1).

The anterior-lateral variant originates from the anterolateral ICA surface as the artery is ascending obliquely to enter the subarachnoid space medial to the ACP. This variant often arises in association with an early OphArt origin, and its clinical and radiographic features may closely resemble the OphArt type of OphSeg aneurysms. The hemodynamic stresses direct the aneurysm anteriorly and superiorly against the OS and undersurface of the ACP and optic canal. As the lesion expands, focal erosion of the optic strut or ACP

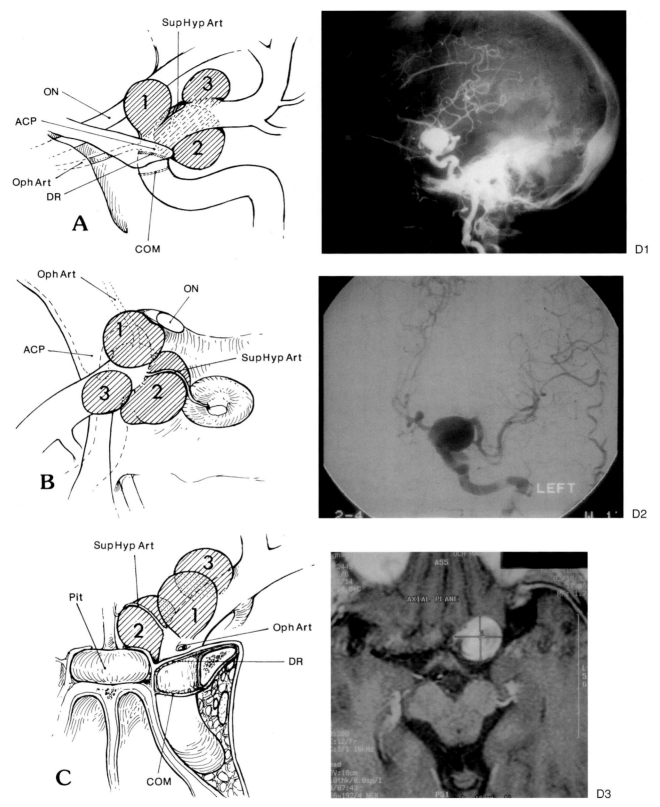

FIG. 3.

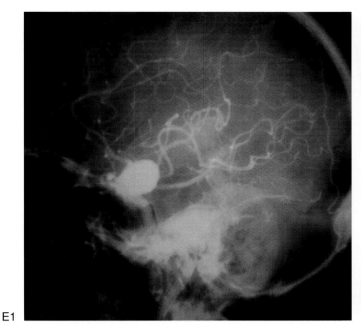

E1

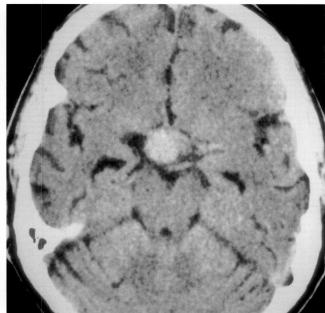

E3

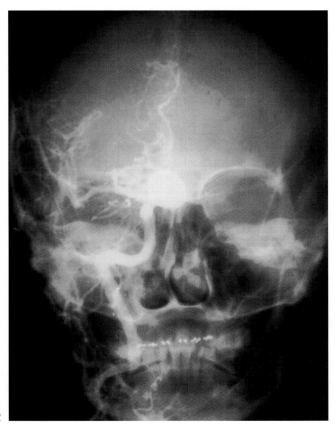

E2

FIG. 3. Ophthalmic segment (OphSeg) aneurysms. **A:** Lateral view (schematic). **B:** dorsal view (schematic). **C:** Anteroposterior (AP) view (schematic). **D:** Ophthalmic artery (OphArt) aneurysm: arteriogram (lateral and AP views). **E:** Superior hypophyseal artery (SupHypArt) aneurysm: arteriogram (lateral and AP views). OphArt aneurysms (1) arise from dorsomedial internal carotid artery (ICA) surface just distal to the OphArt origin. SupHypArt lesions (2) arise from the inferomedial ICA surface independent of the OphArt origin, in close association with the perforators that supply the optic chiasm and parasellar dura. SupHypArt aneurysms may burrow down toward the carotid cave above the dural ring (DR), deflected ventrally by the dura of the lateral sellar wall (paraclinoid variant), or may exceed the ventral confines and expand directly into the suprasellar space below the optic chiasm (suprasellar variant). Dorsal OphSeg aneurysms (3) are rare and arise from the dorsal ICA surface well distal to the OphArt origin. ACP, anterior clinoid process; ON, optic nerve; COM, carotid-oculomotor membrane; Pit, pituitary gland; AN, aneurysm.

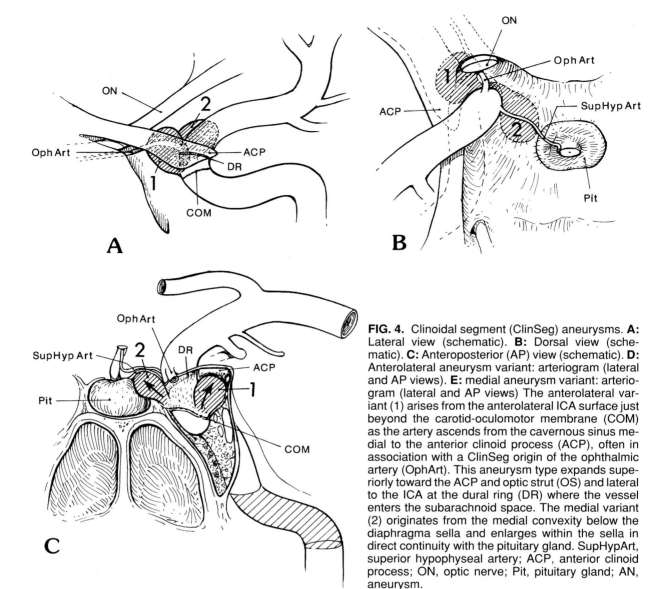

FIG. 4. Clinoidal segment (ClinSeg) aneurysms. **A:** Lateral view (schematic). **B:** Dorsal view (schematic). **C:** Anteroposterior (AP) view (schematic). **D:** Anterolateral aneurysm variant: arteriogram (lateral and AP views). **E:** medial aneurysm variant: arteriogram (lateral and AP views) The anterolateral variant (1) arises from the anterolateral ICA surface just beyond the carotid-oculomotor membrane (COM) as the artery ascends from the cavernous sinus medial to the anterior clinoid process (ACP), often in association with a ClinSeg origin of the ophthalmic artery (OphArt). This aneurysm type expands superiorly toward the ACP and optic strut (OS) and lateral to the ICA at the dural ring (DR) where the vessel enters the subarachnoid space. The medial variant (2) originates from the medial convexity below the diaphragma sella and enlarges within the sella in direct continuity with the pituitary gland. SupHypArt, superior hypophyseal artery; ACP, anterior clinoid process; ON, optic nerve; Pit, pituitary gland; AN, aneurysm.

demonstrable on CT or MRI marks the lesion's proximal origin—findings not seen with OphArt aneurysms.

The medial type of ClinSeg aneurysm extends medially toward the sphenoid sinus or sella and more closely resembles the superior hypophyseal artery variant of OphSeg aneurysms. This variant, however, initially expands below the diaphragma sella, whereas SupHypArt aneurysms primarily enlarge in the suprasellar space above the diaphragma sella.

Because both types of ClinSeg aneurysms originate outside of the subarachnoid space (they are actually interdural, between the two periosteal leaves covering the ACP), small lesions do not pose significant hemorrhage risks, as a thick layer of overlying dura (the roof of the cavernous sinus) restrains their fundus from subarachnoid extension. With enlargement, however, either type may erode through the dura adjacent to the dural ring (medially or anterolaterally) and project secondarily into the subarachnoid space.

CLINICAL PRESENTATION

Ophthalmic Segment Aneurysms

OphSeg aneurysms present with visual symptoms, hemorrhage, and incidental discovery in roughly equal proportions. Multiplicity is common, and 40–50% of patients with one OphSeg lesion harbor at least one other intracranial aneurysm (4,5,22,24–26). Those presenting with visual loss are almost always giant lesions greater than 2.5 cm in external diameter. The high frequency reaching large or giant proportions (one third of cases) without bleeding is probably explained by the reinforcement of the aneurysm's fundus by adjacent structures. An OphArt aneurysm expands upward and medially into the optic nerve, whereas SupHypArt aneurysms initially project into the dura of the lateral sellar wall and cavernous sinus. Small SupHypArt lesions that remain

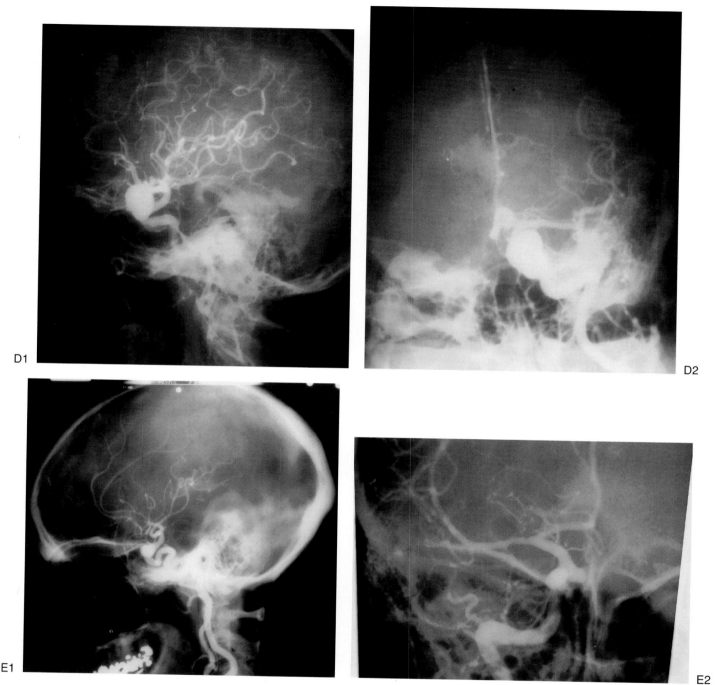

D1

D2

E1

E2

FIG. 4D–E.

purely parasellar have a very low hemorrhage rate compared to those at other locations. Larger aneurysms or those with medial suprasellar extension appear to bleed with higher frequency.

Visual loss from expanding OphArt aneurysms occurs as the lesion elevates the lateral portion of the optic nerve superiorly and medially, angulating the nerve against the sharp edge of the falciform ligament. An inferior nasal field defect may go unnoticed but eventually, as the lesion reaches giant

proportions, the entire nasal field is affected, followed by a superior temporal field loss in the contralateral eye. The stretched optic nerve tethers extension across the midline until late in the clinical course, by which time severe ipsilateral visual loss or blindness has occurred. The overlying optic nerve also impedes superior expansion and enlarging lesions will tend to close the carotid siphon.

Enlarging SupHypArt aneurysms do not produce such a sharp angulation of the optic nerve against the falciform ligament but instead tend to elevate the chiasm, producing visual field deficits more closely akin to those seen with pituitary tumors (27–29). Once these lesions reach the suprasellar space, they tend to extend across the midline beneath the chiasm, above the diaphragma sella. Expansion from their ventromedial origin tends to open the carotid siphon and gives an often erroneous appearance that they are projecting downward into the cavernous sinus.

Clinoidal Segment Aneurysms

ClinSeg aneurysms originate below the dural ring, and small lesions are usually asymptomatic. Once a size of 1 cm is reached, however, the likelihood that the aneurysm has eroded through the dural roof into the subarachnoid space is high, at which time rupture to produce subarachnoid hemorrhage becomes a possibility. The anterior-lateral variant may compress the optic nerve either within the optic canal extradurally or within the subarachnoid space after penetrating the dura. The resultant visual loss is monocular, and the pattern of field loss is more variable than that seen with OphArt aneurysms. The medial type may erode through the lateral sphenoid sinus wall to cause epistaxis (rare) or into the lateral sella beneath the diaphragma sella to mimic a pituitary tumor.

PREOPERATIVE EVALUATION

Arteriography

Four-vessel cerebral angiography is essential in the evaluation of patients with paraclinoid aneurysms, both to define the vascular anatomy and to rule out additional aneurysms elsewhere. Several projections may be needed to differentiate small aneurysms from a vessel bend and to more precisely define the aneurysm neck. If ICA ligation is contemplated as a treatment option, a trial ICA balloon occlusion test under local anesthesia followed by a cerebral blood flow study (SPECT or xenon CT) should be considered to more accurately assess ischemia risks.

OphArt aneurysms typically arise above the posterior ICA bend, just beyond the OphArt takeoff (Fig. 3D). Anterolateral ClinSeg lesions may closely mimic OphArt aneurysms, but originate below the plane of the OphArt and ACP, frequently creating a ''double density'' overlying the anterior siphon region as the aneurysm expands alongside the ICA (Fig. 4D).

Large or giant SupHypArt aneurysms have two scalloped basal surfaces, reflecting the parasellar origins and suprasellar expansion, and their necks are typically quite broad, seemingly incorporating the entire OphSeg (Fig. 3E). The aneurysm neck in medial variant ClinSeg aneurysms is usually quite small, being somewhat restricted by the two planes of dura (the dural ring and carotid-oculomotor membrane) that mark its origin (Fig. 4E).

Computed Tomography and Magnetic Resonance Imaging

CT evaluation can be of great assistance in the management of paraclinoid aneurysms. Any hemorrhage usually appears in the chiasmatic cisterns, and in patients with multiple lesions the pattern of the bleed can be invaluable in determining which aneurysm bled. Calcium seen within the aneurysm wall may forewarn of intraoperative difficulties with clipping and the potential need for more prolonged temporary trapping of the affected ICA segment. The paraclinoid region should be carefully studied for signs of erosion indicating a more proximal (ClinSeg) origin or for actual extension of the aneurysm through the ACP (anterolateral variant). An osseous bridge between the anterior and middle clinoid processes or a pneumatized anterior clinoid process can also be anticipated. MRI may be helpful in revealing luminal thrombosis and can often delineate the optic nerve position relative to the aneurysm.

SURGICAL TREATMENT

With proper exposure and a firm understanding of parasellar and vascular anatomy, most paraclinoid aneurysms are clippable with low risks to the brain or visual apparatus. Carotid ligation or endovascular treatments should in most instances be considered secondary alternatives, as the risks of stroke are higher from parent vessel sacrifice, the visual system is not as effectively decompressed, and complete thrombosis of the aneurysm is not assured. Endovascular coils work best when the aneurysm neck is small. By the time they become symptomatic, however, most paraclinoid aneurysms have large necks that communicate widely with the parent vessel. ClinSeg aneurysms, especially the medial variant, are more likely to have narrower necks and may be, at least in theory, more amenable to this technology. Detachable balloons are generally not effective treatments unless the parent vessel is simultaneously sacrificed.

Patient Selection

If bleeding has occurred, surgery is performed on the earliest day possible following the hemorrhage, as long as the patient is not a poor medical risk or has not sustained significant and irreversible brain injury. Since nearly half of patients with one paraclinoid lesion have at least one other intracranial aneurysm, the surgeon often must decide which lesion bled. Small SupHypArt that remain purely paraclinoid or ClinSeg lesions have lower hemorrhage rates than larger lesions or those at other locations, and asymptomatic lesions can often be treated electively unless intervention is planned for other reasons.

Preoperative Preparation

Bleeding from paraclinoid aneurysms is managed in the same fashion as subarachnoid hemorrhage from other aneurysm locations and includes such measures as bed rest, calcium channel blockers, hydration, ventricular drainage (when indicated), steroids, and anti-convulsants. Prophylactic antibiotics are given to all patients when they enter the operating suite and are continued for 24 hours. Pre-operative bedside testing of visual fields, often overlooked in the subarachnoid hemorrhage patient, documents any significant visual deterioration preoperatively and also provides key knowledge to the surgeon about the anatomy likely encountered in the operating room.

Anesthetic Technique and Monitoring

The ispilateral cervical carotid region should be unencumbered by any anesthetic equipment. Mild hypothermia is maintained throughout the procedure, but cardiac standstill and profound hypothermia are rarely indicated for lesions in this area. If temporary ICA clipping is anticipated, intravenous barbiturates are administered and titrated until burst suppression is achieved on EEG and continued until patency in the carotid system is restored. Blood pressure, monitored with an indwelling radial artery catheter, is generally maintained at normal levels and mildly elevated during the time of temporary clipping. Continuous evoked potential and EEG monitoring are also utilized and the blood pressure further elevated during ICA clipping if focal changes are noted. Spinal drainage is not routinely utilized, but mannitol is administered at the beginning of the case to facilitate brain relaxation and for its potential cerebral protectant effects.

Operative Positioning

The patient is placed in the supine position with the head elevated above the heart to promote good venous drainage. The head is turned 45° toward the opposite side with the vertex lowered to allow gravitational distraction of the frontal and temporal lobes from the skull base. A shoulder roll is used to minimize distortion of the cervical carotid bifurcation. The head is draped to permit visualization of the frontal and temporal regions from the midline to below the zygoma. The cervical region is also draped into the field to allow sterile access to the carotid bifurcation for proximal control or a bypass source as desired.

Operative Procedure

A cervical incision paralleling the anterior margin of the sternocleidomastoid muscle is marked. This incision is opened to expose and isolate the ICA for proximal control whenever a complicated or large\giant paraclinoid aneurysm is being approached. As proximal control for ClinSeg aneurysms lies within the cavernous sinus, and as the intracranial exposure carries significant risks of intraoperative rupture, the threshold for opening the cervical incision

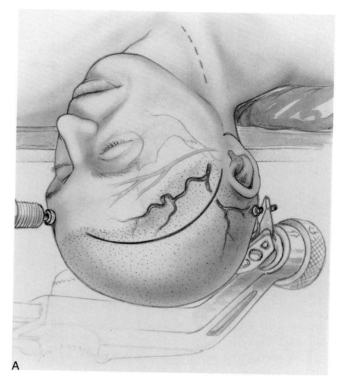

A

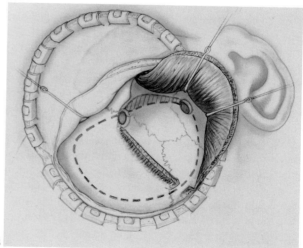

B

FIG. 5. Scalp and temporalis incisions (schematics). **A:** The scalp incision *(solid line)* extends from the midline to the zygoma and is gently curved to stay approximately 1 cm behind the hairline. The inferior part of the incision stays within 1 cm of the tragus to avoid injury to the frontalis branch of the facial nerve and to spare the anterior branch of the superficial temporal artery. The cervical carotid bifurcation region is marked *(dotted line)*, prepped, and draped into the field. **B:** The scalp is reflected anteriorly, independent of the temporalis muscle until the fat pad carrying the frontalis nerve is encountered. The fat pad and its investing fascia are then swept forward, and the temporalis muscle is detached and retracted posteriorly and inferiorly . After two burr holes are placed on each side of the sphenoid wing and connected with a rongeur and high-speed drill, a free bone flap is elevated that includes several centimeters of frontal extension to allow direct subfrontal and orbital roof access without the need for significant brain retraction.

should be low for such lesions regardless of size, especially in the presence of recent hemorrhage.

The skin incision for craniotomy extends from the midline to the zygoma, just behind the hairline (Fig. 5A). The temporalis muscle and fascia are reflected inferiorly and posteriorly to expose the pterional region, using great care to spare the frontal branch of the facial nerve (Fig. 5B). A frontotemporal free bone flap is elevated, opening low enough anteriorly so that 2–3 cm of the posterior frontal fossa floor is exposed. The sphenoid ridge and anterior temporal bone are extensively removed to allow an unobstructed view of the orbital roof and anterior aspect of the middle cranial fossa.

At this point a decision is made as to whether the entire sphenoid ridge and ACP should be removed and whether such removal should be done extradurally or in combination with intradural bony resection (Fig. 6A–C). While not always necessary for smaller lesions, clinoidal removal is invariably required for safe and accurate clipping of large or giant lesions and for all ClinSeg lesions. Extensive removal of the posterior orbital roof and entire sphenoid wing further enhances the exposure. With unruptured OphSeg aneurysms, extradural clinoid removal can usually be done quite safely without exposing the subarachnoid space to bony debris. Because ClinSeg aneurysms are adherent to and may actually erode through the ACP, however, the most medial extent of the lesser wing should be removed intradurally, as extradural removal risks avulsion of part of the aneurysm fundus prior to adequate exposure of the ICA and subarachnoid space. For most paraclinoid aneurysms, we prefer to remove the final vestiges of the ACP intradurally, while visualizing its relationship to the aneurysm, especially if there has been prior hemorrhage.

The posterior roof of the orbit and the lesser wing of the sphenoid bone covering the superior and medial surface of the superior orbital fissure, if resected extradurally, are removed with a rongeur. As the base of the ACP and optic nerve is approached, a high-speed diamond drill is utilized to thin the bone, which is fractured away with microcurettes. The ACP is then grasped with a hemostat, gently rocked free of any remaining attachments, and removed. Bleeding is quite easily controlled with bone wax and gel foam. The dura is opened and reflected to expose the proximal portions of the Sylvian fissure. The fissure is then split widely to allow an unobstructed view of the optic nerve, ICA, and aneurysm with minimal retraction.

When the ACP is removed intradurally, a 2- to 3-cm cruciate incision is made into the dura covering the ACP and optic canal roof (Fig. 6B, C). The ACP, OS, and optic canal roof and lateral wall are then carefully thinned and removed with small rongeurs and a high-speed drill. This removal should be done gently to avoid injury to the oculomotor nerve, which courses within the superior aspect of the cavernous sinus dura, thinly covered by the carotid-oculomotor membrane. Optic nerve displacement, if not already done by the aneurysm, is often necessary to visualize the proximal

neck. The falciform ligament is therefore sectioned and the dural sheath overlying the optic nerve opened before any aneurysm dissection is undertaken, as mobilization of the nerve against the intact ligament's knife-like edge may further increase visual morbidity.

Before beginning the final aneurysm neck dissection, the dural ring should be clearly delineated and the ClinSeg clarified should temporary clipping become necessary (Fig. 6C). Circumferential section of the dural ring allows ICA mobilization and greatly facilitates accurate identification of the OphArt, ClinSeg, and aneurysm anatomy. Exposure of the cervical ICA should be completed if indicated, but this maneuver should not be considered a substitute for extensive clinoidal and optic strut removal.

Ophthalmic Segment Aneurysms

The proximal neck of OphArt aneurysms is isolated by gentle retraction of the aneurysm base and spreading dissection just distal to the OphArt (Fig. 7). The distal neck is usually unencumbered by major branch attachments, but any perforators to the optic nerves, chiasm, or hypophysis should be dissected free. Gently curved or side-angled clips, directed parallel to the ICA and sparing the OphArt, satisfactorily secure most OphArt lesions.

As SupHypArt aneurysms enlarge, their walls become adherent to the parasellar dura, diaphragma, and lateral cavernous sinus wall (Fig. 8). Although the arteriogram may suggest otherwise, these lesions do not project into the cavernous sinus, and the walls of the two structures can be separated. By carefully sectioning the dural ring, the ICA and the inferomedial aneurysm wall are mobilized and separated from the clinoidal dura, thus freeing up the proximal neck. With larger lesions, the ICA is displaced slightly laterally and superiorly toward the surgeon, and the entire carotid wall appears incorporated into the aneurysm neck. The hypophyseal stalk is usually adherent to the posteromedial aneurysm surface, and the posterior communicating artery and its anterior thalamoperforating branches are often draped over the distal end of the aneurysm. These structures must be identified and separated from the aneurysm, and one or more fenestrated clips whose blades encircle and then run parallel to the ICA is placed, spanning the distance between the posterior communicating artery and the dural ring and carefully sparing all ICA branches and perforators (Fig. 8B). Some of the SupHypArt perforators may supply the optic chiasm, and every attempt should be made to spare them from the surgical clip.

Both OphArt and SupHypArt aneurysms may be associated with arteriosclerosis in the ICA and/or adjacent aneurysm neck. The bulk of these aneurysms and the thickness of their necks often causes the initial clip to slip downward and partially obstruct the parent artery lumen. A second clip, applied more distally on the neck and in the same direction as the first, is often helpful in keeping the neck and aneurysm

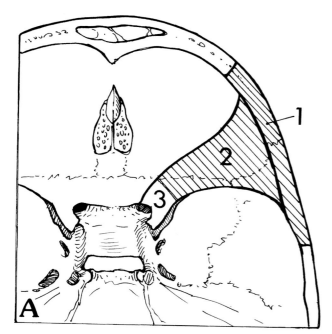

FIG. 6. Stages of sphenoid ridge and clinoidal removal (schematic). **A:** The extradural bone removal includes the craniotomy (no. 1 striped area) and most of the sphenoid ridge and posterior orbital roof (no. 2 striped area) until the optic nerve is encountered at the back of the orbit. The remainder of the exposure is done intradurally (no. 3) while the aneurysm is directly visualized. **B:** The dotted lines mark the dural incision overlying the anterior clinoid process (ACP) and includes a limb to section the falciform ligament to release any compression on the optic nerve prior to its mobilization. **C:** ACP removal and drilling of the optic strut (OS) allows isolation of the clinoidal segment (ClinSeg) of the internal carotid artery, a segment that may then be used for proximal control if necessary. OphArt, ophthalmic artery; SupHypArt, superior hypophyseal artery; PComArt, posterior communicating artery; ON, optic nerve; III, oculomotor nerve; COM, carotid-oculomotor membrane; DR, dural ring; OphSeg, ophthalmic segment.

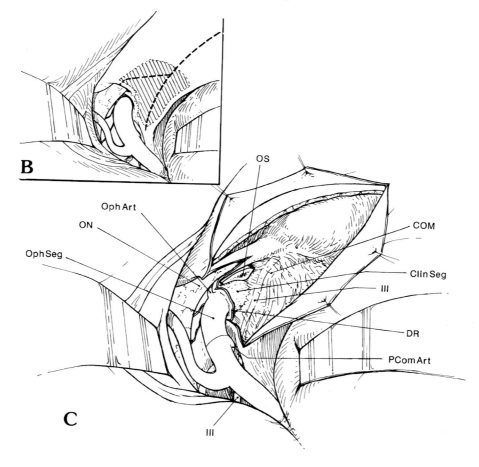

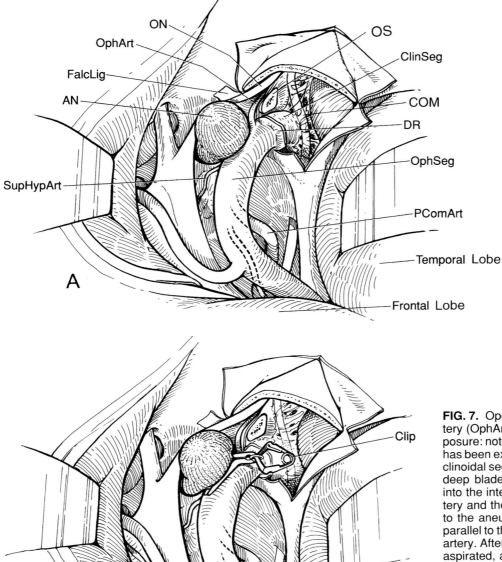

FIG. 7. Operative view of the ophthalmic artery (OphArt) aneurysm (schematic). **A:** Exposure: note that the anterior clinoid process has been extensively removed to expose the clinoidal segment (ClinSeg). **B:** Clipping: the deep blade of a side-angled clip is placed into the interval between the ophthalmic artery and the aneurysm, then rotated medial to the aneurysm, ending in a plane closely parallel to the long axis of the internal carotid artery. After clip placement, the aneurysm is aspirated, and the parent vessel and perforators are inspected for patency. SupHypArt, superior hypophyseal artery; PComArt, posterior communicating artery; ON, optic nerve; III, oculomotor nerve; COM, carotid-oculomotor membrane; DR, dural ring; OS, optic strut; FalcLig, falciform ligament; OphSeg, ophthalmic segment; AN, aneurysm.

collapsed. If placement of the first two clips results in a compromised ICA lumen, a third clip is applied distal to the second and the original clip removed. This process is repeated until wide carotid patency is assured. The lesion is then opened and its contents evacuated without bleeding. The entire aneurysm wall does not need to be removed.

With good exposure, almost all OphSeg lesions judged "unclippable" can be effectively and safely treated with clipping, despite very large and complicated shapes, intraluminal thrombosis, or marked calcification within their walls.

Using barbiturate anesthesia and burst suppression, the OphSeg can be temporarily isolated by placing temporary clips on the cervical ICA, the distal OphSeg proximal to the posterior communicating artery, and the OphArt. The aneurysm is then opened and any calcification or thrombus removed. A hemostat can be used to crush an atheroma and facilitate creation of a surgical neck, but this instrument must be applied distal enough so as not to injure the parent vessel. Debris and air should be thoroughly irrigated from the parent vessel lumen before final clip placement. Fenestrated clips

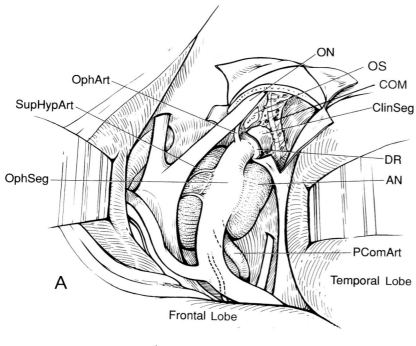

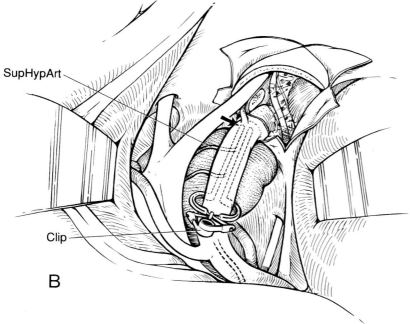

FIG. 8. Operative view: superior hypophyseal artery aneurysm (schematic) **A:** Exposure: note the aneurysm's inferior and medial position and the multiple perforators (superior hypophyseal arteries) intimately associated with its origin. **B:** Clipping: a fenestrated clip is placed parallel to the internal carotid artery to reconstruct the carotid lumen. The dural ring (DR) has been circumferentially sectioned to allow access of the clip blades to the clinoidal segment (ClinSeg) as needed. The butt of the clip must spare the posterior communicating artery, while the tips are advanced proximally beyond the dural ring. The aneurysm is then aspirated, and the parent vessel and perforators inspected for patency. OphArt, ophthalmic artery; SupHypArt, superior hypophyseal artery; PComArt, posterior communicating artery; ON, optic nerve; III, oculomotor nerve; COM, carotid-oculomotor membrane; DR, dural ring; OS, optic strut; FalcLig, falciform ligament; OphSeg, ophthalmic segment; AN, aneurysm.

encircling the atheroma while compressing more pliant portions of the aneurysm neck can also be quite useful.

A catheter placed into the cervical ICA distal to the temporary clip allows gentle aspiration of the blood within the trapped segment and can collapse the aneurysm without opening it directly. This maneuver risks injury to the cervical ICA intima (which may be quite arteriosclerotic or stenotic) and is most valuable for large or giant aneurysms that do not contain intraluminal thrombus or calcific walls that prevent its collapse. The catheter may then be used for intraop-

erative arteriography to validate complete aneurysm obliteration and parent vessel lumen preservation.

Small OphArt aneurysms can often be clipped from a contralateral approach between or behind the optic nerves, a capability that may be quite important when deciding which side to treat first in a patient harboring bilateral lesions, one of which is an OphSeg type. In general, the craniotomy should be done on the side of the symptomatic aneurysm. The surgeon may then choose to explore the opposite ICA, with plans to obliterate a contralateral lesion if feasible. Attempted clipping of large or giant OphSeg lesions from a contralateral approach should be avoided except in emergent situations.

Clinoidal Segment Aneurysms

ClinSeg lesions can often be quite thin and lack an atheromatous wall. Because these aneurysms originate below the dural ring and require extensive ACP and OS removal before any type of clip can be placed, the risk of intraoperative rupture during the exposure is higher, and we advocate prophylactic exposure of the cervical ICA for most lesions. The lateral sphenoid ridge and posterior orbital roof bone removal is performed extradurally, but the ACP tip is always resected from an intradural approach. The OS must thereafter be drilled down flush to the wall of the sphenoid sinus.

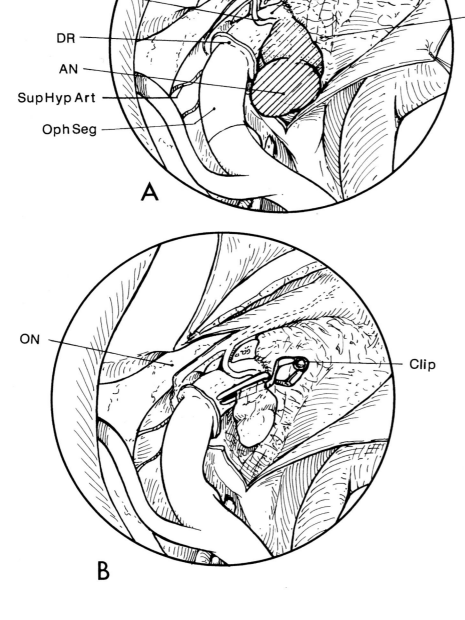

FIG. 9. Operative view: clinoidal segment aneurysm—anterolateral variant (schematic). **A:** Exposure: the anterior clinoid process has been carefully removed to expose the neck of the aneurysm originating within the clinoidal segment (ClinSeg). Note the constriction or "waisting" of the aneurysm at the point where it has eroded through the dura adjacent to the dural ring to enter the subarachnoid space. **B:** Clipping: a gently curved clip is placed along a plane paralleling the curve of the internal carotid artery. After clip placement, the aneurysm is aspirated and the parent vessel inspected for patency. SupHypArt, superior hypophyseal artery; PComArt, posterior communicating artery; ON, optic nerve; III, oculomotor nerve; COM, carotid-oculomotor membrane; DR, dural ring; OS, optic strut; FalcLig, falciform ligament; OphSeg, ophthalmic segment; AN, aneurysm.

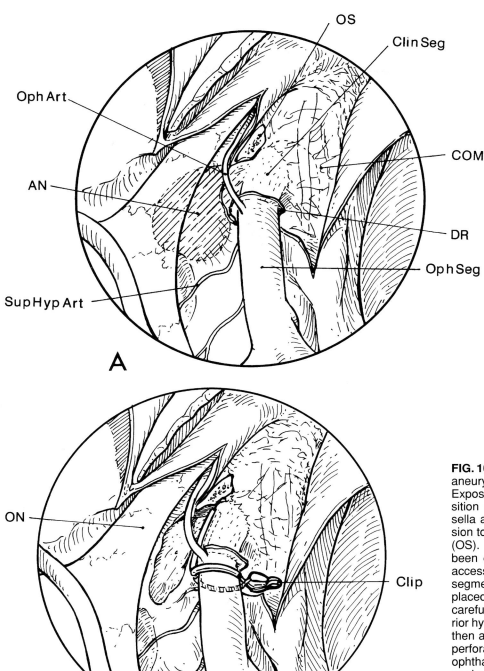

FIG. 10. Operative view: clinoidal segment aneurysm—medial variant (schematic). **A:** Exposure: note the aneurysm's medial position below the plane of the diaphragma sella and the close relationship of this lesion to the medial margin of the optic strut (OS). **B:** Clipping: the dural ring (DR) has been circumferentially sectioned to allow access of the clip blades to the clinoidal segment (ClinSeg). A fenestrated clip is placed parallel to the internal carotid artery, carefully sparing the ophthalmic and superior hypophyseal vessels. The aneurysm is then aspirated, and the parent vessel and perforators inspected for patency. OphArt, ophthalmic artery; SupHypArt, superior hypophyseal artery; PComArt, posterior communicating artery; ON, optic nerve; III, oculomotor nerve; COM, carotid-oculomotor membrane; DR, dural ring; OphSeg, ophthalmic segment; AN, aneurysm.

After mobilization of the optic nerve and identification of the OphSeg branches, the ICA attachments at the dural ring are sectioned circumferentially, permitting complete ClinSeg mobilization and allowing the surgeon unimpeded access to the aneurysm neck for clip placement.

The type of clip used is dependent on the variant of aneurysm being treated (Figs. 9 and 10). The anterolateral variant is usually best managed with a gently curved clip, whereas the medial variant requires a right-angled fenestrated clip that encircles the ICA and reconstructs the vessel lumen. Good ICA patency and aneurysm obliteration may be difficult to ascertain by direct external visualization alone, and we routinely use intraoperative angiography to document proper clip placement.

Temporary occlusion and trapping may be necessary in some cases in which the aneurysm neck is difficult to define and is performed in a fashion similar to that described for OphSeg lesions. During the exposure or clip application, care must be taken to avoid injury to the oculomotor nerve, which courses in the lateral edge of the carotid-oculomotor membrane. Sympathetic fibers from the carotid plexus exit the ICA in the ClinSeg, and extensive dissection in this region can often result in a mild ptosis and miosis without facial anhydrosis.

Once the aneurysm is clipped and aspirated, the dura is closed, including the opening over the ACP. Any communications with the sphenoid sinus must be identified and carefully sealed with muscle and methyl methacrylate to prevent cerebrospinal fluid leakage. A drain is left in the epidural space and brought out posterior to the skin incision through a separate stab wound. If the frontal sinus is violated by the craniotomy, the mucosa is removed, the space packed with gel foam soaked with antibiotics, and the sinus obliterated with methyl methacrylate (and in questionable cases oversewn with periosteum). The bone flap is then anchored in position, and the temporalis muscle and skin are closed in traditional fashion.

POSTOPERATIVE CARE

Patients are managed according to their presenting symptoms. Unruptured aneurysm patients are mobilized the following day, with rapid normalization of medications and fluid intake. Subarachnoid hemorrhage patients with high vasospasm potential are aggressively hydrated for the duration of their risks.

Transient or fixed postoperative hemibody deficits may be an indication of carotid compromise and occur with higher frequency in patients with calcified or partially thrombosed aneurysms with atherosclerosis within the ICA wall. Arteriography must be strongly considered whenever parent vessel patency or embolization is questioned.

Postoperative visual deterioration may be due to intraoperative overmanipulation of the optic nerve already distorted medially and superiorly against the falciform ligament by the underlying aneurysm or by perforator compromise. Unimproved or somewhat worsened visual loss following surgery can be caused by obstruction of either the SupHypArt or OphArt, and exploration and clip repositioning should be strongly considered if intraoperative events do not adequately explain the deficit.

Postoperative diplopia may be due to either an abducens or oculomotor nerve paresis. When the dural ring is opened, these nerves lie in a relatively superficial position within the wall of the clinoidal space. They may be disturbed within the cavernous sinus either by clinoid removal or by the clip blades as they are advanced proximally beyond the aneurysm neck.

REFERENCES

1. Day AL, Masson RL, Knego RS. Surgical management of aneurysms and fistulas invloving the cavernous sinus. In: Schmidek HH, Sweet WH, eds. *Operative Neurosurgical Techniques*. Philadelphia: WB Saunders, 1995;975–984.
2. Drake CG, Vanderlinden RG, Amacher AL. Carotid ophthalmic aneurysms. *J Neurosurg* 1968;29:24–36.
3. Fox J. Microsurgical treatment of ventral (paraclinoid) internal carotid artery aneurysms. *Neurosurgery* 1988;22:32–39.
4. Guidetti B, La Torre E. Management of carotid-ophthalmic aneurysms. *J Neurosurg* 1975;42:438–442.
5. Kothandran P, Dawson BH, Kruyt RC. Carotid ophthalmic aneurysms. A study of 19 patients. *J Neurosurg* 1971;34:544–548.
6. Nutik S. Ventral paraclinoid carotid aneurysms. *J Neurosurg* 1988;69:340–344.
7. Yasargil MG, Gasser JC, Hodosh RM, et al. Carotid-ophthalmic aneurysms: direct microsurgical approach. *Surg Neurol* 1977; 8:155–165.
8. Yasargil MG. Inferior wall aneurysms of the internal carotid artery. In: Yasargil MG, ed. *Microneurosurgery*. Stuttgart: Thieme, Verlag, 1984;60–70.
9. Inoue T, Rhoton AL, Theele D, et al. Surgical approaches to the cavernous sinus: a microsurgical study. *Neurosurgery* 1990;26:903–932.
10. Nutik SL. Removal of the anterior clinoid process for exposure of the proximal intracranial carotid artery. *J Neurosurg* 1988;69:529–534.
11. Perneczky A, Knosp E, Vorkapic P, et al. Direct surgical approach to infraclinoid aneurysms. *Acta Neurochir* 1985;76:36–44.
12. Dolenc VV. A combined epi- and subdural direct approach to carotid—ophthalmic artery aneurysms. *J Neurosurg* 1985; 62:667–672.
13. Knosp E, Muller G, Perneczky A. The paraclinoid carotid artery: anatomical aspects of a microsurgical approach. *Neurosurgery* 1988; 22:896–901.
14. Kobayashi S, Kyoshima K, Gibo H, et al. Carotid cave aneurysms of the internal carotid artery. *J Neurosurg* 1989;70:216–221.
15. Gibo H, Lenkey C, Rhoton A. Microsurgical anatomy of the supraclinoid portion of the internal carotid artery. *J Neurosurg* 1981;560–574.
16. Hayreh S. The ophthalmic artery. In: Newton TH, Potts DG, eds. *Radiology of the Skull and Brain*. St Louis: CV Mosby, 1974;1333–1350.
17. Nishio S, Matsushima T, Fukui M, et al. Microsurgical anatomy around the origin of the ophthalmic artery with reference to contralateral pterional surgical approach to the carotid-ophthalmic aneurysm. *Acta Neurochir* 1985;76:82–89.
18. Dawson BH. The blood vessels of the human optic chiasma and their relation to those of hypophysis and hypothalamus. *Brain* 1958;81:207–217.
19. Gibo H, Kobayashi S, Kyoshima K, et al. Microsurgical anatomy of the arteries of the pituitary stalk and gland as viewed from above. *Acta Neurochir* 1988;90:60–66.
20. Rosner S, Rhoton A, Ono M, et al. Microsurgical anatomy of the anterior perforating arteries. *J Neurosurg* 1984;61:468–485.
21. Rhoton AL. Anatomy of saccular aneurysms. *Surg Neurol* 1980;43:59–66.
22. Almeida GM, Shibata MK, Bianco E. Carotid-ophthalmic aneurysms. *Surg Neurol* 1976;5:41–45.
23. Day AL. Aneurysms of the ophthalmic segment. A clinical and anatomical analysis. *J Neurosurg* 1990;72:677–691.
24. Kodama N, Mineura K, Fujiwara S, Suzuki J. Surgical treatment of the carotid-ophthalmic aneurysm. In: Suzuki J, ed. *Cerebral Aneurysms*. Tokyo: Neuro, 1979;269–274.
25. Weir B. Carotid ophthalmic aneurysm. In: Weir B, ed. *Aneurysms Affecting the Nervous System*. Baltimore: Williams and Wilkins, 1987;447–451.
26. Yasargil MG. Carotid-ophthalmic aneurysms. In: Yasargil MG, ed. *Microneurosurgery*. Stuttgart: Theime Verlag, 1984;43–55.
27. Shibuya M, Sugita K. Surgery of paraclinoid aneurysms. In: Schmidek H, Sweet W, eds. *Operative Neurosurgical Techniques, Indications, Methods, and Results*. Philadelphia: WB Saunders, 1995;993–1002.
28. Raymond LA, Tew J. Large suprasellar aneurysms imitating pituitary tumor. *J Neurol Neurosurg Psychiatry* 1978;41:83–87.
29. White JC, Ballantine HT. Intrasellar aneurysms simulating hypophyseal tumours. *J Neurosurg* 1961;18:34–50.

Cerebrovascular Disease, edited by H. Hunt Batjer.
Lippincott-Raven Publishers, Philadelphia © 1997.

CHAPTER 78

Posterior Carotid Wall Aneurysm: Surgical Techniques

Thomas A. Kopitnik, Jr.

GENERAL BACKGROUND

Cerebral aneurysms of the posterior carotid wall typically arise in conjunction with the origin of the posterior communicating artery (PcomA) and are among the most prevalent aneurysms encountered by neurosurgeons. One third of all intracranial aneurysms occur on the internal carotid artery (ICA) and the majority of these arise at the PcomA origin (1) (Fig. 1). Aneurysms in this location share the seemingly paradoxical distinction of relative ease of exposure compared to most other intracranial aneurysms but are notoriously hazardous and severely disabling if not treated appropriately. PcomA aneurysms are anecdotally underestimated in both their difficulty and their potential morbidity by neurosurgeons and neurosurgery residents. Premature intraoperative rupture, irreparable injury to the ICA, inadvertent sacrifice of the PcomA, injury or compromise of the anterior choroidal artery, or injury of the thalamic perforators arising from the PcomA can lead to disastrous consequences and possible neurologic devastation. Although anatomic variations frequently exist along all intracranial vessels, meticulous adherence to a standard conceptual approach to aneurysms associated with the PcomA can reduce some of the potential hazard with the surgical treatment of these common lesions. This chapter will focus on the surgical techniques and rational used to treat PcomA aneurysms using contemporary microsurgical techniques.

Many intracranial aneurysms are erroneously referred to as PcomA aneurysms and often include any aneurysm distal to the ophthalmic artery. Batjer et al. have helped elucidate the terminology and the sites of origin of paraclinoidal ICA aneurysms by describing three anatomic aneurysm locations associated with proximal ICA aneurysms (2). These include ophthalmic, superior hypophyseal, and posterior carotid wall

aneurysms arising proximal to the PcomA. By convention, PcomA aneurysms are those aneurysms that arise from the ICA at or distal to the origin of the PcomA and proximal to the origin of the anterior choroidal artery (AchA). PcomA aneurysms are intimately associated with the PcomA origin and may grow to incorporate the Pcom vessel into the aneurysm neck in some circumstances. A precise understanding of the microsurgical anatomy of the PcomA is important to ensure optimal surgical planning and intraoperative decision making when surgically treating these lesions.

The PcomA originates from the posterolateral surface of the ICA and curves posterior and medial to anastomose with the posterior cerebral artery (PCA) at the P1/P2 junction. The PcomA forms the lateral boundary of the circle of Willis in which various vascular anomalies are commonly found. The majority of patients have a PcomA that is patent but smaller in diameter than the ipsilateral PCA. The PcomA is larger than the P1 artery in approximately 20% of patients and is referred to as fetal in this circumstance (3,4). As the PcomA courses posteriorly it is invested by a sleeve of arachnoid adherent to the arachnoid investing the oculomotor nerve. The PcomA pierces the arachnoid of the interpeduncular cistern and forms a vascular anastomosis with the PCA at the P1/P2 junction. The PcomA gives rise to multiple arterial perforate vessels that penetrate the posterior perforated substance in the periinfundibular, perimammillary, and retrooptic perforator zones (5). The perforators in this region are anterior thalamoperforators and may arise at any site along the course of the PcomA. These perforating vessels supply the posterior hypothalamus, anterior thalamus, posterior limb of the internal capsule, subthalamus, optic tract, and mammillary bodies (6). A prominently large perforating vessel can often be identified and is called the premammillary or tuberoinfundibular artery (7). This large perforating vessel can easily be mistaken for the PcomA when dissecting through fresh hemorrhage medial to the carotid artery in the opticocarotid triangle during attempted exposure of the

T. A. Kopitnik, Jr.: Department of Neurological Surgery, University of Texas Southwestern Medical Center, Dallas, TX 75235.

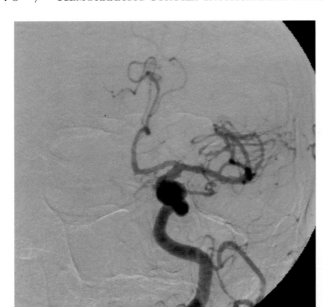

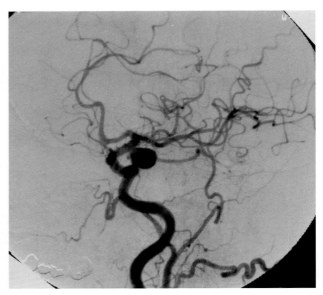

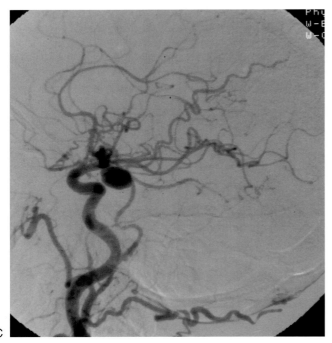

FIG. 1. Left anteroposterior **(A)**, transorbital oblique **(B)**, and lateral **(C)** internal carotid artery arteriogram demonstrating internal carotid artery aneurysm arising at the origin of the posterior communicating artery.

PcomA. Identification of the P1/P2 junction during this medial dissection will ensure the correct differentiation of the PcomA from a large PcomA perforate vessel.

PREOPERATIVE ASSESSMENT

Preoperative assessment of both the patient's condition and the radiographic studies is an important component of the surgical treatment of intracranial aneurysms. One of the most important variables dictating patient outcome has been the neurologic grade at the time of surgery (8). The chance of a good outcome is significantly improved if the patient is Hunt–Hess grade 0–3, whereas patients who are grade 4–5 tolerate an operative procedure, especially temporary arterial occlusion, extremely poorly (9,10). Some controversy exists regarding the optimal treatment of patients who are Hunt–Hess grade 4 following subarachnoid hemorrhage (11). If significant intracerebral hematoma is present, significant hydrocephalus is present, or the configuration of the aneurysm is such that a relatively quick, uncomplicated operative procedure could be reasonably expected, surgery would then be performed despite a Hunt–Hess grade of 4.

PERTINENT NEUROLOGIC AND VASCULAR ANATOMY AND VARIATIONS

Preoperative scrutiny of the arteriogram is important to determine the type of aneurysm present, adjunctive maneuvers that can reasonably be anticipated, the presence of other aneurysms, and to assess the specific cerebral circulation of the patient. The arteriographic appearance of generous collateral circulation may predict tolerance to periods of temporary arterial occlusion during the procedure. The location of the aneurysm and the PcomA origin in relation to the anterior clinoid process may predict difficulty obtaining proximal vascular control early in the operative procedure (Fig. 2). Rarely, a PcomA aneurysm is found arising from a very proximal segment of the ICA such that partial resection of the anterior clinoid process may be necessary to adequately visualize the aneurysm neck. In this situation, cervical carotid exposure should be considered, especially if treating a ruptured lesion. The arteriographic size and relationship of the PCA to the PcomA is another important piece of information that should be evaluated prior to surgery. If the PCA proximal (P1) to the junction with the PcomA is smaller than the PcomA, the circulation pattern is considered fetal. The circle of Willis is highly variable and it is not unusual that atretic or hypoplastic segments, especially regarding the PCA, may be encountered. The inadvertent sacrifice of a nonfetal PcomA is usually an inconsequential event, provided that the anterior thalamoperforators emanating from the PcomA are preserved (12,13). Sacrifice of the PcomA when a fetal circulation or hypoplastic P1 segment is present may result in disastrous complications from insufficient blood flow to the distribution otherwise supplied by the PCA (Fig. 3). The location of the AchA is also important information that can be determined from the arteriogram. The size and location of the AchA should also be determined when planning the operative procedure to ensure that this vital artery remains uncompromised. The most definitive method to prevent inadvertent injury to the AchA is with precise identification of the vessel pre- and intraoperatively. The AchA arises from the ICA in 75% patients, but it may arise from either the PcomA or the middle cerebral arteries (14–16). Inadvertent sacrifice of the AchA is generally poorly tolerated and can produce contralateral hemiparesis, hemianesthesia, and hemianopsia (17). The AchA is usually intimately associated with the distal neck of the aneurysm and must be carefully dissected free prior to attempts at clip application.

SCALP AND BONY EXPOSURE

Posterior communicating artery aneurysms are approached through a standard pterional frontotemporal crani-

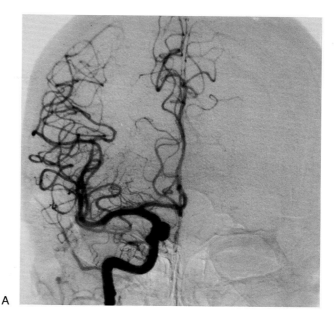

A

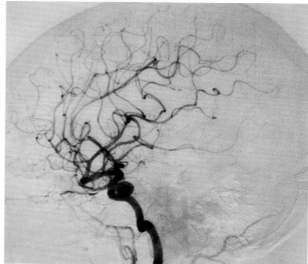

B

FIG. 2. Right anteroposterior **(A)** and lateral **(B)** carotid arteriogram demonstrating proximal internal carotid artery aneurysm consistent with superior hypophyseal artery aneurysm.

otomy approach. The patient is positioned supine with the head rotated toward the contralateral side approximately 30°, the neck extended, and the head translated forward with respect to the axis of the body. The skin incision begins at the level of the zygomatic arch, approximately 1 cm anterior to the tragus, and ends at the midline where the hairline of the scalp meets the bare skin of the forehead. The contour of the incision is generally a gentle curve within the hair-bearing portion of the scalp. The scalp flap is elevated in a submuscular plane and held under gentle retraction with fishhooks. A standard pterional craniotomy free bone flap is fashioned with a pneumatic drill and is elevated and fractured from the attachment to the lateral sphenoid wing. For PcomA aneurysms, a generous resection of the lateral sphenoid wing is

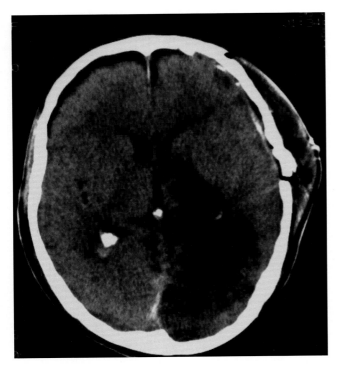

FIG. 3. Computed tomographic scan demonstrating large posterior cerebral territory infarction secondary to inadvertent sacrifice of a fetal posterior communicating artery (PcomA) during aneurysm repair.

performed with rongeurs and the pneumatic drill. A generous subtemporal craniectomy is performed and provides useful working space should aneurysm rupture occur and necessitate rapid mobilization of the temporal lobe. After scrutiny of the systemic blood pressure, the dura is opened with a gentle curved incision based on the sphenoid wing and secured tightly over the scalp flap to minimize epidural bleeding. Using a previously described technique, a ventriculostomy catheter is placed to decompress the ventricular system and facilitate brain relaxation (18). Diuretics should have been administered at the start of the procedure and brain relaxation should be at its maximum.

MICROSURGICAL DISSECTION AND PRINCIPLES

The operative microscope is brought onto the operative field and microdissection is begun. Dissection is first directed to the chiasmatic cistern directly overlying the optic nerve. The arachnoidal adhesions bridging from the frontal lobe to the optic nerve are divided, usually with the use of a microarachnoid knife (Fig. 4). Dissection is then continued sharply with the microscissors along the base of the frontal lobe to divide any arachnoid attachments that prevent elevation of the frontal lobe or exert traction on the optic nerve during retraction of the frontal lobe. Once the arachnoid has been opened over the optic nerve and the base of the frontal

lobe is free of arachnoidal adhesions, a small self-retaining retractor is introduced into the operative field and used to gently elevate the frontal lobe. The purpose of frontal lobe elevation is not solely to create working room but to make the frontal arachnoid adhesions more evident so that they can be divided by sharp dissection. The temporal lobe should not be retracted at this stage of the procedure as that may result in aneurysm rupture early in the dissection. With the use of the microarachnoid knife or the microscissors, the arachnoid is opened into the carotid cistern along the medial border of the ICA and dissection is developed proximally along the medial carotid border to the anterior clinoid process. Once the anterior clinoid process is reached, dissection is carried laterally across the ICA such that proximal vascular control of the ICA is clearly established. Once proximal control has been confirmed, the path of dissection is then redirected to the distal portion of the medial border of the ICA in order to establish distal vascular control (Fig. 4). An important landmark in the dissection is the identification of the ICA distal to the aneurysm neck and the origin of the AchA.

Often at this stage of the operative procedure, the proximal portion of the Sylvian fissure must be opened in order to visualize the distal aspect of the ICA. When a large subarachnoid hemorrhage has occurred, gentle dissection with the

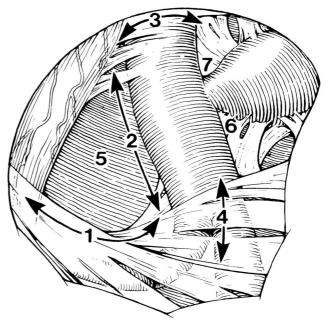

FIG. 4. Order of arachnoid microdissection in the right pericarotid region: (1) arachnoid bridging the optic nerve to the frontal lobe; (2) medial border of the internal carotid artery (ICA); (3) proximal ICA at the anterior clinoid process for proximal vascular control; (4) distal ICA and identification of the anterior choroidal artery; (5) posterior to the ICA to identify the posterior communicating artery (PcomA) and P1/P2 junction; (6) distal aneurysm neck–AchA origin; (7) proximal aneurysm neck.

microarachnoid knife along the blood-filled proximal Sylvian cistern will separate the frontal opercula from the temporal lobe without disturbing the position of the temporal lobe. It is advisable to leave the temporal lobe undisturbed until complete vascular control of the aneurysmal segment has been established, due to risks of disturbing the unstable dome of the aneurysm and producing rupture. The aneurysm dome is often adherent to the medial aspect of the temporal lobe or tentorial incisura and retraction of the temporal lobe not infrequently produces intraoperative rupture in these lesions.

After distal vascular control has been established, it is advisable to dissect deep to the carotid artery between the optic nerve and the ICA in order to identify the PcomA, rather than proceed to aneurysm neck dissection. This is especially important if the PcomA is of large caliber, which may not always be apparent on arteriography. If aneurysm rupture occurs, proximal and distal vascular control may not abate the hemorrhaging if significant blood flow through the PcomA is present. Control of the PcomA can usually be obtained safely by dissecting in the opticocarotid triangle. Early identification of the PcomA will also give the surgeon an idea of the general course and location of the Pcom vessel, whose origin is typically obscured behind the carotid or aneurysm neck.

After the PcomA has been identified, dissection of the proximal and distal neck of the aneurysm is performed. Quite often the AchA is adherent to the distal aneurysm neck or a portion of the aneurysm sac (Fig. 5). The anterior choroidal artery must be spared during the dissection and must not be inadvertently included in the aneurysm clip. The best way

to avoid inadvertent injury to the anterior choroidal artery is by precise anatomic identification. The anterior choroidal may rarely originate from the proximal middle cerebral artery or arise from a common trunk along with the PcomA.

After the aneurysm neck has been dissected using high magnification, an appropriate aneurysm clip is applied under direct vision. A straight aneurysm clip is optimal, although if the brain is swollen and the tips of a straight clip cannot be clearly visualized, a bayoneted clip may provide added visualization during aneurysm clip application. This is especially true when clipping PcomA aneurysms contralateral to the dominant hand of the surgeon, in which the hand used to apply the clip passes in front of the field of vision. Use of an aneurysm clip of appropriate length is important to minimize risk of inadvertent injury to other nearby structures. Excessively long clips may pose a hazard due to torquing after the craniotomy has been closed from local brain tissue swelling and distorting the aneurysm clip. I have seen one case in which an aneurysm clip was actually torn from the side of the ICA several days following surgery from temporal lobe swelling distorting an aneurysm clip of inappropriately excessive length.

After clip application the aneurysm is punctured to ensure that no further filling of the aneurysm occurs and that the clip is in the appropriate position. Intraoperative puncture and deflation of the aneurysm mitigates the need for postoperative angiography with PcomA aneurysms in most circumstances.

Correct clip selection and application is an important component of the surgical treatment of PcomA aneurysms. A large selection of clip shapes, sizes, and brands are available and the preferential use of a particular style or brand depends primarily on the personal preferences of the surgeon. We use only Aesculap Yasargil (Aesculap Inc., San Francisco, CA) aneurysm clips and are satisfied with the available clip configurations and reliability. For clipping nongiant PcomA aneurysms, small straight clips are usually optimal. If the tips of the clip blade are obstructed by the clip applier during application (which can be the case when a right-handed surgeon is applying an aneurysm clip to a left PcomA aneurysm), a small bayonet-shaped clip will usually offset the clip applier enough that the clip blades can be adequately visualized during application. The effort by some surgeons to use curved aneurysm clips to closely mirror the shape of the ICA can be a dangerous maneuver. This maneuver is especially dangerous when carried out by surgeons who only occasionally operate on intracranial aneurysms. Suboptimal clip application may be asymptomatic in this region, or infarction in the anterior thalamus may only be minimally symptomatic. This may cause one to pass curved clips blindly posterior to the ICA until such time as a significant neurologic deficit occurs. Inadvertent clipping of the PcomA or the anterior thalamoperforate vessel may result in significant neurologic deficit. This occurs with curved clips where the precise location of the tips cannot be clearly visualized

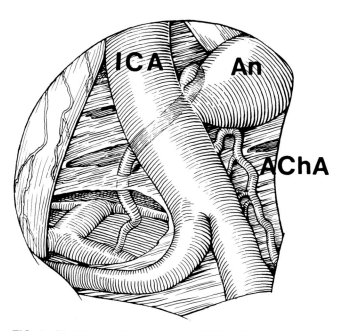

FIG. 5. Right internal carotid artery (ICA) following extensive arachnoid dissection. Anterior choroidal artery (AchA) is often adherent to the aneurysm (An) dome.

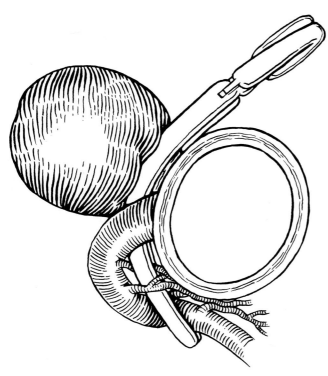

FIG. 6. Incorrectly placed curved aneurysm clip compromising both the posterior communicating artery and the anterior thalamic perforators.

posterior to the carotid artery (Fig. 6). After clip application, careful inspection medial and posterior to the carotid may reveal if the clip blades are across the PcomA or the perforate vessels.

COMPLICATIONS AND THEIR MANAGEMENT

Not infrequently, the dome of a previously ruptured PcomA aneurysm ruptures during closure of the aneurysm clip. This occurs because the dome is commonly adherent to either the medial temporal lobe or to the tentorial incisura. Attempts at subsequent removal of a poorly placed aneurysm clip and replacement with a clip of appropriate configuration may be much more difficult once a clip has been initially applied. The best method to prevent such a complication is to not blindly apply aneurysm clips posterior to the carotid artery and to use straight clip blades if possible (Fig. 7). If clip repositioning is necessary, especially in the event of aneurysm rupture during initial clip placement, the clip should be readjusted under total temporary arterial occlusion, including the PcomA itself. This provides the optimal chance of clear, unobstructed visualization of the clip blades and allows precise clip placement.

Other clip-related problems associated with PcomA aneurysms relate to injury of adjacent structures by clip application. Excessively long clips passed deep to the carotid may injure the oculomotor nerve, inadvertently occlude the poste-

rior cerebral or superior cerebellar artery, or injure the basilar artery. Incomplete dissection of the distal neck of the aneurysm and failure to precisely locate the path and origin of the anterior choroidal artery can lead to injury of this small but vital vessel. Closure of an aneurysm clip on small PcomA perforator vessels, such as the tuberoinfundibular artery, can crush the intima of a small-caliber vessel and result in vessel thrombosis despite subsequent prompt clip removal and repositioning.

Intraoperative aneurysm rupture is an inescapable component of the surgical treatment of intracranial aneurysms and should be anticipated at each step of the surgical procedure. The most common phase of dissection in which rupture of the aneurysm is likely to occur is during final microdissection of the aneurysm neck (19,20). Strict attention to principles of sharp microdissection and elimination of blunt dissection techniques will minimize the occurrence of intraoperative rupture. Inexperienced surgeons may be wary of disturbing the delicate aneurysm tissue and resort to blunt dissection of the aneurysm neck with microdissectors or bipolar coagulation forceps; however, rupture is less likely to occur if the aneurysm neck is sharply dissected, and bleeding with sharp dissection techniques is more controllable than bleeding with blunt dissection techniques. A common maneuver that conventionally increases the likelihood of PcomA aneurysm rupture is aggressive retraction of the temporal lobe early in the operative procedure. A PcomA aneurysm is often adherent to the medial aspect of the temporal

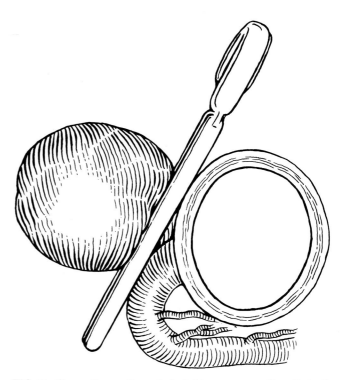

FIG. 7. Correctly positioned straight aneurysm clip with both the posterior communicating artery (PcomA) and perforators clear of the clip.

lobe. Even slight retraction of the temporal lobe can shear the dome from the aneurysm neck. The conventional wisdom has been that temporal lobe retraction should be minimized when surgically treating a ruptured PcomA aneurysm to decrease the chance of early disruption of an unstable segment of the aneurysm dome.

PcomA aneurysms are also prone to hemorrhage during closure of the aneurysm clip. This occurs because the fragile aneurysm tissue can be adherent to the medial temporal lobe, the tentorial incisura, or the oculomotor nerve, which tears from stretch during closure of the aneurysm clip. If bleeding occurs during clip closure, a quick determination of the position of the clip blades should be made without withdrawing the clip. If the surgeon is reasonably certain that the clip blades have not pierced the wall of the aneurysm and are completely across the neck of the aneurysm, controlled closure of the clip blades will usually abate the hemorrhage. If a clip blade has penetrated the aneurysm sac, the aneurysm clip should not be closed as this will likely enlarge the tear. In this case, the clip should be carefully withdrawn and temporary arterial occlusion instituted. The injured region of the aneurysm can then be closely inspected and decisions regarding the best solution to the problem instituted. If a tear occurs in the aneurysm neck close to the ICA, a good option is to include the origin of the Pcom vessel into the aneurysm clip provided that a patent P1 vessel exists and that the posterior cerebral perfusion territory is not critically dependent on the Pcom arterial input.

OVERVIEW

Aneurysms associated with the origin of the PcomA remain a common source of subarachnoid hemorrhage and are encountered in most neurosurgical practices. An understanding of the hazards associated with aneurysms in this region combined with an organized, planned, surgical attack can lead to one of the more successful surgical outcomes associated with the surgical treatment of ruptured intracranial aneurysms. In a similar fashion, complacency and inadequate surgical planning can lead to devastating results with what superficially seems to be a relatively straightforward neurosurgical condition.

REFERENCES

1. Fox JL. *Intracranial Aneurysms.* New York: Springer-Verlag, 1983; 949.
2. Batjer HH, Kopitnik TA, Giller CA, Samson DS. Surgery for paraclinoidal carotid artery aneurysms. *J Neurosurg* 1994;80:650–658.
3. Padget DH. The circle of Willis. Its embryology and anatomy. In: Dandy WE, ed. *Intracranial Arterial Aneurysms.* New York: Hafner, 1944;67–90.
4. Yasargil MG. Operative anatomy. In: Yasargil MG, ed. *Microneurosurgery.* Stuttgart: Thieme Verlag, 1984;60–66.
5. Yasargil MG. Operative Anatomy. In: Yasargil MG, ed. *Microneurosurgery.* Stuttgart: Thieme Verlag, 1984;145–155.
6. Saeki N, Rhoton AL. Microsurgical anatomy of the upper basilar artery and the posterior circle of Willis. *J Neurosurg* 1977;46:583–578.
7. Stephens RB, Stilwell DL. *Arteries and Veins of the Human Brain.* Springfield, IL: Charles C Thomas, 1969.
8. Hunt WE, Hess RM. Surgical risk as related to time of intervention in the repair of intracranial aneurysms. *J Neurosurg* 1968;28:14–20.
9. Batjer HH, Frankfurt AI, Purdy PD, Smith SS, Samson DS. Use of Etomidate, temporary arterial occlusion, and intraoperative angiography in surgical treatment of large and giant cerebral aneurysms. *J Neurosurg* 1988;68:234–240.
10. Kopitnik TA, Samson DS, Batjer HH, White J. The risk of brainstem infarction with temporary arterial occlusion during surgery for basilar apex aneurysms. *J Neurosurg* 1995;82:347A.
11. Bailes JE, Spetzler RF, Hadley MN, Baldwin HZ. Management morbidity and mortality of poor-grade aneurysm patients. *J Neurosurg* 1990; 72:559–566.
12. Kopitnik TA, Batjer HH, Samson DS. Combined transsylvian-subtemporal exposure of cerebral aneurysms involving the basilar apex. *Microsurgery* 1994;15:534–540.
13. Yasargil MG, Antic J, Laciga R, Jain KK, Hodosh RM, Smith RD. Microsurgical pterional approach to aneurysms of the basilar bifurcation. *Surg Neurol* 1976;6:83–91.
14. Carpenter MB, Noback CR, Moss ML. The anterior choroidal artery. Its origin, distribution, and variations. *Arch Neurol Psychiatry* 1954; 71:714–722.
15. Herman LH, Fernando BU, Gurdjian ES. The anterior choroidal artery. An anatomic study of its area of distribution. *Anat Rec* 1966;154: 95–102.
16. Otomo E. The anterior choroidal artery. *Arch Neurol* 1965;13:656–658.
17. Abbie AA. The clinical significance of the anterior choroidal artery. *Brain* 1933;56:233–246.
18. Paine JT, Batjer HH, Samson DS. Intraoperative ventricular puncture. *Neurosurgery* 1988;22:1107.
19. Batjer HH, Samson DS. Intraoperative aneurysm rupture: incidence, outcome, and suggestions for surgical management. *Neurosurgery* 1986;18:701–706.
20. Kopitnik TA, Batjer HH, Samson DS. Surgical management of intraoperative aneurysmal rupture. In: Schmidek HH, Sweet WH, eds. *Operative Neurosurgical Techniques,* 3rd ed. Philadelphia: WB Saunders, 1995;985–991.

Cerebrovascular Disease, edited by H. Hunt Batjer.
Lippincott-Raven Publishers, Philadelphia © 1997.

CHAPTER 79

Internal Carotid Bifurcation Aneurysm: Surgical Techniques

Michihiko Osawa, Shigeaki Kobayashi, and Yuichiro Tanaka

GENERAL BACKGROUND

Of 1544 aneurysms that have been operated on in the past 6 years at Shinshu University and its affiliated hospitals, 25 were internal carotid bifurcation aneurysms (IC bifurcation aneurysm) accounting for 1.6% of all aneurysms. One grade 5 (Hunt and Kosnik) case had only ventricular drainage and the others underwent clipping operation via the frontotemporal approach. The incidence of IC bifurcation aneurysm was smaller than that in another series (1–4). In our series, aneurysms located at the origin of perforators of the proximal M1 or A1 segment were categorized as M1- or A1 aneurysm, respectively. Some of them may be included in the IC bifurcation aneurysms in other series. These aneurysms appear similar in the operating field but there are some differences between them from the technical point of view, as will be described later. We had no experience of intraoperative premature bleeding from the IC bifurcation aneurysm. Mortality and morbidity rates were 2 and 3, respectively, in our series of 24 cases with direct surgery.

PERTINENT NEUROLOGIC AND VASCULAR ANATOMY AND VARIATIONS

An understanding of the microsurgical anatomy around the internal carotid bifurcation, especially that of the perforating arteries, which are often difficult to see on the angiogram (Fig. 1), is indispensable.

Posterior Communicating Artery

About seven or eight perforators originate from the superolateral side of the posterior communicating artery. The

M. Osawa, S. Kobayashi, and Y. Tanaka: Department of Neurosurgery, Shinshu University School of Medicine, Matsumoto, Japan

most important arteries in this group are the premamillary artery or the anterior thalamoperforating artery (5,6). These critical perforating arteries commonly originate from the middle one-third portion of the posterior communicating artery.

Anterior Choroidal Artery

The anterior choroidal artery is known to be one of the most important branches of the internal carotid artery. Its origin is from the posterior wall of the internal carotid artery, more laterally than that of the posterior communicating artery (7–10). Wider critical areas perfused by the artery, which is about half the size of the posterior communicating artery, include the optic tract, lateral geniculate body, and cerebral peduncles (11). This artery should never be sacrificed. Symptoms due to occlusion of the anterior choroidal artery are well known as Abbie's syndrome, and it is quite rare that aplasia or hypoplasia of this critical artery occurs (9). Even if the artery is confirmed in the operative field, the surgeon still has to be careful not to overlook a possible second anterior choroidal artery. Occasionally the artery duplicates or gives off a smaller branch and in some cases one of the double anterior choroidal arteries is hidden behind the carotid artery (8).

Perforators of the A1 Segment

The majority of A1 perforators originate from the superior or posterior wall of the proximal A1 segment near the internal carotid bifurcation (12,13). The area of distribution of the A1 perforators overlaps to some extent with that of the perforators of the M1 segment. When M1 perforators are found to be poorly developed during the initial approach, one may encounter many well-developed A1 perforators.

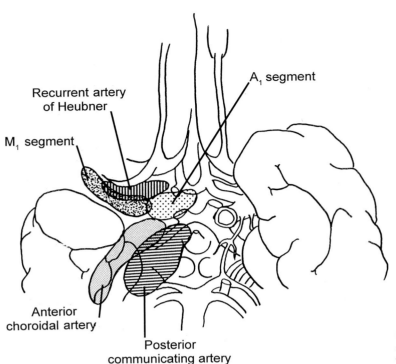

FIG. 1. Schema of the basal view of the brain demonstrating penetrating areas of the perforators around the carotid bifurcation.

Recurrent Artery of Heubner

The recurrent artery of Heubner takes superior or posterior position in relation to the A1 segment, loops over the internal carotid bifurcation, and penetrates the anterior perforating substance (12,14). The proximal portion of the recurrent artery can be found in the space between the frontal lobe and distal A1 segment on the optic nerve. It sometimes passes behind the internal carotid artery below the level of the carotid bifurcation. According to an anatomic study, two thirds of the course of the recurrent arteries are classified as the superior type, as they course over the superior wall of the A1, passing the internal carotid artery below the level of the carotid bifurcation (15). In some cases, the course may be higher than the bifurcation level and hidden behind the aneurysm (Fig. 2).

Perforators of the Proximal M1 Segment

The middle cerebral artery gives off some perforators from its proximal portion (the proximal group of lateral lenticulostriate arteries), which are less in number than the distal group of lateral lenticulostriate arteries.

GENERAL SURGICAL PRINCIPLES AND STRATEGIES

Hemodynamic stress of cerebral blood flow on the wall of the internal carotid bifurcation is thought to be larger than on other bifurcations in the anterior circulation. If premature rupture should occur intraoperatively, the bleeding can be violent, leading easily to a poor result as the aneurysm is located in the basal cistern. The IC bifurcation aneurysm is often surrounded by critical structures such as the optic tract and perforators with adhesion to its dome. Therefore, careful dissection is required at surgery.

Strategies for IC bifurcation aneurysm surgery are summarized in the following three points: (a) how to confirm critical structures, especially perforators hidden behind the aneurysm and to spare them during clip application; (b) how to prevent premature bleeding; and (c) how to prevent iatrogenic damage to the brain.

PATIENT POSITIONING

The patient is placed on the operating table with the upper half of the body elevated about 15–30° to keep the head above the heart level. The head is placed and fixed in the head frame with rotation about 30° to the contralateral side. The vertex is placed about 15° below the horizontal line, which is a reasonable position for adequate illumination for keeping the microscope in a comfortable position during surgery and permitting the brain to fall away from the skull base. This positioning is beneficial when opening the Sylvian fissure. It is the best angle to approach the aneurysm perpendicularly to its neck. However, the initial approach requires different angles. It is important to adjust the head position or angle of rotation as the approach advances to the critical area (16).

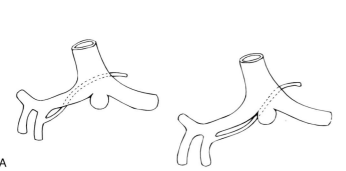
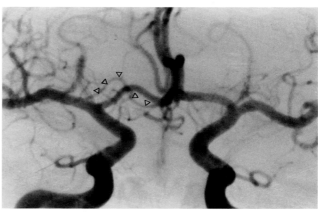

A   B

FIG. 2. A: Anatomic relation between the recurrent artery of Heubner and the carotid bifurcation as seen in the right pterional approach. About two thirds of the recurrent arteries course behind the A1 segment and pass the carotid artery below the level of the bifurcation *(left)*. In some cases, the recurrent artery is located near the bifurcation and may be hidden behind the aneurysm with adhesion *(right)*. **B:** An angiogram (anteroposterior view) demonstrating the course of the recurrent artery of Heubner *(arrowheads)*.

SCALP AND BONY EXPOSURE

Frontotemporal craniotomy is performed for a pterional approach. The bone window is extended further medially than for middle cerebral artery aneurysms. According to the projection of the aneurysm and location of perforators, which are often difficult to see in detail on the preoperative angiogram, the surgeon has to apply a clip from the medial side or subfrontal direction. It can also be convenient to dissect and follow the anterior cerebral artery behind the neck. Retraction of the temporal lobe is not as needed because it is always possible to get enough space for application from the lateral side by widely opening the Sylvian fissure. It is most important to remove the bony edge substantially at the frontal base and sphenoid wing. The bony edge will disturb the microscopic view, interfere with the applier or other surgical instruments, and cause unnecessary retraction of the brain. If the frontal air sinus is opened, the inner table is removed completely. This process is advantageous because the created sinus cavity can be turned into a working space.

In case of severe subarachnoid hemorrhage, ventricular drainage is implemented prior to craniotomy. It is often useful to reduce intracranial pressure by removing cerebrospinal fluid (CSF) via ventricular tap, with the tap kept in place postoperatively for several days for ventricular irrigation by anticoagulant drugs.

MICROSURGICAL DISSECTION AND PRINCIPLES

Widely opening the Sylvian fissure in safe and gentle fashion is one of the basic techniques of neurosurgery. Which is better for opening the Sylvian fissure: the proximal or the distal side? What causes excessive brain retraction? When the Sylvian fissure is opened violently without cutting the arachnoid membrane and trabeculae sharply and carefully, intraoperative brain edema develops during the subsequent procedures. Arachnoid trabeculae are fine but are also traction-resistant, like an anchor. Spatulas on the frontal lobe are always placed from the parietal side to the frontal base. When we begin to open the Sylvian fissure from the deep side, the arachnoid membrane in the parietal side is left untouched and the brain is compressed unnecessarily until the process is completed. On the other hand, when the process is performed from the distal side or surface of the Sylvian fissure to the deeper side, spatulas can be placed on the area where arachnoid membrane and trabeculae between the frontal and temporal lobes had disappeared. The process of beginning deeply and following toward the surface is, however, of some advantage in securing the parent artery at an early stage. In our series, the surface of the Sylvian fissure was opened initially, the middle cerebral artery confirmed, and dissection followed retrogradely toward the internal carotid bifurcation. The internal carotid artery was secured before the final dissection of the aneurysm complex was made in the carotid bifurcation area.

Tapered spatulas are placed on the frontal and temporal lobes across the Sylvian fissure, giving minimum tension to the arachnoid membrane, which is then cut by microscissors. Fine trabeculae in the cistern is also cut carefully. Assistant surgeons should intermittently irrigate the subarachnoid space by saline solution, which facilitates aspiration of the clots. Position of the spatula is changed frequently toward the deeper Sylvian fissure.

It is not very difficult to spare veins which sometimes cross the Sylvian fissure. It is useful to lengthen the free segment of a vein in the Sylvian fissure by dissecting the surrounding arachnoid membrane (Sugita method) (16).

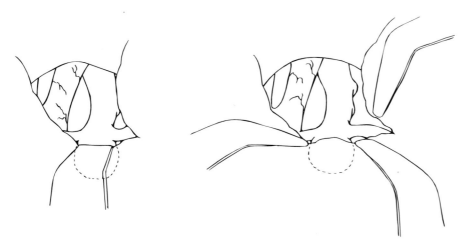

FIG. 3. Use of a wider spatula *(left)* and multiple tapered spatulas *(right)*. When a wide spatula is applied, not only an unnecessary large portion of the brain but also the critical area near the aneurysm neck is retracted.

Special care should be taken not to tear these free veins in the final step of clipping. This can be done by an assistant surgeon seeing the field under low magnification, while the surgeon concentrates on a narrow microscopic field under a higher magnification.

Brain retraction is one of the essential techniques of neurosurgery but only a few clinical studies have been reported. Techniques to reduce compression pressure to the brain and to minimize the brain damage are summarized as follows: (a) drainage of cerebrospinal fluid, (b) intermittent retraction, and (c) use of multiple retractors (17).

Ventricular drainage from the anterior horn in the contralateral side of the approach or lumbar spinal drainage is often placed prior to craniotomy. When the retraction pressure or intracranial pressure increases above the critical level, aspiration of a small amount of CSF, always 5–10 ml in our experiences, can reduce and normalize the pressure rapidly. It is a simple technique but helpful for brain protection. The CSF can be intermittently aspirated but continuous drainage after setting the fluid level below the critical pressure is more recommended. The drainage can be used for continuous intraventricular pressure monitoring and the route for postoperative irrigation therapy.

The usefulness of multiple retractors to reduce retraction pressure and obtain a wide view has been reported (17) (Fig. 3). Intermittent retraction has to be kept in mind also. The spatulas should be replaced or reduced within every 5–10 minutes (18). This process may be troublesome for surgeons who want to maintain a smooth or "rhythmic" flow of operation. Quick reactions of the assistant surgeons are required. Self-retraining retractors are always utilized in aneurysm surgery (19). Proper fixation is obtained when the flexible arm is arranged in a semicircular shape with a diameter of about 20 cm (20). The tapered retractor made of light-weight titanium alloy is superior to the retractor of the same shape made of stainless steel. Correct use of each spatula is required for the safe and efficient operation. The axis of the distal side of the self-retaining retractor where the spatula is connected should be set in the aimed direction of the brain. It is important to avoid accidental touch of the surgeon's hand or other surgical instruments to the retractors (Fig. 4).

The cotton patty is one of the important tools to protect brain tissue. The soft cotton patties made from pure cellulose (Bemsheet R) are also used for dissection, hemostasis, and protection against tissue injury with the suction tip. Silicone rubber sheets or split silicone tubes have been introduced for intraoperative protection of cranial nerves and perforating arteries. The silicone materials are thin and smooth providing the advantage of tissue protection from injury by electrical current of bipolar forceps (21,22).

The middle cerebral artery is followed proximally to the optic nerve and the internal carotid artery in the microscopic field. The surgeon has to observe the local appearance of subarachnoid hemorrhage around the carotid bifurcation. Location of hard clots indicates not only direction but also the rupture site of the aneurysm, which is difficult to prede-

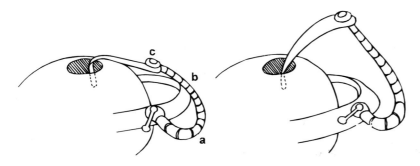

FIG. 4. Setting of a spatula and a self-retaining retractor. *Left:* A correct use of the instruments. The base side of the retractor, making a semicircular shape with a diameter of about 20 cm **(A)**, is touched or placed on the base frame **(B)** to make it steadier. The retractor and spatula are connected in a natural shape **(C)**, which is advantageous to conduct the retraction power and get free space. *Right:* An example of an incorrect setting.

termine from preoperative angiograms or computed tomography (CT) scans. When these thick clots are removed, a wide subarachnoid space is created, which is advantageous for work with microsurgical instruments. Commonly the IC bifurcation aneurysm is directed superiorly or superoposteriorly, and buried or adherent to the inferior aspect of the frontal lobe. Therefore, retraction of the temporal lobe is recommended initially. The carotid cistern is sharply opened to minimize mechanical stress to the aneurysm, and clots are aspirated. The arachnoid membrane superior to the optic nerve is cut off and the chiasmatic cistern is opened in the same manner, beyond the optic nerve to the medial side as far as possible. Satisfactory dissection may reduce the retraction pressure and make it possible to obtain a wider field in which to continue further procedures. The horizontal portion of the anterior cerebral artery, occasionally with the recurrent artery of Heubner, is confirmed at this point.

Fine trabeculae between the optic nerve and the internal carotid artery are cut off to evacuate clots, with special care not to injure small perforators. The perforators here, including small branches from the posterior-communicating, anterior choroidal, and superior hypophyseal arteries are important and can easily be injured. Aspiration pressure of suction, always held in the left hand, has to be kept within an appropriate level to evacuate clots. Saline irrigation is also important during this procedure. Liliequist's membrane is opened to drain CSF to reduce the intracranial pressure and restore CSF flow.

The origins of the posterior communicating and anterior choroidal arteries are commonly confirmed in the posterolateral side of the internal carotid artery. Running medially behind the carotid artery and passing through the subarachnoid space near the bifurcation, they penetrate the lateral perforated substances. If possible, the course and branching pattern of these major perforators should be confirmed through the optico-carotid space. In some cases, the wall of the parent artery is so hard with arteriosclerosis that use of a clip for temporary occlusion is difficult. In our experience, even in such a case, the wall of the carotid artery close to the bifurcation is not too hard, and a clippable region can be secured before the final step.

When aneurysm puncture is required, several clips are used to trap the aneurysm by occluding the internal carotid artery M1 and A1 segments. Temporary clips for M1 segment and carotid artery can be placed away from the carotid bifurcation with the heads of the clips tilted to the opposite side of the neck to obtain sufficient working space around the aneurysm. Bayonet clips serve to the same purpose. The temporary clip on the A1 segment, however, sometimes disturbs the microscopic field because the space to insert it is so narrow.

When the aneurysm dome is directed superiorly, a careless movement of the spatula may introduce laceration of the neck. Application of two tapered spatulas and sharp dissection of the arachnoid membrane will help disperse direct traction power to the critical point.

Orientation of the aneurysm complex is sometimes confused by a tortuous A1 and/or irregular neck (Fig. 5). It is often difficult to get correct information prior to surgery from the preoperative angiogram in these unusual cases because arteries and aneurysm are seen overlapping each other. In such complicated cases, the surgeon should not hesitate to utilize temporary clipping on the parent arteries to dissect the whole body of the aneurysm.

Tightly adherent perforators to the aneurysm are sometimes encountered. These arteries should be separated from the aneurysm to render enough space to insert blades without causing perforator occlusion. Safe dissection requires understanding that IC bifurcation aneurysms are divided into two main groups. The first of these is "true" bifurcation aneurysms, protruding from the junction between A1 and M1, ie, from the summit of the terminal internal carotid artery. The second is aneurysms originating from the base of a perforator of A1 or M1 segment near the summit (Fig. 6). The three-dimensional relationships between the A1 or M1 segment and internal carotid artery are different in each case and hemodynamic stress is not always largest at the summit. In our series, about 2.5% of the total aneurysms were located at the origin of a perforator and classified as an M1 or A1 aneurysm. Some of these aneurysms are located very close to the IC summit showing similar appearance to the true IC bifurcation aneurysm. Technical aspects of clipping these two groups are almost the same, but a surgeon trying to dissect around the neck should keep the distinction in mind.

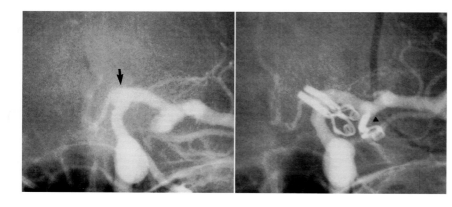

FIG. 5. Angiograms (anteroposterior view) of a case of multiple aneurysms. *Left (preoperative)*: The internal carotid artery and bifurcation aneurysm associated overlap with A1 aneurysm *(arrow)*. *Right (postoperative)*: Two clips are applied to these two aneurysms. The third clip is applied to an incidentally found middle cerebral artery aneurysm *(arrowhead)*.

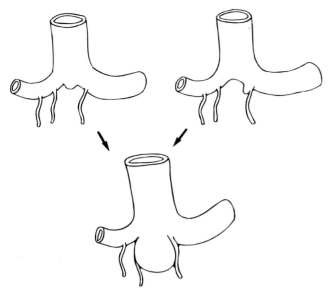

FIG. 6. Drawing to illustrate the origins of the aneurysm protruded from the carotid summit *(upper left)* and the aneurysm originated from the base of a perforator near the summit *(upper right)*, both developing to a bifurcation aneurysm *(lower)*.

However tight the adhesion between the neck and a perforator might be, there must be some distance between the origin of the perforator and true IC bifurcation aneurysm. On the other hand, in some cases of the second group, the base of the perforator originated from the neck. However, it is sometimes quite difficult to distinguish between these two groups even by intraoperative direct observation, although certain information about it can be obtained from the preoperative angiogram. When the angle between the axis of internal carotid artery and the A1 segment on the anteroposterior view is the same as that between M1 seguement, ie, when the pattern of the carotid bifurcation is symmetric on the AP view of the angiogram, the aneurysm is likely the true IC bifurcation aneurysm. When the pattern is asymmetric, it may be an A1 or M1 aneurysm.

Dissection of the neck is carried out carefully. A pair of tapered spatulas are applied on the both sides of the brain close to the neck (Fig. 3). They should not be placed on the aneurysm dome buried in the frontal lobe. Confirmation of possible perforators behind the aneurysm complex is sometimes difficult or dangerous before the whole body has been dissected, freed, and made movable. The subpial dissection method is useful when the aneurysm is small or the wall is thin. After small corticotomy, the subpial space is dissected and the aneurysm is separated away from the brain with pia mater left on the surface of the dome.

The surgeon must choose the best clip for complete clipping, without leaving residual neck and occluding perforators (2,3,4,23,24). Clips that were thought to be most beneficial or convenient are sometimes difficult to use because they might injure critical structures during application. Many

special techniques such as multiple clipping, shank clipping, compression clipping, tentative clipping, applicator changing, rotation advance, as well as others, have been reported to achieve complete clipping (25). It is also important to use a correct applier with an adequate shape to obtain an appropriate microscopic view. Before the final step, the surgeon should be prepared for unexpected bleeding or other possible accidents and pay attention to general condition of the patient including blood pressure and microscope position.

A straight or bayonet clip is commonly applied to an IC bifurcation aneurysm (Fig. 7a,b,c,8). While placing a clip, the surgeon should try to confirm perforators behind the aneurysm as the procedure creates some space around the aneurysm. Bayonet clips are helpful for seeing the critical point clearly and are also useful for performing shank clipping, which is a technique to utilize the angle portion of the bayonet clip when the aneurysm involves part of the parent artery (26).

When a curved clip is applied with the blades placed parallel to the axis made by A1 and M1 segment, it sometimes matches the natural shape of the bifurcation. To apply a curved clip in such a way, the reverse side of the dome must be dissected completely and the Sylvian fissure opened widely enough to obtain working space (Fig. 7d,e). Applying a ring clip is one of the more useful options, with the ring encircling major arteries or perforators (27) (Fig. 7f,g). A wider space around the aneurysm complex is required to apply a ring clip than other clips. The space is necessary not only to insert blades but to facilitate their removal safely when needed.

After placing the clip, it is important to ascertain that residual neck is not left behind and that the perforators are not misclipped. Microsurgical mirrors are helpful for seeing the reverse side, and micro-Doppler probes are often utilized to confirm the blood flow. In the case of larger aneurysm, it is also useful to puncture the aneurysm dome to reduce its size. But when the aneurysm is small, especially with a thin wall, additional dissection after aneurysm puncture may be dangerous for the following two reasons. The first is that a small hole, made by a needle on a small aneurysm with a thin component, easily develops to a laceration that involves the aneurysm neck. The second is that dissection between the surrounding normal structures and slackened thin aneurysm wall often injures the slackened side. One should know that there is a significant difference technically between separating or dissecting a tense aneurysm and a slackened one.

When a perforator is found to be originating from the aneurysm body or dome, this can be sacrificed, provided the perforator is small and there are other perforators nearby that do not originate from the aneurysm and can be spared (25).

COMPLICATIONS AND THEIR MANAGEMENT

In our series, there were some complications such as premature bleeding, perforator occlusion, and misclipping. A

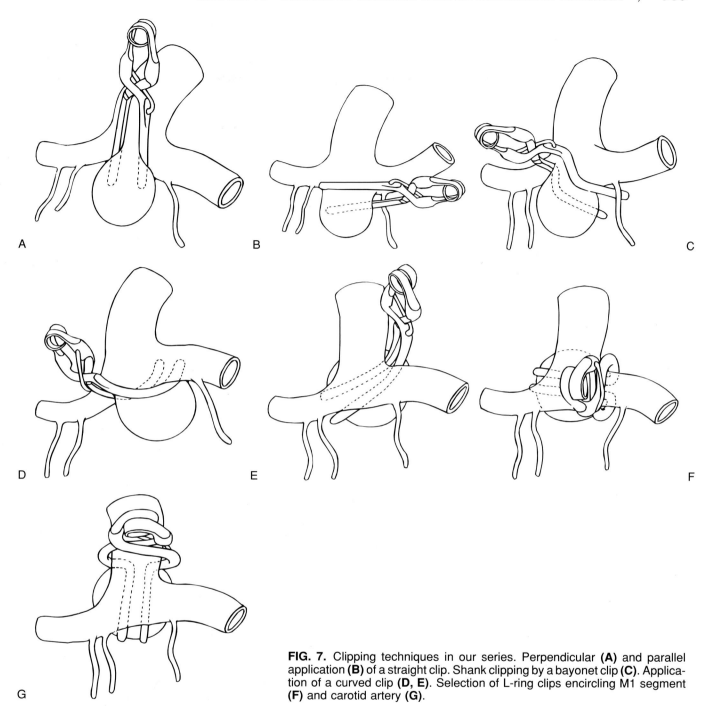

FIG. 7. Clipping techniques in our series. Perpendicular **(A)** and parallel application **(B)** of a straight clip. Shank clipping by a bayonet clip **(C)**. Application of a curved clip **(D, E)**. Selection of L-ring clips encircling M1 segment **(F)** and carotid artery **(G)**.

perforator was sacrificed in two cases by clipping because intraoperative bleeding occurred before the perforators had been completely separated. One of the aneurysms was giant with calcified wall and tight adhesion; the temporary clipping was not effective to control the bleeding. A small bleb on the other aneurysm adherent to the optic tract ruptured during dissection in a narrow space. A wider working space, enough to accomplish further dissection with a temporary clip, should have been obtained.

The third case of irregular aneurysm was instructive for us (Fig. 9). The aneurysm, demonstrated as dumbbell-shaped on the preoperative angiogram, proved to be a combined double aneurysm with a wide neck, after the initial clipping. The surgeon mistook half of the aneurysm as the proximal portion of the A1, and only one half of the aneurysmal neck was clipped. Misclipping, due to the disorientation, was found on exploration after clipping, and reclipping was performed immediately. Two of the 25 IC bifurcation aneu-

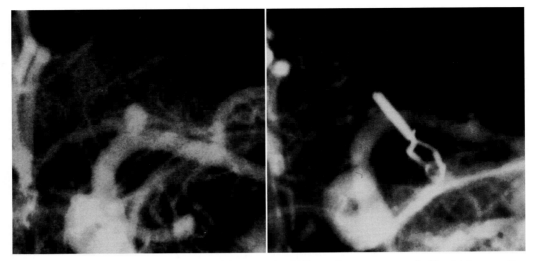

FIG. 8. Angiographic appearance of usual intracerebral bifurcation aneurysm *(left)*, which was clipped by straight clip *(right)*.

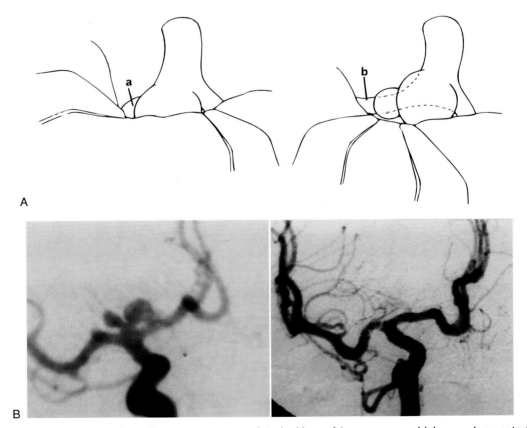

FIG. 9. A case of a bifurcation aneurysm associated with an A1 aneurysm, which was demonstrated as a dumbbell shape on the preoperative angiogram *(lower left)*. Drawing of aneurysm prior to initial clipping *(upper left)* and final clipping *(upper right)*. What was thought to be the A1 segment **(A)** was actually a half of the aneurysm and A1 segment **(B)** was confirmed behind it. Two aneurysms were clipped by a straight clip *(lower right)*.

rysms were associated with an A1 aneurysm. Their shapes were irregular with combined domes and it was quite impossible to demonstrate the exact shape on the preoperative angiogram.

OVERVIEW

Technical principles and strategies for surgical treatment of internal carotid bifurcation aneurysms are described in summary as follows:

1. Create enough working space, with special care to protect the brain tissue.
2. Determine anatomic relations, which might be different from those made on the basis of the preoperative information.
3. Prepare many options for possible premature rupture.
4. Confirm critical structures well before clip application.
5. Never skip final inspection after clipping.

REFERENCES

1. Kodama N, Koshu K, Mineura K, Suzuki J. Surgical treatment of internal carotid bifurcation aneurysms. In: Suzuki J, ed. *Cerebral Aneurysms. Experiences with 1000 Directly Operated Cases.* Tokyo: Neuron Publishing, 1979;263–268.
2. Ogilvy C, Crowell RM. Carotid bifurcation aneurysms. In: Appuzo MLJ, eds. *Brain Surgery: Complication Avoidance and Management.* vol 1. New York: Churchill Livingstone, 1993;970–983.
3. Flamm ES. Aneurysms of internal carotid and anterior communicating arteries. In: Wilkins RH, Rengachary SS, eds. *Neurosurgery.* vol 2. New York: McGraw-Hill, 1985;1394–1404.
4. Yasargil MG. Aneurysms of the internal carotid artery bifurcation (ICBi-aneurysms). In: Yasargil MG, ed. *Microneurosurgery.* vol 2. New York: Thieme Verlag, 1984;109–123.
5. Pedroza A, Dujovny M, Cabezudo-Artero J, Umansky F, Berman SK, Diaz FG, Ausman JI, Mirchandani G. Microanatomy of the premamillary artery. *Acta Neurochir (Wien)* 1987;86:50–55.
6. Saeki N, Rhoton AL Jr. Microsurgical anatomy of the upper basilar artery and the posterior circle of Willis. *J Neurosurg* 1977;46:563–578.
7. Yasargil MG. Operative anatomy, internal carotid artery. In: Yasargil MG, ed. *Microneurosurgery.* vol 1. New York: Thieme Verlag, 1984; 56–71.
8. Yasargil MG, Yonas H, Gasser JC. Anterior choroidal artery aneurysms: their anatomy and surgical significance. *Surg Neurol* 1978;9: 129–138.
9. Rhoton AL Jr, Fujii K, Fradd B. Microneurosurgical anatomy of the anterior choroidal artery. *Surg Neurol* 1979;12:171–187.
10. Gibo H, Lenkey C, Rhoton AL Jr. Microsurgical anatomy of the supraclinoid portion of the internal carotid artery. *J Neurosurg* 1981;55: 560–574.
11. Rosner SS, Rhoton AL Jr, Ono M, Barry M. Microsurgical anatomy of the anterior perforating arteries. *J Neurosurg* 1984;61:468–485.
12. Marinkovic S, Milisavljevic M, Kovacevic M. Anatomical bases for surgical approach to the initial segment of the anterior cerebral artery, Microanatomy of Heubner's artery and perforating branches of the anterior cerebral artery. *Surgical Radiologic Anatomy* 1986;8:7–18.
13. Gomes FB, Dujovny M, Umansky F, et al. Microanatomy of the anterior cerebral artery. *Surg Neurol* 1986;26:129–141.
14. Kribs M, Kleihues P. The reccurent artery of Heubner. In: Zulch AJ, ed. *Cerebral Circulation and Stroke.* New York: Springer-Verlag, 1971; 40–56.
15. Gomes FB, Dujovny M, Umansky F, Ausman JI, Diaz FG, Ray WJ, Mirchandani HG. Microsurgical anatomy of the recurrent artery of Heubner. *J Neurosurg* 1984;60:130–139.
16. Sugita K. General considerations. In: *Microneurosurgical Atlas.* Sugita K, ed. Berlin: Springer-Verlag, 1985;1–2.
17. Hongo K, Kobayashi S, Yokoh A, Sugita K. Monitoring retraction pressure on the brain. An experimental and clinical study. *J Neurosurg* 1987;66:270–275.
18. Yokoh A, Sugita K, Kobayashi S. Intermittent versus continuous brain retraction. *J Neurosurg* 1983;58:918–923.
19. Sundt TM Jr, Kobayashi S, Fode NC, Whisnant JP. Result and complications of surgical management of 809 intracranial aneurysms in 722 cases. *J Neurosurg* 1982;56:753–765.
20. Tada T, Kobayashi S, Sugita K. Dynamic properties of self-retaining retractors under load. Technical note. *Neurosurgery* 1991;28:914–917.
21. Shibuya M, Sugita K, Kobayashi S. Intraoperative protection of cranial nerves and perforating arteries by silicone rubber sheets. *J Neurosurg* 1991;74:677–679.
22. Tanaka Y, Kobayashi S, Hongo K, Oikawa S. Intraoperative protection of cranial nerves and arteries by split silicone tube. *Neurosurgery* 1993; 33:523–525.
23. Sugita K. Instrumentation. In: *Microneurosurgical Atlas.* Berlin: Springer-Verlag, 1985;3–9.
24. Fox JL. Aneurysms at the bifurcation of the internal carotid artery. In: Fox JL, ed. *Intracranial Aneurysms.* vol 2. New York: Springer-Verlag, 1983;969–975.
25. Kobayashi S, Tanaka Y. Aneurysm clip design, selection, and application. In: Appuzo MLJ, eds. *Brain Surgery: Complication Avoidance and Management.* vol 1. New York: Churchill Livingstone, 1993; 825–846.
26. Osawa M, Obinata C, Kobayashi S, Tanaka Y. Newly designed bayonet clips for complicated aneurysms. Technical note. *Neurosurgery* 1995; 36:425–427.
27. Sugita K, Kobayashi S, Kyoshima K, Nakagawa F. Fenestrated clips for unusual aneurysms of the carotid artery. *J Neurosurg* 1982;57: 240–246.

Cerebrovascular Disease, edited by H. Hunt Batjer.
Lippincott-Raven Publishers, Philadelphia © 1997.

CHAPTER 80

Middle Cerebral Aneurysm: Surgical Techniques

Alberto Pasqualin, Renato Scienza, and Renato Da Pian

GENERAL BACKGROUND

Aneurysms of the middle cerebral artery (MCA) are quite common, accounting for approximately 20% of all cerebral aneurysms (1). In the majority of cases, they are located on the main branching of the MCA, although some are located on the first tract of the MCA (the M1 tract), and a few on the secondary branches of the MCA. Due to these different points of origin, the variable length of the M1 tract, and the anatomic configuration of the Sylvian fissure, these aneurysms pose more difficulties in the surgical localization than aneurysms in the rest of the anterior circulation.

Another feature that makes the surgical approach slightly different from that employed for other aneurysms is the frequent association with large intracerebral hematomas. In this case, recognition of the vascular structures in the Sylvian fissure may be difficult, owing to the abundance and adherence of the clots and to the absence of circulating cerebrospinal fluid (CSF).

Finally, the MCA is a terminal artery, and the sacrifice of any of its branches may result in severe disability. This is particularly true for those aneurysms that "sit" on the main trunks of division of the MCA and need to be excluded with full respect to these vessels: the anatomic configuration of these aneurysms is often complex, and surgical exclusion may require multiple clips, arranged in various ways.

PERTINENT NEUROLOGIC AND VASCULAR ANATOMY AND VARIATIONS

The Sylvian fissure is the "anatomic container" of a large part of the MCA. At approximately the bifurcation of the internal carotid artery, the first part of the MCA is covered

A. Pasqualin, R. Scienza, and R. Da Pian: Department of Neurosurgery, Verona City Hospital, 37100 Verona, Italy.

by thickened arachnoid fibers, which represent a "door" between the carotid cistern and the Sylvian cistern. These fibers connect the fronto-orbital to the temporal gyrus. Often one large (or a few smaller) anastomotic fronto-orbital vein(s) run(s) above these fibers from the anterior perforated substance to the mesial temporal lobe. Distally to this point, the first tract of the MCA, known as the M1 tract, or "sphenoidal segment" of the MCA, according to Gibo et al (2), enters the depth of the Sylvian fissure, covered by the frontal and temporal opercula through loose arachnoidal fibers. The M1 tract runs adjacent to the anterior perforated substance, posterior to the division of the olfactory tract, posterior and parallel to the sphenoid ridge. The first part of the Sylvian fissure, which contains the M1 tract, is called the "sphenoidal compartment" (2) and ends at the limen insulae (or genu). The frontal and temporal opercula—which form the walls of this compartment—may lie in juxtaposition, parallel to one another; alternatively one operculum (most often the lateral orbital gyrus of the frontal operculum) indents the other operculum, concealing the deep portion of the cistern and the M1 tract.

The M1 tract can be considered the direct continuation of the internal carotid artery, and in 70% of cases is larger than the anterior cerebral artery, ranging between 2.4 and 4.6 mm at the origin (1). Its length is approximately 14–16 mm (1,3) but may vary widely, if the main division of the MCA is proximal or distal to the limen insulae. According to Gibo et al, the main division is slightly proximal to the limen in 86% of the hemispheres (2). Depending on the length of the internal carotid artery, the proximal M1 tract can vary in depth within the fissure, whereas the depth of the distal M1 tract depends only on the individual configuration of the vessel and is expressed on angiography by the distance from the sphenoid wing (4). For example, a pronounced inferior loop of the distal MCA is often seen in the elderly and corresponds to a superficial location in the fissure.

In the sphenoidal compartment, various vessels originate

from the M1 tract: (a) the inferolateral group of vessels and (b) the superomedial group of vessels. The group of vessels arising from the *inferolateral* wall of the M1 tract (according to the angiographic and anatomic projection) are the uncal artery, the temporopolar artery, and the anterior temporal artery (usually the largest artery of the M1 tract). Whereas the uncal artery can arise also from the distal internal carotid artery, the temporopolar artery is often hypoplastic or absent, and there can also be a common trunk of the temporal arteries. Very rarely, the temporal arteries arise from the inferior (temporal) trunk of division of the MCA, not from the M1 tract. When the anterior temporal artery or the common temporal trunk is quite large, it can give the impression of an early bifurcation, known as "pseudobifurcation," of the MCA. In extreme cases, a large common temporal trunk can arise directly from the terminal portion of the internal carotid artery, giving the impression of a "double" or "accessory" MCA (Fig. 1) (3,5,6). It should be noted that in a few cases a temporal artery can arise from the anterosuperior wall of the M1 tract and run inferiorly toward the temporal operculum, creating a loop.

The group of vessels arising from the *superomedial* wall of the M1 tract is the lateral lenticulostriate arteries (in various numbers) and occasionally a lateral fronto-orbital artery (generally close to the main division of the MCA). A common stem of the striate arteries with the lateral fronto-orbital artery is rarely found but when present can be mistaken for a false bifurcation of the MCA. One large striate artery is more often observed than two striate arteries, whereas the observation of many small striate arteries is a rare occurrence. According to their site of origin along the M1 tract, they have been divided into proximal and distal lateral striate

arteries by some authors (1,7). A more suitable division into three groups of striate arteries—medial, intermediate, and lateral—has been proposed by Rosner et al (8). According to these authors, the intermediate group has a distinctive "candelabra" appearance, possessing at least one major artery with complex distal arborization, whereas the arteries of the lateral group have an S-shaped course (8). Further along their course, the three groups of lenticulostriate arteries penetrate the middle and posterior portion of the lateral half of the anterior perforated substance (8), and supply the body and head of the caudate nucleus, the lateral segment of the globus pallidus, the superior half of the internal capsule, and most of the putamen (5,7,8). Very rarely, a common fronto-orbital/striate trunk can arise from the anterior cerebral artery and run parallel and superior to the M1 tract; this trunk can be identified as an accessory MCA (1,3,9). Thus, the accessory MCA can originate from the internal carotid artery and run inferior to the M1 tract, or from the anterior cerebral artery and run superior to the M1 tract (3,6,9).

As mentioned above, at or proximal to the limen insulae the M1 tract bifurcates, giving rise in most cases to an inferior (temporal) trunk and a superior (frontal) trunk. These trunks bend 90° backward exactly along the limen insulae, and after diverging at the bifurcation they converge in the depth of the Sylvian fissure, 1–2 cm distal to the MCA bifurcation. Whereas the frontal trunk is more superficial, generally the temporal trunk is hidden under the temporal operculum along its proximal course. The part of the Sylvian fissure distal to the limen insulae is called the "operculo-insular compartment" (2) and is wide and covered by bridging veins, generally anastomosing with one or more large temporosphenoidal vein(s). While these veins form the group of the superficial Sylvian veins, one (and very rarely more than one) deep Sylvian vein is commonly encountered on the insular cortex, adjacent and posterior to the distal M1 tract and to the MCA bifurcation. The superficial Sylvian veins generally drain toward the sphenoparietal sinus and rarely backward to the vein of Labbé. For the deep Sylvian vein, the vein of Rosenthal is the main drainage (4). The "operculoinsular compartment" of the Sylvian cistern is further divided into a more superficial horizontally oriented cleft (the opercular cleft, between the opposing fronto-parietal and temporal opercula) and a deep vertically oriented cleft (the insular cleft, perpendicular to the opercular cleft, between the insula and the opercula) (2). The insular cleft in turn is composed of a superior limb (between the insula and the frontoparietal operculum) and an inferior limb (between the insula and the temporal operculum): the greatest branching of the MCA occurs mainly in the insular cleft, over the anterior part of the insula, just distal to the genu. The distal branches of the MCA emerge through the opercular cleft to nourish the temporal, occipital, parietal, and frontal hemispheres. The vessels directed superiorly undergo a "double flexion" (two 180° turns), while those directed inferiorly follow a less tortuous course when exiting from the fissure (2).

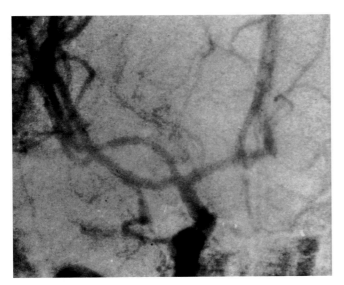

FIG. 1. Right carotid angiography in a patient with an "accessory" MCA: both trunks of division of the MCA (frontal and temporal) originate from the internal carotid bifurcation, with the temporal trunk bifurcating distally into two large secondary branches.

Regarding the main division of the MCA, an equal bifurcation with both trunks of the same caliber is a relatively rare occurrence, whereas more often one trunk (the temporal trunk) (2) is dominant over the other. In rare cases, one trunk of division is small, and its area of vascular supply is partially covered by a larger artery originating from the M1 tract. There is some controversy on the concept of trifurcation or tetrafurcation of the MCA. While other authors have described more than two trunks of division in 22–30% of cases (2,3), Yasargil has pointed out that most of these cases represent very proximal secondary divisions of the temporal or frontal trunks (1). Although the concept expressed by Yasargil is true in most cases of supposed tri- or tetrafurcation, we have observed a few cases with a true trifurcation or tetrafurcation (Fig. 2). Very rarely [in 6% of cases, according to Umanski et al. (3)] there is no bifurcation of the MCA, and the M1 tract continues along the Sylvian fissure, giving rise to the various cortical arteries and ending in the angular artery.

The proximal portion of the temporal and frontal trunks may give rise to distal striate vessels, which due to their course are identified as "recurrent" perforating arteries

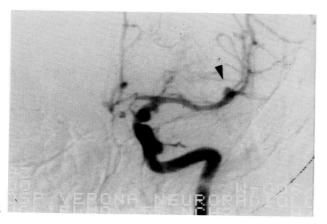

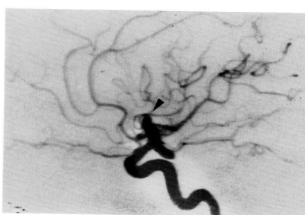

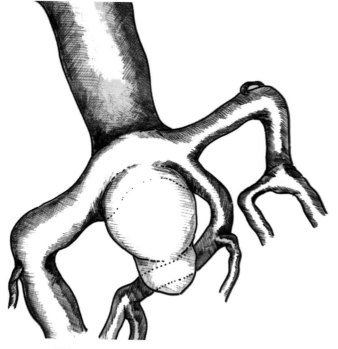

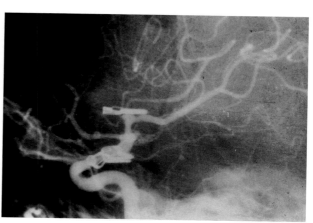

FIG. 2. A, B: Left carotid angiography in a patient with a bleeding left posterior communicating artery aneurysm, a small left anterior choroidal artery aneurysm (faintly seen on the anteroposterior view), and a left middle cerebral artery aneurysm *(arrow)*. This aneurysm originates at the trifurcation of the MCA (two frontal trunks and one temporal trunk). **C:** Operative sketch, showing a true trifurcation, with the aneurysm between the lateral frontal trunk and the temporal trunk. **D:** Postoperative angiography, documenting the exclusion of all three aneurysms and the preservation of the three trunks of division of the MCA (two frontal and one temporal).

(5,7,8); moreover, a lateral fronto-orbital artery can arise from the frontal trunk, with a recurrent (medially directed) course. The recurrent perforating arteries are not rarely observed, being present in 21% of cases according to Umanski et al (7) and in 20% of cases according to Rosner et al (8). They may arise from the frontal trunk (8.5% of cases), from the temporal trunk (6% of cases), and also from secondary temporal (5.3% of cases) or frontal (0.4% of cases) branches of the main division trunks, originating very close to the MCA bifurcation (7). As expected, these recurrent perforating arteries are more often observed when the MCA bifurcation is proximal to the usual point of division (8).

As for the course of the secondary branches arising from the MCA division trunks, the frontal trunk generally supplies the inferior frontal cortex, the frontal opercular cortex, the parietal and the central cortex, and the temporal trunk supplies the middle and posterior temporal cortex, the temporo-occipital, the angular and the posterior parietal areas. The vascular supply of the posterior part of the hemisphere and the origin of the posterior branches of the MCA (the posterior parietal, angular, and temporo-occipital arteries) may vary according to the dominance of the temporal or frontal trunk (2); the angular artery is the largest cortical branch of the MCA (3).

Apart from the previously mentioned variations of branching of the MCA along its course in the Sylvian fissure, a very rare anomaly, described by Yasargil and observed once in our surgical series, is the fenestration of the MCA, generally occurring along the proximal M1 tract (1).

GENERAL SURGICAL PRINCIPLES AND STRATEGIES

Aneurysms of the middle cerebral artery are located mostly in the Sylvian fissure at the main branching of the MCA or, less frequently, along the M1 tract. Very rarely, they originate from secondary divisions of the MCA, still inside the Sylvian fissure; a peripheral location outside the fissure is extremely rare. The surgical approach to these aneurysms is generally trans-Sylvian, although some authors have also advocated a transcortical (temporal) approach (10,11). In short, three approaches listed below can be used, depending on the location and direction of the aneurysm, the association with an intracerebral hematoma, the presence of vasospasm, and other conditions:

1. A *proximal approach,* starts from the bifurcation of the internal carotid artery and proceeds distally along the M1 tract up to the main MCA division. This approach is gained through exposure of the proximal Sylvian fissure and is generally defined as the "subfrontal approach" because it requires elevation of the frontal lobe.
2. A *distal approach,* starts from the secondary branches of the MCA exposed in the distal part of the fissure, and proceeds proximally along these branches and the main trunks, up to the MCA division. Because this approach requires the surgeon to work in the depth of the fissure between the opposing opercula, it is defined as the "trans-Sylvian approach."
3. A *transcortical approach,* proceeds through the superior temporal gyrus (generally 2–3 cm long and parallel to the Sylvian fissure). Through this approach the Sylvian veins are left undisturbed and the deeper part of the Sylvian fissure is penetrated, encountering the main trunks of division of the MCA. From this point, the surgeon proceeds backward to the main MCA division, as in the distal approach.

For both the proximal and distal approaches, an adequate opening of the Sylvian fissure is necessary. This is not easy in many acute cases, with clots very adherent to the arachnoid of the opercula: in these cases, penetration under the arachnoid layer of the fissure into the parenchyma should be avoided, although it can occur easily. When the brain is swollen, it is sometimes difficult to superficially identify the proximal part of the Sylvian fissure. This is also due to the frequent overlapping of one operculum over the other. However, when the arachnoid of the fissure is finally identified, further opening of the fissure is easily accomplished. Although small bridging veins over this proximal part of the fissure can be sacrificed, larger bridging veins (encountered over the distal part of the fissure) should be preserved whenever possible.

The depth of the aneurysm within the Sylvian fissure is difficult to predict and requires a "spatial" understanding of the vascular architecture as well as of the bony structures (most important, the shape of the sphenoid wing). In general, a long internal carotid artery (with a distal internal carotid bifurcation) will keep the first tract of the MCA deep in the fissure; however, the depth of the distal M1 tract and the MCA division will also depend on the architectural configuration of the whole MCA complex (4). It should be pointed out that some aneurysms can be very superficial in the fissure—especially when the sac is large and anteriorly projecting—and may even be attached to the dura of the sphenoid wing.

In the absence of rules for easy identification of the aneurysm within the fissure, it is wise to plan the surgical approach carefully considering the projection of the dome in order to avoid the premature rupture of the sac before exposure of the main vessels in the fissure. When the aneurysm is projecting anteriorly or inferiorly, a proximal approach can be dangerous, whereas a distal approach allows the surgeon to reach the aneurysm from behind, controlling the main trunks of division, and very often also the distal portion of the M1 tract, which can be conveniently exposed and clipped (transiently) from behind, when needed (4). Conversely, when the aneurysm is projecting posteriorly or superiorly, the proximal approach is safe and allows easy control of the proximal vasculature, whereas the distal approach is more tedious and does not allow the surgeon to control the distal M1 tract (4). When the aneurysm has a lateral projection, the proximal and distal approaches can be employed indifferently, and often in combination, in order to better control the proximal and distal vessels. When needed, a combined approach also allows the surgeon to relax the brain through opening of the basal cisterns.

The transcortical approach through the superior temporal gyrus has the advantage of giving the surgeon a circumferential view of the aneurysm and consequently better opportunities for clipping the aneurysm from many directions, according to its shape. However, it is not suitable for aneurysms located proximally to the limen insulae (as for aneurysms on the M1 tract or located on a proximal MCA bifurcation) or for MCA bifurcation aneurysms projecting posteriorly (10). An advantage of the transcortical temporal approach in patients with a swollen brain is the minimal brain retraction required to expose the vessels, while more retraction is needed for the distal approach and even more for the proximal approach. These considerations should be taken into account, especially in patients operated on soon after the hemorrhage. Another advantage of the transcortical approach is the adequate exposure of the temporal (inferior) trunk of division, which is frequently hidden beneath the temporal operculum when a distal trans-Sylvian approach is performed.

In the approach to MCA aneurysms, inadvertent occlusion of major Sylvian veins can in some cases has severe consequences for the patient. In particular, closure of the deep Sylvian vein can lead to large areas of fronto-opercular infarction, possibly as a result of brain retraction and particularly in the presence of few superficial Sylvian veins. Because the consequences of venous occlusion are often unpredictable, particular care should be paid to spare the major venous trunks.

Before clipping, exposure of the M1 tract proximal to the aneurysm is very important, allowing placement of a temporary clip when needed. In particular, temporary clipping can be used to control a significant hemorrhage from aneurysmal rupture, deflate a large sac with continuous aspiration before placement of the clip, and open a large thrombosed sac and remove intraaneurysmal thrombi before clip exclusion. Temporary occlusion of the MCA is generally safe for up to 5 minutes (12) and should be performed under cerebral protection, because the MCA is a terminal artery. Moreover, special care should be paid to avoid injury to perforators (especially recurrent distal lenticulostriate arteries) when positioning the clip on the M1 tract.

The final procedure of clip exclusion must respect the configuration of the MCA bifurcation, as will be discussed later. Moreover, the presence of endoluminal thrombi close to the neck may cause the clip to slide proximally over the main trunks, and in this case a staged technique with a second clip positioned distally and removal of the first clip should be used. Sometimes, it is even necessary to position a second clip in parallel in order to reinforce the action of the first clip and to obtain complete exclusion of the aneurysm. Alternatively, the sac should be opened during temporary M1

clipping and the thrombi should be removed. This is often unavoidable for giant partially thrombosed aneurysms, as will be described later.

When in spite of various attempts a proximally located bulging area cannot be excluded with a clip, its coarctation with low bipolar current is advised. A piece of muscle can be positioned over these areas after coarctation. Progressive coarctation with bipolar current is also advised for large sacs in order to reduce aneurysmal size, especially in proximity of the neck, and facilitate exclusion by the clip (1). Wrapping with muscle is still advised for truly unclippable aneurysms or for microaneurysms that are too small to accept even a miniclip (1).

In patients with large hematomas, the brain can be extremely swollen and not allow adequate exposure of the Sylvian vessels unless the hematoma is partially evacuated. Partial evacuation can be obtained through a small incision in the superior temporal or inferior frontal gyrus. It is, however, very important to leave a portion of the hematoma around the suspected location of the aneurysm in order to avoid a premature aneurysmal rupture. When the aneurysm is safely excluded, further evacuation of the hematoma is needed; for large temporal hematomas, evacuation should extend to the temporal horn of the lateral ventricle.

ANESTHETIC CONSIDERATIONS

Perioperative anesthesiologic management of MCA aneurysms, in addition to smooth induction, appropriate monitoring, hemodynamic stability, and prevention of hypertensive episodes, requires a slack brain, especially for superiorly projecting aneurysms, and protection against intraoperative cerebral ischemia during temporary clipping. The choice of the anesthetic technique should take into account the possibility of elevated intracranial pressure (ICP) and low cerebral compliance. When large hematomas cause intracranial hypertension, early aggressive treatment is required; hyperventilation, mannitol, and intravenous anesthetic agents may promote ICP reduction. In spite of the increased risk of rebleeding, adequate perfusion pressure should be reached, decreasing ICP and/or increasing blood pressure by vasoactive drugs, until the dura is opened.

In the absence of intracranial hypertension, a slack brain should be obtained in order to facilitate the isolation of the aneurysm and to avoid secondary compressive damage, using a safe balanced anesthesia in a normovolemic and moderately hypocapnic patient. Meticulous titration of arterial blood pressure is mandatory, both to maintain adequate cerebral perfusion and to avoid hyperemic edema, since disruption of cerebral autoregulation frequently occurs after subarachnoid hemorrhage (SAH). Preoperative administration of captopril or clonidine may facilitate blood pressure control (13). Complete intravenous anesthesia (thiopental, opioids, propofol or etomidate, lidocaine) may be used, particularly before clipping the aneurysm, in order to avoid vasodilatation due to volatile anesthetic drugs (13–15). Hyperventilation, mannitol, and cerebrospinal fluid drainage may facilitate brain retraction. Monitoring of jugular bulb venous saturation may identify the optimum level of hypocapnia and cerebral perfusion pressure, which should be determined in each patient during the different steps of the procedure.

Cerebral protection during temporary clipping of the parent vessel depends on a multifaceted strategy aimed to preserve adequate regional blood flow to meet metabolic demand (15–17). The brain should be prepared in advance to sustain critical regional reduction in blood flow; rheology and oxygen delivery can be improved by moderate hemodilution (which ameliorates flow through collateral circuits), carefully avoiding hyponatremia and reduced osmolality, which may cause cerebral edema. Hyperglycemia (claimed to worsen the ischemic lesion by increasing intracellular lactic acidosis) should be avoided. A moderate increase in mean blood pressure can maximize regional cerebral perfusion, and adequate hyperventilation can improve the redistribution of flow, during temporary artery clipping, by the inverse steal effect. In order to decrease the cerebral metabolic request, mild hypothermia (between 33 and 35°C) offers the best risk–benefit ratio. Cautious rewarming after aneurysm clipping should be performed in order to obtain normothermia before extubation (15). There is experimental evidence that barbiturates might be beneficial for focal ischemia (14). If temporary vessel occlusion is anticipated, loading doses of thiopental should be administered before clipping in order to achieve an EEG pattern of burst suppression, which indicates maximum metabolic reduction. A continuous infusion should be titrated to maintain stable suppression on the EEG. During vessel occlusion, additional boluses of barbiturate may only increase hemodynamic instability, since the uptake and wash-out are minimized by the reduced blood flow in the ischemic region (14). Other drugs have been proposed and used; propofol may provide a quicker awakening (13) and etomidate may have less hypotensive effect, in addition to experimentally demonstrated ''protective'' properties (16). To preserve stable and adequate perfusion pressure during infusion of intravenous anesthetic agents, dopamine or other vasoactive drugs may be safely used, particularly when vessel occlusion has consistently deflated the aneurysmal sac (15).

PATIENT POSITIONING

As for other anterior circulation aneurysms, the patient with an MCA aneurysm should be positioned with the plane of the sphenoid ridge roughly perpendicular to the horizontal plane of the floor. In order to obtain this result, the patient is positioned supine, with its head secured to a 3-pin headrest and rotated 40–45° to the side contralateral to the aneurysm. The chin should be gently flexed toward the clavicle. Particular care should be taken to avoid positions that can compro-

mise the jugular venous return, especially in patients with large hematomas, who are expected to have a swollen brain. The level of the head is maintained slightly above the level of the thorax in order to maximize the venous return throughout the operative procedure.

For the rare patients with distal MCA aneurysms, it may be advisable to rotate the head toward the contralateral side by 60° or more, positioning a cushion under the ipsilateral shoulder and still maintaining the patient in a supine position, so that the whole Sylvian fissure can be adequately exposed, together with the adjacent opercular areas. In the presence of very peripheral aneurysms located on the parieto-occipital cortex, a rare occurrence in our experience, the patient can be positioned on the lateral side or in the park-bench position, with the head conveniently rotated in order to place the surgical flap exactly over the cortical area where the aneurysm is located.

Before positioning the patients according to these guidelines, a lumbar drainage is inserted in all patients operated soon after SAH, provided that the ventricular system is on the midline. A lumbar drainage is also used for patients with posteriorly projecting aneurysms, which are expected to be ''buried'' in the depth of the fissure and often require significant retraction of the frontal and temporal lobes for exposure. Finally, lumbar drainage is also useful for giant aneurysms because the surgical maneuvers around the dome are facilitated by a wider exposure, and the danger of ischemia is minimized by less retraction.

SCALP AND BONY EXPOSURE

For most patients with MCA aneurysms, the standard frontotemporal skin flap proposed by Yasargil (1) is adopted. The incision begins immediately anterior to the tragus, over the superior edge of the zygoma, and runs superiorly and medially, with an anterior curve up to the midline just posterior to the hairline. With this incision, it is possible to spare the frontalis branch of the facial nerve and also to preserve at least one branch of the superficial temporal artery. The scalp flap is reflected anteriorly in a single layer, together with the temporalis muscle, and retained with fishhook retractors. Thus, the deeper layer of the reflected muscle will constitute the antero-inferior wall of the surgical exposure. In patients with large hematomas, the flap is extended posteriorly along the projected line of the Sylvian fissure, in order to have enough room for evacuation of intracerebral and especially subdural hematomas.

Once the bone is exposed with the superior temporal line in the middle of the approach, the frontal and temporal edges of the zygomatic bone should be visualized. One burr hole should be placed immediately superior to the frontozygomatic suture (the so-called key hole) and one on the temporal squama just above the zygoma, while the two remaining burr holes should be placed one on the posterior edge of the superior temporal line and one on the forehead, taking care to avoid the frontal sinus. Once the free bone flap has been removed with a limited craniectomy performed in the subtemporal region, the lateral third of the sphenoid ridge is resected with a drill and flattened as far medially as to the lateral aspect of the superior orbital fissure. Also, the inner table of the frontal bone between the key hole and the forehead hole is flattened with a drill in order to minimize retraction of the frontal lobe.

If the frontal sinus is penetrated during the bony exposure, its mucosa should be extensively cauterized and the hole filled with muscle and covered with a periosteal flap of adequate size, sutured to the dura. Small openings in the orbit with minimal protrusion of orbital fat do not require surgical repair. Lacerations of the frontal dura frequently occur in the elderly. If these are extensive, they should be repaired with a pedunculated periosteal flap, and/or with pieces of muscle sutured to the intact dura and to the bony edge.

Opening of the dura is performed in a semilunar fashion over the Sylvian fissure. The dura is covered with moist gel foam to avoid its shrinking and secured with stitches against the scalp flap and the reflected temporalis muscle.

MICROSURGICAL DISSECTION AND PRINCIPLES OF EXCLUSION

In order to discuss dissection and exclusion of MCA aneurysms in detail, aneurysms of the M1 tract are dealt with separately from aneurysms at the main MCA division. Additional remarks will also be made for giant MCA aneurysms and distal MCA aneurysms.

Aneurysms of the M1 Tract

Aneurysms of the M1 tract account for 2.2% of all aneurysms, according to Yasargil (1). The approach to these an-

eurysms is somewhat complicated by the vertical direction of the M1 tract during surgery, compelling the surgeon to expose this region from an oblique anterior view. These aneurysms are often deeply located, especially when projecting superiorly, and require significant retraction of the frontal lobe for adequate exposure. In the dissection of the proximal Sylvian fissure, the small fronto-orbital bridging veins can be sectioned. A larger fronto-orbital vein, often present above the internal carotid bifurcation, can also be sectioned whenever control of the initial M1 tract is needed, as for the rare aneurysms at the origin of the uncal or temporopolar arteries. In this region it is important to maintain the dissection within the arachnoidal boundaries of the fissure in order to minimize surgical trauma. In the progressive opening of the fissure, the first vessel to be encountered is the anterior temporal artery, following which the M1 tract can be visualized and adequately exposed.

When the aneurysm is *projecting inferiorly (or infero-anteriorly)*, it is generally surrounded by the anterior temporal (or the temporopolar) artery, and the dome is projecting toward the surgeon (Fig. 3). In this case, it is advisable to first expose the distal M1 tract, then identify the origin of the aneurysm moving retrogradely along the tract, and finally apply particular care in the exposure of the proximal M1 tract, owing to the possible adhesions of the sac with the opercula and to the superficial location of some of these aneurysms in the fissure. The aneurysm can also extend with its dome into the temporal lobe, and suction of a limited amount of brain tissue adjacent to the neck may be required before application of the clip. In all cases, but especially when the anterior temporal artery is large, mimicking a proximal bifurcation of the MCA, the branching vessel must be spared. When the vessel is completely hidden by the sac, a clip is positioned distally and suitably repositioned when the

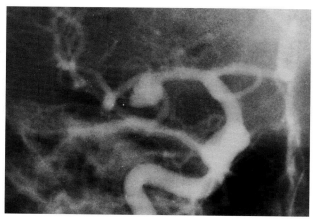

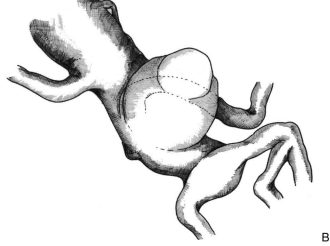

A   B

FIG. 3. A: Right carotid angiography in a patient with a bleeding aneurysm of the right M1 tract, at the origin of a large anterior temporal artery, with inferior projection. **B:** Operative sketch, illustrating the shape of the aneurysm and the anatomic relation with the anterior temporal artery; the main division of the middle cerebral artery is distal to the origin of the aneurysm.

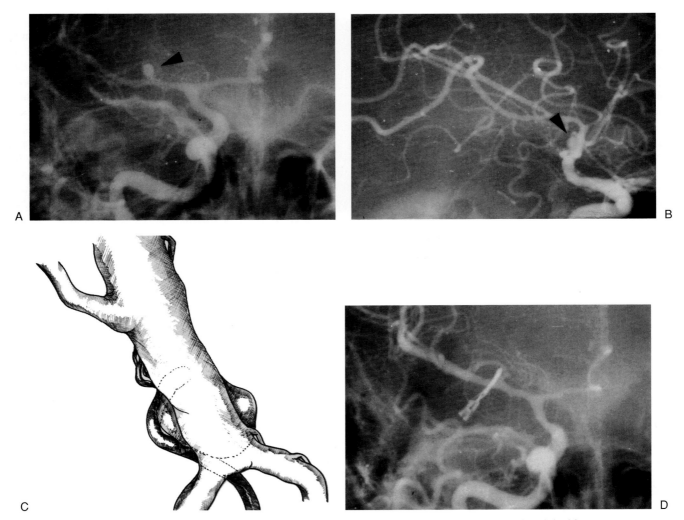

FIG. 4. A, B: Right carotid angiography in a patient with a bleeding aneurysm of the right M1 tract, projecting superiorly. The aneurysm *(arrow)* is located at the origin of a large fronto-orbital artery. **C:** Operative sketch, showing the base of the aneurysm covered by the M1 tract, and the origin of the fronto-orbital artery. A few lenticulostriate vessels are proximal to the neck of the aneurysm. **D:** Postoperative angiography, showing the exclusion of the aneurysm and the preservation of the fronto-orbital artery.

origin of the vessel is visualized. Alternatively, when the dome is large, the aneurysm can be deflated with continuous aspiration before clipping. In rare cases, the aneurysm can present an inferoposterior projection. In this situation, although the branching vessel is still the anterior temporal artery, the dome may also have adherences with the lenticulostriate arteries and with the deep Sylvian vein.

When the aneurysm is *projecting superiorly (or superoposteriorly)* (Fig. 4), it is generally located at the origin of a lenticulo-striate vessel or at the origin of a common frontoorbital/striate trunk. In a few cases, a temporal artery can originate from the superior wall of the M1 tract, enwrap the aneurysm, and then proceed inferiorly toward the temporal lobe. In the most common situation, the dome of the aneurysm is directed toward, or buried within, the anterior perforated substance and surrounded by lenticulostriate vessels

(Fig. 4). These vessels must be gently separated from the neck of the aneurysm before application of the clip. Since the M1 tract itself can hide the aneurysmal neck when the aneurysm has a true posterior direction, fenestrated clips are very useful in order to "jump over" the M1 tract and exclude the aneurysm, obviously after careful inspection of the portion of the neck superior or inferior to the M1 tract. In some cases, the aneurysm is located on the distal M1 tract, at the origin of a true fronto-orbital artery (Fig. 4), and can have extensive adherences to the perforating vessels if the lateral group of the lenticulostriate arteries is well represented. In many cases, these aneurysms also have adherences to the deep Sylvian vein. When the superficial Sylvian veins are scant or absent, this vein should be spared. In rare cases, the aneurysm can present a supero-anterior projection, and hide the proximal M1 tract and the origin of the lenticulostriate arteries. In this situation, the first clip application must be adjusted after visualization of the branching artery, if the latter has been caught in the clip.

Aneurysms of the Main MCA Division

Aneurysms of the main MCA division account for 15% of all aneurysms, according to Yasargil (1). As previously mentioned, the approach to these aneurysms can be trans-Sylvian (either proximal or distal) or temporal transcortical. A trans-Sylvian approach has been used in most of our cases, consisting of the opening of the basal cisterns after elevation of the frontal lobe, and then in a distal trans-Sylvian approach to the MCA bifurcation, following the main branches of division in the Sylvian fissure (4). The trans-Sylvian approach requires the surgeon to preserve the large superficial veins (generally lying on the temporal edge of the fissure) and when needed to sacrifice only the bridging veins to the frontal operculum. In most cases, except in the rare condition of a posteriorly projecting aneurysm, the area of the Sylvian fissure overlying the main MCA division, generally at a distance of about 2 cm from the sphenoid ridge, is left untouched in order to avoid premature aneurysmal rupture, and the distal Sylvian fissure is opened by sharp dissection, following (retrogradely) the first artery that leaves the fissure at that level. Although this technique is easy in many cases, the possible presence of thick and adherent intracisternal clots makes the progressive opening of the fissure difficult during acute surgery, leading the surgeon away from the fissure into the adjacent nervous parenchyma.

When a main trunk is exposed in the fissure (generally the frontal trunk), it is useful to localize the other trunk before advancing backward to the main division. This is generally done by gentle retraction of the temporal operculum in order to expose the temporal trunk (frequently hidden under the lateral edge of the Sylvian fissure). Further dissection along the main trunks is better achieved when both trunks are progressively exposed ''in parallel.'' Thereby the surgeon avoids following only one trunk and losing the spatial orientation of the MCA division.

Approaching the aneurysm, it is important to be familiar with the individual anatomic configuration of the MCA branching, drawn from a careful angiographic evaluation; in particular, the presence of a trifurcation (or even a tetrafurcation) must be recognized at an early stage of dissection around the aneurysmal area, and the approach along the main trunks must reach their origin from the MCA division because many trifurcations prove to be very proximal secondary divisions of the frontal or temporal trunks (Fig. 5). Recognition of unusual shapes of MCA bifurcation bear a surgical importance. For example, an arrow-shaped bifurcation makes the use of multiple clips almost compulsory, whereas an asymmetric T-shaped bifurcation demands particular care in order to avoid stenosis of one trunk during clipping (Fig. 6). On the contrary, a symmetric T-shaped

bifurcation does not require particular attention during clipping, and a V-shaped bifurcation causes problems only when one or both trunks are adherent to the sac.

When a portion of the aneurysm (generally the back) is finally visualized, it is important to expose not only the origin of the main trunks from the MCA division but also the last portion of the M1 tract (frequently seen from behind) before attempting further dissection of the aneurysm. If the last portion of the M1 tract cannot be visualized from behind, as for many laterally projecting aneurysms, it is advisable to jump over the aneurysmal area and expose the M1 tract in the proximal part of the fissure in order to accomplish a temporary M1 occlusion, if needed. Before dissection of the aneurysmal neck, the spatulas are conveniently positioned over the opposing opercula in order to facilitate application of the clip. Further maneuvers around the aneurysm depend on its projection.

When the aneurysm is *projecting inferiorly or inferoanteriorly,* the last portion of the M1 tract is hidden under the sac (Fig. 7). Sometimes the origin of the temporal trunk is also hidden, particularly when the dome of the aneurysm is inside the temporal operculum and not free in the fissure. In this case, a circumferential approach to the aneurysm can be adopted, advancing along the frontal edge of the aneurysm to expose the distal M1 tract and along the temporal edge to expose the origin of the temporal trunk. This may require a limited suction of nervous tissue adjacent to the sac in order to avoid direct dissection on the dome. The proximal portion of the temporal trunk may be very adherent to the aneurysm in a few cases. This condition requires careful dissection of the vessel up to its origin in order to avoid significant stenosis when the clip is applied. When these aneurysms are large and extend into the temporal operculum, they are often covered by anterior temporal branches, which can be very adherent to the dome. Their dissection is not always required, and when it is needed, it should be delayed until clip exclusion. These aneurysms can also be adherent to the dura of the sphenoid ridge, and when this condition is suspected at angiography, the utmost care should be applied during opening of the superficial part of the Sylvian fissure. In these cases, exposure of the distal M1 tract can be difficult. Not rarely, these aneurysms have an associated anterior or posterior extension, which makes exclusion with a single clip very difficult. A good compromise is exclusion of the larger part of the aneurysm with a straight clip, positioned in an oblique posteroanterior direction perpendicular to the axis of the bifurcation and application of an additional fenestrated clip in order to exclude the remaining part (with the fenestration over the blades of the main clip). If the aneurysm is not very large, also a single clip transversally applied along the axis of the bifurcation can be an adequate option, provided that the origin of the frontal or temporal trunk is respected. Coarctation of a small residual bulging area with low bipolar current can also be performed in this case. A few aneurysms with anterior (but not anteroinferior) projection can extend into the frontal operculum, and in this condi-

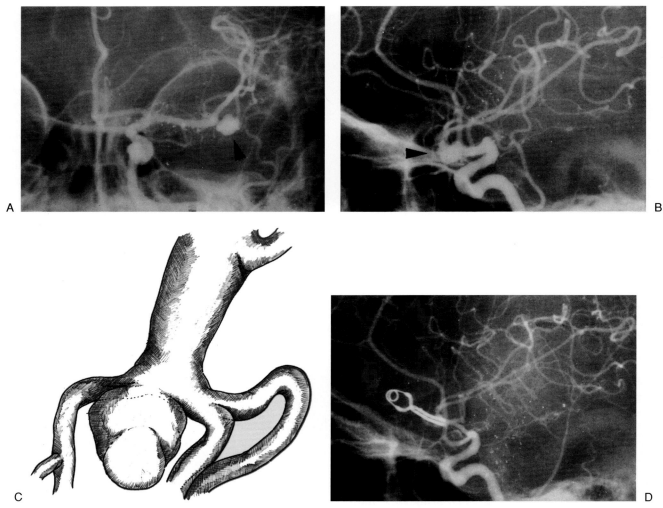

FIG. 5. A, B: Left carotid angiography in a patient with a bleeding aneurysm at the main division of the left middle cerebral artery. The sac *(arrow)* projects laterally and seems to be located at a trifurcation of the middle cerebral artery. **C:** The operative sketch shows that the aneurysm is located at a pseudotrifurcation, since the frontal trunk of division bifurcates very proximally into two secondary branches. **D:** Postoperative angiography, showing the exclusion of the aneurysm.

tion the frontal trunk can be adherent to (or even hidden by) the sac.

When the aneurysm is *projecting laterally,* both trunks of division can frequently be adherent to the sac and need to be dissected with great care (Fig. 5). If large, the aneurysm can cover one or both trunks with its dome or with its secondary lobes. The aneurysm can be free in the fissure, or buried in the temporal or, more frequently, in the frontal operculum. Very few of these aneurysms are adherent to the sphenoid wing. When exposure of one or both trunks is hindered by the main sac or by a secondary lobe, the sac can be deflated before clipping by continuous aspiration, or gently pushed away with the aspirator, or even intentionally ruptured (with or without temporary clipping). Alternatively, limited suction of the nervous tissue adjacent to the aneurysm can be performed as previously discussed in order to expose the origin of the hidden trunk from a different angle. When the

aneurysm has a lateral projection, the M1 tract is easier to visualize and can be exposed either anteriorly or posteriorly to the sac. In these cases, proximal branches originating from the M1 tract (fronto-orbital or, rarely, anterior temporal arteries) and secondary branches originating on the proximal portion of the frontal or temporal trunk can also be adherent to the sac and need to be dissected. This is particularly important when recurrent perforating (lenticulostriate) arteries leave the frontal (or temporal) trunk close to the aneurysmal wall. The adherence of the main trunks or secondary vessels to the dome is frequently observed with V-shaped configurations of the main MCA division, whereas adherences are scant in the presence of T-shaped configurations. Obviously, only the proximal portion of the adherent vessel needs to be dissected in order to have enough space for introduction of the clip blades and cause minimal injury to the vessel. The identification of very proximal secondary divisions along

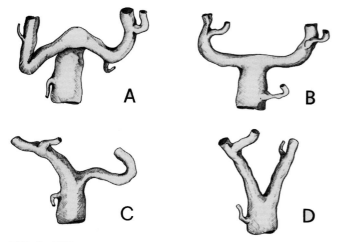

FIG. 6. Different shapes of bifurcation of the middle cerebral artery. **A:** "Arrow-shaped" bifurcation, with the trunks of division at more than 180° from one another. **B:** "Symmetrical" T-shaped bifurcation, with the trunks of division at around 180° from one another. **C:** "Asymmetric" T-shaped bifurcation, with one trunk of division originating at a different level than the other trunk. **D:** V-shaped bifurcation.

the main trunks ("pseudo-trifurcations") is very important especially for this aneurysmal projection (Fig. 5) because the proximal portion of the trunk is very frequently hidden or adherent to the sac, and the third (unexpected) vessel can be missed and caught up inadvertently during clipping. Also for aneurysms with this projection, anterior and/or posterior extensions can be observed. In this situation, multiple clips should be applied or a single transversal clip should be positioned (with or without coarctation of the base), as previously discussed.

Very rarely, *double aneurysms* of the main MCA division, with parallel or divergent projection (generally inferoanterior and lateral) are observed (1). In these cases, one sac is buried in the temporal operculum and one is free in the fissure. In general, each aneurysm needs to be clipped separately, and the problems encountered in the dissection depend on the projection of the sac. However, sometimes one aneurysm is adherent to the other for a long tract and they need to be separated, at least close to the neck, in order to facilitate separate clipping of each aneurysm.

When the aneurysm is projecting posteriorly or posterosuperiorly, the sac is partially covered by the distal M1 tract, the MCA bifurcation, and/or the main trunks of division,

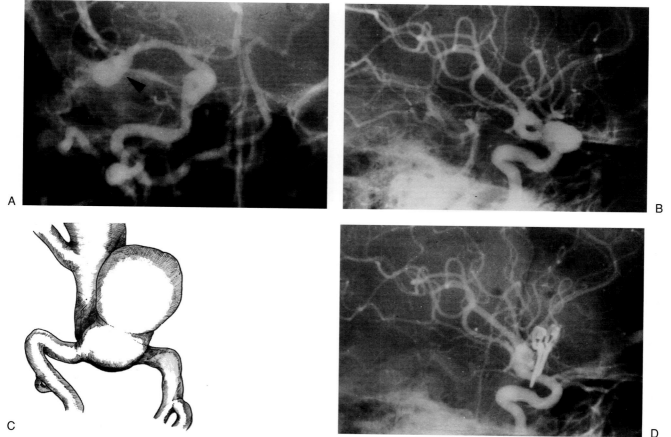

FIG. 7. A, B: Right carotid angiography in a patient with a bleeding aneurysm at the main division of the right middle cerebral artery, with inferoanterior projection *(arrow)*. **C:** The operative sketch shows the large sac partially hiding the M1 tract and the origin of the temporal trunk. **D:** Postoperative angiography, showing the exclusion of the aneurysm.

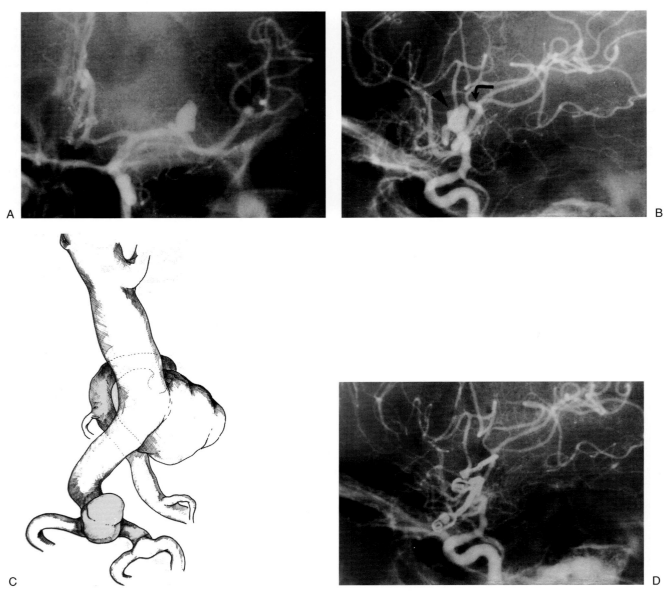

FIG. 8. A: Left carotid angiography in a patient with two aneurysms of the left middle cerebral artery, one at the main bifurcation of the middle cerebral artery (which is proximally located) and one at a secondary division of the temporal trunk *(arrow)*. **B:** Lateral view, showing the larger aneurysm at the main bifurcation, projecting superiorly *(straight arrow)* and the smaller aneurysm in a distal position *(curved arrow)*. **C:** Operative sketch, illustrating the position of both aneurysms along the middle cerebral artery complex; note the course of the frontal trunk, the projection of the larger aneurysm against the frontal operculum, and the location of the smaller aneurysm at a secondary division of the temporal trunk. **D:** Postoperative angiography, showing the exclusion of both aneurysms.

and extends into the frontal operculum (Fig. 8), into the insula or, occasionally, into the temporal operculum. The neck of the aneurysm may be adherent to the deep Sylvian vein. In our experience, aneurysms with this projection often originate from a proximal MCA division, resulting in a deep location inside the Sylvian fissure (Fig. 8). This condition may require, in some cases, significant retraction on the frontal lobe in order to expose the aneurysm. When recurrent lenticulostriate arteries leave one trunk of division, they may

be adherent to the dome. Even the lateral lenticulostriate arteries originating from the distal M1 tract may be adherent to the sac. The exclusion of these aneurysms often requires the use of fenestrated clips in order to jump over the MCA division trunks and/or the distal M1 tract. Alternatively, a limited suction of the limen insulae may be required to expose the neck of the aneurysm before direct clipping. Some of these aneurysms have an associated lateral extension, and this part of the sac can be adherent to one trunk of the MCA division. In this case, multiple clips are often needed for exclusion. Adherence to the frontal trunk is also sometimes observed for aneurysms with a simple posterosuperior projection.

Giant MCA Aneurysms

As for other aneurysmal locations, *giant MCA aneurysms* pose particular problems in the surgical approach and exclusion. Very often, their dome reaches the superficial part of the fissure and can be prematurely lacerated in the opening of the fissure if care is not applied. In these cases, recognition of the proximal and distal vasculature is often hampered by the large dome, which almost always sits on the main division. These lesions are not infrequently thrombosed to a large degree and require generous removal of thrombi for adequate exclusion. As previously mentioned, transient occlusion of the M1 tract is very useful, allowing the deflation of large non-thrombosed aneurysms or aneurysm endoarterectomy (with removal of thrombi) when needed. Due to the volume of the sac, one or both trunks of the MCA division may be adherent for a long tract to the aneurysmal walls, requiring extensive dissection. Application of the adequate clip (or clips) on the neck can be very difficult, and requires a staged clipping and complex combinations, comprehending fenestrated clips, and in spite of this, "dog ears" may remain on the base of the aneurysm, close to the neck. In a few cases of large thrombosed aneurysms, clip exclusion can prove impossible without the sacrifice of one MCA division trunk. In these cases, vascular reconstruction can be performed using two main techniques: (a) reimplantation of the threatened trunk on the other trunk, as suggested by Yokoh and Coll (18), or (b) vein graft anastomosis between the superficial temporal (or the external carotid) artery and the MCA trunk distal to the main division (19). Although we do not have direct experience with these techniques in exclusion of MCA aneurysms, good results have been reported by others in a few cases (12).

Distal MCA Aneurysms

Distal MCA aneurysms are very rare, accounting for 1.0% of all aneurysms, according to Yasargil (1). For practical purposes, they should be divided into (a) aneurysms located on a secondary division and (b) peripheral aneurysms, located on a cortical branch. The first type is still hidden inside the Sylvian fissure and is adjacent to the main MCA division. Often its distal location is discovered only at surgery, and its exclusion requires the same precautions and poses the same problems as for more proximal aneurysms. In our experience, these aneurysms are not infrequently associated with MCA bifurcation aneurysms (Fig. 8). In one case with a giant sac, temporary clipping has been used, followed by aneurysmectomy and preservation of a central canal with parallel clips. The second (peripheral) type is extremely rare,

generally located outside the Sylvian fissure, and frequently inside a cortical sulcus. Not infrequently, this peripheral type of aneurysm is large or giant, and not implanted on a vascular branching. While its surgical localization can sometimes be difficult, its exclusion can often be accomplished through simple closure of the parent artery or trapping, without consequences for the patient. If the aneurysm is large or giant, aneurysmectomy is advised.

COMPLICATIONS AND THEIR MANAGEMENT

As for other aneurysmal locations, surgery on MCA aneurysms may be followed by postoperative complications. Some are common to all other cranial procedures, such as epidural or subdural hematomas and infection, and will not be discussed here. A few are relatively independent from the surgical procedure itself, such as hydrocephalus, epilepsy, and vasospasm, and some are strictly related to the surgical technique and to this anatomic area.

Hydrocephalus is also observed in patients operated on for MCA aneurysms, although the subarachnoid collection of blood is often asymmetric, and ventricular blood is scant or absent (except in the rare cases with large hematomas extending into the ventricles). Its frequency in patients with MCA aneurysms has been estimated at around 5%, according to Yasargil (1), and at around 25% in our experience, when considering only patients admitted within 3 days of hemorrhage. Whenever hydrocephalus becomes symptomatic, insertion of a ventriculoperitoneal (or lumboperitoneal) shunt is advised (in 9% of cases, in our experience).

Epilepsy is rare—6% for Yasargil (1)—but relatively frequent in patients who underwent evacuation of large intracerebral and/or subdural hematomas. In these patients, a cortical hole may be observed during surgery in the area where the intracerebral clot has "broken" into the subdural space. If epilepsy develops postoperatively, prolonged pharmaceutical control with antiepileptic drugs is advised because the trend toward repeated seizures is common in these cases.

Vasospasm is a well-known complication of, and may be worsened by, surgery in the acute or subacute stage. Since vasospasm can be prevalent on the Sylvian vessels, especially in patients with thick layers of blood in the insular cistern, development of motor deficits is frequent. Prophylactic treatment with calcium antagonists (20,21) and with hypervolemia is indicated in all cases with significant layers of blood in the Sylvian/insular cisterns. If subacute clinical deterioration develops, additional treatment with hypertension (23,24) and with transluminal angioplasty in selected cases (25,26) may be advisable. Unfortunately, vasospasm may develop in patients with large hematomas, already in a poor neurologic condition, and in these cases the probability of a useful survival is scant in spite of treatment.

Complications strictly related to the surgical procedure are distal ischemia, venous infarction, and persistent brain swelling. *Distal ischemia* may develop postoperatively, due to sliding of the clip on one trunk of division or on the distal M1 tract. This complication is particularly observed in patients with large partially thrombosed MCA aneurysms. In other cases, distal ischemia is caused by spasm or inadvertent occlusion of a small perforator during the surgical procedure. For treatment of both complications, pharmacologically induced hypertension may be a reasonable choice, provided that it is started very early after ischemia. In selected cases, prompt surgical exploration and replacement of the clip may be advisable after angiographic documentation.

Venous infarction is luckily a complication observed only in a minority of patients subjected to surgical occlusion of a major venous trunk. It is possibly more common after occlusion of the deep Sylvian vein, particularly when the superficial veins are scant. In these cases, the infarcted area (frequently the frontobasal operculum) may act as an expanding mass lesion, requiring prompt surgical evacuation to halt the neurologic deterioration.

Persistent brain swelling is not rare in patients operated on in coma, with large intracerebral hematomas. In spite of careful evacuation of the clot, "infiltration" of blood into the insular or parietal operculum may be associated with large areas of perilesional edema. When brain swelling is anticipated in the postoperative period, intraoperative or postoperative ventricular drainage may be of help to reduce intracranial pressure, together with mannitol and adequate ventilation.

A very rare complication after surgical exclusion of MCA aneurysms is *aneurysmal regrowth*. We have recently observed one such case, with the development of a large aneurysm a few months after clip exclusion of a laterally projecting MCA bifurcation aneurysm of standard size. This phenomenon is rarely observed for this and other aneurysmal locations, with a frequency of 1.2% in the surgical series of Yasargil (1). Although direct surgical correction has been advocated (1), an alternative approach with an endovascular procedure and coil exclusion (27) may be equally satisfactory and better accepted by the patient.

OVERVIEW

In summary, surgery of MCA aneurysms requires a thorough understanding of the anatomic area of the Sylvian cistern, the modality of branching of the MCA, and the projection of the sac. During the surgical approach, the utmost care should be paid to avoid premature rupture of the aneurysm, adopting a strategy that allows exposure of the main vessels before manipulation of the dome. Clip exclusion may be demanding in many cases, especially in the presence of large aneurysms and when the MCA bifurcation has an unfavorable shape. Lenticulostriate vessels are often encountered during the dissection of the aneurysm and need to be spared in order to avoid severe ischemic deficits. In patients with large hematomas, the second purpose of surgery after clip

exclusion should be avoidance of postoperative brain swelling. Unexpected postoperative deterioration should be investigated thoroughly, and adequate measures to correct identified complications should be adopted promptly.

ACKNOWLEDGMENTS

We thank Dr. Francesco Procaccio for invaluable advice on the anesthetic management of patients with MCA aneurysms.

REFERENCES

1. Yasargil MG. Middle cerebral artery aneurysms. In: Yasargil MG, ed. *Microneurosurgery.* vol 2. Stuttgart: Thieme Verlag, 1984;124–213.
2. Gibo H, Carver CC, Rhoton AL, Lenkey C, Mitchell R. Microsurgical anatomy of the middle cerebral artery. *J Neurosurg* 1981;54:151–169.
3. Umansky F, Montoya Juarez S, Dujovny M, et al. Microsurgical anatomy of the proximal segments of the middle cerebral artery. *J Neurosurg* 1984;61:458–467.
4. Scienza R, Da Pian R, Pasqualin A. Aneurismi della cerebrale media. In: Da Pian R, Pasqualin A, Scienza R, eds. *Aneurismi e Angiomi Cerebrali: Principi di Trattamento.* Verona: Edizioni Libreria Cortina, 1986;111–121.
5. Grand W. Microsurgical anatomy of the proximal middle cerebral artery and the internal carotid artery bifurcation. *Neurosurgery* 1980;7:215–218.
6. Stabler J. Two cases of accessory middle cerebral artery, including one with an aneurysm at its origin. *Br J Radiol* 1970; 43:314–318.
7. Umansky F, Gomes FB, Dujovny M, et al. The perforating branches of the middle cerebral artery. A microanatomical study. *J Neurosurg* 1985;62:261–268.
8. Rosner SS, Rhoton AL, Ono M, Barry M. Microsurgical anatomy of the anterior perforating arteries. *J Neurosurg* 1984;61:468–485.
9. Handa J, Shimizu Y, Matsuda M, et al. The accessory middle cerebral artery: report of further two cases. *Clin Radiol* 1970;21:415–416.
10. Heros RC, Ojemann RG, Crowell RM. Superior gyrus approach to middle cerebral artery aneurysms: technique and results. *Neurosurgery* 1982;10:308–313.
11. Ojemann RG, Crowell RM. Middle cerebral aneurysms. In: Ojemann RG, Crowell RM, eds. *Surgical Management of Cerebrovascular Disease.* Baltimore: Williams and Wilkins, 1983;201–209.
12. Samson DS, Batjer HH. *Intracranial Aneurysm Surgery: Techniques.* Mount Kisco, NY: Futura Publishing, 1990.
13. Stone DJ. Anesthesia in aneurysm surgery. In: Pasqualin A, Da Pian R, eds. *New Trends in Management of Cerebrovascular Malformations.* Wien: Springer-Verlag, 1994;159–163.
14. Michenfelder JD. *Anesthesia and the Brain.* New York: Churchill Livingstone, 1988.
15. Young WL, Stone JD. Special anesthetic considerations for management of cerebral aneurysm clipping. In: Pasqualin A, Da Pian R, eds. *New Trends in Management of Cerebrovascular Malformations.* Wien: Springer-Verlag, 1994;164–173.
16. Batjer HH. Cerebral protective effects of etomidate: experimental and clinical aspects. *Cerebrovasc Brain Metab Rev* 1993;5:17–32.
17. Warner DS. Perioperative neuroprotection. *Curr Opin Anesthesiol* 1994;7:416–420.
18. Yokoh A, Ausman JI, Dujovny M, et al. Anterior cerebral artery reconstruction. *Neurosurgery* 19;26–35, 1986.
19. Diaz FG, Umansky F, Metha B, et al. Applications of deep middle cerebral artery anastomosis in the Sylvian fissure. In: Spetzler RF, Selman WR, Carter LP, et al, eds. *Cerebral Revascularization for Stroke.* Stuttgart: Thieme Verlag, 1985:337–341.
20. Pasqualin A, Barone G, Scienza R, et al. Clinical effects of nimodipine in prevention of vasospasm after subarachnoid hemorrhage. In: Pasqualin A, Da Pian R, eds. *New Trends in Management of Cerebro-Vascular Malformations.* Wien: Springer-Verlag, 1994;107–112.
21. Pickard JD, Murray GD, Illingworth R, et al. Effect of oral nimodipine

on cerebral infarction and outcome after subarachnoid hemorrhage: British aneurysm nimodipine trial. *Br Med J* 1989;298:636–642.

22. Pritz MB, Giannotta SL, Kindt GW, McGillicuddy JE, Prager RL. Treatment of patients with neurological deficits associated with cerebral vasospasm by intravascular volume expansion. *Neurosurgery* 1978;3:364–368.

23. Kassell NF, Peerless SJ, Durward QJ, Beck DW, Drake CG, Adams HP. Treatment of ischemic deficits from vasospasm with intravascular volume expansion and induced arterial hypertension. *Neurosurgery* 1982;11:337–343.

24. Levy ML, Giannotta SL: Cardiac performance and hypervolemic ther-apy in the treatment of cerebral vasospasm. *J Neurosurg* 1991;75: 27–31.

25. Higashida RT, Halbach VV, Cahan LD, et al. Transluminal angioplasty for treatment of intracranial arterial vasospasm. *J Neurosurg* 1989;71: 648–653.

26. Newell DW, Eskridge JM, Mayberg MR, Grady HS, Winn RH. Angioplasty for the treatment of symptomatic vasospasm following subarachnoid hemorrhage. *J Neurosurg* 1989;71:654–660.

27. Guglielmi G, Vinuela F, Dion J, Duckwiler G. Electrothrombosis of saccular aneurysms via endovascular approach. Part 2: Preliminary clinical experience. *J Neurosurg* 1991;75:8–14.

Cerebrovascular Disease, edited by H. Hunt Batjer.
Lippincott-Raven Publishers, Philadelphia © 1997.

CHAPTER 81

Anterior Communicating Artery Aneurysms: Surgical Techniques

Peter D. Le Roux and H. Richard Winn

GENERAL BACKGROUND

Aneurysms located at the anterior communicating artery (ACoA) are common and represent a third of aneurysms associated with subarachnoid hemorrhage (SAH) (1) or that are operated on (2). Direct surgical obliteration (3) or wrapping (4) of ACoA aneurysms was first reported in the 1930s. Early results were poor; indirect approaches, such as proximal dominant A1 (5) or common carotid artery ligation (6), were therefore favored for the next 30 years. Following SAH, however, these procedures do not provide patients any benefit over bed rest alone (7). In 1961, Pool (8) described a bifrontal approach and routine temporary clip use to obliterate ACoA aneurysms, but until the advent of the operating microscope, surgical results remained disappointing (9—11). For example, in the first Cooperative Study 34% of patients in good clinical grade undergoing repair of ACoA aneurysms died (11). With advances in anesthesiology and since the introduction of the operating microscope, refinements in microsurgical techniques, and appreciation of microvascular anatomy, excellent surgical results have been reported for direct surgical obliteration of ACoA aneurysms (2,12,13). Two surgical approaches—pterional or interhemispheric—are most frequently used; which provides the optimum results, however, is unclear.

PERTINENT NEUROLOGIC AND VASCULAR ANATOMY AND VARIATIONS

Aneurysms located at the ACoA present a difficult technical challenge, in part because of the complex arterial anatomy in this region. In addition, the operative field, surrounded by the anterior skull base and orbital surface of the frontal lobe, is narrow and deep. Successful surgical treatment of ACoA aneurysms requires a thorough three-dimensional understanding of the microsurgical anatomy and frequent anatomic variations of the arterial complex. The important vascular anatomy is illustrated in Fig. 1.

The anterior cerebral artery (ACA) is bilateral and arises at the internal carotid artery (ICA) bifurcation as the medial and smaller ICA termination. From its origin to the ACoA the ACA, or A1 segment, averages 13 mm in length. The proximal A1 diameter varies between 0.2 and 3.4 mm in diameter (14). Approximately 2 mm from its origin, the A1 courses anteromedially in a horizontal plane between the optic chiasm and olfactory trigone where it lies in the subarachnoid space medial to the olfactory tract and in contact with the posterior orbital surface of the frontal lobe. At the posterior aspect of the gyrus rectus, the A1 is applied to the superior aspect of the optic nerve which it then crosses. Near the midline, where it approximates the optic chiasm, the A1 begins a gentle superior medial curve, inferomedial to the gyrus rectus, and heads between 2 and 4 mm into the interhemispheric fissure. Here, anterior to the lamina terminalis, the A1 joins the opposite A1 through a short anastomotic vessel, the ACoA.

The anterior communicating artery is a conducting vessel surrounded by the chiasmatic cistern inferiorly, the lamina terminalis cistern superiorly, the pial surface of the lamina terminalis posteriorly, and laterally by the pial surface of the adjacent gyri of the medial frontal lobe. The ACoA varies in size; on average it is 2.5–3 mm in length and is slightly smaller than the A1 in diameter (14–17). From the A1 and ACoA junction, the A2 segment represents the rostral continuation of the ACA in the interhemispheric fissure. The A2 segment runs toward the splenium of the corpus callosum, in close association with the opposite A2, and irrigates the medial cerebral hemisphere. The A2 is the least variable of the

P. D. Le Roux: Department of Neurosurgery, New York University, New York, New York 10016.

H. R. Winn: Department of Neurosurgery, Harborview Medical Center, University of Washington, Seattle, Washington 98104.

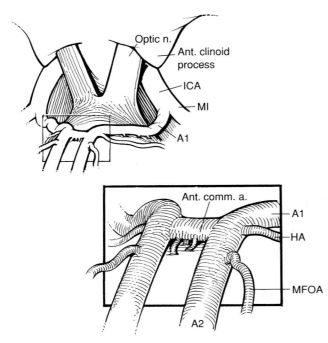

FIG. 1. Diagrammatic illustration of anterior communicating artery microvasculature. HA, recurrent artery of Heubner; MFOA, medial frontal orbital artery.

anterior cerebral vessels; the right and left A2's are of similar diameter, between 1.5 and 2 mm in 90% of patients.

There are several branches and perforators that emanate from the ACoA arterial complex. Identification and preservation of these vessels is critical to successful aneurysm surgery. Several perforators arise from the inferior and posterior aspects of the A1 segment (15). These branches are usually identified on the lateral half of the A1 and supply the anterior perforated substance, the dorsal optic chiasm and optic tract, the suprachiasmatic hypothalamus, the inferior frontal lobe, and, rarely, the optic nerve (14). Occasionally the A1 perforators may arise as a common trunk, the medial proximal striae artery (15). Two vessels, the medial frontal orbital artery and the recurrent artery of Heubner, arise at the junction of the A1 and A2. A common origin may be found in some patients (14, 15). The recurrent artery of Heubner is the most important and identifiable perforator. Typically, the recurrent artery arises from the superolateral aspect of the ACA at the level of the ACoA, or within millimeters of the ACoA from the very distal A1 or proximal A2 (18). In approximately 80% of patients, the recurrent artery originates from the lateral aspect of the very proximal A2 and then runs parallel to the A1, across the orbital cortex toward the carotid bifurcation. Branches enter the lateral anterior perforated substance and the medial Sylvian fissure to supply the head of the caudate, the anterior putamen, the globus pallidus externa, and the anterior limb of internal capsule (14,19). The medial frontal orbital artery collateralizes with the frontal polar artery, which exits the anterior inferior aspect of the A2 a variable distance from the ACoA.

The frontal polar artery runs anterior and inferior to exit the interhemispheric fissure toward the frontal pole. During a gyrus rectus resection, it may sometimes be necessary to divide the medial frontal orbital artery. The frontal polar artery, however, is generally not in the operative field. Between 3 and 10 perforators emanate from the superior and posterior surfaces of the ACoA (15,17). These perforators pass directly posteriorly within the interhemispheric fissure to supply the suprachiasmatic region of the hypothalamus, the optic chiasm, and the anterior perforated substance (17,19). Frequently two large ACoA branches, the median artery of the corpus callosum or the subcallosal artery, may be identified (14–17,20). Perforators from the proximal A2 that pass posteriorly in the interhemispheric fissure to the anterior hypothalamus may sometimes be found.

Variations in ACoA vascular anatomy are common (18,20–23). The most frequent variation is unilateral hypoplasia of the A1 segment, which may be observed in up to 85% of patients (15,18,21–23). Fenestration, duplication or triplication of the ACoA, may be observed in 10–40% of patients, the incidence depending in part on the diagnostic method used to evaluate the ACoA (14,16–18,20). When the ACoA is duplicated or triplicated, one vessel appears dominant whereas the others appear vestigial. Small perforators can arise from any branch, but generally arise from the larger. A third A2 segment, the median artery of the corpus callosum (MACC), or accessory ACA, may be identified in 2–13% of patients. Less common anomalies include a duplicated A1 or azygous A2 (18,20). Some vascular anomalies, such as the MACC, may be difficult to identify on preoperative angiogram (20). The presence of vascular anomalies, however, does not appear to influence surgical exposure or outcome (18).

Aneurysms usually take origin from the anterior communicating artery and A1 junction (23,24). The association between a dominant A1 and ACoA aneurysms is common (14,21–23). For example, Charbel et al (23) studied 51 patients with ACoA aneurysms and 50 matched controls; a dominant A1 was observed angiographically in 57% of aneurysm patients and 14% of control patients. Exclusive filling of the aneurysm from one A1 occurred in 78% of aneurysm patients. It is postulated that hemodynamic stress from a dominant A1 may contribute to aneurysm formation because the aneurysm most commonly arises with its neck at the bifurcation of the dominant A1 and ACoA and points contralaterally in the direction of dominant segment flow (13–15,24). In the presence of a median artery of the corpus callosum, the aneurysm may arise at the ACoA, A1, and MACC junction, making it difficult to identify (13). Projection of the ACoA aneurysm dome is variable and can be oriented inferiorly, anteriorly, superiorly, or posteriorly. Approximately 80% of ACoA aneurysm project into the interhemispheric fissure (13–15,24).

An understanding of cisternal anatomy is important during the surgical approach for cerebrospinal fluid drainage, brain relaxation, and exposure. The ICA is surrounded by the carotid cistern. Through the pterional approach for ACoA aneurysms the carotid cistern will be the most posterior and inferior cistern in the operative field. The carotid cistern shares arachnoid partitions with the olfactory cistern superiorly, the Sylvian cistern posterior and laterally, and the chiasmatic cistern medially. Following the ICA in the carotid cistern will lead into the Sylvian cistern, which contains the proximal MCA. In the posterior aspect of the chiasmatic cistern over the optic chiasm, the ACA origin is found usually near thick arachnoid shared with the carotid cistern. Superior to the chiasmatic cistern the ACoA, perforators and recurrent artery of Heubner are found in the lamina terminalis cistern whereas the proximal A2's run in the callosal cisterns.

GENERAL SURGICAL PRINCIPLES AND STRATEGIES

A thorough radiographic evaluation of the aneurysm and surrounding anatomy is necessary before surgery is undertaken. Computed tomography (CT) is the investigation of choice to diagnose SAH, which following rupture of ACoA aneurysms is frequently seen in the interhemispheric fissure. In addition, intraventricular hemorrhage is common. Intracerebral hemorrhage (ICH) may be observed in the medial frontal lobe, the location of which can influence the surgical approach. Occasionally the aneurysm may be visualized on CT scan. Additional information may be obtained from infusion CT scan, 3D spiral CT, magnetic resonance imaging (MRI), or magnetic resonance angiography (MRA). These radiologic tests are particularly useful for giant aneurysms to delineate the aneurysm and adjacent structures, and to determine whether calcification or thrombosis is present in the aneurysm. To accurately delineate ACoA aneurysms angiography is required in all patients and should demonstrate (a) the aneurysm sac and the direction in which it points, (b) the aneurysm neck, and (c) the relationship of the lesion to the parent vessels. Frequently special views, such as those afforded by oblique or base film, are required. In addition, cross-compression of the contralateral carotid during injection of the ipsilateral ICA is necessary to visualize the ACoA. The posterior circulation should also be evaluated to exclude other aneurysms. Angiography should be repeated a week later if the first angiogram following SAH is negative.

When should ruptured ACoA aneurysms be operated? Early surgery, within 72 hours of SAH, provides patients, particularly those in good clinical grade, the most reasonable chance of a favorable outcome (25). In addition, several studies comparing cohorts of patients or historical controls suggest that the incidence and severity of surgical complications or surgical morbidity is similar in patients undergoing early or delayed surgery (26–31). Although cerebral swelling is more common in poor grade patients, we have found that the incidence of surgical complications is no different in

these patients or patients in good clinical grade (32). We have also found that the ability to predict outcome in poor grade patients based on admission clinical and radiographic findings is unreliable (33,34). Consequently, we prefer early surgery on all patients, including those in poor clinical grade, following ACoA aneurysm rupture. Patients who harbor giant ACoA aneurysms, however, are generally operated on in a delayed fashion. Rapidly deteriorating patients with ICH may be treated by immediate surgery based on the CT infusion scan alone (35). In patients with symptomatic intraventrilcular hemorrhage (IVH) and hydrocephalus, judicious ventricular drainage is used to stabilize patients for surgery. Finally, we do not delay surgery on patients with vasospasm because several lines of evidence suggest that mechanical manipulation of the vessels does not exacerbate arterial narrowing (36–38). Furthermore, several treatment modalities, including angioplasty, that can ameliorate vasospasm or its deleterious consequences are best performed after aneurysm occlusion (39–41).

Anterior communicating artery aneurysms can be operated on through lateral, anterior, or skull base exposures. Lateral approaches include pterional (13) or temporal approaches (42) through a frontal temporal craniotomy. Anterior approaches include anterior interhemispheric, using a bifrontal craniotomy (2), midline trephine (43), or basal interhemispheric approach (44). Skull base approaches are midway between lateral and anterior exposures and include supraorbital (45), subfrontal and transorbital (46), and orbit-ocranial-zygomatic (47) exposures. The pterional or interhemispheric approaches are the most frequently used exposures for ACoA aneurysms.

Several factors, including aneurysm location, size, and orientation, and time from rupture, may influence the decision to use a particular approach. First, acute surgery may be better performed using a pterional (48) or a basal interhemispheric approach rather than an anterior interhemispheric approach (44). Second, aneurysms located more than 13 mm above the anterior clinoid process may be best treated through an interhemispheric approach (49). Third, skull base approaches may be suited to giant ACoA aneurysms, particularly if they project superiorly (46). Finally, aneurysms that project inferiorly may be best approached through a pterional exposure, whereas an anterior exposure may be preferable for aneurysms that project superiorly or posteriorly deep into the interhemispheric fissure (2). Whether there is any advantage to a particular approach is unclear since the ability to identify pertinent vascular anatomy and surgical outcome does not appear to be associated with the approach used (18, 49). Most surgeons decide on a particular approach to ACoA aneurysms according to their experience and familiarity with that exposure.

Anterior communicating artery aneurysms may be approached through a right or left pterional exposure; laterality is determined by a variety of factors. For example, for a right-handed surgeon, it may be technically easier to approach ACoA aneurysms from the right. For some surgeons, this consideration may override other factors (50,51). A right-sided approach also avoids retraction on the dominant left frontal lobe. In contrast, other surgeons determine their approach based on the side of the dominant A1 to provide access to the feeding vessel. There are several indications for a left-sided approach: (a) the right A1 is not visible angiographically, (b) multiple aneurysms that may be safely occluded at the same operation are located on the left, (c) the aneurysm arises from the lateral aspect of the left A2–ACoA junction, (d) the angiogram demonstrates a giant aneurysm that only fills from left, or (e) a hematoma is present in the left frontal lobe. If a left-sided approach is used it is useful for the right-handed surgeon to bring the anterior medial extent of the craniotomy closer to the midline because this affords greater operative maneuverability during clip application.

Several surgeons advocate an anterior interhemispheric approach to ACoA aneurysms (2,8,20,52). For this approach the patient is positioned supine and the head dorsiflexed 15°. A bifrontal craniotomy, adjacent to the upper orbital ridge, is performed and the dura opened in a "W" fashion and reflected anteriorly. The superior sagittal sinus is then coagulated, ligated at its most anterior location to divide the falx, and the interhemispheric fissure opened. The ACoA is then identified by following the A2's from the genu of the corpus callosum and by elevation of the frontal lobe to expose the A1's (2,52).

There are two less commonly performed variations of the anterior interhemispheric approach: basal interhemispheric (44,53) and midline trephine (43). In both procedures, the interhemispheric fissure is opened to identify the A2's at the genu. In the basal interhemispheric approach the bifrontal craniotomy is extended by a bone chisel into the anterior midsection of the frontal base toward each supraorbital notch and into the nasal bones. This approach is more complicated and time consuming than the anterior interhemispheric approach and always requires opening of the frontal sinus. The basal approach provides an additional 20° lower approach and some advantage over the anterior interhemispheric approach: (a) there is less frontal lobe retraction, particularly for aneurysms located in a high position, (b) venous anatomy may be better preserved, and (c) the olfactory nerves may be preserved (44). The midline trephine approach involves a low anterior midline trephine approximately 4 cm in diameter that is placed close to the orbital ridge and a unilateral dural opening that does not compromise the sagittal sinus and requires traction on only one frontal lobe (43). However, this approach is not popular for the following reasons: (a) access is limited, (b) <80% of aneurysms can be directly obliterated through this approach, and (c) cosmetic results may be unappealing because a transverse forehead skin incision is used and bone resorption is common unless cranioplasty is used.

The midline or interhemispheric approach has several potential disadvantages: (a) both frontal lobes are at risk, (b) disorientation during subpial dissection can lead to avulsion of cortical vessels, (c) sacrifice of bridging veins can lead to venous infarction particularly during acute surgery (48), (d) the olfactory tract may be injured, and (e) an open frontal sinus significantly increases the risk of infection. Proponents of a midline approach, however, cite two major advantages over the pterional approach: less brain retraction and full visualization of the ACoA. In our experience we have found that during the pterional approach there is both limited brain retraction and excellent visualization of the ACoA if the patient is correctly positioned, the skull base is drilled down, and maximal brain relaxation is achieved.

The pterional approach through a frontotemporal craniotomy is the most widely used exposure for ACoA aneurysms. In this approach the dura is opened around the Sylvian fissure and by following the ipsilateral A1 the ACoA is identified. A limited gyrus rectus resection is often required. The pterional exposure provides a tangential approach to the aneurysm and avoids opening of the frontal sinus as well as injury to the olfactory tract (13,50,51,54,55). We prefer the standard pterional exposure, with some minor modifications, for ACoA aneurysms; our approach is described in detail below.

ANESTHETIC CONSIDERATIONS FOR ANTERIOR COMMUNICATING ARTERY ANEURYSMS

Following rupture of ACoA aneurysms, patients should be admitted to the intensive care unit to provide normovolemia, hemodynamic stability, adequate oxygenation, and intracranial pressure (ICP) control prior to surgery. Some poor grade patients, particularly those with massive ICH, may go directly to the operating room. In addition to a full radiographic evaluation each patient should undergo a standard preoperative laboratory evaluation including complete blood count, coagulation profile, electrolytes, chest X ray, and electrocardiogram (ECG). Four units of blood should be crossmatched. Anticonvulsants, calcium channel antagonists, and steroids are administered. Additional premedication should be individualized. Patients in good clinical grade, particularly if anxious or hypertensive, receive morphine, 1–5 mg or midazolam, 1–5 mg titrated in 1-mg increments, whereas patients who are in poor clinical condition and are intubated receive larger doses of morphine (1–20 mg) or midazolam (5–10 mg). Muscle relaxants may be required during transport of intubated patients. In some patients, a preoperative visit by the anesthesiologist and thorough preoperative explanation may preclude the need for premedication and so allow continued accurate assessment of the preoperative clinical condition.

Careful anesthetic technique is central to the successful surgical treatment of ACoA aneurysms. Induction can be achieved with a variety of agents; we prefer thiopental 3–5 mg/kg combined with fentanyl 2–3 μg/kg. The goal of induction is to minimize transmural pressure and reduce the risk of aneurysm rupture while simultaneously maintaining cerebral perfusion pressure. Consequently, an arterial line to monitor blood pressure is established in all patients and an ICP monitor placed in poor grade patients prior to induction. The hypertensive response to intubation can be controlled by a several techniques including (a) a second dose of thiopental (100 mg) administered immediately before laryngoscopy, (b) lidocaine, 1.5 mg/kg, given 2–3 minutes before intubation, (c) deep inhalational anesthesia using isoflurane or desflurane, (d) a small dose of labetolol (10 mg) or esmolol (500 μg/kg), and (e) additional narcotics (fentanyl 5–10 μg/kg). In good grade patients, we generally use deep isoflurane anesthesia and a second dose of thiopental, whereas in poor grade patients we administer additional narcotics and thiopental and avoid inhalational agents. The choice of muscle relaxant depends, in part, on the nature and response of other drugs used during induction. We generally prefer a nondepolarizing agent because succinylcholine has been reported to increase ICP in some patients or result in excess potassium release in the plegic patient. Usually we use vecuronium (1.0 mg/kg) as a muscle relaxant because atracrurium may cause systemic hypotension and pancuronium may cause tachycardia and hypertension.

Following induction and intubation using a reinforced endotracheal tube, additional monitors, including ECG, noninvasive blood pressure cuff, pulse oximetry, end-tidal capnograph, urinary catheter, and esophageal stethoscope and temperature monitor are placed. Intravenous access is important; at least one 16- or 14-gauge peripheral catheter is inserted. In addition, all patients undergoing surgery should have insertion of a central venous catheter or, if in poor clinical grade, a Swan–Ganz catheter. Central venous or Swan– Ganz catheters may be useful for several reasons: (a) hypovolemia is common after rupture of ACoA aneurysms, (b) fluid shifts may occur from the use of osmotic and loop diuretics for brain relaxation, and (c) myocardial dysfunction or autonomic instability may result from hemorrhage into the hypothalamus. Other monitors, such as jugular bulb oxygen saturation cerebral oximetry, transcranial Doppler (TCD), electroencephalogram (EEG), and somatosensory evoked potential (SSEP) may be used in selected patients. Analysis of jugular bulb oxygen may prove useful to determine the optimum level of hyperventilation or to detect early ischemia through detecting increased oxygen extraction. Continuous TCD may improve the safety of induced hypotension by correlating changes in systemic blood pressure with blood flow velocity changes. Finally, EEG and SSEP may prove helpful, in some patients, to predict tolerable occlusion time of temporary clips or the effectiveness of cerebral protectants.

There are several important goals during the maintenance of anesthesia: (a) provide a relaxed brain, (b) maintain cerebral perfusion pressure, (c) reduce transmural aneurysm pressure, and (d) facilitate prompt neurologic assessment when surgery is complete. There are no data about the influence of anesthetic agents on brain condition or outcome for aneurysm surgery; in our experience 0.5–1.0 minimal alveolar concentration (MAC) isoflurane and a fentanyl infusion

(1–2 μg/kg/hr) has proved satisfactory. We generally omit nitrous oxide when isoflurane is used because the former is a cerebral vasodilator and may increase cerebral metabolic rate. Normovolemia is maintained during surgery and once the aneurysm is clipped slight hypervolemia is induced. We prefer solutions such as Plasmalyte or normal saline, and avoid glucose-containing solutions or hetastarch. Patients in good clinical grade who undergo an uneventful clipping are awakened and extubated in the operating room. Consequently, the narcotic infusion is stopped 1 hour before the procedure end. Patients in poor clinical grade are kept intubated at the end of surgery using an intravenous-based anesthetic technique.

A relaxed brain that allows minimal retraction is essential. In our experience, a combination of techniques provides maximal brain relaxation. First, a lumbar subarachnoid drain is placed to reduce cerebrospinal fluid (CSF) volume. We use a commercially available kit (Cordis, Lumbar Catheter Accessory Kit) that has a soft flexible catheter with multiple orifices and carefully drain about 100 ml during bone work. Second, to reduce brain tissue volume a 20% mannitol (0.5–2 mg/kg) infusion, augmented with furosemide (0.1–0.5 mg/kg), is administered over 30–45 minutes during positioning and skin preparation. Third, cerebral blood volume can be reduced through hyperventilation that is individualized to operating conditions. We aim for mild hypocapnia ($Paco_2$ 30–35 mm Hg) before the dura is opened. Moderate hypocapnia ($Paco_2$ 25–30 mm Hg) after the dura is open and normocapnia during induced hypotension and once the aneurysm is occluded. In poor grade patients CO_2 reactivity may be impaired. In these patients, estimation of jugular oxygen extraction may be useful to optimize operating conditions. The following steps are taken if the brain remains tight: (a) evaluate for hypoxemia or hypertension, (b) ensure there is no venous obstruction in the neck, (c) discontinue nitrous oxide, (d) tilt the head up, (e) readminister a mannitol bolus (1 mg/kg) after checking serum osmolarity, and (f) administer thiopental (150–200 mg). If relaxation improves, an infusion of 4–5 mg/kg/hr is continued. Alternatively, shorter acting drugs such as etomidate (0.2–0.3 mg/kg/hr) or propofol (150–200 μg/kg/hr) can be used.

The risk of intraoperative aneurysm rupture may be reduced by induced hypotension or temporary arterial occlusion. Close communication between surgeon and anesthesiologist is necessary. We do not favor routine hypotension because autoregulation, especially in poor grade patients, may be impaired after SAH (56–58). Furthermore, a recent study using historical controls suggests that intraoperative hypotension does not provide protection against rupture and can significantly worsen outcome if rupture occurs (59,60). To facilitate aneurysm dissection, however, we occasionally use moderate hypotension in young, good grade patients with no evidence of vasospasm. Moderate hypotension (systolic blood pressure, or SBP, 90–100 mm Hg) can be achieved by a slight increase in the amount of isoflurane or by titrated nitroprusside.

We prefer judicious use of temporary arterial occlusion

rather than systemic hypotension to facilitate aneurysm dissection. We attempt to occlude the dominant A1 only; however, occlusion on all ACoA complex vessels, including a hypoplastic A1, is sometimes required. Tolerable occlusion time is difficult to predict; 5–7 minutes is generally well tolerated but this is insufficient time to occlude difficult aneurysms. To extend tolerable occlusion time, we use an additional infusion of 20% mannitol, elevate the blood pressure (SBP 160 mm Hg) to augment collateral flow, and carefully control temperature prior to clip application. If the preoperative angiogram demonstrates that the collateral circulation is poor, we also administer etomidate (0.4 mg/kg) or thiopental (5–6 mg/kg) intravenously until EEG burst suppression is observed. In these patients, scalp needles are placed in a bihemispheric fronto-occipital montage for routine compressed spectral analysis of EEG prior to surgery. Electrophysiologic monitoring, such as SSEP, may also be used to determine the upper limit of tolerable occlusion. However, the false-negative and false-positive rate for ACA occlusion is fairly high in most reported series (61–64). Therefore we do not routinely use SSEP monitoring during ACoA aneurysm surgery.

PATIENT POSITIONING

For the pterional approach, the patient is positioned supine with the ipsilateral shoulder slightly elevated. Anterior communicating artery aneurysms are located at the level of the planum sphenoidale and tuberculum sella. It is important, therefore, to carefully position the patient to minimize brain retraction. The head is positioned with the ipsilateral maxilla uppermost, the vertex slightly below the horizontal plane, and the frontal fossa floor perpendicular to the body axis. Since the aneurysm lies anteriorly in the sagittal plane, some authors advocate turning the head 60° from the incision side (50). Head rotation too far laterally, however, can obscure the opposite A2. Consequently, we prefer a more subfrontal approach with approximately 30° of head rotation to provide better identification of the opposite A2. The head is secured in the Mayfield 3 point head holder after infiltrating the pin sites with 1% lidocaine; we place the single pin behind the ipsilateral pinna level to the mastoid process. Before draping, bony prominences are padded, pneumatic compression stockings placed, the endotracheal tube is checked, and head and neck position inspected to ensure that no venous obstruction can occur. Similarly, to prevent venous obstruction, we secure the endotracheal tube with tape rather than a tie around the neck.

SCALP AND BONE EXPOSURE

The scalp and bony exposure is designed to provide an unobstructed lateral subfrontal view anterior to the lesser wing of the sphenoid (Fig. 2). During the initial exposure loupe magnification and headlight illumination are used. A

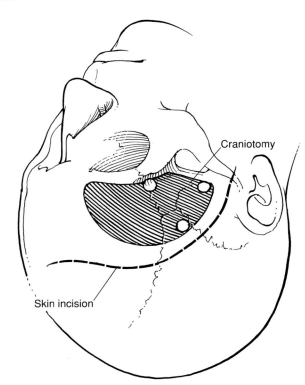

FIG. 2. The craniotomy created for anterior communicating artery aneurysms is slightly larger than that for other anterior circulation aneurysms and is cut low on the anterior fossa floor beyond the midpupillary line. The frontal bone inner table is removed and the orbital roof flattened.

curvilinear frontotemporal incision, just behind the hairline, that extends from the root of the zygoma, superior and anterior to the tragus and over the midline is made after infiltration with 1% lidocaine without epinephrine. Care is taken to preserve the superficial temporal artery, and hemostatic Raney clips are applied to the skin edges. Using a combination of monopolar electrocautery and elevators, the temporalis muscle is separated from the frontal and temporal bones and, with the scalp, is reflected anterolaterally to identify the orbitofrontal angle. The supraorbital ridge should also be defined to just beyond the supraorbital nerve. The scalp and muscle flap is covered with a Bacitracin-soaked sponge and then retracted over a sponge, to prevent ischemic complications, using small towel clips secured with rubber bands to a Greenberg secondary bar or the Layla bar positioned flat over the patient's face from the contralateral side. If the muscle remains bulky at the orbitofrontal angle it can be dissected from the fascia and separately reflected in a posterolateral direction. Care is taken to preserve the frontalis branch of the facial nerve. The periosteum is elevated separately and preserved.

The bone flap used to approach ACoA aneurysms is larger than for other aneurysms located in the anterior circulation. Careful lumbar CSF drainage is initiated during bone work. In patients <55 years old a single burr hole is placed in the squamous temporal bone behind the sphenotemporal suture, whereas in older patients three burr holes are placed: (a) posterior to the orbital rim and superior to the frontozygomatic suture, (b) at the junction of the coronal suture and linea temporalis, and (c) in the squamous temporal bone. We avoid placing an inferomedial burr hole in the orbital rim for cosmetic reasons. After separating the dura from the skull, using a Penfield 3, a frontotemporal craniotomy is created with the Midas Rex craniotome. The bone flap is carried anteriorly and low along the anterior fossa floor to the midpupillary line about 4 cm from the zygomatic frontal junction. The cut follows the temporal line into the temporal region. Bone over the temporal tip is removed; a subtemporal craniectomy, however, is unnecessary. The edges of the craniotomy should be beveled to prevent later sinking; however, if microplate and screw fixation is used to close the craniotomy, sunken flaps are not a problem. In older patients dural tears may occur in the inferior medial frontal region or close to the zygomatic frontal burr hole. These tears can be repaired with a series of sutures that are placed through drill holes in the skull edge. Occasionally, the frontal sinus may be opened during creation of the bone flap. When this happens, preoperative prophylactic antibiotics should be supplemented with anaerobic coverage. The defect can be covered with bone wax, on a Surgicel scaffold, if the mucosa is intact. However, if the mucosa is violated, exenteration of the frontal sinus is necessary. In both circumstances a vascularized pericranial flap is secured over the sinus opening during closure.

Operative exposure and access is enhanced by additional bone work using rongeurs and a high-speed burr to flatten the orbital roof and lesser sphenoid wing, and partly remove the inner table of the frontal bone across the inferior aspect of the craniotomy. These maneuvers should provide unobstructed access anterior to the lesser sphenoid wing. The bone edges are then waxed, lined with Oxycel and 2-inch cottonoids, and 4-0 silk dural tackups placed around the periphery of the craniotomy to achieve epidural hemostasis and divert blood from the dural opening. Before opening the dura the operative field is lined with moist laparotomy sponges to cover exposed tackups or instruments that may snare suction tubing during the microscopic dissection. A small dural flap is then opened in a curvilinear direction extending from the anterior aspect of the bone flap across the Sylvian fissure into the temporal region. The dural flap is covered with Surgicel and held flush against the inferior aspect of the craniotomy with tackup sutures.

MICROSURGICAL DISSECTION AND PRINCIPLES

The distal ICA and ICA bifurcation is first exposed. After opening the dura, the brain surface is inspected and covered with moist gel foam to protect it from inadvertent injury while using the microscope. Under loupe magnification, a retractor is placed on the orbital surface of the frontal lobe, immediately anterior to the Sylvian fissure and advanced along the sphenoid ridge to elevate the frontal lobe gently. The brain surface is protected by moist telfa. The olfactory tract, a few millimeters posterior to the optic nerve region, is identified and the arachnoid veil over the medial Sylvian fissure and parasellar area is opened, CSF drained, and the optic nerve and proximal ICA identified. A site for proximal control on the ICA is established and the vessel followed to its bifurcation using sharp microdissection. In some patients the ICA is long and to see the bifurcation and proximal A1 would require excessive frontal lobe retraction. Rather than follow the ICA in these patients, the medial fissure is opened on the frontal side of the veins, and the proximal M1 identified and followed lateral to medial to the carotid bifurcation. Alternatively, the gyrus rectus can be resected (see below). In most cases, the temporal tip bridging veins are divided allowing the exposed temporal lobe, protected by telfa, to fall away posteriorly.

The next stage in dissection is ipsilateral A1 exposure (Fig. 3). The operating microscope is now used with the surgeon comfortably seated and the assistant positioned to his right. First, the olfactory tract is dissected from the optic nerve and the retractor advanced until it almost touches the optic nerve to further elevate the frontal lobe. The retractor blade should be carefully sized so that the retractor arm can lie flush to the patient's skull and prevent inadvertent motion. Frontal lobe elevation places the arachnoid binding the gyrus rectus to the optic nerve under tension; this arachnoid is sharply divided. Next, dissection is advanced medially across the optic nerve to free the gyrus rectus from the optic

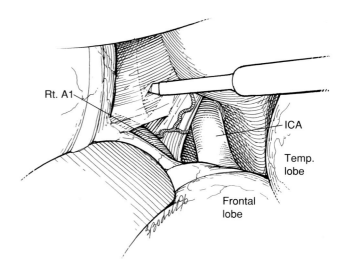

FIG. 3. The initial stage of dissection includes identification of the internal carotid artery and proximal A1. The A1 is exposed by elevation of the frontal lobe and sharp dissection of the arachnoid between the gyrus rectus and the optic nerve. The olfactory tract is behind the retractor blade. The opposite A1 may be identified by continuing sharp dissection across the optic chiasm where the ipsilateral A1 turns away from the optic nerve.

nerve and chiasm. Finally, the retractor blade is deepened in an anterior and medial direction to expose the A1 as it crosses the optic nerve. In many instances, however, proximal A1 exposure requires partial resection of the ipsilateral gyrus rectus (see below). The A1 is prepared to accept a temporary clip, and the retractor further advances, parallel to the A1, to continue dissection across the optic chiasm.

Exposure of the opposite A1 depends in part on aneurysm orientation. The opposite A1 can be exposed before dissection of the ACoA when the aneurysm is directed superiorly into the interhemispheric fissure. To do this sharp dissection is continued across the optic chiasm, rather than on the A1, when the ipsilateral vessel diverges from the optic nerve. The chiasmatic cistern is also opened and CSF drained. At the opposite optic nerve and chiasm juncture the contralateral A1 is identified as it heads toward the interhemispheric fissure. Arachnoid is dissected from the vessel and it is prepared for a temporary clip. Alternatively, the ipsilateral A1 can be followed across the anterior and ventral surface of the ACoA to identify the opposite A1. We generally prefer to identify both A1's first because this establishes proximal control before dissection of the ACoA. When the aneurysm points forward onto the optic chiasm, the contralateral A1 may be best exposed after the ipsilateral gyrus rectus has been resected by finding the opposite A2 in the interhemispheric fissure and following it retrograde to the opposite A1; access to the opposite A1, therefore, is behind the lesion. It is important during dissection and exposure of the A1's to identify and protect the recurrent artery of Heubner and other perforators. In addition, the opposite recurrent artery of Heubner should not be mistaken for the contralateral A1.

In most instances, full exposure of the A1 requires that the ipsilateral gyrus rectus be removed (Fig. 4). The lamina terminalis cistern between the two gyri recti may be opened allowing better visualization across the midline. The ipsilateral frontal lobe is then retracted away from the interhemispheric fissure. The retractor blade is withdrawn slightly and positioned where the ipsilateral A1 turns into the interhemispheric fissure. Beneath the retractor about 5 mm of gyrus rectus lateral to interhemispheric fissure is exposed. After coagulating the arachnoid with bipolar electrocautery, it is sharply opened and the gyrus rectus removed in a subpial fashion. The pia-arachnoid on the medial aspect of the gyrus rectus in the interhemispheric fissure is initially preserved and then cauterized and sharply divided to expose the distal A1 in the interhemispheric fissure, the ACoA, and the ipsilateral A2 takeoff. Posterior pointing aneurysms generally require more extensive retraction and gyrus rectus resection. Occasionally, the A1 can be easily followed to the ACoA and the aneurysm exposed without a gyrus rectus resection or frontal lobe retraction.

Following the gyrus rectus resection, the ipsilateral A2 origin and the ACoA area are well seen. The next goal is to fully delineate and expose the inferior and superior aspects of the distal ipsilateral A1, the proximal ipsilateral A2, and the ACoA before aneurysm dissection (Fig. 5). Retraction may be increased to demonstrate the contralateral A1. Careful preoperative angiographic evaluation and full appreciation of 3D anatomy and knowledge of any variants will significantly guide the next step in dissection: demonstration of the opposite A2 origin. Aneurysm orientation determines how the opposite A2 is exposed (Fig. 6). For an aneurysm oriented superiorly, or superiorly and posteriorly, dissection first proceeds across the ACoA's inferior aspect to the contralateral A1 and is then continued distally, superior to the ipsilateral A2 origin and anterior to the aneurysm neck to expose the contralateral A2. The aneurysm neck is dissected

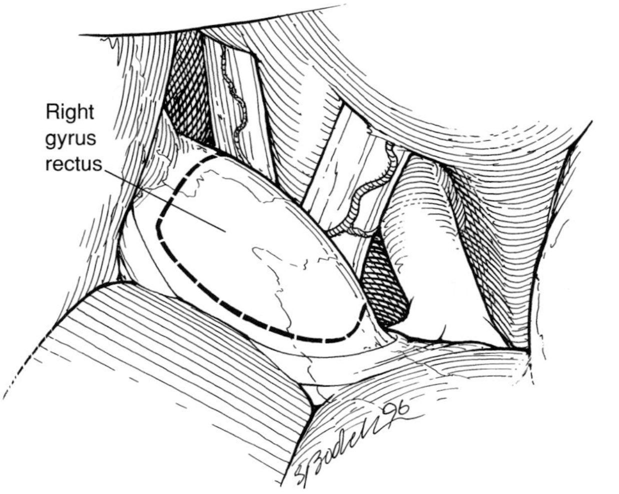

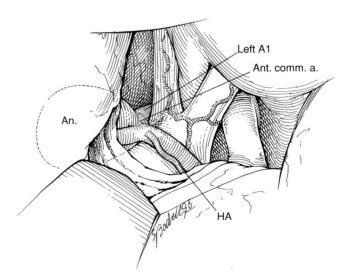

FIG. 4. Once the proximal A1 is identified, the ipsilateral gyrus rectus is removed. The arachnoid in the lamina terminals cistern may be first incised to separate the two gyri recti. The retractor is then withdrawn slightly to lie over the ACoA complex. A careful subpial resection of the gyrus rectus is performed *(hatched line).*

FIG. 5. After gyrus rectus resection, the ipsilateral A1, the proximal A2, and the ACoA are exposed. Dissection is continued to identify the opposite distal A1 and proximal A2.

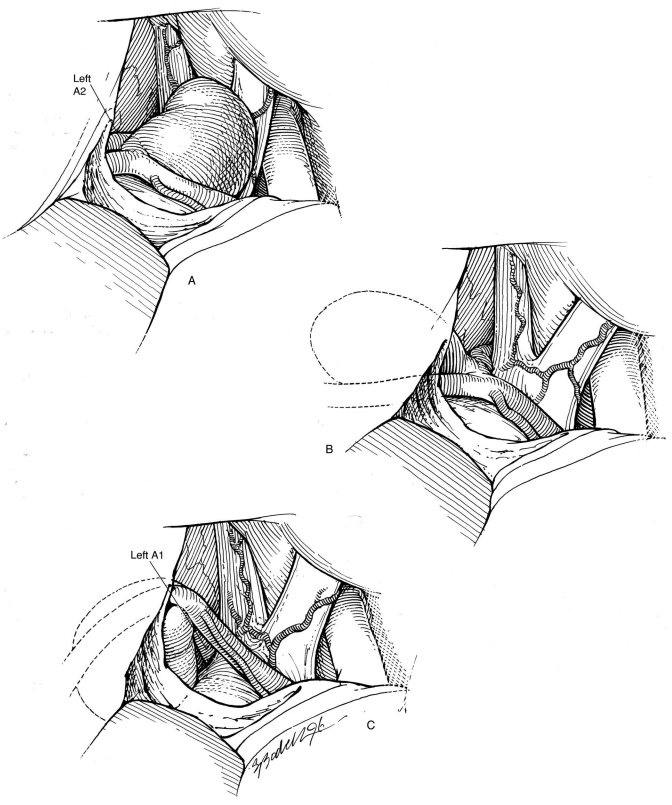

FIG. 6. Aneurysm orientation in part determines how the ACoA complex exposure is accomplished. **A:** When the aneurysm is oriented inferiorly, dissection is continued medially along the anterior-inferior aspect of the ipsilateral A2 to expose the opposite A2. **B:** Dissection along the inferior origin of the aneurysm neck where it joins the ACoA will delineate the opposite A2 for anterior-superior oriented aneurysms. **C:** Further gyrus rectus resection and gentle mobilization of the aneurysm neck is required to expose the ACoA complex and opposite A2 when the aneurysm projects posteriorly.

at its origin inferiorly to expose the contralateral A2 origin if the aneurysm is directed anterior and superior. Sharp dissection is started on the inferior aspect of the ipsilateral A2 and carried medially through the interhemispheric fissure, superior and anterior to the aneurysm to see the opposite A2 when the aneurysm projects in an inferior direction. Further gyrus rectus resection and mobilization of the aneurysm may be required to delineate the opposite A2 when the aneurysm projects superior and posterior superior. To allow aneurysm mobilization, the arachnoid in the interhemispheric fissure is sharply divided and the ipsilateral vessels mobilized to expose the aneurysm neck.

Aneurysm dissection is started once the ACoA complex is defined. Ideally, both A1's and A2's should first be clearly delineated. The goal of aneurysm dissection is to define the neck and create a free cleavage plane between the ventral posterior surface and the perforators that arise from the posterior ACoA surface. There are a variable number of perforators, and care should be taken to identify and preserve all perforators, since during clip application visualization is frequently compromised by the clip applier. There should therefore be no hurry to place a clip on an inadequately dissected ACoA complex and aneurysm. Aneurysm orientation determines in part how the perforators are defined. Manipulation of the aneurysm may be necessary. Generally, it can be held with a microsucker and cottonoid or a blunt microdissector. However, to free the aneurysm from adherent structures it is preferable to use sharp dissection because blunt dissection is more frequently associated with severe intraoperative aneurysm rupture (65). From the pterional approach it may be difficult to identify the perforators when the aneurysm is oriented posteriorly. In addition, perforators may be adherent to the ventral posterior aneurysm wall. Using careful microdissection the aneurysm and A2 can be reflected superiorly, to view its ventral plane. Similarly, when the aneurysm projects superiorly it can be mobilized in an anterior direction and its ventral surface observed over the ipsilateral A2. Most problems with perforator identification occur when a superior- or posterior-oriented aneurysm has a large or broad neck. Temporary clip application and suction decompression can be useful in this circumstance. The temporary clips should preferably be applied at the ACoA origins rather than on the afferent and efferent vessels. This same technique may be useful if aneurysm rupture occurs and may be used to occlude large-necked aneurysms provided no perforators arise from the ACoA.

Aneurysm obliteration is attempted only when all of the vessels and their relationship to the aneurysm neck are defined. A wide neck may be reconfigured by bipolar coagulation applied at a low setting under constant gentle irrigation. In addition, the bipolar blades should pass completely across the neck and be intermittently released and applied. The selected clip should extend across the entire neck and not include any vessels. A sucker or blunt dissector can be used to manipulate the aneurysm neck into the clip blades. In addition, the variangle Sano clip applier may help preserve

visibility (66). Aneurysm size, shape, and orientation dictate in part which clip is used, and how, as follows (Fig. 7): (a) For aneurysms that project inferiorly, the clip may be passed over the ipsilateral A2 and beneath the contralateral A2. Alternatively, a fenestrated clip, with the aperture around the ipsilateral A1 or A2, can be passed under and parallel to the ACoA. (b) For anterior-oriented aneurysms, the clip can be introduced parallel to the ACoA with the posterior blade anterior to A2 segments and the anterior blade above the optic apparatus. (c) Aneurysms that project superiorly may require anterior mobilization to separate the lesion from perforators. This retraction can obscure the aneurysm neck behind the A2 or kink the A2 origin when the clip is passed superior to ACoA. To prevent these problems, a fenestrated clip that encircles the proximal ipsilateral A2 can be applied when the aneurysm is retracted anteriorly. (d) The clip can be applied perpendicular to the ACoA between the A2's when the aneurysm projects in a posterior direction. (e) Giant aneurysms are frequently multilobulated and distort anatomy. To occlude these lesions, temporary clips to isolate the aneurysm from the circulation and suction decompression can be useful. Giant aneurysms often require two clips or booster clips, and occasionally may be opened to perform aneurysmorrhaphy.

When a fenestrated clip is applied it is important to ensure that the distal ACoA is reconstructed and that the encircled vessel is not compromised. Fenestrated clips, including blade-deviated fenestrated clips (67), are less likely to leave a small residual neck than curved clips. During clip application, the blades should be moist and advanced gently using slow rotational movements. If resistance is felt, the dissection is incomplete and the clip should be withdrawn. Once the clip is applied it should be carefully inspected to confirm patency of the circulation and perforators and occlusion of the entire aneurysm neck. A small spinal needle mounted on a 2-ml syringe should be used to puncture the aneurysm dome, away from the neck, and confirm aneurysm obliteration. A collapsed aneurysm also allows further dissection and inspection of the ACoA complex. In some complex aneurysms intraoperative angiography or microvascular Doppler may be useful to confirm vessel patency and aneurysm occlusion. Neither test, however, can evaluate perforator patency; this can only be done by direct inspection. We generally wrap the clip blades in cotton wisps to promote scarring and prevent potential aneurysm growth at its base. The clip should be positioned to prevent torque on the neck or pressure on the chiasm. Finally, we prefer long clips because we have observed a few cases in which small clips unrestrained by the skull base have inadvertently compressed the optic nerve.

After checking that the aneurysm is occluded and vessels are patent the craniotomy is closed. Close communication between the anesthesiologist and surgeon is necessary to ensure an uneventful immediate postoperative course. The retractors are removed, and after blood pressure and Pa_{CO_2} are returned to normal levels, meticulous hemostasis is ob-

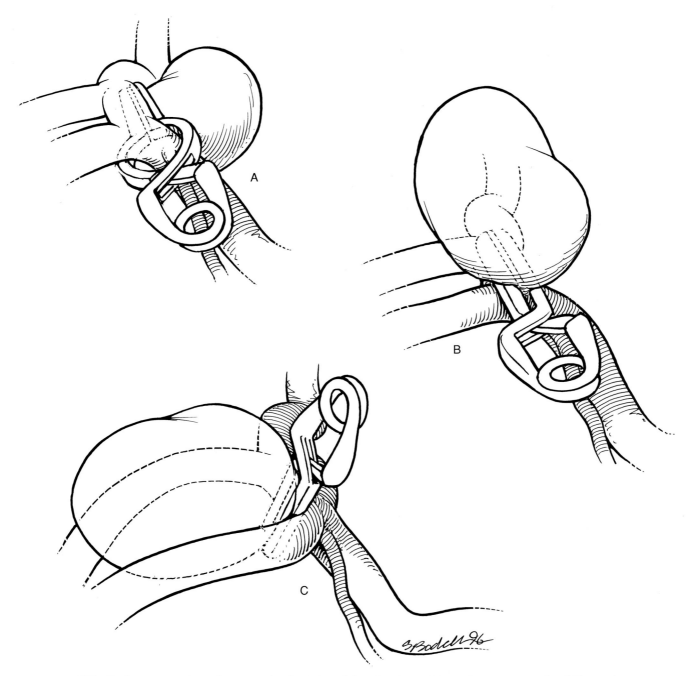

FIG. 7. Aneurysm size, shape, and orientation determine in part how the aneurysm is obliterated. Schematic illustrations representing occlusion of **(A)** inferior, **(B)** anterior-superior, and **(C)** posterior-superior projecting aneurysms.

tained. The gyrus rectus resection is lined with Surgicel. Dura is then closed using a running 4-0 silk suture, after irrigating the subdural space with saline, and tackup sutures are inserted to obliterate the epidural space. The bone is replaced using a microplate and screw fixation system and the muscle and galea reapproximated using 2-0 or 3-0 Dexon sutures. Skin is closed with a running 3-0 nylon suture and an intracranial pressure monitor is routinely placed.

Immediate postoperative management depends in part on the patient's clinical grade and the complexity of surgery. A patient in good grade who undergoes uneventful surgery can be awakened and extubated in the operating or recovery room. Lidocaine (1.5 mg/kg) can be administered to minimize cough. Moderate hypertension (<180 mm Hg) is tolerated; if the systolic blood pressure is >180 mm Hg labetelol in 5- to 10-mg increments is administered. Grade III patients are extubated provided the brain is well relaxed, surgery was uncomplicated, laryngeal reflexes are intact, and the patient can maintain ventilation. Other grade III patients and all poor grade patients are kept intubated. In the recovery room, frequent neurologic assessment and careful control of ventilation, fluid status, and blood pressure are necessary. All patients are subsequently managed in the intensive care unit. A postoperative CT scan and bilateral carotid angiograms are routinely obtained.

COMPLICATIONS AND THEIR MANAGEMENT

In addition to the general complications of anesthesia, craniotomy, and SAH, there are several intraoperative technical mishaps or postoperative surgical complications that are related to surgical occlusion of ACoA aneurysms. Complications commonly associated with repair of ACoA aneurysms include intraoperative aneurysm rupture, vessel occlusion or perforator injury, and poor neuropsychological outcome. In addition, complications such as venous infarction, frontal lobe contusion, anosmia, and meningitis are more frequently associated with repair of ACoA aneurysms through an interhemispheric approach. Some series suggest that surgical complications are related to aneurysm location and occur most frequently when ruptured basilar bifurcation or ACoA aneurysms are repaired (60,68–70). Other series, however, suggest that the ruptured aneurysm's size rather than location is associated with complications (30,71,72). Similarly, size rather than location appears to be the more important determinant of complications when unruptured aneurysms are repaired (73,74).

There are several complications that are more frequently associated with the interhemispheric approach to ACoA aneurysms, although they may also occur with the pterional approach. First, venous infarction may occur and is eightfold more common when the bridging veins are sacrificed (48). Second, frontal lobe contusion may result from excessive lateral retraction (44). Third, the olfactory tract is at risk during the interhemispheric approach and olfactory disturbance or anosmia is common even when the olfactory tract is preserved anatomically (44,75). Finally, infection, including brain abscess or meningitis, can occur because the frontal sinus is opened. For example, Yasui et al. (44) observed that 17% of patients undergoing either a basal or an interhemispheric approach to ACoA aneurysms developed meningitis.

New postoperative neurologic abnormalities are primarily related to vessel occlusion but should be differentiated from postoperative hematomas, hydrocephalus, vasospasm, or metabolic disorders. It is important, therefore, to identify and preserve all vessels and perforators of the ACoA complex. The resulting clinical syndromes depend largely on which vessel is compromised and include leg weakness when the ACA is involved, facial and upper extremity hemiparesis from injury to the recurrent artery of Heubner, speech disturbance after occlusion of the dominant recurrent artery

of Heubner, and hypokinesis, visual field defects, Korsakoff's syndrome, affective disorders, abulia, and diabetes insipidus from perforator injury. Several principles such as adequate operative exposure and brain relaxation, access to key vessels, judicious temporary arterial occlusion, and sharp dissection may reduce or help correct inadvertent vessel or perforator occlusion. Finally, visual disturbances, including blindness, may result from direct injury to the optic chiasm or nerve. In addition, blindness may result from optochiasmal arachnoiditis, which may complicate muslin wrapping. Some patients suffering from optochiasmal arachnoiditis respond to steroid therapy (76).

Neuropsychological and cognitive morbidity affects approximately half of survivors of ruptured ACoA aneurysms (77,78). Some studies suggest that ACoA aneurysms are associated with a greater incidence of poor neuropsychological outcome than aneurysms at other locations (69,79,80); however, this association is not observed in all series (77,81). There is a wide range of neuropsychological deficits ranging from discrete memory defects to a Korsakoff-like syndrome or global amnesia. Intellect is usually not impaired, although some patients may have difficulties in conceptual learning (78). Memory loss appears to be associated with structural lesions in the basal forebrain and striatum (82), and appears to be primarily related to the effects of the initial hemorrhage, hydrocephalus, and vasospasm rather than surgery (78,83–85). For example, Sengupta et al (85) evaluated 26 patients after direct occlusion of ruptured ACoA aneurysms; personality changes demonstrated a significant correlation with clinical grade. In addition, many deficits observed postoperatively in patients undergoing repair of ruptured ACoA aneurysms are also observed preoperatively (84). Nevertheless, it is critical to preserve all vessels and perforators at surgery to reduce the risk of disabling neuropsychological sequelae.

OVERVIEW

Anterior communicating artery aneurysms are common but may pose problems related to their location and complex vascular anatomy. Since the introduction of the operating microscope, excellent technical results can be obtained and an operative mortality <5% can be expected in select patients undergoing repair of ACoA aneurysms (2,13). Clinical grade is the primary determinant of outcome following ACoA aneurysm rupture (18,43,44,49,52); factors such as the surgical approach, aneurysm orientation, or the presence of ACoA vascular anomalies do not appear related to outcome (8,18,20,49). Several surgical approaches have been described for ACoA aneurysms; however, successful surgical treatment depends on (a) careful preoperative radiographic assessment, (b) neuroanesthesia, (c) maximal brain relaxation, (d) accurate dissection and isolation of the aneurysm neck without premature rupture, (e) preservation of both cerebral hemispheres and judicious gyrus rectus resection, (f) preservation and patency of the A1 and A2 segments, the recurrent artery of Heubner, and all perforators, and (g) pre- and postoperative intensive care efforts (86).

REFERENCES

1. Sahs AL, Perret GE, Locksley HB. *Intracranial aneurysms and subarachnoid hemorrhage.* Philadelphia: JB Lippincott, 1969.
2. Suzuki J, Mizoi K, Yoshimoto T. Bifrontal interhemispheric approach to anterior communicating artery aneurysms. *J Neurosurg* 1986;64:183–190.
3. Russel CK. Spontaneous subarachnoid hemorrhage following rupture of a congenital aneurysm of the anterior communicating artery of the circle of Willis; report of a case in which the aneurysm was excised. *Trans Am Neurol Assoc* 1939;65:130–134.
4. Tonnis W. Erfolgreiche behandling eines aneurysmader art. commun. ant. cerebri. *Zentralbl Neurochir* 1936;1:39–42.
5. Logue V. Surgery in spontaneous subarachnoid hemorrhage. Operative treatment of aneurysms on the anterior cerebral and anterior communicating artery. *Br Med J* 1956;1:473–479.
6. Shenkin HA, Polakoff P, Finneson BE. Intracranial internal carotid artery aneurysms. Results of treatment by cervical carotid ligation. *J Neurosurg* 1958;15:183–191.
7. McKissock W, Richardson A, Walsh L. Anterior communicating aneurysm, a trial of conservative and surgical treatment. *Lancet* 1965;1:873–876.
8. Pool JL. Aneurysms of the anterior communicating artery. Bifrontal craniotomy and routine use of temporary clips. *J Neurosurg* 1961;18:98–111.
9. French LA, Zarling ME, Schilz EA. Management of aneurysms of the anterior communicating artery. *J Neurosurg* 1962;19:870.
10. Hook O, Norlen G. Aneurysms of the anterior communicating artery. *Acta Neurol Scand* 1964;40:219.
11. Graf CJ, Nibbelink DW. Cooperative study of intracranial aneurysms and subarachnoid hemorrhage. Report on a randomized treatment study III. Intracranial surgery. *Stroke* 1974;5:559.
12. Hori S, Suzuki J. Early and late results of intracranial direct surgery of anterior communicating artery aneurysms. *J Neurosurg* 1979;50:433–440.
13. Yasargil MG. Anterior cerebral and anterior communicating artery aneurysms. In: Yasargil MG, ed. *Microneurosurgery.* vol 2. Stuttgart: Thieme Stratton, 1984;165–231.
14. Perlmutter D, Rhoton AL. Microsurgical anatomy of the anterior cerebral and anterior communicating recurrent artery complex. *J Neurosurg* 1976;45:259–272.
15. Yasargil MG. Anterior cerebral artey complex. In: Yasargil MG, ed. *Microneurosurgery.* vol 1. Stuttgart: Thieme Stratton, 1984;92–116.
16. Gomes FB, Dujovny M, Umansky F. Microanatomy of the anterior cerebral artery. *Surg Neurol* 1986;26:129–141.
17. Marinkovic S, Milisavljevic M, Marinkovic Z. Branches of the anterior communicating artery. Microsurgical anatomy. *Acta Neurochir* 1990;106:78–85.
18. Nathal E, Yasui N, Sampei T, Suzuki A. Intraoperative anatomical studies in patients with aneurysms of the anterior communicating artery complex. *J Neurosurg* 1992;76:629–634.
19. Rosner SS, Rhoton AL, Ono M, Barry M. Microsurgical anatomy of the anterior perforated arteries. *J Neurosurg* 1984;61:468–485.
20. Ogawa A, Suzuki M, Sakurai Y, Yoshimoto T. Vascular anomalies associated with aneurysms of the anterior communicating artery: microsurgical observations. *J Neurosurg* 1990;72: 706–709.
21. Wilson G, Riggs H, Rupp C. The pathologic anatomy of ruptured cerebral aneurysms *J Neurosurg* 1954;11:128–134.
22. Kirgis HD, Fischer WI. Llewellyn RC, Peebles EM. Aneurysms of the anterior communicating artery and gross anomalies of the circle of Willis. *J Neurosurg* 1966;25:73–78.
23. Charbel FT, Seyfried D, Mehta B, Dujovny M, Ausman J. Dominant A1: angiographic and clinical correlations with anterior communicating artery aneurysms. *Neurol Res* 1991;13:253–256.
24. Vander Ark GD, Kempe LC. Classification of anterior communicating aneurysms as a basis of surgical approach. *J Neurosurg* 1970;32:300–303.
25. Haley EC, Kassell NF, Torner JC. The international cooperative study on the timing of aneurysm surgery: the North American experience. *Stroke* 1992;23:205–214.
26. Milhorat TH, Krautheim M. Results of early and delayed operations for ruptured intracranial aneurysms in two series of 100 consecutive patients. *Surg Neurol* 1986;26:123–128.
27. Disney L, Weir B, Petruk K. Effect on management mortality of a deliberate policy of early operation on supratentorial aneurysms. *Neurosurgery* 1987;20:695–701.
28. Chyatte D, Fode NC, Sundt TM Jr. Early versus late intracranial aneurysm surgery in subarachnoid hemorrhage. *J Neurosurg* 1988;69:326–331.
29. Kassell NF, Torner JC, Haley C, Jane J, Adams HP, Kongable BSN: the international cooperative study on the timing of aneurysm surgery: Part 1: overall management results. *J Neurosurg* 1990;73:18–36.
30. Kassell NF, Torner JC, Jane J, Haley EC, Adams HP. The international cooperative study on the timing of aneurysm sugery. 2. Surgical results. *J Neurosurg* 1990;73:37–47.
31. Deruty R, Mottolese C, Pelissou-Guyotat I, Soustiel JF. Management of the ruptured intracranial aneurysm—early surgery, late surgery, or modulated surgery? *Acta Neurochir (Wien)* 1991;113:1–10.
32. Le Roux P, Elliott JP, Winn HR. The incidence of surgical complications is similar in good and poor grade patients undergoing repair of ruptured anterior circulation aneurysms: a retrospective review of 355 patients. *Neurosurgery.* 1996;38:837–895.
33. Le Roux P, Winn HR. The poor grade aneurysm patient. In: Salcman M, ed. *Current Techniques in Neurosurgery.* Philadelphia: Current Medicine, 1993;10.1–10.28.
34. Le Roux P, Elliott JP, Newell DW, Grady MS, Winn HR. Predicting outcome in poor grade subarachnoid hemorrhage: a retrospective review of 159 aggressively managed patients. *J Neurosurg.* In press.
35. Le Roux PD, Dailey AT, Newell DW, Grady MS, Winn HR. Emergent aneurysm clipping without angiography in the moribund patient with intracerebral hemorrhage: the use of infusion computed tomography scans. *Neurosurgery* 1993;33:189–197.
36. Origitano TC, Wascher TM, Reichman OH, Anderson DE. Sustained increased cerebral blood flow with prophylactic hypertensive hypervolemic hemodilution (Triple-H therapy) after subarachnoid hemorrhage. *Neurosurgery* 1990;27: 729–740.
37. Findlay JM, MacDonald RL, Weir BKA, Grace MGA. Surgical manipulation of primate cerebral arteries in established vasospasm. *J Neurosurg* 1991;75:425–532.
38. MacDonald RL, Wallace MC, Coyne TJ. The effect of surgery on the severity of vasospasm. *J Neurosurg* 1994;80:433–439.
39. Newell DW, Eskridge JM, Mayberg MR, Grady MS, Winn HR. Angioplasty for the treatment of symptomatic vasospasm following subarachnoid hemorrhage. *J Neurosurgery* 1989;71:654–660.
40. Le Roux P, Mayberg M. Management of vasospasm: angioplasty. In: Ratcheson R, Wirth F, eds. *Ruptured Cerebral Aneurysms: Perioperative Management.* Baltimore: Williams and Wilkins, 1994;155–167.
41. Le Roux PD, Newell DW, Eskridge J, Mayberg MR, Winn HR. Severe symptomatic vasospasm: the role of immediate postoperative angioplasty. *J Neurosurg* 1994;80: 224–229.
42. Poletti CE. A temporal approach to anterior communicating artery aneurysms. *J Neurosurg* 1989;71:144–146.
43. Keogh AJ, Sharma RR, Vanner GK. The anterior interhemispheric trephine approach to anteriro midline aneurysms: results of treatment in 72 consecutive patients. *Br J Neurosurg* 1993;7:5–12.
44. Yasui N, Nathal E, Fujiwara H, Suzuki A, Ohta H. The basal interhemispheric approaches for acute anterior communicating artery aneurysms. *Acta Neurochir* 1991;118:91–97.
45. Jane JA, Park TS, Pobereskin LH, Winn HR, Butler AB. The supraorbital approach: technical note. *Neurosurgery* 1982;11:537–542.
46. Sekhar LN, Kalia KK, Yonas H, Wright DC, Ching H. Cranial base approaches to intracranial aneurysms in the subarachnoid space. *Neurosurgery* 1994;35:472–483.
47. Origitano TC, Anderson DE, Tarassoli Y, Reichman OH, Al-Mefty O. Skull base approaches to complex cerebral aneurysms. *Surg Neurol* 1993;40:339–346.
48. Tsutsumi K, Shiokawa Y, Sakai T, Aoki N, Kubota M, Saito I. Venous infarction following interhemispheric approach in patients with acute subarachnoid hemorrhage. *J Neurosurg* 1991;74;715–719.
49. Diraz A, Kobayashi S, Toriyama T, Ohsawa M, Hokoma M, Kitazama K. Surgical approaches to the anterior communicating artery aneurysm and their results. *Neurol Res* 1993;15:273–280.

50. Samson DS, Batjer HH. Aneurysms of the anterior communicating artery. In: Samson D, Batjer HH, eds. *Intracranial Aneurysm Surgery: Techniques.* New York: Futura, 1990;7–120

51. Sundt TM. Anterior communicating artery. In: Sundt TM, ed. *Surgical Technique for Saccular and Giant Intracranial Aneurysms.* Baltimore: Williams and Wilkins, 1990;153–172.

52. Ito Z. The microsurgical anterior interhemispheric approach suitable applied to ruptured aneurysms of the anterior communicating artery in the acute stage. *Acta Neurochir* 1982;63:85–99.

53. Yasui N, Suzuki A, Ohta H. Microneurosurgical anterior and basal interhemispheric approaches for lesions in and around the third ventricle. In: Sami M, ed. *Surgery in and around the Brainstem and the Third Ventricle.* Berlin: Springer-Verlag, 1986;39–345.

54. Kempe LC, Vander Ark GD. Anterior communicating artery aneurysms. Gyrus rectus approach. *Neurochirgia* 1971;–70.

55. Yasargil MG, Fox Jl, Ray MW. The operative approach to aneurysms of the anterior communicating artery. In: Krayenbuhl H, ed. *Advances and Technical Standards in Neurosurgery.* vol 2. New York: Springer-Verlag, 1975;113–170.

56. Dernbach PD, Little JR, Jones SC, Ebrahim ZY: Altered cerebral autoregulation and CO_2 reactivity after aneurysmal subarachnoid hemorrhage. *Neurosurgery* 1988;22:822–826.

57. Tenjin H, Hirakawa K, Mizukawa N, Yano I, Ohata T, Uchibori M. Dysautoregulation in patients with ruptured aneurysms: cerebral blood flow measurements obtained during surgery by a temperature-controlled thermoelectrical method. *Neurosurgery* 1988;23:705–709.

58. Klingelhöfer J, Sander D. Doppler CO_2 test as an indicator of cerebral vasoreactivity and prognosis in severe intracranial hemorrhages. *Stroke* 1992;23:962–966.

59. Hitchcock ER, Tsementzis SA, Dow AA. Short and long trem prognosis of patients with a subarachnoid hemorrhage in realtion to intraoperative period of hypotension. *Acta Neurochir* 1984;70:235–241.

60. Giannotta SL, Oppenheimer JH, Levy ML, Zelman V. Management of Intraoperative Rupture of Aneurysm without Hypotension. *Neurosurgery* 1991;28:531–536.

61. Kidooka M, Nakusau Y, Watanabe K, Matsuda M, Handa J. Monitoring of somatosensory evoked potential during aneurysm surgery. *Surg Neurol* 1987;27:69–76.

62. Momma F, Wang AD, Symon L. Effects of arterial occlusion on somatosensory evoked responses in aneurysm surgery. *Surg Neurol* 1987;27:343–352.

63. Mizoi K, Yoshimoto T. Intraoperative monitoring of the somatosensory evoked potentials and cerebral blood flow during aneurysm surgery. *Neurol Med Chir (Tokyo)* 1991;31:318–325.

64. Schramm J, Koht A, Schmidt G, Pechstein U, Taniguchi M, Fahlbusch R. Surgical and electrophysiological observations during clipping of 134 aneurysms with evoked potential monitoring. *Neurosurgery* 1990; 26:61–70.

65. Batjer H, Samson D. Intraoperative aneurysmal rupture: incidence, outcome and suggestions for surgical management. *Neurosurgery* 1986; 18:701–707.

66. Sano K. A multipurpose all-angle clip applier for aneurysm surgery. Technical note. *J Neurosurg* 1980;53:260–261.

67. Fujita S, Kawaguchi T, Shose Y. Blade deviated fenestrated clips for anterior communicating artery aneurysms. *Surg Neurol* 1993;39: 204–209.

68. Sundt TM, Whisnant JP. Subarachnoid hemorrhage from intracranial aneurysms. Surgical management and natural history of disease. *N Engl J Med* 1978;299:116–122.

69. Ljunggren B, Saveland H, Brandt L. Causes of unfavorable outcome after early aneurysm operation. *Neurosurgery* 1983;13:629–633.

70. Schramm J, Cedzich C: Outcome and management of intraoperative aneurysm rupture. *Surg Neurol* 1993;40:26–30.

71. Drake CG, Friedman AH, Peerless SJ. Failed aneurysm surgery. *J Neurosurg* 1984;61:848–856.

72. Pasqualin A, Battaglia R, Sciencza R, Da Pian R. Italian cooperative study on giant intracranial aneurysms. Results of treatment. *Acta Neurochir Suppl* 1988;42:65–70.

73. Wirth FP, Laws ER Jr, Piepgras D, Scott RM. Surgical treatment of intracranial aneurysms. *Neurosurgery* 1983;12:507–511.

74. Solomon RA, Fink M, Pile-Spellman J. Surgical management of unruptured intracranial aneurysms *J Neurosurg* 1994;80:440–446.

75. Suzuki J, Yoshimoto T, Mizoi K. Preservation of the olfactory tract in bifronatl craniotomy for anterior communicating artery aneurysms and the functional prognosis. *J Neurosurg* 1981;54:342–345.

76. McFadzean RM, Hadley DM, McIlwaine GG. Optochiasmal arachnoiditis following muslin wrapping of ruptured anterior communicating artery aneurysms. *J Neurosurg* 1991;75:393–396.

77. Laiacona M, De Santis A, Barbarotto R, Basso A, Spagnoli D, Capitani E. Neuropsychological follow-up of patients operated for aneurysms of anterior communicating artery. *Cortex* 1989;25:261–273.

78. Stenhouse LM, Knight RG, Longmore BE, Bishara SM. Longterm cognitive deficits in patiernts after surgery of the anterior communicating artery. *J Neurol Neurosurg Psychiatry* 1991;54:909–914.

79. Bornstein RA, Weir BKA, Petruk KC, Disney LB. Neuropsychological function in patients after subarachnoid hemorrhage. *Neurosurgery* 1987;21:651–654.

80. Sonesson B, Ljunggren B, Saveland H, Brandt L. Cognition and adjustment after late and early operation for ruptured aneurysms *Neurosurgery* 1987;21:279–287.

81. Hutter BO, Gilsbach JM. Cognitive deficits after rupture and early repair of anterior communicating artery aneurysms. *Acta Neurochir* 1992;116:6–13.

82. Irle E, Wowra B, Kunert HJ, Hampl J, Kunze S. Memory disturbances following anterior communicating artery aneurysm rupture. *Ann Neurol* 1992;31:473–480.

83. Logue V, Durward M, Pratt RTC. The quality of survival after rupture of an anterior cerebral aneurysm. *Br J Psychiatry* 1968;114:137–160.

84. Storey PB. Brain damage and personality after subarachnoid hemorrhage *Br J Psychiatry* 1970;117:129–142.

85. Sengupta RP, Chiu JSP, Brierly H. Quality of survival following direct surgery for anterior communicating artery aneurysms. *J Neurosurg* 1975;43:58–64.

86. Le Roux P, Elliott JP, Downey L, Newell DW, Grady MS, Mayberg MR, Winn HR. Improved outcome following rupture of anterior circulation aneurysms: a retrospective 10 year review of 224 good grade patients. *J Neurosurg* 1995;83:394–402.

Cerebrovascular Disease, edited by H. Hunt Batjer.
Lippincott-Raven Publishers, Philadelphia © 1997.

CHAPTER 82

Distal Anterior Cerebral Artery Aneurysms

Michael A. Murphy and H. Hunt Batjer

GENERAL BACKGROUND

Distal anterior cerebral artery (DACA) aneurysms are uncommon, composing 2.1–9.2% of large aneurysm series (1–6). They have several unique features and are treated through various surgical approaches based on their individual anatomy and location.

DACA aneurysms are diverse in etiology and may be mycotic, tumorous, traumatic, or "congenital" in origin. The most common site of bacterial aneurysm formation is distally along cerebral vessels, with the middle cerebral artery being the most frequent, followed by the anterior cerebral artery (ACA) (7). The aneurysms may or may not be saccular and have an irregular angiographic outline with thin friable walls. They arise from the deposition of emboli in vessel walls, invoking an inflammatory response with polymorphonuclear leukocytic infiltration and later, loss of intima, and destruction of elastic tissue are characteristic findings. Importantly, the inflammatory process often involves a large percentage of the wall circumference; this finding carries obvious therapeutic implications as direct clipping of the aneurysm is rarely possible. These emboli usually originate from bacterial vegetations in the heart. Tumorous aneurysms arise from emboli from atrial myxomas. Traumatic aneurysms are rare lesions that may occur on the distal pericallosal artery in association with closed head injuries due to the production of shearing forces at the level of the inferior margin of the falx.

The DACAs are the second most common site for multiple aneurysms (after paraclinoidal carotid aneurysms). The incidence of multiplicity is 25–50% in several large series (5,8,9). The other aneurysms associated with multiplicity most commonly occur at the middle cerebral and internal carotid artery bifurcations (7) and have significant implications in determining which aneurysm has bled and which

operative approach should be used. Several vascular anomalies have been associated with DACA aneurysms (10–14). These include azygous A2, triplication of A2 segment, bihemispheral A2, and vascular malformations (presumably from hemodynamic changes). Finally, DACA aneurysms are often small and broad-based with many ruptured aneurysms being less than 5 mm in diameter (6,9,15). Giant aneurysms in this region are very rare (14,16–18).

PERTINENT NEUROLOGIC AND VASCULAR ANATOMY

The anterior cerebral arteries (ACAs), after being connected by the anterior communicating artery, ascend anterior to the lamina terminalis in the interhemispheric fissure between the medial aspect of the frontal lobes. They then curve around the genu of the corpus callosum, where they divide into the callosomarginal arteries, which ascend around the cingulate sulcus, and pericallosal (true continuation of the ACA) arteries, which pass over the body of the corpus callosum to anastomose with the splenial branches of the posterior cerebral arteries (19).

The DACAs have been subdivided into four segments, A2–A5. A2 refers to that part of the artery from the anterior communicating artery to the junction of the rostrum and genu of the corpus callosum, with the orbitofrontal and frontopolar arteries arising from this segment as well as several small unnamed orbital branches proximally. A3 extends from that point around the genu of the corpus callosum to a point where the artery turns sharply posterior above the genu, and the callosomarginal arise from this segment. A4 extends to a point bisected by the coronal suture. A5 extends distally to the anastomosis with the splenial arteries (19) (Fig. 1).

Saccular aneurysms most commonly arise from the junction of the callosomarginal and pericallosal arteries, and less commonly from the orbitofrontal and frontopolar arteries. Aneurysms occurring distal to the origin of the callosomarginal and pericallosal arteries are uncommon and may occur unrelated to branching points. Under such circumstances,

M. A. Murphy: Department of Neurological Surgery, University of Texas, Southwestern Medical Center, Dallas, Texas 75235.

H. H. Batjer: Division of Neurosurgery, Northwestern University Medical School, Chicago, Illinois 60611.

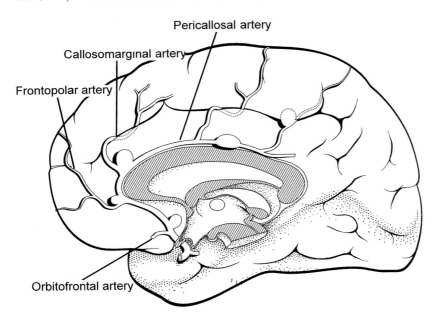

FIG. 1. Main branches of the distal anterior cerebral artery involved with aneurysms.

a diagnosis of mycotic or traumatic aneurysms should be considered (20). In the case of the latter, the traumatic incident does not have to be major (21).

GENERAL SURGICAL PRINCIPLES AND STRATEGIES

DACA aneurysms may present in one of three ways. First, the aneurysm may rupture, producing a subarachnoid, intracerebral (particularly if the aneurysm is adherent to the adjacent cingulate gyrus), or intraventricular hemorrhage. The subarachnoid hemorrhage (SAH) may be local or diffuse, but in either case the computed tomography (CT) scan demonstrates a predominance of blood in the interhemispheric fissure. Focal intracerebral hemorrhage may produce memory deficits or mutism, or, if occurring distally, a monoparesis. Second, they may be diagnosed as an incidental finding on an angiogram of a patient who has had a SAH from another aneurysm, as indicated by the location of the hemorrhage and/or local spasm. In some cases, we prefer to secure the DACA aneurysm in the same operation. Therefore, the operative position, skin incision, and craniotomy should be fashioned accordingly. However, if the patient has a poor clinical grade or it is difficult to achieve satisfactory brain relaxation, then only the ruptured aneurysm should be secured, particularly if a separate craniotomy is required for the DACA aneurysm. If these patients develop vasospasm, it should be treated aggressively with volume expansion, hypertension, and angioplasty if necessary (assuming the spasm is remote from the DACA), as the risk of the unsecured aneurysm rupturing with hyperdynamic therapy is minimal (22,23). Third, an aneurysm may be an incidental finding in the investigation of neurologic symptoms. These aneurysms are often small, and despite the fact that in other areas small

aneurysms may be watched due to their size (<5 mm), we would advise against that in this area unless surgery is contraindicated due to the large number of hemorrhages we have seen from small lesions at this site. These aneurysms have been associated with a worse prognosis than other anterior circulation aneurysms in the past (4,24), although improvement in surgical outcome has been noted with modern anesthesia and microsurgical techniques (25,26). Four-vessel angiography should be performed in all patients and carefully studied for the presence of other aneurysms. Magnetic resonance imaging (MRI) may also be useful in determining the relationship of the dome of the aneurysm to the cingulate gyrus.

Patients who present in good clinical grade are usually operated on within 24 hours of admission to our center. Patients in poor grade are medically treated until their neurologic condition has improved. The exception to this general rule is the presence of an intracerebral hemorrhage, which may be contributing to the patient's altered conscious state. In this case the hematoma should be evacuated and the aneurysm secured. Intraventricular hemorrhage may require ventricular drainage, as may significant hydrocephalus.

Preoperatively the patient is kept normovolemic and normotensive. A central venous catheter is used to monitor the central venous pressure (CVP), with the aim of 10–12 torr, using crystalloid and/or colloidal solutions. A mild dilutional anemia is thus usually produced. Corticosteroids and anticonvulsants are given prophylactically and antibiotics administered upon call to the operating room.

ANESTHETIC CONSIDERATIONS

Anesthesia is similar to that employed for other aneurysms. Mannitol, hyperventilation, and cerebrospinal fluid (CSF) drainage (via ventriculostomy at our center) are used for brain relaxation. If temporary occlusion is anticipated we prefer to utilize cerebral protection in the form of hypothermia and pharmacologically induced burst suppression. Patients are cooled to approximately 32°C and electroencephalographic activity is monitored bilaterally. In the setting of normovolemia and normotension, sodium thiopental, propofol, or etomidate is titrated to maintain burst suppression during temporary occlusion.

PATIENT POSITIONING

The approach chosen depends on the location of the DACA aneurysm. If a patient has multiple aneurysms and the surgeon intends to secure all aneurysms, then the position of the patient, skin incision, and craniotomy are based on consideration of the location of the other aneurysms. As these are often middle cerebral or internal carotid artery aneurysms, a separate craniotomy is required. The ruptured aneurysm has first priority and is secured first. The head is then repositioned for treatment of the secondary aneurysms.

DACA aneurysms arising from the proximal 1.5 cm of the A2 can be approached either through a pterional or interhemispheric approach, whereas those distal to this point are best approached interhemispherically, with the position of the patient and craniotomy depending on the exact location of the aneurysm. In the pterional approach the side chosen should be ipsilateral to the aneurysm unless the multiple aneurysm circumstance mandates an alternative approach.

Pterional Approach

Scalp and Bony Exposure

This approach is reserved for aneurysms arising from the junction of the ACA and the orbitofrontal arteries. The patient's head is placed in the Mayfield head fixation system with the head rotated about 60° and extended to bring the malar eminence uppermost. Flexion of the head toward the nonoperative shoulder brings the floor of the frontal fossa perpendicular to the long axis of the body.

The skin incision, which lies immediately behind the hairline, extends superiorly from the zygomatic process 1 cm anterior to the tragus, curving gently anteriorly to the midline. A myocutaneous flap is performed and held in position with fish hooks. Burr holes are placed over the "key hole," temporal squamous bone, and posterior and inferior to the superior temporal line, and a free bone flap elevated. This flap is carried more anteriorly than the standard pterional craniotomy, with the flap as close as possible to the floor of the anterior cranial fossa. The frontal sinus may be entered and, if so, should be obliterated. The rongeurs and the cutting drill are used to remove the lateral aspect of the sphenoidal wing and the inner table of the exposed frontal bone inferiorly. The dura is then opened in a curvilinear fashion based on the sphenoidal wing. The frontal horn of the lateral ventricle is then cannulated (if necessary, for brain relaxation) using an equilateral right triangle with sides of 2.5 cm constructed with one edge at the sphenoidal ridge and the other

on the Sylvian fissure passing the catheter perpendicular to the cortex (27).

Microsurgical Dissection and Principles

The microscope is then brought in and self-retaining retractor is introduced along the line of the sphenoidal wing, and the frontal lobe is gently elevated until the optic nerve is identified. The arachnoid over the nerve, medial aspect of the Sylvian fissure, carotid cistern, and prechiasmatic cistern are opened in a lateral-to-medial direction using sharp dissection, and the CSF is aspirated. Further retraction of the frontal lobe and sharp dissection separates the gyrus rectus from the optic nerve until the ipsilateral A1 is seen crossing the nerve. The recurrent artery of Heubner may be identified lying posterosuperiorly to the A1. Dissection is then carried medially along the anteroinferior aspect of the A1 segment, avoiding the posteriorly placed medial lenticulostriate vessels. This dissection leads to the interhemispheric fissure and anterior communicating artery. As the A1 leaves the optic nerve/chiasm to enter the interhemispheric fissure, the surgeon continues his dissection above the optic chiasm to identify the contralateral A1 as it crosses the contralateral optic nerve. With this dissection, the arachnoidal adhesions between the contralateral gyrus rectus and optic nerve are divided. Proximal control is thus obtained (Fig. 2A).

The ipsilateral gyrus rectus is then resected in a subpial fashion and this tissue removal is carried more anterosuperiorly than for an anterior communicating artery aneurysm so as to reveal the distal A2 segment, orbitofrontal artery (rarely seen on angiogram), and the aneurysm. The contralateral A2 is identified prior to clipping in order to avoid it being trapped in the ends of the clip blade. The pia-arachnoid is then divided over the ipsilateral A1/2 junction, and the remainder of the anterior communicating artery and the origin of the recurrent artery of Heubner are all identified. The proximal A2 is then dissected, leading to the orbitofrontal branch and the neck of the aneurysm. The A2 is then dissected distally to the aneurysm, yielding both proximal and distal control (Fig. 2B). The aneurysm neck is dissected free and the aneurysm clipped. Aneurysms with narrow necks may be clipped perpendicular to the parent artery. However, if the neck is broad-based, then it should be clipped parallel to the artery, as perpendicular clipping may produce a stenosis of the parent artery (Fig. 2C). In large or broad-based aneurysms temporary occlusion may be necessary, although these are very rare.

Interhemispheric Approach

Scalp and Bony Exposure

This approach is used for all aneurysms arising distal to the frontopolar branches. The skin incision and craniotomy depend on the location of the aneurysm. The aneurysm should be approached from the right, unless otherwise indi-

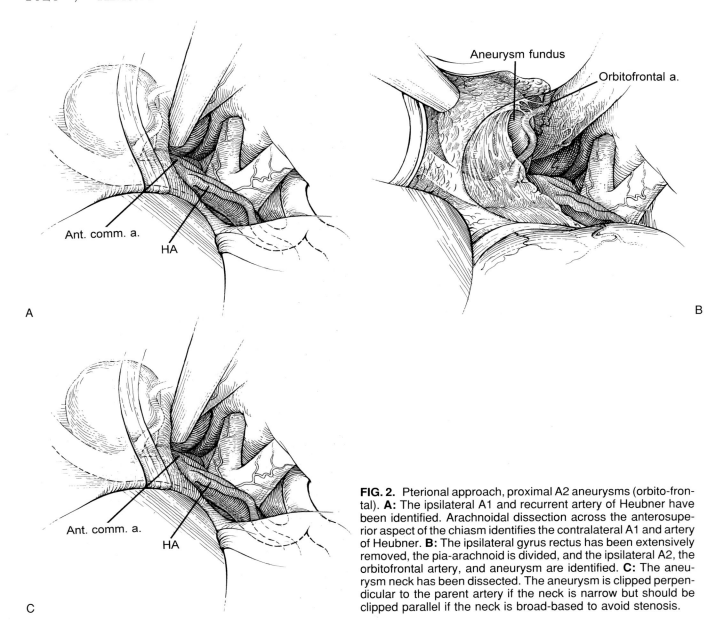

FIG. 2. Pterional approach, proximal A2 aneurysms (orbito-frontal). **A:** The ipsilateral A1 and recurrent artery of Heubner have been identified. Arachnoidal dissection across the anterosuperior aspect of the chiasm identifies the contralateral A1 and artery of Heubner. **B:** The ipsilateral gyrus rectus has been extensively removed, the pia-arachnoid is divided, and the ipsilateral A2, the orbitofrontal artery, and aneurysm are identified. **C:** The aneurysm neck has been dissected. The aneurysm is clipped perpendicular to the parent artery if the neck is narrow but should be clipped parallel if the neck is broad-based to avoid stenosis.

cated, as with multiple aneurysms or if it is a large aneurysm with the dome buried in the right cingulate gyrus in which retraction of that gyrus may result in aneurysm rupture. The interhemispheric approach may be difficult in acute aneurysm surgery, as the callosal cistern is small and often only minimal amounts of CSF are present; therefore we would recommend a ventriculostomy prior to microsurgical dissection. If the aneurysm arises from a frontopolar or callosomarginal artery, which is inferior to the genu of the corpus callosum, a modified bicoronal skin incision with a parasagittal craniotomy centered one third of the way between the nasion and bregma, and crossing the midline, should be performed. The head is placed in the Mayfield head holder in the supine position in 15° of extension. For those aneurysms in which the callosomarginal artery originates at the level of the genu,

the head is placed in the neutral position and the craniotomy is placed midway between the nasion and bregma. A horseshoe skin incision crossing the midline is used. If the aneurysm is more distally located, a similar skin incision is used, with the position of the craniotomy depending on the exact location of the aneurysm, and draining veins as indicated by the preoperative angiogram. In these cases the patient's head is positioned in 15° of flexion to optimize the approach for the seated surgeon. The size of the craniotomy flap should be generous as unexpected draining veins may limit interhemispheric access.

Microsurgical Dissection and Principles

After the craniotomy has been performed the dural flap is hinged on the superior sagittal sinus. The flap should be taken right up to the sinus and reflected without occluding the sinus. An area of access between bridging veins is then identified and the microscope is positioned. A self-retaining retractor is introduced and the frontal lobe retracted laterally. The surgeon needs to be careful not to stretch bridging veins such that they become occluded, which can lead to ischemia/infarction. Arachnoidal adhesions between the falx and medial frontal lobes are divided as the retraction is deepened. The cingulate gyri may be adherent and must be dissected free of one another. If particularly adherent, they may be mistaken for the corpus callosum, with the callosomarginal being mistaken for the pericallosal arteries. Dissection in this area should be done sharply and carefully as the aneurysm may be embedded in one or both cingulate gyri (Fig. 3A). Many small veins are located here, and are coagulated

and divided. If there is a hematoma in the cingulate gyrus it may be partially decompressed, providing further brain relaxation and access to the aneurysm during this maneuver. A layer of pia-arachnoid should be separating the surgeon from the dome of the aneurysm, but extreme care should be used, as vascular control is not yet accomplished.

The pericallosal arteries are seen deep to the transverse arachnoidal fibers of the callosal cistern, which are divided. Often only one pericallosal artery is initially seen, particularly in the presence of hydrocephalus, but both need to be dissected free, as it is often difficult to determine which is the ipsilateral and which is the contralateral unless both are seen. In an interhemispheric approach the distal vessels are located first and followed proximally to the aneurysm. This differs from the usual approach to aneurysm surgery, where

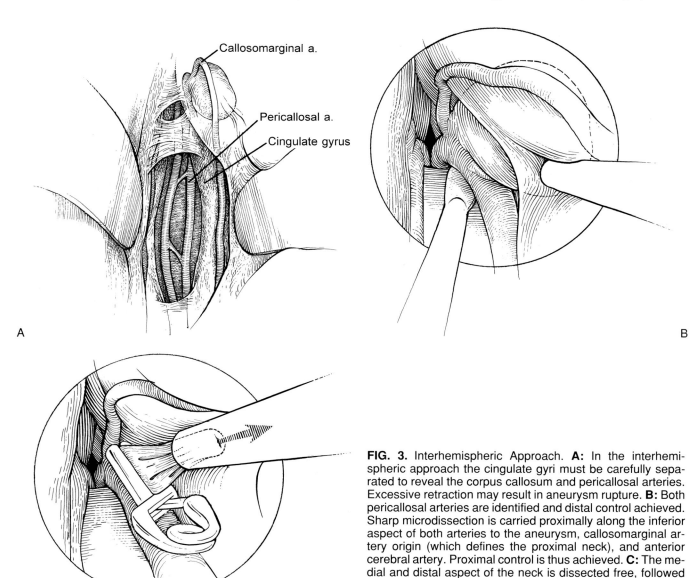

FIG. 3. Interhemispheric Approach. A: In the interhemispheric approach the cingulate gyri must be carefully separated to reveal the corpus callosum and pericallosal arteries. Excessive retraction may result in aneurysm rupture. B: Both pericallosal arteries are identified and distal control achieved. Sharp microdissection is carried proximally along the inferior aspect of both arteries to the aneurysm, callosomarginal artery origin (which defines the proximal neck), and anterior cerebral artery. Proximal control is thus achieved. C: The medial and distal aspect of the neck is dissected free, followed by the lateral aspect. The aneurysm is then clipped parallel to the pericallosal artery, as perpendicular clipping may result in stenosis due to the broad neck of these aneurysms. Complex aneurysms may require temporary occlusion.

proximal control is obtained first. Aneurysms arising at the callosomarginal artery origin at the genu arise in the crotch between the callosomarginal and pericallosal arteries. Therefore, in order to obtain proximal control, dissection should be carried along the posterior aspect of the pericallosal artery to the anterior cerebral artery (Fig. 3B). Once proximal control has been obtained, attention should be turned to the proximal neck of the aneurysm, which is dissected free of the callosomarginal artery. The distal neck is then dissected. Temporary occlusion of the anterior cerebral, callosomarginal, and pericallosal arteries is used if necessary. Occlusion of the anterior cerebral artery alone may soften the aneurysm, but rupture will result in significant bleeding without distal control, as collateral flow is robust. As mentioned previously, aneurysms in this area are often small and broad-based; therefore the clip, where possible, should be placed parallel to the parent artery, as perpendicular clip placement may produce a stenosis in the pericallosal artery or shearing of the neck. The lateral aspect of the aneurysm neck should be dissected free with parallel clip placement as to avoid trapping the callosomarginal artery in the clip blades (Fig. 3C).

Modifications of the above technique have been described in the literature. Resection of part of the anterior 2.5 cm of the genu of the corpus callosum to provide exposure of the anterior cerebral artery and proximal control has been advocated (20,28). A transfalcine approach, approaching a left callosomarginal artery from the right, has also been described, but in our opinion it offers no advantage over the above-described approaches (29).

COMPLICATIONS AND THEIR MANAGEMENT

Specific operative complications can be divided into two groups with the interhemispheric operation: approach and clipping. With the approach, the bridging veins may be damaged, which may result in venous infarction and/or hemorrhage, and excessive retraction may lead to ischemia in the cingulate gyrus, which may produce memory problems and/or akinetic mutism. In the latter case, the complications are usually only transient. Careful clip placement is important to avoid stenosis of the parent artery and neurologic deficit, particularly if the aneurysm is not clipped along the long axis of the parent artery.

The extravasated blood associated with a hemorrhage from a DACA aneurysm is often confined to the interhemispheric fissure, producing focal vasospasm. Prophylactic removal of clot at the time of the operation, if within 48 hours of hemorrhage, may be of benefit. This may be done either by suction or by the injection of thrombolytic agents such as tissue-type plasminogen activator (t-PA) substance, although the latter is still experimental. Postoperatively, a combination of hypervolemia and hypertensive therapy is used if symptomatic vasospasm develops. If symptoms are unresponsive to these measures, then intraarterial injection

of papaverine or angioplasty may be used, although success may be limited due to the distal location of the vessels. Fortunately, collateral flow to the distal anterior cerebral territory is usually excellent, minimizing the long-term consequences of symptomatic ischemia. Infarction, should it develop and be localized to this territory, is usually not as disabling as that from more proximal locations, and the leg deficits tend to improve over time.

Intraoperative ruptures have been reported with varying frequency with DACA aneurysms in the literature (1,6,15,24,25). In the authors' opinion, the use of sharp dissection minimizes the risk of rupture, and when it does occur it is easier to manage. Blunt dissection often results in a rent in the proximal aneurysm sac, which may extend into the neck. Bleeding from sharp dissection, on the other hand, produces only small rents and may be managed with coagulation or tamponading. Whichever method is used, in the authors' opinion, the definitive treatment of intraoperative rupture is early temporary occlusion, so as to avoid damage to adjacent structures, including the parent artery, and allow for definitive clipping without compromise.

As mentioned previously, DACA aneurysms are often small and broad-based. Therefore suction aspiration or blunt dissection may result in serious neck shearing, placing the parent vessel at risk. This may be managed with either a right angle fenestrated clip (if some neck remains) or a Sundt encircling clip placed around the parent artery. If these methods cannot be used without producing significant stenosis, then a trapping procedure sparing the callosomarginal artery can be performed. There is usually a rich collateral supply to the territories supplied by the DACA that can be evaluated by removing the distal temporary clip and assessing the back bleeding.

OVERVIEW

DACA aneurysms are not an infrequent cause of subarachnoid hemorrhage (SAH) and more particularly are not an uncommon incidental finding in patients who have had an SAH from aneurysm rupture at another site. Often they are small lesions that in other locations would be observed but at this site are prone to hemorrhage. The operative approach is dependent on the location of the aneurysm along the DACA. These lesions should be definitively clipped but in cases of traumatic shearing or with mycotic aneurysm on the DACA, trapping is an acceptable alternative due to the rich collateral supply.

REFERENCES

1. Hernesniemi J, Tapaninacho A, Vapalahti M, Niskanen M, Kari A, Luukkonen M. Saccular aneurysms of the distal anterior cerebral artery and its branches. *Neurosurgery* 1992;31:994–999.
2. Laitinen L, Snellman A. Aneurysms of the pericallosal artery. A study of 14 cases verified angiographically and treated mainly by direct surgical attack. *J Neurosurg* 1968;17:447–459.

3. McKissock W, Paine KWE, Walsh LS. An analysis of the results of treatment of ruptured intracranial aneurysms. Report of 772 consecutive cases. *J Neurosurg* 1960;17:62–76.

4. Nishioka H. Report on the cooperative study of intracranial aneurysms and subarachnoid hemorrhage. 1. Evaluation of the conservative management of ruptured aneurysms. *J Neurosurg* 1966;25:574–592.

5. Ohno K, Monma S, Suzuki R, Masaoka H, Matsushima Y, Hirakewa K. Saccular aneurysms of the distal anterior cerebral artery. *Neurosurgery* 1990;27:908–913.

6. Yasargil MG, Carter LP. Saccular aneurysm of the distal anterior cerebral artery. *J Neurosurg* 1974;39:218–223.

7. Samson DS, Batjer HH. Aneurysms of the anterior cerebral artery. In: Samson DS, Batjer HH: *Intracranial Aneurysm Surgery: Techniques.* Mount Kisco, NY: Futura, 1990;108–120.

8. Weir B. Specific sites and results of series: distal anterior cerebral aneurysms. In: Weir B, ed. *Aneurysms Affecting the Nervous System.* Baltimore: Williams and Wilkins, 1987;464–468.

9. Yasargil MG. Anterior cerebral and anterior communicating artery aneurysms. In: Yasargil MG. *Microneurosurgery.* Vol 2. Stuttgart: Thieme Verlag, 1984;224–231.

10. Baptista AG. Studies on the arteries of the brain. 2. The anterior cerebral artery: some anatomic features and their clinical implications. *Neurology* 1963;13:825–835.

11. Huber P, Braun J, Hirschmann D, Agyeman JF. Incidence of berry aneurysm of unpaired pericallosal artery: Angiographic study. *Neuroradiology* 1980;19:143–147.

12. LeMay M, Gooding CA. The clinical significance of the azygous anterior cerebral artery. *Am J Roetgenol Radium Ther Nucl Med* 1966;98:602–610.

13. Nardi PV, Esposito S, Greco R, Massari A, Patricolo A. Aneurysm of the azygous anterior cerebral artery. Report of two cases treated by surgery. *J Neurosurg Sci* 1990;34:17–20.

14. Preul M, Tampieri D, LeBlanc R. Giant aneurysm of the distal anterior cerebral artery: associated with an anterior communicating artery aneurysm and a dural arteriovenous fistula. *Surg Neurol* 1992;38:347–352.

15. Shucart W. Distal anterior cerebral artery aneurysms. In: Apuzzo M, ed. *Brain Surgery: Complications Avoidance and Management.* New York: Churchill-Livingstone, 1993;1035–1040.

16. Hashizuma K, Nukui H, Horikoshi T, Kanako M, Fukamachi A. Giant aneurysm of the azygos anterior cerebral artery associated with acute subdural hematoma. Case Report. *Neurol Med Chir (Tokyo)* 1992;32:693–697.

17. Maiuri F, Corriero G, D'Amico L, Somonetti L. Giant aneurysm of pericallosal artery. *Neurosurgery* 1990;26:703–706.

18. Pozzati E, Nuzzo G, Gaist G. Giant aneurysm of the pericallosal artery. Case Report. *J Neurosurg* 1982;57:566–569.

19. Perlmutter D, Rhoton AL. Microsurgical anatomy of the distal anterior cerebral artery. *J Neurosurg* 1978;49:204–228.

20. Dickey PS, Bloomgarden GM, Arkins TJ, Spencer DD. Partial callosal resection for pericallosal aneurysms. *Neurosurgery* 1992;30:136–137

21. Senegor M. Traumatic pericallosal aneurysm in a patient with no major trauma. Case Report. *J Neurosurg* 1991;75:475–477.

22. Kassell NF, Peerless SJ, Durward QJ, Beck DW, Drake CG, Adams HP. Treatment of ischemic deficits from vasospasm with intravascular volume expansion and induced arterial hypertension. *Neurosurgery* 1982;11:337–343.

23. Swift DM, Solomon RA. Unruptured aneurysms and postoperative volume expansion. *J Neurosurg* 1992;77:908–910.

24. Snyckers FD, Drake CG. Aneurysms of the distal cerebral artery. A report of 24 verified cases. *South Afr Med J* 1973;47:1787–1791.

25. Mann KS, Yue CP, Wong G. Aneurysms of the pericallosal-callosomarginal junction. *Surg Neurol* 1984;21:261–266.

26. Sindou M, Pelissou-Guyotat I, Mertens P, Karavel Y, Athayde AA. Pericallosal aneurysms. *Surg Neurol* 1988;30:434–440.

27. Paine JT, Batjer HH, Samson DS. Intraoperative ventricular puncture. *Neurosurgery* 1988,22:1107–1109.

28. Traynelis VC, Dunker RO. Interhemispheric approach with callosal resection for distal anterior cerebral artery aneurysms. Technical note. *J Neurosurg* 1992;77:481–483.

29. Ellenbogen RG, Scott RM. Transfalcine approach to a callosomarginal artery aneurysm. *Neurosurgery* 1991;29:140–143.

Cerebrovascular Disease, edited by H. Hunt Batjer.
Lippincott-Raven Publishers, Philadelphia © 1997.

CHAPTER 83

Vertebral Aneurysms: Surgical Management

Christopher J. Baker and Robert A. Solomon

GENERAL BACKGROUND

The first clinical description of a vertebral–PICA saccular aneurysm was that of Cruveilhier in 1829. Early operative experiences with these lesions, however, were largely accidental. In 1937, Tonnis inadvertently opened a giant vertebral artery (VA) aneurysm presumed to be a tumor. He was able to control the bleeding by packing the interior of the sac and the patient survived. A few years later, Dandy treated a vertebral aneurysm with vessel ligation by tying off the atlanto-axial portion of the artery. Logue was the first to describe the intracranial ligation of the VA just proximal to fusiform vertebral aneurysms. Routine surgery for vertebral–PICA aneurysms was slow to develop because of the lack of vertebral angiography and the intimate relationship of the vessel to the brainstem and lower cranial nerves. Schwartz in 1948 described the surgical approach of a posterior fossa aneurysm diagnosed by a bloody spinal fluid, not by angiography. Intraoperative rupture was followed by the successful trapping of a small saccular lesion. Rizzoli and Hayes had similarly excised a PICA aneurysm the year before. It was not until 1958 that DeSaussure reported the trapping of two PICA aneurysms diagnosed angiographically. By the mid-1960s, the results of Drake and the microsurgical advances in the region espoused by Rand ushered in the modern age of VA aneurysm surgery.

PERTINENT NEUROLOGIC ANATOMY AND VARIATIONS

The extracranial suboccipital portion of the VA runs around the lateral mass of the atlas in the horizontal groove above the posterior arch of C1. It then turns anterosuperiorly to pierce the atlanto-occipital membrane and enter the dura in the lateral aspect of the foramen magnum about 15 mm

from the midline. The vessel's periosteal sheath is in continuity with the dura and extends intracranially for 4–6 mm.

The intracranial portion of the VA averages 2.5 mm in diameter. Forty percent of the time the left VA is dominant, 30% of the time the right one is dominant, and the remainder of individuals have symmetric vessels (1). Rarely, a VA will be hypoplastic or fenestrated around a lower cranial nerve. In both instances, the chance of aneurysm formation in the vertebral system is greater. The VA enters the perimedullary cistern and moves anteromedially as it courses rostrally along the lateral medulla (Fig. 1). As it reaches the pontomedullary sulcus, it joins the opposite VA anterior to the rostral medulla forming the basilar artery. Lateral medullary, anterior spinal, and posterior inferior cerebellar branches all arise from the VA along its course. The anterior spinal arteries arise symmetrically from the midportion of the vertebral arteries and join in the premedullary cistern.

The posterior inferior cerebellar artery is the largest and most distal branch of the VA. It is a single vessel in 90%, duplicated in 6%, and absent in 4% of cases (1). Its origin is variable but it typically arises 10 mm above the foramen magnum and 15 mm proximal from the origin of the basilar artery in the anterior medullary cistern. It may arise as low as the extracranial vertebral segment or as high as the basilar origin.

PICA can be divided into five segments: anterior medullary, lateral medullary, tonsillomedullary, telovelotonsillar, and cortical (2). The anterior medullary segment begins at the PICA origin and is intimately related to the hypoglossal nerve. The artery passes superior to or through the hypoglossal nerve as it heads posteriorly to form the lateral medullary segment. The lateral medullary segment heads caudally passing around the inferior aspect of the olive and supplying branches to the lateral medulla. The caudal extension, passing between the branches of IX, X, and XI, is the tonsillomedullary segment that loops around the cerebellar tonsil. This caudal loop extends a few millimeters below the tonsil to the foramen magnum in one third of patients. The cranial loop, which follows behind IX, X, and XI, is the teloveloton-

C. J. Baker and R. A. Solomon: Department of Neurosurgery, Columbia University College of Physicians and Surgeons, Columbia-Presbyterian Medical Center, New York, New York 10032.

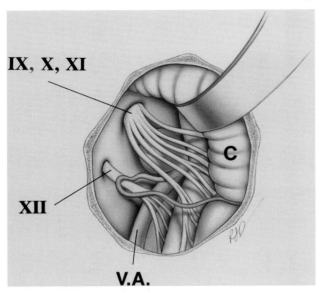

FIG. 1. Relationship of the VA, PICA, and cranial nerves IX–XII as viewed from a lateral suboccipital approach.

sillar segment. As PICA reaches the posterior medullary velum it supplies the choroid plexus of the fourth ventricle and the tonsil. The tonsillomedullary and telovelotonsillar segments supply a number of posterolateral medullary branches to the medulla. The telovelotonsillar segment passes between the tonsil and the vermis to form the cortical segment. Medial branches supply the vermis and lateral branches supply the inferior cerebellar hemispheres. PICA and AICA reciprocally share supply of the cerebellar hemispheres. The size of these vessels is highly variable and rarely equal.

CLINICAL PRESENTATION

Published series of vertebral aneurysms reveal a clear patient profile for these lesions. There is roughly a 2 : 1 ratio of females to males with presentation closely clustered between 45 and 55 years of age (1–10). Most vertebral aneurysms reaching medical attention are less than 1 cm in size (2,5,10). The left VA is more commonly dominant with a greater blood flow than the right vertebral. Hudgins et al (2) found more left-sided saccular vertebral–PICA aneurysms supporting a flow-related aneurysm etiology. In contrast, series of Andoh and Kitanaka contained more right-sided vertebral aneurysms (8,10). Most series demonstrate a correlation between the dominant VA and aneurysm formation.

VA aneurysms present with subarachnoid hemorrhage in 75–90% of cases (6,7,10). The specific clinical signs and symptoms that accompany this event referrable to the posterior fossa are few. In good-grade patients, occipital headaches and acute neck stiffness from meningismus can be localizing. A higher proportion of vertebral aneurysms present with acute hydrocephalus secondary to IIIrd and IVth

ventricular blood. Direct injury to the brainstem and lower cranial nerves with subarachnoid hemorrhage (SAH) localize the lesion in a minority of cases. There are many reports of limb dysesthesias, Horner's syndrome, VIth nerve palsy, dysarthria, and even cardiac arrest after medullary injury following aneurysm rupture.

The presentation of a VA aneurysm depends to some extent on the type of lesion. Vertebral aneurysms are roughly 60% saccular, 20% fusiform, and 20% dissecting in nature (3,10). In contrast to the more common saccular lesions, fusiform aneurysms are less likely to rupture and are seen in atherosclerotic populations. These lesions more often present as large aneurysms with signs of brainstem compression (10). Dissecting aneurysms occur in a slightly younger population because of a subset of dissections that are traumatic in etiology. Brainstem infarction is seen in 30% of these lesions because of sacrifice of perforating vessels (8).

A CT scan of a suspected SAH patient correctly diagnoses a posterior fossa aneurysm with about 90% sensitivity (Fig. 2) (6,10). Blood is seen surrounding the medulla or in the cerebellopontine angle. It may also track up to the basilar cisterns. Intraventricular blood is common, predominantly in the fourth and third ventricle (4). The CT scan also allows the diagnosis of acute obstructive hydrocephalus. The sensitivity of CT scan in this area is somewhat impaired by bony artifact. If suspicion is high, a lumbar puncture can diagnose aneurysmal rupture or venous perimesencephalic rupture.

VA aneurysms are diagnosed with conventional angiography. Unfortunately, aneurysms in this location have an unusual number of negative initial angiograms (Fig. 2). Any clinical suspicion necessitates repeat angiogram utilizing bilateral vertebral injections and multiple views. Angiography provides vital information about the size, shape, and anatomic location of the aneurysm in question. Multiple views usually allow differentiation between saccular, fusiform, and dissecting lesions based on morphology. At surgery, aneurysms felt to be saccular angiographically can actually be fusiform or dissecting lesions. Dissecting aneurysms are often fusiform in shape but can be distinguished from true fusiform lesions. Fusiform dilatation associated with proximal or distal narrowing ("pearl and string sign") suggests a dissecting aneurysm. An intraluminal linear defect, contrast retention, or a double lumen all also suggest an aneurysmal dissection.

Magnetic resonance imaging (MRI) scans are being obtained increasingly frequently, particularly in unruptured symptomatic individuals with aneurysms. Saccular aneurysms show up on T1-weighted images as dilated flow voids adjacent to the VA. Partially thrombosed saccular aneurysms can also be well defined along with the aneurysms relationship to other brainstem structures. Extensive enlarged flow voids of the VA indicate a fusiform lesion. MRI scans can also be useful in differentiating between fusiform and dissecting intracranial vertebral lesions. A hyperintense signal within the vessel that enhances with gadolinium on T1-weighted imaging is the characteristic finding in vertebral

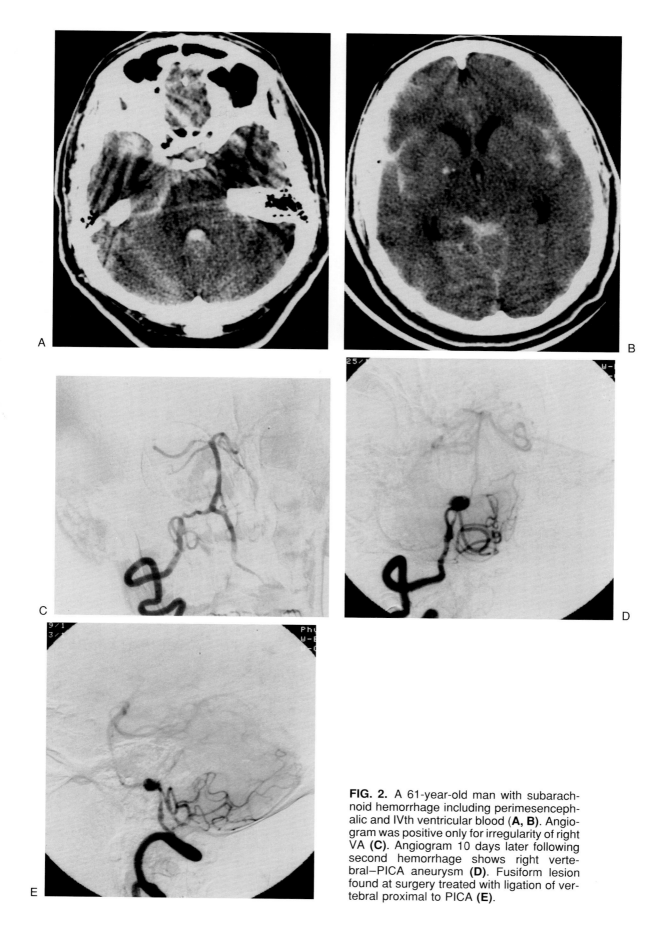

FIG. 2. A 61-year-old man with subarachnoid hemorrhage including perimesencephalic and IVth ventricular blood (**A, B**). Angiogram was positive only for irregularity of right VA (**C**). Angiogram 10 days later following second hemorrhage shows right vertebral–PICA aneurysm (**D**). Fusiform lesion found at surgery treated with ligation of vertebral proximal to PICA (**E**).

dissections. The dissection may also present as an isointense (acute) or hyperintense (chronic) hematoma or thickening of the vessel wall (11,12). Clear intraluminal hyperintense cords are seen less frequently but are thought to represent the actual intimal flap (13). The lateral medullary infarcts that accompany these lesions can also be seen with MRI. Finally, the rapid advances in MR angiography technology promise to allow these noninvasive methods of aneurysm diagnosis to replace angiography in the near future.

OPERATIVE EXPERIENCE

Direct Clipping

Aneurysms of the VA–PICA complex compose 1–3% of all intracranial aneurysms and 20% of posterior fossa aneurysms (14). Seventy-five percent of the aneurysms in this area arise at the distal wall of the VA–PICA bifurcation. In fact, VA–PICA bifurcation aneurysms are second only to basilar bifurcation aneurysms in frequency in the posterior fossa (15). The remainder of VA region aneurysms consist of distal PICA, VA proper, and VA–BA lesions in descending order of frequency (2,3,5,16,17). There are three distinct types of vertebral–PICA aneurysms: saccular, dissecting, and fusiform. Roughly 60% of lesions are saccular, 20% fusiform atherosclerotic, and 20% dissecting (3,10). The majority of VA–PICA aneurysms are 10 mm or less on presentation (2,17). Less than 5% of lesions are giant aneurysms (2.5 cm) at the time of presentation (3,4,15).

The majority of conservatively treated ruptured posterior fossa aneurysms sustain fatal reruptures within one year (18). Despite this fact, early surgery for vertebral aneurysms lagged behind such surgery for anterior circulation lesions. Reports of the hazards of delaying surgery and increased surgeon comfort in the posterior fossa have largely changed this practice. The rate of early rebleeding in vertebral aneurysms is at least as high as in the anterior circulation. Andoh and Yamaura separately found a rebleed rate of 24%, largely within the first two weeks (3,10). Lang and Herniesnemi found a more conservative rehemorrhage rate in the same time period (4,5). Salcman et al confirmed that perihemorrhage cerebral swelling was not a problem around the brainstem and cranial nerves of the posterior fossa (17).

With the majority of lesions both saccular and less than 10 mm, direct clipping of the aneurysm base is possible in a large number of cases (Fig. 3). Yamaura was able to clip 90% of saccular vertebral aneurysms operated upon (3). Most vertebral aneurysms can be successfully reached via a lateral suboccipital craniectomy. Giant and VA-BA vertebral aneurysms may require a far lateral or retrolabyrinthine presigmoid approach. Direct clipping of saccular lesions results in 80–90% good/excellent outcomes in major series (1,3,4,15–17,19–22). There remains a minority of giant saccular aneurysms and fusiform lesions that cannot be directly clipped. These lesions are either wrapped or treated with proximal ligation with slightly poorer results (3,9,10). Dissecting aneurysms are typically thin-walled, friable, and have no discernible neck. These also frequently require proximal vertebral occlusion.

Proximal Ligation and Trapping

Giant, dissecting, or fusiform VA aneurysms are often unclippable. If this is clear angiographically before surgery, endovascular occlusion of the artery proximal to the lesion is now routinely carried out. Frequently, the decision that an aneurysm is unclippable is made intraoperatively. In these cases, direct clip occlusion of the VA proximal to aneurysm is performed. Ideally, the proximal surgical clip can be placed more precisely at the origin of the aneurysm than vertebral balloon occlusion allows (23). This decreases the likelihood of perforator injury and more consistently alters the flow dynamics in the aneurysm. The PICA can often be saved by clipping the VA distal to it. Salvage of this vessel is not usually possible with endovascular techniques. Occlusion of the VA leads to aneurysm thrombosis in the majority of instances while incurring a small risk of immediate or delayed cerebral ischemia. Proximal ligation is used most commonly for dissecting vertebral aneurysms. Kitanaka found it necessary to proximally occlude 15 of 20 dissecting aneurysms because of unclippable aneurysm necks (8).

Most dissections originate immediately distal to the origin of PICA (8,24). In these patients, proximal clipping of the VA leads to thrombosis of the aneurysm due to near–flow arrest with little risk of rehemorrhage. There is a small risk of embolic complications from the thrombosed vertebral cul-de-sac in these patients (25). Proximal occlusion of VA dissections where the dissection involves PICA do not exclude this vessel from the vertebral circulation. As a result, many of these patients maintain sufficient retrograde PICA flow to hamper thrombosis. These individuals may still be at risk for rehemorrhage (8,25). Batjer suggests that VA dissections which begin proximal to PICA should be treated with trapping procedures to eliminate the risk of rebleeding (26). PICA–PICA revascularization grafts should be considered in those not tolerating PICA or vertebral occlusion. In fact, scattered reports support VA bypasses, when the contralateral artery is inadequate, using radial artery or saphenous vein grafts.

Steinberg and Drake's long-term evaluation of basilar and VA occlusion for unclippable posterior circulation aneurysms provides the best data on this mode of treatment (9). Seventy-two of the 201 patients in the series had vertebral or vertebrobasilar artery aneurysms. The long-term outcome in these patients was good/excellent in 87% of cases. Those presenting with subarachnoid hemorrhage fared better than those with signs of brainstem compression. Acute neurologic deterioration caused by vertebrobasilar ischemia, surgical trauma, or rehemorrhage occurred in only 5.4% of VA ligations. The 3% of individuals suffering from vertebrobasilar

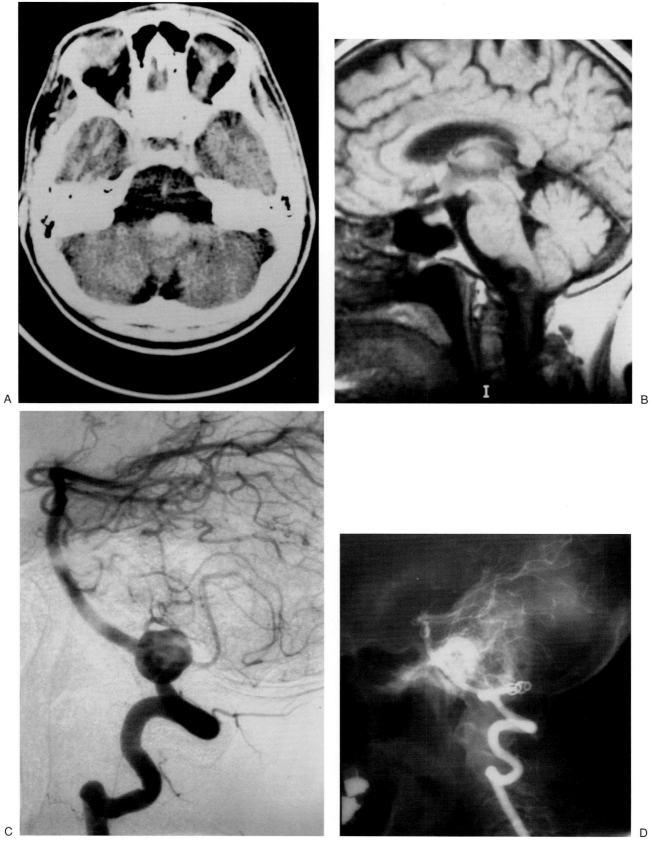

FIG. 3. A 67-year-old woman with large left vertebral–PICA aneurysm visualized on contrast CT scan **(A)**, sagittal T1-weighted MRI **(B)**, and angiogram **(C)**. The aneurysm was successfully clipped via lateral suboccipital approach **(D)**.

1035

ischemia had either temporary hemodynamic insufficiency or more serious thromboembolic sequelae. The small risk of rerupture has been seen by others as well.

Aneurysm thrombosis was achieved in 87% of instances and these patients had only a 4% risk of late neurologic complications. Unfortunately, incomplete aneurysm thrombosis carried a 45% late complication risk with the majority of these being fatal. The smaller experience in other series supports these findings.

Isolation of a vertebral aneurysm by trapping has proven useful in two instances. Giant VA aneurysms with neurologic signs secondary to brainstem compression have a poor prognosis (9,27). Trapping of these lesions followed by aneurysmorrhaphy and removal of thrombotic material allows for decompression of the brainstem and improvement in select cases.

Trapping is also used in a subset of dissecting and fusiform VA aneurysms (3,8,9,24). It can be used to isolate a

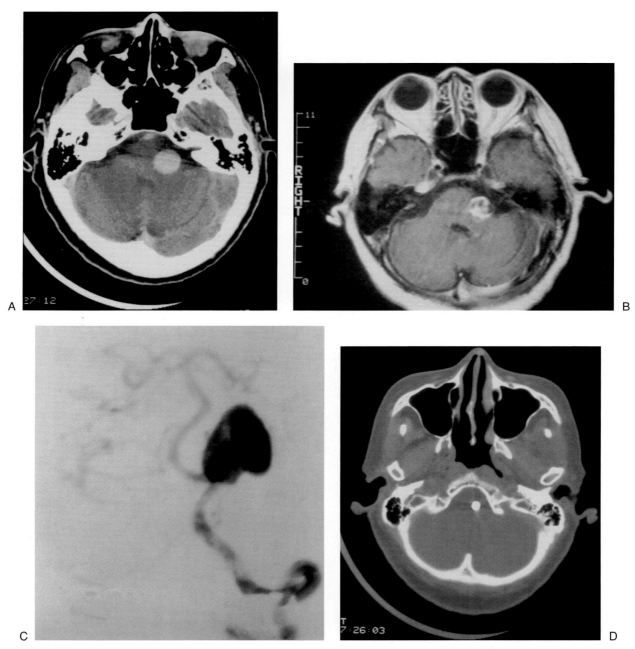

FIG. 4. A 38-year-old woman with lesion of left pontomedullary junction seen on contrast CT **(A)** and T1-weighted MRI **(B)**. Giant left vertebral–PICA aneurysm diagnosed on angiogram **(C)**. Endovascular proximal balloon occlusion of vessel **(D)** led to angiographic obliteration of lesion as viewed from right vertebral injection **(E)**. (Films courtesy of Dr. John Pile-Spellman.)

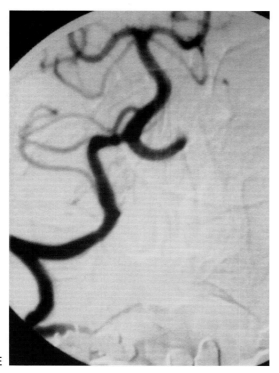

FIG. 4. *(Continued.)*

vertebral segment after tearing of the aneurysm neck or parent artery (17). It may also be used in those cases that fail endovascular proximal ligation. Trapping of a dissected segment precludes the possibility of postoperative rehemorrhage. Trapping procedures are more likely to compromise important brainstem perforators leading to ischemic symptoms. Unfortunately, Kitanaka found this procedure to be associated with a higher incidence of severe lower cranial nerve palsies than proximal occlusion (8). Others have found higher mortality rates in vertebral aneurysms treated via trapping procedures (10,24).

Endovascular Techniques

The relatively high morbidity of posterior fossa aneurysm surgery and the ease with which vertebrobasilar vessels are approached endovascularly suggests a role for transluminal techniques in the posterior fossa. In fact, endovascular treatment of VA lesions is becoming increasingly popular. Ideally, these techniques provide aneurysm obliteration without the brainstem and cranial nerve manipulation inherent in open procedures. Detachable balloon occlusion of the proximal VA for VA dissections and inoperable fusiform lesions has been shown to be a reliable treatment with acceptable risk (28,29). Furthermore, in medically unstable or poor-grade patients, endovascular coiling of the aneurysmal dome can turn a ruptured aneurysm into an ''unruptured'' lesion. In this way, aggressive initial medical and hypervolemic therapy may be pursued with less chance of acute rerupture.

In cases of endovascular VA occlusion, the angiogram is first examined to ensure an adequate contralateral VA to supply the basilar artery. Awake patients initially undergo a 30-minute balloon occlusion test with a provocative blood pressure lowering to induce ischemic neurologic symptoms. Cerebral blood flow studies (xenon-CBF) are performed during this time to confirm adequate perfusion of the regions at risk. A cerebral blood flow drop of more than 30% indicates insufficient collateral flow. Xenon-CBF has some limitations in the posterior fossa making careful neurologic evaluation paramount. Successful temporary occlusion is followed by permanent occlusion of the VA just proximal to the dissection or fusiform aneurysm. Care is taken to avoid dislodging any thrombus. Heparinization continues for 24 hours to maintain perforator patency and collateral flow in the region.

More recently, direct endovascular obliteration of saccular vertebral aneurysms has begun using electrolytically detachable platinum coils (30). When fed into the dome of the aneurysm, the coils conform to the aneurysm shape and induce thrombosis from dome to neck. Results with detachable coils in saccular aneurysms shows significantly less morbidity than the treatment of these aneurysms with detachable balloons. There have now been many reports of angiographic obliteration of giant vertebral aneurysms and even relief of symptoms of brainstem compression with coiling of saccular aneurysms (30).

Unfortunately, there are also problems related to endovascular coils in saccular vertebral aneurysms. The most serious problem is the subtotal thrombosis of many giant aneurysms by this technique. We have now seen a large number of cases where residual aneurysm necks after endovascular coiling have caused continued aneurysm growth resulting in either rupture or worsening mass effect. Even successfully coiled aneurysms often do not provide symptomatic relief because aneurysm dome thrombosis may not remove the mass effect of the aneurysm. Lastly, in a number of giant aneurysms that have continued to grow after endovascular coiling we have found surgical clipping of the aneurysm neck more difficult due to the presence of coils in the lesion.

Despite these reservations, endovascular techniques remain a good alternative to aneurysms not amenable to direct surgical clipping. When ligation of the VA proximal to PICA is contemplated, endovascular techniques are superior to surgery. Trial occlusion in the awake patient can be performed and postprocedure anticoagulation safely instituted (Fig. 4).

SURGICAL PRINCIPLES AND STRATEGIES

Lateral Suboccipital Approach

The surgical approach to vertebral aneurysms is tailored to the morphology of the specific lesion. Most aneurysms of the VA and vertebral–PICA junction can be approached via a lateral suboccipital craniotomy. Vertebrobasilar junction or distal vertebral aneurysms may require a far lateral approach to the foramen magnum or a presigmoid retrolabyrinthine approach. Giant vertebral aneurysms and telovelotonsillar PICA lesions may clipped via these latter methods as well. The rare distal PICA aneurysm may be approached via a more standard suboccipital approach.

The lateral suboccipital craniotomy has replaced paramedian suboccipital craniotomies in the sitting position as the standard approach to vertebral–PICA aneurysms (31,32). This craniotomy gives wide exposure of the medulla and lateral pons but only limited access to more distal, medial vertebral aneurysms. In a patient with a supple neck, the patient can be placed supine with the head turned 90° to the opposite side. Alternatively, the patient can be placed in the straight lateral or park bench position with the chin slightly flexed. A shoulder roll is placed under the contralateral axilla to prevent brachial plexus injury. The ipsilateral shoulder is taped downward to move it out of the field. The head is tilted 10–20° to the contralateral shoulder. Reverse Trendelenberg positioning of the bed now allows the head to be elevated above the heart for venous return while remaining parallel to the floor. Mannitol and spinal drainage are used to improve cerebellar relaxation.

A gentle S-shaped incision is begun 0.5 cm medial to the mastoid notch. This is extended 5 cm rostrally curving laterally at its superior extent. The inferior margin of the incision curves medially to end at the spinous process of C2. Careful electrocautery is used to dissect down to the occipital bone and the arch of C1. Blunt subperiosteal dissection is used on the occiput and mastoid but sharp dissection of the occiput-C1 region is recommended to avoid proximal VA injury. Curved cerebellar retractors are used to hold open the incision.

The superior and lateral borders of the suboccipital craniectomy are the transverse and sigmoid sinuses, respectively. Inferiorly, the foramen magnum should be rongeured open from the midline to the occipital condyle. If desired, removal of C1 can allow a more inferior approach with less retraction on the cerebellar hemisphere. The dura is next opened in a K-shaped fashion. It is important that the superior and lateral dural leaves are opened to the sinus edge. Tacking of these leaves to the lateral occipital musculature elevates the sigmoid sinus, slightly improving access to the lateral brainstem. In the lateral position, the cerebellum tends to fall away from the field and requires only gentle retraction. Before a retractor is placed, the cisterna magna should be opened widely to drain CSF, improve cerebellar relaxation, and help bring the VA and lower cranial nerves into view. The first dentate ligament may be cut to allow the medulla to fall away and improve access to the VA.

The cerebellar tonsil is now gently lifted upward and medially with a self-retaining retractor. The arachnoid adhesions between the tonsil and the spinal portion of the XIth nerve are cut. Careful dissection around this nerve reveals the VA deep to it. It is important at this stage to dissect clear a portion of the proximal VA for potential temporary clip placement. Once proximal VA control is ensured, the tonsil

may be retracted further revealing the vertebral–PICA junction. Cranial nerves VII and VIII will be seen in the upper portion of the operative field at this point and are covered with gel foam for protection. The IXth, Xth, and XIth nerve complex has an intimate relationship with the VA in this area. Extensive dissection of the arachnoid trabeculations between these nerves may be necessary to create space for aneurysm dissection and clip placement. In many cases, however, the aneurysm can be approached below these delicate structures. Vertebral–PICA aneurysms almost always arise just beyond the PICA origin in the angle between the vessels. Following the VA distally, this bifurcation can be located. The origin of the hypoglossal nerve courses immediately dorsal to the vertebral–PICA junction serving as a good landmark. Typically the aneurysm dome is projecting superiorly and medially allowing dissection of the distal VA. A clear temporary clip site is next dissected out allowing distal VA control if necessary. Once the aneurysm is delineated in this fashion, the distal PICA can be dissected proximally toward the aneurysm neck. The hypoglossal nerve is carefully mobilized off the most proximal portion of the PICA. If the neck of the aneurysm remains unclear, gentle retraction on the medulla just proximal to PICA allows visualization of the medial portion of the VA at the aneurysm origin.

At this point definitive clipping of the aneurysm should be possible. Aneurysms that are located on the more distal segments of the VA require significant hemispheric retraction with this technique and visualization of the VIIth and VIIIth cranial nerves for proper exposure.

Far Lateral Approach

Yamaura found that vertebral aneurysm necks located <10 mm from the midline or >13 mm from the clivus had an increased operative morbidity and mortality with a lateral suboccipital approach (3). Giant aneurysms also have higher operative complications when approached in this fashion. The far lateral approach to the medulla and proximal VA has a number of advantages for difficult VA aneurysms. The more lateral dural entry improves the anterior exposure of the inferior brainstem, VA, and vertebrobasilar junction. The additional bony removal provides this view without additional cerebellar or medullary retraction. Finally, control of the C1 portion of the VA proves useful for giant vertebral or vertebral–PICA aneurysms.

Patients may be positioned in the lateral or park bench position. The chin is maximally flexed (two finger breadths space to chest), the head tilted laterally 30° toward the opposite shoulder, and the head rotated 30° away from the side of the lesion. In this position, the mastoid process on the operative side should be the highest point. Rotation of the bed is used for small adjustments. The inferior clivus is now perpendicular to the floor allowing a lateral approach to the brainstem. A hockey stick incision begins at the base of the mastoid curving rostrally and medially under the superior nuchal line. At the midline the incision heads downward ending at the spinous process of C3. The posterior skin flap is elevated taking care to avoid the accessory nerve traveling from the posterior aspect of the sternomastoid to the trapezius (33,34). The sternomastoid attachment to the posterior mastoid is detached. The exposed splenius capitis, splenius cervicis, and levator scapulae are divided close to their anterior attachments. A cuff of nuchal fascia should be left to allow muscle approximation with closure. This muscle is retracted inferolaterally. Subperiosteal dissection of the occiput and ipsilateral lamina of C1 and C2 is performed. Blunt dissection caudal to the inferior oblique muscle between C1 and C2 will locate the ventral ramus of C2. This nerve crosses the C1–C2 portion of the VA. The oblique muscle is now detached from the transverse process of C2 and the VA followed from the sulcus arteriosus of C1 to its dural entry. The venous plexus around the artery is cauterized as necessary. A C1 hemilaminectomy is performed with a cutting burr on a high-speed drill.

A standard retromastoid craniectomy follows with removal to the foramen magnum. The high-speed drill is used to remove the mastoid as far as the vertical segment of the facial canal unroofing the sigmoid sinus. Lateral exposure inferiorly is obtained by rongeuring the remaining rim of the foramen magnum to the occipital condyle. The inner portion of the posterior third of the condyle is drilled away taking care to protect the extradural VA. Drilling stops on reaching the condylar veins and the outer cortex of the posterior condyle is removed with a mastoid. The dura is now opened at the lateral margin of the bony opening in a curvilinear fashion and tacked up to the lateral paraspinal musculature. Wide access to the VA is possible at this point.

Combined Retrolabyrinthine Presigmoid Approach

Large VA aneurysms near the vertebrobasilar junction often require a transpetrosal approach for adequate visualization of the lateral pons and medulla. The exposure of the distal VA can be greatly enhanced when combining this with a supratentorial approach. We prefer the retrolabyrinthine presigmoid approach because it provides excellent exposure to the cerebellopontine angle and lateral brainstem while preserving hearing and facial nerve function. Translabyrinthine and transcochlear techniques improve exposure to the anterior brainstem but cause hearing loss and endanger the VIIth nerve.

Patients have a spinal drain placed and receive mannitol. They are placed in the supine position with the table elevated 20° and a sandbag placed under the ipsilateral shoulder. The head is fixed in a Mayfield head holder and maximally turned away from the aneurysm side making sure there is no jugular venous compression. The chin is flexed downward slightly and the head tilted 20° toward the floor. This brings the clivus parallel to the floor. Intraoperative adjustments can be made by rotating the table (35,36).

A reverse question mark incision begins at the root of the zygoma. This continues posteriorly 1–2 cm above the pinna and descends below and 1 cm posterior to the mastoid. The incision ends around C1. The scalp flap is retracted inferiorly using towel clips and a Leyla bar. The temporalis muscle is retracted anteriorly and the sternomastoid insertion is separated from the mastoid groove and retracted inferiorly. The periosteum of the exposed posterior temporal and occipital bones is reflected inferiorly revealing the temporal fossa, mastoid, and lateral posterior fossa.

Using the asterion as a landmark, first a lateral suboccipital craniectomy is performed. The bone over the transverse sinus is thinned with a high-speed burr. Careful removal of this bone from the adherent underlying sinus allows entry into the supratentorial compartment. In the area of the sinodural angle, a temporal craniotomy based on the floor of the temporal fossa is begun. This extends anteriorly as far forward as the internal auditory meatus allowing the removal of a 2- to 3-cm-wide bone flap. A complete mastoidectomy is performed after thinning of the bone overlying the sigmoid sinus down to the jugular bulb. After the sigmoid sinus is skeletonized, the large burr should be changed to a small diamond bit for the high-speed drill.

The sinodural angle, the lateral and posterior semicircular canals, and the endolymphatic sac are now exposed. Drilling continues along the pyramid to thin the petrous bone toward the apex. The facial canal is left intact. Unroofing of the sigmoid sinus is completed and emissary veins coagulated. All mastoid air cells are waxed at this point. A horizontal temporal dural opening is begun 1 cm from the petrous floor and carried posteriorly to the sinodural angle taking care to avoid the vein of Labbé. The posterior fossa dura is opened a few millimeters in front of the sigmoid sinus from the jugular bulb to the superior petrosal sinus. The superior petrosal sinus is then cauterized and divided. A dural opening may be made behind the sigmoid sinus as well if necessary to improve exposure (36). We rarely transect the sigmoid sinus even if it is nondominant. Opening the tentorium improves rostral exposure, but more important for vertebral aneurysms is that it improves the capability for retracting the cerebellum. The tentorium is transected from the sinodural angle to the incisura. The IVth nerve is visible here before it enters the tentorial edge. The dura is tacked laterally allowing clear exposure of the vertebrobasilar system, the lateral pons, medulla, and cranial nerves V–XI.

Closure of these lesions must be meticulous to prevent CSF leaks. The dura is closed primarily with a fascia lata patch from the thigh. After careful rewaxing of all bony surfaces, fat from the thigh is packed into the bony defect. Fibrin glue may also be used at this stage. A good muscle and scalp closure follows. The spinal drain is left in for 2 days postoperatively to lessen the chance of CSF leak.

POSTOPERATIVE COMPLICATIONS AND THEIR MANAGEMENT

Surgical treatment of vertebral aneurysms carries with it the same risks of wound infection, posterior fossa syndrome,

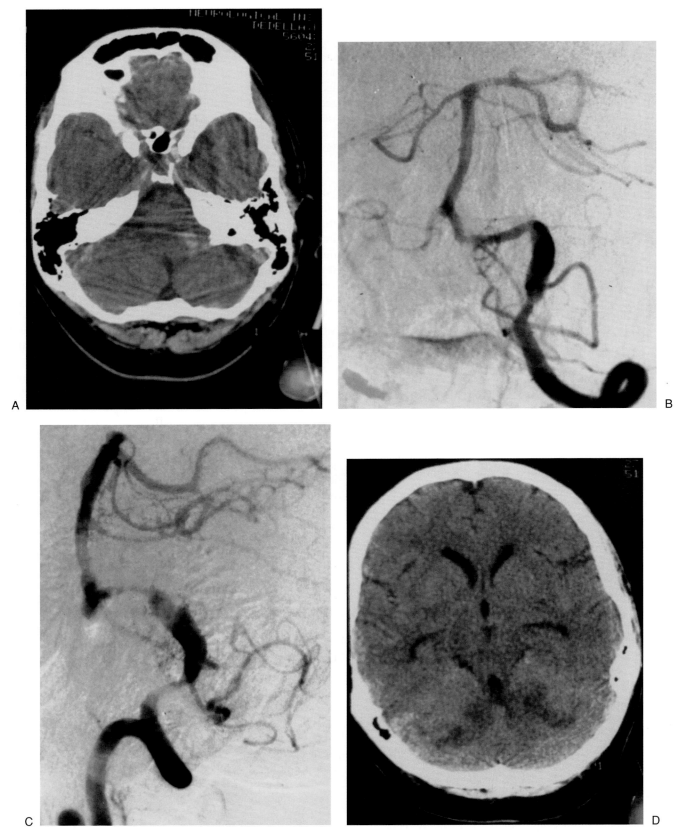

FIG. 5. A 45-year-old man with left fusiform distal VA aneurysm seen on CT scan **(A)** and on vertebral angiogram **(B, C)**. Successful balloon occlusion was followed 48 hours later by acute embolism of VA thrombus leading to bilateral cerebellar infarcts **(D)**.

and postoperative CSF leaks seen in other posterior fossa surgeries. Postoperative hematomas in this region are more serious because of the intolerance of the brainstem to compression. There are other complications more specific to aneurysm surgery in this area.

Most vertebral aneurysms present after subarachnoid hemorrhage and are therefore at risk for hydrocephalus, vasospasm, and rebleeding. Rebleeding does not occur with definitive clipping of aneurysms but is seen infrequently in fusiform and dissecting lesions treated with proximal ligation, trapping, or wrapping (8). Hydrocephalus is a common sequelae resulting from obstruction of the IVth ventricular foramina or intraventricular blood. Typically transient in nature, perioperative CSF diversion with an external lateral ventricular drain is usually sufficient. Persistent hydrocephalus is treated with a ventriculoperitoneal shunt.

Brainstem ischemia may result for a number of reasons. Intraoperative injury or sacrifice of portions of the vertebral–PICA complex or its medullary branches can be asymptomatic, cause a lateral medullary syndrome, or lead to coma depending on the size of the brainstem infarct. Lateral medullary syndrome (Wallenberg's syndrome) involving long tract signs, sympathetic disturbances, and motor deficits occurred in 20% of Kitanaka's series. These symptoms were more common in trapping and clipping of aneurysms than those treated by proximal VA ligation. Thrombosis of arterial cul-de-sacs created after proximal clipping or trapping of the VA is another source of postoperative stroke. Debate now centers on whether placing a clip proximal to a PICA–VA dissection, which fosters embolism formation, is more dangerous than the increased risk of brainstem ischemia and thrombosis with clips placed distal to the PICA.

Lower cranial nerve palsies are the most common postoperative complication after VA aneurysm surgery occurring in up to 75% of cases (7). The intimate relationship of IX, X, and XI to the vascular anatomy in this area makes intraoperative injury during dissection and clip placement difficult to avoid. Abducens and hypoglossal nerve injuries are infrequent and rarely serious. Lower cranial nerve symptoms range from hoarseness to dysarthria to dysphagia. Palatal dysfunction dramatically increases the risk of aspiration pneumonia. Patients should remain intubated postoperatively until fully conscious and able to protect their airway. Most instances of lower cranial nerve dysfunction are mild and can be treated with a few days to a week of oral feeding tubes and airway protection. More severe cases tend to resolve over 3–6 months. In these patients, tracheostomy and gastrostomy feeding tubes are indicated.

Finally, occlusion of the VA carries with it the risk of thrombus propagation into the basilar artery with disastrous consequences. Endovascular techniques allow for immediate heparinization after the procedure and therefore minimize this problem. In addition to thrombus formation, clot from the site of open or endovascular vessel occlusion can embolize into the posterior circulation (Fig. 5).

REFERENCES

1. Yasargil MG. Vertebrobasilar system. In Yasargil MG, ed. *Microneurosurgery.* New York: Thieme Verlag, 1984;128–131.
2. Hudgins RJ, Day AL, Quisling RG, Rhoton AL Jr, Sypert GW, Garcia-Bengochea C. Aneurysms of the posterior inferior cerebellar artery. *J Neurosurg* 1983;58:381–387.
3. Yamaura A. Diagnosis and treatment of vertebral aneurysms. *J Neurosurg* 1988;69:345–349.
4. Herniesnemi J, Vapalahti M, Niskanen M, Kari A. Management outcome for vertebrobasilar artery aneurysms by early surgery. *Neurosurgery* 1992;31:857–862.
5. Lang DA, Galbraith SL. The management outcome of patients with a ruptured posterior circulation aneurysm. *Acta Neurochir (Wien)* 1993;125:9–14.
6. Lanzino G, Andreoli A, Limoni P, Tognetti F, Testa C. Vertebro-basilar aneurysms: does delayed surgery represent the best surgical strategy? *Acta Neurochir (Wien)* 1993;125:5–8.
7. Solomon RA, Stein BM. Surgical approaches to aneurysms of the vertebral and basilar arteries. *Neurosurgery* 1988;23:203–208.
8. Kitanaka C, Sasaki T, Eguchi T, Teraoka A, Nakane M, Hoya K. Intracranial vertebral artery dissections: Clinical, radiological features, and surgical considerations. *Neurosurgery* 1994;34:620–627.
9. Steinberg GK, Drake CG, Peerless SJ. Deliberate basilar or vertebral artery occlusion in the treatment of intracranial aneurysms. *J Neurosurg* 1993;79:161–173.
10. Andoh T, Shirakami S, Nakashima T, Nishimura Y, Sakai N, Yamada H, Ohkuma A, Tanabe Y, Funakoshi T. Clinical analysis of a series of vertebral aneurysm cases. *Neurosurgery* 1992;31:987–993.
11. Arroyo S, Munoz A, Vazquez A, Hernandez A, Varela de Seijas E. Magnetic resonance imaging of acute spontaneous dissection of the vertebral artery. *Stroke* 1991;22(12):1606–1607.
12. Hoffman M, Sacco RL, Chan S, Mohr JP. Noninvasive detection of vertebral artery dissection. *Stroke* 1993;24:815–819.
13. Fujiwara S, Yokoyama T, Matsushima T, Matsubara T, Fukui M. Repeat angiography and magnetic resonance imaging (MRI) of dissecting aneurysms of the intracranial vertebral artery. *Acta Neurochir (Wien)* 1993;121:123–129.
14. Weir B. *Aneurysms Affecting the Nervous System.* Baltimore: Williams and Wilkins, 1984;489–491.
15. Peerless SJ, Drake CG. Posterior circulation aneurysms. In: Wilkins RH, Rengachary SS, eds. *Neurosurgery.* New York: McGraw-Hill, 1985;1422–1437.
16. Lee KS, Gower DJ, Branch CL Jr, et al. Surgical repair of aneurysms of the posterior inferior cerebellar artery: a clinical series. *Surg Neurol* 1989;31:85–92.
17. Salcman M, Rigamonte D, Numaguchi Y, et al. Aneurysms of the posterior inferior cerebellar artery-vertebral artery complex: variations on a theme. *Neurosurgery* 1990;27:12.
18. Batjer HH, Kopitnik TA, Purdy PD, Samson DS. Vertebral and PICA aneurysms. In: Carter LP, Spetzler RF, eds. *Neurovascular Surgery.* New York: McGraw-Hill, 1995;763–776.
19. Ausman JI, Sadasivan B. Posterior inferior cerebellar artery—vertebral artery aneurysms: infratentorial procedures. In: Apuzzo MLJ, ed. *Brain Surgery.* vol 2. New York: Churchill Livingstone, 1993;1875–1889.
20. Heros RC. Lateral suboccipital approach for vertebral and vertebrobasilar artery aneurysms. *J Neurosurg* 1986;64:559–562.
21. Marsh WR, Sundt TM Jr. Posterior circulation aneurysms. In: Suzuki J, ed. *Advances in Surgery for Cerebral Stroke.* Tokyo: Springer-Verlag, 1988;67–68.
22. Ojemann RG, Heros RC, Crowell RM. Basilar trunk and vertebral artery aneurysms. In: *Surgical Management of Cerebrovascular Disease.* 2nd ed. Baltimore: Williams and Wilkins, 1988;232–295.
23. Standard SC, Hopkins LN. Comment in: Tsukahara T, Wada H, Satake K, Yaoita H, Takahashi A. Proximal balloon occlusion for dissecting vertebral aneurysms accompanied by subarachnoid hemorrhage. *Neurosurgery* 1995;36:914–920.
24. Mizutani T, Aruga T, Kirino T, Miki Y, Saito I, Tsuchida T. Recurrent subarachnoid hemorrhage from untreated ruptured vertebrobasilar dissecting aneurysms. *Neurosurgery* 1995;36:905–913.
25. Yamada K, Hayakawa T, Ushio Y, Iwata Y, Koshino K, Bitoh S, Takimoto N. Therapeutic occlusion of the vertebral artery for unclipable vertebral aneurysm. Relationship between site of occlusion and clinical outcome. *Neurosurgery* 1984;15:834–838.

26. Batjer HH. Comment in, Kitanaka C, Sasaki T, Eguchi T, Teraoka A, Nakane M, Hoya K. Intracranial vertebral artery dissections: Clinical, radiological features, and surgical considerations. *Neurosurgery* 1994; 34:620–627.

27. Nagahiro S, Takada A, Goto S, Kai Y, Ushio Y. Thrombosed growing giant anerysms of the vertebral artery: growth mechanism and management. *J Neurosurg* 1995;82:796–801.

28. Aymard A, Gobin YP, Hodes JE, Bien S, Rufenacht D, Reizine D, George B, Merland JJ. Endovascular occlusion of vertebral arteries in the treatment of unclipable vertebrobasilar aneurysms. *J Neurosurg* 1991;74:393–398.

29. Higashida RT, Halbach VV, Dowd CF. Intracranial aneurysms: treatment with detachable ballons: results in 215 cases. *Radiology* 1991; 178:663–671.

30. Halbach VV, Higashida RT, Dowd CF, Fraser KW, Smith TP, Teitelbaum GP, Wilson CB, Hieshima GB. Endovascular treatment of vertebral artery dissections and pseudoaneurysms. *J Neurosurg* 1993;79: 183–191.

31. Diaz FG, Fessler RD. Vertebral artery and posterior inferior cerebellar artery aneurysms: surgical management. *Neurosurgical Operative Atlas.* vol 3. Baltimore: Williams and Wilkins, 1991;355–361.

32. Tew JM Jr, Scodary DJ. Surgical positioning: infratentorial procedures. In: Apuzzo MLJ, ed. *Brain Surgery.* vol 2. New York: Churchill Livingstone, 1993;1609–1620.

33. Hamilton MG, Kraus GE, Daspit CP, Zabramski JM, Spetzler RF. Giant aneurysms: infratentorial. In: Carter LP, Spetzler RF, eds. *Neurovascular Surgery.* New York: McGraw-Hill, 1995;829–850.

34. Sen CN, Sekhar LN. An extreme lateral approach to intradural lesions of the cervical spine and foramen Magnum. *Neurosurgery* 1990;27: 197–204.

35. Al-Mefty O, Schenk MP, Smith RR. Petroclival meningiomas. In: Rangachary SS, Wilkins RH, eds. *Neurosurgical Operative Atlas.* vol 1. Baltimore: Williams and Wilkins, 1991;339–350.

36. Gianotta SL, Maceri DR. Retrolabyrinthine transsigmoid approach to basilar trunk and vertebrobasilar artery junction aneurysms. *J Neurosurg* 1988;69:461–466.

Cerebrovascular Disease, edited by H. Hunt Batjer.
Lippincott-Raven Publishers, Philadelphia © 1997.

CHAPTER 84

Basilar Trunk Aneurysms: Surgical Techniques

Neil A. Martin

GENERAL BACKGROUND

Aneurysms of the basilar artery can be divided into three groups: those arising at the basilar artery apex (or basilar bifurcation), those arising at the junction of the superior cerebellar artery with the basilar artery, and those arising from the basilar artery trunk. Basilar trunk aneurysms include those that originate from the region of the vertebrobasilar junction to the origin of the superior cerebellar artery: vertebrobasilar junction aneurysms, aneurysms arising at the site of a basilar artery fenestration, basilar trunk–anterior inferior cerebellar artery (AICA) aneurysms, upper basilar trunk aneurysms (not arising at the AICA origin), and fusiform basilar trunk aneurysms.

Posterior circulation aneurysms make up 10–20% of the aneurysms seen in most surgical series. The majority of posterior circulation aneurysms arise at the basilar artery bifurcation, with the next most common location being the origin of the posterior inferior cerebellar artery (PICA) from the vertebral artery. Basilar trunk aneurysms are rare and compose only 1–2% of intracranial aneurysms. Subarachnoid hemorrhage is usually the mode of presentation. While giant basilar trunk aneurysms may also cause subarachnoid hemorrhage, many of the large lesions present with cranial nerve deficits, hemiparesis, ataxia, or bulbar palsy due to mass effect. Subarachnoid hemorrhage from posterior circulation aneurysms appears to carry a much graver prognosis than that from anterior circulation aneurysms. A recent review from Rochester, Minnesota of patients diagnosed with aneurysmal subarachnoid hemorrhage indicated that the mortality rate within 48 hours of hemorrhage was 68% for patients with posterior circulation aneurysms and only 23% for patients with anterior circulation aneurysms (1). Furthermore, the clinical grade on admission to the hospital was significantly worse in patients with posterior circulation aneurysms.

These aneurysms are among the most difficult to approach, isolate, and separate from adjacent cranial nerves, basilar artery branch vessels, and critical brainstem perforating vessels. The corridor of surgical approach to these lesions is characteristically narrow, deep, and restricted by cranial nerves. The surgical difficulty of treating basilar trunk aneurysms is compounded by their rarity, a factor that limits the acquisition of experience in treating these lesions by any individual neurosurgeon. However, recent advances in neuroanesthesiology and cerebral protection, neurosurgical instrumentation (narrow profile clip appliers and temporary clips), and the development of innovative skull base approaches for exposure of the ventral brainstem/clival area have dramatically improved the success rate for the surgical treatment of basilar trunk aneurysms. This chapter reviews the relevant surgical anatomy, the general operative management, and the specific aspects of the surgical approaches to these aneurysms.

PERTINENT NEUROLOGIC AND VASCULAR ANATOMY AND VARIATIONS

The basilar artery trunk is formed by the confluence of the vertebral arteries, generally at the level of the junction of the lower and middle thirds of the clivus (near or just above the level of the jugular foramen). Although the origins of the AICAs are quite variable, they generally are found near the level of the internal auditory canal, and at or below the junction of the middle and upper third of the clivus (below the level of the floor of the sella turcica). The upper limit of the basilar trunk, as it will be considered in this chapter, is the origin of the superior cerebellar arteries, which are found at the level of the upper third of the clivus, in the region of the floor of the sella turcica.

The vertebrobasilar junction occurs at or just above the level of the pontomedullary junction (2). The basilar artery lies in the prepontine cistern and travels in a shallow groove along the ventral surface of the pons until it enters the interpeduncular cistern anterior to the midbrain. It is important to

N. A. Martin: Division of Neurosurgery, Section of Neurovascular Surgery, UCLA School of Medicine, Los Angeles, California 90095.

note that the basilar artery is frequently tortuous and may deviate significantly from the midline, especially in elderly patients. It has a perfectly straight course in only about 25% of cases. The length of the entire basilar artery trunk falls in the range of approximately 25–35 mm. The average diameter of the basilar artery is approximately 4 mm but may be slightly larger in elderly patients with atherosclerosis. The most common basilar artery anomaly of clinical significance is that of a focal duplication, or fenestration. This anomaly has been identified in 1–5% of autopsies, usually involves the lower half of the basilar artery, and generally extends no more than 3–4 mm (3,4). In addition to the AICAs (which are described below), there are two groups of small arterial branches that supply the pons: the median branches, and the transverse or circumferential branches. The median branches arise almost at a right angle from the posterior surface of the basilar artery trunk, penetrate the median groove of the pons, and extend to the region of the floor of the fourth ventricle. The transverse branches are slightly larger and are found in four to six pairs that originate from the posterolateral aspect of the basilar artery. These vessels give off small perforating branches that penetrate the surface of the pons (2). Occlusion of these pontine branches may give rise to a syndrome similar to pontine lacunar infarction (pure motor hemiplegia, dysarthria–clumsy hand syndrome, or ataxic hemiparesis), or it may cause ocular movement deficits or nystagmus.

The origin of the AICA is variable: it originates from the lower third of the basilar artery in approximately 75% of cases and above this level in the remainder (Fig. 1) (5). The main trunk of the AICA travels laterally along the surface of the pons, where it generally lies in close approximation to the proximal portion of the abducens nerve. The AICA then travels through the cerebellopontine cistern where it is found ventromedial to the roots of cranial nerves VII and VIII. In the vicinity of these nerves, the AICA bifurcates into medial and lateral cerebellar branches. The medial branch also supplies the middle cerebellar peduncle and nearby regions of the pons. Generally, the proximal portion of the AICA also gives rise to the internal auditory artery, which supplies both the nerve roots and the sensory organs of the inner ear. Occlusion of the AICA may cause hemiplegia, Horner's syndrome, facial paralysis, deafness, nystagmus, ataxia, and sensory deficit.

Cranial nerves V–XI play a role in surgery for aneurysms of the basilar artery trunk because they may traverse the avenues of surgical approach (5). The Vth, VIIth, and VIIIth nerves may present obstacles for an approach from a superior direction (the subtemporal, transtentorial approach). The VIIth and VIIIth nerve complex is always somewhat of an impediment to lateral approaches (petrosal and transsigmoid approaches). The Vth nerve serves as the superior limit, whereas the nerves at the jugular foramen define the inferior limit of the lateral approaches. The caudal approach to the lower basilar trunk (far lateral transcondylar approach) requires working around or through the IXth, Xth, and XIth cranial nerves. The VIth cranial nerve is often adjacent or adherent to aneurysms arising from the basilar artery trunk.

PREOPERATIVE EVALUATION

The first clue as to the presence of a basilar artery aneurysm is the definition of posterior fossa subarachnoid hemorrhage by cranial computed tomography (CT) scanning. The resolution of the subarachnoid spaces in the posterior fossa by CT scanning is poor enough that the origin of hemorrhage in such cases can seldom be defined clearly. Only giant basilar trunk aneurysms can be imaged directly by CT. CT scanning may be helpful in planning the surgical approach, however, as it defines the size of the mastoid air cells, and may indicate the side of the dominant sigmoid sinus by the size of the sigmoid groove and jugular foramen.

Magnetic resonance imaging (MRI) is particularly helpful for the evaluation of patients with giant basilar trunk aneurysms. The presence or absence of intraluminal thrombus, as well as the degree and direction of brainstem displacement are well defined by MRI. These findings are valuable in planning the surgical strategy and approach.

Cerebral angiography is the critical preoperative diagnostic technique for basilar trunk (or any) aneurysms. It is critically important that the angiographer take great pains to define the site of origin, size, projection, and relationship to the basilar artery and AICA. The angiogram must be carefully evaluated for the presence of a basilar artery fenestration, so that this is recognized before surgery. It is important that lateral and anteroposterior projections be filmed (a) with subtraction so that the arterial anatomy can be seen precisely and (b) without subtraction so that the relationship of the basilar artery and the aneurysm to the level of the clivus (on the lateral view) and the midline (on the anteroposterior, or AP, view) can be determined. The nonsubtracted views are often important for determining the optimal angle and side of surgical approach. The angiographic studies should also include complete delineation of the dural sinuses. In some cases the lateral approach to the basilar artery trunk requires ligation and division of the sigmoid sinus, which can only be considered if the two transverse sinuses communicate through the torcula and the contralateral transverse sinus is of adequate size. The location and size of the veins of Labbé should be defined, so that these critical vessels can be protected when a subtemporal approach is required. The patency and size of the two posterior communicating arteries should be demonstrated in patients with giant or fusiform aneurysms when vertebral or basilar artery ligation is considered as a treatment option. This may require performance of the vertebral artery injection with simultaneous carotid artery compression in order to fill the posterior communicating artery (the Allcock test) (6).

GENERAL ANESTHETIC AND SURGICAL PRINCIPLES

In order to prevent early rebleeding, we have generally preferred urgent surgical treatment of acutely ruptured basi-

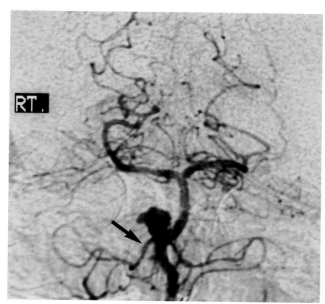

A

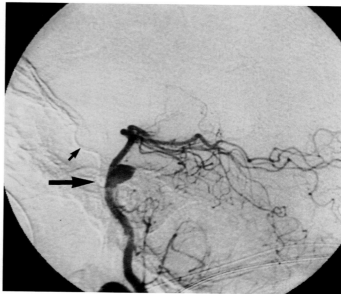

B

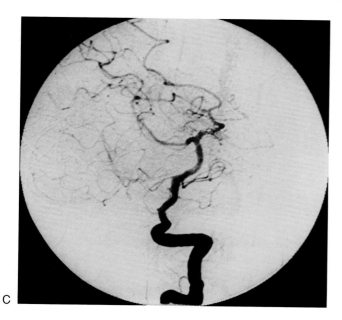

C

FIG. 1. Ruptured anterior inferior cerebellar artery (AICA) aneurysm. **A:** The Towne projection demonstrates an irregular aneurysm projecting superiorly and laterally from the lower basilar trunk adjacent to the origin of the AICA *(arrow)*. Note that the aneurysm projects from the convex side of a region of tortuosity and is eccentric toward the right. **B:** The lateral view shows that the neck of the aneurysm arises well below the level of the floor of the sella *(small arrow)*, above the midpoint of the clivus *(large arrow)*. This aneurysm is ideally situated for the petrosal approach from the side of origin *(right)* of the aneurysm. This approach will provide access to the proximal basilar trunk and will allow visualization of the origin of the AICA. **C:** This patient, who had neurogenic pulmonary edema after her subarachnoid hemorrhage, was initially successfully treated endovascularly by Guglielmi detachable coil occlusion of the aneurysm. Although the aneurysm was near totally occluded, a follow-up angiogram 6 months later demonstrated compaction of the coils with refilling of the base of the aneurysm. At that point the patient had recovered medically from the subarachnoid hemorrhage and a surgical approach was carried out. By the petrosal approach with division of the sigmoid sinus, the aneurysm was exposed and clipped. The origin of the AICA could clearly be seen and was preserved.

lar trunk aneurysms. We have found that adequate brain relaxation can be achieved for the rather mild extent of cerebellar retraction required by the petrosal or transsigmoid approach, or the far lateral transcondylar approach to the basilar trunk. However, the more extensive degree of temporal lobe retraction required for the transtentorial approach to the upper basilar trunk may be more injurious in patients with acutely ruptured aneurysms. It may be reasonable to delay surgery, or consider early endovascular therapy, when this approach is required.

The choice of surgical approach is a key component in the successful management of basilar trunk aneurysms. The surgical approach should be selected to provide the widest possible access to the region of the neck of the aneurysm, the proximal basilar artery, and the adjacent branch arteries,

without, if possible, working over or around the dome of the aneurysm. Particularly germane to planning of the approach to basilar trunk aneurysms is the fundamental principle of skull base surgery: to sacrifice noncritical structures (bone, dura, tentorium, and in some cases dural sinuses) in order to facilitate preservation of cranial nerves and critical vascular structures, and to minimize brain retraction.

Brain monitoring and cerebral protection are key components of successful surgical treatment. Electroencephalography is monitored in order to titrate barbiturate coma and to aid in the electrophysiologic assessment of occipital cortex. Somatosensory evoked potentials are monitored to assess the integrity of sensory pathways in the brainstem, and auditory evoked potentials are monitored in order to measure function of the VIIIth cranial nerve, as well as the mid- and upper brainstem. As is the routine for all procedures done on acutely ruptured or complex intracranial aneurysms, mild hypothermia (to 32–33°C) is employed to reduce cerebral metabolic requirements and provide protection from cerebral ischemia. Barbiturate cerebral protection is employed whenever temporary arterial occlusion is planned or is likely (as during dissection of an acutely ruptured aneurysm). Barbiturates are preferred over etomidate, as etomidate provides a lesser degree of metabolic protection for the brainstem and cerebellum (7).

A critical step in the management of any acutely ruptured aneurysm, and particularly in the case of ruptured posterior circulation aneurysms, is the discussion between surgeon and anesthesiologist regarding the strategies to be employed in the event of crisis. We make it a habit to discuss the likelihood of barbiturate coma, temporary clipping, and the appropriate levels for maintenance of arterial Pco_2, and arterial blood pressure (without and with temporary arterial occlusion). When the surgical approach will involve the region of the Xth cranial nerve, it is important that the anesthesiologist be prepared to treat sudden episodes of bradycardia, or even asystole, due to mechanically induced vagal discharge.

The general principles of intracranial aneurysm surgery are followed. These include: (a) minimal retraction of brain, (b) protection of cranial nerves, (c) early proximal and distal arterial control, (d) approach to the aneurysm from the region of the neck with avoidance of the dome (rupture site), (e) planned temporary clipping if manipulation of the fundus or dome is required, (f) complete occlusion of the aneurysm at its neck, and (g) preservation of the parent artery, major branches, and small perforating arteries. Because it may be difficult to establish with certainty that aneurysm clip placement is perfect in the tight confines of the prepontine space, intraoperative digital subtraction angiography is routinely performed before closure (8). With the insertion of a femoral artery sheath at the beginning of the case and careful planning during patient positioning, it is possible to allow for transfemoral angiography with virtually any patient position.

SURGICAL APPROACHES

The large number of innovative, ingenious, and complex approaches employed for the approach of basilar trunk aneurysms bears testimony to the difficulties encountered in exposing this region. Only over the last 10 years has international neurosurgical experience with skull base approaches, particularly those involving the petrous bone, brought the development of highly satisfactory approaches to aneurysms of the basilar artery trunk. Charles Drake and his colleagues opened the door to the field of treatment of basilar trunk aneurysms and achieved laudable results with some of the most complex lesions imaginable in their remarkable series (9). While Dr. Drake achieved remarkable results using the subtemporal transtentorial approach for upper basilar trunk aneurysms, and the caudal lateral suboccipital approach for

vertebral artery and lower basilar trunk aneurysms, it became clear to less experienced aneurysm surgeons that these approaches were not optimal for aneurysms between the vertebral artery confluence and the superior cerebellar artery. These approaches resulted in a deep narrow view of the aneurysm origin and necessitated substantial brain, brainstem, and cranial nerve retraction. Drake and others experimented with transoral/transclival approaches with the thought of avoiding brain retraction altogether. However, the basilar artery exposure remained deep and suboptimal, and the complications with CSF leakage and infection caused these approaches to be largely abandoned for aneurysms.

Kawase et al modified the subtemporal-transtentorial approach by entering the posterior fossa from an anterolateral angle, extradurally through the defect created by removing the apex of the petrous bone (10,11). Although this minimized the need for temporal lobe and brainstem retraction, the resultant exposure was very tight, and the bone removal came uncomfortably close to the petrous carotid artery and the cochlea.

In 1979, Kasdon and Stein pointed the way to the currently employed lateral approaches to the basilar trunk (12). They employed a combined suboccipital and temporal craniotomy, with exposure, ligation, and division of the sigmoid sinus (much as Malis described for the treatment of petroclival neoplasms) (13). This approach has been refined by a series of surgeons, resulting in the techniques that are currently employed. Hashi et al extended the bone removal forward to expose the junction of the superior petrosal sinus with the sigmoid sinus and the dura anterior to the sigmoid sinus (14). By ligating and dividing the superior petrosal sinus, dividing the tentorium, and opening the posterior fossa dura anterior to the sigmoid sinus, this dural sinus could be preserved. Samii, Al-Mefty, and others have reported variations and refinements of this technique for the treatment of ventral posterior fossa neoplasms (15–17). Giannotta combined retrolabyrinthine petrous bone removal with sigmoid sinus transection to treat basilar trunk aneurysms (18). Spetzler et al extended the petrosal and retrolabyrinthine transsigmoid approaches by removing more of the posterior aspect of the petrous bone, including the region of the labyrinth and cochlea (19). This extension further widened exposure of the ventral posterior fossa, clivus, and basilar artery, albeit at the cost of auditory function. Variations of these lateral posterior petrosal/presigmoid or transsigmoid approaches now provide the most effective avenue for exposure for the great majority of basilar trunk aneurysms (20). The posterior petrosal approaches will be the focus of much of the discussion in this chapter.

Fukushima and Sekhar et al have described variations on the supra- and transtentorial approaches to the upper portion of the basilar artery trunk (21–23). Heros et al have refined the inferior lateral posterior fossa approach for exposure of the lower region of the basilar artery trunk (24). A discussion of these two approaches to the upper and lower limits of the basilar artery trunk will complete this chapter.

SUBTEMPORAL TRANSTENTORIAL APPROACH

The subtemporal transtentorial approach is an extension of the standard subtemporal approach to the incisura and is employed to provide exposure of the upper basilar artery trunk below the level of the basilar artery apex. This approach allows visualization of the interpeduncular area and basilar artery apex, and the upper prepontine cistern and upper basilar trunk. Exposure of the mid- and lower basilar trunk through this approach requires significant retraction of cerebellum, cranial nerves, and brainstem. The subtemporal approach can be extended to improve access to the mid- and lower basilar artery by intradural or extradural resection of the ridge of the petrous bone. Drake et al were the first to make extensive use of this approach for basilar trunk aneurysms (9). Kawase, Harsh, Sekhar, and Day have more recently described variations and extensions of the subtemporal approach (11,21–23).

Operative Procedure

In most cases, this approach is made from the right (nondominant) side. A lumbar subarachnoid drain, inserted after induction of anesthesia, is employed for CSF drainage to provide maximal brain relaxation during temporal lobe retraction. The patient is positioned supine with the right shoulder elevated and the head rotated toward the left until it is within 10° of horizontal. The vertex is dropped slightly in order to improve access beneath the temporal lobe. We have employed a curving incision that begins below the level of the zygomatic arch, curves 2–3 cm posteriorly to the external auditory canal above the pinna, and then curves forward to the hairline above the level of the superior temporal line. The scalp flap is elevated, taking care to avoid the frontal branch of the facial nerve. The lateral surface of the zygomatic arch is exposed by subperiosteal dissection. The zygomatic arch is divided anteriorly and posteriorly, and then reflected inferiorly along with the temporalis muscle. Removal of the zygomatic arch allows a more anterior approach parallel to the floor of the middle cranial fossa. The free temporal craniotomy flap extends from the temporal pole posteriorly to a point 2–3 cm posterior to the external auditory canal. The temporal bone is drilled flush with the floor of the middle cranial fossa. The removal of this bone markedly reduces the need for temporal lobe retraction.

The dura is opened along the inferior aspect of the temporal lobe. At this point, CSF is drained through the lumbar subarachnoid catheter, and the temporal lobe is gently elevated to expose the tentorium and incisura. The edge of the tentorium is elevated and retracted in order to identify the trochlear nerve. A traction suture is placed into the edge of the tentorium just behind the entry of the IVth cranial nerve into its dural tunnel. The tentorial edge is then coagulated approximately 2 cm posterior to the entry point of the IVth cranial nerve into the tentorial edge, and the tentorial incision is initiated and extended laterally to the superior petrosal sinus. The superior petrosal sinus is clipped and divided, and the dural incision is then carried along the apex of the petrous bone to the region of the dura overlying Meckel's cave. The dural incision is extended into the region of Meckel's cave to allow far anterior retraction of this tentorial flap. The superior petrosal vein beneath the tentorium must be avoided, or coagulated and divided. The tentorial flap is reflected anterolaterally in order to expose the posterior fossa. The retraction of the tentorial flap is limited by the trochlear nerve, and additional retraction may be permitted by dissecting the IVth cranial nerve from its dural tunnel on the edge of the tentorium. The tentorial opening provides exposure to the ventrolateral surface of the upper pons, the trigeminal root entry zone, and the upper basilar artery trunk for a distance of 1–2 cm below the origin of the superior cerebellar artery. In most cases, the origin of the AICA cannot be seen without retraction of the Vth nerve, the VIIth and VIIIth nerve complex, and the brainstem. This approach provides excellent access to the upper part of the basilar artery trunk. This is appropriate for high-lying AICAs and for aneurysms arising from the ventral surface of the upper part of the basilar artery. For lower basilar trunk aneurysms, the petrosal approach is preferable.

THE PETROSAL APPROACH

Surgical treatment of basilar trunk aneurysms has been advanced remarkably by the use of petrosal skull base approaches, originally designed for surgical treatment of neoplasms involving the posterior petrous and clival region (15–19). Resection of the petrous bone, and opening of the dura anterior to the sigmoid sinus or transection of the sigmoid sinus, provides a shortened operative distance to the ventral brainstem, basilar artery, and clivus. Spetzler et al divided the posterior petrosal approaches into variations based on the amount of petrous bone removed (19). The most conservative approach is the retrolabyrinthine technique as described by Samii and Al Meftly (15,17). The petrosal approach may be extended by more complete removal of the temporal bone with sacrifice of hearing (translabyrinthine approach). Maximal exposure is achieved by extensive petrous drilling with transposition of the facial nerve (transcochlear approach) (19).

We have found that exposure of the basilar trunk from the vertebrobasilar junction to the origin of the superior cerebellar arteries is best achieved by the posterior petrosal/retrolabyrinthine approach, with division of the sigmoid sinus. It must be recognized that the sigmoid sinus can be sacrificed only if the two transverse sinuses communicate through the torcula (an anatomic feature that must be defined on the preoperative angiogram). If the transverse sinuses do not communicate, the sigmoid sinus must be preserved. Reasonably good exposure can be attained by preserving the sigmoid sinus, but dividing the superior petrosal sinus and the tentorium as well as retracting the sigmoid sinus posteriorly along with the cerebellar hemisphere.

Operative Technique

The patient is positioned supine on the operating table with the head turned parallel to the floor. A periauricular incision is made, and the scalp is reflected in the subgaleal plane (Fig. 2). The muscle and pericranium are reflected with the scalp flap or dissected separately. A complete mastoidectomy is performed with the pneumatic drill, and a self-irrigating high-speed drill is used for the detailed skeletonization of the bony labyrinth.

The prominence of the lateral (horizontal) semicircular canal within the mastoid antrum is identified early during the drilling and is used as a point of reference during the remainder of the mastoid dissection (16). Bone is removed to expose the inferior temporal lobe, sigmoid sinus, and posterior fossa dura anterior and posterior to the sigmoid sinus. The anterior extent of the posterior fossa dural exposure is determined by identifying the endolymphatic duct that pierces the temporal bone adjacent to the posterior semicircular canal. In the event of inadvertent opening of the semicircular canal, bone wax is immediately applied to the exposed canal. A combined temporal and suboccipital craniotomy extending across the transverse sinus is then turned. The dura can be incised anterior to the sigmoid sinus and along the inferior surface of the temporal lobe. Care is taken to define and protect the vein of Labbé, which at times must be dissected from its arachnoidal covering on the cortex

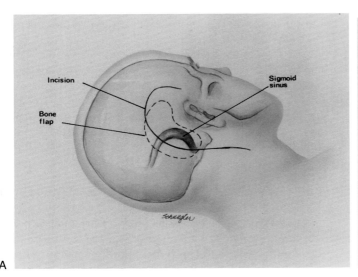

A

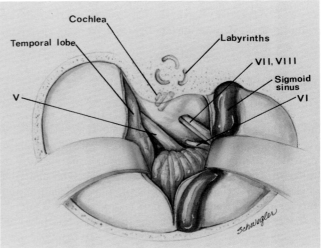

B

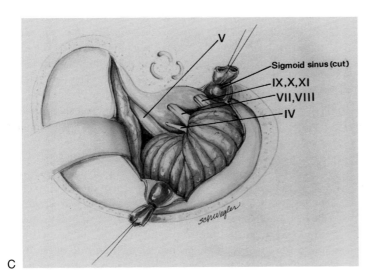

C

FIG. 2. The petrosal approach to the basilar artery trunk (without and with sacrifice of the sigmoid sinus). **A:** The patient is positioned supine with the head rotated away from the side of surgery. The skin incision and bone flap are indicated. **B:** The mastoidectomy has been completed and the posterior petrosal area has been drilled to the level of the semicircular canals. The bone flap exposes the posterior inferior temporal region and the anterolateral posterior fossa. The dura has been opened along the inferior aspect of the temporal lobe and anterior to the sigmoid sinus. The superior petrosal sinus, which is not demonstrated, has been ligated and divided. The tentorium has been divided through the incisura. **C:** The exposure is expanded by ligation and division of the sigmoid sinus. This can only be performed when the ipsilateral transverse sinus communicates through the torcula with a normal-sized contralateral transverse sinus. **D:** *(next page)* Retraction of the cerebellum to expose the interval between the Vth cranial nerve, and the VIIth and VIIIth cranial nerve complex is demonstrated. This angle of approach is employed for aneurysms arising from the mid- to upper part of the basilar trunk. In this case an AICA aneurysm is demonstrated.

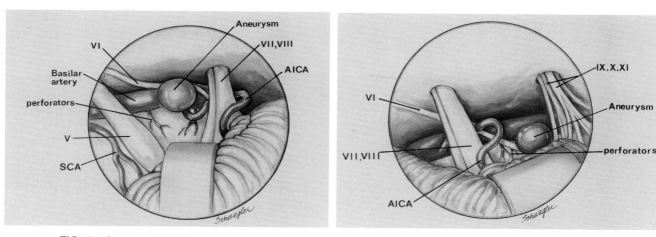

FIG. 2. *Continued.* **E:** This demonstrates exposure of a vertebrobasilar junction aneurysm through the space between nerves VII and VIII, and the nerves at the jugular foramen. Often it is necessary to work through both of the intervals between the groups of cranial nerves.

to allow safe retraction of the temporal lobe. The superior petrosal sinus is identified, ligated, and cut, allowing division of the tentorium to the incisura. The trochlear nerve can usually be seen covered by arachnoid adjacent to the tentorial edge by elevating the tentorium prior to completing its division. The temporal lobe and cerebellum are then gently retracted to expose the petroclival region, the ventral pons, and the basilar artery.

If preoperative angiography has demonstrated that the torcula provides communication for both transverse sinuses and the sigmoid sinus on the operative side is not markedly dominant, it can be doubly ligated and divided. This increases exposure to the cerebellopontine angle and clival region and allows additional cerebellar retraction. We prefer to incorporate sinus transection whenever possible in order to maximize exposure.

The AICA is identified adjacent to cranial nerves VII and VIII and followed to the basilar artery trunk. Care is taken not to disturb the dome of the aneurysm until the basilar artery is identified and isolated both proximal and distal to the aneurysm. The basilar artery trunk is prepared for temporary clipping should this become necessary. The approach to the upper basilar trunk can be carried out in the interval between the Vth and the VIIth and VIIIth cranial nerves. The lower basilar trunk can be exposed by working through the interval between the VIIth and VIIIth cranial nerves, and the IXth–XIth cranial nerves at the jugular foramen. Care must be taken to avoid stretching or traction on any of these nerves. Excessive traction or stretching of the VIIIth cranial nerve can result in deafness. Compression or traction of the Xth cranial nerve may cause bradycardia or even asystole. It is usually necessary to insert one instrument, such as a suction in the left hand, through the interval between the Vth and VIIth/VIIIth nerves, and another instrument, such as the clip applier, through the more caudal space between the VIIth/VIIIth cranial nerves and the nerves of the jugular foramen.

The neck of a basilar trunk aneurysm that projects anteriorly or posteriorly can be exposed from either side. In such cases, the side of approach is determined both by the position of the basilar artery and by the anatomy of the dural sinuses. If the basilar trunk is tortuous and swings far to one side, the approach is made from that side. If the other factors are equal, the approach is made from the side of the nondominant transverse/sigmoid sinus. If the aneurysm projects laterally, we approach it from that side. If one approaches from the opposite side, it can be difficult to see the origin of the aneurysm and the adjacent AICA origin from the lateral surface of the basilar artery. By approaching the neck of the aneurysm initially from the caudal and rostral directions, one can isolate the neck without undue dissection of the dome of the aneurysm. However, in some cases it is necessary to separate the dome of the aneurysm from the ventral surface of the pons in order to visualize the AICA origin adequately. This generally should be done with temporary clips in place. The basilar artery can safely be occluded for a matter of a few minutes, if one employs barbiturate cerebral protection with moderate hypothermia.

The VIth cranial nerve may be adherent to the dome of the aneurysm. Often, one can isolate and clip the neck without disturbing the VIth cranial nerve. In some cases, however, the VIth nerve runs over the region of the neck of the aneurysm and must be dissected free. This may cause a transient postoperative cranial nerve VI palsy. In each case where this has occurred we have noted complete resolution over 1–3 months postoperatively.

After clipping of the aneurysm and completion of the intraoperative angiogram, primary closure of the dura should be attempted in all cases. This can be difficult in some cases, and the dura may be reinforced with autologous fibrin glue and fascia lata. A small piece of muscle is used to occlude the antrum of the middle ear, and the mastoid sinus is obliterated with autologous fat taken from the abdomen or thigh.

Routinely, spinal CSF drainage is employed for 3 days postoperatively.

INFERIOR LATERAL (TRANSCONDYLAR) SUBOCCIPITAL APPROACH

This approach, very much as it is generally employed now, was described by Heros in 1986 for the treatment of vertebral/posterior inferior cerebellar artery or vertebrobasilar junction aneurysms (24). This approach has also been employed with success for the treatment of ventrally located foramen magnum neoplasms, and for intracranial vertebral endarterectomy. We employ this approach for vertebrobasilar junction aneurysms when they are low lying, and when the projection of the dome makes the approach from a petrosal approach undesirable.

Several choices are available for the skin incision. A number of surgeons have advocated the use of a hockey-stick incision, with the horizontal limb beginning at the mastoid and coursing to the region of the inion, where a vertical extension travels down the posterior midline to the level of C-2. We have employed this incision in certain cases and have found that the bulk of the suboccipital and posterior cervical musculature can serve as an impediment to the far-lateral angle, which is desirable. We have generally employed the ''lazy S'' incision described by Heros. This vertically oriented incision begins posterior to the base of the mastoid and curves gently to the posterior midline midway between the level of the inion and the spinous process of C-2, where it then continues vertically down the midline. This incision requires cutting across the suboccipital and posterior cervical musculature on the side of the approach but leaves a much smaller mass of muscle laterally at the level of the foramen magnum. This facilitates the inferior lateral angle of approach, which is most advantageous. Although this incision through the muscle causes a modest increase in postoperative neck pain and stiffness, we have not found it to result in any permanent discomfort or limitation in the range of neck movement.

The occipital bone is exposed from the midline laterally to the posterior edge of the mastoid process and inferolaterally to the joint capsule of the atlanto-occipital joint. The spinous process and lamina of C-2 and the posterior arch of C-1 are exposed. The vertebral artery is exposed above the arch of C-1 and elevated from its bony groove. A single burr hole is placed approximately 1.5 cm posterior and inferior to the level of the base of the mastoid process, and a pneumatic craniotome is used to cut the craniotomy. In many cases it is possible to include the rim of the foramen magnum in the bone flap, but in some cases it is necessary to remove this separately with rongeurs. The key step in this exposure is bone removal laterally at the level of the foramen magnum. In order to obtain optimal exposure of the vertebral artery, the PICA origin, and the vertebrobasilar junction, we have found it necessary to extend the bone removal far enough laterally that the posterior one third of the occipital condyle is removed. One often encounters bleeding from a complex of veins associated with an emissary foramen just above the occipital condyle. These vessels can be controlled with bipolar coagulation, and packing of the small foramen with bone wax or Surgicel. The tubercle and ipsilateral posterior arch of C-1 are then removed laterally to the level of the pedicle. The lateral C-1 arch and occipital condyle removal provides an inferior, posterolateral approach that is parallel to the course of the intradural vertebral artery. Often this angle allows one to work below rather than through the nerves at the jugular foramen, which reduces the risk of postoperative dysphagia and aspiration.

The dural incision extends from the superior/lateral corner of the posterior fossa craniotomy to the foramen magnum and down the midline of the spinal dura to C-2. When the arachnoid of the cisterna magna is opened, the intradural segment of the vertebral artery, and the XIth and XIIth cranial nerves are seen. Retraction of the cerebellar tonsil medially and superiorly allows the exposure of the PICA origin and the vertebrobasilar junction. In some cases, the vertebral basilar junction can be exposed by working beneath the nerves at the jugular foramen, and in other cases it is necessary to work carefully between these nerves.

It may be necessary to retract the medulla gently with a small brain retractor in order to expose the vertebrobasilar junction. The base of the aneurysm is carefully cleared of arachnoid, and the anterior spinal artery must be identified and freed in order to ensure that it is cleared from the aneurysm. Clipping of the aneurysm often requires use of a low-profile aneurysm clip applier or a long-bladed clip in order to work in the narrow confines of this space. The closure is routine, and no special precautions are required for postoperative cervical immobilization.

MANAGEMENT OF FUSIFORM BASILAR TRUNK ANEURYSMS

It is important to distinguish the two predominant types of fusiform basilar trunk aneurysms. Congenital fusiform aneurysms are found as an isolated vascular abnormality in younger patients, and aneurysmal dolichoectasia of the basilar trunk is found in older atherosclerotic patients (Figs. 3 and 4) (6,9,25). Isolated fusiform aneurysms in younger patients may present with symptoms due to mass effect or aneurysm rupture. Charles Drake pioneered the treatment of these lesions by surgical occlusion of the vertebral or basilar artery (9). Proximal arterial occlusion (Hunterian ligation) precipitates thrombosis of the aneurysm by reducing or eliminating anterograde flow, which results in intraaneurysmal stasis. This form of treatment is effective if the distal basilar artery territory is adequately supplied through the posterior communicating arteries. Sufficient collateral flow is almost guaranteed when both posterior communicating arteries are larger than 1 mm in diameter and is likely when at least one of the

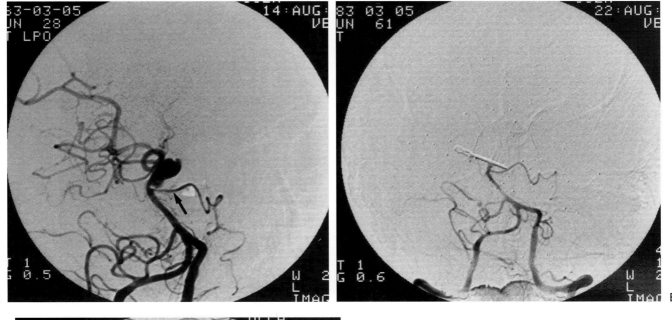

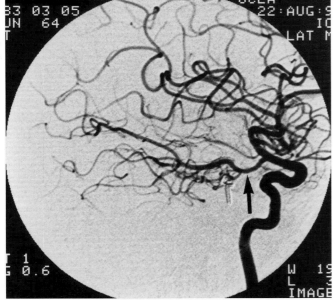

FIG. 3. Ruptured fusiform aneurysm of the upper basilar trunk. **A:** An oblique projection demonstrates a fusiform aneurysm involving the basilar trunk above the origin of the anterior inferior cerebellar artery *(arrow)*. This patient was 22 years old and had sustained a minor subarachnoid hemorrhage. **B:** The aneurysm was exposed through a subtemporal/transtentorial approach, and the basilar artery trunk was occluded at the origin of the aneurysm. **C:** Occlusion of the basilar artery was possible in this case because the patient had a large posterior communicating artery *(arrow)* that supplied the upper basilar territory. The patient tolerated the basilar artery occlusion without difficulty and recovered completely.

posterior communicating arteries is of this size (Fig. 3) (6,9). If collateral flow through the posterior communicating arteries is inadequate, proximal arterial occlusion can only be performed after construction of an arterial bypass to the posterior cerebral or superior cerebellar artery. We have treated four patients with fusiform basilar trunk aneurysms, and absent or tiny posterior communicating arteries. Preliminary extracranial/intracranial bypass to the posterior cerebral artery is completed before planning basilar or vertebral artery occlusion. The proximal occlusion was carried out successfully in three cases, precipitating complete or near-complete aneurysm thrombosis in all of them. However, one of these three patients later expired from fatal rupture due to high-pressure retro-

grade flow down the basilar artery trunk into the aneurysm from a large saphenous vein graft to the posterior cerebral artery. One other patient expired 4 days after the performance of a saphenous vein graft to the posterior cerebral artery even before planned proximal vertebral artery occlusion was carried out, again presumably due to bypass-induced flow or pressure changes in the aneurysm. If this treatment is to be employed in the future, it is clear that the aneurysm should be completely isolated from the circulation by proximal and distal arterial occlusion (''trapping'').

There have been reports of successful treatment of fusiform basilar artery aneurysms by endovascular proximal arterial occlusion (26). As is the case for surgical proximal

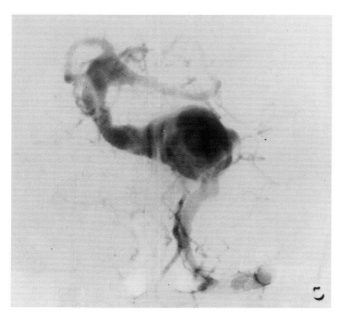

FIG. 4. Atherosclerotic fusiform basilar artery aneurysm (dolichoectasia). This 60-year-old hypertensive patient presented with a history of recurrent episodes of brainstem ischemia and cranial nerve compression. He was treated with antiplatelet therapy in order to reduce the risk of future ischemic events, which in cases such as this are generally related to intraluminal thrombosis.

arterial occlusion, adequate distal collateral circulation must be present for this to be feasible and safe.

Dolichoectatic aneurysms of the basilar artery generally defy treatment. Most attempts to treat these lesions with proximal occlusion, with or without bypass, have resulted in disastrous brainstem ischemia from extensive basilar artery thrombosis (9,27).

ENDOVASCULAR TREATMENT OF BASILAR TRUNK ANEURYSMS

Because of the surgical difficulties associated with the treatment of basilar trunk aneurysms, there has been substantial interest in the application of endovascular techniques to these lesions. Intrasaccular balloon embolization has been employed successfully for the treatment of certain high-risk basilar trunk aneurysms, but the high morbidity and mortality rate associated with this particular endovascular technique has led to its being abandoned in favor of newer methods (28). Currently, the most successful technique for endosaccular embolization of aneurysms involves occlusion with detachable platinum coils (Guglielmi detachable coils, GDCs). This technique, which has by now been employed in thousands of patients worldwide and recently received FDA approval in the United States, has proved to be an effective technique for occluding posterior circulation aneurysms in many cases (29). It is clear that this technique provides a significant degree of protection from aneurysmal bleeding and has a much lower technique-related complication rate than balloon embolization. This technique is particularly valuable in patients who are poor candidates for microsurgical treatment, ie, those who are very elderly or who are medically or neurologically unstable. However, this technique has certain significant limitations; complete aneurysm occlusion is seldom possible in wide-neck aneurysms. Furthermore, the rate of refilling or recurrence of the aneurysms is substantially higher than for microsurgical clipping (30). At UCLA, in 1996, this technique is generally reserved for the immediate postrupture treatment of basilar trunk aneurysms in patients whose medical or neurologic condition renders them unacceptable candidates for general anesthesia and surgery, for treatment of aneurysms which upon exploration are found to be unclippable, or for patients of advanced age.

COMPLICATIONS

The predominant cause of postoperative complications is ischemic brain damage related to inadvertent small branch artery occlusion by the clip (9). This is much more of a problem with basilar apex aneurysms than with basilar trunk aneurysms. In most cases of non-giant basilar trunk aneurysms, meticulous high-magnification sharp dissection allows one to visualize the neck of the aneurysm sufficiently so that critical small perforating vessels are not occluded during clip application. The final clip position must be inspected very carefully to ensure that no branch vessels have been accidentally included in the clip blades. Ischemic injury may also occur if the basilar artery itself or the AICA becomes occluded. It may be difficult to judge visually the degree of stenosis caused to vessels at the neck of the aneurysm by clip placement, particularly in larger aneurysms. The use of intraoperative digital subtraction angiography allows one to be certain that the final anatomic result is acceptable.

Intraoperative aneurysm rupture is an unusual complication during surgery for basilar trunk aneurysms, if the principle of early exposure of the parent artery proximal and distal to the aneurysm is followed. This allows one to approach the aneurysm generally from the region of its neck and to use temporary arterial clipping in order to reduce the risk of rupture should dissection or manipulation of the dome be required. If the aneurysm ruptures during the dissection, the bleeding can generally be controlled by tamponading the rent. Temporary clips can then be applied to trap the aneurysm. It is important to remember that *trapping* of an aneurysm that ruptures intraoperatively is optimal because proximal temporary occlusion alone allows bleeding out of the distal collateral circulation.

The surgical approach to basilar trunk aneurysms often requires working in constricted spaces between the cranial nerves. Post-operative cranial nerve deficits are not uncommon. In our experience, the most common postoperative deficit has been a VIth nerve palsy. This has been caused by dissection of the nerve from the neck or base of an aneurysm, or retraction of the nerve in order to approach the basilar trunk. Generally, the postoperative VIth nerve palsy recovers completely over 6–12 weeks. We have had one patient develop a permanent deafness. This was related to extensive retraction of the VIIIth nerve required to introduce a large clip into the ventral posterior fossa. The most serious postoperative cranial nerve deficits involve the glossopharyngeal and vagal nerves. Deficits related to these nerves can cause dysphagia, impaired airway protection, and aspiration. After any procedure that involves manipulation or retraction of these nerves, vocal cord and swallowing function must be evaluated carefully and proper precautions taken to prevent aspiration. A patient with evidence of severe lower cranial nerve dysfunction may require the performance of a tracheotomy and feeding tube insertion in order to protect them from aspiration pneumonia until swallowing function improves.

Cerebrospinal fluid leakage may occur, particularly after the posterior petrosal approaches. It is important that exposed mastoid air cells be waxed thoroughly and that the middle ear be sealed carefully with a muscle pledget at the end of the procedure. Although it is occasionally not possible to achieve a water-tight primary closure when the presigmoid dura has been opened, it is important to seal meticulously this area with pericranium, fascia lata, fat, and autologous fibrin glue.

OVERVIEW

Basilar trunk aneurysms continue to present a substantial technical challenge. However, the use of skull base surgical techniques has provided dramatically improved exposure of these lesions. The surgical approach may involve the combined efforts of an otologic surgeon and a neurosurgeon. Wider appreciation and use of these approaches is destined to improve the surgical results for basilar trunk aneurysms.

REFERENCES

1. Schievink WI, Wijdicks EF, Piepgras DG, et al. The poor prognosis of ruptured intracranial aneurysms of the posterior circulation. *J Neurosurg* 1995;82:791–795.
2. Takahashi M. The basilar artery. In: Newton TH, Potts DG, eds. *Radiology of the Skull and Brain*. Great Neck, NY: Medibooks, 1986.
3. Hoshimaru M, Hashimoto N, Kikuchi H, et al. Aneurysm of the fenestrated basilar artery: report of two cases. *Surg Neurol* 1992;37:406–409.
4. Sanders WP, Sorek PA, Mehta BA. Fenestration of intracranial arteries with special attention to associated aneurysms and other anomalies. *Am J Neuroradiol* 1993;14:675–680.
5. Rhoton A. Anatomic foundations of aneurysm surgery. *Clin Neurosurg* 1993;41:289–324.
6. Pelz DM, Vinuela F, Fox A, et al. Vertebrobasilar occlusion therapy of giant aneurysms. Significance of angiographic morphology of the posterior communicating arteries. *J Neurosurg* 1984;60:560–565.
7. Batjer H. Cerebral protective effects of etomidate: experimental and clinical aspects. *Cerebrovasc Metab Rev* 1993;5:7–32.
8. Martin NA, Bentson J, Vinuela F, et al. Intraoperative digital subtraction angiography and the surgical treatment of intracranial aneurysms and vascular malformations. *J Neurosurg* 1990;73:526–533.
9. Drake CG. The treatment of aneurysms of the posterior circulation. *Clin Neurosurg* 1979;26:96.
10. Kawase T, Shipbara R, and Toya S. Anterior transpetrosal-transtentorial approach for sphenopetroclival meningiomas: surgical method and results in 10 patients. *Neurosurgery* 1991;28:868–875.
11. Kawase T, Toya S, Shiobara R, et al. Transpetrosal approach for aneurysms of the lower basilar artery. *J Neurosurg* 1985;63:857.
12. Kasdon DL, Stein BM. Combined supratentorial and infratentorial exposure for low-lying basilar aneurysms. *Neurosurgery* 1979;4:422–426.
13. Malis LI. Surgical resection of tumors of the skull base. In: Wilkins RH, Rengachary SS, eds. *Neurosurgery*. vol 1. New York: McGraw-Hill, 1985;1011–1021.
14. Hashi K, Nin K, Shimotake K. Transpetrosal combined supratentorial and infratentoral approach for midline vertebrobasilar aneurysms. In: Brock M, ed. *Modern Neurosurgery*. vol 1. Berlin: Springer-Verlag, 1982;442–448.
15. Al-Mefty O, Ayoubi S, Smith R. The petrosal approach: indications, technique, and results. *Acta Neurochir Suppl (Wien)* 1991;53:166–170.
16. Canalis RF, Black K, Martin N, et al. Extended retrolabyrinthine transtentorial approach to petroclival lesions. *Laryngoscope* 1991;101:6–13.
17. Samii M, Ammiriati M, Mahran A, et al. Surgery of petroclival meningiomas: report of 24 cases. *Neurosurgery* 1989;24:12–17.
18. Giannotta SL, Maceri DR. Retrolabyrinthine transsigmoid approach to basilar trunk and vertebrobasilar junction aneurysms. *J Neurosurg* 1988;69:461.
19. Spetzler RJ, Daspit CP, Pappas CTE. The combined supra- and infratentorial approach for lesions of the petrous and clival regions: experience with 46 cases. *J Neurosurg* 1992;76:588.
20. King W, Black K, Martin N, et al. The petrosal approach with hearing preservation. *J Neurosurg* 1993;79:508–514.
21. Day J, Fukushima T, Giannotta S. Microanatomical study of the extradural middle fossa approach to the petroclival and posterior cavernous sinus region: description of the rhomboid construct. *Neurosurgery* 1994;34:1009–1016.
22. Harsh G.R. IV, Sekhar L. The subtemporal, transcavernous, anterior transpetrosal approached upper brain stem and clivus. *J Neurosurg* 1992;77:709–717.
23. Sekhar L, Kalia K, Yonas H, et al. Cranial base approaches to intracranial aneurysms in the subarachnoid space. *Neurosurgery* 1994;35:472–483.
24. Heros RC. Lateral approach for vertebral and vertebrobasilar artery lesions. *J Neurosurg* 1986;64:559.
25. Nishizaki T, Tamiki N, Takeda N, et al. Dolichoectatic basilar artery: a review of 23 cases. *Stroke* 1986;17:1277.
26. Aymard A, Gobin Y, Hodes J, et al. Endovascular occlusion of vertebral arteries in the treatment of unclippable vertebrobasilar aneurysms. *J Neurosurg* 1991;74:393–398.
27. Sundt T, Piepgras D, Houser O. Interposition saphenous vein grafts for advanced occlusive disease and large aneurysms in the posterior circulation. *J Neurosurg* 1982;56:205–215
28. Higashida R, Halback V, Cahan L, et al. Detachable balloon embolization therapy of posterior circulation intracranial aneurysms. *J Neurosurg* 1989;71:512–519.
29. Guglielmi G, Vinuela F, Duckwiler G, et al. Endovascular treatment of posterior circulation aneurysms by electrothrombosis using electrolytically detachable coils. *J Neurosurg* 1992;77:515–524.
30. Gurian JH, Martin NA, King WA, et al. Neurosurgical management of cerebral aneurysms following unsuccessful or incomplete endovascular embolization. *J Neurosurg* 1995;83:843–853.

Cerebrovascular Disease, edited by H. Hunt Batjer.
Lippincott-Raven Publishers, Philadelphia © 1997.

CHAPTER 85

Distal Basilar Artery Aneurysm: Surgical Techniques

Jacques J. Morcos and Roberto C. Heros

INTRODUCTION

The following statement by Kenneth Jamieson, made in 1967, has been widely quoted: "It is clear that the basilar bifurcation is no place for the faint of heart. Only time and greater experience will indicate whether it is a place for neurosurgeons at all." This quotation, at least the first half of it, rings true for many reasons. Seated deep in the interpeduncular cistern, the basilar top presents a major difficulty in access. One has to study carefully the angle of approach and maneuverability around other vascular structures as well as the IIIrd and IVth nerves. Once exposed, an aneurysm of this region has to be dissected off a very important set of perforators that will be described below. None of these small vessels is forgiving. As end arteries, their occlusion can result in a plethora of clinical stroke syndromes that affect somatic, visceral, and higher mental functions. Surgery of the basilar top aneurysm allows no room for error.

The history of the treatment of posterior circulation aneurysms in general dates back to 1932 when Olivecrona is said to have performed the first unplanned trapping of a PICA aneurysm. Tonnis in 1937 inadvertently opened a cerebellopontine (CP) angle aneurysm having made the assumption that it was a tumor preoperatively (1). Dandy in 1944 performed the first vertebral artery ligation at C1–C2 for the treatment of an intracranial aneurysm, whereas Schwartz in 1948 performed the first direct surgical approach to trap a posterior fossa aneurysm (2). Gillingham in 1957 described the surgical treatment of five patients, three of whom died and one of whom was left in a vegetative state (3). Logue introduced intracranial vertebral artery ligation in 1958 (4). Mount described basilar artery ligation in 1962 (5). Drake,

J. J. Morcos: Department of Neurosurgery, University of Miami/Mount Sinai Medical Center, Miami Beach, FL 33140.

R. C. Heros: Department of Neurosurgery, University of Miami, Miami, FL 33136.

who pioneered the field, published his initial experience with four surgical cases in 1961, and Jamieson reported 19 surgical cases in 1964, 10 of whom had died and 5 were left with severe morbidity (6,7). With the advent of microneurosurgical techniques in the late 1960s and their propagation in the 1970s, the surgical treatment of nongiant basilar bifurcation aneurysms resulted in significantly improved outcomes from the 1960s to the 1970s to the 1980s and into the early 1990s. Worldwide reported surgical mortality rates have dropped from 37% to 6.9% to 5.1% to 2.3%, respectively, whereas morbidity has averaged between 9.5% and 13.3% (8).

In this chapter we will address the surgical microanatomy of the top of the basilar region, discuss surgical indications, and detail both conventional and skull base approaches, with an emphasis on surgical pitfalls and complication avoidance. The use of Hunterian ligation, circulatory arrest for complex/giant aneurysms, as well as results of endovascular interventional techniques are beyond the scope of this chapter and are covered fully elsewhere.

VASCULAR ANATOMY OF THE BASILAR ARTERY

The basilar artery generally begins at the pontomedullary sulcus caudally and ends at the level of the interpeduncular fossa rostrally. Becoming more tortuous and elongated with age, it generally acquires a lateral curvature convex away from the dominant vertebral artery, which is generally the left one.

The basilar artery develops from the coalescence of bilateral longitudinal vascular trunks (9). These are supplied initially by the embryonic trigeminal arteries, subsequently by input from posterior communicating and other caroticobasilar anastomoses and finally and more permanently by the developing vertebral arteries. The basilar bifurcation into both posterior cerebral arteries occurs at a variable point in relation to the clivus. It occurs at the level of the posterior clinoid process in half of the cases, higher in 30% and lower in 20% (10). The basilar tip lies within 1 cm from the clivus in 87% of cases. On an anteroposterior (AP) angiogram, the takeoff of the posterior cerebral arteries creates a W-shaped configuration when the bifurcation is high and a V-shaped configuration when it is low. The shorter and older the patient, the higher the basilar bifurcation tends to be. Relative to the brain, the basilar bifurcation ends between 0 and 40 mm from the mamillary bodies with an average of 8.1 mm (11).

The basilar artery ontogeny is complex and thus subject to anatomic variations. The posterior communicating artery and the P1 segment of the posterior cerebral artery originate from the caudal division of the internal cerebral artery (ICA). The remaining portions of the posterior cerebral artery (PCA) originate from the diencephalic and mesencephalic arteries, whereas the superior cerebellar artery (SCA) arises from the mesencephalic artery. Since the vertebral arteries arise as the result of fusion of intersegmental cervical arteries, it is not surprising that the basilar artery is the most common site for intracranial arterial fenestration (9). This most commonly occurs at the vertebrobasilar rather than the basilar bifurcation zone and is associated with a high propensity for aneurysm formation at the proximal end of the fenestrated segment.

Common aneurysm sites at the top of the basilar region are the basilar bifurcation proper, the P1 segment, and the SCA origin. The proper study of the anatomic relations of these aneurysms requires a detailed understanding of the course of the PCA and SCA. The sizes of the posterior communicating artery and the P1 segment are inversely related. Saeki and Rhoton identified a persistent large fetal posterior communicating artery in 20% of cases unilaterally and 2% bilaterally, with respectively atretic P1's (12). The persistent fetal posterior communicating artery is more common on the right side. The PCA successively traverses the interpeduncular, crural, ambient, and quadrigeminal cisterns before it becomes cortical (13). The cisternal segment of the PCA thus courses parallel and below the level of the basal vein of Rosenthal, which closely hugs the midbrain but above the IIIrd nerve and the free edge of the tentorium. The P2 segment starts at the junction with the posterior communicating artery and ends at the takeoff of the inferior temporal branches. It is predominantly in the ambient cistern. P3 starts at the temporal branches takeoff and ends at the bifurcation into calcarine and parieto-occipital arteries, usually at the level of the isthmus of the cingulate gyrus. P3 is therefore predominantly in the quadrigeminal cistern.

Branches of the PCA have predominantly four destinations: thalamus, midbrain, choroid plexus, and cerebral cortex. The P1 segment gives rise to posterior thalamoperforator and mesencephalic arteries that predominantly arise from its superior and posterior surfaces (11,13–15). In addition to these perforating branches, the quadrigeminal artery that supplies the quadrigeminal plate is a constant long circum-

flex branch of the inferior surface of P1 (11,14,15), while the medial posterior choroidal artery may arise from either P1 or P2, travels medial to the cisternal segment of the PCA supplying the quadrigeminal plate, and passes lateral to the pineal body to reach the tela choroidea in the roof of the third ventricle. According to Saeki and Rhoton, the most medial branch of P1 was also the largest in 56% of the cases and was almost always a posterior thalamoperforator (12). The number of posterior thalamoperforators can range between 1 and 13 branches and these are predominantly directed vertically upward to penetrate the posterior perforated substance (12,14). They can either arise as individual branches of P1 or as a large stem that immediately branches. Thus stems are found in close to 70% of cases (15,16). More importantly, in 8% of specimens one P1 is found to have no thalamoperforators whereas the other carries a large stem that supplies both sides (16). It was also pointed out that a hypoplastic P1, found in 17% of cases, was frequently more than twice the length of the contralateral normal P1 and frequently bore larger perforators (15). Posterior thalamoperforators supply anterior and part of the posterior thalamus, posterior limb of the internal capsule, hypothalamus, subthalamic nucleus, substantia nigra, and red nucleus. The medial posterior choroidal artery arises predominantly from P2 (in 71% of cases), but it can arise from P1, P3, or P4 (17). It is frequently duplicated along its long path to the foramen of Monroe. It may supply the peduncle, tegmentum, geniculate bodies, colliculi, pulvinar, pineal gland, roof of third ventricle, habenula, and dorsal medial thalamus (13). The lateral posterior choroidal artery generally arises distal to its medial counterpart and in 50% of the cases from P2 (17). It enters the lateral choroidal fissure within a few millimeters of the entrance of the anterior choroidal artery, supplies the temporal horn, and then courses beneath the column of the fornix into the medial choroidal fissure to supply pulvinar, body of fornix, and dorsomedial thalamus. The thalamogeniculate artery generally arises from the midportion of P2. Several branches arise and course superoposteriorly to supply medial and lateral geniculate bodies, posterolateral thalamus, and posterior limb of internal capsule.

The superior cerebellar arteries arise from the top of the basilar just proximal to its bifurcation. This is the most common configuration and, unlike the other cerebellar arteries, the superior cerebellar artery is always present on both sides. Its main trunk is divided into three segments: anterior pontine, ambient, and quadrigeminal. It commonly terminates in three named branches: medial, lateral, and superior vermian. Along its course, the SCA supplies the superolateral pons, the midbrain, and the superior cerebellar surface (10). The SCA contributes perforators to the posterior perforated substance at the depth of the interpeduncular fossa. During its course, it travels caudal to the IIIrd and IVth cranial nerves as well as caudal and parallel to the free edge of the tentorium and the PCA. Collaterals form via the superior vermian branch with the inferior vermian branch off the PICA; via the medial branch with the quadrigeminal branches off the

PCA; and via the lateral branch with the cortical branches of the AICA. The SCA is frequently duplicated or triplicated, and this merely represents a separate origin for its medial and lateral branches from the basilar artery. In addition, it can originate from the P1 segment in up to 18% of cases, particularly in the presence of a low bifurcation with a steep vertical takeoff for the PCAs (13).

Besides the posterior cerebral and superior cerebellar arteries, the rostral basilar artery is itself a source of perforators. According to Zeal and Rhoton, its upper centimeter gives rise to an average of eight perforating branches, 50% of which are from the posterior surface and 50% from the sides (17). No perforating branches arose from the anterior surface of the basilar (15,17). These perforators are destined to the midbrain, the caudal thalamus, and the upper pons. Caruso et al confirmed that the basilar summit itself does not give rise to perforators and that, unlike the vertically ascending posterior thalamoperforators of P1, distal basilar origin perforators are very nearly horizontal (15).

Surgical Implications of Vascular Anatomy

Based on the anatomy discussed above, the following factors can be considered key elements in surgical decision making and techniques:

1. *Level of the basilar top.* With low-lying basilar bifurcation aneurysms, the P1's will follow a vertically ascending course and therefore partially obstruct access to the aneurysm from a subtemporal approach, necessitating the use of a fenestrated clip. A high aneurysm, on the other hand, will not in general be obscured by the P1, but will present a high degree of complexity on account of its intimate adherence to the interpeduncular fossa and its relative inaccessibility without undue brain retraction through conventional surgical approaches.

2. *Distance from clivus.* Because trans-Sylvian approaches to the basilar top involve a downward directed surgical angle, the closer the aneurysm neck is to clivus the more hidden it becomes from the surgeon's view. On the other hand, while it may be more desirable to the surgeon that the aneurysm be distanced from the clivus, the more posterior it is, the more it becomes intimately adherent to the brain stem.

3. *P1 perforators.* These remain the nemesis of top of the basilar aneurysm surgery. The surgeon, however, can at least rely on the constancy of the following anatomical facts: A hypoplastic P1 carries as many and as vital perforators as a normal-sized P1 and therefore demands equal respect and preservation. If the ipsilateral P1 carries no perforators, then the contralateral P1 almost certainly carries perforators that supply both sides. The direction that the perforators take is dependent on the level at which they arose. With a low-lying P1 segment, the perforators climb vertically upward, aiming for the posterior perforated substance, whereas they remain rela-

tively more horizontal with a high bifurcation. The former scenario implies that the perforators would be intimately adherent to the back wall of the basilar bifurcation aneurysm and clip application has to take this into consideration.

4. *Posterior communicating artery perforators.* The anterior thalamoperforators leaving the posterior communicating artery do so generally from its medial-dorsal aspect and ascend rostroposteriorly. The decision to divide a small posterior communicating artery to improve exposure cannot be made without first confirming that the ipsilateral P1 is not atretic or that the ipsilateral P1 will definitely not be compromised by the clip placement as this would result in an ipsilateral PCA territory ischemia.

5. *Superior cerebellar artery perforators.* In the setting of an SCA origin aneurysm, the surgeon has to be on the lookout for possible perforators leaving the SCA near its origin and supplying the interpeduncular group of the posterior perforated substance. Although less numerous than their P1 counterparts, these perforators can still result in significant brainstem strokes if compromised.

6. *Basilar top perforators.* It is important to realize that these do not arise from the exact apex of the basilar artery but usually at a point more proximal and never from the anterior surface. Thus, these perforators become significant in the presence of a posterior pointing aneurysm with a caudally hanging sac. The surgeon thus has to contend with and separate not only these but also the P1 perforators.

CLINICAL VASCULAR SYNDROMES

Posterior Cerebral Artery

Occlusion of the PCA can result in a variety of clinical syndromes depending on the exact site of occlusion and the extent of collateral flow. Thus, there are two general categories: brainstem and cortical syndromes.

Cortical syndromes arise from the occlusion of temporal or occipital branches. The unilateral occipital infarct results in contralateral homonymous hemianopsia with macular sparing. Visual hallucinations may occur in the hemianopic field (Cogan's syndrome). Dominant infarction involving both the dominant occipital lobe and the splenium of the corpus callosum results in a disconnection syndrome characterized by alexia without agraphia, and color anomia. Bilateral occipital lobe lesions result in cortical blindness often accompanied by lack of awareness of the patient (Anton's syndrome), or by oculomotor apraxia and visual inattention (Balint's syndrome). Occlusion of branches supplying the medial inferior dominant temporal lobe or both temporal lobes results in a variety of memory defects, including Korsakoff's syndrome.

Occlusion of the posterior thalamoperforators most commonly results in a contralateral hemiballismus or hemichoreoathetosis. Occlusion of the interpeduncular perforators may result in Weber's syndrome (ipsilateral IIIrd nerve palsy and contralateral hemiplegia) or Claude's syndrome (ipsilateral IIIrd nerve palsy and contralateral cerebellar ataxia and tremor due to the involvement of the brachium conjunctivum and the red nucleus, respectively). Occlusion of the thalamogeniculate arteries results in the thalamic syndrome of Dejerine with contralateral hemisensory loss which is gradually replaced in time by pain and hyperpathia. Homonymous hemianopsia from lateral geniculate involvement may also be present.

Superior Cerebellar Artery

Occlusion in this territory most commonly results in ipsilateral cerebellar ataxia. Less common findings, due to the inconsistency of brainstem perforator supply, are contralateral hemianesthesia and partial deafness among others.

There is in addition a variety of top of the basilar syndromes due to occlusion of the most rostral basilar artery and/or its branches, causing various combinations of drowsiness, memory deficits, visual hallucinations, delirium, visual deficits, and disorders of ocular movement (18).

SURGICAL PRINCIPLES

Indications and Timing of Surgery

The most frequent and compelling indication for surgical treatment of a distal basilar aneurysm is a recent subarachnoid hemorrhage (SAH). Under such circumstance, the only reasonable relative contraindications to surgery are poor neurologic grade, poor medical condition, very old age, or the availability of a more effective and/or safer form of treatment. We generally do not operate while patients are in poor neurologic grades (grades 4 and 5) unless the neurologic condition can be improved with such maneuvers as ventriculostomy, excision of an intracerebral hematoma, medical treatment of increased intracranial pressure, etc. If the patient stabilizes but remains in poor neurologic condition, the decision as to whether to treat the aneurysm or not is a difficult one that needs to be resolved on a case-by-case basis after attending to many factors such as the family's wishes, the presumed wishes of the patient, age, and so forth. Medical contraindications are almost always relative, although some conditions such as a recent myocardial infarction, end-stage liver or pulmonary disease, and widespread malignancies are generally absolute contraindications. Old age is another relative contraindication, but there are some reports indicating that the morbidity in individuals in their late 60s and 70s in good medical condition is comparable to that to be expected in the younger age group.

Another strong indication for treatment is the appearance or progression of symptoms and signs of brainstem and/or cranial nerve (usually oculomotor) compression by the aneurysm. Some of the specific syndromes that are seen with these aneurysms were discussed above. Less commonly, a patient with a distal basilar aneurysm develops ischemic signs from thrombotic or embolic occlusion of the posterior cerebellar arteries or the distal basilar perforators. These syndromes, however, are much more common with fusiform, partially thrombosed basilar trunk aneurysms.

A more complicated and as-yet-unresolved issue is that of the relative merit of endovascular vs. open surgical aneurysmal occlusion. Technically, these basilar aneurysms are not more difficult and perhaps easier to treat by endovascular methods than aneurysms at any of the other common locations. This is in contradistinction to open surgery, which clearly carries a higher morbidity in most hands than surgery for an equivalent-sized aneurysm at any other location. It appears that either complete or even subtotal occlusion of the aneurysm with coils introduced by endovascular technique offers significant protection against subarachnoid hemorrhage, at least for the first year, which is, of course, the period of maximal risk for rebleeding. Whether these results will hold on longer follow-up is presently unknown, but if they do, they will make endovascular occlusion a reasonable alternative to open microsurgical treatment of aneurysms in this difficult location.

The issue of timing of surgery for distal basilar aneurysms is a difficult one that has not been settled. Clearly, the trend has been toward early surgery. However, the approach to the distal basilar artery always requires brain retraction, regardless of the particular surgical approach used. The larger the aneurysm, the more exposure will be necessary and therefore the more retraction will be required. Very high basilar bifurcation aneurysms also require additional brain retraction. Clearly, a patient in relatively poor neurologic grade could be harmed by such retraction, and it may be prudent in such patients to wait until the intracranial pressure has normalized before entertaining surgery. The experience of the surgeon is also important and as experience with these aneurysms increases, the surgeon will require less retraction and the retraction will need to be applied for a shorter time, which is the reason that most experienced aneurysm surgeons are now operating early in the majority of patients in good neurologic condition with less than giant basilar aneurysms. However, an aneurysm in this location makes it perfectly justifiable to delay surgery when the aneurysm is large or complex, when the patient shows signs of increased intracranial pressure or when the surgeon does not have extensive experience with surgery in this region.

Preoperative Preparation

The general management of patients with SAH from a distal basilar aneurysm is no different than for other patients with aneurysmal SAH. As with other difficult aneurysms that are relatively deep, brain relaxation at the time of surgery is important. With the frontotemporal approach, we generally do not use a lumbar catheter because enough cerebrospinal fluid (CSF) can be withdrawn from the cisterns, after opening the dura, to achieve relaxation. Occasionally, once the dura is open, the surgeon encounters a very swollen brain that makes it difficult to reach the medial cisterns to withdraw CSF. In these cases, we have inserted a ventricular needle directly through the frontal lobe using the landmarks suggested by Paine et al (a perpendicular insertion of the needle for about 5–6 cm at the point of the right angle formed by 2.5-cm lines drawn perpendicularly from the Sylvian fissure and from the base of the frontal fossa (19). Whenever we use the subtemporal approach, we insert a lumbar catheter after induction of anesthesia. It is important not to lose too much fluid to prevent premature rupture of the aneurysm. After the dura is opened, we release an average of 60 cm³, which usually is adequate to allow comfortable temporal lobe retraction. Regardless of the approach, at the beginning of the craniotomy, we infuse 100 g of mannitol and, depending on the urine output, we use Lasix to promote osmotic diuresis.

In many patients, temporary clipping of the basilar artery is utilized to soften the aneurysm during the final stages of dissection and clipping. Unless prolonged temporary clipping is anticipated, we use no special precautions other than maintaining a normal blood pressure in most instances because usually the temporary clipping is kept to a period of less than a few minutes. However, if prolonged temporary clipping is anticipated because of the difficulty of dissection or because there is planned opening of the aneurysm, special precautions need to be taken. When this is the case, we use an additional bolus infusion of 50 g of mannitol given about 15 minutes prior to cross-clamping. During this time we also elevate the blood pressure moderately, by approximately 15–20 mm Hg over the baseline pressure. Body temperature is allowed to fall spontaneously during anesthesia by 2–3°C. A bolus of thiopental (10 mg/kg) is used immediately prior to cross-clamping. In exceptional cases, when the anticipated period of cross-clamping is likely to exceed 25 minutes, arrangements are made for cardiac arrest with extracorporeal circulation.

SURGICAL APPROACHES

The first successful approach to distal basilar aneurysms is the subtemporal approach as elaborated and perfected by Drake (6). The advantages of this approach are the shorter working distance; the direct lateral approach along what is usually the widest axis of the neck of the aneurysm which allows the use of a fenestrated clip that leaves the PCA on the fenestration; the enhanced ability to see the posterior aspect of the aneurysm and the critical perforators; and the enhanced ability, by folding or dividing the tentorium, to see below the tentorium inferiorly, which is necessary for

proximal control of relatively low-lying aneurysms. The main disadvantages of the subtemporal approach are the need for temporal retraction, which makes it very difficult to approach relatively high-lying aneurysms; and the limited angle of vision, which allows only a lateral surgical corridor and makes it difficult, particularly with relatively broad-necked aneurysms, to see the opposite PCA and its critical early perforators.

The second approach to the basilar bifurcation is the frontotemporal–trans-Sylvian approach popularized by Yasargil (20). The frontotemporal approach has been modified and elaborated by several other surgeons in an effort to increase the angle of vision mostly by extending the anterior temporal exposure (21–24). The main advantage of the frontotemporal trans-Sylvian approach is the more oblique approach, which when combined with the wider angle of vision allows better visualization of the opposite PCA and its perforators and application of the clip from in front between the true neck of the aneurysm and the two posterior cerebral arteries. Additionally, the frontotemporal approach reduces significantly the need for brain retraction; allows the surgeon to withdraw CSF from the medial cisterns without need for a lumbar drain; offers a better visualization of the entire anterior circle of Willis, which permits clipping of additional aneurysms; and provides a wider field with several different surgical corridors, which may be necessary to approach complex and giant aneurysms. The main disadvantage of the frontotemporal approach is the relative difficulty in visualizing the posterior aspect of the aneurysm and the perforators in that region, particularly when the base of the aneurysm is relatively broad in the lateral direction. Additionally, the working distance with the frontotemporal approach is greater and the ability to work in this relatively deep field, between important structures such as the optic nerve, the carotid artery and its branches, and the IIIrd nerve, requires considerable microsurgical expertise. Furthermore, although ideal for high-lying basilar aneurysms, the frontotemporal approach is inadequate for very low-lying aneurysms and additional modifications such as drilling of the posterior clinoid, or of the anterior petrous apex, are necessary in order to reach low-lying aneurysms with the frontotemporal exposure.

Our own preferences have evolved gradually through the years. Initially, we approached every basilar aneurysm by the subtemporal approach. However, because of the relative difficulty in visualizing the anatomy of the opposite side of the neck of the aneurysm with the subtemporal approach, we encountered a few cases where the opposite PCA was "pinched" and/or one of its early perforators was occluded by the clip with significant neurologic consequence.

We then tried the classical pterional approach, as originally described by Yasargil, in a few cases but found it very confining because of the relative lack of anterior temporal exposure and the relatively restricted angle of vision. For this reason, we started to modify the frontotemporal approach to include a better anterior temporal exposure (21). Nowadays we use this extended frontotemporal approach, which we call a "combined pterional/anterior temporal approach" for practically all aneurysms of the basilar bifurcation. For relatively high-lying basilar bifurcation aneurysms, we modify this approach by adding an orbitozygomatic resection, which allows a more inferior angle of vision with less need for brain retraction. For low-lying aneurysms, we have frequently drilled the posterior clinoid and have occasionally used an anterior petrosectomy as described by Kawase (25, 26). We still use the subtemporal approach occasionally for small aneurysms that are relatively low lying, for low-lying aneurysms that project anteriorly and appear to be stuck to the clivus, and for aneurysms that project directly posteriorly toward the brainstem.

We will proceed to elaborate the two most commonly used surgical approaches as utilized by the authors for basilar bifurcation aneurysms; however, these approaches can also be used for all other distal basilar and proximal PCA aneurysms. We will then describe in detail the skull base approaches to the distal basilar.

The Subtemporal Approach

Preparation and Positioning

In the subtemporal approach, the patient is positioned in the full lateral with the head elevated and the vertex dipped slightly, to permit the temporal lobe to fall away from the skull base. As mentioned earlier, we always use a lumbar drain for this approach and the drain is opened immediately after the beginning of dural opening.

Soft Tissue and Bony Exposure

Although a vertical "tic" incision has been used extensively for this approach, we have found that if we keep the incision above the zygoma, we cannot get a broad enough base of our craniotomy inferiorly, where the exposure is needed. The linear incision cannot be carried below the zygoma without injuring the frontalis branch of the facial nerve. For this reason, we now use a modified pterional incision that is carried a bit posteriorly over the ear. The skin flap is then turned down at the layer superficial to the temporalis fascia; the flap is held down with fishhooks. The temporalis fascia and muscle are then opened on an inverted T fashion with the short limb of the T being approximately 1 cm on each direction just under the zygoma to allow maximal exposure of the base of the temporal bone at the level of the floor of the temporal fossa. The muscle is then dissected from the temporal bone and retracted to each side, along the long limb of the T with fishhooks A low craniotomy is then made through a burr hole using a high-speed craniotome. The base of the craniotomy is then rongeured away along the floor of the temporal fossa to allow a broad inferior exposure along the entire length of the zygoma, which allows a wider angle of vision, particularly inferiorly,

to be able to see the opposite PCA both from in front and from behind the aneurysm. This relatively broad-based craniotomy allows the surgeon to work either in front of the third nerve (between the IIIrd nerve and the carotid artery) (Fig. 1) or behind the IIIrd nerve (between the IIIrd nerve and the edge of the tentorium) (Fig. 2). After withdrawal of approximately 50–65 cm³ of CSF from the lumbar catheter, the temporal lobe can generally be gradually retracted off the floor of the temporal fossa to expose the tentorial incisura. This temporal lobe retraction has to be done gradually and carefully looking for small bridging veins which generally can be taken provided that the surgeon is sure that this is not a major part of the drainage of the temporal lobe, which, of course, usually is more posteriorly along the vein of Labbé. When the vein of Labbé drains more anteriorly, the surgeon must be extremely careful not to injure it. Occasionally, when the anterior temporal fossa is relatively hollow and the brain is swollen, which is frequent with recently ruptured aneurysms, it is preferable to resect a small portion of the anterior-inferior temporal lobe to facilitate retraction rather than to exert vigorous deep retraction of the temporal lobe, which can transmit pressure to deep structures and result in morbidity from temporal lobe swelling postoperatively (Fig. 3). The uncus can usually be gently elevated on the retractor being very careful with the IIIrd nerve, which is normally adherent to the uncus. Occasionally, the uncus projects inferiorly medial to the tentorial incisura and it may be preferable to resect part of it subpially rather than to exert excessive retraction.

To increase the exposure of the proximal basilar artery, we routinely retract the edge of the tentorium by placing a suture or two from the edge of the tentorium, between the IIIrd nerve and the point at which the fourth nerve goes under the edge of the tentorium, to the dura more laterally along the floor of the temporal fossa.

Microdissection

Under the microscope, the arachnoid is initially opened below the IIIrd nerve, with care taken not to injure the SCA, which of course runs below the nerve and may be difficult to identify through the arachnoid in cases where the cistern is filled with blood. Frequently, the entire dissection can be carried out without separating the IIIrd nerve from the uncus by working inferior and posterior to the IIIrd nerve. It is in these cases in which we have not had to separate the IIIrd nerve from the uncus that we usually see intact IIIrd nerve function after surgery. More commonly, we need to separate the IIIrd nerve from the uncus to develop the visual corridor above the IIIrd nerve. In these cases there is most frequently some dysfunction of the IIIrd nerve postoperatively, but excellent recovery within a period of weeks to months almost invariably occurs.

In cases without recent hemorrhage, the surgeon immediately sees the basilar artery and the aneurysm. When the

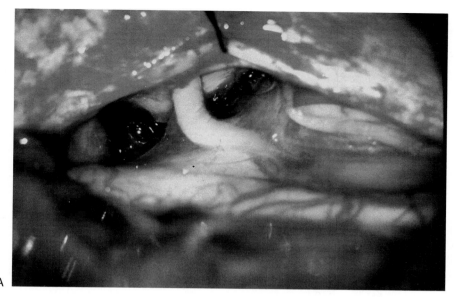

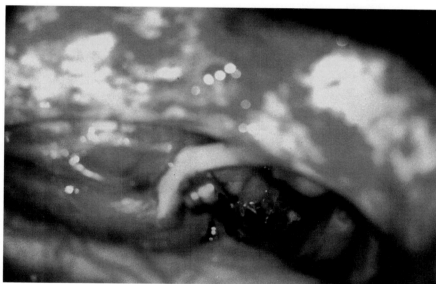

FIG. 1. Right-sided subtemporal exposure. Note the suture at the edge of the tentorium just behind the IIIrd nerve. With this relatively broad exposure, the surgeon can choose to work in front or behind the IIIrd nerve (**A**). In this particular case, the aneurysm was clipped from in front of the IIIrd nerve (**B**).

prepontine cistern is full of blood, dissection must proceed more slowly by using the superior cerebellar and the posterior cerebral arteries as landmarks. These arteries can be identified laterally in relation to the IIIrd nerve which they straddle and they then can be followed medially towards the base of the aneurysm. For as long as the surgeon is working below the PCA, he will not encounter the dome of the aneurysm before identifying its base.

An alternative when the landmarks are obscured by blood is to identify the posterior communicating artery anteriorly and open the membrane of Lielquist below and parallel to the posterior communicating artery where there are no perforators (they run superiorly). Once the membrane is opened, the surgeon can usually suction enough blood to see the posterior cerebral and superior cerebellar arteries more posteriorly. When the surgeon identifies the base of the aneu-

rysm, a decision is made as to whether to dissect posterior or anterior to the aneurysm first. In the rare aneurysms that project forward towards the clivus, it is important to carry out all of the dissection posteriorly first. The main danger in these cases is to retract the aneurysm posteriorly and rupture it when the dome is stuck to the dura of the clivus or the dorsum sella. Unfortunately, this type of projection, which is by far the easiest to deal with, is much less common. The reason anterior projection makes the dissection easier is that the posterior cerebral arteries can be readily identified behind the aneurysm and the perforators run backward, away from the aneurysm. In most instances, however, the aneurysm projects straight upward and backward between the posterior cerebral arteries. In these cases, we prefer to dissect first anterior to the aneurysm by coming along the base of the aneurysm and gently depressing the top of the basilar

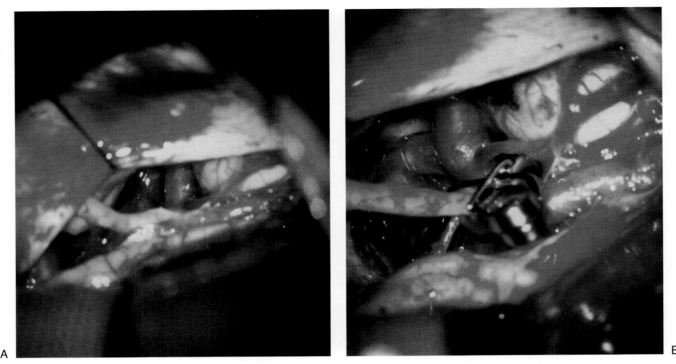

A   B

FIG. 2. Right subtemporal exposure. Note the wide exposure both in front and behind the IIIrd nerve **(A)**. In this particular case, the aneurysm was clipped in the space behind the IIIrd nerve **(B)**.

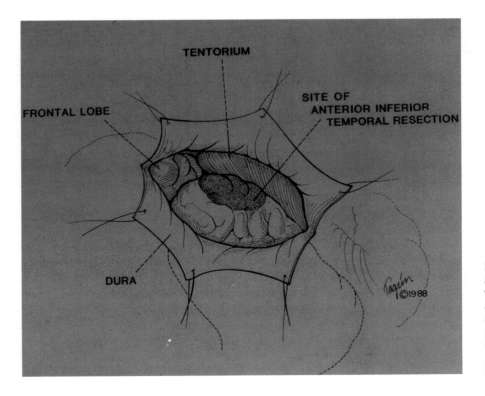

FIG. 3. Area of possible resection in the anterior-inferior temporal lobe in cases where there is a deep temporal fossa and retraction would have to be excessive without some brain resection. (With permission from Ojemann RG, Heros RC, Crowell RM. *Surgical Management of Cerebrovascular Disease.* 2nd ed. New York: Williams and Wilkins, 1988.)

backwards to identify the posterior cerebral on the other side. It is with this maneuver that the wider field of vision that can be obtained by a relatively wide-based temporal craniotomy is useful. The critical maneuver at this stage is to dissect free the distal aspect of the neck, separating the important early perforators from the initial portion of the contralateral PCA (P1). Once this is done, the surgeon has a good view of the width of the aneurysm and can begin to select a clip with blades of the appropriate length to go exactly across the neck, which is extremely important in cases where a fenestrated clip, to be applied over the ipsilateral P1, is chosen.

Clipping

Unfortunately, the array of clips available may not always provide the exact blade length required; when this is the case, we use a wire cutter to shorten a longer clip to the appropriate size and then polish the ends with the diamond drill. After the anterior aspect of the base of the aneurysm is defined and the opposite side of the neck is prepared, the surgeon proceeds to prepare the proximal neck separating the proximal perforators of the ipsilateral P1 from the neck. At this point, the surgeon decides whether the anatomy calls for the use of a fenestrated clip or, less commonly, a straight clip that can be placed from anteriorly between the two P1's or, in the rare case of the difficult aneurysms that project straight backward, from posteriorly leaving the P1's above the clip.

With a clip already preselected, the surgeon proceeds with the critical and most dangerous aspect of the dissection, which is to develop the plane posterior to the aneurysm between the base of the aneurysm and the perforators on the back. This maneuver is particularly difficult in those fortunately rare aneurysms that project straight backward toward the brainstem. Also, the lower the basilar bifurcation the more difficult this dissection is because the perforators tend to be adherent to the back of the aneurysm because they run upward along the same direction than the aneurysm. High-lying basilar aneurysms present a bit more difficulty with temporal retraction but are generally much easier because the perforators run straight backward away from the generally upward projecting aneurysm. The posterior dissection has to continue until the surgeon has seen the opposite side of the neck. With broad-based aneurysms, it is a problem to hold a space between the perforators and the aneurysm for placement of the clip. Sometimes the surgeon can keep the perforators separated with a fine suction tip or with a dissector, but because frequently the surgeon has to use one hand to suction and the other to apply the clip, as the clip is advanced, the only solution is to use the posterior blade of the clip to gradually push the dome of the aneurysm forward, away from the perforators, as the perforators are held backward with the suction tip in a dynamic fashion as the clip is gently advanced. This maneuver is greatly facilitated by

softening the base of the aneurysm by the use of a temporary clip. We use such a temporary clip whenever we have sufficient proximal exposure, except in cases of small aneurysms where the clipping is relatively straight-forward.

In our experience, the initial clip placement is generally successful only in the smaller and less complex aneurysms. In larger more complex aneurysms, more often than not we find upon inspection that either there is a perforator or more in the clip or that the clip is either not completely across the neck or too far into the opposite P1 and its initial perforators. Also, with the use of a fenestrated clip, one frequently finds that either there is too much neck inside the fenestration, which leaves the aneurysm open, or part of the ipsilateral P1 has been pinched by the beginning of the blades distal to the fenestration. The surgeon must proceed to reposition the clip until there is certainty that no perforators are included in the clip, that all of the neck is clipped and that the two P1's are free. This sometimes calls for several repositionings of the clip in the more complex aneurysms. Not infrequently, the surgeon must use a different length of clip than the one initially used.

Closure

Once the surgeon is satisfied with the clipping, he is ready to close after thorough irrigation of the subarachnoid spaces and insurance that hemostasis is perfect. The stitch from the tentorium is removed, and the area of the temporal lobe under the retractor is lined with Surgicel. The dura is then closed in a water-tight fashion and the bone flap replaced and secured with wires or microplates. The muscle is then reapproximated in the normal anatomic position and the rest of the wound closed in layers in the usual fashion.

The Combined Pterional/Anterior Temporal (Extended Frontotemporal Trans-Sylvian) Approach

Preparation and Positioning

We described our modification of the standard frontotemporal approach in a recent publication (21). The patient is placed in the supine position with the head turned approximately 45° to the opposite side.

Soft Tissue and Bony Exposure

We use a standard pterional skin incision, which is modified slightly in two ways. First, the incision starts about 0.5 cm below the zygoma right in front of the tragus to avoid injury to the temporal branches of the facial nerve, which cross the zygoma about 2 cm anterior to the tragus. Second, the incision extends upward in a straight line for about 4 or 5 cm before gradually curving forward; this allows a slightly larger craniotomy to expose the anterior temporal lobe and the anterolateral aspect of the Sylvian fissure (Fig. 4). The

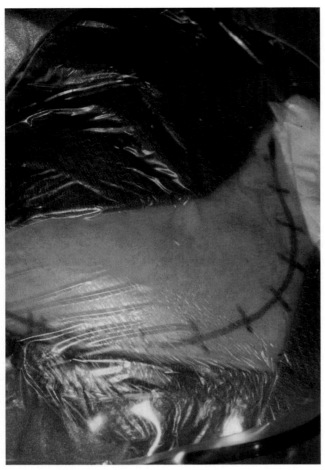

FIG. 4. Skin incision for the combined pterional/anterior temporal approach. The ear is covered with a piece of telfa and the incision starts about 1cm below the zygoma just in front of the tragus.

skin flap is turned down at a level superficial to the periosteum and the superficial temporalis fascia and it is held down with fishhooks. About 1.5–2 cm superior to the zygoma, the surgeon encounters a small fat pad as he is turning the skin flap down. At this level, the superficial layer of the temporalis fascia is incised horizontally in a direction parallel to the zygoma. This incision is carried down to the deeper, fascial layer, which is intimately adherent to the temporalis muscle itself. This is possible because at this point the superficial temporalis fascia divides into two layers leaving an interfascial space that contains fat, a few blood vessels, and the frontalis branch of the facial nerve. By continuing the retraction of the skin flap at this level, the surgeon preserves the frontalis branch in the process of exposing the zygoma. We proceed to completely expose the zygoma and the zygomaticofrontal process (Fig. 5). The skin flap, which now includes the superficial layer of the temporalis fascia with its fat pad and the frontalis branch of the facial nerve, is then forcefully held anteriorly with fishhooks to maintain the exposure of the zygoma and the zygomaticofrontal process. At this point, the surgeon has the choice of leaving the zygoma intact, as we do in most cases, or proceeding with an orbitozygomatic resection, as will be described later, which we generally reserve for cases of complex, giant, or very high-lying aneurysms. When the zygomatic arch is going to be left intact, we open the muscle in such a fashion as to be able to turn it backwards over the ear and away from the anterior temporal region which is critical for good exposure in this area. If one turns the temporalis muscle down over the zygoma, the bulk of the muscle prevents the deep anterior inferior temporal exposure that makes this approach so versatile. To retract the muscle posteriorly, we cut it along its superior and anterior insertions leaving a cuff of temporalis fascia that is continuous with the periosteum to which the muscle can be reattached at closure. After dividing

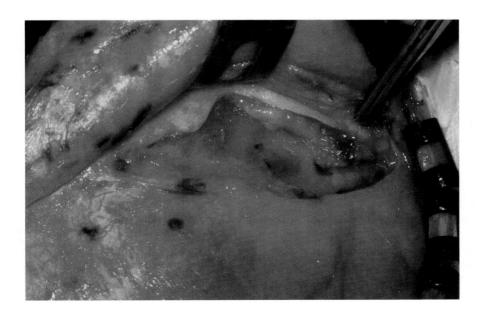

FIG. 5. Right combined pterional/anterior temporal exposure. The skin flap has been taken down at a level superficial to the temporalis fascia up to a point about 2 cm above the zygoma where the superficial layer of temporalis fascia has been incised so that it can be taken down with the skin flap to completely expose the zygoma and the zygomaticofrontal process without injuring the frontalis nerve. The retractor is at the junction of the zygomatic body with the zygomaticofrontal process.

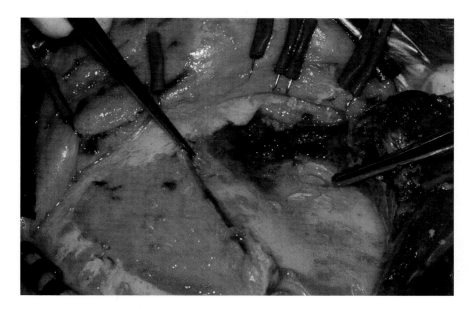

FIG. 6. Right combined pterional/anterior temporal approach. The skin flap, containing the superficial layer of the temporalis fascia inferiorly, is held down with fishhooks. The muscle has been divided, as explained in the text, so that it can be retracted backwards over the ear (right side of the exposure).

sharply the anterior insertion line, the muscle is cut inferiorly for about 2 cm under the anterior aspect of the zygoma. With this cut, a small artery that runs anteriorly under the zygoma is usually transected and has to be controlled. By leaving the posterior aspect of the muscle intact, one preserves the posterior vascular pedicle and we have had no problem with unsightly atrophy of the muscle postoperatively. The muscle is then retracted backward with fishhooks producing an excellent anterior inferior temporal exposure (Fig. 6).

The standard burr holes are used as for the classical pterional approach. We use one burr hole just behind the lateral orbital ridge in the "keyhole" region and one posteriorly and inferiorly, behind the pterion. We then use the high-speed craniotome to cut a free craniotomy flap that is essentially the same as the standard pterional flap but with an additional temporal extension. The bone flap is then fractured at the pterion and the bone in the temporal region rongeured or drilled down to the floor of the temporal fossa below the zygoma. Using rongeurs and the high-speed air drill, the pterion and the lesser wing of the sphenoid are thoroughly removed with particularly aggressive bone removal of the posterior aspect of the pterion and part of the greater sphenoid wing to completely expose the dura over the anterior aspect of the tip of the temporal pole. This bone removal in the anterior temporal region is the key to this approach. The dura is then tented all around the bone flap and opened with a semi-circular incision based inferiorly at the pterion. The anterior-inferior leaf of the dural flap is then sutured forcibly upward to offer a flat line of vision inferiorly all the way to the base of the anterior clinoid with minimal retraction. When more posterior subtemporal exposure is desired, a second dural flap can then be developed with a perpendicular cut that extends backward and inferiorly from the initial curvilinear cut. The second flap can then

be tented upward over the zygoma to afford good anterior subtemporal exposure. Since retraction of the temporal pole is necessary, we proceed at this point to coagulate and divide one or more small bridging temporopolar veins. To our knowledge, we have never had a problem with this maneuver, although we are aware of the fact that other surgeons condemn it. The frontal and temporal self-retaining retractors are then placed at right angles to each other to facilitate opening of the Sylvian fissure and the microscope is brought into the field (Fig. 7).

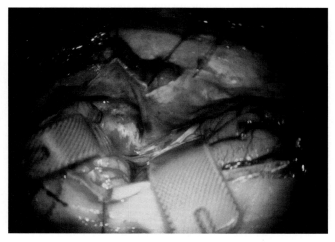

FIG. 7. Right combined pterional/anterior temporal approach. The dura has been opened and tented forward after removing the pterion and the lesser wing of the sphenoid as well as part of the greater wing as explained in the text. The self-retaining retractors in the frontal lobe *(left)* and the temporal lobe *(right)* have been positioned so as to place the lowest aspect of the Sylvian fissure under slight stretch to facilitate its opening.

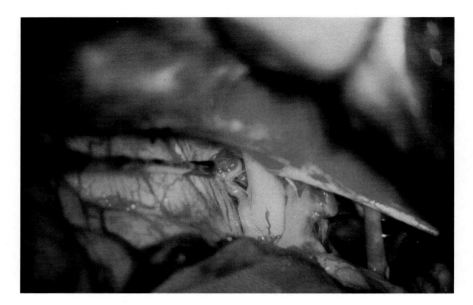

FIG. 8. Right combined pterional/anterior temporal approach. Under the microscope, the arachnoid of the medial cisterns has been opened widely so as to expose the opposite A-1, the anterior communicating complex (notice the small anterior communicating aneurysm under the small retractor), the right A-1, the right carotid artery, and, more posteriorly, the IIIrd nerve seen as it goes just under the edge of the tentorium and below it and behind it the distal basilar artery.

Microdissection

Under the microscope, we open the medial cisterns extensively to completely separate the frontal lobes from the optic chiasm and to expose first the opposite carotid artery and the origin of the ophthalmic artery under the opposite optic nerve. Next we identify the opposite anterior cerebral artery, which ensures good arachnoidal separation of the opposite frontal lobe from the opposite optic nerve. The opposite proximal anterior cerebral artery (A1) can usually be followed to the anterior communicating complex (Fig. 8). At this point, we proceed with the opening of the Sylvian fissure. The decision as to whether to open the fissure from lateral to medial or from medial to lateral depends on its appearance at surgery. In cases without recent hemorrhage,

it is usually easier to open the fissure from lateral to proximal, but in cases of recent hemorrhage, the anatomy is frequently distorted and the surgeon has to proceed with the more tedious medial to lateral dissection following the distal carotid artery to the middle cerebral. The endpoint is to expose all of the middle cerebral artery trunk down to the limen insula, which is usually the point of the bifurcation of the middle cerebral artery. The temporal lobe is then very carefully separated from the middle cerebral artery to avoid avulsion of small temporal branches from the middle cerebral artery once the temporal pole is retracted backward. At this point, the surgeon completes the opening of the medial cisterns by freeing up the IIIrd nerve, the posterior communicating artery, and the anterior choroidal artery (Fig. 9). To obtain better exposure lateral and posterior to the oculomotor

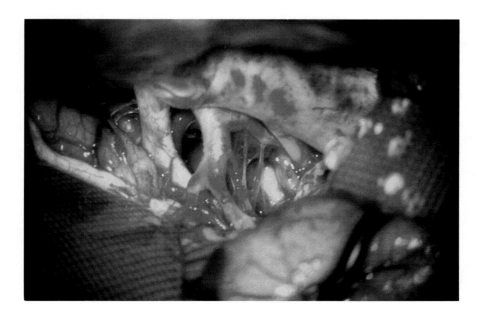

FIG. 9. Right combined pterional/anterior temporal approach in a different case. The field is centered on the right carotid artery. The arachnoid has been opened widely in this case with fresh hemorrhage to reveal the posterior communicating artery (just under the tentorial edge in front of the IIIrd nerve) with its perforators and the anterior choroidal artery a bit more superiorly. The Sylvian fissure has been opened to expose the middle cerebral artery to its first bifurcation.

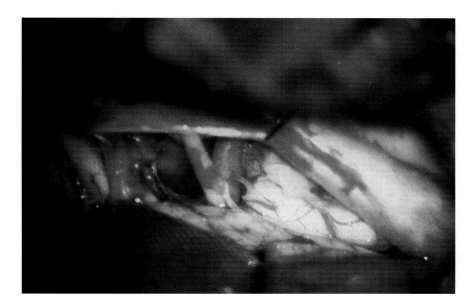

FIG. 10. Right combined pterional/anterior temporal approach. In a different case, the IIIrd nerve is at the center of the surgical field. A stitch has been placed behind the IIIrd nerve to gain better exposure of the proximal basilar artery, which is clearly seen immediately posterior to the IIIrd nerve.

nerve, we frequently suture the edge of the tentorium laterally behind the IIIrd nerve in the same fashion as with the subtemporal approach (Fig. 10). This last maneuver allows an additional corridor of vision posterolateral to the IIIrd nerve. At this point, the microscope is moved more laterally to come from a more anterior temporal direction so as to have the IIIrd nerve essentially in the middle of the field, giving the surgeon the opportunity to work along three different corridors: between the optic nerve and the carotid artery, between the carotid artery and the IIIrd nerve, and between the IIIrd nerve and the tentorium (Fig. 11). In this fashion, the surgeon has all of the advantages offered by both the pterional and the subtemporal approaches in terms of the angle of vision. It should be emphasized that the anterior temporal exposure, lateral to the carotid artery, is ob-

tained by posterolateral retraction of the temporal pole rather than by elevation of the temporal lobe. It is our impression that posterolateral retraction of the temporal pole is much better tolerated, in terms of postoperative temporal edema, than the temporal lobe elevation that is required for the subtemporal approach. In other words, the exposure obtained in the manner described is a combined subfrontal (over the lesser wing of the sphenoid) and pretemporal (along the posterior aspect of the greater wing of the sphenoid) exposure.

Clipping

The subsequent steps of aneurysmal approach and clipping are essentially identical to those described for the sub-

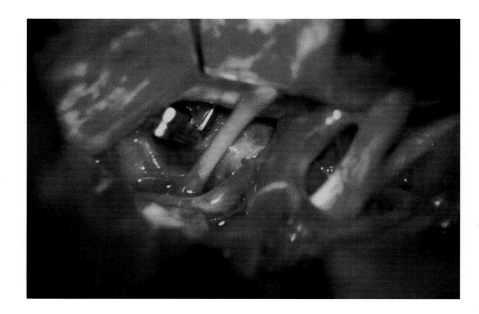

FIG. 11. Left combined pterional/anterior temporal approach. In this case of a left-sided exposure, the IIIrd nerve is seen going below the tentorium in the center of the field. The clip has been applied in the space between the IIIrd nerve and the edge of the tentorium in a direction comparable to the usual lateral direction of the subtemporal approach. The optic chiasm, partially covered by blood in this case of fresh subarachnoid hemorrhage, is seen to the right of the exposure.

temporal approach. However, more often than not, the surgeon ends up applying a clip, when this combined approach is used, from an oblique anterolateral direction with the posterior blade of the clip going between the ipsilateral P1 and the aneurysm and then between the posterior aspect of the aneurysm and the perforators. The anterior blade goes between the contralateral P1 and the aneurysm carefully preserving the early perforators from the P1. Nevertheless, by slightly increasing the degree of temporopolar retraction, a more lateral line of vision can be obtained which allows the placement of a fenestrated clip leaving the ipsilateral P1 in the fenestration, much as in the subtemporal approach. To obtain this more lateral exposure, between the IIIrd nerve and the edge of the tentorium, it is helpful to resect subpially a bit of the uncus, which we prefer to uncal retraction, which would require that the retractor be placed medial to the edge of the tentorium—a somewhat dangerous situation in our opinion. In other words, we prefer to have the retractor resting on the tentorium so that it cannot accidentally be pushed against vital structures.

Skull Base Approaches to the Distal Basilar Artery

During the last decade, new neurosurgical techniques were introduced in an effort to expand the limits of resectability of skull base tumors. It became clear that enlarging the exposure resulted in several advantages:

1. The more bone one drills, the less brain retraction is necessary.
2. The surgeon is brought closer to the pathology.
3. The surgical corridor is wider.
4. Illumination and visibility are enhanced at the depth of the field.
5. Areas previously inaccessible by conventional approaches become accessible.

These elements were promptly extrapolated to aneurysm surgery and particularly to the basilar bifurcation lesion. It would be fair to state that none of the various newer techniques advocated for the treatment of difficult basilar aneurysms were original contributions per se. What follows is a historical, chronological description of applicable skull base approaches as originally described in the literature.

In 1979, Kasdon and Stein described the combined *supratentorial/infratentorial approach* for the treatment of lower basilar trunk aneurysms in two patients (27). They used the lateral position with lumbar spinal drainage. The incision was extended from the temporal area into the posterior fossa midway between mastoid and inion. The temporal bone flap was created and suboccipital craniectomy completed. The dura was opened above and below the tentorium and then test occlusion of the transverse sinus carried out. After confirming tolerance to the occlusion by lack of brain swelling, the sinus was divided and the tentorium transected to the

incisura. It is interesting that the authors described in addition drilling the petrous bone between the Vth nerve and the internal auditory meatus for increased exposure, an area that was subsequently recognized by Kawase and is presently known as Kawase's triangle or rhomboid. The approach gave the authors full view of the entire basilar artery and the aneurysms were clipped satisfactorily.

With the advent of transpetrosal approaches, the need for the combined supratentorial-infratentorial approach with sacrifice of the transverse sinus has become exceedingly rare. It is, however, a procedure that one needs to be familiar with as it provides a panoramic view from foramen magnum to petrous apex and thus would be theoretically suitable for basilar trunk or very low-lying basilar bifurcation aneurysms. When we have had to use this approach, we have relied on a preoperative angiogram in the venous phase to demonstrate a patent contralateral transverse sinus and we have used intraluminal pressure measurements of the transverse sinus using a 23-gauge butterfly with a temporary clip placed laterally. The lack of a dramatic rise in pressure following clipping reassured us the patient would tolerate permanent division of the sinus.

The *supraorbital approach* revived and modified an older extended frontal approach for the exposure of tumors in the floor of the frontal fossa, aneurysms of the anterior communicating artery complex, as well as lesions of the orbit (28). However, the indications for this approach were subsequently extended by Al-Mefty, through the so-called *tailored cranio-orbital approach*, to treat lesions such as basilar bifurcation aneurysms located above the level of the posterior clinoids (29). As originally described, the technique involves a bicoronal skin incision and elevation of the scalp including the underlying periosteum. The periorbita, continuous with the pericranium at the level of the superior orbital ridge, is separated from the bony orbital roof after freeing the supraorbital nerve from the supraorbital notch. The notch can be a complete or an incomplete bony tunnel and a small osteotome can be used to open the tunnel and release the nerve, which is then displaced with the skin flap. One burr hole is placed in the midline over the glabella and the other in the keyhole area just behind the curve of the zygomatic process. The underlying dura is stripped through both burr holes and the Gigli saw is used to connect both holes with a cut placed as posterior as possible on the orbital roof. This is made possible only by depressing the orbital contents for direct visualization of the path of the saw. Thus, the free frontal bone flap is elevated with the superolateral orbital rim and anterior orbital roof as a single piece. Following a low dural incision, the base of the frontal lobe can be accessed with minimal retraction. The surgical corridor can be deepened subfrontally to access the frontal fossa floor, the chiasm, the suprasellar area, as well as the opticocarotid space that leads to the interpeduncular cistern and the basilar bifurcation. At closure, a vascularized pedicle flap of pericranium is turned down to cover the breached frontal sinus and sutured to the dura.

We do not advocate the use of this approach for accessing aneurysms of the rostral basilar artery because although the removal of the orbital rim provides a lower vantage point and therefore a higher angle of view in the AP plane, the width of the approach is limited to the subfrontal surface that is tethered by the olfactory tract, the optic chiasm, and, to a certain degree, the supraclinoid carotid artery. In addition, the exposure of the basilar artery at the depth is at the mercy of the available width of the opticocarotid space. Thus, the approach in most instances will prove too deep and confining.

Anterior Transpetrosal Approach

This approach has its roots in the original simple middle fossa approach introduced by Bill House at the House Ear Institute in the 1960s. The simple approach provides an excellent view from above of the contents of the internal auditory canal. It became clear in the 1970s that extending that approach anteriorly by drilling into the anterior petrous pyramid would provide excellent access to cerebellopontine angle tumors (30,31). The so-called extended middle fossa approach was born. Kawase was the first, however, to utilize it for the treatment of basilar aneurysms (25). His first two patients actually harbored lower basilar trunk lesions. We prefer utilizing the posterior transpetrosal approaches, which will be described in other chapters, for midbasilar trunk and high vertebrobasilar junction aneurysms. Kawase's approach, however, is an excellent alternative for the unusually low-lying basilar top aneurysm where either the aneurysm neck or proximal control of the basilar artery cannot be secured despite the splitting of the tentorium through a subtemporal approach. For this reason, we will describe a modification of this approach in detail.

Anatomical Considerations

Kawase's area has been variously described as a triangle, a rhomboid, or a pyramid. From a technical point of view, it is most helpful to visualize it in its three dimensions as a pyramidal block of bone whose summit is the petrous apex. Three lines leave from this summit or its immediate vicinity: the line of the petrous ridge, the line of the greater superficial petrosal nerve, and the line of the inferior petrosal sinus. A bony surface is thus defined by each pair of these lines for a total of three surfaces forming the three sides of the pyramid. The base is an imaginary plane lying perpendicular to the floor of the middle fossa and containing the internal auditory canal. From the perspective of a middle fossa approach, the surgeon can identify a rhomboid surface demarcated by the following landmarks: posteriorly, the axis of the internal auditory canal; anteriorly, the posterior border of the trigeminal ganglion; laterally, the greater superficial petrosal nerve; and medially, the petrous ridge. This rhomboid can be expanded into a triangle by retracting and elevat-

ing the trigeminal ganglion to expose the trigeminal bony impression and apex proper. The greater superficial petrosal nerve overlies the horizontal portion of the petrous carotid artery, which can often be seen prior to any drilling due to frequent dehiscence of its bony roof. Lateral and parallel to this carotid segment lies the tensor tympani muscle, which has a thin bony shelf separating it from its medial and lateral relations, the carotid artery and the eustachian tube, respectively. In the posterolateral corner of the rhomboid area, in the axilla formed by the posterior part of the greater superficial petrosal nerve emerging from the geniculate ganglion, and the lateral part of the canalicular portion of the VIIth nerve, lies the cochlea. Thus, besides the medial bulge of the horizontal petrous carotid artery and the cochlea, the bony pyramid as defined above is exclusively made of cortical and cancellous bone and can be drilled in its entirety.

Indications

We favor using the subtemporal anterior transpetrosal approach when a subtemporal transtentorial approach fails to provide adequate exposure to the basilar top aneurysm. This generally implies an aneurysm lying below the level of the petrous ridge but above the midpoint of the clivus. It is important to realize that because of the kyphotic shape of the skull base whereby the clivus makes an angle of about 120° with the anterior fossa floor, anterior approaches are more favorable for rostral lesions and posterior approaches for caudal lesions. Thus, although complete drilling of the anterior petrous apex will expose the upper three fourths of the clivus, the more proximal the lesion, the more the surgeon needs to angulate downward, at the expense of further temporal lobe retraction.

Preparation and Positioning

The same principles that apply to the classic subtemporal approach apply here. After the induction of general anesthesia, a lumbar drain is placed and anywhere between 30 and 70 cm^3 of CSF are drained throughout the procedure. We position the patient supine with as much ipsilateral shoulder elevation on a sandbag as necessary to allow complete contralateral head rotation with the sagittal sinus parallel to the floor. The vertex is inclined about 15° down to facilitate the initial subtemporal exposure. A single dose of broad-spectrum prophylactic antibiotic is given with induction, along with mannitol (1 g/kg) and Decadron. The goal of hyperventilation is an arterial Pco$_2$ of 28–30 mm Hg. The anterior transpetrosal approach can be combined with either the subtemporal approach or the combined pterional/anterior temporal approach. However, the first scenario is much more likely because it would be preselected in the setting of a very low-lying basilar top aneurysm. We will therefore limit our description to the subtemporal transpetrosal approach.

Soft Tissue and Bony Exposure

For this approach we prefer using a modified pterional skin incision in a question mark fashion. It starts just in front of the tragus at the lower border of the root of the zygoma, curves in front then above the ear and then forward to the hairline at the level of the superior temporal line. The temporalis muscle is split leaving a muscle cuff on the superior temporal line for reattachment during closure. The temporalis muscle is retracted with fish hooks antero-inferiorly to the maximum degree. This generally requires a subperiosteal dissection of the zygomatic arch, which can be partially drilled superiorly to provide a flatter angle. The free bone flap is elevated with its base equally extending in front and behind the root of the zygoma. The bone is drilled down to the level of the floor of the middle fossa over the entire anteroposterior extent of the base of the bone flap. At this point the microscope is brought in and the self-retaining retractor applied extradurally. With the benefit of spinal drainage retraction is advanced gradually medially. It is important to start the dural elevation posteriorly down to the level of the arcuate eminence and then proceed anteriorly from that point. This is because the greater superficial petrosal nerve courses in an anteromedial direction as it emerges from the facial hiatus. Thus, it is easier to first identify and then separate it from the dura at the hiatus. Early identification is necessary to prevent inadvertent traction from being transmitted to the geniculate ganglion and resulting in facial paralysis. When identified, it is best transected and followed anteriorly where it is important to locate foramen spinosum posterolateral to foramen ovale and coagulate and divide the middle meningeal artery to allow further untethering of the dura from the middle fossa floor. The trigeminal ganglion and V3 are identified as the anterior limit of the partially exposed rhomboid and complete stripping of the superior petrosal sinus off the petrous ridge from arcuate eminence to trigeminal ganglion completes the exposure. The dura becomes tougher to elevate the more medial one goes and it is often helpful to wedge the tip of the retractor between the elevated superior petrosal sinus and the petrous ridge for a more optimal hold. One can tailor the extent of drilling according to the exposure needed. For maximum drilling, it is important to identify the horizontal petrous carotid and uncover its superomedial quadrant to establish the lateral limit of drilling. This can be achieved with a low-speed cutting and subsequently a diamond drill bit. The posterolateral corner of the rhomboid should be avoided to preserve the cochlea. Drilling proceeds medially and caudally. The axis of the internal auditory canal, though not seen at this early stage, is estimated as the bisector of the angle formed by the axis of the superior arcuate eminence and the greater superficial petrosal nerve (method of Fisch). Because the internal auditory canal is deeper in the petrous bone at the porus than at Bill's bar, more bone needs to be drilled medially. The trigeminal ganglion and V3 can be elevated with a dissector and drilling of the petrous tip can be completed.

Exposure of the inferior petrosal sinus in the occipitopetrous fissure indicates complete drilling of the pyramid. The surgeon could certainly proceed with the drilling into the clivus proper but, for the purpose of basilar artery access, there is no more exposure to be gained by further drilling.

Unlike the original description of Kawase, we will at this point open the dura over the temporal lobe in a V-shape fashion based inferiorly and elevate the anterior temporal lobe intradurally. The dura is then incised starting from the free edge of the tentorium behind the entrance of the IVth nerve proceeding laterally to the superior petrosal sinus, which is coagulated and divided, or, alternatively, clipped with metal clips. At this point, the dura splits into the middle fossa and posterior fossa layers with an empty cavity created by the bony drilling left in between. An incision into both of these layers completes the tentorial split. The free edge of the dural leaflets can be stitched back to maintain the exposure. Cranial nerves III to VIII should be in full view along with the anterolateral aspect of the pons, basilar trunk, posterior cerebral and superior cerebellar arteries. Dissection can proceed on either side of the trigeminal root.

Harsh and Sekhar added three modifications to the original Kawase approach and introduced the *subtemporal transcavernous anterior transpetrosal approach* (32,33), ie, intradural (not extradural) removal of petrous apex, complete division (not fenestration) of the tentorium, and mobilization of the trigeminal root, ganglion, and V3 to access the inferoposterolateral cavernous sinus. They feel that this technique avoids exposing the petrous ICA, sacrificing the greater superficial petrosal nerve, retracting extradurally against the tethered middle fossa dura, while at the same time providing a shorter and less oblique view of the basilar top and the retrosellar area. These modifications come at the cost of frequent intentional sacrifice of the IVth nerve and inducing cavernous venous bleeding and possible IIIrd nerve injury from packing. In addition, we believe that visualizing the ICA extradurally is a superior measure of protection. For these reasons and for the purpose of aneurysm exposure and clipping, extradural drilling followed by a tentorial split and only modest mobilization of the Vth nerve is more than adequate exposure.

Zygomatic, Orbitozygomatic Approaches and Their Variants

Anatomic Considerations

The interpeduncular cistern contains the upper third of the basilar artery. It is flanked by uncus on each side, guarded anteriorly by dorsum sella and upper clivus and contained posteriorly by a bulging upper pons. It is roofed by an inverted V-shaped surface, formed anteriorly by the forward-downward sloping of the floor of the third ventricle (infundibulum, tuber cinereum, and mamillary bodies) and posteriorly by the downward-backward sloping of the cerebral peduncles. The highest summit in the cistern is the apex of the inverted V and consists of the interpeduncular group of the posterior perforated substance (13). It is among the deepest intracranial cisterns. Except for its lateral recess, which contains the IIIrd nerve and the posterior communicating artery, it is completely concealed from the surgeon's view by other overlying cisterns that are, from anterior to lateral to inferior, as follows: chiasmatic (separated from it by Liliequist's membrane and containing optic nerve, chiasm, and pituitary stalk), carotid (containing supraclinoid carotid), crural (containing anterior choroidal artery and basal vein of Rosenthal), ambient (containing P2 and the basal vein of Rosenthal), and, lastly, prepontine (containing the lower two thirds of the basilar artery and the VIth nerve). All surgical approaches previously described in this chapter rely on establishing surgical corridors around these various structures and each offers a distinct but partial visualization of the interpeduncular cistern. None of the procedures already described offers a face-on view of the sloping roof top. The only anatomically viable surgical approaches to the roof are either directly from above or directly from below.

From above implies an *interhemispheric transcallosal approach* to and then through the floor of the third ventricle to reach very high basilar top aneurysms as has already been described in a few case reports (34,35). This is an extremely unusual and undesirable approach: a long and narrow corridor, encountering the dome of the aneurysm prior to its neck and lack of proximal basilar control. Access from below can be achieved by lowering the surgical line of view, making it steeper and bringing the surgeon closer to the center. There are three surgically viable alternatives: anteriorly, anterolaterally, or laterally. The *transmaxillary-transclival approach* provides a midline anterior view of the interpeduncular fossa. Its disadvantages, however, are numerous. The line of sight is such that the sella and the pituitary gland are completely in the way, obscuring the so-called blind spot behind the dorsum sella. The risk of CSF leakage and meningitis is too high, let alone the fact that vital perforators are diametrically opposite to the surgeon from the aneurysm. We generally do not recommend transfacial-transclival approaches to intradural pathology. The anterolateral inferior angle can be provided by removal of the lateral orbital rim and the body of the zygoma, while the lateral inferior angle is achieved by zygomatic arch resection. We will detail these two types of approaches below.

History

Fujitsu and Kuwabara initiated an interest in these types of approaches by publishing their *zygomatic approach* in 1985 (36). The operation they described started with a 45° head rotation with a downward tilt of 30°. After a pterional skin incision, the zygomatic arch was subperiosteally exposed and sectioned as a free bone flap allowing the temporalis muscle to be retracted more inferiorly. The craniotomy

followed as usual. Pitelli et al described an identical technique, except for leaving the sectioned zygomatic arch attached to the masseter and temporalis muscle (37). Later, Shiokawa et al (38) combined the zygomatic arch resection with the temporopolar approach of Sano (23) and called the technique the *zygomatic temporopolar approach.* Attempts to modify this approach from lateral to anterolateral started with Hakuba et al (39) in their *orbitozygomatic infratemporal approach.* The entire frontotemporal bone flap is kept attached to the orbitozygomatic bar, thus removing roof, lateral wall and rim of orbit, posterior body of zygoma, and the entire zygomatic arch and frontotemporal bone flap as one unit kept attached to the mobilized temporalis muscle. Although suggested by the designation of the approach, the exposure does not involve the infratemporal fossa. In the so-called *zygomaticotemporal* (40) or *transzygomatic approach* (41), the osteotomy on the orbital rim instead is made just above the frontozygomatic suture line and the orbitozygomatic bar is reflected on the masseter. The frontotemporal bone flap is taken free. The advantages of Sano's temporopolar and Hakuba's orbitozygomatic approaches were combined by Ikeda et al. (42) who reported on the *orbitozygomatic temporopolar approach* and described two cases of high basilar tip aneurysms with a short supraclinoid carotid artery. Because this approach utilizes several techniques used in most other skull base approaches and because it has become our preferred approach for high and complex lesions of the basilar top, we will describe our version of it in detail.

Indications

We prefer to use this approach with basilar top aneurysms that are 1 cm or more higher than the posterior clinoids or that are normally located aneurysms whose degree of complexity can be lessened by improved visualization and maneuverability, such as large, giant, incompletely coiled, or recurrent aneurysms. It remains to be proven as to whether the minimized brain retraction would also benefit all acutely ruptured cases with Hunt–Hess grade 3 or higher.

Preparation and Positioning

After induction of general anesthesia, we place the head in a Mayfield head holder, tilt the vertex down by about 30°, and turn the head contralaterally by 30°. The degree of initial head turn is not crucial as different stages of the procedure require a different amount of head rotation. We tape the patient circumferentially around the operating table to allow airplaning the table intraoperatively. The initial full Sylvian fissure splitting is best done with the head turned 30° because the fissure slants temporally, but subsequent cisternal dissection may require rotations up to 60° depending on the length of the supraclinoid ICA, the relative width of the optico-carotid and carotico-oculomotor spaces, and the size and location of the posterior communicating artery. Hyperventilation (arterial P_{CO_2} of 28 mm Hg), mannitol (1 g/kg), and Decadron are instituted.

Soft Tissue and Bony Exposure

The incision starts just in front of the tragus, 0.5 cm below the inferior border of the posterior zygomatic root. It extends straight up vertically, curving smoothly anteriorly to end at the midline of the hairline. Galea is separated from superficial temporalis fascia up to a point no closer than 2 cm from the superolateral orbital rim to avoid injury to the temporal branch of the facial nerve. It should be remembered that this branch generally leaves the facial nerve and crosses the zygomatic arch at a point 2 cm in front of the tragus and stays within 2 cm of the orbital rim, traveling in between the two leaflets of the superficial temporalis fascia before supplying orbicularis and frontalis muscles. Another method of estimating its course is to consider that a line drawn from the ear lobe to the midline of the hairline demarcates the safe zone posteriorly from the danger zone anteriorly. The superficial temporalis fascia is then incised in a crescentic fashion starting just below the posterior zygomatic root, coming across it and then gradually curving forward, crossing the superior temporal line at the origin of the temporalis muscle at a point about 3 cm (no less) from the zygomatic process of the frontal bone, then continuing onto the periosteum of the forehead. This incision in the fascia is deepened down to but not through the temporalis muscle fibers and this entire fascial/periosteal continuous layer is gradually elevated from the orbital rim and zygomatic arch. This subperiosteal dissection gets tougher due to increased soft tissue resistance as one approaches the body of the zygoma. Several fishhooks anchored on a Leyla bar are used to maintain scalp retraction and the completed exposure achieves visualization of the entire zygomatic arch with the upper masseter fibers, the posterosuperior part of the zygoma, and the entire superolateral orbital rim. The supraorbital nerve is released from its notch or complete bony foramen by the use of a small osteotome and mallet and is allowed to be retracted with the skin flap. The periorbita are freed from the bony roof and lateral wall of the orbit to a depth of at least 3 cm. The temporalis muscle is then incised posteriorly along the line of the skin incision, then forward just below its superior temporal line attachment, leaving a small muscle cuff for reapproximation during closure. The anterior fibers are simply detached from the frontozygomatic process down to the extracranial opening of the inferior orbital fissure, which is at the axial level of the orbital floor. The bulk of the temporalis muscle is detached from the skull with minimal use of coagulation to avoid irreversible injury to the nerve and blood supply that run on its undersurface. The temporalis is kept attached to the coronoid process of the mandible.

A generous frontotemporal free bone flap is created by using a single squamous temporal burr hole. A high-power drill with a drill guard makes the inferior cut as low as possi-

ble on the frontal and temporal floors. The lesser wing of the sphenoid is drilled very thoroughly and generally includes the unroofing of the superior orbital fissure. All cancellous bone should be drilled away and only a "cortical egg shell" corresponding to the orbital roof and lateral wall should remain. The dura is stripped generously off the anterior orbital floor back to the planum sphenoidale. Next the osteotomies to remove the orbitozygomatic bar are started. A reciprocating saw with a straight-tapered blade is used to make the first cut across the superior orbital rim, generally just lateral to the supraorbital notch. We like to slant the cut in a superomedial to inferolateral direction to ensure a proper wedging during reconstruction. This cut is carried posteriorly, parallel to the sagittal midline and then across the orbital roof laterally along a line 3 cm posterior to the rim to preserve enough orbital roof and prevent postoperative pulsating exophthalmus. The surgical assistant is instrumental in placing one retractor to depress the orbital contents and one retractor to elevate the frontal dura and guide the primary surgeon as to the depth and location of the sawing blade in the orbit. The osteotomy cut continues laterally and inferiorly paralleling the orbital rim until it emerges at the inferior orbital fissure. The second cut is made at the posterior zygomatic root in a V-shaped fashion to again ensure proper wedging during reconstruction and avoid leaving a protuberant zygomatic root that can hinder exposure. The third and last osteotomy line is a V-shaped cut across the body of the zygoma. The posterior limb of the V is shallow and fairly easy to make whereas the anterior limb has to be deepened all of the way back to the intraorbital aspect of the inferior orbital fissure. This last cut completes the circuit and the orbitozygomatic bar can be detached from the masseter fibers and elevated free. The temporalis muscle can now be further mobilized inferiorly making the exposure 1–2 cm lower. We generally drill the greater wing of the sphenoid to achieve a completely tangential view of the floor and anterior wall of the middle fossa. The remaining posterior orbital roof is excised with rongeurs. We have not encountered postoperative cosmetic defects due to this maneuver. It is important to realize that the added exposure, as compared to that afforded by a low pterional craniotomy, is not only the measure of the width of the orbital rim but an extra 1 cm or so gained after opening the dural flap and anchoring it in such a way as to depress further the orbital contents. Any orbital fat that may have herniated due to inadvertent rupture of the periorbita will be contained by the taut dural flap. The dural opening should take full advantage of the bony exposure and expose the Sylvian fissure completely. The subsequent microsurgical dissection is identical to what was described with the combined approach. One redeeming factor with a high basilar lesion is the availability of a long segment of distal basilar for proximal control.

Closure

The orbitozygomatic bar is wedged back in place and secured with plates and screws. Care must be taken not to trap

TABLE 1. *Summary of approaches to the distal basilar artery*

Line of sight	Conventional	Outer drilling	Inner drilling	Outer and inner
Lateral	Subtemporal (Drake)	Zygomatic (Fujitsu; Pitelli) Orbitozygomatic infratemporal (Hakuba)	Anterior transpetrosal (Kawase; Sekhar)	Anterior transpetrosal with zygomatic orbitozygomatic
Anterolateral	Pterional (Yasargil)	Supraorbital (Jane) Cranioorbital (Al-Mefty)	Transclinoid (Dolenc)	Transclinoid with cranioorbital or orbitozygomatic
Both	Combined (Sano)	Zygomatic temporopolar (Shiokawa) Oribozygomatic temporopolar (Ikeda)	Temporopolar transpetrous Temporopolar transclinoid	Orbitozygomatic with anterior transpetrosal and transclinoid

Surgical approaches to the distal basilar can be classified based on the line of sight used and the degree of bone removal achieved.

orbital tissue between bone edges to prevent postoperative restrictive ophthalmopathy. The bone flap is secured similarly with plates and screws.

Table 1 summarizes the various approaches that have been described over the years in an attempt to continuously improve surgical access to the distal basilar artery. They can be categorized by the angle of approach, the use of a skull base modification, and, when such a modification is used, whether it consisted of removing bone from the outer circle (ie, the surface of the craniofacial skeleton) or the inner circle (ie, the depth of the bony exposure). Outer osteotomies are usually attempts at maximizing access while minimizing brain retraction. Inner drilling usually improves exposure in the immediate vicinity of the aneurysm.

SELECTION OF A SURGICAL APPROACH: SUMMARY

In the final analysis, after a decision is made to approach an aneurysm of the basilar top, selection of the particular route depends on the following:

1. Site and size of aneurysm
2. Projection of fundus
3. Clival level of the basilar bifurcation
4. Distance from sagittal midline
5. Surgeon's familiarity with specific approaches

Side of Approach

Posterior cerebral and superior cerebellar artery aneurysms are almost always approached from the ipsilateral side. Although the dome of the aneurysm may be encountered before the neck is fully exposed, the advantage of visualizing the neck first via a contralateral approach is greatly offset by the poor dome exposure that is obtainable due to the narrow confines of the surgical space. With midline basilar bifurcation aneurysms, an approach from the right side is almost always chosen, except when there is already a left IIIrd nerve palsy or associated aneurysms on the left side.

Clival Level of the Aneurysm

More than its exact site of origin, the relation of the aneurysm to the clivus essentially dictates the optimal surgical angle of approach. We have found it convenient to divide the clival length in quarters with the bottom rim of the internal auditory meatus defining roughly the midpoint. The upper two quarters are separated by the level of the petrous ridge whereas the lower two quarters are separated by the line of the jugular tubercles. Figure 12 summarizes our choice of approaches across the clival spectrum.

The usual basilar bifurcation aneurysm will be level with the posterior clinoids and our bias toward the combined pterional/anterior temporal approach has already been discussed. We will use this approach up to a point 1 cm above the posterior clinoids. Higher lesions necessitate combining the approach with an orbitozygomatic osteotomy. In the lower region of the upper quarter, the subtemporal approach becomes gradually more favorable as the posterior clinoid obscures the aneurysm from an anterolateral line of sight. For the rare basilar bifurcation aneurysm located in the second quarter below the level of the petrous ridge, a subtemporal transtentorial approach combined with an anterior petrosectomy provides an excellent exposure. More caudal basilar trunk, vertebrobasilar and vertebro-PICA aneurysms will be covered in other chapters.

SPECIAL ANEURYSMS

Superior Cerebellar Artery Aneurysms

A discussion of distal basilar artery aneurysms is incomplete without specific reference to aneurysms arising at the origin of the SCA. These are considerably rarer than aneurysms of the basilar bifurcation. They present frequently

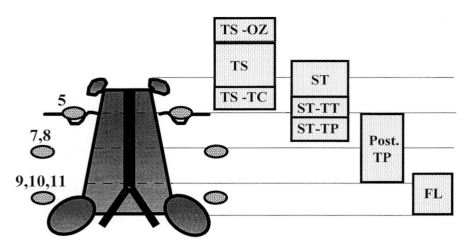

FIG. 12. The clivus is depicted as viewed from behind. Note the posterior clinoids, the petrous ridge and trigeminal impression, the occipital condyles and the vertebrobasilar complex, as well as Meckel's cave, porus acousticus and jugular foramen. The clivus is divided in quarters. Note the overlap in indications for some of the surgical approaches. TS, Transsylvian; ST, Subtemporal; TS-OZ, Extended transsylvian with orbitozygomatic; TS-TC, Transsylvian with posterior transclinoid; ST-TT, Subtemporal transtentorial; ST-TP, Subtemporal with anterior petrosectomy; Post. TP, Posterior petrosectomy approaches; FL, Far lateral approach.

with SAH or, when giant, with signs of brainstem compression. In addition, they can present with an isolated IIIrd nerve palsy; in fact, this is the second most common aneurysmal site for this type of presentation.

The surgical approach is identical to that used for aneurysms of the basilar bifurcation, ie, they can be approached either subtemporally or by the frontotemporal approach. We use the extended frontotemporal approach almost exclusively for these aneurysms. We have used the subtemporal approach but, with this latter approach, one comes directly upon the dome of the aneurysm, which is a significant disadvantage. The more oblique frontotemporal approach is, in our opinion, ideal for these aneurysms because the surgeon has a perfect view of the neck anteriorly and because the main disadvantage of the frontotemporal approach with aneurysms of the basilar bifurcation, the difficulty dissecting behind the aneurysm, is not a major factor with the superior cerebellar aneurysms. The reason for this is that the perforators of concern with basilar tip aneurysms take origin superiorly, usually from the PCA and from the tip of the basilar bifurcation, and are rarely a problem with superior cerebellar aneurysms. In fact, because of the lack of difficulty in sparing perforating vessels, we consider superior cerebellar aneurysms in a different class from basilar tip aneurysms in terms of difficulty. Our results with aneurysms at this site have been considerably superior to our results with aneurysms of the basilar tip, as will be discussed later. One particular difficulty that needs to be kept in mind with superior cerebellar aneurysms is that they can be intimately related to the IIIrd nerve, particularly when they are large. However, the surgeon can usually dissect free the neck of these aneurysms without disturbing the IIIrd nerve, which is usually in relation to the dome (43,44).

Proximal Posterior Cerebral Aneurysms

Aneurysms of the proximal segment of the PCA (P1) are amenable to the same surgical approaches utilized for basilar tip aneurysms. We prefer the extended frontotemporal (combined pterional/anterior temporal) approach for these aneurysms. The subtemporal approach is adequate for many, but because the proximal portion of the PCA usually rises above the level of the basilar bifurcation, these aneurysms tend to be relatively high and considerable temporal retraction is necessary when the subtemporal approach is used. These aneurysms have a propensity for being fusiform and half of the small number that we have encountered have been giant. However, in our experience the results with this group of aneurysms is superior to the results with large and giant basilar tip aneurysms because P1 aneurysms are usually distal to the early critical perforators from the PCA, which can ordinarily be spared when clipping these aneurysms. Additionally, even with giant aneurysms, trapping is frequently possible because the P1 segment distal to the origin of the important early perforators can be trapped if there is adequate distal flow through a posterior communicating artery. In fact, in Drake's experience, proximal ligation of the P1, distal to the earliest perforators and the origin of the medial posterior choroidal, which commonly has an early origin from the P1, was well tolerated. Drake suggested that puncturing the aneurysm after proximal ligation may give a clue as to the adequacy of collateral circulation through the posterior communicating artery. If the flow is poor, Drake recommended using a tourniquet on the P1 distal to the early perforators in order to perform the occlusion with the patient awake. His results with these aneurysms were generally good (45).

Giant and Large Complex Aneurysms of the Basilar Artery

Giant aneurysms of the tip of the basilar artery can present either with SAH or with mass effect. When located at the basilar tip, these aneurysms project superiorly into the diencephalon and sometimes produce obstructive hydrocephalus (46,47). These aneurysms may also grow posteriorly into the interpeduncular fossa producing pseudobulbar palsy, ataxia, and quadriparesis. This latter syndrome is more common with aneurysms of the basilar trunk, but it certainly can be seen with aneurysms at the basilar tip, particularly when the origin is relatively low. Large and giant basilar tip aneurysms can also grow asymmetrically and compress the cerebral peduncle and the IIIrd nerve, resulting in a Weber's syndrome with contralateral hemiparesis and ipsilaterally oculomotor paralysis. As stated earlier, however, isolated IIIrd nerve compression is more common with aneurysms originating from the basilar-superior cerebellar junction.

Giant and large complex aneurysms of the distal basilar artery present one of the most difficult neurosurgical challenges. Drake, however, has had success with direct occlusion of the neck of many of these aneurysms (45). He has also introduced basilar artery ligation and unilateral or bilateral vertebral artery ligation for the treatment of these aneurysms (48). Basilar artery ligation can be accomplished by a tourniquet, as described by Drake, which has the advantage of allowing the surgeon to turn down the tourniquet under direct radiographic control with the patient awake (45). Alternatively, when the surgeon is satisfied with the adequacy of collateral circulation, the distal basilar artery can be clipped directly at surgery. It would be ideal to clip the basilar artery between the superior cerebellar and the posterior cerebral arteries, but this is almost never possible with large aneurysms because their base incorporates the SCA. A prerequisite to this basilar artery occlusion is the demonstration of at least one normal-sized posterior communicating artery by the Alcock maneuver (injection of a vertebral artery while each internal carotid is sequentially occluded) (45). If both posterior communicating arteries are very small, the surgeon must consider a distal extracranial to intracranial bypass graft before occlusion. Drake has used prophylactic bypass only occasionally in a large series of basilar artery ligations (45,48). Others have preferred to use a bypass graft, usually a saphenous vein graft to the proximal PCA, whenever basilar occlusion is contemplated (49). The planned arterial occlusion should be done, in our opinion, immediately after establishment of the bypass graft, particularly if the bypass is a high-flow conduit such as a saphenous vein graft. Otherwise one runs the risk of having the aneurysm rupture at the time when the basilar artery is still open and the bypass is patent, as happened in one of our cases (50).

Basilar-superior cerebellar artery giant aneurysms are more amenable to clipping, but they are quite rare and we have encountered only four such lesions.

We now recommend the extended frontotemporal approach, usually with an orbitozygomatic osteotomy, for all giant and large complex aneurysms of the distal basilar artery. This approach clearly offers the surgeon a wider angle of vision and the ability to use multiple temporary clips, which are frequently necessary when the surgeon plans to open the aneurysm in order to facilitate clipping. It goes without saying that at least proximal temporary occlusion is mandatory during the final stages of dissection and clipping of these aneurysms. Therefore, adequate proximal control is essential and frequently the surgeon has to remove additional

bone either in the posterior clinoid region or the anterior petrous tip (Kawase's approach) or both in order to ensure the adequacy of proximal control.

The problem with these aneurysms, of course, is that their neck is usually wide enough to incorporate the origin of the superior cerebellar and the posterior cerebral arteries; consequently, clipping attempts frequently result in the clip slipping down over the origin of at least the posterior cerebral arteries. The neck above the posterior cerebral arteries is usually too broad to allow the clip to be placed between the P1 and the aneurysm, even under temporary proximal occlusion. Aneurysmorrhaphy, which is of course a very useful maneuver with giant aneurysms elsewhere, is extremely difficult in the confining space of the interpeduncular fossa, and obtaining control of the distal basilar and both superior cerebellar and posterior cerebral arteries is difficult even with the best of exposures.

Even though we have not had significant experience with this technique, we are of the opinion that nowadays most giant and very large complex aneurysms of the distal basilar artery should probably be operated with the surgeon at least prepared to use circulatory arrest. There have been several detailed reports of this technique and because our experience is limited we will not expand in this respect (51–60). Initially, this technique resulted in very significant morbidity related mostly to systemic problems after extracorporeal circulation (45). However, modern techniques, which take advantage of our better understanding of the coagulation problems attending circulatory arrest, have added considerable safety to this technique and very encouraging reports have emerged from a few centers (56,61,62).

RESULTS AND COMPLICATIONS

Our own results are indicated in Table 2. Of note is that in our hands only half of the giant aneurysms at the tip of the basilar artery have done well. In contrast, we have had better results with giant aneurysms of the superior cerebellar and the P1 segment. Since we have been operating early on basilar aneurysms only for the last few years and then only in good grade patients, the poor results indicated in Table 2 are mostly due to surgical complications rather than to vasospasm or other factors. This is in contrast with aneu-

TABLE 2. *Distal basilar artery aneurysms: surgical results*

	Number	Good	Poor	Dead
Basilar tip	124 (12)	102 (6)	18 (4)	4 (2)
Superior cerebellar	15 (4)	12 (2)	2 (1)	1 (1)
Proximal PCA	6 (3)	5 (2)	1 (1)	0 (0)
Totals	145 (19)	119 (10)	21 (6)	5 (3)

Numbers in parentheses represent giant aneurysms. "Good" refers to an independent patient who is neurologically intact or has a mild deficit. "Poor" refers to patients with a moderate to severe permanent deficit.

rysms of the anterior circulation where the number of complications directly attributable to the operation is considerably smaller. Most of our poor results in basilar tip aneurysms are due to perforator injury or to intraoperative rupture with less than optimal clipping. The one death with a giant SCA aneurysm was actually due to a tear at the junction of the carotid artery and the anterior cerebral artery when the clip applier, which had been inserted through the narrow space between the optic nerve and the carotid artery, was forcibly opened to release the clip.

Drake and colleagues have reported by far the largest series of basilar artery aneurysms. Their results reflect a 30-year experience with these lesions and they have maintained careful follow-up over the years. In a report of 102 unruptured small (<12 mm) distal basilar aneurysms surgically treated, there were 90 excellent and 8 good results (63). Among the 46 unruptured large (12–25 mm) lesions, there were 36 excellent and 7 good results (63). In a more recent appraisal of 113 basilar bifurcation (excluding SCA and PCA lesions) ruptured aneurysms operated on within 7 days, good/moderate outcomes were obtained in 82% with 8% mortality (64). Among 83 cases where Hunterian ligation had to be utilized, 64% had a good/moderate outcome, with a 31% mortality (65).

The Dallas group has also had significant experience with these aneurysms. In a recent article analyzing their complications, Batjer and Samson reported 126 patients of whom 102 had a good outcome, 14 had a poor outcome, and 10 died (66). Yasargil, Sundt, Spetzler, and others have also reported a satisfactory experience with these aneurysms (24,62,67).

The most common surgical complication with aneurysms of the distal basilar artery is a IIIrd nerve palsy which, fortunately, is almost always transient. We have encountered this problem perhaps with two thirds of patients operated by the subtemporal approach and with about one third to one half of the patients operated by the combined pterional/anterior temporal approach. Obviously, the larger the aneurysm, the more likely it is that a IIIrd nerve palsy will result. Also, we have found that the use of a temporary clip is likely to increase the incidence of IIIrd nerve palsy because of the extra need for manipulation of the IIIrd nerve to apply the temporary clip so that it is away from the critical field of the neck of the aneurysm.

The most common source of permanent morbidity with these aneurysms is, of course, perforator injury or occlusion. We mentioned the early problems we had with the perforators from the origin of the opposite P1 when using the subtemporal approach, which makes it difficult to visualize the opposite side of the neck. We have had three patients who have awakened from surgery with bilateral IIIrd nerve palsies, and in each instance we attributed the ipsilateral IIIrd nerve palsy to manipulation of the nerve and the contralateral palsy to an injury to the oculomotor nucleus from occlusion or damage of an early perforator from the opposite P1. These patients have also had significant ataxia and a pseudobulbar syndrome. In each instance, the ipsilateral IIIrd nerve palsy

has improved earlier and the patient has had a variable degree of recovery from the contralateral palsy. Much of our morbidity from perforator occlusion has involved some degree of pseudobulbar palsy, ataxia, memory loss, and a variable degree of hemiparesis. The likelihood of perforator occlusion is compounded in large and giant aneurysms and with intraoperative rupture where clipping has to take place under less than optimal conditions. We had some morbidity from temporal lobe edema when we used routinely the subtemporal approach, but this was not a major permanent problem except in one patient who developed hemorrhagic infarction of the temporal lobe that we attributed to venous occlusion.

In our opinion, the best and most thoughtful analysis of complications of surgery for these aneurysms is that of Batjer and Samson (66). They encountered an 8% mortality and 11% incidence of permanent neurologic disability in a large series that included many patients with large, giant, and difficult aneurysms. They classify their errors into failed management of initial hemorrhage, timing errors, conceptual errors, technical errors, delayed ischemic deficits, and bad luck. Their article is highly recommended to any surgeon who operates with any frequency on aneurysms in this location.

REFERENCES

1. Tonnis, W. Zur Behandlung intracranieller Aneurysme. *Langenbecks Arch Klin Chir* 1937;189:474.
2. Schwartz HG. Arterial aneurysms of the posterior fossa. *J Neurosurg* 1948;5:312–316.
3. Gillingham, FJ. The management of ruptured intracranial aneurysms. *Ann R Coll Surg* 1958;23:89–117.
4. Logue, V. Posterior fossa aneurysms. *Clin Neurosurg* 1964;11:183–219.
5. Mount, LA, J.M. Taveras. Ligature of the basilar artery in treatment of an aneurysms of the basilar-artery bifurcation. *J Neurosurg* 1962;19:167–170.
6. Drake CG. Bleeding aneurysms of the basilar artery. Direct surgical management in four cases. *J Neurosurg* 1961;18:230–238.
7. Jamieson KG. Aneurysms of the vetebrobasilar system. *J Neurosurg* 1964;21:781–797.
8. Wascher TM, Spetzler RF. Saccular aneurysms of the basilar bifurcation. In: Carter LP, Spetzler RF, Hamilton MG, eds. *Neurovascular Surgery*, New York: McGraw-Hill, 1995;729–752.
9. Mayer PL, Kier EL. The ontogenetic and phylogenetic basis of cerebrovascular anomalies and variants. In: Apuzzo MLJ, eds. *Brain Surgery: Complication Avoidance and Management*. New York: Churchill Livingstone, 1993;691–792.
10. Huber P. Krayenbuhl, Yasargil. *Cerebral Angiography*. Stuttgart: Thieme Verlag, 1982.
11. Rhoton AL, Saeki N, Perlmutter D, Zeal A. Microsurgical anatomy of common aneurysm sites. *Clin Neurosurg* 1979;26:248–306.
12. Saeki N. Rhoton AL Jr. Microsurgical anatomy of the upper basilar artery and the posterior circle of Willis. *J Neurosurg* 1977;46:563.
13. Yasargil M. *Microneurosurgery I. Microsurgical Anatomy of the Basal Cisterns and Vessels of the Brain, Diagnostic Studies, General Operative Techniques and Pathological Considerations of the Intracranial Aneurysms*. New York: Thieme Stratton, 1984.
14. Grand W, Hopkins LN. The microsurgical anatomy of the basilar artery bifurcation. *Neurosurgery* 1977;1:128–130.
15. Caruso G, Vincentelli F, Giudicelli G, Grisoli F, Xu T, Gouaze A. Perforating branches of the basilar bifurcation. *J Neurosurg* 1990;73:259–265.
16. Lang J, Brunner FX. Uber die Ramic Centrles der Aa. Cerebri anterior and Media. *Gengenbaurs Morph JB* 1978;124:364.

17. Zeal AA, Rhoton AL Jr. Microsurgical anatomy of the posterior cerebral artery. *J Neurosurg* 1978;48:534.
18. Adams RD, Victor M. *Principles of Neurology.* New York: McGraw-Hill, 1989.
19. Paine T, Batjer HH, Samson DS. Intraoperative ventricular puncture. Technical note. *Neurosurgery* 1988;22:1107–1109.
20. Yasargil MG, Antic J, Laciga R, Jain KK, Hodosh RM, Smith RD. Microsurgical pterional approach to aneurysms of the basilar bifurcation. *Surg Neurol* 1976;6:83–91.
21. Heros RC, Lee SH. The combined pterional/anterior temporal approach for aneurysms of the upper basilar complex. Technical report. *Neurosurgery* 1993;33:244–251.
22. Symon L. Surgical approaches to tentorial hiatus. *Adv Tech Standards Neurosurg* 1982;9:69–112.
23. Sano K. Temporo-polar approach to aneurysms of the basilar artery at and around the distal bifurcation: technical note. *Neurological Research* 1980;2:361–367.
24. Sundt TM. *Surgical Techniques for Saccular and Giant Intracranial Aneurysms.* Baltimore: William and Wilkins, 1990;212–223.
25. Kawase T, Toya S, Shiobara R, Mine T. Transpetrosal approach for aneurysms of the lower basilar artery. *J Neurosurg* 1985;63:857–861.
26. Kawase T, Shiobara R, Tya S. Anterior transpetrosal-transtentorial approach for sphenopetroclival meningiomas: surgical methods and results in 10 patients. *Neurosurgery* 1991;28:868–875.
27. Kasdon D, Stein B. Combined supratentorial and infratentorial exposure for low-lying basilar aneurysms. *Neurosurgery* 1979;4:422–426.
28. Jane JA, Park TS, Pobereskin LH, Winn HR, Butler AB. The supraorbital approach: technical note. *Neurosurgery* 1982;11:537–542.
29. Al-Mefty O, Smith RR. Tailoring the cranio-orbital approach. *Keio J Med* 1990;39:217–224.
30. Morrison AW, King TT. Experiences with a translabyrinthine-transtentorial approach to the cerebellopontine angle. Technical note. *J Neurosurg* 1973, 38:382–390.
31. Hakuba A. Total removal of cerebello pontium angle tumors with a combined transpetrosal-transtentorial approach. *No Shinkei Geka* 1978, 6:347–354.
32. Harsh GR, Sekhar L. The subtemporal, transcavernous, anterior transpetrosal approach to the upper brain stem and clivus. *J Neurosurg* 1992, 77:709–717.
33. Sekhar LN, Kalia KK, Yonas H, Wright DC, Ching H. Cranial base approaches to intracranial aneurysms in the subarachnoid space. *Neurosurgery* 1994, 35:472–481.
34. Delos Reyes RA, Kantrowitz AB, Boehm FH, Spatola MA. Transcallosal, transventricular approach to a basilar apex aneurysm. *Neurosurgery* 1992, 31:597–601.
35. Canbolat A, Onal C, Kiris T. A high-position basilar top aneurysm approached via third ventricle: case report. *Surg Neurol* 1993, 39:196–199.
36. Fujitsu K, Kuwabara T. Zygomatic approach for lesions in the interpeduncular cistern. *J Neurosurgery* 1985, 62:340–343.
37. Pitelli SD, Almeida GG, Nakagawa EJ, Marchese AJT, Cabral ND. Basilar aneurysm surgery: the subtemporal approach with section of the zygomatic arch. *Neurosurgery* 1986, 18:125–128.
38. Shiokawa Y, Saito I, Aoki N, Mizutani H. Zygomatic temporopolar approach for basilar artery aneurysms. *Neurosurgery* 1989, 25:793–797.
39. Hakuba A, Liu S, Nishimura S. The orbitozygomatic infratemporal approach: a new surgical technique. *Surg Neurol* 1986, 26:271–276.
40. Neil-Dwyer G, Sharr M, Haskell R, Currie D, Hosseini M. Zygomaticotemporal approach to the basis cranii and basilar artery. *Neurosurgery* 1988;23:20–22.
41. Gerber CJ, Neil-Dwyer G, Evans BT. An alternative surgical approach to aneurysms of the posterior cerebral artery. *Neurosurgery* 1993;32:928–931.
42. Ikeda K, Yamashita J, Hashimoto M, Futami K. Orbitozygomatic temporopolar approach for a high basilar tip aneurysm associated with a short intracranial internal carotid artery: A new surgical approach. *Neurosurgery* 1991;28:105–110.
43. Bose B, Northrup B, Osterholm J. Giant basilar artery aneurysm presenting as a third ventricular tumor. *Neurosurgery* 1983;13:699–702.
44. Thron A., Bockenheimer S. Giant aneurysms of the posterior fossa suspected as neoplasms on computed tomography. *Neuroradiology* 1979;18:93–97.
45. Drake CG. Giant intracranial aneurysms: experience with surgical treatment in 174 patients. *Clin Neurosurg* 1979;26:12–95.
46. Koga H, Mori K, Kawano T. Tsutsumi K, Jinnouchi T. Parinaud's syndrome in hydrocephalus due to a basilar artery aneurysm. *Surg Neurol* 1983;19:548–553.
47. Piek J, Lim DP, Bock WJ. Obstructive hydrocephalus caused by a growing, giant aneurysm on the upper basilar artery. *Surg Neurol* 1983; 288–290.
48. Drake CG. Ligation of the vertebral (unilateral or bilateral) or basilar artery in the treatment of large intracranial aneurysms. *J Neurosurg* 1975;43:255–274.
49. Sundt TM Jr, Piepgras DG. Surgical approach to giant intracranial aneurysms. Operative experience with 80 cases. *J Neurosurg* 1979;51:731–742.
50. Heros RC, Ameri AM. Rupture of a giant basilar aneurysm after saphenous vein interposition of graft to the posterior cerebral artery. Case report. *J Neurosurg* 1984;61:387–390.
51. Drake CG, Barr HWK, Coles JC, Gergely NF. The use of extra-corporeal circulation and profound hypothermia in the treatment of ruptured intracranial aneurysm. *J Neurosurg* 1964;21:575–581.
52. Gissen AJ, Matteo RS, Housepian EM, Bowman O Jr. Elective circulatory arrest during neurosurgery for basilar artery aneurysms. *JAMA* 1969;207:1315–1318.
53. Guegan JM, Scarabin JM, LeGuilcher C, Gillou L, Logeais Y, Pecker J. Extracorporeal circulation with deep hypothermia and circulatory arrest in the treatment of intracranial arterial aneurysms. *Surg Neurol* 1985;24:441–448.
54. Housepian EM, Bowman FO Jr, Gissen AJ. Elective circulatory arrest in intracranial surgery. *J Neurosurg* 1967;26:594–597.
55. Michenfelder JD, Kirklin JW, Uihlein A, Svien HJ. Clinical experience with a closed-chest method of producing profound hypothermia and total circulatory arrest in neurosurgery. *Ann Surg* 1984;199:125–158.
56. Silverberg GD, Reitz BA, Ream AK. Hypothermia and cardiac arrest in the treatment of giant aneurysms of the cerebral circulation and hemangioblastoma of the medulla. *J Neurosurgery* 1980;3:301–305.
57. Mount LA. Results of treatment of intracranial aneurysms using the Selverstone clamp. *J Neurosurg* 1959;16:611–618.
58. Sundt TM, Pluth JR, Gronert GA. Excision of giant basilar aneurysm under profound hypothermia. *Mayo Clin Proc* 1972;47:631–634.
59. Uihlein A, MacCarty CS, Michenfelder JD, Terry HR, Daw EF. Deep hypothermia and surgical treatment of intracranial aneurysms. *JAMA* 1966;195:127–129.
60. Woodhall B, Sealy WC, Hall KD, Floyd WL. Craniotomy under conditions of quinidine-protected cardioplegia and profound hypothermia. *Ann Surg* 1959;152:37–44.
61. Solomon RA, Smith CR, Raps EC, Young WL, Stone JG, Fink ME. Deep hypothermic circulatory arrest for the management of complex anterior and posterior circulation aneurysms. *Neurosurgery* 1991;29:732–738.
62. Spetzler RF, Hadley MN, Rigamonti D, Carter LP, Raudzens P. Shedd SA, Wilkinson E. Aneurysms of the basilar artery treated with circulatory arrest, hypothermia, and barbiturate cerebral protection. *J Neurosurg* 1988;68:868–879.
63. Rice BJ, Peerless SJ, Drake CG. Surgical treatment of unruptured aneurysms of the posterior circulation. *J Neurosurg* 1990;73:165–173.
64. Peerless SJ, Hernesniemi JA, Gutman FB, Drake CG. Early surgery for ruptured vertebrobasilar aneurysms. *J Neurosurg* 1994;80:643–649.
65. Steinberg GK, Drake CG, Peerless SJ. Deliberate basilar or vertebral artery occlusion in the treatment of intracranial aneurysms. *J Neurosurg* 1993;79:161–173.
66. Batjer HH, Samson DS. Causes of morbidity and mortality from surgery of aneurysms of the distal basilar artery. *Neurosurgery* 1989;25:904–915.
67. Yasargil MG. Vertebrobasilar aneurysms. *Microneurosurgery.* II. New York: Thieme-Stratton, 1984:232–295.

Cerebrovascular Disease, edited by H. Hunt Batjer.
Lippincott-Raven Publishers, Philadelphia © 1997.

CHAPTER 86

Giant Intracranial Aneurysm: Surgical Techniques

Carlos A. David, Sydney J. Peerless, and Charles G. Drake

Giant intracranial aneurysms are aneurysms with a diameter of greater than 2.5 cm. First critically studied by Morley and Barr in 1969 (1), giant aneurysms continue to be a formidable therapeutic challenge, even with the remarkable progress made in imaging and surgical treatment during the last two decades.

Early experience with giant aneurysms was fraught with disaster. Many were accidentally found at exploration in patients presenting with symptoms of a slow-growing neoplasm. Direct attack was seldom successful and often disastrous. In view of these poor results, many neurosurgeons recommended observation or, at most, proximal arterial occlusion (Hunterian ligation) (1–3).

Drake's pioneering and innovative efforts indicated that many giant aneurysms could be treated by direct surgical methods with fairly good results. In a series of 174 giant aneurysms, he achieved an excellent or good result in approximately 70% (4). The barrier had been breached and in the ensuing years advances in neuroradiology, interventional methods, and microsurgical techniques confirmed that good outcomes could be attained.

In this chapter, we will review the clinical and pathologic features of giant intracranial aneurysms and discuss options and surgical strategies employed for these lesions at various anatomic sites.

EPIDEMIOLOGY

The incidence of giant intracranial aneurysms is thought to be about 5% of all cerebral aneurysms and range from 3% to 13% (1,5–7). These aneurysms typically present dur-

ing the fifth to seventh decades with a slight female predominance (1,5).

Giant aneurysms occur at the same locations as their smaller and more common counterparts. The most frequent sites involve the cavernous and proximal intracranial carotid artery (8), with the former location more commonly seen in males and the latter in females.

NATURAL HISTORY

The natural history of giant intracranial aneurysm has been a subject of dispute for almost three decades. The initial report by Sadik et al (9) in 1965 proposed that due to the commonly found concentric layers of thrombus these lesions were afforded protection from rupture. Subsequent reports of giant aneurysms unchanging or growing smaller in time, as well as reports correlating no relationship between size and incidence of rupture, further bolstered this line of thought. Conservative "observation" became the mainstay of treatment after early disastrous attempts at direct surgical attack.

Drake's report of 31 patients with untreated giant aneurysms suggested a dismal prognosis associated with these lesions. He found a 68% mortality at 2 years and an 85% mortality at 5 years (4). It is now clear that giant intracranial aneurysms, even when largely thrombosed, will continue to enlarge with time at a rate that is quite random. Moreover, more than 50% of these aneurysms will rupture. In recent years, it has even been suggested that the risk of rupture increases with the size of the aneurysm (10). Many giant sacs will declare their presence by mass effect and local compression of neurologic structures. Less often, ischemic injury to brain by occlusion of adjacent branch vessels and distal thromboembolism from the sac may occur. Other reports have substantiated the poor long-term outcome associated with these lesions (11,12).

C. A. David: Department of Neurological Surgery, University of Miami School of Medicine, Miami, Florida 33136.

S. J. Peerless: Mercy Neuroscience Institute, and Department of Neurological Surgery, University of Miami School of Medicine, Miami, Florida 33133.

C. G. Drake: Division of Neurosurgery, University of Western Ontario, London, Ontario, Canada N6A 5A5.

PATHOGENESIS

Giant aneurysms usually arise from small saccular aneurysms that expand and increase in size to eventually reach giant dimensions. The mechanism for this expansion is unknown but may be explained in part by the mechanical factors of pressure and turbulent flow acting on congenital or acquired defects in the arterial media. This combination leads to a weakening of the arterial wall and outpouching usually beginning at a site of bifurcation (13,14). As this outpouching grows there is consequent thinning of the early aneurysm's thin wall. If rupture does not occur, repair mechanisms result in the deposition of a fibrous collagenous layer resulting in thickening and enlargement of the aneurysmal wall. In time, turbulent blood flow and further enlargement disrupts the endothelial lining, resulting in platelet aggregation and the formation of thrombus. Repair mechanisms again come into play with resultant cyclical enlargement of the aneurysm.

Schubiger (15) et al have proposed an alternative growth mechanism for giant intracranial aneurysms analogous to the membranous enlargement of chronic subdural hematomas. Their theory is based on the fact that aneurysmal walls are highly vascularized structures. They propose clinically unrecognized rupture of a small saccular aneurysm as the primary event, followed by the formation of a fibrin and then a collagenous neomembrane over the site of rupture. During this healing process, capillary growth into this membrane occurs. These fragile capillaries may rupture, leading to further intramembranous hemorrhage, formation of new membranes, and continued enlargement of the aneurysm. Of interest is that this theory proposes a growth mechanism independent of blood pressure and may explain the continued growth of largely thrombosed giant aneurysms.

CLINICAL PRESENTATION

Giant intracranial aneurysms generally present in three ways: pseudotumor, hemorrhage, and cerebral ischemia.

Pseudotumoral Syndromes

Giant aneurysms usually present with symptoms caused by mass effect and progressive neurologic dysfunction (16). The exact signs and symptoms are dependent on the location and involved adjacent neural structures. Aneurysms arising from the cavernous and proximal intracranial carotid artery with its branches (ophthalmic, posterior communicating, anterior choroidal arteries) as well as the anterior communicating region may present with dysfunction of ocular movement or vision (17,18). Rarely, a lesion in this location, particularly the anterior communicating region, can present with symptoms referable to hypothalamic-pituitary axis dysfunction (19,20).

Giant aneurysms of the carotid bifurcation and middle cerebral artery (MCA) generally present with symptoms of hemispheric compression, ie, hemiparesis, dysphasia, and complex partial seizures. Rarely, a giant aneurysm in this location can reach enormous dimensions and result in frontal lobe dysfunction as evidenced by personality changes and dementia.

Giant aneurysms of the posterior circulation usually produce variable lower cranial nerve palsies, as well as symptoms of brainstem compression such as bulbar palsies and paresis. Those arising from the basilar bifurcation most often cause dementia and short-term memory disturbances but rarely affect the oculomotor nerve and produce diplopia, which is typical of basilar–superior cerebellar artery (SCA) giant aneurysms. Lesions more caudal on the basilar artery generally affect the abducens nerve, whereas lesions in the vertebral–basilar (V-B) junction and vertebral–posterior inferior cerebellar artery (PICA) junction produce dysfunction of lower cranial nerves, resulting in facial weakness, deafness, tongue weakness and wasting, dysphagia, and hoarseness. On occasion, V-B junction aneurysms may present with obstructive hydrocephalus.

Hemorrhage

Although at one time giant aneurysms were felt to be immune from rupture, it is now known that these lesions frequently present with rupture and subarachnoid hemorrhage (Fig. 1). The true incidence of rupture varies from series to series but generally lies between 20% and 70% (4–6). Subarachnoid hemorrhage has also been found to be the most common cause of death in giant aneurysms managed conservatively. Although rare, it has been observed that even when a giant aneurysm is completely thrombosed rupture may occur (21).

Ischemic Manifestations

Approximately 4% of giant aneurysms present with ischemic symptoms such as transient ischemic attack (TIA) or stroke. This is presumably secondary to distal thromboembolism from thrombi within the sac (22,23). Ischemic presentations are most frequently seen with giant aneurysms that arise from the internal carotid and middle cerebral arteries (22) but have been seen with giant aneurysms in all locations in the series of the senior authors.

NEURORADIOLOGIC FEATURES

Recent advances in diagnostic imaging have markedly improved the preoperative assessment of intracranial aneurysms. Computed tomography (CT), magnetic resonance imaging (MRI), and conventional angiography are necessary in most patients. The great strides in MR technology not only allow better demonstration of cerebral aneurysms but

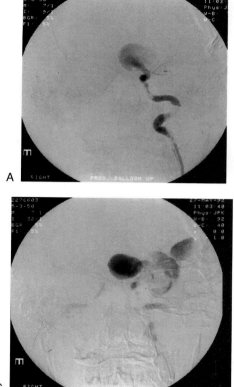

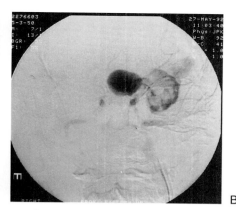

FIG. 1. These dramatic images during attempted proximal balloon occlusion of a giant para-ophthalmic artery aneurysm found to be unclippable at surgery betray the true dismal nature of these lesions. As can be seen, as the aneurysm began filling, massive rupture ensued with almost instantaneous death of the patient.

also permit enhanced understanding of the aneurysmal neck and associated arterial and cerebral anatomy.

Angiography remains the most essential diagnostic test of patients harboring giant intracranial aneurysms. The angiographic evaluation of a giant aneurysm requires high-quality four-vessel visualization of the entire cerebral circulation. The size, shape, and projection of the aneurysm must be obtained (Fig. 2) as well as the relationship of the aneurysmal neck to the parent vessel and the presence of adjacent branches and potential perforators. In addition, information regarding the extracranial circulation is critical in the event that an extracranial-to-intracranial (EC-IC) bypass may be required. Lastly, the degree of collateral circulation must be determined. Flow across the anterior communicating artery to the opposite hemisphere is evaluated by employing contralateral carotid compression. Whereas, evaluation of the carotid–basilar connection via the posterior communicating artery is assessed by ipsilateral carotid compression while a vertebral injection is performed (Allcock's test).

The main limitation of angiography is that it provides only images of the lumen. This may significantly underestimate the true size of the lesion. The use of CT or MRI provides better detail regarding the anatomic location, true size, and the extent of intraaneurysmal thrombosis (Fig. 3).

Typically, the unenhanced CT image of a giant aneurysm is characterized by a partially calcified border surrounding a homogeneous, isointense to slightly hyperintense center

corresponding to the aneurysmal wall and the thrombosed portion of the sac, respectively (Fig. 4). Administration of contrast results in enhancement of the wall and filling lumen. Spiral CT techniques permit three-dimensional reconstructed images of the aneurysm and its neck, which have proven very useful.

MRI and, more recently, MR angiography (MRA) have proved to be valuable in the evaluation of giant aneurysms. Although the appearance of an aneurysm on MR scans can be highly variable and complex, the typical aneurysm with rapid flow will exhibit a signal void on T1- and T2-weighted images (Fig. 5). Partially thrombosed aneurysms have a much more complex image pattern; generally a flow void in the region of the patent lumen is seen surrounded by alternating layers of high- and low-signal intensity due to hemosiderin and methemoglobin within the thrombus. If flow through the patent lumen is turbulent, an isointense signal may be seen, making it difficult to delineate it from the thrombus without contrast administration. Intravenous contrast will commonly enhance the wall of the aneurysm. The use of the above imaging method with MRA has provided exquisite detailed images of the aneurysm and associated cerebral vasculature. This method can image the true size and orientation of the aneurysm and its relationship to the parent artery and incorporation or adherence of important branch vessels to the dome of the aneurysm. More recently, methods for obtaining three-dimensional images of the aneu-

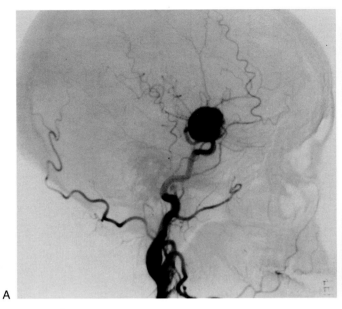

A

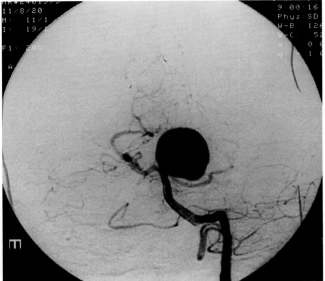

B

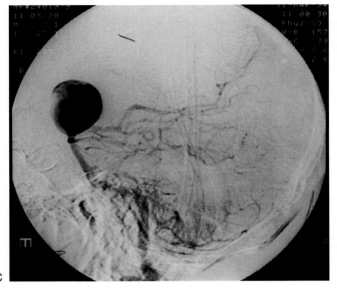

C

FIG. 2. A, Common carotid angiogram demonstrating a giant para-ophthalmic artery aneurysm. B,C, Vertebral angiograms demonstrating a giant basilar bifurcation aneurysm.

rysm and related cerebral vasculature have become available, substantially improving vessel and aneurysm visualization (Fig. 6).

MANAGEMENT STRATEGIES

The successful management of giant intracranial aneurysms rests on the understanding that each lesion is unique and will require a distinct treatment strategy. The operative solution is founded not only on specific techniques and their execution but, most importantly, on proper judgment. A variety of methods and operative approaches have been developed in the treatment of giant intracranial aneurysms. The basic therapeutic principle is to exclude the aneurysmal sac from the arterial circulation while preserving normal flow

in the parent vessel and its branches. The options include direct clipping of the neck, proximal (Hunterian) ligation, trapping, and intraluminal occlusion (coils and balloons).

Direct Clipping of the Aneurysmal Neck

The ideal treatment, as stated above, is usually best achieved by direct clip placement across the aneurysmal neck. This can be a formidable challenge with giant aneurysms, and its feasibility is determined at operation after completely delineating the regional vascular anatomy, as well as the shape, configuration, and location of the aneurysm. Of vital importance is the thickness and compressibility of the neck, the presence of calcified atheromatous plaque, intraluminal thrombosis, and the location and rela-

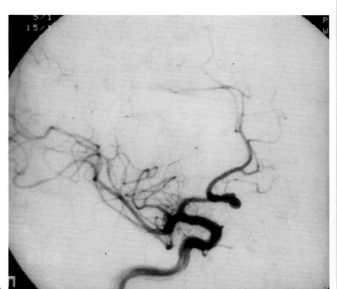

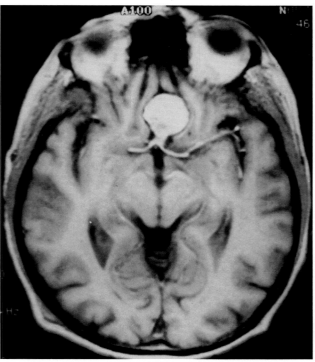

FIG. 3. A, Oblique right internal carotid angiogram revealing what appears to be a small anterior communicating artery aneurysm. B, T1-weighted gradient refocused study revealing the true dimensions of this partially thrombosed aneurysm.

tionships of primary branches and vital perforator vessels to the neck.

The basic steps in preparing the aneurysm for clipping are the same as those used for routine saccular aneurysms. First, proximal and distal control are obtained and the major vessels entering and exiting in the region of the neck of the aneurysm are identified. At this point the aneurysm and its neck are dissected, however, due to the inherent bulk and tension this task can be quite difficult. The use of proximal temporary clipping at this juncture can be quite advantageous. Once the aneurysmal neck, arterial branches, and perforators are well delineated, attempted clipping can be undertaken.

The surgeon must have available a variety of clips: long clips with high closing pressures, long and short fenestrated clips, and multiple short and varied angle clips. A variety of options are available with regard to actual clip application. Rarely will the application of a single clip suffice in obliterating a giant aneurysm. This is due to the fact that the walls and necks of giant aneurysms are commonly broad, thick, and contain calcified atheromatous plaque. If clip occlusion is attempted, the surgeon must be aware of the potential disastrous complications. In cases where the neck contains atheromatous plaque, the clip may not be completely occlusive and may migrate off toward the parent artery resulting in parent artery stenosis or occlusion. If the neck is fragile, the clip may cut and tear the neck. In addition, thromboem-

bolic material propagating from the sac to distal branches may lead to ischemic sequela.

In order to decrease these risks, multiple clipping techniques—booster, tandem, and parallel—have evolved. Booster clipping involves the placement of a second clip across the blades of a primary clip, thereby increasing the closing pressure. Tandem clipping involves the serial application of multiple short fenestrated clips across the base of the aneurysmal sac until a neck is fashioned and occluded. This technique has the added advantage of applying uniformly high closing pressures along the entire length of the aneurysmal base, thus making the possibility of clip migration unlikely. In addition, the parent artery lumen is preserved and reconstructed. Lastly, a less useful method of multiple clipping is the placement of multiple clips perpendicular to the axis of the parent vessel, so-called parallel clipping. This technique can be useful with the smaller giant aneurysms but has the potential problem of leaving a dog ear of thin-walled neck (24). If this situation occurs, these aneurysmal residua should be reinforced with cotton, muscle, or specially designed encircling clips as they may in time lead to the development of aneurysm recurrence.

Commonly, the disproportionate relationship between aneurysm and parent vessel size is so massive that it becomes almost impossible to delineate the aneurysm's neck and adjacent branches. In these situations the use of methods to soften or decrease the bulk of the aneurysm can be advantageous.

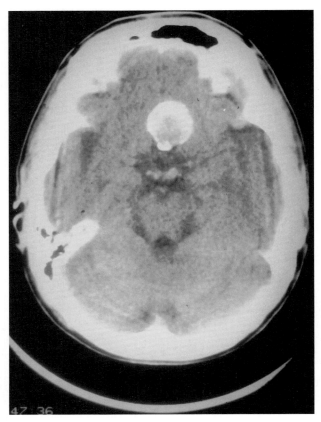

FIG. 4. Non-contrast computed tomographic scan of a giant anterior communicating artery aneurysm. Note the calcified border surrounding the isointense partially thrombosed portion of the sac.

This is most commonly achieved with the use of temporary proximal clipping or trapping. Although quite useful, this technique carries the risk of ischemic injury to the territory of the occluded vessels. In order to lessen this risk, the use of induced hypertension and cerebral protective agents can be employed. Notwithstanding, temporary occlusion must be used within the limits of tissue vulnerability. Samson et al (25) recently reported that temporary occlusion can generally be tolerated for up to 30 minutes. The use of intermittent reperfusion during temporary clipping, however, remains a controversial issue. A trend (which was not statistically significant) for poor outcome was found with intermittent reperfusion in their study. This observation is not in keeping with our experience, and recent experimental evidence suggests that intermittent reperfusion is neuroprotective during focal ischemia.

Temporary clipping may be combined with maneuvers such as suction decompression of the aneurysmal sac either through the dome or via the parent vessel in order to make the neck visible and clip occlusion possible (26,27).

The use of hypothermic cardiac arrest has been advocated for certain difficult giant aneurysms, particularly those of the posterior circulation where a bloodless field and greater exposure are needed. Although these techniques have been available since the early 1950s, recent technical advances have led to a resurgence in their use. Despite this we have rarely found this method necessary. There are major complications associated with hypothermic cardiac standstill, specifically cerebral ischemia, prolonged bleeding during rewarming, postoperative hemorrhage, and cardiac arrhythmias. The reported morbidity in the most experienced hands

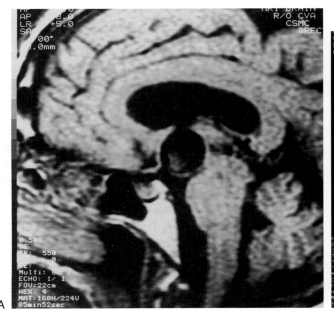

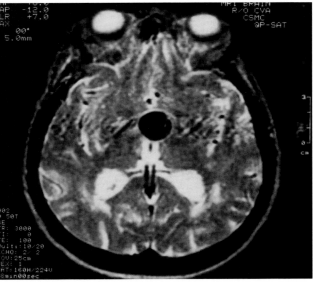

FIG. 5. A, T1-weighted MR image and B, T2-weighted MR image of a giant basilar bifurcation aneurysm demonstrating the hypointense signal void of rapid flow. Note the pulsation artifact on the T2-weighted image (blurred areas of scan on either side of the aneurysm).

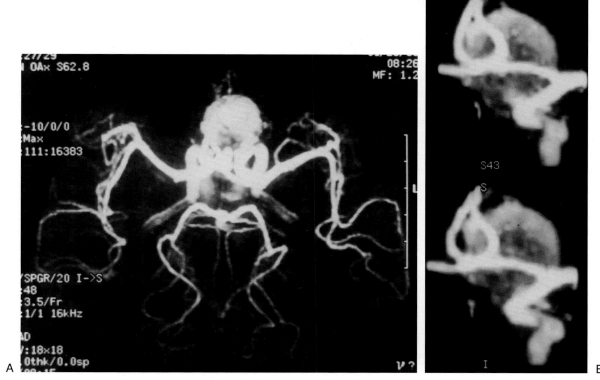

FIG. 6. A, Axial view of an MR angiogram revealing a giant anterior communicating artery aneurysm. B, 3-D MR angiogram delineating the precise location of the A2 vessels draped over the dome of the aneurysm.

is as high as 15%; hence the use of this technique can only be justified in the most extreme situations (28).

Although the desire to clip the aneurysm is strong, the surgeon must realize that for many of these lesions successful clip application is impossible. Perhaps the most important surgical decision the neurovascular surgeon faces is when to abandon attempts at clipping and proceed with an alternative treatment strategy. Slavish devotion to clipping the neck is unwise. In our experience, less than half of giant aneurysms can be clipped directly (4).

Hunterian Ligation or Proximal Occlusion of the Parent Vessel

When a giant aneurysm is not amenable to direct clipping, an often effective alternative is proximal parent artery occlusion or Hunterian ligation. The goal of parent artery occlusion is to decrease the pressure head into the aneurysmal dome and promote sluggish blood flow that will in turn result in thrombosis and permanent obliteration of the giant sac. The occlusion must be performed as close to the giant aneurysm as feasible. Only in this manner will good chance at permanent obliteration of the aneurysm be obtained while decreasing the risk of extension of thrombus into nearby branches or thrombo-embolic complications.

The main risks encountered with this technique are cerebral ischemia and infarction from thrombosis and thromboembolism. In order to lessen these risks, several details must be considered. First, preoperative evaluation of the available collateral blood flow is mandatory. This can be accomplished via angiography as already described; however, other adjuncts must be mentioned. Trial occlusion with a nondetachable proximal balloon has proved invaluable in giant aneurysms of the proximal carotid or vertebral arteries. Xenon-131 blood flow studies with trial occlusion may also be helpful. If after this evaluation the patient is determined to have insufficient natural collaterals, then microvascular bypass is employed prior to proximal artery occlusion.

The use of the Drake microtourniquet has facilitated the use of proximal arterial occlusion. The loop of the tourniquet is applied around the proximal vessel when it has been determined that the aneurysm cannot be clipped. The patient can then undergo trial arterial occlusion after surgery while awake. The clinician is therefore able to observe the patient for ischemic symptoms, reversing the occlusion if not tolerated.

Although Hunterian ligation lacks the finality of a direct reconstructive procedure, it remains a highly effective alternative. In the senior author's extensive experience in London, Ontario with Hunterian ligation, it was noted that 84%

of the patients achieved good clinical outcomes (29a,b). Hence, it remains a safe and clinically effective alternative.

Aneurysm Trapping, Aneurysmorraphy, Wrapping

Aneurysm trapping involves the proximal and distal occlusion of the parent vessel. This technique has the advantages of allowing for decompression of the aneurysmal sac and offering a definitive treatment for a mass lesion. However, in order to be successful, the segment trapped must contain no vital branches, or at least these branches must have collateral potential. In addition, microvascular bypass to the distal segment must frequently be employed. These requisite conditions are usually present only in the posterior cerebral artery where a rich collateral circulation is available.

Aneurysmorraphy, the resection of the aneurysmal dome with reconstruction of the parent vessel, is a technically demanding procedure that requires that the tissues of the neck of the aneurysm and parent vessel not be friable so as to permit suture or clip repair. Although aneurysmorraphy has the advantage of preserving blood flow through the parent artery, successful application of this procedure is seldom achieved in our opinion.

One last alternative, which has been frequently used in the past, is the wrapping and coating of aneurysms in order to reinforce the walls. These methods rarely achieve complete encasement of the aneurysm and its neck, and hence provide little protection from continued growth and hemorrhage. It is our opinion that there is probably little role for this method in the modern treatment of giant aneurysms.

SURGICAL MANAGEMENT OF SPECIFIC ANEURYSMS

Anterior Circulation Aneurysms

Craniotomy and Initial Exposure

The classical pterional craniotomy, as described by Yasargil (30), can be used with few modifications for practically all aneurysms of the anterior circulation. The skin incision is planned to allow adequate exposure of the pterion and floor of the frontal fossa. Generally, a curvilinear incision beginning at the level of the zygoma and extending just behind the hairline to the midline will suffice. The temporalis fascia is sharply incised and the temporalis muscle is detached with electrocautery and reflected forward fashioning a myocutaneous flap. A frontotemporal craniotomy is fashioned. It is essential that this bony opening be flush with the floor of the frontal fossa. Using a high-speed drill, the lesser sphenoid wing is removed as far medially as the superior orbital fissure. Hemostasis is obtained with bone wax and oxycellulose. The dura is then incised in a C shape hinged on the skull base and reflected forward.

At this point the operating microscope is brought into position and the Sylvian fissure is opened widely by sharply dividing the arachnoid. Self-retaining frontal and temporal retractor blades are used to provide gentle retraction and exposure of the carotid and optic cisterns, which are opened, permitting cerebrospinal fluid (CSF) drainage. With adequate retraction and brain relaxation, the parent vessel and its branches are exposed as will be described below.

Giant Aneurysms of the Para-ophthalmic Carotid Segment

Some neurosurgeons have suggested that these aneurysms are unclippable by standard techniques. Their giant size, broad necks, and intimate relationship to the optic nerve under the anterior clinoid posed significant obstacles in the direct attack of these lesions. The majority were treated with Hunterian ligation. However, with the improved understanding of the anatomy of this region and the advent of the retrograde suction decompression technique described by Batjer and Samson (31), most of these lesions can now be effectively treated by direct clipping.

The standard pterional craniotomy is combined with intradural removal of the anterior clinoid process. The dura overlying the clinoid is incised with a dural knife and reflected over the proximal carotid artery and optic nerve. Using a diamond-tipped burr the anterior clinoid is completely removed. Bleeding can be controlled with oxycellulose in addition to bone wax. Once adequate removal of the clinoid has been achieved the falciform ligament is incised, decompressing the optic nerve and exposing the proximal carotid artery and the origin of the ophthalmic artery.

A separate neck incision is made along the medial border of the sternocleidomastoid muscle from the mastoid process to the suprasternal notch. Using sharp dissection, the subcutaneous tissues, platysma, and investing fascia are opened. The common facial vein must usually be ligated and divided. The ansa hypoglossi is identified and followed proximally to expose the hypoglossal nerve, which must be protected. At this point, the carotid sheath is opened and the common, external, and internal carotid arteries are exposed. Vessel loops are placed around these vessels in preparation for occlusion later in the operation.

Completion of aneurysm exposure is then undertaken. The arachnoid investments must be taken down sharply and all perforators, including the ophthalmic artery, should be dissected free. Distally, the internal carotid artery (ICA) should be exposed and the posterior communicating artery identified. Following the complete dissection and exposure of the ICA, aneurysm clip selection and a planned repair are formulated.

A temporary clip is placed on the carotid artery proximal to the posterior communicating and choroidal arteries. The common and external carotid arteries in the neck are clamped, and using an 18-gauge angiocatheter the ICA is punctured and suction applied. The aneurysm will usually soften or collapse completely, allowing precise placement of the clips obliterating the neck of the aneurysm and preserving the parent vessel. The temporary clip is removed and the external and common carotid arteries are unclamped restoring flow. The aneurysm should be observed for some time to ensure that it does not refill.

Giant Aneurysms of the Posterior Communicating Artery

Giant aneurysms of the carotid communicating segment are often amenable to direct clipping. The exposure is as already described; however, some specific points must be made. The head must be rotated 30–45° away from the lesion depending on the aneurysmal projection. Once the brain is exposed and the microscope is brought into the field, the arachnoid of the Sylvian fissure is sharply divided. Retraction should be cautiously applied and mainly on the frontal lobe in order not to avulse the dome of the aneurysm, which may be adherent to the temporal lobe and precipitate catastrophic hemorrhage.

The initial dissection should open the carotid and chiasmatic cisterns and allow egress of CSF. The proximal ICA is then dissected and prepared for the possibility of temporary clipping. Next, the carotid artery is dissected distally, slowly exposing the neck of the aneurysm. Every attempt should be made to identify the posterior communicating and anterior choroidal arteries.

A variety of clips should be available, with the main objective being preservation of the posterior communicating and choroidal arteries and lumen of the carotid artery. Long angled clips and fenestrated clips, which can be applied with the blades parallel to the carotid artery, will usually accomplish this goal. Once clipped, these aneurysms should be punctured and decompressed to ensure adequacy of the repair and to decompress the oculomotor nerve.

Giant Aneurysms of the Carotid Bifurcation

Giant aneurysms of the carotid bifurcation pose particular problems in surgical management. The numerous perforating arteries that arise in this location are frequently draped over or arise from the neck and waist of these aneurysms. The surgeon must be prepared in that the lesion may not be amenable to direct clipping. In the senior author's experience, many of these lesions can be effectively managed by Hunterian ligation, usually with a bypass to the distal MCA.

The basic approach is as already described. Wide splitting of the Sylvian fissure is obligatory. The ICA is exposed and prepared for temporary clipping. Dissection is continued exposing the bifurcation, the M1 and A1. With temporary clipping of the ICA, and frequently the M1 and A1 vessels, the aneurysm is explored and the neck exposed. Attempts should be made to identify and separate perforators from the aneurysmal dome. If the aneurysm has a well-defined neck, the use of a variety of clips, including curved, bayoneted, and fenestrated, may be particularly useful in these situations. With the neck clipped, one must ensure that there is no kinking of the A1 or M1 and that the terminal carotid

artery is open. If clipping is not feasible, an alternative is to perform Hunterian ligation or trapping with distal revascularization to the MCA.

Giant Aneurysms of the Middle Cerebral Artery

The craniotomy is fashioned in a similar manner to the approach for carotid bifurcation aneurysms. After dissection of the Sylvian fissure and exposure of the carotid bifurcation, the proximal M1 is exposed and traced out distally, exposing the aneurysm and other remaining middle cerebral branches. These aneurysms can often be completely dissected in a circumferential manner thus visualizing the parent vessels and providing for proximal control.

Clip reconstruction usually requires multiple fenestrated clips or the tandem clipping technique previously described. During clipping care must be taken not to propagate thromboembolic material into distal branches since these aneurysms commonly are partially thrombosed. If the aneurysm cannot be clipped, MCA occlusion with distal bypass is an effective alternative.

Giant Aneurysms of the Anterior Cerebral Artery

Giant aneurysms of the anterior communicating artery may be approached via the standard pterional craniotomy. However, it is often necessary to remove more frontal bone, as well as generous removal of the lesser wing of the sphenoid.

The dissection should begin along the ipsilateral A1 segment, following it to the region of the anterior communicating artery. The contralateral A1 is then exposed thus allowing for complete proximal control. An attempt is then made to identify both A2 segments. Once all four limbs of the communicating complex are exposed, identified, and prepared for temporary occlusion, the aneurysm can be dissected. It is critical to identify the hypothalamic perforators. Only after the anatomy of this complex is completely understood should one proceed with attempted clipping. Care should be taken during clip application to obliterate the aneurysm and preserve not only the anterior cerebral vessels but also the communicating segment from which many of the vital perforators arise. Perforators may seem to originate from the aneurysm itself as the anterior communicating and A1–A2 junction are incorporated into the sac as it forms.

In many instances, these aneurysms cannot be safely clipped. Tourniquet occlusion of either the A1 or A2 may be a safer alternative in the awake patient. We have a number of examples when proximal Hunterian ligation has completely obliterated the aneurysm with the distal A2 vasculature adequately supported by collateral flow.

Posterior Circulation Aneurysms

Giant aneurysms of the vertebrobasilar circulation are the most difficult of all to treat. The main obstacle is adequate exposure in that these aneurysms are located in a small confined space delimited by bone anteriorly and laterally and the brainstem with the cerebellum posteriorly. The cranial nerves emerging from the brainstem and arcing anteriorly to the cavernous sinus further obscure the surgeon's path to the lesion. Due to these anatomic confines, several surgical approaches and exposures have evolved. Each of these approaches has advantages over others. Some are relatively straightforward whereas others require complicated skull base techniques. The approach utilized should be dictated by the surgeon's familiarity with the involved anatomy and experience with the specific approach.

Approaches that have been proposed include various transpetrosal exposures, which can be subdivided into retrolabyrinthine, translabyrinthine, and transcochlear. These approaches can be combined with supra- and infratentorial dural openings to provide exposure along the entire length of the vertebrobasilar circulation. The far lateral approach has also evolved as an extension of the suboccipital exposure to provide exposure of the more proximal vertebrobasilar circulation. All of the above exposures require extensive skull base resection and mandate a real knowledge of temporal bone anatomy. In addition, there is a significant risk to hearing and facial nerve function in addition to postoperative CSF leak and meningitis.

We have found that the great majority of vertebrobasilar aneurysms can be safely and adequately exposed via the commonly known subtemporal and lateral suboccipital approaches. The choice of approaching these aneurysms from above or below is dependent on the ease of access to the neck. Only rarely have we found it necessary to employ some of the more extensive exposures described above. For specific technical details regarding the approaches listed above, we refer the reader to several excellent monographs listed in the references (28,32–34). The details of the subtemporal and lateral suboccipital approach will be reviewed below.

Subtemporal Approach

Positioning

The lateral position is employed for the subtemporal exposure. The nondominant side is usually exposed, although certain situations such as a right hemiparesis, dense left oculomotor palsy, or the direction and shape of the aneurysm dictate a dominant side exposure. Lumbar drainage is routinely employed in order to facilitate a slack brain and ease the retraction. The drain is placed after anesthetic induction and remains clamped off until the bony exposure is completed. The head is positioned with the anteroposterior axis parallel to the floor and the midsagittal plane directed inferiorly approximately 15–20° below the horizontal.

Scalp Incision and Craniotomy

We commonly employ a linear scalp incision beginning below the zygoma remaining within 1 cm of the tragus and extending just above the temporal squama. This simple incision provides more than adequate bony exposure and has the added advantage of rapid healing. If a larger exposure and division of the tentorium is anticipated, a temporal scalp flap can be fashioned and hinged inferiorly by using the same anterior limb and extending the posterior limb behind the ear.

The initial soft tissue dissection should be low enough to expose the zygomatic arch, which marks the level of the middle fossa floor. A self-retaining retractor is used to retract the soft tissues. We prefer to make one burr hole low in the temporal bone. The dura is then separated from the overlying bone, and using a craniotome, a small ovoid temporal bone flap is fashioned. Any remaining bone obscuring the floor of the middle fossa is removed with rongeurs and a high-speed drill. Care must be taken to wax these bone edges, which are frequently aerated, in order to prevent a postoperative CSF leak. The dura should be tacked up to the bony edges as troublesome epidural bleeding may occur after the lumbar drain is opened.

CSF is allowed to drain by unclamping the spinal drain, and the dura is not opened until it is noted to be flat or concave to the level of the bony opening. The dura is then opened in a Y-shaped manner with the inferior dural flap retracted inferiorly and sutured to the temporalis muscle.

Initial Intradural Exposure

With adequate CSF drainage and brain relaxation, two tapered retractor blades are slowly advanced along the underside of the temporal lobe until the uncus is elevated from the tentorial edge and the arachnoid covering the lateral pontine cistern and oculomotor nerve comes into view. Care must be taken to protect the vein of Labbé, which lies in the posterior reaches of the exposure.

We have found it quite helpful at this juncture to suture the edge of the tentorium back into the middle fossa. This stitch is placed just posterior to the dural penetration of the trochlear nerve and is anchored to the dura of the middle fossa floor. The arachnoid, inferior to the oculomotor nerve, is then incised, exposing the SCA. This vessel is then traced forward along the cerebral peduncle to its origin from the basilar artery, which can then be delineated with further dissection being dictated by the aneurysm's anatomic location and orientation.

Lateral Suboccipital Approach

Positioning

The patient is positioned in the straight lateral or park bench position with the head slightly rotated toward the floor. The neck is flexed but not to a degree that will obstruct venous drainage. The ipsilateral shoulder is taped downward toward the feet, but again care must be taken not to produce excessive tension, which may result in a brachial plexus injury. We prefer to allow the dependent shoulder to rest below the bed with the elbow flexed and the forearm resting on a padded arm side rest. A gel roll is used to protect the axilla.

Scalp Incision and Craniotomy

A paramedian curvilinear, linear, or S-shaped incision is made centered halfway between the mastoid process and the inion. The subcutaneous tissues and muscle mass are divided in a similar manner exposing the underlying occipital bone, mastoid process, and C1 lamina. Careful subperiosteal dissection is then used along the lamina of C1 until the extracranial vertebral artery is delineated at the point of entry into the atlanto-occipital membrane. A craniotomy is then fashioned extending from the midline superiorly to the transverse sinus, laterally to the sigmoid sinus and including the rim of the foramen magnum. On occasion, the lamina of C1 may also be removed. Bone edges are meticulously waxed in order to avoid postoperative CSF leak. The dura is then incised in a curvilinear fashion and hinged toward the sigmoid sinus.

Initial Intradural Exposure

A tiny dural-arachnoid opening into the cisterna magna is made and CSF allowed to escape. Once enough CSF drainage has occurred to allow adequate brain relaxation, the dura is widely opened and a tapered retractor blade is placed so as to elevate the cerebellar tonsil medially and upward thus exposing the lower cranial nerves and caudal loop of PICA. The vertebral artery is easily identified in the lateral gutter and the origin of PICA by its characteristic relationship with the hypoglossal nerve rootlets. The goal of the initial exposure is to prepare the vertebral artery for possible temporary occlusion and proximal control. Further dissection distally along the vertebral artery will expose the vertebrobasilar junction and provide a glimpse of the opposite vertebral artery.

CONSIDERATIONS IN SPECIFIC ANEURYSMS

Aneurysms of the Basilar Bifurcation

The principles of giant basilar bifurcation aneurysm dissection are similar to those used for their smaller counterparts. The initial exposure begins with the SCA along the cerebral peduncle to the basilar artery. The origin of the posterior cerebral artery is easily identified just superior to the takeoff of the SCA.

The first goal at this juncture is preparing a segment of the distal basilar artery for temporary clipping. A 2- to 3-mm segment below the SCA can usually be found free of perforators, which is suitable for temporary clipping. The dissection of the aneurysm is begun along its anterior aspect. The origin of the P1 is followed anteriorly where the anterior neck of the aneurysm becomes apparent. This may necessitate gentle retraction of the cerebral peduncle. With giant

aneurysms in this location, the dome may be adherent to the clivus anteriorly and great care must be taken not to avulse the adherent wall from its attachment precipitating disastrous hemorrhage.

After the ipsilateral SCA, P1, and anterior neck have been delineated, gentle retraction on the neck will usually bring the opposite P1 and SCA into view. The critical aspect of the dissection is then undertaken along the posterior aspect of the aneurysm. These giant aneurysms are buried in the brainstem, making visualization of the vascular anatomy and the vital perforators quite difficult. These perforators, most arising from the proximal P1 segment, must be clearly identified and separated from the aneurysm if clip placement is to be successful or even possible. They can be identified with gentle anterior retraction along the posterior waist of the aneurysm. This maneuver should be continued across the interpeduncular cistern thus exposing the opposite P1 artery and its perforators.

One must have available straight, curved, angled, bayoneted, and fenestrated clips of all sizes and closing pressures. Straight clips will suffice when the aneurysm points forward or backward from the bifurcation. When applying a clip in these situations, one must ensure that the blades do not occlude or kink the origins of the P1 arteries and, most importantly, that no perforators are trapped in the blades of the clip. The more commonly encountered aneurysm, however, arises in line with the origins of the P1 arteries and projects directly upward. In this situation, fenestrated clips can be useful. The ipsilateral P1 artery and adjacent perforators can be enclosed safely within the fenestration, allowing the blades to compress only the neck of the aneurysm. Great care must be taken in selecting the precise blade length that will completely obliterate the aneurysm's neck without occluding the opposite P1 artery or allow continued filling of the aneurysm. One must keep in mind that clipping should always be done so as to preserve the primary axis of the major vessels from which the aneurysm arises. In the case of the basilar bifurcation, the usual axis is along the P1–P1 union. Clip application along this axis is best accomplished when applied from the side, underscoring an advantage of the subtemporal approach.

Due to the size of these aneurysms and the small confines in which they are found, these lesions frequently are not amenable to direct clipping. We have found proximal basilar artery occlusion with the microtourniquet to be very effective in decreasing the risk of rupture and promoting gradual thrombosis of these giant sacs.

Aneurysms of the Posterior Cerebral and Superior Cerebellar Arteries

Giant aneurysms of the posterior cerebral artery arise in order of frequency at the P2–P3 junction followed by the P1–P2 junction and, lastly, the proximal P1 segment. The surgical management of these aneurysms is similar to the approach for basilar bifurcation aneurysms with the critical maneuver again being the delineation of the perforators. Most of these aneurysms cannot be safely clipped. Proximal occlusion and even trapping techniques can be applied. In the senior author's experience, the posterior cerebral territory has a rich potential for collateral supply. Proximal occlusion without bypass has been exceptionally well tolerated.

Giant aneurysms of the SCA tend to grow from the proximal SCA as well as the basilar artery. As these aneurysms enlarge and attain giant dimensions, they incorporate the SCA and curiously even the origin of the posterior cerebral artery. The adjacent oculomotor nerve usually becomes displaced above or laterally as the aneurysmal dome grows into and becomes buried in the cerebral peduncle. The perforators arising from P1 are often associated with the superior aspect of this aneurysm; small branches from the SCA and perforators from the posterior aspect of the basilar artery will have a relationship to the medial and inferior margins of the sac. These vital branches must be identified and protected.

The approach is the same as for basilar bifurcation aneurysms. A subtemporal approach is preferred with initial dissection along the anterior surface of the aneurysm until the origins of the superior cerebellar arteries and posterior cerebral arteries are identified. However, this aneurysm may also be approached from the neck side, opposite the dome. After this perforators must be separated from the aneurysmal dome and the neck prepared for clipping if possible. Curved and gently angled clips are often useful for this type of aneurysm. The oculomotor nerve may be protected by encircling it in the aperture of a fenestrated clip. Care must be taken not to kink the origins of the SCA or PCA or narrow the basilar artery itself. Finally, critical inspection must be made for any perforators that may have been entrapped by the posterior blades of the aneurysm clip. The posterior and medial (hidden) surface of this aneurysm is where the danger lay.

Giant Aneurysms of the Basilar Trunk

These aneurysms can be divided into two groups: those arising at the origin of the anterior inferior cerebellar artery (basilar-AICA) and those arising between the origins of the SCA and AICA (midbasilar trunk). This distinction becomes blurred when these aneurysms attain giant dimensions and in this circumstance are referred to as giant basilar trunk aneurysms. These aneurysms are constrained in a confined space anterior to the pons and are frequently buried in the substance of the pons and medulla or adherent to the clivus.

Due to the location of these aneurysms, we have found that either a subtemporal-transtentorial or suboccipital approach is most useful. The half-and-half approach with division of the tentorium can also be successfully employed and provides a wider angle of view. Using the subtemporal-transtentorial route, the opening is as previously described for the standard subtemporal approach with the modification of centering the bone flap on the petrous bone.

The free edge of the tentorium is split approximately 1–1.5 cm behind the attachment of the trochlear nerve. Once this has been performed, the arachnoid membrane of the posterior fossa is opened and the petrosal vein coagulated and divided. Arachnoidal dissection is continued lateral to the trigeminal nerve and slight retraction of the anterior cerebellum will expose the basilar artery entirely along its length to the vertebrobasilar junction.

Dissection then proceeds along the basilar artery until the neck of the aneurysm is identified. Identification of the origin of the AICA can be particularly difficult with giant aneurysms in this region; however, this vessel and its origin must be clearly delineated. With basilar-AICA aneurysms, the exposure is usually straightforward; however, midbasilar trunk aneurysms can be quite treacherous. Their location frequently incorporates many vital perforators and their exposure is hampered by the overlying trigeminal nerve. Exposure in this region frequently requires retraction of the trigeminal nerve laterally in conjunction with minimal pontine retraction.

Giant basilar trunk aneurysms located near the vertebrobasilar junction are best approached via a suboccipital route and working between and around the lower cranial nerves. This approach can be fraught with hazard, as manipulation of the lower cranial nerve rootlets frequently results in serious morbidity from dysphagia and aspiration pneumonia.

Giant Aneurysms of the Vertebral Artery

These aneurysms can arise from the vertebral–PICA junction, the distal vertebral artery beyond the origin of PICA, or the vertebral–basilar junction, in which case they are frequently associated with a fenestration of the basilar artery. Aneurysms in this location are always anatomically related to cranial nerves IX, X, XI, and XII. In particular, the hypoglossal nerve has an intimate relationship to the origin of PICA from the vertebral artery. As they reach giant dimension, they distort and bury into the medulla and pontomedullary junction. Deformation of the lower cranial nerves and medulla may cause problems with swallowing, tongue movements, and even a Wallenberg syndrome.

These aneurysms are most easily approached via the standard lateral suboccipital approach. Once the vertebral artery is identified, dissection is carried out distally along this vessel toward the origin of the PICA where the aneurysm will be found. The spinal branch of the accessory nerve serves as a key landmark in this regard. It is found posterior to the first dentate ligament as it ascends to join the lower rootlets of the vagus nerve. The aneurysmal neck is then divested of any arachnoid and its relationship to the PICA origin studied. Further dissection is necessary distally along the vertebral artery in order to realize the anatomic relationships of the aneurysm and to gain access should trapping be necessary. The lower cranial nerves are gently separated from the aneurysm, particularly the hypoglossal nerve in preparation for clipping. Great care must be taken in separating the lower cranial nerves from the aneurysm, particularly the glosso-pharyngeal and vagus as problems with swallowing and aspiration constitute the major cause of morbidity.

Clipping usually requires employment of varied aperture clips incorporating the PICA and lower cranial nerves. Great care in manipulating the vital cranial nerves in this region cannot be overstressed. The clip is ideally placed parallel to the axis of the vertebral artery with the fenestration incorporating it. This aneurysm typically takes origin from both the vertebral artery and PICA. Often a length of PICA is involved with the neck, making the PICA appear to originate from the aneurysm. Critical medullary perforators also arise from this segment. Thus the origin of PICA must always be protected in any repair.

CONCLUSIONS

Giant intracranial aneurysms comprise a unique entity that continue to represent a difficult challenge to the neurosurgeon. Major strides have been made in the past three decades in the surgical management of these formidable lesions. Continued advances in the understanding of the underlying pathophysiology as well as development of pharmacologic interventions for brain ischemia will undoubtedly enhance the management of these lesion. More importantly, earlier recognition and repair of aneurysms before they attain giant dimensions will perhaps have the greatest impact.

The rapid development and proliferation of endovascular techniques will almost certainly reduce the number of giant aneurysms available for direct surgical repair. Early attempts to obliterate the lumen of the sacs with balloons were unsatisfactory due to rupture of the sac, continued enlargement, collapse, and migration of the balloons. The more recent experience with metallic coils placed within the sac to promote thrombosis appear to be safer, but only with prolonged follow-up will we know if this intraluminal thrombosis affects a permanent cure.

REFERENCES

1. Morley TP, Barr HWK. Giant intracranial aneurysms: diagnosis, course, and management. *Clin Neurosurg* 1969;16:73–94.
2. McKissock W, Paine KWE, Walsch LS. An analysis of the results of treatment of ruptured intracranial aneurysms. *J Neurosurg* 1960;17:762–776.
3. Miller JD, Jamrad K, Jennett B. Safety of carotid ligation and its role in the management of intracranial aneurysms. *J Neurol Neurosurg Psychiatry* 1977;40:64– 72.
4. Drake CG. Giant intracranial aneurysms: experience with surgical treatment in 174 patients. *Clin Neurosurg* 1979;26:12–96.
5. Bull J. Massive aneurysms at the base of the brain. *Brain* 1969;92:535–570.
6. Locksley HB. Report of the cooperative study of intracranial aneurysms and subarachnoid hemorrhage. Sect V, Part II. Natural history of subarachnoid hemorrhage, intracranial aneurysms and arteriovenous malformations based on 6368 cases in the cooperative study. *J Neurosurg* 1966;23:321–368.
7. Pia HW, Zierski J. Giant cerebral aneurysms. *Neurosurg Rev* 1982;5:117–148.
8. Lawton MT, Spetzler RF. Management strategies for giant intracranial aneurysms. *Contemp Neurosurg* 1994;16(17).
9. Sadik AR, Budzilovich GN, Shulman K. Giant aneurysm of the middle cerebral artery. *J Neurosurg* 1965;22:177–181.
10. McCormick WF, Acousta-Rua GJ. The size of intracranial saccular aneurysms: an autopsy study. *J Neurosurg* 1970;33:422.
11. Michael WF. Posterior fossa aneurysms simulating tumors. *J Neurol Neurosurg Psychiatry* 1974;37:218–223.
12. Ojemann RG. Management of the unruptured intracranial aneurysm. *N Engl J Med* 1981;304:725–726.
13. Ferguson GG. Physical factors in the initiation, growth, and rupture of human intracranial saccular aneurysms. *J Neurosurg* 1972;37:666–677.
14. Jain KK. Mechanism of rupture of intracranial saccular aneurysms. *Surgery* 1963;54:347–350.
15. Schubiger O, Valavanis A, Wichmann W. Growth-mechanism of giant intracranial aneurysms; demonstration by CT and MR imaging. *Neuroradiology* 1987;29:266–271.
16. Heros RC, Kolluri S. Giant intracranial aneurysms presenting with massive cerebral edema. *Neurosurgery* 1984;15:512–577.
17. Hjer-Pedersen E, Hasse J. Giant anterior communicating artery aneurysm with bitemporal hemianopsia: case report. *Neurosurgery* 1981;8:703–706.
18. Peiris JB, Ross Russell RW. Giant aneurysms of the carotid system presenting as visual field defect. *J Neurol Neurosurg Psychiatry* 1980;43:1053–1064.
19. Raymond LA, Tew J. Large suprasellar aneurysms imitating pituitary tumor. *J Neurol Neurosurg Psychiatry* 1978;41:83–87.
20. White JC, Ballantine HT. Intrasellar aneurysms simulating hypophyseal tumors. *J Neurosurg* 1961;18:34–50.
21. Swearingen B, Heros RC. Fatal rupture of a thrombosed giant basilar artery aneurysm. *Surg Neurol* 1985;23:299–302.
22. Busse O, Grote E. Recurrent cerebral embolization from a carotid bifurcation aneurysm. *Acta Neurochir* 1982;62:203–206.
23. Cohen MM, Hemalatha CP, Dadda Rio RT, et al. Embolization from a fusiform middle cerebral artery aneurysm. *Stroke* 1980;11:158–161.
24. Tanaka Y, Kobayashi K, Kyoshima K, Sugita K. Multiple clipping technique for large and giant internal carotid aneurysms and complications: angiographic analysis. *J Neurosurg* 1994;80:635–642.
25. Samson D, Batjer HH, Bowman G, et al. A clinical study of the parameters and effects of temporary arterial occlusion in the management of intracranial aneurysms. *Neurosurgery* 1995;34:22–29.
26. Batjer HH, Frankfurt AI, Purdy PD, et al. Use of etomidate, temporary arterial occlusion, and intraoperative angiography in surgical treatment of large and giant cerebral aneurysms. *J Neurosurg* 1988;68:234–240.
27. Scott JA, Horner TG, Leipzig TJ. Retrograde suction decompression of an ophthalmic artery aneurysm using balloon occlusion. Technical note. *J Neurosurg* 1991;75:146–147.
28. Spetzler RF, Hadley MN, Rigamonti D, et al. Aneurysms of the basilar artery treated with circulatory arrest, hypothermia and barbiturate cerebral protection. *J Neurosurg* 1988;68:868.
29a. Drake CG, Peerless SJ, Ferguson GG. Hunterian proximal arterial occlusion for giant aneurysms of the carotid circulation. *J Neurosurg* 1994;81:656–665.
29b. Drake CG, Peerless SJ, Hernesniemi JA. *Surgery of Vertebrobasilar Aneurysms: London, Ontario Experience on 1767 Patients.* Wien: Springer-Verlag, 1996.
30. Yasargil MG, Gasser JC, Hodosh RM, et al. Carotid-ophthalmic aneurysms: direct microsurgical approach. *Surg Neurol* 1977;8:155–165.
31. Batjer HH, Samson DS. Retrograde suction decompression of giant paraclinoidal aneurysms. Technical note. *J Neurosurg* 1990;73:305–306.
32. Gianotta SL, Maceri DR. Retrolabyrinthine transsigmoid approach to basilar trunk and vertebrobasilar artery junction aneurysms. Technical note. *J Neurosurg* 1988;69:461–466.
33. Solomon RA, Stein BM. Surgical approaches to aneurysms of the vertebral and basilar arteries. *Neurosurgery* 1988;23:203–208.
34. Spetzler RF, Daspit CP, Pappas CTE. The combined supra- and infratentorial approach for lesions of the petrous and clival regions: experience with 46 cases. *J Neurosurg* 1992;76:588–599.

Cerebrovascular Disease, edited by H. Hunt Batjer.
Lippincott-Raven Publishers, Philadelphia © 1997.

CHAPTER 87

Aneurysm Surgery: Timing

Giuseppe Lanzino, Mark E. Shaffrey, Christopher I. Shaffrey,
Scott Henson, and Neal F. Kassell

It is estimated that in the United States as many as 5,000,000 people harbor an intracranial aneurysm, and approximately 28,000 aneurysms will rupture each year, resulting in subarachnoid hemorrhage (SAH) (1). Of these, 10,000 patients will die or be left disabled by the initial insult (1). The majority of the 18,000 patients who survive aneurysmal SAH have the potential for a good functional recovery; however, these potentials are not fully realized. Aneurysmal SAH, in fact, is a peculiar disease. Whereas in other acute disorders, such as traumatic brain injury, the outcome for the most part is established at the time of the primary injury, patients that survive aneurysm rupture are still at risk for further deterioration and death. The major causes of death in patients who survive the primary hemorrhage are rebleeding and vasospasm (each representing 37.5% of cases), followed by medical (12.5%) and surgical (12.5%) complications (2). Therefore, many patients die or are left disabled as a consequence of avoidable complications.

One of the most controversial aspects of the management of aneurysmal SAH is the timing of surgery. For each patient, the treating physician is faced with two choices: (a) secure the aneurysm as early as possible to prevent rebleeding and allow for more aggressive treatment of vasospasm or (b) wait until the patient has stabilized and operate on a more relaxed brain. In this chapter, we will try to objectively analyze the pros and cons of each treatment strategy and then discuss our current approach to the patient with a ruptured aneurysm.

HISTORICAL PERSPECTIVE

The modern treatment of cerebral aneurysms started in 1937 with Walter Dandy, who used a McKenzie silver clip to secure the neck of an unruptured posterior communicating aneurysm that had caused third nerve palsy (3). After Dandy's pioneering efforts, other surgeons tried to clip the sac immediately after rupture in an attempt to prevent the most feared event, rebleeding. Unfortunately, such early attempts were accompanied by prohibitively high mortality and morbidity. During the first attempts at early surgery, it became clear that the technical problems encountered diminished if the intracranial operation was delayed a week or more after the initial bleeding. When the operation was delayed, the brain was slack, the dissection easier, and the phenomenon of arterial spasm (now recognized as a complication of aneurysmal SAH) had subsided in most cases.

In 1953, Norlen and Olivecrona (4) reported on a series of 63 patients with anterior circulation aneurysms who had undergone aneurysm repair 3 weeks or more after the onset of SAH. In this group of patients, they reported a mortality of 3%, as compared with a 53% mortality rate in a subset of 15 patients who were operated on in the "acute stage" (defined as a few hours to 3 weeks following SAH) (4). Based on this observation, they concluded that intracranial operations for ruptured aneurysms were extremely dangerous during the acute phase and suggested that surgery should be delayed for 3 weeks after the acute episode. This report represented a landmark in the controversy of the timing of aneurysm surgery and would greatly influence the attitude of many surgeons in the years to come. Thus, delayed surgery became the modus operandi for the next 20 years (2).

With increasing experience in the surgical treatment of intracranial aneurysms, it was realized that despite improving surgical results overall management outcome was unsatisfactory. The distress and frustration of seeing potentially salvageable patients become disabled or die while waiting for delayed surgery led many neurosurgeons to reevaluate their position on the timing of the operation. At the same time, several technical improvements were taking place that encouraged such changes. With the introduction of the operative microscope, the resolution and accurate visualization it provided made details easily dissectable and visualization

All authors: Department of Neurosurgery, Virginia Neurological Institute, Charlottesville, Virginia, 22908.

of important microstructures possible. In addition, fine microinstruments and removable clips were developed. Progress in neuroanesthesia has also been instrumental in improving the feasibility of operating in the hyperacute phase, providing a slack brain through the use of deep hypotension, controlled ventilation, and osmotic diuretics.

Due to these changes, in the late 1970s, there was a resurgence of the idea of early surgery, prompted in large part by reports from Japanese neurosurgeons showing that combined mortality and morbidity figures were not worse with early surgery (5). These reports have been followed by a vigorous debate about the timing of surgery, and several large series of patients submitted to early surgery after aneurysmal SAH have been published (6–8). These reports have stressed the technical feasibility and good results following early aneurysm surgery (ie, within the first 48–72 hours after hemorrhage). Encouraged by these series, more surgeons have tried the early surgical approach for ruptured aneurysms. The change in management pattern that occurred is demonstrated by the fact that while early surgery (within 7 days of onset) in Japanese centers took place in only 18% of cases between 1974 and 1975 (9), between 1980 and 1983 early surgery (days 0–3) was planned in 75% of the Japanese patients enrolled in the International Cooperative Study on the Timing of Aneurysm Surgery (ICSTAS) (10). Similarly, a randomized trial evaluating the effects of nicardipine in SAH showed that between 1989 and 1991 early surgery was performed in North American centers in more than 60% of the patients eligible for the study (11).

THE INTERNATIONAL COOPERATIVE STUDY ON THE TIMING OF ANEURYSM SURGERY

Due to this controversy, the ICSTAS was initiated in the early 1980s (12,13). The study was a prospective, observational, epidemiologic survey primarily conducted to define the relationship between timing of surgery and outcome in patients with ruptured aneurysms (12). It involved standardized data collection in patients admitted within 3 days after

SAH. Principal outcome measures included the patients' neurologic and disability status at 6 months after SAH, rates of vasospasm and rebleeding, and medical and surgical complications during hospitalization. On completion of the initial admission examination, surgeons were required to specify at which time interval they planned to conduct surgery. The intervals that could be chosen included days 0–3, days 4–6, days 7–10, days 11–14, days 15–32, and no surgery. Between December 1980 and June 1983, 3521 patients eligible for the study were admitted to the 68 participating centers.

Analysis of the individual intervals has indicated that patients who had surgery planned between days 7 and 10 after SAH had the least favorable outcome and the highest mortality (13) (Table 1). Otherwise, the results of surgery for all other intervals were similar (13). When the level of consciousness at admission was taken into account, the most favorable outcome and lowest mortality were observed among alert patients for whom surgery was planned on days 0–3 or 11–14 (13). Among drowsy patients, surgery planned for days 0–3 was not advantageous (13). The surgery interval in drowsy patients that yielded the least favorable results was days 7–10 (13). No significant differences were noted between the various intervals in stuporous or comatose patients (13). The incidence of focal ischemic deficits was higher in planned intervals of days 7–10, 11–14, and 15–32, and the incidence of hydrocephalus was highest in patients with planned surgery at days 15–32 (13) (Table 2).

The overall comparison demonstrated that considerable morbidity and mortality occurred after early surgery and prior to late surgery (13). The mortality associated with intervening events before delayed surgery nearly equaled the postoperative mortality rate following early surgery (13). Surgery planned for days 7–10 had high both pre- and postoperative rates, resulting in an overall higher mortality level (13). It must be emphasized that these patients were cared for in neurosurgical centers with a recognized interest and experience in managing aneurysmal SAH. Most important, this study clearly showed that early surgery was not techni-

TABLE 1. *Good recovery and mortality rates at 6-month follow-up period after subarachnoid hemorrhage (SAH)*[a]

Admission consciousness	Planned surgery interval (days from SAH)					Significance
	0–3	4–6	7–10	11–14	15–32	
Good Recovery Rate (%)						
Alert	78	69	70	76	59	$p = .0132$
Drowsy	54	62	49	57	62	NS
Stuporous	33	29	33	27	33	NS
Comatose	16	10	12	22	17	NS
Overall	63	60	56	62	63	$p = .0459$
Mortality Rate (%)						
Alert	11	17	15	13	15	NS
Drowsy	26	24	31	28	22	NS
Stuporous	40	46	40	41	39	NS
Comatose	56	32	79	55	55	NS
Overall	20	24	28	21	20	$p = .007$

[a] (From ref. 13, with permission). Results are expressed in percentage (adjusted). NS, not significant.

TABLE 2. *Pre- and postoperative complications by planned surgery interval after subarachnoid hemorrhage*

Complication	Planned surgery interval (days from SAH)					Significance
	0–3	4–6	7–10	11–14	15–32	
Rebleeding	91 (5.7%)	35 (9.4%)	79 (12.7%)	60 (13.9%)	53 (21.5%)	$p < .001$
Focal ischemic deficit	427 (26.8%)	106 (28.5%)	201 (32.3%)	133 (30.7%)	82 (33.2%)	$p = .043$
Angiographic complication	24 (1.5%)	11 (3.0%)	18 (2.9%)	11 (2.5%)	6 (2.4%)	NS
Brain swelling	192 (12.0%)	44 (11.8%)	63 (10.1%)	41 (9.5%)	12 (4.9%)	$p = .011$
Epidural hematoma	11 (0.7%)	2 (0.5%)	6 (1.0%)	5 (1.2%)	1 (0.4%)	NS
Hydrocephalus	201 (12.6%)	27 (7.3%)	66 (10.6%)	63 (14.5%)	65 (26.3%)	$p < .001$
Iatrogenic arterial occlusion	32 (2.0%)	7 (1.9%)	9 (1.4%)	1 (0.2%)	5 (2.0%)	NS
Intracerebral hemorrhage	128 (8.0%)	26 (7.0%)	38 (6.1%)	32 (7.4%)	25 (10.1%)	NS
Seizures	62 (3.9%)	15 (4.0%)	33 (5.3%)	22 (5.1%)	11 (4.4%)	NS
Subdural hematoma	24 (1.5%)	6 (1.6%)	14 (2.2%)	7 (1.6%)	7 (2.8%)	NS
Total number of cases	1595	372	623	433	247	

(From ref. 13, with permission); Key: NS, not significant.

cally more difficult than later surgery, even though the incidence of a swollen, tight brain was higher in early surgery (Fig. 1).

In 1992, Haley et al (10) separately analyzed the results of the study in the participating North American centers. In contrast to the results of the overall study, they noted that, when adjusted for prognostic factors and center variability, the good recovery rate was found to be higher in the group that had surgery planned for the interval day 0–3 than that planned for days 11–32 ($p < .01$) (10). This analysis confirmed that the overall outcome was worse in the group of patients that had surgery planned for the day 7–10 period, which is recognized as the period of greatest risk for angiographic and symptomatic vasospasm. While mortality from surgical complications was slightly reduced in those patients assigned to delayed management, surgical morbidity was not. In terms of overall outcome, mortality was significantly worse in the group of patients scheduled for surgery on days 7–10. Mortality in patients planned for surgery during days 0–3 was 15% and was equivalent to that of the later planned surgical intervals. The percentage of patients achieving good recovery at 6 months, however, was significantly better in those patients planned for surgery on days 0–3. Alert pa-

tients generally did well regardless of the planned surgical interval, but drowsy patients had better outcomes if surgery was planned before day 6 or after day 14. Comatose patients with surgery planned for after the first week generally had better outcomes, although the mortality was high in all planned surgical intervals for this group of patients.

In an attempt to explain these improved results, the authors hypothesized that they were a consequence of the more aggressive management of vasospasm in the North American centers (10). Hypervolemia alone or combined with induced hypertension, in fact, were adopted in these centers more frequently than in other participating centers around the world, and these differences were statistically significant (10). The ICSTAS was conducted before intentional hypervolemia, induced hypertension, or calcium antagonist drugs became widely available. It can be speculated that with the current widespread use of these treatment modalities, the advantages of an early surgery policy may be more striking.

FACTORS AFFECTED BY TIMING OF SURGERY

Traditionally, the advantage of early surgery was to secure the aneurysm sac and prevent the feared complication of

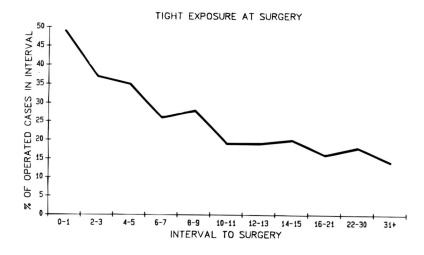

FIG. 1. Percentage of patients with brain tightness during surgical exposure correlated with the day of operation after subarachnoid hemorrhage. (From ref. 13, with permission.)

TABLE 3. *Pros and cons of early surgery*

Pros
Prevention of rebleeding
Aggressive management of vasospasm
  Hypertensive-hypervolemic therapy
  Angioplasty
Removal of subarachnoid clot
  Mechanical removal
  Subarachnoid injection of thrombolytic substances
Reduced hospital stay
More effective prevention of medical complications
  Early mobilization of patients (prevention of pneumonia,
  deep venous thrombosis)
Prevention of hydrocephalus (?)
  Prevention and release of subarachnoid adhesions, re-
  moval of subarachnoid blood, application of rt-PA
Reduced psychosocial stress

Cons
Swollen brain
Unstable patient
Scheduling

rebleeding. However, the availability of novel pharmacologic agents and strategies to counteract vasospasm and its consequences—intraarterial injection of papaverine, hypertensive-hypervolemic therapy, angioplasty of spastic vessels—and a better understanding of the pathophysiology of some of the complications (ie, chronic hydrocephalus and medical complications) would suggest that several factors other than rebleeding may be affected by an early surgical intervention. These factors can be schematically subdivided into hemorrhage-related, aneurysm-related, patient-related, and environment-related factors (14). A summary of these factors in relation to timing of surgery is given in Table 3.

Aneurysm-Related Factors

Rebleeding

Rebleeding is the most deleterious complication of aneurysm rupture, occurring in as many as 30% of all cases (15). The peak period for rebleeding and death is the first two weeks after the initial rupture of an intracranial arterial aneurysm. Kassell and Torner (16) have reported a maximum rebleeding rate of 4% for day 0, with an increase of 1.5% per day totaling a 27% chance in 2 weeks. The rate of rebleeding then decreases to 3% per year after 6 months and persists for the first decade (15,16).

Rerupture carries significant morbidity and mortality. In the ICSTAS, 45% of patients who had rebleeding while taking antifibrinolytics died within 2 weeks. Moreover, in patients with multiple bleeds, the likelihood of further SAH and resulting death is markedly elevated (16). These patients should undergo surgery on an emergency basis. The likelihood of rebleeding appears to be greater in poor-grade patients, those with hypertension, and the elderly (17,18).

Other factors shown to be significantly related to rebleeding include female sex, interval to treatment, and medical condition (17).

One of the major hypothetical advantages of early operation is the elimination of the rebleeding potential during the highest-risk period. The number of patients who suffered rebleeding in the ICSTAS increased progressively with longer intervals of planned surgery from approximately 6% for days 0–3 to approximately 22% for days 15–32 (see Table 2) (13). Additionally, other studies have shown a significantly decreased incidence of rebleeding with early surgery (6–8); however, approximately one patient in 25 will experience aneurysm rerupture before diagnostic studies and subsequent surgery can be completed (16). This impressive early-rebleeding rate implies that if early operation is being considered to decrease the incidence of subsequent SAH, it must be used on an emergency basis with minimal delay (16).

In the late 1960s and the 1970s, when delayed surgery was largely adopted, measures to reduce the incidence of rebleeding, such as hypotension and antifibrinolytic therapy, were proposed with the hope that preventing the lysis of the fibrin-platelet seal would prevent recurrent hemorrhage. The two most commonly used compounds were ϵ-aminocaproic acid and tranexamic acid, which act by competitive inhibition of plasminogen activation. The use of these agents is indeed associated with a decrease in the incidence of rebleeding. In the ICSTAS, patients who received antifibrinolytic therapy had a cumulative 14-day rebleeding risk of 14%, whereas the risk was 26.5% for patients who did not receive therapy (16). Unfortunately, patients on antifibrinolytics continued to rebleed, although at a lower rate. In addition, several studies demonstrate that the use of these agents did not result in overall improvement of outcome because of increased complications from ischemia and hydrocephalus (19). If early surgery is anticipated, there is no definitive role for the use of fibrinolytic therapy. If surgical treatment is to be delayed or not performed, it may be reasonable to employ these agents, despite the potential to develop focal ischemic deficits and hydrocephalus.

Technical Considerations

One of the major obstacles limiting the widespread use of early surgery was that the surgeon was presented with a swollen brain and a confining exposure. Immediately after SAH, autoregulation is impaired and the brain is more swollen, softened, hyperemic, and prone to contusion and laceration. In addition, during the early phase after SAH, the clot in the subarachnoid cisterns is more adherent to the vessels and tends to obscure the smaller perforators. Attempts to mechanically remove the subarachnoid clot may result in bruising of pial banks and injury to small vessels, particularly veins. One of the most striking findings of the ICSTAS was that, in experienced hands, early surgery could be performed without a significantly increased complication rate. In that study, the participating surgeons were asked to report certain aspects of the operative procedure. As might have been expected, the brains of patients operated on early were noted to be more swollen than in the delayed cases (see Fig. 1). In spite of this, there was no greater need for major resections at the time of early surgery than in the delayed cases. Furthermore, the incidence of brain contusions and lacerations was no greater following early surgery. With regard to the aneurysms, the degree of difficulty reported in performing the dissection was equal for both groups. Leak or rupture of the aneurysm was no greater with earlier surgery. Therefore, for experienced surgeons early surgery does not pose any serious obstacles. Dissection of the aneurysm itself with removal of fresh clot, identification of the neck, and separation of the perforators, although somewhat more tedious in the acute phase, is not accompanied by a significantly higher incidence of complications.

Posterior Circulation Aneurysms

Only a few neurosurgeons have extended an early-surgery policy for ruptured posterior circulation aneurysms. Secondary to the less common occurrence of these aneurysms and the combined limited surgical experience and technical difficulty in treating them, there has been a general trend to delay surgery in these cases. Peerless and coworkers (20) recently reported their extensive experience with over 200 such aneurysms operated on in the early phase. In their hands, the frequency of intraoperative rupture was not different in the early- and late-surgery groups. Although temporary clipping was required in 41% of the cases in the early-surgery group as opposed to 19% in the late-surgery group, results in good-grade patients were excellent. Of 66 patients with basilar bifurcation aneurysms classified preoperatively as Botterell grade 1, there were five poor outcomes and two deaths. They recommended early surgery for those patients in good preoperative grade (Botterell grade 1 or 2 or a Hunt and Hess grade I–III) whose aneurysm does not present a particular technical difficulty because of size, configuration, or location. They also advised early surgery for the occasional patients whose lives appear to be in jeopardy because of recurrent hemorrhage. However, due to the highest incidence of poor results, they were "hesitant to recommend early surgery for aneurysms arising from the basilar trunk" (20). This large series showed that the clinical grade of the patient remains the primary determinant of outcome, while aneurysm location is of secondary importance in the comparison of timing of surgery for anterior vs. posterior circulation aneurysms in experienced hands.

Giant Aneurysms

Unless the aneurysm is >25 mm (giant size), aneurysm size does not affect the timing of surgery. If the aneurysm sac is of giant size, the technical complexity of surgical repair is greatly increased. There is often an associated intraluminal clot, the neck can be broad-based, and arterial branches may be partially encased into the neck or base of the aneurysm dome. Surgery in these cases requires significant manipulation and often prolonged periods of temporary occlusion of the parent vessel. Neck clipping in these cases is always difficult and may be even impossible. It seems reasonable to allow the brain to recover as much as possible from the primary insult.

Hemorrhage-Related Factors

Vasospasm

Vasospasm is recognized as the major cause of delayed serious morbidity and mortality after aneurysm rupture. The incidence of vasospasm in SAH varies widely in the available literature, whether angiographic vasospasm or only symptomatic vasospasm is considered. The onset and duration of vasospasm after aneurysmal SAH often follows a precise and well defined timetable. Vasospasm has its onset about day 3 after SAH, is maximal at days 6–8, and has usually subsided by day 12 (21).

There are four possible strategies for the management of vasospasm: (a) prevent arterial narrowing before it occurs, (b) reverse arterial narrowing, (c) antagonize the ischemic consequences of the increased cerebral vascular resistance, and (d) protect the brain from infarction (19).

Prevention of Arterial Narrowing

In 1980, Fisher and coworkers (22) directed attention to the fact that the development of cerebral vasospasm is closely related to the amount and presence of blood in the subarachnoid space as visualized by computed tomography (CT). Reporting on a series of 47 patients, they observed that if subarachnoid blood was not detected or was diffusely distributed, severe vasospasm occurred in only one of 18 cases. If large subarachnoid clots (≥1 mm) were present in the fissures and cisterns, severe vasospasm developed in 23 of 24 patients. In addition, distribution of severe vasospasm was strongly associated with the site of the large subarachnoid clots. From these observations, it was concluded that extravascular blood is the single most significant etiologic factor promoting vasospasm. These clinical observations have been substantiated by experimental work showing that the presence and persistence of large subarachnoid blood collections are associated with vasospasm (19).

Based on these observations, it has been proposed that early and extensive removal of perivascular blood collections should be effective in minimizing the occurrence of vasospasm and delayed ischemic deficits (23). This may be achieved by washout of blood and spasmogenic substances from the basal cisterns at the time of surgery. Irrigation of the subarachnoid space at surgery usually results in partial removal of the subarachnoid blood; overly aggressive lavage should be avoided since it can damage the pial vessels. Less traumatic removal of the extravasated blood can be achieved with intracisternal injection of fibrinolytic agents at the time of surgery. This consists of the irrigation of the subarachnoid space with recombinant tissue plasminogen activator (rt-PA) or urokinase at the time of surgery or postoperatively (24). A double-blind, placebo-controlled efficacy study of intracisternal rt-PA in patients with aneurysmal SAH was recently completed (25). This study evaluated the safety of intrathecal rt-PA and its effects on cerebral vasospasm. The study involved 100 patients who received a single intracisternal instillation of rt-PA or placebo following aneurysm repair 7–72 hours after SAH. The overall incidence of angiographic vasospasm was not significantly different in the two groups; however, there was a trend toward less severe vasospasm in the rt-PA group ($p = .07$) and less common and severe vasospasm in those patients with thick clots on CT scan ($p = .02$). The limiting factor of this approach is related to the possibility of precipitating intracranial bleeding, particularly in patients with significant parenchymal damage following the initial bleed. However, in this study the incidence of intracranial bleeding was not different in the two groups considered (six placebo-treated and nine rt-PA–treated patients, $p = .54$). Although the conclusions were limited by the small sample size, this series suggests that intracisternal rt-PA affords acceptable risk and could benefit patients at high risk for vasospasm (25).

At our institution, most patients are operated on as soon as possible after admission. At surgery, the basal cisterns are widely exposed, and only subarachnoid blood that can be gently removed without damaging the underlying pial banks is removed with suction and irrigation. It is our belief that thick clot removal can be facilitated by the injection of rt-PA at the time of surgery. This therapy may reduce the severity of vasospasm and should be instituted in suitable patients no longer than 2–3 days after SAH in order to be effective.

Reversal of Arterial Narrowing

Reversal of arterial narrowing can be achieved mechanically and pharmacologically. Mechanical dilation of the large spastic vessels can be achieved using endovascular techniques. Angioplasty has been shown to be effective in reversing vessel narrowing and improving cerebral blood flow following the onset of vasospasm, as well as in restoring neurologic function impaired due to vasospasm (26). Up to 66% of the patients who undergo angioplasty in the setting of cerebral vasospasm show a sustained improvement (26). The most dramatic improvements have been observed in those whose treatment was initiated within 6–12 hours of symptom onset (26). The key to successful therapy is to reverse ischemia before infarction ensues. The longer the delay is between the onset of symptoms and treatment, the

higher is the risk of infarction. There are significant complications associated with this procedure if carried out in a patient with an unsecured aneurysm. The marked increase in cerebral perfusion that follows mechanical dilation of the narrowing is likely to increase the risk of rebleeding of an unclipped aneurysm. In a series of over 60 patients treated with angioplasty alone, only two patients had endovascular therapy when the aneurysm had not been secured (26). Both patients rebled and died, while awaiting definitive treatment of the aneurysm (26). It is recommended that a recently ruptured aneurysm should be treated prior to performing angioplasty.

Theoretically, other means of achieving reversal of arterial spasm include inactivation or blockade of spasmogenic substances and use of cerebral vasodilators. Once arterial spasm has occurred, there are no agents that can specifically inactivate or block the spasmogenic substances. Potent vasodilating agents administered intravenously to reverse vasospasm have failed; however, in selected patients, intraarterial and intracisternal injection of papaverine is effective in dilating narrowed arteries and reversing clinical vasospasm (19).

Treatment of the Ischemic Consequences

Cerebral blood flow is directly proportional to the perfusion pressure across the brain and inversely proportional to the viscosity of the blood and the cerebral vascular resistance. Both the perfusion pressure and blood viscosity can be manipulated in order to increase blood flow in patients with vasospasm. The cerebral perfusion pressure is the difference between the mean arterial pressure and the intracranial pressure. In patients with vasospasm, the autoregulatory property of the intracranial vessels is lost, and the flow is strictly dependent on the perfusion pressure. Prevention or reversal of ischemic deficits can be achieved through optimization of the patient's hemodynamic and rheologic status. This approach is often referred to as hypervolemic, hypertensive, hemodilution (or "triple H") therapy. Systemic arterial pressure can be increased through the use of vasopressor agents, increasing the blood volume, or increasing cardiac output. Collateral circulation to potentially ischemic areas can be improved by dilating the leptomeningeal collaterals. Blood viscosity can be decreased by augmenting the blood volume, thereby decreasing cerebrovascular resistance and increasing cerebral blood flow. These measures are better taken if the aneurysm has been secured. In noncontrolled studies, this management strategy has been shown to result in permanent improvement (defined as complete or partial resolution of neurologic deficits within 30 minutes) in approximately 75% of patients (27). In approximately 12%, the improvement was temporary, and in the remaining 12% there was no improvement (27). Aneurysm rebleeding occurred in 50% of patients with an unsecured aneurysm in whom this treatment was employed (27).

Drawbacks of the triple-H therapeutic approach include the cost of intensive critical care, medications and intravenous fluids, and the morbidity associated with extensive invasive hemodynamic monitoring. Iatrogenic elevated arterial pressure could result not only in rebleeding of the unsecured aneurysm but also in rupture of associated aneurysms, intracerebral hemorrhage from ruptured small vessels, hemorrhagic conversion of infarction, exacerbation of cerebral edema, and increased intracranial pressure, in addition to a significant incidence of pulmonary edema (27).

It is our policy to administer intravenously approximately 3 L/d of fluids (one third colloid, two thirds crystalloid) to asymptomatic patients with secured aneurysms in order to achieve mild volume expansion. Induced hypertension is not used at this stage, unless the patient is hypotensive after aneurysm clipping.

If vasospasm is demonstrated by transcranial Doppler ultrasound studies or is present on angiogram but the patient is asymptomatic, a fluid intake of about 3 L/d is continued, but the amount of colloids is increased to two thirds of the total volume. A target hematocrit of 35–40% is achieved. In patients with clinically symptomatic vasospasm, hypervolemia is induced to optimize cardiac output (measured by Swan-Ganz catheter) through infusion of colloid, crystalloid, and packed red blood cells to maintain plasma electrolytes within normal ranges and hematocrit between 30% and 35%. Pulmonary function is closely monitored, and mannitol is administered for its rheologic effect on the microcirculation, as well as for its antioxidant properties. Hypertension is induced with inotropic agents and titrated to the neurologic deficit. If no improvement is seen within 1 hour from initiation of therapy, balloon angioplasty is considered.

Prevention of Cerebral Infarction

The neurologic deficit following cerebral vasospasm is a consequence of neuronal ischemia. Several cytoprotective agents such as nimodipine, naloxone, and monosialoganglioside have been reported in some clinical trials to be effective in reducing the extent of infarction and the ensuing neurologic morbidity and mortality (19). This mode of therapy for vasospasm can be instituted safely whether or not the aneurysm has been clipped and therefore is the modality least affected by the timing of surgery. In particular, the role of the calcium antagonist nimodipine has been extensively reviewed. Most reports show that the incidence of severe neurologic deficits is reduced, despite evidence that there is little effect on the incidence and severity of angiographic vasospasm (19). It has been suggested that the nonvascular, antiischemic effects of nimodipine and other calcium antagonists, such as nicardipine, may occur by limiting neuronal calcium entry, thus reducing cell damage caused by calcium excess. At our institution, calcium channel blocking agents are used in all patients with aneurysmal SAH. Nimodipine, in an oral dose of 60 mg every 4 hours, has no effect on angiographic vasospasm but does appear to reduce clinical vasospasm, whereas nicardipine in a dose of approximately 10 mg/h by continuous intravenous infusion reduces angiographic and clinical vasospasm.

Of the cytoprotective agents that do not act through calcium-influx blockade, the most promising is the 21-aminosteroid, tirilazad mesylate (U-74006F). This agent is attractive because of its potential for reducing cerebral vasospasm and its cytoprotective effects in focal ischemia, possibly related to inhibition of lipid peroxidation. Two recent randomized, prospective, double-blind studies evaluating the effectiveness of tirilazad after aneurysmal SAH have been completed. The results were consistent with a significant reduction in the rate of vasospasm and improvement in favorable outcomes at dosages of 2.0 mg/kg/d and 6.0 mg/kg/d (28). While these results were consistent irrespective of the patient's sex in the European trial, the treatment under study in North American centers was effective only in males (28) (Kassell et al, unpublished data). The effects of an increased dose in the female SAH population are currently under study.

Hydrocephalus

SAH can be complicated by acute or chronic hydrocephalus. Acute hydrocephalus may result from subarachnoid or intraventricular blood that interferes with the absorption and circulation of cerebrospinal fluid (CSF). Chronic hydrocephalus is thought to be induced by adhesions forming in the pia-arachnoid, permanently impeding CSF circulation or its absorption at the arachnoid granulations. Factors such as increasing age, preexisting or postoperative hypertension, elevated blood pressure at admission, admission CT findings of intraventricular hemorrhage or a diffuse collection of subarachnoid blood, and preoperative use of antifibrinolytic drugs are associated with the development of hydrocephalus after aneurysmal SAH (29). It is also known that patients with hydrocephalus after SAH have a poorer prognosis (29). On the basis of some of these associations, one can speculate that mechanical washing of blood in the subarachnoid space (especially at the level of the basal cisterns) at the time of operation and sharp dissection of the arachnoid membrane can result in a lowered incidence of post-SAH hydrocephalus (8). In addition, since antifibrinolytic use has been associated with an increased incidence of post-SAH hydrocephalus, it is possible that intracisternal injection of rt-PA or other fibrinolytics may be helpful in preventing this disturbing complication. It is other authors' opinion that early aneurysm surgery and washout of blood-contaminated CSF lessens the risk of subarachnoid fibrosis and impaired CSF outflow (8).

Associated Hematoma

It has been recommended that in patients with aneurysm rupture and intracerebral hemorrhage (ICH), surgery should be performed immediately and the aneurysm should be secured at the same time as intracerebral hematoma evacuation. Patients treated with evacuation of the ICH without clipping have a mortality rate of 75% as opposed to 29% for those who undergo evacuation and clipping during the same operation (30). The prognosis in these cases, however, remains grim. Only 9% of the patients with SAH and associated intraparenchymal hematoma are discharged without a significant neurologic deficit (30). In these cases, if therapy is to be undertaken at all, the obvious advantages of early operation are removal of the mass and prevention of further bleeding. In cases of rapid deterioration secondary to hematoma and herniation (usually with a temporal lobe clot), emergency surgery must be carried out without an angiogram because of time constraints.

Medical Complications

Although the largest proportion of severe morbidity and mortality following aneurysmal SAH has been attributed to neurologic complications such as rebleeding, vasospasm, and hydrocephalus, medical complications are now widely recognized as a significant contributor (31). According to a recent analysis of a randomized prospective study conducted in North America in the late 1980s, severe medical complications were responsible for about 23% of the deaths registered after SAH, a proportion comparable to patients dying directly from neurologic complications (31). On the basis of these observations, it has become clear that appropriate management of the patients with aneurysmal SAH includes the prevention and treatment of medical complications. Although some of the medical complications observed are not influenced by the choice of time of surgery (ie, hypertension, cardiac arrhythmias, and ischemia), other complications such as deep venous thrombosis (DVT) and pulmonary complications are influenced by the timing of surgery.

Deep Venous Thrombosis and Pulmonary Complications

It is estimated that approximately 2% of patients suffer DVT after aneurysmal SAH, and as many as one half of these patients will develop pulmonary emboli (19). The likelihood of DVT is increased if a neurologic deficit is present. Once diagnosed, DVT cannot be conventionally treated in the neurosurgical patient because of the risk of intracranial bleed. Passive exercise and early mobilization are very important in preventing this complication. These measures are better and more comfortably undertaken in the patient with a secured aneurysm.

Pulmonary complications are a significant contributor to the mortality following SAH and are responsible for 50% of all deaths from medical complications (31). Pneumonia, adult respiratory distress syndrome, and pulmonary embolism are the most frequent causes of respiratory mortality and morbidity in patients with aneurysmal SAH. It can be argued that these worrisome complications are prevented

with early mobilization and the shorter hospital stay associated with early surgery.

Patient-Related Factors

Poor-Grade Patients

Poor-grade patients represent a significant proportion of the total population of patients with ruptured aneurysms. Classically, a more conservative approach has been suggested in these cases. This recommendation is based on the assumption that aneurysm clipping is more easily carried out in neurologically stable patients.

A poor neurologic status and an altered level of consciousness after SAH, however, can be determined by several factors, some of which are amenable to treatment with an acute surgical intervention. After SAH, there is a sudden increase in intracranial pressure that in some patients causes an acute obstruction of the normal CSF outflow, with resulting acute ventricular dilation. In other cases, the sudden loss of consciousness can be a consequence of the accompanying mass effect from a coexisting hematoma, often associated with subarachnoid blood in poor-grade patients. In these circumstances, an acute surgical intervention that includes ventricular decompression and/or hematoma evacuation along with aneurysm clipping can result in significant improvement of the neurologic status in a percentage of patients as high as 54% (32). Early clipping of the aneurysm also allows for a more aggressive treatment of vasospasm, a frequent event in these patients who often have large collections of subarachnoid blood. In addition, results of the ICSTAS have shown that early surgery in poor-grade patients does not result in a significant increase in the rate of surgical complications (13).

Age

Elderly patients constitute a significant proportion of the patients who suffer aneurysmal SAH. Large studies report a frequency of 23–26% in patients older than age 60 years (18). Age is a recognized risk factor for poor outcome after aneurysmal SAH, and wide differences exist in terms of recovery related to the patient's age. In the ICSTAS, it was shown that there was a linear correlation between age and outcome (12). The rate of good recovery decreased from 86% in the 18–29-years age group to 26% in the oldest age group (70–87 years of age) (12). Traditionally, advanced age has been considered a limiting factor in recommending early surgery; however, more recent data show that advanced age should not be considered a contraindication. Indeed, in the recently completed trial evaluating the effects of nicardipine after SAH, there were no significant differences in terms of timing of surgery according to patient age (18). In this study, early surgery (days 0–3) was performed in 63% of patients younger than 40 years, in 60.4% of patients between ages 61 and 70 years, and in 67% of patients older than 70 years (18).

There are several theoretical reasons that support early surgery in elderly patients. The rebleeding rate increases with advancing age (17,18). In addition, after aneurysm rupture elderly patients are more likely to experience intraventricular and intracranial hemorrhage, both of which are amenable to treatment with an early intervention (18). Older patients also have a decreased cerebrovascular reserve and are more likely to suffer symptomatic vasospasm (18). When this occurs, it can be more aggressively treated with triple-H therapy if the aneurysm has been secured.

Although caution has to be exercised with patients older than 70 years, there is evidence that early surgery can be performed in elderly patients as safely as in younger subjects. In the ICSTAS, it was shown that patients older than 65 years who had surgery planned for days 0–3 did not have an especially unfavorable outcome (13).

Length of Stay

Early surgery is also accompanied by a markedly shortened hospital stay. Ljunggren et al (8) reported that the patients with good recoveries in the group operated on early spent an average of 16 days in the hospital in contrast to twice that amount for patients receiving delayed therapy.

Psychosocial Stress

Early exclusion of the aneurysm sac reduces the amount of stress for the patient who lives with the consciousness of having a ''time bomb'' ready to explode in his or her head. It also significantly relieves families and the medical team from the fear of rebleeding.

Associated Medical Conditions

In the presence of serious medically associated conditions, it may be reasonable to delay surgery and try to stabilize the patient as much as possible.

Environment-Related Factors

If early surgery is the strategy of choice, it must be carried out as soon as possible since about one in 25 patients who have suffered aneurysmal rupture will experience rebleeding within 24 hours (16). There are several obstacles, however, to a prompt surgical correction of the aneurysm. Not every center has a referral system so well organized as to have a significant proportion of the aneurysmal SAH population available for surgical treatment within a few hours after the hemorrhage. In addition, surgery on an emergency basis is often performed at night and on weekends, when the best surgical team may not be available. These considerations are especially critical in the case of technically difficult aneurysms, such as posterior circulation aneurysms, and unstable, poor-grade patients.

OUR APPROACH

At our institution, an aggressive early-surgery approach is taken. Patients referred from outside medical facilities are routinely transported by helicopter or fixed-wing aircraft to shorten referral times. Initial stabilization and diagnostic studies such as CT, angiography, and lumbar puncture (if necessary) are conducted in the emergency room. Once aneurysmal SAH has been documented, the patient is prepared for surgery in the neurologic intensive care unit (NICU). Patients who have acute hydrocephalus or an intracerebral hematoma with significant mass effect are taken immediately to the operating room without further preoperative attempts at stabilization.

For other patients who present in poor neurologic condition, especially those with significant medical problems such as uncontrolled hypertension, congestive heart failure, or ischemic heart disease, care is taken to achieve a normotensive state to reduce the likelihood of rebleeding. In addition, morphine sulfate can be used to reduce the stress of severe headache and neck stiffness. A Foley catheter, arterial line, and central venous line are routinely inserted. The average time of preparation from the time the patient arrives at the medical center to the time of operation is less than 12 hours.

Intraoperative lumbar drains are routinely inserted with the exception of cases of middle cerebral artery aneurysms where the CSF aids in the dissection of the aneurysm in the sylvian fissure. Induced hypotension with isoflurane is often used to aid in safe dissection and manipulation of the aneurysm. When temporary clipping is necessary, the blood pressure is elevated. Accessible subarachnoid clot is carefully removed, and the subarachnoid space is well irrigated prior to closure; radical clot removal is not performed.

CT scans are performed on the first postoperative day. Transcranial Doppler ultrasound studies are done at regular intervals and are correlated to angiographic results. Angiograms are performed on day 8 after aneurysm rupture to determine the status of the aneurysmal obliteration and vasospasm (1).

Clinical evidence of vasospasm is treated immediately and aggressively. Patients are monitored in the NICU with a Swan-Ganz catheter. Blood pressure and cardiac output are maximized using hypervolemic doses of plasma protein solutions and often pressor agents. In addition, the patient is maintained on 100% oxygen for the first 24 hours, and mannitol is administered for its rheologic effects.

The exceptions to the policy of early surgery are those patients who are delayed in referral and those with severe angiographic and clinical vasospasm. Surgery is delayed until the time when vasospasm improves and the medical and neurologic condition has stabilized.

CONCLUSIONS

The timing of surgery for ruptured intracranial aneurysms remains controversial. Several advances in microsurgical and neuroanesthesia techniques have made it possible for surgery to be performed in the hyperacute phase following SAH with an acceptable morbidity and mortality, even in the setting of a swollen, tight brain. Early surgery is effective in reducing the rebleeding rate. The subarachnoid clot, which has been causally related to the development and severity of vasospasm, can also be washed out at the time of surgery with the use of fibrinolytics. In addition, once the aneurysm is secured several alternatives such as hypervolemic-hypertensive therapy and intraluminal angioplasty with intraarterial injection of pharmacologically active substances, can be safely adopted in an attempt to prevent or reverse vasospasm and antagonize its consequences. When feasible, early surgery also allows for a better prevention of some of the numerous medical complications that can negatively affect the outcome of the patient with a ruptured aneurysm.

However, several limitations still exist. These are related to the technical difficulty of critically located and giant aneurysms, to problems in scheduling emergency surgery, and to the presence of severe associated medical conditions. In these cases, a flexible strategy tailored to the characteristics and the need of the individual patient is warranted. Since we now have available noninvasive means to diagnose unruptured aneurysms, we agree with Peerless and coworkers (20) that ''there is progress toward the best timing of aneurysms: operation before they rupture.''

ACKNOWLEDGMENTS

The authors wish to acknowledge the kind help of Mrs. Desiree Lanzino and Mrs. Sarah Hudson, who edited the manuscript.

REFERENCES

1. Kassell NF, Shaffrey CI, Shaffrey ME. Timing of aneurysm surgery. In: Wilkins RH, Rengachary SS, eds. *Neurosurgery Update*, vol 2. New York: McGraw-Hill, 1990:95–99.
2. Kassell NF, Drake CG. Timing of aneurysm surgery. *Neurosurgery* 1982;10:514–519.
3. Dandy WE. Intracranial aneurysm of the internal carotid artery. Cured by operation. *Ann Surg* 1938;107:654–659.
4. Norlen G, Olivecrona H. The treatment of anuerysms of the circle of Willis. *J Neurosurg* 1953;10:404–415.
5. Suzuki J, Onuma T, Yoshimoto T. Results of early operations on cerebral aneurysms. *Surg Neurol* 1979;11:407–412.
6. Chyatte D, Fode NC, Sundt TM Jr. Early versus late intracranial aneurysm surgery in subarachnoid hemorrhage. *J Neurosurg* 1988;69: 326–331.
7. Disney L, Weir B, Petruk K. Effect on management mortality of a deliberate policy of early operation on supratentorial aneurysms. *Neurosurgery* 1987;20:695–701.
8. Ljunggren B, Brandt L, Kagstrom E, Sundbarg G. Results of early operations for ruptured aneurysms. *J Neurosurg* 1981;54:473–479.
9. Nishimoto A, Ueta K, Onbe H, et al. Nationwide co-operative study of intracranial aneurysm surgery in Japan. *Stroke* 1985;16:48–52.
10. Haley EC Jr, Kassell NF, Torner JC, et al. The International Cooperative Study on the Timing of Aneurysm Surgery. The North American experience. *Stroke* 1992;23:205–214.
11. Haley EC, Kassell NF, Torner JC, et al. The International Cooperative Study on the Timing of Aneurysm Surgery. A randomized controlled trial of high-dose intravenous nicardipine in aneurysmal subarachnoid hemorrhage. A report of the Cooperative Aneurysm Study. *J Neurosurg* 1993;78:537–547.
12. Kassell NF, Torner JC, Haley EC Jr, et al. The International Cooperative Study on the Timing of Aneurysm Surgery. I: Overall management results. *J Neurosurg* 1990;73:18–36.
13. Kassell NF, Torner JC, Haley EC Jr, et al. The International Cooperative Study on the Timing of Aneurysm Surgery. II: Surgical results. *J Neurosurg* 1990;73:37–47.
14. Batjer HH. Timing of operation for ruptured aneurysms: Early surgery. In: Ratcheson RA, Wirth FP, eds. *Ruptured Cerebral Aneurysms: Perioperative Management*. Baltimore: Williams & Wilkins, 1994:46–53.
15. Jane JA, Winn HR, Richardson AE. The natural history of intracranial aneurysms: Rebleeding rates during the acute and long-term period and implication for surgical management. *Clin Neurosurg* 1977;24: 176–184.
16. Kassell NF, Torner JC. Aneurysmal rebleeding: A preliminary report from the cooperative study. *Neurosurgery* 1983;3:479–481.
17. Torner JC, Kassell NF, Wallace PB, Adams HB. Preoperative prognostic factors for rebleeding and survival in aneurysm patients receiving antifibrinolytic therapy: Report of the Cooperative Aneurysm Study. *Neurosurgery* 1981;9:506–513.
18. Lanzino G, Kassell NF, Germanson TP, et al. Age and outcome following aneurysmal subarachnoid hemorrhage: why do elderly patients fare worse? *J Neurosurg* (In Press).
19. Shaffrey ME, Shaffrey CI, Lanzino G, Kassell NF. Nonoperative treatment of aneurysmal subarachnoid hemorrhage. In: Youmans JR, ed. *Neurological Surgery*, 4th ed. Philadelphia: W.B. Saunders, 1995.
20. Peerless SJ, Hernesniemi JA, Gutman FB, Drake CG. Early surgery for ruptured vertebrobasilar aneurysms. *J Neurosurg* 1994;80:643–649.
21. Weir B, Grace M, Hansen J, Rothberg C. Time course of vasospasm in man. *J Neurosurg* 1978;48:173–178.
22. Fisher CM, Kistler JP, Davis JM. Relation of cerebral vasospasm to subarachnoid hemorrhage visualized by computerized tomography scanning. *Neurosurgery* 1980;6:1–9.
23. Mizukami M, Kawase T, Usami T, Tazawa T. Prevention of vasospasm by early operation with removal of subarachnoid blood. *Neurosurgery* 1982;10:301–307.
24. Stolke D, Seifert V. Single intracisternal bolus of recombinant tissue plasminogen activator in patients with aneurysmal subarachnoid hemorrhage: Preliminary assessment of efficacy and safety in an open clinical study. *Neurosurgery* 1992;30:877–881.
25. Findlay JM, Kassell NF, Weir BKA, et al. A randomized trial of intraoperative, intracisternal tissue plasminogen activator for the prevention of vasospasm. *Neurosurgery* 1995; 37:168–178.
26. Eskridge JM, Newell DW, Winn RH. Endovascular treatment of vasospasm. *Neurosurg Clin N Am* 1994;5:437–448.
27. Kassell NF, Peerlesss SJ, Durward QJ, Beck DW, Drake CG, Adams HP. Treatment of ischemic deficits from vasospasm with intravascular volume expansion and induced arterial hypertension. *Neurosurgery* 1982;11:337–343.
28. Kassell NF, Haley EC, Hansen CA, et al. The International Cooperative Study on the Timing of Aneurysm Surgery. A randomized, double-bind, vehicle-controlled trial of tirilazad mesylate in patients with subarachnoid hemorrhage: A cooperative study in Europe/Australia/New Zealand. *J Neurosurg* 1996;84:221–8.
29. Graff-Radford NR, Torner J, Adams HP, Kassell NF. Factors associated with hydrocephalus after subarachnoid hemorrhage. A report of the Cooperative Aneurysm Study. *Arch Neurol* 1989;46:744–752.
30. Wheelock B, Weir B, Watts R, et al. Timing of surgery for intracerebral hematomas due to aneurysm rupture. *J Neurosurg* 1983;58:476–481.
31. Solenski NJ, Haley CE, Kassell NF, et al. Medical complications of aneurysmal subarachnoid hemorrhage: A report of the cooperative study. *Crit Care Med* 1995;23:1007–1017.
32. Bailes JE, Spetzler RF, Hadley MN, Baldwin HZ. Management morbidity and mortality of poor-grade aneurysm patients. *J Neurosurg* 1990; 72:559–566.

Cerebrovascular Disease, edited by H. Hunt Batjer.
Lippincott-Raven Publishers, Philadelphia © 1997.

CHAPTER 88

The Poor-Grade Aneurysm Patient

Rafael J. Tamargo and Daniele Rigamonti

Patients who suffer an aneurysmal subarachnoid hemorrhage (SAH) and arrive in the hospital devastated neurologically or medically by this event are typically described as "poor grade" patients. The medical management of these patients remains challenging, and their surgical management is controversial. In this chapter, the epidemiology, evaluation, and current trends in the management of poor-grade SAH patients are reviewed.

DEFINITION

We define poor-grade patients as those classified as grade IV or V in either the Hunt and Hess or the World Federation of Neurological Surgeons (WFNS) scales (Tables 1 and 2) In the Hunt and Hess (1) scale, these are patients who are stuporous with a moderate to severe hemiparesis and possibly displaying early extensor posturing (grade IV) or those in a deep coma with extensor posturing and a moribund appearance (grade V). In the WFNS scale (2), based on the Glasgow Coma Scale (GCS) (3), poor-grade patients are those with a GCS score of 7–12 who at best open their eyes to voice, localize a painful stimulus, and are disoriented (grade IV) or those with a GCS score of 3–6 who at best open their eyes to pain, display extensor posturing, and make incomprehensible sounds (grade V).

We also consider as poor grade those patients who, based on their neurologic examination, would be described as grade III by either the Hunt and Hess or the WFNS scales, but instead are classified as grade IV because of medical instability associated with a preexisting systemic condition or because of a medical complication of the SAH. As proposed by Hunt and Hess (1), one should increase the patient's grade by one level if the patient has a serious medical condition that is incapacitating and potentially life-threatening. For instance, these are patients with severe heart disease

showing signs of cardiac insufficiency or with advanced pulmonary, hepatic, renal, or endocrine insufficiency. In the physical status classification of the American Society of Anesthesiologists (ASA) (4), the standard scale used by anesthesiologists to predict the mortality and morbidity of anesthesia independent of the surgical procedure, this description corresponds to an ASA physical status class 4 (Table 3). This degree of systemic impairment is associated with an operative mortality of 7.8% for all surgical procedures (5).

Most series since 1968 have used the Hunt and Hess scale to grade SAH patients (6). In this chapter, unless otherwise stated, the Hunt and Hess grading scale is used. We recently evaluated the outcome of 207 aneurysm patients treated at the Johns Hopkins Hospital between 1992 and 1995 and correlated this outcome with their Hunt and Hess and WFNS grades on admission. We found that both scales are comparable as predictors of mortality and neurologic condition at the time of discharge (Walter KA, Witham TF, Tamargo RJ, unpublished data). In our practice, we currently favor the WFNS scale because its definitions are unequivocal and minimize interobserver variability.

EPIDEMIOLOGY

Using the definitions outlined above, approximately one fifth of SAH patients are classified as poor grade on admission. In the original study by Hunt and Hess (1), 47 (17%) of 275 patients were either grade IV or V. In the recent International Cooperative Study on the Timing of Aneurysm Surgery (ICSTAS) (1980–1983) (7,8), 662 (19%) of 3521 patients were either stuporous or comatose on their initial evaluation. The Cooperative Study did not report the condition of the patients using either the Hunt and Hess or WFNS scales, but it is reasonable to compare the stuporous or comatose patients in the study with grade IV or V patients by either scale. In a review of aneurysm patients treated at the Johns Hopkins Hospital since January 1992, we identified 43 (21%) of 207 WFNS grades IV and V patients.

The comprehensive survey of SAH in King County,

Both authors: Department of Neurosurgery, Division of Cerebrovascular Surgery, The Johns Hopkins University School of Medicine, Baltimore, Maryland, 21287.

TABLE 1. *Hunt and Hess scale of severity of subarachnoid hemorrhage[a]*

Grade	Criteria
I	Asymptomatic, or minimal headache and slight nuchal rigidity
II	Moderate to severe headache, nuchal rigidity, no neurologic deficit other than cranial nerve palsy
III	Drowsiness, confusion, or mild focal deficit
IV	Stupor, moderate to severe hemiparesis, possibly early decerebrate (extensor) rigidity and vegetative disturbances
V	Deep coma, decerebrate (extensor) rigidity, moribund appearance

(From ref. 1, with permission)
[a] Grades IV and V are considered poor grades.

TABLE 3. *American Society of Anesthesiologists (ASA) physical status classification[a]*

Physical status class	Description
I	A normal healthy patient
II	A patient with mild systemic disease
III	A patient with a severe systemic disease that limits activity but is not incapacitating
IV	A patient with an incapacitating systemic disease that is a constant threat to life
V	A moribund patient not expected to survive 24 hours with or without operation

(From ref. 4, with permission)
[a] Class IV is associated with a 7.8% mortality and class V with a 9.4% mortality, independent of the surgical procedure (5).

Washington (1987–1989), however, reported a higher incidence of poor-grade patients. In this survey, 47 (28%) of 166 hospitalized patients were either grade IV or V (9). This higher proportion may be closer to the true incidence of grades IV and V patients within the SAH population, since this was a population-based study. A population-based study attempts to eliminate the referral bias inherent in hospital-based surveys. A higher proportion of poor-grade patients, similar to that noted in the King County study, was reported in an analogous population-based study from Izumo City and Shimane prefecture in Japan (1980–1984), which reported that 157 (25%) of 622 patients were either grade IV or V on admission (10).

After the hemorrhage, poor-grade patients have a higher incidence of medical complications, delayed ischemia associated with vasospasm, and aneurysmal rebleeding as compared with grades I–III patients. The original cooperative study of intracranial aneurysms and SAH (1963–1970) identified a correlation between poor neurologic status and development of severe medical problems (11). This study, which predated the Hunt and Hess scale and used a six-level neurologic grading system, revealed that 66% of patients with a poor neurologic grade were in fair or poor medical condition on admission. By contrast, only 35% of patients with a good neurologic grade were in fair or poor medical condition. This study also identified a correlation between poor neurologic status and vasospasm. The incidence of vasospasm increased with the neurologic grade; the incidence of vasospasm was 22% in the group with the best neurologic status and 73% in the worst group. The correlations between poor neurologic condition and medical complications or vasospasm have been confirmed by subsequent surveys.

A poor neurologic status is also correlated with a higher rate of aneurysmal rebleeding. The report of the Danish Aneurysm Study Group of 1076 SAH patients (1978–1983) revealed a rebleeding rate within the first two weeks of 11.6% for grades I and II patients and 21.6% for grades III–V patients (12).

Furthermore, poor-grade patients are less likely to undergo surgery than patients in good neurologic condition. In the ICSTAS, 83% of all patients were treated surgically, but only 58% of stuporous patients and 35% of comatose patients underwent surgery (7,8).

Although the outcome of grades IV and V patients treated expectantly or surgically has improved over the past three decades, it is still poor. In 1968, Hunt and Hess (1) reported a mortality of 71% for grade IV patients and 100% for grade V patients. The combined results of the three most recent series detailing the outcomes in these patients reveal a mortality of 43% for grade IV patients and 84% for grade V patients (10,13,14). In the ICSTAS, stuporous patients had a 44% mortality and 26% morbidity, and comatose patients had a 72% mortality and 17% morbidity (7,8). In the King County study, 87% of grade IV patients and 100% of grade V patients had a poor outcome, defined as a severe neurologic deficit, vegetative state, or death (9). In our series, we have documented a 34% mortality for WFNS grade IV patients and 71% mortality for WFNS grade V patients.

TABLE 2. *World Federation of Neurological Surgeons (WFNS) scale of severity of subarachnoid hemorrhage[a]*

WFNS grade	GCS score	Motor deficit
I	15	Absent
II	14–13	Absent
III	14–13	Present
IV	12–7	Present or absent
V	6–3	Present or absent

(From ref. 2, with permission)
Key: GCS, Glasgow Coma Scale.
[a] Grades IV and V are considered poor grades.

EVALUATION

The initial evaluation of the poor-grade patient is similar to that of any SAH patient. The patient's neurologic status is assessed, and the GCS score and the WFNS or Hunt and Hess grade are determined. In the WFNS scale, grade IV patients are those with a GCS score of 7–12, and grade V patients are those with a GCS score of 3–6.

Patients who are stuporous and can not protect their airway or those with hypoxemia, hypercarbia, or an impaired respiratory drive should be intubated. Typically, patients with a GCS score ≤10 are candidates for intubation. The intubation should be performed by either an experienced anesthesiologist or an intensivist skilled in airway management of patients with central nervous system disorders. SAH patients about to be intubated should have adequate anesthesia with general anesthetic agents, as well as topical agents. This treatment attempts to minimize laryngeal stimulation that typically results in gagging, coughing, and elevation of the systemic blood pressure, which in turn could lead to aneurysmal rerupture.

Imaging Studies

Computed tomography (CT) is typically the first imaging study performed in a patient suspected of having a SAH. When all SAH patients are considered, the initial CT scan shows the hemorrhage in only 90% of patients (7). In our experience, however, the initial CT scan is invariably positive in poor-grade patients.

The CT scan also identifies patients with significant hydrocephalus or a large intraparenchymal hematoma. In the ICSTAS, 15% of the admission scans revealed hydrocephalus, and 17% revealed an intracerebral or intraventricular hematoma (7). Milhorat (15) evaluated the incidence of hydrocephalus in 200 patients with aneurysmal SAH. In this series, an incidence of hydrocephalus of 20% was documented for the whole group, but it was noted that hydrocephalus was more common in the higher-grade patients; only 3% of grade I but 42% of grade IV patients had hydrocephalus (15). Either hydrocephalus or an intraparenchymal hematoma may be the major cause of a patient's poor neurologic status and may need to be addressed early in the evaluation, either by insertion of an intraventricular catheter or by surgical evacuation, respectively.

If the patient is stable, we typically obtain a four-vessel angiogram on the day of admission. This study is helpful in guiding management even in patients who are clearly not immediate surgical candidates. When an angiogram cannot be done, as in the case of emergent surgery for comatose SAH patients with an intraparenchymal hematoma, localization of the aneurysm can be accomplished with either a preoperative high-resolution infusion CT scan or an intraoperative angiogram. The technique of infusion CT scanning for identification of aneurysms was validated by Newell and colleagues (16) using the following protocol: A constant intravenous infusion of 80–100 ml of diatrizoate sodium was administered during dynamic mode scanning from the floor of the sella turcica to above the level of the anterior commu-

nicating artery. This yielded 15–25 slices, 1.5 mm thick, with images adjusted to an intermediate window (level 80 window, 400 Hounsfield units) to distinguish between blood and enhanced vessels. This technique has been shown to be quick and reliable (16,17). Alternatively, an angiogram can be obtained in the operating room, after the initial evacuation of the hematoma, to guide the clipping of the aneurysm.

Magnetic resonance angiography (MRA) has recently been advocated as a potential substitute for standard angiography. In our opinion, given the current state of this technology, MRA does not at present have a major role in the radiographic evaluation of cerebral aneurysms. In our experience, it is common for this test to miss even large aneurysms and is therefore unreliable.

Medical Complications

Although SAH patients can present with various associated medical complications, we pay particular attention in poor-grade patients to cardiac arrhythmias, neurogenic pulmonary edema, and hyponatremia. Of these three conditions, neurogenic pulmonary edema is typically the most serious and is often present in the most critically ill patients. Cardiac arrhythmias and myocardial dysfunction may not be as clinically obvious as pulmonary edema on physical examination, but they can be equally lethal. Hyponatremia, by contrast, is rarely a life-threatening problem in SAH patients, although it exacerbates an already complicated clinical picture and should be addressed as soon as noted. These medical conditions may influence the decision to delay early surgical intervention in poor-grade patients.

Since the first two reported cases of SAH accompanied by cardiac abnormalities in 1947 (18) and in 1953 (19), numerous other publications have documented the association of aneurysmal SAH with cardiac arrhythmias and cardiac dysfunction (20–24). In some series, more than 50% of SAH patients have displayed electrocardiographic (ECG) abnormalities, the most common being ST-T segment changes, U-wave abnormalities, and a wide range of arrhythmias (24). In a study of SAH patients evaluated with Holter monitoring in the acute period, 29 (41%) of 70 patients had serious arrhythmias and three (4%) had malignant arrhythmias defined as torsade de pointe, ventricular flutter, or ventricular fibrillation (23). The mechanism by which a SAH induces cardiac changes is not known, but there is evidence that either the hypothalamus or the sympathetic nervous system are involved (20,25). Continuous cardiac monitoring with serial ECGs and evaluation of serum myocardial creatine kinase MB isoenzyme levels whenever appropriate should be considered in all poor-grade patients.

Pulmonary edema without apparent cardiac dysfunction has been identified in various intracranial injuries. Since the first report of neurogenic pulmonary edema in the presence of intracranial hemorrhage in 1939 (26) and specifically in SAH in 1972 (27), several other reports have confirmed this association (20). It is currently thought that the intracranial pathology induces a sympathetic discharge that in turn affects the pulmonary circulation, resulting in high pulmonary capillary pressures and abnormally increased permeability (28). In a series of fatal SAH cases, pulmonary edema was identified at the time of autopsy in 55 (71%) of 78 patients, and the condition was clinically evident in 18 (31%) of the 78 patients (29). Neurogenic pulmonary edema is a serious medical complication of SAH that is more common in poor-grade patients and is frequently associated with a fatal outcome. It is easily diagnosed by the patient's clinical appearance, hypoxemia, and the characteristic radiologic findings.

Hyponatremia is another medical complication of SAH that may delay early surgical intervention. It is evident in up to 33% of SAH patients (30). Post-SAH hyponatremia is rarely severe: The serum sodium concentration is usually 125–130 mEq/L, although levels as low as 120 mEq/L have been reported (31). In poor-grade patients, however, even mild hyponatremia can significantly worsen their condition. The etiology of hyponatremia in SAH remains controversial, with some cases being consistent with primary cerebral salt wasting (32) and others suggestive of the syndrome of inappropriate antidiuretic hormone secretion (SIADH) (33). This is an important issue, since the preferred treatment for SIADH is fluid restriction, whereas the preferred treatment of cerebral salt wasting is sodium supplementation. In SAH patients, however, fluid restriction is not an option because it can precipitate or worsen a delayed ischemic deficit from vasospasm (30). Although surgery should not be delayed because of mild hyponatremia, every attempt should be made to at least prevent a further decrease in serum sodium prior to surgery.

SURGICAL MANAGEMENT

The surgical management of the poor-grade patient remains controversial. On the conservative end of the spectrum are those who advocate supportive care initially and reserve surgery for those patients who survive the first 2 or 3 weeks after the SAH and demonstrate meaningful neurologic recovery. On the other end of the spectrum are those who advocate immediate surgical intervention in all poor-grade patients to provide every patient with the best opportunity for recovery. We favor a systematic approach that incorporates elements of both philosophies but still individualizes therapy.

Clinically, poor-grade SAH patients tend to fall into four groups: (a) patients with a poor neurologic examination due to acute hydrocephalus, (b) patients with a poor neurologic examination due to an acute intraparenchymal hematoma with mass effect, (c) patients with a poor neurologic examination due primarily to the SAH, and (d) patients with favorable neurologic function but with medical complications that preclude further intervention. The management of the first

TABLE 4. *Good recovery and mortality rates at 6 months for stuporous and comatose patients in the International Cooperative Study on the Timing of Aneurysm Surgery*

Admission status	Planned surgery interval (days from SAH)				
	0–3	4–6	7–10	11–14	15–32
	Good recovery rate (%)				
Stuporous	33	29	33	27	33
Comatose	16	10	12	22	17
	Mortality rate (%)				
Stuporous	40	46	40	41	39
Comatose	56	32	79	55	55

(From ref. 8, with permission)
Key: SAH, subarachnoid hemorrhage.

two groups is straightforward, but management of the last two is more complicated.

At present, there is no consensus as to when is the best time for surgery in poor-grade SAH patients. Although early surgery in good-grade patients is currently favored by most neurosurgeons, the benefit of early surgery in poor-grade patients is not as obvious. In the ICSTAS, the good recovery and mortality rates for stuporous and comatose patients were similar for the early planned surgery intervals of days 0–3 and 4–6 as compared with the delayed planned surgery intervals of days 11–14 and 15–32 (8) (Table 4). In comatose patients, mortality was highest (79% vs. 32–56%) for the planned surgery interval of days 7–10, although this difference was not significant. Therefore, it is reasonable to conclude that early surgery in poor-grade patients is neither more beneficial nor more harmful than delayed surgery and that surgery during the days 7–10 interval after SAH should probably be avoided.

Immediate surgical intervention in the form of placement of an intraventricular catheter is indicated in poor-grade patients with acute hydrocephalus, since ventricular dilatation can be the major cause of poor neurologic function (Fig. 1). Once the catheter is inserted into the ventricle, CSF should be drained slowly to a pressure no lower than 15–20 cm H$_2$O to avoid an aneurysmal rerupture. The patient's neurologic status after ventricular decompression will then dictate subsequent treatment.

Immediate surgical intervention is indicated in poor-grade patients with a large intraparenchymal hematoma, since the hematoma may be the major reason for the patient's poor neurologic condition (Fig. 2). In 1987, Brandt and colleagues (34) reported on a series of four young females with large intraparenchymal hematomas and middle cerebral artery aneurysms who presented in deep coma after SAH. All four underwent immediate surgical evacuation of the hematomas and clipping of the aneurysms. Three patients recovered and returned home but remained with moderate focal deficits and significant cognitive impairment. One patient died 3 weeks after surgery from a pulmonary embolus. In 1991, Batjer and Samson (35) reported on a series of four comatose

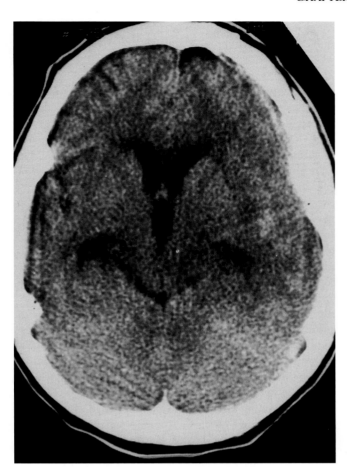

FIG. 1. CT scan of a grade IV patient with hydrocephalus. Because of cerebral swelling and decreased compliance, the size of the ventricles may not be impressive, but a rounded third ventricle, as in this case, is indicative of hydrocephalus with increased intracranial pressure.

SAH patients who underwent emergent surgery without angiography for evacuation of the hematoma, clipping of the aneurysm, and temporal lobectomy. Three of the four patients survived and one was able to participate independently in activities of daily living. In 1993, Le Roux and colleagues (17) reported on a series of 25 patients—all WFNS grade V patients with a GCS score <5—who underwent emergent surgery for evacuation of the hematoma and clipping of the ruptured aneurysm. A lobectomy was performed in eight of the 25 patients, and the bone flap was not replaced in 15 patients. Of the 25 patients, 12 survived, eight of whom were independent but moderately disabled at 6 months. Therefore, there is growing evidence that comatose SAH patients with large intraparenchymal hematomas may benefit from immediate surgical intervention, although further evaluation of outcome is important, particularly in reference to cognitive deficits.

The management of the poor-grade patient without an intraparenchymal hematoma or without severe hydrocephalus, however, is more complicated. We have found the guidelines proposed by Bailes and colleagues (14) from the Barrow Neurological Institute useful in determining the management of these patients. In 1990, these authors reported a series of 54 grades IV and V SAH patients treated both conservatively and surgically. In this study, grades IV and V patients had a mortality of 26.9% and 65.6%, respectively. The authors emphasized the use of intracranial pressure to determine whether a patient should be treated surgically.

We have developed a protocol based on the Barrow Neurological Institute recommendations and used this protocol for WFNS grades IV and V patients since 1992. After completion of the CT scan, the patient is transferred to the intensive care unit. All patients are treated with nimodipine, hydration, steroids, and anticonvulsants. Hypertension is rarely treated in the acute period, particularly in the presence of increased intracranial pressure (ICP). In general, if the patient is able to localize a painful stimulus and has no complicating medical issues, surgery is carried out within the next 12 hours.

If the decision to proceed with surgery is less obvious, because of the patient's neurologic status or medical complications, a frontal intraventricular catheter (IVC) is inserted and drainage set at 15–20 cm H_2O. In the case of patients with an intraventricular hemorrhage, a large diameter IVC

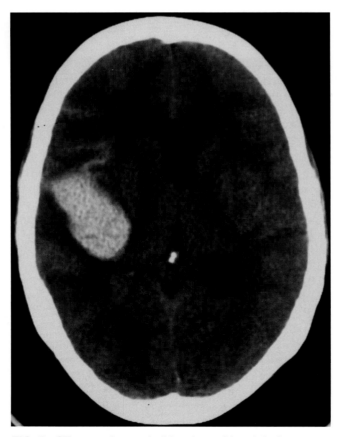

FIG. 2. CT scan of a grade IV patient with a right frontotemporal intraparenchymal hematoma and focal mass effect evidenced by distortion of the right frontal horn.

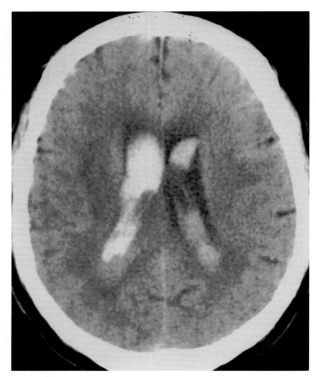

FIG. 3. CT scan of an intraventricular hemorrhage with hydrocephalus. In such cases, a large-diameter intraventricular catheter is used to minimize clogging and facilitate drainage.

(EDM Ventricular Catheter, I.D. 2.6 mm, O.D. 4.9 mm, Pudenz-Schulte Medical, Goleta, CA) is used to minimize clogging and facilitate drainage (Fig. 3). Most poor-grade patients display ventricular dilatation so that IVC placement is possible. If the ventricle cannot be cannulated, a bolt or fiberoptic cable is inserted. If the ICP is >30 cm H_2O and the patient does not show any clinical improvement with ventricular drainage, then surgical intervention is deferred. An angiogram is obtained if the patient is stable. By contrast, if the ICP is <30 cm H_2O and the patient has viable neurologic function, then a four-vessel angiogram is obtained and surgery is carried out within the next 12 hours. Patients who initially do not meet the criteria for surgery are reassessed daily and considered for surgery if their ICP falls below 30 cm H_2O, their neurologic examination improves, and they remain medically stable. We tend to avoid surgery, however, during the 7–10 day interval after SAH or during a period when there is evidence of vasospasm documented either by clinical examination or by transcranial Doppler ultrasound (TCD) studies.

Rarely, we encounter a patient with a good neurologic examination—typically WFNS grade III—but with medical complications that force us to defer surgical intervention. For instance, we treated a patient with a SAH from a giant posteroinferior cerebellar artery aneurysm who presented with a GCS of 14 and mild hemiparesis but with arrhythmias, myocardial infarction, and cardiogenic pulmonary edema.

We deferred surgery for 3 weeks until her cardiac and pulmonary functions improved. She then underwent an uneventful procedure for clipping and debulking of the aneurysm and went on to recover fully.

The Guglielmi detachable coils for endovascular electrothrombosis of aneurysms (36,37) may be a useful adjunct in the management of poor-grade patients whose surgery has to be deferred. Theoretically, the coils may reduce the risk of aneurysmal rebleeding when packed into the dome of the aneurysm. We have used Guglielmi coils for this purpose in three cases. In two patients, subsequent angiography showed growth of the aneurysm and widening of the neck, and the aneurysms were clipped. In the third patient, further evaluation was not possible because of the patient's deteriorating condition. Clipping of an aneurysm after treatment with coils, however, is complicated by the presence of the coils because these have to be evacuated from the dome or at least from the neck of the aneurysm prior to application of the clip. If the coils are protruding from the base of the aneurysm into the lumen of the parent vessel, then the clip may not completely obliterate the neck or, even worse, may shear the wall of the neck as the clip blades close over the coils. Further clinical experience with the coils will determine their role in the management of ruptured aneurysms.

In the operating room, we use the following techniques for aneurysm clipping. We favor continuous electrophysiologic monitoring with somatosensory evoked potentials (SSEPs) and electroencephalography (EEG), mild hypothermia (core temperature of 32–34°C), mannitol, lumbar drainage, and temporary arterial occlusion of afferent vessels under burst suppression with propofol (38) or etomidate (39). We avoid hypotension, hypovolemia, and hyperventilation/hypocarbia. In cases involving giant or complex aneurysms, we routinely utilize intraoperative angiography.

Postoperatively, we maintain high intravenous fluids titrated to a central venous pressure of about 8 mm Hg or to a pulmonary capillary wedge pressure of about 14 mm Hg and monitor cerebral blood flow with TCD. If a delayed ischemic deficit becomes evident, we then initiate hypervolemic-hypertensive therapy (40). In patients in vasospasm but also with a focal injury with mass effect, such as an intraparenchymal hematoma or stroke with surrounding edema, hypertonic saline (2% or 3% sodium chloride solution) can be useful to treat both conditions simultaneously (41,42). In this situation, the treatment of vasospasm with standard intravenous fluids may exacerbate the edema. In the past few years, we have moved from the administration of boluses of hypertonic saline, as described in the literature (41,42), to a continuous infusion of hypertonic saline titrated to a serum osmolality of 310 mOsm/kg H_2O, which corresponds approximately to a serum sodium of 150 mEq/L. The hypertonic solution should be administered through a central venous line and, once the clinical endpoint is reached, tapered slowly over a few days.

CONCLUSION

The management of poor-grade SAH patients remains challenging and controversial. Over the past three decades, however, there has been an improvement in the outcome of grade IV patients and, to a lesser extent, of grade V patients. In addition to the guidelines described above, there are other important socioeconomic considerations that play a role in the management of poor-grade patients. Some of these social issues are advanced age, premorbid condition, and the wishes of the patient and family. A growing economic concern is the social and financial cost of treating conditions such as a grade V SAH, with a reported mortality of 84%.

A systematic approach in the surgical treatment of poor-grade patients may maximize their potential for meaningful recovery. When Hunt and Hess (1) reported their series in 1968, all grade V patients died, grade IV patients had a 71% mortality, and grade III patients had a 37% mortality. In the last 3 years, between January 1992 and December 1994, we have treated at the Johns Hopkins Hospital 43 WFNS grades IV and V patients using the guidelines described above and have obtained a mortality of 34% for grade IV patients and of 71% for grade V patients. When we compare our results with those of Hunt and Hess, it appears that the outcome of poor-grade patients has shifted by one level over the past 30 years; today, grades IV and V patients have a mortality that would have been associated with grades III and IV patients 30 years ago. In the future, further efforts to select adequate surgical candidates and to implement appropriate therapeutic maneuvers may result in improvement in the outcome of poor-grade SAH patients.

ACKNOWLEDGMENTS

The authors would like to thank the following individuals for their thoughtful review of this manuscript: Drs. Henry Brem, Allen K. Sills, Jr, Reid C. Thompson, and John A. Ulatowski.

REFERENCES

1. Hunt WE, Hess RM. Surgical risk as related to the time of intervention in the repair of intracranial aneurysms. *J Neurosurg* 1968;28:14–19.
2. Drake CG. Report of World Federation of Neurological Surgeons Committee on a universal subarachnoid hemorrhage grading scale. *J Neurosurg* 1988;68:985–986.
3. Teasdale G, Jennett B. Assessment of coma and impaired consciousness: A practical scale. *Lancet* 1974;2:81–84.
4. American Society of Anesthesiologists. New classification of physical status. *Anesthesiology* 1963;24:111.
5. Vacanti CJ, VanHouten RJ, Hill RC. A statistical analysis of the relationship of physical status to postoperative mortality in 68,388 cases. *Anesth Analg* 1970;49:564–566.
6. Van Gijn J, Bromberg JEC, Lindsay KW, et al. Definition of initial grading, specific events, and overall outcome in patients with aneurysmal subarachnoid hemorrhage. A survey. *Stroke* 1994;25:1623–1627.
7. Kassell NF, Torner JC, Haley EC, et al. The International Cooperative Study on the Timing of Aneurysm Surgery. I: Overall management results. *J Neurosurg* 1990;73:18–36.
8. Kassell NF, Torner JC, Haley EC Jr, et al. The International Cooperative Study of the Timing of Aneurysm Surgery. II: Surgical results. *J Neurosurg* 1990;73:37–47.
9. Longstreth WT, Nelson LM, Koepsell TD, van Belle G. Clinical course of spontaneous subarachnoid hemorrhage: A population-based study in King County, Washington. *Neurology* 1993;43:712–718.
10. Inagawa T, Takahashi M, Aoki H, et al. Aneurysmal subarachnoid hemorrhage in Izumo City and Shimane Prefecture of Japan. Outcome. *Stroke* 1988;19:176–180.
11. Graf CJ, Nibbelink DW. Cooperative study of intracranial aneurysms and subarachnoid hemorrhage. III. Intracranial surgery. *Stroke* 1974; 5:559–601.
12. Rosenorn J, Eskesen V, Schmidt K, Ronde F. The risk of rebleeding from ruptured intracranial aneurysms. *J Neurosurg* 1987;67:329–332.
13. Petruk KC, West M, Mohr G, et al. Nimodipine treatment in poor-grade aneurysm patients. Results of a multicenter double-blind placebo-controlled trial. *J Neurosurg* 1988;68:505–517.
14. Bailes JE, Spetzler RF, Hadley MN, Baldwin HZ. Management morbidity and mortality of poor-grade aneurysm patients. *J Neurosurg* 1990; 72:559–566.
15. Milhorat TH. Acute hydrocephalus after aneurysmal subarachnoid hemorrhage. *Neurosurgery* 1987;20:15–20.
16. Newell DW, Le Roux PD, Dacey RG, et al. CT infusion scanning for the detection of cerebral aneurysms. *J Neurosurg* 1989;71:175–179.
17. Le Roux PD, Dailey AT, Newell DW, et al. Emergent aneurysm clipping without angiography in the moribund patient with intracerebral hemorrhage: The use of infusion computed tomography scans. *Neurosurgery* 1993;33:189–197.
18. Byer E, Ashman R, Toth LA. Electrocardiograms with large, upright T-waves and long Q-T intervals. *Am Heart J* 1947;33:796–806.
19. Levine HD. Non-specificity of the electrocardiogram associated with coronary artery disease. *Am J Med* 1953;15:344–355.
20. Weintraub BM, McHenry LC Jr. Cardiac abnormalities in subarachnoid hemorrhage: A resume. *Stroke* 1974;5:384–391.
21. Estanol Vidal B, Badui Degal E, Cesarman E, et al. Cardiac arrhythmias associated with subarachnoid hemorrhage: A prospective study. *Neurosurgery* 1979;5:675–680.
22. Rudehill A, Olsson GL, Sundqvist K, Gordon E. ECG abnormalities in patients with subarachnoid hemorrhage and intracranial tumours. *J Neurol Neurosurg Psychiatry* 1987;50:1375–1381.
23. Andreoli A, di Pasquale G, Pinelli G, et al. Subarachnoid hemorrhage: Frequency and severity of cardiac arrhythmias. A survey of 70 cases studied in the acute phase. *Stroke* 1987;18:558–564.
24. Brouwers PJAM, Widjiks EFM, Hasan D, et al. Serial electrocardiographic recording in aneurysmal subarachnoid hemorrhage. *Stroke* 1989;20:1162–1167.
25. Tabbaa MA, Ramirez-Lassepas M, Snyder BD. Aneurysmal subarachnoid hemorrhage presenting as cardiorespiratory arrest. *Arch Intern Med* 1987;147:1661–1662.
26. Weisman SJ. Edema and congestion of the lungs resulting from intracranial hemorrhage. *Surgery* 1939;6:722–729.
27. Ciongoli AK, Poser CM. Pulmonary edema secondary to subarachnoid hemorrhage. *Neurology* 1972;22:867–870.
28. Knudsen F, Jensen HP, Petersen PL. Neurogenic pulmonary edema: Treatment with dobutamine. *Neurosurgery* 1991;29:269–270.
29. Weir BK. Pulmonary edema following fatal aneurysm rupture. *J Neurosurg* 1978;49:502–507.
30. Wijdicks EFM, Vermeulen M, Hijdra A, van Gijn J. Hyponatremia and cerebral infarction in patients with ruptured intracranial aneurysms: Is fluid restriction harmful. *Ann Neurol* 1985;17:137–140.
31. Castel JP. Aspects of medical management in aneurysmal subarachnoid hemorrhage. *Adv Tech Stand Neurosurg* 1991;18:47–110.
32. Nelson PB, Seif SM, Maroon JC, Robinson AG. Hyponatremia in intracranial disease: Perhaps not the syndrome of inappropriate secretion of antidiuretic hormone (SIADH). *J Neurosurg* 1981;55:938–941.
33. Schwartz WB, Bennett W, Curelop S, et al. A syndrome of renal sodium loss and hyponatremia probably resulting from inappropriate secretion of antidiuretic hormone. *Am J Med* 1952;23:529–542.
34. Brandt L, Sonesson B, Ljunggren B, Saveland H. Ruptured middle cerebral artery aneurysm with intracerebral hemorrhage in younger patients appearing moribund: Emergency operation? *Neurosurgery* 1987;20:925–929.
35. Batjer HH, Samson DS. Emergent surgery without cerebral angiography for the comatose patient. *Neurosurgery* 1991;28:283–287.

36. Guglielmi G, Vinuela F, Sepetka I, Macellari V. Electrothrombosis of saccular aneurysms via endovascular approach. Part 1: Electrochemical basis, technique, and experimental results. *J Neurosurg* 1991;75:1–7.

37. Guglielmi G, Vinuela F, Dion J, Duckwiler G. Electrothrombosis of saccular aneurysms via endovascular approach. Part 2: Preliminary clinical experience. *J Neurosurg* 1991;75:8–14.

38. Ravussin P, de Tribolet N. Total intravenous anesthesia with propofol for burst suppression in cerebral aneurysm surgery: Preliminary report of 42 patients. *Neurosurgery* 1993;32:236–240.

39. Batjer HH, Franfurt AI, Purdy PD, et al. Use of etomidate, temporary arterial occlusion, and intraoperative angiography in surgical treatment of large and giant cerebral aneurysms. *J Neurosurg* 1988;68:234–240.

40. Kassell NF, Peerless SJ, Durward QJ, et al. Treatment of ischemic deficits from vasospasm with intravascular volume expansion and induced arterial hypertension. *Neurosurgery* 1982;11:337–343.

41. Worthley LIG, Cooper DJ, Jones N. Treatment of resistant intracranial hypertension with hypertonic saline. *J Neurosurg* 1988;68:478–481.

42. Fisher B, Thomas D, Peterson B. Hypertonic saline lowers raised intracranial pressure in children after head trauma. *J Neurosurg Anesthesiol* 1992;4:4–10.

Cerebrovascular Disease, edited by H. Hunt Batjer.
Lippincott-Raven Publishers, Philadelphia © 1997.

CHAPTER 89

Cerebral Vasospasm: Prevention and Treatment

R. Loch Macdonald and Bryce Weir

In the 40 years since its description, the cerebral vasospasm that complicates aneurysmal subarachnoid hemorrhage (SAH) has been recognized as an important adverse prognostic factor for outcome in SAH patients. There is a growing body of literature that is defining the etiology and pathogenesis of vasospasm, and several therapies have reduced the morbidity and mortality of vasospasm from approximately 30% in the 1960s to 15% in the early 1980s.

Angiographic vasospasm, symptomatic vasospasm, and delayed cerebral ischemia or delayed ischemic neurologic deficit are terms that describe various aspects of vasospasm. Angiographic vasospasm is transient arterial narrowing visualized on a cerebral angiogram 4–12 days after SAH. Symptomatic vasospasm, delayed cerebral ischemia, and delayed ischemic neurologic deficit refer to the cerebral ischemia that may result from the angiographically demonstrable vasospasm.

EPIDEMIOLOGY OF CEREBRAL VASOSPASM

Incidence and Prevalence of Cerebral Vasospasm

Dorsch and King (1) reviewed over 1000 reports on cerebral aneurysms published since 1960. Angiographic vasospasm was documented in 43% of patients. When analysis was restricted to patients with angiography in the second week after SAH, 67% showed vasospasm, and it was believed that if angiography were done every day, the incidence of angiographic vasospasm would approach 100%. Vasospasm is rare within 2 days, peaks in 5–7 days, and resolves by 14 days after a single SAH. Vasospasm earlier than 2 days after SAH should raise suspicion of an earlier SAH or some other cause for arterial narrowing.

Symptomatic vasospasm or delayed cerebral ischemia was reported in 10,445 (32%) of 32,188 patients from 297 references (1). The peak day of onset of delayed ischemia was 7–8 days after SAH or 1–2 days after the mean time of onset of angiographic vasospasm. In a randomized, placebo-controlled trial of nicardipine, 17% of 123 patients in the placebo-treated group who had angiograms 7–11 days post-SAH had no angiographic vasospasm, 28% had mild spasm, 23% had moderate spasm, and 28% had severe vasospasm (2). Neurologic worsening was attributed to vasospasm in 30% of patients.

Other Conditions Associated with Cerebral Vasospasm

Any disease associated with subarachnoid blood may be associated with vasospasm, although the thick SAH in the basal cisterns that occurs with aneurysm rupture and that causes vasospasm is uncommon with conditions other than aneurysm rupture. SAH is observed on computed tomography (CT) in 68% of patients with severe head injury (3). Angiographic vasospasm occurs in 5–40% of patients with closed head injury, and transcranial Doppler ultrasound (TCD) studies suggest vasospasm in 27–89% of these cases (3).

Routine postoperative CT scanning shows that the majority of cases of vasospasm associated with arteriovenous malformation rupture after removal of intracranial tumors and surgery for unruptured aneurysms are due to SAH. There are occasional reports, however, in which SAH does not seem to have been present, and other causes of arterial narrowing, such as infection or arterial trauma, must be considered.

Vasospasm and Prognosis After Aneurysm Rupture

After aneurysmal SAH, there is a general relationship between clinical grade, volume of SAH on CT scan, vaso-

Both authors: Section of Neurosurgery, University of Chicago Medical Center, Chicago, Illinois, 60637.

spasm, acute hydrocephalus, and a variety of other neurologic and systemic indices that are altered in relation to the severity of the SAH. Despite these interrelationships, multivariate analyses show that vasospasm is an important independent predictor of poor outcome after aneurysmal SAH (4–6). A multivariate analysis of the 3521 patients entered into the International Cooperative Study on the Timing of Aneurysm Surgery found that the most important prognostic factors were level of consciousness on admission, age, blood pressure on admission, amount of SAH on CT scan, preexisting medical conditions, aneurysm site, and vasospasm (4). Several other multiple regression analyses reported that the factors that influence outcome after aneurysmal SAH included clinical grade, hypertension, the amount of SAH on the admission CT scan, intracerebral hemorrhage, age, and vasospasm (3,6). The day of admission to hospital is also important in that patients admitted late are a selected population that have a better prognosis by virtue of having survived for several days.

Factors Predicting Development of Vasospasm

The location and volume of subarachnoid blood visualized on a CT scan within 4–5 days of SAH is the most important predictor of the development of vasospasm. Fisher et al (7) classified SAH on CT scan obtained within 5 days of the event into the following groups: 1—no blood detected; 2—diffuse, thin layers of SAH <1 mm thick; 3—localized clots and/or vertical layers of blood >1 mm thick or more than 5 × 3 mm in size in the longitudinal or transverse planes; and 4—intracerebral or intraventricular hemorrhage, with little or no subarachnoid blood (Fig. 1). When no blood or only diffuse, thin layers were observed on CT scan, vasospasm developed in 5.6% of 18 cases. Patients with localized or diffuse, thick clots (group 3) developed severe vasospasm in 96% of 24 cases. Hemorrhage into the intracerebral or intraventricular compartments (group 4) seldom resulted in vasospasm. A prospective study of this classification confirmed its ability to predict vasospasm.

Other criteria used to predict which patients will develop vasospasm after aneurysm rupture include intraventricular hemorrhage, acute hydrocephalus, abnormal electroencephalogram (EEG), increased cerebrospinal fluid fibrin degradation products, decreased blood volume, increased serum complement, increased middle cerebral artery flow velocity on TCD, elevated plasma catecholamines, decreased circulating blood volume and serum sodium, peripheral leukocytosis, and electrocardiogram (ECG) changes (3,5). Many of these parameters will covary with the volume of SAH that has occurred—and therefore with vasospasm—and multivariate statistical techniques are required to demonstrate which factors independently predict vasospasm. The occurrence of vasospasm in proximity to the ruptured aneurysm is probably due to the increased amount of blood deposited around the aneurysm. Others have argued that rupture of the

aneurysm disrupts a portion of the arterial wall and that this causes vasospasm. The low incidence of vasospasm in patients with aneurysms that rupture into the brain or the ventricles argues against this hypothesis.

Treatment of patients with SAH with antifibrinolytic drugs increases the risk of cerebral ischemia, presumably by prolonging the life of the clot and the duration of contact by spasmogens with the vessel wall. In a multicenter, randomized, double-blind, placebo-controlled trial of tranexamic acid for prevention of rebleeding after SAH, there was no significant difference in outcome between the groups at 3 months (8). Rebleeding occurred in 24% of controls and 9% of treated patients, but cerebral ischemia developed in 24% of treated patients and 15% of placebo-treated patients.

Influence of Surgery on Vasospasm

There is a tendency for patients operated on during vasospasm to have a higher risk of developing ischemic neurologic deficits. Observations during surgery indicate that manipulation of arteries and temporary clipping may precipitate acute vessel spasm, and there is concern that aggravation of vasospasm is a cause of perioperative ischemia. Mechanical spasm, however, is short-lived and probably does not contribute significantly to perioperative cerebral ischemia under normal circumstances. It is conceivable, however, that mechanical spasm could have deleterious effects when superimposed on a preexisting degree of vasospasm in arteries supplying already compromised brain. Angiographic and TCD studies of clinical and experimental vasospasm suggest that surgical manipulation of cerebral arteries has minimal effect on the severity of vasospasm and that the increased risk of cerebral ischemia in patients operated on during vasospasm is due to other factors (3). The distinction between preoperative and postoperative vasospasm reflects the time of surgery in relation to the natural history of vasospasm and not an effect of surgery on vasospasm per se.

Relationship Between Vasospasm and Cerebral Infarction

Vasospasm produces cerebral ischemia by predominately hemodynamic mechanisms. There is seldom complete arterial thrombosis or embolization. The Hagen–Pouiseulle equation that describes flow of Newtonian fluids through rigid tubes states that resistance to blood flow is related to the length of the stenosis and the viscosity of the blood and inversely related to the radius of the tube to the fourth power. While there are probably inaccuracies in applying this to the situation in vivo, it is likely that the blood flow through a vasospastic artery is related to severity and length of stenosis, blood viscosity, and factors that alter flow proximal to the stenosis such as the blood pressure, cardiac output, and intravascular volume. The oxygen and glucose content of the blood, the extent of collateral and anastomotic flow,

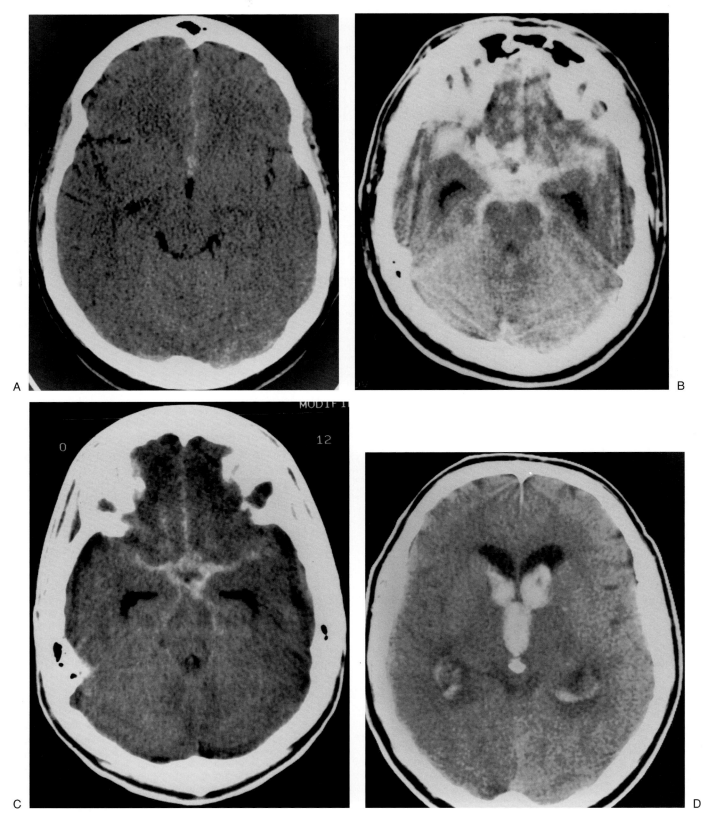

FIG. 1. (A) A CT scan demonstrates a thin, Fisher grade 2 SAH in the anterior interhemispheric fissure from an aneurysm arising at the anterior communicating artery. It is unlikely that this would be associated with clinically significant vasospasm. **(B)** A CT scan shows a diffuse, thick, Fisher grade 3 SAH that would almost certainly be associated with clinically significant vasospasm. **(C)** This diffuse, Fisher grade 3 SAH shows less blood than the last example, and vasospasm would be likely to be less of a problem. **(D)** A CT scan shows a Fisher grade IV intraventricular hemorrhage from a basilar bifurcation aneurysm. Vasospasm would be very unlikely to occur.

1113

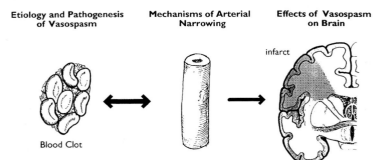

Etiology and Pathogenesis of Vasospasm

1. Subarachnoid blood clot causes vasospasm.
2. Hemolysis and release of spasmogenic erythrocyte cytosol are necessary.
3. Potential spasmogens include hemoglobins, breakdown products of hemoglobin, other red cell stromal proteins or compounds.
4. Pathogenesis of hemoglobin-induced vasospasm may include free radical reactions, inhibition of endothelium-dependent relaxation, increase in endothelin release, alteration of arterial wall eicosanoid release, altered balance of vasodilatory and vasoconstrictor perivascular nerves.
5. Other processes that may be important in vasospasm include inflammation and immunologically mediated processes.
6. Pathogenesis of prolonged vasoconstriction in vasospasm is unclear but may involve non-physiological, prolonged ↑ in intracellular calcium and several contractile processes such as calmodulin-myosin light chain kinase, protein kinase C, calcium-activated proteolysis, a rigor state, or a latch state.

Mechanisms of Arterial Narrowing

1. Majority of arterial narrowing of vasospasm is vasoconstriction that is sensitive to papaverine at least in experimental models early after SAH.
2. With time, papaverine-resistant spasm develops that is associated with ↓ arterial contractility and compliance and ↓ endothelium-dependent relaxation.
3. With time, there is smooth muscle necrosis and arterial wall fibrosis, that may contribute to papaverine-resistant vasospasm.
4. Intimal proliferation occurs late after angiographic vasospasm and does not contribute to arterial narrowing.
5. Myofibroblasts may proliferate in the artery, producing contraction and arterial fibrosis.

Effects of Vasospasm on Brain

1. Vasospasm produces ischemia and infarction by hemodynamic mechanism in majority of cases, thrombosis and embolism are uncommon.
2. Whether infarct develops with a given degree of vasospasm depends on severity and length of stenosis, blood viscosity, blood pressure, cardiac output, blood volume, arterial oxygen and glucose, collateral and anastomotic flow, preexisting arterial stenoses and hypoplasias, brain temperature, therapies for vasospasm that are used like calcium channel antagonists, hemodynamic therapy, angioplasty, and intrarterial papaverine.
3. Other causes of infarction may complicate aneurysmal SAH such as hypoxic-ischemia encephalopathy from ↑ intracranial pressure, major arterial occlusion, perforator injury, retraction or venous injury from surgery, and other causes of stroke.

FIG. 2. A summary of current knowledge of the etiology, pathogenesis, and mechanisms of vasospasm and some of the factors that determine whether or not vasospasm produces cerebral ischemia and infarction of the brain.

preexisting arterial hypoplasias and atherosclerotic narrowings, administration of brain protectants, variations in brain temperature, and therapies for vasospasm will also influence whether a given degree of vasospasm causes cerebral infarction (Fig. 2). In view of these factors, in addition to the other causes of cerebral infarction after SAH and aneurysm surgery, it is not surprising that it is difficult in every case to document a direct and constant relationship between vasospasm and cerebral infarction. In most series, however, there is a significant correlation between severe vasospasm and infarction in the territory of the spastic artery.

ETIOLOGY AND PATHOGENESIS OF VASOSPASM

The ability to produce vasospasm in experimental animals by the subarachnoid placement of blood clot and to prevent it by removal of the clot, both in man and animals, proves that the cause of vasospasm is subarachnoid blood clot. How subarachnoid blood causes vasospasm has not been completely worked out yet, but there is probably an interaction of spasmogenic substances released from the blood clot with

the endothelial and smooth muscle cells of the arterial wall, and possibly with the perivascular nerves (see Fig. 2).

Experiments in several lower species showed that the component of blood necessary for prolonged vasospasm to develop was the erythrocyte (9). Furthermore, intact erythrocytes were not vasoactive, but upon lysis they released vasoconstricting compounds that included oxyhemoglobin or other forms of hemoglobin and its breakdown products and other compounds in erythrocyte stroma. While the exact identity of the substances released from hemolyzing erythrocytes have probably not all been identified, it would seem at present that other blood components such as platelets and fibrin-degradation products and other small molecules such as potassium, magnesium, catecholamines, histamine, serotonin, and eicosanoids play a relatively minor role in the pathogenesis of vasospasm.

Hemoglobin or other unidentified erythrocyte stromal components may produce spasm by generating vasoactive free radicals, damaging perivascular nerves, interacting directly in some way with vascular smooth muscle, and/or influencing the balance of release of vasoconstricting and vasodilating factors from the vascular endothelium. The endothelium plays a critical role in maintenance of blood vessel tone through secretion of vasoconstricting (endothelins, some eicosanoids) and vasodilating (prostacyclin, endothelium-derived relaxing factor) compounds. Processes that may contribute to vasoconstriction during vasospasm include inhibition of endothelium-dependent relaxation and possibly augmentation of release of endothelin from endothelial cells (3,9,10).

The large cerebral arteries affected by vasospasm are innervated by catecholaminergic, cholinergic, and peptidergic nerves, stimulation of which may cause vasoconstriction or vasodilation. The extent to which innervation of the cerebral arteries controls arterial diameter under physiologic conditions, however, is not clear but is probably minor. The time course of denervation observed histologically following clot application in monkeys did not correspond to the time course of angiographic vasospasm (11).

The inability of cyclosporine and FK-506 to prevent experimental vasospasm, coupled with the knowledge that vasospasm is not a clinical problem in patients with meningitis, casts doubt on theories that vasospasm is an inflammatory or immunologically mediated phenomenon (3). Peterson and colleagues (12) suggested that inflammation did not cause vasospasm directly but that complement-mediated reactions and inflammation were important in producing erythrocyte lysis in the subarachnoid space, a process that would release spasmogenic compounds from red cells.

Structural Arterial Wall Changes and Vasospasm

Observation of the pathology of vasospastic arteries and the demonstrated efficacy of intraarterial papaverine shows that the predominant process occurring initially is smooth muscle contraction or vasoconstriction (3,13). The dismal failure of numerous intravenously administered vasodilator drugs to prevent cerebral vasospasm despite their favorable effects on peripheral vasospastic disorders caused some neurosurgeons to discard the idea that vasospasm is vasoconstriction (5). These observations, coupled with the prolonged course of vasospasm and the histopathologic changes in the arterial wall, led to theories that nonmuscle contractile and noncontractile processes contribute to vasospasm (3,5,13). Animal studies have suggested that both processes contribute to vasospasm (13). The exact timing of the changes vary, probably with the severity of the SAH among other things, but within 7–10 days of SAH in dogs and rabbits, the majority of the narrowing is due to vasoconstriction. With increasing time from SAH and with increasingly severe vasospasm, pathologic changes are observed in vasospastic arteries, and these changes are associated with reduced arterial contractility and compliance and reduced endothelium-dependent relaxation (13). Whether the pathologic changes are a cause or consequence of the pharmacologic changes (and the biochemical basis of both) remains open to question. The end result, however, is a decreased ability of vasodilator drugs to reverse the vasospasm. These changes tend to occur and

to progress as the angiographic phase of vasospasm resolves. Morphometric analysis of vasospastic arteries has shown that intimal proliferation does occur in vasospastic arteries but that it is not severe enough in the majority of cases to narrow the arterial lumen significantly and occurs too late after the hemorrhage to be important during the period of symptomatic vasospasm (3).

Evidence has accrued in favor of involvement in vasospasm of the numerous different biochemical pathways of smooth muscle contraction including the calcium–calmodulin–myosin light-chain phosphorylation mechanism, protein kinase C, smooth muscle rigor, calcium-activated neutral proteases (calpains), and other states of loss of intracellular calcium homeostasis (3). We do not yet know how they contribute to the vasoconstriction of vasospasm.

Cerebral Blood Flow and Metabolism in Cerebral Vasospasm

Intracranial pressure rises acutely with aneurysm rupture in proportion to the volume and rate of hemorrhage and may reach the level of systemic blood pressure, causing intracranial circulatory arrest, loss of consciousness, and a global cerebral ischemic insult (14). This insult, in addition to the toxic effects of subarachnoid blood, results in a prolonged decrease in cerebral blood flow after SAH (3,5,14,15). Worse clinical grades and large-volume SAHs are associated with increasingly severe reductions in blood flow and concomitant increases in cerebral blood volume. Vasospasm causes additional regional decreases in cerebral blood flow in the territories of vasospastic arteries. Blood flows are lowest 7 days after SAH, but they may remain significantly decreased for months after SAH in grades 4 and 5 patients. Increased cerebral blood flow or "luxury perfusion" has been observed in clinical grades 4 and 5 patients with SAH, possibly secondary to induced hypertension in the presence of loss of autoregulation.

In common with other acute cerebrovascular disorders, autoregulation (maintenance of normal blood flow in spite of changing blood pressure) and compensatory changes in cerebral blood flow in response to changes in arterial carbon dioxide are progressively impaired with worsening clinical grade and with vasospasm after SAH (14). Detailed studies in animals have documented these changes, which are most marked during the peak of vasospasm 7 days post-SAH. Autoregulation tends to be more sensitive to pathologic alterations in the brain than carbon dioxide reactivity.

Cerebral metabolism falls in the first days after SAH (15). Within 4 days of SAH, there was a significant (25%) reduction in the cerebral metabolic rate for oxygen ($CMRO_2$) and no significant change in oxygen extraction fraction, suggesting relative hyperemia, although the extent to which these changes were related to therapy of vasospasm was unclear (16). During vasospasm, the oxygen extraction fraction increased without an accompanying change in $CMRO_2$, indicating cerebral ischemia without infarction ("misery perfusion"). Infarction is heralded by luxury perfusion or matched falls in metabolism and perfusion (16).

CLINICAL FEATURES

Accurate and early diagnosis and assessment of the amount of SAH on a CT scan within hours or days of the SAH allow the neurosurgeon to know which patients are at risk for vasospasm and to be vigilant for symptoms and signs of delayed cerebral ischemia so that treatment can be initiated early. Few clinical situations offer such a pretreatment possibility for cerebral ischemia.

Clinical deficits from vasospasm occur in relation to the angiographic time of vasospasm between days 4 and 12 after a single SAH (1). The peak time of onset is 7–8 days post-SAH, with earlier onset suggesting more severe or prior SAH. Middle cerebral artery territory ischemia is most common, accounting for 75% of deficits due to vasospasm. Focal deficits may develop in the territory of any other major cerebral artery. In consideration of discharging patients early, it should be kept in mind that large series document onset of ischemic deficits more than 13 days after SAH in 3–4% of patients (5). In addition to focal neurologic deficits, vasospasm is associated with increasing headache and meningismus, decreased level of consciousness, and low-grade fever.

DIAGNOSIS AND DIFFERENTIAL DIAGNOSIS

Computed Tomography, Magnetic Resonance Imaging, Angiography

A CT scan showing focal or diffuse, thick subarachnoid blood clots remains the best test to predict the development and location of vasospasm. Magnetic resonance imaging (MRI) is at least as sensitive and specific for identifying subarachnoid blood as CT scan, although it adds little to the information obtained on CT scan. The large volumes of clot that are important for predicting vasospasm are easily seen on CT scan without the additional time, expense, and difficulty of obtaining MR images in critically ill patients. The angiographic features of vasospasm include the appearance of focal or diffuse, relatively concentric arterial narrowings on an angiogram 4–12 days after aneurysmal SAH; these features resolve after 14 or more days (Fig. 3).

Transcranial Doppler Ultrasound

Transcranial Doppler ultrasound (TCD) may suggest the diagnosis of vasospasm in many cases. Mean cerebral artery flow velocities >120 cm/sec have a sensitivity of 59% and a specificity of 100% for angiographic vasospasm (17). Flow velocities increase during the time of angiographic vaso-

spasm 4–12 days after SAH, and they tend to be higher in patients with more subarachnoid clot in the arteries that are encased in the clot. Velocities in the middle cerebral artery are obtained most reliably, and maximum flow velocities >200 cm/sec are usually associated with severe vasospasm and cerebral ischemia and infarction. Flow velocities are directly related to cerebral blood flow and inversely to the square of the radius of the artery. In the interpretation of flow velocities, it must be remembered that cerebral blood flow is often altered after SAH and other factors alter flow, such as intracranial pressure, arterial carbon dioxide, and blood pressure. Although increased flow velocities often precede development of clinical vasospasm, rapid, early increases in flow velocity >50 cm/sec/d are also ominous (3). Some authors have recently challenged the efficacy of TCD in the evaluation of cerebral hemodynamics (18).

PREVENTION AND TREATMENT OF VASOSPASM

The best method to prevent vasospasm is to prevent the formation of aneurysms and to surgically obliterate known aneurysms before they rupture (Table 1). In perhaps 95% of cases, intracranial saccular aneurysms are acquired lesions resulting from hemodynamically induced degeneration of the cerebral arterial wall at bifurcations. There are few known predisposing factors, and mass screening is not a cost-effective option at this time. Deficiency of type III collagen does not seem to be a reliable systemic marker in these cases (19). Screening for cerebral aneurysms has been simplified by MR angiography, and it is recommended that patients undergo screening if they have two or more first-degree relatives with aneurysms, if an identical twin had an aneurysm, or if there are family members with adult-onset polycystic kidney disease, coarctation of the aorta, or Marfan's syndrome. Other diseases associated with aneurysms include fibromuscular dysplasia, Ehlers-Danlos syndrome, tuberous sclerosis, moyamoya disease, hereditary hemorrhagic telangiectasia, and iatrogenic or spontaneous carotid occlusion.

Cigarette smoking is a serious adverse risk factor for both the development of cerebral aneurysms and their rupture. Smoking was associated with a 2.1–11.1-fold increased relative risk of SAH, depending on the amount smoked and the sex of the patient (20). Although the evidence is less compelling in SAH, logic would dictate that one avoid and treat other stroke risk factors as well, such as hypertension, diabetes, obesity, and excess dietary fat and alcohol. Cocaine probably adversely affects the natural history of cerebral aneurysms by causing acute hypertension and rupture of aneurysms that might not otherwise have burst.

Unruptured aneurysms may be identified when patients with multiple aneurysms have suffered one aneurysm rupture, incidentally when brain imaging is performed for unrelated reasons, or when they cause symptoms prior to rupture.

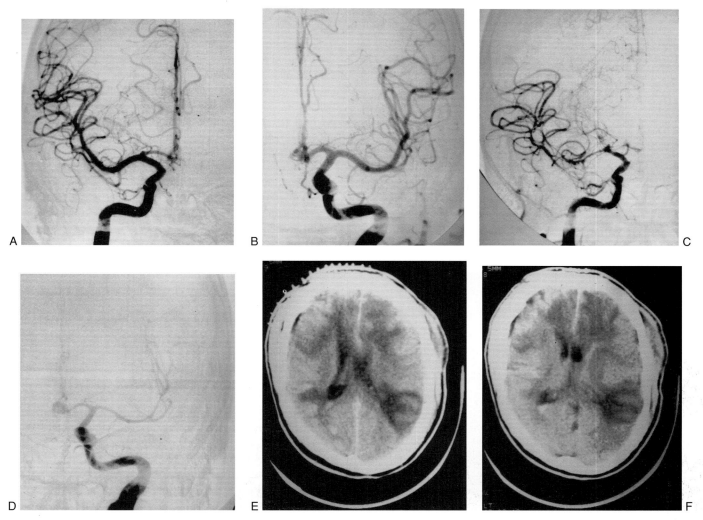

FIG. 3. A typical case of symptomatic vasospasm. The initial CT scan (see Fig. 1B) showed diffuse, thick SAH. The initial anteroposterior view internal carotid angiograms on the right **(A)** and left **(B)** show an anterior communicating artery aneurysm. Seven days later the patient deteriorated and was found to have severe, diffuse vasospasm on anteroposterior view internal carotid angiograms on the right **(C)** and left **(D)**. A subsequent CT **(E,F)** scan showed bilateral anterior and middle cerebral artery territory hypodensities consistent with infarcts from vasospasm.

Symptomatic aneurysms bleed at a rate of about 6% per year and should be obliterated urgently. Since the overall risk of surgery for unruptured aneurysms is approximately 5–10%, we would recommend surgical obliteration of all unruptured aneurysms >4–5 mm in diameter, except when there are overwhelming contraindications to surgery, such as medical illness or advanced biological age.

The symptoms and signs of aneurysm rupture are well known to neurosurgeons, but minor hemorrhages or warning leaks continue to be misdiagnosed in up to 50% of cases. The catastrophic natural history of aneurysm rupture dictates that physicians have a low threshold for investigation of patients with headaches suspicious for SAH.

The important advances in vasospasm treatment include avoiding conditions that increase the risk that angiographic vasospasm will become symptomatic. Antifibrinolytic drugs increase the risk of cerebral ischemia. Their use should probably be reserved for the uncommon circumstance where early surgery is not possible and the patient is not at high risk of vasospasm. Hypovolemia and hyponatremia are common after SAH, and the former adversely affects cerebral blood flow. Hyponatremia should not be treated with fluid restriction, and patients should receive at least 3 L/d of fluid. Treatment of hypertension lowers cerebral blood flow after SAH and increases the risk of cerebral infarction because autoregulation is impaired (3). Increased intracranial pressure should be treated aggressively with mannitol, ventricular drainage, and modest hyperventilation, since increases above levels that reduce cerebral perfusion pressure to <60–70 mm Hg can aggravate cerebral ischemia.

TABLE 1. *Methods for the prevention and treatment of vasospasm*

Methods to prevent vasospasm
Prevent formation and rupture of aneurysms by avoiding smoking and cocaine
Clip unruptured aneurysms that are found incidentally in patients with other ruptured aneurysms, that are symptomatic but unruptured, or that are identified by screening of individuals at risk
Diagnose and treat patients with warning leaks from aneurysms
Remove subarachnoid clots
   Surgical removal of clot
   Pharmacologic removal of clot with t-PA or other fibrinolytic agent(s)
Pharmacologic prevention of vasospasm
   Calcium channel antagonists
   Tirilazad

Methods to treat vasospasm
Facilitate management of vasospasm
   Early aneurysm clipping
Improve cerebral perfusion
   Avoid hypovolemia and hyponatremia, induce hypervolemia, increase cardiac output
   Avoid antifibrinolytics
   Avoid hypotension and antihypertensives, induce hypertension
   Avoid increased intracranial pressure
   Avoid increased hematocrit
Reverse established vasospasm
   Transluminal angioplasty
   Superselective intraarterial papaverine infusion
Protect the brain from cerebral ischemia
   Possible effect of calcium channel antagonists, tirilazad

Calcium Channel Antagonists

Nimodipine is a dihydropyridine compound that blocks calcium entry through L-type voltage-dependent calcium channels. Since the increases in intracellular calcium that underlie vasoconstriction—and therefore vasospasm—may occur through pathways not involving L-type channels, nimodipine does not completely prevent vasospasm. The efficacy of nimodipine as prophylactic treatment is strongly supported by metaanalysis of the seven randomized, double-blind, placebo-controlled trials that showed a highly significant association between nimodipine treatment and good outcome (21). The risk of poor outcome was 42% less for nimodipine-treated patients and the odds ratio for treatment with nimodipine was 0.58, with a 95% confidence interval <1. Adverse effects of nimodipine are limited to hypotension. Because of the minor and statistically insignificant effects on angiographic vasospasm, other modes of action of nimodipine are postulated, including dilation of collateral arteries with improvement of cerebral blood flow to ischemic brain, neuronal protection from ischemia by preventing increased intracellular calcium, and improvement of blood rheology (21). Nimodipine also improved outcome when

administered therapeutically to patients with acute onset of delayed neurologic deterioration after SAH (21).

Nicardipine (0.15 mg/kg/h), another dihydropyridine L-type calcium channel antagonist, significantly reduced symptomatic and angiographic vasospasm and the use of antihypertensive medications and hemodynamic therapy, when compared with placebo in a randomized, blinded clinical trial (2). Despite this, there were no significant differences in overall outcome at 3 months after SAH, with approximately 55% of patients making good recoveries and 17% dead in each group. The reason for this was postulated to be that although nicardipine prevented symptomatic vasospasm, hemodynamic therapy was an equally effective therapy. Lower doses of nicardipine (0.075 mg/kg/h) may be equally efficacious and associated with fewer adverse medical events (22).

HA 1077 (AT-877) is a sulfonamide derivative that antagonizes the action of intracellular calcium by a different mechanism than the dihydropyridines. A dose-escalation study and a double-blind, placebo-controlled, randomized study in humans were conducted and showed that vasospasm was reduced and outcome was improved in patients with aneurysmal SAH (23). Further studies will be necessary to determine the ultimate utility and the mechanism of action of this class of compounds.

Other Pharmacologic Treatments for Vasospasm

The 21-aminosteroid, tirilazad mesylate (U-74006F), was tested in several animal models of SAH and in humans after aneurysm rupture (3). The drugs in this class are steroid derivatives that inhibit iron-dependent lipid peroxidation in vitro but lack glucocorticoid steroid side effects. They may also inhibit iron-independent lipid peroxidation, scavenge hydroxyl free radicals, and stabilize cell membranes. A phase II trial of three doses of tirilazad (0.6, 2, and 6 mg/kg/d IV for 10 days), designed to test safety but not efficacy, found that patients receiving 2 mg/kg were less likely to develop symptomatic vasospasm and more likely to have a favorable outcome, although the differences between groups were not significant (24). There were no serious drug-related adverse effects. A phase III randomized, double-blind, placebo-controlled trial of the same doses was conducted in 1023 patients randomized and treated within 48 hours of SAH (25). In pairwise comparisons of each treatment group vs. placebo, the 6 mg/kg/d group experienced significantly less mortality (12% vs. 21%), less clinical vasospasm (18% vs. 26%) and less need for hemodynamic therapy to reverse vasospasm (9% vs. 15%). This group also had significantly more patients with good recovery than the placebo group.

Although intravenous infusion of vasodilator drugs has seldom been of benefit in patients with established vasospasm, superselective intraarterial infusions of vasodilators, such as papaverine, directly into spastic arteries have shown promise in vasospasm. After infusion of papaverine

100–300 mg into spastic arteries that were not dilatable by angioplasty, angiographic and clinical improvement was observed in up to 75% of patients (3,26). Vasospasm has a tendency to recur after this therapy in 15–20% of patients.

Clot Removal and Clot Lysis

Vasospasm depends largely on the presence of subarachnoid blood clot, and experimental studies suggest that hemolysis of erythrocytes in the clot is necessary for vasospasm to develop. Since hemolysis does not peak for several days after SAH, removal of blood clot before hemolysis might prevent vasospasm. This has been proven in several experimental models, although opinions are divided about the efficacy of surgical clot evacuation for the prevention of spasm in man (3,27). The technical difficulties associated with microsurgical removal of clot from the basal cisterns include prolonged retraction of the already swollen brain, perforator injury, and precipitation of further bleeding—factors that put this procedure beyond the technical prowess of most neurosurgeons.

Pharmacologic fibrinolysis of subarachnoid clots with urokinase or tissue plasminogen activator (t-PA) has been tested in humans (27). The criteria were that patients have thick subarachnoid clots and be at high risk of vasospasm and that the ruptured aneurysm be clipped so that t-PA could be administered within 72 hours of rupture. The t-PA has been injected as a single intracisternal bolus of 10 mg, administered after aneurysm clipping, or as multiple, daily 1–4 mg doses through intracisternal catheters. Among 157 patients treated in phase I/II trials, 91% had thick subarachnoid clots and these often cleared very rapidly after administration of the t-PA (27). Symptomatic vasospasm developed in 7 (4%) of 157 patients and angiographic vasospasm in 47 (35%) of 136 patients. Comparison to historical controls would suggest that 64% of a cohort of patients with a similar degree of SAH would develop severe, diffuse vasospasm (6). Bleeding complications developed in about 25% of patients, although they were serious in fewer that 5%.

In a blinded, placebo-controlled trial of 100 patients given perioperative intracisternal t-PA (10 mg), there was a 56% relative risk reduction in severe vasospasm for patients with thick subarachnoid clots (28). Only 12% of t-PA–treated patients died compared with 23% of placebo-treated patients, and bleeding complications did not differ between the groups. The study demonstrated consistent trends toward less vasospasm and improved outcome in patients treated with t-PA. This treatment would seem worthwhile for patients at high risk for vasospasm when operated on by experienced surgeons.

Balloon Angioplasty

Balloon angioplasty is the use of intravascular balloons to mechanically dilate narrowed arterial segments. The crite-

rion for angioplasty for vasospasm is a new neurologic deficit in the territory of an artery shown by angiography to be in severe vasospasm (3,29). Other causes for neurologic deficit should be excluded by CT scan and appropriate blood tests. Although it would seem prudent to dilate spastic arteries as soon as possible after onset of a deficit, the appropriate timing of angioplasty will be dictated by how quickly medical management can be optimized to determine if the deficit reverses, since the potential complications of angioplasty generally preclude its use except as a salvage therapy. One has to proceed rapidly, however, since a hypodensity on CT scan is a contraindication to angioplasty. Angioplasty is usually reserved for cases in which the ruptured aneurysm has been clipped.

Among 173 patients undergoing dilation of 515 arterial territories for symptomatic vasospasm due to aneurysmal SAH, angiographic improvement was noted in over 95% of cases and clinical improvement was noted in 63% (3). Complications attributed to angioplasty developed in 17 patients (10%) and included nine episodes of aneurysm rebleeding (usually from ruptured but unclipped aneurysms), four arterial ruptures, three arterial occlusions, and one hemorrhagic infarction.

Hypervolemia, Hypertension, and Hemodilution

After SAH and during vasospasm, there is loss of regulation of cerebral blood flow to blood pressure and possibly to blood volume, cardiac output, and viscosity. These parameters can thus be altered to augment cerebral blood flow and prevent cerebral infarction. Of the three components of hemodynamic therapy, induced hypertension has the most sound scientific basis. Vasospasm and SAH are associated with regional and time-dependent impairments in autoregulation. Induction of hypertension will directly augment cerebral blood flow under these circumstances. Although there is some disruption of the blood–brain barrier after SAH, concerns that adrenergic agents used to elevate blood pressure might cause cerebral vasoconstriction are probably exaggerated, and worsening of cerebral edema is usually not a problem.

The effects of hypervolemia on cerebral blood flow in patients with vasospasm are more complex, and it is not known at present what the mechanism of action of hypervolemia is and it is impossible to separate its effects from those induced by alteration of hematocrit (30). Increasing blood volume can increase cerebral blood flow, possibly as an effect of hemodilution that usually accompanies infusion of colloids or crystalloids necessary to increase volume. Alternatively, the associated increases in cardiac output may increase flow to ischemic areas of brain that no longer possess ''autoregulation'' in response to changes in cardiac output. As with induced hypertension, aggravation of cerebral edema and intracranial pressure with hypervolemia seems to be uncommon.

Finally, hemodilution may have beneficial, as well as deleterious, effects in patients with vasospasm. Decreasing hematocrit decreases the oxygen-carrying capacity of the blood and decreases oxygen delivery to the brain. There is no question that reducing hematocrit, either from above normal to normal or from normal to below normal, increases cerebral blood flow. The question is whether the increase in flow is due to reduced oxygen delivery to the brain or to regulation of blood flow by viscosity (ie, lower viscosity improves blood rheology so that less blood flow is required for the same tissue demand). Evidence suggests that in normal animal and human brain, both mechanisms are important, with perhaps the reduction in oxygen content of the blood being more influential (3,30,31). The situation may differ in ischemic brain, and firm recommendations cannot be made, although positron emission tomography studies of SAH patients have concluded that flow may be augmented because less oxygen is getting to the brain (31).

We believe that the most important aspect of hemodynamic therapy is elevation of the blood pressure to >150 mm Hg systolic and often up to a maximum of 200–240 mm Hg systolic if the aneurysm was clipped. If the aneurysm is not clipped, a lower maximum systolic blood pressure is aimed for but the exact level will depend on the overall clinical picture. Maintenance of normo- or hypervolemia is required to induce hypertension, and this is achieved with infusions of crystalloid, albumin, plasma, or packed erythrocytes. The central venous pressure should be maintained at 10–12 mm Hg and the pulmonary capillary wedge pressure at 15–18 mm Hg. A central venous catheter is usually adequate, but a Swan-Ganz catheter is indicated in patients who require inotropes or who have other medical indications for more invasive monitoring. The hematocrit usually drifts down in these patients, but it is recommended to keep it >33%. In patients who are deteriorating from vasospasm, the progressive and rapid implementation of induced hypertension and moderate degrees of hypervolemia will often result in clinical improvement. Complications of hemodynamic therapy develop in up to 25% of patients and include, in order of decreasing frequency, pulmonary edema, aneurysm rebleeding, hemorrhagic infarction, dilutional hyponatremia, coagulopathy, and complications of central venous catheterization.

Summary of Current Vasospasm Treatment

Patients with SAH generally are monitored in an intensive care or stepdown unit especially during the time of risk of vasospasm. Most patients are kept in hospital after SAH for at least 7–10 days. Optimum vasospasm therapy includes aneurysm clipping as soon as possible after SAH. Hypovolemia, hypotension, increased intracranial pressure, hyponatremia, and antifibrinolytics are avoided. Amost all patients receive calcium channel antagonists. Treatment depends on many factors including the time of presentation after SAH,

the risk of vasospasm as assessed by the amount of blood on the CT scan, and the presence on angiography of established vasospasm with or without ischemia.

Treatment Within 3 Days of SAH

Patients with acute hydrocephalus or intracerebral hematomas associated with brain herniation require emergency surgery if they are operative candidates. Otherwise, patients in clinical grades 1–4 undergo urgent surgery for aneurysm obliteration. Delayed surgery or endovascular therapy is preferred for some giant and more difficult posterior circulation aneurysms. Early aneurysm clipping facilitates optimal management of vasospasm and is not associated with an increased risk of surgical complications. If the CT scan does not show SAH, then nimodipine may not be necessary and all that may be required is avoidance of adverse factors. Otherwise, patients receive nimodipine, 60 mg orally every 4 hours and at least 3 L/d fluid. The hematocrit is maintained >33%. The decision to insert a central venous line early should be individualized, since complications occur in up to 10% of cases and there is a progressive increase in infection rate with time. If a Swan-Ganz catheter is placed immediately after SAH, it will already have been in place for 7–8 days by the time it is required for management of symptomatic vasospasm.

In patients with focal or diffuse thick clots on CT scan, particular attention should be paid to keeping the systolic blood pressure >150–160 mm Hg. Transcranial Doppler ultrasound (TCD) recording of middle cerebral artery flow velocities may be obtained daily. It is important to obtain baseline studies soon after SAH and to take into account the intracranial pressure when interpreting the velocities.

Delayed Neurologic Deterioration

A CT scan and a peripheral blood specimen should be obtained to detect causes of deterioration. Intracranial pressure should be normal to optimize cerebral perfusion. Blood pressure should be elevated until the deficit improves. Hypervolemia may be instituted after placing at least a central venous catheter and sometimes a Swan-Ganz catheter. The hematocrit should be >33% to optimize oxygen-carrying capacity. Supplemental oxygen may be used. TCD should confirm that the deficit is due to vasospasm, and if this is not consistent, then the deficit should be confirmed with an angiogram. Intraarterial papaverine and transluminal angioplasty are therapeutic options if a clinically significant deficit does not improve with hypertension and hypervolemia and if there is no hypodensity on the CT scan.

Presentation During Vasospasm (Days 4–12 Post-SAH)

Adverse factors should be avoided and all patients should receive nimodipine. The admission angiogram should be reviewed for evidence of vasospasm. Although surgery has been avoided during this interval, there is little evidence that surgery precipitates vasospasm, and the poor outcome of patients who undergo surgery during this time may be due to the effects of brain retraction and cardiovascular fluctuations on the marginally perfused brain. With fluid loading and attention to blood pressure, immediate aneurysm clipping can be carried out in the face of vasospasm, unless the patient has developed a focal neurologic deficit or is in poor condition from the effects of the SAH or from severe, diffuse vasospasm. In some of these latter cases, immediate surgery, hemodynamic therapy, and angioplasty under the same anesthetic may improve outcome.

REFERENCES

1. Dorsch NWC, King MT. A review of cerebral vasospasm in aneurysmal subarachnoid hemorrhage. Part 1: Incidence and effects. *J Clin Neurosci* 1994;1:19–26.
2. Haley EC Jr, Kassell NF, Torner JC, et al. The International Cooperative Study on the Timing of Aneurysm Surgery. A randomized controlled trial of high-dose intravenous nicardipine in aneurysmal subarachnoid hemorrhage: A report of the cooperative aneurysm study. *J Neurosurg* 1993;78:537–547.
3. Macdonald RL. Cerebral vasospasm. *Neurosurg Quart* 1995;5:73–97.
4. Kassell NF, Torner JC, Haley EC, et al. The International Cooperative Study on the Timing of Aneurysm Surgery. I: Overall mangement results. *J Neurosurg* 1990;73:18–36.
5. Weir BK. *Aneurysms Affecting the Nervous System.* Baltimore: Williams & Wilkins, 1987.
6. Disney L, Weir B, Grace M, and the Canadian Nimodipine Study Group. Factors influencing the outcome of aneurysm rupture in poor grade patients: A prospective series. *Neurosurgery* 1988;23:1–9.
7. Fisher CM, Kistler JP, Davis JM. Relation of cerebral vasospasm to subarachnoid hemorrhage visualized by computerized tomographic scanning. *Neurosurgery* 1980;6:1–9.
8. Vermeulen M, Lindsay KW, Cheah MF, et al. Antifibrinolytic treatment in subarachnoid hemorrhage. *N Engl J Med* 1984;311:432–437.
9. Macdonald RL, Weir BKA. A review of hemoglobin and the pathogenesis of cerebral vasospasm. *Stroke* 1991;22:971–982.
10. Cosentino F, Katusic ZS. Does endothelin-1 play a role in the pathogenesis of vasospasm? *Stroke* 1994;25:904–908.
11. Hara H, Nosko M, Weir B. Cerebral perivascular nerves in subarachnoid hemorrhage: A histochemical and immunohistochemical study. *J Neurosurg* 1986;65:531–539.
12. Peterson JW, Kwun BD, Teramura A, et al. Immunological reaction against the aging human subarachnoid erythrocyte. A model for the onset of cerebral vasospasm after subarachnoid hemorrhage. *J Neurosurg* 1989;71:718–726.
13. Vorkapic P, Bevan RD, Bevan JA. Longitudinal time course of reversible and irreversible components of chronic cerebrovasospasm in the rabbit basilar artery. *J Neurosurg* 1991;74:951–955.
14. Voldby B. Pathophysiology of subarachnoid hemorrhage. Experimental and clinical data. *Acta Neurochir (Wien)* 1988;45(suppl):1–6.
15. Grubb RL Jr, Raichle ME, Eichling JO, Gado MH. Effects of subarachnoid hemorrhage on cerebral blood volume, blood flow, and oxygen utilization in humans. *J Neurosurg* 1977;44:446–452.
16. Carpenter DA, Grubb RL Jr, Tempel LW, Powers WJ. Cerebral oxygen metabolism after aneurysmal subarachnoid hemorrhage. *J Cereb Blood Flow Metab* 1991;11:837–844.
17. Sloan MA, Haley EC Jr, Kassell NF, et al. Sensitivity and specificity of transcranial Doppler ultrasonography in the diagnosis of vasospasm following subarachnoid hemorrhage. *Neurology* 1989;39:1514–1518.
18. Laumer R, Steinmeier R, Gonner F, Vogtmann T, Priem R, Fahlbusch R. Cerebral hemodynamics in subarachnoid hemorrhage evaluated by transcranial Doppler sonography. Part 1. Reliability of flow velocities in clinical management. *Neurosurgery* 1993;33:1–9.
19. Leblanc R, Lozano AM, van der Rest M, Guttmann RD. Absence of collagen deficiency in familial cerebral aneurysms. *J Neurosurg* 1989;70:837–840.
20. Juvela S, Hillbom M, Numminen H, Koskinen P. Cigarette smoking and alcohol consumption as risk factors for aneurysmal subarachnoid hemorrhage. *Stroke* 1993;24:639–646.
21. Tettenborn D, Dycka J. Prevention and treatment of delayed ischemic dysfunction in patients with aneurysmal subarachnoid hemorrhage. *Stroke* 1990;21(suppl IV):IV85–IV89.
22. Haley EC Jr, Kassell NF, Torner JC, et al. A randomized trial of two doses of nicardipine in aneurysmal subarachnoid hemorrhage. A report of the cooperative aneurysm study. *J Neurosurg* 1994;80:788–796.
23. Shibuya M, Suzuki Y, Sugita K, et al. Effect of AT877 on cerebral vasospasm after aneurysmal subarachnoid hemorrhage. Results of a prospective placebo-controlled double-blind trial. *J Neurosurg* 1992;76:571–577.
24. Haley EC, Kassell NF, Alves WW, et al. The International Cooperative Study of the Timing of Aneurysm Surgery. Phase II trial of tirilazad in aneurysmal subarachnoid hemorrhage. A report of the cooperative aneurysm study. *J Neurosurg* 1995;82:786–790.
25. Kassell N, Haley EC Jr, Alves W, Hansen CA. Phase III trial of tirilazad in aneurysmal subarachnoid hemorrhage (abstract). *J Neurosurg* 1994;80:383A.
26. Kassell NF, Helm G, Simmons N, Phillips CD, Cail WS. Treatment of cerebral vasospasm with intra-arterial papaverine. *J Neurosurg* 1992;77:848–852.
27. Macdonald RL, Weir BK. Management of vasospasm: Tissue plasminogen activator. In: Ratcheson RA, Wirth FP, eds. *Ruptured Cerebral Aneurysms: Perioperative Management.* Baltimore: Williams & Wilkins, 1994:168–181.
28. Findlay JM, Kassell NF, Weir BKA, et al. A randomized trial of intraoperative, intracisternal tissue plasminogen activator for prevention of vasospasm. *Neurosurgery* 1995;37:168–178.
29. Eskridge JM, Newell DW, Pendleton GA. Transluminal angioplasty for treatment of vasospasm. In: Winn HR, Mayberg MR, eds. *Cerebral Vasospasm.* Philadelphia: W. B. Saunders, 1990;1:387–399. Neurosurgery Clinics of North America.
30. Tranmer BI, Keller TS, Kindt GW, Archer D. Loss of cerebral regulation during cardiac output variations in focal cerebral ischemia. *J Neurosurg* 1992;77:253–259.
31. Hino A, Mizukawa N, Tenjin H, et al. Postoperative hemodynamic and metabolic changes in patients with subarachnoid hemorrhage. *Stroke* 1989;20:1504–1510.

Cerebrovascular Disease, edited by H. Hunt Batjer.
Lippincott-Raven Publishers, Philadelphia © 1997.

CHAPTER 90

Subarachnoid Hemorrhage: Perioperative Critical Management

Daniel S. Kanter and Philip E. Stieg

Due to advances in operative techniques and the advent of early surgery, most of the mortality and morbidity from subarachnoid hemorrhage (SAH) occurs before the patient arrives at the hospital or in the perioperative intensive care unit (ICU) period. Prehospital injury is very difficult to prevent, but careful ICU care can alleviate deaths and neurologic injury. General guidelines for the overall management of aneurysmal SAH are available (1). In this chapter, we will describe our approach to the basic issues in perioperative care of the patient with SAH.

INITIAL ASSESSMENT AND STABILIZATION

One in four patients with SAH arrives in the emergency room with a depressed level of consciousness (2). Some are intubated in the field, and occasionally patients are pharmacologically paralyzed and/or sedated for air evacuation. All such patients need careful attention to their respiratory and hemodynamic status on arrival. The first minute should be occupied with assessing whether the patient appears to be moving sufficient quantities of air and whether there is a stable heart rate, acceptable blood pressure, and signs of adequate tissue perfusion.

The initial neurologic examination includes assessment of the level of arousal and observation for spontaneous movement. The basic historical information can be quickly elicited, and the patient's orientation, mental coherence, and ability to follow commands determined. Pupillary size, shape, reactivity, and extraocular movements should be noted. Motor tone at this point is usually normal to flaccid

D. S. Kanter: Neurology/Neurosurgery Intensive Care Unit and Department of Neurology, Brigham and Women's Hospital, Harvard Medical School, Boston, Massachusetts 02115.

P. E. Stieg: Cerebrovascular Surgery and Division of Neurosurgery, Brigham and Women's Hospital and Children's Hospital, Harvard Medical School, Boston, Massachusetts 02115.

except in patients who are posturing. Reflexes are often brisk, and the presence of Babinski's sign should be recorded. The motor abilities of poorly responsive patients can be elicited with noxious stimuli such as a nasal tickle, sternal rub, or pressure over the nail beds. At this point, the patient can be graded based on the Hunt and Hess scale provided that the examination is not clouded by sedatives, paralytics, or hydrocephalus.

Once the initial assessment is complete, the blood pressure must be stabilized and the patient's airway-protective abilities evaluated. If oral secretions are pooling in the mouth, aspiration pneumonia is a significant risk and elective intubation is advised. In patients who are somnolent with a weak cough and gag reflex, intubation for airway protection may be helpful, but there are few controlled studies to clarify the risks. Patients who rouse easily and have a vigorous cough and gag can probably be observed closely without intubation.

Initial Blood Pressure Control

There is a legitimate fear of aneurysmal rebleeding in the initial hours after SAH. The rebleeding rate is approximately 4% in the first 24 hours, and almost half of all rebleeding episodes are fatal. There is anecdotal evidence to suggest that some episodes of rebleeding are associated with elevated blood pressures, but recent studies of this issue have been inconclusive and a safe threshold for blood pressure has not been defined. Some suggest that variations in blood pressure may be more deleterious than specific absolute values. It is the practice of many centers to use intravenous antihypertensives to maintain a systolic blood pressure <150 mm Hg and mean arterial blood pressure <100–110 mm Hg in a patient with SAH from an unclipped aneurysm, but there is much variation in these practices. Patients believed to be in symptomatic vasospasm are often maintained at higher

TABLE 1. *Parenteral antihypertensive agents*

Agent	Dose	Actions	Advantages	Cautions
Nitroprusside	0.25–10 μg/kg/min	Direct vasodilator	Potent; onset in seconds, lasts 3–5 min	Could raise ICP or CBF or contribute to "steal" phenomena; cyanide or thiocyanate toxicity may occur with prolonged use
Labetolol	10–80 mg at 10 min intervals; up to 300 mg maximum; or continuous drip of 2–8 mg/min	α- and β-adrenergic blocker	No effect on ICP or CBF	Lasts 2–4 h
Esmolol	500 μg/kg or more as a load; maintenance usually 50–200 μg/kg/min	β_1 antagonist	Half-life of 8 min	Bradycardia and congestive heart failure are potential side effects
Propranolol	1 mg under close monitoring	β-adrenergic blocker	No effect on ICP or CBF; decreases sympathetic tone	Contraindicated in obstructive airway disease or congestive heart failure; 3–5 h half-life
Enalaprilat	0.625–1.25 mg every 6 h	Angiotensin-converting enzyme inhibitor	No effect on ICP	Lasts 4–6 h
Hydralazine	10–20 mg every 4–6 h	Direct arterial vasodilator		May increase CBF and ICP; may last 4–6 h
Morphine sulfate or sedatives	2–5 mg IV	Agonists at opioid receptors	Produces analgesia; may decrease hypertension in response to pain	May depress neurologic and respiratory function

Key: ICP, intracranial pressure; CBF, cerebral blood flow.

blood pressures. Pain, vomiting, and agitation can elevate blood pressure above this range and should be promptly treated. Nursing interventions such as suctioning or medical procedures such as line placement can exacerbate hypertension and should be done carefully with adequate local anesthesia and short-acting sedatives.

Table 1 shows some parenteral drugs that are available for urgent reduction of blood pressure. We prefer sodium nitroprusside due to its rapid onset of action, short half-life, and potency. There is a theoretical concern about cerebral vasodilatation causing increased cerebral blood flow (CBF) and raised intracranial pressure (ICP). In patients with disordered autoregulation, a vasodilator could also cause steal from an area of poor perfusion. We have never seen a clear adverse clinical consequence of nitroprusside use in patients with SAH, but others argue strongly against its use in this setting. Many of our patients have indwelling ICP monitors, and nitroprusside use has not been seen to cause raised ICP. Labetalol is also an excellent drug for use in this context and is preferred by many due to its lack of effect on CBF and ICP. Esmolol is not generally potent enough in reducing blood pressure but does control tachycardia very well. Hydralazine and enalaprilat have half-lives that are too long for close control of labile blood pressure. Hydralazine, like nitroprusside, has the added theoretical risk of vasodilation causing raised ICP and CBF.

Diagnostic Tests

Most emergency departments have the capability to rapidly perform computed tomography (CT). This should be done promptly in any patient suspected of SAH or emergently in poorly responsive patients. Ventricular drainage for acute hydrocephalus can be life-saving, and imaging should not be delayed even if the diagnosis of SAH is clear. Because acute hemorrhage is readily seen on CT scans as hyperintense material, CT is still preferred over magnetic resonance imaging (MRI) as an acute imaging technique in SAH. MRI is superior in delineating anatomy, and MR angiography sequences can show aneurysms >2–3 mm in size. Newer MRI sequences may pick up subtle areas of bleeding, but on standard T1- and T2-weighted sequences, acute blood may be isointense and requires careful scrutiny to discern. MRI is also more readily degraded by patient motion, and extra precautions are necessary to scan patients requiring monitoring equipment or ventilatory support.

In one large series, CT scans were positive in 92% of patients with SAH who were scanned within 24 hours of the ictus. The sensitivity of CT declines with longer intervals from the original bleed. Hence, a lumbar puncture must be performed in patients with a history suspicious for SAH if the initial head CT scan is negative. Such patients usually have small volume bleeds and are awake and can relate an accurate history. Despite their appearance, they remain at risk for serious morbidity and death from rebleeding.

Once the presence of SAH has been established by CT or lumbar puncture, the source of the bleeding must be determined expeditiously. Angiography remains the gold-standard technique for defining intracranial aneurysms. Patients can be studied if they are on ventilators or vasoactive drips, and their medical and neurologic status can be readily monitored. Agitated patients can move excessively and require sedation to reduce the risk of an angiographic complication. Patients in known vasospasm should be studied with caution, as catheterization can induce some proximal vasospasm and the dye load through a stenotic vessel can induce ischemic symptoms. In situations where rapid neurologic deterioration is occurring, an angiogram may not be possible. Spiral CT has been shown to demonstrate aneurysms >3 mm (3). This is a rapid technique that is feasible in intubated and unstable patients who require emergent surgery.

INITIAL ICU MANAGEMENT

On arrival in the ICU, attention should first be directed to the adequacy of respiratory and circulatory function. Patients who are not intubated need to have their oxygenation, ventilation, and airway-protective abilities reassessed, because a patient with SAH can readily deteriorate within the first few hours after admission or during intrahospital transport. Intubated patients should have an arterial blood gas panel, and endotracheal tube position and cuff patency should be checked. Bucking or breathing against the ventilator should be avoided, as it leads to elevated intrathoracic pressures, decreased cardiac output, and increased ICP. Intermittent nasogastric suction should be started to decompress the stomach in all intubated patients.

A more detailed history, general physical examination, and neurologic assessment should be documented. Any changes since the first evaluation need to be carefully explained and identified as being due to either medications, rebleeding, hydrocephalus, seizures, or cerebral ischemia.

Many care decisions depend on an accurate assessment of the timing of the subarachnoid hemorrhage. Most alert patients recall an explosive sudden headache followed by syncope or near syncope. Some patients have a more subacute prodrome with intermittent or chronic headaches over days, and hence the original bleed date may not be known. In cases of uncertain timing, angiography should be performed both to document the vascular anatomy and to determine whether cerebral vasospasm is present. Transcranial Doppler ultrasonography (TCD) can also be used for this purpose, but it is less comprehensive and accurate as a screening test for vasospasm. The presence of vasospasm requires changes in blood pressure control and the initial fluid management to avoid further ischemia. These changes require careful balancing of risks in a patient with an unclipped aneurysm.

Once the patient is stabilized, a diagnosis established, and

the presence or absence of vasospasm determined, a decision can be made on the feasibility and timing of surgical clipping of the aneurysm.

Arterial and Venous Access

Arterial-line placement for continuous blood pressure monitoring is recommended for all patients with acute SAH. This allows continuous recording of blood pressure, with immediate recognition of significant changes by bedside monitoring equipment with appropriate alarms. This also allows ready access for arterial blood gases and other blood samples. The recommended site for arterial cannulation is the radial artery due to its accessibility, compressibility, and the presence of good collateral flow to the hand by ulnar branches. Permanent ischemic complications and catheter infections are rare with regular site changes. Our policy is to change the catheter to a new site every 5 days. Other sites of arterial cannulation are the femoral and axillary arteries. The brachial artery site is not recommended due to limited collaterals to the distal arm. Note that reflected systolic waves from the distal arterial tree can artifactually augment radial artery systolic pressure measurements. Resonance or damping in the circuit can also lead to inaccurate readings. In such cases, blood pressure readings determined with a cuff must be followed.

Central venous access is advisable for all patients who have had a recent aneurysmal SAH and is essential for those likely to require continuous drips of vasoactive medications or rapid manipulation of their volume status. Rebleeding can produce sudden and profound hemodynamic changes and immediate resuscitative measures are facilitated by central venous access.

Complications of central venous cannulation are directly correlated with the experience of the operator. Hence, the operator should choose the site with which he or she is most familiar. The internal jugular site has a low risk of pneumothorax and is compressible. Accidental carotid puncture, however, can occur, and the sterile dressings are harder to maintain in this location. In addition, poorly cooperative patients often require sedation to cannulate the internal jugular vein. The subclavian approach has a higher risk of pneumothorax (1–2% of insertion attempts) but requires less cooperation on the part of the patients and the dressings are easier to keep intact. This site does not allow adequate compression, so patients with coagulopathies should not have a subclavian line placed if other sites are available. Femoral vein sites are readily available in urgent situations but should only be used for a few days due to the risk of infectious and thrombotic complications.

Much controversy still surrounds the issue of whether scheduled changes of central venous lines are necessary to prevent local line infections or bacteremia. Our policy is to leave central venous catheters in place, unless the site looks infected or the patient has an unexplained fever, at which point cultures through the line are drawn. If the cultures are positive or if there remains any doubt about its sterility, the line is changed to a new site.

Prophylaxis Against Seizures

Approximately 10–25% of patients with SAH will have a seizure, with the highest risk in the first 24 hours after SAH. The incidence is higher with thicker cisternal blood and in association with rebleeding (4). A brief, limited seizure in an otherwise stable patient would normally not lead to any permanent injury. However, patients with SAH are at risk from the increased blood pressure, respiratory compromise, increased cerebral blood flow (CBF), and increased ICP associated with generalized seizure activity. The increased blood pressure and CBF may precipitate rebleeding in the presence of an unclipped aneurysm. It is our practice to place all patients with SAH on prophylactic anticonvulsants, until their aneurysm has been clipped and they are out of the ICU. We taper off the anticonvulsant over the next 1–3 months. The incidence of drug fever or rash from phenytoin is fairly common (5%), and if present, we switch to carbamazepine in patients taking oral medications or phenobarbital in patients still requiring intravenous medications.

Gastric Prophylaxis

Recent endoscopic studies in a general population of ICU patients have shown a high incidence of gastritis, but the occurrence of significant hemorrhage is uncommon—roughly less than 5%. Many observers have noted the occurrence of gastrointestinal (GI) bleeding after neurologic catastrophes, but the incidence among all patients with SAH is around 4%. Raised ICP influences gastrin secretion, and mucosal defenses are impaired. Some authors have noted a higher rate of GI bleeding with decreasing Glasgow Coma Scale scores (5). Concomitant use of steroids also impairs mucosal integrity, and decreased splanchnic blood flow from vasopressors can encourage ulcer formation as well. Cushing's ulcer refers to a severe ulcer after a serious neurologic event with a high rate of perforation. For unclear reasons, such events are much rarer in recent years. Gastritis and occult blood loss are common but rarely produce hemodynamic compromise. There is considerable debate about the optimal prophylactic approach to prevent GI bleeding, but we recommend that all patients with SAH receive H₂ blockers or sucralfate. Some feel that H₂ blockers increase the incidence of aspiration pneumonia by interfering with normal gastric acidity and leading to bacterial colonization of the stomach, thus increasing the infectivity of aspirated material. H₂ blockers can on rare occasions cause confusion in susceptible patients, usually the elderly. Once a patient is receiving continuous enteral feeding, continued GI prophylaxis is probably unnecessary.

Prophylaxis Against Deep Venous Thrombosis and Pulmonary Embolism

Pulmonary embolism is a serious threat to all hospitalized patients but especially those undergoing craniotomy or with neurologic impairment. Recent prospective studies in critically ill patients reveal a high incidence of unsuspected deep venous thromboses (DVTs) of the lower and even the upper extremities. The incidence of clinically recognized pulmonary embolism after SAH is approximately 1–2%, and the rate of clinically recognized DVT is approximately 2%. These latter figures include studies of patients receiving standard prophylactic measures. The safety of subcutaneous low-dose heparin has been demonstrated in a general neurosurgical population and did not lead to increased rebleeding in a population with intracerebral hemorrhage (6,7). Since the rebleeding rate is usually low in such patients, one cannot directly apply this experience to patients with SAH. Low-dose subcutaneous heparin should be freely employed after adequate aneurysmal clipping. Pneumatic compression boots should also be placed on all patients with SAH as soon as possible after admission, and their use should be continued in the operating room. If the patients have clinical signs of DVT on admission or have been immobile for a prolonged period, ultrasound screening of the lower-extremity veins should be done before the application of pneumatic compression boots. Given the poor sensitivity of the clinical examination for DVTs, we have recently begun screening all immobile patients in our unit with lower-extremity ultrasound on a weekly basis. Patients with positive studies are treated as described later in the chapter.

Ventricular Drainage and ICP Monitoring

Hydrocephalus develops in 20–25% of patients with SAH and is readily recognized on admission CT scans. However, after an initial scan with normal ventricles, hydrocephalus can develop abruptly, so patients who deteriorate after arrival require a repeat CT scan, even if the interval has only been a few hours. The clinical signs of hydrocephalus include headache and depressed level of consciousness. Hypertension is common, and in severe cases bradycardia, posturing, and respiratory depression can occur. Occasionally, patients will develop downward deviation of the eyes.

Once recognized, hydrocephalus should be promptly treated with insertion of a ventricular catheter. The burr hole is usually placed in the right frontal region 3 cm lateral to the midline just anterior to the coronal suture, and the ventricular catheter is passed into the lateral ventricle. Complications of insertion are uncommon and consist mainly of intraparenchymal hemorrhage. The tubing is generally tunneled under the scalp before exiting. It is then connected to a bag and drip chamber. The height of the outflow orifice dictates the pressure required for cerebrospinal fluid (CSF) to exit the skull via the ventricular drain. Hence, the ventricular drain height is usually set 10–20 cm above the external auditory meatus, which marks the level of the foramen of Monro. Patency of flow can be confirmed by brisk flow of CSF when the bag is momentarily lowered. In addition, the CSF waveform should have a prominent P_1 component, corresponding to systolic pulsations of the choroid plexus. Air in the tubing can dampen the waveform. Similarly, blood clots can impede CSF drainage and dampen the waveform.

Strict sterility of the drainage systems must be maintained at all times. Despite such precautions, infection remains a threat with prolonged use of ventricular catheters. The infection rate appears to rise with duration of catheter use and the presence of intraventricular hemorrhage. The effectiveness of prophylactic systemic or intrathecal antibiotics remains unclear, and local practices vary considerably. Our protocol is to change ventricular catheters to a new site after 5–7 days if prolonged drainage is required. We do not routinely employ intrathecal antibiotics but recommend systemic antibiotics just prior to catheter insertion and for 24 hours thereafter.

Subarachnoid bolts or epidural or subdural catheters are rarely used in patients with SAH. In most cases, patients with raised ICP after SAH require ventricular drainage, and a separate monitor is rarely necessary. Due to ease of use and a low complication rate, fiberoptic ICP monitors are recommended when ICP monitoring alone is desired. These have an extremely low complication rate.

Recording ICP waveforms over time (trend monitoring) can demonstrate cyclic variations in ICP. The most important to recognize are the plateau or A waves, which are ICP elevations >50 mm Hg and generally last 5–30 minutes. These are a hallmark of severely disordered cerebral autoregulation. They can be spontaneous or triggered by a variety of stimuli including suctioning or turning. They are rare after SAH except in grades IV and V patients. Treatment of raised ICP is discussed below.

Risk of Rebleeding

The risk of rebleeding is greatest in the first 24 hours after SAH (approximately 4%) and approaches 20% for the first 2–3 weeks. Rebleeding has a 50–70% mortality, and every effort should be made to avoid this devastating complication. Since most centers now routinely perform early surgery in aneurysm patients, rebleeding is a threat only for the shorter preoperative period in most patients. However, patients with incompletely clipped or inoperable aneurysms and those who are judged too ill to be taken to surgery due to poor neurologic grade or concurrent medical illnesses remain at significant risk for rebleeding. Undue excitement, sudden changes in blood pressure, or increased sympathetic tone due to pain, nursing manipulations, or emotional upset can precipitate rebleeding and should be avoided.

Careful blood pressure control is thought to lessen the risk of rebleeding, but this has not been established in a con-

trolled trial and the target blood pressure range remains a matter of conjecture. Most centers keep the mean arterial pressure <100–110 mm Hg and systolic blood pressure <150 mm Hg in patients with unclipped aneurysms. This becomes problematic if the patient becomes symptomatic from cerebral vasospasm or elevated velocities develop on TCD examinations. The most effective intervention to prevent rebleeding is surgical clipping, but if this is not feasible, some protection can be gained by partial or complete obliteration of the aneurysmal lumen via endovascular techniques. If new neurologic deficits develop secondary to symptomatic vasospasm, an elevated blood pressure may be necessary to prevent severe morbidity, even though the risk of rebleeding may be increased.

Antifibrinolytic therapy was widely used to reduce the risk of rebleeding before early surgery became widespread. By reducing plasmin activity, these agents stabilize fibrin clots including, presumably, the one in the aneurysmal tear. Several studies have shown mixed outcomes from using these agents. Rebleeding rates may be diminished, but overall results are unchanged due to increased ischemic complications (8,9). The adoption of early surgery has rendered these agents unnecessary in the majority of patients. For patients who cannot have early surgery, endovascular techniques are probably a safer means of reducing the risk of rebleeding without causing a generalized antifibrinolytic effect. Aminocaproic acid is the antifibrinolytic agent most widely used in the United States, and the dosing is generally a 5 g IV load followed by an IV infusion of 1–1.5 g/h. Complications besides thrombosis include myopathy, rhabdomyolysis, and possibly an increased risk of hydrocephalus.

Initial Electrolyte Disorders and Fluid Management

Electrolyte derangements in the first 48 hours after SAH are usually associated with disorders of total body water or are iatrogenic. Iatrogenic disorders include hyponatremia due to excessive intravenous fluids, hyperglycemia from glucocorticoids, and hypokalemia and hypophosphatemia due to respiratory alkalosis.

Alterations in total body water are common after SAH. Some patients have depleted total body water due to inadequate fluid intake from a prolonged period of neurologic impairment. This should be considered in any SAH patient found unconscious who has been unobserved for a period of 12 hours or more. The serum sodium level may be low, normal, or high, but there are usually other clues to volume depletion such as an elevated blood urea nitrogen/creatinine ratio, decreased skin turgor, and an elevated urine specific gravity.

The syndrome of inappropriate secretion of antidiuretic hormone (SIADH) and the cerebral salt-wasting syndrome constitute the principal disorders affecting serum sodium levels and osmolality after SAH. SIADH can be precipitated by hydrocephalus or direct injury to the pituitary–hypothalamic axis from the SAH or mass effect from an aneurysm. This is manifest by the continued production of ADH causing resorption of water in the collecting ducts of the kidney despite the development of low serum osmolality and excess total-body free water. The urine osmolality is characteristically higher than the serum osmolality despite the excess total-body free water. Treatment of this condition normally includes free-water restriction, but this can be dangerous in patients with SAH who are at risk for delayed cerebral ischemia. One important study demonstrated an infarction rate due to cerebral vasospasm of 81% in SAH patients with hyponatremia on fluid restriction (<1 L/d), compared with 33% in those with normal fluid intake (10). A safer and more specific approach is to provide isotonic fluids and remove excess free water as needed with furosemide or other diuretics, with careful monitoring of fluid balances. Demeclocycline is a tetracycline antibiotic that antagonizes the renal effects of ADH and can also be employed in these patients. Additionally, sodium chloride can be supplied in a concentrated form orally or via small amounts of IV 3% NaCl.

For SIADH to be truly "inappropriate," the total body water (or extracellular component) should be normal or increased. However, a significant proportion of patients with SAH (30–50%) have reduced extracellular fluid and hypovolemia. In such cases, continued ADH secretion may be appropriate to restore intravascular volume. There is evidence that ADH is secreted both appropriately (to restore extracellular volume) and inappropriately (with low osmolalities) in many patients with SAH and helps explain the mild hyponatremia found even in those patients with normal extracellular volume. One study of SAH patients treated with hypervolemia concluded that poorly understood humoral factors appear to cause both sodium loss and water retention (11).

The cerebral salt-wasting syndrome is difficult to diagnose definitively, and its pathophysiology is poorly understood. It may involve increased glomerular filtration leading to excessive sodium and water excretion in the urine, but elevated atrial natriuretic peptide, which promotes sodium and water excretion by the kidney, may play a role. It does not respond to fluid restriction and is best treated in a similar fashion to SIADH after SAH but with more emphasis on sodium replacement. Thus, fluid restriction should be avoided and isotonic fluids used with diuretics and sodium supplements as needed (12) (Table 2).

Hyponatremia after SAH has been associated with a poor prognosis, but this may reflect its increased occurrence with larger amounts of hemorrhage and with hydrocephalus. Hyponatremia per se can lead to seizures, and low serum osmolality can contribute to cerebral edema by promoting migration of fluid into brain cells. Hypovolemia (with or without hyponatremia) can contribute to worse outcomes by deleterious effects on cerebral perfusion in ischemic areas.

In the preoperative period, we suggest using maintenance intravenous fluids of 0.9% NaCl at 70–100 ml/h. Mild hyponatremia is usually of no consequence at this stage, and vigorous volume resuscitation or free-water compounds (5% dextrose or 0.45% saline) should be avoided. Postoperative fluid management is discussed below.

Iatrogenic hyponatremia may result from excessive administration of 0.45% NaCl with 5% dextrose or simply 5% dextrose solutions. Such fluids are hypotonic, especially after the rapid metabolism of the dextrose, and can lead to excess free water and a modest decline in the serum sodium. This is usually not clinically significant, but

TABLE 2. *Common disorders of sodium and extracellular fluid volume after subarachnoid hemorrhage*

Disorder	Mechanism	Diagnostic clues	Extracellular fluid volume	Serum sodium	Treatment
Volume depletion (dehydration)	Diminished oral intake due to prolonged unconsciousness	↑ BUN/creatinine ratio ↓ Skin turgor ↑ Urine specific gravity	Low	Low, normal, or high	Rehydrate with isotonic fluids NOTE: proceed cautiously with elevated ICP
Syndrome of inappropriate secretion of antidiuretic hormone (SIADH)	Hypothalamic–pituitary dysfunction	Urine osmolality > serum osmolality despite normal ECFV	Normal or high	Low	0.9% saline Furosemide to ↓ free water Demeclocycline 300 mg Q6h NaCl per NG tube IV 3% Saline
Cerebral "salt-wasting" syndrome	? ↑ GFR ? ↑ ANP	Resolves with infusions of isotonic fluids	Low	Low	0.9% saline Furosemide to ↓ free water Demeclocycline 300 mg Q6h NaCl per NG tube IV 3% Saline

Key: ECFV, extracellular fluid volume; GFR, glamerular filtration rate; ANP, atrial natripretic peptide.

this mechanism should be kept in mind in the evaluation of hyponatremia in the SAH patient. Large amounts of hypertonic saline can produce hypernatremia, but this fluid is rarely given except in cases of documented hyponatremia. Dexamethasone and other glucocorticoids are often given after SAH and can lead to hyperglycemia and produce pseudohyponatremia.

Respiratory or metabolic alkalosis produces a shift of potassium into cells as part of a potassium–hydrogen exchange and can lead to hypokalemia without potassium depletion. Diuretic use, excessive nasogastric suctioning, steroids, and diarrhea are the main causes of hypokalemia due to potassium depletion. Hypophosphatemia can be seen in patients who are aggressively hyperventilated for a neurologic catastrophe. This is due to phosphate influx into cells to supply the increased glycolysis associated with intracellular alkalosis.

Pharmacologic Agents to Reduce Delayed Neurologic Deficits

Nimodipine is the only medication specifically licensed for the prevention of delayed cerebral ischemia after SAH. Its use is based on several randomized studies showing improved outcome when given to SAH patients starting within 96 hours of the hemorrhage (13). No angiographic improvement in vasospasm is seen with the use of nimodipine. The mechanism of action presumably relates to reduced calcium entry into ischemic cells, although there could be an antivasospastic effect on collateral vessels that is too small to visualize on angiography. The oral dose is 60 mg every 4 hours. An intravenous form is available in Europe. The 60-mg dose can cause hypotension, which is counterproductive if patients have symptomatic vasospasm. In such cases, splitting the dose to 30 mg every 2 hours is advisable, although on rare occasions the medication has to be stopped altogether for recurrent hypotension.

Nicardipine is another dihydropyridine calcium antagonist and has been shown to reduce the incidence of symptomatic vasospasm after SAH (14). Overall outcomes were similar to placebo, presumably because the hypertensive-hypervolemic therapy was effective in reducing ischemic deficits in symptomatic patients. This therapy was more commonly employed in the placebo group. A recent trial of the 21-aminosteroid free-radical scavenger tirilazad mesylate (U-74006F) showed improved outcomes in some patients with SAH (those given the 2 mg/kg/d dose) (15).

Many neurosurgeons routinely use corticosteroids in patients with SAH, and the rationale for this is based on the role of white blood cells in the production of vasospasm. This approach has never been validated in a controlled trial in humans, and there are some theoretical reasons for caution. Elevated intracellular glucose levels in ischemic cells can promote lactate formation and intracellular acidosis. Other immunosuppressive agents such as

cyclosporine have also been tried in small series with inconclusive results.

Indications for Admission to the ICU

Patients with a recent SAH are at a significant risk for rebleeding, hydrocephalus, and seizures in the first days after their bleed. Such patients should be monitored in an ICU setting with a high nurse-to-patient ratio so that frequent neurologic evaluations can be done. These nurses should have specialized training in neurologic assessments to recognize early and subtle signs of neurologic deterioration so that appropriate interventions can be carried out. Patients with SAH who have depressed levels of consciousness or other significant deficits or who are at high risk for vasospasm are at the greatest risk for deterioration and often require one-to-one ICU nursing. All patients who require ventilatory support, continuous intravenous drips of vasoactive medications, or invasive monitoring need to be in an ICU or intermediate setting. Some patients who have a CT pattern characteristic of angiogram-negative SAH and have undergone angiography with no visible aneurysms can be managed in a less intensive setting. We do not believe that patients with SAH can be safely managed on a routine hospital ward until after their aneurysm is clipped and they are safely out of the period of significant risk of vasospasm.

Communication with Family Members

SAH is a frightening experience for patients and their families. The fact that this disorder strikes suddenly in healthy people makes adjustment to its occurrence that much more difficult. The patients and their families require careful explanations of the risks of this disorder, the treatment options, and possible outcomes. Opportunities to voice their questions and concerns can allay some of the anxieties and stress of this dangerous illness.

POSTOPERATIVE MANAGEMENT

Neurologic Assessment

The presence of anesthetic agents must be kept in mind in assessing the postoperative patient. The prolonged half-lives of anesthetic agents in elderly patients and those with liver and renal disease may lead to prolonged sedation, clouding their neurologic examination. Indeed, sufficiently high doses of anesthetic agents can abolish all visible neurologic functions including pupillary light responses. Of course, neuromuscular junction blockers can produce similar effects, abolishing all motor activity. When in doubt, an electric nerve stimulator can be used to assess for neuromuscular junction block. Similarly, an electroencephalogram may show slow cerebral electrical activity that, although nonspecific, may suggest lingering effects of anesthesia.

Management of Raised Intracranial Pressure

In a recent series, 24% of patients with SAH had evidence of raised intracranial pressure (ICP) (16). Raised ICP can lead to death or severe cerebral injury and must be recognized and aggressively treated. The ICP rises abruptly during aneurysmal ruptures and may lead directly to sudden death or precipitate an arrhythmia or respiratory arrest. The raised ICP can approach the mean arterial pressure and hence greatly diminish or arrest cerebral perfusion. This produces loss of consciousness or the presyncopal feelings experienced by many patients with SAH. If the ICP falls quickly, patients can awaken or recover. Prolonged reductions in cerebral perfusion may lead to permanent ischemic injury. Ischemia secondary to raised ICP may be the mechanism responsible for most of the neurologic impairment present shortly after SAH.

After the initial rupture, subsequent rises in ICP are due to either rebleeding, hydrocephalus, or cerebral edema. Hydrocephalus occurs when blood products or an inflammatory response impair cerebrospinal fluid (CSF) outflow through the ventricular system or the basal foramina or impede CSF resorption through the arachnoid villi. Cerebral edema occurs around parenchymal hematomas, in tissue subjected to ischemia or exposed to blood-breakdown products, or as a result of disordered cerebral autoregulation.

The hallmark of raised ICP is a diminished level of consciousness, but awake patients will almost universally describe the presence of headache. This somnolence is the most common and important finding in raised ICP but is unfortunately nonspecific. It could be due to medication effects, sleep interruption, or medical complications. The recognition of abnormal somnolence is crucial in diagnosing an unstable neurologic examination before a more obvious and perhaps permanent deficit, such as hemiplegia, ensues. Patients who are already comatose may posture or develop abrupt elevations in blood pressure, heart rate, or respirations. Rarely, bradycardia will occur. Posturing may be sufficiently vigorous that some observers mistake it for seizure activity.

These clinical signs are nonspecific and can result from the original SAH alone. The key characteristic will be the tempo and pattern of changes in the clinical examination. Patients with a single SAH should have a relatively stable or improving neurologic examination after admission, unless rebleeding, hydrocephalus, symptomatic vasospasm, cerebral edema, seizures, or medical complications develop. Neurologic worsening must be explained by one of these processes. Raised ICP accompanies many of them.

All patients with unexpected rises in ICP need emergent imaging studies to diagnose rebleeding or hydrocephalus, which may require immediate neurosurgical intervention. Radiographic evidence of raised ICP includes sulcal and cisternal effacement, lateral or vertical tissue shifts, or ventricular compression. However, these signs may be obscured by the presence of subarachnoid blood, which can render sulci and cisterns hyperintense or isodense to brain depending on the age of the blood.

To be successful, therapy for raised ICP must be instituted early—hence the importance of prompt recognition—and directed at the underlying process (eg, hydrocephalus), as well as the raised ICP itself (Table 3).

The range of normal ICP is 60–200 mm H_2O or 5–15 mm Hg. An ICP in the range of 15–20 mm Hg may be well tolerated and probably does not lead to significant cerebral injury. An ICP >20 mm Hg is abnormal and may lead to further ischemia, tissue injury, and herniation. Severely elevated ICP is highly correlated with death or significant neu-

TABLE 3. *Treatments for raised intracranial pressure (ICP) after subarachnoid hemorrhage*

CSF drainage	Works instantly; can titrate to desired ICP; may exacerbate tissue shifts.
Hyperventilation	Reduces ICP for a few hours. Not recommended for long-term or prophylactic use; may exacerbate ischemia by reducing cerebral blood flow Use a stepwise reduction in Pco_2 to the 30–35 mm Hg range and then 25–30 mm Hg, if necessary. Sustained hyperventilation should be tapered off over 8–24 hours
Mannitol	Dose (0.25–1.0 g/kg) every 4–8 h. Hold for serum osmolality >320 mOsm/kg H_2O or acceptable ICPs. When discontinuing use, tapering is advised to avoid a rebound increase in ICP. Furosemide 10–20 mg every 8–12 h only when euvolemia is carefully maintained.
Dexamethasone	Use mainly in cases of vasogenic edema, postsurgical cases.
Pentobarbital	Boluses of 50–100 mg for specific ICP elevations or a drip with 5–15 mg/kg loading dose and then 1–5 mg/kg/h. Hypotension is common and pressors are often necessary, especially to maintain cerebral perfusion pressure. Reductions in blood pressure may be deleterious in patients with vasospasm. Intubation, mechanical ventilation, and arterial and central lines are necessary for continuous infusions.
Head position	ICP generally falls with the head raised 30°. Some patients suffer a fall in cerebral perfusion in this position.
Hypothermia	Mild hypothermia (32–34°C) may reduce ICP with negligible side effects.
Factors that aggravate ICP	Endotracheal suctioning and intubation; pain; fever; "bucking" the ventilator; and occasionally nitrates and calcium channel blockers.

rologic impairment. Hence, every reasonable means should be employed to maintain the ICP <20 mm Hg.

CSF Drainage

Hydrocephalus develops in 20–25% of patients with SAH. In such patients, the quickest and most reliable therapeutic maneuver for raised ICP is CSF drainage. Drainage of several milliliters of CSF can dramatically lower the ICP. In patients with impaired CSF absorption over the arachnoid villi and no focal hematomas or focal swelling, lumbar drainage may be enough to control hydrocephalus and raised ICP.

In most ventricular catheter setups, a stopcock can be turned to switch between CSF drainage or ICP monitoring alone. The height of the reservoir outflow port should be set 10–20 cm above the foramen of Monro (using the external auditory meatus as a landmark) to avoid overdrainage. Drainage of CSF implies that the ICP is rising above the level of the outflow height. Note that most transducer and ventricular drain setups do not allow accurate determinations of ICP with the system open to drainage. It has to be clamped momentarily to allow accurate readings. A low ICP value can be due to occlusions or damping. Thus, it is important to visualize good ICP waveforms and to demonstrate catheter patency and unimpeded flow.

Hyperventilation

Hyperventilation is a very effective short-term treatment for raised ICP. Hyperventilation raises the CSF and extracellular pH, which induces cerebral vasoconstriction. This lowers the cerebral blood volume and hence ICP. Cerebral vasoconstriction may be deleterious in patients with SAH who are at risk for symptomatic vasospasm and should only be used when other approaches fail. Moreover, hyperventilation only lowers ICP for a few hours at most and hence is ineffective in treating persistently elevated ICP. The common practice of prophylactic hyperventilation in the face of coma or possibly rising ICP is now being questioned in view of the short-term effect of hyperventilation and its possibly deleterious effects on cerebral perfusion. A recent randomized trial in head-injury patients showed no benefit from prophylactic hyperventilation (17). In SAH patients, we recommend placement of an ICP-monitoring device and using short episodes of hyperventilation only for specific rises in ICP that cannot be treated with CSF drainage. The extracellular pH equilibrates quickly so that sudden normocapnia (after therapeutic hypocapnia) produces vasodilatation, just as sudden hypercapnia does under normal circumstances. Hence, when prolonged hyperventilation is discontinued, it should be tapered off over hours to prevent a rebound increase in ICP.

Mannitol and Furosemide

Mannitol is an osmotic diuretic that reduces ICP by reducing extravascular fluid and possibly by a vasoconstrictive effect. The latter may be related to its ability to improve perfusion by decreasing blood viscosity and improving red blood cell deformability. These changes can improve tissue perfusion, which can result in an overall decrease in cerebral blood flow by a feedback mechanism. There are few studies of mannitol use after SAH, but there has been a randomized, controlled study of mannitol use in intraparenchymal hematomas that found no benefit. There are some data to suggest that continuous low-dose mannitol may be helpful in ischemia due to mannitol's ability to improve perfusion through decreased blood viscosity and red blood cell deformability (18). Since fluid balance is so tenuous after SAH, the volume status, osmolality, and electrolytes have to be followed extremely closely when mannitol is used in this setting.

The duration of mannitol's effect on ICP varies depending on the dose and clinical situation. Higher doses last longer, but there is a risk of pulmonary edema, hypovolemia, and hypernatremia. Most centers are using lower doses of mannitol and titrating them to measured ICP values, if available, and serum osmolality. The osmotic effects of mannitol cease to be effective in a few days due to production of idiogenic osmoles by cerebral cells. Furosemide potentiates the effect of mannitol on ICP, perhaps in part by lowering CSF production. Furosemide use can be deleterious, however, as it frequently leads to hypovolemia, which can diminish cerebral perfusion. There is a theoretical concern about mannitol use with extensive blood–brain barrier disruption because it could extravasate into tissue and contribute to edema formation.

The diuresis that occurs with mannitol use can be harmful in the setting of vasospasm. Euvolemia or therapeutic hypervolemia must be scrupulously maintained in patients with SAH. We do not advocate routine use of mannitol, but rather it should be employed for specific rises in ICP as an adjunct to other measures.

Dexamethasone for Raised Intracranial Pressure

While there is some evidence in animal models of an effect of steroids on the development of vasospasm, the effects in nonspecific elevations of ICP are more elusive. Overall, there is little evidence that steroids cause a significant reduction in ICP related to trauma or hemorrhage. One randomized study examined steroid effects in patients with intraparenchymal hematomas and found no benefits. SAH is a different disease and may produce a more widespread cortical injury, but at present there are no adequate studies supporting a beneficial effect on ICP. There is empiric evidence that dexamethasone is helpful in reducing vasogenic edema from brain tumors and perhaps edema secondary to surgical manipulation. Some postoperative SAH patients have swelling and hypointensities on CT scan that may be edema or areas of infarction. Many physicians employ dexamethasone in such circumstances to reduce edema or in cases of raised

ICP. This approach may be helpful for postsurgical edema but has never been proven effective for raised ICP in general. There are some theoretical reasons to suspect that it may be harmful to ischemic or injured cells due to elevated intracellular glucose levels that can increase lactate formation and intracellular acidosis. High-dose steroids may also exacerbate gastrointestinal bleeding and predispose patients to infection. (The merits of dexamethasone in treatment or prevention of vasospasm are discussed above.) We recommend dexamethasone mainly for postsurgical edema and not as a general therapy for raised ICP.

Barbiturates

Barbiturates can lower ICP presumably by reducing cerebral metabolism and blood flow. In the operating room, barbiturates are often used to reduce metabolic demands during interruptions of arterial flow or as an adjunct to complete circulatory arrest for complex aneurysm operations. Patients with SAH may have areas of ischemia and disordered autoregulation. Reducing metabolism may reduce the metabolic demands and risk of ischemia, but if the reduction in blood flow is disproportionate, ischemia might be worsened. Barbiturates frequently reduce mean arterial pressures through a myocardial-depressant effect. Such reductions in blood pressure can be detrimental in patients with symptomatic vasospasm. Some have used prolonged barbiturate infusions for patients with raised ICP due to infarcts or intraoperative events after SAH, but clear evidence of benefit is lacking (19). Their presence complicates neurologic assessments and brain-death determinations.

Head Position

There continues to be controversy about the ideal head position for patients with raised ICP. For most patients with head injury, for which we have the best data, the ICP will diminish with head elevation to 30° (20). In some, however, cerebral perfusion pressure may fall disproportionately in this position, which could be harmful. The head should not be turned, and the neck should be free of bindings to prevent impaired jugular venous outflow, which can raise ICP.

Hypothermia

Hypothermia is also employed intraoperatively to reduce ischemic injury during cross-clamping of arteries, and there is experimental evidence for a subsequent reduction in ischemic damage. Several small studies have described the use of mild hypothermia (32–34°C) for patients with raised ICP after head injury. The therapeutic benefits in patients with symptomatic vasospasm in the ICU setting have not been studied, but this may be a helpful technique.

Other Factors Aggravating Raised Intracranial Pressure

Endotracheal suctioning and intubation can cause profound elevations in ICP. Pain, fever, and breathing against the ventilator breaths (''bucking'') can also raise ICP. Certain drugs commonly used in ICUs such as sodium nitroprusside and calcium channel blockers have caused ICP elevations in small groups of patients.

Surveillance for Vasospasm and Assessment of Risk

With the trend toward early surgery, vasospasm has become the major danger of the postoperative period, affecting 20–30% of patients with SAH overall. Symptomatic vasospasm characteristically occurs in the days 4–14 interval after SAH. Maximal symptoms are usually during days 7–10, and this is when vigilance must be highest.

Several studies have correlated the risk of symptomatic vasospasm with the size of blood clots in the basal cisterns and fissures on initial imaging studies. Dense clots greater than 5 mm × 3 mm in the horizontal plane are associated with a much higher risk of delayed cerebral ischemia (21). Hence, the initial CT scan in conjunction with other factors allows clinicians to group patients into broad categories based on their risk of symptomatic vasospasm (see Table 5).

The development of transcranial Doppler (TCD) ultrasound technology has made a major contribution to early identification of patients at risk for vasospasm and has helped guide therapeutic interventions. TCD flow-velocity values that are rising 50 cm/sec/d in the early post-SAH period are highly correlated with the subsequent development of symptomatic vasospasm. The specificity and sensitivity of TCD for middle cerebral artery vasospasm approaches 90%. Most centers with TCD capabilities study patients with SAH on postbleed day 7 and at more frequent or even daily intervals for patients judged to be at higher risk. We recommend TCD evaluation on days 4 and 7 in all low-to-moderate risk patients and daily TCD for high-risk patients from days 4 to 10.

One aspect of surveillance that needs to be emphasized is close neurologic observation. These patients can become hemiplegic over a few minutes, especially with blood pressure changes, and careful scrutiny by skilled nurses and physicians is crucial to prevent disabling deficits or death. Nighttimes are particularly dangerous. A patient who appears to be sleeping may be stirred only to reveal a depressed level of consciousness or new focal deficit. If at all possible, post-SAH patients at risk for symptomatic vasospasm should be cared for in a specialized ICU with extensive experience in recognizing and managing delayed cerebral ischemia.

Treatment and Prophylaxis of Vasospasm

It is now standard at most centers to place patients with symptomatic vasospasm on some form of hypertensive, hypervolemic, and hemodilution ("triple H") therapy, and some forms of this therapy are used prophylactically. Although this approach has never been proven in a randomized, controlled study, most experienced intensivists can attest to its effectiveness, if instituted early, in reversing new deficits from vasospasm. Prospective and retrospective series using historical controls have shown reduced mortality and neurologic deficits with elements of triple-H therapy (hemodilution is used infrequently at most centers) (22). However, there are risks associated with triple-H therapy including pulmonary edema, cardiac ischemia, electrolyte disturbances, coagulopathy, and specific complications of the necessary invasive monitoring lines and vasoactive drugs. Moreover, patients with large infarcts present before institution of hypervolemic therapy may develop severe cerebral edema or hemorrhagic transformation of their infarcts (23). There is also a risk of aneurysmal rebleeding in patients with unclipped aneurysms. Each component of triple-H therapy has not been adequately studied in isolation to determine specific risks and benefits, nor are the risks and benefits of combined approaches well delineated. This therapeutic approach does not alter the constricted diameters of vasospastic vessels but presumably improves cerebral perfusion through the vasospastic vessels or via collaterals. If successfully employed as a prophylactic approach, the patient will remain asymptomatic and only TCD or angiographic data will reveal the extent and course of vasospastic changes.

Hypertension in the Treatment and Prophylaxis of Vasospasm

Hypertension is the most important and most straightforward approach to prophylaxis and treatment of symptomatic vasospasm. It is our impression that this is the most potent bedside treatment that can be used to reverse or prevent delayed cerebral ischemia. The effects are presumably based on the presence of disordered autoregulation in ischemic areas that are then passively subject to changes in perfusion based on systemic blood pressures. The induction of hypertension is more readily accomplished in the setting of hyper-

volemia, so a combined approach is ideal. Institutions vary considerably in their blood pressure targets for hypertensive therapy, and there are no randomized studies favoring one approach. There are studies confirming resolution of cerebral ischemia with induced hypertension, but regional effects can vary (24). Appropriate caution should be exercised when inducing hypertension in patients with unclipped aneurysms and in those with areas of frank infarction. Aneurysmal rupture, hemorrhagic transformation, and cerebral edema are potential complications.

We employ phenylephrine as our first-line agent, which acts via pure α_1-adrenergic effects to cause arterial vasoconstriction. There is often a reflex bradycardia. If this fails to result in an acceptable blood pressure, additional crystalloid or colloid should first be given to make sure that patients have plentiful intravascular volume. We then generally add dopamine, which has dose-dependent β- and α-adrenergic effects and can produce arterial vasoconstriction, increased cardiac output, and an increased heart rate. This agent can produce tachycardia and arrhythmias. Our third-line agent is norepinephrine, and on rare occasions we use boluses or drips of epinephrine to induce hypertension. All of these agents can lead to mesenteric, peripheral, or cardiac ischemia, and these complications are common in medical ICU patients. We have been impressed, however, by the relative safety of phenylephrine in patients with SAH, and serious noncerebral ischemic complications of these agents are quite rare in typical SAH patients. Since vasospasm is so obviously harmful, vasopressors should be employed in a symptomatic patient without hesitation, given the rarity of permanent noncerebral side effects (Table 4).

Hypervolemia in the Treatment and Prophylaxis of Vasospasm

Hypervolemia is an important adjunctive therapy in vasospasm treatment and prevention, but its individual contribution is unclear, as noted above. The basis for its effect could be improved perfusion by decreased blood viscosity and increased cardiac output. Hypervolemia also potentiates the

TABLE 4. *Agents used to induce hypertension in patients with subarachnoid hemorrhage*

Agent	Mechanism	Dose range	Adverse effects
Phenylephrine	α-Adrenergic effect to induce vasoconstriction	2–10 μg/kg/min	Bradycardia mesenteric, cardiac, peripheral ischemia
Dopamine	Dose dependent α-adrenergic arterial vasoconstriction; also β-adrenergic inotropic and chronotropic effects	2–20 μg/kg/min	Tachycardia and arrhythmias; mesenteric, cardiac, and peripheral ischemia
Norepinephrine	α- and β-adrenergic effects	2 μg/min and titrate upwards	Tachycardia and arrhythmias; mesenteric, cardiac, and peripheral ischemia
Epinephrine	α- and β-adrenergic effects	1–4 μg/min	Tachycardia and arrhythmias; mesenteric, cardiac, and peripheral ischemia

effect of vasopressors and results in higher systemic blood pressures. Some argue, however, that isovolemic hemodilution alone can lead to improved cerebral perfusion (25). In clinical settings, hypervolemic therapy is almost always employed with hypertensive therapy. The procedures and targets vary from center to center. We describe our approach below.

Monitoring the volume status is more difficult than it sounds. Readily available information includes daily weight, intake and output measurements, blood urea nitrogen and creatinine values, and urine specific gravities. Since most of our patients have central venous lines, central venous pressure (CVP) measurements are readily available and provide a rough guide to right-heart filling pressures and, by inference, volume status. However, the accuracy of this inference has been questioned based on other direct measurements of blood volume. Pulmonary capillary wedge pressures (PCWPs) may be more accurate measures of volume status than CVPs, but these measurements are more difficult to obtain and are fraught with technical errors in 20–30% of cases. Some use pulmonary artery catheters to monitor cardiac output or guide therapy with inotropic agents in an effort to improve cardiac output. Others place pulmonary artery catheters to detect signs of myocardial ischemia or pulmonary edema, which can be precipitated by aggressive hypertensive-hypervolemic therapy. Given the absence of proven efficacy of combined hypertensive-hypervolemic therapy and its individual components, the relative contribution of pulmonary artery catheters to the care of SAH patients is difficult to delineate. Hence, we do not know whether raising the cardiac output by a certain amount is necessary or effective in specific patients with SAH. Certainly in patients in whom myocardial ischemia, sepsis, or left heart failure are suspected, a pulmonary artery catheter can be essential for diagnostic or therapeutic reasons. We first manipulate volume status based on clinical findings, intake–output charts, and daily weights and manipulate blood pressures based on arterial-line readings. We employ pulmonary artery catheters in patients who have signs of myocardial ischemia or left heart failure, sepsis, or severe pulmonary edema or who remain symptomatic from vasospasm. Other centers routinely use pulmonary artery catheters in patients with vasospasm.

Protocol for the Treatment and Prophylaxis of Symptomatic Vasospasm (Table 5)

We categorize patients based on their perceived risk for delayed cerebral ischemia and adjust their volume status and blood pressure targets accordingly. Patients with minimal amounts of SAH in clinical grades I–II and nonsuspicious findings on TCD are judged to be at low risk for symptomatic vasospasm and are kept hypervolemic with crystalloid solutions. Our protocol is to avoid antihypertensives, and vasopressors are not routinely used in low-risk patients. Moderate-risk patients are those grade I–II patients with moderate-sized blood collections and elevated TCD recordings up to mean middle cerebral artery velocities of 130 cm/sec. Moderate-risk patients are given vasopressors to maintain their systolic blood pressure in the 160–180 mm Hg range, and they are kept hypervolemic with crystalloid and colloid infusions as needed. High-risk patients have extensive clots, are in grades III–V, or have TCD values that are rising by 50 cm/sec/d or have mean middle cerebral artery velocities >130 cm/sec. Our high-risk patients are maintained with a systolic blood pressure around 180 mm Hg, but this is quickly raised to 190–210 mm Hg if there is any question of deterioration. They are also kept hypervolemic with crystalloid and colloid solutions. If symptoms of delayed cerebral ischemia are present in any group, their blood pressure

TABLE 5. *Prophylaxis of symptomatic vasospasm by risk category*

Risk of vasospasm	Clinical criteria	TCD surveillance	Hypervolemia[a]	Induced hypertension
Low	No dense clots Grade I–II TCDs with mean MCA velocities <100 cm/sec	Days 4, 7	Crystalloid (5% dextrose NS or NS) at 100–125 ml/h starting on post-SAH day 3	None, unless symptomatic
Moderate	Grade I–II Thick clots on CT but <5 × 3 mm in horizontal plane TCDs with mean MCA velocities <130 cm/sec	Days 4, 7	Crystalloid 100–125 ml/h plus albumin 5% prn to keep CVP >8 or PCWP >10–14	Keep systolic BP in 160–180 mm Hg range
High	Grades III–V Dense clots >5 × 3 mm TCDs rising 25% or 50 cm/d Mean MCA velocities >130 cm/sec	Days 3–10 or longer	Crystalloid 100–125 ml/h plus albumin 5% prn to keep CVP >10 or PCWP >12–14	Systolic BP around 180 mm Hg; increase to 190–210 mm Hg if necessary

Key: TCD, transcranial Doppler ultrasound; MCA, middle cerebral artery; CVP, cerebral venous pressure; NS, 0.990 NaCl; PCWP, pulmonary capillary wedge pressure.
[a] This table contains prophylactic regimens. Fluids are increased for symptomatic patients. All fluid regimens are adjusted based on weights, intake/outputs, and presence of hyponatremia.

targets are immediately raised in an aggressive fashion. Mean arterial pressures are technically more accurate than systolic pressures, but we have found that systolic pressures are more familiar to the staff and afford adequate reliability and reproducibility.

Hypervolemic-hypertensive therapy is usually begun on post-SAH day 3 and continued through days 7–10 or longer, depending on the clinical course and TCD results. The use of colloid remains debatable but is an easier and quicker (albeit more expensive) way to induce hypervolemia. There is no convincing evidence that isotonic crystalloids cause more brain edema than is seen with the use of colloids. Significant amounts of infused albumin do end up in the extravascular space.

Neurologic deterioration from symptomatic vasospasm can lead to large and devastating infarctions and death. Although the first manifestations of a deterioration are subtle, they should be treated as medical emergencies. Physicians must be in constant attendance until the symptoms resolve and the patients stabilize. If additional volume infusions and aggressive induced hypertension to a systolic blood pressure of 200–210 mm Hg fail to reverse the deficits within 2 hours, interventional neuroradiologic approaches should be used where available. As experience with angioplasty with or without papaverine infusion grows, it is becoming clear that refractory symptomatic vasospasm can be successfully treated by these techniques with a low rate of complications.

Fluid Management

SIADH and the cerebral salt-wasting syndrome are the principal disorders of serum sodium and extracellular fluid volume in the post- and preoperative period (see discussion above). Their treatment involves the use of crystalloid and colloid solutions, as well as diuretics and salt supplements. These fluids are also used in the postoperative period to treat patients who are at risk for symptomatic vasospasm or who have already developed symptoms.

Crystalloid fluids contain sodium, which dictates their distribution in the body. Hence, 80% of crystalloid fluids will be distributed to extravascular extracellular spaces, and 20% will remain in the vascular compartment. Colloids, on the other hand, consist of large-molecular-weight substances, such as albumin, that do not readily cross into the extravascular space. If equivalent amounts of colloid and crystalloid are infused, the colloid will result in a greater intravascular expansion, although colloid does extravasate eventually. Both fluid types can cause pulmonary edema, and patients receiving large amounts of either one need to be monitored carefully. One of the indications for pulmonary artery catheters after SAH is to allow monitoring of PCWPs, which are often close to 20 mm Hg when pulmonary edema develops. Large amounts of colloid infusions can also cause a dilutional hyponatremia. Large amounts of crystalloid infusions

can cause a mild metabolic acidosis. Cerebral edema does not appear more common with one fluid type than another.

Patients after SAH are at risk for cerebral edema and raised intracranial pressure (ICP), and they may have areas of infarction. Hypotonic or free-water infusions may exacerbate edema and should be avoided. The crystalloids we recommend are 0.9% NaCl with or without 5% dextrose. For colloids we use 5% albumin but in urgent situations sometimes choose 25% albumin. We use crystalloid as our main maintenance fluid, as well as for inducing hypervolemia. However, some patients have excessive diuresis due to the salt-wasting syndrome or due to normal homeostatic mechanisms. In such cases, we resort to intermittent colloid infusions to maintain a positive fluid balance and keep the CVP >10 mm Hg or the PCWP 12–14 mm Hg. If a patient develops a new neurologic deficit from vasospasm, we will immediately induce hypertension with pressors and often use 5% albumin to immediately expand the intravascular volume. In rare cases, vasopressin is needed to maintain adequate intravascular volume in patients with severe vasospasm.

These CVP and PCWP goals are arbitrary and, in many cases, inaccurate estimates of intravascular volume. This management approach has not been proven to reduce delayed cerebral ischemia. These pressure values should only be used along with other measures of volume status such as weight and intake–output records. Moreover, younger patients are often very resistant to developing high CVPs or PCWPs, regardless of the fluids used. Hypervolemic therapy should not target a particular CVP or PCWP reading to be achieved at all costs. Instead, in the absence of more elaborate volume studies, we should seek particular numerical goals only if they make sense clinically, while we remain cognizant of the inaccuracies of our invasive measurements in estimating intravascular volume.

We taper off the hypervolemic therapy once a patient has passed postbleed days 7–10 without incident or after TCD and other imaging studies place them in a low-risk category at day 7.

Respiratory Issues

Aspiration pneumonia occurs in approximately 20% of SAH patients and is more common in those with depressed levels of consciousness or bulbar weakness and in those who are intubated. In an intubated patient, the diagnosis can be complicated, since bacterial colonization of the trachea is common and positive sputum cultures alone do not signify a pneumonia requiring treatment. The classic findings of pneumonia include consolidation on physical examination, an infiltrate on chest radiograph, and a positive sputum culture. Since intubated patients may have colonized sputum, other features such as chest X-ray findings, fever, an elevated white blood cell count, increased oxygen requirement, and a change in the character of the sputum are the defining features. After the patient has been hospitalized for more than 48 hours, the pneumonia must be considered hospital-acquired, and broad coverage for gram-negative and anaerobic organisms must be considered. We do not favor prophylactic antibiotics for pneumonia because they tend to select resistant organisms for a subsequent respiratory infection.

Whether pneumonia is present or not, pulmonary toilet is an important feature of the ICU care of patients with SAH. Many have depressed levels of consciousness and oropharyngeal secretions may need to be suctioned by the nursing staff at frequent intervals. The supine posture and shallow breaths contribute to atelectasis, and chest physical therapy and incentive spirometry can address these problems.

Patients with severe bulbar weakness or severely depressed levels of consciousness generally require tracheostomy for continued pulmonary toilet or ventilatory support. The proper timing for tracheostomy varies with each patient, but endotracheal intubation should normally be discontinued by 2–3 weeks after intubation to prevent tracheomalacia and stenosis.

Pulmonary edema has become more common in the SAH patient since the advent of hypervolemic therapy. Its frequency in a recent series was 23%. It is precipitated more readily by colloid than crystalloid infusions, but either fluid type can be the culprit. The classic findings include pink, frothy sputum, an increased oxygen requirement, extensive rales, diaphoresis, dyspnea, a third heart sound, and diffuse bilateral chest film haziness with vascular redistribution. The standard treatments for pulmonary edema include afterload reduction, morphine as a pulmonary vasodilator, and loop diuretics. By reducing the blood pressure and intravascular volume, these maneuvers may be dangerous in patients with vasospasm. Unfortunately, these patients are also the ones at greatest risk for pulmonary edema because of the large volume infusions and vasopressors they are given. This requires a delicate trade-off that weighs the severity of the pulmonary edema against the vasospasm risk or symptoms. If increased oxygen requirements are modest, we recommend small doses of diuretics, with careful attention that the blood pressure does not fall significantly. For life-threatening pulmonary edema, more extensive diuresis is required, but the neurologic examination must be carefully monitored and hypertensive therapy employed if deficits develop.

Neurogenic pulmonary edema is a rare disorder characterized by interstitial pulmonary edema that is thought to be neurally mediated. This is generally seen only with catastrophic intracranial events and may be due to loosening of tight junctions in pulmonary capillary endothelium. Left ventricular function is normal at onset, but cardiac dysfunction later develops in some patients (26). Treatment is supportive, although some advocate empiric trials of β-adrenergic blockers.

Pulmonary embolus remains a feared complication in all neurologically ill ICU patients, although it is diagnosed in fewer than 1%. (Prophylactic measures are described above.) The clinical diagnosis of pulmonary embolism is not highly reliable, as the key findings are fairly nonspecific. A severe alveolar–arteriolar oxygen gradient with a clear chest X-ray film point toward a diagnosis of pulmonary embolism. However, many of our patients have preexisting infiltrates or oxygen requirements, and the changes may be subtle. Mucus plugging is one of the most common causes of transient drops in oxygenation in the ICU, so vigorous suctioning should be done for any patient with sudden changes in oxygenation. Patients who are alert may describe new dyspnea and a new tachycardia, or signs of right heart strain may develop. When the situation is doubtful, a ventilation–perfusion scan or pulmonary angiography needs to be done to clarify the diagnosis, which has serious implications if undiscovered. In a patient with a clipped aneurysm, there is no contraindication to anticoagulation. If there is an unclipped aneurysm, we recommend placement of an inferior vena cava filter to prevent further embolization.

Adult respiratory distress syndrome (ARDS) is characterized by arteriolar hypoxemia from alveolar inflammation and edema in the absence of left heart failure. It is found most often after aspiration pneumonias and has a high mortality rate. This is a rare occurrence after SAH (4% in a recent series) (16). When present, high inspired-oxygen percentages and high amounts of positive end-expiratory pressures (PEEP) are often required. PEEP levels >15 cm H_2O can raise the ICP, and patients with ARDS have decreased pulmonary compliance leading to further elevations in intrathoracic pressure. Such pressures can be transmitted to the intracranial compartment via the venous system. We recommend ICP monitoring in patients with depressed levels of consciousness and high PEEP requirements.

Most patients with SAH require only modest amounts of inspired oxygen (21–40%) while intubated, unless aspiration pneumonia, pulmonary embolism, or ARDS is present. Since delayed cerebral ischemia is a risk, we recommend avoidance of hyperventilation, which produces cerebral vasoconstriction and respiratory alkalosis, unless its short-term use is urgently required for ICP management. In the absence of preexisting lung disease, most patients with SAH have no pulmonary contraindications to early extubation. Standard weaning criteria can be used, such as a negative inspiratory force >25 cm H_2O, a vital capacity >1 L, or a tidal volume of 8–10 ml/kg. The most vexing issue is whether drowsy patients will adequately protect their airway from secretions. Unfortunately, this cannot be determined with certainty while the patient is intubated. We generally look for an excellent cough to tracheal suctioning and manipulation and the presence of limb mobility and spontaneous eye opening. In many cases, one can only determine airway protection by extubating the patient and observing him or her closely.

Cardiac Dysfunction after SAH

It has been well documented that a variety of arrhythmias, conduction disturbances, and electrocardiographic (ECG) changes can be seen after SAH, ranging from intraventricular conduction delays, to T-wave inversions, to atrial and ventricular tachyarrhythmias (27). ECG abnormalities of any type may be present in 50–100% of patients after SAH. The incidence of arrhythmias in one recent series was 35%, but only 5% were described as life-threatening. Another study using 24-hour Holter monitoring detected arrhythmias in 91% of patients, and 41% were described as serious (28). Direct myocardial injury can occur after neurologic catastrophes such as SAH. This subendocardial necrosis is thought to be mediated by catecholamines released from nerve terminals and systemically. Not surprisingly, elevated creatine kinase MB fraction levels after SAH have been shown, and perhaps 10% of all SAH patients without prior cardiac disease have wall motion abnormalities by echocardiography. In our experience, such changes are rarely symptomatic. Ischemia and other standard causes for elevated creatine kinase MB fractions and cardiac dysfunction need to be vigorously sought. SAH-induced creatine kinase MB elevations and cardiac dysfunction should remain a diagnosis of exclusion. The overall incidence of myocardial infarction after SAH is approximately 1%, and this does not appear to be increased by hypervolemic-hypertensive therapy. The most frequent adverse effects from vasopressors are tachyarrhythmias from dopamine. The bradycardia from phenylephrine is rarely symptomatic. In patients with a history of coronary artery disease or diabetes who are at higher risk of silent ischemia, pulmonary artery catheters to monitor PCWP and cardiac outputs may be advisable. There have been some studies of prophylactic medications to prevent SAH-induced arrhythmias or myocardial injury, but more work is needed before such medications become part of the standard approach.

Infectious Disease Issues

Fever is a common occurrence after SAH and is present in at least 30% of patients (16). Initial attention should be focused on respiratory infections (aspiration pneumonia or nosocomial pneumonia) or a cerebrospinal fluid (CSF) or wound infection in patients who have an intracranial device or recently had a craniotomy. Another explanation is a drug fever, and phenytoin is a common culprit. Clues to a drug fever include a diffuse erythematous rash, elevated liver function tests, and an elevated eosinophil count. Despite vigorous efforts, however, there are many patients with fever in whom no cause can be found. This seems to be most common with extensive intraventricular hemorrhage and SAH. Hence, the supposition is that this is due to a chemical meningitis from the blood in the CSF. These patients are most prone to symptomatic vasospasm as well and generally have more indwelling lines and catheters to further complicate the fever work-up.

When an indwelling ventricular catheter is present, cell counts, Gram's stains, and cultures from the catheter must be part of any fever workup. Care should be taken not to flush the contents of the catheter back into the intracranial compartment after the sample is taken. The normal ratio of white blood cells (WBCs) to red blood cells in the CSF is approximately 1:500–700. Since the SAH may produce an elevated CSF WBC count and an elevated protein, the culture result is the most reliable way of determining the presence of a CSF infection. If in doubt, serial samples can be collected, and a rising CSF WBC is a strong indicator of infection since the blood-induced chemical meningitis rarely worsens beyond the first 2–3 days.

Nutritional Support

The intestinal villi begin to atrophy within 24 hours of stopping enteral feeding. Although a brief lack of feeding can be well tolerated in otherwise healthy patients, wound healing and the response to infection are improved by early nutritional support. Enteral feedings are recommended in all patients who are not able to swallow safely or who are intubated. Gastric retention can be treated with cisapride, which does not cause sedation or extrapyramidal side effects as metoclopramide does.

Agitation, Confusion, and Pain Control

Agitation and confusion are common after SAH and can be exacerbated by sedatives for procedures, anesthetic agents, and the sensory stimulation and sleep disruption of the ICU environment. A well meaning but potentially deleterious practice is the vigorous every 30–60-minute neurologic check in an otherwise stable patient. Certainly, vigilance must be maintained for rebleeding and other complications, but in elderly patients, those on multiple medications, or those with preexisting cognitive impairment, such interruptions in sleep can contribute to the agitated, confused state.

One of the first issues to face in the care of awake and alert patients after SAH is what to give them for headache. There is a legitimate fear that sedating medications will obscure the neurologic examination and delay recognition of deterioration. Nevertheless, patients can be safely given narcotics in an escalating fashion, as long as they are carefully assessed before each dose and the minimum dose necessary to make them comfortable is given. We generally start with acetaminophen with codeine by mouth and then proceed to morphine sulfate (2–5 mg IM or IV). This can be rapidly reversed as needed and is generally not too sedating. Occasionally, patients with a severe chemical meningitis will only respond to nonsteroidal antiinflammatory drugs or intravenous or oral steroids.

Agitation that compromises safe care can be difficult to control without oversedation. We favor short-acting sedatives such as fentanyl or midazolam for individual episodes of agitation. Often a longer period of calm is required, and we next use morphine sulfate or lorazepam. Haloperidol is an alternative that is generally very well tolerated in ICU patients (tardive dyskinesia is rarely seen after ICU use) and can be calming without inducing excessive drowsiness.

Timing for Transfer out of the ICU

Patients with SAH require close observation through the period of maximal risk for vasospasm. As a practical matter, an intact patient at low risk for symptomatic vasospasm with a clipped aneurysm after SAH can be watched in an intermediate-level setting if the nurse-to-patient ratio allows frequent neurologic monitoring by nurses experienced in the postoperative care of patients with SAH. In most hospitals, a specialized ICU is the most appropriate setting for all patients with SAH. Since delayed cerebral ischemia is the most serious complication, if patients remain medically and neurologically stable and their TCD studies are not suggestive of developing vasospasm, they can be transferred to a less intensive setting on days 7–10, depending on the particular case. In patients with unclipped aneurysms, we advise continuing ICU care until a definitive treatment for the aneurysm is performed.

REFERENCES

1. Mayberg MR, Batjer HH, Dacey R, et al. Guidelines for the management of aneurysmal subarachnoid hemorrhage. *Stroke* 1994;25: 2315–2328.
2. Kassell NF, Torner JC, Haley EC, et al. The International Cooperative Study on the Timing of Aneurysm Surgery. I: Overall management results. *J Neurosurg* 1990;73:18–36.
3. Schwartz RB, Tice HM, Hooten RT, et al. Evaluation of cerebral aneurysms with helical CT: Correlation with conventional angiography and MR angiography. *Radiology* 1994;192:717–722.
4. Hasan D, Schonck RSM, Avezaat CJJ, et al. Epileptic seizures after subarachnoid hemorrhage. *Ann Neurol* 1993;33:286–291.
5. Muller P, Jirsch D, D'Sousa J, Kerr C, Knapp C. Gastrointestinal bleeding after craniotomy: A retrospective review of 518 patients. *Can J Neurol Sci* 1988;15:384–387.
6. Barnett HG, Clifford JR, Llwellyn RC. Safety of mini-dose heparin administration in neurosurgical patients. *J Neurosurg* 1977;47:27–30.
7. Boeer A, Both E, Henze T, Prange HW. Early heparin therapy in patients with spontaneous intracerebral hemorrhage. *J Neurol Neurosurg Psychiatry* 1991;54:466–467.
8. Kassell NF, Torner JC, Adams HP Jr. Antifibrinolytic therapy in the acute period following aneurysmal subarachnoid hemorrhage: Preliminary observations from the cooperative aneurysm study. *J Neurosurg* 1984;61:225–230.
9. Tsementzis SA, Hitchcock ER, Meyer CH. Benefits and risks of antifibrinolytic therapy in the management of ruptured intracranial aneurysms: A double-blind placebo-controlled study. *Acta Neurochir (Wien)* 1990;102:1–10.
10. Wijdicks EFM, Vermeulen M, van Gijn J. Hyponatremia and cerebral infarction in patients with ruptured intracranial aneurysms: Is fluid restriction harmful? *Ann Neurol* 1985;17:137–140.
11. Diringer MN, Wu KC, Verbalis JG, Hanley DF. Hypervolemic therapy prevents volume contraction but not hyponatremia following subarachnoid hemorrhage. *Ann Neurol* 1992;31:543–550.
12. Mayer SA. Fluid management in subarachnoid hemorrhage. *Neurologist* 1995;1:71–85.
13. Pickard JD, Murray GD, Illingworth R, et al. Effect of oral nimodipine on cerebral infarction and outcome after subarachnoid hemorrhage: British aneurysm nimodipine trial. *BMJ* 1989;298:636–642.
14. Haley EC, Kassell NF, Torner JC, et al. A randomized controlled trial of high-dose intravenous nicardipine in aneurysmal subarachnoid hemorrhage. *J Neurosurg* 1993;78:537–547.
15. Haley EC, Kassell NF, Alves WM, et al. Phase II trial of tirilazad in aneurysmal subarachnoid hemorrhage. *J Neurosurg* 1995;82:786–790.
16. Solenski NJ, Haley EC, Kassell NF, et al. Medical complications of aneurysmal subarachnoid hemorrhage: A report of the multicenter, cooperative aneurysm study. *Crit Care Med* 1995;23:1007–1017.
17. Muizelaar JP, Marmarou A, Ward JD, et al. Adverse effects of prolonged hyperventilation in patients with severe head injury: A randomized clinical trial. *J Neurosurg* 1991;75:731–739.
18. Jafar JJ, Johns LM, Mullan SF. The effect of mannitol on cerebral blood flow. *J Neurosurg* 1986;64:754–759.
19. Kassell NF, Peerless SJ, Drake CG, et al. Treatment of ischemic deficits from cerebral vasospasm with high-dose barbiturate therapy. *Neurosurgery* 1980;7:593–597.
20. Feldman Z, Kanter MJ, Robertson CS, et al. Effect of head elevation on intracranial pressure, cerebral perfusion pressure, and cerebral blood flow in head-injured patients. *J Neurosurg* 1992;76:207–211.
21. Kistler JP, Crowell RM, Davis KR, et al. The relation of cerebral vasospasm to the extent and location of subarachnoid blood visualized by CT scan: A prospective study. *Neurology* 1983;33:424–436.
22. Awad IA, Carter LP, Spetzler RF, et al. Clinical vasospasm after subarachnoid hemorrhage: Response to hypervolemic hemodilution and arterial hypertension. *Stroke* 1987;18:365–372.
23. Shimoda M, Oda S, Tsugane R, Sata O. Intracranial complications of hypervolemic therapy in patients with a delayed ischemic deficit attributed to vasospasm. *J Neurosurg* 1993;78:423–429.
24. Darby JM, Yonas H, Marks EC, et al. Acute cerebral blood flow response to dopamine-induced hypertension after subarachnoid hemorrhage. *J Neurosurg* 1994;80:857–864.
25. Tu YK, Heros RC, Karacostas O, et al. Isovolemic hemodilution in experimental focal cerebral ischemia. Part 2: Effects on regional cerebral blood flow and size of infarction. *J Neurosurg* 1988;69:82–91.
26. Mayer SA, Fink ME, Homma S, et al. Cardiac injury associated with neurogenic pulmonary edema following subarachnoid hemorrhage. *Neurology* 1994;44:815–820.
27. Marion DW, Segal R, Thompson ME. Subarachnoid hemorrhage and the heart. *Neurosurgery* 1986;18:101–106.
28. Andreoli A, di Pasquale G, Pinelli G, et al. Subarachnoid hemorrhage: Frequency and severity of cardiac arrhythmias. *Stroke* 1987;18: 558–564.

Cerebrovascular Disease, edited by H. Hunt Batjer.
Lippincott-Raven Publishers, Philadelphia © 1997.

CHAPTER 91

Subarachnoid Hemorrhage: Concerns of the Neuroanesthesiologist

Eugene Ornstein, Ze'ev Shenkman, and William L. Young

The contribution of modern-day neuroanesthesiologists to the care of patients suffering from acute subarachnoid hemorrhage (SAH) begins with the preoperative period, when we are asked to assist with the medical evaluation and stabilization of the patient to facilitate appropriate early surgical intervention. Intraoperatively, our role is not solely to provide an asleep and immobile patient. Our specialized monitoring techniques and our cardiorespiratory and pharmacologic interventions help provide brain relaxation, a decrease in aneurysmal wall tension, neuroprotection, and the ability to begin or maintain prophylaxis or treatment against vasospasm. After the patient's rapid emergence from anesthesia, we may be asked to participate in intensive care management, with invasive hemodynamic monitoring and aggressive fluid and pharmacologic therapy. The patient with aneurysmal SAH benefits from a team approach in which there is communication between all members of the care team. Neurologists and neurosurgeons with a good understanding of the risks and benefits of the various available anesthetic options are in a better position to provide useful information to the neuroanesthesiologist, so that he or she can develop an anesthetic care plan for each individual patient.

THE PREOPERATIVE PERIOD

Depending on the length of time from hospital admission to surgery, the aneurysm patient may suffer from a wide variety of medical problems, in addition to the neurologic consequences of SAH. Among the disease processes associated with SAH are hypertension, arrhythmia and other electrocardiographic (ECG) abnormalities, pneumonia, pulmonary aspiration, pulmonary edema and other manifestations of cardiac or pulmonary dysfunction, anemia, gastrointestinal bleeding, deep vein thrombosis, syndrome of inappropriate secretion of antidiuretic hormone (SIADH), electrolyte imbalances, and diabetes mellitus.

Following SAH, the timing of aneurysm surgery is more likely to be determined on surgical- rather than anesthesia-based criteria. With the ever increasing appreciation of the benefits of early surgical clipping—specifically, the prevention of rebleeding and the facilitation of prophylaxis against vasospasm—the anesthesiologist is more likely to be faced with a patient whose medical status has not been optimized, or even properly assessed.

The anesthesiologist must utilize all obtainable information from the patient's past medical history, the current physical examination, and any diagnostic studies (complete blood count, electrolyte panel, ECG, and chest X-ray in all patients) from the preoperative period to develop an anesthetic plan that maximizes individual patient safety. For example, if the patient is noted to suffer from significant ischemic heart disease, it may be necessary to compromise the desired goal of rapid postoperative awakening and settle for a more gradual, but myocardially less stimulating, emergence from anesthesia. Similarly, if the patient is known to have had difficulty with intubation of the trachea in the past, an awake fiberoptic intubation following adequate topical anesthesia and suppression of autonomic reflexes might be considered instead of the more conventional intubation following the induction of general anesthesia.

The neuroanesthesiologist must also be aware of the effects of SAH on the pathophysiology of patients' preexisting diseases. For example, aneurysmal rupture is associated with a wide variety of ECG changes in 50–80% of patients (1). These changes usually occur within 14 days of SAH, lasting

E. Ornstein: Department of Anesthesiology Columbia University College of Physicians and Surgeons, New York, New York 10032.

Z. Shenkman: Department of Anesthesiology and Critical Care Medicine, Hadassah University Hospital and The Hebrew University, Jerusalem, Israel.

W. L. Young: Departments of Anesthesiology, Radiology, and Neurological Surgery, Columbia University College of Physicians and Surgeons, New York, New York 10032.

up to 6 weeks, and may include changes suggestive of myocardial ischemia, dysrrhythmias, and conduction abnormalities. ST-segment depression, T-wave inversion, or even new-onset Q waves are not infrequent. These abnormalities may persist, worsen, or first become apparent after surgery (2). Although some postmortem studies have shown microscopic damage to the subendocardium in these patients, ECG changes have also been found in patients with no evidence of cardiac disease. In fact, ECG changes in most patients are not associated with adverse cardiac or neurologic outcome (2) and are postulated to be due to autonomic hyperactivity resulting from hypothalamic dysfunction (3). The differentiation between SAH-associated and myocardial ischemia–related ECG changes can be difficult in a patient with coexisting cardiac disease. Thus, if the cardiac status of the neurosurgical patient is in doubt and it is inadvisable to await serial ECGs or serum myocardial enzyme levels, it may be possible to obtain, in a reasonable period of time, an echocardiographic evaluation of myocardial function. Even so, it should be noted that echocardiographic abnormalities in patients with SAH are more likely to be correlated to a poor neurologic outcome rather than a poor cardiovascular outcome (4).

The anesthesiologist's preoperative evaluation emphasizes the state of the neurologic, cardiovascular, pulmonary, and endocrine systems. Allergies, medications used, and the response to previous anesthetics should all be considered. A brief physical examination stressing the cardiorespiratory and neurologic systems is mandatory, as is assessment of the upper airway for signs of anticipated difficulty in tracheal intubation (5). Neurologic evaluation includes assessment of state of consciousness, presence of signs of meningeal irritation, signs of focal neurologic deficits, and the presence or absence of raised intracranial pressure. Cardiovascular assessment should include notation of the range of blood pressure (particularly neurologic deterioration during periods of hypotension), intravascular blood volume, electrolyte imbalance, and the ECG.

It is often necessary to balance the severity and ease of treatment of the patient's pathophysiologic states against the desire or need to expedite the definitive treatment of the intracranial process. For example, malignant hypertension should certainly be controlled prior to anesthetic induction. The prudence of delaying surgery to control hemodynamically insignificant arrhythmias, on the other hand, is questionable.

It may be difficult to decide whether to proceed with or postpone surgery in a patient with both SAH and active myocardial ischemia. The decision should be made on a case-by-case basis, with consideration of neurologic status and prognosis, the risk of vasospasm, rebleeding, and their sequelae, the complexity of the proposed operation, the impact of intraoperative hemodynamic manipulations, the patient's cardiac functional reserve, and the potential of optimizing processes such as ongoing ischemia, malignant dysrhythmias, and congestive heart failure.

Pulmonary evaluation should include a detailed history, physical examination, and a chest X-ray for detection of pathology particularly related to SAH, such as aspiration pneumonia or neurogenic pulmonary edema. In patients with a past history of significant pulmonary disease, an arterial blood sample for baseline blood gas analysis is useful, although this may be obtained in the operating room when the arterial catheter is placed.

Fever is not uncommon in patients with SAH and may be due to the presence of blood in the subarachnoid space. However, other etiologies should also be explored and treated because even small increases in temperature may have a negative impact on patient outcome (6).

The carotid arteries should be auscultated and gently palpated for the detection of possible occlusive disease. The peripheral vasculature should be assessed to anticipate problems with intravenous or arterial access, which may be common in cases in which antifibrinolytic therapy was used.

The presence of hyperglycemia, which may be due to preexisting diabetes mellitus or the perioperative use of glucocorticoids, should be noted, as high levels of blood glucose have been associated with worsening of ischemic brain damage (7).

The patient's preoperative drug regimen also needs to be considered. Patients receiving calcium channel blockers tend to arrive in the operating room with lower blood pressure than control patients (8), and these drugs may potentiate muscle relaxants and volatile anesthetics. Anticonvulsants will attenuate the effect of muscle relaxants if they have been administered for more than a week (9). Patients receiving carbamazepine, which is not available as an intravenous preparation, must be switched to another anticonvulsant. Vascular access problems, as well as propensity to deep venous thrombosis, may be expected in patients receiving antifibrinolytic drugs, which may also contribute to vasospasm and hydrocephalus. H_2-receptor blocking agents, particularly cimetidine, will delay the elimination of several anesthetic and other drugs metabolized by the liver. Glucocorticosteroids may contribute to hyperglycemia, hypertension, gastrointestinal bleeding, electrolyte imbalance, and inhibition of the hypothalamic–pituitary–adrenal axis.

Although blood pressure is often allowed to drift into the hypertensive range in order to alleviate the risk of vasospasm, it must be remembered that the difference between the systemic arterial pressure and the intracranial pressure is the major determinant of transmural pressure across the aneurysmal wall that promotes rerupture. Preoperative extreme hypertension is best treated with an agent such as labetalol, a combined α- and β-adrenergic receptor antagonist that appears to have no effect on cerebral blood flow (CBF) and intracranial pressure. An alternative drug recently shown to be effective in the treatment of hypertension is the calcium channel blocker, nicardipine (10). Vasodilators, such as sodium nitroprusside and hydralazine, may increase CBF and are best used only after the cranium has been opened, especially in the presence of intracranial hyperten-

TABLE 1. *Anesthetic goals*

1. Smooth rapid induction with minimal hemodynamic changes.
2. Brain relaxation.
3. Rapid and reversible blood pressure reduction, if required.
4. Minimal interference with electrophysiologic monitoring, if desired.
5. Brain protection: pharmacologic or hypothermic.
6. Deliberate hypertension, if needed in cases of collateral failure.
7. Preventive or therapeutic measures against vasospasm.
8. Management of patient with intraoperative rupture.
9. Rapid and smooth recovery from anesthesia, to enable timely neurologic evaluation.

sion. No matter what method is used to reduce blood pressure, one must realize that SAH may be associated with autoregulatory failure attributable to vasospastic vessels, such that CBF may fall to ischemic levels, at otherwise normal or even elevated levels of perfusion pressure. If the patient has a preoperative change in mental status or other neurologic changes as the blood pressure is reduced, the level of blood pressure at which these changes occur should be noted and the blood pressure should not be allowed to approach this level.

The use of preoperative sedation is controversial. Although it has been reported that a thorough preoperative visit has a greater anxiolytic effect than any premedication, many feel that particularly anxious patients may benefit from a small dose of a benzodiazepine, with minimal respiratory depression. Alternatively, incremental doses of a benzodiazepine such as midazolam may be intravenously administered when the patient arrives in operating room. Patients with altered sensorium should receive no sedative premedication.

With all the above considerations, it should be possible to plan an anesthetic that will achieve the goals in Table 1.

INDUCTION OF ANESTHESIA

It is our practice to monitor all patients scheduled for craniotomy with a pulse oximeter, five-lead ECG, capnograph, temperature probe, Foley catheter, peripheral nerve stimulator, and direct transduction of arterial pressure, most commonly from the radial artery. Arterial puncture is generally accomplished before the induction of anesthesia, with mild sedation and local anesthesia. This enables us to monitor blood pressure on a beat-to-beat basis, as well as obtain a baseline sample for blood gas analysis. In very anxious and uncooperative patients who are otherwise healthy, the availability of accurate and rapid noninvasive monitors of arterial pressure, expired carbon dioxide, and oxygen saturation enables us to delay arterial puncture until after the induction of general anesthesia.

A Swan-Ganz pulmonary artery catheter is inserted in patients who have had a recent SAH, especially in those with a poor clinical grade or large amounts of subarachnoid blood, as they are most likely to benefit from prophylactic measures against vasospasm. Since the prophylactic regimen most commonly used is a combination of calcium channel blocker therapy and hypertensive, hypervolemic, hemodilution ("triple H") therapy (11), these patients are at risk for the development of iatrogenic complications. When volume loading is used with or without inotropes such as dopamine or afterload enhancers such as phenylephrine, careful monitoring of cardiac filling pressures can minimize the possibility of fluid overload, dilutional hyponatermia, exacerbation of cerebral edema, congestive heart failure, pulmonary edema, and myocardial ischemia. The choice of pulmonary artery rather than central venous catheterization lies in both the added ability to determine cardiac output and the frequently poor correlation between these two pressures, especially in patients with significant myocardial or pulmonary dysfunction. In our opinion, the beneficial aspects of pulmonary artery catheterization outweigh the potential complications of its insertion.

Transesophageal echocardiography (TEE) is occasionally used in patients with myocardial or valvular heart disease for on-line determination of cardiac performance, cardiac chamber volume, and valvular function. We also find TEE to be a useful tool for verifying proper placement of intracardiac cannulae inserted via the femoral vessels in patients undergoing hypothermic cardiac arrest for complicated aneurysm surgery.

Electrophysiologic monitors such as electroencephalogram (EEG) and evoked potentials are often used to monitor cerebral function, especially during deliberate hypotension and temporary arterial occlusion, as well as the response to large doses of anesthetics administered for brain protection.

Besides these continuous monitors, intermittent determinations are made of hematocrit, serum glucose and electrolytes, and arterial blood gases throughout the surgical period.

The induction of anesthesia represents a critical period in the management of the patient with an unsecured intracranial aneurysm. A smooth induction of anesthesia is desired in order to avoid any hypertensive stress on the aneurysm, because rebleeding is a dramatic complication, second only to vasospasm as a cause of morbidity. Rupture during induction and tracheal intubation has been reported in up to 2% of patients (12). In fact, rebleeding may lead to an even greater increase in intracranial pressure (ICP) than the initial bleed, as blood spread is limited by the presence of adhesions and clot. Rerupture during anesthetic induction is associated with a markedly poorer prognosis than intraoperative rupture (12,13). It is equally important to avoid prolonged hypotension that may lower cerebral perfusion, particularly in patients with elevated ICP, vasospastic vessels and in areas with autoregulatory failure (see discussion of deliberate hypotension below).

The patient is precurarized with a small dose of a nondepolarizing muscle relaxant such as curare. This helps attenuate the rise in ICP and the development of fasciculations from succinylcholine chloride, if succinylcholine will be used to facilitate intubation. If, on the other hand, the trachea is to be intubated after a paralyzing dose of a nondepolarizer, precurarization decreases the onset time of relaxation, rapidly optimizing intubating conditions. Because we prefer a well controlled, gradual increase in anesthetic depth, it is our preference not to use succinylcholine, which has a rapid onset, short duration, and several undesirable side effects, except when airway patency and ease of intubation are somewhat in doubt. If intubation fails in these situations, succinylcholine will allow rapid recovery from paralysis, enabling spontaneous ventilation, after which fiberoptic intubation may be accomplished. It must be remembered that succinylcholine is contraindicated in patients with recent or progressive motor deficits, because the proliferation of extrajunctional cholinergic receptors predisposes the patient to possibly fatal hyperkalemia.

Our choice of nondepolarizing muscle relaxant is guided by the desire to avoid hemodynamic compromise. Thus, pancuronium bromide, which is associated with tachycardia and hypertension, and atracurium besylate, which may lead to histamine release and increased ICP, are generally not used. Several relaxants, such as vecuronium bromide, pipecuronium bromide, and doxacurium chloride lack significant cardiovascular effects.

In reasonably calm patients, a 3-minute period of preoxygenation by facemask is desirable as a means to denitrogenate the functional residual capacity and fill it with as much oxygen as possible. This increases the length of the apneic period before which oxygen desaturation begins, and thus attenuates the risk of hypoxemia in patients who are difficult both to intubate and to ventilate by facemask.

Induction of anesthesia is generally accomplished with one of the rapid-acting intravenous agents. We choose to use thiopental, with etomidate reserved for patients particularly at risk for hypotension. Propofol, benzodiazepines, and opioids may be used as supplementary or primary induction agents. Occasionally, in the patient with significant cardiac disease, a ''cardiac induction'' is used, whereby hemodynamic stability is achieved with large doses of opioids such as fentanyl citrate or fentanyl derivatives, thus sacrificing the goal of early emergence from anesthesia.

Anesthetic depth is adjusted either by additional induction agent with or without supplementary opioid analgesics or, alternatively, by a potent volatile anesthetic such as isoflurane. Graded stimulation is used to assess the depth of anesthesia, so that the response to oral airway insertion, bladder catheterization, and so on is noted before laryngoscopy. A variety of drugs may be administered to blunt the tachycardic, hypertensive response to intubation. Most commonly, intravenous lidocaine hydrochloride is used for this purpose, although additional anesthetics or an adrenergic antagonist (eg, esmolol, labetalol) may also be used. The patient is manually ventilated in the normocarbic range by bag and mask while the muscle relaxant takes effect (as assessed by peripheral nerve stimulation, thereby preventing bucking and coughing that may increase ICP), after which the patient is intubated. If it is noted that the blood pressure rises significantly at any point during laryngoscopy, the laryngoscope is removed, ventilation is resumed by bag and mask, and autonomic reflexes are suppressed with anesthetics or supplementary drugs (as mentioned above), before intubation is undertaken.

ANESTHESIA MAINTENANCE

Many factors enter into the choice of anesthetic agent to be used for the maintenance of anesthesia. Rapidity of onset and recovery and the effects on cerebral blood flow (CBF), autoregulation, cerebral metabolic rate, ICP, and the interpretability of the EEG and evoked potentials are all to be considered (see Chapter 11). In most cases, however, it should be noted that the choice of currently available agents, in and of itself, is probably inconsequential to the outcome of surgery, so that it is more important that the anesthesiologist use those agents with which he or she is most familiar and comfortable.

Those unfamiliar with neuroanesthesia are often surprised by how low the anesthetic requirements are for neurosurgery. Most of the neurosurgical procedure, with the exception of application of the head holder, skin incision and closure, craniotomy, and dural and cranial nerve manipulation, does not provide much somatic stimulation. Hence, blood pressure has a tendency to decrease as a result of the vasodilatory effects of the anesthetics. The pre- and intraoperative use of calcium channel blockers with rather long half-lives such as nimodipine, nicardipine (10,11), and diltiazem (14) may synergistically enhance the hypotensive effect.

Some anesthetic drugs, most notably thiopental, may offer brain protection during focal temporary ischemia by reducing cerebral metabolic rate or redistributing CBF (11). This may be most important when temporary arterial occlusion is being planned or if there is a focal decrease in regional CBF (eg, vasospasm).

Although opioid analgesics such as fentanyl or sufentanil citrate and volatile potent anesthetic agents such as isoflurane, halothane and, more recently, desflurane are most commonly used as supplements to nitrous oxide, there is some interest in the more widespread use of other intravenous anesthetics. As opposed to isoflurane, propofol, an agent used with or without a short-acting opioid such as alfentanil hydrochloride in total intravenous anesthesia, reduces CBF and ICP and maintains cerebral autoregulation (11,15). In addition, propofol combined with alfentanil is less likely to interfere with the interpretation of evoked-potentials data. Another intravenous agent, etomidate, may be neuroprotective but has not enjoyed widespread use due to concerns regarding adrenocortical suppression, which is more likely to be seen following prolonged continuous infusions.

Because recovery from anesthesia should be rapid, drugs with short half-lives and rapid dissipation of effect are desirable. In addition, these drugs are readily titratable to permit dose adjustment according to level of stimulation. Thus, desflurane with a faster recovery profile than other volatile anesthetics has been proposed as a suitable anesthetic for neurosurgical procedures (16). However, the use of desflurane during induction has been associated with significant increases in blood pressure (17). Continuous infusion of propofol has also been shown to be associated with more rapid recovery than either isoflurane or thiopental (11). Similarly, remifentanil, a new opioid with a very short half-life independent of the duration of infusion, is currently being evaluated for neuroanesthesia (18).

Although there is no need for muscle relaxation in a properly anesthetized patient during craniotomy, it is the practice of many anesthesiologists to maintain complete muscle relaxation during surgery to insure that there is no coughing or patient movement that can have devastating effects during microsurgery. Patients are mechanically ventilated, except in rare cases when spontaneous respiration is being used to monitor brainstem function (19). The $Paco_2$ is generally kept in the mildly hypocapnic range, at least until the neck of the aneurysm or the feeding vessel becomes accessible. This prevents a significant decrease in ICP and its associated increase in transmural pressure (with the skull closed), as well as preventing cerebral vasoconstriction in areas where perfusion pressure may already be near the ischemic threshold.

Fluid administration is determined by calculated maintenance requirements, blood loss, and urine output. Hypoosmolar solutions, such as 0.45% saline, are avoided so as to prevent cerebral edema, while glucose-containing solutions are no longer used because hyperglycemia potentiates brain injury following brain ischemia (7). The patient is kept normovolemic before clip application, after which the patient's filling pressures are raised into the high normal range to assist in the management or prevention of vasospasm.

One of the goals of neuroanesthesia is to provide a relaxed brain to minimize the brain-retraction pressure required to obtain adequate exposure of the aneurysm. Besides mannitol, furosemide, and lumbar cerebrospinal fluid (CSF) drainage, some of the intravenous anesthetics such as thiopental and propofol are known to decrease cerebral blood volume (11). The timing of mannitol administration is important but controversial. Commencement of infusion may be delayed until after removal of bone flap or dural reflection because of concerns for tearing of bridging veins, a potential increase in cerebral blood volume and flow, or a rapid decrease in ICP. It should be noted that although the onset is within 5 minutes, the peak effect occurs after 45 minutes. The cerebrovascular and central hemodynamic consequences of rapid administration of hypertonic mannitol should also be considered. Hypocarbia is also effective, although profound hypocarbia may lead to cerebral ischemia by increasing cerebrovascular resistance without a compensatory decrease in cerebral metabolic rate. Occasionally, when ICP seems high and difficult to treat, repositioning the patient in a slightly more head-up position with care that there is no impediment

to venous drainage may be more effective in lowering ICP than any pharmacologic maneuver. ICP should not be decreased too aggressively in light of the fact that a drop in ICP may have the same effect on transmural pressure as an increase in arterial pressure. Of note, mannitol may increase transmural pressure by affecting both ICP and arterial pressure. Similarly, too rapid removal of CSF may lead to a hypertensive and bradycardic response that will potentiate the increase in transmural pressure resulting from the decrease in ICP.

When the aneurysm is being approached, and before application of the clip, measures may be taken to reduce the transmural pressure across the aneurysmal wall. This decreases the risk of rupture, as well as the rate of bleeding if rupture should occur. In order to reduce the pressure within the dome of the aneurysm, the systemic arterial pressure may be reduced, or the surgeon may apply a temporary clip across the vessel feeding the aneurysm.

Until recently, deliberate controlled hypotension was in widespread use during aneurysm clipping and was considered a major advance in neurosurgery that improved outcome in the surgical management of intracranial aneurysms (20). Concerns regarding the risk of perioperative cerebral ischemia and infarction, however, have led to the abandonment of this technique in many centers (21). Even so, with meticulous attention to detail and the application of modern cardiovascular and neurophysiologic monitoring techniques, hypotension may still be indicated in selected patients. In fact, a recent survey of 41 North American aneurysm centers revealed that this technique is still utilized by approximately 48% of neuroanesthesiologists (22).

The ideal hypotensive agent is one that has a rapid onset and short duration and is readily titratable. One of the first drugs to be used for deliberate hypotension, trimethaphan camsylate, has lost popularity due to tachyphylaxis and the potential for vasoconstriction with regional disruption of CBF (23). Although sodium nitroprusside remains the most frequently used hypotensive drug, the presence of tachyphylaxis, rebound hypertension, reflex tachycardia, increased cerebral blood volume, increased pulmonary dead space, shunt, and the potential for cyanide toxicity have been impetus for the use of other drugs (24). High doses of isoflurane provide hypotension and may contribute to cerebroprotection. Unfortunately, although the onset is reasonably rapid, the hypotension occasionally persists for longer than the desired time, and a delayed emergence from anesthesia may be expected. Similarly, experiments with prostaglandin E_1, which does not lower regional CBF have revealed a persistent (60 minutes) effect despite rapid elimination from the circulation (23). Nitroglycerin, like nitroprusside may increase cerebral blood volume and ICP. Adenosine, studied extensively in Scandinavia, is extremely rapid in both onset and offset and has little effect on CBF in hyperventilated patients (25). Adenosine however is an extremely potent coronary vasodilator and may theoretically promote myocardial steal in some patients suffering from coronary artery disease, leading to ischemia. Esmolol, a cardioselective β-adrenergic receptor antagonist with a half-life of 9 minutes, is effective as a hypotensive agent, although the mechanism of action is via a decrease in cardiac output that may far exceed the decrease in blood pressure (26). A short-acting agent that possesses both α- and β-adrenergic antagonism would of course be preferable. Unfortunately, the only clinically available combined antagonist, labetalol, which has no direct effect on CBF, has a plasma half-life of approximately 5 hours and occasionally causes bradycardia postoperatively, limiting its usefulness intraoperatively when moment-to-moment blood pressure control is needed. Of note, most of the limitations of nitroprusside may be alleviated, if not eliminated, by the concurrent use of β-adrenergic blocking agents.

Of importance equal to or greater than the choice of hypotensive agent is the lowest level of blood pressure that will be tolerated. Unfortunately, the ischemic threshold for any individual patient cannot be predicted with certainty. The tolerance to hypotension is diminished in the presence of raised ICP, intracerebral hematoma, excessive brain retraction, vasospasm, or other states of depressed cerebral autoregulatory function. Other patients with a relative contraindication for deliberate hypotension include patients with chronic hypertension, especially when severe and uncontrolled, elderly patients, patients with cerebrovascular atherosclerotic disease, and those with pulmonary, hepatic, or renal dysfunction, anemia, and fever. In healthy patients with a good clinical grade, normal autoregulation is probably present. Thus, CBF should not decrease if mean arterial pressure is maintained >60 mm Hg. If necessary, it may be possible to allow mean arterial pressure to decrease as low as 40 mm Hg for short periods of time. The resulting decrease in CBF, theoretically, should not lead to cerebral ischemia. The speed with which hypotension is attained is also important. With a gradual drop in blood pressure, a lower mean arterial pressure may be tolerated. In hypertensive patients, with a rightward shift of their autoregulation curve, many believe that mean arterial pressure should not be allowed to decrease to levels lower than 60% of the baseline blood pressure.

Whether or not deliberate hypotension is planned, hypotensive agents should be readily available in case of aneurysmal rupture. The prognosis following intraoperative bleeding appears to be related to the speed with which hemostasis is achieved. Mean arterial pressure may need to be rapidly decreased to 50 mm Hg, or even 40 mm Hg, in order to decrease bleeding and facilitate surgical exposure to gain control of the aneurysm and its feeding vessels. It may be helpful to manually compress the ipsilateral common carotid artery. Thus, it is advisable to assure that these vessels are accessible when the patient is positioned. Fluid and blood should be rapidly administered as necessary to maintain hemodynamic stability.

Recently, temporary occlusion of the aneurysm's feeding vessel has become the more commonly used method to lower the pressure stress within the aneurysm. With temporary clipping, blood pressure is generally kept above awake levels, in order to reduce the likelihood of collateral circulatory failure. Because of the hypotensive effect of most anesthetics, it is occasionally necessary to augment the blood pressure pharmacologically. The α-adrenergic agonist, phenylephrine, is the most commonly used agent for this purpose. Despite the maintenance of normotension, temporary occlusion may be associated with the risk of cerebral ischemia that may progress to infarction (27). Thus, various cerebroprotective measures have been suggested. These include deliberate hypothermia, additional intravenous or inhalational anesthetics, lumbar CSF drainage, deliberate hypertension, and the administration of agents such as mannitol, phenytoin, and calcium channel blockers.

Approximately 24% of neuroanesthesiologists report using cerebral protective pharmacotherapy in all patients undergoing temporary vascular occlusion, while others selectively use these agents based either on surgical assessment of risk, changes in intraoperative EEG or evoked-potentials recordings, or metabolic changes such as jugular bulb oxygen saturation (22).

Currently, the most commonly used neuroprotective anesthetic is thiopental. Just before application of the temporary clip, thiopental is titrated to a deep burst suppression or isoelectric pattern on the EEG. Limiting the dose to burst suppression may preserve the ability to detect cerebral ischemia on the basis of progressive EEG changes. Although the utility of EEG analysis during aneurysm surgery has been challenged on the basis of poor sensitivity, the number of false negatives may be reduced by using cortical EEG electrodes that survey the area at greatest risk (28) (Fig. 1). Alternatively, evoked potentials may be used for detection of ischemia after large doses of thiopental (15). Thiopental in large doses has been thought to be a strong myocardial depressant. However, recent studies have shown that myocardial function and blood pressure are well maintained, provided that the patient is reasonably well hydrated (29). Even so, in patients with significant myocardial dysfunction or severe ischemic heart disease, etomidate is suggested as the agent of choice.

Hypothermia may be a greater factor in brain protection than the choice of anesthetic agent used. Various animal models have shown a direct correlation between brain or systemic temperature and histopathologic cerebral damage resulting from temporary global brain ischemia (30,31). Conversely, mild hyperthermia caused an increase in ischemic infarct volume and edema in animal models (6). Although both hypothermia and certain anesthetics are neuroprotective, the link between the cerebral metabolic depression and brain protection has recently been questioned (32).

In extremely complicated aneurysms, such as giant aneurysms of the vertebrobasilar system, there is renewed interest in the use of cardiopulmonary bypass and deep hypothermic circulatory arrest, whereby brain temperature is reduced to approximately 16°C. More commonly, temperature is main-

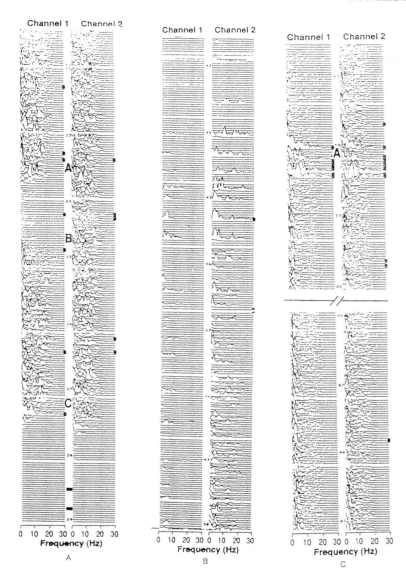

FIG. 1. EEG compressed spectral array from cortical electrodes in a patient with a middle cerebral artery (MCA) aneurysm. Each line depicts a 2-second epoch. **(A)** Trial occlusion of a main MCA branch at point *A* results in an immediate decrease in EEG power in posterior lead *(Ch. 1)*. Anterior lead *(Ch. 2)* is essentially unchanged probably due to collateral flow from the anterior cerebral artery. Ischemic change is rapidly reversed at point *B* after the release of occlusion. At point *C*, thiopental 400 mg is given, resulting in EEG isoelectricity, and the MCA was reoccluded for approximately 7 minutes. **(B)** Thiopental effect is beginning to dissipate with burst suppression. Even so, the amplitude in Ch. 1 is significantly lower than in Ch. 2. By minute 48, the asymmetry is unequivocal. The surgeons were informed, at which time it was noted that one of the permanent clips was partially occluding one of the main MCA branches. **(C)** Clip repositioning was completed at point *A*, immediately followed by resolution of the asymmetry. (From ref. 28, with permission.)

tained in the mildly hypothermic range (32–34°C), especially when temporary cerebrovascular occlusion is planned. Even this degree of hypothermia may suppress metabolism by 25–30%. The use of cooling blankets facilitates the drop of temperature to this level and may even result in more profound hypothermia than desired. It is thus prudent to terminate active cooling once a temperature of 34°C is reached. However, it has recently been shown that brain temperature may not be reflected by esophageal, blood, or tympanic membrane temperature (Fig. 2). The degree of discrepancy seems to be related to the rapidity of the temperature drop (33). Some difficulty has been noted in rewarming these patients to normothermic levels even with the use of heating blankets (34). Moreover, the brain may warm at a different rate than is reflected by the systemic temperature (33). Other potential disadvantages to hypothermia are postoperative shivering, delayed awakening, possible aggravation of myocardial ischemia, and coagulation and platelet disorders.

Deliberate hypertension may improve blood flow in cases of collateral failure during temporary clipping or in the presence of abnormalities in autoregulation, wherein regional CBF may become pressure passive (35) (Fig. 3). It may be necessary to elevate mean arterial pressure to levels >100 mm Hg and pulmonary capillary wedge pressure to 15 mm Hg (11). The benefits of this course of action must be balanced against the risk of rupture of this and other unsecured aneurysms that may be present, as well as against the effect on coexisting significant heart disease.

Whether or not deliberate hypotension or temporary clipping of the feeding vessel is utilized, extreme hypocarbia is to be avoided in order to avoid further vasoconstriction and ischemia in already compromised brain regions (11).

Once the aneurysm is clipped, more aggressive therapy toward the prevention or treatment of vasospasm may be instituted. Intravascular volume is increased, blood pressure is raised to the high-normal range by intravascular volume

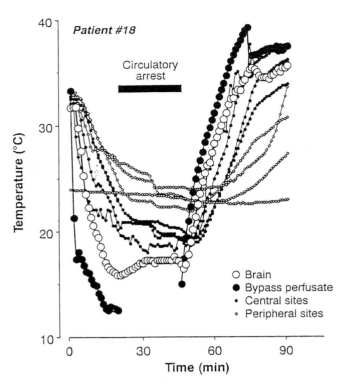

FIG. 2. Temperature vs. time relationship in a patient with giant aneurysm undergoing cardiopulmonary bypass and deep hypothermic arrest. Central sites are nasopharynx, tympanic membrane, esophagus, and pulmonary artery. Peripheral sites are bladder, rectum, axilla, and sole of foot. The slowest cooling sites were tympanic membrane and esophagus. (From ref. 33, with permission.)

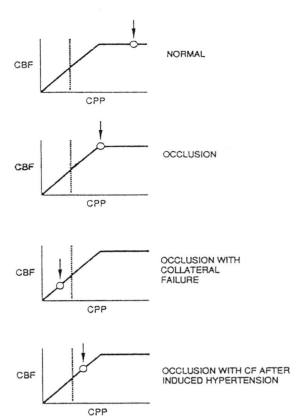

FIG. 3. Induced hypertension model. **(A)** Operating state during normal autoregulation. **(B)** With temporary occlusion, input pressure drops in the resistive bed to a level determined by the number and caliber of collateral vascular pathways. In this example, perfusion pressure is maintained just above the threshold of the pressure-passive range. **(C)** In this example with collateral failure, the patient is in the pressure passive range with CBF below the ischemic threshold, requiring treatment. **(D)** With deliberate hypertension, the increased pressure is transmitted across the collateral pathways. Although not sufficient to restore normal pressure in the ischemic bed, the pressure augmentation is sufficient to increase CBF above the ischemic threshold. (From ref. 36, with permission.)

loading and/or the administration of cardiotonic or vasopressor agents. Blood loss is not replaced unless the decrease in hematocrit or red cell mass is great enough to compromise tissue perfusion and oxygen delivery.

RAPID EMERGENCE FROM ANESTHESIA

Rapid return of consciousness, providing the means for early neurologic evaluation, is crucial. In case of a malpositioned clip, early detection may facilitate timely surgical intervention that may prevent a neurologic catastrophe.

The administration of anesthetic agents is stopped toward the end of the surgical procedure. Timing is dependent on the pharmacokinetic and pharmacodynamic profiles of the drugs that were used. The benefit of a more tranquil emergence, which may be afforded by any residual opioid analgesic effect following a recent bolus or continued opioid infusion, must be balanced against the risk of hypoventilation and possible delay in awakening. Lidocaine may be administered intravenously just before removal of the head holder and application of the head dressing in order to suppress airway reflexes due to endotracheal tube movement, although this too may delay awakening. Marked hypertension

is treated with sympatholytic agents. The inspired oxygen concentration is raised to 100%, and any residual muscle-relaxant effect is reversed with a cholinesterase inhibitor (eg, neostigmine) administered with an antimuscarinic agent (eg, glycopyrrolate). The upper airway is suctioned, and the trachea is extubated when the patient begins to regain consciousness. The goal is to permit a neurologic examination encompassing assessment of mental status, cranial nerve function, and motor and verbal function.

Delayed awakening may not be solely due to residual anesthetic. The intraoperative use of deliberate hypotension or hypothermia, excessive retractor pressure, and the patient's baseline neurologic status are all compounding factors.

The patient is transported in a 30° head-up position with oxygen supplementation to the intensive care unit for at least 12 hours of intensive monitoring. Oxygen therapy is continued, and analgesics are administered in doses small enough not to interfere with serial neurologic examinations.

REFERENCES

1. Andreoli A, di Pasquale G, Pinelli G, et al. Subarachnoid hemorrhage: Frequency and severity of cardiac arrhythmias. *Stroke* 1987;18:558–564.
2. Manninen PH, Lam AM, Gelb AW. Electrocardiographic changes during and after isoflurane-induced hypotension for neurovascular surgery. *Can J Anaesth* 1987;34:549–554.
3. Cruickshank JM, Neil-Dwyer G, Stott AW. Possible role of catecholamines, corticosteroids, and potassium in production of electrocardiographic abnormalities associated with subarachnoid haemorrhage. *Br Heart J* 1974;36:697–706.
4. Davies KR, Gelb AW, Manninen PH, et al. Cardiac function in aneurysmal subarachnoid haemorrhage: A study of electrocardiographic and echocardiographic abnormalities. *Br J Anaesth* 1991;57:58–63.
5. Benumoff JL. Management of the difficult adult airway. *Anesthesiology* 1991;75:1087–1110.
6. Haraldseth O, Gronas T, Southon T, et al. The effects of brain temperature on temporary global ischemia in rat brain: A 31-phosphorous NMR spectroscopy study. *Acta Anaesthesiol Scand* 1992;36:393–399.
7. Pulsinelli WA, Levy DE, Sigsbee B, et al. Increased damage after ischemic stroke in patients with hyperglycemia with or without established diabetes mellitus. *Am J Med* 1983;74:540–544.
8. Warner DS, Sokoll MD, Maktabi M, Godersky JC, Adams HP. Nicardipine HCl: Clinical experience in patients undergoing anaesthesia for intracranial aneurysm clipping. *Can J Anaesth* 1989;36:219–223.
9. Ornstein E, Matteo RS, Schwartz AE, Silverberg PA, Young WL, Diaz J. The effect of phenytoin on the magnitude and duration of neuromuscular blockade following atracurium or vecuronium. *Anesthesiology* 1987;67:191–196.
10. Abe K, Iwanaga H, Shimada Y, Yoshiya I. The effect of nicardipine on carotid blood flow velocity, local cerebral blood flow, and carbon dioxide reactivity during cerebral aneurysm surgery. *Anesth Analg* 1993;76:1227–1233.
11. Ravussin P, de Tribolet N. Total intravenous anesthesia with propofol for burst suppression in cerebral aneurysm surgery: Preliminary report of 42 patients. *Neurosurgery* 1993;32:236–240.
12. Tsementzis SA, Hitchcock ER. Outcome from "rescue clipping" of ruptured intracranial aneurysms during induction anaesthesia and endotracheal intubation. *J Neurol Neurosurg Psychiatry* 1985;48:160–163.
13. Schramm J, Cedzich C. Outcome and management of intraoperative aneurysm rupture. *Surg Neurol* 1993;40:26–30.
14. Abe K, Iwanaga H, Inada E. Effect of nicardipine and diltiazem on internal carotid artery blood flow velocity and local cerebral blood flow during cerebral aneurysm surgery for subarachnoid hemorrhage. *J Clin Anesth* 1994;6:99–105.
15. Taniguchi M, Nadstawek J, Pechstein U, Schramm J. Total intravenous anesthesia for improvement of intraoperative monitoring of somatosensory evoked potentials during aneurysm surgery. *Neurosurgery* 1992;31:891–897.
16. Ornstein E, Young WL, Fleischer L, Ostapkovich N. Desflurane and isoflurane have similar effects on cerebral blood flow in patients with intracranial mass lesions. *Anesthesiology* 1993;79:498–502.
17. Fleischer L, Young WL, Ornstein E, Smiley RS. Systemic hemodynamic changes of desflurane vs. isoflurane during anesthetic induction (abstract). *Anesthesiology* 1992;77:A334.
18. Baker KZ, Ostapkovich N, Jackson T, Ornstein E, Young WL. Cerebral blood flow reactivity is intact during remifentanil/N₂O anesthesia. *Anesth Analg* 1995;80:S27.
19. Manninen PH, Cuillerier DJ, Nantau WE, Gelb AW. Monitoring of brainstem function during vertebral basilar aneurysm surgery. The use of spontaneous ventilation. *Anesthesiology* 1992;77:681–685.
20. Wilson CB, Spetzler RF. Factors responsible for the improved results in the surgical management of intracranial aneurysms and vascular malformations. *Am J Surg* 1977;134:33–38.
21. Drummond JC. Deliberate hypotension for intracranial aneurysm surgery: Changing practices (letter). *Can J Anaesth* 1991;38:935.
22. Craen RA, Gelb AW, Eliasziw M, Lok P. Current anesthetic practices and use of brain protective therapies for cerebral aneurysm surgery at 41 North American centers (abstract). *Anesthesiology* 1994;81:209.
23. Abe K, Demizu A, Yoshiya I. Effect of prostaglandin E₁-induced hypotension on carbon dioxide reactivity and local cerebral blood flow after subarachnoid hemorrhage. *Br J Anaesth* 1992;68:268–271.
24. Ornstein E, ed. *Deliberate Hypotension in Anesthesia and Surgery.* Philadelphia: JB Lippincott, 1993. Problems in Anesthesia, vol 7.
25. Owall A, Gordon E, Lagerkranser M, et al. Clinical experience with adenosine for controlled hypotension during cerebral aneurysm surgery. *Anesth Analg* 1987;66:229–234.
26. Ornstein E, Young WL, Ostapkovich N, Matteo RS, Diaz J. Deliberate hypotension in patients with intracranial arteriovenous malformations: Esmolol compared with isoflurane and with sodium nitroprusside. *Anesth Analg* 1991;72:639–644.
27. Samson D, Batjer HH, Bowman G, et al. A clinical study of the parameters and effects of temporary arterial occlusion in the management of intracranial aneurysms. *Neurosurgery* 1994;34:22–29.
28. Young WL, Solomon RA, Pedley TA, et al. Direct cortical EEG monitoring during temporary vascular occlusion for cerebral aneurysm clipping. *Anesthesiology* 1989;71:794–799.
29. Stone JG, Young WL, Marans ZS, et al. Cardiac performance preserved despite thiopental loading. *Anesthesiology* 1993;79:36–41.
30. Sano T, Drummond JC, Patel PM, Grafe MR, Watson JC, Cole DJ. A comparison of the cerebral protective effects of isoflurane and mild hypothermia in a model of incomplete forebrain ischemia in the rat. *Anesthesiology* 1992;76:221–228.
31. Busto R, Dietrich WD, Globus MYT, et al. Small differences in intraischemic brain temperature critically determine the extent of ischemic neuronal injury. *J Cereb Blood Flow Metab* 1987;7:729–738.
32. Todd MM, Warner DS. A comfortable hypothesis reevaluated: Cerebral metabolic depression and brain protection during ischemia. *Anesthesiology* 1992;76:161–164.
33. Stone JG, Young WL, Smith CR, et al. Do standard monitoring sites reflect true brain temperature when profound hypothermia is rapidly reduced and reversed? *Anesthesiology* 1995;82:344–351.
34. Baker KZ, Young WL, Stone JG, Kader A, Baker CJ, Solomon RA. Deliberate mild hypothermia for craniotomy. *Anesthesiology* 1994;81:361–367.
35. Young WL, Cole DJ. Deliberate hypertension: Rationale and application for augmenting cerebral blood flow. In: Ornstein E, ed. *Deliberate Hypotension in Anesthesia and Surgery.* Philadelphia: JB Lippincott, 1993:140–153. Problems in Anesthesia, vol 7.
36. Young WL. Clinical Neuroscience Lectures. Munster, IN: Cathenart Publishing, 1996 (in press).

Cerebrovascular Disease, edited by H. Hunt Batjer.
Lippincott-Raven Publishers, Philadelphia © 1997.

CHAPTER 92

Protection of the Brain from Iatrogenic Ischemia

H. Hunt Batjer, R. Tyler Frizzell, Jing Guo, Thomas A. Kopitnik, and Duke S. Samson

The goal of therapy for intracranial aneurysm is the complete obliteration of the aneurysmal sac after its isolation from the cerebral circulation with preservation of all afferent and efferent vasculature. Modern microsurgical technique allows exquisite clip occlusion of the overwhelming majority of small, straightforward intracranial aneurysms. A number of clinical circumstances, however, render the accomplishment of this ideal difficult and, in some cases, impossible. As aneurysms enlarge, a greater portion of the circumference and length of the parent artery becomes involved in the disease process, and simple clipping is not possible; clip exclusion of the aneurysmal tissue involves true reconstruction of the parent artery. Unfortunately, many of these lesions become extremely atherosclerotic, calcific, and filled to varying extent with intraluminal thrombosis; and precise closure by placement of a clip across the neck of an aneurysm cannot be achieved due to the aneurysm's intrinsic turgor and wall characteristics. Typically, a clip placed on this type of lesion migrates proximally onto the true wall of the parent vessel, producing stenosis and, potentially, intimal damage. While the management of giant intracranial aneurysms has been favorably affected by the availability of long and strong multiangled and fenestrated clips and booster clips (1–4), the use of temporary arterial occlusion as a direct surgical adjunct has proven extremely beneficial in our practice.

Temporary clips are available from many vendors in a variety of sizes and configurations and with closing pressures insufficient to cause permanent endothelial and intimal damage (5). Following Pool's (6) work, temporary clips can be applied to the proximal afferent trunk to soften an aneurysm for final dissection or clip application, or more complex strategies can be invoked. Complete afferent and efferent temporary clipping can be used to deflate the aneurysmal tissue or to open the aneurysmal sac widely for evacuation of thrombotic material.

The temporary interruption of blood flow for short periods of time in virtually all intracranial vessels is well tolerated. Unfortunately, as the complexity of the anatomic situation increases and the time required to reconstruct vascular anatomy becomes prolonged, the brain tissue rendered ischemic by the vascular interruption is at risk for the development of permanent infarction (7). While the physiology and pathophysiology of the conversion of ischemic to infarcted tissue is complex and dependent on many interacting variables, the neurosurgeon confronted with a difficult neurovascular problem must consider (a) what the safe limits of temporary arterial occlusion are in the specific anatomic region under consideration and (b) whether there are therapeutic manipulations that can extend this safe interval if prolonged temporary occlusion is anticipated. It is extremely difficult to answer the first question. Anecdotal evidence suggests wide ranges of tolerance up to 1 hour in several vascular distributions. It is also well known that permanent vessel sacrifice in many circumstances is without risk of even temporary ischemia. Nevertheless, the clinician is often left in a circumstance in which a patient requires prolonged temporary vascular interruption and thus has to assume that the distal cerebral tissue is at risk during the procedure. Several strategies designed to protect ischemic brain tissue during this type of procedure have been developed, based on three general

H. H. Batjer: Division of Neurological Surgery, Northwestern University Medical School, Chicago, Illinois 60611.
R. T. Frizzell: Division of Neurosurgery, University of Alabama at Birmingham, Birmingham, Alabama 35294.
J. Guo: Department of Neurosurgery, Beijing General Railway Hospital, Beijing 100038, Peoples Republic of China.
T. A. Kopitnik, Jr.: Department of Neurological Surgery, The University of Texas Southwestern Medical School, Dallas, Texas 75235.
D. S. Samson: Department of Neurological Surgery, The University of Texas Southwestern Medical School, Dallas, Texas 75235.

precepts: (a) increase supply of substrate, (b) decrease metabolic demand, or (c) eliminate toxic metabolic substances. Arguably, the most successful approaches to this problem have been concerned with decreasing the metabolic requirements of the brain and therefore decreasing the demand for blood flow.

Due to their multiple pharmacologic actions, barbiturates were studied early as potential cerebral protectants. These agents have been shown to protect the brain in numerous animal models of hypoxia and ischemia and have suggested a benefit in a number of clinical situations (8–14). Unfortunately, the cardiac depressant effects of barbiturates at required dosage not infrequently decrease mean arterial pressure to levels that impair collateral flow into the ischemic territory. The properties of etomidate, an intravenously administered carboxylated imidazole derivative that produces significant depression of cerebral metabolism with minimal cardiac toxicity, led us to begin using this agent during aneurysm procedures (7,15–24). Since approximately 60% of the cerebral metabolic rate is concerned with the electrical generation of impulses (a function that can be monitored with the electroencephalogram [EEG]) and approximately 40% is concerned with the maintenance of cellular homeostasis, it seems reasonable to assume that the use of a pharmacologic agent such as a barbiturate, etomidate, or propofol, each of which abolishes electrical generation, should extend the ischemic tolerance of the brain by roughly one half.

Early studies of etomidate showed a comparable level of metabolic suppression with barbiturates, as well as a coincident and dramatic decrease in cerebral blood flow, resulting in favorable protective properties that met or exceeded those noted with the barbiturates (23,24). While remarkable systemic and cardiovascular stability was noted even with high doses of etomidate (21), certain untoward side effects were described. Even with brief use of this agent, endogenous cortisol production was found to be substantially diminished (19,25). In addition, some activation of the EEG was noted in patients with preoperative epilepsy (17). Nevertheless, in clinical practice high doses of steroids are commonly employed over the perioperative period in patients with intracranial vascular disease. This steroid coverage essentially negates the most important adverse affect of the drug, and etomidate remains a very attractive clinical means of reducing the cerebral metabolic rate and, hopefully, extending ischemic tolerance. Over the past several years, a number of laboratory and clinical studies have been performed through our department to evaluate some of the issues related to the tolerance of the brain to iatrogenic ischemia; the subsequent discussion will consider some of this work.

INCOMPLETE GLOBAL CEREBRAL ISCHEMIA

A canine model of incomplete global ischemia was developed using induced severe hypotension with sodium nitro-

prusside and trimethaphan camsylate (26). Cerebral blood flow (CBF) was monitored in this preparation with global (Kety-Schmidt nitrous oxide washout) and cortical (thermal diffusion probe) techniques. Arterial sampling was derived from the femoral artery, and cerebral venous sampling was obtained by catheterization of the torcular Herophili. The required craniectomy also allowed cortical EEG monitoring and cortical CBF monitoring. A standard general anesthetic was employed with induction by a short-acting barbiturate and maintenance with 1.5% inspired isoflurane and 5–10% nitrous oxide. Paralysis was maintained with vecuronium bromide (0.1 mg/kg/h). The anesthetic technique employed was felt to mimic the clinical setting as closely as possible. After the induction and maintenance of anesthesia and the creation of an appropriate craniectomy with arterial and venous cannulation, a 45-minute period of stabilization was followed by 30 minutes of severe hypotension to approximately 30 mm Hg. A final 45-minute period of recovery was then observed after cessation of the hypotensive agents. Three groups of animals were studied: control, low-dose etomidate, and high-dose etomidate. In the control series, no ischemic protection was employed. In the low-dose etomidate group, a 1 mg/kg bolus was infused followed by 0.5 mg/kg/min during the study interval. In the high-dose etomidate group, burst suppression was induced and maintained with a 3 mg/kg bolus followed by 0.1 mg/kg/min, with additional supplementation as necessary to maintain burst suppression.

The initial studies conducted by Frizzell et al (26) lowered the mean arterial pressure to similar levels in each study group (approximately 30 mm Hg). The mean cerebral oxygen extraction fraction (OEF) increased in the control animals tested from 0.23 ± 0.02 to 0.55 ± 0.08 ($p < .05$). These data are graphically illustrated in Fig. 1. In the low-dose etomidate group, the OEF rose from 0.33 ± 0.02 to 0.53 ± 0.02 ($p < .05$). In the high-dose etomidate group, the OEF did not increase during hypotension. Mean global CBF levels decreased in all groups during the hypotensive insult: It decreased $52\% \pm 12\%$ in the control group, $56\% \pm 13\%$ in the low-dose etomidate group, and $60\% \pm 4\%$ in the high-dose etomidate group. Global CBF levels during hypotension ranged from 21–24 ml/100 g/min. Frizzell et al (26) concluded that this experiment suggested that burst-suppressive doses of etomidate were required to maintain the cerebral metabolic state during incomplete cerebral ischemia. This study certainly suggests that EEG monitoring is critical during clinical use of cerebral metabolic depressants and that empiric dosage, if too low, may be completely ineffective. In subsequent studies utilizing this model (unpublished data), thiopental was compared with etomidate in the types of metabolic responses elicited by hypotension. Thiopental behaved identically to etomidate in these studies, with the exception that significant decreases in mean arterial blood pressure were noted as a direct effect of thiopental administration.

Hypothermia has been considered and studied for several decades as a means of protecting the brain from a number of

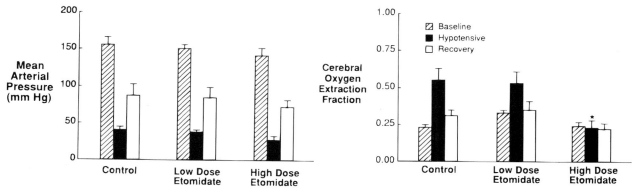

FIG. 1. Effect of hypotension on mean arterial blood pressure **(A)** and cerebral oxygen extraction fraction **(B)** without etomidate (control), with low-dose etomidate, or with high-dose etomidate. *Asterisk* indicates that the data for the high-dose etomidate group were significantly less than for the control and low-dose etomidate groups ($p < .05$). (From ref. 26, with permission.)

physical and ischemic insults. Physiologic evidence would suggest that hypothermia decreases the metabolic rate by a combined effect on electrical generation as well as the slowing of homeostatic and enzymatic mechanisms. Therefore, it is possible that synergism could exist between pharmacologic metabolic suppression and mild hypothermia, in which EEG activity remains to further diminish the cerebral metabolic rate, thus theoretically extending ischemic tolerance. Frizzell et al (27) conducted additional experiments using the above described canine model of incomplete global ischemia and studied four groups: control, etomidate, hypothermia (28°C), and combined etomidate with hypothermia. In this series of studies, etomidate did not affect the animals' mean arterial pressure but did lower the heart rate. Hypothermia, with or without etomidate, lowered both mean arterial pressure and heart rate significantly. Etomidate administration did not result in a change in the esophageal, brain parenchymal, or subdural temperature. Cerebral metabolic rate (ml/100 g/min) decreased ($p < .05$) during etomidate administration (3.2 ± 0.4 to 1.7 ± 0.2) and hypothermia (3.5 ± 0.2 to 1.1 ± 0.2), but the addition of etomidate to hypothermia did not further reduce the cerebral metabolic rate (3.1 ± 0.5 to 1.3 ± 0.2) despite decreasing brain hemispheric electrical activity to a burst-suppressive state. During hypotension, the cerebral arteriovenous difference in oxygen increased ($p < .05$) in the control group but not in the other experimental groups. Thus, etomidate was found not to possess the adverse cardiovascular effects associated with moderate hypothermia. However, in this model at 28°C etomidate did not further reduce cerebral metabolism despite decreasing brain hemispheric electrical activity. Etomidate, hypothermia, and the combination of etomidate and hypothermia were all successful at blunting the hypotension-induced increased oxygen extraction.

SPECIFIC VASCULAR TERRITORIES

It is very likely that specific arterial territories react to temporary vascular interruption in differing ways. The ana-

tomic substrate for this feature is likely the very different collateral resources available to vessels such as the proximal carotid or vertebral arteries and other regions such as the terminal basilar artery or middle cerebral artery, in which terminal endarteries (perforators) are a vital component. It is well known that carotid endarterectomy can be performed safely with temporary occlusion of the common, internal, and external carotid arteries in excess of 45 minutes. This is not surprising based on the findings of modern endovascular techniques, which have allowed trial occlusion of the internal carotid artery as an adjunct to the management of skull base vascular and neoplastic problems. Our experience with these techniques has been that roughly 80% of patients provocatively studied can tolerate the loss of a single internal carotid artery without developing hemodynamic evidence of distal hypoperfusion or ischemia.

To further complicate the situation, it is likely that various types of pharmacologic therapy may have activity based on receptor interactions. Those receptors may be variably distributed throughout the supra- and infratentorial components of the brain. Thus, their activity might well be severely limited in one region and quite important in another. Our clinical familiarity with etomidate suggests that such a problem might be present in this drug. Abundant clinical and laboratory experience suggests that minimal or no cardiovascular instability develops with even high doses of this agent. Such cardiovascular stability is obviously not the rule with high doses of thiopental. Thus, it is at least possible that brainstem metabolic activity is significantly more affected by the barbiturates than by etomidate. It is also obvious that doses of both drugs, which eliminate cortical electrical activity, do not eliminate brainstem auditory evoked potentials (BAEPs). Davis et al (28) performed animal studies that demonstrated that etomidate was clearly effective at reducing the cerebral metabolic rate supratentorially but that its impact on the hindbrain was negligible. Dr. Jing Guo worked in our department in the early 1990s with an interest in producing an animal model of brainstem ischemia that was analogous to the clinical circumstance of temporary arterial occlusion involving the vertebrobasilar system. He went through a number of preliminary studies, attempting to produce brainstem ischemia in the dog. Monitoring local CBF with laser Doppler flowmetry and BAEPs, he confirmed that basilar artery ligation alone failed to produce physiologically measurable alterations. In addition, ligation of the vertebral arteries and ventrospinal artery, as well as the distal basilar artery, resulted in the mean basilar arterial pressure decreasing by only one third. Vigorous collateral flow into the basilar artery during this preparation maintained cardiovascular stability, regional CBF, and BAEPs. Simply eliminating collateral flow from the anterior circulation by occluding the posterior communicating arteries was insufficient in eliminating this collateral. Ultimately, he achieved profound brainstem ischemia by embolizing the terminal basilar artery and its branches with acrylic glue.

Canine Brainstem Ischemic Model

This canine preparation was accomplished by a standard anesthetic using acepromazine maleate as a preanesthetic followed by induction with thiamylal sodium (20 mg/kg IV) and maintenance with isoflurane at 2–3% inspired volume during surgery and at 1–1.5% during the ischemia and reperfusion periods of the experiment. Ventilation was accomplished with a Harvard pump (Harvard Apparatus, Millis, MA) to maintain arterial oxygenation (Pao_2) of 200 ± 50 mm Hg and a $Paco_2$ of 40 ± 3 mm Hg. Vecuronium was given to facilitate muscle relaxation. The dog was placed in the supine position with the head hyperextended. Catheters were placed in the femoral artery and vein for the purposes of arterial blood pressure measurement and blood sampling. Fluid administration was accomplished with 0.9% sodium chloride at 2–3 ml/min. Esophageal temperature was monitored throughout the experiments.

An incision was made from the midpoint of the mandible to the midpoint of the neck just lateral to the trachea. The incision was then continued between the carotid sheath and sternohyoid muscles. Midline structures were separated, and the larynx and esophagus were retracted contralaterally, allowing the surgeon easy access to the longus colli and rectus capitis ventralis muscles. These muscles were detached from the cranial base and C-1. After removal of the joint capsule and anterior arch of C-1, the anterior rim of the foramen magnum and the occipital condyles were removed with an electric drill. Bone resection was continued rostrally to the joint of the clivus and basisphenoid body. The dura was opened in the midline, exposing the basilar artery from its origin to within 1 cm of its bifurcation. This exposure also demonstrated the ventrospinal artery circle and the vertebral arteries bilaterally. Polyethylene tubing with an outer diameter of 0.6 mm was inserted between the ventrospinal bifurcation and the junction of the left vertebral artery in such a way that blood flow from the right vertebral artery and ven-

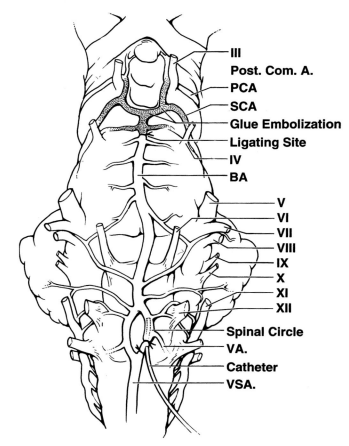

FIG. 2. Ventral view showing canine brainstem. The illustration shows the sites of glue embolization and catheter insertion (*Post. Com. A.*, posterior communicating artery; *PCA*, posterior cerebral artery; *SCA*, superior cerebellar artery; *BA*, basilar artery; *III–XII*, cranial nerves; *VA*, vertebral artery; *VSA*, ventrospinal artery). (From ref. 30, with permission.)

trospinal artery to the basilar artery was not jeopardized. The basilar artery perfusion pressure was then monitored with a Space Labs 90603A surgical monitor (Space Labs, Inc., Redmond, WA). The basilar artery was ligated just proximal to its bifurcation and punctured distally with a 22-gauge needle in order to inject cyanoacrylate glue 0.05 ml for embolization of the distal collateral bed (Fig. 2).

Regional cerebral blood flow (rCBF) was measured with a laser Doppler flowmeter (Vasamedics, Inc., St. Paul, MN) placed on the brainstem surface near the emergence of the hypoglossal nerve. BAEPs were monitored with a Neuropak Four EMG evoked-response measuring system (Model MEM-4104K, Nihon Kohden America, Inc., Irvine, CA) with platinum needle electrodes to evaluate brainstem ischemia. Both reference electrodes and the active electrode were placed on the skull base just beside the brainstem, with one reference electrode being placed on the ventral surface of the basisphenoid bone near the midbrain and the other caudally at the rim of the foramen magnum. Click stimuli of 80-dB, 10-Hz, and 0.1-ms duration were presented to both ears with a headphone set.

After baseline measurement of rCBF and BAEPs, a control group and three experimental groups were studied. The control group received no further surgical manipulation except the surgical procedures and the distal basilar embolization. The three experimental groups underwent occlusion of the ventrospinal arteries and vertebral arteries by temporary clipping for various durations (10, 20, and 30 minutes). After clip removal, reperfusion was allowed for 5 hours, with rCBF and BAEP measurements being obtained at 5 and 10 minutes during the ischemic challenge and at 10 minutes, 30 minutes, 1 hour, 3 hours, and 5 hours during reperfusion. Initial studies evaluated the use of Evans blue dye as a means of quantitating permanent cerebral injury. Unfortunately, this technique failed to differentiate the various severities of ischemic challenge. Interestingly, the pattern of BAEPs was exquisitely sensitive to induced ischemia and variable recovery rates.

During the ischemic challenge, rCBF decreased significantly from baseline to <10 ml/100 g/min during clipping ($p < .0001$). After reperfusion, rCBF reached its highest value almost at once. There was some degree of hyperemia lasting for about 30 minutes. In the animals subjected to ischemia for 10 and 20 minutes, the brainstem rCBF recovered promptly to control levels and remained at those levels throughout the period of reperfusion observation. In the animals undergoing 30 minutes of brainstem ischemia, a progressive decrease in rCBF to levels <10 ml/100 g/min was noted after 5 hours of reperfusion. This group was significantly different from the behavior of the other experimental groups ($p = .0012$). Thus, some evidence of a no-reflow phenomenon was observed after 30 minutes of brainstem ischemia. As mentioned, the BAEP measurements proved exquisitely sensitive in identifying the severity of the ischemic injury. Within seconds of institution of temporary clipping, the third peak of the BAEP dropped to essentially zero amplitude and remained at that level until reperfusion was initiated. For animals undergoing 10 minutes of brainstem ischemia, rapid recovery of BAEPs to baseline level

occurred, and they remained normal during the 5 hours of observation (Fig. 3). Dogs subjected to a 30-minute challenge suffered a permanent obliteration of BAEPs, which did not recover during the period of observation. Interestingly, the 20-minute ischemic challenge resulted in an injury of intermediate severity with initial loss of amplitude followed by some degree of recovery that remained substantially less than 50% of baseline (see Fig. 3). A significant difference was thus demonstrated between these intervals of temporary brainstem ischemia ($p < .0001$)(29).

We were intrigued by the potential of this 20-minute ischemic challenge, as it provided in this animal model a measurable and quantifiable physiologic parameter of insult severity and the time duration of the involved insult was roughly appropriate to suspected time limits of brainstem ischemia during human aneurysm surgery. In addition, many complex aneurysms of the vertebrobasilar system require at least 20 minutes of temporary arterial occlusion for surgical correction. We felt that this 20-minute insult was potentially a very valuable model for the evaluation of various protective strategies of clinical importance. Subsequent studies with that model have been performed with etomidate (30). Interestingly, the therapeutic doses of etomidate failed to suppress BAEPs or brainstem cardiovascular responses to the ischemic challenge. When animals receiving etomidate were compared with control animals, both subjected to 20 minutes of brainstem ischemia, a significant but only temporary recovery in BAEPs was noted in the etomidate group. In addition, etomidate failed to have any significant impact on animals rendered ischemic for 30 minutes. This finding was felt to be important, as the dose of etomidate used was adequate for the induction of EEG-documented burst suppression, yet BAEPs were preserved and minimal if any brainstem protective activity was noted. Thus, the value of etomidate in temporary vertebral or basilar artery occlusion based on these studies and on previous laboratory work (28) is highly questionable.

Next, Guo et al (31) reproduced this model and studied

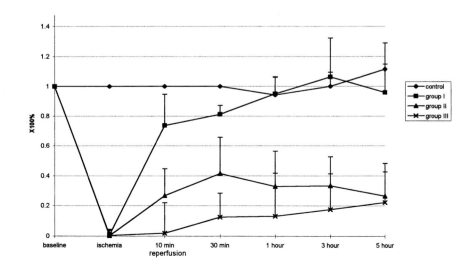

FIG. 3. Amplitude changes of brainstem auditory evoked potentials (BAEPs) as percentages of the baseline value. The *vertical bars* show the standard deviation in each group. The BAEP amplitude of group 1 (10-minute ischemia) returned to the baseline level after 1 hour of reperfusion, but those of group 2 (20-minute ischemia) and group 3 (30-minute ischemia) remained at a low level. The changes in groups 2 and 3 differed significantly from changes in group 1 and the control group ($p < .05$). (From ref. 29, with permission.)

the effects of thiopental. Interestingly, during the therapeutic trial, BAEPs were preserved after thiopental administration as they were with etomidate. During the ischemic challenge, both control and thiopental-treated animals experienced a dramatic decrease in BAEP amplitude to <10% of baseline. On reperfusion for 30 minutes, the BAEPs increased in both groups to near 40% of baseline. In the untreated animals, a progressive decrease in amplitude was noted for the duration of reperfusion observation. In the thiopental-treated animals, however, the BAEPs continued to recover progressively over time to a mean of 70% of baseline at 5 hours of reperfusion. This improvement was clearly different from the etomidate-treated animals in the previous study. In light of the preservation of BAEPs during drug administration, the actual mechanism of thiopental's protective effect remains a significant question.

Perflubron (Oxygent; Alliance Pharmaceutical Corp., San Diego, CA) is a second generation perfluorocarbon emulsion. This agent has superior oxygen delivery characteristics and greater stability than previous perfluorochemicals, as well as a significantly more rapid clearance than the first-generation agents and therefore presumably less reticuloendothelial toxicity. Guo et al (32) evaluated this agent in the canine model of brainstem ischemia. Animals were pretreated by ventilation with 100% oxygen followed by an intravenous dose of perflubron at 1.5 ml/kg. Similarly severe BAEP changes were noted in both control and perflubron-treated animals during the ischemic insult. In the early period of reperfusion, the BAEPs increased in both control and perflubron groups to 50–70% of baseline. In the perflubron-treated group, however, BAEPs continued to recover to a final sustained level of well over 80% of baseline (Fig. 4). The control animals suffered a progressive decrease in BAEPs to 23% of baseline after the brief postischemic peak.

This clear beneficial effect was found not to relate to hyperoxygenation per se, and the pattern demonstrated suggests some beneficial effect on a reperfusion injury. This markedly positive result with perflubron in doses that should be clinically tolerable, and with a protocol that is analogous to what could be used intraoperatively, may hold significant promise in the treatment of giant vertebrobasilar aneurysms in humans requiring prolonged temporary occlusion.

CLINICAL TEMPORARY ARTERIAL OCCLUSION STUDY

Etomidate, as mentioned earlier, became routinely employed in our clinical practice several years ago. Due to the large volume of aneurysm patients treated at our center, it seemed possible to investigate the variables associated with the ultimate development of infarction to determine the safest and most effective utilization of temporary arterial occlusion. During a 2-year period, 121 patients from a group of 234 consecutive aneurysm cases were treated by elective temporary arterial occlusion. Of this initial group, 21 patients were excluded due to intraoperative aneurysm rupture before the institution of temporary clipping, operative sacrifice of afferent or efferent arteries, or pre- or postocclusion performance of an extracranial-to-intracranial arterial bypass. These exclusions left 100 patients for study. This study was not a trial of any specific therapeutic modality but was simply an investigation to determine what the safe limits were in our particular practice with our protocol and which clinical factors had a positive or negative impact on tolerance. The dosage of etomidate to maintain burst suppression during this study was 1 mg/kg followed by 10 μg/kg/min. Patient parameters studied included age, Hunt–Hess clinical grade,

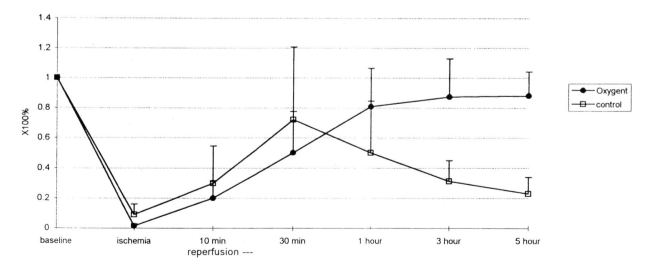

FIG. 4. Graphic representation of the amplitude of peak III of the BAEP comparing treated and untreated animals. Both groups experience a large drop in BAEP during ischemia, with subsequent recovery during early reperfusion. Beginning 1 hour postreperfusion, perflubron-treated animals continued to increase in peak III amplitude and untreated animals continued to decay. (From ref. 32, with permission.)

presence or absence of subarachnoid hemorrhage, vasospasm, aneurysm size, and vascular territory. The technical parameters included the total duration of occlusion, the degree of temporary occlusion, and the use of intermittent vs. sustained arrest. All patients were treated using our standard anesthetic technique of etomidate-induced burst suppression during elective temporary clipping under normotension, normothermia, and normovolemia. Mannitol (1 g/kg) was administered at the time of skin incision. Temporary occlusion was considered complete if all afferent and efferent vessels were clipped and incomplete if one or more efferent vessels was left patent. A separate subcategory was designed for those cases in which only proximal-vessel occlusion was used. Postoperative follow-up evaluations included computed tomography in 100% of the cases, angiography in 87%, and magnetic resonance imaging in 48%. Clinical follow-up was obtained to a minimum of 6 months with a mean of 19 months. Outcome parameters measured included final clinical condition and clinical or radiographic evidence of cerebral infarction in the appropriate vascular territory. Simple proximal occlusion was utilized in 39 patients, incomplete trapping in 21, and complete trapping in 40.

Of the patients treated in the above protocol, 19 could be defined as having suffered cerebral infarction following surgery; 81 patients had no clinical or radiographic evidence of ischemia or infarction in the distribution of the arteries occluded intraoperatively. As noted in our report of this work (33), analysis was hindered by the often difficult assessment of temporary ischemia, perforator injury, vasospasm, and direct effect of subarachnoid hemorrhage as the most important contributor to an untoward clinical event.

Several parameters were found to be statistically significantly related to the postoperative development of clinical or radiographic cerebral infarction in the anatomical distribution of the arteries temporarily occluded. This correlation with poor ischemic tolerance was noted with advanced patient age, poor preoperative clinical grade, protracted duration of temporary clipping, and the use of incomplete (as opposed to complete) local arrest. These findings can be summarized as follows:

1. Patients older than age 61 years tolerated temporary arterial occlusion poorly, developing clinical and radiographic evidence of infarction at time durations shorter than those tolerated in younger patients.
2. Patients in more advanced clinical grades (Hunt–Hess grades III and IV) demonstrated a higher incidence of ischemic complications than patients in better clinical grades. Additionally, these complications were found to occur at shorter intervals of temporary occlusion than those tolerated by patients in better condition. The 95% confidence level for the tolerance of temporary occlusion in patients in grades I and II was 19 minutes; the 95% confidence level for poor-grade patients was 15 minutes.
3. All patients undergoing temporary arterial occlusion for >31 minutes had both radiographic and neurologic evidence of infarction in the postoperative period. Patients occluded for periods between 21 and 30 minutes routinely had both radiographic and clinical evidence of ischemia, although in a number of cases neurologic recovery was significant. Patients occluded for durations between 14 and 21 minutes had largely satisfactory clinical and radiographic outcomes, although several patients in the 18–21 minute interval developed deficits. All patients occluded for <14 minutes had no clinical or radiographic sequelae of the iatrogenic ischemia.
4. The degree of local arterial arrest could be judged as either complete, incomplete, or simple proximal occlusion. These modalities were compared both in the entire patient population and in those occluded for periods >14 minutes. In patients undergoing protracted occlusion (>14 minutes), a strong statistical trend suggested a close relationship between incomplete arrest and the development of postoperative neurologic deficit and/or infarction.

Two additional parameters were found to have suggestive but not statistically significant relationship to the above-mentioned endpoints.

1. Of the specific vascular territories undergoing temporary occlusion, the distribution of perforating arteries appeared to be uniquely sensitive to ischemic injury. While the number of distal basilar artery aneurysms treated in this population was substantially higher than that of middle cerebral artery aneurysms, a similar sensitivity was suggested for the thalamoperforating vessels and the lenticulostriate arteries.
2. A suggestive but not significant relationship was identified between increasing episodes of temporary occlusion and the postoperative development of ischemia. This finding was weighted by the use of multiple episodes of occlusion in patients treated with incomplete local arrest, suggesting that the relative technical inefficiency of incomplete occlusion mandated more extended periods of ischemia to achieve the desired technical result. It should also be noted that our practice differs from many others in the way we employ temporary occlusion. Patterned after Drake (34), many centers employ extremely brief periods of temporary occlusion (1–2 minutes) to perform a particular dissection maneuver. This process may then be repeated many times. Our practice, on the other hand, operates under the unproven assumption that a single episode of protracted ischemia is better tolerated than multiple episodes of brief occlusion. Due to this characteristic of our practice, we typically occlude the involved vessel and perform as much of the dissection and reconstruction as possible without restoring flow. If it becomes obvious that aneurysmal exclusion cannot be accomplished within a reasonable period of time and aneurysmal opening has not been

performed, flow is restored for a period of 10–15 minutes.

3. Interestingly, several factors failed to demonstrate a significant or suggestive relationship to the outcome measures of the study. No correlation could be found between the patient's sex, the preoperative presence of subarachnoid hemorrhage, the presence of angiographic vasospasm, or the size of the aneurysm and the risk of development of postoperative neurologic or radiographic evidence of infarction.

DISCUSSION

Despite the limitations of our clinical and laboratory investigations, it is our feeling that several tentative conclusions can be made. First, the use of pharmacologic brain protection with etomidate is extremely safe for the aneurysm patient, and a substantial body of evidence suggests that supratentorial cerebral tolerance of iatrogenic ischemic insults will be prolonged with use of metabolic suppression. For procedures involving brainstem ischemia, it is likely that etomidate will be much less effective than thiopental or other experimental strategies. Second, it is clear that in our practice the limits of cerebral tolerance for temporary arterial occlusion for many vascular territories are between 15 and 20 minutes. It is clear that many outliers exist; yet for the population at large this interval is potentially very significant. Third, the addition of induced hypothermia to pharmacologic metabolic suppression offers potential synergism. The laboratory studies of Frizzell et al (27) employed 28°C as the target for a noncirculatory arrest procedure. In clinical practice, however, induced hypothermia <32°C seems to induce some degree of coagulopathy, as well as a threat to cardiovascular stability. It is certainly possible that the use of surgically induced hypothermia to 32°C could prove synergistic with pharmacologic metabolic suppression.

The use of deep hypothermia (16°C) and complete circulatory arrest for the treatment of giant cerebral aneurysms has been under investigation for some time (35–37). Early attempts with this technique at extending cerebral tolerance of ischemia were complicated by hemorrhagic problems postoperatively. Improvements in the overall systemic safety of this procedure and the use of low-flow states as opposed to vascular decompression have precipitated a resurgence of interest in this methodology for intracranial aneurysm surgery (38). It is clear that the addition of deep hypothermia allows circulatory arrest intervals of up to 50 minutes with full neurologic recovery. Massive and thrombotic giant aneurysms can be successfully reconstructed within this time frame.

As a result of our experience, we are currently approaching the aneurysm patient with three strategies for brain protection. For patients in whom we anticipate occlusion times of <15 minutes, we routinely employ normothermia, normotension, and EEG burst suppression with etomidate, barbitu-

rate, or propofol. In cases of vertebrobasilar aneurysm, thiopental is used in place of these other agents. In cases with anticipated occlusion times of between 15 and 25 minutes, we utilize the previously mentioned pharmacologic approach with the addition of mild hypothermia to 32°C. We have not noted hemorrhagic complications with this technique to date. When occlusion times >25 minutes are anticipated, we employ deep hypothermia and circulatory arrest to enhance the tolerance of the ischemic interval and expand the spectrum of intracranial aneurysms that can be safely treated. This procedure is clearly experimental and consumes a large amount of health care resources to perform. It is becoming safer for the patient and the use of low flow as opposed to blood evacuation has greatly reduced the risk of air embolism as a major complication.

REFERENCES

1. Sugita K, Kobayashi S, Inoue T, Banno T. New angled fenestrated clips for fusiform vertebral artery aneurysms. *J Neurosurg* 1981;54: 346–350.
2. Sugita K, Kobayashi S, Inoue T, Takehae T. Characteristics and use of ultra-long aneurysm clips. *J Neurosurg* 1984;60:145–150.
3. Sugita K, Kobayashi S, Kyoshima K, Takemae T. Fenestrated clips for unusual aneurysms of the carotid artery. *J Neurosurg* 1982;57: 240–246.
4. Sundt TM Jr, Piepgras DG, Marsh WR. Booster clips for giant and thick-based aneurysms. *J Neurosurg* 1984;60:751–762.
5. Jabre A, Symon L. Temporary vascular occlusion during aneurysm surgery. *Surg Neurol* 1987;27:47–63.
6. Pool JL. Aneurysms of the anterior communicating artery, bifrontal craniotomy, and routine use of temporary clips. *J Neurosurg* 1961;18: 98–112.
7. Batjer HH, Samson DS. Limits of temporary arterial occlusion. In: Pasqualin A, Da Pian R, eds. *New Trends in Management of Cerebrovascular Malformations.* Wien, New York: Springer-Verlag, 1994: 356–363.
8. Goldstein A Jr, Wells BA, Keats AS. Increased tolerance to cerebral anoxia by pentobarbital. *Arch Int Pharmacodyn Ther* 1966;161: 138–143.
9. Michenfelder JD, Milde JH. Influence of anesthetics on metabolic, functional and pathological responses to regional cerebral ischemia. *Stroke* 1975;6:405–410.
10. Michenfelder JD, Milde JH, Sundt TM Jr. Cerebral protection by barbiturate anesthesia. *Arch Neurol* 1976;33:345–350.
11. Michenfelder JD, Theye RA. Cerebral protection by thiopental during hypoxia. *Anesthesiology* 1973;39:510–517.
12. Smith AL, Hoff JT, Nielsen SL, Larson CP. Barbiturate protection in acute focal cerebral ischemia. *Stroke* 1974;5:1–7.
13. Steen PA, Michenfelder JD. Cerebral protection with barbiturates. Relation to anesthetic effect. *Stroke* 1978;9:140–142.
14. Yatsu FM, Diamond I, Graziano C, Lindquist P. Experimental brain ischemia: Protection from irreversible damage with a rapid acting barbiturate (methohexital). *Stroke* 1972;3:726–732.
15. Batjer HH. Cerebral protective effects of etomidate: Experimental and clinical aspects. *Cerebrovasc Brain Metab Rev* 1993;5:17–32.
16. Batjer HH, Frankfurt AI, Purdy PD, Smith SS, Samson DS. Use of etomidate, temporary arterial occlusion, and intraoperative angiography in surgical treatment of large and giant cerebral aneurysm. *J Neurosurg* 1988;68:234–240.
17. Ebrahim ZY, DeBoer GE, Luders H, Hahn JF, Lesser RP. Effect of etomidate on the electroencephalogram of patients with epilepsy. *Anesth Analg* 1986;65:1004–1006.
18. Ghoneim MM, Yamada T. Etomidate: A clinical and electroencephalographic comparison with thiopental. *Anesth Analg* 1977;56:479–485.
19. Kenyon CJ, McNeil LM, Fraser R. Comparison of the effects of etomidate, thiopentone, and propofol on cortisol systhesis. *Br J Anaesth* 1985;57:509–511.

20. Milde LN, Milde JH. Preservation of cerebral metabolites by etomidate during incomplete cerebral ischemia in dogs. *Anesthesiology* 1986;65: 272–277.

21. Milde LN, Milde JH, Michenfelder JD. Cerebral functional, metabolic, and hemodynamic effects of etomidate in dogs. *Anesthesiology* 1985; 63:371–377.

22. Renou AM, Vernhiet J, Macrez P, Constant P, Billerey E, Khadaroo MY, Caille FM. Cerebral blood flow and metabolism during etomidate anesthesia in man. *Br J Anaesth* 1978;50:1047–1051.

23. Wauquier A. Brain protective properties of etomidate and flunarizine. *J Cereb Blood Flow Metab* 1982;2[suppl 1]:S53–S56.

24. Wauquier A, Ashton D, Clincke G. Anti-hypoxic effects of etomidate, thiopental, and methohexital. *Arch Int Pharmacodyn Ther* 1981;249: 330–334.

25. Moore RA, Allen MC, Wood PJ, Rees LH, Sear JW. Peri-operative endocrine effects of etomidate. *Anaesthesia* 1985;40:124–130.

26. Frizzell RT, Meyer YJ, Borchers DJ, et al. The effects of etomidate on cerebral metabolism and blood flow in a canine model for hypoperfusion. *J Neurosurg* 1991;74:263–269.

27. Frizzell RT, Fichtel FM, Jordan MB, et al. Effects of etomidate and hypothermia on cerebral metabolism and blood flow in a canine model of hypoperfusion. *J Neurosurg Anesthesiol* 1993;51:104–110.

28. Davis DW, Mans AM, Biesbuyck JF, Hawkins RA. Regional brain glucose utilization in rats during etomidate anesthesia. *Anesthesiology* 1986;64:751–757.

29. Guo J, Liao JJ, Preston JK, Batjer HH. A canine model of acute hindbrain ischemia and reperfusion. *Neurosurgery* 1995;36:986–993.

30. Guo J, White JA, Batjer HH. Limited protective effects of etomidate during brainstem ischemia in dogs. *J Neurosurg* 1995;82:278–283.

31. Guo J, White JA, Batjer HH. The protective effects of thiopental on brainstem ischemia. *Neurosurgery* 1995;37:490–495.

32. Guo J, White JA, Batjer HH. Intravenous perflubron emulsion administration improves the recovery of auditory evoked potentials after temporary brainstem ischemia in dogs. *Neurosurgery* 1995;36:350–357.

33. Samson DS, Batjer HH, Bowman G, Mootz L, Krippner W, Meyer YJ, Allen B. A clinical study of the parameters and effects of temporary arterial occlusion in the management of intracranial aneurysms. *Neurosurgery* 1994;34:22–29.

34. Drake CG. Giant intracranial aneurysms: Experience with surgical treatment in 174 patients. *Clin Neurosurg* 1979;26:12–95.

35. Baumgartner WA, Silverberg GD, Ream AK, Jamieson SW, Takaber J, Reitz BA. Reappraisal of cardiopulmonary bypass with deep hypothermia and circulatory arrest for complex neurosurgical operations. *Surgery* 1983;94:242–249.

36. Silverberg GD, Reitz BA, Ream AK. Hypothermia and cardiac arrest in the treatment of giant aneurysms of the cerebral circulation and hemangioblastoma of the medulla. *J Neurosurg* 1981;55:337–346.

37. Silverberg GD, Reitz BA, Ream AK, Taylor G, Enzmann DR. Operative treatment of a giant cerebral artery aneurysm with hypothermia and circulatory arrest: Report of a case. *Neurosurgery* 1980;6:301–305.

38. Spetzler RF, Hadley MN, Rigamonti D, Carter LP, Raudzens PA, Shedd SA, Wilkinson E. Aneurysms of the basilar artery treated with circulatory arrest, hypothermia, and barbiturate cerebral protection. *J Neurosurg* 1988;68:868–879.

Cerebrovascular Disease, edited by H. Hunt Batjer.
Lippincott-Raven Publishers, Philadelphia © 1997.

CHAPTER 93

Management of Carotid Cavernous Fistula

Phillip D. Purdy

GENERAL BACKGROUND

Carotid cavernous fistulae (CCFs) represent a group of disorders that are collectively characterized by abnormal shunting from the external and/or internal carotid artery into the cavernous sinus (CS). Under normal circumstances, the CS also provides venous drainage from the orbit by way of the superior orbital vein. Thus, the drainage from the vitreous of the eye is into the CS by way of the venous drainage from the orbit. Maintenance of a normal intraocular pressure is a function of maintenance of normal venous pressure in the orbit, among other factors.

In the presence of an arteriovenous shunt into the CS, flow becomes reversed in the orbital vein and becomes anteriorly directed. Because outflow tracts for venous drainage are diminished under normal circumstances over the scalp, venous congestion occurs in the territory drained by the orbital vein. This gives rise to many of the classic symptoms of CCF.

Patients with CCF present with a combination of proptosis caused by edema in the orbital fat, chemosis caused by conjunctival edema, scleral injection from increased venous pressure on the globe, and conjunctival hemorrhage from venous rupture due to increased pressure.

Diminished visual acuity can result not only from retinal detachment but from the production of glaucoma due to decreased drainage of vitreous into the pressurized venous system. Further visual decline may be secondary to production of papilledema, again secondary to the increased venous pressure. Visual decline can be fulminant and necessitate emergent therapy. Thus, close ophthalmologic monitoring and participation is an important component in the management of this family of disorders. Pharmacologic management of glaucoma requires close monitoring of intraocular pressure by the ophthalmologic members of the team. Also, acute rise in intraocular pressure or worsening proptosis may necessitate canthotomy. In patients with impaired ocular perfusion, this may assist visual preservation until successful treatment of the fistula is achieved.

Headaches may be related to stretching of dural structures in the CS, venous thrombosis, venous hemorrhage, or pathologic involvement in the Vth cranial nerve, the latter either by way of pressure in the CS or by pulsatile trauma from abnormal arterial flow in the CS.

Another common complaint, diplopia, may be secondary either to direct compression or pulsation on the IIIrd or VIth cranial nerves in the CS, or due to ischemic injury from decreased venous drainage of the nerves from the elevated venous pressure (1).

Halbach et al. reported a pulse synchronous bruit (2) in approximately 50% of 30 patients with dural fistulas involving the CS. I suspect the incidence is higher in those with traumatic CCF. The bruit can often be heard on examination with a stethoscope, either over the involved eye or elsewhere on the cranium. Observation of a bruit is an important component in management, as it represents a noninvasive means for rapid assessment of either the possible elimination or recurrence of a fistula during treatment. Its presence or absence should be recorded at the time of the initial examination so that subsequent examiners will be able to check for it.

Though cerebral symptoms are unusual in CCF, they are a particular risk in high-flow fistulas. They may occur secondary to increased pressure in cerebral cortical veins, resulting in cerebral edema or hemorrhage. They may also be secondary to cerebral ischemia due to arterial steal into the fistula, resulting in deprivation of flow to the brain. Subdural or subarachnoid hemorrhage may also occur when the arterialized blood drains pathologically into dural or cortical veins.

Understanding both the symptomatology and treatment of CCFs requires understanding the vascular and neural anatomy in and around the CS. Though it is assumed that readers of this text already understand that anatomy, a brief review is in order prior to discussion of therapeutic intervention, as the vascular channels are the major pathway for that therapy.

P. D. Purdy: Division of Neuroradiology, Department of Radiology, University of Texas Southwestern Medical Center, Dallas, TX 75235.

PERTINENT NEUROLOGIC AND VASCULAR ANATOMY AND VARIATIONS

The carotid artery exits the carotid canal of the temporal bone at its medial aspect and ascends into the CS from that point. This is at approximately the level of the posterior clinoid processes. After ascending approximately 1–1.5 cm, it makes a right-angle bend anteriorly and traverses the space between the posterior and anterior clinoid processes in the so-called horizontal segment. At the anterior clinoid process, it makes an acute bend posteromedially and enters the sub-arachnoid space as it ascends medial to the anterior clinoid process. This segment of the carotid artery has been labeled the siphon, and segments have been numbered for anatomic identification from 1 to 5, with 1 being the supraclinoid segment, 2 the portion as it enters the CS and turns poste-riorly, 3 the horizontal segment, 4 the segment as it angles inferiorly, and 5 the segment descending into the petrous carotid canal into the CS. It makes no particular sense, but the numbering goes from higher to lower as you progress from proximal to distal along the carotid.

Branches from the cavernous carotid include the meningo-hypophyseal trunk, arising from the fourth segment of the carotid siphon and coursing posteriorly to give branches to the hypophysis (the inferior hypophyseal artery) and to the meninges (including the artery to the tentorium, or the artery of Bernasconi and Cassinari). The lateral main stem artery arises from the posterior aspect of the third segment, giving branches to the meninges in the wall of the CS, and can anastomose with the middle meningeal artery. There are anterior capsular arteries arising from the anterior third and second portions of the carotid that contribute to blood supply

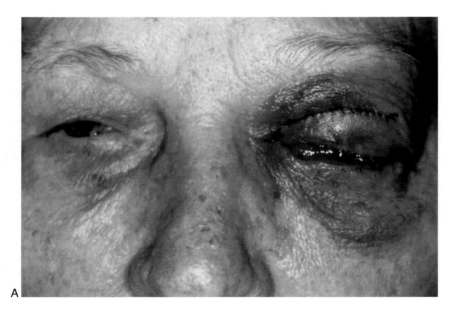

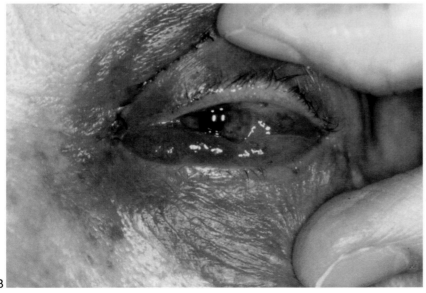

FIG. 1. A patient with a known carotid cavernous fistula presented with proptosis and chemosis. **A:** Baseline view shows the patient to be status post orbital surgery with the suture line in the eyelid. Note discoloration and edema around the affected orbit. Also, edematous conjunctiva is seen protruding from the proptotic, closed eyelid. **B:** The eye is held open and discoloration in the sclera as well as further evidence of conjunctival edema can be seen. (Case courtesy of Joe Hise, M.D.)

to the pituitary gland and sella but are rarely seen on an arteriogram. The ophthalmic artery arises from the distal second portion of the siphon. Between the ophthalmic artery and the intracranial carotid bifurcation, the superior hypophyseal, posterior communicating, and anterior choroidal arteries arise. Though a posterior communicating artery aneurysm has been reported to rupture into the CS to cause a CCF (3), this is a rare event and will not be discussed further.

The CS is a space bounded laterally and superiorly by dura. Inferiorly and medially, the walls of the sella turcica and greater wing of the sphenoid bone form the boundary. The CS is composed of multiple venous channels that surround the cavernous carotid (4) and receive contribution from the orbital venous drainage, the sphenoparietal sinus, and potential anastomoses with the pterygopalatine vessels by way of the inferior ophthalmic vein. Venous anastomotic channels routinely allow communication between the left and right sides of the CS and provide an important potential pathway for accessing a CS from a contralateral venous approach. Egress from the CS is by way of the superior petrosal sinus into the sigmoid sinus and by way of the inferior petrosal sinus into the internal jugular vein at the jugular foramen. In the pathologic state, egress occurs via the orbital veins owing to a reversal of the normal flow toward the sinus.

Cranial nerves traversing the CS include the IIIrd and IVth cranial nerves laterally, the VIth cranial nerve adjacent to the carotid artery at its inferolateral aspect, and the V1 and V2 segments of the Vth cranial nerve. The IIIrd, IVth, and VIth nerves traverse the sinus from posterior to anterior and exit via the superior orbital fissure. The V1 segment of the Vth cranial nerve exits via the superior orbital fissure as well. The V2 segment exits via the foramen rotundum and supplies sensation to the midface. Thus, pathology involving the CS can present with dysfunction of one or all of those cranial nerves.

The diagnosis of CCF can usually be made clinically. In the absence of a history of trauma, patients present because they have complaints related to the effect on the eye of increased venous pressure (Fig. 1). Imaging studies with either computed tomography or magnetic resonance confirm the diagnosis by the presence of the distended superior orbital vein. The diagnosis is confirmed by angiography, which should be performed with an eye toward the ultimate treatment of the disease. Therefore, maneuvers to elucidate the site and size of the CCF should be undertaken, including rapid sequence digital filming. Compression of the ipsilateral carotid during injection helps to slow the flow and better allows contrast to fill the fistula site prior to obliteration by the diffuse stain of the CS. Ipsilateral carotid compression during contralateral carotid or vertebral injection helps to create retrograde flow into the fistula. Multiple views are needed to try to demonstrate the anatomy of any ruptured aneurysm with consideration of demonstration of the aneurysm neck for therapeutic planning via an endovascular approach (5). The diagnostic arteriogram, therefore, is best performed by those who are charged with the ultimate

treatment of the disease rather than by the local radiologist prior to patient transfer. In many instances in our institution, patients have arrived with an inadequate diagnostic arteriogram, though the arteriogram amply demonstrated the presence of the fistula, only to have the arteriogram repeated for therapeutic planning purposes.

In addition, selective study of the external carotid should be performed in every case. Although traumatic fistulas and ruptured aneurysms are obvious as to their etiology, the collateral pathways between the extracranial and the intracranial circulation at the level of the CS are such that it is probably better to plan a thorough study of all of the anatomy rather than trying to select the patients in whom that bit of information can be excluded. In one case in our experience, for instance, the horizontal segment of the cavernous carotid contained multiple disruptions, necessitating carotid sacrifice. Retrograde flow in the ophthalmic artery, demonstrated on the external carotid arteriogram, was used to show the necessary location for distal occlusion beyond the fistula but proximal to the ophthalmic artery collateral.

GENERAL SURGICAL PRINCIPLES AND STRATEGIES

Treatment of a CCF is directed to relief of symptoms. In the case of most direct CCFs, this also involves elimination of the fistula. In the case of indirect CCFs, although elimination of the fistula is the goal, cure is sometimes difficult to achieve. In those cases, symptomatic relief can sometimes be achieved by elimination of the venous outflow to the orbit. A secondary goal in each case is preservation of the carotid artery flow to the brain. In some patients this is a necessity insofar as carotid sacrifice would not be tolerated.

In direct CCFs, treatment is therefore directed to the venous side of the pathology. Historically, the most successful and well-established treatment modality involved the placement of a detachable balloon across the CCF using flow direction from the arterial side. The balloon was then inflated such that it was wedged in the CS against the fistula. The balloon thereby created a tamponade of the CCF, eliminating flow and permitting healing across the orifice of the fistula (Fig. 2). In particularly large CCFs or in fistulas in which the CS was distended, multiple balloons were sometimes needed. The goal again was to position the balloons such that the last one placed was wedged against the arterial rent, causing the cessation of flow across it.

It has been said to be possible to cure 90% of all CCFs using an intraarterial approach and detachable balloons (6). However, if one is constricted to the use of intraarterial therapy and detachable balloons, carotid preservation is not possible in all situations.

Use of a transvenous approach (7) or a surgical approach to the CS (8) increases the rate of cure of CCFs without decreasing the rate of carotid preservation. However, detachable balloons can present substantial technical difficulties

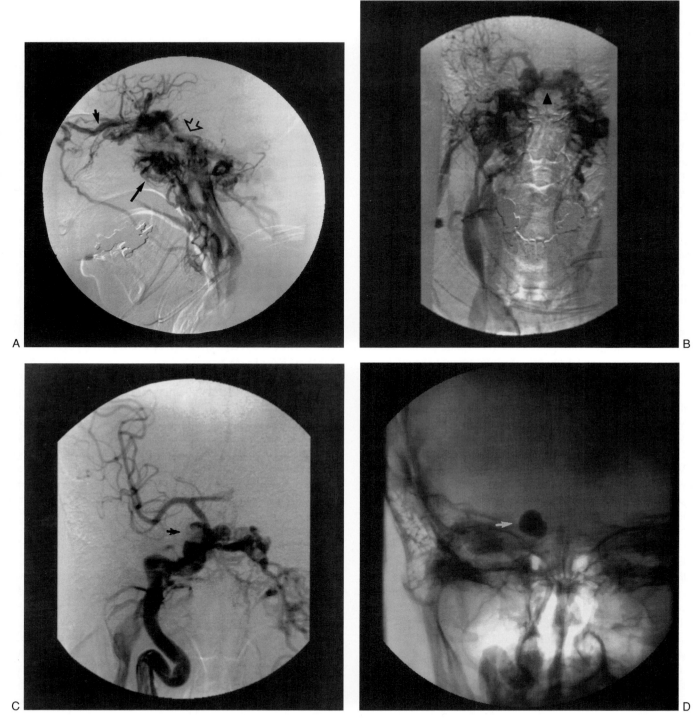

FIG. 2A–D.

when these approaches are used. Also, even in the case of direct CCF, it is not always possible to get a balloon to cross the arterial defect.

With indirect CCF, the problem is even greater for production of cure. Halbach et al. have reported the use of carotid jugular compression to create flow restriction in the carotid circulation to encourage thrombosis of fistulas. This conservative approach yielded cure in 34% of cases (1). In cases not requiring urgent treatment, we prefer a 4- to 6-week trial of carotid compression therapy with either direct or indirect CCFs. However, by the time of their referral, many patients present with elevated intraocular pressure, visual decline, or

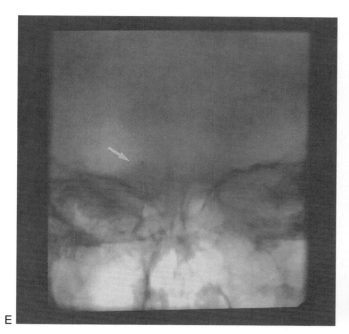

E

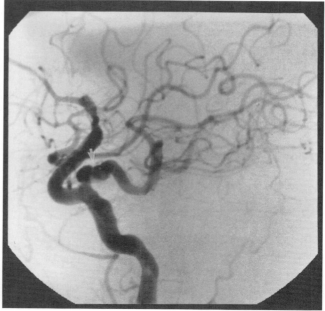

F

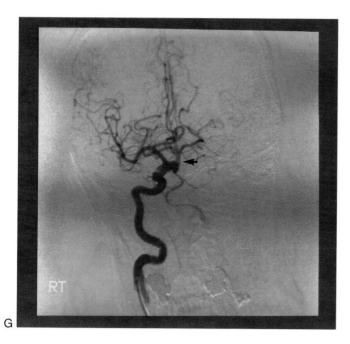

G

FIG. 2. Elderly female presented with a spontaneous occurrence of severe eye pain associated with fulminant proptosis and chemosis which awakened her from sleep. **A:** Lateral view pretreatment demonstrates venous drainage from the cavernous sinus. The orbital vein *(short arrow)*, the pterygopalatine venous plexus *(long arrow)*, and the inferior petrosal sinus *(open arrow)* are well demonstrated in this view. The majority of flow is diverted into the fistula and only a small amount is seen superiorly in the normal middle cerebral vessels. **B:** In this anteroposterior view, drainage is shown to be bilateral with cross-filling via the coronary sinus system *(arrowhead)*, which surrounds the pituitary fossa in the sella turcica. **C:** The occlusion of the carotid cavernous fistula (CCF) is regulated such that arterial patency is preserved. This is achieved via partial balloon inflation and test injection. In this view, the partially inflated balloon is seen *(arrow)*. The CCF remains patent. The balloon is a filling defect within the arterial shadow. Compare this to the appearance of that region in Part B. **D:** When inflated with contrast material, the balloon is readily apparent at fluoroscopy or on radiographs. However, hydroxyethyl methacrylate (HEMA), a polymerizing solution used to help prevent balloon deflation, is not radiopaque. **E:** The platinum marker at the tip of the catheter *(arrow)* is much more visible than the faintly opacified balloon, which is filled primarily with HEMA. **F:** Following balloon detachment, lateral view shows no further filling of the abnormal venous structures. However, a persistent trigeminal artery is shown at the balloon site *(arrow)*. **G:** The anteroposterior view shows retrograde filling into the basilar artery by way of the persistent trigeminal artery *(arrow)*.

cerebral symptoms necessitating a more urgent approach. In other cases, cosmetic symptoms are so severe that the patient is unwilling to participate in a conservative trial of therapy.

Again, indirect CCFs can be treated from an arterial, venous, or surgical approach. The surgical approach is reserved for cases in which the arterial and venous approaches either are unavailable or fail. Achievement of cure is often much more difficult with indirect than with direct CCFs. Transarte-

rial embolization can sometimes produce improvement in symptoms. However, as with other arteriovenous malformations, partial embolization often provides only temporary relief. It is rarely possible to cross an arterial fistula to the venous side from an arterial approach. In one case in our experience, placement of coils on the venous side of a fistula from that approach resulted in elimination of the fistula. However, under most circumstances the feeders are numer-

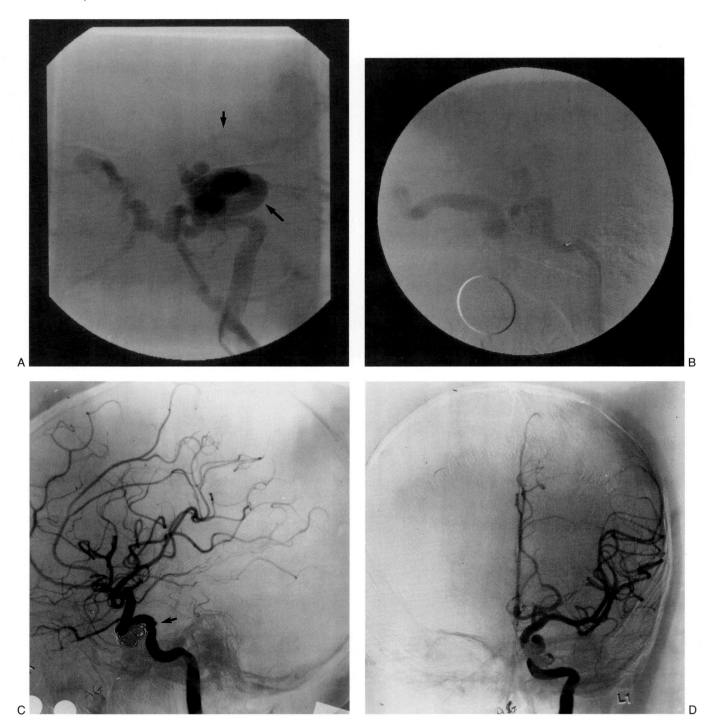

FIG. 3. This 7-year-old boy was poked in his left eye 2 months prior to the study when he fell and broke a fiberglass fishing rod. The rod tip missed his globe but punctured his orbit, giving him a through-and-through puncture wound in his cavernous carotid. **A:** Anteroposterior arteriogram of the left internal carotid reveals minimal flow in the intracranial circulation *(short arrow)*. Large orbital vein on the left is filling *(long arrow)*. Note also contrast flowing into the contralateral orbital vein via the venous sinus encircling the sella turcica. **B:** Lateral view during microcatheter placement of a detachable platinum coil demonstrates the large orbital vein draining anteriorly. **C, D:** Lateral (C) and anteroposterior (D) views following treatment demonstrate the platinum coil in the cavernous sinus with no further filling of the orbital vein. A small pseudoaneurysm *(arrow)* on the lateral view is seen at the posterior puncture site on the cavernous carotid.

ous and quite small. In symptomatic CCFs supplied in this fashion, the venous approach is often more rewarding.

In either direct or indirect CCFs, symptoms of elevated ophthalmic venous pressure are the primary problem. In those cases, our approach is generally by way of the inferior petrosal sinus to the CS. The goal is to advance the catheter to the posterior aspect of the superior orbital vein, beyond the CS. At that point, we begin packing coil material into the orbital vein and back the catheter slowly through the CS, depositing coils along the way. If the ipsilateral inferior petrosal sinus is occluded, as is often the case, it is sometimes possible to catheterize the contralateral inferior petrosal sinus and to access the ipsilateral orbital vein by way of the rich basilar plexus of veins that lies along the clivus or by way of the circular sinus that surrounds the infundibulum.

Though balloons can be advanced in the inferior petrosal sinus if the channel is widely patent and direct, advancement of catheters over guide wires is much simpler and allows a much more tortuous course to be navigated successfully. Thus, our first choice from the transvenous route has always been coils. Likewise, the flexibility offered with catheters and guide wires in the subtemporal transdural approach favors coils in that application, though the use of balloons has been reported (8).

Other materials can be used for embolization of CCFs. However, it must be remembered that the drainage from the orbit is normally retrograde to the CS. This is reversed in the setting of CCF. Particles or surgical silk are sometimes effective for use in conjunction with coils, where the particles are used for final occlusion in a vein with a basket of coils already in place. However, if small particles or liquid embolic material are used, the tendency will be for flow to carry the particles anteriorly, where they may occlude alternate venous drainage pathways from the orbit. We have seen acute deterioration in some patients using particulate or liquid embolic material and believe its indication to be unusual in light of improvements in available coil selection. Specifically, we have utilized ethanol in the successful treatment of several fistulas. Initially, we feared visual decline without anatomic justification of the belief that the retina might be exposed to ethanol. No retinal toxicity has been encountered. However, experience in at least two cases with acute rise in intraocular pressure and transient secondary decline in visual acuity causes us to believe this should be used with extreme caution and conservatism.

With the advent of more stringent regulatory control over intravascular devices, detachable silicone balloons that were once widely used with considerable success are now largely unavailable in the United States. We have used standard platinum microcoils as well as Guglielmi detachable coils (GDC) (Target Therapeutics, Fremont, CA) with success that we believe competes with that encountered with balloons (Fig. 3). In some ways, the control offered by GDC coils and the advantage of navigating tortuous anatomy with microcatheters makes detachable coils the material of choice.

When carotid sacrifice is contemplated or anticipated as a possible complication of a procedure, it is often desirable to assess the patient's potential for neurologic tolerance of that maneuver. Balloon occlusion testing is complicated by the hemodynamics of the fistula, which can produce cerebral steal via retrograde flow into the fistula when only proximal occlusion is achieved. We often perform temporary occlusion testing using a nondetachable balloon placed distal to the fistula. Though this may increase flow into the venous side of the fistula by temporarily cutting off distal carotid outflow, it should not affect the cerebral hemodynamics. If necessary, a balloon can also be placed proximally, temporarily trapping the fistula while neurologic testing is performed. We occlude the carotid for 15 minutes for routine temporary occlusion testing.

UNIQUE ANESTHETIC CONSIDERATIONS FOR THIS SPECIFIC CASE

Embolization of CCF can normally be done with the patient awake but sedated. This allows better monitoring of the patient's vision and neurologic condition. In some cases, such as acute occlusion of high-flow fistulas in which normal perfusion pressure breakthrough may be a concern, performance of the procedure with the patient awake may be specifically necessitated for monitoring purposes. However, when prolonged procedures are expected or where patient cooperation is questionable due to age, mental status, or anxiety, general anesthesia may assist considerably in the successful and efficient performance of a procedure.

The difficulty with these guidelines is that these embolizations are punctuated by unanticipated events and procedure time is, as a rule, unpredictable. Generally speaking, however, most of our procedures in adults are performed in the awake state.

I know of no specific sophisticated anesthetic considerations in these cases. We pretreat patients with broad-spectrum antibiotics prior to placement of intravascular foreign material. We also tend to pretreat with calcium channel blockers (nimodipine 60 mg PO or SL) and dexamethasone (Decadron), and embolizations are performed under systemic heparinization, particularly when originating on the arterial side. Routine placement of a Foley catheter decreases interruptions and increases patient comfort.

COMPLICATIONS AND THEIR MANAGEMENT

During treatment, complications may be encountered involving either the eye or the cerebral circulation. As mentioned earlier, use of particulate or liquid embolic material can cause acute venous outflow obstruction, resulting in worsening of the elevation of intraocular pressure. In one patient alluded to earlier, visible progression of proptosis and acute monocular blindness due to fulminant worsening of glaucoma necessitated emergent canthotomy for relief of intraocular pressure. The patient subsequently recovered normal vision and the worsened proptosis was transient, but the case underscored for us the need for close collaboration with the neuro-ophthalmology service in treatment of these patients.

Other routes of transvenous access might include percutaneous catheterization of the angular vein on the scalp to the superior orbital vein or retrograde catheterization by way of the facial vein. Direct placement of a cannula in the orbital vein may be performed under surgical exposure (9) (Fig. 4).

Neurologic decline during balloon embolization of a high-flow fistula has been reported that was relieved with partial balloon deflation (10). This was attributed to normal perfu-

sion pressure breakthrough following reestablishment of intracranial arterial pressurization when the fistula was relieved. This was successfully treated with graded occlusion. We have not seen this with coils nor have we seen it reported because coils tend to produce a slightly more gradual occlusion by their nature.

As is the case with any transarterial procedure, embolic complications are possible that could result in stroke. However, routine use of heparin during these procedures limits the incidence of that complication. The use of smaller introducer catheters for microcatheters than for balloons may also limit the incidence of intimal injury from the introducer cath-

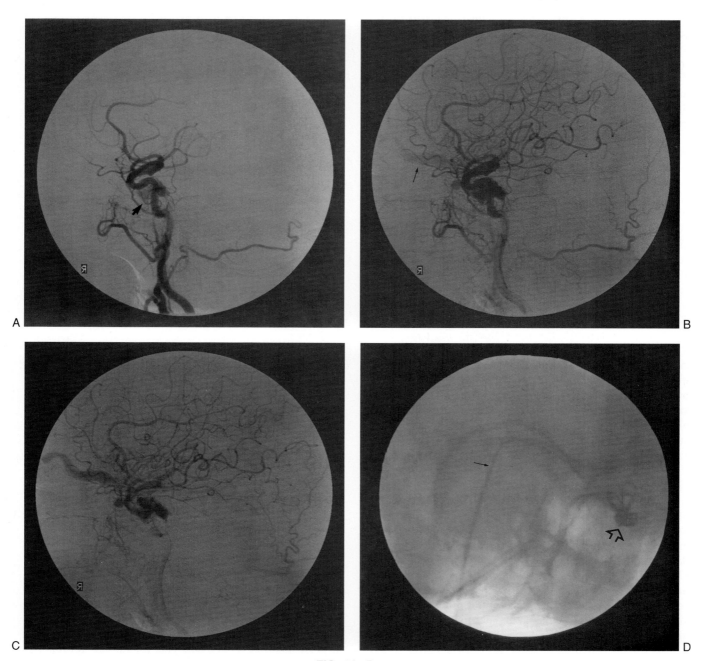

FIG. 4A–D.

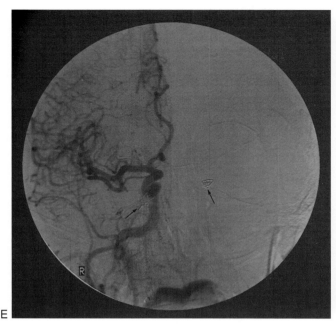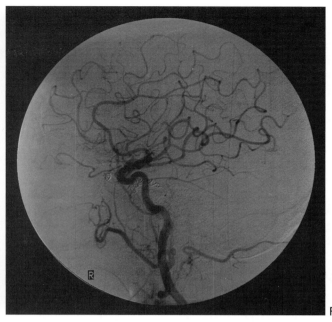

E   F

FIG. 4. This patient with a posttraumatic fistula presented with proptosis and chemosis. **A–C:** Sequential films from a lateral carotid arteriogram demonstrate flow into the fistula. In (A), there is hazy opacification of the cavernous sinus (CS) around the carotid *(arrow)*. In (B), the orbital vein is filling *(arrow)* as the cortical arteries are also filling. In the late arterial phase (C), the venous opacification in the CS in the orbital vein continues even as the carotid artery is washed out. **D:** Attempts at arterial and venous catheterizations from a femoral approach were unsuccessful. Direct surgical exposure of the orbital vein was undertaken. The catheter is seen traversing the bony orbit *(arrow)*. Platinum coils are being placed in the CS by way of retrograde catheterization of the superior orbital vein *(arrowhead)*. **E, F:** Successful catheterization of both orbital veins was achieved by way of the unilateral approach. Anteroposterior (E) and lateral (F) arteriograms obtained postoperatively reveal coils bilaterally *(arrows)*. Note lack of venous filling with preservation of arterial flow. (Case courtesy of Joe Hise, M.D.)

eter. Also, newer generations of introducer catheters are hydrophilic and have softer distal segments.

Special mention should be made of the hazards inherent in treatment of patients with Ehlers–Danlos syndrome. The arteries are extremely fragile in those patients, and venous packing is difficult to achieve. Halbach et al noted this vascular fragility in their report of treatment in four patients with this disease (11). In one patient, transarterial treatment with carotid preservation was successful. In another, carotid sacrifice was required. In another, a massive cervical carotid hematoma ensued during direct carotid puncture. The fourth patient died of pontine hemorrhage from presumed diversion of arterial flow to pontine venous channels. Whether there is increased compliance in such patients' venous systems or whether there is some other factor at work remains to be elucidated.

OVERVIEW

CCFs can result from direct trauma or developmental anomaly, both congenitally and secondarily. They can involve either the internal or external carotid. Those involving the internal carotid and resulting usually from trauma or ruptured intracavernous aneurysm are called direct fistulas, whereas those involving the external carotid and usually representing more complex vascular anomalies are called indirect fistulas. Either direct or indirect fistulas may result in visual compromise, ophthalmoparesis, or signs of venous hypertension in the orbit, such as proptosis and chemosis. Headaches are common, and neurologic deficit from arterial steal, venous hypertension, or cerebral hemorrhage are less common.

Both direct and indirect CCFs are treated primarily by endovascular means. The goal with a direct CCF is to seal the fistula from the venous side while preserving the carotid artery flow. Failing that, carotid sacrifice may be required, necessitating occlusion not only below but also above the fistula site in order to prevent recurrence of the fistula via retrograde flow. The goal with an indirect CCF may be the same if it is a relatively simple and straightforward fistula. However, often the goal with an indirect CCF is to provide relief of symptoms with or without elimination of the fistula. Those symptoms may include tinnitus, but the more frequent and more urgent problems relate to orbital or cerebral venous hypertension and complications thereof.

In the case of indirect CCFs, arterial embolization can sometimes give symptomatic relief, but venous embolization with occlusion of the involved portions of the CS and orbital vein are frequently needed. This is most often achieved from an inferior petrosal sinus approach, but the embolization must begin on the orbital side of the fistula in order not to cut off access while redirecting flow away from the posterior drainage, which is usually more benign.

The diminished availability of detachable balloons has removed a major ally in the treatment of this difficult problem. However, advances in coil technology, particularly with the availability of detachable coils, have filled much of the void left by the unavailability of balloons. Combinations of coils and particulate emboli are often effective to eliminate residual flow where coils alone produce incomplete occlusion. Symptomatic relief or angiographic cure should still be possible in approximately 90% of patients with carotid preservation.

ACKNOWLEDGMENTS

The author thanks Leslie Mihal for her assistance in the preparation of this manuscript.

REFERENCES

1. Halbach V, Higashida RT, Hieshima GB, Dowd CF. Endovascular therapy of dural fistulas. In: Vinuela F, Halbach V, Dion J, eds. *Interventional Neuroradiology: Endovascular Therapy of the Central Nervous System*. New York: Raven Press, 1992;29–49.
2. Halbach VV, Higashida RT, Hieshima GB, Reicher M, Norman D, Newton TH. Dural fistulas involving the cavernous sinus: results of treatment in 30 patients. *Radiology* 1987;163:437–442.
3. Kinugasa K, Higashi H, Ohmoto T. Fistula of the posterior communicating artery and cavernous sinus. *AJNR* 1995;16:1626–1628.
4. Hacker H. Superficial supratentorial veins and dural sinuses. In: Newton TH, Potts DG, eds. *Radiology of the Skull and Brain*, vol 2, book 3. St. Louis: CV Mosby, 1974;1861.
5. Guglielmi G, Vinuela F, Briganti F, Duckwiler G. Carotid cavernous fistula caused by a ruptured intracavernous aneurysm: endovascular treatment by electrothrombosis with detachable coils. *Neurosurgery* 1992;31:591–594.
6. Debrun G. Management of traumatic carotid cavernous fistulas. In: Vinuela F, Halbach V, Dion J, eds. *Interventional Neuroradiology: Endovascular Therapy of the Central Nervous System*. New York: Raven Press, 1992;107–112.
7. Halbach VV, Higashida RT, Hieshima GB, Hardin CW, Yang PJ. Transvenous embolization of direct carotid-cavernous fistulas. *AJNR* 1988;9:741–747.
8. Batjer HH, Purdy PD, Neiman M, Samson D. Subtemporal transdural use of detachable balloons for traumatic carotid cavernous fistulas. *Neurosurgery* 1988;22:290–296.
9. Monsein LH, Debrun GM, Miller NR, Nauta HJW, Chazaly JR. Treatment of dural carotid cavernous fistulas via the superior ophthalmic vein. *AJNR* 1991;12:435–439.
10. Halbach VV, Higashida RT, Hieshima GB, Norman D. Normal perfusion pressure breakthrough occurring during treatment of carotid and vertebral fistulas. *AJNR* 1987;8:751–756.
11. Halbach VV, Higashida RT, Dowd CF, Barnwell SL, Hieshima GB. Treatment of carotid-cavernous fistulas associated with Ehlers–Danlos syndrome. *Neurosurgery* 1990;26:1021–1027.

Cerebrovascular Disease, edited by H. Hunt Batjer.
Lippincott-Raven Publishers, Philadelphia © 1997.

CHAPTER 94

Vascular Complications of Head Injury

Mark D. D'Alise, Caetano Coimbra, and H. Hunt Batjer

In this chapter, we will attempt to categorize and describe a very heterogenous group of patients suffering blunt and penetrating head trauma in whom acute, subacute, or markedly delayed clinical complications develop as a result of injuries to the arterial or venous system. The heterogeneity of this group is obvious, not only from the variable time course of the neurovascular symptoms but also from the fact that injury to the vascular tree may produce minor or massive hemorrhage, as well as thromboocclusive events leading to cerebral ischemia. These injuries share the tendency to produce injury in predictable vascular territories with other forms of cerebrovascular disease.

Much of the information on which traditional teachings are based derives from the era before computed tomography (CT). As a result, the actual incidence of these complications cannot be accurately deduced from early published data. Because many of the sequelae of arterial or venous injury only become manifest days or weeks after the initial trauma, vascular injuries were underestimated when diagnostic angiography was the primary means of diagnosing head trauma. In recent decades, the immediate availability of CT and magnetic resonance imaging (MRI) diagnostic equipment has perhaps complicated rather than simplified the diagnosis of vascular injuries.

From a clinical standpoint, the fact that many intracranial vascular injuries occur in association with blunt or penetrating cerebral damage may mask the presence or significance of the vascular insult. The recent innovations of noninvasive technology including regional cerebral blood flow measurements, transcranial Doppler ultrasound measurements, and, more recently, CT angiography may help screen patients with much more certainty than in the past.

In the following discussion, we will attempt to categorize intracranial vascular injuries by location and pathophysiology. Emphasis will be placed on optimizing diagnosis for complex patients and identification of rational therapeutic approaches whenever possible.

VASCULAR INJURIES AT THE SKULL BASE

The unique anatomy of the internal carotid artery (ICA) in the petrous bone and cavernous sinus renders these segments of the ICA vulnerable to blunt and penetrating trauma. Knowledge of the anatomy of this area is important for understanding the mechanisms of injury associated with trauma to the ICA in this region. Before entering the petrous bone, the ICA is firmly adherent to the skull base via a dense fibrous ring. In the petrous bone, the vertical and horizontal segments of the ICA are confined to the bony carotid canal. After exiting the petrous bone, the ICA runs through the foramen lacerum and is fixed to the skull base by a layer of connective tissue. Inside the cavernous sinus, the ICA is relatively mobile, although still tethered to its intracavernous branches and the trabeculae of the sinus. The clinoidal segment of the ICA is in continuity with the intracavernous ICA and attached to the skull base dura by the proximal and distal dural rings. This peculiar situation—fixed and mobile segments in close relation to osseous and venous structures—makes this portion of the ICA particularly susceptible to shear forces and fractures during trauma to this region. Injury to the ICA at the skull base can lead to occlusion, arterial transection, aneurysm formation, or more commonly carotid cavernous fistula.

Aarabi and McQueen (1) reviewed a large group with traumatic ICA occlusion at the skull base and found that most of the injuries were associated with severe craniocerebral trauma and skull base fractures. In these cases, the artery tends to be crushed in the carotid canal by fractured bone fragments. In a small percentage of patients, occlusion of the ICA followed minor head trauma and was not related to skull fracture. In the former cases, the likely mechanism of injury is shear force applied at the points where the artery

M. D. D'Alise and C. Coimbra: Department of Neurological Surgery, The University of Texas Southwestern Medical Center, Dallas, Texas 75235.

H. H. Batjer: Division of Neurological Surgery, Northwestern University Medical School, Chicago, Illinois 60611.

is fixed to bony structures adjacent to more mobile segments. Traumatic occlusion of the ICA in the skull base involves intimal disruption, subintimal and medial dissection, and subsequent thrombosis. The commonly associated distal embolic showering is often the source of life-threatening neurologic injury, and the hemodynamic changes associated with acute vessel loss are less commonly symptomatic.

Occlusive lesions of this type are extremely difficult to manage, partially due to the frequent association with primary brain injury. When an altered level of consciousness is present or the CT scan demonstrates traumatic hematoma or evolving infarction, the occlusion should simply be reinforced with surgical ligation or endovascular techniques. For patients with intact consciousness, normal CT findings, and a very recent focal deficit, revascularization may be contemplated if reflow can be accomplished within 4 hours of the onset of deficit. It is critical to insure that the patient's neurologic deficit is not due to distal embolization at the time of occlusion. The contralateral carotid injection or vertebral injection with filling of the ipsilateral middle cerebral territory must be carefully studied to evaluate this possibility. In the absence of hemorrhagic brain lesions in these cases, anticoagulation, local thrombolytic therapy, or even embolectomy may be considered to reestablish flow.

Traumatic ICA aneurysms at the skull base can occur in the intracavernous and petrous segments of the carotid. The intracavernous variety is more common and frequently has a silent initial presentation that may later present with life-threatening epistaxis. Most of these hemorrhages occur within 3 weeks of trauma, but rare cases have been reported years later. Interestingly, the initial episode of epistaxis can be minor, only to be followed by massive hemorrhage leading to exsanguination and death (2,3). Such deaths are often the result of diagnostic and therapeutic delays. The clinical triad of monocular blindness, past head injury, and severe epistaxis should warn the physician of the possibility of skull-base false aneurysm.

Treatment for the patient who is actively bleeding must be undertaken emergently with the realization that a life-threatening complication exists. When no radiographic studies have been performed to clarify which carotid is injured, alternate carotid compression may be tried to determine which side lessens the flow. If this measure is not diagnostic, nasal packing should be attempted en route to the angiography suite. Rapid common carotid injection should clarify the offending site rapidly, and definitive endovascular balloon (3) or coil occlusion can be performed for proximal control. Distal trapping of this type of injury is recommended following the proximal procedure and can be done in a more controlled fashion during subsequent craniotomy. Alternatively, it is sometimes possible to place endovascular occlusive balloons across the aneurysmal segment, effectively trapping the ruptured aneurysm. If a surgical strategy is selected for achieving distal control—and assuming the carotid sacrifice is well tolerated—the surgeon should make every attempt at craniotomy to clip ligate the clinoidal seg-

ment of the carotid proximal to the origin of the ophthalmic artery to preserve important collateral potential.

For the patient whose bleeding has stopped, treatment is urgent but should consist of thorough diagnostic angiography with careful assessment of the site of injury, as well as sources of collateral flow. For the patient failing temporary trial occlusion, a number of alternatives exist, including graded clamp occlusion or distal revascularization followed by repeat trial occlusion and proximal sacrifice.

INTRACRANIAL VASCULAR OCCLUSIVE LESIONS

The majority of intracranial occlusive lesions result from nonpenetrating trauma. The extent of the arterial damage can be divided into intimal damage alone, intimal and medial damage, or complete transection (4). A nidus for thrombus formation and subsequent embolization may be formed after laceration of the intima without involvement of the media or the adventitia. Dissection and its anterograde propagation occurs with the violation of the intima and splitting of the internal elastic lamina. The likely hemorrhage between the internal elastic lamina and media may lead to either stenosis, occlusion, or embolization. When the media is damaged, leaving the adventitia intact, a "true" aneurysm may develop. However, this situation appears to be less frequent than rupture of the vessel or "false" aneurysm formation.

Epidemiologic evidence suggests that the majority of patients with intracranial traumatic vascular dissections are young. The peak occurrence occurs in the third decade of life, with a large number having been reported in children (5). The minor nature of the primary injury has been emphasized in the literature (4). It is possible that the delicate nature of the intima and the internal elastic lamina in humans and the entire vessel wall in the young could predispose to dissection following relatively minor injury.

The location of injury along the course of the artery is dependent on shearing forces applied at points of change in arterial mobility. Intracranially, these sites of maximal vulnerability are the point of dural ICA penetration, the ICA immediately distal to the posterior communicating artery, the carotid bifurcation, the point of the dural vertebral artery penetration, and distal to the origin of posterior inferior cerebellar artery. Damage to the intradural ICA is also associated with fracture of the anterior clinoid process.

A time interval between head injury and the first ischemic episode is a feature of traumatic ICA dissection. While patients occasionally develop acute neurologic deficit or subarachnoid hemorrhage (SAH), the majority either remain silent or present with symptoms in a delayed fashion a few hours to a few weeks after the original insult (4). The outlook is relatively poor for symptomatic patients with these injuries. Loar et al (6) reviewed patients with middle cerebral artery traumatic occlusions and found that one third were dead and a high percentage of the survivors had severe neurologic deficits. This high morbidity as well as the youth of the vulnerable individuals suggests a major need for vigilance in pursuing this diagnosis and for the development of more accurate noninvasive diagnostic methods.

Reported therapeutic alternatives have included no therapy, anticoagulation, stellate block, hypothermia, thrombolytic agents, steroids, and hyperbaric oxygen. Several factors intrinsic to this condition complicate or preclude rational therapy. First, most patients develop neurologic deficits prior to the diagnosis of any vascular injury and occasionally are not even in the hospital at the time of onset. This factor makes it extremely unlikely that any form of therapy could be instituted prior to the evolution of established infarction. Second, the nature of a dissection channel itself often jeopardizes vital penetrating arteries, including the anterior choroidal, lenticulostriates, and pontine perforators. No form of therapy would be expected to be beneficial when the origins of these vessels have been destroyed by a dissection channel. The third factor relates to the definite risk of SAH in these patients. Even those without SAH as a presenting feature may be at risk for this potentially fatal complication if anticoagulant or thrombolytic therapy were instituted.

The choice of therapy for these unfortunate patients must be well thought out, and our current thinking relies on angiographic criteria, the nature and severity of the patient's deficit, and whether SAH has occurred. For the asymptomatic patient or one who has a focal deficit attributable to perforating artery occlusion with angiographically mild stenosis, either no specific therapy or platelet suppression may be appropriate. Careful follow-up with angiographic confirmation should be performed. In the patient with a severely stenotic lesion and dense neurologic deficit, anticoagulation may be cautiously recommended to prevent thrombosis within the residual lumen or distal embolization. Transluminal angioplasty has been mentioned in this setting in hopes of widening the true lumen, although its use must be considered experimental and potentially dangerous in a patient with a weakened arterial wall. If incomplete occlusion is either found initially or develops in a delayed fashion, no specific therapy may be required if the neurologic course is stable and distal collaterals appear adequate. A fluctuating neurologic course would suggest that anticoagulation be initiated after adequate blood volume is insured. In very rare patients with obvious hemodynamic compromise of the distal vascular territory such that postural changes or fluctuations in the blood pressure produced neurologic compromise, maximal medical therapy with flat bed position, volume expansion, hemodilution, and pressor support should be offered. If this measure proves inadequate or weaning from the hemodynamic therapy is not tolerated, distal revascularization may be considered.

Once SAH has occurred, our impression is that definitive therapy should be undertaken as these patients appear to have a malignant natural history. In the ideal situation involving a vertebral artery dissection distal to the posterior inferior cerebellar artery (PICA) origin that results in SAH,

clip ligation of the vertebral artery distal to the PICA origin with or without trapping of the segment is usually curative and well tolerated. Patients treated by proximal ligation alone have a small but definite risk of rebleeding, especially if the dissection occurs proximal to the PICA origin, as retrograde flow across the vertebral confluens may reenter the dissection channel.

Occlusion of the anterior cerebral artery, posterior cerebral artery, and PICA is not rare following traumatic cerebral herniation syndromes. Infarction is quite common subsequent to these life-threatening crises. However, therapy is obviously directed at the cause of the herniation. In this context, the residual vascular insult, if present, is often relatively unimportant. Rarely, a false aneurysm may develop at the site of contact between the involved vessel and the skull base or dural reflection and produce symptoms days or weeks later.

POSTTRAUMATIC SUBARACHNOID HEMORRHAGE AND VASOSPASM

Posttraumatic SAH documented by the initial CT is currently accepted as an indicator of poor prognosis in head injured patients (7,8). In a prospective multicenter study, data derived from the initial CT scans of 753 patients with severe head injury documented subarachnoid blood in 39% of the cases. Furthermore, this study described an association between subarachnoid blood after severe head injury, elevated intracranial pressure (ICP), and mortality. Patients with SAH had a 2:1 increase in risk of death across all centers participating in the referred study (7). It remains unclear, however, how SAH influences the final outcome of severe head-injury patients. It is likely that SAH may not only reflect the extent of the injury but also act in ways similar to aneurysmal SAH and that vasospasm may be a common mechanism (7,9).

Posttraumatic vasospasm has remained controversial in a number of respects. Clearly the thickness of blood characteristically found in the subarachnoid space following head injury is quite different from that found after aneurysmal SAH. Thus, it would be anticipated that the incidence of vasoactive complications might be substantially less in trauma patients. It is also possible, however, that vascular injury at the time of head trauma may increase the sensitivity of the damaged vasculature to vasoactive compounds. Another hypothesis is that increased ICP could be primarily responsible for arterial narrowing in head-injury patients. However, vasospasm has recently been demonstrated in patients with normal ICP (10,11).

In the older literature, when the predominant method of investigation was angiography, the reported incidence of vasospasm following head trauma varied from 5% to 40% (7). More recently, a study using transcranial Doppler ultrasound (TCD) documented an incidence of vasospasm as high as 40% in severely head-injured patients. Vasospasm was found mainly in patients with a large amount of cisternal blood seen on CT scan (12). Another study employing similar techniques demonstrated a significant correlation between the TCD maximum mean flow velocity of the middle cerebral artery and the quantity of blood seen on CT scan of patients with posttraumatic SAH. This same study showed earlier occurrence of TCD high mean flow velocity compared with patients with aneurysmal SAH (11). Martin et al. (10) used TCD in conjunction with cerebral blood flow monitoring and angiography to follow head-injury patients and found vasospasm in 27% of the cases and SAH in all cases of severe vasospasm. The time course of spasm in this study was similar to that noted in aneurysmal SAH. In addition, the degree of arterial narrowing seen on the angiograms was comparable with that seen in aneurysmal SAH patients and correlated with the degree of reduction in the cerebral blood flow. An uncharacteristic, short vasospastic course (1.25 days) was noted in patients who developed vasospasm not associated with SAH. These findings led the authors to conclude that a different pathophysiology unrelated to toxic breakdown of blood products might be operant in this subgroup (10). It is possible that direct vascular injury may be an important event leading to vasospasm.

Although posttraumatic vasospasm is a well accepted entity, its clinical and prognostic importance is yet to be clarified. It is conceivable that some patients do develop ischemic symptoms referable to vasospasm after head injury. The diagnosis of these ischemic deficits is rendered difficult, if not impossible, due to coincident direct cerebral injury. We expect that the widespread use of TCD and other noninvasive techniques will allow us to learn more about the clinical significance of this condition. Furthermore, it is critical to determine whether treating vasospasm in head injury offers any benefit in terms of the patient's ultimate disability. In a multicenter trial, intravenous nimodipine was associated with a trend toward a more favorable outcome in patients who exhibited traumatic SAH on initial CT scan (8). On the other hand, damaged cerebral tissue may not tolerate hyperdynamic therapy routinely used to treat aneurysm-induced vasospasm. At the present time, we recommend careful monitoring to determine when vasospasm is developing. In the unusual circumstance where new deficits or neurologic deterioration can only be attributable to vasospasm, we recommend cautious volume and pressor support. This strategy should be abandoned if ICP increases or if there is an increase in low-density or mass effect on sequential CT scans.

TRAUMATIC INTRACRANIAL ANEURYSM

The development of cerebral aneurysm following head trauma is a rare event, particularly when measured against the high incidence of traumatic brain lesions. Despite this rarity, the probability of aneurysmal rupture combined with a possible surgical cure makes early diagnosis an imperative

goal. Unfortunately, the anatomy and pathophysiology of these lesions make repair with preservation of the parent vessel extremely unlikely.

Direct or indirect trauma to the cerebral vessels can lead to aneurysm formation. Direct injuries result from in-driven bone fragments or from a variety of missiles and weapons. Iatrogenic vascular injury as a cause of direct traumatic aneurysm following brain surgery or endovascular procedures is well documented in the literature and lately has become an increasingly important entity. Indirect injuries are generally associated with serious closed head injury and marked acceleration–deceleration distortion of the brain. Cerebral vessels can be damaged by striking the falx, the tentorium, or the sphenoidal ridge or by arterial laceration at tethering points of the circle of Willis during major brain shift. Surface arterioles, particularly those adherent to the dura, may be injured during sliding rotatory movements of the brain during trauma. This mechanism may explain peripherally located middle cerebral artery aneurysm occurring in absence of skull fracture (13). More commonly, however, traumatic aneurysmal lesions in this location are associated with linear skull fracture. The proposed mechanism is momentary trapping of surface vessels in the fracture lines.

Traumatic aneurysms may be classified based on the severity of vessel wall injury and resultant loss of structural integrity. True, false, and mixed aneurysms have all been carefully identified histologically. True aneurysms occur with disruption of the intima, internal elastic lamina, and media, with preservation of the adventitia. The distended adventitia thus forms the aneurysmal wall. False aneurysms are the most common type. They occur when the intima, internal elastic lamina, media, and adventitia are all disrupted, resulting in extravasation contained only by clot, arachnoidal plane, or brain parenchyma. A mixed traumatic aneurysm is defined by rupture of a true aneurysm, so that circulating blood is restrained only by hematoma or brain tissue at some site.

By far, the most common location for traumatic cerebral aneurysm is the distal middle cerebral branches (14) (Fig. 1). The second most common location is the distal anterior cerebral branches. In this location, the participation of the falx in the genesis of these lesions is well accepted (14). Supraclinoid ICA traumatic aneurysms are less common but can occur in association with fractures of the orbital roof and anterior clinoid process (13). Alternatively, lesions of the carotid artery at the origin of the posterior communicating artery can follow sudden brain shifts during head trauma.

Several reports in the literature have dealt with traumatic cerebral aneurysm in military practice. Aarabi (15) reported 223 patients who had been studied with cerebral angiography after injury with missiles during the Iran-Iraq war. It was reported that 3.6% of these patients ultimately developed traumatic aneurysms. Aarabi did note a higher risk of aneurysm formation with lesions caused by shell fragments, particularly when involving the pterional region or crossing the midline near branches of the anterior cerebral artery. Addi-

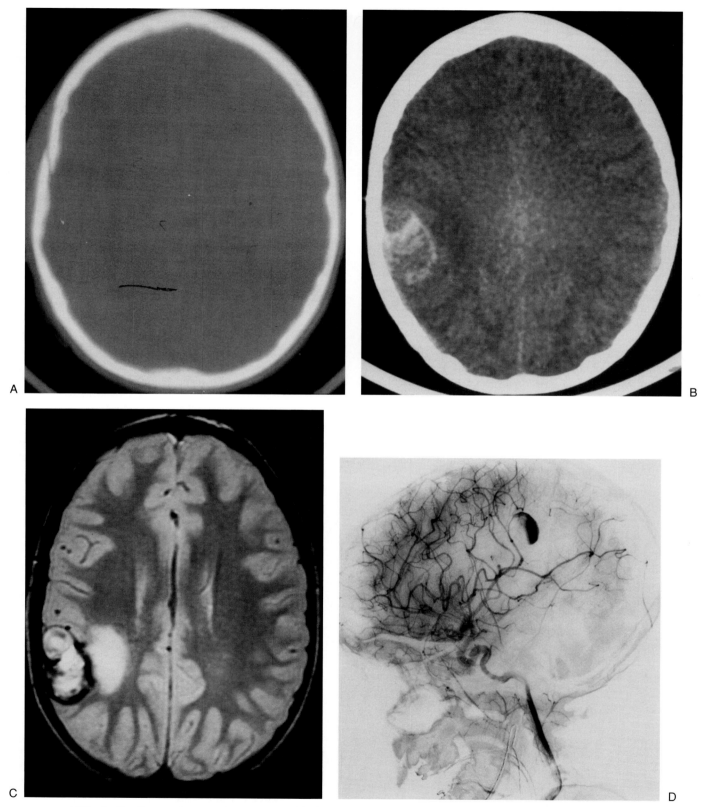

FIG. 1. Posttraumatic pseudoaneurysm. **(A)** Initial bone window CT scab of an 8-year-old boy who suffered a mild head injury from a fall. The only finding on the initial workup was the minimally displaced right temporal skull fracture. **(B)** He presented again 1 year later with a seizure and decreased level of consciousness and was found to have intra parenchymal hemorrhage on noncontrast CT. **(C)** T1-weighted noncontrast MRI demonstrates a false aneurysm with adjacent hematoma and edema. **(D)** Right carotid arteriogram shows filling of the distal middle cerebral pseudoaneurysm. The patient underwent craniotomy for clip sacrifice of the lesion.

tionally, the presence of significant intracerebral hematoma was considered indicative of traumatic aneurysm. Haddad et al (16) reviewed patients injured in the Beirut, Lebanon, conflict and described 15 patients with intracranial aneurysms secondary to missile injury. The vast majority of these lesions resulted from shrapnel wounds and involved the middle cerebral artery territory. Intracerebral hematoma or acute subdural hematoma was present in a high percentage of the patients.

Leavy et al (9) subjected 30 patients with craniocerebral penetrating gunshot injury and SAH in a civilian population to cerebral angiogram and documented only one cerebral aneurysm. It is postulated that bullets having high velocity and high energy are more likely to transect an artery. Nevertheless, shrapnel or shell fragments with low energy and cutting edges are more prone to injure the wall of a vessel and cause the formation of an aneurysm (16).

Penetrating stab wounds to the head carry a significant risk of vascular lesions. In a large series of patients with this kind of injury, duTrevou and van Dellen (17) documented cerebral aneurysm in 12% of cases and advocated cerebral angiography as early as possible in all patients with stab wounds to the head.

Traumatic cerebral aneurysms, as opposed to traumatic arterial dissections discussed earlier in this chapter, are almost always associated with evidence of additional, significant brain injury. The prognosis for these lesions is intimately related to the extent of the initial craniocerebral trauma. A large volume of experience is available from which to study the natural history of traumatic aneurysms. There is remarkable similarity between reported series and our own experience in Dallas, Texas, and there is every indication that these lesions are highly unstable and pose an immediate threat to life. The classical presentation of traumatic aneurysm is sudden neurologic deterioration associated with SAH or intracerebral hematoma several days after head injury. In Fleischer and colleagues' (14) review, 43% of patients presented with delayed SAH. While immediate rupture of traumatic aneurysms has certainly been reported, in general, hemorrhage occurs a few days after injury. Roughly 90% of aneurysms have ruptured within 3 weeks of injury and about one half of these ruptures are fatal (14). A current mortality of 18% for surgically treated patients contrasts with a mortality of 41% for medically managed patients (14). While these data undoubtedly reflect some selection bias, it is clear that these lesions are inherently unstable and an aggressive surgical posture is advised.

Traumatic aneurysms may be angiographically evident as early as 2 hours after the initial injury, although it has yet to be clarified how late these lesions can form after trauma. Cerebral angiogram should be contemplated in every head-trauma patient with evidence of unexplained late deterioration in conjunction with SAH or cerebral hematoma. In addition, patients with penetrating brain injury must have an angiogram when a significant cerebral hematoma is present in the territory of the middle cerebral or anterior cerebral artery. Several features may help in angiographically differentiating traumatic aneurysms from congenital ones; the former generally lack a discrete neck and their sac has an irregular contour. In addition, delayed filling and emptying of the aneurysm is commonly seen with traumatic lesions.

While scattered reports of spontaneous regression of traumatic aneurysms are to be found, the literature is replete with documented radiographic enlargement of these lesions over time (13). In light of the evidence from the literature and our own experience, we recommend immediate surgical exclusion of these injured segments of the circulation. Due to their mechanism of formation, they are rarely amendable to definitive clip ligation, at least in the acute phase. The surgeon should anticipate a true laceration of the vessel and plan on definitive trapping. Due to the overwhelming likelihood of vessel sacrifice, thought needs to be given to the issue of available collateral flow. In general, the urgency of the procedure itself helps dictate whether flow augmentation can be contemplated. For comatose patients with an immediate life-threatening intracranial hematoma, trapping of the diseased segment and evacuation of the mass is routinely performed. The majority of traumatic aneurysms involve the distal middle cerebral branches and as such do not often require revascularization. When the aneurysm involves an eloquent segment, however, planned bypass into the distal segment is appropriate. In general, the distal anterior cerebral artery has excellent collateral potential from the posterior pericallosal artery. After temporary isolation of the aneurysmal segment and opening of the aneurysm, brisk back bleeding is the rule. To date, we have not revascularized a pericallosal artery. In stable patients with lesions involving the proximal carotid or vertebral arteries, it is now possible to perform trial occlusion in the awake patient. In our experience, however, these patients are typically critically ill and unconscious with major brain injuries or severe SAH. Therefore, some distinction is made between the acutely ruptured cerebral artery and the somewhat more stable traumatic aneurysm. The acute arterial laceration is typically much more severe in its consequences, and treatment is emergent and directed at the attempt to save the patient's life. For the patient who suffers a survivable SAH several days after injury, the considerations are much more directed toward careful preoperative evaluation and preservation of function.

TRAUMATIC ARTERIOVENOUS FISTULAS

Fistulous connections between the arterial and venous systems may occur as a result of extremely minor or quite major arterial disruptions. Fistulas may be found to involve vessels of the neck, skull base, scalp, dura, or cortex. These fistulas may remain silent for many days, weeks, or years after the injury, before becoming symptomatic. The most common traumatic arteriovenous (AV) fistula is the carotid cavernous fistula (CCF) (Figs. 2 and 3). Traumatic CCF generally results from direct communication between the carotid artery

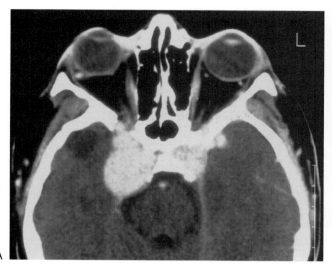

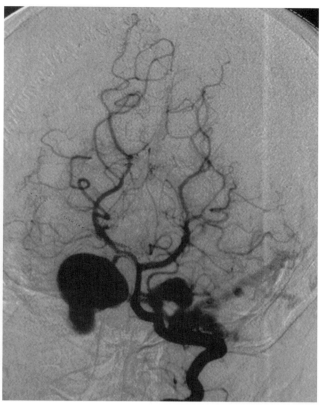

A · B

FIG. 2. Carotid cavernous fistula with pseudoaneurysm. **(A)** Contrast-enhanced CT scan of a 12-year-old girl who suffered a severe head injury 1 year earlier and presented with a 1-week history of chemosis, proptosis, and ophthalmoplegia of the right eye. Note the medial gaze of right eye demonstrated on CT. **(B)** Anteroposterior and lateral vertebral arteriograms show high-flow carotid cavernous fistula with bilateral cavernous sinus involvement and associated right cavernous carotid pseudoaneurysm. She underwent a trial balloon occlusion, which was tolerated clinically and by qualitative blood flow study, and was treated with a trapping procedure that included cervical internal carotid ligation and right fronto-temporal craniotomy for clipping of the intracranial carotid artery proximal to the ophthalmic artery.

and the cavernous sinus as a result of blunt or penetrating trauma. The unique anatomic position of the cavernous carotid artery within a myriad of venous channels provides the proper substrate for fistula development. Direct lesions of the intracavernous carotid by fractured osseous fragments or missiles are the most common causal mechanism of traumatic CCF. On rare occasions, avulsion or laceration of a meningeal branch of the cavernous ICA may lead to CCF. External carotid artery branches tend to be involved in spontaneous CCF, but occasionally they may also participate in traumatic CCF, mainly after late recurrence of the fistula following successful treatment.

Traumatic CCF can be divided into high- and low-flow fistulas, the former being by far the more common variety. The typical clinical manifestation of traumatic CCF is represented by the triad of pulsating exophthalmos with audible bruit, conjunctival chemosis, and visual deficit on the side of the fistula. Extraocular movement dysfunction may also be present. Characteristically, these clinical symptoms and signs are frequently delayed by days or even weeks after the traumatic injury (18). The size of the arterial injury and the

individual venous anatomy of the cavernous sinus are important determinants of the clinical presentation in CCF. For example, large fistulas in the presence of a cavernous sinus with dominant posterior venous drainage may present with minimal ocular signs. On the other hand, small fistulas with minimal posterior outflow may display prominent ocular signs. Several CCF angiographic findings may be associated with an unusual clinical course. Halbach et al (19) studied 155 patients with CCF and concluded that when CCF is associated with cavernous sinus varix or pseudoaneurysm extending into the subarachnoid space, massive SAH may occur with grave consequences. Cortical venous drainage, often connected with poor cavernous sinus outflow, may lead to cortical venous hypertension and/or intracerebral bleeding. Life-threatening epistaxis complicating CCF is frequently the result of a pseudoaneurysm or venous pouch entering the sphenoidal sinus through a basal skull fracture (19).

High-flow fistulas often demand prompt treatment. The most common neurologic sequela requiring urgent therapy is progressive visual failure due to elevation of intraocular

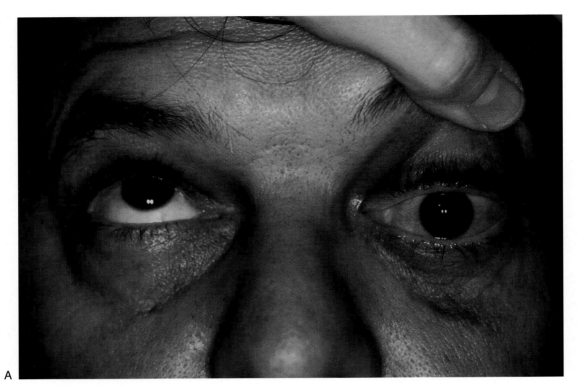

A

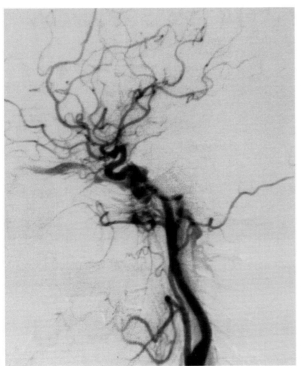

B

FIG. 3. Carotid-cavernous fistula. **(A)** A 45-year-old male with ophthalmoplegia, chemosis and proptosis following a minor head injury. **(B)** Left carotid arteriogram demonstrating carotid cavernous fistula.

venous pressure. Other complications of CCF that dictate less urgent intervention are intolerable bruit and/or headache and proptosis with corneal exposure. The treatment of CCF has made tremendous progress over the last 20 years. The therapeutic armamentarium includes a large variety of direct surgical techniques (20–22), interventional endovascular ra-

diologic procedures (18,21,23), and combined approaches (24). Less aggressive maneuvers such as intermittent external carotid and jugular compression have also been utilized as an initial approach to low-flow fistulas. The ideal treatment of CCF should produce eradication of the fistula, preservation of the ICA flow, and resolution of the fistula-related symptoms. Visual function is almost always salvageable when preoperative visual loss is only mild. Severe visual loss, on the other hand, is consistently irreversible and tends to progress to blindness.

Interventional radiology has currently assumed a dominant role in the management of these patients. The initial transvascular approaches employing a Fogarty catheter with permanent occlusion of the fistula and carotid have been replaced by more contemporary techniques involving detachable silicone balloons, particulate emboli, liquid adhesive, and more recently platinum coils (18,21,23). Arterial and/or venous navigation to the cavernous sinus has been employed with these techniques according to the individual location and anatomy of the fistula. Recently, alternative techniques to access the cavernous sinus through the superior orbital fissure, superior orbital vein, or angular vein of the forehead have been proposed, mainly as a rescue option when initial treatment failed or when the arterial opening involves the anteroinferior compartment of the cavernous sinus (25,26). These combined techniques have made it possible to cure the fistula and preserve the artery in the overwhelming majority of patients with lesions. Careful follow-up of these patients is mandatory, and we have good documentation of apparently perfect angiographic resolution of the fistulas, only to be followed by the delayed development of giant false aneurysm. At present, open surgical procedures should be reserved for patients failing endovascular attempts.

Orbital venous varix is generally thought of as a congenital lesion that presents with positional or exertional exophthalmos. It can, however, be related to penetrating orbital trauma (Fig. 4). To the unfamiliar examiner, this lesion can be mistaken for an AV fistula. The natural history is very benign, and treatment is considered only in situations where the periodic exophthalmos is a cosmetic concern. Although transorbital surgical excision has been reported, it is a technical challenge; therefore, if available, supraorbital, transvenous endovascular obliteration is the treatment of choice.

Scalp AV fistulas are surprisingly rare considering the intense vascularity of the scalp and the high frequency of trauma to this region. Nevertheless, they can occur following relatively minor blunt or penetrating head trauma (27). The clinical picture generally consists of a soft focal area of swelling on the scalp with associated audible bruit and/or headache. These lesions often involve the occipital and superficial temporal arteries but can also recruit feeding vessels from vertebral and subclavian arteries and other branches of the external carotid. The fistula consists of multiple endothelial-lined channels between the involved artery and vein. Internal and external carotid angiography, as well as vertebral system evaluation in more posterior lesions, is recommended for detailed demonstration of the arterial feeders. Recommendation for treatment should be tailored to each case. Asymptomatic small fistulas can be followed, but large ones, symptomatic or not, should be treated to prevent increasing shunting and recruitment of new feeders. Another concern is the possibility of exsanguination following a

minor trauma to the area of the lesion. Complete surgical excision with ligation of all the feeders is curative. Endovascular embolization is an option but, if incomplete, will result in later recurrence.

In a systematic review of cerebral angiograms in 446 head trauma patients, Freckmann et al (28) found a 1.8% incidence of AV fistula involving the middle meningeal artery. These fistulas generally involve a communication between the middle meningeal artery and neighboring veins or the sphenoparietal sinus; they are often associated with linear skull fractures over the involved region. This particular type of dural AV fistula is generally asymptomatic, and spontaneous closure has been reported. Treatment is not mandatory, but follow-up is recommended since the natural history of these lesions is not completely understood. Middle meningeal AV fistulas can rarely be complicated by cortical and scalp feeders and/or cortical drainage (29–31). The clinical course in these cases tends to be less benign and patients may present with hemorrhage, seizures, or focal neurologic signs. Surgical resection with or without endovascular embolization is the treatment of choice for such cases. Traumatic AV fistulas involving dural sinuses present a more complex problem. It is our impression that most of these lesions represent a late complication of thrombosis of a major venous sinus and behave similarly to their spontaneous AV malformation counterpart. These fistulas may recruit cortical venous drainage and pose a risk of SAH or intracerebral hemorrhage. Elevation of the venous pressure in the major sinuses is a possibility. This untoward event may produce intracranial hypertension or progressive neurologic deficit. Our strategy for these complex fistulas involves preoperative embolization followed by surgical skeletonization of the sinus and occasionally excision of the sinus itself, if located favorably. For sigmoid sinus fistulas associated with venous occlusions or anomalies without cortical drainage, therapy is often worse then the condition itself. The typical complaints of audible bruit can be improved by asking the patient to sleep with some radio static (white noise) in the room and by carefully informing them of the magnitude of a complete excision.

Rarely, vertebral artery–vertebral plexus fistulas can present with intracranial hemorrhage when associated with a fracture of the foramen magnum (Fig. 5). Because of the ability of pressurized blood to track through injured tissue planes, noncontrast CT should always be utilized in patients with high-cervical penetrating vascular injuries.

Pure, traumatic cortical AV fistulas are rare and not well documented in the literature. It is possible that this type of lesion can develop following a penetrating head wound or depressed skull fracture. Our feeling is that, when diagnosed, they should be excised, as they carry some risk of subarachnoid or intraparenchymal hemorrhage.

VENOUS SINUS INJURY

Dural venous sinus injuries present a potential life-threatening complication of head trauma. The superficial anatomi-

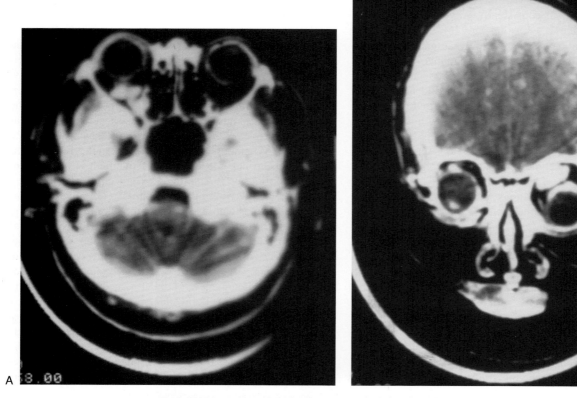

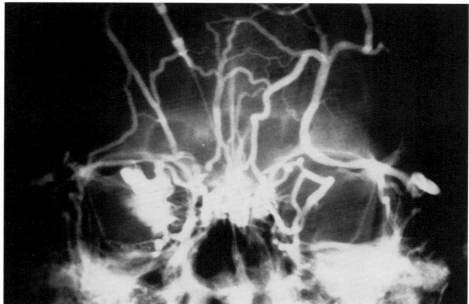

FIG. 4. Orbital varix. Supine **(A)** and prone **(B)** CT scans show orbital varix in a 45-year-old male who suffered a shrapnel wound 25 years earlier and complained of positional, right proptosis. **(C)** Supraorbital venogram demonstrates the varix. The patient elected observation with annual ophthalmologic evaluation.

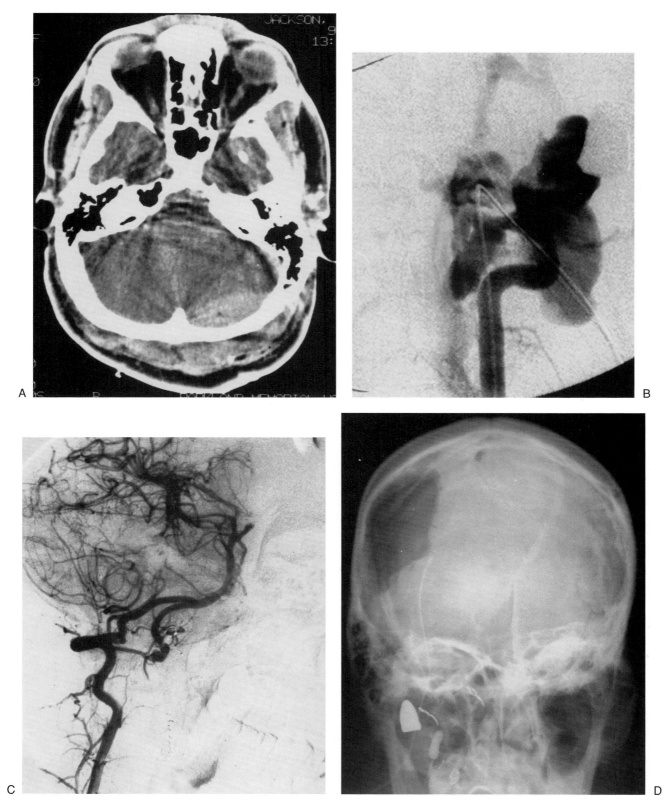

FIG. 5. Vertebral arteriovenous fistula. **(A)** Initial CT scan of a 21-year-old male with a gunshot wound to the posterior midcervical spine. Note the large left posterior fossa epidural hematoma. **(B)** Left vertebral arteriogram demonstrates an AV fistula at the level of the foramen magnum. **(C,D)** Surgical exploration demonstrated a complete transection of the left vertebral artery. It was sacrificed with proximal balloon embolization followed by proximal and distal clip placement. The distal clip was placed through a far lateral suboccipital craniotomy, just proximal to the posteroinferior cerebellar artery.

cal position of these large venous conduits renders them highly susceptible to penetrating injury and depressed skull fracture. In a recent report from Germany, dural sinus injury was reported in 4% of operated patients with severe head injury. The mortality rate was as high as 40% (32). Fatal massive hemorrhage and uncontrolled intracranial pressure (ICP) elevation secondary to sinus obstruction are the most grave consequences of venous sinus injury.

Hemorrhage following sinus injury is usually into the epidural or subdural space or externally if the wound is compound. Bilateral epidural hematoma can occur with superior sagittal sinus injury. In the posterior fossa, the majority of extradural hematomas are associated with a fracture overlying the transverse sinus or the torcular (33). Epidural lesions can affect the patient by compression of the underlying brain and/or the sinus wall followed by venous congestion (33). Compound wound fractures over a venous sinus can cause severe blood loss and hypovolemic shock. The importance of expeditious recognition and treatment of this situation cannot be overemphasized. Initial treatment consists of cautious elevation of the head and local packing to control the hemorrhage. Careful attention to avoid air embolism is mandatory.

Depressed skull fracture over a sinus may result in laceration and/or occlusion of the sinus with subsequent develop-

ment of cerebral venous congestion and increased ICP (34). It is our opinion that not all midline depressed skull fractures should be elevated. The ones located in the anterior third of the sagittal sinus should be left undisturbed, unless hemorrhage can not be controlled by others means. Stable patients with depressed fractures over the posterior two thirds should initially undergo angiography. If the sinus is patent, elevation of bone fragments over the midline should be avoided. When the angiogram demonstrates occlusion of the sinus or severe flow compromise, the fracture should be reduced and the sinus reconstructed as necessary. Patients with copious uncontrolled hemorrhage should not await angiography, and the surgeon should be prepared to repair a potential sinus laceration.

Much of our current surgical standards on venous sinus injury stem from the military experience during the second half of this century. Meirowsky (35) reported 112 cases of sinus injury during the Korean War with a 11.6% overall mortality rate and a 20% mortality when only sigmoid sinus injuries were considered. The majority of the technical repairs in this report consisted of sutures tied over muscle stamps and oversewing of the sinus laceration. Experiences with sinus injury during the Vietnam War saw the introduction of repair with autologous vein patches or grafts (36) and the use of a temporary indwelling shunt during periods

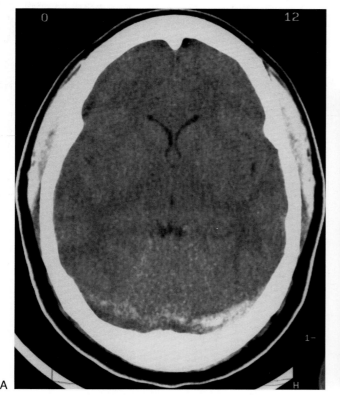

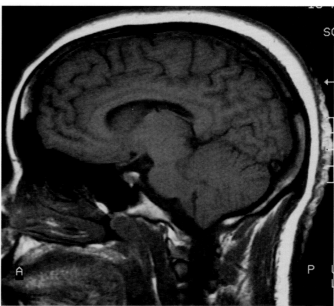

FIG. 6. Sagittal sinus thrombosis. A 25-year-old female with a history of a minor motor vehicle collision 3 weeks earlier presented with progressive headache and memory loss. **(A)** Nonenhanced CT scan demonstrates thrombosis within both transverse sinuses and the torcular. **(B)** Sagittal MRI confirms the absence of superior sagittal sinus flow void and clot within torcular.

of temporary occlusion (37). Reporting on sinus injury during the same conflict, Kapp et al (37) showed the evolution of treatment and its impact on patient outcome. During the 1968–1970 time period, the overall mortality rate was 27%, with a substantial improvement seen during the 1971–1972 interval when only one death in 16 cases was reported (6%).

Concepts of repair of sinus injuries must take into consideration the unique anatomy of these structures, formed by separation of inextensible dural leaves and suspended in their deepest extension by the falx or the tentorium. To overcome these anatomic barriers, extensive exposure proximal and distal to the anticipated site of injury should be obtained early during the procedure. This allows definitive trapping of the involved segment if major hemorrhage develops at the time of final bone removal. We have found it helpful to open the dura on both sides of the sinus proximal and distal to the injured segment to facilitate this maneuver. After careful inspection, if the injury involves a simple outer leaflet laceration, the edges of the sinus can simply be oversewn. When a portion of the sinus wall is missing, however, a dural flap can be fashioned to reconstitute luminal patency. This maneuver is easy and can be quickly performed, but clearly does not leave an intimal surface in contact with the flowing venous blood. Although late thrombosis is a risk, it is surprising how often this tactic is successful in the long term. When a significant portion of the sinus wall has been lost, placement of a venous patch graft is recommended. We agree with Kapp's recommendation that no grafting is necessary if 50% of the sinus lumen can be preserved by direct repair (37). In extensive sinus injury, however, either wide-patch grafting or venous-interposition grafting is required. Fogarty catheters can be inserted into the proximal and distal sinus lumina and inflated to facilitate hemostasis. If temporary occlusion is anticipated to be protracted, shunting can be performed during the reconstructive procedure (37). It is possible that morbidity associated with interposition grafts to the superior sagittal sinus is primarily related to loss of cortical venous structure entering this segment of the sinus.

Thrombosis of the sagittal sinus or transverse/sigmoid sinuses can develop after mild closed-head injury with or without fracture (38–40) (Fig. 6). Several theories have attempted to explain the pathogenesis of this condition. They include intramural hemorrhage caused by rupture of small sinusoids, injury to the endothelial lining, and alteration of blood coagulation after head trauma. The clinical picture generally develops 2–10 days after head trauma and varies according to the severity of trauma, the patient's age, and the location of the occlusion. It may involve signs and symptoms of posterior fossa–cerebellar dysfunction (40) or increased ICP and venous congestion with or without seizures (38,39). Some cases can have a protracted course and develop a pseudotumor-like syndrome. The treatment is controversial and should be individualized for each patient according to the severity of the symptoms. Therapies include general supportive care, cerebrospinal fluid shunt, surgical or endovascular thrombectomy, or thrombolytic therapy. In

TABLE 1. *Thrombolytic technique*

1. 6F sheath placed into ipsilateral common femoral vein and contralateral femoral artery.
2. Perform cerebral arteriography, filming late into venous phase.
3. Advance 5F catheter into internal jugular vein to C-1 level.
4. Advance microcatheter and guidewire through diagnostic catheter and into sigmoid sinus.
5. Advance wire into appropriate sinus. May need to rotate wire tip to macerate clot in order in advance the wire tip.
6. During advancement through clot, infuse 50,000 IU urokinase every 15 min to bathe the thrombus as it is traversed.
7. 250,000–500,000 IU urokinase given during each sitting.
8. Position catheter near distal end of the thrombus, with careful attention paid to not leaving it at a point where the urokinase will preferentially drain through venous collaterals.
9. Secure catheter to patient's thigh with an occlusive dressing and place patient on infusion of 60,000–100,000 IUs/hr.
10. 18–24 hours later repeat the angiography. If thrombolysis is inadequate, reposition the catheter as needed and continue the overnight infusion of urokinase.
11. When the superior sagittal sinus and at least one transverse sinus are open, one may consider terminating the infusion. Aim for opening both transverse sinuses.
12. Convert patient from heparin to warfarin and continue warfarin for 3–6 mos.

our institution, aggressive attempts toward thrombolytic therapy are made in patients diagnosed within 48 hours of occlusion (Table 1). Chances of restoring sinus patency after 48 hours of occlusion are much lower.

CONCLUSION

These relatively infrequent and clearly heterogeneous arterial and venous injuries represent an important cause of major morbidity and mortality following mild and severe head trauma. New diagnostic techniques are becoming available that are less and less invasive and offer a high degree of accuracy in terms of patient screening. Judicious use of these diagnostic tools will result in a higher likelihood of more accurate and earlier diagnoses and should provide the clinician with an opportunity to intervene in selected cases before the evolution of permanent cerebral injury.

REFERENCES

1. Aarabi B, McQueen JD. Traumatic internal carotid occlusion at the base of the skull. *Surg Neurol* 1978;10:233–236.
2. Chambers EF, Rosemblum AE, Norman D, et al. Traumatic aneurysms of cavernous internal carotid artery with secondary epistaxis. *Am J Neuroradiol* 1981;2:167–173.
3. Simpson RK, Haper RL, Bryan RN. Emergency balloon occlusion for massive epistaxis due to traumatic carotid-cavernous aneurysm. Case report. *J Neurosurg* 1988;68:142–144.

4. Morgan MK, Besser M, Johnson I, Chaseling R. Intracranial carotid artery injury in closed head trauma. *J Neurosurg* 1987;66:192–197.

5. Frantzen E, Jacobsen HH, Therkelsen J. Cerebral artery occlusions in children due to trauma to the head and neck. *Neurology* 1961;11:695–700.

6. Loar CR, Chadduck WM, Nugent GR. Traumatic occlusion of the middle cerebral artery. *J Neurosurg* 1973;39:753–759.

7. Eisenberg HM, Gary HE Jr, Aldrich EF, et al. Initial CT findings in 753 patients with severe head injury: A report from the NIH Traumatic Coma Data Bank. *J Neurosurg* 1990;73:688–698.

8. The European Study Group on Nimodipine in Severe Head Injury. A multicenter trial of efficacy of nimodipine on outcome after severe head injury. *J Neurosurg* 1994;80:797–804.

9. Leavy LL, Rezai A, Masri LS, Litofsky SN, Giannnota SL, Apuzzo MLJ, Weiss MH. The significance of subarachnoid hemorrhge after penetrating craniocerebral injury: Correlations with angiography and outcome in civilian population. *Neurosurgery* 1993;32:532–540.

10. Martin NA, Doberstein C, Zane C, Caron MJ, Thomas K, Becker DP. Posttraumatic cerebral arterial spasm: Transcranial Doppler ultrasound, cerebral flow, and angiographic findings. *J Neurosurg* 1992;77:575–583.

11. Sander D, Klingerlhofer J. Traumatic vasospasm following post-traumatic subarachnoid hemorrhage evaluated by transcranial Doppler ultrasonography. *J Neurol Sci* 1993;119:1–7.

12. Grolimund P, Weber M, Seiler RW, Reulen HJ. Time course of cerebral vasospasm after severe head injury (letter). *Lancet* 1988;2:1173.

13. Bernoit BG, Wortzman G. Traumatic cerebral aneurysms. Clinical features and natural history. *J Neurol Neurosurg Psychiatry* 1973;36:127–138.

14. Fleischer AS, Patton JM, Tindall GT. Cerebral aneurysms of traumatic origin. *Surg Neurol* 1975;1:200–203.

15. Aarabi B. traumatic aneurysm of brain due to high velocity missile head wounds. *Neurosurgery* 1988;22:1056–1063.

16. Haddad FS, Haddad GF, Taha J. Traumatic intracranial aneurysms caused by missiles; their presentation and management. *Neurosurgery* 1991;28:1–7.

17. duTrevou MD, van Dellen JR. Penetrating stab wound to the brain: The timing of angiography in patients presenting with the weapon already removed. *Neurosurgery* 1992;31:905–912.

18. Debrum GM. Treatment of traumatic carotid-cavernous fistula using detachable balloon catheters. *Am J Neuroradiol* 1983;4:355–356.

19. Halbach VV, Hieshima GB, Higashida RT, Reicher M. Carotid cavernous fistulae: Indications for urgent treatment. *Am J Neuroradiol* 1987;8:627–633.

20. Dolenc VV. Direct microsurgical repair of intracavernous vascular lesions. *J Neurosurg* 1983;58:824–831.

21. Goto K, Hieshima GB, Higashida RT, et al. Treatment of direct carotid cavernous sinus fistulae. Various therapeutic approaches and results in 148 cases. *Acta Radiol Suppl* 1986;369:576–579.

22. Mullan S. Treatment of carotid-cavernous fistulas by cavernous sinus occlusion. *J Neurosurg* 1979;50:131–144.

23. Halbach VV, Higashida RT, Barnwell SL, et al. Transarterial platinum coil embolization of carotid-cavernous fistulas. *Am J Neuroradiol* 1991;12:429–433.

24. Batjer HH, Purdy PD, Neiman M, Samson D. Subtemporal transdural use of detachable balloons for traumatic carotid-cavernous fistula. *Neurosurgery* 1988;22:290–296.

25. Morsein LH, Debrum GM, Miller NR, et al. Treatment of dural carotid-cavernous fistulas via the superior ophthalmic vein. *Am J Neuroradiol* 1991;12:435–439.

26. Teng MM, Lirng JF, Chang T, et al. Embolization of carotid cavernous fistula by means of direct puncture through the superior orbital fissure. *Radiology* 1995;194:705–711.

27. Hyshaw C, DiTulio M, Renaudin J. Superficial temporal arteriovenous fistula. *Surg Neurol* 1979;12:46–48.

28. Freckmann N, Sator K, Hermann HD. Traumatic fistulae of the middle meningeal artery and neighbouring veins or dural sinuses. *Acta Neurochir (Wien)* 1981;55:273–281.

29. Bitoh S, Hasegawa H, Fujiwara M, Nakata M. Traumatic arteriovenous fistula between the middle meningeal artery and cortical vein. *Surg Neurol* 1980;14:355–358.

30. Feldman RA, Hieshima G, Giannota SL, Gade GF. Traumatic dural arteriovenous fistula supplied by scalp, meningeal, and cortical arteries: Case report. *Neurosurgery* 1980;6:670–674.

31. Ishiguro S, Kimura A, Munemoto S, et al. Traumatic arteriovenous fistula with feeders of the scalp, dura mater and pia mater: Case report [in Japanese]. *No Shinkei Geka. Neurol Surg (Tokyo)* 1987;15:677–681.

32. Meier U, Gartner F, Knopf W, et al. The traumatic dural sinus injury: A clinical study. *Acta Neurochir (Wien)* 1992;119:91–93.

33. Schmidek HH, Auer LM, Kapp JP. The cerebral venous system. *Neurosurgery* 1985;17:663–678.

34. duPlessis JJ. Depressed skull fracture involving the superior sagittal sinus as a cause of persistent raised intracranial pressure: A case report. *J Trauma* 1993;34:290–292.

35. Meirowsky AM. Wounds of dural sinuses. *J Neurosurg* 1953;10:496–514.

36. Rish BL. The repair of dural venous sinus wounds by autogenous venorraphy. *J Neurosurg* 1971;35:392–395.

37. Kapp JP, Gielchinsky I, Deardourff SL. Operative tachniques for management of lesions involving the dural venous sinuses. *Surg Neurol* 1977;7:339–242.

38. Hesselbrock R, Sawaya R, Tomsick T, Wadhwa S. Superior sagittal thrombosis after closed head injury. *Neurosurgery* 1985;16:825–828.

39. Satoh H, Uozumi T, Kiya K, et al. Venous thrombosis after closed head injury: A report of two cases presenting as intracranial hypertension [in Japanese]. *No Shinkei Geka. Neurol Surg (Tokyo)* 1993;21:953–957.

40. Taha JM, Crone KR, Berger TS, et al. Sigmoid sinus thrombosis after closed head injury in children. *Neurosurgery* 1993;32;541–545.

Cerebrovascular Disease, edited by H. Hunt Batjer.
Lippincott-Raven Publishers, Philadelphia © 1997.

CHAPTER 95

Infectious Intracranial Aneurysms

Randolph C. Bishop, Winfield S. Fisher III, and Richard B. Morawetz

Infectious intracranial aneurysms are uncommon but life-threatening and carry a poor prognosis (1). They can be divided into two main groups based on etiology. The more common group, bacterial, is usually associated with bacterial endocarditis and is historically termed *mycotic* aneurysm (2). The second, less common group includes fungal or true mycotic aneurysms. This chapter will review the incidence, pathogenesis, and treatment of these unusual lesions and propose guidelines for their management based on the existing literature.

BACTERIAL ANEURYSMS

Eppinger (3) described intracranial aneurysms associated with endocarditis as ''mycotic'' and ''embolic.'' Later, Bohmfalk et al (4) further defined the association of bacterial endocarditis with intracranial aneurysms and used the term *bacterial* aneurysms. Most recently, Frazee et al (5) completed a literature review of reported cases of bacterial aneurysms and noted that nearly all patients had a predisposing medical condition that might have led to bacterial endocarditis.

It has been estimated that bacterial intracranial aneurysms constitute 4% of all intracranial aneurysms (4), although with improved antibiotic therapy this incidence may be decreasing. Clinical series have reported that patients with bacterial endocarditis treated with antibiotics have a 4–15% risk of an intracranial aneurysm (6,7). These figures probably underestimate the true incidence, as some, if not most, aneurysms remain asymptomatic and undiagnosed. In addition, the evolution and resolution of bacterial aneurysms occur

over days to weeks (8), and thus early angiographic studies may miss lesions.

The most common bacterial pathogens associated with these aneurysms are streptococci, followed by staphylococci. In 1984, Ojemann et al (9) reviewed 81 cases of bacterial aneurysms occurring in patients with endocarditis and found the following incidence of causative organisms: streptococci (44%), staphylococci (18%), multiple organisms (4.8%), and negative cultures (10%). The incidence of staphylococcal endocarditis is increasing, whereas that of alpha-hemolytic streptococcal and pneumococcal endocarditis is diminishing.

Karsner (10) classified infectious aneurysms into two types. The first and most common type has an intravascular source and is the result of embolization of bacteria-laden vegetations from an infected heart valve. The second type has an extravascular source, resulting from direct extension of a neighboring infection such as meningitis, osteomyelitis, cavernous sinus thrombophlebitis, or postoperative infection. Embolic (intravascular-source) aneurysms are more likely to occur in the periphery of the vascular tree and are likely to be multiple. The causative, infected emboli are quite friable, and additional aneurysms may result from the distal break up and lodgment of the fragments. The high incidence of these aneurysms in the distal branches of the middle cerebral artery is related to laminar flow. If the aneurysm originates extravascularly, it tends to be located near the base of the skull and in larger vessels due to direct extension of a basal infection.

PATHOGENESIS

In 1968, Nakata et al (11) published experimental results showing that vascular wall destruction due to bacterial infection began in the vasa vasorum after infusion of bacteria into a dog aorta. They concluded that stasis and sepsis in the vasa vasorum was a necessary initiating event for the formation of a bacterial aneurysm.

Molinari et al (12) pointed out that although the original

R. C. Bishop: Division of Neurosurgery, University of Alabama—Birmingham, Birmingham, Alabama 35294.

W. S. Fisher III: Division of Neurosurgery, University of Alabama—Birmingham, Birmingham, Alabama 35294.

R. B. Morawetz: Division of Neurosurgery, University of Alabama—Birmingham, Birmingham, Alabama 35294.

site of infection may be the vasa vasorum in extracranial vessels, vasa vasorum are rarely present in cerebral arteries, particularly in distal branches where bacterial aneurysms are most common. Using experimental dog models, they concluded that aneurysms consistently appeared at the site of lodgment of the infected embolus and that the early changes in the vessel walls appeared in the adventitial layer and involved the media. They proposed that in the absence of the vasa vasorum bacteria could spread through the occluded origins of thin-walled penetrating vessels to the Virchow-Robin spaces and then to the adventitia of the parent vessel. Aneurysm enlargement was produced either by pulsation against the necrotic wall of the occluded vessel or by the same pulsation against the weakened wall of a recanalized vessel. This latter process may explain the observed late appearance of an aneurysm during antibiotic treatment for bacterial endocarditis. Molinari et al (12) stressed the short time (1–3 days) between the lodging of the infected embolus in the cerebral vessel and aneurysm formation in animals not treated with antibiotics. Of those animals that had been treated with antibiotics, aneurysm rupture did not occur despite the presence of aneurysms at sacrifice 7 days after embolization, strongly suggesting that appropriate antibiotic therapy altered the natural history of the lesion.

CLINICAL PRESENTATION

The great majority of patients harboring bacterial intracranial aneurysms present with symptoms from bacterial endocarditis (1,4,5,8), although embolic cerebral infarction, subarachnoid hemorrhage, and intraparenchymal hemorrhage can also occur. Of patients with bacterial endocarditis, 17% suffer a major cerebral infarction, and a significant percentage is thought to develop bacterial intracranial aneurysms (6,7). In Ojemann's (9) review of patients with bacterial intracranial aneurysms and endocarditis, 52% presented with hemorrhage. In the series reported by Roach and Drake (13), all five patients (100%) presented with hemorrhage. In his report of 13 patients from one institution, Frazee and colleagues (5) found all to have suffered various premonitory symptoms or signs suggestive of cerebral ischemic disease and recommended angiography for patients with bacterial endocarditis who develop sudden and severe headache, focal neurologic deficits, or seizures. The prognosis is extremely poor once the aneurysm ruptures, with mortality in the 60–90% range (1,4).

DIAGNOSIS

Clinical suspicion should be high in patients with predisposing conditions. In addition to patients with bacterial endocarditis, there is an increased incidence of these lesions in immunocompromised patients (eg, acquired immunodeficiency syndrome [AIDS]) and intravenous drug users. Neurologic changes in these patients warrant further evaluation.

Laboratory examination and cultures of cerebrospinal fluid and blood are useful in identifying the responsible pathogen, as well as subarachnoid hemorrhage. Patients with suspected infectious aneurysm should undergo echocardiography for the diagnosis of endocarditis.

Computed tomography (CT), due to its sensitivity to intracranial blood, can be used to diagnose subarachnoid hemorrhage and localize hematoma. Magnetic resonance imaging (MRI) and MR angiography (MRA) can visualize larger aneurysms and can be used to follow these lesions if needed. The sensitivity of MRI/MRA in diagnosing small infectious aneurysms has not been established, and thus angiography is recommended to achieve a diagnosis in equivocal cases and to gain knowledge that may affect further management (Fig. 1).

TREATMENT

Improved understanding of the time course of the evolution and resolution of bacterial intracranial aneurysms has resulted from multiple careful angiograms performed in patients with bacterial aneurysms over time (8). In 1965, Roach and Drake (13) commented that infectious aneurysms not treated with appropriate antibiotic therapy carried a high risk of rupture. The following year Cantu and LeMay (14) documented the disappearance of intracranial bacterial aneurysms during antibiotic therapy and recommended serial arteriography in patients with proximally located aneurysms, such as those at the middle cerebral bifurcation. Surgical obliteration was recommended for distally located and easily accessible lesions and for those seen to enlarge on serial studies. Further documentation of the resolution of such lesions led Bingham (1) to recommend using serial angiographic studies in all patients with unruptured bacterial intracranial aneurysms to determine any surgical treatment. Enlargement or lack of reduction in the size of aneurysms after a full course of antibiotic therapy was thought to be an indication for operation. Bohmfalk et al (4) discussed CT scanning, as well as serial angiography, in the evaluation of such patients and concluded that patients with intact proximal aneurysms and multiple aneurysms should be treated nonsurgically, whereas patients with symptomatic mass lesions (hematoma), single peripheral aneurysms, and perhaps multiple superficial aneurysms should undergo surgical obliteration of such lesions. Thus, the indications for operative treatment of bacterial aneurysms, to some extent, are based on the ease of approach to a given lesion and the success or failure of antibiotic treatment.

Morawetz and Karp (8) showed that bacterial intracranial aneurysms may enlarge over 6 weeks despite antibiotic therapy and then resolve over several months, at a time when parenteral antibiotic therapy has been stopped (Fig. 2). The most important step in the treatment of patients with bacterial intracranial aneurysms is the eradication of infection through institution of appropriate antibiotic therapy and cor-

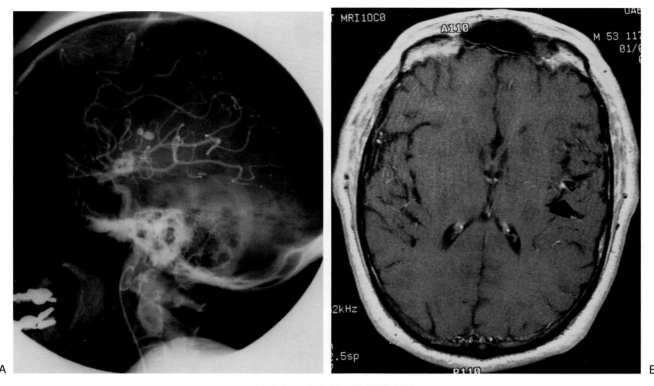

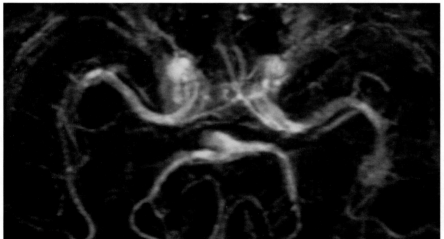

FIG. 1. Bacterial aneurysm of the left middle cerebral artery is seen on angiography **(A)**, MRI **(B)**, and MRA **(C)** in a patient presenting with subarachnoid hemorrhage following dental extraction for caries.

rection of the responsible cardiac lesion as necessary. Apparent enlargement of a bacterial intracranial aneurysm may be a function of the timing of angiography rather than the inefficacy of antibiotic treatment. The production of a cerebral infarction by an infected embolus seemingly depends on the size of the vessel occluded, the duration of the occlusion, and the availability of collateral flow. Analysis of serial angiograms in patients with bacterial aneurysms suggests that whereas cerebral infarction develops over hours, the development of bacterial intracranial aneurysms probably requires days to weeks. Little information is available concerning the natural history of bacterial aneurysms that persist for many months.

The nonsurgical resolution of bacterial intracranial aneurysms appears to involve thrombosis of the involved vessels resulting in angiographic disappearance. The thrombosis extends both distally to the aneurysm and proximally to the first feeding-artery branch point. The loss of such vessels can occur silently with no clinical indication that thrombosis has occurred, presumably because of the presence of adequate collateral flow that prevents cerebral infarction. Thus, recognition of bacterial intracranial aneurysms and documentation of their size and location depend on careful serial angiography and, to some extent, on favorable timing. Early angiography may demonstrate a ragged vessel, indicating the lodgment and breakup of an embolus, usually at a bifur-

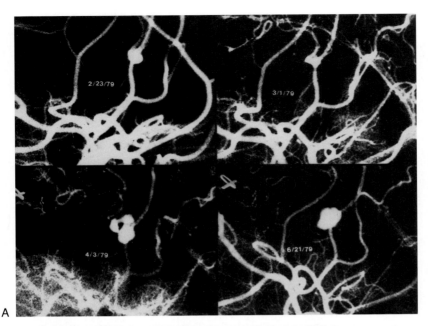

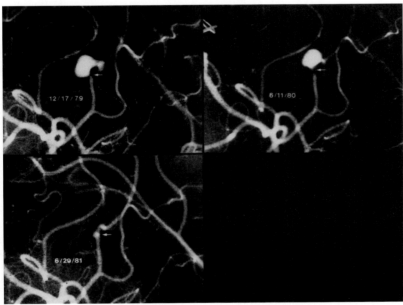

FIG. 2. Sequential angiograms following antibiotic therapy of a bacterial aneurysm of the left distal middle cerebral artery. Note the gradual resolution of the aneurysm from 2/23/79 to 6/29/81.

cation of a vessel. Over the next few weeks, an aneurysm may appear and enlarge even with antibiotic treatment. If it does not rupture (no data are available regarding the propensity to do so), it may resolve, with preservation of the involved vessel in some cases and its loss in others. It may be that an aneurysm more distally located is more likely to resolve by loss of the parent vessel; this loss may or may not be accompanied by a clinical deficit. The lodgment of an embolus at a vessel bifurcation may lead to occlusion of one branch and preservation of the other. The occluded stump may give rise to an aneurysm, thus giving the appearance of an aneurysm with a neck.

Patients harboring bacterial intracranial aneurysms who require urgent cardiac valve replacement should undergo cardiac operation before the repair of intracranial aneurysms, unless they are threatened by mass effect due to intracerebral hematoma or brain abscess. No exacerbation of neurologic deficit associated with cardiopulmonary bypass and cardiac valve replacement in patients with bacterial intracranial aneurysm has been observed (6). Despite the heparinization necessary for cardiopulmonary bypass, rupture of an aneurysm during the perioperative period is rare. The goal of the cardiac operation is to remove actively infected tissue, debride necrotic tissue, drain abscesses, and correct the hemodynamic defect. Surgery effectively removes the source of cerebral emboli, thus protecting the brain from further

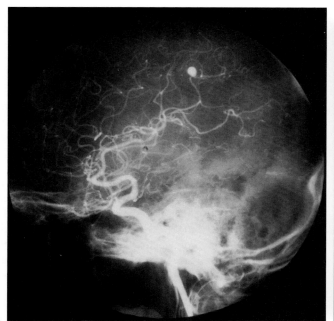
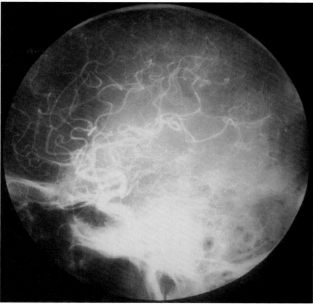

A   B

FIG. 3. This bacterial aneurysm left distal middle cerebral artery **(A)** was treated with embolization coils with resultant obliteration of the aneurysm **(B)**.

embolic events and formation of new bacterial intracranial aneurysms. In patients with bacterial intracranial aneurysms identified preoperatively, the operative procedure is altered in that a bioprosthetic (tissue) valve is used to obviate postoperative anticoagulation. For this reason, patients with bacterial endocarditis requiring cardiac valve replacement should be considered for cerebral angiography preoperatively if there is evidence that cerebral embolization has occurred or if intracranial bacterial aneurysms are thought to be present.

Because the resolution of bacterial intracranial aneurysms during and after antibiotic treatment has been clearly demonstrated, the presence per se of such an aneurysm does not mandate operation. If operation is elected, delayed operation after the institution of antibiotic therapy might reduce the dangers attendant to an acutely inflamed brain and a friable aneurysm wall. The common fusiform nature of the more proximal bacterial intracranial aneurysm precludes obliteration without the sacrifice of the involved vessel and the risk of cerebral infarction. The use of extracranial-to-intracranial (EC-IC) bypass grafting in dealing with the more proximally located lesions has been proposed to circumvent such hazards. However, a relatively long segment of thickened, friable vessel wall in the vicinity of the bacterial intracranial aneurysm may make the vessel a poor recipient for a bypass graft. Other therapies including endovascular approaches (Fig. 3) have been reported and may hold promise for the future (15).

FUNGAL ANEURYSMS

The first case of fungal aneurysm was reported in 1968, and since that time sporadic case reports have been pub-

lished. The rarity of the disease is obvious, but the widespread use of corticosteroids and immunosuppressive drugs and the emergence of AIDS would suggest that fungal infections, including those of the cerebral arteries, may become more common in the future.

The majority of cases are caused by *Aspergillus* organisms, with a minority caused by *Candida, Nocardia,* and *Penicillium* species. The sources of infection in these patients are direct extension and hematogenous spread. The site of infection usually involves the proximal major vessels such as the internal carotid or basilar arteries. Unlike patients with bacterial intracranial aneurysm, who have strong cardiac histories, those with fungal aneurysms appear to lack significant early warning symptoms or signs that would suggest intracranial disease. The disease in these patients appears to progress rapidly and is universally lethal. Similar guidelines for the treatment of bacterial aneurysms can be applied to aneurysms of fungal etiology, although the prognosis for the latter patients remains grim.

RECOMMENDED THERAPEUTIC GUIDELINES

We have adopted the following guidelines for the treatment of patients with bacterial intracranial aneurysms:

1. Any patient with known bacterial endocarditis who develops a neurologic deficit suggestive of cerebral embolization should be considered for four-vessel cerebral angiography. The decision whether or not to perform angiography depends on how the angiographic information will be used. If identification of an aneurysm will

not lead to operation, which is reasonable given current information, then angiography is not indicated. Patients not known to have bacterial endocarditis who present with subarachnoid hemorrhage from peripherally located or fusiform cerebral aneurysms should be evaluated for possible presence of bacterial intracranial aneurysms and bacterial endocarditis. High-resolution CT or MRI scans should be obtained to detect sites of embolization and to delineate surgical mass lesions, infarcts, and aneurysms.

2. Appropriate wide-spectrum antibiotic therapy should be started as soon as the diagnosis of bacterial intracranial aneurysm is made and should be modified accordingly when blood cultures are obtained. Therapy for 4–6 weeks is required regardless of whether or not surgery is undertaken.

3. The correction of any underlying cardiac disorder carries a high priority. Patients with bacterial endocarditis with or without bacterial intracranial aneurysms are often critically ill and may require emergency cardiac valve replacement for intractable cardiac failure despite their neurologic condition. We advise the use of bioprosthetic (tissue) valves in patients with bacterial intracranial aneurysms to eliminate the need for postoperative anticoagulation.

4. A clear indication for operation includes the presence of an intracerebral hematoma with significant mass effect. If surgical treatment for intracerebral hematoma is undertaken, the responsible aneurysm will often present in the wall of the clot cavity and should be dealt with. The friable nature of the aneurysm and surrounding vasculature makes it difficult to maintain flow in the parent artery after clipping and may result in distal occlusion. Good results have been reported with EC-IC bypass procedures in these patients (16), but EC-IC bypass must be carried out before aneurysm obliteration and may not be possible in the acute phase of the disease. The decision to obliterate other aneurysmal lesions at the same time, when multiple aneurysms are present, will depend on the location and accessibility of the lesions.

In a significant number of patients, initial cerebral angiography will demonstrate occlusion of the artery distal to the aneurysm. In these patients in whom distal flow has been lost, endovascular occlusion techniques have been described to obliterate the aneurysm with good success (15).

5. The presence of an unruptured bacterial intracranial aneurysm is in itself not a definite indication for operation. As discussed, no natural history data regarding the likelihood of rupture vs. resolution of infectious aneurysms

are available, but complete resolution without operation has been reported (8). A clinical decision must be made in each case regarding the frequency of reassessment with appropriate serial radiography. In the presence of nonoperated aneurysms, we consider performing repeat radiographic studies based on changes in the patient's clinical condition and after completion of a full course of antibiotic therapy. During the first 4–6 weeks of therapy, new aneurysms may appear and existing ones may enlarge. Neither of these situations mandates surgical intervention.

6. In view of the propensity for spontaneous resolution of bacterial intracranial aneurysms, we think that surgical obliteration is mandatory only after demonstration of a causative aneurysm following intracerebral or subarachnoid hemorrhage or when an aneurysm enlarges after completion of a full course of antibiotic therapy. Surgical obliteration of unruptured aneurysms has not been shown to be necessary.

REFERENCES

1. Bingham WF. Treatment of mycotic intracranial aneurysms. *J Neurosurg* 1977;46:428–437.
2. Osler W. Gulstonian lectures on malignant endocarditis. *Lancet* 1885; 1:415–418, 459–464, 505–508.
3. Eppinger H. Pathogenesis der Aneurysmen einschliesslich der Aneurysma equi verminosum. *Arch Klin Chir* 1887;35:1–553.
4. Bohmfalk GL, Story JL, Wessenger JP. Bacterial intracranial aneurysm. *J Neurosurg* 1978;48:369–382.
5. Frazee JG, Cahan LD, Winter J. Bacterial intracranial aneurysms. *J Neurosurg* 1980;53:633–641.
6. Richardson JV, Karp RB, Kirklin JW, Dismukes WE. Treatment of infective endocarditis: A ten year comparative analysis. *Circulation* 1978;58:589–597.
7. Jones HR, Siekert RG, Geraci JE. Neurological manifestations of bacterial endocarditis. *Ann Intern Med* 1969;71:21–28.
8. Morawetz RB, Karp RB. Evolution and resolution of intracranial bacterial (mycotic) aneurysms. *Neurosurgery* 1984;15:43–49.
9. Ojemann RG. Infectious intracranial aneurysms. In: Fein JM, Flamm ES, eds. *Cerebrovascular Surgery.* New York: Spinger-Verlag, 1984; 3:1047–1060.
10. Karsner HT. *Acute Inflammation of Arteries.* Springfield, IL: Charles C Thomas, 1947:16.
11. Nakata Y, Shionoya S, Kamiya K. Pathogenesis of mycotic aneurysm. *Angiology* 1968;19:593–601.
12. Molinari GF, Smith L, Goldstein MN. Pathogenesis of cerebral mycotic aneurysms. *Neurology* 1972;23:325–332.
13. Roach M, Drake CG. Ruptured cerebral aneurysms caused by microorganisms. *N Engl J Med* 1965;273:240–244.
14. Cantu RC, LeMay M. The importance of repeated angiography in the treatment of mycotic-embolic intracranial aneurysms. *J Neurosurg* 1966;25:189–193.
15. Frizzell RT, Vitek JJ, Fisher WS III. Treatment of bacterial (mycotic) intracranial aneurysm using an endovascular approach. *Neurosurgery* 1993;32:852–854.
16. Hadley MN, Spetzler RF. Middle cerebral artery aneurysm due to *Nocardia asteroides:* Case report of aneurysm excision and extracranial-intracranial bypass. *Neurosurgery* 1988;22:923–925.

SECTION V
Socioeconomic and Ethical Issues

As this volume was organized to provide a comprehensive approach to clinical cerebrovascular conditions for neuroscientists worldwide, it may seem inappropriate to conclude with a section pertaining to socioeconomic issues. Clearly, much of the information in the following chapters has been generated with regard to the major health care system upheavals underway in the United States. On the other hand, practitioners in all countries must deliver care under the constraints applied by their government and local societal pressures. The physician's role and obligation is to determine what defines optimal care, to attempt to secure the resources necessary to deliver that level of care, and to utilize to the best of his or her ability the technology and environment made available by that society. When viewed in that context, each country's health care system faces the same fundamental problems.

Chapters in this section will consider cerebrovascular conditions in the context of the requirements of high-technology subspecialty care, dealing with governmental and societal pressures to reduce overall costs. The reader will note a number of potential options, including centers of special expertise, clinical trials, and guidelines that can help to sequester the most expensive resources and develop methods to determine which patients clearly benefit from that technology.

The ethical issues unique to catastrophic neurological illness will also be considered with the question of whether significant cost savings can be acquired without sacrificing societal and moral ethical considerations.

H. Hunt Batjer, M.D.

Cerebrovascular Disease, edited by H. Hunt Batjer.
Lippincott-Raven Publishers, Philadelphia © 1997.

CHAPTER 96

Cerebrovascular Care in the Next Decade: Cost, Prudence, Progress, and Rationing

H. Hunt Batjer

Quality and accessibility of medical care for all citizens have been concerns in the American health care debate that began in 1992, but without question the touchstone for all deliberations and potential interventions has remained cost containment. Health care spending, which represents 14% of the gross domestic product and is rapidly growing, notably surpasses expenditures in other developed nations and is felt by the public and policy makers to be excessive. Advanced technology and expensive surgical procedures have been targeted as major cost offenders. A reduction in their use and reimbursement devaluation are felt to offer a means toward substantial savings.

Several features contribute to the high cost of treating cerebrovascular disease, which encompasses a broad spectrum of disorders ranging from primarily medical to primarily surgical conditions. First, the types of diagnostic procedures commonly used are highly technical and extremely expensive. Second, the majority of patients afflicted with cerebrovascular disorders require at least one admission to a high-cost critical care environment. Third, those conditions requiring open surgical or interventional radiologic procedures typically require the most complex and demanding operations, consuming substantial resources from providers, hospitals, and payers. Given that ischemic stroke alone affects huge numbers of people each year and remains the third leading cause of death and disability in the United States (1,2), the magnitude of the economic drain is obvious.

Undoubtedly, the new trends and mandates currently being implemented in our transforming health care system will impact on physicians and surgeons caring for cerebrovascular patients. Whether incremental gains by the managed care market will lead to the prominence of these large groups or whether some alternative centralized structure will

be established remains to be seen. Nevertheless, the guiding principle of these groups, and one that will almost certainly persist, is that complex technical procedures and examinations are considered to be consumers of major resources rather than generators of revenue. This shift will influence physicians' interactions with payers and policy makers and the care of patients with cerebrovascular disease.

The purpose of this essay is to attempt to place in perspective the potential strategies for managing complex clinical problems in a very new environment, while recognizing the diversity of clinical philosophies from the profoundly nihilistic to the radically activist articulated by the physician experts in these fields. Before consideration of the specific issues of cost, prudence, progress, and rationing, several points should be made about the unique modifiers that preclude lumping cerebrovascular disease with other medical conditions in the attempt to insure optimal care for our patients:

1. *Young age.* Many types of cerebrovascular disease, particularly hemorrhagic stroke conditions, affect a relatively youthful population. Thus, loss of life or productivity for these patients exacts an even higher toll on the families and work force than diseases primarily affecting the aged. The health-spending issue is compounded in this context, as we are much more willing to offer very costly and even heroic forms of therapy to those with expected longevity.

2. *Nonmalignant.* Virtually all forms of primary cerebrovascular disease are not neoplastic or cancerous and are therefore potentially survivable. This has major implications regarding the expectations of patients and their families, as well as the emotional and ethical concerns surrounding withdrawal of support for irreversibly damaged patients.

3. *Extreme risk.* The overwhelming majority of conditions considered to be ischemic or hemorrhagic stroke are

H. H. Batjer: Division of Neurological Surgery, Northwestern University Medical School, Chicago, Illinois 60611.

attended by extreme risks of death or disability, if a major clinical event occurs as part of the natural history or as a complication of treatment.

4. *Necessity for tertiary care.* While all neurologists, neurosurgeons, vascular surgeons, and even primary care physicians treat the common forms of cerebrovascular disease, the most complex cases, such as giant aneurysms, vascular malformations, and intracranial stenoses, are referred to regional centers for subspecialty evaluation and care.

5. *Treatment is usually prophylactic.* While considerable progress in the realm of neuronal salvage is being made by molecular biologists and pharmacologists, the overwhelming majority of patients suffer a clinical event or deficit. Thus, our therapeutic strategy is aimed at preventing recurrence or progression of neurologic compromise. This even applies to most forms of hemorrhagic stroke, as medical, surgical, or endovascular care is designed primarily to prevent rebleeding or secondary brain damage. This has relevance to the current discussion, as the guideline authors, gatekeepers, payers, and medicolegal community may ask, ''What is the real risk of recurrence of this condition and does a relatively modest natural history risk (as in the case of arteriovenous malformation) justify a highly expensive and potentially dangerous therapeutic approach?''

6. *Deceptive early results.* Since most of the therapeutic alternatives for cerebrovascular patients are prophylactic, the environment is ripe for seductive inadequate remedies to be proposed due to ''cost effectiveness.'' The initial results may appear favorable as judged by lack of recurrent symptoms; however, time and continued natural history risks may show that these strategies are terribly dangerous to patients and ultimately much more costly. As an example, consider the patient suffering from a ruptured giant intracranial aneurysm who is in good neurologic condition. Definitive surgical treatment would mandate extensive surgical exposure under ideal anesthetic conditions, temporary arterial occlusion and aneurysm deflation, precise clipping and vessel reconstruction, and tedious postoperative care, possibly requiring extended rehabilitative care and a delayed return to work. An ''attractive'' alternative would be to cautiously expose the lesion and discover that it is difficult or ''unclippable'' and to proceed with wrapping portions of the aneurysm with gauze. Ideally, the patient could make a rapid recovery from surgery and be discharged from the hospital within a week. Rehemorrhage and sudden death at home days or weeks later would be inexpensive for the medical examiner to handle. While the ''health care system'' may have benefited by this strategy, the patient and his family certainly did not.

7. *Inadequacy of treatment standards and basic research.* In many respects, care of cerebrovascular patients remains empiric and often seriously inadequate. Scientists and clinicians studying issues of neurogenetics, growth factors, neural regeneration, and ischemic salvage are poised on the threshold of major new advances, but continued and revitalized financial support will be required to move out of the therapeutic dark ages.

In the following discussions, I will attempt to make specific recommendations and reiterate the theme of optimizing current patient care while creating an environment in which future scientific progress can be forged.

COST

The pivotal concern about health care funding in the United States is brought home by the fact that in 1990 nearly $670 billion were spent, which translates to $2,566 per citizen (3). It is possible to estimate the fraction of this staggering sum that is consumed by patients with cerebrovascular disorders, although it is difficult to quantitate the nonhospital-related expenses, including nursing home care, inpatient and outpatient rehabilitation services, hospice care, family support when the primary wage earner is lost, and the monetary value of lost years of productivity. The enormity of direct costs due to cerebrovascular disease arise from the fact that more than 500,000 Americans suffer ischemic stroke each year (1,2). The American Heart Association calculates current expenditures on ischemic stroke by extrapolating from the methodology used and reported by the National Center for Health Statistics in 1984 (4). With use of this technique, it is estimated that ischemic stroke costs the United States $19.7 billion annually (5). Hemorrhagic stroke is also a substantial contributor to the problem, as 30,000 Americans suffer nontraumatic subarachnoid hemorrhage each year (6). The incidence of spontaneous intracerebral hemorrhage may be substantially higher than aneurysmal hemorrhage. In a recent study, Broderick et al (7) reported the prevalence of cerebral hemorrhage in the greater Cincinnati area. These investigators found that the annual incidence of intracerebral hemorrhage was 15 cases per 100,000 people, which was more than twice the incidence of aneurysmal rupture. In addition, the mortality rates were virtually identical: 44% for intracerebral hemorrhage and 46% for subarachnoid hemorrhage.

While the concept of ''brain attack'' and the emphasis on early triage and acute intervention holds significant promise for several forms of cerebrovascular disease, particularly in light of new therapeutic innovations becoming available, it must be kept in mind that these advances may in fact be very cost *in*effective. Indeed, from a purely economic viewpoint the ''saved lives'' are not really saved at all. Although these patients may return to their previous functional capacity for some time, they still become ill, disabled, and die. At that point the health care system will have paid for two (or more) catastrophic illnesses for that person instead of one. While, arguably, some may have benefited society because the individual returned to the work force after the initial neurologic illness, this benefit only applies to those affected before retirement. This callous example illustrates the profound deception of applying economic principles to health care considerations and underscores the fact that good or great health care does not *save* money, it *costs* money.

In light of the clear need to reduce expense and in keeping with the belief that compassionate and excellent care must continue to be offered in an environment conducive to future scientific advances, I envision several areas in which substantial savings can be made, as detailed in the following sections.

Diagnostic Tests

Clinicians must be increasingly reminded of the staggering cost of the modern diagnostic armamentarium. We can no longer afford the luxury of highly expensive confirmatory studies. These studies are helpful clinical adjuncts but should be ordered judiciously and only when a therapeutic decision is likely to be influenced. Magnetic resonance imaging (MRI) can beautifully confirm a small pontine infarction due to penetrating-arterial disease, but the clinician should ask, ''Will the MRI obviate the need for further diagnostic workup or allow specific treatment to be initiated or will it simply confirm a clinical impression?'' If the clinical diagnosis is clear and angiography is planned for evaluating potential therapeutic intervention, then there appears little justification for MRI.

As another example, MR angiography (MRA) represents a wonderful technical advance—and a highly expensive one—that for a variety of reasons is plagued by a high incidence of false positive and false negative findings. In my practice, MRA has never provided adequate information to plan surgical intervention or to clearly obviate the need for conventional angiography. Indeed, many MRA studies have been interpreted as showing lesions that led to angiography but would have otherwise not been indicated, which demonstrates that the MRA ''finding'' was spurious. There may well be reasonable indications to use MRA for follow-up of known vascular lesions, but I do not believe that this modality should be included in any standard diagnostic work-up. The potential benefit has not justified the expense.

When hospital bills for critically ill patients with cerebrovascular disease are scrutinized, it can be seen that an impressive amount of money has been spent on follow-up diagnostic studies. For many forms of hemorrhagic stroke, especially in the postoperative period, great comfort can be obtained (for the physician, not the patient) by the ordering of daily CT scans. This practice is a luxury that is no longer justifiable except in extremely rare situations. An argument for these sequential studies can be made in situations where the patient is not examinable due to barbiturate therapy or therapeutic muscle relaxants, but in virtually all other situations these studies should be requested only when the clinical situation changes.

Most neurosurgeons over the past 30 years have requested postoperative angiography for most patients treated for vascular malformations and for many treated for intracranial aneurysms. The immediate risk of leaving residual arteriovenous malformations behind (which may be de-efferented) justifies the use of these studies in many, if not most, patients. However, in the aneurysm patient, modern microsurgical illumination and visualization allow exquisite understanding of the anatomy before and after clipping. In addition, the aneurysm can be aspirated postclipping to confirm successful treatment. The use of routine postoperative angiography is therefore questionable. This modality should be reserved for situations in which an unexplained neurologic deficit arises or when a specific surgical question (with relevance to subsequent treatment plans) remains unanswered.

Embolization Procedures

Enormous strides have been made in recent years by our endovascular colleagues. These surgical procedures often directly benefit the patient and serve as either primary therapy or surgical adjuncts, although their specific roles and indications have not been completely clarified. It is clear that these procedures carry substantial expense and are definitely not without risk.

Preliminary experience with coiling procedures for aneurysms has suggested that this concept is unlikely to provide definitive long-term protection. Aneurysm recurrence requires either a repeat endovascular procedure or an open surgical procedure. Any modest cost savings over an initial direct surgical approach would be more than offset by the need for a second procedure. However, I believe that aneurysm embolization is extremely useful in the following three situations:

1. Treatment of an aneurysm deemed unclippable by an experienced cerebrovascular surgeon;
2. Treatment of a patient who is not an acceptable risk for standard neuroanesthesia and operation due to medical complications (eg, pulmonary, cardiac, etc.);
3. Treatment (even if palliative) of the poor-grade subarachnoid hemorrhage patient to protect against early rebleeding and allow treatment for vasospasm.

Embolization of arteriovenous malformations is virtually never definitive, as the procedure is usually incomplete and recanalization is common. In addition, each embolization procedure is attended by a 5–10% risk of serious ischemic or hemorrhagic complication (8). On the other hand, it is my view that these procedures have allowed significant improvement in treatment outcome for many patients with complex vascular lesions. My argument is simply that an expensive and hazardous procedure should not be offered to a patient as a reflex but rather should be judiciously employed for specific clinical indications (9). A list of these indications, which should be individualized for every situation, includes the following:

1. Palliation. A markedly symptomatic elderly patient who suffers progressive ischemic symptoms may represent an indication.
2. Large high-flow malformations. Embolization clearly makes surgical therapy safer in these cases.
3. Deep feeding vessels. When it will be technically difficult for the neurosurgeon to access deep vascular pedicles, the interventional radiologist can be of great help. The recruitment of feeding perforating arteries into a malformation represents perhaps the best indication for embolization, as they are difficult to manage surgically. The point is that superficial cortical vessels are easily accessible surgically and in the absence of a large high-flow lesion, no attention should be given to them endovascularly.

Withdrawal of Support

Major expenditures are made on behalf of critically ill patients, including those who have no real hope for recovery. Approximately 52% of the overall expense of caring for stroke victims is consumed by hospital care alone (4). Medicare data are extremely revealing in this regard. Between 27.2% and 30.6% of the total Medicare budget is devoted to individuals in their last year of life, and this fraction has remained constant over many years (10). Of this sum, over one half (52%) is consumed during the last 60 days of life (10). Many policy analysts have carefully scrutinized the type of care provided for individuals during their final hospital admission, in the hope that eliminating "futile" care would achieve major savings.

The American public has repeatedly stated in surveys that they do not desire needless prolongation of life (11). An argument can be made that the use of advance directives, wider use of hospice care, and judicious elimination of high-technology strategies could serve our patients more humanely and at the same time benefit the public concern over health expenditures.

Two studies have addressed the impact of advance directives on ultimate hospital charges in dying patients. Both studies found no real impact by the use of these instruments (12,13). Teno et al (13) found that the average hospital bill for patients without an advance directive was $56,300 compared with $61,589 for patients with a living will and $58,346 for those with a durable power of attorney.

Several studies have suggested that the use of hospice care for terminally ill patients may save as much as 31–64% of medical costs (14–16). However, the National Hospice Study found that the longer hospice care was utilized, the more likely it was that costs would ultimately exceed conventional care costs (17). In addition, for a variety of reasons, the earlier quoted studies may overstate the actual savings available (11). Most hospice patients are from high-socioeconomic backgrounds and thus have a better intrinsic support system. In addition, the majority of patients in these studies suffered from malignancies, a problem that may jeopardize the generalization of these data to cerebrovascular patients.

As mentioned earlier, the avoidance of "futile" care at the end of life also represents a potential opportunity for savings. Unfortunately, definitive data are lacking. In a study of patients dying at a tertiary care hospital, it was found that patients with do-not-resuscitate (DNR) orders incurred similar hospital costs to patients without DNR orders (18).

Emanuel and Emanuel (11) presented a very thoughtful analysis of the potential savings available by avoiding expensive alternatives in terminally ill patients. They suggest that the maximal savings may have totaled $18.1 billion in 1988, which amounts to only 3.3% of all health care spending. While 3.3% of health care expenses is much less than original projections, the impact of savings at this level should not be overlooked. The implementation of these principles in cerebrovascular patients is, unfortunately, difficult. These patients are not dying from a malignant disease, and therefore family expectations are for survival. Many of them arrive at the terminal state after a series of therapeutic and often surgical interventions. Furthermore, a sense of "defeat" by the physician or surgeon is an intrinsic part of the treatment of patients with clinical and radiographic evidence of massive cerebral damage; the period of introspection and often self-criticism, in my own experience, frequently delays the appropriate weaning of the patient from critical support. Despite the inherent difficulties, it is my feeling that if the physician carefully evaluates the clinical situation, including CT evidence of damage, and makes recommendations to the patient's family identical to those the physician would make for an irreversibly ill family member, compassionate and ethical care would result and some (probably modest) health care savings would arise.

Minimizing Administrative Costs

Our peculiar system (or nonsystem) results in a huge amount of intrinsic waste from a variety of regulatory and other factors. The result is that an astounding 20% of health care expenditures arises from administrative costs (19). While the individual practicing physician cannot be blamed for—or significantly affect—the systemic ills that generate these figures, the physician can scale down his or her own clinical operation to maximize efficiency and minimize cost shifting. This streamlining must include the elimination of employees who perform the laborious and costly function of interacting with third-party carriers and managed plans. Although the absence of these individuals will increase the workload of remaining employees, most practices cannot afford the luxury of their services. In my view, this change is mandatory for survival over the next decade.

The issue of tort reform should be considered at this point. Progress in this area has ramifications for several aspects of cost, in addition to administrative overhead. While an ethical system must distribute resources to individuals injured by medical negligence, we must push to see that it is the patients themselves who receive these rewards. Frivolous lawsuits based on poor clinical results and not on negligence must be controlled. Defensive care is quite costly, impacts the use of high-expense diagnostic equipment, and certainly increases cost in the case of some terminally ill patients. Some progress has been made in this area, particularly in California, but it is clearly an uphill battle that will require substantial resources if we hope to achieve a truly equitable environment for delivery of medical care.

Regional Centers

It remains to be seen how changes in the American health care system will have an impact on the survival (or development) of regional centers of expertise in highly specialized areas. It seems logical to assume, however, that such dedicated facilities have the potential to markedly improve the quality of care for patients with uncommon and "high-end" cerebrovascular diseases and to aggregate highly technical personnel and equipment to a few areas, thus avoiding duplication of effort and systemic redundancy. It seems unwise to offer treatment for giant intracranial aneurysms, giant arteriovenous malformations, and such high-technology adjuncts as radiosurgery in multiple sites within the same city, except in the largest metropolitan areas. The prevalence of these diseases in the population simply does not justify such redundancy. There is little doubt that physicians and hospitals that deal routinely with these complex illnesses do so with superior clinical results in contrast to those who treat these problems sporadically. It is of concern that some of the recently implemented outcome parameters might provide gravely incorrect feedback to funding agencies and oversight bodies, in the process causing the loss of some of our great health care centers. Consider, for example, the comparison of outcome parameters such as mortality rate, length of stay, and total cost for subarachnoid hemorrhage patients treated at two hospitals in the same city. Hospital A treats five to ten patients with aneurysms each year and refers all poor-grade and complex cases to hospital B. Hospital B serves as a regional referral resource for many hospitals like hospital A. The resulting case load at hospital B includes some 200 aneurysm patients annually, with a marked skew toward the more high-risk patients. The payer and analyst would discover that hospital A had outperformed hospital B in terms of cost, length of stay, return to work, and other measurable parameters. The erroneous conclusion that hospital A should treat all aneurysm patients included in that region or plan would seem to be a logical conclusion.

PRUDENCE

The concept of prudence in handling our interactions with cerebrovascular diseases, patients, hospitals, payers, and agencies is particularly relevant at this time. While standard definitions of this term imply careful management or economical restraint, a broader definition "implies not only caution but the capacity for judging in advance the probable results of one's actions" (20). This applies especially well to cerebrovascular problems. The issue of prudence includes the potentially difficult and untenable position in which physicians are forced to make decisions and recommendations when the best interest of the individual patient is in direct conflict with the best interest of the public. This conflict could arise if by scientific testing a specific medication or procedure was found to improve outcome but was challenged by the gatekeepers or payers because the expense of the treatment was not felt to be offset by the return of a patient's productivity, eg, a disease that affects only the elderly or a correctable condition (ruptured aneurysm) in the aged patient. This problem will be discussed in subsequent sections, but clearly the issue of prudent decision making surfaces in each portion of this essay. It is clear that we must exercise our considerable power carefully and wisely to avoid selling ourselves out morally and selling our patients out by supporting inadequate treatments simply for cost containment.

PROGRESS

Despite noteworthy progress in certain areas, that stroke remains the third leading killer in the United States and that only one half of subarachnoid hemorrhage victims return to useful life suggest that much of our current therapy remains inadequate. Huge progress must be made to confront these elusive illnesses; this will require training, commitment, time, and funding. An element of the "culprit" of cost shifting that seems lost to our policy makers is that a large portion of current clinical research, including multiinstitutional studies in cerebrovascular disease, is conducted on clinical revenues. Academic departments use clinic revenues to support these efforts, often to the financial detriment of the faculty (reimbursement) and to the hospital (increased cost from "extra" diagnostic studies). Obviously studies of this type are jeopardized by spending caps and many other aspects of managed care negotiations.

It is also vital to remember that while this type of research is critical, many of our most fundamental advances have come from technological disciplines: CT, MRI, the surgical microscope, and so on. In both biomedical and biotechnological research, restraints on innovation due to cost concerns must not jeopardize the power of talented individuals to push their ideas from concept to available public service.

Our cerebrovascular patients are in serious need of carefully constructed outcome studies that will clarify in subtle subgroups the natural history course and the results of our various therapeutic interventions. In my opinion, this process will be facilitated by accumulating the highest-risk patients who need the most intensive evaluation and treatment in tertiary regional referral centers.

In light of federal efforts to contain health care spending as well as scientific spending, where will the money come from? It is clear that many of the pharmaceutical corporations and other industrial sponsors have been major supporters of scientific efforts, and not just a few have remained ethical and neutral, allowing the investigations to proceed to whatever conclusion they may. This source of support is vital and must continue. Universities currently raise major resources from community-based philanthropists. It is my perception that in many circumstances the bulk of this money was used to support basic molecular biological research efforts over the past 10–15 years. While these actions have been rewarded with substantial progress, it is now time for some reprioritization to occur. In the context of current clinical funding restraints, unless a more substantial portion of the philanthropic dollar is directed at clinically based research and outcome studies, such studies simply will not be possible.

RATIONING

Rationing in many forms is practiced in each hospital in the world. Expensive technology is not offered to patients in which there is no hope of altering the natural course of their illnesses (eg, patients dying of metastatic cancer are not resuscitated and placed on life support when the end of life is imminent). Rationing is destined to become much more prevalent over the next decade as spending caps are instituted. This evolution does not necessarily mean that a medical posture of ''meanness'' or ''cold hostility'' will confront patients who are told that they cannot have an MRI scan. To the contrary, the burden will be on us as clinical neurologists, neurosurgeons, neuroradiologists, and vascular surgeons to educate our policy makers about which investigations and treatments are valid and which are wasteful. Similarly, we must educate the public (our patients) about these same concerns, as well as creating a new perception of modern medical technology as a finite national resource, not a purchasable and unlimited commodity. Indeed, the challenges that face us offer great opportunities to focus our remarkable technology on the individuals who most need it. That this process must by definition be arbitrary or unfair is clearly refuted by the track record established by the organ procurement and transplantation effort (21). The public and individual good has been highly regarded and well served by effectively allocating this particular resource.

Specific measures that can be considered under the name of rationing have been previously alluded to: avoidance of major prophylactic procedures in patients with less than 10 years to live (unruptured aneurysm), withdrawal of critical care modalities in hopeless situations, and the use of measures such as circulatory arrest in surgical procedures and major interventional radiologic techniques only when less expensive conventional measures have no hope for success.

SUMMARY

I have attempted to characterize the challenges that have arisen in recent years in the management of one of our worst ailments—cerebrovascular disease. I hope that we will look to these new challenges and envision new opportunities for success in the battle with these difficult disorders. We stand on the threshold of great progress in the areas of neuronal preservation and salvage, particularly as new molecular techniques implemented in the field will minimize treatment delay. Thus, the clinician activists supporting the ''brain attack'' message can support (and be supported by) basic science colleagues for the immediate benefit of their patients.

We have the responsibility to exercise sound judgment and recommend scientifically valid measures to patients and their families, gatekeepers, payers, and government agencies. Implicit in this position of responsibility is the goal of minimizing futile or hopeless interventions.

Finally, as practicing physicians, we must get back to our roots. We may have positions as administrators, policy advisors, scientists, or entrepreneurs but must not lose sight of the fact that it is our fundamental privilege and obligation to be patient advocates. Our goals of optimizing outcome from miserable diseases and ensuring fertile ground for future development will not be realized if we abrogate this fundamental position. In modern practice, we will be increasingly placed in the untenable position of approving (recommending) or denying (failing to recommend) certain types of care to individual patients. To successfully confront this situation, the physician must hold in highest esteem the nonpecuniary intrinsic value of life and neurologic function. If, when making difficult recommendations, we think of each patient as a family member, we will be doing the right thing.

REFERENCES

1. Adams HP Jr, Caplan LR, Feussner JR, et al. Management dilemmas in carotid artery disease. *Patient Care* 1990;24:14–46.
2. Fayad PB, Brass LM. Transient ischemic attacks: Clinical clues that will influence your diagnosis and management decisions. *Consultant* 1990;30:25–36.
3. Schieber GJ, Poullier J-P, Greenwald LM. U.S. health expenditure performance: An international comparison and data update. *Health Care Financ Rev* 1992;13:1–15.
4. Hodgson TA, Kopstein AN. Health care expenditures for major diseases in 1980. *Health Care Financ Rev* 1984;5:1–12.
5. American Heart Association. *Heart and Stroke Facts, 1994 Statistical Supplement*. Dallas, TX: American Heart Association, 1994.
6. Mayberg MR, Batjer HH, Dacey R, et al. Guidelines for the management of aneurysmal subarachnoid hemorrhage. A statement for health care professionals from a special writing group of the Stroke Council of the American Heart Association. *Stroke* 1994;25:2315–2328.
7. Broderick JP, Brott T, Tomsick T, et al. Intracerebral hemorrhage more than twice as common as subarachnoid hemorrhage. *J Neurosurg* 1993; 78:188–191.
8. Purdy PD, Batjer HH, Samson DS. Management of hemorrhagic com-

plications from preoperative embolization of arteriovenous malformations. *J Neurosurg* 1991;74:205–211.

9. Batjer HH. Preoperative AVM embolization: Is it for everyone? In: Hadley MN, ed. *Perspectives in Neurological Surgery.* St. Louis, MO: Quality Medical Publishing, 1993;4(No 1):30–43.

10. Lubitz JD, Riley GF. Trends in Medicare payments in the last year of life. *N Engl J Med* 1993;328:1092–1096.

11. Emanuel EJ, Emanuel LL. The economics of dying. The illusion of cost savings at the end of life. *N Engl J Med* 1994;330:540–544.

12. Schneiderman LJ, Kronick R, Kaplan RM, Anderson JP, Langer RD. Effects of offering advance directives on medical treatments and costs. *Ann Intern Med* 1992;117:599–606.

13. Teno J, Lynn J, Phillips R, et al. Do advance directives save resources? (abstract) *Clin Res* 1993;41:551A.

14. Kidder D. The effects of hospice coverage on Medicare expenditures. *Health Serv Res* 1992;27:195–217.

15. Spector WD, Mor V. Utilization and charges for terminal cancer patients in Rhode Island. *Inquiry* 1984;21:328–337.

16. Mor V, Kidder D. Cost savings in hospice; final results of the National Hospice Study. *Health Serv Res* 1985;20:407–422.

17. Greer DS, Mor V. An overview of National Hospice Study findings. *J Chronic Dis* 1986;39:5–7.

18. Maksond A, Jahnigen DW, Skibinski CI. Do not resuscitate orders and the cost of death. *Arch Intern Med* 1993;153:1249–1253.

19. Angell M. How much will health care reform cost? *N Engl J Med* 1993;328:1778–1779.

20. Morris W, ed. *The American Heritage Dictionary of the English Language.* Boston: American Heritage Publishing Co, Inc, and Houghton Mifflin Co, 1970:1054.

21. Benjamin M, Cohen C, Grochowski E. What transplantation can teach us about health care reform. *N Engl J Med* 1994;330:858–860.

Cerebrovascular Disease, edited by H. Hunt Batjer.
Lippincott-Raven Publishers, Philadelphia © 1997.

CHAPTER 97

Regional Centers of Expertise: Are They Feasible?

Richard A. Roski

The constant evolution of the American health care system necessitates a reassessment of the feasibility of developing regional centers of expertise in the future. Regionalization of medical care has been commonplace throughout this country for many years. This concept was greatly expanded in a 1964 Presidential Commission on Heart Disease, Cancer, and Stroke (the Debakey Commission), which recommended government funding for the establishment of a national network of regional centers, local diagnostic and treatment stations, and medical complexes designed to unite the worlds of scientific research, medical education, and medical care (1). Although the recommendations of the commission were focused on the specific areas of heart disease and stroke, the notion of regionalizing isolated areas of medical care has continued to grow. Regional centers of expertise have been developed by physicians and/or hospitals to market a wide spectrum of specialized medical or surgical services. Historically, the most common types of regional centers have been for the treatment of trauma, cancer, burns, neonatal intensive care, rehabilitation, drug rehabilitation, heart disease, and stroke. As our health care system faces increasing pressure for cost containment from both managed care and government regulation, the question arises as to whether or not regional centers of expertise will remain a practical component of our health care system. In order to address the future role of regional centers of expertise, we need first to understand the financial evolution of our present health care system. Upon that framework, we can see how regional centers developed and flourished. We then must contrast the financial climate of the past with our present health care environment, so that we can see how centers of expertise may be able to survive in the future. There are also two issues that require discussion in order to understand our present health care environment and the future role of these

regional centers. These are (a) the change in reimbursement to health care providers that has come about because of actions taken by both the federal government and the health insurance industry and (b) the impact that managed care and clinical outcome data presently have on patient access to specialty care. The success of any regional center will be dependent on how well these issues are addressed in their planning for the future.

FINANCIAL EVOLUTION OF OUR HEALTH CARE SYSTEM

At the turn of the century, physicians received their reimbursement for medical services directly from patients. That once personal interaction has been profoundly affected by the insurance industry and the federal government throughout this century. Early forms of health insurance provided reimbursement for medical expenses directly to patients who were responsible for payment to the physician and for hospital charges. Hospitals were the first to ask the insurance industry to reimburse them directly for their charges rather than have payments made to patients. Although physicians opposed the idea at first, they too eventually accepted direct payment from the insurance companies. As payments increasingly were made directly to the health care providers and not to patients, patients became less aware of the actual costs that were accrued during an illness. Subsequently, they became increasingly insensitive to the rising cost of medical care, as long as they were insured. Cost effectiveness and medical appropriateness were not concepts that were discussed when referring to limiting the treatment of a patient. Outcome data were not available to compare treatment results, and often some physicians were considered superior to others because of their reputation or simply because of the higher charges for their services. Patients became even more removed from concerns of the costs of medical care

R. A. Roski: Genesis Medical Center, Davenport, Iowa 52804.

when the federal government made health insurance a tax-deductible item for corporations. This shielded patients not only from the actual costs of medical care but also from the escalating price of health insurance. Not being active cost-conscious consumers, patients were then more willing to undergo extensive diagnostic and medical treatments with little concern for the costs involved.

The federal government enacted several regulations that helped mold our health care system through the middle of this century (2). After World War II, there was a movement to expand the medical infrastructure in this country. This was prompted by the great successes that the medical profession had shown in handling injured soldiers during the war. Society wanted to increase both the number of physicians trained and the number of hospitals built. In 1946, the Hospital Survey and Construction Act was signed into law. This legislation, better known as the Hill–Burton Act, provided funds to hospitals to expand their facilities and purchase expensive new equipment. These funds contributed greatly to the expansion and modernization of hospitals across the country, as they were able to purchase the latest in high technology equipment, while increasing the size and capacity of their inpatient facilities.

Another major impact of the federal government came in 1965 when the Medicare Act was signed into law by President Lyndon Johnson. This law was designed to cover medical expenses for the elderly. After its implementation, Medicare regional carriers negotiated rates with the hospital providers. These rates were calculated on a cost-plus basis. Depreciation of assets bought with funds from the Hill–Burton Act were also included in the cost analysis. Medicare dollars were therefore used to help pay for the expanding costs of hospital care without any significant restrictions on how those costs were incurred. Medicare had no plan at its inception to control the cost of hospitalization or the fees charged by physicians. Most commercial health insurance plans did not have any mechanism for controlling hospital or physician charges or for regulating the appropriateness of treatment. In this type of environment, it was easy for hospitals and physicians to develop regional centers of expertise. Money was easily available through Hill–Burton funds, Medicare, commercial insurance carriers, and hospital foundations. Hospitals were not required to meet criteria to indicate the need for new facilities in the community, especially if they were for a center of expertise that had not been previously available in the region.

Federal laws at that time were much more lenient in allowing hospitals to recruit physicians and pay salaries in their regional centers. There were no restrictions preventing physicians from owning centers or from having a financial interest in a center to which they referred their own patients. Although primary care physicians could refer into these centers, there were usually avenues available for patients to have direct access to the system. Preapproval and mandatory primary care physician authorization were uncommon at that time.

The success of regional centers was based primarily on the maximum volume of paying patients who could be treated. The larger the number of patients, the higher the profits, because charges were generated for any and all services rendered. Advertising and reputation played an important role, since outcome results were often not available to provide comparison with other centers. The most significant issue was that there were no constraints placed on how much could be charged or how elaborate a treatment plan could be prescribed. Again, cost had not yet become a driving force in our health care system.

The cost of our health care system is now a major political and economic issue. It is difficult to define whether or not the health care system in the United States is in a serious financial crisis, as many would suggest. The numbers, however, do indicate that we may have problems. The total health care expenditure for the United States in 1970 was $69 billion. In just 10 years, it more than tripled to $230 billion. By 1992, it had tripled yet again to $800 billion, and expenditure predictions for the year 2000 are now estimated to be $1.7 trillion. Another way to calculate changes in the cost of health care in the United States is to look at its cost as a percentage of the gross domestic product (GDP). In 1970, health care expenditures made up 7.3% of the GDP. By 1992, this had increased to 14.5%, and it is projected to reach 19% by the year 2000 (3). At present, most other industrialized nations have maintained their health care expenditures at or below 12% of their GDP. Despite the difficulty in defining the crisis, there are ongoing attempts to curtail our spiraling health care costs. Both the federal government and the insurance industry are presently striving to contain the increasing costs of health care. These attempts will significantly influence the feasibility of regional centers of expertise.

CHANGE IN PROVIDER REIMBURSEMENT

In the first half of this century, reimbursement for health care services was generally lucrative and unrestricted. This made it safer to take the financial risks associated with developing a new regional center of expertise. Capitation and global payment schemes had not yet been developed. In the second half of this century, however, reimbursement to health care providers has gone through dramatic changes.

When the Medicare program was signed into law in 1965, projections were made to estimate its future cost to the country. The projected costs for Part A of Medicare was $5.7 billion by the year 1980; instead, the costs reached $25.6 billion. With the federal government already providing construction funds through the Hill–Burton Act, it was becoming a major financial contributor to the entire health care system. As expenditures skyrocketed past predictions, the government tried several methods to control the costs. These included the signing of the National Health Planning and Resources Development Act in 1974 and implementation of the Medicare Prospective Payment System in 1983 and the Medicare fee schedule in 1992.

Since the Hill–Burton Act did not have stringent criteria for hospitals to obtain funds, it was not difficult for hospitals to obtain money for modernization and expansion of their facilities. In an attempt to control the widespread excessive use of those funds, the Congress finally enacted the National Health Planning and Resources Development Act in 1974 (4). This law encouraged states to pass certificate of need (CON) laws in an attempt to place tighter controls on the expansion of hospital facilities and excessive duplication of high technology equipment. In most regions of the country, it is now impossible to build a new medical facility or to purchase an expensive piece of equipment, such as a CT scanner, without getting approval from a local or state CON board. Although designed as a means of saving money for the community and the federal government, the CON boards can often provide political roadblocks to the development of competing regional centers. Even when financing is fully obtainable for a regional center project, getting approval from a CON board may prove to be the biggest hurdle to cross.

The Medicare Prospective Payment System was implemented in 1983. This provided reimbursement to Medicare-providing hospitals based on patient's admitting diagnosis. A large group of diagnosis-related groups (DRGs) were established so that every patient admission could be categorized by a DRG code. The impact of this type of reimbursement system is threefold. It forces hospitals to minimize the length of hospital stays, move more diagnostic and surgical care to the outpatient area, and decrease the use of unnecessary testing. This reimbursement plan has had varying impacts on hospitals throughout the country. Some larger hospitals were able to average out the costs from their Medicare patients and were able to develop revenue-producing outpatient facilities, while other hospitals were forced to close. This type of hospital-reimbursement system has already spilled over into the managed care and health maintenance organization (HMO) markets, where hospital contracts often define reimbursement based on DRGs. The large cuts in hospital reimbursement by Medicare alone have made most hospitals wary of taking on financial projects that include expanding inpatient facilities, and many are unable to take on any new projects that require significant cash expenditures.

The Congress addressed the issue of how to control physician costs by asking the Health Care Financing Administration (HCFA) to develop a national fee schedule to be used by the Medicare program. The Resource-Based Relative Value Scale (RBRVS) was developed by Professor Hsiao at Harvard University and was used as the basis for the development of the Medicare fee schedule. The RBRVS-based fee schedule was subsequently enacted by Congress in 1992. Although designed as a way to standardize physician fees for Medicare, the RBRVS has now become a widely used tool in the managed care arena as well. The significant drop in Medicare reimbursement to physicians has had a measura-

ble effect on physician incomes. With managed care insurance plans also implementing the Medicare fee schedule for physician reimbursement, doctors are not as able to afford the financing necessary to establish a regional center of expertise. More important, with the standardization of fees, physicians are unable to charge more for services just because they are provided within in a center of expertise.

The Congress has also passed legislation designed to address the perceived abuse by physicians who were referring patients to their own treatment or diagnostic centers. The initial law prohibited physicians from referring Medicare patients to a clinical laboratory if the physician or his or her immediate family had a financial relationship with that laboratory. The Omnibus Budget Reconciliation Act for 1993 (OBRA 1993) significantly expanded this self-referral ban (5). The law presently restricts the ability of a physician to refer Medicare or Medicaid patients for designated health services to a facility in which the physician has a financial interest. Designated health services include clinical laboratories; radiology or diagnostics centers; physical, occupational, or radiation therapy; durable medical equipment; parenteral and enteral nutrients; equipment and supplies; prosthetics, orthotics, and prosthetic devices; home health services; outpatient prescription drugs; and inpatient and outpatient hospital services. Group practices are also limited from providing physician compensation that is based directly or indirectly on the volume of referrals for designated health services that the physician generates. The laws also place restrictions on the financial relationships that can be established between a physician and a hospital. These self-referral laws, commonly referred to as Stark I and Stark II after one of the authors, United States Representative Pete Stark of California, will likely continue to go through an evolving process of change over the coming years. They will certainly have a significant impact on how regional centers of expertise are owned and controlled in the future. Physicians and hospitals must be extremely careful in both how they structure their relationship and how they define reimbursement parameters.

The federal government has not been alone in starting to limit expenditure payments for health care. Large industries in this country have pressured their insurance carriers to contain expenditures, as the cost of providing health insurance benefits for employees started to escalate at an unacceptable rate. In an effort to solve the problem, the insurance industry attempted to manage how health care was being delivered to their members. The idea of managed care has continued to grow and expand across the country. Although HMOs and other managed care plans have existed in this country since 1926, the idea is now far more prevalent. However, there are still no good guidelines on how to manage the delivery of health care. Like the federal government, the insurance industry has focused much of their attention on how to cut costs, and thus cut payments to hospitals and physicians. When an insurance company insured a significant number of people in a medical community, it realized that it could approach hospitals and physicians to provide exclusive medical services at discounted fees. Numerous physician relationships, such as preferred provider organizations (PPOs) and independent practice associations (IPAs), have developed to provide the negotiating entity to contract with insurance carriers. The exclusive right to provide care, however, has come at the price of reduced fees for physician services. With a surplus of hospital beds in this country, hospitals, attempting to maintain acceptable patient census levels, have been especially hard hit with significant charge discounts for inpatient services.

Even with the decrease in reimbursement that has come from the federal government and the insurance industry, physicians could try to maintain their incomes by providing more services. This usually meant performing more procedures or operations. In many areas of the country, that has been addressed by reimbursing physicians on a capitated vs. a fee-for-service basis. Under the capitation system, physicians are paid a fixed amount of money per enrolled life that is to be used to cover the costs of physician services. In some markets, the capitation is paid to cover all physician services, and in more sophisticated markets it is broken down to cover individual specialty areas such as cardiology, general surgery, or neurosurgery. The incentive under a capitated reimbursement system is to provide as few procedures as possible and focus on preventive treatment. The old idea of a regional center making money based on a large volume of expensive tests and procedures does not hold up well in a capitated reimbursement environment.

The cost controls used by Medicare and the managed care insurance industry have had a significant impact on the potential reimbursement to a regional center of expertise. The federal government is no longer the generous provider of funds for new construction or modernization projects. Although other sources of funding can be found, it is certainly much more difficult than in the past. State certificate of need boards are often much more strict in the present environment, making it difficult, if not sometimes impossible, for a hospital or group of physicians to build new facilities. With the implementation of the Stark laws, it is becoming increasingly difficult for hospitals and physicians, as well as physician groups, to legally structure the types of relationships that were commonplace with regional centers in the past. It is most important in today's environment to understand how reimbursement for services is going to be structured. A regional center of expertise will need to be structured much differently in a heavily capitated market from how it was structured in a fee-for-service market.

MANAGED CARE AND CLINICAL OUTCOME DATA

The effects of managed care on the health care system in the United States include more than the impact on reimbursement. The issue of specialty-care access has produced some major concerns for physicians, although it may also provide some opportunities to physicians with good clinical outcome data. With attempts to constrain health care costs even further, managed care plans have often turned to gatekeeper models of managed care. In a gatekeeper model, the decision for referral to specialty care lies in the hands of a primary care physician. There may be a significant financial interest in keeping a patient from obtaining specialty care, especially if reimbursement is paid on a capitated basis, with all of the money being paid to the primary care physician or gatekeeper. If the money that is paid to specialists must come from the capitated pool that is controlled by primary care physicians, there is a significant financial disincentive for them to refer to specialty physicians. These types of plans have raised concern about whether managed care can protect the quality of care and unduly restrict access to appropriate care, as well as whether it suppresses innovation in medical care (6). Managed care plans may therefore place significant obstructions in the path of a patient who wishes to obtain the services of a regional center of expertise. The center must be prepared to negotiate for the managed care contracts in its region of the country to ensure adequate patient volumes. Such situations, however, may become a benefit to a well run center of expertise. Managed care plans in most areas of the country have focused primarily on cost savings. As competition increases in the managed care marketplace, quality and efficiency will become more important. As centers of expertise begin providing clinical outcome data that demonstrate that they can treat certain illness at less cost, more efficiently, and with better outcome, then they will be in the best position to negotiate for exclusive care or carve out managed care contracts. Some centers have already taken this approach in the treatment of patients undergoing carotid endarterectomy. When attention was focused on how to cut the costs of carotid endarterectomy surgery in a teaching institution, the mean discharge time decreased from 3.4 to 1.5 days, costs were cut by $750,000 over 300 cases, and the overall complication rate decreased from 10% to 2% (7). That type of management will provide the necessary data for a potential regional center of expertise to compete well in the managed care market.

Managed care has produced several changes in the health care marketplace that significantly impact the feasibility of a regional center of expertise. In general, managed care plans have decreased the level of reimbursement to all providers of health care, including hospitals and physicians. Tightly controlled managed care plans that have physician gatekeepers can severely restrict or deny access to certain facilities or specialty care. They may also not pay for experimental or unproven treatments. If a regional center of expertise is not contracted with a particular managed care plan, patients from that plan will have no access to the services offered by the facility. Managed care plans are not only replacing many of the indemnity insurance plans but are also contracting for Medicare and Medicaid patients. The overall effect of managed care on a regional center of expertise is to decrease revenues and restrict patient access. By responding proactively to the concerns presented by managed care plans, ie, lower costs and better clinical outcome data, a regional center of expertise may be able to strongly position itself in the marketplace.

CONCLUSION

Regional centers of expertise can survive in the future. Their challenge in our evolving health care environment will be their ability to show cost effectiveness and efficacy of their treatment plans. Accurate collection of clinical outcome data will be critical for regional centers to justify their existence and eventually compete against other centers. To be successful, they must carefully analyze their patient population base. They need to understand how the majority of their revenues will be funded. Only a careful business plan will help to predict whether or not the decreasing revenues in health care will continue to surpass expenses in the future. It is essential that regional centers of expertise plan their product or services so as to meet the needs of a heavily managed care market. As more medical care is being reimbursed on a capitation basis, the providers of truly cost-effective care will do well financially. If, on the other hand, the business plan is based on a large volume of self-referred patients and an unnecessarily extensive diagnostic work-up of patient complaints without solid medical justification, then such a regional center will fail.

The opportunities for a regional center of expertise to succeed are very real in today's market. Just as with any form of business, however, those centers must be prepared to adapt to the changing marketplace. Innovative planning and careful preparation can produce a successful center.

REFERENCES

1. President's Commission on Heart Disease, Cancer and Stroke. *Report to the President: A National Program to Conquer Heart Disease, Cancer and Stroke*. Washington, DC: US Government Printing Office, 1964;1: viii.
2. Starr P. *The Social Transformation of American Medicine*. New York: Basic Books, 1982.
3. Physician Payment Review Commission. *Annual Report to Congress*. Washington DC: US Government Printing Office, 1993.
4. Feldstein PJ. *Health Care Economics*. New York: Delmar Publishers, 1993.
5. *Omnibus Budget Reconciliation Act 1993. Conference Report of the Committee on the Budget House of Representatives*. Washington DC: US Government Printing Office, 1993.
6. Teisberg EO, Porter ME, Brown GB. Making competition in health care work. *Harvard Business Review* July-August 1994:131–141.
7. Harbaugh RE, Harbaugh KS, Perron AD. Increasing the value of carotid endarterectomy: Experience of a neurosurgical training program. In press.

Cerebrovascular Disease, edited by H. Hunt Batjer.
Lippincott-Raven Publishers, Philadelphia © 1997.

CHAPTER **98**

Ethical Aspects of Cerebrovascular Care

Howard Morgan and Ralph G. Greenlee, Jr.

Cerebrovascular insult to the brain, besides disturbing neurologic functioning, results in an immediate and intimate disturbance of the afflicted patient's personhood and personal autonomy. Physicians who treat patients with cerebrovascular diseases are almost daily confronted with the ethical aspects of treatment decisions. It is the physician's role to assist patients and their families in making difficult decisions regarding treatment options in settings where the patient's decision-making ability is frequently impaired. This chapter serves as a broad guide to understanding medical ethics as applied to cerebrovascular disease, brain death, and the persistent vegetative state as well as when and how to forego life-sustaining treatment.

Medical ethics is a practical discipline in which ethical problems having to do with the practice of medicine or biomedical research are identified and analyzed in an orderly fashion in an effort to guide decision making or resolve conflict. Since the 1970s, the field of medical ethics, also termed biomedical ethics or bioethics, has burgeoned into a relatively autonomous discipline. Most medical schools now require an introductory course in medical ethics for students and many college and university philosophy departments offer courses for undergraduate and graduate students. Besides the clinician, experts in biomedical ethics have emerged from the fields of law, nursing, academic philosophy, and the clergy. Most hospitals now have ethics committees and many have human experimentation review boards. Institutes have come into existence for the purpose of studying ethical problems encountered in contemporary health care delivery, eg, the Hastings Center in Briarcliff, New York, and the Kennedy Institute of Ethics at Georgetown University in Washington, D.C. Specific cases of patients and their families caught in seemingly insoluble and sometimes absurd encounters in hospitals and nursing homes have

become topics of public interest and the subject of newspaper and magazine articles as well as television and radio reports.

Ethics has to do with right and wrong human conduct, good and evil, and the conforming of members of certain groups, such as the professions, to standards of behavior. Although the term *morality* connotes a social institution dealing with right and wrong human conduct and the term *ethics* connotes a study of morality, the two terms are commonly used interchangeably, which will be the case in this chapter.

HISTORY

The importance of a moral basis for the practice of medicine was recognized in antiquity. For example, almost 4000 years ago the code of the Babylonian king Hammurabi set standards for medical practitioners. In ancient Athens where Western scientific medicine is generally thought to have originated, the Hippocratic Oath dates back to the fourth or fifth century B.C. Codes of medical ethics also were formulated by ancient Indian, Chinese, and Persian writers. The basis for these and subsequent codes of ethics for medical practice is the societal recognition that patients seeking medical assistance are in a temporary position of vulnerability and in need of help, often powerless and open to exploitation. This aspect of medical practice is the basis of medicine as a profession, not just a trade.

In 1803 the prominent English physician Thomas Percival published *Medical Ethics; Or, A Code of Institutes and Precepts Adapted to the Professional Conduct of Physicians and Surgeons,* which was in contrast to and served as a response for the troublesome conduct of some British practitioners of the day. In 1847 the fledgling American Medical Association adopted a Code of Ethics in response to a similar lack of respect for the profession by the American public due to the conduct of some of those who practiced medicine and surgery (1).

Starting in the late 1950s, several decades of social revolution and scientific advancement helped to bring into public

H. Morgan: Department of Neurological Surgery, University of Texas Southwestern Medical Center, Dallas, TX 75235.

R. G. Greenlee, Jr.: Department of Neurology, University of Texas Southwestern Medical Center, Dallas, TX 75235.

focus ethical problems facing modern health care delivery. Technological breakthroughs such as long-term hemodialysis, mechanical ventilators, newer antimicrobial and chemotherapeutic cancer drugs, and the introduction of intensive care units gave medicine the ability to prolong life but engendered questions concerning whether and when such technology could be withheld or withdrawn and who should make those decisions. Besides scientific advances, social upheaval during the 1960s contributed to evolution of medical ethics. The public became better informed as a consequence of broader education and telecommunications. Encouraged by the civil rights movement, the protest movement against the Vietnam War, and consumerism, the public demanded to participate more in the decision-making process. Distrust of authority, starting with government officials and the military, spread to include all authority figures, even doctors. The ''patients' rights movement,'' which demanded that the patient be included in decisions concerning health care delivery, was born. Until just a few decades ago, physicians generally practiced in a paternalistic manner, striving to benefit their patients and not harm them but rarely involving the patient or the patient's family in the decision making process. Spawned by public demand and well-publicized cases as well as by a few court decisions, a radical transformation occurred in medical ethics in the 1960s and 1970s. The right of the patient to make health care decisions, even if those decisions seemed unreasonable to medical experts and likely to cause death, came to be recognized as an important value and principle itself, on an equal and possibly higher moral footing than the traditional principles of the physician benefiting and not harming his or her patients.

HOW TO MAKE MORAL DECISIONS IN MEDICAL PRACTICE

When making ethical decisions dealing with patient care, the physician goes through a process that in some ways is similar to, and in some ways is different from, that used for making nonethical decisions. For example, when deciding what antibiotic to use in the treatment of a pneumonia, the physician wants to have available the pertinent facts about the case, including the organism cultured or most likely to be the causative agent, the antibiotic sensitivity test results if available, the chest X-ray, and a list of the patient's drug allergies. Better factual information usually leads to better treatment, and knowing all the facts of the case will lead the physician on a relatively straightforward, logical path toward making a good decision regarding treatment. When making ethical decisions, however, one cannot derive what ought to be from what is the case. This ''is/ought'' dichotomy is sometimes called Hume's dictum (named after the 18th century British philosopher David Hume) or the naturalistic fallacy according to the early 20th century British philosopher George Moore. Simply stated, it means that factual information alone is insufficient when making moral evaluations (2,

3). It does help to have available the pertinent medical and nonmedical information when making an ethical decision dealing with patient care, but the facts alone will not lead to an appropriate solution. Physicians in the process of making a decision of ethical consequence often look repeatedly at the patient's chart or order more and more tests in hope of finding the answer to an ethical dilemma. The answer is not to be found in the data alone. At some point the physician must decide what is the right course of action. What guidelines, then, can the doctor use? Some writers in the field of biomedical ethics have tried to adapt ethical theories not designed for medical situations to the clinical encounter. Others have tried to develop a theory, code of conduct, or set of principles specifically for the medical profession. Whether or not any of the classical ethical theories are fully applicable to medical situations remains in question. Some familiarity with the general concepts of ethical theory is usually helpful in resolving ethical dilemmas, reviewing problem cases, and formulating health care policy.

Utilitarianism

Utilitarianism is an ethical theory that judges actions according to their consequences. The British philosophers Jeremy Bentham (1748–1832) and John Stuart Mill (1806–1873) conceived utilitarianism, Bentham evaluating actions according to the production of pleasure and Mill according to the production of happiness. For example, using Mill's greatest happiness principle the totality of happiness of all involved for different courses of action can be weighed and compared, and, according to utilitarianism, the course of action that maximizes net happiness is right. Arguments against utilitarianism say that it demands too much if practiced rigidly (to maximize the overall good might require some individuals to give up considerable comfort and gain) and that it permits too much (some individuals' rights could be trampled to maximize the good of others).

Deontology

Deontological ethical theories are characterized by the idea that actions are right or wrong according to some feature of the act itself independent of consequences and that an action is right when it is in accordance with duty. The biblical golden rule, ''Do unto others as you would have them do unto you,'' is an example. The best known deontological ethical theory was formulated by the German philosopher Immanuel Kant (1724–1804). Kant argues that what he terms the categorical imperative best guides rational persons in making moral decisions. The better known formulation of the categorical imperative is sometimes called the principle of universality: ''Act only according to that maxim whereby you can at the same time will that it should become a universal law'' (4). In other words, you should act only according to a rule of conduct that can be applied to all other individuals in similar circumstances. Will universalizing the maxim defeat your purpose? If so, the act is immoral. If not, it is morally permissible. Kant's second formulation of the categorical imperative is sometimes called the principle of humanity and may be more applicable to medical ethics: "Act in such a way that you treat humanity, whether in our own person or in the person of another, always at the same time as an end and never simply as a means" (4). In other words, never treat people exclusively as a means to your own ends; always respect them as persons. Kant is often criticized for not recognizing and for not suggesting a method of solution when moral duties are in conflict.

Virtue Ethics

Unlike utilitarian and deontological theories, virtue ethics does not focus on what act we ought to do or ought not to do. Rather, virtue-based ethics focuses on the character traits and dispositions of the person involved. Good acts are defined as the acts of a virtuous individual. This type of ethical theory dates back to and follows the teachings of Plato and Aristotle. In the biomedical arena, virtue ethics consists of defining the kind of person the good physician should be and defining those virtues that work toward the ends of medicine (eg, integrity, compassion, honesty, knowledge, and skill).

Principle Theory

Beauchamp and Childress in *Principles of Biomedical Ethics,* now in its fourth edition, base their approach to biomedical ethics on what they see as the commonly held moral traditions and common sense moral beliefs of members of society (5). Although not an ethical theory in the strict sense, these ideas and traditions are brought together in the form of principles that assist in ethical decision making and reflection. The principles are not absolute; they are prima facie binding, meaning that they are binding unless they can be overridden by strong, sound reasoning. A principle is most commonly overridden when two or more principles conflict. In such a case, the course of action in accordance with the principle that makes the strongest argument is held to be the best moral choice.

There are four principles of biomedical ethics according to Beauchamp and Childress: beneficence, nonmaleficence, respect for autonomy, and justice.

Beneficence is the principle that obligates one person to endeavor to benefit another. Generally one citizen is not bound to help another, but individuals may be in special situations or occupy special roles when they are expected to work for the benefit of others. For example, we expect parents to provide for their children even if it means the parents have to make some sacrifices for their offspring. We expect policemen and firemen to take some risks in protecting the public. In a similar way, society expects the physician to

work for the benefit of his or her patient even if it requires some self-effacement of the physician's interests and even some risk. A point of contention obviously is how much self-effacement and how much risk should society rightfully expect.

The principle of *nonmaleficence* is the obligation not to intentionally inflict harm and is similar to the long-held medical rule *primum non nocere* ("above all do no harm").

Respect for autonomy is the principle that binds one person to respect the right of another person to be self-governing. It requires that we treat with deference the right of other persons to make their own decisions and act independently without constraint. For an individual to act autonomously, he or she must have the capacity to make decisions, must be free from coercion, must have available and understand pertinent factual information, and must be able to express and follow through with his or her choice. A major problem in biomedical ethics during the past two decades has been how to respect the autonomy of individuals who no longer possess the capacity to act autonomously. In such situations, we appeal to surrogate decision-making and advance directives that will be discussed later.

The principle of *justice* has to do with distributive justice, not legal justice, and involves the fair distribution of benefits and burdens--who should receive medical care, how much care should each receive, and who pays for the care. In the decade of the 1990s, issues of justice in health care have taken center stage (eg, questions of rationing, access to care, cost containment, and managed care).

Other Theories

In *situational ethics*, each case is weighed on its own merits without regard for preconceived rules or principles. Each situation is looked at as a unique occurrence, but this isolated approach does not do justice to our moral experience, which is more than just a series of segregated, discontinuous events (6). *Casuistry* is an approach to ethics that focuses on the detailed understanding of a particular case, practical decision-making, and the historical account of similar cases. Casuistry is similar to legal proceedings where the precedent of past case decisions carries great weight. Both situational ethics and casuistry reject the idea that ethics can be generalized in the form of a theory or a set of universal rules or principles that apply in all situations.

Communitarian ethics looks at communal values and the common good as being paramount. Communitarianism renounces the primacy of the concepts of individuality and rights that are held as fundamental by most liberal Western ethical theories. *Ethics of care,* which recently has been espoused by some feminist writers, also rejects the importance of individuality and rights and stresses intimate personal relationships and responsibilities similar to that of the family.

Two ethical views that work contrary to ethical problem solving and deny the social nature of morality are *moral absolutism* and *moral relativism* (6). Moral absolutism is seen in the individual who holds rigidly to a moral rule allowing no room for reflection and deliberation. The individual works from a solution and not toward a solution. He or she already knows the answer. Moral relativism is the attitude that moral choices are no more than subjective opinions or preferences of an individual or a society that cannot be substantiated or negated. If moral relativism were the case, there would be no justification in condemning another person or another society for a course of action if that course were in keeping with the existing moral attitude of the society and no basis to believe that individuals or communities could progress or reform their moral standing (7). To enter into ethical reflection and problem solving is to engage in reasoned deliberation and to be able to justify a course of action. When examining an ethical problem, a helpful starting place often is to examine one's own ethical assumptions (6). Are your moral beliefs and convictions more than just moral hunches and intuitions, and can they withstand critical evaluation?

ETHICAL ISSUES IN CEREBROVASCULAR DISEASE

The moral questions that confront the physician treating patients with cerebrovascular disease are the same or very similar to those he or she confronts when treating patients with other disorders of the nervous system, such as head injury or brain tumors. Some issues may be similar to those surrounding patients with other vascular diseases, such as coronary artery insufficiency, or general medical conditions, such as diabetes mellitus. In fact, all of the issues seen in the wide field of biomedical ethics can be found in patients with cerebrovascular disorders including many of those dealing with maternal-fetal and neonatal medicine and pediatrics. In no other area of medicine are matters of competency and personhood more frequently encountered than they are in stroke patients.

Foregoing Life-Sustaining Treatment and Advanced Directives

In the past three decades trends in medical ethics and court decisions have affirmed the concept that competent individuals have the right to decide whether or not to submit to any and all medical treatment, including that which is life sustaining. Life-sustaining treatment refers to medical intervention that is used to prolong the biological life of the patient without reversing the underlying disease process. The terminology "foregoing treatment" refers to abating treatment and can mean either to withhold treatment not already begun or to withdraw treatment once started. Although there may be some practical differences for the practicing physician, most ethicists stress that there is no moral distinction between stopping life-sustaining treatment and not starting

that same treatment. Examples of treatments that may be life sustaining include mechanical ventilation, renal dialysis, the administration of blood products, antibiotic therapy, chemotherapy, and the administration of fluids and nutrition by artificial means such as a nasogastric or gastrostomy tube.

When a patient who has previously been autonomous is no longer capable of making health care decisions and when that patient's biological life processes require sustaining treatment, making the decision to forego treatment is more problematic. Physicians caring for stroke patients are often faced with dilemmas regarding abatement of treatment in patients who have suffered a severe subarachnoid hemorrhage, a massive cerebral infarction or intracerebral hemorrhage, or a major brainstem stroke. Using the principle of respect for patient autonomy, physicians are obligated to abide by the decisions of competent patients who opt to forego life-sustaining treatment. When faced with such a situation, the physician should ascertain that the decision is indeed autonomous, ie, that the patient is capable of making a reasoned decision, that no coercion is involved, and that the patient is not merely expressing depression or feelings of abandonment. More frequently, however, the patient who has suffered a cerebrovascular catastrophe has also lost consciousness and consequently is unable to make any decision. At such times, accurate information regarding prognosis is frequently helpful for the decision makers as well as for the attending physician, ie, what is the likelihood that even with treatment the patient will survive and not be severely disabled (eg, see ref. 8). These decision makers are usually the patient's family who are assisted by the attending physician and other health care providers, their clergy, and occasionally by ethics committees or ethicists. This decision making process is facilitated by advanced directives that provide a means for the patient's autonomy to be expressed and for the patient to play a part in making decisions regarding his or her own life even if he or she is incapacitated at the time the situation arises.

There are two basic types of advanced directives; the first is frequently termed the "living will" in which the patient indicates the types of treatment he or she does or does not want, and the second is the "durable power of attorney for health care" in which the patient appoints in advance a proxy or surrogate to make health care decisions just in case he or she loses decision making capacity. Presumably, such a decision maker knows the patient well, has knowledge of the patient's values and desires, and will use this information to reconstruct the decision the patient would make if able, rather than merely inflict his or her own opinions on the patient. Many advanced directives combine features of both the living will and the durable power of attorney for health care. The Patient Self-Determination Act of 1991 mandates that hospitals in the United States acquaint patients with their right to execute advance directives.

The situation becomes more difficult when the patient does not leave clear instructions, the patient's values are not known, there is no family or close friend, there is disagreement among family members, or the proxy appears not to be acting in the patient's best interest. These types of cases are usually best managed with the assistance of an institutional ethics committee. On rare occasions, the assistance of the courts should be sought. In keeping with the tenets of beneficence in biomedical ethics and the deliverance of sound medical care, the physician caring for the stroke patient should strive to render to his or her patient all of the treatment that reasonably may be beneficial. When life-sustaining treatment becomes futile, any or all of it may be withdrawn or withheld. The physician must be careful not to impose his or her own value system on the patient or on the patient's proxy when such decisions are made. The physician should also be careful not to confuse or conflate the issue of foregoing life-sustaining treatment, which in appropriate circumstances is legal and generally considered ethical, with the issues of active euthanasia and assisted suicide, which are illegal and, according to time-honored medical tradition, unethical.

Early Prediction of Neurologic Impairment and Death

With increasing frequency and very early in the course of an illness that causes unconsciousness or other serious impairment, the physician is being asked to predict the eventual outcome. For the most part, the pathophysiology of the insult determines the ability to predict the clinical outcome. The Glasgow Coma Scale has been validated to predict the outcome of the traumatic brain-injured patient based on the score at a certain time following the injury but is less reliable in cases of subarachnoid hemorrhage or ischemia. In nontraumatic coma, Levy et al found simple clinical criteria most useful to predict disability and death, ie, the absence of corneal, pupillary, and vestibular responses combined with severe impairment of motor and verbal abilities at 24 hours to be associated with a very poor outcome as far as functional survival is concerned (9). The Study to Understand Prognosis and Preferences for Outcomes and Risks of Treatment (SUPPORT) identified five variables at day 3 after the insult that are associated with a poor outcome or death. These include abnormal brainstem response (absent pupillary response, absent corneal response, or absent or dysconjugate roving eye movements), absent verbal response, absent withdrawal response, creatinine level ≥1.5 mg/dl, and age 70 years or older. Mortality at 2 months for patients with four of these five risk factors was 97%. Patients with either abnormal brainstem response or absent motor response had a 96% rate of death or severe disability at 2 months (8). Such information is useful to the physician caring for such afflicted patients, especially when asked by the family to predict whether the patient will recover. In such circumstances, the physician should present the probabilities and uncertainties with honesty and compassion. Unfortunately, no clearly useful group of criteria have been developed that are as reliable in cases involving children and young adults.

Brain Death

The theological, philosophical, medical, and legal definition of death has a long and sometimes confusing history. However, the past 30 years has imposed a pragmatic approach among many of the parties interested in this debate. Because it is now possible to maintain the cardiopulmonary function of many permanently apneic, irreparably brain-damaged persons, physicians in particular and society in general have become aware of the complexities associated with the care of persons with severe neurologic damage. For example, the cases of Karen Quinlan, Paul Brophy, Elizabeth Bouvia, and others have been discussed in the news media as well as in biomedical articles.

In 1968, the Harvard Ad Hoc Committee published a seminal paper describing a framework for declaring a person legally dead by virtue of irreparable brain damage (10). Since that time, close collaboration between the medical and legal professions has helped state legislatures achieve definitions of brain death that are morally acceptable to most of their constituents. Similar definitions have become accepted in most other Western societies. In 1978, the President's Commission for the Study of Ethical Problems in Medicine and Biomedical and Behavioral Research articulated a definition of death that emphasized that the human organism functions as an integrated whole rather than the directionless sum of its parts (11). The Commission argued persuasively that the whole brain, not just the brainstem or cerebral cortex, was necessary for the maintenance of the ''organism as a whole.'' The brain was recognized as the necessary coordinating organ for biological existence of the entire organism as well as for consciousness and learning. In essence, the human organism can function purposefully without its limbs and many other structures and can function with some transplanted organs. Individual portions of the brain may be destroyed with the person still surviving and functioning. However, destruction of the whole brain results invariably in death within a few days or weeks even though biological life may be maintained temporarily by artificial means.

The reasons for determining brain death include the need to make organs such as the kidneys and the heart available for transplantation before injury by ischemia and hypoxia, which would occur if the traditional cardiac and pulmonary criteria were used, the desire to not have the families of these patients wait needlessly hoping for recovery when none can possibly be forthcoming, the realization that the patient in an intensive care unit is subjected to procedures and treatments that many consider undignified, and the need to conserve and best use scarce resources.

Physicians who care for patients suspected of fulfilling the criteria for brain death must be acquainted with the law of the state in which they practice as well as with the criteria suggested by national and local authorities on the subject. For example, the President's Commission states that a person can be declared dead if he or she presents with findings of irreversible cessation of circulatory and respiratory function or the neurologic findings of irreversible cessation of all functions of the entire brain, including the brainstem (11). The cause of the coma and whether or not it is irreversible should be established with absolute confidence, and the absence of brain function should persist for a predefined period of observation. Complicating conditions must be eliminated including drug intoxication, metabolic or endocrine derangement, hypothermia, and shock.

The clinical examination for brain death includes the documentation that the patient is unconscious; has no motor response to painful stimulation (with the possible exception of primitive spinal reflexes); has no brainstem reflexes, especially those to cold caloric stimulation of the vestibular system; and is apneic without response to apnea testing (Tables 1 and 2). In most instances, a confirmatory examination is usually recommended after a another predetermined period of observation (usually 12–24 hours). Recently, detailed guidelines for the determination of brain death in adults and children have been published (12–15). In cases of cerebrovascular disease causing coma, a computed tomography (CT) or magnetic resonance (MR) scan of the head is usually helpful and probably mandatory in documenting diagnosis as well as in determining the severity of the stroke. In cases in which the cerebral insult does not produce anatomic abnormality on the CT or MR scan to explain the patient's condition, electroencephalogram, evoked potential monitoring, cerebral angiography, and radioisotope brain blood flow studies may be helpful in proving that the brain is irreparably damaged. Special considerations and criteria are required when a child is the patient due to the potential for reorganization in the immature brain. The confidence in the clinical neurologic tests used in adults is less in children due to the ability of the young child's brain to withstand some injuries that an adult brain cannot. Finally, the physician who makes the determination of brain death should have no direct interest in any possible organ harvesting process.

Persistent Vegetative State

Patients who survive an insult to the brain that produces coma may emerge from the coma into a state of apparent wakefulness without awareness. This condition is termed the vegetative state, and when it lasts more than a month the condition is defined as persistent (16–18). Such patients have suffered extensive damage to their cerebral hemispheres but incomplete injury to their brainstems. The persistent vegetative state can be considered permanent 3 months after a nontraumatic brain injury. Recovery after that period of time is extremely rare, and those few cases in which consciousness has been regained are associated with severe disability (19,20). The biological life of patients in a permanent vegetative state may last for years at considerable emotional and financial expense to their loved ones. Because most people would not choose to exist under such circumstances, termination of life-sustaining treatment including the with-

TABLE 1. *Suggested protocol for determining brain death*

The etiology of the patient's coma must be defined.
The presence of endogenous toxins must be excluded.
Hypothermia (less than 32°C) and hypotension (less than 90 mm systolic) should be corrected.
The duration of the coma must be
  a. 6 hr if a structural lesion is present.
  b. 24 hr if a metabolic alteration is responsible.
There should be no signs of eye opening, no spontaneous movement, and no movement elicited by painful stimulation to the face or trunk (eg, supraorbital pressure, sternal rub, or pinching the nipple) other than spinal cord reflex movement.
Brainstem reflexes should be absent, including
  a. Pupillary light reflex (in a semidark room, a strong light shone in each eye sequentially causes no pupillary constriction in either eye).
  b. Corneal reflex (a sterile piece of cotton or soft tissue is lightly touched to the patient's cornea, not the conjuctiva. Any movement of the eyelid during this maneuver which is performed bilaterally suggests some preservation of brainstem function).
  c. Gag reflex (a tongue depressor or other similar object is pressed against the back of the pharynx or the endotracheal tube is moved against the pharynx. Movement of the uvula or retching indicates preservation of brainstem function).
  d. Cough reflex (a cannula is passed down the endotracheal tube into the tracheobronchial tree or the endotracheal tube is irrigated with a small amount of sterile saline. Any movement or coughing excludes the diagnosis of brain death).
  e. Extraocular movements (these may initially be tested with the oculocephalic or doll's eyes maneuver—turning the patient's head from side to side with the head elevated 30°. If there is no response, the patient's ears should be irrigated with ice water in the cold caloric or oculovestibular response test. The ears must be free of significant wax and the ear drums must be intact. The head is elevated 30° and the ear canal is irrigated with 50 cm³ of iced water over a period of 30–45 sec. The eyes should be observed for movement over a period of 3 min. After the one ear is tested, the contralateral is also tested. Any movement demonstrates some preservation of brainstem functioning.
Spontaneous respiratory movements should be absent and the apnea test brings about no respiratory effort (see Table 2).
Confirmatory Tests (optional in massive, untreatable brain trauma. Only used to shorten the period of observation):
For structural lesions: documentation of absence of cerebral blood flow by radioisotopic or angiographic means, *or* electrocerebral silence on a single EEG
For metabolic coma: Two EEGs separated by at least 12 hr demonstrating electrocerebral silence, *or* documentation of absence of cerebral blood flow by radioisotope or angiographic means

drawal of food and fluids administered by nasogastric or gastrostomy tubes comes into question. A legal and ethical consensus has emerged in the United States that families or other proxies may authorize the foregoing of life-sustaining treatment, including artificial feeding, for patients in a permanent vegetative state (21–23). But a consensus has not

TABLE 2. *Suggested protocol for apnea testing*

1. An arterial line should be in place for rapid blood gas measurements.
2. Adjust the ventilator to deliver 100% oxygen. Adjust the rate and volume to a pCO_2 of approximately 40 mm Hg.
3. Obtain arterial blood gas measurement.
4. Remove the patient from the ventilator and deliver oxygen at 6–8 L/min through a cannula placed 3–4 in. down the endotracheal tube. Assume a 3 mm Hg rise in pCO_2 per minute and continue off the ventilator for a sufficient time to achieve a pCO_2 of approximately 60 mm Hg or greater (approximately 5 min). Utilizing this technique will assure no significant change in oxygenation while allowing for pCO_2 to rise sufficiently to stimulate respiration.
5. Observe the patient for respiratory movement. Monitor heart rate and blood pressure carefully. Any evidence of bradycardia or hypotension necessitates discontinuance of the test and immediate mechanical ventilation and blood gas determination.
6. At the end of the estimated time to reach a pCO_2 of 60 mm Hg, draw an arterial blood gas and place the patient back on the ventilator.
7. A rise in pCO_2 to approximately 60 mm Hg or higher without evidence of spontaneous respirations establishes apnea for the purpose of this protocol.
8. Goose bumps, shivering, extensor movements of the arms, rapid flexion of the elbows, elevation of the arms above the bed, crossing the hands, reaching of the hands toward the neck, forced exhalation, and thoracic respiratory-like movements can all occur. These are considered spinal cord release phenomena and do not mean that the patient is not dead.
9. Chronic pulmonary or cardiac diseases may alter the response to hypercarbia.

been reached in the case of a patient who is in a permanent vegetative state and for whom the patient's proxy wants continued treatment even though health care providers argue for termination of treatment on the grounds of futility. While there is no need for the physician to provide treatment in the case of a patient who fulfills the criteria of death either by cardiopulmonary or brain death standards, a consensus has not emerged concerning the case of the patient in a permanent vegetative state for whom the proxy wants continued life-sustaining treatment and for whom the health care providers believe that treatment should be abated. To extend the definition of brain death to include the patient in a permanent vegetative state, as some have argued, is problematic for a number of reasons (24). Angell has suggested that society move toward a consensus assumption that patients in the permanent vegetative state would not want to be kept alive indefinitely (21). If the family or proxy of a patient in the permanent vegetative state is in opposition to the termination of life-sustaining treatment, then it would be their burden to prove that the patient would not want the treatment terminated. If that burden were met, health care providers would be obligated to continue treatment. Otherwise, life-sustaining treatment could be abated in spite of opposition. In the meantime, such cases should be dealt with through discussion and negotiation with the patient's family or proxy.

The assistance of institutional ethics committees and ethics consultants can be helpful to the attending physician in cases where decisions regarding limiting life-sustaining treatment are being considered. Occasionally, a court decision may be requested. Hopefully, we can avoid termination of life-sustaining treatment decisions being made by third-party payers on purely economic grounds.

Managed Care

Since World War II, medical care in the United States as well as in most of the Western world has undergone major advancement in terms of being more effective in combating human maladies and in being more and more in demand as well as becoming very expensive. In the United States in particular, this has resulted in an ever-increasing part of the nation's resources being spent on health care. While 5% of the gross national product for the United States was spent on health care in 1950, the figure was 13% in 1992. The 1990s have seen the establishment of managed care coverage to control the ever-rising health care costs, which consequently limit the access of patients to health care providers as well as procedures and treatments. The physician is placed in a conflict between the traditional obligation to serve the patient and society's new duty to conserve dollars. It is one thing to talk of rationing care to benefit society as a whole and quite another to ration care for the benefit of stockholders, CEOs, and entrepreneurs. Unfortunately, this is the case in the United States today. Many traditional not-for-profit third-party payers have become for-profit corporations resulting in lower percentages of premium dollars spent on direct patient care, increased and sometimes astronomical salaries for corporate chiefs, and more premium dollars utilized for administration and for the rewarding of stockholders. Physicians are pressured to provide their services at ever-decreasing reimbursement rates and see their professional autonomy diminishing. The more troublesome ethical problems for physicians in the managed care era are that the physician's advocacy for the patient is at odds with the utilization review usually performed by insurance company employees who are not physicians and the practice of gatekeepers who are primary care physicians rewarded for denying services. The patient with a stroke often requires a period of observation in the hospital before a course of treatment can be finalized or a prognosis determined. During this time, the utilization reviewers may incessantly demand to know what is being done for the patient and threaten to deny coverage. Stroke patients frequently require expensive tests and procedures for diagnosis and treatment that third-party payers may or may not be willing to cover. At times such as these, it is helpful for the physician to remember the gold standard of medical ethics—"the primacy of the patient's well-being" (25). That in a nutshell is what the physician should hold as his or her first and highest obligation, ie, that the patient's well-being must be the foremost consideration.

Physicians should be cautious about moving from an ethical basis of being an advocate for the patient to one of being an allocator of resources.

REFERENCES

1. Konald D. Codes of medical ethics: history. In: Reich WT, ed. *Encyclopedia of Bioethics*. New York: Free Press, 1978;162–171.
2. Rachels J. *Created from Animals. The Moral Implications of Darwinism*. New York: Oxford University Press, 1990.
3. Raphael DD. *Moral Judgement*. Westport, CT: Greenwood Press, 1978.
4. Kant I. *Grounding for the Metaphysics of Morals*. Ellington JW, trans. Indianapolis: Hackett, 1987.
5. Beauchamp TL, Childress JF. *Principles of Biomedical Ethics*, 4th ed. New York: Oxford University Press, 1994.
6. Churchill LR, Smith HL, Frey JJ. Ethical decisions. In: McGaghie W, Frey J, eds. *Handbook for the Academic Physician*. New York: Springer-Verlag, 1986.
7. Rachels J. *The Elements of Moral Philosophy*. New York: Random House, 1986.
8. Hamel MB, Goldman L, Teno J, et al. Identification of comatose patients at high risk for death or severe disability. *JAMA* 1995;273:1842–1848.
9. Levy DE, Caronna JJ, Singer BH, Lapinski RH, Frydman H, Plum F. Predicting outcome from hypoxic ischemic coma. *JAMA* 1985;233:1420–1426.
10. Ad Hoc Committee of the Harvard Medical School to Examine the Definition of Brain Death. A definition of irreversible coma. *JAMA* 1968;205:337–340.
11. President's Commission for the Study of Ethical Problems in Medicine and Biomedical and Behavioral Research. *Defining Death: Medical, Legal, and Ethical Issues in the Determination of Death*. Washington, DC: Government Printing Office, 1981.
12. American Academy of Pediatrics. Report of special task force: guidelines for the determination of brain death in children. *Pediatrics* 1987;80:298–300.
13. Lynch J, Eldadah MK. Brain-death criteria currently used by pediatric intensivists. *Clin Pediatrics* 1992;31:457–460.
14. Wijdicks EFM. Determining brain death in adults. *Neurology* 1995;45:1003–1011.
15. Report of the Quality Subcommittee of the American Academy of Neurology (Summary Statement). Practice parameters for determining brain death in adults. *Neurology* 1995;45:1012–1014.
16. Council of Scientific Affairs and Council on Ethical and Judicial Affairs. Persistent vegetative state and the decision to withdraw or withhold life support. *JAMA* 1990;263:426–430.
17. The Multi-Society Task Force on PVS. Medical aspects of the persistent vegetative state (first of two parts). *N Engl J Med* 1994; 330:1499–1508.
18. Report of the Quality Standards Subcommittee of the American Academy of Neurology. Practice parameters: assessment and management of patients in the persistent vegetative state (Summary Statement). *Neurology* 1995;45:1015–1018.
19. The Multi-Society Task Force on PVS. Medical aspects of the persistent vegetative state (second of two parts). *N Engl J Med* 1994; 330:1572–1579.
20. Ashwal S, Cranford RE, Rosenberg JH. Commentary on the practice parameters for the persistent vegetative state. *Neurology* 1995;45:859–860.
21. Angell M. After Quinlan: the dilemma of the persistent vegetative state. *N Engl J Med* 1994;330:1524–1525.
22. President's Commission for the Study of Ethical Problems in Medicine and Biomedical and Behavioral Research. *Deciding to Forego Life-Sustaining Treatment: A Report on the Ethical, Medical, and Legal Issues in Treatment Decisions*. Washington, DC: Government Printing Office, 1983.
23. Cruzan *v.* Harmon, 760 S.W. 2d 408 (1988).
24. Bernat JL. Brain death. Occurs only with destruction of the cerebral hemispheres and the brain stem. *Arch Neurol* 1992;49:569–570.
25. Pellegrino ED. Ethics. *JAMA* 1994;271:1668–1669.

Cerebrovascular Disease, edited by H. Hunt Batjer.
Lippincott-Raven Publishers, Philadelphia © 1997.

CHAPTER 99

The Role of Clinical Trials and Outcomes Research in Cerebrovascular Practice

Stephen J. Haines

Cerebrovascular disease in its many manifestations is one of the most common and potentially devastating conditions treated by neurosurgeons. Death and disability caused by ischemic and hemorrhagic stroke and subarachnoid hemorrhage are a leading cause of death and disability in the United States and therefore merit significant attention from public health authorities. This focuses attention, public interest, and public resources on these problems. It can, however, complicate individual neurosurgical practices because of societal demands for proof of the efficiency, efficacy, and cost effectiveness of surgical intervention on both a societal and individual level.

Cerebrovascular surgery has been the subject of important clinical trials and outcome studies and provides an excellent example of how we may expect to integrate such studies and information into other areas of neurosurgical practice in the future. There are also lessons to learn about the importance of understanding and embracing the concepts underlying outcomes research and analysis as a way of stabilizing and expanding the role of neurosurgery in the management of these important and complicated problems.

DEFINITIONS

There is controversy as to just what constitutes outcomes research. Outcomes research does not refer to a specific type of study design but to a strategy that stresses the assessment of four major impacts of medical intervention: medical effectiveness, patient functional status, patient satisfaction, and cost effectiveness. For example, in a traditional study of treatment of aneurysmal subarachnoid hemorrhage, one would measure success of clipping rates, rebleeding rates,

morbidity, and mortality. The outcomes researcher would be interested in all of these measures of medical effectiveness but would add global measures of patient functional status such as the Karnofsky scale or SF-36 (1a), the frequency with which patients return to their premorbid employment, a measure of how satisfied patients and their families were with the outcome of their treatment, and a measure of the cost of treatment as compared with the long-term outcome in patient function and satisfaction.

Studies with such a focus can be done with many different research designs. Traditional retrospective designs such as case–control and retrospective cohort studies, prospective cohort studies and even randomized clinical trials can incorporate such outcome measures and truly be considered outcomes research. In addition, studies of variations in the application of medical interventions and their outcomes between small geographic areas can be illuminating (small-area variation studies). Large data bases, such as those maintained by the Medicare system and several large insurance companies, may provide useful outcomes data. The parameters affecting the application of some of this information to clinical decision making may best be identified in a decision-analysis model. In many ways, outcomes research is simply an extension of what clinicians have traditionally done to assess the value of their interventions. The outcomes movement has tended to focus on nonrandomized studies because they are easier to conduct and can obtain results more quickly and less expensively than large-scale randomized clinical trials. The outcomes movement has emphasized that it is necessary to conduct such retrospective studies with much greater scientific rigor than has traditionally been the case in clinical reports. In addition, the outcomes movement is in the process of developing and validating measures of functional status and patient satisfaction that can be applied to specific diseases.

In short, outcomes research is more an attitude than a specific methodology. It represents a commitment to rigor-

S. J. Haines: Department of Neurosurgery, University of Minnesota, Minneapolis, Minnesota 55455.

ous examination of multiple dimensions of the outcome of medical interventions. Outcomes research therefore represents an opportunity for physicians who treat cerebrovascular disease to simultaneously meet professional needs for better information on the medical effectiveness of their interventions and societal demands for better information on patient functional outcome and cost effectiveness.

CEREBROVASCULAR SURGERY LEADS THE WAY

The earliest neurosurgical randomized clinical trials were done in the field of cerebrovascular surgery. In London in the early 1960s, Wiley McKissock conducted controlled trials of the surgical treatment of ruptured intracranial aneurysm and intracerebral hemorrhage, in which patients were randomly allocated between surgical and nonsurgical management (1,2). Like the operations they studied, these trials were at a crude level of technical development and were flawed in many respects. They did not provide evidence favoring surgical intervention and, probably for that reason, were disregarded by the neurosurgical community. These studies do, however, express an attitude of wanting to know the effectiveness of neurosurgical intervention, as accurately as possible. In that sense, these trials are a landmark in that they show a neurosurgeon willing to submit this attitude to scientific testing.

The controlled trial of carotid endarterectomy carried out by Fields and associates (3) in the 1960s was similarly flawed. While the primary analysis in this study did not show a clear benefit for surgery, refinements of analysis suggest that technically successful endarterectomy was indeed effective in reducing subsequent stroke risk. The study was not effective in constraining the proliferation of carotid endarterectomy in the subsequent two decades but did form a basis for skepticism, mostly within the neurology community, that ultimately expressed itself in well designed controlled trials of the procedure.

In 1968, Donaghy and Yasargil (4) reported the first extracranial-to-intracranial (EC-IC) bypass procedures for revascularizing ischemic cerebral cortex. The logic of the procedure was appealing, and the technical prowess it required led to its rapid acceptance by neurosurgeons as a major advance. Around the world, several thousand procedures were carried out and hundreds reported in consecutive series that seemed to suggest the effectiveness of the operation. As always, there were differences in indications and results between various neurosurgical centers, and uncertainty as to the precise indications and outcomes arose. An international multicenter trial of the operation was carried out with great technical success (5). The trial enrolled 1377 patients, who were carefully followed. The technical success with the operation was documented at excellent levels. No demonstrable advantage for the surgically treated patients could be identified.

The EC-IC bypass trial results were embraced by antisur-

gical neurologists who had never believed in the operation. They were accepted by third-party payers, who now had a strong reason to refuse to pay for the procedure. These results influenced research funding organizations to deny funding for further studies to refine the indications for the operation and identify subgroups of patients who might benefit.

The study came in for excoriating criticism from the neurosurgical community. On sober reflection, however, several facts emerged that showed that the neurosurgical community can be justifiably proud of having (a) conducted the study, (b) implemented its primary findings, and (c) resisted the efforts of those outside of the neurosurgical community who would overinterpret the results in an attempt to completely eliminate the procedure from the neurosurgeons' armamentarium.

The study was a technically excellent one that demonstrated no benefit of surgery for the patients enrolled in the study. The characteristics of those patients closely resembled those of the largest proportion of patients to whom the operation was being offered at the time of the study, and therefore the study results are generalizable to the group of patients that is similar to that in the study (ie, those with inaccessible internal carotid or middle cerebral artery stenosis or occlusion presenting with transient ischemic attacks [TIAs] or minor stroke). However, the study results are not generalizable to any other population.

The inappropriate overgeneralization of the negative result of the EC-IC bypass study has denied researchers the opportunity to better define groups of patients who may benefit. Such groups might include patients with moyamoya disease and those who can be demonstrated by some physiologic test such as positron emission tomography or cerebral blood flow imaging to have significant cerebral ischemia. In addition, patients undergoing deliberate occlusion of certain vessels may well benefit from prophylactic or immediate postocclusion bypass. None of these patient groups is large enough that we can expect a study of a comparable technical quality to be performed, but the patient groups are sufficiently different that the results of the EC-IC bypass study are not directly transferable.

CAROTID ENDARTERECTOMY TRIALS

Unfortunately, we did not learn quite the right lesson from the EC-IC bypass trial. The frequency of carotid endarterectomy rose rapidly during the 1970s and 1980s without clear scientific evidence of its effectiveness. A significant portion of the neurology community was unconvinced of the effectiveness of the operation, and there was evidence that complication rates, at least in some settings, were much higher than those being reported in the literature (6,7). A concerted effort to create uncertainty about the scientific bases for the operation ensued. There was a resultant decline in the utilization of the operation concurrent with the formation of three studies for symptomatic patients and two for asymptomatic patients.

This time the surgeons were right. Both the European Carotid Surgery Trial (8) and the North American Symptomatic Carotid Endarterectomy Trial (9) reached a clear conclusion that surgery is beneficial to patients who both have a >70% stenosis of the appropriate internal carotid artery and have had TIAs or minor strokes in the distribution of that vessel. The Veterans Administration (VA) study confirmed these findings (10). Recently, the Asymptomatic Carotid Atherosclerosis Study (11) reported similar findings in asymptomatic patients with significant internal carotid artery stenosis. Findings from the VA study are compatible with this (12).

Not surprisingly, the surgical and neurosurgical communities have embraced the results of these studies. However, the lesson is not that we should be happy with studies that support our practices and unhappy with those that refute them but that good studies, properly interpreted, advance the practice of cerebrovascular surgery and improve the care we deliver to our patients. Indeed, when we look at carotid endarterectomy, we see that persuasive argument, force of personality, and appeals to authority could not resolve the question of the value of the operation. Careful study of a few thousand patients (after years of operating on hundreds of thousands of patients) placed the operation on sound footing and caused the opposition to melt away. How many thousands of patients could have been offered the operation and saved from stroke had we performed those studies on a few thousand patients at an earlier time? We should recognize that we can bring innovative surgical procedures into common practice faster by putting them through a rigorous controlled trial than by simply introducing them sporadically into the practice of a few physicians.

Cerebrovascular surgery has a proud tradition of subjecting its interventions to controlled clinical trials. For the future, studies of interventional neuroradiologic procedures, various procedures for the treatment of intracerebral hemorrhage, and stereotactic radiosurgery for arteriovenous malformations provide great opportunities to continue the tradition of excellent clinical science and cerebrovascular surgery.

OTHER TYPES OF OUTCOME STUDIES

When the complication rate of a procedure as applied in community practice is studied, the results are sometimes remarkable. This is true of the study by Brott and Thalinger (13) of community complication rates for carotid endarterectomy. A wide range of variation was identified, far exceeding the accepted standards of roughly 6% mortality plus morbidity. Such a study accomplishes many things: it creates local impetus for improvement and monitoring of individual surgeon's complication rates, highlights the importance of such quality control measures, and emphasizes the fact that pub-

lished complication rates cannot substitute for valid individual complication rates. The results of the previously discussed carotid endarterectomy trials, obtained with low mortality and morbidity, are certainly not generalizable to surgeons who have combined mortality and morbidity rates of 10–20%.

Studies of neuropsychological outcome following subarachnoid hemorrhage have shown that the ultimate effect on patient functional status is not nearly as beneficial as the clear medical effectiveness of successfully clipping the aneurysm and excluding it from the circulation (14). Such patients may appear to be normal to the neurosurgeon's clinical examination but be unable to return to their former occupation, particularly if it requires significant cognitive skill. They may also have important personality disturbances affecting their interpersonal and family relationships. Such abnormalities must be looked for in order to be found and clearly have a negative impact on the total benefit of the surgical procedure.

Decision analyses have been published for several neurosurgical problems, most prominently, that of electing surgical treatment for arteriovenous malformations (15,16). These analyses highlight the fact that decision analysis is a tool for identifying important factors in clinical decision making and for investigating the effect of varying those factors on the ultimate decision. Decision analysis produces a model of the decision-making process; it is not complete or definitive. It has not reached a point where it can substitute for individual patient and surgeon judgment. It can be extremely useful in demonstrating the impact of varying certain parameters on the decision to be made. Such exercises may influence the formulation of policy, but they cannot substitute for it.

COST-EFFECTIVENESS STUDIES

Studies of cost effectiveness bring to the fore a number of factors foreign to much of medical decision making. It becomes necessary to identify financial values for things such as life, avoiding stroke, living without fear, and so on that we ordinarily consider priceless. It is easy to ignore certain factors that can have a profound influence on the results of the cost–benefit analysis. For example, if one simply looks at costs during hospitalization and ignores both costs and lost income during the recovery period, results can be badly skewed. As this is a new area of investigative research for neurosurgeons, it is strongly recommended that a qualified health economist participate in such studies.

INDIVIDUAL OUTCOME ANALYSIS

As patients and others who pay for neurosurgeons' services begin to apply the results of outcome studies to the selection of individual surgeons to provide services, it becomes essential that the individual surgeons have detailed and valid information about their own practices. It is no longer unusual to be asked what your stroke and death rates are by a patient contemplating a carotid endarterectomy. It is very common to be asked how many arteriovenous malformations you have operated on and what the results were.

It is not as easy to collect this information as it sounds. Mortality rates are relatively objective and easily retrieved. Nonetheless, I suspect that most neurosurgeons know of colleagues who explain away some of their postoperative deaths as unrelated to surgery. Unless this is done in an identical way by all the surgeons whose rates are being compared, the comparisons are invalid. With infection, the problem of the clinically definite infection with purulent drainage from a wound or perhaps abscess formation but a negative culture can lead to different interpretations and therefore different quoted infection rates. The problem becomes more difficult when postoperative stroke is assessed. Some surgeons will religiously include the most subtle postoperative numbness or sensory change as a stroke, while others will not count a patient who has made full recovery from an obvious stroke by 6 months after surgery. It is obviously possible to manipulate postoperative complication rates in a way that shows the surgeon in the best possible light. Therefore, if a surgeon is to embark on a detailed recording of his or her own complication rates, the definitions must be clearly established. Unfortunately, there are no nationally agreed-on definitions for such data collection. This is an urgent item for the profession. In the meantime, we can look to published literature for commonly accepted definitions (ie, mortality = any death within 30 days of surgery regardless of cause). It is also appropriate to turn to those who wish to use the data, such as major health plans, for their own definitions.

It is suggested that each neurosurgeon identify a limited number of outcome measures that can be compared with readily available or published norms, eg, mortality, infection, length of stay, stroke in the case of cerebrovascular surgery, and so on. These outcomes should be recorded for every patient. The system of keeping data should be flexible enough so that when newly validated outcome measures come along, they can be added without too much difficulty.

We need to recognize and be prepared for the fact that many neurosurgical outcomes include highly subjective components. In such cases, the evaluation of the patients and surgeons may not be accurate, and we may have to have the assessment of the outcome measured made by a third party.

This process of collecting individual outcome data is a very important but potentially difficult one. Preliminary efforts are currently underway by national neurosurgical organizations to create systems that will standardize and simplify this process for the individual neurosurgeon. It is hoped that not only will each neurosurgeon be able to collect useful outcome information, but that comparability of these data will allow it to be combined and used to promote national quality standards.

CONCLUSIONS

Cerebrovascular surgery has a long tradition of willingness to engage in a scientific evaluation of its outcomes. This is by no means universally accepted and is rarely accomplished without a good deal of discomfort on the part of the surgeons involved. Nonetheless, it is becoming increasingly evident that maintaining the widespread acceptance of the neurosurgeon's role in the treatment of cerebrovascular disease requires that we generate high-quality clinical evidence of the effectiveness of what we do. Cerebrovascular surgery is in an outstanding position to lead neurosurgery in this arena.

In a world of limited resources, neurosurgeons will increasingly be required to justify their interventions on the basis of demonstrative medical effectiveness, impact on patient functional status and satisfaction, and cost effectiveness. Individual neurosurgeons need to understand the value and interpretation of these various kinds of outcomes assessment both for research purposes and for assessing their own practice. Neurosurgeons can expect to be asked to document their own performance on outcome measures used in published studies. Doing this prospectively would be wise. Neurosurgeons should learn to demand high-quality evidence before incorporating new procedures into their practice. The practicing neurosurgeon should become part of studies designed to accomplish this. Outcomes research is best accomplished in actual clinical practice settings. While these are available in academic centers, results may be even more generalizable if they also come from private-practice settings. Such studies can and should be designed to interfere as little as possible with ordinary clinical practice, for it is in the setting of ordinary clinical practice that new procedures must be effective if they are to be of value.

An expanded role for neurosurgery in the treatment of cerebrovascular disease can be assured and achieved more quickly by conducting good outcomes research rather than by the traditional method of doing large numbers of operations and sorting out the results later.

ACKNOWLEDGMENTS

Supported in part by a grant from the Congress of Neurological Surgeons for the COSIN project.

REFERENCES

1a. Ware J. The MOS 36-item short-form health survey (SF-36): conceptual framework and item selection. *Medical Care* 1992;3:473–483.
1. McKissock W, Richardson A, Taylor J. Primary intracerebral hemorrhage. A controlled trial of surgical and conservative treatment in 180 unselected cases. *Lancet* 1961;2:221–226.
2. McKissock W, Richardson A, Walsh L. Posterior-communicating aneurysms. A controlled trial of the conservative and surgical treatment of ruptured aneurysms in the internal carotid artery at or near the point of origin of the posterior communicating artery. *Lancet* 1960;1: 1203–1206.

3. Fields WS, Maslenikov V, Meyer JS, Hass WK, Remington RD, MacDonald M. Joint study of extracranial arterial occlusion. V. Progress report of prognosis following surgery or nonsurgical treatment for transient cerebral ischemic attacks and cervical carotid artery lesions. *JAMA* 1970;211:1993–2003.

4. Donaghy RMP, Yasargil MG. Extra-intracranial blood flow diversion. Presented at the American Association of Neurological Surgeons, Chicago, IL, April 11, 1968; abstract 52.

5. EC/IC Bypass Study Group. Failure of extracranial-intracranial arterial bypass to reduce the risk of ischemic stroke. Results of an international randomized trial. *N Engl J Med* 1985;313:1191–1200.

6. Barnett HJM, Plum F, Walton JN. Carotid endarterectomy—An expression of concern. *Stroke* 1984;15:941–943.

7. Warlow C. Carotid endarerectomy: Does it work? *Stroke* 1984;15:1068–1076.

8. European Carotid Surgery Trialists' Collaborative Group. MRC European carotid surgery trial: Interim results for symptomatic patients with severe (70%–99%) or with mild (0%–29%) carotid stenosis. *Lancet* 1991;337:1235–1243.

9. North American Symptomatic Carotid Endarterectomy Trial Collaborators. Beneficial effect of carotid endarterectomy in symptomatic patients with high-grade carotid stenosis. *N Engl J Med* 1991;325:445–453.

10. Mayberg MR, Wilson SE, Yatsu F, et al. Carotid endarterectomy and prevention of cerebral ischemia in symptomatic carotid stenosis. *JAMA* 1991;266:3289–3294.

11. Executive Committee for the Asymptomatic Carotid Atherosclerosis Study. Endarterectomy for asymptomatic carotid artery stenosis. *JAMA* 1995;273:1421–1428.

12. Hobson RW II, Weiss DG, Fields WS, et al. Efficacy of carotid endarterectomy for asymptomatic carotid stenosis. *N Engl J Med* 1993;328:221–227.

13. Brott T, Thalinger K. The practice of carotid endarterectomy in a large metropolitan area. *Stroke* 1984;15:950–955.

14. Ljunggren B, Sonesson B, Saveland H, Brandt L. Cognitive impairment and adjustment in patients without neurological deficits after aneurysmal SAH and early operation. *J Neurosurg* 1985;62:673–679.

15. Auger RG, Wiebers DO. Management of unruptured intracranial arteriovenous malformations: A decision analysis. *Neurosurgery* 1992;30:561–569.

16. Fisher WS III. Decision analysis: A tool of the future: An application to unruptured arteriovenous malformations. *Neurosurgery* 1989;24:129–134.

Cerebrovascular Disease, edited by H. Hunt Batjer.
Lippincott-Raven Publishers, Philadelphia © 1997.

CHAPTER 100

Practice Guidelines for Stroke: Enforceable? Meaningful?

Michael Salcman

The Institute of Medicine defines practice guidelines as "systematically developed statements to assist practitioner and patient decisions about appropriate health care for specific clinical circumstances" (1). More than 30 different names have been identified for such clinical management tools, including critical paths, practice parameters, clinical guidelines, clinical protocols or algorithms, and standards of care (2). In the United States, increased interest in the development and application of practice guidelines has been fueled by at least two concerns, namely, the rising cost of health care and a demonstrable and significant regional variability in the utilization of specific procedures and interventions. In one famous study, residents in New Haven, Connecticut, were twice as likely as residents of Boston to undergo coronary artery bypass surgery, but Bostonians were twice as likely to undergo carotid endarterectomy (3). It is believed that variability in health care delivery may contribute to unnecessary costs and may reflect lack of quality. Widespread uncertainty in regard to what health care dollars buy has focused the debate on "value" in health care. "To make any type of judgement regarding the 'value' of services purchased, some notion of what is necessary and appropriate to treat medical conditions (or to prevent them) is required" (2); hence, the hope that practice guidelines can identify appropriate types of treatment and eliminate variability. As Menken (4) has stated, variability in delivery has been "identified as a symptom that the science of health care has lagged behind the science of its biomedical foundation." A major component of variability is overutilization, itself a function of many societal expectations and economic forces. Practice guidelines are viewed as a possible mechanism for reducing the extent of medical practice variation and the amount of "inappropriate" care. The potential importance of this strategy was explicitly recognized by the

federal government when it established the Agency for Health Care Policy and Research (AHCPR) in 1989. Prioritization of guideline development within the AHCPR is often determined by the global economic impact of a diagnostic category or therapeutic intervention (5). As of 1993, it was estimated that more than 30 different commissions and 80 different professional societies were at work on more than 1400 sets of guidelines (2).

GUIDELINE DEVELOPMENT

The development of a medical practice guideline is usually carried out by an expert panel convened by a government agency or a private organization with official standing. The methodology used by such panels usually consists of four analytic steps: (a) definition of the goals and methods of the project, including the target condition and relevant patient population, the interventions that will or will not be examined, and the user population for which the guideline is intended; (b) assessment of clinical benefits and risks (ie, outcomes analysis) and development of a preliminary recommendation for alternative clinical interventions; (c) assessment of practice feasibility for the various proposed interventions, including an analysis of the economic costs, the concerns of relevant parties, and the impact of patient variability, cost effectiveness, societal values, medical ethics, local resources, liability issues, and other factors; and (d) preparation of a draft document for external review and pretesting by clinical practitioners (6). After further revision, the final document is usually delivered to the AHCPR.

A critical step in the initial stage of guideline development is the elaboration of a management model or flowchart, in which the linkages between each intervention and each potentially beneficial or harmful outcome are explicitly recognized. The panel then decides whether some or all of the linkages need to undergo data analysis and which of the

M. Salcman: Private practice, Towson, Maryland 21204.

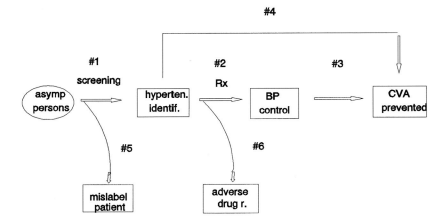

FIG. 1. Linkage diagram for a management model in regard to hypertension screening to prevent stroke. For each linkage, a literature search and metaanalysis are carried out to determine the effectiveness and side effects of each numbered intervention. A linkage diagram is very similar to a decision tree, and many of the figures used in it in regard to efficacy, sensitivity, specificity, and complications are equivalent to probabilities. (Modified from ref. 6, with permission.)

linkages will be the subject of a final recommendation in the guideline. A hypothetical example of a management model that might be used by a panel to develop guidelines on screening an asymptomatic population for hypertension in order to prevent stroke is illustrated in Fig. 1. Note that both the bad and good outcomes of each intervention are clearly identified. It is important that the management model accurately reflect the complexity of clinical decision making; otherwise, the final guideline developed from it will not be relevant to the realities of medicine, and its intended audience will not accept it (6).

Outcomes research is essential to the development of clinical guidelines and is specifically mandated to the AHCPR. The Patient Outcomes Research Teams (PORTs) are considered the showcase investments of the AHCPR. PORTs are large-scale, long-term, multifaceted, multisite, and multidiscipilinary grants and contracts. "The goals of a PORT project are to identify and analyze the outcomes and costs of alternative interventions for a given clinical condition, in order to determine the most effective and cost-effective means to prevent, diagnose, treat, or manage it and to develop and test methods for reducing inappropriate or unnecessary variations" (5). The data so gathered are to be used by independent expert panels in the development of practice guidelines. Most of the conditions studied in the initial PORTs are among the 20 most frequent Medicare and Medicaid inpatient diagnoses. A multicenter PORT project has been initiated in stroke at Duke University. Given the prevalence of stroke in the elderly population, continued funding by the AHCPR is to be expected.

PRACTICE GUIDELINES AND THE LAW

Practice guidelines have enormous legal implications and not just for malpractice liability (2). This is because practice guidelines are directly relevant to the growing body of law and public policy required to deal with a wide variety of countervailing forces that are external to the doctor–patient relationship. In both the public and private sector, these forces include large organizations that determine the nature of benefit packages, the utilization of services, and the medical necessity of reimbursable interventions. In the managed care paradigm, underutilization or the failure to deliver appropriate or enough services has become as important an issue as overutilization (7). The shift from utilization review as a postdelivery means of cost containment to utilization management raises the specter of denying access to care as a means of lowering costs. In this rapidly changing environment, determining who and what represents appropriate care is a central issue, and practice guidelines become important, not just to the federal government but to many state legislatures struggling with their own health care reform initiatives.

From a regulatory standpoint, the history of practice guidelines is quite clear. In 1972, the Professional Standards Review Organization (PSRO) law was enacted in order to develop regional norms for medical care. Physician compliance was to be achieved by denying Medicare and Medicaid payment for services not meeting the standards. As an added incentive, federal law explicitly protected practitioners from malpractice liability in regard to services rendered according to the norms of a PSRO. The next stage in the evolution of guidelines arrived in 1982 when this local system was replaced by the statewide Peer Review Organization (PRO) program, and the Congress simultaneously introduced diagnosis-related groups (DRGs) as the basis for Medicare payment to hospitals. Soon generic quality screens became an important tool, and PRO review became a clinical-problem detection and correction program. Interest in a national standard for appropriate care grew with awareness of regional variability in health care delivery and the report of the Physician Payment Review Commission (PPRC) that volume performance standards would be needed to help institute physician-payment reform (2).

It was in response to these forces that the AHCPR was created in 1989. Its mandate is as follows:

> The purpose of the Agency is to enhance the quality, appropriateness and effectiveness of health care services, and access to such services, through the establishment of a broad base of scientific research and through the promotion of

improvements in clinical practice and in the organization, financing and delivery of health care services (42 USC §299).

Within the AHCPR, the Forum for Quality and Effectiveness in Health Care was specifically created to arrange for the development, periodic review, and updating of practice guidelines. One of the stated goals of developing a common standard of behavior was to reduce variation among physicians; this consideration was to be used in prioritizing the agenda of the Forum. With this congressional mandate in hand, the AHCPR then turned to the Institute of Medicine to provide guidance on how to implement its authority. As a result of the Institute's deliberations, practice guidelines were clearly separated from medical-review criteria, the first being defined as aids to practitioners during the delivery of care and the second as tools applied after the fact to assess the appropriateness of health care decisions, services, and outcomes (1).

Once the first six AHCPR guidelines were published, the very next group of topics selected included two of immediate interest to the neuroscience community, low back pain (8) and poststroke rehabilitation. In addition, the AHCPR funded a Stroke PORT Study (9), organized in 1991 and headquartered at Duke University, to identify the most effective approaches to stroke prevention and to examine patterns of care and cost of care for both the prevention and treatment of stroke. In summary, guideline development is no longer a purely local or professional responsibility; it is established in federal law through the creation of the AHCPR and funded by millions of Public Health Service and Medicare dollars.

There are two types of potential legal liabilities in the use of clinical practice guidelines: (a) those that relate to the development and implementation (ie, antitrust issues) of guidelines and (b) those faced by practitioners who apply the guidelines in a particular setting. Despite an exemption from liability under the PRO program that has been on the books in some form for 20 years, as of 1994 "no case law . . . . has explicitly dealt with guideline adherence, as such, as a basis for protection from malpractice liability" (2). However, recent health care reform proposals have provided for such a link, chiefly because of the potential cost savings involved with a decrease in defensive medicine. In addition, physicians who follow practice guidelines appear to perform fewer unnecessary or inappropriate procedures. Be that as it may, among the states, only Maine and Minnesota have established the use of guidelines as an affirmative defense and then only in the case of some specialties. In addition, a guideline in Maine may not be used by the plaintiff to establish liability (10). However, a recent Harvard School of Public Health study indicates that guidelines are three times more likely to be used against physicians than in their defense (11,12).

In the future, clinicians may be held liable for their ignorance concerning the existence of a guideline or their failure to discuss treatment options included in the guideline. Informed consent may become an especially difficult area. In the case of some guidelines, public dissemination and awareness have been especially rapid; witness the release of the AHCPR guidelines on the management of pain in patients with cancer (13). Organizations, as well as individual practitioners, face the risk of malpractice litigation; a developing body of case law has begun to establish that managed care organizations, as well as utilization review companies, can be held liable for bad outcomes if their management of care delivery through systems and incentives is not consistent with the standard of care (2). On the other hand, once the appropriate guideline has been discussed with the patient or, better yet, once the patient is in physical possession of it, the physician may find guidelines a useful defense for a complication arising from a properly performed procedure. Of 399 personal-injury lawyers surveyed in the Harvard study, 27% reported that a guideline helped convince them to drop a case or settle out of court (11,12).

In addition to malpractice litigation, other future legal applications of guidelines pertain to the antidumping and premature discharge provisions of Medicare law; at present, PRO review of such incidents occurs without a specific clinical basis. Increased use of guidelines for utilization management is likely to affect payment decisions in Medicare and in the private sector. Blue Cross and Blue Shield has made adherence to practice guidelines part of its contract with physicians in their Managed Care Network Preferred. Perhaps half of all managed care networks are now using some clinical guidelines (14). These documents come from a variety of sources, the interests of which are sometimes in conflict (Table 1). As this trend becomes normative, a host of legal issues is certain to arise in regard to contractual liability, industry standards, guidelines as a basis for capitation, and access to the guideline development process (15).

> Guidelines, then, are no panacea. They cannot cover every conceivable situation. They are not going to assure a successful outcome, even if followed resolutely on a course of treatment with a high probability of success. They must allow room for the individual physician to exercise judgement and practice the art of medicine. But they also must have enough teeth to leave their impact in a world where Medicare and other payers are already dictating every day to physicians through their coverage decisions how they should practice medicine (15).

One can also foresee hospital credentialing and selective contracting with health delivery networks as other potential areas of conflict involving the use of guidelines. Since guidelines are used for clinical decision making, medical-review criteria and standards of quality can be derived from them to assess and evaluate performance by the practitioner in conformity with the guidelines after the care has been delivered. Performance measures are simply numerical statements of the extent of conformity (1,2).

The legal enforceability of guidelines is probably directly dependent on their quality. If they are drawn up in accordance with the recommendations of the Institute of Medicine, approved and accepted by specialty societies and the

TABLE 1. *Sources of practice guidelines used by managed care plans in 1994*[a]

Guideline source	Extent of use[b]			
	Always	Sometimes	Rarely	Never
Federal agencies	60	35	3	2
National professional societies	77	23	0	0
Parent company	37	23	17	23
Plan's medical staff	75	20	3	2
Contract with other organizations	11	15	8	66
Other	36	16	0	48

(Adapted from ref. 14, 1995 Physician Payment Review Commission report to Congress, p. 377)
[a] Based on PPRC 1995 survey of group and staff HMOs, network and independent practice association HMOs, and preferred provider organizations (n = 65).
[b] Percentage of responding plans.

AHCPR, directed at a specific condition in a specific population, and based on the best available scientific data, then they are likely to be very enforceable. Hence, the desirable attributes of clinical practice guidelines include validity, reliability, reproducibility, clinical applicability, clinical flexibility, clarity, multidisciplinary development, scheduled review, and documentation (16). When these features are present, the problems attributed to clinical guidelines by physicians are denied by legal authorities (17). The legal ramifications of practice guidelines are further discussed in the proceedings of a recent conference (15); an annotated guide to the literature on this subject is also available (18).

ECONOMICS OF STROKE

Stroke is one of the most expensive medical problems in the United States. Application of practice guideline methodology to patients with stroke is an almost inevitable consequence of our national preoccupation with the perfectability and costs of health care. Further impetus to this trend is provided by certain clinical attributes of cerebrovascular diseases, including their dramatic personal impact and ready quantification. Each year there are approximately 550,000 new strokes, causing 150,000 deaths and leaving 300,000 disabled survivors (9). There are more than 3 million survivors of stroke in the United States (19). In the 1987 Medicare population, cerebral artery occlusion was the eighth most frequent inpatient diagnosis, accounting for nearly 200,000 discharges and was the sixth-highest condition in billing charges, representing $1.44 billion (5). Cerebrovascular diseases are the third leading cause of death in the United States and a major cause of occupational disability. Indeed, stroke is the leading cause of adult disability in the United States. Beyond the costs of the initial hospitalization (43%), rehabilitation and hospital readmissions contribute 16% and 14%, respectively, to the total cost of stroke care; physician costs represent another 14%. In 1993, the nonmedical costs of stroke, including the dollar value of lost productivity, represented 43% of the societal cost of stroke, or $13 billion. Direct medical costs, including hospitalization, physician

services, rehabilitation services, nursing homes, and durable medical equipment represented 57% of the total economic impact, or $17 billion (9). In 1993, the United States population was projected to included 3 million stroke survivors, with 31% requiring assistance with care, about 20% needing help with walking, and 16% being institutionalized (20). Seven years after their stroke, 71% of survivors still have some degree of impaired vocational capacity (20). Thirty-five percent of the survivors were between 35 and 65 years of age and were unemployable.

Such economic and societal costs are formidable, and the sums involved provide considerable motivation to physicians and laymen who advocate prevention and early intervention. In addition, virtually every public official personally knows some friend or relative who has been emotionally and functionally devastated by a stroke. For these and other reasons, there has been considerable interest in the early application of practice guideline methodology to stroke. Furthermore, the clinical features of cerebrovascular diseases lend themselves to quantification and facilitate the development of guidelines. For example, unlike the insidious progression of a disease like cancer, the onset of a stroke is easily identified and its clinical course, in terms of neurologic disability, can be rated. Furthermore, the AHCPR is specifically charged with health care technology evaluation and assessment and the repetitive use of expensive imaging technology is central to the diagnosis and management of the stroke patient. Finally, there is considerable evidence that manipulation of risk factors for atherosclerosis is likely to reduce the incidence of stroke. In manifold ways, therefore, cerebrovascular diseases readily lend themselves to an analysis of outcomes and costs, and such an analysis is central to the development of practice guidelines. Whether the guidelines that result from such analyses are beneficial, enforceable, or dangerous is the subject of this chapter.

HISTORY OF GUIDELINES FOR STROKE

As early as 1973, linkage of cerebrovascular disorders with cardiovascular diseases resulted in the promulgation of guidelines for stroke facilities and management (21). Such general recommendations did not directly impact on the day-to-day decision making of individual practitioners. Improvements in data gathering and the advent of randomized trials soon resulted in more specific and potentially restrictive recommendations. An example of the latter would be the interim assessment of carotid endarterectomy by the American Academy of Neurology in 1989, in which it was strongly suggested that surgeons operating on asymptomatic patients should have a combined perioperative morbidity and mortality rate due to stroke of less than 3% and that "formal ongoing audits" should be carried out in all institutions where the operation was performed (22). In 1992, the AHCPR awarded a 5-year, $5.6 million PORT contract to Duke University to determine the most effective methods of preventing strokes in people who are at high risk or those who have had transient ischemic attacks (TIAs). In addition, the study is designed to examine patterns of care and costs of care for both the prevention and treatment of stroke. This PORT study involves 11 major institutions. It is intended that guidelines developed from this study in regard to prevention be widely disseminated to the public, as well as to physicians.

Initial guidelines in stroke were based on outcomes analysis without regard to cost. For example, published algorithms for the evaluation and treatment of TIA and minor ischemic stroke have been reported to be "cost-effective and scientifically based" without provision of a specific economic analysis (23). Recent guidelines developed by the Stroke Council of the American Heart Association for the management of patients in the first 24 hours after an acute ischemic stroke do not contain a cost–benefit analysis (24). However, the authors did use rules of evidence in developing their recommendations; the use of such rules has been encouraged by the AHCPR (Table 2). The Stroke Council included in its recommendations an educational program for the general public and emergency medical system personnel in addition to the education of physicians. It strongly recommended that patients be admitted to specialized units under the care of medical teams devoted to the emergency treatment of strokes. These recommendations are in concert with the recent emphasis on the concept of "brain attack" within the neuroscience community. Geographic and resource factors must be taken into account when such guidelines are promulgated and their efficacy is evaluated. A geographic variability in stroke outcome has been identified. In the 1991 Medicare population, the 90-day mortality for ischemic stroke varied from a low of 19.4% in New England to a high of 24.3% in the Mountain region (9). The average rural mortality was 46% higher than urban mortality within the first 90 days.

A pioneering attempt to compare the cost effectiveness of aspirin and ticlopidine suffered from major methodologic problems (25,26). Marginal risk reductions achieved by ticlopidine were counterbalanced by its high cost, a high dropout rate due to its side effects, and the need for monitoring blood cell counts biweekly for the first 3 months of use. Since ticlopidine was more effective than aspirin in reducing the incidence of fatal and nonfatal strokes during the first year after a TIA or minor stroke, should it be used in aspirin-tolerant patients for a limited period of time? Are the costs of even limited use justified by savings in additional patient years of survival, decreased disability, and increased patient productivity? We simply do not know. For every 20 patients treated with ticlopidine instead of aspirin, an aggregate of 1 year of good-quality life was achieved at an expenditure of about $40,000 (26). Almost all such "economic" analyses in the literature have been carried out by physicians without specific training in the appropriate analytic methodology. Almost all claims for savings are based on the general public health care costs of a completed stroke without regard to whether society is willing to expend any and all resources in the prevention and treatment of disease in any and all of its members.

For example, in the absence of outcome and cost-based guidelines, it might be argued that all adults should be afforded the benefits of carotid Doppler ultrasound or magnetic resonance angiography screening and prophylactic carotid endarterectomy. The routine screening of half the adults in the 60–75-year age group might cost $7.1 billion; if 3% of these patients were to undergo carotid endarterectomy, a further cost of $4.3 billion would ensue (27). This relatively crude example of estimating the potential economic impact of a stroke protocol does not take into account the clinical effectiveness of the procedure. It does, however, indicate the magnitude of costs involved in the diagnosis and treatment of cerebrovascular diseases. Therefore, the routine application of a clinical rule can have tremendous economic impact.

The estimate of this impact can be sharpened through use of data from the recently completed carotid endarterectomy trials (28) (Fig. 2). Calculation of the marginal cost-effectiveness ratio (MCER) of carotid endarterectomy clarifies an important impetus behind the development of clinical guidelines, ie, the linkage between cost, safety, and clinical efficacy. David B. Matchar, the head of the PORT team at Duke University, has presented the preliminary results of such an evaluation (27).

The clinical effectiveness of any medical procedure depends on a large number of variables, including the morbid-

TABLE 2. Levels of evidence in developing guidelines

Level	Definition
1	Data from randomized trials with low false-positive (α) and low false-negative (β) errors.
2	Data from randomized trials with high false-positive (α) and high false-negative (β) errors.
3	Data from nonrandomized concurrent cohort studies.
4	Data from nonrandomized cohort studies using historical controls.
5	Data from anecdotal case studies.

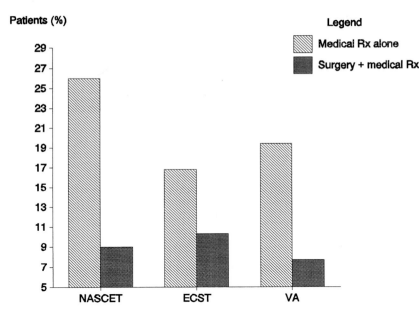

Patients (%)

Legend

Medical Rx alone

Surgery + medical Rx

FIG. 2. Reduction in risk of stroke for patients receiving surgery plus medical therapy in three clinical trials. Values are for ipsilateral stroke at 2 years in patients with 70% stenosis who have experienced a TIA or minor stroke in the North American Symptomatic Carotid Endarterectomy Trial *(NASCET)*, for ipsilateral stroke at 3 years in the European Carotid Surgery Trial *(ECST)*, and for stroke or crescendo TIAs at 1 year in the Veterans Affairs Cooperative Studies Program *(VA)*. Note that these values do not indicate the number of additional years of useful survival provided or their cost (Modified from ref. 20, with permission.)

ity and mortality of the acute intervention, demonstrated efficacy in decreasing long-term disability and death relative to the natural history of the disease, the clinical impact of side effects and complications, the age of the population at risk, and the number of available years of additional useful survival. Within the first 90 days after an ischemic stroke, 20% of patients older than 65 years die and the average 90-day cost to Medicare in 1991 was $15,000 (9). Since the average cost of a new stroke in the first year is approximately $50,000, a treatment might be considered cost effective if it is less expensive than $50,000 per year of additional useful survival. The MCER is a method by which the cost per additional health benefit (ie, years of additional survival) can be calculated and compared for each of two treatments (A and B):

$$MCER = (Cost\ A - Cost\ B)\ /\ (Effectiveness\ A - Effectiveness\ B)$$

In the carotid endarterectomy study, best medical therapy (B) was compared with medical therapy plus carotid endarterectomy, and the data apparently indicate a favorable MCER for endarterectomy of less than $50,000 for each additional year of useful survival. However, the carotid endarterectomy trial was carried out in centers by experienced cerebrovascular teams and surgeons with combined surgical morbidity and mortality rates of less than 3%.

Since one can expect some variability in different clinical settings, it is necessary to subject the overall favorable MCER to a sensitivity analysis in order to determine which variables or factors might affect the value of the MCER. A hypothetical example of a sensitivity analysis is presented in Fig. 3.

Matchar performed such an analysis and discovered that the only signficant factors were: (a) the underlying risk of stroke in the population under study, (b) the surgical effectiveness of carotid endarterectomy relative to the natural his-

tory and medical therapy (ie, the percentage reduction in death and stroke), (c) the durability of surgical effectiveness (ie, the duration of the beneficial effect or years of protection), and (d) the morbidity and mortality of the surgical procedure. Conversely, he found that the acute medical and hospital costs of the procedure did not affect the MCER. The obvious conclusion is that demonstrated safety and efficacy in the delivery of stroke care is of greater importance than the acute charges associated with such care. An independent calculation of the data in the North American Symptomatic Carotid Endarterectomy Trial indicates that if the surgical complication rate rises from 5.8% to 10%, all the clinical value of the operation is lost (20). The implication is clear. Third-party payers and medical managers are likely to become extremely interested in the development of clinical guidelines that promote safety and efficacy in the delivery of health care.

EVALUATION OF STROKE GUIDELINES

In general, evaluation of the impact of practice guidelines on individual practitioner behavior has been given much less attention than guideline development and implementation (4,16). For example, a survey of obstetricians and hospitals in Ontario, Canada, revealed only a modest effect on practice behavior after the wide dissemination of national consensus guidelines for the use of cesarean section (29). In the field of stroke, an exception has been the guidelines for the hospital management of stroke in the United Kingdom, developed by the King's Fund and the Royal College of Surgeons (30). A series of 15 specific standards covering initial assessment and management, rehabilitation, discharge, and secondary prevention was developed from these guidelines and evaluated in a series of 100 consecutive patients. The interobserver agreement on their use in practice was quite good

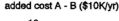

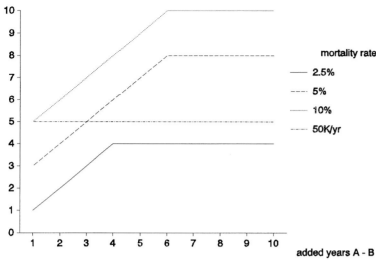

FIG. 3. Hypothetical sensitivity analysis for surgery plus medical therapy vs. medical therapy alone in stroke. The additional cost of A over B in increments of $10,000 per year is plotted against years of additional survival conferred by A over B for three different surgical mortality rates: 2.5%, 5%, and 10%. The lowest mortality rate is cost effective (ie, less than the $50,000/yr line) for all durations of therapy. The intermediate mortality rate is cost effective only in the first few years. The highest mortality rate is never cost effective. The slope of each line is the MCER (see text).

(≥80%). Certain standards were well met (adequate social history, routine investigation, prevention of pressure sores, and monitoring of blood pressure), whereas others were poorly met (diagnosis, rapid referral to therapists, functional reassessment, liaison with general practitioners, documentation of multidisciplinary rehabilitation programs, and communication with patients and relatives.) In the British study, several standards, especially those central to the rehabilitation process, were met significantly more frequently in patients managed by geriatricians than by general physicians (30). Some of this success was due to the geographic concentration of patients and rehabilitation programs directed by consultants trained in stroke management. The authors concluded that these standards were verifiable measures that could be used more widely to audit the process of care. Compliance with practice guidelines is enforced by a majority of managed care systems that utilize such documents to assist decision making (Table 3).

Of course, the outcomes observed by specialists in a particular disease entity not only depend on geographic variability of patients and the resources of an individual service in a specific hospital but also on the capabilities of other services within the institution. A four-center study of anesthetic outcomes in Canada has done much to reveal the complexity of clinical analysis (31). Data on 27,184 patients were collected, and the analysis of outcomes determined for the intraoperative, postanesthetic care unit and postoperative time periods. Across the three time periods, wide variations in minor outcomes were found across the four hospitals, but the rate of deaths and major events were similar. Possible reasons advanced to explain the variability in outcomes included compliance in recording events, inadequate case-mix adjustment, differences in the interpretation of variables "despite guidelines," and institutional differences in monitoring and charting protocols. The authors concluded that "measuring quality of care in anesthesia by comparing major outcomes is unsatisfactory since the contribution of anesthesia to perioperative outcomes is uncertain and that variations may be explained by institutional differences which are beyond the control of the anesthetist" (31). Could not each neurosurgeon, neurologist, vascular specialist, and neuroradiologist say the same?

TABLE 3. *Use of practice guidelines by managed care plans by type of plan in 1994[a]*

Use of practice guidelines	All plans (n = 108)	Group/staff HMOs (n = 29)	Network/IPA HMOs (n = 50)
Extent of use of formal written guidelines			
Fairly extensive	32	34	40
In a few areas only	31	41	36
Not used	37	24	24
Guideline follow-up			
Compliance monitored[b]	87	91	81
Meet with physician to review results[c]	80	80	87

(Adapted from ref. 14, Physician Payment Review Commission 1995 Report to Congress, p. 382)
[a] Based on PPRC 1995 survey (see note to Table 2).
[b] Only plans reporting guideline use answered this question.
[c] Only plans reporting monitoring of compliance responded to this item.

CONCLUSION

The proponents of practice guidelines hope that they will reduce regional variations in care, the preponderance of which are due to overuse. It is estimated that the elimination of as much as 25% of total hospital days and procedures, and perhaps 40% of all medications, would actually improve the overall quality of medical care (32). Whether this can actually be achieved in a society in which the expectations of consumers are exceedingly high and the threshold for litigious activity is exceedingly low is a doubtful proposition. The Institute of Medicine has noted that

> guidelines for the provision of clinical care have been linked in recent years to almost every major problem and proposed solution on the American health policy agenda. Practice guidelines have been tied in some way, by some individual or organization, to costs, quality, access, patient empowerment, professional autonomy, medical liability, rationing, competition, benefit design, utilization variation, bureaucratic micro-management of health care and more. The concept has acted as a magnet for the hopes and frustrations of practitioners, patients, payers, researchers and policymakers (16).

At the very least, however, one can expect that expensive procedures and protocols of marginal effectiveness will be eliminated by prudent health care system managers. In addition to the goals of reducing cost and improving the quality of care, practice guidelines will be used to resolve difficult ethical dilemmas, foster risk management, and reduce malpractice premiums. The latter clearly have served as the goals of practice guidelines developed by American and Canadian anesthesiology societies (31). When such guidelines are written by expert panels using explicit rules of evidence, they are likely to receive federal support and achieve strong legal standing. It is vital that consensus guidelines be flexible enough to account for outlier patients and a wide variety of practice situations, lest physicians find themselves more frequently assailed rather than protected in court by their adherence to guidelines. Many aspects of stroke care are unlikely to lend themselves to definitive statements; it is critical therefore that physicians participate in the development of guidelines to properly reflect scientific uncertainty and the realities of clinical practice. Indeed, the complexity of some subjects precludes, at present, the elaboration of a straightforward management model (see Fig. 1), and available guidelines do little more than collect all of the evidence in regard to good clinical practice (33). Some uncertainty can be reduced through a properly conducted economic analysis. Lack of sufficient flexibility in guidelines may result in a loss of professional autonomy and may act as a brake on clinical and scientific innovation. On the other hand, lack of specificity is unlikely to achieve the societal goal of a normative quality of care at reasonable cost with some degree of legal protection for individual neurologists and neurosurgeons. During the next few years, attaining an Aristotelian mean between these two extremes will prove an important challenge for all of us involved in the care of patients with stroke.

REFERENCES

1. Field MJ, Lohr KN. *Clinical Practice Guidelines: Directions for a New Program.* Washington, DC: Institute of Medicine, National Academy Press, 1990.
2. Gosfield AG. Clinical practice guidelines and the law: Applications and implications. In: Gosfield AG, ed. *Health Law Handbook, 1994 Edition.* Deerfield, IL: Clark Boardman & Callaghan, 1994:65–99.
3. Wennberg JE, Freeman JL, Culp WJ. Are hospital services rationed in New Haven or over-utilized in Boston? *Lancet* 1987:8543:1185–1189.
4. Menken M. Practice guidelines in neurology. Will they get us where we want to go? *Arch Neurol* 1992;49:193–195.
5. Raskin IE, Maklan CW. Medical treatment effectiveness research. A view from inside the Agency for Health Care Policy and Research. *Evaluation and the Health Profession,* June 1991:161–186.
6. Woolf SH. *Manual for Medical Practice Guideline Development: A Draft Protocol for Expert Panels Convened by the Office of the Forum for Quality and Effectiveness in Health Care.* Washington, DC: US Government Agency for Health Care Policy and Research, 1990:37.
7. Hirshfeld EB. Should ethical and legal standards for physicians be changed to accommodate new models for rationing health care? *University of Pennsylvania Law Review* 1992;140(5).
8. Agency for Health Care Policy and Research. Development of clinical guidelines for low back disorders. *Federal Register* March 18, 1991; 56(52):11452–11453.
9. Matchar DB, Duncan PW. Cost of stroke. *Stroke: Clinical Update* 1994;V(3):9–12.
10. General Accounting Office. *Medical Malpractice, Maine's Use of Practice Guidelines to Reduce Costs.* Washington, DC: General Accounting Office, 1993. GAO/HRD-94-8.
11. Felsenthal E. Doctors' own guidelines hurt them in court. *Wall Street Journal* October 10, 1994:B1.
12. Hyams AL, Brandenburg JA, Lipsitz, Brennan TA. *Report to the Physician Payment Review Commission: Practice Guidelines and Malpractice Litigation.* Washington DC: Harvard School of Public Health, January 25, 1994.
13. Jacox A, Carr DB, Payne R. New clinical-practice guidelines for the management of pain in patients with cancer. *N Engl J Med* 1994;330: 651–655.
14. Physician Payment Review Commission. *Annual Report to Congress.* Washington, DC: 1995:377, 382.
15. *Legal Issues Related to Clinical Practice Guidelines.* Washington, DC: National Health Lawyers Association, 1995:31.
16. Field MJ, Lohr KN, eds. *Guidelines for Clinical Practice: From Development to Use.* Washington, DC: Institute of Medicine, National Academy Press, 1992:1,44–45.
17. Kapp MB. "Cookbook" medicine: A legal perspective. *Arch Intern Med* 1990;150:496–500.
18. Kapp MB. The legal status of clinical practice parameters: An annotated bibliography. *Am Coll Med Quality* 1993;8:24–27.
19. *1989 Stroke Facts.* Dallas, TX: American Heart Association, 1989.
20. Easton JD. Preventing stroke. An overview of medical and surgical options. In: Reducing the Odds of Stroke: A Special Report. *Postgraduate Medicine* February, 1995:5–15.
21. Joint Committee for Stroke Facilities. Table of organization, I. Epidemiology for stroke facilities planning. *Stroke* 1972;3:351–371; and VII. Medical and surgical management of stroke. *Stroke* 1973;4:269–320.
22. Caplan LR, Easton JD. Interim assessment: Carotid endarterectomy. Presented at the American Academy of Neurology, Minneapolis, MN, 1989.
23. Brown RD, Evans BA, Wiebers DO, Petty GW, Meissner I, Dale AJD. Transient ischemic attack and minor ischemic stroke: An algorithm for evaluation and treatment. *Mayo Clin Proc* 1994;69:1027–1039.
24. Adams HP, Brott TG, Crowell RM, et al. Management of patients with acute ischemic stroke: Special writing group of the Stroke Council, American Heart Association (draft document). 1994.
25. Hass WK, Easton JD, Adams HP, Pryse-Phillips W, Molony BA, Anderson S, Kamm B. A randomized trial comparing ticlopidine hydrochloride with aspirin for the prevention of stroke in high-risk patients. *N Engl J Med* 1989;321:501–507.
26. Oster G, Huse DM, Lacey MJ, et al. Cost-effectiveness of ticlopidine in preventing stroke in high risk patients. *Stroke* 1994;25: 1149–1156.

27. Matchar DB. Oral presentation, 1994.

28. North American Symptomatic Carotid Endarterectomy Trial Collaborators. Beneficial effect of carotid endarterectomy in symptomatic patients with high-grade stenosis. *N Engl J Med* 325:445–453, 1991.

29. Lomas J, Anderson GM, Domnick-Pierre K, Vayda E, Enkin MW, Hannah WJ. Do practice guidelines guide practice? *N Engl J Med* 1989; 321:1306–1311.

30. Stone SP, Whincup P. Standards for the hospital management of stroke patients. *J R Coll Physicians Lond* 1994;28:52–58.

31. Cohen MM, Duncan PG, Pope WD, Biehl D, et al. The Canadian four-centre study of anaesthetic outcomes: II. Can outcomes be used to assess the quality of anaesthesia care? *Can J Anaesth* 1993;40:79–81.

32. Brook RH. Practice guidelines and practicing medicine: Are they compatible? *JAMA* 1989;262:3027–3030.

33. Mayberg MR, Batjer HH, Dacey R, et al. Guidelines for the management of aneurysmal subarachnoid hemorrhage. A statement for health care professionals from a special writing group of the Stroke Council, American Heart Association. *Stroke* 1995. In press.

Subject Index

for middle cerebral artery stenosis, 484
for venous thrombosis, 561–564,
562–563t
Hereditary cerebral hemorrhage with
angiopathy of Dutch type, 629
Hereditary cerebral hemorrhage with
angiopathy of Icelandic type, 629
Herpesvirus thymidine kinase gene, gene
therapy for stroke and, 131–132
Heubner's artery, 10
carotid bifurcation aneurysm and, 984,
985i
occlusion of, ischemic syndromes
caused by, 342
Hexokinase, in brain energy metabolism,
25
HH. See Hemiataxia-hypesthesia
HHS. See Homonymous horizontal
sectoranopia
HI. See Hemorrhagic infarction
High-flow intracranial arteriovenous
malformations. See also Carotid
cavernous fistula
endovascular treatment of, 697–699
High intensity transient signals (HITS),
275, 277, 281
HK. See Hexokinase
HLA. See Human leukocyte antigens
Hollenhorst plaque, carotid
endarterectomy in patients with,
413–414
Holter monitoring
in cardioembolism diagnosis, 378
after subarachnoid hemorrhage, 1137
Homocysteine
gene therapy for stroke and, 130
stroke risk and, 594
Homonymous horizontal sectoranopia,
stroke evaluation and, 154
Homonymous quadrantanopia, stroke
evaluation and, 154
Hormone therapy, postmenopausal, stroke
risk and, 596
Horner's syndrome
in cervical internal carotid artery
dissection, 387
in lateral upper medulla lesions, 358i,
358t, 359
partial, in carotid occlusive disease, 341
stroke evaluation and, 154
HSPs. See Heat shock proteins
HTN. See Hypertension
Human gene therapy trials, 135, 136i
Human leukocyte antigens (HLA), in
moyamoya disease, 495
Hunt—Hess Clinical Grading Scale, for
subarachnoid hemorrhage, 891,
891t
poor-grade aneurysm patient and, 1103,
1104t
Hunterian ligation, for giant aneurysms,
1085–1086
Hyaline atherosclerosis/hyaline
change/hyalinosis. See
Lipohyalinosis
Hydralazine
for eclampsia, 100

for subarachnoid hemorrhage, 1124,
1124t
Hydrocephalus
after arteriovenous malformation
resection, 786, 797
in dural arteriovenous fistulas, 804
hemorrhage of arteriovenous
malformations and, 663, 664i
middle cerebral artery aneurysm
surgery and, 1005
subarachnoid hemorrhage and, 895,
1126–1127
cerebrospinal fluid drainage for,
1131
timing of aneurysm surgery and,
1099
ventricular drainage for, 1126–1127,
1131
in vein of Galen aneurysms, 826
Hydrogen, white matter concentrations of,
anoxia affecting, 311
Hydrogen peroxide
in ischemic neuronal damage, 321–324
in stroke pathophysiology, 304
Hydroxyl radical
in ischemic neuronal damage, 321–324
in stroke pathophysiology, 304
Hypercapnia, hyperventilation-induced, for
elevated intracranial pressure and
brain edema in stroke patient, 527
Hyperemia
arteriovenous malformation surgery and,
857–861
after carotid endarterectomy, 337
transcranial Doppler ultrasound in
evaluation of, 279
Hyperglycemia
hemorrhagic infarction and, 653
stroke magnitude and, 303, 303i
in stroke patient, management of, 526
after subarachnoid hemorrhage, 1140
Hyperhidrosis, transient unilateral, stroke
evaluation and, 154
Hyperhomocystinemia, stroke risk and,
594
Hyperlipidemias, familial, gene therapy
for stroke and, 131
Hypernatremia, in stroke patient,
management of, 525
Hyperperfusion syndrome, after carotid
endarterectomy, 100–101
Hypersensitivity reactions, to radiocontrast
media in angiography, 212
Hypertension
aneurysm formation and, 69
aneurysmal subarachnoid hemorrhage
and, 889, 1140–1141
arteriovenous malformation surgery and,
864
carotid endarterectomy and, 440–441
cerebral angiopathy and, 85–95
arterial and arteriolar, 85–86, 86i
fibrinoid necrosis, 87–88
lipohyalinosis, 86–87, 88i, 89i
microaneurysm, 88–91, 90i, 91i
microatheroma, 86, 87i
cerebrovascular disease and, 79–83

cervical internal carotid artery
dissection and, 387
deliberate
for aneurysm surgery, 1145, 1146i
arteriovenous malformation
embolization and, 854
arteriovenous malformation surgery
and, 864–865
for carotid endarterectomy, 336
in cerebral vasospasm prevention and
treatment, 1119, 1133, 1133t
for progressive stroke, 531–532, 532t
encephalopathy and. See Hypertensive
encephalopathy
in extracranial vertebral artery
dissection, 391
hemorrhagic infarction and, 653
intracerebral hemorrhage and, 81,
92–93, 606, 607–608, 614–615.
See also Intracerebral/intracranial
hemorrhage
computed tomography in detection
of, 174, 175i
in intracranial vertebral artery
dissection, 393
lacunar infarcts and, 57, 81, 91–93, 92i
microcirculatory pathophysiology and,
93–94
parenchymal brain lesions and, 91–93,
92i
pathophysiology of, 80–81
as small deep infarct risk factor, 57
in stroke patient, management of,
524–525, 525t
stroke risk and, 57, 144–145, 145t, 146,
592–593
modification in stroke prevention
and, 596–597
subcortical leukoencephalopathy and, 93
treatment of, 81–82
Hypertensive encephalopathy, 93, 97–102
cerebrovascular support for patients
with, 296
clinical presentation of, 97–98
eclampsia and, 99–100, 100i
hyperperfusion syndrome after carotid
endarterectomy and, 100–101
imaging studies in, 99
computed tomography, 99, 174, 176i
magnetic resonance imaging, 99
pathology and pathophysiology of,
98–99
treatment of, 99
Hypertensive-hypervolemic therapy
in cerebral vasospasm, 1119, 1133,
1133–1134, 1133t
in progressive stroke, 531–532, 532t
Hypertensive intracranial hemorrhage. See
Intracerebral/intracranial
hemorrhage
Hyperventilation
for brain edema, in stroke patient,
527
for elevated intracranial pressure
in stroke patient, 527
after subarachnoid hemorrhage,
1130t, 1131

ISBN 0-397-51661-4

9 780397 516612